Clinical Gynecologic Endocrinology and Infertility

Sixth Edition

Clinical Gynecologic Endocrinology and Infertility

Sixth Edition

Leon Speroff
Robert H. Glass
Nathan G. Kase

Illustration and Page Design
by Lisa Million

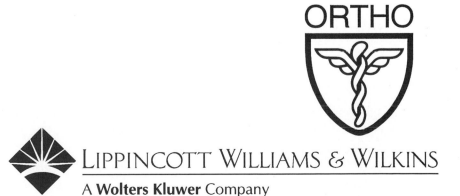

LIPPINCOTT WILLIAMS & WILKINS
A **Wolters Kluwer** Company

Editor: Charles Mitchell
Managing Editor: Ray Reter
Marketing Manager: Joy Stewart
Production Editor: Robert D. Magee

Copyright © 1999 Lippincott Williams & Wilkins

351 West Camden Street
Baltimore, Maryland 21201-2436 USA

227 East Washington Square
Philadelphia, PA 19106

Printed in the United States of America

First Edition, 1973

Library of Congress Cataloging-in-Publication Data

Speroff, Leon, 1935–
    Clinical gynecologic endocrinology and infertility / Leon Speroff, Robert H. Glass, Nathan G. Kase ; illustration and page design by Lisa Million. —6th ed.
        p.   cm.
    Includes bibliographical references and index.
    ISBN 0-683-30379-1
    1. Endocrine gynecology. 2. Infertility—Endocrine aspects. I. Glass, Robert H., 1932– II. Kase, Nathan G., 1930–   III. Title.
    RG159.S62 1999
    618.1—dc21   98-36104
                                                                          CIP

The publishers have made every effort to trace the copyright holders for borrowed material. If they have inadvertently overlooked any, they will be pleased to make the necessary arrangements at the first opportunity.

To purchase additional copies of this book, call our customer service department at **(800) 638-3030** or fax orders to **(301) 824-7390**. International customers should call **(301) 714-2324.**

99 00 01 02 03
1 2 3 4 5 6 7 8 9 10

Preface

A quarter of a century later, the millennium and our 6th edition! The impact of our book has been one of the most gratifying experiences in our careers. We know it has helped many readers to successfully overcome examinations, but, most rewarding of all, is the recognition of the effect on patient care derived from the clinical usefulness of our text. An appreciation for this impact carries with it a profound sense of obligation. We have always understood the importance of "getting it right" and "causing no harm." For that reason, every edition is the culmination of a tremendous effort, an effort increasingly difficult with the amazing growth of knowledge and communications. In 1972, it was a Royal portable typewriter. At the millennium, we are armed with a personal computer and a modem, Word 97 for the text, EndNote for references, and MEDLINE for searches,

The book grows progressively thicker, reflecting the explosion of knowledge in reproductive biology and medicine. Nevertheless, we believe we have stayed true to our objective: to provide both factual knowledge and systematic approaches to clinical problems. Our text continues to be an expression and formulation of our collective professional activities as teachers, investigators, and most importantly, as clinicians in the field of reproductive endocrinology and infertility. We have tried to retain the style and clinical relevance of our first edition, but at the same time to provide all the new information. This basic knowledge is the foundation for the physiologic principles that in turn are the foundation for our methods of clinical management.

As always, our book is dedicated to the improvement of patient care, and we hope that it will aid all readers in accomplishing that goal. We are grateful to those who have taught us, and most of all, we thank our patients, who are our best teachers.

Leon Speroff, M.D.
Portland, Oregon

Robert H. Glass, M.D.
San Francisco, California

Nathan G. Kase, M.D.
New York, New York

P.S. The cover color of the 6th edition is a nostalgic return to Yale blue. The symbol on the cover is the Macedonian Star, from the days of Philip of Macedon and Alexander the Great.

Contents

Part I

Reproductive Physiology

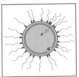

1 Molecular Biology for Clinicians

GCAGCCGTATTTCTACTGCGACGAGGAG
GAGAACTT**SPEROFF**CTACCAGCAGCAG
AGCGAGCTGGC**GLASS**AGCCCCGGCGC
CCAGGGATATCTGGAA**KASE**GAAATTCGA
GCTGCTGCCGCCCTGTCCCTAGCCGCG

The above DNA sequence is obviously a mutant. But the fact that we can recognize this cryptogram as a nucleotide sequence and diagnose a mutant change illustrates the incredible progress made in the understanding of human biology. Molecular biology is the subspecialty of science devoted to understanding the structure and function of the genome, the full complement of DNA (desoxyribonucleic acid), the macromolecule which contains all the hereditary information.

The Austrian monk, Gregor Mendel, studied his garden of peas for much of his life at his monastery and was the first to express the principles of heredity in the 1860s. He described dominant and recessive traits and the "laws" of transmission governing the homozygous and heterozygous inheritance of these traits. Mendel's theories remained unknown until 1900, when they were discovered. Unfortunately, Mendel died 16 years before recognition of his work.

The pairing and splitting of chromosomes at cell division was proposed in 1903, but it was not until 1946 that Edward Tatum and Joshua Lederberg at Yale University demonstrated in bacteria that DNA carried hereditary information. James Watson and Francis Crick, working at the Cavendish Laboratories in Cambridge, proposed in 1953, the structure of DNA by creating a model based on the parameters provided by Maurice Wilkins and Rosalind Franklin obtained with x-ray crystallography. Crick, Watson, and Wilkins received the Nobel Prize in 1962; Franklin died in 1958, and Nobel prizes are not awarded posthumously.

DNA replication involves many enzyme systems. DNA polymerase was isolated in 1958, and RNA polymerase in 1960. In 1978, Werner Arber, Hamilton Smith, and Daniel Nathans received the Nobel prize for their discovery, in the 1960s, of the enzymes for joining or cutting DNA. The use of ligase and restriction endonuclease enzymes permitted the production of recombinant DNA molecules, first accomplished by Paul Berg at Stanford University in 1972.

E.M. Southern of Edinburgh University developed in 1975 the technique to transfer (to blot) DNA from agarose gels onto nitrocellulose filters, enabling DNA fragments to be joined with radiolabeled RNA probes and thus isolated. The cloning of genes or DNA fragments followed the breakthrough discovery that plasmids carrying foreign DNA molecules could be inserted into bacteria, leading to the replication of the foreign DNA.

We have entered the age of molecular biology. It won't be long before endocrine problems will be explained, diagnosed, and treated at the molecular level. Soon the traditional hormone assays will be a medical practice of the past. The power of molecular biology will touch us all, and the many contributions of molecular biology will be perceived throughout this book. But unfortunately, molecular biology has its own language, a language that is almost unintelligible to the uninitiated. We offer this chapter as a guide for the new molecular medicine.

To begin a clinical book with a chapter on molecular biology and a chapter on biochemistry only serves to emphasize that competent clinical judgment is founded on a groundwork of basic knowledge. On the other hand, clinical practice does not require a technical and sophisticated proficiency in a basic science. The purpose of these first two chapters, therefore, is not to present an intensive course in a basic science, but rather to review the most important principles and information necessary for the development of the physiological and clinical concepts to follow. It is further intended that certain details, which we all have difficulty remembering, will be available in these chapters for reference.

The Chromosomes

We are *eukaryotes,* organisms with cells having a true nucleus bounded by a nuclear membrane, with multiplication by mitosis. Bacteria are *prokaryotes,* organisms without a true nucleus, with reproduction by cell division. With the exception of DNA within mitochondria, all of our DNA is packaged in a nucleus surrounded by a nuclear membrane. Mitochondria are believed to be descendants of primitive bacteria engulfed by our ancestors, and they still contain some important genes.

Chromosomes are packages of genetic material, consisting of a DNA molecule (which contains many genes) to which are attached large numbers of proteins that maintain chromosome structure and play a role in gene expression. Human somatic cells contain 46 chromosomes, 22 pairs of autosomes, and 1 pair of sex chromosomes. All somatic cells are diploid—23 pairs of chromosomes. Only gametes are haploid with 22 autosome chromosomes and 1 sex chromosome. The chromosomes vary in size, and all contain a pinched portion called a centromere, which divides the chromosome into two arms, the shorter p arm and the longer q arm. The two members of any pair of autosomes are homologous, one homologue derived from each parent. The number of chromosomes does not indicate the level of evolutionary sophistication and complexity; the dog has 78 chromosomes and the carp has 104!

A single gene is a unit of DNA within a chromosome that can be activated to transcribe a specific RNA. The location of a gene on a particular chromosome is designated its locus. Because there are 22 pairs of autosomes, most genes exist in pairs. The pairs are homozygous when similar and heterozygous when dissimilar.

The usual human karyotype is an arrangement of the chromosomes into pairs, usually after proteolytic treatment and Giemsa staining to produce characteristic banding patterns allowing a blueprint useful for location. The staining characteristics divide each arm into regions, and each region into bands that are numbered from the centromere outward. A given point on a chromosome is designated by the following order: chromosome number, arm symbol (p for short arm, q for long arm), region number, and band number. For example, 7q31.1 is the location for the cystic fibrosis gene.

Mitosis

All eukaryotes, from yeasts to humans, undergo similar cell division and multiplication. The process of nuclear division in all somatic cells is called mitosis, during which each chromosome divides into two. For normal growth and development, the entire genomic information must be faithfully reproduced in every cell.

Mitosis consists of the following stages.

Interphase

During this phase, all normal cell activity occurs except active division. It is during this stage that the inactive X chromosome (the Barr body or the sex chromatin) can be seen in female cells.

Prophase

As division begins, the chromosomes condense, and the two chromatids become visible. The nuclear membrane disappears. The centriole is an organelle outside the nucleus that forms the spindles for cell division; the centriole duplicates itself, and the two centrioles migrate to opposite poles of the cell.

Metaphase

The chromosomes migrate to the center of the cell, forming a line designated the equatorial plate. The chromosomes are now maximally condensed. The spindle, microtubules of protein that radiate from the centrioles and attach to the centromeres, is formed.

Anaphase

Division occurs in the longitudinal plane of the centromeres. The two new chromatids move to opposite sides of the cell drawn by contraction of the spindles.

Telophase

Division of the cytoplasm begins in the equatorial plane, ending with the formation of two complete cell membranes. The two groups of chromosomes are surrounded by nuclear membranes forming new nuclei. Each strand of DNA serves as a template, and the DNA content of the cell doubles.

Meiosis

Meiosis is the cell division that forms the gametes, each with a haploid number of chromosomes. Meiosis has two purposes: *reduction* of the chromosome number and *recombination* to transmit genetic information. In meiosis I, homologous chromosomes pair and split apart. Meiosis II is similar to mitosis as the already divided chromosomes split and segregate into new cells.

The First Meiotic Division (Meiosis I)
Prophase:

Lepotene: Condensation of the chromosomes.

Zygotene: Pairing of homologous chromosomes (synapsis).

Pachytene: Each pair of chromosomes thickens to form four strands. This is the stage in which **crossing over** or **recombination** can occur (DNA exchange of homologous segments between two of the four strands). Chiasmata are the places of contact where cross-overs occur (and can be visualized). This movement of blocks of DNA is a method for creating genetic diversity. On the other hand, genetic diseases can result from the insertion of sequences during gametogenesis. Transpositional recombination, utilizing enzymes that recognize specific nucleic acid sequences, allows the insertion of a genetic element into any region of a chromosome. This is a method used by viruses (such as the human immunodeficiency virus) to transform host cells.

Diplotene: Longitudinal separation of each chromosome.

Metaphase, Anaphase, and Telophase of Meiosis I

The nuclear membrane disappears, and the chromosomes move to the center of the cell. One member of each pair goes to each pole, and the cells divide. Meiosis I is often referred to as reduction division because each new product now has the haploid chromosome number. It is during the first meiotic division that mendelian inheritance occurs. Cross-overs, that occur prior to metaphase, result in new combinations of genetic material, both favorable and unfavorable.

The Second Meiotic Division (Meiosis II)

The second division follows the first without DNA replication. In the oocyte, meiosis II occurs after fertilization. The end result is the production of 4 haploid cells.

The Structure and Function of DNA

DNA is the material of the gene responsible for coding the genetic message as transmitted through specific proteins. Thus, it is the most important molecule of life and the fundamental mechanism for evolution. Genes are segments of DNA that code for specific proteins, together with flanking and intervening sequences that serve controlling and regulating functions. Each molecule of DNA has a deoxyribose backbone, identical repeating groups of deoxyribose sugar linked through phosphodiester bonds. Each deoxyribose is attached in order (giving individuality and specificity) to one of 4 nucleic acids, the nuclear bases:

  A purine — adenine or guanine.
  A pyrimidine — thymine or cytosine.

A nucleotide is the basic building block of DNA. It consists of 3 major components: the deoxyribose sugar, a phosphate group, and a nucleic acid base. The phosphate-sugar linkages are asymmetric; the phosphorous is linked to the 5-carbon of one sugar and to the 3-carbon of the following sugar. Thus, one end is the 5' (5 prime) end and the other the 3' (3 prime) end. By convention, DNA and its nuclear acid sequences are written from left to right, from the 5' end to the 3' end, the direction of the transcription process. The 5' end leads to the formation of the amino end of the protein; the 3' end forms the carboxy end of the protein.

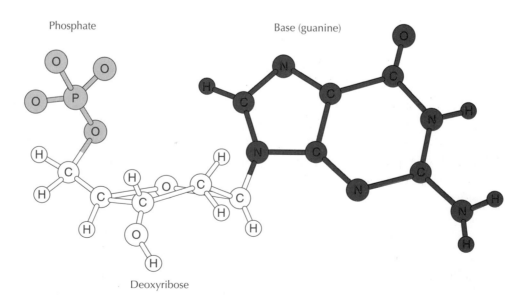

Deoxyribose

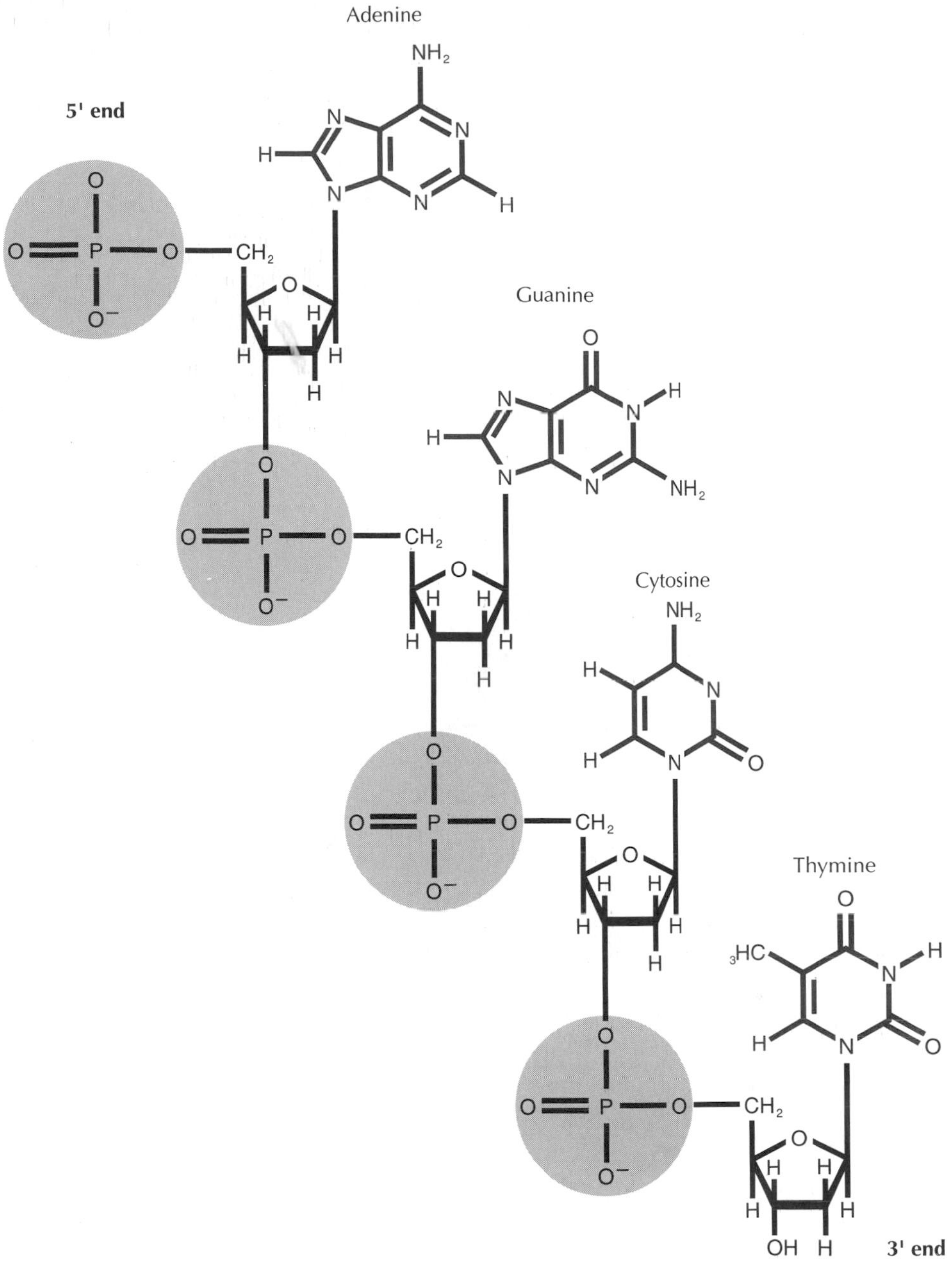

Adenine

5' end

Guanine

Cytosine

Thymine

3' end

DNA consists of two deoxyribose strands twisted around each other clockwise in a double helix, with the nucleic acids on the inside and the nuclear bases paired by hydrogen bonding, adenine with thymine and cytosine with guanine. RNA differs from DNA in that it is single stranded, its sugar moiety is ribose, and it substitutes uracil for thymine.

How can a cell's DNA, which stretched out measures nearly 2 meters long, fit into a cell? Watson and Crick figured this out when they proposed a tightly coiled two-stranded helix, the double helix. Like the centimeter is a measure of length, the base pair (bp) is the unit of measure for DNA. The base pair is either adenine-guanine or cytosine-thymine, the nucleic acid of one chain paired with the facing nucleic acid of the other chain. A fragment of DNA is, therefore, measured by the number of base pairs, e.g., a 4800-bp fragment (a 4.8 kb fragment). It is estimated that we have 3 billion bp of DNA, only a small portion of which actually codes out for proteins.

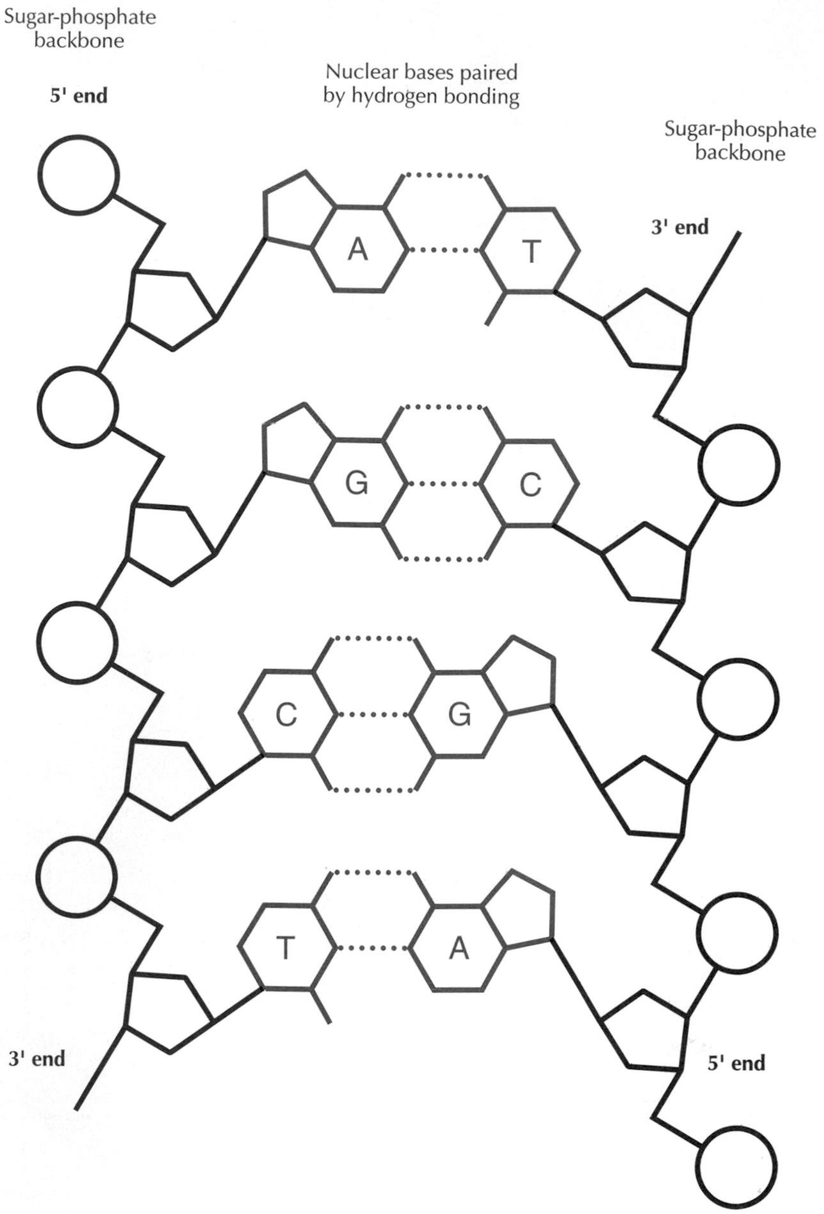

Sugar-phosphate
backbone

Nuclear bases paired
by hydrogen bonding

5' end

Sugar-phosphate
backbone

3' end

A ········ T

G ········ C

C ········ G

T ········ A

3' end

5' end

DNA does not exist within the cell as a naked molecule. The nucleotide chains wind about a core of proteins (histones) to form a nucleosome. The nucleosomes become condensed into many bands, the bands that are recognized in karyotype preparations. This condensation is another important mechanism for packing the long DNA structure into a cell. Many other proteins are associated with DNA, important for both structure and function.

The process of DNA replication begins with a separation of the double-stranded DNA helix, initiated at multiple steps by enzyme action. As the original DNA unwinds into template strands, DNA polymerase catalyzes the synthesis of new duplicate strands, which reform a double helix with each of the original strands (this is called replication). Each daughter molecule, therefore, contains one of the parental strands. It is estimated that the original DNA molecule present in the fertilized zygote must be copied approximately 10^{15} times during the course of a human lifetime. Rapidity and accuracy are essential. By combining precision with error correction systems, errors that affect the function of the gene's protein are surprisingly rare.

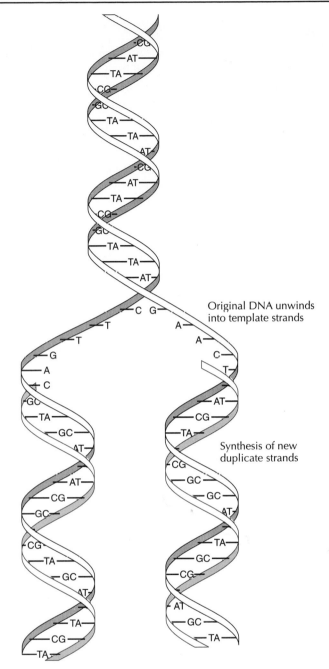

Original DNA unwinds into template strands

Synthesis of new duplicate strands

The **homeobox** is a DNA sequence, highly conserved throughout evolution, that encodes a series of 60 amino acids, called a homeodomain. Homeodomain protein products function as transcription factors by binding to DNA. The homeobox influences specific tissue functions that are critical for growth and development of the embryo.

The Human Genome

The genome for each species consists of the complete set of DNA sequences on all the chromosomes. There are 3 billion base pairs in each haploid human genome; in the double stranded helix DNA, there are 6 billion nucleotides, and there are an estimated 60,000 to 150,000 genes, the smallest functional unit of inherited information. Genes account for only about 3% of human DNA. Although enormously complex at first glance, the entire genetic language is written with only four letters: A, C, G, and T (U in RNA). Furthermore, the language is limited to only 3 letter words, codons. Finally, the entire genetic message is fragmented into the 23 pairs of chromosomes. With four nucleotides, reading groups of three, there are 64 possible combinations. Essentially all living organisms use this code. The genome changes only by new combinations derived from parents or by mutation.

The 20 Amino Acids in Proteins

Amino Acid	Three-Letter Abbreviation	Single-Letter Code
Glycine	Gly	G
Alanine	Ala	A
Valine	Val	V
Isoleucine	Ile	I
Leucine	Leu	L
Serine	Ser	S
Threonine	Thr	T
Proline	Pro	P
Aspartic acid	Asp	D
Glutamic acid	Glu	E
Lysine	Lys	K
Arginine	Arg	R
Asparagine	Asn	N
Glutamine	Gln	Q
Cysteine	Cys	C
Methionine	Met	M
Tryptophan	Trp	W
Phenylalanine	Phe	F
Tyrosine	Tyr	Y
Histidine	His	H

The mRNA Genetic Code

First Position (5' end)	Second Position				Third Position (3' end)
	U	C	A	G	
U	Phe	Ser	Tyr	Cys	U
	Phe	Ser	Tyr	Cys	C
	Leu	Ser	Stop	Stop	A
	Leu	Ser	Stop	Trp	G
C	Leu	Pro	His	Arg	U
	Leu	Pro	His	Arg	C
	Leu	Pro	Gln	Arg	A
	Leu	Pro	Gln	Arg	G
A	Ile	Thr	Asn	Ser	U
	Ile	Thr	Asn	Ser	C
	Ile	Thr	Iys	Arg	A
	Met	Thr	Lys	Arg	G
G	Val	Ala	Asp	Gly	U
	Val	Ala	Asp	Gly	C
	Val	Ala	Glu	Gly	A
	Val	Ala	Glu	Gly	G

Reading across the first row of the table, the codon UUU specifies Phenylalanine, the codon UCU specifies Serine, the codon UAU specifies Tyrosine, and the codon UGU specifies Cysteine. UAA, UAG, and UGA are stop codons.

Gene Structure and Function

The linear arrangement of many genes forms a chromosome. A gene is composed of a segment of DNA containing exons separated by introns, the coding and noncoding codons of nucleotides, respectively. Intron–exon patterns tend to be conserved during evolution. The alpha- and beta-globin genes are believed to have arisen 500 million years ago, with the introns in the same location as they are today.

Exon
The segment of a gene that yields a messenger RNA product that codes for a specific protein.

Intron
The segment of a gene not represented in mature RNA and, therefore, noncoding for protein.

Codon
A sequence of 3 bases in RNA or DNA that codes for a specific amino acid; the triplet codon.

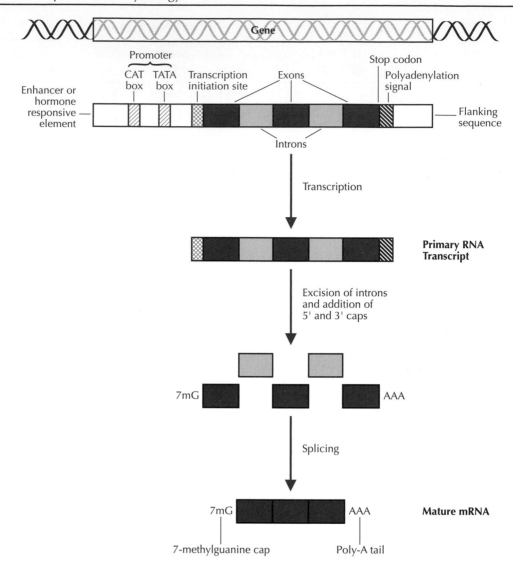

With some exceptions, essentially one gene yields one protein. As noted above, the introns are not translated into protein products. Only the DNA sequences in the exons (the part that "exits" the nucleus) are transcribed into messenger RNA and then translated into proteins. Genes also include flanking sequences important for gene transcription. The area that will initiate DNA action (e.g., DNA binding to the hormone-receptor complex) is called an ***enhancer*** region. The actual area where transcription begins is the ***promoter*** region. Only a few relatively short nucleotide sequences are promoters, such as the T-A-T-A-A sequence, or TATA box, and the C-C-A-A-T sequence, or CAT box. The promoter sites (the binding sites for RNA polymerase and numerous cofactors) are usually near the start of the coding region of the gene. Enhancer sites are larger than promoter sites and can be located anywhere, even far from the gene, but usually are in the 5' flanking end. At the 3' end, a coding sequence is usually present for the polyadenine tail common for most messenger RNA molecules.

The enhancer sites bind proteins (regulatory proteins) that serve as signals to regulate gene expression by either increasing or repressing the binding of RNA polymerase in the promoter region. This is one method of creating unique cellular functions. For example, a hormone target tissue can respond to the hormone because it contains a specific receptor protein that, on binding to the hormone, will bind to a DNA enhancer site. Specific proteins (called transcription factors) bind to enhancer sites and activate transcription. The regulation of gene transcription usually involves DNA sequences in the 5' flanking upstream region of a gene.

Three codons (UAG, UAA, UGA) are called **stop codons,** because they specify a stop to translation of RNA into protein (like a period at the end of a sentence). By contrast, an **open reading frame** is a long series of base pairs between two stop codons; therefore, an open reading frame encodes the amino acid sequence of the protein product. Finding and identifying an open reading frame is an important step in analyzing DNA sequences because such a long sequence is usually encountered only in an active gene.

Gene expression is composed of the following steps: transcription of DNA to RNA, RNA processing to produce functional messenger RNA by splicing out introns, translation of messenger RNA on a ribosome to a peptide chain, and protein structural processing to the functional form.

Transcription

Transcription is the synthesis of single-stranded messenger RNA from a gene (double-stranded DNA). The amino acid sequence of the protein is coded in the DNA by codons; a single amino acid is coded by each codon, a triplet of 3 nucleic acid bases. RNA polymerase constructs the messenger RNA by reading the DNA strand (the "antisense" strand) that is complementary to the RNA; thus, the RNA is an exact copy of the other DNA strand (the "sense" strand), which is also called the complementary strand of the DNA molecule (remember, important differences are that thymine in DNA is replaced by uracil and ribose replaces deoxyribose in RNA).

Molecular complementarity is both a difficult and a simple concept to grasp. The simple aspect is the concept of one thing being like another. The difficult part is the necessity to understand and visualize that the complementary molecule is not identical to its template, but more like the place where the template goes in, the complementary molecule goes out. Thus, the strands of the double helix are not identical. Each DNA strand has a complementary structure, in a sense, one positive template and one negative template, each specifying the other. Each strand, therefore, serves as a template for its complementary DNA (in the process of replication) or complementary RNA (in the process of transcription). Thus, messenger RNA is synthesized from the negative template, the "antisense" strand, so that it will have the same structure as the positive template, the "sense" strand. Molecular biologists have to think in three dimensions!

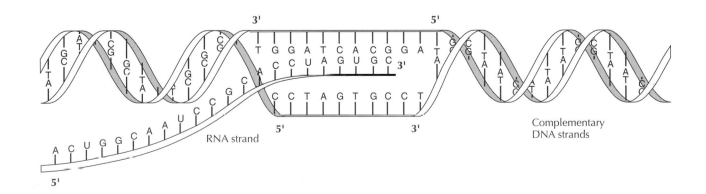

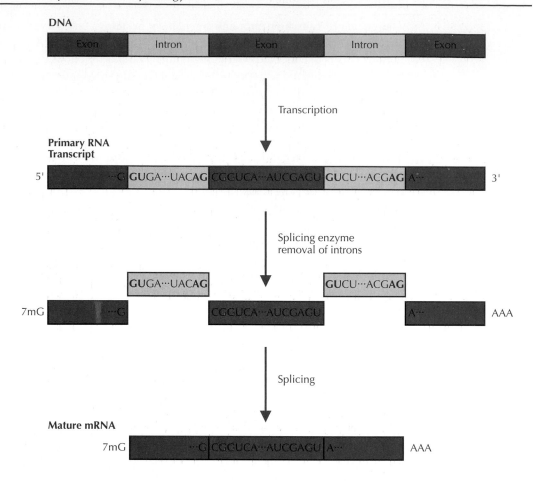

Transcription is initiated at the upstream start site, the 5' untranslated flanking region where the two strands of the double helix come apart. The process continues downstream, copying one of the strands until a specific codon is reached, which provides a stop message. RNA synthesis continues with the addition of a long chain of adenines, the poly-A tail; this is the 3' untranslated region that is believed to stabilize RNA by preventing degradation. After transcription from a gene, the RNA moves into the cytoplasm where the intron regions are excised, and the exons are joined together *(RNA splicing)* to produce a complete, mature RNA molecule. The start and end of each exon and intron have sequences that when copied onto the RNA, signal an enzyme to remove the intervening parts. Almost all introns begin with GU and end with AG (GT and AG in the DNA intron). Introns are of varying lengths; a single intron can be longer than the final RNA product. The mature RNA molecule has an addition at one end ("capping," by the addition of a modified nucleotide, 7-methyl guanosine) to protect against RNAases and at the other end, a polyadenine tail (the poly A tail) is added (in addition to a stabilizing factor, perhaps a signal to direct exit from the nucleus). Both ends are untranslated in the ribosomes.

Transcription Factors. Transcription factors are proteins that bind to regulatory elements in DNA (enhancers and promoters) and thus influence gene expression. The steroid hormone receptors are transcription factors. Gene transcription and the formation of messenger RNA can be either stimulated or inhibited through direct interactions with DNA. Transcription factors can further interact with other factors (coactivators and corepressors, also called adapter proteins) to produce cooperative effects. The activity of these proteins can also be affected by phosphorylation triggered by signals from cell-surface receptors (often growth factors). An important concept is to view the final result of hormonal activity and gene expression as a reflection of *cellular context*, the nature and activity of transcription factors as influenced by specific intracellular adapter proteins. This explains how similar agents (and similar transcription factors, e.g., the estrogen receptor) can have different actions in different tissues.

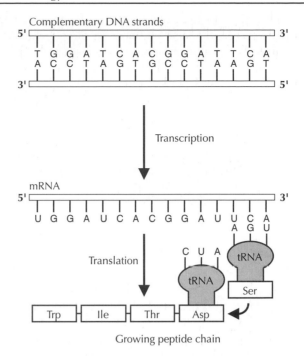

Translation

The messenger RNA travels from the chromosome on which it was synthesized to a ribosome in the cytoplasm, where it directs the assembly of amino acids into proteins (translation). Amino acids are brought into the process by specific transfer RNA molecules. The specific sequence of 3 bases at one end of the transfer RNA is complementary to the codon coding for the specific amino acid. Binding of this area to the messenger RNA codon places the specific amino acid at the other end into the proper sequence for the protein. The amino acids are placed one at a time as the transfer RNA molecules read the RNA template, beginning at the amino acid end (the 5' end) and finishing at the carboxy end (the 3' end). The process begins at the first AUG triplet and continues until a stop codon (UAA, UAG, or UGA) is reached, whereupon the messenger RNA falls off the ribosome and degenerates. The specific linear sequence of amino acids is specified by the genetic coding; in turn, this sequence determines the 3-dimensional form of the protein, the folded structure necessary for function.

The final expression of a gene may not end with the translation process. Further (posttranslational) processing of proteins occurs, such as glycosylation (the gonadotropins) or proteolytic cleavage (conversion of proopiomelanocortin to ACTH).

The mechanisms that produce proteins from genes are similar throughout the biologic world. This means that important knowledge regarding human function can be gained by studying simple organisms, and microbes can be engineered to produce human proteins.

Mutations

Any change in DNA sequence constitutes a mutation. Substitution refers to a change in a single nucleic acid base. A substitution in a codon can result in the incorporation of the wrong amino acid into a protein, leading to a change or loss in function. Insertion or deletion of amino acids into the final protein product can result from improper RNA splicing. Because of great redundancy in the genetic code (many triplet codons code out for the same amino acid, and there are only 20 amino acids), not all substitutions produce an effect. A clinical example of a single base substitution (point mutation) is the sickle mutation, in which thymine is substituted for adenine in the beta-globin gene. If homologous regions of DNA are misaligned, unequal crossover can occur, resulting in deletions and insertions (additions). Deletions and insertions can involve single bases, up to entire exons, or genes or several genes. Recombination or exchange of genetic material usually occurs in meiosis. Even a change at the junction of a coding and noncoding region can lead to abnormal messenger RNA.

Chromosomal Abnormalities

Numerical Abnormalities

Numerical abnormalities usually are due to nondisjunction, a failure of separation at anaphase, either during mitotic division or during meiosis. *Aneuploidy* is a chromosome number that is not an exact multiple of the haploid number, e.g., monosomy (45,X Turner syndrome) or trisomy (trisomy 13 Patau syndrome, trisomy 18 Edward syndrome, trisomy 21 Down syndrome, 47,XXY Klinefelter syndrome). *Mosaicism* indicates one or more cell lines with a different karyotype, usually arising from nondisjunction during early mitosis (failure of two paired chromosomes to separate). *Polyploidy,* multiples of the haploid number of chromosomes, is a significant cause of spontaneous miscarriage.

Structural Abnormalities

Structural abnormalities are usually due to chromosomal breaks induced by radiation, drugs, or viruses. The resulting abnormality depends on the rearrangement of the broken pieces. Thus, in a *translocation* there is interchange of material between two or more nonhomologous chromosomes. A balanced translocation is associated with neither gain nor loss of genetic material, and such an individual is a translocation carrier.

Single-Gene Defects

Single-gene defects are due to mutations in specific genes. These mutations are transmitted according to mendelian inheritance: autosomal dominant, autosomal recessive, X-linked recessive, and rarely X-linked dominant.

Autosomal Dominance. Transmission is not linked to the sex of an individual, and homozygous and heterozygous children are affected (only one allele needs to be abnormal). With two heterozygous parents, each child has a 75% risk of being affected. With one heterozygous parent, each child has a 50% risk of being affected. The effect is subject to variable expression. Examples of autosomal dominant conditions include Huntington disease, neurofibromatosis, and Marfan syndrome.

Autosomal Recessive. These conditions are phenotypically expressed only in homozygotes (both alleles must be abnormal). With heterozygote parents, each child has a 25% risk of being affected and a 50% chance of being a carrier. Examples of autosomal recessive conditions are cystic fibrosis, sickle cell disease, and adrenal hyperplasia due to a deficiency in 21-hydroxylase.

X-Linked Recessive Inheritance. An affected father can transmit the condition only to daughters. Only homozygous females are affected when the condition is recessive. Red–green color blindness and hemophilia A are examples.

Genomic Imprinting

Genomic imprinting indicates persisting influences on genome function by the male and female parental contributions. For example, placental development is controlled mostly by paternally derived genes. Thus, a hydatidiform mole has a normal karyotype, but all of its chromosomes are derived from the father. Experiments in nature and animal experiments indicate that the maternal contribution to the genome is more important for embryonic development. In certain autosomal recessive conditions, the expression, severity, and age of onset will be influenced by the gender of the parent providing the mutant gene or chromosome.

Techniques of Molecular Biology

An enzyme that breaks the phosphodiester bonds and cuts the DNA molecule into fragments is an endonuclease; a ***restriction enzyme*** (restriction endonuclease) will cut only at sites with specific nucleic acid sequences. Restriction enzymes were discovered in bacteria in which they form a defense mechanism to cut (and thus inactivate) any foreign DNA (from invading viruses) introduced into the bacterial cell. As part of this protection mechanism, bacteria also contain methylases that methylate recognition sites in native DNA, directing the action of the restriction enzyme to the nonmethylated foreign DNA. Different bacteria have different restriction enzymes with specific action sites . Restriction enzymes are available that cut DNA into pieces (restriction fragments), ranging from many small fragments to a few large pieces, depending on the number of nucleotides in the recognition sequence. They are named for the organism and strain from which they are derived. The combination of restriction fragments, the merger of two cut pieces of DNA, yields ***recombinant DNA.***

DNA polymerase is an enzyme that brings single nucleotides into a DNA molecule. A DNA polymerase can form DNA only in the presence of a DNA template; the synthesized DNA will be complementary to the template. RNA polymerase can make RNA also only in the presence of a DNA template.

A ***DNAase*** can remove nucleotides. By combining DNAase treatment with DNA polymerase action, radiolabeled nucleotides can be introduced into a DNA molecule, producing a ***DNA probe.*** A DNA probe can be compared with the antibody used in immunoassays. The antibody is specific and recognizes the hormone against which it is formed. The DNA probe specifically detects a sequence of DNA.

Reverse transcriptase is DNA polymerase that is RNA dependent. It is called reverse transcriptase because the flow of information is from RNA to DNA, the reverse of the usual direction of flow. This enzyme permits the copying of essentially any RNA molecule into single-stranded DNA; such DNA is called ***complementary DNA*** because it is a mirror image of the messenger RNA. Complementary DNA probes are limited by their reading only the exons (remember that introns are excised from RNA), and thus these probes read only large areas.

DNA and RNA are charged molecules and, therefore, will migrate in an electrical field. Fragments can be analyzed by gel (agarose or polyacrylamide) electrophoresis, the largest fragments migrating the slowest. By convention, the gels are read from top to bottom, with the smallest fragments at the bottom.

Southern blot analysis

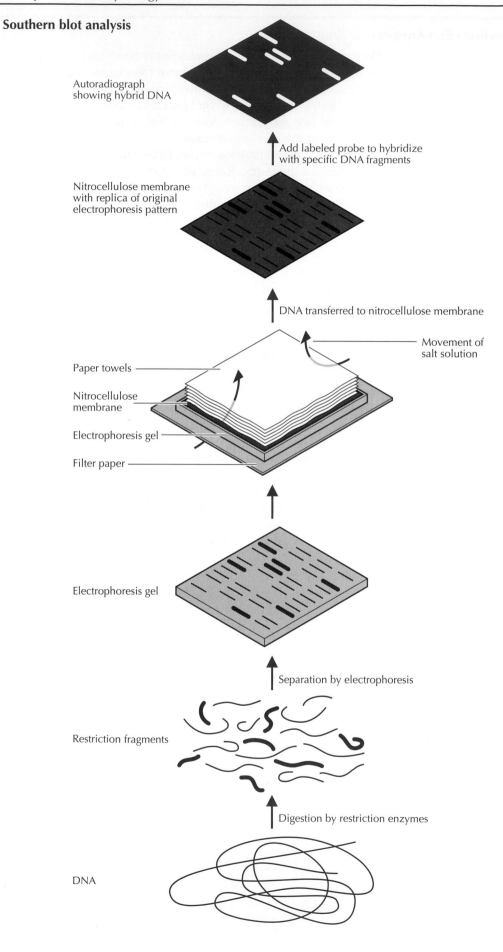

Autoradiograph
showing hybrid DNA

Add labeled probe to hybridize
with specific DNA fragments

Nitrocellulose membrane
with replica of original
electrophoresis pattern

DNA transferred to nitrocellulose membrane

Movement of
salt solution

Paper towels

Nitrocellulose
membrane

Electrophoresis gel

Filter paper

Electrophoresis gel

Separation by electrophoresis

Restriction fragments

Digestion by restriction enzymes

DNA

Southern Blot Analysis

DNA is first denatured to separate the two strands, then digested by restriction enzymes to produce smaller fragments. The Southern blot method, named after E.M. Southern, determines the fragment sizes. The fragments are separated by electrophoresis. The electrophoresis gel is placed over a thick piece of filter paper with its ends dipped in a high-salt solution. A special membrane (nitrocellulose) is placed over the gel, and over this is placed a stack of paper towels compressed by a weight. The salt solution rises by wick action into the filter paper; it moves by capillary action through the gel carrying the DNA with it. The DNA is carried to the nitrocellulose membrane to which it binds. The salt solution keeps moving and is absorbed by the paper towels. The nitrocellulose membrane thus creates a replica of the original electrophoresis pattern. The DNA is fixed to the membrane either by high-temperature baking or by ultraviolet light. Specific labeled probes then can be introduced for hybridization. *Hybridization* means that a specific probe anneals to its complementary sequence. The fragments with this sequence are then identified by autoradiography.

Northern blotting refers to RNA processing, Northern because RNA is the opposite image of DNA. Extracted RNA is separated by electrophoresis and transferred to a cellulose membrane as in Southern blotting for hybridization with probes (complementary DNA). Northern blotting would be used, for example, to determine whether hormone stimulation of a specific protein in a tissue is mediated by messenger RNA, i.e., gene expression.

Electrophoresis to separate proteins is called *Western blotting,* and antibodies are used for the hybridization identification process. Like Northern blotting, Western blotting tests gene expression, not just the presence of a gene. Northern and Western represent intentional witticisms (a rare event in science) in response to Southern blotting. Hybridization without electrophoresis by placing a drop of the cell extract directly on filter paper is called *dot or slot blotting.*

Hybridization

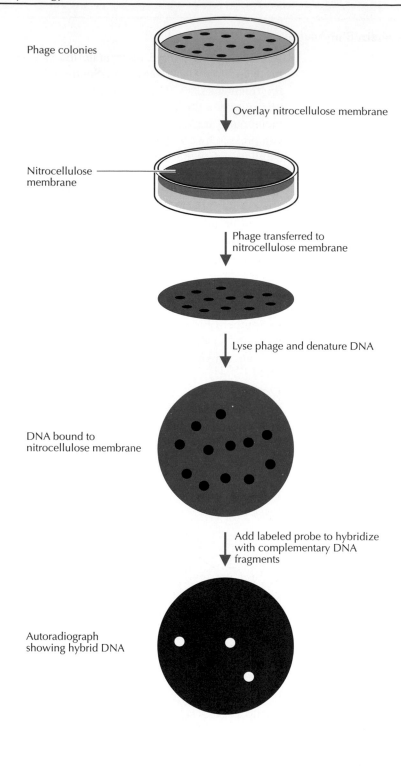

Phage colonies

Overlay nitrocellulose membrane

Nitrocellulose membrane

Phage transferred to nitrocellulose membrane

Lyse phage and denature DNA

DNA bound to nitrocellulose membrane

Add labeled probe to hybridize with complementary DNA fragments

Autoradiograph showing hybrid DNA

Hybridization

When two complementary strands of DNA reassociate, the process is called hybridization. Hybridization allows a specific area of the DNA to be studied using a radiolabeled DNA probe that is specific (a complementary sequence). The nitrocellulose membrane produced after Southern blotting is first treated to block nonspecific binding sites. The membrane is then treated (hybridized) with the labeled probe. The location of bound probe is then identified by autoradiography (for radiolabeled probes) or by colorimetric methods. The sequence of the probe, therefore, determines the sequence at the site of binding. Whenever two products are complementary, hybridization occurs. Thus, complementary DNA can be hybridized to its template messenger RNA.

In situ hybridization is the technique in which labeled DNA or RNA probes are placed directly on a slide of tissue or cells. A piece of cloned DNA labeled with a fluorescent marker can be utilized; the method is referred to as *FISH*, fluorescence in situ hybridization. The region corresponding to the cloned DNA lights up under fluorescent illumination unless the region has been deleted from one of the chromosomes. Several microdeletion syndromes have been discovered with the FISH technique, e.g., the Prader-Willi syndrome.

Polymerase Chain Reaction (PCR)

The polymerase chain reaction (PCR) is a technique to amplify (relatively quickly) small fragments or areas of DNA into quantities large enough to be analyzed with electrophoresis and blotting methods. This technique produces enormous numbers of copies of a specific DNA sequence without resorting to cloning. The sequence to be amplified must be known. Specific markers (synthesized short sequences of DNA corresponding to each end of the sequence to be studied) are selected that will delineate the region of DNA to be amplified. These flanking sequences are called primers. The DNA sample, the primers, and an excess of free single nucleotides are incubated with a DNA polymerase.

The first step involves separating DNA into its single strands by denaturation with heat (92°C), then the temperature is lowered (40°C), causing the primers to stick (anneal) to their complementary regions on the DNA. The temperature is raised to 62°C, and DNA polymerase then synthesizes a new strand beginning and ending at the primers, forming a new double-stranded DNA. Repeating the cycle many times (by alternating the reaction temperature) amplifies the amount of DNA available for study (more than 1 million-fold); the increase occurs exponentially. Thus, DNA can be analyzed from a single cell, and genes can be visualized by blotting without labeled probes.

Because the process requires alternate heating and cooling, a DNA polymerase resistant to heat is an advantage in that periodic replenishment is not necessary. This problem was solved with the discovery of DNA polymerase (Taq polymerase) in a microorganism (*Thermus aquaticus*) that is a thermophile (a hot water microbe) and was found in an out-of-the-way Yellowstone National Park hot spring called Mushroom Pool. This high-temperature polymerase allows automation of the process.

The technique of polymerase chain reaction has made possible the study of incredibly small amounts of DNA. Most impressive is the amplification of small amounts of degraded DNA from extinct and rare species preserved in museums. DNA from fossils has been amplified and sequenced (e.g., from an 18-million-year-old magnolia plant).

Cloning DNA

Cloning means isolating a gene and making copies of it. A DNA library is a collection of DNA molecules derived from cloning methods. A complementary DNA library is the DNA counterpart of all of the messenger RNA isolated from a particular cell or tissue. By starting with messenger RNA, the search for the gene of interest can be focused (instead of searching the entire genome). Such a library is made using reverse transcriptase. The DNA molecules then can be inserted into an appropriate vector (described below) and replicate molecules can be produced. Using probes, the complementary DNA can be selected that matches the gene of interest (keeping in mind that complementary DNA only includes the exons of a gene). Cloning the DNA simply means the production of many identical copies of a specified fragment of DNA. Cloning can also be performed using the polymerase chain reaction. As indicated above, complementary DNA cloning focuses on the DNA counterpart of messenger RNA; genomic DNA cloning, using a restriction endonuclease, copies the DNA in genes. Cloning also can be used to make multiple copies of probes or unknown DNA fragments.

Identification of specific DNA by hybridization with known oligonucleotide sequences

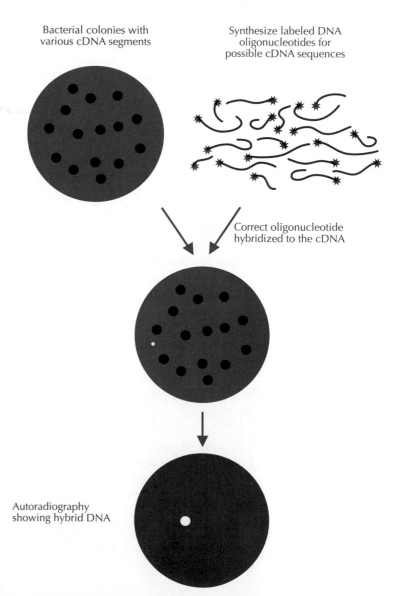

Known amino acid sequence　Met — Tyr — Lys — Asp — Trp — Gln — Cys

Possible cDNA sequence	ATG	TAT	AAA	GAT	TGG	CAA	TGT
		TAC	AAG	GAC		CAG	TGC

Bacterial colonies with various cDNA segments

Synthesize labeled DNA oligonucleotides for possible cDNA sequences

Correct oligonucleotide hybridized to the cDNA

Autoradiography showing hybrid DNA

If the amino acid sequence is unknown, one can work backward. Knowing the specific protein product, antibodies can be produced against the protein. When complementary DNA is inserted into certain vectors, production of the protein can be identified with the antibodies; thus, the DNA fragment will be isolated.

A vector is an entity in which foreign DNA can be inserted. The vector plus the foreign DNA are inserted into a host cell; the host cell produces both the vector and the foreign DNA. The first vectors were bacterial plasmids, circular DNA molecules (minichromosomes) that coexist in the cytoplasm with the bacterial chromosomal DNA. Most noteworthy, they carry genes that code for antibiotic resistance. This enables the bacterial cells that contain the plasmid to be selected by appropriate antibiotic treatment. Plasmid vectors have also been developed that allow selection by color. A variety of bacterial strains have been developed, each for a specific use.

Disruption of the plasmid DNA with restriction enzymes, followed by incorporation of foreign DNA with DNA ligase, produces plasmid DNA molecules (recombinant DNA containing the foreign DNA) that can be replicated. Plasmid vectors can incorporate foreign DNA fragments up to 10 kb in size. Digestion of recovered plasmids with restriction enzymes releases the desired DNA fragment, which can then be recovered by electrophoresis.

Other vectors exist. Bacteriophages (or phages) are viruses that infect and replicate within bacteria. Phage vectors can incorporate larger DNA inserts, up to 20 kb. Cloning DNA with phage vectors follows the same basic design as with plasmids. Larger fragments of foreign DNA are cloned with cosmid vectors, artificially produced combinations of phage and plasmid vectors. Very large fragments, up to 1000 kb, can be cloned using yeast artificial chromosomes. This method can work with whole genes.

Basic Steps for Cloning

1. Choose a DNA source: either genomic DNA or complementary DNA.

2. Fragment the DNA by restriction endonucleases.

3. Insert the fragments into vectors.

4. Introduce the vectors into bacteria.

5. Collect the cloned DNA propagated in the bacteria to form a library.

6. Screen the library for the desired sequence. Possible methods include the use of complementary nucleotide probes for fragments that hybridize or the detection of a specific protein produced with antibodies to the protein or by assaying the function of the protein.

Knockout Animal Models

Animal models for the function of a gene employ the method of "knocking out" a specific gene. In a straightforward, but important demonstration, it can be determined whether a specific gene and its protein are essential for life, or for a function (such as pregnancy).

**Identification of
specific DNA by
detecting a known
protein product**

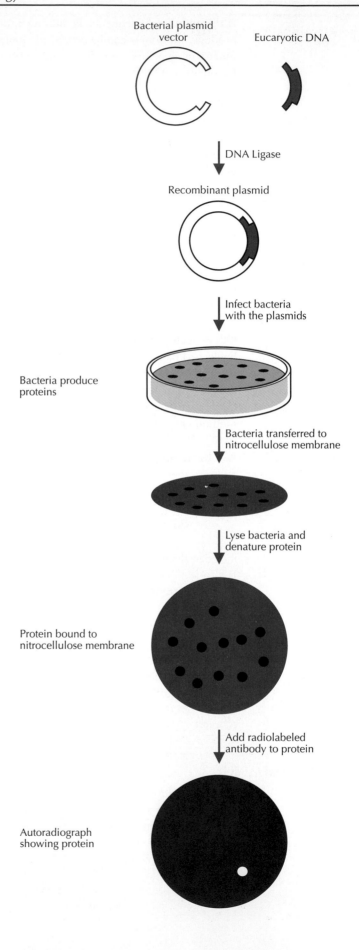

Bacterial plasmid
vector

Eucaryotic DNA

DNA Ligase

Recombinant plasmid

Infect bacteria
with the plasmids

Bacteria produce
proteins

Bacteria transferred to
nitrocellulose membrane

Lyse bacteria and
denature protein

Protein bound to
nitrocellulose membrane

Add radiolabeled
antibody to protein

Autoradiograph
showing protein

The Identification of Genes

To clone an entire gene whose protein product is known, a complementary DNA library is produced. The specific DNA fragment is identified by linking it to the protein. Once identified, the total gene can be screened using the identified complementary DNA, indicating the introns and exons. Another strategy is to synthesize an oligonucleotide probe, basing the sequence on the known amino acid sequence in the protein product (from the peptide sequence, the DNA sequence that codes for that protein can be predicted). This method can be used with just a relatively small piece of the peptide. As more and more genes are cloned, the codon frequency for particular amino acids is being established. Complementary DNA can be cloned without producing a library by using the polymerase chain reaction to amplify complementary DNA made from messenger RNA by reverse transcriptase. Overlapping sequences of the genome can be cloned, using a piece of DNA from each succeeding product, to work across a chromosome in a systematic manner to search for a gene; this is called *chromosome walking.*

The entire sequencing process can be performed by a computer, even searching for open reading fames. Once the sequence of a DNA fragment has been identified, the computer can utilize DNA and protein data bases to predict sequence, recognition site, protein translation, and homology with known sequences. The scientist can then select restriction fragment sizes for cloning. Once a gene has been analyzed, it has to be compared with the gene in the disease state. If a mutation is of large size, this can be detected by Southern blotting. Minor alterations require comparisons in DNA sequences, which is possible by using polymerase chain amplification to produce specific gene sequences in amounts readily studied.

A gene can be localized to a specific chromosome when its protein product is unknown by studies involving chromosome rearrangements and linkage analysis. Specific diseases are associated with karyotypic changes. Thus, the specific chromosome can be targeted for gene localization. Linkage analysis utilizes restriction fragment length polymorphisms.

DNA Polymorphism

Southern blotting reveals specific patterns of bands that reflect the varying lengths of the DNA fragments produced by restriction enzyme action. A specific site can exhibit a mutation by having a different pattern (a different length of the DNA fragment on Southern blotting due to sequence difference). These differences in DNA sequences are called restriction fragment length polymorphisms, or simply polymorphisms, usually a benign variation. A polymorphism will be governed by the mendelian regulations of inheritance, and if by chance, a polymorphism is identified in a patient with a specific disease, the transmission of the disease can be studied. The polymorphism, which is linked to the disease by chance, can be used to study the inheritance of a disease when the genes are unknown. The polymorphism is like a flag that marks specific areas of chromosomes. This method of study requires DNA from at least one affected individual and a sufficient number of family members to trace the polymorphism, either by Southern blotting (for long sequences) or with the polymerase chain reaction (best for short sequences).

Minisatellites are a form of polymorphisms. Minisatellites are noncoding areas of DNA that repeat in variable numbers, so-called variable number *tandem repeat sequences*, distributed throughout the length of every human chromosome. These areas can be followed by DNA probes, providing a "fingerprint" for specific individuals. This uniqueness is applied in forensic medicine. Microsatellites, as the name implies, are smaller than minisatellites. Usually, microsatellites consist of repetitions of only two nucleotides.

DNA polymorphisms now number in the thousands and allow genetic mapping with great precision. A polymorphism can serve as a genetic marker for a medically important gene.

The Human Genome Project

All of the human genes are collectively known as the genome. Begun in 1990, the goal of the international human genome project is to sequence the 3 billion base pairs of the human genome, enough information to occupy 10,000 conventional floppy disks. Using the standard thin-layer vertical gel electrophoresis followed by autoradiographs of gel blots, it would require tens of millions of gels to accomplish this project. Shared data and computer analysis are necessary, and high speed automated sequencing technology must be utilized. Each laboratory will determine its small part of the sequence and then have to figure out where it fits in the big picture. When the computer finds an open reading frame, the probable amino acid sequence and the function can be predicted for the gene's protein. A genetic linkage map can serve as a foundation for locating disease sites and for integrating the genetic sequencing with biologic functions. Remember that there are anywhere from 60,000 to 150,000 genes. By the end of 1997, more than 60 million (of the total 3 billion) base pairs had been analyzed, and an electronic version is available on the World Wide Web at http://www.ncbi.nlm.nih.gov/. This represents about 50,000 genes, The complete genomic sequences had been determined for 141 viruses, 51 organelles, 2 eubacteria, and one eukaryote. A complete map of the human genome is predicted to be available by 2005. Soon, we will be able to have in our possession a personal CD that contains our individual complete genetic blueprint.

The U.S. Department of Energy maintains a Web site that provides basic information and useful links to other sites regarding the human genome project:

http://www.ornl.gov/techresources/human_genome/publicat/publictions.html

Genetic Maps. By 1997, about 6000 polymorphic markers had been identified to localize genes that predispose to disease. Using this method, a gene can be targeted for more specific localization.

Physical Maps. Genes of interest are localized by comparing overlapping DNA fragments. This isolates chromosomal segments for sequencing.

Sequence Maps. The challenge of the Human Genome Project can be appreciated by considering that technology is capable of reading about 36,000 DNA letters per day, and there are about 130 million DNA letters in the average human chromosome. Although the genetic and physical maps are nearing completion, complete sequence maps will take many more years.

The chromosomal locations of genes responsible for hormone production are rapidly being mapped. From the cloned DNA sequences, the amino acid sequences can be predicted. Every protein product of a gene represents a potential diagnostic or therapeutic target. And of course, inherited disorders will be subject to characterization and, eventually, gene therapy. However, even after a gene has been identified and genetically mapped, its full characterization remains a difficult and time-consuming task. Full understanding of disorders that involve the interactions of multiple genes will be even more complicated.

But molecular progress is inexorable. The future will see preventive medicine by prediction. By knowing an individual's genetic constitution, appropriate and intensive screening can be directed to predisposed conditions. This kind of knowledge will also require social and political considerations. It is not far-fetched to envision marriages and children avoided because of a bad match of genetic predispositions. Society will have to develop guidelines regarding the use of this information: by individuals, by employers, by health organizations, and by the government. Scientific progress must be matched by public and professional education to appropriately manage this knowledge.

Clinical Applications

The molecular diagnosis of genetic disorders requires only a small sample of DNA, obtainable from any cells that are nucleated, such as white blood cells or epithelial cells. Polymerase chain reaction carried out by automatic machinery allows speedy DNA diagnosis with material amplified from a single cell. This is an important advantage in prenatal genetic analysis and in preimplantation sexing and diagnosis. PCR makes it possible to perform DNA diagnosis from a single cell removed from embryos fertilized in vitro.

Molecular diagnosis is limited by the prevalence of heterogeneic genetic changes. In other words, many disorders involve different mutations in different people. In contrast, some (like sickle cell disease) always involve the same change. With cystic fibrosis, 70% of patients (of northern European ancestry) have the same 3-base deletion, whereas the remaining 30% have an extremely heterogeneous collection of mutations. Molecular diagnosis is further challenged by the need to not only find a subtle change in a gene but to distinguish important changes from benign variations (polymorphisms). Ingenious PCR-based methods have been developed for rapid screening and detection of mutations. The significance of detected mutations requires segregation of the mutation with an identified disease in a family.

At least one type of growth hormone deficiency is inherited in an autosomal recessive pattern. The cloning of growth hormone DNA complementary to its messenger RNA permitted localization of the growth hormone gene. The growth hormone gene is in a cluster that also includes the gene for human placental lactogen. This cluster of genes contains multiple units of DNA that are homologous and prone to recombination, which leads to deletion on one chromosome and duplication on another. Similar mechanisms operate for other protein products governed by genes in clusters, such as the globins.

The commercial production of proteins from cloned genes inserted into bacteria is rapidly increasing. The production of insulin (the first) and growth hormone are good examples. Glycosylation does not occur in bacterial systems, and therefore the commercial production of recombinant glycoproteins requires a mammalian cell line for the process. This has been accomplished, and recombinant gonadotropins are now available. The gene for gonadotropin-releasing hormone on the short arm of chromosome 8 has been isolated and cloned. Molecular technology was important in the characterization of inhibin, the ovarian follicular hormone that inhibits follicle-stimulating hormone (FSH) secretion. The inhibin gene has been sequenced and found to be homologous to the gene for antimüllerian hormone. The alpha-subunit common to gonadotropins, thyroid-stimulating hormone, and human chorionic gonadotropin (HCG) has been traced to a gene that has been isolated, sequenced, and localized on chromosome 6.

The Y chromosome carries a genetic locus responsible for differentiation of the testes, called the testes-determining factor. The theory that this is a male-specific histocompatibility antigen (the H–Y antigen) has been abandoned. Using material from intersex patients, maps of the Y chromosome have placed the testes determining factor on the short arm, and it is now believed that this activity resides specifically with the SRY gene. Certain intersex disorders, therefore, result from an exchange of X and Y DNA when the short arms of the X and Y chromosomes pair and crossover during meiosis. The exact locus (or loci) of the ovarian determinants on the X chromosomes has not yet been identified.

Because of the importance of X-linked disease, the X chromosome is one of the most studied of all human chromosomes. By 1993, about 40% of the 160 million base pairs of the X chromosome DNA had been cloned; in addition, 26 inherited disease genes had been cloned, and more than 50 other genes had been localized by linkage analysis.

Insertion of a foreign gene into an embryo results in a transgenic animal. The inserted foreign gene will be present in many tissues, and if the animal is fertile, it will be inherited. There are many applications for transgenic animals. Transgenic animals provide animal models for inherited diseases and malignant tumors and provide a means to carry out experiments in gene therapy. The transfer of new or altered genes is an important method to study gene function. Transgenic plants can even be developed to produce new pharmaceuticals, and the introduction of genes conferring resistance to insects may solve the problem of insecticide contamination.

The human genome contains many genes with the potential to cause cancer. Other genes have the ability to block malignant growth. Cancer is a genetic disease in that tumors can be said to be clonal; all the cells are genetically related. ***Oncogenes***, discovered in tumor viruses, are genes that transform cells from normal to abnormal growth by encoding proteins that are involved in signal transduction, specifically the transmission of growth-regulatory messages. There are many oncogenes and many different pathways of action, all of which result in a proliferative state. The mutations that activate these genes either lead to protein activity independent of incoming signals or to activity at the wrong place at the wrong time. The bottom line is the turning on (by an altered oncogene) of persistent growth.

There are also antioncogenes in normal cells, growth-suppressing genes that must be inactivated before tumors can grow. Inherited susceptibility for cancer can also result from a mutation in tumor suppresser genes. Although activation of an oncogene is a dominant effect, tumor suppresser mutations are recessive and can be carried and transmitted, but are not active as long as pairing occurs with a normal antioncogene.

Cancer, therefore, is a genetic disease, but regulation of normal growth involves a complex system that takes a long time to overcome. During this time period, the technology of recombinant DNA may be able to achieve diagnosis sufficiently early to yield cures. Knowing the specific oncogene involved in a given tumor also offers therapeutic possibilities. For example, an antimetabolite can be attached to antibody for an oncogene, targeting the cancer cells.

Molecular biology is changing both diagnosis and therapy. Viral and bacterial DNA can be identified. The automated PCR process can produce electrophoretic patterns that can be read automatically. With this technique, a single human papillomavirus DNA molecule can be detected among 10,000 or more human cells.

Faulty endogenous protein production can be corrected by replacing the problematic mechanism. There are two strategies: foreign cells that produce the missing protein could be introduced, or the faulty gene could be replaced (or more accurately, adding a complementary-corrected DNA). Thus, recessive single-gene disorders are potentially amenable to gene therapy, as are acquired diseases such as cancer and infections. Gene therapy is broadly defined as the enlistment of the patient's own cellular machinery to produce a therapeutic agent. A gene delivered to a cell can either replace a defective or missing gene or produce a protein with a desired effect. However, this is a field in its infancy.

Specific guidelines for gene therapy have been developed requiring several levels of review. One class of human therapy is the use of retroviral vectors to transfer marker genes into cultured human cells that are returned to patients of origin. For example, this allows tracking of tumor-infiltrating lymphocytes, donor hepatocytes, or killer T cells that are specific for the human immunodeficiency virus. These transferred genes can also be crafted to provide a function in patients with single-gene inherited disorders. Another class of therapy involves the transfer of genes that encode for factors that destroy tumor cells, such as tumor necrosis factor or interleukin. Retroviral vectors are viruses that have been altered so that no viral proteins can be made by cells infected by the vectors. Thus, viral replication and spread are prevented, but gene transfer into replicating cells can take place. Other transfer methods being developed include the use of adenovirus vectors and specifically targeted plasmid DNA.

References

Dib CS, Faure S, Fizames C, Samson D, Drouot N, Vignal A, Millasseau P, Marc S, Hazan J, Seboun E, Lathrop M, Gyapay G, Morissette J, Weissenbach J, A comprehensive genetic map of the human genome based on 5,264 microsatellites, Nature 380:152, 1996.

Rowen L, Mahairas G, Hood L, Sequencing the human genome, *Science* 278:605, 1997.

Schuler GD, Boguski MS, Stewart EA, Stein LD, Gyapay, G, Rice K, White RE, et al, A gene map of the human genome, *Science* 274:540, 1996.

Watson JD, Gilman M, Witkowski J, Zoller M, *Recombinant DNA,* 2nd ed, New York, Scientific American Books,1992.

Online Resources

List of biochemical genetics tests by diseases, produced by the University of California, San Diego: *http://biochemgen.ucsd.edu/wbgtests/dz-tst.htm*

The U.S. National Library of Medicine search service for MEDLINE and other databases, including genomes, and DNA and protein sequences: *http://www.ncbi.nlm.nih.gov*

Database of inherited disorders: *http://www.ncbi.nlm.nih.gov/Omim*

2 Hormone Biosynthesis, Metabolism, and Mechanism of Action

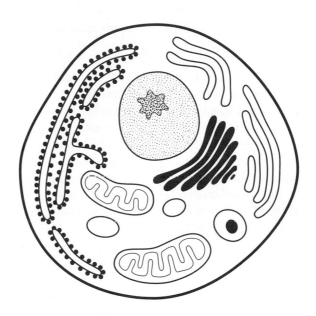

The classical definition of a hormone is a substance that is produced in a special tissue, where it is released into the bloodstream, and travels to distant responsive cells in which the hormone exerts its characteristic effects. What was once thought of as a simple voyage is now appreciated as an odyssey that becomes more complex as new facets of the journey are unraveled in research laboratories throughout the world. Indeed, the notion that hormones are products only of special tissues has been challenged.

Complex hormones and hormone receptors have been discovered in primitive, unicellular organisms, suggesting that endocrine glands are a late development of evolution. The widespread capability of cells to make hormones explains the puzzling discoveries of hormones in strange places, such as gastrointestinal hormones in the brain, reproductive hormones in intestinal secretions, and the ability of cancers to unexpectedly make hormones. Hormones and neurotransmitters were and are a means of communication. Only when animals evolved into complex organisms did special glands develop to produce hormones that could be used in a more sophisticated fashion. Furthermore, hormones must have appeared even before plants and animals diverged because there are many plant substances similar to hormones and hormone receptors. Therefore, it is not surprising that, because every cell contains the genes necessary for hormonal expression, cancer cells, because of their dedifferentiation, can uncover gene expression and, in inappropriate locations and at inappropriate times, make hormones.

Hormones, therefore, are substances that provide a means of communication and should now be viewed broadly as chemical regulatory and signaling agents. The classic endocrine hormones travel through the bloodstream to distant sites, but cellular communication is also necessary at local sites. Words that are now encountered frequently are paracrine, autocrine, and intracrine, depicting a more immediate form of communication.

Paracrine Communication

Intercellular communication involving the local diffusion of regulating substances from a cell to nearby (contiguous) cells.

Autocrine Communication

Intracellular communication whereby a single cell produces regulating substances that in turn act upon receptors on or within the same cell.

Intracrine Communication

This form of intracellular communication occurs when unsecreted substances bind to intracellular receptors.

Let us follow an estradiol molecule throughout its career and in so doing gain an overview of how hormones are formed, how hormones work, and how hormones are metabolized. Estradiol begins its lifespan with its synthesis in a cell specially suited for this task. For this biosynthesis to take place, the proper enzyme capability must be present along with the proper precursors. In the adult human female the principal sources of estradiol are the granulosa cells of the developing follicle and the corpus luteum. These cells possess the ability to turn on steroidogenesis in response to specific stimuli. The stimulating agents are the gonadotropins, follicle-stimulating hormone (FSH) and luteinizing hormone (LH). The initial step in the process that will give rise to estradiol is the transmission of the message from the stimulating agents to the steroid-producing mechanisms within the cells.

Messages that stimulate steroidogenesis must be transmitted through the cell membrane. This is necessary because gonadotropins, being large glycopeptides, do not ordinarily enter cells but must communicate with the cell by joining with specific receptors on the cell membrane. In so doing they activate a sequence of communication. A considerable amount of investigation has been devoted to determining the methods by which this communication takes place. E. M. Sutherland received the Nobel Prize in 1971 for proposing the concept of a second messenger.

Gonadotropin, the first messenger, activates an enzyme in the cell membrane called adenylate cyclase. This enzyme transmits the message by catalyzing the production of a second messenger within the cell, cyclic adenosine 3',5'-monophosphate (cyclic AMP). The message passes from gonadotropin to cyclic AMP, much like a baton in a relay race.

Cyclic AMP, the second messenger, initiates the process of steroidogenesis, leading to the synthesis and secretion of the hormone estradiol. This notion of message transmission has grown more and more complex with the appreciation of new physiologic concepts, such as the heterogeneity of peptide hormones, the up- and down-regulation of cell membrane receptors, the regulation of adenylate cyclase activity, and the important roles for autocrine and paracrine regulating factors.

Secretion of estradiol into the bloodstream directly follows its synthesis. Once in the bloodstream, estradiol exists in two forms, bound and free. A majority of the hormone is bound to protein carriers, albumin and sex steroid hormone-binding globulin. The purpose of this binding is not totally clear. The biologic activity of a hormone may be limited by binding in the blood, thereby avoiding extreme or sudden reactions. In addition, binding may prevent unduly rapid metabolism, allowing the hormone to exist for the length of time necessary to ensure a biologic effect. This reservoir-like mechanism avoids peaks and valleys in hormone levels and allows a more steady state of hormone action.

The biologic and metabolic effects of a hormone are determined by a cell's ability to receive and retain the hormone. The estradiol that is not bound to a protein, but floats freely in the bloodstream, readily enters cells by rapid diffusion. For estradiol to produce its effect, however, it must be grasped by a receptor within the cell. The job of the receptor is to aid in the transmission of the hormone's message to nuclear gene transcription. The result is production of messenger RNA leading to protein synthesis and a cellular response characteristic of the hormone.

Once estradiol has accomplished its mission, it is eventually released back into the bloodstream. It is possible that estradiol can perform its duty several times before being cleared from the circulation by metabolism. On the other hand, many molecules will be metabolized without ever having the chance to produce an effect. Unlike estradiol, other hormones, such as testosterone, are metabolized and altered within the cell in which an effect is produced. In the latter case, a steroid is released into the bloodstream as an inactive compound. Clearance of steroids from the blood varies according to the structure of the molecules.

Cells that are capable of clearing estradiol from the circulation accomplish this by biochemical means (conversion to estrone and estriol, moderately effective and very weak estrogens, respectively) and conjugation to products that are water soluble and excreted in the urine and bile (sulfo and glucuro conjugates).

Thus, a steroid hormone has a varied career packed into a short lifetime. We are now ready to review the important segments of this lifespan in greater detail.

Nomenclature

All steroid hormones are of basically similar structure with relatively minor chemical differences leading to striking alterations in biochemical activity. The basic structure is the perhydrocyclopentanephenanthrene molecule. It is composed of three 6-carbon rings and one 5-carbon ring. One ring is benzene, two rings naphthalene, and three rings phenanthrene; add a cyclopentane (5-carbon ring), and you have the perhydrocyclopentanephenanthrene structure of the steroid nucleus.

The sex steroids are divided into 3 main groups according to the number of carbon atoms they possess. The 21-carbon series includes the corticoids and the progestins, and the basic structure is the *pregnane* nucleus. The 19-carbon series includes all the androgens and is based on the *androstane* nucleus, whereas the estrogens are 18-carbon steroids based on the *estrane* nucleus.

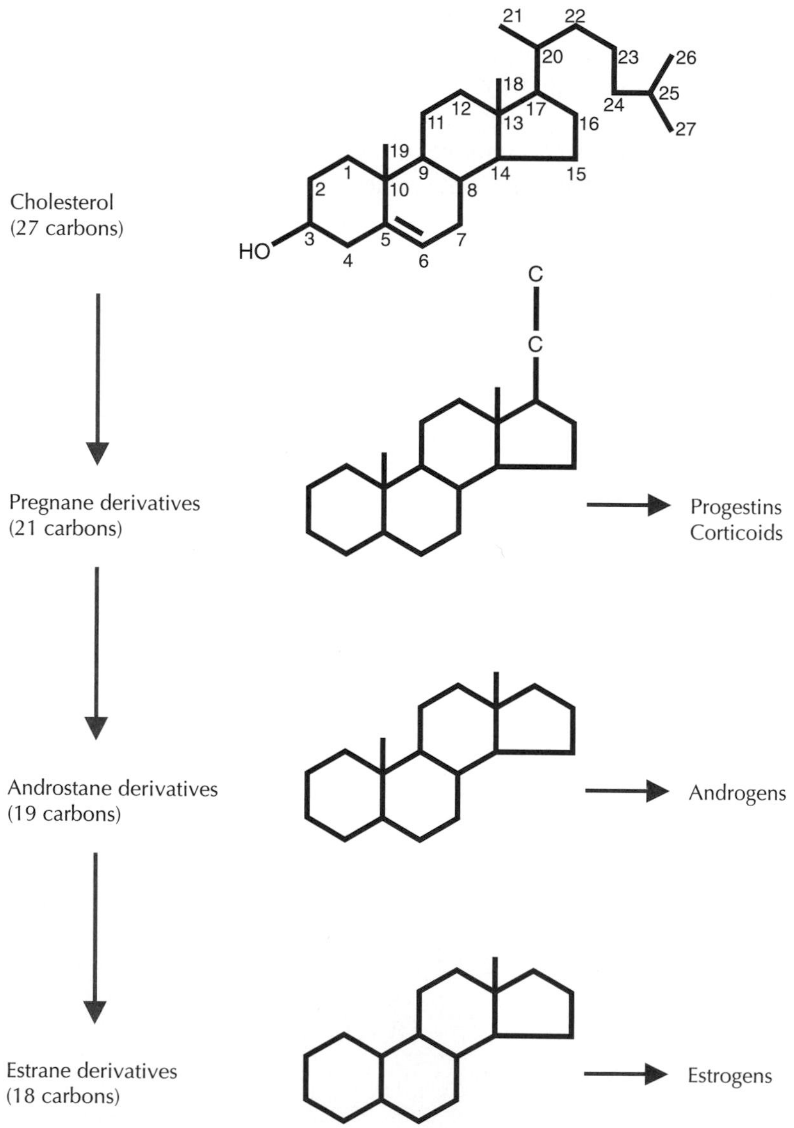

Cholesterol
(27 carbons)

Pregnane derivatives
(21 carbons) → Progestins
Corticoids

Androstane derivatives
(19 carbons) → Androgens

Estrane derivatives
(18 carbons) → Estrogens

There are 6 centers of asymmetry on the basic ring structure, and there are 64 possible isomers. Almost all naturally occurring and active steroids are nearly flat, and substituents below and above the plane of the ring are designated alpha (α) (dotted line) and beta (β)(solid line), respectively. Changes in the position of only one substituent can lead to inactive isomers. For example, 17-epitestosterone is considerably weaker than testosterone; the only difference being a hydroxyl group in the α position at C-17 rather than in the β position.

Progesterone

Top View

Side View

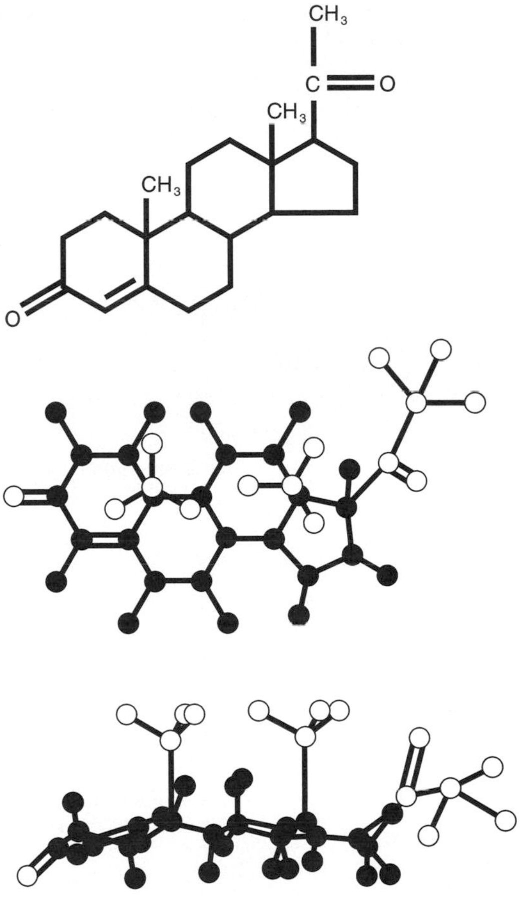

The convention of naming steroids uses the number of carbon atoms to designate the basic name (e.g., pregnane, androstane, or estrane). The basic name is preceded by numbers that indicate the position of double bonds, and the name is altered as follows to indicate 1, 2, or 3 double bonds: -ene, -diene, and -triene. Following the basic name, hydroxyl groups are indicated by the number of the carbon attachment, and 1, 2, or 3 hydroxyl groups are designated -ol, -diol, or -triol. Ketone groups are listed last with numbers of carbon attachments, and 1, 2, or 3 groups designated -one, -dione, or -trione. Special designations include: dehydro, elimination of 2 hydrogens; deoxy, elimination of oxygen; nor, elimination of carbon; delta or Δ, location of double bond.

Estrone
1,3,5(10)-Estratriene-3β-ol-17-one

Testosterone
4-Androstene-17β-ol-3-one

Progesterone
4-Pregnene-3,20-dione

Lipoproteins and Cholesterol

Cholesterol is the basic building block in steroidogenesis. All steroid-producing organs except the placenta can synthesize cholesterol from acetate. Progestins, androgens, and estrogens, therefore, can be synthesized in situ in the various ovarian tissue compartments from the 2-carbon acetate molecule via cholesterol as the common steroid precursor. However, in situ synthesis cannot meet the demand, and, therefore, the major resource is blood cholesterol that enters the ovarian cells and can be inserted into the biosynthetic pathway or stored in esterified form for later use. The cellular entry of cholesterol is mediated via a cell membrane receptor for low-density lipoprotein (LDL), the bloodstream carrier for cholesterol.

Lipoproteins are large molecules that facilitate the transport of nonpolar fats in a polar solvent, the blood plasma. There are 5 major categories of lipoproteins according to their charge and density (flotation during ultracentrifugation). They are derived from each other in the following cascade of decreasing size and increasing density.

Chylomicrons

Large, cholesterol (10%)- and triglyceride (90%)-carrying particles formed in the intestine after a fatty meal.

Very Low-Density Lipoproteins (VLDL)

Also carry cholesterol, but mostly triglyceride; more dense than chylomicrons.

Intermediate-Density Lipoproteins (IDL)

Formed (for a transient existence) with the removal of some of the triglyceride from the interior of VLDL particles.

Low-Density Lipoproteins (LDL)

The end products of VLDL catabolism, formed after further removal of triglyceride leaving approximately 50% cholesterol; the major carriers (2/3) of cholesterol in the plasma and thus a strong relationship exists between elevated LDL levels and cardiovascular disease.

High-Density Lipoproteins (HDL)

The smallest and most dense of the lipoproteins with the highest protein and phospholipid content; HDL levels are inversely associated with atherosclerosis (high levels are protective). HDL can be further separated into a lighter fraction (HDL_2) and a denser fraction (HDL_3). HDL_2 is strongly associated with cardiovascular disease.

The lipoproteins contain 4 ingredients: 1) cholesterol in two forms: free cholesterol on the surface of the spherical lipoprotein molecule and esterified cholesterol in the molecule's interior; 2) triglycerides in the interior of the sphere; 3) phospholipid, and 4) protein: electrically charged substances on the surface of the sphere and responsible for miscibility with plasma and water. The surface proteins, called *apoproteins,* constitute the sites that bind to the lipoprotein receptor molecules on the cell surfaces. The principal surface protein of LDL is apoprotein B, and apoprotein A-1 is the principal apoprotein of HDL.

Lipids for peripheral tissues are provided by the secretion of VLDL by the liver. Triglycerides are liberated from VLDL by lipoprotein lipase located in the capillary endothelial cells as well as a lipase enzyme located on the endothelial cells in liver sinusoids. In this process, the surface components (free cholesterol, phospholipids, and apoproteins) are transferred to HDL. Finally, the VLDL is converted to LDL, which plays the important role of transporting cholesterol to cells throughout the body. The hepatic lipase enzyme is sensitive to sex steroid changes: suppression by estrogen and stimulation by androgens.

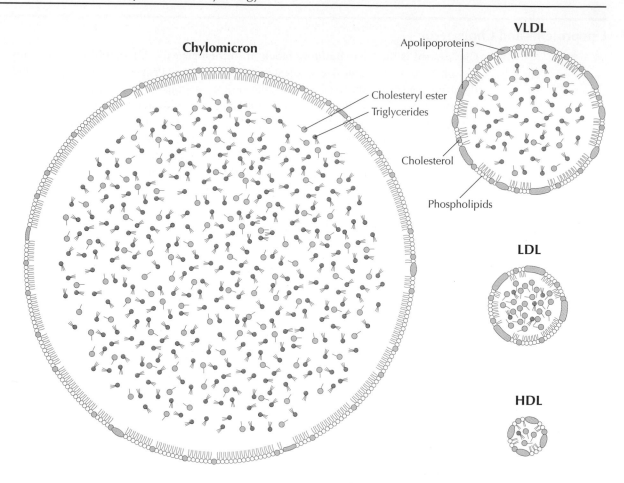

Chylomicron

VLDL

Apolipoproteins

Cholesteryl ester

Triglycerides

Cholesterol

Phospholipids

LDL

HDL

LDL is removed from the blood by cellular receptors that recognize one of the surface apoproteins. The lipoprotein bound to the cell membrane receptor is internalized and degradated. Intracellular levels of cholesterol are partly regulated by the up- and down-regulation of cell membrane LDL receptors. When these LDL receptors are saturated or deficient, LDL is taken up by "scavenger" cells (most likely derived from macrophages) in other tissues, notably the arterial intima. Thus, these cells can become the nidus for atherosclerotic plaques.

HDL is secreted by the liver and intestine or is a product of the degradation of VLDL. Cholesteryl ester molecules move to form a core in a small spherical particle, the HDL_3 particle. These particles accept additional free cholesterol, perhaps mediated by receptors that recognize apoprotein A-1. With uptake of cholesterol, the particle size increases to form HDL_2, the fraction that reflects changes in diet and hormones. HDL_3 levels remain relatively stable.

The protein moieties of the lipoprotein particles are strongly related to the risk of cardiovascular disease, and genetic abnormalities in their synthesis or structure can result in atherogenic conditions. The lipoproteins are a major reason for the disparity in atherosclerosis risk between men and women. Throughout adulthood, the blood HDL-cholesterol level is about 10 mg/dL higher in women, and this difference continues through the postmenopausal years. Total and LDL-cholesterol levels are lower in premenopausal women than in men, but after menopause they rise rapidly.

The protective nature of HDL is due to its ability to pick up free cholesterol from cells or other circulating lipoproteins. This lipid-rich HDL is known as HDL_3, which is then converted to the larger, less dense particle, HDL_2. Thus, HDL converts lipid-rich scavenger cells (macrophages residing in arterial walls) back to their low-lipid state and carries the excess cholesterol to sites (mainly liver) where it can be metabolized. Another method by which HDL removes cholesterol from the body focuses on the uptake of free cholesterol from cell membranes. The free cholesterol is esterified and moves to the core of the HDL particle. Thus, HDL can remove cholesterol by delivering cholesterol to sites for utilization (steroid-producing cells) or metabolism and excretion (liver).

Understanding the role of the cell surface receptors for the homeostasis of cholesterol (discussed later in this chapter), the work of the 1985 Nobel Laureates, Michael S. Brown and Joseph L. Goldstein, revolutionized our concepts of cholesterol, lipoprotein metabolism, and hormone action at the cell membrane.[1] In their Nobel lecture, Brown and Goldstein paid tribute to cholesterol as the most highly decorated small molecule in biology.

For good cardiovascular health, the blood concentration of cholesterol must be kept low, and its escape from the bloodstream must be prevented. The problem of cholesterol transport is solved by esterifying the cholesterol and packaging the ester within the cores of plasma lipoproteins. The delivery of cholesterol to cells is in turn solved by lipoprotein receptors. After binding the lipoprotein with its package of esterified cholesterol, the complex is delivered into the cell by receptor-mediated endocytosis (discussed later in this chapter), in which the lysosomes liberate cholesterol for use by the cell.

Major protection against atherosclerosis depends on the high affinity of the receptor for LDL and the ability of the receptor to recycle multiple times, thus allowing large amounts of cholesterol to be delivered while maintaining a healthy low blood level of LDL. Cells can control their uptake of cholesterol by increasing or decreasing the number of LDL receptors according to the intracellular cholesterol levels. Thus, a high cholesterol diet influences the liver to reduce the number of LDL receptors on its cells, causing an elevated blood level of LDL. Brown and Goldstein postulate that the LDL receptor evolved under dietary conditions of a lower fat intake, and that the high-fat, high-cholesterol modern diet suppresses the production of LDL receptors, thereby allowing cholesterol to rise to levels associated with cardiovascular disease.

Steroidogenesis

The overall steroid biosynthesis pathway shown in the figure is based primarily on the pioneering work of Kenneth. J. Ryan and his coworkers.[2, 3] These pathways follow a fundamental pattern displayed by all steroid-producing endocrine organs. As a result, it should be no surprise that the normal human ovary produces all 3 classes of sex steroids: estrogens, progestins, and androgens. The importance of ovarian androgens is appreciated, not only as obligate precursors to estrogens, but also as clinically important secretory products. The ovary differs from the testis in its fundamental complement of critical enzymes and, hence, its distribution of secretory products. The ovary is distinguished from the adrenal gland in that it is deficient in 21-hydroxylase and 11β-hydroxylase reactions. Glucocorticoids and mineralocorticoids, therefore, are not produced in normal ovarian tissue.

During steroidogenesis, the number of carbon atoms in cholesterol or any other steroid molecule can be reduced but never increased. The following reactions can take place.

1. Cleavage of a side chain (desmolase reaction).

2. Conversion of hydroxyl groups into ketones or ketones into hydroxyl groups (dehydrogenase reactions).

3. Addition of OH group (hydroxylation reaction).

4. Creation of double bonds (removal of hydrogen).

5. Addition of hydrogen to reduce double bonds (saturation).

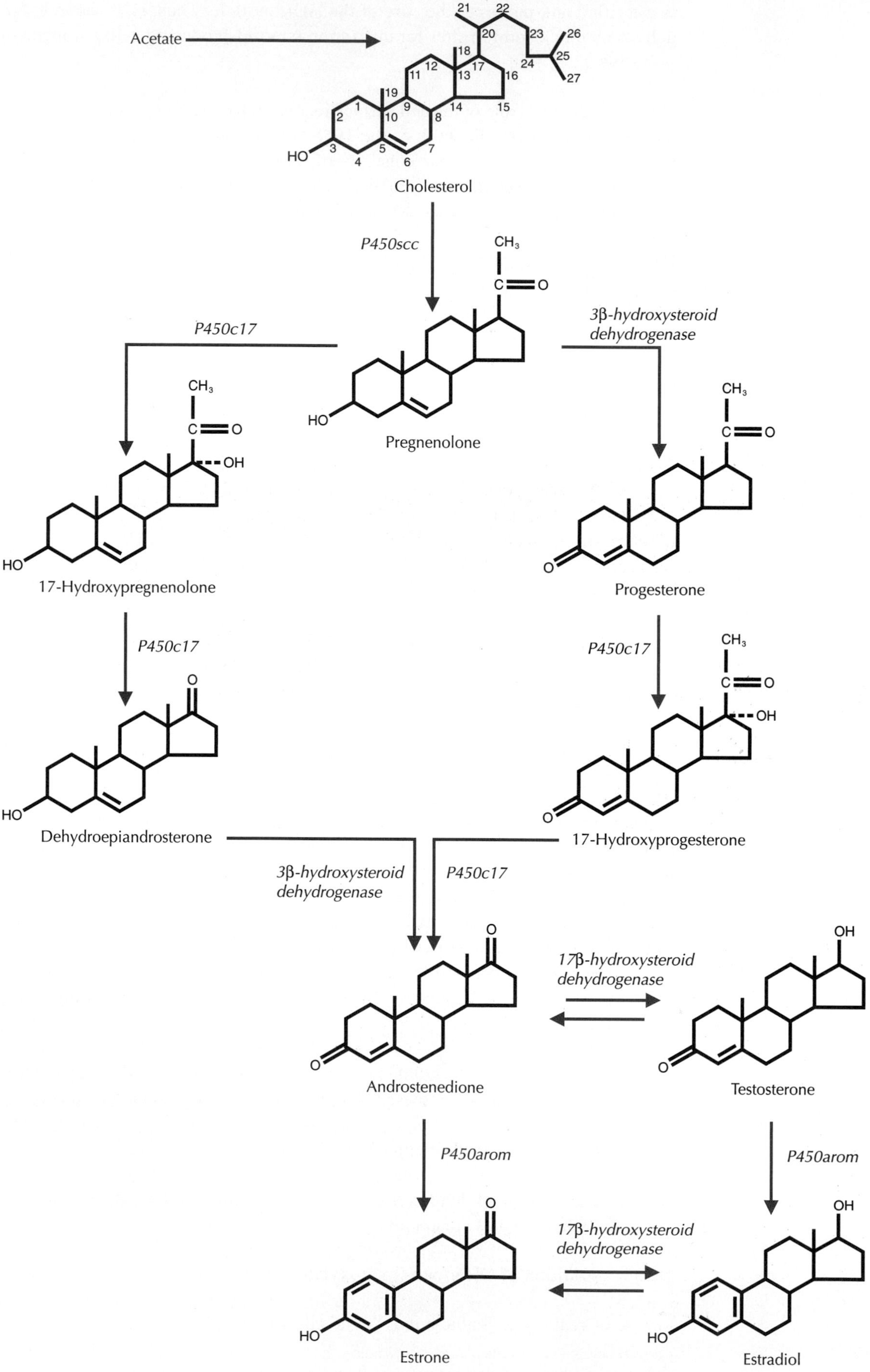

Acetate

Cholesterol

P450scc

Pregnenolone

P450c17

17-Hydroxypregnenolone

3β-hydroxysteroid dehydrogenase

Progesterone

P450c17

Dehydroepiandrosterone

P450c17

17-Hydroxyprogesterone

3β-hydroxysteroid dehydrogenase

P450c17

Androstenedione

17β-hydroxysteroid dehydrogenase

Testosterone

P450arom

P450arom

Estrone

17β-hydroxysteroid dehydrogenase

Estradiol

The traditional view of steroidogenesis was that each step was mediated by many enzymes, with differences from tissue to tissue. A fundamental simplicity to the system emerged when the responsible complementary DNAs and genes were cloned.[4, 5]

Steroidogenic enzymes are either dehydrogenases or members of the cytochrome P450 group of oxidases. Cytochrome P450 is a generic term for a family of oxidative enzymes, termed 450 because of a pigment (450) absorbance shift when reduced. P450 enzymes can metabolize many substrates; e.g., in the liver, P450 enzymes metabolize toxins and environmental pollutants. The following distinct P450 enzymes are identified with steroidogenesis: P450scc is the cholesterol side chain cleavage enzyme; P450c11 mediates 11-hydroxylase, 18-hydroxylase, and 19-methyloxidase; P450c17 mediates 17-hydroxylase and 17,20-lyase; P450c21 mediates the 21-hydroxylase; and P450arom mediates aromatization of androgens to estrogens. Marked differences in the exon–intron organization of the P450 genes are compatible with an ancient origin; thus, the superfamily of P450 genes diverged more than 1.5 billion years ago.

Enzyme	Cellular Location	Reactions
P450scc	Mitochondria	Cholesterol side chain cleavage
P450c11	Mitochondria	11-hydroxylase 18-hydroxylase 19-methyloxidase
P450c17	Endoplasmic reticulum	17-hydroxylase, 17,20-lyase
P450c21	Endoplasmic reticulum	21-hydroxylase
P450arom	Endoplasmic reticulum	Aromatase

The structural knowledge of the P450 enzymes that has been derived from amino acid and nucleotide sequencing studies demonstrated that all the steps between cholesterol and pregnenolone were mediated by a single protein, P450scc, bound to the inner mitochondrial membrane. Cloning data indicate the presence of a single, unique P450scc gene on chromosome 15. These experiments indicated that multiple steps did not require multiple enzymes. Differing activity may reflect posttranslational modifications. These genes contain tissue-specific promoter sequences which is at least one reason that regulatory mechanisms can differ in different tissues (e.g., placenta and ovary).

Conversion of cholesterol to pregnenolone involves hydroxylation at the carbon 20 and 22 positions, with subsequent cleavage of the side chain. Conversion of cholesterol to pregnenolone by P450scc takes place within the mitochondria. It is one of the principal effects of tropic hormone stimulation, which also causes the uptake of the cholesterol substrate for this step. The tropic hormones from the anterior pituitary bind to the cell surface receptor of the G protein system, activate adenylate cyclase, and increase intracellular cyclic AMP. Cyclic AMP activity leads to gene transcription that encodes the steroidogenic enzymes and accessory proteins. More acutely, cyclic AMP stimulates the hydrolysis of cholesteryl esters and the transport of free cholesterol to the mitochondria.

Most of the cholesterol used for steroid synthesis is derived from the mobilization and transport of intracellular stores.[6, 7] Indeed, the rate-limiting step in steroidogenesis is the transfer of cholesterol from the outer mitochondrial membrane to the inner mitochondrial membrane where fully active P450scc waits for substrate. The rate-limiting transfer of hydrophobic cholesterol through the aqueous space between the outer and inner mitochondrial membranes is mediated by protein activation stimulated by the tropic hormone. Long-term, chronic steroidogenesis requires gene transcription and protein synthesis, but short-term, acute responses occur independently of new RNA synthesis, although protein synthesis is still necessary, specifically the proteins that regulate cholesterol transfer across the mitochondrial membrane.

Several proteins have been characterized and proposed as regulators of acute intracellular cholesterol transfer. Sterol carrier protein 2 (SCP2) is able to bind and transfer cholesterol between compartments within a cell. Another candidate is a small molecule, steroidogenesis activator polypeptide (SAP), and still another is peripheral benzodiazepine receptor (PBR), which affects cholesterol flux through a pore structure. But the most studied and favored protein as a regulator of acute cholesterol transfer is ***steroidogenic acute regulator (StAR) protein***.[8, 9] StAR messenger RNA and protein are induced concomitantly with acute steroidogenesis in response to cyclic AMP stimulation; StAR increases steroid production; and StAR is imported and localized in the mitochondria. But most impressively, congenital lipoid adrenal hyperplasia (an autosomal recessive disorder) has been demonstrated to be a failure in adrenal and gonadal steroidogenesis due to a mutation in the StAR gene, which results in premature stop codons.[10, 11] With this mutation, a low level of steroidogenesis is possible, even permitting feminization at puberty, but continuing tropic hormonal stimulation results in an accumulation of intracellular lipid deposits that destroy steroidogenic capability.[12]

StAR mediates the transport of cholesterol into mitochondria in adrenal and gonadal steroidogenesis, but not in the placenta and brain. It is synthesized in a precursor form as a 285-amino acid protein that has a 25-residue sequence cleaved from the NH_2-terminal after transport into mitochondria.[13] The mutant forms of StAR undergo premature truncation that prevents this proteolytic cleavage. Mutations of the StAR gene, located on chromosome 8p11.2, are the only inherited disorder of steroidogenesis not caused by a defect in one of the steroidogenic enzymes. The absence of StAR expression in placenta and brain indicates the presence of different mechanisms for cholesterol transport in those tissues.

It is important to note that once pregnenolone is formed further steroid synthesis in the ovary can proceed by one of 2 pathways, either via Δ^5-3β-hydroxysteroids or via the Δ^4-3-ketone pathway. The first (the Δ^5 pathway) proceeds by way of pregnenolone and dehydroepiandrosterone (DHA) and the second (the Δ^4 pathway) via progesterone and 17α-hydroxyprogesterone.

The conversion of pregnenolone to progesterone involves two steps: the 3β-hydroxysteroid dehydrogenase and Δ^{4-5} isomerase reactions that convert the 3-hydroxyl group to a ketone and transfer the double bond from the 5–6 position to the 4–5 position. The 3β-hydroxysteroid dehydrogenase enzyme catalyzes both the dehydrogenation and isomerization reactions, and exists in 2 forms (type I and type II), encoded by two separate genes on chromosome 1 (the type II gene is expressed in the gonads and the adrenal glands). Once the Δ^{4-5} ketone is formed, progesterone is hydroxylated at the 17 position to form 17α-hydroxyprogesterone. 17α-Hydroxyprogesterone is the immediate precursor of the C-19 (19 carbons) series of androgens in this pathway. By peroxide formation at C-20, followed by epoxidation of the C-17, C-20 carbons, the side chain is split off, forming androstenedione. The 17-ketone may be reduced to a 17β-hydroxyl to form testosterone by the 17β-hydroxysteroid dehydrogenase reaction. Both C-19 steroids (androstenedione and testosterone) are rapidly converted to corresponding C-18 phenolic steroid estrogens (estrone and estradiol) by microsomal reactions in a process referred to as aromatization. This process includes hydroxylation of the angular 19-methyl group, followed by oxidation, loss of the 19-carbon as formaldehyde, and ring A aromatization (dehydrogenation).

As an alternative, pregnenolone can be directly converted to the Δ^5-3β-hydroxy C-19 steroid, DHA, by 17α-hydroxylation followed by cleavage of the side chain. With formation of the Δ^4-3-ketone, DHA is converted into androstenedione. It is thought that conversion of each of the Δ^5 compounds to their corresponding Δ^4 compounds can occur at any step; however, the principal pathways are via progesterone and DHA. Regardless of the precursor source, C-19 Δ^4-3-ketone substrates proceed to estrogens as noted above.

The four reactions involved in converting pregnenolone and progesterone to their 17-hydroxylated products are mediated by a single enzyme, P450c17, bound to smooth endoplasmic reticulum, regulated by a gene on chromosome 10. 17-Hydroxylase and 17,20 lyase were traditionally regarded as separate enzymes. These two different functions of a single enzyme, P450c17, are not genetic or structural but represent the effect of local influencing factors.

Characterization of the P450c21 protein and gene cloning indicate that there is only one 21-hydroxylase enzyme, the P450c21 in the smooth endoplasmic reticulum. Two human P450c21 genes (the A and B genes) have been cloned (on chromosome 6p), and the evidence indicates that only one (the B gene) is active. The molecular genetics of 21-hydroxylase deficiency indicate that the syndrome can be due to gene conversions of material in the active B gene to resemble material in the inactive A gene, as well as deletions in the P450c21 B gene. A conversion is similar to a cross-over in genetic effect. However, rather than appearing as a deletion or addition, the gene changes, but the number of gene copies does not change.

Aromatization is mediated by P450arom found in the endoplasmic reticulum.[14] The human genome has one P450arom gene, located on chromosome 15q21.1, and designated as the CYP19 gene, denoting oxidation of the C-19 methyl group. Aromatization in different tissues with different substrates is the result of the single P450arom enzyme encoded by the single gene. Aromatase transcription is regulated by several promotor sites that respond to cytokines, cyclic nucleotides, gonadotropins, glucocorticoids, and growth factors. Tissue-specific expression is regulated by tissue-specific promoters. Thus, this gene has alternative promoters that allow the extremes of highly regulated expression in the ovary and nonregulated expression in the placenta and adipose. Very specific inhibitors of P450arom have been developed which allow intense blockage of estrogen production, with clinical applications that include the treatment of breast cancer (e.g., anastrozole) and dysfunctional uterine bleeding. The aromatase complex also includes NADPH-cytochrome P450 reductase, a ubiquitous flavoprotein for transferring reducing equivalents.

The 17β-hydroxysteroid dehydrogenase and 5α-reductase reactions are due to non-P450 enzymes. The 17β-hydroxysteroid dehydrogenase is bound to the endoplasmic reticulum and the 5α-reductase to the nuclear membrane. The 17β-hydroxysteroid dehydrogenase enzymes convert estrone to estradiol, androstenedione to testosterone, and DHA to androstenediol, and vice versa. Four different isozymes have been identified, types I–IV.[15] The type I enzyme is active in the placenta, converting estrone to estradiol. The type II and type IV enzymes form androstenedione and estrone from testosterone and estradiol, respectively, and the type III enzyme in the testis reduces androstenedione to testosterone.

The Two-Cell System

The two-cell system is a logical explanation of the events involved in ovarian follicular steroidogenesis.[16] This explanation, first proposed by Falck in 1959,[17] brings together information on the site of specific steroid production, along with the appearance and importance of hormone receptors. The following facts are important:

1. FSH receptors are present on the granulosa cells.

2. FSH receptors are induced by FSH itself.

3. LH receptors are present on the theca cells and initially absent on the granulosa cells, but, as the follicle grows, FSH induces the appearance of LH receptors on the granulosa cells.

4. FSH induces aromatase enzyme activity in granulosa cells.

5. The above actions are modulated by autocrine and paracrine factors secreted by the theca and granulosa cells.

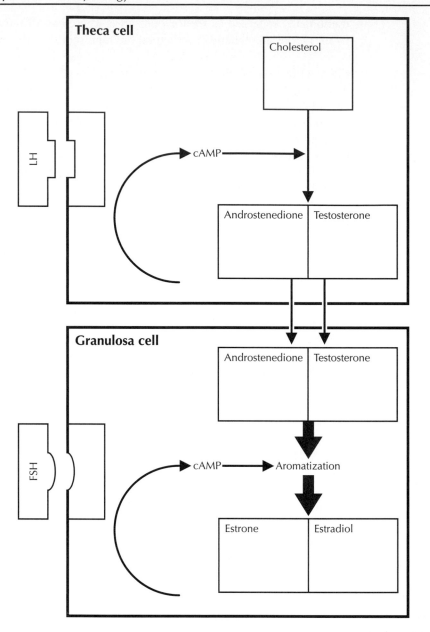

These facts combine into the two-cell system to explain the sequence of events in ovarian follicular growth and steroidogenesis. The initial change from a primordial follicle to a preantral follicle is independent of hormones, and the stimulus governing this initial step in growth is unknown. Continued growth, however, depends on FSH stimulation. As the granulosa responds to FSH, proliferation and growth are associated with an increase in FSH receptors, a specific effect of FSH itself, but an action that is enhanced very significantly by the autocrine and paracrine peptides. The theca cells are characterized by steroidogenic activity in response to LH, specifically resulting in androgen production, by transcription of the P450scc, P450c17, and 3β-hydroxysteroid dehydrogenase genes. Aromatization of androgens to estrogens is a distinct activity within the granulosa layer induced by FSH by activation of the P450arom gene. Androgens produced in the theca layer, therefore, must diffuse into the granulosa layer. In the granulosa layer they are converted to estrogens, and the increasing level of estradiol in the peripheral circulation reflects release of the estrogen back toward the theca layer and into blood vessels.

The theca and granulosa cells secrete peptides that operate as both autocrine and paracrine factors.[18] Insulin-like growth factor (IGF) is secreted by the theca and enhances the LH stimulation of androgen production in the theca cells as well as FSH-mediated aromatization in the granulosa. Evidence indicates that the endogenous insulin-like growth factor in the human ovarian follicle is IGF-II in both the granulosa and the thecal cells.[19] Studies indicating activity of IGF-I with human ovarian tissue can be explained by the fact that both IGF-I and IGF-II activities can be mediated by the type I IGF receptor which is structurally similar to the insulin receptor. Theca production of transforming growth factor can promote the growth of granulosa cells and FSH induction of LH receptors on the granulosa. The regulation of FSH receptors on granulosa cells is relatively complex. Although FSH increases the activity of its own receptor gene in a cyclic AMP-mediated mechanism, this action is influenced by inhibitory agents, such as epidermal growth factor, fibroblast growth factor, and even a gonadotropin-releasing hormone (GnRH)-like protein. Inhibin and activin are produced in the granulosa in response to FSH, and activin has the important autocrine role of enhancing FSH actions, especially the production of FSH receptors. Inhibin enhances LH stimulation of androgen synthesis in the theca to serve as substrate for aromatization to estrogen in the granulosa, whereas activin suppresses androgen synthesis. This important paracrine regulation of androgen production in thecal cells by inhibin and activin is exerted primarily through modification of the expression of steroidogenic enzymes, especially P450c17.[20]

After ovulation, the dominance of the luteinized granulosa layer is dependent on preovulatory induction of an adequate number of LH receptors, and, therefore, dependent on adequate FSH action. Prior to ovulation the granulosa layer is characterized by aromatization activity and conversion of the theca androgens to estrogens, an FSH-mediated activity. After ovulation the granulosa layer secretes progesterone and estrogens directly into the bloodstream, an LH-mediated activity.

Granulosa and theca cells each have an androgen aromatase system that can be demonstrated in vitro. However, in vivo, the activity of the granulosa layer in the follicular phase is several hundred times greater than the activity of the theca layer, and, therefore, the granulosa is the main biosynthetic source of estrogen in the growing follicle.[21] Because granulosa cells lack P450c17, the rate of aromatization in the granulosa layer is directly related to and dependent on the androgen substrate made available by the theca cells. Hence, estrogen secretion by the follicle prior to ovulation is the result of combined LH and FSH stimulation of the two-cell types, the theca and the granulosa. After ovulation, it is believed the two-cell types continue to function as a two-cell system; luteal cells derived from theca produce androgens for aromatization into estrogens by luteal cells derived from granulosa.

Blood Transport of Steroids

While circulating in the blood, a majority of the principal sex steroids, estradiol and testosterone, is bound to a protein carrier, known as sex hormone-binding globulin (SHBG) produced in the liver. Another 10–30% is loosely bound to albumin, leaving only about 1% unbound and free. A very small percentage also binds to corticosteroid-binding globulin. Hyperthyroidism, pregnancy, and estrogen administration all increase SHBG levels, whereas corticoids, androgens, progestins, growth hormone, insulin, and IGF-I decrease SHBG.

	Free (Unbound)	**Albumin-Bound**	**SHBG-Bound**
Estrogen	1%	30%	69%
Testosterone	1%	30%	69%
DHA	4%	88%	8%
Androstenedione	7%	85%	8%
Dihydrotestosterone	1%	71%	28%

From Mendel[22]

The circulating level of SHBG is inversely related to weight, and, thus, significant weight gain can decrease SHBG and produce important changes in the unbound levels of the sex steroids. Another important mechanism for a reduction in circulating SHBG levels is insulin resistance and hyperinsulinemia (independent of age and weight).[23] Thus, increased insulin levels in the circulation lower SHBG levels, and this may be the major mechanism that mediates the impact of increased body weight on SHBG. This relationship between the levels of insulin and SHBG is so strong that SHBG concentrations are a marker for hyperinsulinemic insulin resistance, and a low level of SHBG is a predictor for the development of type II diabetes mellitus.[24]

The distribution of body fat has a strong influence on SHBG levels. Android or central fat is located in the abdominal wall and visceral-mesenteric locations. This fat distribution is associated with hyperinsulinemia, hyperandrogenism, and decreased levels of SHBG.[25] The common mechanism for these changes is probably the hyperinsulinemia.

SHBG is a glycoprotein that contains a single binding site for androgens and estrogens, even though it is a homodimer composed of two monomers. Its gene has been localized to the short arm (p12–13) of chromosome 17.[26] Genetic studies have revealed that the SHBG gene also encodes the androgen-binding protein present in the seminiferous tubules, synthesized by the Sertoli cells.[27, 28] Dimerization is believed to be necessary to form the single steroid-binding site. Specific chromosomal abnormalities with decreased or abnormal SHBG have not been reported. However, SHBG gene expression has now been identified in other tissues (brain, placenta, and endometrium), although a biologic significance has not been determined.

Transcortin, also called corticosteroid-binding globulin, is a plasma glycoprotein that binds cortisol, progesterone, deoxycorticosterone, corticosterone, and some of the other minor corticoid compounds. Normally about 75% of circulating cortisol is bound to transcortin, 15% is loosely bound to albumin, and 10% is unbound or free. Progesterone circulates in the following percentages: 2% unbound, 80% bound to albumin, 18% bound to transcortin, and less than 1% bound to SHBG. Binding in the circulation follows the law of mass action: the amount of the free, unbound hormone is in equilibrium with the bound hormone. Thus, the total binding capacity of SHBG will influence the amount that is free and unbound.

The biologic effects of the major sex steroids are largely determined by the unbound portion, known as the free hormone. In other words, the active hormone is unbound and free, whereas the bound hormone is relatively inactive. This concept is not without controversy. The hormone-protein complex may be involved in an active uptake process at the target cell plasma membrane.[29] The albumin-bound fraction of steroids may also be available for cellular action because this binding has low affinity. Because the concentration of albumin in plasma is many-fold greater than that of SHBG, the contribution of the albumin-bound fraction is significant. Routine assays determine the total hormone concentration, bound plus free, and special steps are required to measure the active free level of testosterone, estradiol, and cortisol.

Estrogen Metabolism

Androgens are the common precursors of estrogens. 17β-Hydroxysteroid dehydrogenase activity converts androstenedione to testosterone, which is not a major secretory product of the normal ovary. It is rapidly demethylated at the C-19 position and aromatized to estradiol, the major estrogen secreted by the human ovary. Estradiol also arises to a major degree from androstenedione via estrone, and estrone itself is secreted in significant daily amounts. Estriol is the peripheral metabolite of estrone and estradiol and not a secretory product of the ovary. The formation of estriol is typical of general metabolic "detoxification," conversion of biologically active material to less active forms.

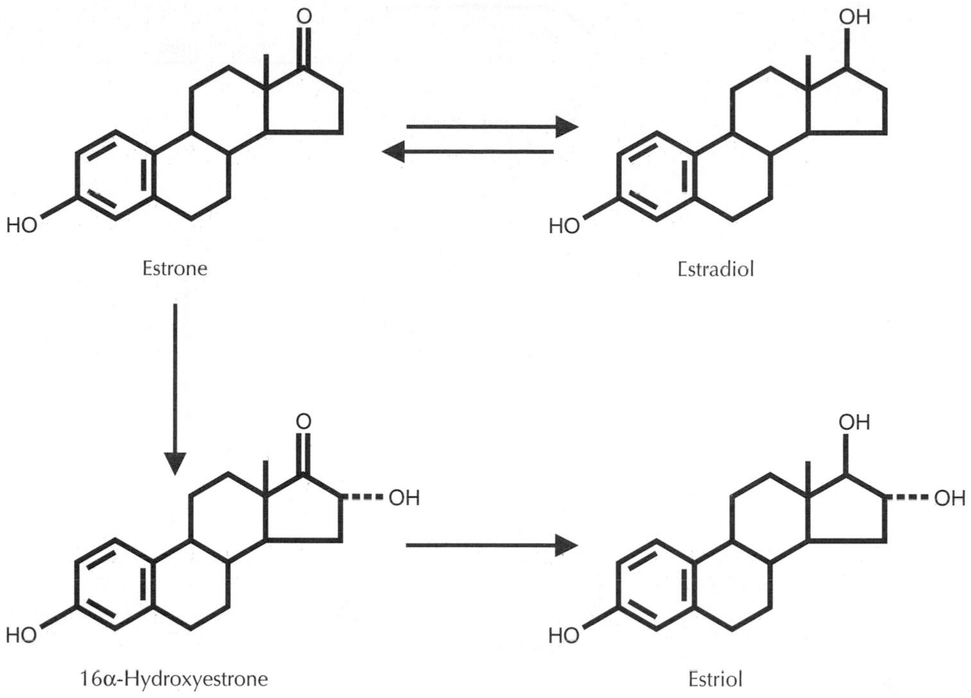

Estrone   Estradiol

16α-Hydroxyestrone   Estriol

The conversion of steroids in peripheral tissues is not always a form of inactivation. Free androgens are peripherally converted to free estrogens, for example, in skin and adipose cells. The location of the adipose cells influences their activity. Women with central obesity (the abdominal area) produce more androgens.[30] The work of Siiteri and MacDonald[31] demonstrated that enough estrogen can be derived from circulating androgens to produce bleeding in the postmenopausal woman. In the female the adrenal gland remains the major source of circulating androgens, in particular androstenedione. In the male, almost all of the circulating estrogens are derived from peripheral conversion of androgens.

It can be seen, therefore, that the pattern of circulating steroids in the female is influenced by the activity of various processes outside the ovary. Because of the peripheral contribution to steroid levels, the term *secretion rate* is reserved for direct organ secretion, whereas *production rate* includes organ secretion plus peripheral contribution via conversion of precursors. The *metabolic clearance rate (MCR)* equals the volume of blood that is cleared of the hormone per unit of time. The *blood production rate (PR)* then equals the metabolic clearance rate multiplied by the concentration of the hormone in the blood.

MCR = Liters/Day

PR = MCR x Concentration

PR = Liters/Day x Amount/Liter = Amount/Day

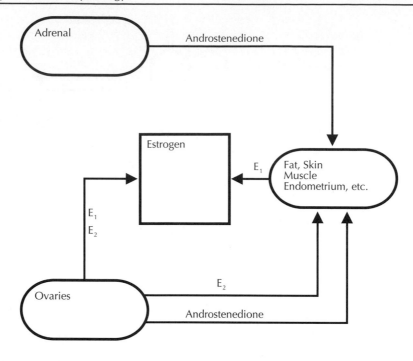

In the normal nonpregnant female, estradiol is produced at the rate of 100–300 µg/day. The production of androstenedione is about 3 mg/day, and the peripheral conversion (about 1%) of androstenedione to estrone accounts for about 20–30% of the estrone produced per day. Because androstenedione is secreted in milligram amounts, even a small percent conversion to estrogen results in a significant contribution to estrogens, which exist and function in microgram amounts. Thus, the circulating estrogens in the female are the sum of direct ovarian secretion of estradiol and estrone, plus peripheral conversion of C-19 precursors.

Premenopausal Peripheral Conversion

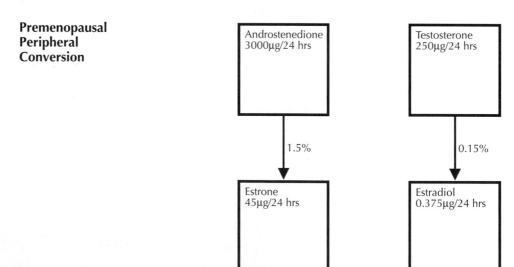

Progesterone Metabolism

Peripheral conversion of steroids to progesterone is not seen in the nonpregnant female; rather, the progesterone production rate is a combination of secretion from the adrenal and the ovaries. Including the small contribution from the adrenal, the blood production rate of progesterone in the preovulatory phase is less than 1 mg/day. During the luteal phase, production increases to 20–30 mg/day. The metabolic fate of progesterone, as expressed by its many excretion products, is more complex than estrogen. About 10–20% of progesterone is excreted as pregnanediol.

Pregnanediol glucuronide is present in the urine in concentrations less than 1 mg/day until ovulation. Postovulation pregnanediol excretion reaches a peak of 3–6 mg/day, which is maintained until 2 days prior to menses. The assay of pregnanediol in the urine now has little use, except in home test kits that allow women to self-test for ovulation.

In the preovulatory phase in adult females, in all prepubertal females, and in the normal male, the blood levels of progesterone are at the lower limits of immunoassay sensitivity: less than 100 ng/dL. After ovulation, i.e., during the luteal phase, progesterone ranges from 500 to 2000 ng/dL. In congenital adrenal hyperplasia, progesterone blood levels can be as high as 50 times above normal.

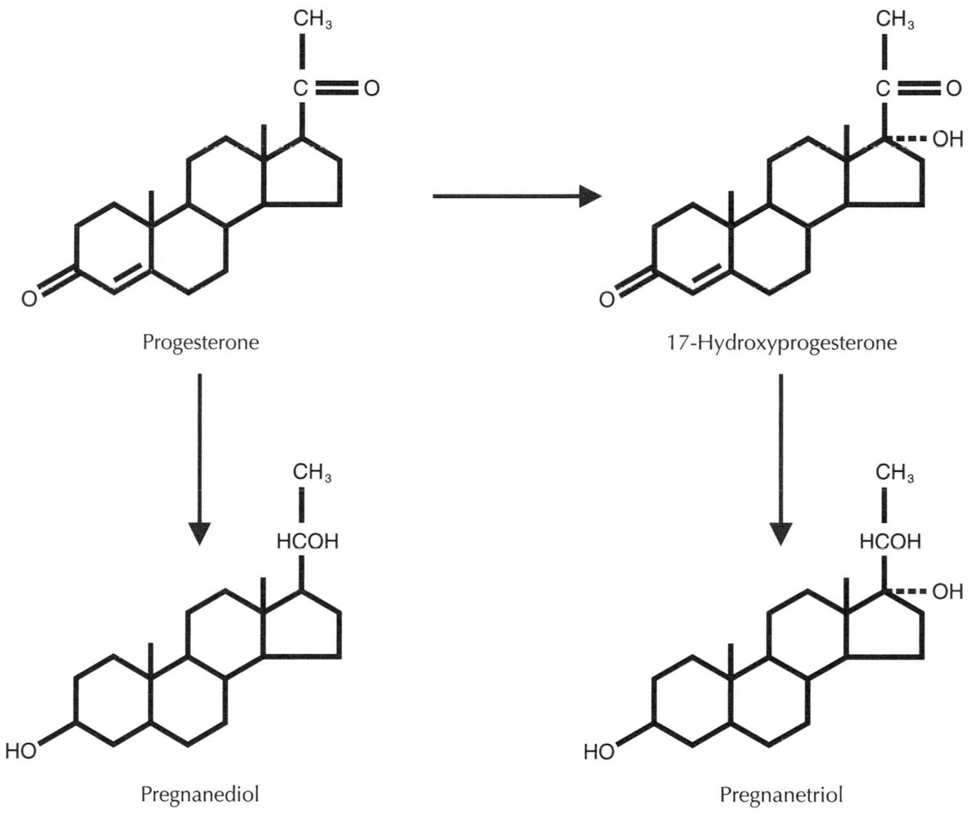

Progesterone

17-Hydroxyprogesterone

Pregnanediol

Pregnanetriol

Pregnanetriol is the chief urinary metabolite of 17α-hydroxyprogesterone and has clinical significance in the adrenogenital syndrome, in which an enzyme defect results in accumulation of 17α-hydroxyprogesterone and increased excretion of pregnanetriol. The plasma or serum assay of 17α-hydroxyprogesterone is a more sensitive and accurate index of this enzyme deficiency than measurement of pregnanetriol. Normally, the blood level of 17α-hydroxyprogesterone is less than 100 ng/dL, although after ovulation and during the luteal phase of a normal menstrual cycle, a peak of 200 ng/dL can be reached. In syndromes of adrenal hyperplasia, values can be 10–400 times normal.

Androgen Metabolism

The major androgen products of the ovary are dehydroepiandrosterone (DHA) and androstenedione (and only a little testosterone), which are secreted mainly by stromal tissue derived from theca cells. With excessive accumulation of stromal tissue or in the presence of an androgen-producing tumor, testosterone becomes a significant secretory product. Occasionally, a nonfunctioning tumor can induce stromal proliferation and increased androgen production. The normal accumulation of stromal tissue at midcycle results in a rise in circulating levels of androstenedione and testosterone at the time of ovulation.

The adrenal cortex produces 3 groups of steroid hormones, the glucocorticoids, the mineralocorticoids, and the sex steroids. The adrenal sex steroids represent intermediate byproducts in the synthesis of glucocorticoids and mineralocorticoids, and excessive secretion of the sex steroids occurs only with neoplastic cells or in association with enzyme deficiencies. Under normal circumstances, adrenal gland production of the sex steroids is less significant than gonadal production of androgens and estrogens. About one-half of the daily production of DHA and androstenedione comes from the adrenal gland; the other half of androstenedione is secreted by the ovary, but the other half of DHA is split almost equally between the ovary and peripheral tissues. The production rate of testosterone in the normal female is 0.2–0.3 mg/day, and approximately 50% arises from peripheral conversion of androstenedione (and a small amount from DHA) to testosterone, whereas 25% is secreted by the ovary and 25% by the adrenal. The major androgens are excreted in the urine as 17-ketosteroids.

There is no circadian cycle of the major sex steroids in the female. However, short-term variations in the blood levels due to episodic secretion require multiple sampling for absolutely accurate assessment. ***Although frequent sampling is necessary for a high degree of accuracy, a random sample is sufficient for clinical purposes to determine whether a level is within a normal range.***

The testosterone-binding capacity is decreased by androgens; hence, the binding capacity in men is lower than that in normal women. The binding globulin level in women with increased androgen production is also depressed. Androgenic effects are dependent on the unbound fraction that can move freely from the vascular compartment into the target cells. Routine assays determine the total hormone concentration, bound plus free. Thus, a total testosterone concentration can be in the normal range in a woman who is hirsute or even virilized, but because the binding globulin level is depressed by the androgen effects, the percent free and active testosterone is elevated. The need for a specific assay for the free portion of testosterone can be questioned because the very presence of hirsutism or virilism indicates increased androgen effects. In the face of hirsutism, one can reliably interpret a normal testosterone level as compatible with decreased binding capacity and increased active free testosterone.

Both total and unbound testosterone are normal in only a few women with hirsutism. In these cases, the hirsutism, heretofore regarded as idiopathic, most likely results from excessive intracellular androgen effects (specifically increased intracellular conversion of testosterone to dihydrotestosterone).

Reduction of the Δ^4 unsaturation (an irreversible pathway) in testosterone is very significant, producing derivatives very different in their spatial configuration and activity. The 5β-derivatives are not androgenic, and this is not an important pathway; however, the 5α-derivative (a very active pathway) is extremely potent. Indeed, dihydrotestosterone (DHT), the 5α-derivative, is the principal androgenic hormone in a variety of target tissues and is formed within the target tissue itself.

In men, the majority of circulating DHT is derived from testosterone that enters a target cell and is converted by means of 5α-reductase to DHT. In women, because the production rate of androstenedione is greater than testosterone, blood DHT is primarily derived from androstenedione and partly from dehydroepiandrosterone.[32] Thus, in women, the skin production of DHT may be predominantly influenced by androstenedione. DHT is by definition an intracrine hormone, formed and acting within target tissues.[33] The 5α-reductase enzyme exists in two forms, type I and II, each encoded by a separate gene, with the type I enzyme found in skin and the type II reductase predominantly expressed in reproductive tissues.[34]

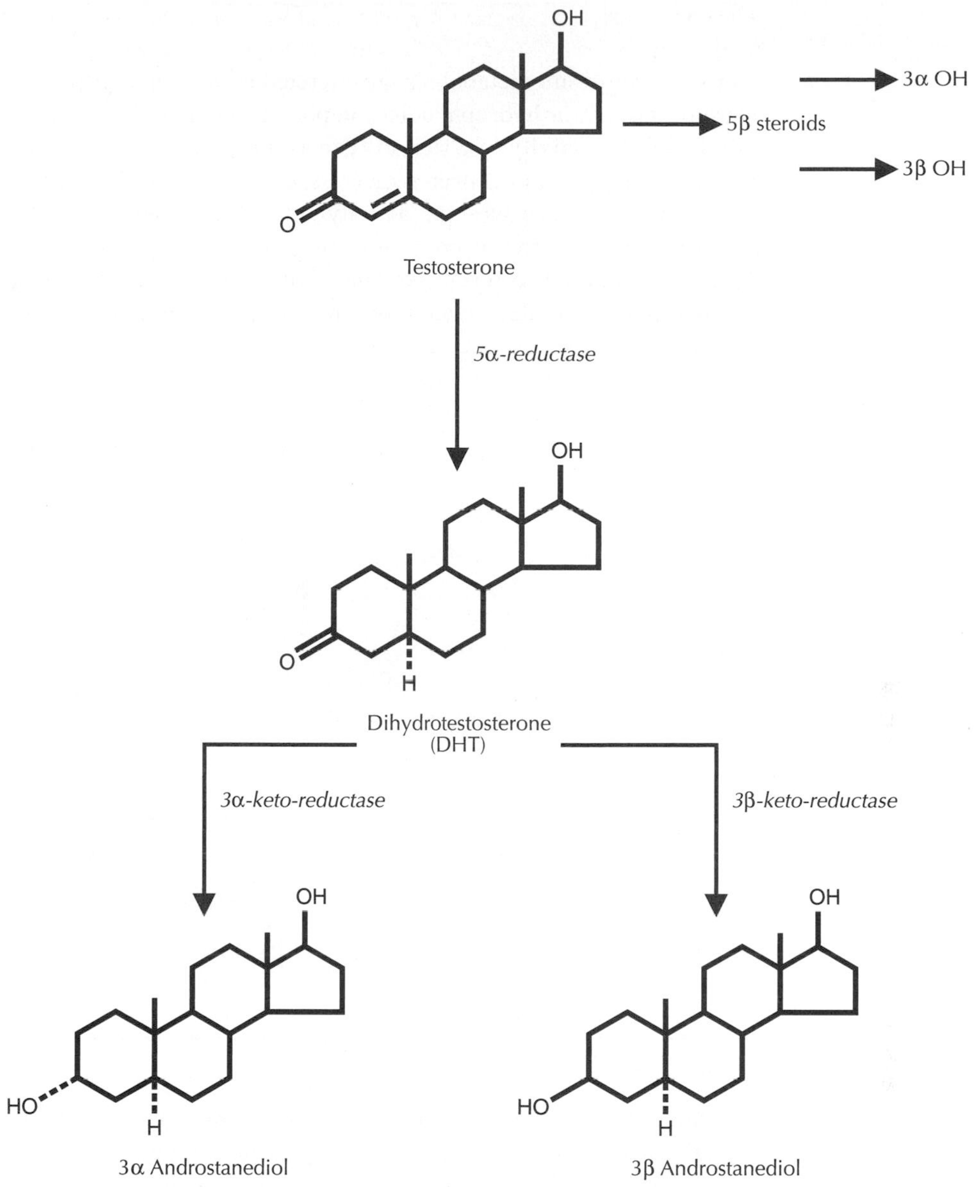

Testosterone

5α-reductase

Dihydrotestosterone
(DHT)

3α-keto-reductase   3β-keto-reductase

3α Androstanediol   3β Androstanediol

DHT is largely metabolized intracellularly; hence, the blood DHT is only about one-tenth the level of circulating testosterone, and it is clear that testosterone is the major circulating androgen. In tissues sensitive to DHT (which includes hair follicles), only DHT enters the nucleus to provide the androgen message. DHT also can perform androgenic actions within cells that do not possess the ability to convert testosterone to DHT. DHT is further reduced by a 3α-keto-reductase to androstanediol, which is relatively inactive. The metabolite of androstanediol, 3α-androstanediol glucuronide, is the major metabolite of DHT and can be measured in the plasma, indicating the level of activity of target tissue conversion of testosterone to DHT.

Not all androgen-sensitive tissues require the prior conversion of testosterone to DHT. In the process of masculine differentiation, the development of the wolffian duct structures (epididymis, the vas deferens, and the seminal vesicle) is dependent on testosterone as the intracellular mediator, whereas development of the urogenital sinus and urogenital tubercle into the male external genitalia, urethra, and prostate requires the conversion of testosterone to DHT.[35] Muscle development is under the direct control of testosterone. Testosterone is also aromatized to a significant extent in the brain, liver, and breast; and in some circumstances (e.g., in the brain) androgenic messages can be transmitted via estrogen.

Excretion of Steroids

Active steroids and metabolites are excreted as sulfo and glucuro conjugates. Conjugation of a steroid converts a hydrophoboic compound into a hydrophilic one and generally reduces or eliminates the activity of a steroid. This is not completely true, however, because hydrolysis of the ester linkage can occur in target tissues and restore the active form. Furthermore, estrogen conjugates can have biologic activity, and it is known that sulfated conjugates are actively secreted and may serve as precursors, present in the circulation in relatively high concentrations because of binding to serum proteins. Ordinarily, however, conjugation by liver and intestinal mucosa is a step in deactivation preliminary to, and essential for, excretion into urine and bile.

Glucosiduronate

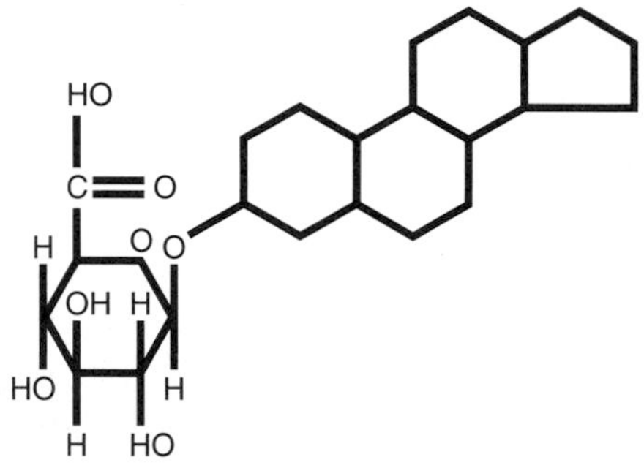

Sulfate

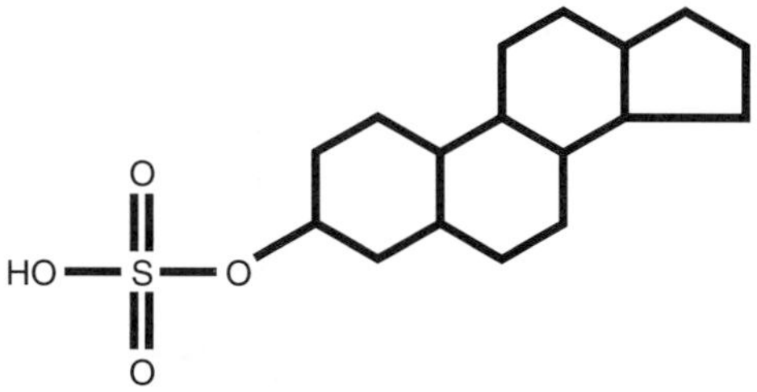

Cellular Mechanism of Action

Hormones circulate in extremely low concentrations and, in order to respond with specific and effective actions, target cells require the presence of special mechanisms. There are 2 major types of hormone action at target tissues. One mediates the action of tropic hormones (peptide and glycoprotein hormones) with receptors at the cell membrane level. In contrast, the smaller steroid hormones enter cells readily, and the basic mechanism of action involves specific receptor molecules within the cells. It is the affinity, specificity, and activity of the receptors, together with the large concentration of receptors in cells, that allow a small amount of hormone to produce a biologic response. The many different types of receptors can be organized into the following basic categories.

Intracellular Receptors

Receptors in the nucleus lead to transcription activation. Examples include the receptors for estrogen and thyroid hormones.

G Protein Receptors

These receptors are composed of a single polypeptide chain that spans the cell membrane. Binding to a specific hormone leads to interaction with G proteins that, in turn, activate second messengers. Examples include receptors for tropic hormones, prostaglandins, light, and odors. The second messengers include the adenylate cyclase enzyme, the phospholipase system, and calcium ion changes.

Ion Gate Channels

These cell surface receptors are composed of multiple units, that after binding, open ion channels.

The influx of ions changes the electrical activity of the cells. The best example of this type is the acetylcholine receptor.

Receptors With Intrinsic Enzyme Activity

These transmembrane receptors have an intracellular component with tyrosine or serine kinase activity. Binding leads to receptor autophosphorylation and activity. Examples include the receptors for insulin and growth factors (tyrosine kinase) and the receptors for activin and inhibin (serine kinase).

Other Receptors

Receptors that do not fit the above categories include the receptors for LDL, prolactin, growth hormone, and some of the growth factors.

Mechanism of Action for Steroid Hormones

The specificity of the reaction of tissues to sex steroid hormones is due to the presence of intracellular receptor proteins. Different types of tissues, such as liver, kidney, and uterus, respond in a similar manner. The mechanism includes: 1) steroid hormone diffusion across the cell membrane, 2) steroid hormone binding to receptor protein, 3) interaction of a hormone-receptor complex with nuclear DNA, 4) synthesis of messenger RNA (mRNA), 5) transport of the mRNA to the ribosomes, and finally, 6) protein synthesis in the cytoplasm that results in specific cellular activity.[36] The steroid hormone receptors primarily affect gene transcription, but also regulate post transcriptional events and nongenomic events. ***Steroid receptors regulate gene transcription through multiple mechanisms, not all of which require direct interactions with DNA.***

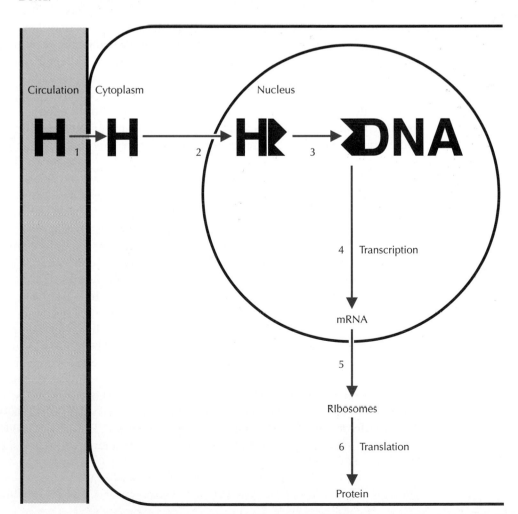

Each of the major classes of the sex steroid hormones, including estrogens, progestins, and androgens, has been demonstrated to act according to this general mechanism. Glucocorticoid, mineralocorticoid, and probably androgen receptors, when in the unbound state, reside in the cytoplasm and move into the nucleus after hormone-receptor binding. Estrogens and progestins are transferred across the nuclear membrane and bind to their receptors within the nucleus.

Steroid hormones are rapidly transported across the cell membrane by simple diffusion. The factors responsible for this transfer are unknown, but the concentration of free (unbound) hormone in the bloodstream seems to be an important and influential determinant of cellular function. Once in the cell, the sex steroid hormones bind to their individual receptors.[37–39] During this process, ***transformation or activation*** of the receptor occurs. Transformation refers to a conformational change of the hormone-receptor complex revealing or producing a binding site that is necessary in order for the complex to bind to the chromatin. In the unbound state, the receptor is associated with heat shock proteins that stabilize and protect the receptor and maintain the DNA binding region in an inactive state. Activation of the receptor is driven by hormone binding that causes a dissociation of the receptor-heat shock protein complex.

The hormone-receptor complex binds to specific DNA sites (***hormone-responsive elements***) that are located upstream of the gene. The specific binding of the hormone-receptor complex with DNA results in RNA polymerase initiation of transcription. Transcription leads to translation, mRNA-mediated protein synthesis on the ribosomes. The principal action of steroid hormones is the regulation of intracellular protein synthesis by means of the receptor mechanism.

Biologic activity is maintained only while the nuclear site is occupied with the hormone-receptor complex. The dissociation rate of the hormone and its receptor as well as the half-life of the nuclear chromatin-bound complex are factors in the biologic response because the hormone response elements are abundant and, under normal conditions, are occupied only to a small extent.[40] Thus, an important clinical principle is the following: ***duration of exposure to a hormone is as important as dose.*** One reason only small amounts of estrogen need be present in the circulation is the long half-life of the estrogen hormone-receptor complex. Indeed, a major factor in the potency differences among the various estrogens (estradiol, estrone, estriol) is the length of time the estrogen-receptor complex occupies the nucleus. The higher rate of dissociation with the weak estrogen (estriol) can be compensated for by continuous application to allow prolonged nuclear binding and activity. Cortisol and progesterone must circulate in large concentrations because their receptor complexes have short half-lives in the nucleus.

An important action of estrogen is the modification of its own and other steroid hormone activity by affecting receptor concentrations. Estrogen increases target tissue responsiveness to itself and to progestins and androgens by increasing the concentration of its own receptor and that of the intracellular progestin and androgen receptors. This process is called ***replenishment***. Progesterone and clomiphene, on the other hand, limit tissue response to estrogen by blocking the replenishment mechanism, thus decreasing over time the concentration of estrogen receptors. Replenishment is very responsive to the available amount of steroid and receptors. Small amounts of receptor depletion and small amounts of steroid in the blood activate the mechanism.

Replenishment, the synthesis of the sex steroid receptors, obviously takes place in the cytoplasm, but with estrogen and progestin receptors, synthesis must be quickly followed by transportation into the nucleus. There is an incredible nuclear traffic.[41] The nuclear membrane contains 3000 to 4000 pores. A cell synthesizing DNA imports about one million histone molecules from the cytoplasm every 3 minutes. If the cell is growing rapidly, about 3 newly assembled ribosomes will be transported every minute in the other direction. The typical cell can synthesize 10,000 to 20,000 different proteins. How do they know where to go? The answer is that these proteins have localization signals. In the case of steroid hormone receptor proteins, the signal sequences are in the hinge region.

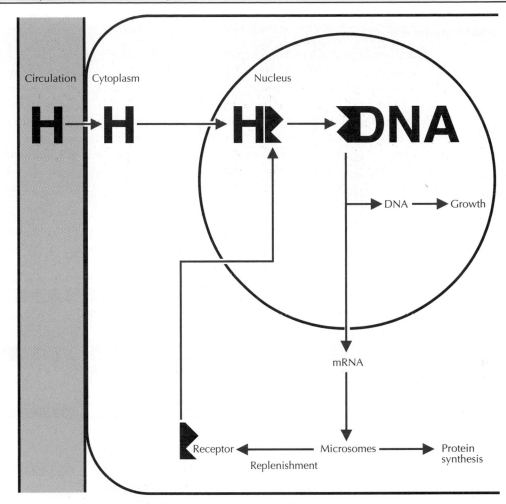

Estrogen and progestin receptors exit continuously from the nucleus to the cytoplasm and are actively transported back to the nucleus. This is a constant shuttle; constant diffusion into the cytoplasm is balanced by the active transport into the nucleus. This raises the possibility that some diseases are due to poor traffic control. This can be true of some acquired diseases as well; e.g., Reye's syndrome, an acquired disorder of mitochondrial enzyme function.

The fate of the hormone-receptor complex after gene activation is referred to as hormone-receptor *processing.* In the case of estrogen receptors, processing involves the conversion of high-affinity estrogen receptor sites to a rapidly dissociating form followed by loss of binding capacity, which is completed in about 6 hours. The rapid turnover of estrogen receptors has clinical significance. The continuous presence of estrogen is an important factor for continuing response.

The best example of the importance of these factors is the difference between estradiol and estriol. Estriol has only 20–30% affinity for the estrogen receptor compared with estradiol; therefore, it is rapidly cleared from a cell. But if the effective concentration is kept equivalent to that of estradiol, it can produce a similar biologic response.[42] In pregnancy, where the concentration of estriol is very great, it can be an important hormone, not just a metabolite.

The depletion of estrogen receptors in target tissues by progestational agents is the fundamental reason for adding progestins to estrogen treatment programs. The progestins accelerate the turnover of pre-existing receptors, and this is followed by inhibition of estrogen-induced receptor synthesis. Using monoclonal antibody immunocytochemistry, this action has been pinpointed to the interruption of transcription in estrogen-regulated genes. The mechanism is different for androgen antiestrogen effects. Androgens do not involve depletion of estrogen receptors but in some way decrease estrogen-induced RNA activity in the cytoplasm.[43]

The Receptor Superfamily

Recombinant DNA techniques have permitted the study of the gene sequences that code for the synthesis of nuclear receptors. Steroid hormone receptors share a common structure with the receptors for thyroid hormone, 1,25-dihydroxy vitamin D_3, and retinoic acid; thus, these receptors are called a superfamily.[44] Each receptor contains characteristic domains that are similar and interchangeable. Therefore, it is not surprising that the specific hormones can interact with more than one receptor in this family. Analysis of these receptors suggests a complex evolutionary history during which gene duplication and swapping between domains of different origins occurred.[45] This family now includes about 150 proteins, present in practically all species, from worms to insects to humans. Many are called *orphan receptors* because specific ligands for these proteins have not been identified.

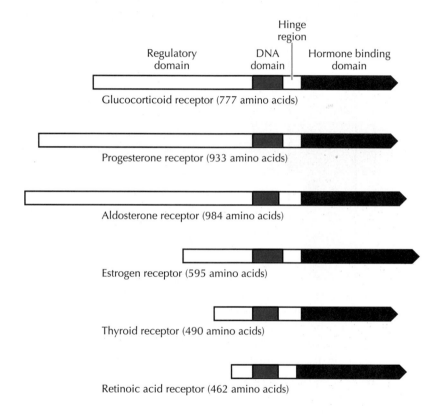

The Estrogen Receptors

Two estrogen receptors have been identified, designated as estrogen receptor-alpha (ER-α) and estrogen receptor-beta (ER-β).[46, 47] The estrogen receptor-alpha was discovered about 1960, and the amino acid sequence was reported in 1986.[48–50] The estrogen receptor-alpha is translated from a 6.8-kilobase mRNA that contains 8 exons derived from a gene on the long arm of chromosome 6.[51] It has a molecular weight of approximately 66,000 with 595 amino acids. The receptor alpha half-life is approximately 4–7 hours, thus the estrogen receptor-alpha is a protein with a rapid turn over. The more recently discovered estrogen receptor-beta is encoded by a gene localized to chromosome 14,q22-q24, in close proximity to genes related to Alzheimer's disease.[52]

The Estrogen Receptor-Alpha

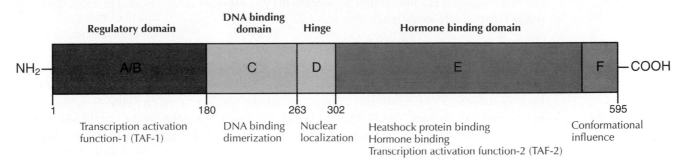

The Estrogen Receptor-Beta

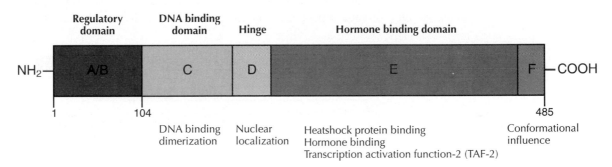

The estrogen receptors are divided into 6 regions in 5 domains, labeled A to F. The ER-β is 97% homologous in amino acid sequence with the alpha estrogen receptor in the DNA binding domain and 59% homologous in the hormone-binding domain.[47] The full comparison is as follows:[52]

	ER-α and ER-β Homology
The regulatory domain	17.5%
The DNA-binding domain	97%
The hinge	30%
The hormone-binding domain	59.1%
The F region	17.9%

The following discussion represents information derived from studies of the ER-α. The hormone binding characteristics of the ER-α and the ER-β are similar, indicating that they respond in a comparable manner to the same hormones.[53] There are differences, however; for example, phytoestrogens have a greater affinity for ER-β than for ER-α. Different genetic messages can result not only because of differences in binding affinity, but through variations in the mechanisms to be discussed, notably differences in conformational shape and cellular contexts. In addition, because the regulatory domains differ in the two receptors, ER-β may not be capable of activating gene transcription by means of TAF 1 (discussed below).

A/B Region, The Regulatory Domain

The amino acid terminal is the most variable in the superfamily of receptors, ranging in size from 20 amino acids in the Vitamin D receptor, to 600 amino acids in the mineralocorticoid receptor. In the ER-α, it contains several phosphorylation sites and the ***transcription activation function*** *called TAF-1*. TAF-1 can stimulate transcription in the absence of hormone binding. The regulatory domain is considerably different in the two estrogen receptors, and in ER-β, TAF-1 is either significantly modified or absent.

C Region, The DNA-Binding Domain

The middle domain binds to DNA and consists of 100 amino acids with 9 cysteines in fixed positions, the two *zinc fingers*. This domain is essential for activation of transcription. Hormone binding induces a conformational change that allows binding to the hormone-responsive elements in the target gene. This domain is very similar for each member of the steroid and thyroid receptor superfamily; however, the genetic message is specific for the hormone that binds to the hormone-binding domain. The DNA-binding domain controls which gene will be regulated by the receptor and is responsible for target gene specificity and high-affinity DNA binding. The specificity of receptor binding to its hormone responsive element is determined by the zinc finger region, especially the first finger. The specific message can be changed by changing the amino acids in the base of the fingers. Substitutions of amino acids in the fingertips lead to loss of function. Functional specificity is localized to the second zinc finger in an area designated the d (distal) box. Different responses are due to the different genetic expression of each target cell (the unique activity of each cell's genetic constitution allows individual behavior).

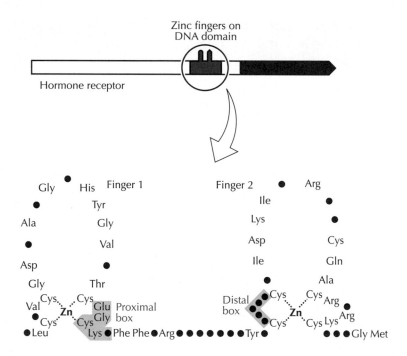

D Region, The Hinge

The region between the DNA-binding domain and the hormone-binding domain contains a signal area that is important for the movement of the receptor to the nucleus following synthesis in the cytoplasm. This nuclear localization signal must be present for the estrogen receptor to remain within the nucleus in the absence of hormone. This region is also a site of rotation (hence the hinge designation) in achieving conformational change.

E Region, The Hormone-Binding Domain

The carboxy end of the estrogen receptor-alpha is the hormone-binding domain (for both estrogens and antiestrogens), consisting of 251 amino acids (residues 302–553). In addition to hormone binding, this region is responsible for *dimerization* and contains the *transcription activation function called TAF-2*. This is also the site for binding by heat shock proteins (specifically hsp 90), and it is this binding to the heat shock proteins that prevents dimerization and DNA binding. In contrast to TAF-1 activity, TAF-2 depends on hormone binding for full activity. The hormone-binding domain of the steroid receptors contains a characteristic structure, containing helices that form a pocket (also referred to as a sandwich fold).[54] After binding with a hormone, this pocket undergoes a conformational change that creates new surfaces with the potential to interact with co-activator and co-repressor proteins.

F Region

The F region of ER-α is a 42 amino acid C-terminal segment. This region modulates gene transcription by estrogen and antiestrogens, having a role that influences antiestrogen efficacy in suppressing estrogen-stimulated transcription.[55] The conformation of the receptor-ligand complex is different with estrogen and antiestrogens, and this conformation is different with and without the F region. The F region is not required for transcriptional response to estrogen; however, it affects the magnitude of ligand-bound receptor activity. It is speculated that this region affects conformation in such a way that protein interactions are influenced. Thus, it is appropriate that the effects of the F domain vary according to cell type and protein context. The F region affects the activities of both TAF-1 and TAF-2, which is what one would expect if the effect is on conformation.[56]

Mechanism of Action

The steroid family receptors are predominantly in the nucleus even when not bound to a ligand, except for the androgen, mineralocorticoid, and glucocorticoid receptors where nuclear uptake depends on hormone binding. But the estrogen receptor does undergo what is called ***nucleocytoplasmic shuttling.*** The estrogen receptor constantly diffuses out of the nucleus and is rapidly transported back in. When this shuttling is impaired, receptors are more rapidly degraded in the cytoplasm. Agents that inhibit dimerization (e.g., the pure estrogen antagonists) inhibit nuclear translocation and thus increase cytoplasmic degradation.

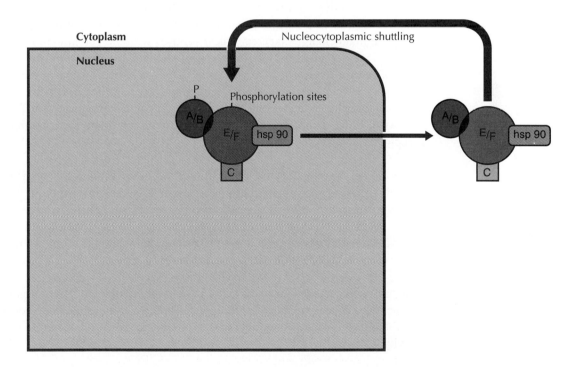

Prior to binding, the estrogen receptor is an inactive complex that includes a variety of proteins, including the heat shock proteins. Heat shock protein 90 appears to be a critical protein, and many of the others are associated with it. This heat shock protein is not only important for maintaining an inactive state, but also for causing proper folding for transport across membranes. "Activation" or "transformation" is the dissociation of heat shock protein 90.[57]

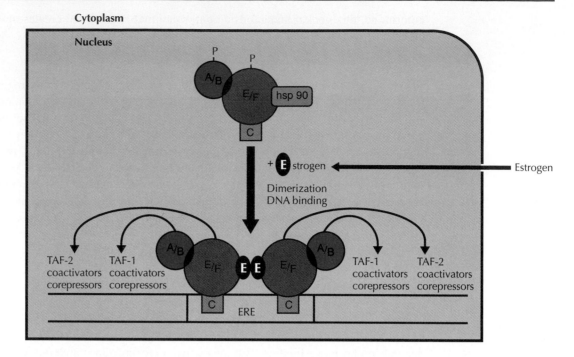

Imagine the unoccupied steroid receptor as a loosely packed, mobile protein complexed with heat shock proteins. The steroid family of receptors exists in this complex and cannot bind to DNA until union with a steroid hormone liberates the heat shock proteins and allows dimerization. The conformational change induced by hormone binding involves a dissociating process to form a tighter packing of the receptor. The hormone-binding domain contains helices that form a pocket (also referred to as a sandwich fold).[54] After binding with a hormone, this pocket undergoes a conformational change that creates new surfaces with the potential to interact with co-activator and co-repressor proteins. ***Conformational shape is an important factor in determining the exact message transmitted to the gene.*** Conformational shape is slightly but significantly different with each ligand; estradiol, tamoxifen, and raloxifene each induce a distinct conformation that contributes to the ultimate message of agonism or antagonism.[58, 59] The weak estrogen activity of estriol is because of its altered conformation shape when combined with the estrogen receptor in comparison with estradiol.[60]

The hormone-binding domain of the estrogen receptors contains a cavity surrounded by a wedge-shaped structure, and it is the fit into this cavity that is so influential in influencing the genetic message. The size of this cavity on the estrogen receptor is relatively large, larger than the volume of an estradiol molecule, explaining the acceptance of a large variety of ligands. Thus, estradiol, tamoxifen, and raloxifene each bind at the same site within the hormone binding domain, but the conformational shape with each is not identical.

Conformational shape is a major factor in determining the ability of a ligand and its receptor to interact with coactivators and corepressors. Conformational shapes are not simply either "on" or "off," but intermediate conformations are possible providing a spectrum of agonist/antagonistic activity.

Members of the thyroid and retinoic acid receptor subfamily do not exist in inactive complexes with heat shock proteins. They can form dimers and bind to response elements in DNA, but without ligand, they act as repressors of transcription.

Estrogen receptor mutants can be created that are unable to bind estradiol. These mutants can form dimers with natural estrogen receptor (wild type), and then bind to the estrogen response element, but they cannot activate transcription.[61] This indicates that transcription is dependent on the result after estradiol binding to the estrogen receptor, an estrogen-dependent structural change. Dimerization by itself is not sufficient to lead to transcription; neither is binding of the dimer to DNA sufficient.

Molecular modeling and physical energy calculations indicate that binding of estrogen with its receptor is not a simple key and lock mechanism. It involves conversion of the estrogen-receptor complex to a preferred geometry dictated to a major degree by the specific binding site of the receptor. The estrogenic response depends on the final bound conformation and the electronic properties of functional groups that contribute energy. The final transactivation function is dependent on these variables.[62]

Estrogen, progesterone, androgen, and glucocorticoid receptors bind to their response elements as dimers, one molecule of hormone to each of the two units in the dimer. The estrogen receptor-alpha can form dimers with other alpha receptors (homodimers) or with an estrogen receptor-beta (heterodimer). Similarly, the estrogen receptor-beta can form homodimers or heterodimers with the alpha receptor. This creates the potential for many pathways for estrogen signaling, alternatives that are further increased by the possibility of utilizing various response elements in target genes. Cells that express only one of the estrogen receptors would respond to the homodimers; cells that express both could express to a homodimer and a heterodimer.

The similar amino acid sequence of the DNA-binding domains in this family of receptors indicates evolutionary conservation of homologous segments. An important part of the conformational pattern consists of multiple cysteine-repeating units found in two structures, each held in a finger like shape by a zinc ion, the so-called zinc fingers.[63] The zinc fingers on the various hormone receptors are not identical. These fingers of amino acids are thought to interact with similar complementary patterns in the DNA. Directed changes (experimental mutations) indicate that conservation of the cysteine residues is necessary for binding activity, as is the utilization of zinc.

The DNA binding domain is specific for an enhancer site (called the hormone responsive element) in the gene promoter, located in the 5' flanking region. The activity of the hormone-responsive element requires the presence of the hormone-receptor complex. Thus, this region is the part of the gene to which the DNA-binding domain of the receptor binds. There are at least four different hormone-responsive elements, one for glucocorticoids/progesterone/androgen, one for estrogen, one for vitamin D_3, and one for thyroid/retinoic acid.[64] These sites significantly differ only in the number of intervening nucleotides.

Binding of the hormone-receptor complex to its hormone-responsive element leads to many changes, only one of which is a conformational alteration in the DNA. Although the hormone-responsive elements for glucocorticoids, progesterone, and androgens mediate all of these hormonal responses, there are subtle differences in the binding sites, and there are additional sequences outside of the DNA-binding sites that influence activation by the three different hormones. The cloning of complementary DNAs for steroid receptors has revealed a large number of similar structures of unknown function. It is believed that the protein products of these sequences are involved in the regulation of transcription initiation that occurs at the TATA box.

There are 3 different RNA polymerases (designated as I, II, and III), each dedicated to the transcription of a different set of genes with specific promoters (the site of polymerase initiation of transcription). ***Transcription factors are polypeptides, complexed with the polymerase enzyme, that modulate transcription either at the promoter site or at a sequence further upstream on the DNA.***[36] The steroid hormone receptors, therefore, are transcription factors. The polymerase transcription factor complex can be developed in sequential fashion with recruitment of individual polypeptides, or transcription can result from interaction with a preformed complete complex. The effect can be either positive or negative, activation or repression.

In most cases, therefore, the steroid hormone receptor activates transcription in partnership with several groups of polypeptides.[36]

1. Other transcription factors — peptides that interact with the polymerase enzyme and DNA.

2. Coactivators and corepressors — peptides that interact with the TAF areas of the receptor, also called adaptor proteins.

3. Chromatin factors — structural organizational changes that allow an architecture appropriate for transcription response.

The steroid-receptor complex regulates the amount of mRNA transcripts emanating from target genes. The estrogen-occupied receptor binds to estrogen response elements in the 5' flanking regions of estrogen-regulated genes, allowing efficient induction of RNA transcription. This can occur by direct binding to DNA and interaction with the estrogen response element or by protein interactions with ***coactivators*** between the estrogen receptor and DNA sites. ***Coactivators and corepressors are intracellular proteins (called adaptor proteins) that activate or suppress the TAF areas, either by acting on the receptors or on DNA.***[65–67] Most of the genes regulated by estrogens respond within 1–2 hours after estrogen administration. Only a few respond within minutes. This time requirement may reflect the necessity to synthesize regulating proteins.[68]

One of the aspects of activation, for example with the estrogen receptor, is an increase in affinity for estrogen. This is an action of estrogen, and it is greatest with estradiol and least with estriol. This action of estradiol, the ability of binding at one site to affect another site, is called ***cooperativity***. An increase in affinity is called positive cooperativity. The biologic advantage of positive cooperativity is that this increases the receptor's ability to respond to small changes in the concentration of the hormone. One of the antiestrogen actions of clomiphene is its property of negative cooperativity, the inhibition of the transition from a low-affinity to a high-affinity state. The relatively long duration of action exhibited by estradiol is due to the high-affinity state achieved by the receptor.

TAF (transcriptional activation function) is the part of the receptor that activates gene transcription after binding to DNA. Ligand binding produces a conformation that allows TAFs to accomplish its tasks. TAF-1 can stimulate transcription in the absence of hormone when it is fused to DNA; however, it also promotes DNA binding in the intact receptor. TAF-2 is affected by the bound ligand, and the estrogen receptor depends on estrogen binding for full activity. TAF-2 consists of a number of dispersed elements that are brought together after estrogen binding. The activities of TAF-1 and TAF-2 vary according to the promoters in target cells. These areas can act independently or with one another.

Thus the differential activities of the TAFs account for different activities in different cells. In addition to the binding of the dimerized steroid receptor to the DNA response element, steroid hormone activity is modulated by other pathways (other protein transcription factors and coactivators/corepressors) that influence transcription activation.[69]***This is an important concept: the concept of cellular context. The same hormone can produce different responses in different cells according to the cellular context of protein regulators.***

The concentration of coactivators/corepressors can affect the cellular response, and this is another explanation for strong responses from small amounts of hormone. A small amount of receptor but a large amount of coactivator/corepressor and the cell can be very responsive to a weak signal.

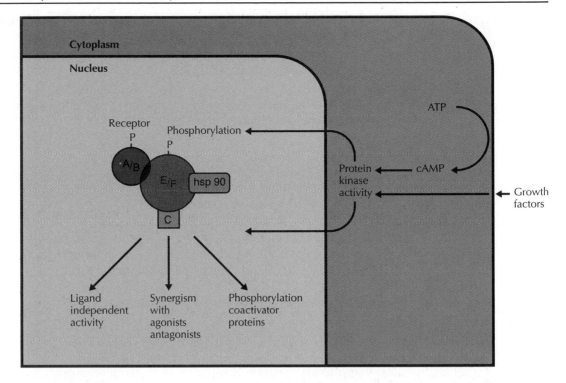

Phosphorylation of specific receptor sites is an important method of regulation, as well as phosphorylation of other peptides that influence gene transcription. Phosphorylation can be regulated by cell membrane receptors and ligand binding, thus establishing a method for cell membrane-bound ligands to communicate with steroid receptor genes.

Cyclic AMP and protein kinase A pathways increase transcriptional activity of the estrogen receptor by phosphorylation. In some cases phosphorylation modulates the activity of the receptor; in other cases, the phosphorylation regulates the activity of a specific peptide or coactivator/corepressor that, in turn, modulates the receptor. The steroid receptor superfamily members are phosphoproteins. Phosphorylation follows steroid binding and occurs in both the cytoplasm and nucleus. This phosphorylation is believed to enhance activity of the steroid receptor complex.

Phosphorylation of the receptor increases the potency of the molecule to regulate transcription. Growth factors can stimulate protein kinase phosphorylation that can produce synergistic activation of genes or even ligand-independent activity. Epidermal growth factor (EGF), IGF-I, and TGF-α can activate the estrogen receptor in the absence of estrogen. This response to growth factors can be blocked by pure antiestrogens (suggesting that a strong antagonist locks the receptor in a conformation that resists ligand-independent pathways). The exact mechanism of growth factor activation is not known, but it is known that a steroid receptor can be activated by means of a chemical signal (a phosphorylation cascade) originating at the plasma membrane. ***The recruitment of kinase activity is specific for specific ligands; thus not all ligands stimulate phosphorylation.***

Another explanation for strong responses from small amounts of steroids is a positive feedback relationship. Estrogen activates its receptor, gene expression stimulates growth factors (EFG, IGF-I, TGF-α, FGF), and the growth factors in an autocrine fashion further activate the estrogen receptor.[70]

Summary — Steps in the Steroid Hormone–Receptor Mechanism

1. Binding of the hormone to the hormone-binding domain that has been kept in an inactive state by various heat shock proteins.

2. Activation of the hormone-receptor complex, by *conformational change*, follows the dissociation of the heat shock proteins.

3. Dimerization of the complex.

4. Binding of the dimer to the hormone-responsive element on DNA by the zinc finger area of the DNA-binding domain.

5. Stimulation of transcription, mediated by transcription activation functions (TAFs), and influenced by the protein (other transcription factors and coactivators/corepressors) *context of the cell*, and by *phosphorylation*.

Summary — Factors that Determine Biologic Activity

1. Affinity of the hormone for the hormone-binding domain of the receptor.

2. Target tissue differential expression of the receptor subtypes (e.g., ER-α and ER-β).

3. Conformational shape of the ligand-receptor complex, with effects on two important activities: dimerization and modulation of adapter proteins.

4. Differential expression of target tissue adaptor proteins and phosphorylation.

Different Roles for ER-α and ER-β

Male and female mice have been developed that are homozygous for disruption of the alpha estrogen receptor gene, "estrogen receptor-alpha knockout mice."[71] Both sexes with this knockout are infertile. Spermatogenesis in the male is reduced and the testes undergo progressive atrophy, a result of a testicular role for estrogen, because gonadotropin levels and testicular steroidogenesis remain normal. Sexual mounting behavior is not altered, but intromission, ejaculation, and aggressive behaviors are reduced. Female mice with the alpha estrogen receptor gene disrupted do not ovulate, and the ovaries do not respond to gonadotropin stimulation. These female animals have high levels of estradiol, testosterone, and LH. FSH β-subunit synthesis is increased, but FSH secretion is at normal levels, indicating different sites of action for estrogen and inhibin. Uterine development is normal (due to a lack of testosterone in early life), but growth is impaired. Mammary gland ductal and alveolar development is absent. Female mice with absent alpha estrogen receptor activity do not display sexual receptive behaviors. This genetically engineered line of mice demonstrates essential activities for the alpha estrogen receptor. Relatively normal fetal and early development suggests that the beta estrogen receptor plays a primary role in these functions. For example, the fetal adrenal gland expresses high levels of ER-β and low levels of ER-α.[72] However, nongenomic actions of estrogen are also possible and can explain some of the estrogenic responses in a knockout model.

Differential expression of the alpha and beta receptors is likely in various tissues (e.g., ER-β is the prevalent estrogen receptor in certain areas of the brain and the cardiovascular system) resulting in different and selective responses to specific estrogens. Human granulosa cells from the ovarian follicle contain *only* ER-β mRNA; the human breast expresses both ER-α and ER-β.[52] Some parts of the rat brain contain only ER-β, others only ER-α, and some areas contain both receptors.[73]

The estrogen story is further complicated by the fact that the same estrogen binding to the alpha and beta receptors can produce opposite effects. For example, estradiol can stimulate gene transcription with ER-α and a given site of the estrogen response element, whereas estradiol inhibits gene transcription with ER-β in this same system.[74] Different and unique messages, therefore, can be determined by the specific combination of (1). a particular estrogen, (2) the alpha or beta receptor, and (3) the targeted response element. To some degree, differences with ER-α and ER-β are influenced by activation of TAF-1 and TAF-2; agents that are capable of mixed estrogen agonism and antagonism produce agonistic messages via TAF-1 with ER-α, but because ER-β lacks a similar TAF-1, such agents can be pure antagonists in cells that respond only to ER-β. ER-α and ER-β affect the peptide context of a cell, especially coactivators and corepressors, differently.

The Progesterone Receptor

The progesterone receptor is induced by estrogens at the transcriptional level and decreased by progestins at both the transcriptional and translational levels (probably through receptor phosphorylation).[75] The progesterone receptor (in a fashion similar to the estrogen receptor) has two major forms, designated the A and B receptors.[76] The two forms are expressed by a single gene; the two forms are a consequence of transcription from distinctly different promoters, in a complex system of transcription regulation.[77] Each form is associated with additional proteins, which are important for folding of the polypeptide into a structure that allows hormone binding and receptor activity.[78] The molecular weight of A is 94,000 and B, 114,000, with 933 amino acids, 164 more than A. The B receptor has a unique upstream segment (164 amino acids) referred to as the B-upstream segment (BUS).

The Progesterone Receptor-A

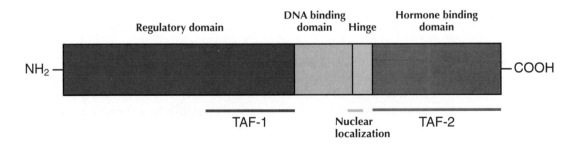

The Progesterone Receptor-B

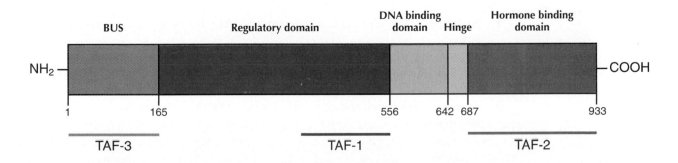

On the progesterone receptor, TAF-1 is located in a 91-amino acid segment just upstream of the DNA-binding domain. TAF-2 is located in the hormone-binding domain. A fragment missing the hormone-binding domain activates transcription to levels comparable to full-length hormone-activated B receptors, and higher than that with the A receptor, thus beyond that of TAF-1 alone. In appropriate cells, therefore, BUS contains a third activation domain, TAF-3, and can autonomously activate transcription or it can synergize with the other TAFs.[79] In the absence of hormone binding, the C-terminal region of the progesterone receptor exerts an inhibitory effect on transcription.[80] Progesterone agonists induce a conformational change that overcomes the inherent inhibitory function within the carboxy tail of the receptor. Binding with a progesterone antagonist produces a structural change that allows the inhibitory actions to be maintained.

Progestational agents can elicit a variety of responses determined by target tissue production and activity of the two receptor forms with dimerization as AA and BB (homodimers) or AB (heterodimer). The progesterone receptors function in the mechanism shared by this superfamily of receptors: an unbound complex with heat shock proteins, hormone binding, dimerization, DNA binding to a progesterone response element, and modulation of transcription by phosphorylation and various proteins.[59, 81]

A and B are expressed in approximately equal amounts in breast cancer and endometrial cancer cell lines. Studies indicate that the two receptors can be regulated independently; e.g., the relative levels differ in endometrium during the menstrual cycle.[82] Tissue specificity with the progesterone receptor is influenced by which receptor and which dimer is active, and in addition, the transcriptional activities of A and B depend on target cell differences, especially in promoter context. However, in most cells, B is the positive regulator of progesterone-responsive genes, and A inhibits B activity. Mutations within the carboxy terminus of B affect the transcriptional activity of B. But mutations in A have no effect on its transcriptional inhibitory activity. This indicates two separate pathways for transcription activation and repression by the progesterone receptor. Thus, repression of human estrogen receptor transcriptional activity (as well as glucocorticoid, mineralocorticoid, and androgen transcription) is dependent on the expression of A.[83, 84]

The broad activity of A in regards to all steroids suggests that A regulates steroid hormone action wherever it is expressed. A does not form a heterodimer with the estrogen receptor. A does not prevent the estrogen receptor from binding with DNA. A does not change the structure of the estrogen receptor. Therefore, A either competes with the estrogen receptor for a critical protein; in this case A would inhibit the estrogen receptor only in cells that contain the critical factor. Or the target is a critical protein, again an essential transcription activator.[78, 82]

The Androgen Receptor

The cellular mechanism is more complex for androgens. Androgens can work in any one of three ways.

1. By intracellular conversion of testosterone to dihydrotestosterone (DHT), intracrine activity.

2. By testosterone itself, endocrine activity.

3. By intracellular conversion of testosterone to estradiol (aromatization), intracrine activity.

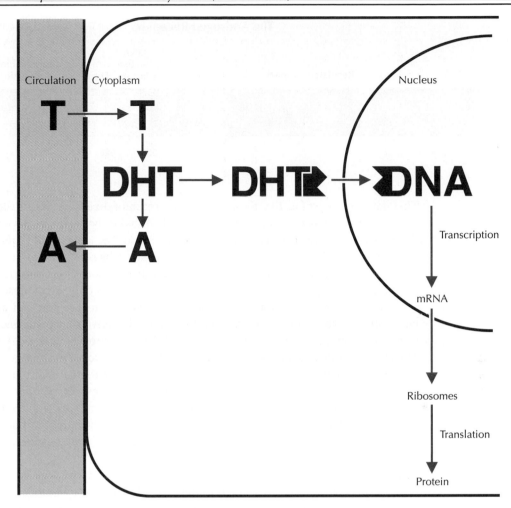

Tissues that exclusively operate via the testosterone pathway are the derivatives of the wolffian duct, whereas hair follicles and derivatives of the urogenital sinus and urogenital tubercle require the conversion of testosterone to DHT. The hypothalamus actively converts androgens to estrogens; hence, aromatization may be necessary for certain androgen feedback messages in the brain.

In those cells that respond only to DHT, only DHT will be found within the nucleus activating messenger RNA production. Because testosterone and DHT bind to the same high-affinity androgen receptor, why is it necessary to have the DHT mechanism? One explanation is that this is a mechanism for amplifying androgen action, because the androgen receptor preferentially will bind DHT (greater affinity). The antiandrogens, including cyproterone acetate and spironolactone, bind to the androgen receptor with about 20% of the affinity of testosterone.[85] This weak affinity is characteristic of binding without activation of the biologic response.

The Androgen Receptor

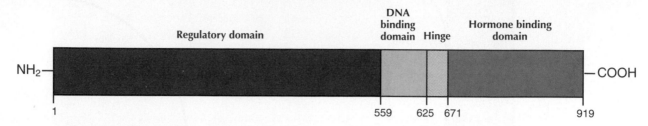

The androgen receptor, like the progesterone receptor, exists as the full-length B form and a shorter A form.[86] It is likely that the A and B forms of the androgen receptor have functional differences; however, this remains to be characterized. The amino acid sequence of the androgen receptor in the DNA-binding domain resembles that of the receptors for progesterone, mineralocorticoids, and glucocorticoids but most closely that of the progesterone receptor.[87] Androgens and progestins can cross react for their receptors but do so only when present in pharmacologic concentrations. Progestins not only compete for androgen receptors but also compete for the metabolic utilization of the 5α-reductase enzyme. The dihydroprogesterone that is produced, in turn, also competes with testosterone and DHT for the androgen receptor. A progestin, therefore, can act both as an antiandrogen and as an antiestrogen. Androgen-responsive gene expression can also be modified by estrogen; it has been known for years that androgens and estrogens can counteract each other's biologic responses. These responses of target tissues are determined by gene interactions with the hormone-receptor complexes, androgen with its receptor and estrogen with its receptor. The ultimate biologic response reflects the balance of actions of the different hormones with their respective receptors, modified by various transcription regulators.

The syndrome of testicular feminization (androgen insensitivity) represents a congenital abnormality in the androgen intracellular receptor (about 200 unique mutations have been identified).[88] The androgen receptor gene is localized on the human X chromosome at Xq11-12, the only steroid hormone receptor to be located on the X chromosome.[89] Thus, testicular feminization is an X-linked disorder. Molecular studies of patients with testicular feminization have indicated a deletion of amino acids from the steroid-binding domain due to nucleotide alterations in the gene that encodes the androgen receptor.[90] What was once a confusing picture is now easily understood as a progressive increase in androgen receptor action. At one end, there is a complete absence of androgen binding—complete testicular feminization. In the middle is a spectrum of clinical presentations representing varying degrees of abnormal receptors and binding. While at the other end, it has been suggested that about 25% of infertile men with normal genitalia and normal family histories have azoospermia due to a receptor disorder.[91] The androgen receptor also plays a role in motor neuron physiology, because a specific mutation in the androgen receptor is responsible for Kennedy's disease (X-linked spinobulbar muscular atrophy), a condition associated with motor neuron degeneration.[92]

Nongenomic Actions of Steroid Hormones

The genomic effects of steroid hormones are characterized by a relatively slow response time of 1 hour or longer. However, some steroid hormone effects are immediate, within a few seconds, and nongenomic mechanisms must be operative in order to achieve such rapid responses.[93] These rapid responses are also unaffected by inhibitors of gene transcription or protein synthesis. Rapid actions have been reported for all steroid hormones and include calcium and sodium transport across membranes, neural effects, and certain oocyte and sperm reactions. The messenger and effector systems utilized vary from cell to cell and from steroid to steroid. Specific cell membrane receptors have been identified for various steroids; however, it has been difficult to demonstrate physiologic roles for these binding sites. Nevertheless, investigation thus far indicates that steroid hormones can bind to membrane receptors and trigger rapid changes in electrolyte transport systems.[94] Estrogen-induced vasodilatation in the coronary arteries is believed to be mediated, at least in part, through a nongenomic calcium flux mechanism.[95]

Agonists and Antagonists

An agonist is a substance that stimulates a response. An antagonist completely inhibits the actions of an agonist. Agonistic activity follows receptor binding which leads to stimulation of the message associated with that receptor. Antagonistic activity follows receptor binding and is characterized by blockage of the receptor message or nontransmission of the message. Most compounds used in this fashion that bind to hormone nuclear receptors have a mix of agonist and antagonist responses, depending on the tissue and hormonal milieu. Examples of antagonists include tamoxifen, RU486, and the histamine receptor antagonists.

Short-Acting Antagonists

Short-acting antagonists, such as estriol, are actually a mixed combination of agonism and antagonism depending on time. Short-term estrogen responses can be elicited because estriol binds to the nuclear receptor, but long-term responses do not occur because this binding is short-lived. Antagonism results when estriol competes with estradiol for receptors. However, if a constant presence of the weak hormone, estriol, can be maintained, then long-term occupation is possible, and a potent estrogen response can be produced.

Long-Acting Antagonists

Clomiphene and tamoxifen are mixed estrogen agonists and antagonists. The endometrium is very sensitive to the agonistic response, whereas the breast is more sensitive to the antagonistic behavior. The antagonistic action is the result of nuclear receptor binding with an alteration in the normal receptor-DNA processing and a failure to replenish hormone receptors, resulting in eventual depletion.

Alteration of the GnRH molecule has produced both agonists and antagonists. GnRH is a decapeptide; antagonists have substitutions at multiple positions, while agonists have substitutions at the 6 or 10 positions. The GnRH agonist molecules first stimulate the pituitary gland to secrete gonadotropins, then because of the constant stimulation, down-regulation and desensitization of the cell membrane receptors occur, and gonadotropin secretion is literally turned off. The antagonist molecules bind to the cell membrane receptor and fail to transmit a message and thus are competitive inhibitors. Various GnRH agonists are used to treat endometriosis, uterine leiomyomas, precocious puberty, cancer of the prostate gland, ovarian hyperandrogenism, and the premenstrual syndrome.

Physiologic Antagonists

Strictly speaking, a progestin is not an estrogen antagonist. It modifies estrogen action by causing a depletion of estrogen receptors. There is also evidence that a progestin can inhibit transcription activation by the estrogen receptor.[96] In addition, progestins induce enzyme activity that converts the potent estradiol to the impotent estrone sulfate, which is then secreted from the cell.[97] Androgens do block the actions of estrogen, but the mechanism is not entirely clear. Rather than a direct impact on estrogen receptor levels, the action is directed to gene activity subsequent to estrogen-receptor binding.[43] High levels of androgen can produce estrogen and progestational effects by binding to the estrogen and progesterone receptors.

Triphenylethylene derivatives

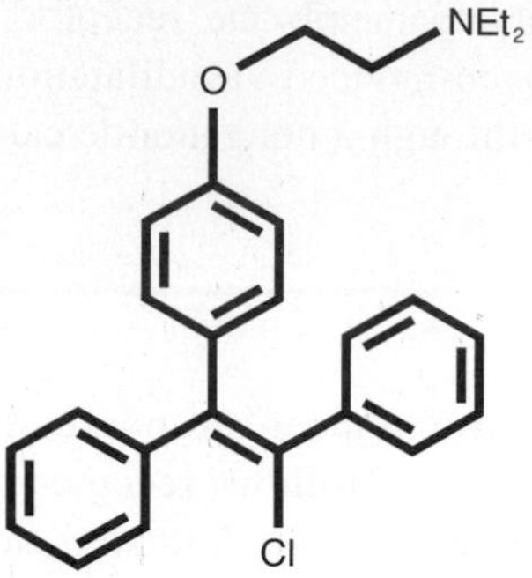

Clomiphene

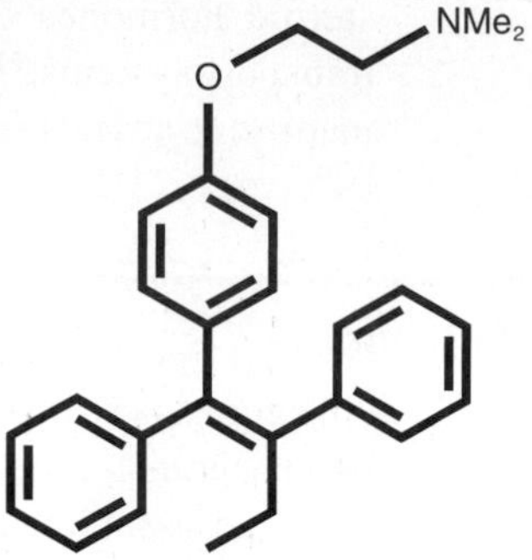

Tamoxifen

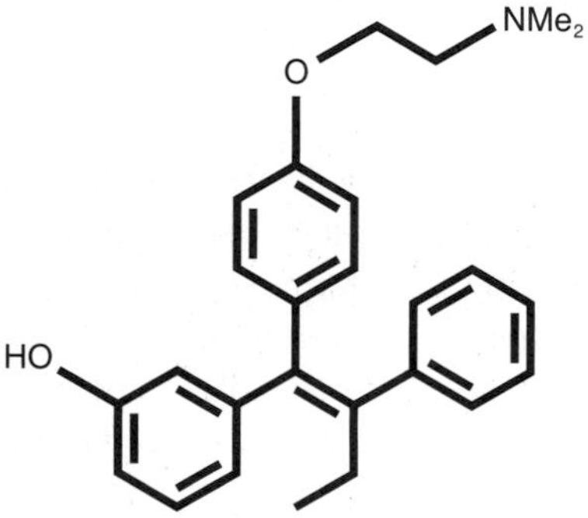

Droloxifene

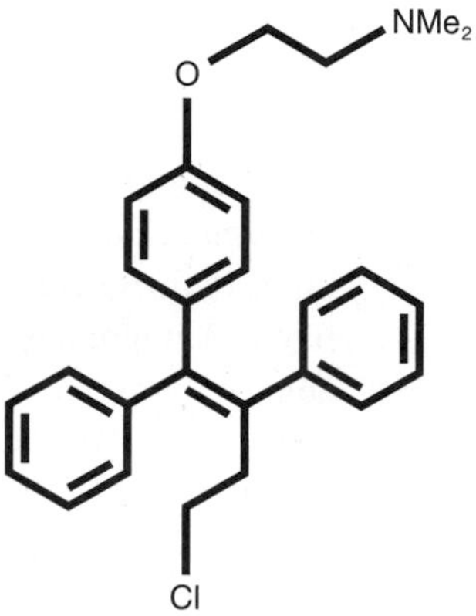

Toremifene

Benzothiphene derivative

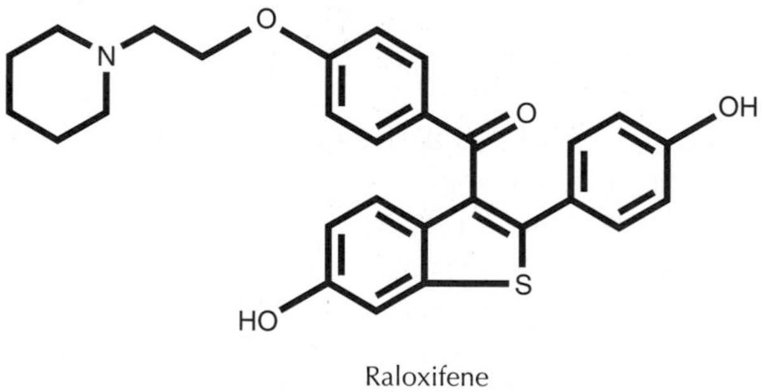

Raloxifene

Pure antiestrogens

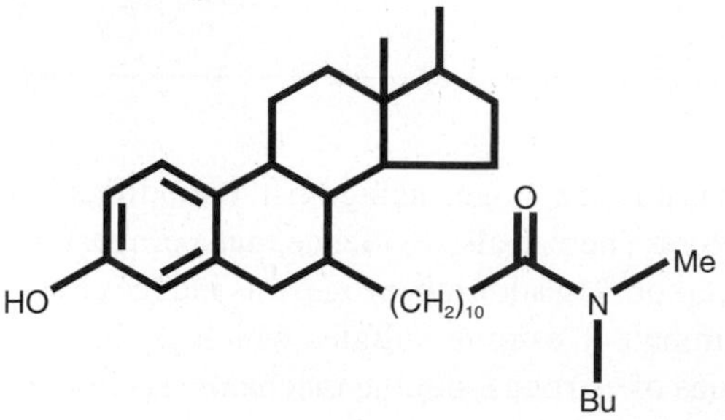

ICI 164,384

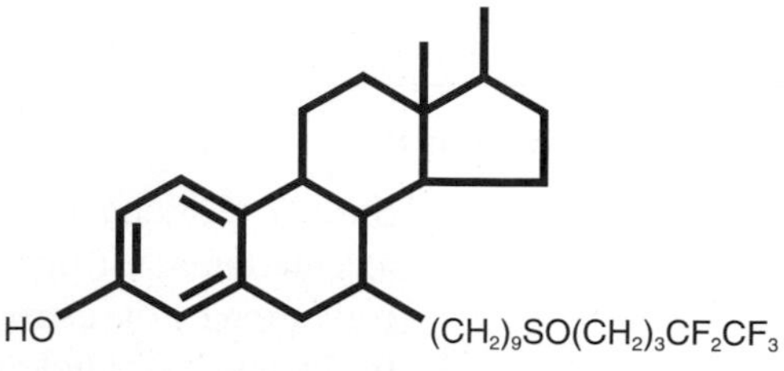

ICI 182,780

Antiestrogens

Currently, there are two groups of antiestrogens: pure antiestrogens and compounds with both agonistic and antagonistic activities. The mixed agonist–antagonist compounds include both the triphenylethylene derivatives (the nonsteroidal estrogen relatives such as clomiphene and tamoxifen) and the nonsteroidal sulfur-containing agents (the benzothiophenes, such as raloxifene). The pure antiestrogens have a bulky side chain that, with only a little imagination, can be pictured as an obstruction to appropriate conformational changes. An ideal antiestrogen would have the following properties:

1. A compound that would be a pure antagonist on proliferating breast carcinoma cells

2. Development of resistance would be rare or require long exposure.

3. High affinity for the estrogen receptor so that therapeutic doses could be easily achieved.

4. No interference with the beneficial actions of estrogens.

5. No toxic or carcinogenic effects.

The Antiestrogen Tamoxifen

Tamoxifen is very similar to clomiphene (in structure and actions), both being nonsteroidal compounds structurally related to diethylstilbestrol. Tamoxifen, in binding to the estrogen receptor, competitively inhibits estrogen binding. In vitro, the estrogen binding affinity for its receptor is 100–1000 times greater than that of tamoxifen. Thus, tamoxifen must be present in a concentration 100–1000 times greater than estrogen to maintain inhibition of breast cancer cells. In vitro studies demonstrate that this action is not cytocidal, but, rather, cytostatic (and thus its use must be long-term). The tamoxifen-estrogen receptor complex binds to DNA, but whether an agonistic, estrogenic message or an antagonistic, antiestrogenic message predominates is determined by what promoter elements are present in specific cell types.

There have been many clinical trials with adjuvant treatment of breast cancer with tamoxifen, and many are still on going.[98] Overall, the impact of tamoxifen treatment on breast cancer can be summarized as follows: disease-free survival is prolonged. There is an increased survival at 5 years of approximately 20%, most evident in women over age 50. Response rates in advanced breast cancer are 30–35%, most marked in patients with tumors that are positive for estrogen receptors, reaching 75% in tumors highly positive for estrogen receptors.

Serum protein changes reflect the estrogenic (agonistic) action of tamoxifen. This includes decreases in antithrombin III, cholesterol, and LDL-cholesterol, while HDL-cholesterol and sex hormone-binding globulin (SHBG) levels increase (as do other binding globulins). The estrogenic activity of tamoxifen, 20 mg daily, is nearly as potent as 2 mg estradiol in lowering FSH levels in postmenopausal women, 26% versus 34% with estradiol.[99] The estrogenic actions of tamoxifen include the stimulation of progesterone receptor synthesis, an estrogen like maintenance of bone, and estrogenic effects on the vaginal mucosa and the endometrium. Tamoxifen increases the frequency of hepatic carcinoma in rats at very large doses. This is consistent with its estrogenic, agonistic action, but this effect is unlikely to be a clinical problem (and it has not been observed) at doses currently used.[98] Tamoxifen causes a decrease in antithrombin III, and there has been a small increase in the incidence of thrombo-embolism observed in tamoxifen-treated patients compared with controls.[100, 101] However, in the world overview of randomized trials, no significant cardiac or vascular increase in mortality was noted in tamoxifen-treated women.[98]

All too often, the antagonistic, antiestrogenic action of tamoxifen is featured, and the estrogenic, agonistic action is ignored. In the 1980s, it was reported that human endometrial cancer transplanted into mice would grow more rapidly during tamoxifen therapy, although the growth of breast cancer cells would be inhibited. This growth in response to tamoxifen can be duplicated in laboratory culture preparations of endometrial cancer cells.

There now have been many reports of endometrial hyperplasia, endometrial polyps, and endometrial cancer occurring in women receiving tamoxifen treatment.[102, 103] In addition, tamoxifen has been associated with major flare-ups in endometriosis. Tamoxifen, therefore, has a variety of side effects that indicate both estrogenic activity and antiestrogenic activity. How can tamoxifen be both an estrogen agonist and an estrogen antagonist?

Tamoxifen Mechanism of Action

TAF-1 and TAF-2 areas can both activate transcription, but TAF-2 activates transcription only when it is bound by estrogen. The individual transactivating abilities of TAF-1 and TAF-2 depend on the promoter and cell context. Tamoxifen's agonistic ability is due to activation of TAF-1; its antagonistic activity is due to competitive inhibition of the estrogen-dependent activation of TAF-2.

An estrogen-associated protein binds to the right hand side of TAF-2. Estrogen binding induces binding of this protein, which then activates transcription. This protein recognizes only an activated conformation of the estrogen receptor, the result of estrogen binding. Tamoxifen binding to the TAF-2 area does not activate this domain because, in at least one explanation, the conformational change does not allow binding of the estrogen-associated protein, the activating factor.[65, 104]

The activity of TAF-2 is negligible in the presence of tamoxifen. In cells where TAF-1 and TAF-2 function independently of each other, tamoxifen would be chiefly an antagonist in cells where TAF-2 predominates, and an agonist where TAF-1 predominates, and in some cells a mixed activity is possible.[105]

The contact sites of estrogens and antiestrogens with the estrogen receptor are not identical.[106] When an antiestrogen binds to the estrogen receptor, the conformational changes that are induced alter the ability of the estrogen receptor-antiestrogen complex to modulate transcriptional activity. The relative agonist–antagonist activity is determined by the specific conformation achieved by the specific antiestrogen.

Even though tamoxifen can block estrogen-stimulated transcription of many genes, its degree of antagonistic activity varies among different animals, different cell types, and with different promoters within single cells. These differences are due to differences in the relative activities of the TAFs. Thus, the extent to which an antiestrogen inhibits an estrogen-mediated response depends on the degree to which that response is mediated by TAF-2 activity as opposed to TAF-1 activity, or mixed activity.[107] In some cell lines TAF-1 is dominant, in others, both are necessary. No cells have yet been identified where TAF-2 is dominant.

In most cell types, TAF-1 is too weak to activate transcription by itself, but, of course, there are now well-known exceptions: endometrium, bone, and liver. In these tissues, the promoter context is right. Tamoxifen is a significant activator of estrogen receptor-mediated induction of promoters that are regulated by the TAF-1 site. Antiestrogens have no effects on TAF-1 dependent transcription in breast cells.[108]

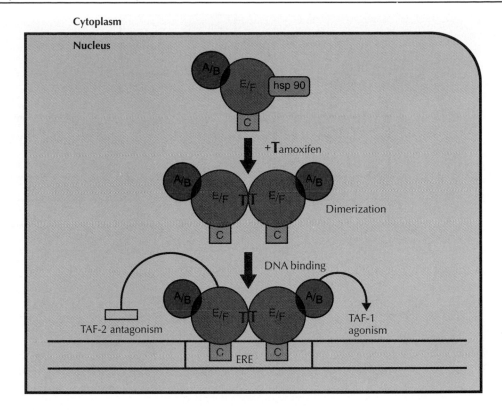

This explanation may not be the same for other mixed agonists and antagonists. Raloxifene may activate an estrogen-responsive gene through a response element separate from the estrogen response element, an action that requires specific activating peptides.[109] Estrogen metabolites also can interact with response elements other than the classical estrogen response element. The bottom line is that there are multiple pathways to gene activation. The estrogen receptor, depending on the ligand, can regulate more than one response element. Thus, estrogen and antiestrogen actions in various tissues can reflect the presence of different response elements.

Summary — The Response of Cells to Estrogens and Antiestrogens Depends on:

1. **The nature of the estrogen receptor.**

2. **The estrogen response elements and nearby promoters.**

3. **The cell context of protein coactivators and corepressors.**

4. **The properties of the ligand.**

5. **Modulation by growth factors and agents that affect protein kinases and phosphorylation.**

Tamoxifen Treatment of Breast Cancer

Tamoxifen treatment achieves its greatest effect (50% reduction in recurrent disease) in estrogen receptor-positive tumors, but it is also effective in estrogen receptor-negative tumors. Most importantly, it is now recognized that acquired resistance eventually develops. Therefore, there are two important questions. *Why is tamoxifen treatment effective with estrogen receptor-negative tumors? How does tamoxifen resistance develop?*

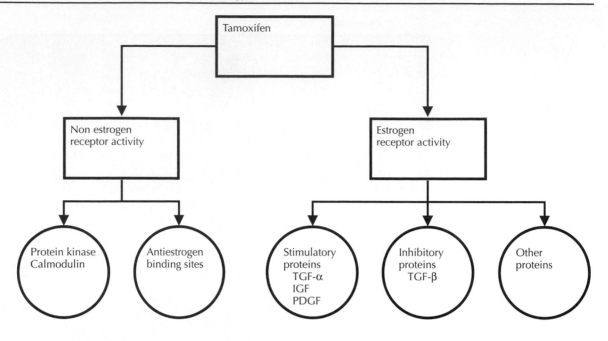

Efficacy of Tamoxifen With Estrogen Receptor-Negative Tumors. Besides binding to the estrogen receptor and providing competitive inhibition, tamoxifen has the following actions:

1. Tamoxifen and clomiphene inhibit protein kinase C activity (phosphorylation).

2. Tamoxifen inhibits calmodulin-dependent cyclic AMP phosphodiesterase, by binding to calmodulin.

3. Tamoxifen and estrogen have opposing effects on growth factors:[110, 111] Tamoxifen stimulates secretion of TGF-β in breast cancer cells as well as in fibroblasts and stromal cells, and TGF-β inhibits growth of breast cancer cells, whereas estrogen and insulin decrease the secretion of TGF-β in cancer cells. Tamoxifen decreases and estrogen increases IGF-I and IGF-II production in stromal fibroblasts.

Some of these actions (especially inhibition of protein kinase activity and stimulation of TGF-β production) occur independently of tamoxifen binding to the estrogen receptor, and thus, estrogen receptor-negative tumors can be affected by these actions.

Mechanisms for Tamoxifen Resistance. The results of randomized clinical trials have indicated that there is little reason to extend tamoxifen treatment of breast cancer patients beyond 5 years.[101, 112] Indeed, the data suggested that survival and recurrence rates worsened with longer therapy, probably due to the emergence of tamoxifen-resistant tumors. There are several possible explanations for resistance, and whichever of these are operative, it is believed that a subpopulation resistant to tamoxifen is present from the beginning, and over time grows to be clinically apparent.[113]

1. Loss of estrogen receptors

Generally it is believed that estrogen receptor expression is not a permanent phenotype of breast cancer cells; thus, tumors can change from receptor-positive to receptor-negative. But more than 50% of resistant tumors retain estrogen receptors.[114] The conventional wisdom has been that progression is associated with loss of cellular control and loss of estrogen receptor expression. However, the correlation between metastatic disease and estrogen receptor-negative state is not strong. Indeed, metastatic disease with estrogen receptor-positive cells despite an estrogen receptor-negative primary lesion has been reported. In addition, the rate of estrogen receptor expression is about the same in *in situ* disease and invasive disease. Most normal breast cells are estrogen receptor-negative, and in vitro, cell lines maintain their receptor status. Thus, there is little reason to believe that tamoxifen-resistant tumors lose receptor expression. *The importance of this is that resistance is not a wild, potentially uncontrollable dedifferentiation.*[115]

2. Variant and mutant estrogen receptors

Mutations in resistant breast tumors are infrequent and are unlikely to account for resistance.[116] Studies of breast tumors from tamoxifen-resistant patients indicate that most express wild type normal estrogen receptor; very few mutated estrogen receptors have been described.

3. Changes in coactivators

If a breast cancer cell were to begin expressing these factors in a fashion similar to endometrium or bone, then agonistic actions would occur.

4. Cross talk between signaling pathways

Because of the synergism between the estrogen receptor and protein kinase pathways, stimulation of protein kinase pathways can change an antagonist message to agonism. [117] This mechanism operates through the phosphorylation of the estrogen receptor or proteins involved in estrogen receptor-mediated transcription. Stimulation of this protein kinase phosphorylation activates the agonist activity of tamoxifen-like antiestrogens. Furthermore, the lack of response of pure antiestrogens to this phosphorylation may be part of the reason for the response of resistant tumors to pure antiestrogens.

5. Binding to other proteins

A remote possibility is the prevention of action by binding to other proteins, such as antiestrogen binding sites, microsomal proteins that bind to tamoxifen with high affinity but do not bind estrogen.[118]

6. Differential cellular transport

Overexpression of the transmembrane efflux pump that excretes compounds from cells could diminish the intracellular amount of tamoxifen present.

7. Differential metabolism

Changes in pharmacology and metabolism of tamoxifen might occur so that cells acquire the ability to metabolize the antagonist to greater agonist activity. Some breast cancer patients develop tumors that regress when tamoxifen is withdrawn. However, estrogenic metabolites of tamoxifen have been reported in only one study of patients with resistant tumors.[119]

The Pure Antiestrogens

The pure antiestrogens are derivatives of estradiol with long hydrophobic side chains at the 7 position. Binding with the pure antiestrogens prevents DNA binding. Because the site responsible for dimerization overlaps with the hormone-binding site, it is believed that pure antiestrogens sterically interfere with dimerization, and thus inhibit DNA binding. In addition, these compounds increase the cellular turnover of estrogen receptor, and this action contributes to its antiestrogen effectiveness. Estrogen and progesterone receptors exit the nucleus but are rapidly transported back. When this shuttling is impaired, receptors are more rapidly degraded in the cytoplasm. Agents that inhibit dimerization inhibit nuclear translocation and thus increase cytoplasmic degradation. The half-life of the estrogen receptor when occupied with estradiol is about 5 hours, when occupied with a pure antiestrogen, it is less than 1 hour. This mechanism may be due to interference with nuclear localization exerted by the hinge region. Thus, newly synthesized receptors cannot be efficiently transported into the nucleus and those in the nucleus will leak back into the cytoplasm.

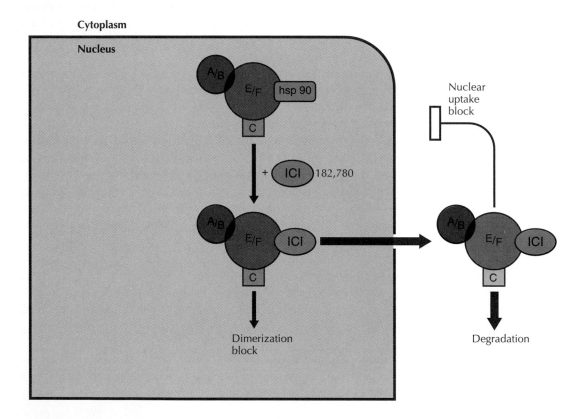

Another possible mechanism for pure antiestrogens involves a binding protein for the insulin-like growth factors. In a breast cancer cell line, ICI 182,780 inhibited growth and increased transcription of the IGFBP-3 gene. Estradiol did the opposite. In the uterus, tamoxifen and estrogen suppress IGFBP-3 production, while the ICI antagonist markedly increases IGFBP and causes uterine involution.[120]

Because these agents function in a different manner than tamoxifen, it is not surprising that tamoxifen-resistant tumors respond to these agents.[121]

Selective Estrogen Agonists/Antagonists (Selective Estrogen Receptor Modulators)

Agents such as raloxifene and droloxifene have antiestrogenic activity in the uterus as well as in the breast, and at the same time exert agonistic effects in certain target tissues.[122–124] Ralxoifene inhibits bone resorption and improves lipids (although there is no effect on HDL-cholesterol). By virtue of variations in conformational changes in the drug-receptor complex and the cellular context of specific tissues, drugs such as these can be developed to produce beneficial effects in certain target systems (such as bone) and to avoid unwanted actions (such as endometrial stimulation).

The Antiprogestin RU486

Both progesterone and the antiprogestins, RU486 (mifepristone) and ZK98299 (onapristone), form hormone-responsive element-receptor complexes that are similar, but the antiprogestin complex has a slightly different conformational change (in the hormone-binding domain) that prevents full gene activation.[125] RU486 has some agonistic activity due to its ability to activate certain, but not all, of the transcription activation functions on the progesterone receptor. New antiprogestins are in development that bind to the progesterone receptor and prevent the subsequent binding of the receptor to gene response elements.

The search for inhibitors of progesterone binding began many years ago, in the late 1960s, but it wasn't until the early 1980s that RU486, the first successful antiprogestin was produced by scientists at Roussel Uclaf, a pharmaceutical company in Paris. RU486 is a 19-nortestosterone derivative. The dimethyl (dimethylaminophenyl) side chain at carbon 11 is the principal factor in its antiprogesterone action. There are three major characteristics of its action which are important: a long half-life, high affinity for the progesterone receptor, and active metabolites.

The affinity of RU486 for the progesterone receptor is 5 times greater than that of the natural hormone. In the absence of progesterone, it can produce an agonistic (progesterone) effect. It does not bind to the estrogen receptor, but it can act as a weak antiandrogen because of its low-affinity binding to the androgen receptor. RU486 also binds to the glucocorticoid receptor, but higher doses are required to produce effects. The binding affinity of RU486 and its metabolites for the glucocorticoid receptor is very, very high. The reason why it takes such a high dose to produce an effect is because the circulating level of cortisol is so high, 1000-fold higher than progesterone. This allows titration of clinical effects by adjustments of dose.

Both progesterone and RU486 induce conformational changes with the progesterone receptor, especially in the hormone-binding domain.[126, 127] Thus, the antiprogestin not only competes with progesterone for the progesterone receptor, but after binding to the hormone-binding domain, the receptor structure is altered in such a way that the transcription activity of the B progesterone receptor is inhibited. In cells where the A progesterone receptor is expressed, antiprogestin binding stimulates A receptor-induced inhibition of transcription activity for all steroid hormone receptors (this would explain the antiestrogen activity of RU486).

RU486 is most noted for its abortifacient activity and the political controversy surrounding it. However, the combination of its agonistic and antagonistic actions can be exploited for many uses, including contraception, therapy of endometriosis, induction of labor, treatment of Cushing's syndrome, and, potentially, treatment of various cancers. Hopefully, new antiprogestins will be free of political and emotional constraints, and the many potential applications will be pursued.

Androgen Antagonists

The two most commonly used androgen antagonists are cyproterone acetate and spironolactone. Cyproterone and spironolactone bind to the androgen receptor and exert mixed agonism–antagonism. In the presence of significant levels of androgens, the antagonism predominates, and these agents are effective for the treatment of hirsutism. Flutamide is a nonsteroidal pure antiandrogen, effectively blocking androgenic action at target sites by competitive inhibition.

Mechanism of Action for Tropic Hormones

Tropic hormones include the releasing hormones originating in the hypothalamus and a variety of peptides and glycoproteins released by the anterior pituitary gland and placenta. The specificity of the tropic hormone depends on the presence of a receptor in the cell membrane of the target tissue. Tropic hormones do not enter the cell to stimulate physiologic events but unite with a receptor on the surface of the cell.

The receptor protein in the cell membrane can either act as the active agent and, after binding, operate as an ion channel or function as an enzyme. Alternatively, the receptor protein is coupled to an active agent, an intracellular messenger. The major intracellular messenger molecules are cyclic AMP, inositol 1,4,5-triphosphate (IP_3), 1,2-diacylglycerol (1,2-DG), calcium ion, and cyclic GMP.

Receptors from this membrane family are also found in the membranes of lysosomes, endoplasmic reticulum, Golgi complex, and in nuclei. The regulation of these intracellular organelle receptors differs from those of the cell surface membranes.

The Cyclic AMP Mechanism

Cyclic AMP is the intracellular messenger for FSH, LH, human chorionic gonadotropin (HCG), thyroid-stimulating hormone (TSH), and ACTH. Union of a tropic hormone with its cell membrane receptor activates the adenylate cyclase enzyme within the membrane wall leading to the conversion of adenosine 5'-triphosphate (ATP) within the cell to cyclic AMP. Specificity of action and/or intensity of stimulation can be altered by changes in the structure or concentration of the receptor at the cell wall binding site. In addition to changes in biologic activity due to target cell alterations, changes in the molecular structure of the tropic hormone can interfere with cellular binding and physiologic activity.

The cell's mechanism for sensing the low concentrations of circulating tropic hormone is to have an extremely large number of receptors but to require only a very small percentage (as little as 1%) to be occupied by the tropic hormone. The cyclic AMP released is specifically bound to a cytoplasm receptor protein, and this cyclic AMP-receptor protein complex activates a protein kinase. The protein kinase is present in an inactive form as a tetramer containing 2 regulatory subunits and 2 catalytic subunits. Binding of cyclic AMP to the regulatory units releases the catalytic units, with the regulatory units remaining as a dimer. The catalytic units catalyze the phosphorylation of serine and threonine residues of cellular proteins such as enzymes and mitochondrial, microsomal, and chromatin proteins. The physiologic event follows this cyclic AMP-mediated energy-producing event. Cyclic AMP is then degraded by the enzyme phosphodiesterase into the inactive compound, 5'-AMP.

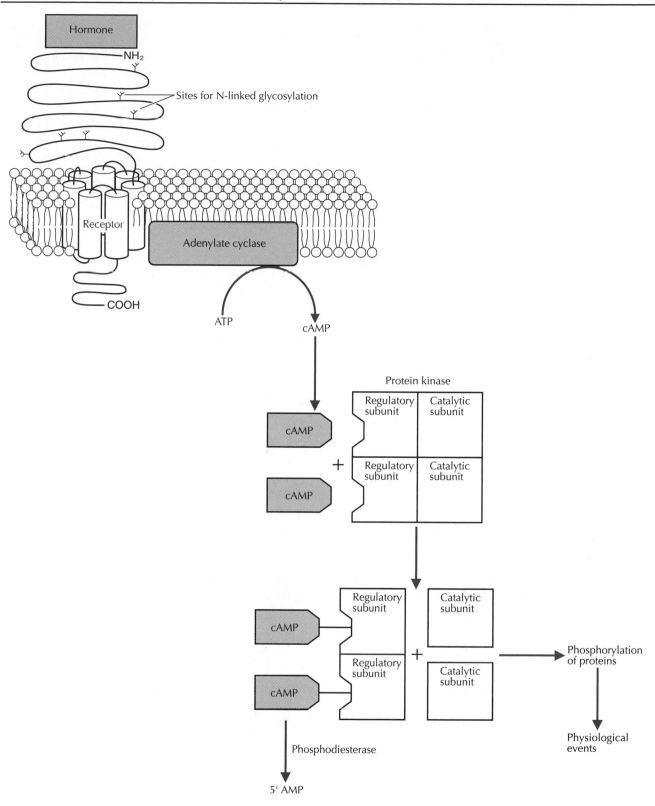

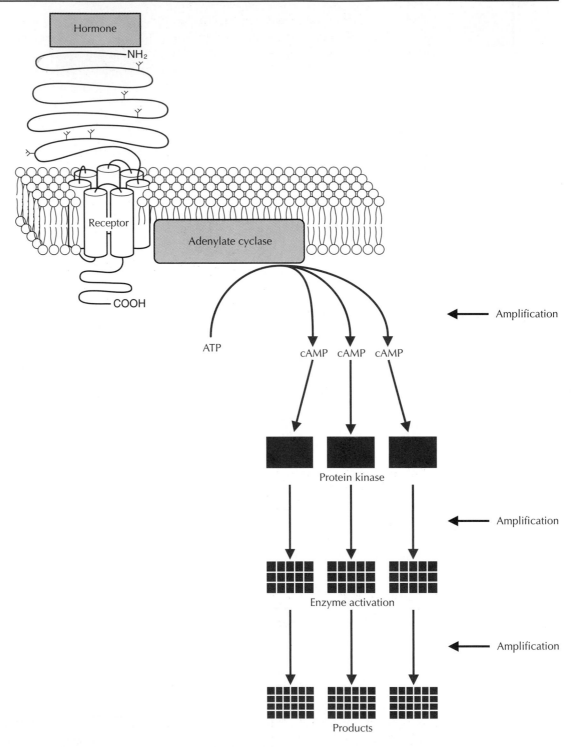

Most noteworthy, DNA contains responsive elements that bind proteins phosphorylated by the catalytic units, thus leading to activation of gene transcription. The ***cyclic AMP responsive element (CRE)*** functions as an enhancer element upstream from the start of transcription.[128] A large family of transcription factors interact with the CRE, creating an important regulatory unit for gene transcription. Cyclic AMP activates a specific transcription factor, cyclic AMP regulatory element-binding protein (CREB); the binding of CREB to CRE activates many genes. This system can also involve DNA sequences upstream from the CRE site.

Because LH can stimulate steroidogenesis without apparent changes in cyclic AMP (at low hormone concentrations), it is possible that an independent pathway exists; i.e., a mechanism independent of cyclic AMP. Mechanisms independent of cyclic AMP could include ion flow, calcium distribution, and changes in phospholipid metabolism.

The cyclic AMP system can be regarded as an example of evolutionary conservation. Rather than developing new regulatory systems, certain critical regulators have been preserved from bacteria to mammals. How is it that a single intracellular mediator can regulate different events? This is accomplished by turning on different biochemical events governed by the different gene expression in individual cells. In addition, the adenylate cyclase enzyme exists in several isoforms, which respond either with stimulation or inhibition to various systems and agents.[129]

The cyclic AMP system provides a method for amplification of the faint hormonal signal swimming in the sea of the bloodstream. Each cyclase molecule produces a lot of cyclic AMP; the protein kinases activate a large number of molecules that in turn lead to an even greater number of products. This is an important part of the sensitivity of the endocrine system. This is a major reason why only a small percentage of the cell membrane receptors need be occupied in order to generate a response.

Prostaglandins stimulate adenylate cyclase activity and cyclic AMP accumulation. Despite the effect on adenylate cyclase, prostaglandins appear to be synthesized after the action of cyclic AMP. This implies that tropic hormone stimulation of cyclic AMP occurs first; cyclic AMP then activates prostaglandin synthesis and, finally, intracellular prostaglandin moves to the cell wall to facilitate the response to the tropic hormone. In addition to actions mediated by cyclic AMP, prostaglandins can also operate through changes in intracellular concentrations of calcium.

Prostaglandins and cyclic GMP (cyclic guanosine 3'5'-monophosphate) may participate in an intracellular negative feedback mechanism governing the degree of, or direction of, cellular activity (e.g., the extent of steroidogenesis or shutting off of steroidogenesis after a peak of activity is reached). In other words, the level of cellular function may be determined by the interaction among prostaglandins, cyclic AMP, and cyclic GMP.

There are differences among the tropic hormones. Oxytocin, insulin, growth hormone, prolactin, and human placental lactogen (HPL) do not utilize the adenylate cyclase mechanism. Receptors for prolactin, growth hormone, and a number of cytokines (including erythropoietin and interleukins) belong to a single transmembrane domain receptor family.[130] Studies of this receptor family indicate that prolactin operates through various signal transduction mechanisms, including ion channels and nuclear kinase activation.

Gonadotropin releasing hormone (GnRH) is calcium dependent in its mechanism of action and utilizes IP_3 and 1,2-DG as second messengers to stimulate protein kinase activity.[131] These responses require a G protein and are associated with cyclical release of calcium ions from intracellular stores and the opening of cell membrane channels to allow entry of extracellular calcium.

The Calcium Messenger System

The intracellular calcium concentration is a regulator of both cyclic AMP and cyclic GMP levels.[132] Activation of the surface receptor either opens a channel in the cell membrane that lets calcium ions into the cell, or calcium is released from internal stores (the latter is especially the case in muscle). This calcium flux is an important intracellular mediator of response to hormones, functioning itself as a second messenger in the nervous system and in muscle.

The calcium messenger system is linked to hormone-receptor function by means of a specific enzyme, phospholipase C, that catalyzes the hydrolysis of polyphosphatidylinositols, specific phospholipids in the cell membrane. Activation of this enzyme by hormone binding to its receptor leads to the generation of 2 intracellular messengers, inositol triphosphate (IP_3) and diacyl glycerol (DAG), which initiate the function of the 2 parts of the calcium system. The first part is a calcium activated protein kinase responsible for sustained cellular responses, and the second part involves a regulator called calmodulin responsible for acute responses. These responses are secondary to alterations in enzyme activity and in transcription factors.

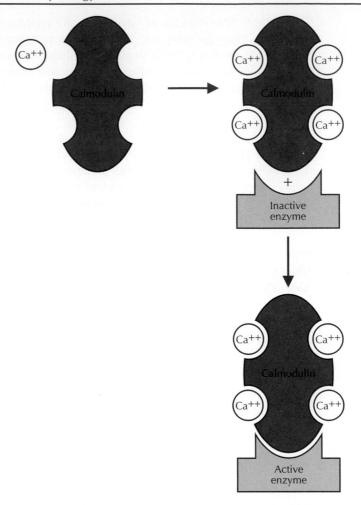

Calmodulin has been identified in all animal and plant cells that have been examined. Therefore, it is a very ancient protein. It is a single polypeptide chain of 148 amino acid residues whose sequence and structural and functional properties are similar to those of troponin C, the substance that binds calcium during muscle contractions, facilitating the interaction between actin and myosin. The calmodulin molecule has 4 calcium-binding sites, and binding with calcium gives a helical conformation which is necessary for biologic activity. A typical animal cell contains more than 10 million molecules of calmodulin, constituting about 1% of the total cell protein. As a calcium regulatory protein, it serves as an intracellular calcium receptor and modifies calcium transport, enzyme activity, the calcium regulation of cyclic nucleotide and glycogen metabolism, and such processes as secretion and cell motility. Thus, calmodulin serves a role analogous to that of troponin C, mediating calcium's actions in noncontractile tissues, and cyclic AMP works together with calcium and calmodulin in the regulation of intracellular metabolic activity.

Kinase Receptors

The cell membrane receptors of insulin, insulin-like growth factor, epidermal growth factor, platelet-derived growth factor, and fibroblast growth factor are tyrosine kinases. All tyrosine kinase receptors have a similar structure: an extracellular domain for ligand binding, a single transmembrane domain, and a cytoplasmic domain. The unique amino acid sequences determine a 3-dimensional conformation that provides ligand specificity. The transmembrane domains are not highly conserved (thus differing in make up). The cytoplasmic domains respond to ligand binding by undergoing conformational changes and autophosphorylation. The structure of the receptors for insulin and insulin-like growth factor is more complicated, with two alpha- and two beta-subunits, forming two transmembrane domains connected extracellularly by disulfide bridges. The receptors for the important autocrine and paracrine factors, activin and inhibin, function as serine-specific protein kinases.

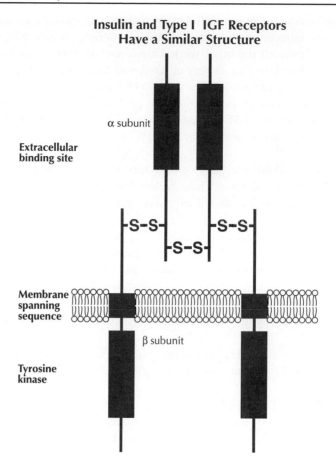

**Insulin and Type I IGF Receptors
Have a Similar Structure**

α subunit

**Extracellular
binding site**

-S-S-   -S-S-

-S-S-

**Membrane
spanning
sequence**

β subunit

**Tyrosine
kinase**

Kinase activation requires distinctive sequences; thus there is considerable homology among the kinase receptors in the cytoplasmic domain. Many of the substrates for these kinases are the enzymes and proteins in other messenger systems; e.g., the calcium messenger system. Thus, the kinase receptors can cross talk with other receptor regulated systems that involve the G proteins.

Regulation of Tropic Hormones

Modulation of the peptide hormone mechanism is an important biologic system for enhancing or reducing target tissue response. The regulation of tropic hormone action can be divided into 4 major components.

1.   Autocrine and paracrine regulation factors.

2.   Heterogeneity of the hormone.

3.   Up- and down-regulation of receptors.

4.   Regulation of adenylate cyclase.

Autocrine and Paracrine Regulation Factors

Growth factors are polypeptides that modulate activity either in the cells in which they are produced or in nearby cells; hence, they are autocrine and paracrine regulators. Regulation factors of this type (yet another biologic family) are produced by local gene expression and protein translation, and they operate by binding to cell membrane receptors. The receptors usually contain an intracellular component with tyrosine kinase activity that is energized by a binding-induced conformational change that induces autophosphorylation. However, some factors work through the other second messenger systems, such as cyclic AMP or IP_3. Growth factors are involved in a variety of tissue functions, including mitogenesis, tissue and cellular differentiation, chemotactic actions, and angiogenesis. The growth factors involved in reproductive physiology include activin, inhibin, insulin-like growth factor-I (IGF-I), insulin-like growth factor-II (IGF-II), transforming growth factor-β (TGF-β), fibroblast growth factor (FGF), and epidermal growth factor (EGF).

In addition to the growth factors, various immune factors, especially cytokines, modulate ovarian steroidogenesis. These factors, including interleukin-1, tumor necrosis factor, and interferon, are found in human follicular fluid and, in general, inhibit gonadotropin stimulation of steroidogenesis.

For mitogenesis to occur, cells may require exposure to a sequence of growth factors, with important limitations in duration and concentrations. Growth factors are important for the direction of embryonic and fetal growth and development. In cellular differentiation, growth factors can operate in a cooperative, competitive, or synergistic fashion with other hormones. For example, IGF-I plus FSH, but not IGF-I alone, increases the number of LH receptors, progesterone synthesis, and aromatase activity in granulosa cells.[133]

Activin and inhibin are disulfide-linked dimers composed of peptide subunits (one alpha subunit and two beta subunits) as follows:[134]

The 3 Forms of Activin:

Activin A:	$Beta_A$-$Beta_A$
Activin AB:	$Beta_A$-$Beta_B$
Activin B:	$Beta_B$-$Beta_B$

The 2 Forms of Inhibin:

Inhibin A:	Alpha-$Beta_A$
Inhibin B:	Alpha-$Beta_B$

Each of the subunits is encoded by separate genes that produce precursor proteins that are cleaved to form the subunits. In addition, the free subunits and related monomeric products can be secreted. Despite the structural similarity between activin and inhibin, they function as antagonists in some systems (e.g., activin stimulates and inhibin inhibits FSH secretion). Activins, inhibins, and TGF-β come from the same gene family, which also includes antimüllerian hormone, and proteins active during insect and frog embryogenesis. The activity of activin is regulated by protein binding, specifically to follistatin. Follistatin is a single-chain glycosylated peptide, structurally unrelated to inhibin and activin, that regulates the activin-inhibin system. Signaling by this family of peptides is accomplished by several receptor isoforms that are transmembrane serine kinases.

TGF-β can either stimulate or inhibit growth and differentiation, depending on the target cell and the presence or absence of other growth factors. In the ovary, TGF-β promotes granulosa cell differentiation by enhancing the actions of FSH (especially in expression of FSH and LH receptors) and antagonizing the down-regulation of FSH receptors. TGF-β and the insulin-like growth factors are required for the maintenance of normal bone mass. EGF is a structural analog of TGF-α and is involved in mitogenesis. In the ovary, EGF, secreted by theca cells, is important for granulosa cell proliferation, an action opposed by TGF-β that is also secreted by the theca cells. The most potent mitogens are the two forms of FGF. Additional roles for FGF, secreted by the granulosa, include modulation of enzyme activity involved in the physical act of ovulation and angiogenic function during the development of the corpus luteum.

The Insulin-Like Growth Factors

The insulin-like growth factors (also called somatomedins) are single-chain polypeptides that resemble insulin in structure and function.[133] These factors are widespread and are involved in growth and differentiation in response to growth hormone, and as local regulators of cell metabolism. IGF-II is more prominent during embryogenesis, while IGF-I is more active postnatally. Only the liver produces more IGF-I than the ovary. According to animal studies, both IGF-I and IGF-II are secreted by granulosa cells. IGF-I amplifies the action of gonadotropins and coordinates the functions of theca and granulosa cells. IGF-I receptors on the granulosa are increased by FSH and LH and augmented by estrogen. In the theca, IGF-I increases steroidogenesis. In the granulosa, IGF-I is important for the formation and increase in numbers of FSH and LH receptors, steroidogenesis, the secretion of inhibin, and oocyte maturation. It should be noted that the endogenous insulin-like growth factor in the human ovarian follicle is IGF-II in both the granulosa and the thecal cells.[19] Studies indicating activity of IGF-I with human ovarian tissue can be explained by the fact that both IGF-I and IGF-II activities can be mediated by the type I IGF receptor that is structurally similar to the insulin receptor.

Granulosa cells also contain receptors for insulin, and insulin can bind to the IGF-I receptor. The IGF-I receptor is a heterotetramer with two alpha- and two beta-subunits in a structure similar to that of the insulin receptor. Insulin can bind to the alpha-subunit ligand-binding domain and activate the beta-subunit, which is a protein kinase. Thus, insulin can modulate ovarian cellular functions either through its own receptor or through the IGF-I receptor.

The biologic potency and availability of the insulin-like growth factors are further modulated by a collection of IGF-binding proteins that bind circulating insulin-like growth factors and also alter cellular responsiveness. Six insulin-like growth factor binding proteins (IGFBP-1 through IGFBP-6) have been detected in serum and various tissues.[135] IGF-I and IGF-II circulate in the blood in a concentration 1000 times greater than insulin; however, largely all of the circulating IGFs are bound to IGFBPs. The multiple IGFBPs and their proteases provide a mechanism for tissue-specific activities of IGFs. The various IGFBPs differ in their actions and individual expression, depending upon the specific cell type and tissue. The principal IGFBP that regulates IGF biologic availability can vary according to metabolic changes. There are many possible permutations because the IGFBPs are not simply transport proteins; there are inhibitory and stimulatory IGFBPs that inhibit or potentiate IGF actions. Tissue-specific regulation of IGFBP protease activity can change the bioavailability of IGFs at specific sites. In addition, the IGFBPs have been demonstrated to have direct effects of their own, independent of IGF. Therefore, this is a complex regulatory system that provides both endocrine signals and autocrine and paracrine functions.

Orphan Receptors Involved in Steroidogenesis

Steroidogenic factor-1 (SF-1) and DAX-1 (a name that represents: **D**osage-sensitive sex reversal-**A**drenal hypoplasia congenita critical region on the **X** chromosome) are nuclear receptors for which specific ligands have not been identified ("orphan receptors"). SF-1 influences the expression of genes that encode steroidogenic enzymes, and when genetic expression of SF-1 is disrupted in mice, gonads and adrenal glands fail to develop.[136, 137] In addition, SF-1 regulates transcription of the StAR gene.[138] Mutations in the DAX-1 gene result in adrenal hypoplasia, and DAX-1 is believed to work with SF-1 in regulating development and function of steroid-producing tissues.[139] SF-1 also regulates genes that encode the gonadotropin subunits, as well as the GnRH receptor.[137] Thus, SF-1 is involved at all levels: the hypothalamus, the pituitary, and in the steroid-producing organs. These proteins function as transcription factors (as are the traditional nuclear hormone receptors such as the estrogen receptor) in the complex mechanisms being unraveled by molecular biologists.

Heterogeneity

The glycoproteins, such as FSH and LH, are not single proteins but should be viewed as a family of heterogeneous forms of varying immunologic and biologic activity.[140] The various forms (isoforms) arise in various ways, including different DNA promoter actions, alterations in RNA splicing, point mutations, and post-translational carbohydrate changes.[141] The impact of the variations is to alter structure and metabolic clearance, thus affecting binding and activity. The isoforms have different molecular weights, circulating half-lives, and biologic activities. Throughout the menstrual cycle, the amazing number of at least 20–30 isoforms of both FSH and LH are present in the bloodstream.[142] *The overall activity of a glycoprotein, therefore, is due to the effects of the mixture of forms that reach and bind to the target tissue.*

The nonglycosylated subunit precursors of glycoprotein hormones are synthesized in the endoplasmic reticulum, followed by glycosylation. The glycosylated subunits combine and then are transported to the Golgi apparatus for further processing of the carbohydrate component. The units combine to form a compact heterodimer. The protein moiety binds to specific target tissue receptors, while the carbohydrate moiety plays a critical role in coupling the hormone-receptor complex to adenylate cyclase (perhaps by determining the necessary conformational structure).

The preciseness of the chemical make up of the tropic hormones is an essential element in determining the ability of the hormone to mate with its receptor. The glycopeptides (FSH, LH, TSH, and HCG) are dimers composed of two glycosylated polypeptide subunits, the α- and β-subunits. The α- and β-subunits are tightly bound in a noncovalent association. The three-dimensional structure and the active conformation of the subunits are maintained by internal disulfide bonds.[143] All of the glycopeptides of the human species (FSH, LH, TSH, and HCG) share a common α-chain, an identical structure containing 92 amino acids. The β-chains (or the β-subunits) differ in both amino acid and carbohydrate content, conferring the specificity inherent in the relationship between hormones and their receptors. Therefore, the specific biologic activity of a glycopeptide hormone is determined by the β-subunit; hypogonadism has been reported due to single amino acid substitution in the LH β-subunit.[144]

β-HCG is the largest β-subunit, containing a larger carbohydrate moiety and 145 amino acid residues, including a unique carboxyl-terminal tail piece of 24 amino acid groups. It is this unique part of the HCG structure that allows the production of highly specific antibodies and the utilization of highly specific immunologic assays. The extended sequence in the carboxy-terminal region of β-HCG contains 4 sites for glycosylation, the reason why HCG is glycosylated to a greater extent than LH, a difference that is responsible for the longer circulating half-life for HCG.

These differences in structure are associated with a different promoter and transcriptional site that is located upstream in the HCG β-subunit gene compared with the site in the LH β-subunit gene. The HCG β-subunit site does not contain a hormone response element, allowing HCG secretion to escape feedback regulation by the sex steroids, in contrast to FSH and LH.

The rate-limiting step in the synthesis of gonadotropins and TSH is the availability of β-subunits, because excess α-units can be found in blood and in tissue. Furthermore, the three dimensional structure of the β-subunit, accomplished by folding the subunit by the formation of the disulfide bonds, is an important conformational step that is essential for assembly with the α-subunit.[145] This conformational change is not completed until the subunits are fully united to produce the final whole hormone.

The half-life of α-HCG is 6–8 minutes, that of whole HCG from the placenta about 24 hours. All human tissues appear to make HCG as a whole molecule, but the placenta is different in having the ability to glycosylate the protein, thus reducing its rate of metabolism and giving it biologic activity through a long half-life. The carbohydrate components of the glycoproteins are composed of fructose, galactose, mannose, galactosamine, glucosamine, and sialic acid. Although the

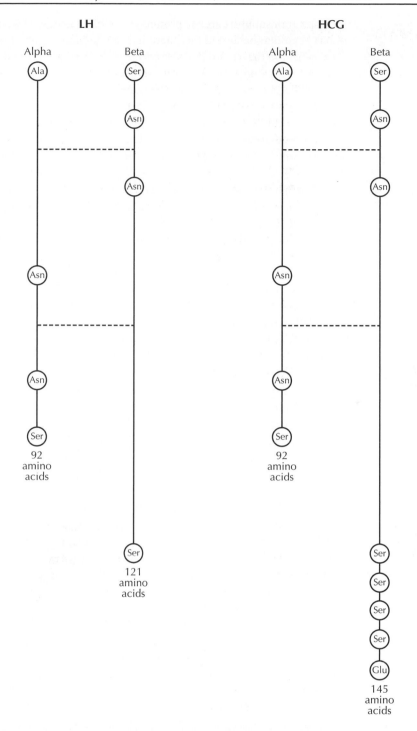

other sugars are necessary for hormonal function, sialic acid is the critical determinant of biologic half-life. Removal of sialic acid residues in HCG, FSH, and LH leads to very rapid elimination from the circulation.

FSH consists of the α-subunit of 92 amino acids and a β-subunit of 118 amino acids. It has four carbohydrate side chains, two on each subunit. The β-subunit of LH consists of 121 amino acids. LH has 3 carbohydrate side chains with a single glycosylation site (with less than half of the sialic acid in FSH). The initial half-life of LH is approximately 20 minutes, compared with the initial half-life of FSH of 3–4 hours.

Genes for tropic hormones contain promoter and enhancer or inhibitor regions located in the 5'-flanking regions upstream from the transcription site. These sites respond to second messengers (cyclic AMP) as well as steroids and other yet unknown regulators. The protein cores of the two glycoprotein subunits are the products of distinct genes.[146] Using recombinant DNA technology, it has been demonstrated that there is a single human gene for the expression of the α-subunit. The gene for the α-subunit shared by FSH, LH, HCG, and TSH is located on chromosome 6p21.1–23. A single promoter site subject to multiple signals and hormones regulates transcription of the α-gene in both placenta and pituitary. The α-subunit gene is expressed in several different cell types, but the β-subunit genes are restricted in cell type. The TSH β-gene is expressed only in thyrotropes regulated by thyroid hormone; the FSH β-gene is expressed in gonadotropes regulated by GnRH, activin, inhibin and gonadal steroids; the LH β-gene, also expressed in gonadotropes, is regulated by GnRH and unaffected by activin and inhibin.[147]

The α-subunit gene requires the activation of distinct regulatory elements in thyrotrope and gonadotrope cells, as well as in the placenta. It is the activation of these cell-specific elements that produces tissue specificity for α-gene expression. In gonadotropes, the GnRH signaling pathway for α-gene transcription utilizes phosphorylase stimulation of diacyl glycerol (DAG) and inositol triphosphate (IP_3) that leads to a release of intracellular calcium stores. GnRH also stimulates the influx of calcium at the cell membrane. DAG, IP_3, and calcium work together to stimulate protein kinase C activity. Protein kinase regulation of the α promoter is a principal part of the overall mechanism. This pituitary process is influenced by multiple factors, including growth factors and gonadal steroids. In the placenta, the mechanism also utilizes specific regulatory elements, but the primary signal is mediated by the cyclic AMP-protein kinase A pathway.

The gene for the FSH β-subunit is on chromosome 11p13, and in the pituitary, it is markedly influenced by activin.[148] Although FSH and LH both require GnRH stimulation, the FSH β-gene is unique in that response to GnRH is dependent on activin.[149] With increasing GnRH stimulation, the role of activin is increasingly repressed by its binding protein, follistatin, the secretion of which is also stimulated by GnRH and activin. Activin is further antagonized by inhibin, the first of these factors recognized to suppress FSH secretion.[150]

The genes that encode for the β-subunits of LH, HCG, and TSH are located in a cluster on chromosome 19q13.3. There are 6 genes for the β-subunit of HCG, and only one for β-LH.[151] Transcription for the 6 HCG genes, each with different promoter activity, varies, and it is not certain why HCG requires multigenic expression (perhaps this is necessary to reach the extremely high level of production in early pregnancy). It is thought that β-HCG evolved relatively recently from β-LH, and the unique amino acid terminal extension of β-HCG arose by a read through mutation of the translation stop codon in the β-LH gene; the DNA sequences of the β-HCG genes and the β-LH gene are 96% identical.[151] Only primates and horses have been demonstrated to have genes for the β-subunit of chorionic gonadotropin. In contrast to human chorionic gonadotropin, equine chorionic gonadotropin exerts both LH and FSH activities in many mammalian species because it contains peptide sequences in its β-subunit that are homologous to those in the pituitary gonadotropins of other species. The equine β-chorionic gonadotropin gene is identical to the equine β-LH gene, and although the primate β-HCG gene evolved from the same ancestral β-LH gene, the horse chorionic gonadotropin gene evolved in a different way. The β-LH gene is not expressed in the placenta.

A specific immunological LH variant is relatively common. This variant is due to two point mutations in the LH β-subunit gene and is more common in people of northern European descent, reaching a carrier frequency of 41.9% in Lapps of northern Finland.[152]. The clinical significance of this mutation is not known; however, routine immunoassays can provide falsely low readings because this variant is not detected.

The placenta-specific expression of β-HCG is due to several differences in DNA sequences between the β-HCG and β-LH genes.[147] The cyclic AMP-mediated enhancement of the β-HCG promoter is influenced by several regulatory proteins. The study of the β-subunit genes has been hampered by difficulties in maintaining glycoprotein-producing cell lines. The availability of choriocarcinoma cell lines, however, has allowed greater investigation of the β-HCG genes.

Although the β-subunit specifies the biologic activity of an individual glycoprotein, the combination of the α- and β-subunits is necessary for full hormonal expression. Furthermore, the α-subunit also plays an important role in accomplishing normal receptor binding and activation.[153, 154] Neither subunit alone can effectively bind to the receptor with high affinity or exert biologic effect. In other words, binding and activation occur only when the hormone is in the combined α-β form.

Variations in Carbohydrate

The glycopeptide hormones can be found in the pituitary existing in a variety of forms, differing in their carbohydrate (oligosaccharides) make up. The isoform mixture of gonadotropins is influenced both quantitatively and qualitatively by GnRH and the feedback of the steroid hormones, producing post translational carbohydrate modifications.[155, 156] This heterogeneity in structure (which is also associated with heterogeneity in charge) represents a mechanism under endocrine control that modulates half-lives and bioactivity.

Certain clinical conditions may be associated with alterations in the usual chemical structure of the glycopeptides, resulting in an interference with the ability to bind to receptors and stimulate biological activity. In addition to deglycosylation and the formation of antihormones, gonadotropins can be produced with an increased carbohydrate content. A low-estrogen environment in the pituitary gland, for example, favors the production of so-called big gonadotropins, gonadotropins with an increased carbohydrate component and, as a result, decreased biological activity.[157] Immunoassay in these situations may not reveal the biologic situation; an immunoassay sees only a certain set of molecules but not all. Therefore, immunologic results do not always indicate the biologic situation.

Bioactive levels of FSH and LH are very low in women receiving oral contraceptives and during the luteal and late follicular phases. The highest values are during the midcycle surge and in postmenopausal women (including women with premature ovarian failure).[158] The levels of bioactive FSH parallel those of immunoactive FSH with a constant ratio throughout the cycle. The greater bioactivity of FSH at midcycle is associated with less sialyated, shorter-lived isoforms. These changes are effects of both GnRH and estrogen.

The carbohydrate component, therefore, affects target tissue response in two ways: 1) metabolic clearance and half-life and 2) biologic activity. The latter action focuses on two functions for the hormone-receptor complex: binding and activation. One structural domain is important for binding and another for triggering the biologic response. Carbohydrate residues, especially the sialic acid residues, are less important in binding. Indeed, experimental data indicate that the carbohydrate chains have no role in the binding of gonadotropins to their receptors.[159] Nevertheless, removal of the carbohydrate moiety of either subunit diminishes gonadotropic activity. Therefore, the carbohydrate component affects the biologic activity of the hormone-receptor complex after binding. Specific studies indicate that the carbohydrate component plays a critical role in activation (coupling) of the adenylate cyclase system.[160]

The circulating half-life of a gonadotropin is mainly proportional to the amount of sialic acid present.[161] The higher content of sialic acid in FSH compared with LH accounts for the more rapid clearance of LH from the circulation (FSH half-life is several hours; LH half-life is about 20 minutes). HCG is highly sialylated, and accordingly, has a half-life of many hours. However, clearance of gonadotropins as measured by half-lives is not explained totally by carbohydrate differences. Differences in amino acid sequences also contribute, and most importantly, the stability of the complete hormone (resisting dissociation into the rapidly cleared subunits) is a major factor.

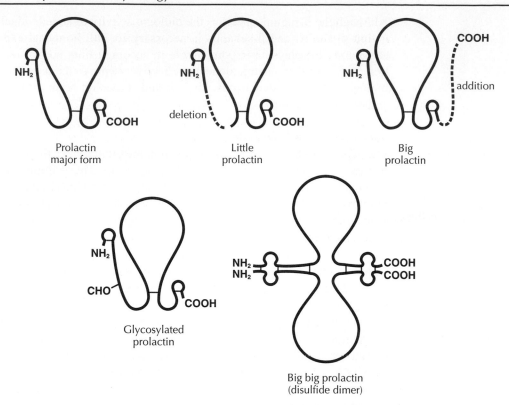

Heterogeneity of Prolactin

In most mammalian species, prolactin is a single-chain polypeptide of 199 amino acids, 40% similar in structure to growth hormone and placental lactogen.[162] All three hormones are believed to have originated in a common ancestral protein about 400 million years ago. Many hormones, growth factors, and neurotransmitters affect the prolactin gene.

Simultaneous measurements of prolactin by both bioassay and immunoassay reveal discrepancies. At first, differences in prolactin were observed based on size, leading to the use of terms such as little, big, and the wonderfully sophisticated term, big big prolactin. Further chemical studies have revealed structural modifications that include glycosylation, phosphorylation, and variations in binding and charge. This heterogeneity is the result of many influences at many levels: transcription, translation, and peripheral metabolism.[163, 164]

Prolactin is encoded by a single gene on chromosome 6, producing a molecule that in its major form is maintained in 3 loops by disulfide bonds.[162] Most, if not all, variants of prolactin are the result of posttranslational modifications. Little prolactin probably represents a splicing variant resulting from the proteolytic deletion of amino acids. Big prolactin can result from the failure to remove introns; it has little biologic activity and does not cross-react with antibodies to the major form of prolactin. The so-called big big variants of prolactin are due to separate molecules of prolactin binding to each other, either noncovalently or by interchain disulfide bonding. Some of the apparently larger forms of prolactin are prolactin molecules complexed to binding proteins.

Other variations exist. Enzymatic cleavage of the prolactin molecule yields fragments that may be capable of biologic activity. Prolactin that has been glycosylated continues to exert activity; differences in the carbohydrate moities can produce differences in biologic activity and immunoreactivity. However, the nonglycosylated form of prolactin is the predominant form of prolactin secreted into the circulation.[165] Modification of prolactin also includes phosphorylation, deamidation, and sulfation.

The prolactin receptor is encoded by a gene on chromosome 5 that is near the gene for the growth hormone receptor. However, there is evidence for more than one receptor, depending upon the site of action (e.g., decidua and placenta).[166] The prolactin receptor belongs to the receptor family that includes many cytokines and some growth factors, supporting a dual role for prolactin as a classic hormone and as a cytokine. The prolactin signal is mediated through a cytoplasmic tyrosine kinase pathway.

At any one point of time, the bioactivity (e.g., galactorrhea) and the immunoactivity (circulating level by immunoassay) of prolactin represent the cumulative effect of the family of structural variants. Remember, immunoassays do not always reflect the biologic situation (e.g., a normal prolactin level in a women with galactorrhea).

Up- and Down-Regulation

Positive or negative modulation of receptors by homologous hormones is known as up- and down-regulation. Little is known regarding the mechanism of up-regulation; however, hormones such as prolactin and GnRH can increase the cell membrane concentrations of their own receptors.

Theoretically, deactivation of the hormone-receptor complex could be accomplished by dissociation of the complex or loss of receptors from the cell, either by shedding (externally) or by internalization of the receptors into the cell. It is the process of ***internalization*** which is the major biologic mechanism by which polypeptide hormones down-regulate their own receptors and thus limit hormonal activity. As a general rule, an excess concentration of a tropic hormone, such as LH or GnRH, will stimulate the process of internalization, leading to a loss of receptors in the cell membrane and a decrease in biological response. We now understand that the principal reason for the episodic (pulsatile) secretion of hormones is to avoid down-regulation and to maintain, if not up-regulate, its receptors. The pulse frequency is a key factor, therefore, in regulating receptor number; however, further effects on target tissue response also occur at sites distal to receptors.[167]

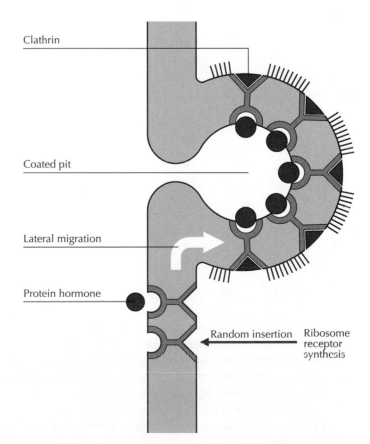

Clathrin

Coated pit

Lateral migration

Protein hormone

Random insertion   Ribosome receptor synthesis

It is believed that receptors are randomly inserted into the cell membrane after intracellular synthesis. The receptor may be viewed as having 3 important segments, an external binding site that is specific for a polypeptide hormone, the transmembrane region, and an internal site that plays a role in the process of internalization. When the receptor is bound to a polypeptide hormone and when high concentrations of the hormone are present in the circulation, the hormone-receptor complex moves through the cell membrane in a process called lateral migration. Lateral migration carries the complex to a specialized region of the cell membrane, *the coated pit.* Each cell in target tissues contains from 500 to 1500 coated pits. Lateral migration, thus, concentrates hormone-receptor complexes in the coated pit (*clustering*), allowing increased internalization of the complex via the special mechanism of receptor-mediated endocytosis.[168] The time course for this process (minutes rather than seconds) is too slow to explain the immediate hormone-induced responses, but other cellular events may be mediated by this mechanism that circumvents the intracellular messenger, cyclic AMP.

The coated pit is a lipid vesicle hanging on a basket of specific proteins, called *clathrins* (from the Latin "clathra" meaning "lattice"). The unit is a network of hexagons and pentagons, thus looking like a soccer ball. The internal margin of the pit has a brush border, hence the name coated pit. The clathrin protein network serves to localize the hormone-receptor complexes by binding to the internal binding site on the receptor.

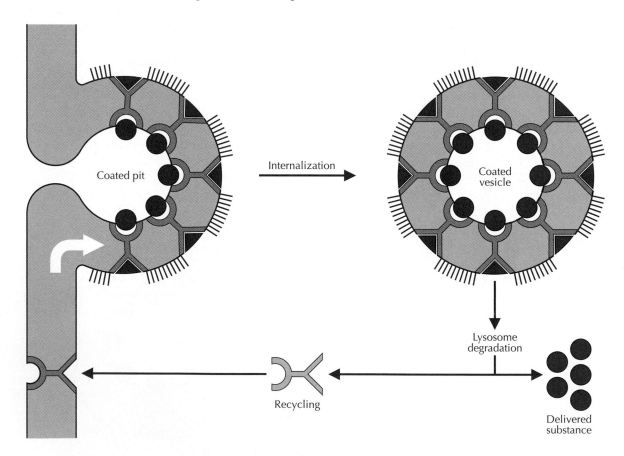

When fully occupied, the coated pit invaginates, pinches off, and enters the cell as a coated vesicle also called a receptosome. The coated vesicle is delivered to the lysosomes in which the structure then undergoes degradation, releasing the substance (e.g., a polypeptide hormone) and the receptor. The receptor may be recycled; i.e., it may be reinserted into the cell membrane and used again. On the other hand, the receptor and the hormone may be metabolized, thus decreasing that hormone's biologic activity. The internalized hormones may also mediate biologic response by influencing cellular organelles such as the Golgi apparatus, the endoplasmic reticulum, and even the nucleus. For example, nuclear membranes from human ovaries bind HCG and LH and there follows an enzyme response that is involved in the transfer of mRNA from nucleus to the cytoplasm.[169]

A similar process, called ***potocytosis***, utilizes cholesterol-rich membrane invaginations called ***caveolae*** (far fewer in number and smaller in structure than the clathrin coated pits) for the internalization of small molecules and ions.[170] This is another method of intracellular signaling in response to hormones, and many proteins involved in cell signaling have been detected in caveolae; e.g., G proteins, kinases, and growth factor receptors. Caveolin is the major protein structural component of caveolae. Nitric oxide, the important mediator of vascular events, resides in caveolae and is regulated by tyrosine phosphorylation and interaction with caveolin.[171, 172] Caveolae also facilitate endocytosis and exocytosis of substances, by the recycling of caveolin between the cell surface and the Golgi network.[173]

Besides down-regulation of polypeptide hormone receptors, the process of internalization can be utilized for other cellular metabolic events, including the transfer into the cell of vital substances such as iron or vitamins.

Cell membrane receptors can be randomly distributed in the cell membrane and transmit information to modify cell behavior.[174] For these receptors, internalization is a method for down-regulation by degradation in lysosomes. Because of this degradation, recycling is usually not a feature of this class of receptors. Hormones that utilize this category of receptors include FSH, LH, HCG, GnRH, TSH, TRH, and insulin. For these hormones, the coated pit can be viewed as a trap to immobilize hormone-receptor complexes. The fate of the hormone, however, can vary from tissue to tissue. In some target tissues, HCG is internalized and the HCG-receptor complex is transferred intact from the coated vesicle into the lysosomes for dissociation and degradation. In other tissues, especially the placenta, it is thought that the HCG-receptor complex is recycled back to the cell surface as a means of transporting HCG across the placenta into both maternal and fetal circulations.[175]

Cell membrane receptors, located in the coated pits, when bound to ligands lead to internalization, thus providing the cell with required factors, the removal of noxious agents from the biologic fluid bathing the cell, or the transfer of substances through the cell (transendocytosis). These receptors are spared from degradation and can be recycled. Examples of this category include low-density lipoproteins (LDL), which supply cholesterol to steroid-producing cells, cobalamin and transferrin, which supply vitamin B_{12} and iron, respectively, and the transfer of immunoglobulins across the placenta to provide fetal immunity.

A closer look at LDL and its receptor is informative. The low-density lipoprotein particle is a sphere. It contains in its center about 1500 molecules of cholesterol which are attached as esters to fatty acids. This core is contained by a bilayer lipid membrane. Protein-binding proteins (the apoproteins) project on the surface of this membrane, and it is these proteins that the receptor must recognize.

Remember, this is an important story, because all cells that produce steroids must use cholesterol as the basic building block. Such cells cannot synthesize enough cholesterol and, therefore, must bring cholesterol into the cell from the bloodstream. LDL is the principal messenger delivering the cholesterol. Experimental evidence, however, indicates that HDL-cholesterol as well as LDL can provide cholesterol to steroid-producing cells.[176] Indeed, human ovarian granulosa cells use HDL-cholesterol in a system that differs from the LDL-cholesterol pathway: the lipoproteins are not internalized, but rather, the cholesteryl esters are extracted from the lipoproteins at the cell surface and then transferred into the cell.[177]

Different cell surface receptors and proteins contain similar structural parts.[178] For example, the receptor for LDL contains a region that is homologous to the precursor of epidermal growth factor and another region that is homologous to a component of complement. The LDL receptor is a "mosaic protein." There are regions of proteins derived from the exons of different gene families. This is an example of a protein that evolved as a new combination of pre-existing functional units of other proteins.

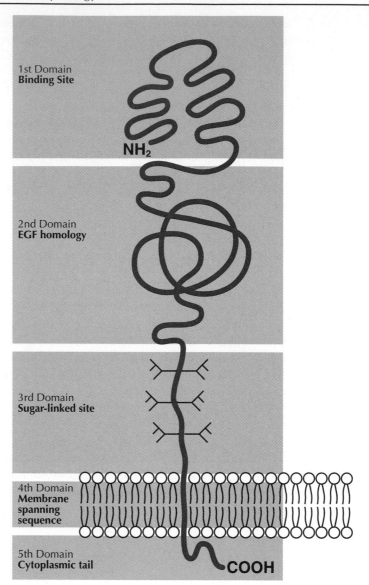

The LDL receptor is synthesized as a precursor of 860 amino acids. The precursor includes 21 amino acids that constitute a hydrophobic signal sequence that is cleaved prior to its insertion into the cell surface. This signal sequence presumably directs the protein where to go in the cell. This leaves an 839 amino acid protein that has 5 recognizable domains.

1. NH$_2$-terminal of 292 amino acids, composed of a sequence of 40 amino acids repeated with some variation 7 times. This domain is the binding site for LDL and is located on the external surface of the cell membrane.

2. Approximately 400 amino acids 35% homologous to epidermal growth factor precursor.

3. The sugar-linked site.

4. 22 Hydrophobic amino acids that cross the cell membrane. Deletion of the transmembrane signal sequence (found in a naturally occurring mutation) results in an LDL receptor that is secreted from the cell instead of being inserted into the membrane.

5. Cytoplasmic tail of 50 amino acids that is located internally and serves to cluster LDL receptors in coated pits.

When the coated pit is fully occupied with LDL, a coated vesicle is delivered into the cell in the process called endocytosis. The vesicle moves to the Golgi system and then is routed by an unknown mechanism (although a similar coated pit system in the Golgi appears to be involved) to the lysosomes in which the structure undergoes degradation, releasing cholesterol esters and the receptor. The receptor may be recycled or degraded. The intracellular level of free cholesterol influences the following important activities: the rate-limiting enzyme for cholesterol synthesis, the reesterification of excess cholesterol for storage as lipid droplets, and the synthesis of LDL receptors. The cholesterol derived from the LDL transport process can have any one of the following fates: utilization in the mitochondria for steroidogenesis, reesterification for storage, use in membrane structures, or excretion.[179] Excretion (release of free cholesterol into the circulation by means of the HDL mechanism) involves the cell surface caveolae.[170, 173] Thus, entry is via coated pits (endocytosis) and efflux from endoplasmic reticulum to the cell membrane is via caveolae (exocytosis).

Synthesis and insertion of new LDL receptors are a function of LH in the gonads and ACTH in the adrenal. This process is relatively fast. It has been calculated that the coated pit system turns over an amount of cell surface equivalent to the total amount of plasma membrane every 30–90 minutes.[179] The LDL receptor makes one round trip every 10 minutes during its 20-hour lifespan for a total of several hundred trips.[1] Genetic defects in receptors for LDL lead to a failure in internalization and hyperlipidemia.

Regulation of Adenylate Cyclase

The biologic activity of polypeptide or glycoprotein hormones (such as FSH or LH) can be altered by autocrine and paracrine regulators, the heterogeneity of the molecules, up- and down-regulation of the receptors, and, finally, by modulation of the activity of the enzyme, adenylate cyclase.

The G Protein System

The 1994 Nobel Prize in Medicine and Physiology was awarded to Alfred G. Gilman and Martin Rodbell for the discovery and description of G proteins. Adenylate cyclase is composed of 3 protein units: the receptor, a guanyl nucleotide regulatory unit, and a catalytic unit.[180] The regulatory unit is a coupling protein, regulated by guanine nucleotides (specifically GTP), and therefore it is called GTP binding protein or G protein for short.[181, 182] The catalytic unit is the enzyme itself which converts ATP to cyclic AMP. The receptor and the nucleotide regulatory unit are structurally linked, but inactive until the hormone binds to the receptor. Upon binding, the complex of hormone, receptor, and nucleotide regulatory unit is activated leading to an uptake of guanosine 5'-triphosphate (GTP) by the regulatory unit. The activation and uptake of GTP result in an active enzyme that can convert ATP to cyclic AMP. This result can be viewed as the outcome of the regulatory unit ***coupling*** with the catalytic unit, forming an intact complete enzyme. Enzyme activity is then terminated by hydrolysis of the GTP to guanosine 5'-diphosphate (GDP) returning the enzyme to its inactive state. Quick action and acute control of adenylate cyclase are assured because the G protein is a GTPase that self-activates upon binding of GTP.

The G protein has been purified. From the amino acid sequence, complementary DNA clones have been produced. These studies have indicated that a family of G proteins exists that couples receptors to active proteins, playing roles in signal transduction, intracellular transport, and exocytosis. The ability of the hormone-receptor complex to work through a common messenger (cyclic AMP) and produce contrasting actions (stimulation and inhibition) is thought to be due to the presence of both stimulatory nucleotide regulatory G proteins and inhibitory nucleotide regulatory G proteins.[183, 184] However, the G protein system is not limited to the cyclic AMP signal, but can activate other messenger-generating enzymes, as well as ion channels.

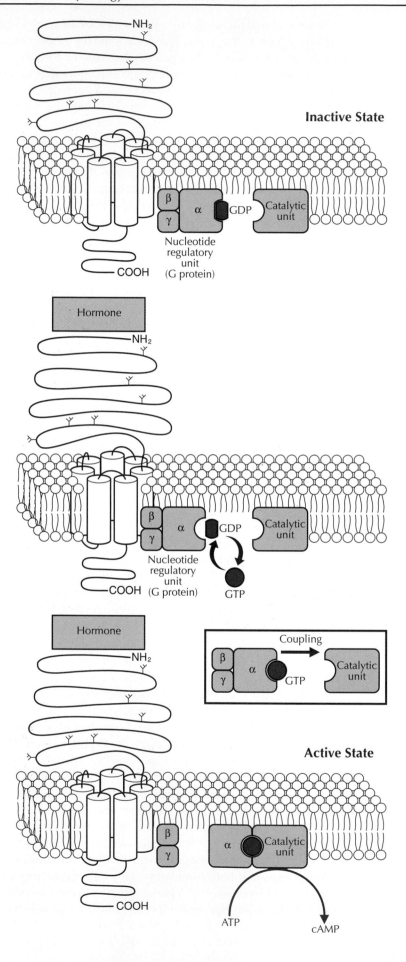

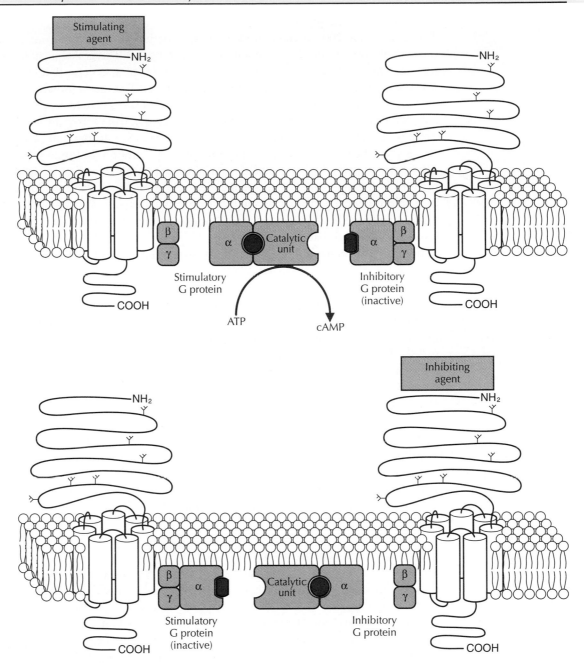

The G proteins are composed of α-, β-, and γ-subunits, each the product of many distinct genes.[185] The β- and γ-subunits are not all alike, and they exhibit selectivity for specific receptors. Each G protein has a unique α-subunit, and there are 16 mammalian α-subunit genes. Based on amino acid similarities, they are grouped into 4 subfamilies: $G_s\alpha$, $G_q\alpha$, $G_i\alpha$, G_{i2}. G_s and G_q proteins mediate stimulatory events such as hormone secretion, whereas G_i proteins exert inhibition. The role of the G_{i2} group is not yet certain. These multiple subunits allow great variability in function to be expressed by many different combinations.

In the inactive state GDP is bound to the α-subunit. Hormone-receptor interaction and binding change the α-subunit conformation. GTP replaces GDP on the α-subunit, freeing the β- and γ-subunits, which allows the GTP-α-subunit to bind to the catalytic unit of adenylate cyclase, forming the active enzyme. The GTP-α-subunit can also activate other messengers, such as ion channels. Intrinsic GTPase activity quickly hydrolyzes the GTP-α to GDP-α, which leads to reassociation with the β- and γ-subunits, reforming the G protein complex for further activation. The functional specificity is due to the α-subunit which differs for each G protein, and therefore there are many different α-subunits encoded by different genes.

The G protein Receptors

The more than 200 receptors linked to G proteins are derived from a supergene family, presumably originating from a common ancestral gene. The gonadotropin receptor contains a transmembrane region that has the structural features of a receptor that couples with G protein and a large extracellular domain.[186] Receptors that utilize the G proteins are inserted in membranes and consist of a long polypeptide chain that folds into 7 helixes, the amino acid loops that connect the helixes extend either into the cytoplasm or into the extracellular space. The amino end extends outside the cell, and the carboxyl end extends into the cell. The large extracellular segment is the site for specific gonadotropin recognition and binding. Binding changes the conformation (which is associated with phosphorylation), leading to interaction with the G proteins, which in turn activate second messengers, either enzymes or ion channels. These are ancient proteins; e.g., they are used by yeast to detect mating pheromones (perhaps this is why this protein is the basic structure for sight and smell in higher organisms; rhodopsin is a G protein located in the light-sensitive rod of the retina). Thus, the G receptors can be activated by hormones, neurotransmitters, growth factors, odorants, and photons of light.

LH and HCG bind to a common receptor, encoded by a gene on chromosome 2. The LH/HCG receptor is highly conserved in mammals; the human receptor is very similar to that of rat and bovine receptors.[187] It is likely that expression of the LH/HCG receptor is regulated by many factors, including endocrine, paracrine, and autocrine mechanisms, but the primary requirement is FSH. In addition to the G protein pathway, activation of the LH/HCG receptor stimulates the calcium messenger system. Actually, two LH/HCG receptor genes have been isolated (Gene I and Gene II), Gene I from a lymphocyte library and Gene II from a human placental library.[188, 189] Gene II appears to be the major form expressed in the ovary.

The receptor for FSH is very similar to the LH/HCG receptor, but it is structurally distinct.[190, 191] Appropriately (for specificity), the extracellular segment contains the major sequence divergence. The FSH receptor gene is located on chromosome 2p21, near the LH/HCG receptor gene. The FSH receptor is also regulated by its hormone environment, especially by FSH and estradiol. Other members of this family include receptors for TSH, catecholamines, vasopressin, angiotensin II, and dopamine.

Mutations in the G protein System

Mutations that alter the structure and activity of G proteins can result in disease.[182, 192] Loss of function mutations of a G protein or a given receptor will result in hormone deficiency syndromes; e.g., the TSH receptor and hypothyroidism, the LH receptor and male pseudohermaphroditism, and pseudohypoparathyroidism due to a $G_s\alpha$ mutation. The McCune-Albright syndrome (sexual precocity, polyostotic fibrous dysplasia, café-au-lait skin pigmentation, and autonomous functioning of various endocrine glands) is due to unregulated activity (gain in function) of the adenylate cyclase system because of a mutation in the $G_s\alpha$ gene. $G_s\alpha$ protein mutations have also been found in adrenal and ovarian tumors, growth hormone-secreting pituitary adenomas, and thyroid adenomas. It is possible that alterations in the G protein system may ultimately explain abnormalities in endocrine-metabolic functions, as well as oncogenic mutations.[183, 184, 193]

Some Genetic Diseases Due to Specific G Protein System Mutations

Mutation	Disorder
Activating LH receptor	Precocious puberty in boys
Inactivating LH receptor	Male pseudohermaphroditism
Inactivating FSH receptor	Premature ovarian failure
$G_s\alpha$ (stimulatory)	McCune-Albright syndrome
$G_i\alpha$ (inhibitory)	Hypothyroidism
Rhodopsin	Retinitis pigmentosa
Vasopressin	Diabetes insipidus

Coupling and Uncoupling, Desensitization

Another way to explain stimulating and inhibiting actions at the adenylate cyclase level focuses on the mechanism of coupling. LH stimulates steroidogenesis in the corpus luteum and works through the coupling of stimulatory regulatory units to the catalytic units of adenylate cyclase. Prostaglandin $F_{2\alpha}$ is directly luteolytic, inhibiting luteal steroidogenesis through a mechanism that follows binding to specific receptors. This luteolytic action may be exerted via an inhibitory regulatory unit that leads to uncoupling with the catalytic unit, thus interfering with gonadotropin action.

Increasing concentrations of tropic hormones, such as gonadotropins, are directly associated with desensitization of adenylate cyclase independent of the internalization of receptors. Desensitization is a rapid, acute change without loss of receptors in contrast to the slower process of internalization and true receptor loss. The desensitization process after prolonged agonist exposure involves receptor phosphorylation (which uncouples the receptor from the G protein). The LH/HCG receptor, a member of the G protein family, undergoes desensitization/uncoupling in response to LH or HCG in a process that involves phosphorylation of the C-terminal cytoplasmic tail of the receptor.[194] Decreased gonadotropin secretion in the presence of prolonged continuous GnRH stimulation is a desensitization response that can occur followed by recovery within the time frame of a normal endogenous GnRH secretory pulse.[195]

Summary of Down-Regulation

Down-regulation is a decrease in response in the presence of continuous stimulation. It involves the following 3 mechanisms:

1. *Densensitization by autophosphorylation of the cytoplasmic segment of the receptor.*

2. *Loss of receptors by internalization, a relatively slow mechanism.*

3. *Uncoupling of the regulatory and catalytic subunits of the adenylate cyclase enzyme.*

References

1. **Brown MS, Goldstein JL,** A receptor-mediated pathway for cholesterol homeostasis, *Science* 232:34, 1986.

2. **Ryan KJ,** Biological aromatization of steroids, *J Biol Chem* 234:268, 1959.

3. **Ryan KJ, Smith OW,** Biogenesis of steroid hormones in the human ovary, *Recent Prog Hor Res* 21:367, 1965.

4. **Miller WL,** Mitochondrial specificity of the early steps in steroidogensis, *J Steroid Biochem Mol Biol* 55:607, 1995.

5. **Stocco DM, Clark BJ,** Regulation of the acute production of steroids in steroidogenic cells, *Endocr Rev* 17:221, 1996.

6. **Liscum L, Dahl NK,** Intracellular cholesterol transport, *J Lipid Res* 33:1239, 1992.

7. **Reaven E, Tsai L, Azhar S,** Cholesterol uptake by the 'selective' pathway of ovarian granulsoa cells: early intracellular events, *J Lipid Res* 36:1602, 1995.

8. **Clark BJ, Wells J, King SR, Stocco DM,** The purification, cloning, and expression of a novel LH-induced mitochondrial protein in MA-10 mouse Leydig tumor cells: characterization of the steroidogenic acute regulatory protein (StAR), *J Biol Chem* 269:28314, 1994.

9. **Clark BJ, Soo SC, Caron KM, Ikeda Y, Parker KL, Stocco DM,** Hormonal and developmental regulation of the steroidogenic acute regulatory (StAR) protein, *Mol Endocrinol* 9:1346, 1995.

10. **Lin D, Sugawara T, Strauss III JF, Clark BJ, Stocco DM, Saenger P, Rogol A, Miller WL,** Role of steroidogenic acute regulatory protein in adrenal and gonadal steroidogenesis, *Science* 267:1828, 1995.

11. **Tee M, Lin D, Sugaware T, Holt JA, Guiguen Y, Buckingham B, Strauss III JF, Miller WL,** T-A transversion 11 bp from a splice acceptor site in the human gene for steroidogenic acute regulatory protein causes congenital lipoid adrenal hyperplasia, *Hum Mol Genet* 4:2299, 1995.

12. **Bose H, Pescovitz OH, Miller WL,** Spontaneous feminization in a 46,XX female patient with congenital lipoid adrenal hyperplasia due to a homozygous frameshift mutation in the steroidogenic acute regulatory protein, *J Clin Endocrinol Metab* 82:1511, 1997.

13. **Sugawara T, Holt JA, Driscoll D, Strauss III JF, Lin D, Miller WL, Patterson D, Clancy KP, Hart IM, Clark BJ, Stocco DM,** Human steroidogenic acute regulatory protein: functional activity in COS-1 cells, tissue-specific expression, and mapping of the gene to 8p11.2 and a pseudogene to chromosome 13, *Proc Natl Acad Sci USA* 92:4778, 1995.

14. **Simpson ER, Mahendroo MS, Means GD, Kilgore MW, Hinshelwood MM, Graham-Lorence S, Amarneh B, Ito Y, Fisher CR, Michael MD, Mendelson CR, Bulun SE,** Aromatase cytochrome P450, the enzyme responsible for estrogen biosynthesis, *Endocr Rev* 15:342, 1994.

15. **Penning TM,** Molecular endocrinology of hydroxysteroid dehydrogenases, *Endocr Rev* 18:281, 1997.

16. **Erickson GF,** Physiologic basis of ovulation induction, *Seminars Reprod Endocrinol* 14:287, 1996.

17. **Falck B,** Site of production of oestrogen in the rat ovary as studied in microtransplants, *Acta Physiol Scand* 163(Suppl 47):1, 1959.

18. **Kol S, Adashi EY,** Intraovarian factors regulating ovarian function, *Curr Opin Obstet Gynecol* 7:209, 1995.

19. **Voutilainen R, Franks S, Mason HD, Martikainen H,** Expression of insulin-like growth factor (IGF), IGF-binding protein, and IGF receptor messenger ribonucleic acids in normal and polycystic ovaries, *J Clin Endocrinol Metab* 81:1003, 1996.

20. **Sawetawan C, Carr BR, McGee E, Bird IM, Hong TL, Rainey WE,** Inhibin and activin differentially regulate androgen production and 17α-hydroxylase expression in human ovarian thecal-like cells, *J Endocrinol* 148:213, 1996.

21. **Hillier SG, Reichert Jr LE, Van Hall EV,** Control of preovulatory follicular estrogen biosynthesis in the human ovary, *J Clin Endocrinol Metab* 52:847, 1981.

22. **Mendel C,** The free hormone hypothesis: a physiologically based mathematical model, *Endocr Rev* 10:232, 1989.

23. **Preziosi P, Barrett-Connor E, Papoz L, Roger M, Saint-Paul M, Nahoul K, Simon D,** Interrelation between plasma sex hormone-binding globulin and plasma insulin in healthy adult women: the Telecom study, *J Clin Endocrinol Metab* 76:283, 1993.

24. **Lindstedt G, Lundberg P-A, Lapidus L, Lundgren H, Bengtsson C, Bjorntorp P,** Low sex hormone-binding globulin concentration as independent risk factor for development of NIDDM. 12-year follow-up of population study of women in Gothenburg, Sweden, *Diabetes* 40:123, 1991.

25. **Peiris AN, Sothmann MS, Aiman EJ, Kissebah AH,** The relationship of insulin to sex hormone binding globulin: role of adiposity, *Fertil Steril* 52:69, 1989.

26. **Bérubé D, Séralini GE, Gagné R, Hammond GL,** Localization of the human sex hormone-binding globulin gene (SHBG) to the short arm of chromosome 17 (17p12-13), *Cytogenet Cell Genet* 54:65, 1990.

27. **Hammond GL, Underhill DA, Rykse HM, Smith CL,** The human sex hormone-binding globulin gene contains exons for androgen-binding protein and two other testicular messenger RNAs, *Mol Endocrinol* 3:1869, 1989.

28. **Hammond GL, Bocchinfuso WP,** Sex hormone-binding globulin: gene organization and structure/function analyses, *Horm Res* 45:197, 1996.

29. **Rosner W,** The functions of corticosteroid-binding globulin and sex hormone-binding globulin: recent advances, *Endocr Rev* 11:80, 1990.

30. **Kirschner MA, Samojlik E, Drejda M, Szmal E, Schneider G, Ertel N,** Androgen-estrogen metabolism in women with upper body versus lower body obesity, *J Clin Endocrinol Metab* 70:473, 1990.

31. **Siiteri PK, MacDonald PC,** Role of extraglandular estrogen in human endocrinology, In: Geyer SR, Astwood EB, Greep RO, eds. *Handbook of Physiology, Section 7, Endocrinology,* American Physiology Society, Washington, DC, 1973, p 615.

32. **Silva PD, Gentzschein EEK, Lobo RA,** Androstenedione may be a more important precursor of tissue dihydrotestosterone than testosterone in women, *Fertil Steril* 48:419, 1987.

33. **Horton R,** Dihydrotestosterone is a peripheral paracrine hormone, *J Androl* 13:23, 1992.

34. **Russell DW, Wilson JD,** Steroid 5α-reductase: two genes/two enzymes, *Ann Rev Biochem* 63:25, 1994.

35. **Mooradian AD, Morley JE, Korenman SG,** Biological actions of androgens, *Endocr Rev* 8:1, 1987.

36. **Beato M, Sánchez-Pacheco A,** Interaction of steroid hormone receptors with the transcription initiation complex, *Endocr Rev* 17:587, 1996.

37. **King WJ, Greene GL,** Monoclonal antibodies localize oestrogen receptor in the nuclei of target cells, *Nature* 307:745, 1984.

38. **Welshons WV, Lieberman ME, Gorski J,** Nuclear localization of unoccupied oestrogen receptors, *Nature* 307:747, 1984.

39. **Press MF, Greene GL,** Localization of progesterone receptor with monoclonal antibodies to the human progestin receptor, *Endocrinology* 122:1165, 1988.

40. **Webb P, Lopez GN, Greene GL, Baxter JD, Kushner PJ,** The limits of the cellular capacity to mediate an estrogen response, *Mol Endocrinol* 6:157, 1992.

41. **Gerace L,** Molecular trafficking across the nuclear pore complex, *Curr Opin Cell Biol* 4:637, 1992.

42. **Katzenellenbogen BS,** Biology and receptor interactions of estriol and estriol derivatives in vitro and in vivo, *J Steriod Biochem* 20:1033, 1984.

43. **Hung TT, Gibbons WE,** Evaluation of androgen antagonism of estrogen effect by dihydrotestosterone, *J Steroid Biochem* 19:1513, 1983.

44. **Evans RM,** The steroid and thyroid hormone receptor family, *Science* 240:889, 1988.

45. **Laudet V, Hanni C, Coll J, Catzeflis F, Stehelin D,** Evolution of the nuclear receptor gene superfamily, *EMBO J* 11:1003, 1992.

46. **Kuiper G, Enmark E, Pelto-Huikko M, Nilsson S, Gustafsson J,** Cloning of a novel estrogen receptor expressed in rat prostate and ovary, *Proc Natl Acad Sci USA* 93:5925, 1996.

47. **Mosselman S, Polman J, Dijkema R,** ER-β: identification and characterizaiton of a novel human estrogen receptor, *FEBS Letters* 392:49, 1996.

48. **Jensen EV, Jacobson HI,** Basic guides to the mechanism of estrogen action, *Recent Prog Hor Res* 18:387, 1962.

49. **Green S, Walter P, Greene G, Krust A, Goffin C, Jensen E, Scrace G, Walterfield M, Chambon P,** Cloning of the human oestrogen receptor cDNA, *J Steroid Biochem* 24:77, 1986.

50. **Greene GL, Gilna P, Walterfield M, Baker A, Hort Y, Shine J,** Sequence and expression of human estrogen receptor cDNA, *Science* 231:1150, 1986.

51. **Parker MG,** Structure and function of the oestrogen receptor, *J Neuroendocrinol* 5:223, 1993.

52. **Enmark E, Pelto-Huikko M, Grandien K, Lagercrantz S, Lagercrantz J, Fried G, Nordenskjöld M, Gustafsson J-Å,** Human estrogen receptor β-gene structure, chromosomal localization, and expression pattern, *J Clin Endocrinol Metab* 82:4258, 1997.

53. **Kuiper GGJM, Carlsson B, Grandien K, Enmark E, Häggblad J, Nilsson S, Gustafsson J,** Comparison of the ligand binding specificity and transcript tissue distribution of estrogen receptors α and β, *Endocrinology* 138:863, 1997.

54. **Wurtz JM, Bourguet W, Renaud JP, Vivat V, Chambon P, Moras D, Gronemeyer H,** A canonical structure for the ligand-binding domain of nuclear receptors, *Nat Struct Biol* 3:87, 1996.

55. **Teutsch G, Nique F, Lemoine G, Fouchoux F, Cérède E, D G, Philibert D,** General structure-activity correlations of antihormones, *Ann NY Acad Sci* 761:5, 1995.

56. **Montano MM, Müller V, Trobaugh A, Katzenellenbogen BS,** The carboxy-terminal F domain of the human estrogen receptor: role in the transcriptional activity of the receptor and the effectiveness of antiestrogens as estrogen antagonists, *Mol Endocrinology* 9:814, 1995.

57. **Parker MG,** Structure and function of estrogen receptors, *Vitamins Hormones* 51:267, 1995.

58. **Brzozowski AM, Pike ACW, Dauter Z, Hubbard RE, Bonn T, Engström O, Öhman L, Greene GL, Gustafsson JÅ, Carlquist M,** Molecular basis of agonism and antagonism in the oestrogen receptor, *Nature* 389:753, 1997.

59. **Tanenbaum DM, Wang Y, Williams SP, Sigler PB,** Crystallographic comparison of the estrogen and progesterone receptors ligand binding domains, *Proc Natl Acad Sci USA* 95:5998, 1998.

60. **Melamed M, Castraño E, Notides AC, Sasson S,** Molecular and kinetic basis for the mixed agonist/antagonist activity of estriol, *Mol Endocrinol* 11:1868, 1997.

61. **Zhuang Y, Katzenellenbogen BS, Shapiro DJ,** Estrogen receptor mutants which do not bind 17β-estradiol dimerize and bind to the estrogen response element *in vivo, Mol Endocrinol* 9:457, 1995.

62. **Wiese TE, Brooks SC,** Molecular modelling of steroidal estrogens: novel conformations and their role in biological activity, *J Steroid Biochem Mol Biol* 50:61, 1994.

63. **Freedman LP,** Anatomy of the steroid receptor zinc finger region, *Endocr Rev* 13:129, 1992.

64. **O'Malley BW, Tsai M-J,** Molecular pathways of steroid receptor action, *Biol Reprod* 46:163, 1992.

65. **Halachmi S, Marden E, Martin G, MacKay H, Abbondanza C, Brown M,** Estrogen receptor-associated proteins: possible mediators of hormone-induced transcription, *Science* 264:1455, 1994.

66. **Cavaillès V, Dauvois S, L'Horset F, Lopez G, Hoare S, Kushner PJ, Parker MG,** Nuclear factor RIP140 modulates transcriptional activtion by the estrogen receptor, *EMBO J* 14:3741, 1995.

67. **Horwitz KB, Jackson TA, Bain DL, Richer JK, Takimoto GS, Tung L,** Nuclear receptor coactivators and corepressors, *Mol Endocrinol* 10:1167, 1996.

68. **Ciocca DR, Vargas Roid LM,** Estrogen receptors in human nontarget tissues: biological and clinical implications, *Endocr Rev* 16:35, 1995.

69. **Hyder SM, Shipley GL, Stancel GM,** Estrogen action in target cells: selective requirements for activation of different hormone response elements, *Mol Cell Endocrinol* 112:35, 1995.

70. **O'Malley BW, Schrader WT, Mani S, Smith C, Weigel NL, Conneely OM, Clark JH,** An alternative ligand-independent pathway for activation of steroid receptors, *Recent Prog Hor Res* 50:333, 1995.

71. **Lindzey J, Korach KS,** Developmental and physiological effects of estrogen receptor gene disruption in mice, *Trends Endocrinol Metab* 8:137, 1997.

72. **Brandenberger AW, Tee MK, Lee JY, Chao V, Jaffe RB,** Tissue distribution of estrogen receptors alpha (ER-α) and beta (ER-β) mRNA in the midgestational human fetus, *J Clin Endocrinol Metab* 82:3509, 1997.

73. **Shughrue PJ, Lane MV, Merchenthaler I,** Comparative distribution of estrogen receptor-alpha and -beta mRNA in the rat central nervous system, *J Comp Neurol* 388:507, 1997.

74. **Paech K, Webb P, Kuiper GG, Nilsson S, Gustafsson J, Kushner PJ, Scanlan TS,** Differential ligand activation of estrogen receptors ERalpha and ERbeta at AP1 sites, *Science* 277:1508, 1997.

75. **Horwitz KB, Tung L, Takimoto GS,** Novel mechanisms of antiprogestin action, *J Steroid Biochem Mol Biol* 53:9, 1995.

76. **Read LD, Katzenellenbogen BS,** Characterization and regulation of estrogen and progesterone receptors in breast cancer, *Cancer Treat Res* 61:277, 1992.

77. **Kastner P, Krust A, Turcotte B, Stropp U, Tora L, Gronemeyer H, Chambon P,** Two distinct estrogen-regulated promoters generate transcripts encoding the two functionally different human progesterone receptor forms A and B, *EMBO J* 9:1603, 1990.

78. **Wen DXL, Xu Y-F, Mais DE, Goldman ME, McDonnell DP,** The A and B isoforms of the human progesterone receptor operate through distinct signaling pathways within target cells, *Mol Cellular Biol* 14:8356, 1994.

79. **Sartorius CA, Melville MY, Hovland AR, Tung L, Takimoto GS, Horwitz KB,** A third transactivation function (AF-3) of human progesterone receptors located in the unique N-terminal segment of the B-isoform, *Mol Endocrinol* 8:1347, 1994.

80. **Vegeto E, Allan GF, Schrader WT, Tsai MJ, McDonnell DP, O'Malley BW,** Mechanism of RU486 antagonism is dependent on the conformation of the carboxyl-terminal tail of the human progesterone receptor, *Cell* 69:703, 1992.

81. **Williams SP, Sigler PB,** Atomic structure of progesterone complexed with its receptor, *Nature* 393:392, 1998.

82. **Feil PD, Clarke CL, Satyaswaroop PG,** Progestin-mediated changes in progesterone receptor forms in the normal human endometrium, *Endocrinology* 123:2506, 1988.

83. **McDonnell DP, Goldman ME,** RU486 exerts antiestrogenic activities through a novel progesterone receptor A form-mediated mechanism, *J Biol Chem* 269:11945, 1994.

84. **McDonnell DP, Shahbaz MS, Vegeto E, O'Malley BW,** The human progesterone receptor A-form functions as a transcriptional modulator of mineralocorticoid receptor transcriptional activity, *J Steroid Biochem Mol Biol* 48:425, 1994.

85. **Tindall DJ, Chang CH, Lobl TJ, Cunningham GR,** Androgen antagonists in androgen target tissues, *Pharmacol Ther* 24:367, 1984.

86. **Wilson CM, McPhaul MJ,** A and B forms of the androgen receptor are present in human genital skin fibroblasts, *Proc Natl Acad Sci USA* 91:1234, 1994.

87. **Jenster G, van der Korput JAGM, Trapman J, Brinkmann AO,** Functional domains of the human androgen receptor, *Mol Cell Endocrinol* 86:187, 1992.

88. **Gottlieb B, Trifiro M, Lumbroso R, Pinsky L,** The androgen receptor gene mutations database, *Nucleic Acids Res* 25:158, 1997.

89. **Lubahn DB, Joseph DR, Sullivan PM, Willard HF, French FS, Wilson EM,** Cloning of human androgen receptor complementary DNA and localization to the X chromosome, *Science* 240:327, 1988.

90. **Brinkman AO, Jenster G, Kuiper GGJM, Ris C, van Laar JH, van der Korput JAGM, Degenhart HJ, Trifiro MA, Pinsky L, Romalo G, Schweikert HU, Veldscholte J, Mulder E, Trapman J,** The human androgen receptor: structure/function relationship in normal and pathological situations, *J Steroid Biochem Mol Biol* 41:361, 1992.

91. **Griffin JE, Wilson JD,** Disorders of androgen receptor function, *Ann NY Acad Sci* 438:61, 1984.

92. **MacLean HE, Warne GL, Zajac JD,** Spinal and bulbar muscular atrophy: androgen receptor dysfunction caused by a trinucleotide repeat expansion, *J Neurol Sci* 135:149, 1996.

93. **Revelli A, Massobrio M, Tesarik J,** Nongenomic actions of steroid hormones in reproductive tissues, *Endocr Rev* 19:3, 1998.

94. **Morley P, Whitfield JF, Vanderhyden BC, Tsang BK, Schwartz JL,** A new, nongenomic estrogen action: the rapid release of intracellular calcium, *Endocrinology* 131:1305, 1992.

95. **Chester AH, Jiang C, Borland JA, Yacoub M, Collins P,** Oestrogen relaxes human epicardial coronary arteries through non-endothelial-dependent mechanisms, *Coron Artery Dis* 6:417, 1995.

96. **Kirkland JL, Murthy L, Stancel GM,** Progesterone inhibits the estrogen-induced expression of *c-fos* messenger ribonucleic acid in the uterus, *Endocrinology* 130:3223, 1992.

97. **Tseng L, Lui HC,** Stimulation of arylsulfotransferase activity by progestins in human endometrium in vitro, *J Clin Endocrinol Metab* 53:418, 1981.

98. **Early Breast Cancer Trialists' Collaborative Group,** Tamoxifen for early breast cancer: an overview of the randomised trials, *Lancet* 351:1451, 1998.

99. **Helgason S, Wilking N, Carlstrom K, Damber MG, von Schoultz B,** A comparative study of the estrogenic effects of tamoxifen and 17β-estradiol in postmenopausal women, *J Clin Endocrinol Metab* 54:404, 1982.

100. **Saphner T, Tormey DC, Gray R,** Venous and arterial thrombosis in patients who received adjuvant therapy for breast cancer, *J Clin Oncol* 9:286, 1991.

101. **Fisher B, Dignam J, Bryant J, DeCillis A, Wickerham DL, Wolmark N, Costantino J, Redmond C, Fisher ER, Bowman DM, Deschênes L, Dimitrov NV, Margolese RG, Robidoux A, Shibata H, Terz J, Paterson AHG, Feldman MI, Farrar W, Evans J, Lickley HL,** Five versus more than five years of tamoxifen therapy for breast cancer patients with negative lymph nodes and estrogen receptor-positive tumors, *J Natl Cancer Inst* 88:1529, 1996.

102. **Kedar RP, Bourne TH, Powles TJ, Collins WP, Ashley SE, Cosgrove DO, Campbell S,** Effects of tamoxifen on uterus and ovaries of postmenopausal women in a randomized breast cancer prevention trial, *Lancet* 343:1318, 1994.

103. **Fisher B, Costantino JP, Redmond CK, Fisher ER, Wickerham DL, Cronin WM, Other NSABP Contributors,** Endometrial cancer in tamoxifen-treated breast cancer patients: findings from the National Surgical Adjuvant Breast and Bowel Project (NSABP) B-14, *J Natl Cancer Inst* 86:527, 1994.

104. **Landel CC, Kushner PJ, Greene GL,** The interaction of human estrogen receptor with DNA is modulated by receptor-associated proteins, *Mol Endocrinology* 8:1407, 1994.

105. **Berry M, Metzger D, Chambon P,** Role of the two activating domains of the oestrogen receptor in the cell type and promoter context dependent agonistic activity of the antioestrogen 4-hydroxytamoxifen, *EMBO* 9:2811, 1990.

106. **Katzenellenbogen BS, Montano MM, Le Goff P, Schodin DJ, Kraus WL, Bhardwaj B, Fujimoto N,** Antiestrogens: mechanisms and actions in target cells, *J Steroid Biochem Mol Biol* 53:387, 1995.

107. **Tzukerman MT, Esty A, Santisomere D, Danielian P, Parker MG, Stein RB, Pike JW, McDonnell DP,** Human estrogen receptor transactivational capacity is determined by both cellular and promoter context and mediated by two functionally distinct intramolecular regions, *Mol Endocrinol* 8:21, 1994.

108. **Webb P, Lopex GN, Uht RM, Kushner PJ,** Tamoxifen activation of the estrogen receptor/AP-1 pathway: potential origin for the cell-specific estrogen-like effects of antiestrogens, *Mol Endocrinol* 9:443, 1995.

109. **Yang NN, Venugopalan M, Hardikar S, Glasebrook A,** Identification of an estrogen response element activated by metabolites of 17ß-estradiol and raloxifene, *Science* 273:1222, 1996.

110. **Murphy LC,** Antiestrogen action and growth factor regulation, *Breast Cancer Res Treat* 31:61, 1994.

111. **Colletta AA, Benson JR, Baum M,** Alternative mechanisms of action of anti-oestrogens, *Breast Cancer Res Treat* 31:5, 1994.

112. **Stewart HJ, Forrest AP, Everington D, McDonald CC, Dewar JA, Hawkins RA, Prescott RJ, George WD, on behalf of the Scottish Cancer Trials Breast Group,** Randomized comparison of 5 years of adjuvant tamoxifen with continuous therapy for operable breast cancer, *Br J Cancer* 74:297, 1996.

113. **Horwitz KB,** Hormone-resistant breast cancer or "feeding the hand that bites you," *Prog Clin Biol Res* 387:29, 1994.

114. **Encarnación CA, Ciocca DR, McGuire WL, Clark GM, Fuqua SAW, Osborne CK,** Measurement of steroid hormone receptors in breast cancer patients on tamoxifen, *Breast Cancer Res Treat* 26:237, 1993.

115. **Robertson JFR,** Oestrogen receptor: a stable phenotype in breast cancer, *Br J Cancer* 73:5, 1996.

116. **Mahfoudi A, Roulet E, Dauvois S, Parker MG, Wahli W,** Specific mutations in the estrogen receptor change the properties of antiestrogens to full agonists, *Proc Natl Acad Sci USA* 92:4206, 1995.

117. **Fujimoto N, Katzenellenbogen BS,** Alteration in the agonist/antagonist balance of antiestrogens by activation of protein kinase A signaling pathways in breast cancer cells: antiestrogen selectivity and promoter dependence, *Mol Endocrinol* 8:296, 1994.

118. **Pavlik EJ, Nelson K, Srinivasan S, Powell DE, Kenady DE, DePriest PD, Gallion HH, van Nagell JRJ,** Resistance to tamoxifen with persisting sensitivity to estrogen: possible mediation by excessive antiestrogen binding site activity, *Cancer* 52:4106, 1992.

119. **Wiebe VJ, Osborne CK, Mcguire WL, DeGregorio MW,** Identification of estrogenic tamoxifen metabolite(s) in tamoxifen-resistant breast tumors, *J Clin Oncol* 10:990, 1992.

120. **Huynh H, Yang X, Pollak M,** Estradiol and antiestrogens regulate a growth inhibitory insulin-like growth factor binding protein-3 autocrine loop in human breast cancer cells, *J Biol Chem* 271:1016, 1996.

121. **Howell A, DeFriend D, Robertson J, Blamey R, Walton P,** Response to a specific antioestrogen (ICI 182780) in tamoxifen-resistant breast cancer, *Lancet* 345:29, 1995.

122. **Hasman M, Rattel B, Löser R,** Preclinical data for droloxifene, *Cancer Letters* 84:101, 1994.

123. **Jordan VC,** Alternate antiestrogens and approaches to the prevention of breast cancer, *J Cellular Biochem* Suppl 22:51, 1995.

124. **Geisler J, Haarstad H, Gundersen S, Raabe N, Kvinnsland S, Lønning PE,** Influence of treatment with the anti-oestrogen 3-hydroxytamoxifen (droloxifene) on plasma sex hormone levels in postmenopausal patients with breast cancer, *J Endocrinology* 146:359, 1995.

125. **Gronemeyer H, Benhamous B, Berry M, Bocquel MT, Gofflo D, Garcia T, Lerouge T, Metzger D, Meyer D, Meyer ME, Tora L, Vergezac A, Chambon P,** Mechanisms of antihormone action, *J Steroid Biochem Mol Biol* 41:217, 1992.

126. **Allan GF, Leng X, Tsai S-T, Weigel NL, Edwards DP, Tsai MJ, O'Malley BW,** Hormone and antihormone induce distinct conformational changes which are central to steroid receptor activation, *J Biol Chem* 267:19513, 1992.

127. **Vegeto E, Shahbaz MM, Wen DX, Goldman ME, McDonnell DP, O'Malley BW,** Human progesterone receptor A Form is a cell- and promoter-specific repressor of human progesterone B function, *Mol Endocrinol* 7:1244, 1993.

128. **Roesler WJ, Vandenbark GR, Hanson RW,** Cyclic AMP and the induction of eukaryotic gene transcription, *J Biol Chem* 263:9063, 1988.

129. **Sunahara RK, Dessauer CW, Gilman AG,** Complexity and diversity of mammalian adenylyl cyclases, *Ann Rev Pharmacol Toxicol* 36:461, 1996.

130. **Kelly PA, Djiane J, Edery M,** Different forms of the prolactin receptor: insights into the mechanism of prolactin action, *Trends Endocrinol Metab* 3:54, 1992.

131. **Tse A, Hille B,** GnRH-induced Ca^{2+} oscillations and rhythmnic hyperpolarizations of pituitary gonadotropes, *Science* 255:462, 1992.

132. **Rasmussen H,** The calcium messenger system, *New Engl J Med* 314:1164, 1986.

133. **Giudice L,** The insulin-like growth factor system in normal and abnormal human ovarian follicle development, *Am J Med* 16:48S, 1995.

134. **Matthews LS,** Activin receptors and cellular signaling by the receptor serine kinase family, *Endocr Rev* 15:310, 1994.

135. **Mohan S, Baylink DJ,** Editorial: insulin-like growth factor (IGF)-binding proteins in serum—do they have additional roles besides modulating the endocrine IGF actions? *J Clin Endocrinol Metab* 81:3817, 1996.

136. **Luo X, Ikeda Y, Parker KL,** A cell-specific nuclear receptor is essential for adrenal and gonadal development and sexual differentiation, *Cell* 77:481, 1994.

137. **Parker KL, Schimmer BP,** Steroidogenic factor 1: a key determinant of endocrine development and function, *Endocr Rev* 18:361, 1997.

138. **Sugawara T, Holt JA, Kiriakidou M, Strauss III JF,** Steroidogenic factor 1-dependent promoter activity of the human steroidogenic acute regulatory protein (StAR) gene, *Biochemistry* 35:9052, 1996.

139. **Burris TP, Guo W, McCabe ER,** The gene responsible for adrenal hypoplasia congenita, DAX-1, encodes a nuclear hormone receptor that defines a new class within the superfamily, *Recent Prog Horm Res* 51:241, 1996.

140. **Lambert A, Talbot JA, Anobile CJ, Robertson WR,** Gonadotrophin heterogeneity and biopotency: implications for assisted reproduction, *Mol Hum Reprod* 4:619, 1998.

141. **Beitins IZ, Padmanabhan V,** Bioactive follicle-stimulating hormone, *Trends Endocrinol Metab* 2:145, 1991.

142. **Wide L, Bakos O,** More basic forms of both follicle-stimulating hormone and luteinizing hormone in serum at midcycle compared with the follicular or luteal phase, *J Clin Endocrinol Metab* 76:885, 1993.

143. **Lapthorn AJ, Harris DC, Littlejohn A, Lustbader JW, Canfield RE, Machin KJ, Mogan FJ, Isaacs NW,** Crystal structure of human chorionic gonadotropin, *Nature* 369:455, 1994.

144. **Weiss J, Axelrod L, Whitcomb RW, Harris PE, Crowley WF, Jameson JL,** Hypogonadism caused by a single amino acid substitution in the β-subunit of luteinizing hormone, *New Engl J Med* 326:179, 1992.

145. **Huth JR, Mountjoy K, Peini F, Ruddon RW,** Intracellular folding pathway of human chorionic gonadotropin beta subunit, *J Biol Chem* 267:8870, 1992.

146. **Gharib SD, Wierman ME, Shupnik MA, Chin WW,** Molecular biology of the pituitary gonadotropins, *Endocr Rev* 11:177, 1990.

147. **Albanese C, Colin IM, Crowley WF, Ito M, Pestell RG, Weiss J, Jameson JL,** The gonadotropin genes: evolution of distinct mechanisms for hormonal control, *Recent Prog Hormone Res* 51:23, 1996.

148. **Weiss J, Guendner MJ, Halvorson LM, Jameson JL,** Transcriptional activation of the follicle-stimulating hormone beta-subunit gene by activin, *Endocrinology* 136:1885, 1995.

149. **Besecke LM, J GM, L SA, Bauer-Dantoin AC, Jameson JL, Weiss J,** Gonadotropin-releasing hormone regulates follicle-stimulating hormone-ß gene expression through an activin/follistatin autocrine or paracrine loop, *Endocrinology* 137:3667, 1996.

150. **Bilezikjian LM, Corrigan AZ, Blount AL, Vale WW,** Pituitary follistatin and inhibin subunit messenger ribonucleic acid levels are differentially regulated by local and hormonal factors, *Endocrinology* 137:4277, 1996.

151. **Jameson JL, Hollenberg AN,** Regulation of chorionic gonadotropin gene expression, *Endocr Rev* 14:203, 1993.

152. **Nilsson C, Pettersson K, Millar RP, Coerver KA, Matzuk MM, Huhtaniemi IT, International Collaborative Research Group,** Worldwide frequency of a common genetic variant of luteinizing hormone: an international collaborative research, *Fertil Steril* 67:998, 1997.

153. **Hwang J, Menon KMJ,** Spatial relationships of the human chorionic gonadotropin (hCG) subunits in the assembly of the hCG-receptor complex in the luteinized rat ovary, *Proc Natl Acad Sci USA* 81:4667, 1984.

154. **Merz WE, Dorner M,** Studies on structure-function relationships of human choriogonadotropins with C-teminally shortened alpha subunits. I. Receptor binding and immunologic properties, *Biochem Biophys Acta* 844:62, 1985.

155. **Wide L, Naessen T,** 17ß-oestradiol counteracts the formation of the more acidic isoforms of follicle-stimulating hormone and luteinizing hormone after menopause, *Clin Endocrinol* 40:783, 1994.

156. **Wide L, Albertsson-Wikland K, Phillips DJ,** More basic isoforms of serum gonadotropins during gonadotropin-releasing hormone agonist therapy in pubertal children, *J Clin Endocrinol Metab* 81:216, 1996.

157. **Mason M, Fonseca E, Ruiz JE, Moran C, Zarate A,** Distribution of follicle-stimulating-hormone and luteinizing-hormone isoforms in sera from women with primary ovarian failure compared with that of normal reproductive and postmenopausal women, *Fertil Steril* 58:60, 1992.

158. **Anobile CJ, Talbot JA, McCann SJ, Padmanabhan V, Robertson WR,** Glycoform composition of serum gonadotrophins through the normal menstrual cycle and in the post-menopausal state, *Mol Hum Reprod* 4:631, 1998.

159. **Combarenous Y,** Molecular basis of the specificity of binding of glycoprotein hormones to their receptors, *Endocr Rev* 13:670, 1992.

160. **Galway AB, Hsueh AJ, Keene JL, Yamoto M, Fauser BC, Boime I,** In vitro and in vivo bioactivity of recombinant human follicle-stimulating hormone and partially deglycosylated variants secreted by transfected eukaryotic cell lines, *Endocrinology* 127:93, 1990.

161. **De Leeuw R, Mulders J, Voortman G, Rombout F, Damm J, Kloosterboer L,** Structure-function relationship of recombinant follicle stimulating hormone (Puregon), *Mol Hum Reprod* 2:361, 1996.

162. **Bole-Feysot C, Goffin V, Edery M, Binart N, Kelly PA,** Prolactin (PRL) and its receptor: actions, signal transduction pathways and phenotypes observed in PRL receptor knockout mice, *Endocr Rev* 19:225, 1998.

163. **Sinha YN,** Structural variants of prolactin: occurrence and physiological significance, *Endocr Rev* 16:354, 1995.

164. **Ben-Jonathan N, Mershon JL, Allen DL, Steinmetz RW,** Extrapituitary prolactin: distribution, regulation, functions, and clinical aspects, *Endocr Rev* 17:639, 1996.

165. **Brue T, Caruso E, Morange I, Hoffmann T, Evrin M, Gunz G, Benkirane M, Jaquet P,** Immunoradiometric analysis of circulating human glycosylated and nonglycosylated prolactin forms: spontaneous and stimulated secretions, *J Clin Endocrinol Metab* 75:1338, 1992.

166. **Maaskant RA, Bogic LV, Gilger S, Kelly PA, Bryant-Greenwood GD,** The human prolactin receptor in the fetal membranes, decidua, and placenta, *J Clin Endocrinol Metab* 81:396, 1996.

167. **Katt JA, Duncan JA, Herbon L, Barkan A, Marshall JC,** The frequency of gonadotropin-releasing hormone stimulation determines the number of pituitary gonadotropin-releasing hormone receptors, *Endocrinology* 116:2113, 1985.

168. **Goldstein JL, Anderson RGW, Brown MS,** Coated pits, coated vesicles, and receptor-mediated endocytosis, *Nature* 279:679, 1979.

169. **Toledo A, Ramani N, Rao CV,** Direct stimulation of nucleoside triphosphatase activity in human ovarian nuclear membranes by human chorionic gonadotropin, *J Clin Endocrinol Metab* 65:305, 1987.

170. **Smart EJ, Ying Y, Donzell WC, Anderson RGW,** A role for caveolin in transport of cholesterol from endoplasmic reticulum to plasma membrane, *J Biol Chem* 271:29427, 1996.

171. **García-Cardeña G, Fan R, Stern DF, Liu J, Sessa WC,** Endothelial nitric oxide synthase is regulated by tyrosine phosphorylation and interacts with caveolin-1, *J Biol Chem* 271:27237, 1996.

172. **Liu J, García-Cardeña G, Sessa WC,** Palmitoylation of endothelial nitric oxide synthase is necessary for optimal stimulated release of nitric oxide: implications for caveolae localization, *Biochem* 35:13277, 1996.

173. **Fielding PE, Gielding CJ,** Intracellular transport of low density lipoprotein derived free cholesterol begins at clathrin-coated pits and terminates at cell surface caveolae, *Biochem* 35:14932, 1996.

174. **Kaplan J,** Polypeptide-binding membrane receptors: analysis and classification, *Science* 212:14, 1981.

175. **Ascoli M,** Lysosomal accumulation of the hormone-receptor complex during receptor-mediated endocytosis of human chorionic gonadotropin, *J Cell Biol* 99:1242, 1984.

176. **Parinaud J, Perret B, Ribbes H, Chap H, Pontonnier G, Douste-Blazy L,** High density lipoprotein and low density lipoprotein utilization by human granulosa cells for progesteone synthesis in serum-free culture: respective contributions of free and esterified cholesterol, *J Clin Endocrinol Metab* 64:409, 1987.

177. **Azhar S, Tsai L, Medicherla S, Chandrasekher Y, Giudice L, Reaven E,** Human granulosa cells use high density lipoprotein cholesterol for steroidogenesis, *J Clin Endocrinol Metab* 83:983, 1998.

178. **Sudhof TC, Goldstein JL, Brown MS, Russell DW,** The LDL receptor gene: a mosaic of exons shared with different proteins, *Science* 228:815, 1985.

179. **Reinhart MP,** Intracellular sterol trafficking, *Experientia* 46:599, 1990.

180. **Gilman AG,** Guanine nucleotide-binding regulatory proteins and dual control of adenylate cyclase, *J Clin Invest* 73:1, 1984.

181. **Neer EJ,** Heterotrimeric G proteins: organizers of transmembrane signals, *Cell* 80:249, 1995.

182. **Spiegel AM,** Genetic basis of endocrine disease. Mutations in G proteins and G protein-coupled receptors in endocrine disease, *J Clin Endocrinol Metab* 81:2434, 1996.

183. **Rodbell M,** The role of GTP-binding proteins in signal transduction: from the sublimely simple to the conceptually complex, *Curr Top Cell Regul* 32:1, 1992.

184. **Neubig RR,** Membrane organization in G-protein mechanisms, *FASEB J* 8:939, 1994.

185. **Wall MA, Coleman DE, Lee E, Iniguez-Lluhi JA, Posner BA, Gilman AG, Sprang SR,** The structure of the G protein heterotrimer Gi alpha 1 beta 1 gamma 2, *Cell* 83:1047, 1995.

186. **Segaloff DL, Ascoli M,** The lutropin/choriogonadotropin receptor. . . 4 years later, *Endocr Rev* 14:324, 1993.

187. **Alpaugh K, Indrapichate K, Abel JA, Rimerman R, Wimalasena J,** Purification and characterization of the human ovarian LH/hCG receptor and comparison of the properties of mammalian LH/hCG receptors, *Biochem Pharmacol* 40:2093, 1990.

188. **Atger M, Misrahi M, Sar S, LeFlem A, Dessen P, Milgrom E,** Structure of the human LH/cG receptor gene, *Mol Cell Endocrinol* 111:113, 1995.

189. **Tsai-Morris C-H, Geng Y, Buczko E, Dufau ML,** A novel human luteinizing hormone receptor gene, *J Clin Endocrinol Metab* 83:288, 1998.

190. **Minegishi T, Nakamura K, Takakura Y, Ibuki Y, Igarashi M,** Cloning and sequencing of human FSH receptor cDNA, *Biochem Biophys Res Commun* 175:1125, 1991.

191. **Simoni M, Gromoll J, Nieschlag E,** The follicle-stimulating hormone receptor: biochemistry, molecular biology, physiology, and pathophysiology, *Endocr Rev* 18:739, 1997.

192. **van Biesen T, Luttrell LM, Hawes BE, Lefkowitz RJ,** Mitogenic signaling via G protein-coupled receptors, *Endocr Rev* 17:698, 1996.

193. **Loganzo Jr F, Fletcher PW,** Follicle-stimulating hormone increases guanine nucleotide-binding regulatory protein subunit α_{i-3} mRNA but decreases α_{i-1} and α_{i-2} mRNA in Sertoli cells, *Mol Endocrinol* 6:1259, 1992.

194. **Hipkin RW, Wang Z, Ascoli M,** Human chorionic gonadotropin (CG) — and phorbol ester-stimulated phosphorylation of the luteinizing hormone/CG receptor maps to serines 635, 639, 649, and 652 in the C-terminal cytoplasmic tail, *Mol Endocrinol* 9:151, 1995.

195. **Weiss J, Cote C, Jameson JL, Crowley Jr WF,** Homologous desensitization of gonadotropin-releasing hormone (GnRH)-stimulated luteinizing hormone secretion in vitro occurs within the duration of an endogenous GnRH pulse, *Endocrinology* 136:138, 1995.

3 The Ovary — Embryology and Development

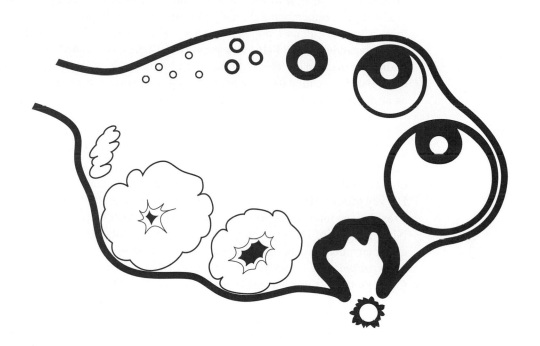

The great names of early Western medicine were Hippocrates, Soranus, and Galen. Although Aristotle (384–322 BC) referred to castration as a common agricultural practice, it was Soranus who provided the first anatomical description of the ovaries. Soranus of Ephesus (a city founded by Greeks on the coast of what is now Turkey) lived from 98 to 138 AD and has often been referred to as the greatest gynecologist of antiquity.[1] He studied in Alexandria and practiced in Rome. His great text was lost for centuries and was not published until 1838.

Galen was born in 130 AD in Pergamum, a Greek city in eastern Turkey, studied in Alexandria and became a famous practitioner and teacher of medicine in Rome. He lived 70 years and wrote about 400 treatises, 83 of which are still in existence. Galen preserved in his own writings (in Greek) Aristotle's descriptions of reproduction. He was a true scholar and was regarded as the ultimate authority on anatomy and physiology until the sixteenth century.[2] It was Galen who established bleeding as the appropriate treatment for almost every disorder. Although in retrospect Galen's conclusions and teachings contained many errors, how many other individuals have been able to satisfy the needs of scholars and physicians for hundreds of years?

After Galen, no further thoughts or advances were recorded for well over 1000 years as the dark weight of the medieval ages descended on western civilization. During the medieval years, it was safe to copy Galen's works but literally dangerous to contribute anything original. Medieval scholars believed it was impossible to progress in knowledge beyond Galen. The doctrine according to Galen was not challenged until the introduction of printing made Galen's works available to scholars.

Although Leonardo da Vinci (1452–1519) drew accurately the anatomy of the uterus and the ovaries, the major advances in anatomical knowledge can be traced to the University of Padua, the famed Italian university where a succession of anatomists made important contributions.[3] It was Andreas Vesalius (1514–1564), who while still in his 20s, because of his own human dissections, realized that Galen described only animals. Appointed Professor of Surgery and Anatomy at the University of Padua at the age of 23, he published *De Humani corporis Fabrica*, his authoritative, illustrated book on human anatomy, in 1543, at the age of 29. Vesalius was harshly attacked by the medical establishment, and one year after the publication of his book, he left Padua to become the court physician in Spain.

Vesalius was the first to describe ovarian follicles and probably the corpus luteum. Fallopius (1534–1562), remembered for his description of the fallopian tubes, was a pupil of Vesalius, and then a successful and popular teacher of anatomy at Padua. Fabricius (Girolamo Fabrici d'Acquapendente, 1533–1619), a pupil of Fallopius, succeeded Fallopius as chair of anatomy at Padua and made major contributions to embryology. Studying the organ in the bird that contained eggs, Fabricius called it the "ovary." During this period of time, the ovaries came to be recognized as structures, but their function remained a mystery.

William Harvey published the first original English book on reproductive anatomy and physiology in 1651, at the age of 69, 35 years after his discovery of the circulation of blood. He obtained his medical education at the University of Padua where he learned to describe accurately his own observations, a practice he was to continue and that culminated in his writings. Unfortunately, Harvey promoted and maintained the Aristotelian belief that the egg was a product of conception, a result of an interaction between semen and menstrual blood. This view was corrected by Bishop Niels Stensen of Denmark in 1667, and in 1672, at the age of 31, the Dutch physician Regnier de Graaf published his great work on the female reproductive organs, *De Mulierum Organis Generationi Inservientibus Tractatus Novus* (A New Treatise on the Female Reproductive Organs), that established the ovary as the source of the ovum.

Ovarian follicles had been described by Vesalius and Fallopius, but the impact of his publication earned de Graaf eternal recognition as the ovarian follicle became known as the Graafian follicle, even though de Graaf believed that the whole follicle was the egg. de Graaf was the first to accurately describe the corpus luteum, although Malpighi, whose works were published posthumously in 1697, invented the name "corpus luteum."

With the discovery of mammalian spermatozoa by van Leeuwenhoek in 1677, it became possible to speculate that fertilization resulted from the combination of a spermatozoon and the Graafian follicle. It would be another 150 years before it was appreciated that the oocyte resides within the follicle (described in 1827 by Carl Ernst von Baer), and that there is a relationship between the ovaries and menstruation. The process of fertilization was described by Newport in 1853–54, bringing to a close the era of descriptive anatomy of the ovary and marking the beginning of scientific explorations into physiology and endocrinology.

The Human Ovary

The physiologic responsibilities of the ovary are the periodic release of gametes (eggs) (oocytes) and the production of the steroid hormones, estradiol and progesterone. Both activities are integrated in the continuous repetitive process of follicle maturation, ovulation, and corpus luteum formation and regression. The ovary, therefore, cannot be viewed as a relatively static endocrine organ whose size and function expand and contract, depending on the vigor of stimulating tropic hormones. Rather, the female gonad is a heterogeneous ever-changing tissue whose cyclicity is measured in weeks, rather than hours.

The ovary consists of three major portions, the outer cortex, the central medulla, and the rete ovarii (the hilum). The hilum is the point of attachment of the ovary to the mesovarium. It contains nerves, blood vessels, and hilus cells, which have the potential to become active in steroidogenesis or to form tumors. These cells are very similar to the testosterone-producing Leydig cells of the testes. The outermost portion of the cortex is called the tunica albuginea, topped on its surface by a single layer of cuboidal epithelium, the germinal epithelium. The oocytes, enclosed in complexes called follicles, are in the inner part of the cortex, embedded in stromal tissue. The stromal tissue is composed of connective tissue and interstitial cells which are derived from mesenchymal cells, and have the ability to respond to luteinizing hormone (LH) or human chorionic gonadotropin (HCG) with androgen production. The central medullary area of the ovary is derived largely from mesonephric cells.

The Fetal Ovary

During fetal life, the development of the human ovary can be traced through four stages.[4] These are 1) the indifferent gonad stage, 2) the stage of differentiation, 3) the period of oogonal multiplication and oocyte formation, and finally 4) the stage of follicle formation.

The Indifferent Gonad Stage

At approximately 5 weeks of gestation, the paired gonads are structurally consolidated coelomic prominences overlying the mesonephros, forming the gonadal ridges. At this point, the gonad is morphologically indistinguishable as a primordial testis or ovary. The gonad is composed of primitive germ cells intermingled with coelomic surface epithelial cells and an inner core of medullary mesenchymal tissue. Just below this ridge lies the mesonephric duct. This indifferent stage lasts about 7–10 days. Together, the mesonephros and the genital ridge are called the urogenital ridge, indicating the close association of the urinary and reproductive systems.

The origin of the gonadal somatic cells is still not certain. The earliest recognizable gonad contains, besides the germ cells, somatic cells derived from at least 3 different tissues: coelomic epithelium, mesenchyme, and mesonephric tissue. In one model, the gonad is formed by the invasion of the "germinal epithelium" into the underlying mesenchyme. The germinal epithelium is simply that part of the coelomic epithelium that gives rise to gonadal tissue. The invading cells form the primary sex cords that contain the germ cells surrounded by somatic cells (the cells destined to form the tissue that holds the germ cells). In a newer model, the somatic cells of the gonad are believed to arise from the mesonephros and not the coelomic epithelium.[5] Ultrastructural studies have even suggested that both coelomic epithelial and underlying mesonephric cells provide the somatic cells that are destined to become follicular cells.[6]

The primordial germ cells originate within the primitive ectoderm, but the specific cells of origin cannot be distinguished. The germ cells are first identified at the end of the 3rd week after fertilization in the primitive endoderm at the caudal end and in the dorsal wall of the adjacent yolk sac, and, soon, they also appear in the splanchnic mesoderm of the hindgut.[7] The gonadal ridge is the one and only site where the germ cells can survive. By displacement because of growth of the embryo and also by active ameboid movement along the dorsal mesentery of the genital ridges, the germ cells "migrate" from the yolk sac through the hindgut to their gonadal sites between weeks 4 and 6 of gestation. The factors that initiate and guide the migration of the germ cells are not known, although chemotactic and adhesive peptides are involved. In rodents, germ cell migration involves stem cell factor and the expression of its receptor (kit) encoded by the C-kit proto-oncogene. In gonads obtained from individuals with intersex disorders that have a high risk of testicular tumors, the expression of kit protein was detected at a later gestational age than in normal controls, consistent with both later germ cell migration and a change in the oncogene expression.[8]

The germ cells begin their proliferation during their migration.[6] The germ cells are the direct precursors of sperm and ova, and by the 6th gestational week, on completion of the indifferent state, these primordial germ cells have multiplied by mitosis to a total of 10,000. By the 6th week of gestation, the indifferent gonads contain the germ cells and supporting cells derived from the coelomic epithelium and the mesenchyme of the gonadal ridge.

The Stage of Differentiation

If the indifferent gonad is destined to become a testis, differentiation along this line will take place at 6–9 gestational weeks. The absence of testicular evolution (formation of medullary primary sex cords, primitive tubules, and incorporation of germ cells) gives implicit evidence of the existence of a primitive, albeit momentarily quiescent, ovary. In contrast to the male, female internal and external genitalia differentiation precedes gonadal maturation. These events are related to the genetic constitution and the territorial receptivity of the mesenchyme. If either factor is deficient or defective, improper development occurs. As has been noted, primitive germ cells are unable to survive in locations other than the gonadal ridge. If partial or imperfect gonadal tissue is formed, the resulting abnormal nonsteroidal and steroidal events have wide ranging morphologic, reproductive, and behavioral effects.

The Testes

The factor that determines whether the indifferent gonad will become a testis is called, appropriately, the testes-determining factor (TDF), a product of a gene located on the Y chromosome.[9] Currently, the best candidate for the testicular determining factor gene is located within a region named SRY, the sex-determining region on the Y chromosome.[10] The protein product of the SRY gene contains a DNA-binding domain to activate gene transcription.[11] Normal testis development requires not only the presence of the SRY gene but its interaction with other genes.[12] Genes similar to SRY have been named SOX genes (the similarity is with the <u>SR</u>Y b<u>ox</u> region that contains the DNA-binding sequence).[11] The expression of the SRY gene is confined to the genital ridge during fetal life, but the gene is also active in the germ cells of the adult, perhaps playing a role in spermatogenesis.[9] The traditional view assigns active gene control and expression for testicular differentiation and a more passive, "default" mode of development for the ovary. However, any process of differentiation requires gene expression, and therefore ovarian development, too, must involve genes and gene products.

When the Y chromosome containing the testes-determining region is present, the gonads develop into testes. The male phenotype is dependent on the products (anti-müllerian hormone and testosterone) of the fetal testes, while the female phenotype is the result of an absence of these fetal gonadal products.[13] Anti-müllerian hormone (AMH), which inhibits the formation of the müllerian ducts, is secreted at the time of Sertoli cell differentiation, beginning at 7 weeks. AMH expression is altered only by mutations in the AMH gene.[14] Regression of the müllerian ducts is dependent on the presence of an adequate number of Sertoli cells, and probably the regulation of AMH receptor.[15] After involution of the müllerian system, AMH continues to be secreted, but there is no known function. However, evidence in the mouse suggests a role in early germ cell transformation during spermatogenesis.[16] In the ovary, very small amounts of AMH mRNA are present early in life, and although there may be no role in female development, its production later in life by the granulosa cells raises the possibility of autocrine and paracrine actions in oocyte maturation and follicular development.[17]

The testis begins its differentiation in week 6–7 of gestation by the appearance of Sertoli cells that aggregate to form the testicular cords. The primordial germ cells are embedded in the testicular cords that will form the Sertoli cells and spermatogonia. The mature Sertoli cells are the site of production of ABP (androgen binding protein, important in maintaining the high local androgen environment necessary for spermatogenesis) and inhibin.

The Leydig cells differentiate (beginning week 8) from mesenchymal cells of the interstitial component surrounding the testicular cords. Thus, secretion of AMH precedes steroidogenesis in Leydig cells. Shortly after the appearance of the Leydig cells, secretion of testosterone begins. Androgen secretion increases in conjunction with increasing Leydig cell numbers until a peak is reached at 15–18 weeks. At this time, Leydig cell regression begins, and at birth, only a few Leydig cells are present.

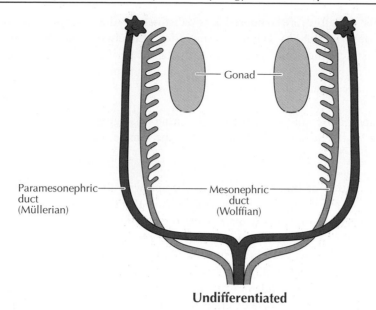

Undifferentiated

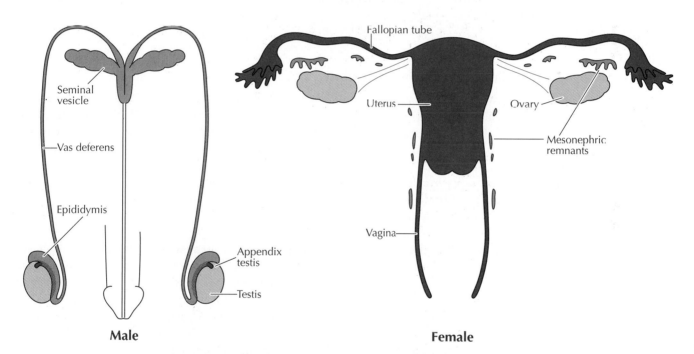

Male   **Female**

The cycle of fetal Leydig cells follows the rise and decline of fetal human chorionic gonadotropin (HCG) levels during pregnancy. This relationship and the presence of HCG receptors in the fetal testes indicate a regulatory role for HCG.[4] The pattern of HCG in the fetus parallels that of the mother, peaking at about 10 weeks and declining to a nadir at 20 weeks of gestation, but the concentrations are only 5% of maternal concentrations.

Testosterone synthesis in human fetal testes begins at the 8th week of gestation, reaches a peak between 15–18 weeks, and then declines. Testicular function in the fetus can be correlated with the fetal hormonal patterns. Although the initial testosterone production and sexual differentiation are in response to the fetal levels of HCG, further testosterone production and masculine differentiation are maintained by the fetal pituitary gonadotropins. Decreased testosterone levels in late gestation probably reflect the decrease in gonadotropin levels. The fetal Leydig cells, by an unknown mechanism, avoid down-regulation and respond to high levels of HCG and LH by increased steroidogenesis and cell multiplication. This generation of cells is replaced by the adult generation of Leydig cells that becomes functional at puberty and responds to high levels of HCG and LH with down-regulation and decreased steroidogenesis.

Leydig cells, therefore, are composed of two distinct populations, one active during fetal life and one active during adult life. The regression of fetal Leydig cells and the appearance of morphologically distinct adult cells during the peripubertal period raise many questions: what is the relationship between these two types, what is the mechanism for the regression and for the new appearance, and what is the origin of the adult cells?

The fetal spermatogonia, derived from the primordial germ cells, are in the testicular cords, surrounded by the Sertoli cells. In contrast to the female, male germ cells do not start meiotic division before puberty.

The differentiation of the wolffian system begins with the increase in testicular testosterone production. The classic experiments by Jost indicate that this effect of testosterone is due to local action, probably explaining why male internal genitalia in true hermaphrodites are only on the side of the testis.[13] Not all androgen-sensitive tissues require the prior conversion of testosterone to dihydrotestosterone (DHT). In the process of masculine differentiation, the development of the wolffian duct structures (epididymis, the vas deferens, and the seminal vesicle) is dependent on testosterone as the intracellular mediator, whereas development of the urogenital sinus and urogenital tubercle into the male external genitalia, urethra, and prostate requires the conversion of testosterone to DHT.[18] In the female, the loss of the wolffian system is due to the lack of locally produced testosterone.

The Stage of Oogonal Multiplication and Oocyte Formation

At 6–8 weeks, the first signs of ovarian differentiation are reflected in the rapid mitotic multiplication of germ cells, reaching 6–7 million oogonia by 16–20 weeks.[7, 19] This represents the maximal oogonal content of the gonad. From this point in time, germ cell content will irretrievably decrease until, some 50 years later, the store of oocytes will be finally exhausted.

By mitosis, the germ cells give rise to the oogonia. The oogonia are transformed to oocytes as they enter the first meiotic division and arrest in prophase. This process begins at 11–12 weeks, perhaps in response to a factor or factors produced by the rete ovarii.[20] Progression of meiosis to the diplotene stage is accomplished throughout the rest of pregnancy and completed by birth. Arrest of meiosis at the end of the first stage is probably maintained by inhibiting substances produced by granulosa cells. A single ovum is formed from the two meiotic divisions of the oocyte, one just before ovulation and the second (forming the haploid ovum) at the time of sperm penetration. The excess genetic material is extruded as one polar body at each meiotic division. Gonadotropins and various growth factors (but not sex steroids) can induce resumption of meiosis in vitro, but only in oocytes enclosed by cumulus-granulosa cells. A family of sterols is present in follicular fluid, presumably secreted by the cumulus cells, that activates oocyte meiosis.[21]

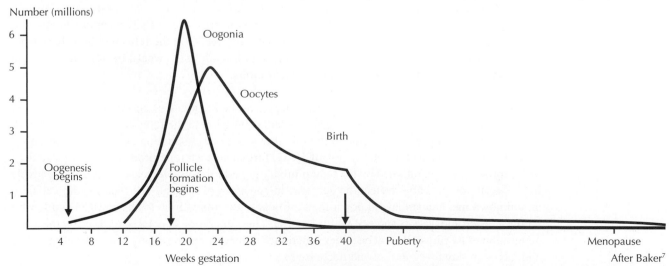

After Baker[7]

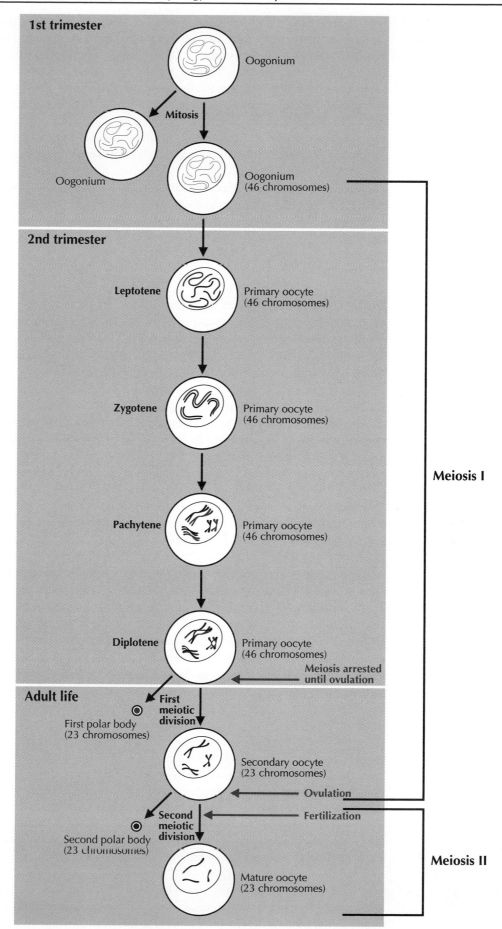

Loss of germ cells takes place throughout all of these events: during mitosis of germ cells, during the various stages of meiosis, and finally, after follicle formation. The massive loss of oocytes during the second half of pregnancy is the consequence of several mechanisms. Besides follicular growth and atresia, substantial numbers of oocytes regress during meiosis, and those oogonia that fail to be enveloped by granulosa cells undergo degeneration. This process is influenced by genes that actively repress germ cell death.[22] In addition, germ cells (in the cortical area) migrate to the surface of the gonad and become incorporated into the surface epithelium or are eliminated into the peritoneal cavity.[23, 24] In contrast, once all oocytes are encased in follicles (shortly after birth), the loss of oocytes will be only through the process of follicular growth and atresia.

Chromosomal anomalies can accelerate germ cell loss. Individuals with Turner syndrome (45,X) experience normal migration and mitosis of germ cells, but the oogonia do not undergo meiosis, and rapid loss of oocytes leaves the gonad without follicles by birth, and it appears as a fibrous streak.

The Stage of Follicle Formation

At 18–20 weeks, the highly cellular cortex is gradually perforated by vascular channels originating in the deeper medullary areas, and this marks the beginning of follicle formation.[25] As the finger like vascular projections enter the cortex, it takes on the appearance of secondary sex cords. As blood vessels invade and penetrate, they divide the previously solid cortical cell mass into smaller and smaller segments. Drawn in with the blood vessels are perivascular cells that are either mesenchymal or epithelial in origin. These cells surround the oocytes that have completed the first stage of meiosis. The resulting unit is the ***primordial follicle — an oocyte arrested in prophase of meiosis, enveloped by a single layer of spindle-shaped pregranulosa cells, surrounded by a basement membrane.*** Eventually all oocytes are covered in this fashion. Residual mesenchyme not utilized in primordial follicle formation is noted in the interstices between follicles, forming the primitive ovarian stroma. The granulosa cells differentiate from coelomic epithelial or mesenchymal precursors (their specific origin is still disputed). This process of primordial follicular development continues until all oocytes in the diplotene stage can be found in follicles, some time shortly after birth.

As soon as the oocyte is surrounded by the rosette of pregranulosa cells, the entire follicle can undergo variable degrees of maturation before arresting and becoming atretic. The formation of a ***primary follicle*** is marked by a change of the pregranulosa layer to a cuboidal layer of granulosa cells. Further differentiation into a ***preantral follicle*** is expressed as more complete granulosa proliferation. Call–Exner body formation (coalescence to form an antrum) and occasionally a minor thecal layer system that differentiates from surrounding mesenchymal cells can be seen. Preantral follicles can be found in the 6th month of gestation, and ***antral follicles*** (the Graafian follicle, characterized by a fluid filled space) are present by the end of pregnancy, but not in large numbers. It is only during the last third of gestation that theca cells can be found surrounding follicles.[19]

Even in fetal life the cycle of follicle formation, variable ripening, and atresia occurs. Although these steps are precisely those typical of adult reproductive life, full maturity, as expressed in ovulation, does not occur. Estrogen production does not occur until late in pregnancy when follicular development takes place, and even then steroidogenesis is not significant. Unlike the male, gonadal steroid production is not required for development of a normal phenotype. The development of the müllerian duct into the fallopian tubes, the uterus, and the upper third of the vagina is totally independent of the ovary.

The ovary at birth and in the first year of life can contain cystic follicles of varying size, undoubtedly stimulated by the reactive gonadotropin surge accompanying the withdrawal of the neonatal hypothalamus and pituitary from the negative feedback of fetoplacental steroids.[26] Ovarian cysts can also be occasionally detected in fetuses by ultrasonography.

The anterior pituitary begins development between 4 and 5 weeks of fetal life. The median eminence is apparent by week 9 of gestation, and the hypothalamic-pituitary portal circulation is functional by the 12th week. Pituitary levels of follicle-stimulating hormone (FSH) peak at 20–23 weeks, and circulating levels peak at 28 weeks. Levels are higher in female fetuses than in males until the last 6 weeks of gestation. Ovaries in anencephalic fetuses which lack gonadotropin-releasing hormone (GnRH) and gonadotropin secretion lack antral follicles and are smaller at term, but progression through meiosis and development of primordial follicles occur, apparently not dependent upon gonadotropins.[4] The ovary develops receptors for gonadotropins only in the second half of pregnancy. Thus, the loss of oocytes during fetal life cannot be solely explained by the decline in gonadotropins. The follicular growth and development observed in the second half of pregnancy, however, is gonadotropin dependent.[27] Hypophysectomy of a fetal monkey is followed by an increase in oocyte loss by atresia.[28]

The Neonatal Ovary

The total cortical content of germ cells falls to 1–2 million by birth as a result of prenatal oocyte depletion.[29] This huge depletion of germ cell mass (close to 4–5 million) has occurred over as short a time as 20 weeks. No similar rate of depletion will be seen again. Because of the fixed initial endowment of germ cells, the newborn female enters life, still far from reproductive potential, having lost 80% of her oocytes.

The ovary is approximately 1 cm in diameter and weighs about 250–350 mg at birth, although sizable cystic follicles can enlarge the total dimensions. Intriguingly, the gonad on the right side of the body in both males and females is larger, heavier, and greater in protein and DNA content than the gonad on the left side.[30] Compartmentalization of the gonad into cortex and a small residual medulla has been achieved. In the cortex, almost all the oocytes are involved in primordial follicle units. Varying degrees of maturation in some units can be seen as in the fetal state.

There is a sex difference in fetal gonadotropin levels. There are higher pituitary and circulating FSH and pituitary LH levels in female fetuses. The lower male levels are probably due to testicular testosterone and inhibin production. In infancy, the postnatal FSH rise is more marked and more sustained in females, whereas LH values are not as high. The FSH levels are greater than the levels reached during a normal adult menstrual cycle, decreasing to low levels usually by one year of age, but sometimes later.[31] LH levels are in the range of lower adult levels. This early activity is accompanied by inhibin levels comparable to the low range observed during the follicular phase of the menstrual cycle. Follicular response to the antral stage is relatively common in the first 6 months of life in response to these elevated gonadotropin levels. The most common cause of abdominal masses in fetuses and newborns is ovarian cysts, a consequence of gonadotropin stimulation.[32]

Interference with the postnatal rise in gonadotropins in monkeys is associated with disturbances in normal hypothalamic-pituitary function at puberty.[33] Indeed, in male monkeys, the administration of a GnRH analogue in the neonatal period has an adverse impact on subsequent immunologic and behavioral functions as well as normal reproduction.[33] After the postnatal rise, gonadotropin levels reach a nadir during early childhood (by about 6 months of age in males and 1–2 years in females) and then rise slightly between 4 and 10 years.

The Ovary in Childhood

The childhood period is characterized by low levels of gonadotropins in the pituitary and in the blood, little response of the pituitary to GnRH, and maximal hypothalamic suppression. The ovary, however, is not quiescent during childhood. Follicles begin to grow at all times and frequently reach the antral stage. Ultrasonography can commonly demonstrate ovarian follicular cysts during childhood, ranging in size from 2 to 15 mm.[34] These small unilocular ovarian cysts are not clinically significant.[35] The process of atresia with an increasing contribution of follicular remnants to the stromal compartment yields progressive ovarian enlargement during childhood, about a ten-fold increase in weight.[36] Of course, the lack of gonadotropin support prevents full follicular development and function. There is no evidence that ovarian function is necessary until puberty. However, the oocytes during this time period are active, synthesizing mRNAs and protein. Furthermore, ovariectomy in prepubertal monkeys indicates that the prepubertal suppression of GnRH and gonadotropins is partially dependent on the presence of ovaries, suggesting some functional activity of the ovary in childhood.[37]

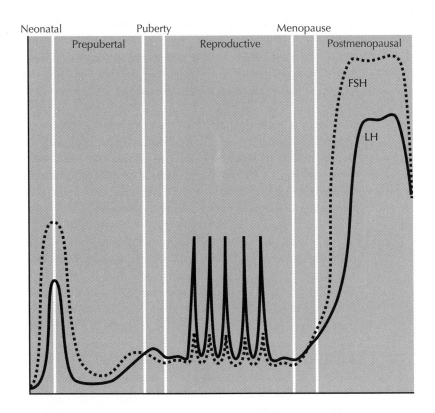

The Adult Ovary

At the onset of puberty, the germ cell mass has been reduced to 300,000 to 500,000 units.[7, 38] During the next 35–40 years of reproductive life, 400 to 500 will be selected to ovulate, and the primary follicles will eventually be depleted to a point at menopause when only a few hundred remain.[39] In the last 10–15 years before menopause, there is an acceleration of follicular loss.[40, 41] This loss correlates with a subtle but real increase in FSH and decrease in inhibin B as well as insulin-like growth factor-I (IGF-I).[42–46] The accelerated loss is probably secondary to the increase in FSH stimulation. Fewer follicles grow per cycle as a woman ages, and cycles are at first shorter due to more rapid follicular growth prior to ovulation (because of the elevated FSH levels) and then longer as anovulation becomes more common.[47–49] These changes, including the increase in FSH (which is probably due to the decrease in inhibin B), all reflect the reduced quality and capability of aging follicles. However, the rise in FSH due to a decrease in inhibin B may be the consequence of a decreasing number of follicles in each cohort of active follicles.[50]

The loss of oocytes (and follicles) through atresia is a response to changes in many factors. Certainly gonadotropin stimulation and withdrawal are important, but ovarian steroids and autocrine and paracrine factors are also involved. The consequence of these unfavorable changes, atresia, is a process called *apoptosis*, programmed cell death. This process is heralded by alterations in mRNAs required for cell proteins that maintain follicle integrity.[51] Indeed, the process is a consequence of an orderly expression of key gene products that either promote or repress the apoptotic events.

Unlike nonprimate species, human ovaries and nonhuman primate ovaries are innervated by sympathetic and sensory neurons.[52] This neuronal network innervates the ovarian vasculature, interstitial tissue, and developing follicles. These neuronal cells produce catecholamines and nerve growth factor. The precise function for this unique primate ovarian nervous system is not known. However, nerve fibers (not in an organized network) are present in nonprimate ovaries. Vasoactive intestinal peptide derived from these nerve fibers suppresses follicular atresia (apoptosis) in a mechanism that also involves IGF-I.[53]

During the reproductive years, the typical cycle of follicle maturation, including ovulation and corpus luteum formation, will be realized. This results from the complex but well defined sequence of hypothalamic-pituitary-gonadal interactions in which follicle and corpus luteum steroid hormones, pituitary gonadotropins, and autocrine and paracrine factors are integrated to yield ovulation. These important events are described in detail in Chapters 5 and 6. For the moment, our attention will be exclusively directed to a description of the events as the gonad is driven inexorably to final and complete exhaustion of its germ cell supply. The major feature of this reproductive period in the ovary's existence is the full maturational expression of some follicle units in ovulation and corpus luteum formation and the accompaniment of varying steroid output of estradiol and progesterone. For every follicle that ovulates, close to 1000 will pursue abortive growth periods of variable length.

Follicular Growth

In the adult ovary, the stages of follicle development observed even in the prenatal period are repeated but to a more complete degree. Initially, the oocyte enlarges and the granulosa cells proliferate markedly. A solid sphere of cells encasing the oocyte is formed. At this point, the theca interna is noted in initial stages of formation. The zona pellucida begins to form.

It is now believed that the time that elapses in progressing from a primary follicle to ovulation is approximately 85 days.[54, 55] The majority of this time passes in development that is independent of gonadotropins, achieving a state of readiness that will yield further growth in response to FSH stimulation. If gonadotropin increments are available, as can be seen early in a menstrual cycle, a further FSH-dependent stage of follicle maturation is seen. The number of follicles that mature is dependent on the amount of FSH available to the gonad and the sensitivity of the follicles to the gonadotropins. FSH receptor expression is greatest in granulosa cells, but significant expression can be detected in ovarian surface epithelium and fallopian tube epithelium, where the function is uncertain, but a role in epithelium-derived tumors is possible.[56]

The antrum first appears as a coalescence of numerous intragranulosa cavities called Call–Exner bodies, that were described by Emma Call and Siegmund Exner in Vienna, in 1875. Emma Call was one of the first woman physicians in the United States.[57] After receiving her medical degree from the University of Michigan, in 1873, she went to Vienna as Exner's postgraduate student. She returned to Boston and practiced as an obstetrician for more than 40 years. Emma Call was the first woman elected to the Massachusetts Medical Society (in 1884). Her description of the Call-Exner bodies was her only publication.

Whether Call–Exner bodies represent liquefaction or granulosa cell secretion is uncertain. At first, the cavity is filled with a coagulum of cellular debris. Soon a liquor accumulates, which is essentially a transudation of blood filtered through the avascular granulosa from the thecal vessels. With antral formation, the theca interna develops more fully, expressed by increased cell mass, increased vascularity, and the formation of lipid-rich cytoplasmic vacuoles within the theca cells. As the follicle expands, the surrounding stroma is compressed and is called the theca externa.

The granulosa cells that surround the oocyte are avascular and separated from the surrounding stroma by a basement membrane. Deprived of a vascular supply until after ovulation, the granulosa cells depend on specialized gap junctions that connect cells and communicate with the oocyte for the purpose of metabolic exchange and the transport of signaling molecules. It is this structure that allows repression and stimulation for the correct timing of meiosis. The granulosa cells differ in function and activity; e.g., LH receptor concentrations are highest in those cells closest to the basement membrane and lowest in those that surround the oocyte.[58]

At any point in this development, individual follicles become arrested and eventually regress in the apoptotic process known as atresia. At first the granulosa component begins to disrupt. The antral cavity constituents are resorbed, and the cavity collapses and obliterates. The oocyte degenerates in situ. Finally, a ribbon-like scarred streak surrounded by theca is seen. Eventually this theca mass loses its lipid and becomes indistinguishable from the growing mass of stroma. Thus, the process of apoptosis is extensive in the granulosa, and the thecal layer is largely spared to be incorporated into the interstitial tissue. Prior to regression, cystic follicles can be retained in the cortex for variable periods of time.

Ovulation

If gonadotropin stimulation is adequate, one of the several follicle units propelled to varying degrees of maturity will advance to ovulation. Morphologically, these events include distension of the antrum by increments of antral fluid and compression of the granulosa against the limiting membrane separating the avascular granulosa and the luteinized, vascularized theca interna. In addition, the antral fluid increment gradually pinches off the cumulus oophorous, the mound of granulosa enveloping the oocyte. The mechanisms of the thinning of the theca over the surface of the now protruding, distended follicle, the creation of an avascular area weakening the ovarian capsule, and the final acute dissension of the antrum with rupture and extrusion of the oocyte in its cumulus, are multiple and complex (discussed in Chapter 6). Repeated evaluation of intrafollicular pressures has failed to indict an explosive factor in this crucial event.

As demonstrated in a variety of animal experiments, the physical expulsion of the oocyte is dependent on a preovulatory surge in prostaglandin synthesis within the follicle. Inhibition of this prostaglandin synthesis produces a corpus luteum with an entrapped oocyte. Both prostaglandins and the midcycle surge of gonadotropins are thought to increase the concentration and activity of local proteases, such as plasminogen conversion to plasmin. As a result of generalized tissue weakening (loss of intercellular gap junction integrity and disruption of elastic fibers), there is swift accumulation of antral fluid followed by rupture of the weakened tissue envelope surrounding the follicle.

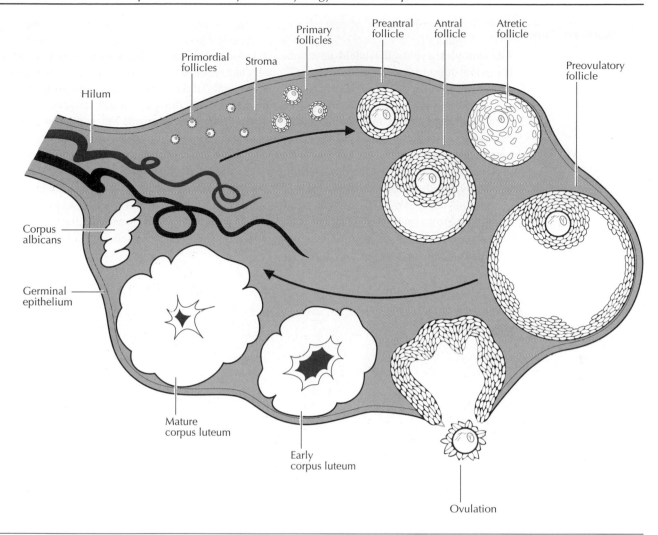

Corpus Luteum

Shortly after ovulation, profound alterations in cellular organization occur in the ruptured follicle that go well beyond simple repair. After tissue integrity and continuity are retrieved, the granulosa cells hypertrophy markedly, gradually filling in the cystic, sometimes hemorrhagic, cavity of the early corpus luteum. In addition, for the first time, the granulosa becomes markedly luteinized by incorporation of lipid-rich vacuoles within its cytoplasm. Both these properties had been the exclusive features of the theca prior to ovulation. For its part, the theca of the corpus luteum becomes less prominent, vestiges being noted eventually only in the interstices of the typical scalloping of the mature corpus luteum. As a result, a new yellow body is formed, now dominated by the enlarged, lipid-rich, fully vascularized granulosa. In the 14 days of its life, dependent on the low but important quantities of LH available in the luteal phase, this unit produces estradiol and progesterone. Failing a new enlarging source of LH-like human chorionic gonadotropin (HCG) from a successful implantation, the corpus luteum rapidly ages. Its vascularity and lipid content wane, and the sequence of scarification (albicantia) ensues.

Modulators of Function

The complex events that yield an ovum for fertilization and ovarian structures that provide hormonal support are the products of essentially every regulating mechanism in human biology. This includes classic endocrine signals, autocrine and paracrine/intracrine regulation, neuronal input, and immune system contributions. Representatives of the white blood cell series constitute a major component of the ovarian stromal (interstitial) compartment. Macrophages present in permanent, noncyclic numbers may influence ovarian function through the secretion of regulatory cytokines.[59] During the adult ovarian cycle, there is an infiltration of white blood cells in a pattern characterized by increasing numbers of mast cells culminating in degranulation and release of histamine that is associated with hyperemia at ovulation.[60] The corpus luteum attracts eosinophils and T lymphocytes, that signal and activate monocytes and macrophages involved in luteolysis. However, this immune mechanism should not be viewed just as a healing and resolving response, but also as an important regulatory system (involving the secretion of cytokines and growth factors) for ovarian function.[59]

References

1. **Graham H,** *Eternal Eve, The History of Gynaecology & Obstetrics,* Doubleday & Company, Inc., Garden City, NY, 1951.

2. **Magner LN,** *A History of Medicine,* Marcel Dekker, Inc., New York, 1992.

3. **Short RV,** The discovery of the ovaries, In: Zuckerman S, Weir BJ, eds. *The Ovary,* 2nd ed, Vol. 1, Academic Press, New York, 1977, p 1.

4. **Rabinovici J, Jaffe RB,** Development and regulation of growth and differentiated function of human and subhuman primate fetal gonads, *Endocr Rev* 11:532, 1990.

5. **Yoshinaga K, Hess DL, Hendrickx AG, Zamboni L,** The development of the sexually indifferent gonad in the prosimian, Galago *crassicaudatus crassicaudatus, Am J Anat* 181:89, 1988.

6. **Motta PM, Makabe S, Nottola SA,** The ultrasructure of human reproduction. I. The natural history of the female germ cell: origin, migration and differentiation inside the developing ovary, *Hum Reprod Update* 3:281, 1997.

7. **Baker TG,** A quantitative and cytological study of germ cells in human ovaries, *Proc Roy Soc Lond* 158:417, 1963.

8. **Meyts ER, Jorgensen N, Muller J, Skakkebaek NE,** Prolonged expression of the c-kit receptor in germ cells of intersex fetal testes, *J Pathol* 178:166, 1996.

9. **Sinclair AH, Berta P, Palmer MS, Hawkins JR, Griffiths BL, Smith JJ, Foster JW, Frischauf A-M, Lovell-Badge R, Goodfellow PN,** A gene from the human sex-determining region encodes a protein with homology to a conserved DNA-binding motif, *Nature* 346:240, 1990.

10. **Tho SPT, Layman LC, Lanclos DK, Plouffe Jr L, Byrd JR, McDonough PG,** Absence of the testicular determining factor gene SRY in XX true hermaphrodites and presence of this locus in most subjects with gonadal dysgenesis caused by Y aneuploidy, *Am J Obstet Gynecol* 167:1794, 1992.

11. **Whitfield LS, Lovell-Badge R, Goodfellow PN,** Rapid sequence evolution of the mammalian sex-determing gene SRY, *Nature* 364:713, 1993.

12. **Foster JW, Dominguez-Steglich MA, Guioli S, Kowk G, Weller PA, Stevanovic M, Weissenbach J, Mansour S, Young ID, Goodfellow PN, et al,** Campomelic dysplasia and autosomal sex reversal caused by mutations in an SRY-related gene, *Nature* 372:525, 1994.

13. **Jost A, Vigier B, Prepin J, Perchellet JP,** Studies on sex differentiation in mammals, *Recent Prog Hormone Res* 29:1, 1973.

14. **Rey R, Al-Attar L, Louis F, Jaubert F, Barbet P, Nihoul-Fekete C, Chaussain JL, Josso N,** Testicular dysgenesis does not affect expression of anti-müllerian hormone by Sertoli cells in premeiotic seminiferous tubules, *Am J Pathol* 148:1689, 1996.

15. **Teixeira J, He WW, Shah PC, Morikawa N, Lee MM, Catlin EA, Hudson PL, Wing J, Maclaughlin DT, Donahoe PK,** Developmental expression of a candidate müllerian inhibiting substance type II receptor, *Endocrinology* 137:160, 1996.

16. **Zhou B, Hutson JM,** Human chorionic gonadotropin (hCG) fails to stimulate gonocyte differentiation in newborn mouse testes in organ culture, *J Urol* 153:501, 1995.

17. **Kim JH, Seibel MM, MacLaughlin DT, Donahoe PK, Ransil BJ, Hametz PA, Richards CJ,** The inhibitory effects of müllerian-inhibiting substance on epidermal growth factor induced proliferation and progesterone production of human granulosa-luteal cells, *J Clin Endocrinol Metab* 75:911, 1992.

18. **Mooradian AD, Morley JE, Korenman SG,** Biological actions of androgens, *Endocr Rev* 8:1, 1987.

19. **Gondos B, Bhiraleus P, Hobel C,** Ultrastructural observations on germ cells in human fetal ovaries, *Am J Obstet Gynecol* 110:644, 1971.

20. **Gondos B, Westergaard L, Byskov A,** Initiation of oogenesis in the human fetal ovary: ultrastructural and squash preparation study, *Am J Obstet Gynecol* 155:189, 1986.

21. **Byskov AG, Andersen CY, Nordholm L, Thogersen H, Xia G, Wassmann O, Andersen JV, Guddal E, Roed T,** Chemical structure of sterols that activate oocyte meiosis, *Nature* 374:559, 1995.

22. **Ratts VS, Flaws JA, Kolp R, Sorenson CM, Tilly JL,** Ablation of bcl-2 gene expression decreases the numbers of oocytes and primordial follicles established in the post-natal female mouse gonad, *Endocrinology* 136:3665, 1995.

23. **Motta PM, Makabe S,** Germ cells in the ovarian surface during fetal development in humans. A three-dimensional microanatomical study by scanning and transmission electron microscopy, *J Submicrosc Cytol Pathol* 18:271, 1986.

24. **Speed RM,** The possible role of meiotic pairing anomalies in the atresia of human fetal oocytes, *Hum Genet* 78:260, 1988.

25. **Ammini AC, Pandey J, Vijyaraghavan M, Sabherwal U,** Human female phenotypic development: role of fetal ovaries, *J Clin Endocrinol Metab* 79:604, 1994.

26. **Cohen HL, Shapiro MA, Mandel FS, Shapiro ML,** Normal ovaries in neonates and infants: a sonographic study of 77 patients 1 day to 24 months old, *Am J Roentgenol* 160:583, 1993.

27. **Thomas GB, McNeilly AS, Gibson F, Brooks AN,** Effects of pituitary-gonadal suppression with a gonadotrophin-releasing hormone agonist on fetal gonadotrophin secretion, fetal gonadal development and maternal steroid secretion in the sheep, *J Endocrinol* 141:317, 1994.

28. **Gulyas BJ, Hodgen GD, Tullner WW, Ross GT,** Effects of fetal or maternal hypophysectomy on endocrine organs and body weight in infant rhesus monkeys *(Macaca mulatta)* with particular emphasis on oogenesis, *Biol Reprod* 16:216, 1977.

29. **Himelstein-Braw R, Byskov AG, Peters H, Faber M,** Follicular atresia in the infant human ovary, *J Reprod Fertil* 46:55, 1976.

30. **Mittwoch U, Mahadevaiah S,** Comparison of development of human fetal gonads and kidneys, *J Reprod Fertil* 58:463, 1980.

31. **Burger HG, Famada Y, Bangah ML, McCloud PI, Warne GL,** Serum gonadotropin, sex steroid, and immunoreactive inhibin levels in the first two years of life, *J Clin Endocrinol Metab* 72:682, 1991.

32. **Hengster P, Menardi G,** Ovarian cysts in the newborn, *Pediatr Surg Int* 7:372, 1992.

33. **Mann DR, Akinbami MA, Gould KG, Tanner JM, Wallen K,** Neonatal treatment of male monkeys with a gonadotropin-releasing hormone agonist alters differentiation of central nervous system centers that regulate sexual and skeletal development, *J Clin Endocrinol Metab* 76:1319, 1993.

34. **Cohen HL, Eisenberg P, Mandel F, Haller JO,** Ovarian cysts are common in premenarchal girls: a sonographic study of 101 children 2–12 years old, *Am J Radiol* 159:89, 1992.

35. **Millar DM, Blake JM, Stringer DA, Hara H, Babiak C,** Prepubertal ovarian cyst formation: 5 years' experience, *Obstet Gynecol* 81:434, 1993.

36. **Bridges NA, Cooke A, Healy MJ, Hindmarsh PC, Brook CG,** Standards for ovarian volume in childhood and puberty, *Fertil Steril* 60:456, 1993.

37. **Pohl CR, de Ridder CM, Plant TM,** Gonadal and nongonadal mechanisms contribute to the prepubertal hiatus in gonadotropin secretion in the female rhesus monkey (Macaca mulatta), *J Clin Endocrinol Metab* 80:2094, 1995.

38. **Block E,** Quantitative morphological investigations of the follicular system in women, *Acta Anat* 14:108, 1952.

39. **Richardson SJ, Senikas V, Nelson JF,** Follicular depletion during the menopausal transition — evidence for accelerated loss and ultimate exhaustion, *J Clin Endocrinol Metab* 65:1231, 1987.

40. **Faddy MJ, Gosden RG, Gougeon A, Richardson SJ, Nelson JF,** Accelerated disappearance of ovarian follicles in mid-life: implications for forecasting menopause, *Hum Reprod* 7:1342, 1992.

41. **Gougeon A, Echochard R, Thalabard JC,** Age-related changes of the population of human ovarian follicles: increase in the disappearance rate of non-growing and early-growing follicles in aging women, *Biol Reprod* 50:653, 1994.

42. **Metcalf MG, Livesay JH,** Gonadotropin excretion in fertile women: effect of age and the onset of the menopausal transition, *J Endocrinol* 105:357, 1985.

43. **Lee SJ, Lenton EA, Sexton L, Cooke ID,** The effect of age on the cyclical patterns of plasma LH, FSH, oestradiol and progesterone in women with regular menstrual cycles, *Hum Reprod* 3:851, 1988.

44. **Hughes EG, Robertson DM, Handelsman DJ, Hayward S, Healy DL, de Kretser DM,** Inhibin and estradiol responses to ovarian hyperstimulation: effects of age and predictive value for in vitro fertilization outcome, *J Clin Endocrinol Metab* 70:358, 1990.

45. **Klein NA, Battaglia DE, Fujimoto VY, Davis GS, Bremmer WJ, Soules MR,** Reproductive aging: accelerated ovarian follicular development associated with a monotropic follicle-stimulating hormone rise in normal older women, *J Clin Endocrinol Metab* 81:1038, 1996.

46. **Klein NA, Illingworth PJ, Groome NP, McNeilly AS, Battaglia DE, Soules MR,** Decreased inhibin B secretion is associated with the monotropic FSH rise in older, ovulatory women: a study of serum and follicular fluid leavels of dimeric inhibin A and B in spontaneous menstrual cycles, *J Clin Endocrinol Metab* 81:2742, 1996.

47. **Treloar AE, Boynton RE, Borghild GB, Brown BW,** Variation of the human menstrual cycle through reproductive life, *Int J Fertil* 12:77, 1967.

48. **Lenton EA, Landgren B, Sexton L, Harper R,** Normal variation in the length of the follicular phase of the menstrual cycle: effect of chronological age, *Br J Obstet Gynaecol* 91:681, 1984.

49. **Cha KY, Koo JJ, Ko JJ, Choi DH, Han SY, Yoon TK,** Pregnancy after IVF of human follicular oocytes collected from nonstimulated cycles, their culture in vitro and their transfer in a donor oocyte program, *Fertil Steril* 55:109, 1991.

50. **Klein NA, Battaglia DE, Miller PB, Branigan EF, Giudice LC, Soules MR,** Ovarian follicular development and the follicular fluid hormones and growth factors in normal women of advanced reproductive age, *J Clin Endocrinol Metab* 81:1946, 1996.

51. **Tilly JL, Kowalski KI, Schomberg DW, Hsueh AJ,** Apoptosis in atretic ovarian follicles is associated with selected decreases in messenger ribonucleic acid transcripts for gonadotropin receptors and cytochrome P450 aromatase, *Endocrinology* 131:1670, 1992.

52. **Dees WL, Hiney JK, Schultea TD, Mayerhofer A, Danilchik M, Dissen GA, Ojeda SR,** The primate ovary contains a population of catecholaminergic neuron-like cells expressing nerve growth factor receptors, *Endocrinology* 136:5760, 1995.

53. **Flaws JA, De Santi A, Tilly KI, Javid RO, Kugu K, Johnson AL, Hirshfield AN, Tilly JL,** Vasoactive intestinal peptide-mediated suppression of apoptosis in the ovary: potential mechanisms of action and evidence of a conserved antiatretogenic role through evolution, *Endocrinology* 136:4351, 1995.

54. **Gougeon A,** Dynamics of follicular growth in the human: a model from preliminary results, *Hum Reprod* 1:81, 1986.

55. **Gougeon A,** Regulation of ovarian follicular development in primates: facts and hypotheses, *Endocrin Rev* 17:121, 1996.

56. **Zheng W, Magid MS, Kramer EE, Chen YT,** Follicle-stimulating hormone receptor is expressed in human ovarian surface epithelium and fallopian tube, *Am J Pathol* 148:47, 1996.

57. **Speert H,** *Obstetric & Gynecologic Milestones Illustrated,* The Parthenon Publishing Group, New York, 1996.

58. **Lawrence TS, Dekel M, Beers WH,** Binding of human chorionic gonadotropin by rat cumuli, oophori and granulosa cells: a comparative study, *Endocrinology* 106:1114, 1980.

59. **Adashi EY,** Cytokine-mediated regulation of ovarian function: encounters of a third kind, *Endocrinology* 124:2043, 1989.

60. **Krishna A, Beesley K, Terranova PF,** Histamine, mast cells and ovarian function, *J Endocrinol* 120:363, 1989.

4   The Uterus

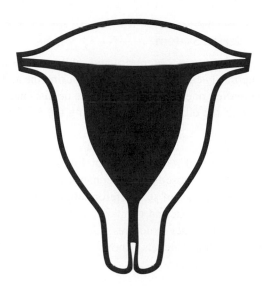

Anatomical knowledge of the uterus was slow to accumulate.[1, 2] Papyrus writings from 2500 BC indicate that the ancient Egyptians made a distinction between the vagina and uterus. Because the dead had to be embalmed, dissection was precluded, but prolapse was recognized because it was important to return the uterus into its proper place prior to mummification. Next to the Egyptian papyri in antiquity were Hindu writings in which descriptions of the uterus, tubes, and vagina indicate knowledge gained from dissections. This was probably the earliest description of the fallopian tubes.

There is little information in Greek writings about female anatomy; however, Herophilus (4th century BC), the great anatomist in Alexandria and the originator of scholarly dissection, recorded the different positions of the uterus. Soranus of Ephesus (98–138 AD) accurately described the uterus (probably the first to do so), obviously from multiple dissections of cadavers. He recognized that the uterus is not essential for life, acknowledged the presence of leiomyomata, and treated prolapse with pessaries.

Herophilus and Soranus were uncertain about the function of the fallopian tubes, but Galen, Rufus, and Aetisu guessed correctly their function. Galen promoted the practice of bleeding for the treatment of almost every disorder. In his argument that nature prevented disease by discharging excess blood, Galen maintained that women were healthier because their superfluous blood was eliminated by menstruation.[3] The writings of Galen (130–200 AD) represented the knowledge of medicine for over 1000 years until the end of the medieval dark ages. Galen's description of the uterus and tubes indicates that he had only seen the horned uteri of animals.

In the 16th century, Berengarius, Vesalius, Eustachius, and Fallopius made significant contributions to the anatomical study of the female genitalia. Berengarius (Giacomo Berengario da Carpi) was the first anatomist to work with an artist. His anatomical text, published in 1514, depicted dissected subjects as if they were still alive.

Gabriele Fallopio (or Fallopius) published his work, *Observationes Anatomicae,* in Venice in 1561, one year before his death from pleurisy at age 40. He provided the first descriptions of the clitoris and the hymen, and the first exact descriptions of the ovaries and the tubes. He named the vagina and the placenta and called the tubes the uteri tuba (the trumpet of the uterus), but soon they were known universally as the fallopian tubes. It was his professor and mentor at the University of Padua, however, Andreas Vesalius, who was the first to accurately reveal the presence of the endometrial cavity.

Development of the Müllerian System

The wolffian (mesonephric) and müllerian (paramesonephric) ducts are discrete primordia that temporarily coexist in all embryos during the ambisexual period of development (up to 8 weeks). Thereafter, one type of duct system persists normally and gives rise to special ducts and glands, whereas the other disappears during the 3rd fetal month, except for nonfunctional vestiges.

Hormonal control of mammalian somatic sex differentiation was established by the classic experiments of Alfred Jost.[4] In Jost's landmark studies, the active role of male determining factors, as opposed to the constitutive nature of female differentiation, was defined as the directing feature of sex differentiation. This principle applies not only to the internal ducts but to the gonad, external genitalia, and perhaps even the brain. The critical factors in determining which of the duct structures stabilize or regress are the secretions from the testes: AMH (anti-müllerian hormone, also known as müllerian inhibiting substance or müllerian inhibiting factor) and testosterone.

AMH is a member of the transforming growth factor-β family of glycoprotein differentiation factors that include inhibin and activin. The gene for AMH has been mapped to chromosome 19. AMH is synthesized by Sertoli cells soon after testicular differentiation and is responsible for the ipsilateral regression of the müllerian ducts by 8 weeks. Despite its presence in serum up to puberty, lack of regression of the uterus and tubes is the only consistent expression of AMH gene mutations. In the absence of AMH, the fetus will develop fallopian tubes, uterus, and upper vagina from the paramesonephric ducts (the müllerian ducts). This development requires the prior appearance of the mesonephric ducts, and for this reason, abnormalities in development of the tubes, uterus, and upper vagina are associated with abnormalities in the renal system.

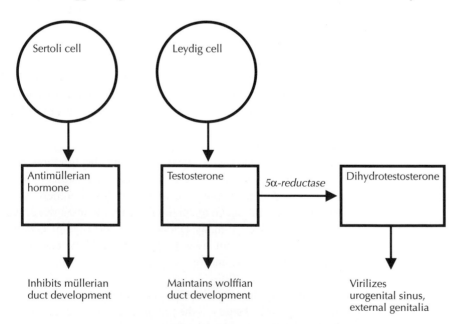

The internal genitalia possess the intrinsic tendency to feminize. In the absence of a Y chromosome and a functional testis, the lack of AMH allows retention of the müllerian system and development of fallopian tubes, uterus, and upper vagina. In the absence of testosterone, the wolffian system regresses. In the presence of a normal ovary or the absence of any gonad, müllerian duct development takes place.

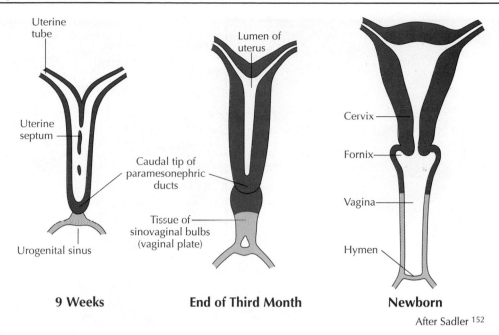

9 Weeks   End of Third Month   Newborn

After Sadler [152]

The paramesonephric ducts come into contact in the midline to form a Y-shaped structure, the primordium for the uterus, tubes, and the upper one-third of the vagina.[5] The fallopian tubes, uterus, and the upper portion of the vagina are created by the fusion of the müllerian ducts by the 10th week of gestation. Canalization to create the uterine cavity, the cervical canal, and the vagina is complete by the 22nd week of gestation. Under the epithelium lies mesenchymal tissue that will be the origin of the uterine stroma and smooth muscle cells. By the 20th week of pregnancy, the uterine mucosa is fully differentiated into the endometrium.

The endometrium, derived from the mucosal lining of the fused müllerian ducts, is essential for reproduction and may be one of the most complex tissues in the human body. It is always changing, responding to the cyclic patterns of estrogen and progesterone of the ovarian menstrual cycle, and to a complex interplay among its own autocrine and paracrine factors.[6]

The Histologic Changes in Endometrium During an Ovulatory Cycle

The sequence of endometrial changes associated with an ovulatory cycle has been carefully studied by Noyes in the human and Bartlemez and Markee in the subhuman primate.[7–11] From these data a description of menstrual physiology has developed based upon specific anatomic and functional changes within glandular, vascular, and stromal components of the endometrium.[12] These changes will be discussed in five phases: 1) the menstrual endometrium, 2) the proliferative phase, 3) the secretory phase, 4) preparation for implantation, and finally 5) the phase of endometrial breakdown. Although these distinctions are not entirely arbitrary, it must be recalled that the entire process is an integrated evolutionary cycle of endometrial growth and regression, which is repeated some 400 times during the adult life of the human female.

The endometrium can be divided morphologically into an upper two-thirds "functionalis" layer and a lower one-third "basalis" layer. The purpose of the functionalis layer is to prepare for the implantation of the blastocyst and, therefore, it is the site of proliferation, secretion, and degeneration. The purpose of the basalis layer is to provide the regenerative endometrium following menstrual loss of the functionalis.

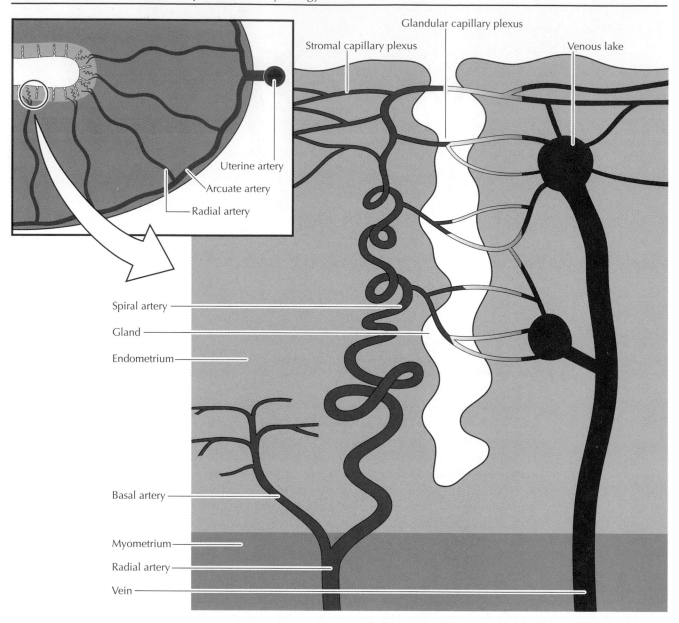

The Uterine Vasculature

The two uterine arteries that supply the uterus are branches of the internal iliac arteries. At the lower part of the uterus, the uterine artery separates into the vaginal artery and an ascending branch that divides into the arcuate arteries. The arcuate arteries run parallel to the uterine cavity and anastomose with each other, forming a vascular ring around the cavity. Small centrifugal branches (the radial arteries) leave the arcuate vessels, perpendicular to the endometrial cavity, to supply the myometrium. When these arteries enter the endometrium, small branches (the basal arteries) extend laterally to supply the basalis layer. These basal arteries do not demonstrate a response to hormonal changes. The radial arteries continue in the direction of the endometrial surface, now assuming a corkscrew appearance (and now called the spiral arteries), to supply the functionalis layer of the endometrium. It is the spiral artery (an end artery) segment that is very sensitive to hormonal changes. One reason the functionalis layer is more vulnerable to vascular permutations is that there are no anastomoses among the spiral arteries. The endometrial glands and the stromal tissue are supplied by capillaries that emerge from the spiral arteries at all levels of the endometrium. The capillaries drain into a venous plexus and eventually into the myometrial arcuate veins and into the uterine veins. This unique vascular architecture is important in allowing a repeated sequence of endometrial growth and desquamation.

The Menstrual Endometrium

The menstrual endometrium is a relatively thin but dense tissue. It is composed of the stable, nonfunctioning basalis component and a variable, but small, amount of residual stratum spongiosum. At menstruation, this latter tissue displays a variety of functional states including disarray and breakage of glands, fragmentation of vessels and stroma with persisting evidence of necrosis, white cell infiltration, and red cell interstitial diapedesis. Even as the remnants of menstrual shedding dominate the overall appearance of this tissue, evidence of repair in all tissue components can be detected. The menstrual endometrium is a transitional state bridging the more dramatic proliferative and exfoliative phases of the cycle. Its density implies that the shortness of height is not entirely due to desquamation. Collapse of the supporting matrix also contributes significantly to the shallowness. Reticular stains in rhesus endometrium confirm this "deflated" state. Nevertheless, as much as two-thirds of the functioning endometrium is lost during menstruation. The more rapid the tissue loss, the shorter the duration of flow. Delayed or incomplete shedding is associated with heavier flow and greater blood loss.

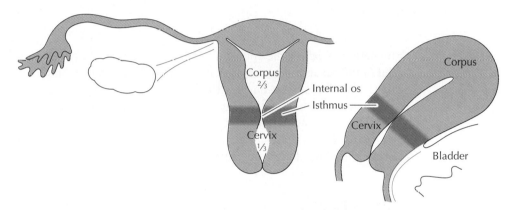

DNA synthesis is occurring in those areas of the basalis that have been completely denuded by day 2–3 of the menstrual cycle (the endometrium in the isthmic area, the narrow area between the cervix and the corpus, and the endometrium in the cornual recesses at the ostia of the tubes remain intact). The new surface epithelium emanates from the flanks of stumps of glands in the basalis layer left standing after menstrual desquamation.[13] Rapid reepithelialization follows the proliferation of the cells in the basalis layer and the surface epithelium in the isthmic and tubal ostial endometrium. This epithelial repair is supported by underlying fibroblasts. The stromal fibroblast layer forms a compact mass over which the resurfacing epithelium can "migrate." In addition, it is likely that the stromal layer contributes important autocrine and paracrine factors for growth and migration. Because hormone levels are at their nadir during this repair phase, the response may be due to injury rather than hormone mediated. However, the basalis layer is rich in its content of estrogen receptors. This "repair" is fast; by day 4 of the cycle, more than two-thirds of the cavity is covered with new epithelium.[13] By day 5–6, the entire cavity is reepithelialized, and stromal growth begins.

The Proliferative Phase

The proliferative phase is associated with ovarian follicle growth and increased estrogen secretion. Undoubtedly as a result of this steroidal action, reconstruction and growth of the endometrium are achieved. The glands are most notable in this response. At first they are narrow and tubular, lined by low columnar epithelium cells. Mitoses become prominent and pseudo stratification is observed. As a result, the glandular epithelium extends peripherally and links one gland segment with its immediate neighbor. A continuous epithelial lining facing the endometrial cavity is formed. The stromal component evolves from its dense cellular menstrual condition through a brief period of edema to a final loose syncytial-like status. Coursing through the stroma, spiral vessels extend (unbranched and uncoiled in the early proliferative phase) to a point

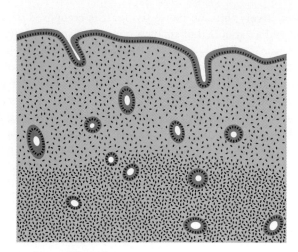

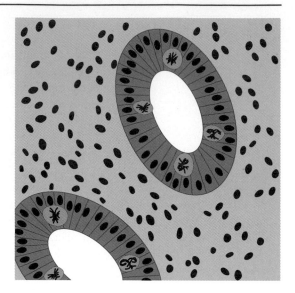

Early Proliferative

immediately below the epithelial binding membrane. Here they form a loose capillary network. All of the tissue components (glands, stromal cells, and endothelial cells) demonstrate proliferation, which peaks on days 8–10 of the cycle, corresponding to peak estradiol levels in the circulation and maximal estrogen receptor concentration in the endometrium.[14] This proliferation is marked by increased mitotic activity and increased nuclear DNA and cytoplasmic RNA synthesis, that is most intense in the functionalis layer in the upper two-thirds of the uterus, the usual site of blastocyst implantation.

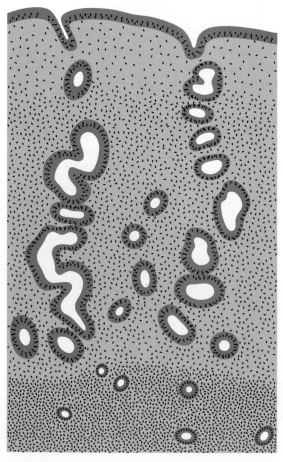

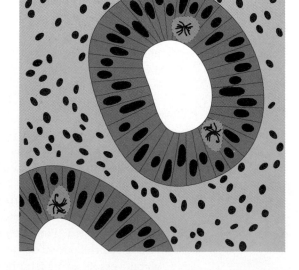

Late Proliferative

During proliferation, the endometrium grows from approximately 0.5 mm to 3.5–5.0 mm in height. This proliferation is mainly in the functionalis layer. Restoration of tissue constituents has been achieved by estrogen-induced new growth as well as incorporation of ions, water, and amino acids. The stromal ground substance has reexpanded from its menstrual collapse. Although true tissue growth has occurred, a major element in achievement of endometrial height is "reinflation" of the stroma.

An important feature of this estrogen dominant phase of endometrial growth is the increase in ciliated and microvillous cells. Ciliogenesis begins on days 7–8 of the cycle.[13] This response to estrogen is exaggerated in hyperplastic endometrium that is the result of hyperestrogenism. The concentration of these ciliated cells around gland openings and the ciliary beat pattern influence the mobilization and distribution of endometrial secretions during the secretory phase. Cell surface microvilli, also a response to estradiol, are cytoplasmic extensions and serve to increase the active surface of cells.

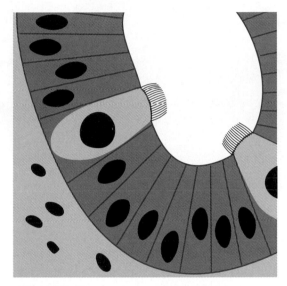

Ciliated Cells

At all times, a large number of cells derived from bone marrow are present in the endometrium. These include lymphocytes and macrophages, diffusely distributed in the stroma.

The Secretory Phase

After ovulation, the endometrium now demonstrates a combined reaction to estrogen and progesterone activity. Most impressive is that total endometrial height is fixed at roughly its preovulatory extent (5–6 mm) despite continued availability of estrogen. Epithelial proliferation ceases 3 days after ovulation.[15] This restraint or inhibition is believed to be induced by progesterone. This limitation of growth is associated with a decline in mitosis and DNA synthesis, significantly due to progesterone interference with estrogen receptor expression and progesterone stimulation of 17β-hydroxysteroid dehydrogenase and sulfotransferase, which convert estradiol to estrone sulfate (which is rapidly excreted from the cell).[16, 17] In addition, estrogen stimulates many oncogenes that probably mediate estrogen-induced growth. Progesterone antagonizes this action by suppressing the estrogen-mediated transcription of oncogene mRNA.[18]

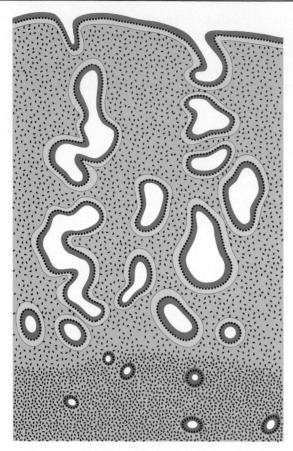

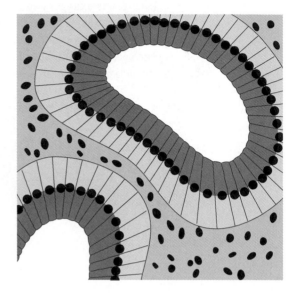

Early Secretory

Individual components of the tissue continue to display growth, but confinement in a fixed structure leads to progressive tortuosity of glands and intensified coiling of the spiral vessels. The secretory events within the glandular cells, with progression of vacuoles from intracellular to intraluminal appearance, are well known and take place over a 7-day postovulatory interval. At the conclusion of these events, the glands appear exhausted, the tortuous lumina variably distended, and individual cell surfaces fragmented in a sawtooth appearance. Stroma is increasingly edematous, and spiral vessels are prominent and densely coiled.

The first histologic sign that ovulation has occurred is the appearance of subnuclear intracytoplasmic glycogen vacuoles in the glandular epithelium on cycle days 17–18. Giant mitochondria and the "nucleolar channel system" appear in the gland cells. The nucleolar channel system has a unique appearance due to progesterone, an infolding of the nuclear membranes. Individual components of the tissue continue to display growth, but confinement in a fixed structure leads to progressive tortuosity of glands and intensified coiling of the spiral vessels. These structural alterations are soon followed by active secretion of glycoproteins and peptides into the endometrial cavity. Transudation of plasma also contributes to the endometrial secretions. Important immunoglobulins are obtained from the circulation and delivered to the endometrial cavity by binding proteins produced by the epithelial cells. The peak secretory level is reached 7 days after the midcycle gonadotropin surge, coinciding with the time of blastocyst implantation.

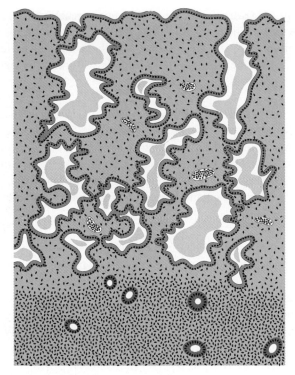

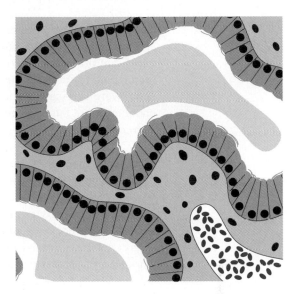

Late Secretory

The Implantation Phase

Significant changes occur within the endometrium from the 7th to the 13th day postovulation (days 21–27 of the cycle). At the onset of this period, the distended tortuous secretory glands have been most prominent with little intervening stroma. By 13 days postovulation, the endometrium has differentiated into three distinct zones. Something less than one-fourth of the tissue is the unchanged basalis fed by its straight vessels and surrounded by indifferent spindle-shaped stroma. The midportion of the endometrium (approximately 50% of the total) is the lace like ***stratum spongiosum***, composed of loose edematous stroma with tightly coiled but ubiquitous spiral vessels and exhausted dilated glandular ribbons. Overlying the spongiosum is the superficial layer of the endometrium (about 25% of the height) called the ***stratum compactum***. Here the prominent histologic feature is the stromal cell, which has become large and polyhedral. In its cytoplasmic expansion one cell abuts the other, forming a compact, structurally sturdy layer. The necks of the glands traversing this segment are compressed and less prominent. The subepithelial capillaries and spiral vessels are engorged.

At the time of implantation, on days 21–22 of the cycle, the predominant morphologic feature is edema of the endometrial stroma. This change may be secondary to the estrogen- and progesterone-mediated increase in prostaglandin production by the endometrium. An increase in capillary permeability is a consequence of this local increase in prostaglandins. Receptors for the sex steroids are present in the muscular walls of the endometrial blood vessels, and the enzyme system for prostaglandin synthesis is present in both the muscular walls and the endothelium of the endometrial arterioles. Mitoses are first seen in endothelial cells on cycle day 22. Vascular proliferation leads to the coiling of the spiral vessels, a response to the sex steroids, the prostaglandins, and to autocrine and paracrine factors produced in response to estrogen and progesterone.

During the secretory phase, so-called K (Körnchenzellen) cells appear, reaching a peak concentration in the first trimester of pregnancy. These are granulocytes that have an immunoprotective role in implantation and placentation. They are located perivascularly and are believed to be derived from the blood. By day 26–27, the endometrial stroma is infiltrated by extravasated polymorphonuclear leukocytes.

The stromal cells of the endometrium respond to hormonal signals, synthesize prostaglandins, and, when transformed into decidual cells, produce an impressive array of substances, some of which are prolactin, relaxin, renin, insulin-like growth factors (IGFs), and insulin-like growth factor binding proteins (IGFBPs). The endometrial stromal cells, the progenitors of decidual cells, were originally believed to be derived from the bone marrow (from cells invading the endometrium), but they are now considered to emanate from the primitive uterine mesenchymal stem cells.[6]

The decidualization process begins in the luteal phase under the influence of progesterone and mediated by autocrine and paracrine factors. On cycle days 22–23, predecidual cells can be identified, initially surrounding blood vessels, characterized by cytonuclear enlargement, increased mitotic activity, and the formation of a basement membrane. The decidua, derived from stromal cells, becomes an important structural and biochemical tissue of pregnancy. Decidual cells control the invasive nature of the trophoblast, and the products of the decidua play important autocrine and paracrine roles in fetal and maternal tissues.

Lockwood assigns a key role to decidual cells in both the process of endometrial bleeding (menstruation) and the process of endometrial hemostasis (implantation and placentation).[19] Implantation requires endometrial hemostasis and the maternal uterus requires resistance to invasion. Inhibition of endometrial hemorrhage can be attributed, to a significant degree, to appropriate changes in critical factors as a consequence of decidualization; e.g., lower plasminogen activator levels, reduced expression of the enzymes that degrade the stromal extracellular matrix (such as the metalloproteinases), and increased levels of plasminogen activator inhibitor-1. Withdrawal of estrogen and progesterone support, however, leads to changes in the opposite directions, consistent with endometrial breakdown.

The Phase of Endometrial Breakdown

Predecidual transformation has formed the "compacta" layer in the upper part of the functionalis layer by day 25 (3 days before menstruation). In the absence of fertilization, implantation, and the consequent lack of sustaining quantities of human chorionic gonadotropin from the trophoblast, the otherwise fixed life span of the corpus luteum is completed, and estrogen and progesterone levels wane.

The withdrawal of estrogen and progesterone initiates important endometrial events: vasomotor reactions, the process of apoptosis, tissue loss, and finally, menstruation. The most prominent immediate effect of this hormone withdrawal is a modest shrinking of the tissue height and remarkable spiral arteriole vasomotor responses. The following vascular sequence has been constructed from direct observations of rhesus endometrium.[7, 8] With shrinkage of height, blood flow within the spiral vessels diminishes, venous drainage is decreased, and vasodilatation ensues. Thereafter, the spiral arterioles undergo rhythmic vasoconstriction and relaxation. Each successive spasm is more prolonged and profound, leading eventually to endometrial blanching.

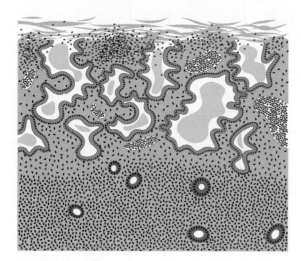 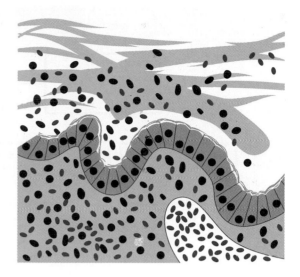

Menstruation

Within the 24 hours immediately preceding menstruation, these reactions lead to endometrial ischemia and stasis. White cells migrate through capillary walls, at first remaining adjacent to vessels, but then extending throughout the stroma. During arteriolar vasomotor changes, red blood cells escape into the interstitial space. Thrombin-platelet plugs also appear in superficial vessels. The prostaglandin content ($PGF_{2\alpha}$ and PGE_2) in the secretory endometrium reaches its highest levels at the time of menstruation. The vasoconstriction and myometrial contractions associated with the menstrual events are believed to be significantly mediated by $PGF_{2\alpha}$ from glandular cells and the potent vasoconstrictor, endothelin-1, derived from stromal decidual cells.

In the first half of the secretory phase, acid phosphatase and potent lytic enzymes are confined to lysosomes. Their release is inhibited by progesterone stabilization of the lysosomal membranes. With the waning of estrogen and progesterone levels, the lysosomal membranes are not maintained, and the enzymes are released into the cytoplasm of epithelial, stromal, and endothelial cells, and eventually into the intercellular space. These active enzymes will digest their cellular constraints, leading to the release of prostaglandins, extravasation of red blood cells, tissue necrosis, and vascular thrombosis. This process is one of *apoptosis*, (programmed cell death, characterized by a specific morphologic pattern that involves cell shrinkage and chromatin condensation culminating in cell fragmentation) mediated by cytokines.[20] An important step in this breakdown is the dissolution of cell to cell adhesion by key proteins. Binding of endometrial epithelial cells utilizes transmembrane proteins, *cadherins*, that link intercellularly with each other and intracellularly with catenins that are bound to actin filaments.[21]

Endometrial tissue breakdown also involves a family of enzymes, matrix metalloproteinases, that degrade components (including collagens, gelatins, fibronectin, and laminin) of the extracellular matrix and basement membrane.[22] The metalloproteinases include collagenases that degrade interstitial and basement membrane collagens, gelatinases that further degrade collagens, and stromelysins that degrade fibronectin, laminin, and glycoproteins. The expression of metalloproteinases in human endometrium follows a pattern correlated with the menstrual cycle, indicating a sex steroid response as part of the growth and remodeling of the endometrium, with a marked increase in late secretory and early menstrual endometrium.[23] Progesterone withdrawal from endometrial cells induces matrix metalloproteinase secretion, which is followed by the breakdown of cellular membranes and the dissolution of extracellular matrix.[24]

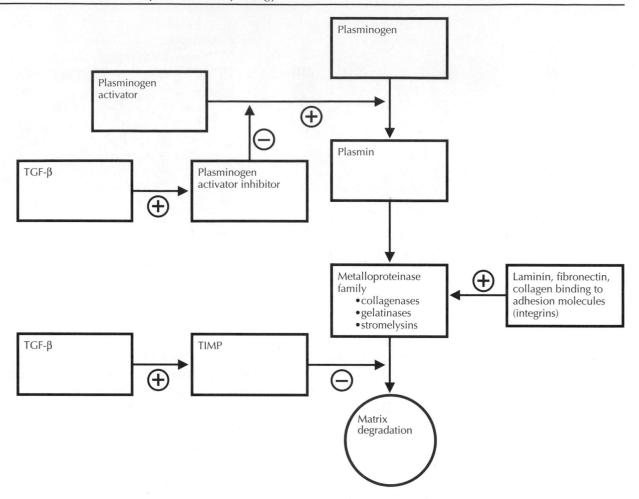

Appropriately, this enzyme expression increases in the decidualized endometrium of the late secretory phase, during the time of declining progesterone levels. With the continuing progesterone secretion of early pregnancy, the decidua is maintained and metalloproteinase expression is suppressed, in a mechanism mediated by TGF-β.[25] In a nonpregnant cycle, metalloproteinase expression is suppressed after menses, presumably by increasing estrogen levels. Metalloproteinase activity is restrained by specific tissue inhibitors designated as TIMP. Thus, progesterone withdrawal can lead to endometrial breakdown through a mechanism that is independent of vascular events (specifically ischemia), a mechanism that involves cytokines.[20] During bleeding, both normal and abnormal, there is evidence indicating that specific genes are activated in the endometrium; one such gene has the structural features of the TGF-β family.[26]

There is considerable evidence to support a major role for a cytokine, tumor necrosis factor-α (TNF-α) in menstruation.[20] TNF-α is a transmembrane protein whose receptor belongs to the nerve growth factor/TNF family for inducing apoptotic signals. The key change is an increase in secretion because TNF-α secretion by endometrial cells reaches a peak at menstruation, but there is no cycle change in receptor content. TNF-α inhibits endometrial proliferation and induces apoptosis; this cytokine causes a loss of adhesion proteins (the cadherin-catenin-actin complex) and induces cell-to-cell dissolution. In addition to endometrial cells, TNF-α also causes damage to vascular endothelium.

Eventually, considerable leakage occurs as a result of diapedesis, and finally, interstitial hemorrhage occurs due to breaks in superficial arterioles and capillaries. As ischemia and weakening progress, the continuous binding membrane is fragmented, and intercellular blood is extruded into the endometrial cavity. New thrombin-platelet plugs form intravascularly upstream at the shedding surface, limiting blood loss. Increased blood loss is a consequence of reduced platelet numbers and inadequate hemostatic plug formation. Menstrual bleeding is influenced by activation of clotting and fibrinolysis. Fibrinolysis is principally the consequence of the potent enzyme, plasmin, formed from its inactive precursor, plasminogen. Endometrial stromal cell tissue factor (TF) and plasminogen activators and inhibitors are involved in achieving a balance in this process. TF stimulates coagulation, initially binding to factor VII. TF and plasminogen activator inhibitor-1 (PAI-1) expression accompanies decidualization, and the levels of these factors may govern the amount of bleeding.[27] PAI-1, in particular, exerts an important restraining action on fibrinolysis and proteolytic activity.[28]

With further tissue disorganization, the endometrium shrinks even more and coiled arterioles are buckled. Additional ischemic breakdown ensues with necrosis of cells and defects in vessels adding to the menstrual effluvium. A natural cleavage point exists between basalis and spongiosum, and, once breached, the loose, vascular, edematous stroma of the spongiosum desquamates and collapses. The process is initiated in the fundus and inexorably extends throughout the uterus. In the end, the typical deflated, shallow, dense, menstrual endometrium results. Within 13 hours, the endometrial height shrinks from 4 mm to 1.25 mm.[12] Menstrual flow stops as a result of the combined effects of prolonged vasoconstriction, tissue collapse, vascular stasis, and estrogen-induced "healing." In contrast to postpartum bleeding, myometrial contractions are not important for control of menstrual bleeding. Thrombin generation in the basal endometrium in response to extravasation of blood is essential for hemostasis. Thrombin promotes the generation of fibrin, the activation of platelets and clotting cofactors, and angiogenesis.

The basalis endometrium remains during menses, and repair takes place from this layer. This endometrium is protected from the lytic enzymes in the menstrual fluid by a mucinous layer of carbohydrate products that are discharged from the glandular and stromal cells.[29]

Normal Menses

Approximately 50% of the menstrual detritus is expelled in the first 24 hours of menstrual flow. The menstrual fluid is composed of the autolysed functionalis, inflammatory exudate, red blood cells, and proteolytic enzymes (at least one of which, plasmin, lyses fibrin clots as they form). The high fibrinolytic activity advances emptying of the uterus by liquefaction of tissue and fibrin. If the rate of flow is great, clotting can and does occur.

Most women (90%) have menstrual cycles with an interval of 24 to 35 days (Chapter 6).[30, 31] Menarche is followed by approximately 5–7 years of increasing regularity as cycles shorten to reach the usual reproductive age pattern. In the 40s, cycles begin to lengthen again. The usual duration of flow is 4–6 days, but many women flow as little as 2 days and as much as 8 days. The normal volume of menstrual blood loss is 30 mL; greater than 80 mL is abnormal (Chapter 15).

Dating the Endometrium

The postovulatory endometrium can be dated according to the histologic changes throughout a hypothetical 28-day menstrual cycle. These changes were described by Noyes, Hertig, and Rock in the lead article of the first volume of *Fertility and Sterility* in 1950.[9] Dating of the endometrium is most accurately accomplished with biopsy specimens obtained 2–3 days before the onset of menses. This method continues to be the most accepted way to diagnose an inadequate luteal phase (endometrium inadequate to sustain a pregnancy because of deficient progesterone secretion by the corpus luteum).

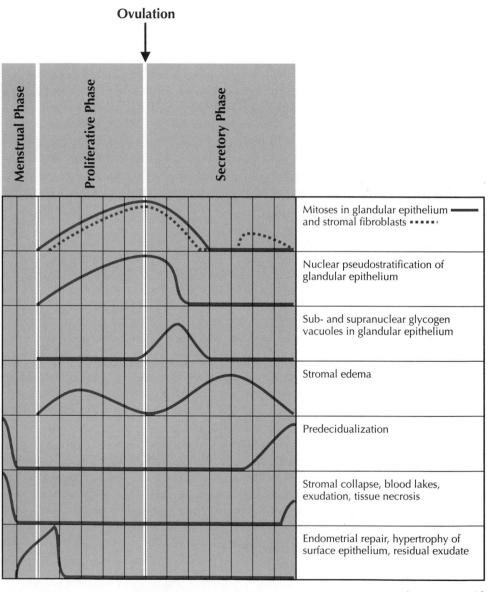

After Noyes, et al [9]

A Teleologic Theory of Endometrial-Menstrual Events

Menstruation is a very recent phenomenon in the evolutionary time line. It occurs in very few species, even among viviparous animals. An unabashedly teleologic view of menstrual events was offered by Rock et al.[32] The basic premise of this thesis is that every endometrial cycle has, as its only goal, nourishing support of an early embryo. Failure to accomplish this objective is followed by orderly elimination of unutilized tissue and prompt renewal to achieve a more successful cycle.

The ovum must be fertilized within 12–24 hours of ovulation. Over the next 2 days, it remains unattached within the tubal lumen utilizing tubal fluids and residual cumulus cells to sustain nutrition and energy for early cellular cleavage. After this stay, the solid ball of cells (morula) which is the embryo leaves the tube and enters the uterine cavity. Here the embryo undergoes another 2–3 days of unattached but active existence. Fortunately, by this time endometrial gland secretions have filled the cavity and they bathe the embryo in nutrients. This is the first of many neatly synchronized events that mark the conceptus-endometrial relationship. By 6 days after ovulation, the embryo (now a blastocyst) is ready to attach and implant. At this time, it finds an endometrial lining of sufficient depth, vascularity, and nutritional richness to sustain the important events of early placentation to follow. Just below the epithelial lining, a rich capillary plexus has been formed and is available for creation of the trophoblast-maternal blood interface. Later, the surrounding zona compactum, occupying more and more of the endometrium, will provide a sturdy splint to retain endometrial architecture despite the invasive inroads of the burgeoning trophoblast.

Failure of the appearance of human chorionic gonadotropin, despite otherwise appropriate tissue reactions, leads to the vasomotor changes associated with estrogen-progesterone withdrawal and menstrual desquamation. However, not all the tissue is lost, and, in any event, a residual basalis is always available, making resumption of growth with estrogen a relatively rapid process. Indeed, even as menses persists, early regeneration can be seen. As soon as follicle maturation occurs (in as short a time as 10 days), the endometrium is ready once again to perform its reproductive function.

The Uterus Is an Endocrine Organ

The uterus is dynamic. It not only responds and changes in a sensitive fashion to classic hormonal signals (the endocrine events of the menstrual cycle), but it is also composed of complex tissues, with important autocrine and paracrine functions that serve not only the uterus but the contiguous tissues of the fetoplacental unit during pregnancy. The most dynamic component of the uterus is the endometrium.

Endometrial Products

The endometrium secretes many substances, the functions of which (and their interrelationships) represent a major investigative challenge.[33] In addition to producing a nourishing, supportive environment for the early embryo, the endometrium plays an important role in suppressing the immune response within the pregnant uterus. The mechanisms controlling the immune response in decidual cells are not understood, but hormonal influence is undoubtedly important.

Lipids	Cytokines	Peptides
Prostaglandins	Interleukin-1α	Prolactin
Thromboxanes	Interleukin-1β	Relaxin
Leukotrienes	Interleukin-6	Prorenin and renin
	Interferon-γ	Endorphin
	Colony-stimulating factor-1	Endothelin-1
	Tumor necrosis factor-α	Corticotropin-releasing hormone
	Leukemia-inhibiting factor	Fibronectin
		Uteroglobin
		Lipocortin-1
		Parathyroid hormone-like protein
		Integrins
		Epidermal growth factor family
		EGF
		Heparin-binding EGF
		TGF-α
		Insulin-like growth factor family
		IGF-I
		IGF-II
		IGFBPs 1–6
		Platelet-derived growth factor
		Transforming growth factor-β
		Fibroblast growth factor
		Vascular endothelial growth factor

The presence of the cytokine family, involved in inflammation and immune responses, is not surprising in a tissue that undergoes cyclic degeneration. The interleukins stimulate prostaglandin production as well as other cytokines.[34] Colony-stimulating factor-1 is a cytokine that influences cellular proliferation and the presence of macrophages. Interferon-γ is produced by activated T-lymphocytes and inhibits endometrial epithelial proliferation. Leukemia-inhibiting factor (LIF) is expressed in response to a variety of other cytokines and growth factors. Like the interleukins, LIF is most abundant during the progesterone-dominated secretory phase and early decidua, and may have a role in embryo implantation.[35, 36] Tumor necrosis factor-α (TNF-α) gene expression is present in endometrium, and its activity is increased during the proliferative phase, decreased early in the secretory phase, and increased again in the midsecretory phase.[37] TNF-α exerts multiple influences on cellular growth.

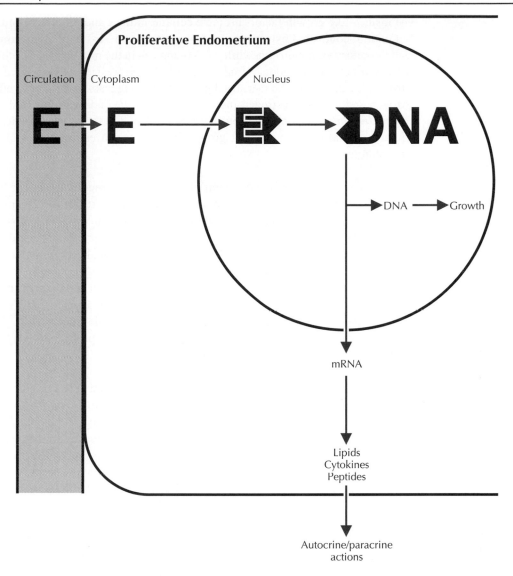

Growth factors are peptides that bind to specific cell membrane receptors and initiate intracellular signaling pathways. Because the growth factors are potent mitogens, it is also not surprising that the follicular phase of the cycle, associated with proliferative activity of the endometrium, is marked by dramatic alterations in growth factors. Estrogen stimulates gene expression for epidermal growth factor (EGF) (and its receptor) and insulin-like growth factor (IGF) production. In turn, EGF elicits estrogen-like actions by interacting with the estrogen receptor mechanism.[38] EGF, a potent mitogen, is present in endometrial stromal and epithelial cells during the follicular phase of the cycle and in the stromal cells during the luteal phase.[39] Transforming growth factor-α (TGF-α) and EGF work through the same receptor and are important mediators of estrogen-induced growth of the endometrium. TGF-α levels peak at midcycle, in contrast to EGF levels, which are relatively stable and noncyclic.[40–42] Platelet-derived growth factor is a potent mitogen localized to stromal cells.

The insulin-like growth factors promote cellular mitosis and differentiation. They are expressed in a pattern controlled by estrogen and progesterone. IGF-I is predominant in proliferative and early secretory endometrium, while IGF-II appears in the mid to late secretory phase and persists in early pregnancy decidua.[43] Endometrial IGF-I expression is correlated with the circulating estrogen levels during the menstrual cycle.[44] This suggests that IGF-I synthesis is regulated by estrogen and mediates estrogen-induced growth of the endometrium, and IGF-II is involved in differentiation in response to progesterone. Evidence in the monkey indicates that IGF-I is the primary regulator of myometrial growth in response to estrogen as well as to estrogen plus progesterone.[45]

As elsewhere in the body, the myometrial IGF activity is modulated by the IGF binding proteins, which respond to the sex steroids in a differential manner; IGFBP-2 parallels IGF-I response, whereas IGFBP-3 is decreased in muscle but increased in vascular endothelium by estrogen.[46] IGFBP-4 and IGFBP-5 respond to estrogen but are unaffected by the addition of progesterone. IGFBP-1, as discussed later, is a major product of decidualized endometrium.

Human myometrial smooth muscle and endometrial stromal cells express mRNA for parathyroid hormone-like protein, the function of which is unknown.[47] Transforming growth factor-β (TGF-β) stimulates the production of the parathyroid hormone-like protein. TGF-β production is greatest in the secretory phase and may inhibit cellular proliferation by increasing IGFBP-3 synthesis.

Prostaglandins are produced by both epithelial and stromal cells, and the prostaglandin content in the endometrium reaches a peak level in late secretory endometrium. The predominant prostaglandin produced by endometrium is prostaglandin $F_{2\alpha}$, a potent stimulus for myometrial contractions.[48] Endometrial prostaglandin production decreases dramatically after implantation, suggesting the presence of an active mechanism for suppression.[49] The production of prostaglandins requires estrogen support, but the increased production by secretory endometrium suggests progesterone enhancement, and acute withdrawal of progesterone promotes a further increase.[48] Endometrial stromal cells produce prostacyclin and thromboxane in response to estrogen, a response that can be blocked by progestins.[50] The myometrium principally produces prostacyclin, utilizing precursors derived from the endometrium. However, receptors for all members of the prostaglandin family are present on human myometrial cells, and contraction of the myometrium is a major consequence of prostaglandin $F_{2\alpha}$.[51]

Thromboxane is synthesized by uterine tissues. Gene expression for the thromboxane synthase and for the thromboxane receptor can be identified in endometrial glands, stromal cells, myometrial smooth muscle, and uterine blood vessels.[52] Thromboxane A_2 is a potent vasoconstrictor and stimulator of smooth muscle cells. Because of its rapid metabolism, it is limited to autocrine and paracrine activity.

Women with excessive menstrual bleeding have alterations in the normal rates of prostaglandin production. For this reason, effective reductions in menstrual blood loss can be achieved with treatment utilizing one of the nonsteroidal anti-inflammatory agents that inhibit prostaglandin synthesis. These agents are also effective treatment for prostaglandin-mediated dysmenorrhea.

Fibronectin and laminin are extracellular matrix substances that are secreted by stromal cells of the endometrium in response to progesterone.[53] These proteins are important adhesion molecules during implantation. Integrins are a family of glycoproteins that function as receptors for proteins such as collagen, fibronectin, and laminin. The integrins are highly expressed in endometrium and are important for cell-to-cell and cell-to-matrix interactions.[54] The expression of integrins appears to be regulated by cytokines and growth factors, not estrogen and progesterone.[55]

Uteroglobin is a small protein expressed in endometrial epithelial cells.[56] The physiologic function of uteroglobin is uncertain. Uteroglobin, with high affinity, binds progestins and may play a role in immunosuppression. Uteroglobin gene expression is stimulated by estrogen, and this response is enhanced by progesterone. Human endometrium can secrete β-endorphin, yet another candidate for involvement in endometrial immunologic events, and its release is inhibited by both estrogens and glucocorticoids.[57]

Endothelins are potent vasoconstrictors produced in the vascular endothelial cells. The vasoconstrictor activity of endothelin-1, present in the endometrium, is balanced by the fact that it promotes the synthesis of the vasodilators, nitric oxide and prostacyclin. Endothelin-1 is synthesized in endometrial stromal cells and the glandular epithelium, stimulated by both TGF-β and interleukin-1α.[58] Endothelin-1 is at least one agent responsible for the vasoconstriction that shuts off menstrual bleeding. It is also a potent stimulator of myometrial contractions and can contribute to dysmenorrhea. Finally, endothelin-1 is a mitogen and can promote the healing reepithelialization of the endometrium. Human decidual cells also synthesize and secrete endothelin-1, from where it may be transported into the amniotic fluid.[59]

Angiogenesis, the formation of new blood vessels, is an essential process in tissue growth and development. Angiogenesis is necessary for tumor growth, and in normal tissues, it is usually kept in check by regulating factors. The female reproductive tissues (specifically ovarian follicles, the trophoblast, and the endometrium), however, must experience periodic and rapid growth and regression. In these tissues, angiogenesis is part of normal events. The endometrium is a major source for angiogenic factors during the menstrual cycle and during pregnancy.[60] Vascular endothelial growth factor, a specific mitogen for endothelial cells, is abundantly expressed in human endometrium, reaching a peak that correlates with the maximal angiogenesis reached during the secretory phase.[61] Angiogenesis is also influenced by many of the growth factors, and other substances such as fibronectin and prostaglandins. Fibroblast growth factor, in particular, is highly mitogenic for endothelial cells as well as endometrial stromal cells.

In all types of endometrial and myometrial cells, estrogen receptor expression reaches a maximum in the late follicular phase.[62, 63] The concentration is greatest in the glandular epithelium. During the early luteal phase, estrogen receptor expression declines, followed by an increase in the mid and late luteal phases. These changes reflect the cyclic changes in estradiol (which increases estrogen receptor expression) and progesterone (which decreases estrogen receptor expression).

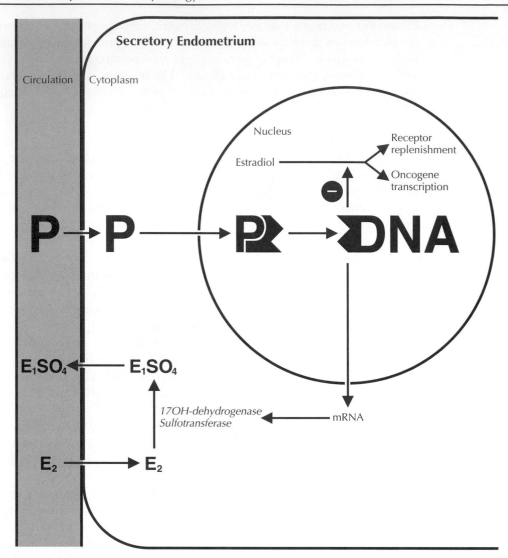

Progesterone receptor expression in endometrial glandular epithelium reaches a maximum in the late follicular and early luteal phases (reflecting induction of progesterone receptor by estrogen), and then declines to nearly undetectable levels by the midpoint of the secretory phase. Stromal cells in the endometrium show only minor fluctuations in progesterone receptors during the menstrual cycle. Decidualizing stromal cells exhibit strong progesterone receptor expression, although progesterone receptors are absent from decidual epithelial cells. Smooth muscle cells of the uterus demonstrate strong progesterone receptor expression throughout the menstrual cycle. Many of the events in uterine growth and function are regulated by the interplay between estrogen and progesterone. In general, progesterone antagonizes estrogen stimulation of proliferation and metabolism. This antagonism can be explained by the effects of progestins on the estrogen receptor (a decrease in levels) and on the enzymes that lead to excretion of estrogen from cells and by progesterone suppression of estrogen-mediated transcription of oncogenes.

Androgen receptor is present in endometrium at all stages of the menstrual cycle, in postmenopausal endometrium, and in the decidua of pregnancy.[64] Surprisingly, the androgen receptor concentration is constant throughout the cycle.

The Decidua

The decidua is the specialized endometrium of pregnancy. The biochemical dialogue between the fetoplacental unit and the mother must pass back and forth through the decidua. The classic view of the decidua conformed to its designation as a thin line in anatomical diagrams, a minor, inactive structural component. We now know that the decidua is a vigorous, active tissue.

The glycoprotein α-subunit, common to follicle-stimulating hormone (FSH), luteinizing hormone (LH), thyroid-stimulating hormone (TSH), and HCG, is secreted into the circulation by the pituitary and placenta. A specific role for the α-subunit has not been apparent; however, gonadotropin receptors are present in the endometrium and in vitro, α-subunit acts synergistically with progesterone to induce decidualization of endometrial cells.[65] In addition, the α-subunit stimulates decidual prolactin secretion.[66]

Decidual cells are derived from the stroma cells of the endometrium, under the stimulation of progesterone. Thus, they appear during the luteal phase and continue to proliferate during early pregnancy, eventually lining the entire uterus, including the implantation site. The decidual cell is characterized by the accumulation of glycogen and lipid droplets and the new expression of a host of substances, including prolactin, relaxin, renin, insulin-like growth factors (IGFs), and insulin-like growth factor binding proteins (IGFBPs). There is no evidence that these proteins are secreted into the circulation, therefore they serve as autocrine and paracrine agents.[67, 68]

Riddick was the first to detect prolactin in the decidualizing endometrium of the late luteal phase.[69] The amino acid sequence and the chemical and biological properties of decidual prolactin are identical to those of pituitary prolactin. Decidual prolactin synthesis and release are controlled by the placenta, fetal membranes, and decidual factors. Dopamine, bromocriptine, and thyroid-releasing hormone (TRH), in contrast to their action in the pituitary, have no effect on decidual synthesis and release of prolactin. A protein named decidual prolactin-releasing factor has been purified from the placenta, and an inhibiting protein, which blocks the stimulatory activity of the releasing factor, has been purified from decidua.[68] IGF-1, relaxin, and insulin all stimulate decidual prolactin synthesis and release, each through its own receptor. The same decidual cells produce both prolactin and relaxin.

Lipocortin-1 is a calcium and phospholipid binding protein, present in the placenta and decidua, that inhibits phospholipase A_2 and responds to glucocorticoids. Lipocortin-1 inhibits decidual prolactin release but in a mechanism independent of phospholipase action and independent of glucocorticoids. The prostaglandin system is not involved in decidual prolactin production, and corticoid steroids do not affect decidual prolactin release.[70]

There is good reason to believe that the amniotic fluid prolactin is derived from the decidua. In vitro experiments indicate that the passage of prolactin across the fetal membranes is in the direction of the amniotic cavity. The amniotic fluid concentration correlates with the decidual content, not maternal circulating levels. Amniotic fluid prolactin reaches peak levels in the first half of gestation (about 4000 ng/mL) when maternal plasma levels are approximately 50 ng/mL and fetal levels about 10 ng/mL. Maternal circulating prolactin reaches maximal levels near term. Finally, amniotic fluid prolactin is unaffected by bromocriptine treatment (which reduces both fetal and maternal circulating levels to baseline levels).

It is believed that decidual prolactin regulates amniotic fluid volume and electrolyte concentrations. It can be demonstrated that prolactin regulates water and ion transport in lower animals, and prolactin binds to amniotic membranes. Disorders in human pregnancy associated with abnormal amniotic fluid volumes may be explained by this mechanism, especially idiopathic polyhydramnios (which is associated with a decrease in the number of prolactin receptors in the membranes). Prolactin may be involved in the regulation of surfactant synthesis in the fetus, and prolactin may inhibit uterine muscle contractility. Prolactin suppresses the immune response and contributes to the prevention of immunologic rejection of the conceptus. Prolactin can also function as an autocrine and paracrine growth factor in the uterus.[71]

Fibroblast growth factor, derived from decidua, stimulates blood vessel growth in early pregnancy. Another factor, endothelial-cell-stimulating angiogenesis factor (a nonprotein mitogen), is also derived from decidua and contributes to the vascularization of the decidua during the first trimester of pregnancy.[72] The expression of corticotropin-releasing hormone (CRH) has been demonstrated in human decidua, and many actions for decidual CRH are possible: activation of prostaglandins, stimulation of myometrial contractions, and a contribution to both maternal and fetal stress responses during pregnancy and labor.[73]

Prorenin (the inactive precursor of renin) is produced in decidua in response to IGF-1, insulin, endothelin, and relaxin.[74, 75] A uterine role for renin has not been determined. The insulin-like growth factor binding proteins, IGFBP-1, -2, -3, and -4, are produced by endometrial stromal cells.[76] Large amounts of IGFBP-1 are present in amniotic fluid. The IGFBPs appear to be regulated by insulin, the IGFs, and relaxin.[77] Relaxin is related structurally to insulin and the IGFs. However, in contrast to insulin and IGF, it stimulates IGFBP-1 production in endometrial stromal cells.[78]

IGFBP-1 begins to appear in midluteal phase endometrium and reaches a level of major production in decidua by late in the first trimester of pregnancy. IGFBP-1, when first identified, was known as placental protein 12 and then as pregnancy-associated α-globulin. By the second trimester of pregnancy, high levels of IGFBP-1 are present in the amniotic fluid and the circulation, which then fall significantly during the third trimester. The decidual production of IGFBP-1 is correlated with the morphologic and histologic changes induced by progesterone and regulated by progesterone, relaxin, insulin, IGF-I, and IGF-II. Binding of the insulin-like growth factors to the IGFBPs would limit further mitogenic activity in the endometrium in the secretory phase and during pregnancy. In addition, decidual IGFBP-1 may contribute to the limitation of trophoblast invasion.

The continuous stimulation of IGFBP-1 production by human endometrium can be maintained in women as long as they retain an intrauterine device that releases a progestin into the endometrial cavity.[79] In endometrial samples from these women, areas of endometrial atrophy correlate with intense staining for IGFBP-1. This makes a strong argument for the importance of insulin-like growth factors for endometrial growth and the potential for prevention of endometrial growth by providing IGFBP-1.

The chorion laeve, villous trophoblast, and decidua are all sites of TGF-β production.[80] TGF-β can signal its own production; thus, TGF-β can be a messenger from fetal tissues to decidua. TGF-β is also believed to play a role in limiting trophoblastic invasion.[81] This may be accomplished by stimulating the production of plasminogen activator inhibitor and the factor that causes tissue inhibition of metalloproteinases.[82]

Summary: The Uterus Is an Endocrine Organ

One cannot dispute the fact that the uterus is an endocrine organ, but the vast array of active substances can be bewildering and overwhelming. It is helpful to keep in mind a fundamental and relatively simple description: the endometrium is necessary for reproduction, and the synchronous, complex cycle of events is dependent on the endocrine guidance of estradiol and progesterone, modulated and mediated by the plethora of locally produced biochemical agents. Each and every signaling substance utilizes one of the pathways discussed in Chapter 2, and makes a contribution to the dynamic sequence of morphological and biochemical events repeatedly dedicated to nourishing and supporting an early embryo.

Anatomical Abnormalities of the Uterus

Congenital abnormalities of the müllerian ducts are relatively common and contribute to the problems of infertility, recurrent pregnancy loss, and poor outcome in pregnancy (encountered in approximately 25% of women with uterine anomalies).[83–86] The problems encountered in pregnancy include preterm labor, breech presentations, and complications that lead to interventions and greater perinatal mortality. Cervical cerclage is often indicated for prevention of preterm labor due to these anomalies. In addition, these abnormalities can produce the symptoms of dysmenorrhea and dyspareunia, and even amenorrhea. Because the embryologic origin of the ovaries is separate and distinct from that of the müllerian structures, patients with müllerian anomalies have normal ovaries and ovarian function.

Incidence of Müllerian Defects[87]

Overall	5%
Fertile women	2–3%
Infertile women	3%
Women with recurrent miscarriages	5–10%
Women with late miscarriages and preterm deliveries	>25%

Anomalies can originate in the failure of the müllerian ducts to fuse in the midline, to connect with the urogenital sinus, or to create the appropriate lumen in the upper vagina and uterus by resorption of the central vaginal cells and the septum between the fused müllerian ducts. Because fusion begins in the midline and extends caudally and cephalad, abnormal results can exist at either end. Formation of the uterine cavity begins at the lower pole and extends cephalad with dissolution of midline tissue; hence, incomplete resorption of tissue commonly yields persistence of the midline uterine wall intruding into the cavity. The molecular pathophysiology of these abnormalities has been insufficiently studied; however, the association with other somatic anomalies and occasional reports of familial transmission suggest genetic linkages.

Vaginal outflow tract obstruction can be minimal with a transverse septum or complete due to agenesis. A septum is the result of a defect in the connection of the fused müllerian ducts to the urogenital sinus or a failure of canalization of the vagina. The location of the septum varies, although it is usually in the upper or middle third of the vagina. Vaginal agenesis is the result of a complete failure in canalization; these patients present with amenorrhea or pain due to accumulated menstrual effluvium. Surgical correction is frequently necessary to relieve the relative constriction (and obstruction) of the vaginal canal. An absent vagina is usually accompanied by an absent uterus and tubes, the classic müllerian agenesis of the Mayer-Rokitansky-Kuster-Hauser syndrome (discussed in Chapter 11).

Distribution of Specific Anomalies[87]

Bicornuate uterus	37%
Arcuate uterus	15%
Incomplete septum	13%
Uterus didelphys	11%
Complete septum	9%
Unicornuate uterus	4.4%

Uterine anomalies can be organized into the following categories.[88] Each of these can be associated with obstructions that present during adolescence with amenorrhea and cyclic pain.[89]

Unicornuate Uterus

An abnormality that is unilateral obviously is due to a failure of development in one müllerian duct (probably a failure of one duct to migrate to the proper location). The altered uterine configuration is associated with an increase in obstetrical complications (early spontaneous miscarriage, ectopic pregnancy, abnormal presentations, intrauterine growth retardation, and

Classification of Müllerian Anomalies [88]

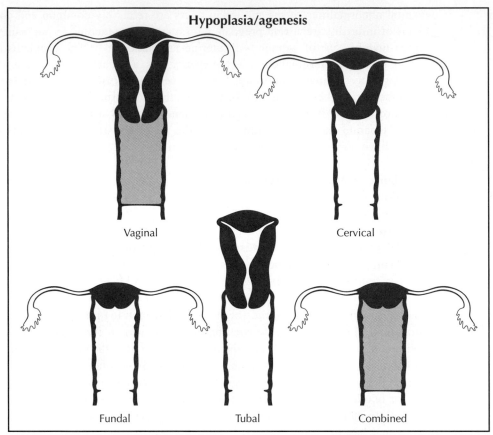

Hypoplasia/agenesis

Vaginal

Cervical

Fundal

Tubal

Combined

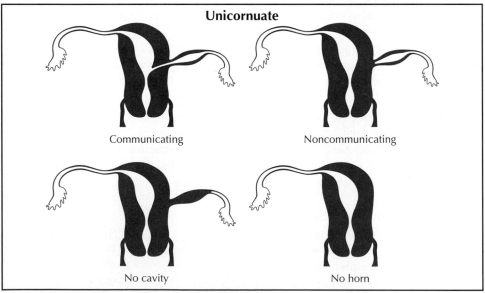

Unicornuate

Communicating

Noncommunicating

No cavity

No horn

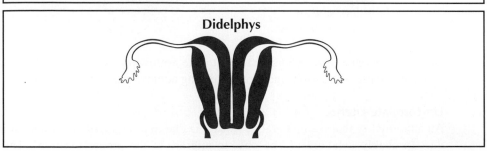

Didelphys

Classification of Müllerian Anomalies [88]

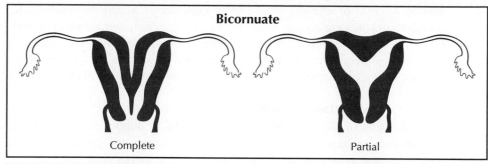

Bicornuate

Complete   Partial

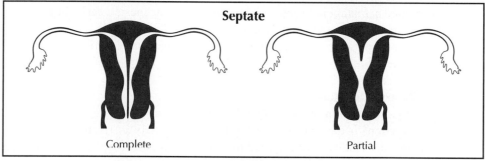

Septate

Complete   Partial

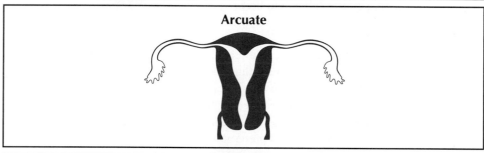

Arcuate

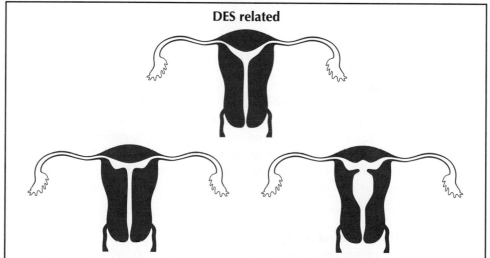

DES related

premature labor).[90–92] There may be a rudimentary horn present, and implantation in this horn is followed by a very high rate of pregnancy wastage or tubal pregnancies. A rudimentary horn can also be a cause of chronic pain, and surgical excision may be worthwhile. However, most rudimentary horns are asymptomatic because they are non-communicating, and the endometrium is not functional. Because of the potential for problems, prophylactic removal of the rudimentary horn is recommended when it is encountered during a surgical procedure. Approximately 40% of patients with a unicornuate uterus will have a urinary tract anomaly (usually of the kidney).[93]

Uterus Didelphus (Double Uterus)

Lack of fusion of the two müllerian ducts results in duplication of corpus and cervix. These patients usually have no difficulties with menstruation and coitus. Occasionally, one side is obstructed and symptomatic. In addition, a double uterus is occasionally associated with an obstructed hemivagina (often with ipsilateral renal agenesis); early diagnosis and excision of the obstructing vaginal septum will preserve fertility. Pregnancy is associated with an increased risk of malpresentations and premature labor, although many patients will have no reproductive difficulties.[92]

The Bicornuate Uterus

Partial lack of fusion of the two müllerian ducts produces a single cervix with a varying degree of separation in the two uterine horns. This anomaly is relatively common, and pregnancy outcome has usually been reported to be near normal. Some, however, find a high rate of early miscarriage, preterm labor, and breech presentations.[86, 92]

The Septate Uterus

Partial lack of resorption of the midline septum between the two müllerian ducts results in defects that range from a slight midline septum (the arcuate, heart-shaped cavity) to a significant midline division of the endometrial cavity. A total failure in resorption can leave a longitudinal vaginal septum (a double vagina). This defect is not a cause of infertility, but once pregnant, the greater the septum the greater the risk of recurrent spontaneous miscarriage. The complete septate uterus is associated with a high risk of preterm labor and breech presentation.[86] Outcomes are excellent with treatment by hysteroscopy.[94, 95] Posttreatment miscarriage rates are approximately 10% in contrast to the 90% pretreatment rates. A longitudinal vaginal septum usually does not have to be excised (unless dyspareunia is a problem). In some reports, the arcuate uterus had no adverse impact on reproductive outcome.[92]

Very Rare Anomalies

Isolated agenesis of the cervix or the endometrium is incredibly rare. Absence of the cervix can lead to so much pain and obstruction that hysterectomy is the best solution. Attempts to preserve fertility by creating a fistulous communication between uterus and vagina have achieved little success, and repeat surgery due to reappearance of obstruction is common.[96] In asymptomatic patients, consideration should be given to preservation of structures for the possibility of pregnancy that can be achieved by means of one of the techniques of assisted reproduction. (Chapter 31)

The Diethylstilbestrol-Associated Anomaly

We are still encountering women whose mothers were treated with high doses of estrogen during their pregnancies. Exposure to these high levels of estrogen during müllerian development caused a variety of anomalies, ranging from the hypoplastic "T" shaped uterus to irregular cavities with adhesions.[97] Women with uterine abnormalities usually also have cervical defects. In these individuals, the chance of term pregnancy is decreased because of higher risks of ectopic pregnancy, spontaneous miscarriage, and premature labor. An incompetent cervix is common. Poor outcome is correlated with an abnormal uterus on hysterosalpingography. No treatment is available beyond cervical cerclage.

Accurate Diagnosis of Anomalies

In the past, full diagnosis has required surgical intervention, first laparotomy and then, more recently, laparoscopy. Today, vaginal ultrasonography and magnetic resonance imaging are highly accurate, and surgical intervention is usually not necessary.[98] Hysterosalpingography is relatively inaccurate, and decisions should not be based upon hysterosalpingography alone. Congenital anomalies of the müllerian ducts are frequently accompanied by abnormalities in the urinary tract. Renal agenesis is often present on the same side as a müllerian defect.

Leiomyomata (Uterine Fibroids)

Uterine leiomyomas are benign neoplasms that arise from uterine smooth muscle. It is hypothesized that leiomyomas originate from somatic mutations in myometrial cells, resulting in progressive loss of growth regulation.[99, 100] The tumor grows as genetically abnormal clones of cells derived from a single progenitor cell (in which the original mutation took place). Studies indicate that leiomyomas are monoclonal. Different rates of growth can reflect the different cytogenetic abnormalities present in individual tumors. Multiple myomas within the same uterus are not clonally related; each myoma arises independently. The presence of multiple myomas (which have a higher recurrence rate than single myomas) argues in favor of a genetic predisposition for myoma formation; however, the familial inheritance of uterine myomas has not been well studied. It is not certain whether leiomyosarcomas arise independently or from leiomyomas. However, the incidence of leiomyosarcomas in patients with leiomyomata is very low (less than 1%).[101]

If surgical specimens are serially sectioned, about 77% of women who come to hysterectomy will have myomas, many of which are occult.[102] Overall, about 17% of hysterectomies are performed for myomas in the U.S. (44% in women 45–54 years old).[103] The peak incidence for myomas requiring surgery occurs around age 45, approximately 8 cases per 1000 women each year. In the U.S., approximately 10–15% of women require hysterectomy for myomas. For unknown reasons, uterine leiomyomas are 2–3 times more prevalent in black women compared with white, Hispanic, and Asian women.[104] The major symptoms associated with myomas are menorrhagia and the physical effects produced by large myomas.

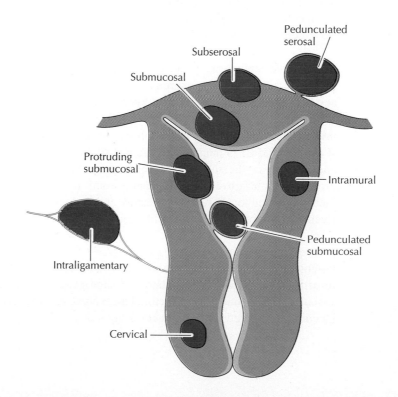

Myomas will be encountered in about 1% of pregnant women. The risk of myoma is decreased with increasing parity and with increasing age at last term birth.[105] Women with at least two full term pregnancies have half the risk for myomas. Smoking decreases the risk (presumably by decreasing estrogen levels), and obesity increases the risk (presumably by increasing estrogen levels). Although a lower risk for myomas is associated with factors that decrease estrogen levels, including leanness, smoking, and exercise, the use of oral contraceptives is not associated with an increased risk of uterine myomas, although the Nurses' Health Study reported a slightly increased risk when oral contraceptives were first used in early teenage years.[105–107]

The hormone sensitivity of leiomyomas is indicated by the following clinical observations. Leiomyomas develop during the reproductive (hormonally active) years and regress after menopause. Occasionally, leiomyomas grow during pregnancy, and the hypogonadal state induced by treatment with gonadotropin-releasing hormone (GnRH) agonists often causes shrinkage of myomas.

The environment within the leiomyoma is hyperestrogenic. The estradiol concentration is increased, and leiomyomas contain more estrogen and progesterone receptors.[108–110] Aromatase gene and enzyme expression are present in significant levels in leiomyomata.[111] Indeed, leiomyoma tissue is hypersensitive to estrogen and appears to have lost a regulatory influence that limits estrogen response.[112] Endometrial hyperplasia is frequently observed at the margins of submucous myomas.[113] In the myometrium and in leiomyomas, peak mitotic activity occurs during the luteal phase, and mitotic activity is increased by the administration of high doses of progestational agents.[114, 115] These facts indicate that progesterone stimulates mitotic activity in leiomyomas, but animal studies indicate both stimulation and inhibition of myometrial growth. Similarly, clinicians have reported both regression and growth with progestational treatment. Nevertheless, most of the evidence supports a growth-promoting role for progestins (the association with estrogen can be explained by the estrogen enhancement of progesterone receptor expression).[116, 117] Treatment with RU486, the progesterone antagonist, is associated with a reduction in leiomyomata size.[118]

The *bcl-2* protooncogene, presumably a cell survival gene, produces a protein that prevents apoptosis and promotes cell replication. Bcl-2 protein expression is increased in leiomyoma cells, and markedly increases in response to progesterone.[119] In contrast, normal myometrial cells do not respond to estradiol or progesterone with Bcl-2 protein expression, and there is no cyclic change throughout the menstrual cycle. This further supports a key role for progestins in leiomyoma growth.

As in the normal uterus, the effects of estrogen and progestins on leiomyomata are mediated by growth factors.[120] EGF is overexpressed in myomas, EGF receptors are present in leiomyomata, and GnRH agonist treatment (and hypogonadism) decreases EGF concentration in myomas (but not in normal myometrium).[121, 122] IGF-I and IGF-II and their receptors are abundant in myometrium, and actively overexpressed in leiomyomas.[123, 124] Leiomyomas express more IGF-II and less IGFBP-3 than myometrium, a situation that would enhance growth factor availability and activity in the tumor.[125] Leiomyomata cells express more parathyroid hormone-related protein (another growth factor) than normal myometrium.[126] Like the endometrium and myometrium, leiomyomas secrete prolactin, and prolactin functions in the uterus as a growth factor.[71] Even hematopoiesis is possible in a leiomyoma.[127]

One of the consequences of altered growth factor expression in myomas is an abnormal vasculature, characterized by a dilated venous plexus.[128] This morphologic feature may be the result of specific vascular regulators of angiogenesis, such as basic fibroblast growth factor and vascular endothelial growth factor. These changes probably contribute to the heavy menstrual bleeding associated with submucosal myomas.

Reproductive Function and Leiomyomata

Leiomyomas are an infrequent cause of infertility, either by mechanical obstruction or distortion (and interference with implantation).[129] When a mechanical obstruction of fallopian tubes, cervical canal, or endometrial cavity is present and no other cause of infertility or recurrent miscarriage can be identified, myomectomy is usually followed by a prompt achievement of pregnancy in a high percentage of patients (usually within the first year).[130] Submucous myomas are best treated by hysteroscopic resection. Preoperative visualization is important, and mapping of myomas by magnetic resonance imaging (MRI) is superior to ultrasonography (which is relatively inaccurate).[131] It is difficult to distinguish between submucous myomas and endometrial polyps with ultrasonography.[132] Very large myomas (greater than 4–5 cm) and myomas that do not have greater than 50% protrusion into the cavity are not good candidates for hysteroscopic removal.

The short-term recurrence rate after myomectomy (either abdominal myomectomy or hysteroscopic resection) is about 15%, with subsequent hysterectomy necessary in 1–5% of patients.[133] In a series with long-term follow-up, the recurrence rate over 10 years reached 27%.[134] Women who gave birth after myomectomy had a recurrence rate (over 10 years) of 16%, compared to a rate of 28% in those who did not give birth. In an Italian study of recurrence, the rate at 5 years reached 55% in those who did gave birth after surgery and 42% in those with no childbirth.[135] These differences may reflect the diligence and sensitivity of the ultrasonographic assessments.

An increased incidence of spontaneous miscarriage because of myomas has not been definitively documented in the literature. Myomectomy for infertility or recurrent miscarriage requires a deliberate and careful decision after all factors have been considered. Intracavitary myomas, however, usually require surgery. Because of the rapid regrowth of myomas following cessation of GnRH agonist therapy, medical therapy for infertility is not recommended.

Myomas are present (diagnosed by ultrasonography) in about 1–2% f pregnancies.[136] Most myomas do not grow during pregnancy.[137] When they do, most of the growth is in the first trimester, and most myomas regress in size after the pregnancy. The size of a myoma will not predict its course; large myomas will not necessarily grow more than small ones. Most pregnancies, in the presence of myomas, will, therefore, be uncomplicated (although a higher incidence of cesarean section has been observed).[136] So-called red degeneration of myomas is occasionally observed during late pregnancy, a condition due to central hemorrhagic infarction of the myoma. Pain is the hallmark of this condition, occasionally associated with rebound tenderness, mild fever, leukocytosis, nausea, and vomiting. Usually pain is the only symptom and resolution follows rest and analgesic treatment.[138] Surgery should be a last resort. The larger the myoma, the greater the risk of premature labor.[139]

Medical Therapyof Leiomyomata

The goals of medical therapy for leiomyomas are to ***temporarily*** reduce symptoms and to reduce myoma size, and the therapy of choice is treatment with a GnRH agonist.[140]

The short half-life of GnRH is due to rapid cleavage of the bonds between amino acids 5-6, 6-7, and 9-10. By altering amino acids at these positions, analogues of GnRH can be synthesized with different properties. Substitution of amino acids at the 6 position or replacement of the C-terminal glycine-amide (inhibiting degradation) produces agonists. An initial agonistic action (the so-called flare effect) is associated with an increase in the circulating levels of follicle-stimulating hormone (FSH) and luteinizing hormone (LH). This response is greatest in the early follicular phase when GnRH and estradiol have combined to create a large reserve pool of gonadotropins. After 1–3 weeks, desensitization and down-regulation of the pituitary produce a hypogonadotropic, hypogonadal state. The initial response is due to desensitizatiion, the uncoupling of the receptor from its effector system, whereas the sustained response is due to a loss of receptors by down-regulation and internalization. Furthermore, postreceptor mechanisms lead to secretion of biologically inactive gonadotropins, which, however, can still be detected by immunoassay.

The GnRH analogues cannot escape destruction if administered orally. Higher doses administered subcutaneously can achieve nearly equal effects as observed with intravenous treatment; however, the smaller blood peaks are slower to develop and take longer to return to baseline. Other forms of administration include nasal spray, sustained release implants, and intramuscular injections of biodegradable microspheres.

Treatment With GnRH Agonists

Summarizing the experience with GnRH agonist treatment of leiomyomata, the mean uterine size decreases 30–64% after 3–6 months of treatment.[140] Maximal response is usually achieved by 3 months. The reduction in size correlates with the estradiol level and with body weight. Menorrhagia, anemia, pelvic pressure, and urinary requency all respond favorably to GnRH agonist treatment. A decrease in operative blood loss can be achieved when the pretreatment uterus is as large or larger as a 16-week pregnancy. Why is there a variation in response? When one considers the many factors involved in myoma growth (estrogen, progesterone, growth factors, and receptors), it makes sense that not every myoma is the same. After cessation of GnRH agonist therapy, menses return in 4–10 weeks, and myoma and uterine size return to pretreatment levels in 3–4 months. The rapid regrowth is consistent with the fact that reduction in size is not due to a cytotoxic effect.

Preoperative GnRH agonist therapy offers several advantages for hysteroscopic removal of submucous tumors. In addition to a decrease in myoma size, endometrial atrophy will improve visualization, and decreased vascularity will reduce blood loss.

Leiomyomatosis Peritonealis Disseminata is a condition in which multiple small nodules of benign smooth muscle are found throughout the abdominal cavity, and occasionally in the pulmonary cavity. This condition appears to be sensitive to estrogen because it has been aggravated by postmenopausal estrogen treatment, and regression has been achieved with GnRH agonist treatment.[141]

Adenomyosis is the ectopic presence of endometrial glands within the myometrium. This diagnosis can be made by magnetic resonance imaging, and successful treatment with a GnRH agonist has been reported.[142, 143]

Side Effects With GnRH Agonists

Hot flushes are experienced by more than 75% of patients, usually in 3–4 weeks after beginning treatment. Approximately 5–15% of patients will complain of headache, vaginal dryness, joint and muscle stiffness, and depression. About 30% of patien will continue to have irregular (although light) vaginal bleeding. It is useful to measure the circulating estradiol level. If the level is greater than 30 pg/mL, suppression is inadequate. On the other hand, Friedman and colleagues have suggested that maintaining the estradiol level in the early follicular phase range (30–50 pg/mL) can protect against osteoporosis and reduce hot flushes, but not allow the growth of myomas.[144] The efficacy of this titration of response requires validation by clinical studies.

A small number (10%) of patients will experience a localized allergic reaction at the site of injection of depot forms of GnRH analogues. More serious reaction is rare, but immediate and delayed anaphylaxis can occur, requiring intense support and management.[145]

Bone loss occurs with GnRH therapy, but not in everyone, and it is reversible (although it is not certain if it is totally reversible in all patients). A significant vaginal hemorrhage 5–10 weeks after beginning treatment is encountered in about 2% of treated women, due to degeneration and necrosis of submucous myomas.[146] A disadvantage of agonist treatment is a delay in diagnosis of a leiomyosarcoma. Keep in mind that almost all leiomyosarcmas present as the largest or only uterine mass. Close monitoring is necessary and surgery has been the usual recommendation when either enlargement or no shrinkage of myomas occurs during GnRH agonist treatment.[147] The use of Doppler ultrasonography or magnetic resonance imaging offers greater accuracy of evaluation. However, the incidence of leiomyosarcoma, even in patients with "rapidly growing leiomyomata," is very low (less than 0.5%) and almost unheard of in premenopausal women.[101] In premenopausal women, a conservative approach is warranted.

Escape of suppression an result in an unexpected pregnancy. No adverse effects of fetal exposure to GnRH agonists have been reported, even when exposure has persisted throughout the early weeks of pregnancy.[148]

GnRH Agonists and Steroid Add-Back

Treatment with a GnRH agonist with steroid add-back has been explored to permit long-term therapy without bone loss.[140] Two strategies have been employed: simultaneous agonist and steroid add-back treatment or a sequential regimen in which the agonist is used alone for 3 months, followed by the combination of the agonist and steroid add-back. This long-term treatment is attractive for women who are perimenopausal, perhaps avoiding surgery. In addition, long-term treatment would be useful for women with coagulopathies, and in women with medical problems who need to postpone surgery.

Simultaneous treatment with agonist and medroxyprogesterone acetate (20 mg daily) or norethindrone (10 mg daily) effectively reduced hot flushing, but was less effective (consistent with a major supportive role for progestins in myomas) in reducing uterine volume.[140, 149] A sequential program, adding a traditional postmenopausal hormone regimen (0.625 mg conjugated estrogens on days 1–25 and 10 mg medroxyprogesterone acetate on days 16–25) effectively reduced uterine volume and maintained the reduced volume for 2 years (and avoided any loss in bone density)/[140] A daily 2.5 mg dose of tibolone also prevents bone loss and inhibits vasomotor symptoms without reducing the therapeutic efficacy of GnRH agonist treatment.[150]

We recommend 1 month of GnRH agonist treatment followed by agonist treatment combined with a daily, continuous add-back of estrogen and progestin using one of the available postmenopausal daily regimens. In view of the sensitivity of leiomyomata tissue to progestational agents, it makes sense to keep the dose of progestin relatively low.

Summary of Clinical Advantages With GnRH Agonist Treatment

Reduction in menstrual blood loss.
Improvement in anemia prior to surgery.
Time for autologous blood donation.
Less operative blood loss.
Hysterectomy less likely.
More likely to allow laparoscopic technique.
Possible conversion from abdominal to vaginal hysterectomy.

Treatment with a GnRH Antagonist

GnRH antagonist treatment can suppress pituitary-gonadal function without the initial stimulatory (flare) response observed with GnRH agonists. Results with depot Cetrorelix preoperative treatment of uterine fibroids are similar to those with GnRH agonist treatment; however, the response is faster (a maximal reduction in size within 14 days), probably because there is no initial flare response.[151]

References

1. **Graham H,** *Eternal Eve, The History of Gynaecology & Obstetrics,* Doubleday & Company, Inc., Garden City, NY, 1951.

2. **Medvei VC,** *The History of Clinical Endocrinology,* The Parthenon Publishing Group, New York, 1993.

3. **Magner LN,** *A History of Medicine,* Marcel Dekker, Inc., New York, 1992.

4. **Jost A, Vigier B, Prepin J, Perchellet JP,** Studies on sex differentiation in mammals, *Recent Prog Hormone Res* 29:1, 1973.

5. **Acién P,** Embryological observations on the female genital tract, *Hum Reprod* 7:437, 1992.

6. **Ferenczy A, Bergeron C,** Histology of the human endometrium: from birth to senescence, In: Bulletti C, Gurpide E, eds. *The Primate Endometrium,* The New York Academy of Sciences, New York, 1991, p 6.

7. **Markee JE,** Menstruation in intraocular endometrial transplants in the rhesus monkey, *JAMA* 250:2167, 1946.

8. **Markee JE,** Morphological basis for menstrual bleeding: relation of regression to the initiation of bleeding, *Bull NY Acad Med* 24:253, 1948.

9. **Noyes RW, Hertig AW, Rock J,** Dating the endometrial biopsy, *Fertil Steril* 1:3, 1950.

10. **Bartelmez GW,** The form and the function of the uterine blood vessels in the Rhesus monkey, *Carnegie Inst Contrib Embryol* 36:153, 1957.

11. **Bartlemez GW,** The phases of the menstrual cycle and their interpretation in terms of the pregnancy cycle, *Am J Obstet Gynecol* 74:931, 1957.

12. **Christiaens GCML, Sixma JJ, Haspels AA,** Hemostasis in menstrual endometrium: a review, *Obstet Gynecol Survey* 37:281, 1982.

13. **Ludwig H, Spornitz UM,** Microarchitecture of the human endometrium by scanning electron microscopy: menstrual desquamation and remodeling, In: Bulletti C, Gurpide E, eds. *The Primate Endometrium,* The New York Academy of Sciences, New York, 1991, p 28.

14. **Bergeron C, Ferenczy A, Shyamala G,** Distribution of estrogen receptors in various cell types of normal, hyperplastic, and neoplastic human endometrial tissues, *Lab Invest* 58:338, 1988.

15. **Tabibzadeh SS,** Proliferative activity of lymphoid cells in human endometrium throughout the menstrual cycle, *J Clin Endocrinol Metab* 70:437, 1990.

16. **Gurpide E, Gusberg S, Tseng L,** Estradiol binding and metabolism in human endometrial hyperplasia and adenocarcinoma, *J Steroid Biochem* 7:891, 1976.

17. **Falany JL, Falany CN,** Regulation of estrogen sulfotransferase in human endometrial adenocarcinoma cells by progesterone, *Endocrinology* 137:1395, 1996.

18. **Kirkland JL, Murthy L, Stancel GM,** Progesterone inhibits the estrogen-induced expression of *c-fos* messenger ribonucleic acid in the uterus, *Endocrinology* 130:3223, 1992.

19. **Lockwood CJ, Schatz F,** A biological model for the regulation of peri-implantational hemostasis and menstruation, *J Soc Gynecol Invest* 3:159, 1996.

20. **Tabibzadeh S,** The signals and molecular pathways involved in human menstruation, a unique process of tissue destruction and remodelling, *Mol Hum Reprod* 2:77, 1996.

21. **Tabibzadeh S, Babaknia A, Kong QF, Zupi E, Marconi D, Romanini C, Satyaswaroop PG,** Menstruation is associated with disordered expression of Desmoplakin I/II, cadherin/catenins and conversion of F to G actin in endometrial epithelium, *Hum Reprod* 10:776, 1995.

22. **Salamonsen LA,** Matrix metalloproteinases and endometrial remodelling, *Cell Biol Int* 18:1139, 1994.

23. **Rodgers WH, Matrisian LM, Giudice LC, Dsupin B, Cannon P, Svitek C, Gorstein F, Osteen KG,** Patterns of matrix metalloproteinase expression in cycling endometrium imply differential functions and regulation by steroid hormones, *J Clin Invest* 94:946, 1994.

24. **Irwin JC, Kirk D, Gwatkin RBL, Navre M, Cannon P, Giudice LC,** Human endometrial matrix metalloproteinase-2, a putative menstrual proteinase. Hormonal regulation in cultured stromal cells and messenger RNA expression during the menstrual cycle, *J Clin Invest* 97:438, 1996.

25. **Bruner KL, Rodgers WH, Gold LI, Korc M, Hargrove JT, Matrisian LM, Osteen KG,** Transforming growth factor beta mediates the progesterone suppression of an epithelial metalloproteinase by adjacent stroma in the human endometrium, *Proc Natl Acad Sci USA* 92:7362, 1995.

26. **Kothapalli R, Buyuksal I, Wu S-Q, Chegini N, Tabibzadeh S,** Detection of *ebaf,* a novel human gene of the transforming growth factor β superfamily, *J Clin Invest* 99:2342, 1997.

27. **Lockwood C, Krikun G, Papp C, Toth-Pal E, Markiewicz L, Wang EY, Kerenyi T, Zhou X, Hauskenecht V, Papp Z,** The role of progestionally regulated stromal cell tissue factor and type-1 plasminogen activator inhibitor (PAI-1) in endometrial hemostasis and menstruation, *Ann NY Acad Sci* 734:57, 1994.

28. **Schatz F, Aigner S, Papp C, Toth-Pal E, Hauskenecht V, Lockwood CJ,** Plasminogen activator activity during decidualization of human endometrial stromal cells is regulated by plasminogen activator inhibitor 1, *J Clin Encrinol Metab* 80:1504, 1995.

29. **Wilborn WH, Flowers Jr CE,** Cellular mechanisms for endometrial conservation during menstrual bleeding, *Seminars Reprod Endocrinol* 2:307, 1984.

30. **Treloar AE, Boynton RE, Borghild GB, Brown BW,** Variation of the human menstrual cycle through reproductive life, *Int J Fertil* 12:77, 1967.

31. **Belsey EM, Pinol APY, and Task Force on Long-Acting Systemic Agents for Fertility Regulation,** Menstrual bleeding patterns in untreated women, *Contraception* 55:57, 1997.

32. **Rock J, Garcia CR, Menkin M,** A theory of menstruation, *Ann NY Acad Sci* 75:830, 1959.

33. **Tazuke SI, Giudice LC,** Growth factors and cytokines in endometrium, embryonic development, and maternal:embryonic interactions, *Seminars Reprod Endocrinol* 14:231, 1996.

34. **Tabibzadeh SS, Kaffka KL, Satyaswarrop PG, Kilian PL,** IL-1 regulation of human endometrial function: presence of IL-1 receptor correlates with IL-1 stimulated PGE_2 production, *J Clin Endocrinol Metab* 70:1000, 1990.

35. **Arici A, Engin O, Attar E, Olive DL,** Modulation of leukemia inhibitory factor gene expression and protein biosynthesis in human endometrium, *J Clin Endocrinol Metab* 80:1908, 1995.

36. **Cullinan EB, Abbondanzo SJ, Anderson PS, Pollard JW, A LB, Stewart CL,** Leukemia inhibitory factor (LIF) and LIF receptor expression in human endometrium suggests a potential autocrine/paracrine function in regulating embryo implantation, *Proc Natl Acad Sci USA* 93:3115, 1996.

37. **Hunt JS, Chen H-L, Hu X-L, Tabibzadeh S,** Tumor necrosis factor-α messenger ribonucleic acid and protein in human endometrium, *Biol Reprod* 47:141, 1992.

38. **Ignar-Trowbridge DM, Nelson KG, Bidwell MC, Curtis SW, Washburn TF, McLachlan JA, Korach KS,** Coupling of dual signaling pathways: epidermal growth factor action involves the estrogen receptor, *Proc Natl Acad Sci USA* 89:4658, 1992.

39. **Hofmann GE, Scott Jr RT, Bergh PA, Deligdisch L,** Immuno-histochemical localization of epidermal growth factor in human endometrium, decidua, and placenta, *J Clin Endocrinol Metab* 73:882, 1991.

40. **Troche V, O'Connor DM, Schaudies RP,** Measurement of human epidermal growth factor receptor in the endometrium during the menstrual cycle, *Am J Obstet Gynecol* 165:1499, 1991.

41. **Prentice A, Thomas EJ, Weddell A, McGill A, Randall BJ, Horne CH,** Epidermal growth factor receptor expression in normal endometrium and endometriosis: an immunohistochemical study, *Br J Obstet Gynaecol* 99:395, 1992.

42. **Horowitz GM, Scott Jr RT, Drews MR, Navot D, Hoffman G,** Immunohistochemical localization of transforming growth factor-α in human endometrium, decidua, and trophoblast, *J Clin Endocrinol Metab* 76:786, 1993.

43. **Giudice LC, Dsupin BA, Jin IH, Vu TH, Hoffman AR,** Differential expression of messenger ribonucleic acids encoding insulin-like growth factors and their receptors in human uterine endometrium and decidua, *J Clin Endocrinol Metab* 76:1115, 1993.

44. **Zhou J, Dsupin BA, Giudice LC, Bondy CA,** Insulin-like growth factor system gene expression in human endometrium during the menstrual cycle, *J Clin Endocrinol Metab* 79:1723, 1994.

45. **Adesanya OO, Zhou J, Bondy CA,** Sex steroid regulation of IGF system gene expression and proliferation in primate myometrium, *J Clin Endocrinol Metab* 81:1967, 1996.

46. **Adesanya OO, Zhou J, Bondy CA,** Cellular localization and sex steroid regulation of insulin-like growth factor binding protein messenger ribonucleic acids in the primate myometrium, *J Clin Endocrinol Metab* 81:2495, 1996.

47. **Casey ML, Mibe M, Erk A, MacDonald PC,** Transforming growth factor-ß stimulation of parathyroid hormone-related protein expression in human uterine cells in culture: mRNA levels and protein secretion, *J Clin Endocrinol Metab* 74:950, 1992.

48. **Eldering JA, Nay MG, Hoberg LM, Longcope C, McCracken JA,** Hormonal regulation of prostaglandin production by Rhesus monkey endometrium, *J Clin Endocrinol Metab* 71:596, 1990.

49. **Maathuis JB, Kelly RW,** Concentrations of prostaglandin $F_{2\alpha}$ and E_2 in the endometrium throughout the human menstrual cycle after the administration of clomiphene or an oestrogen-progesterone pill and in early pregnancy, *J Endocrinol* 77:361, 1978.

50. **Levin JH, Stancyzk FZ, Lobo RA,** Estradiol stimulates the secretion of prostacyclin and thromboxane from endometrial stromal cells in culture, *Fertil Steril* 58:530, 1992.

51. **Senior J, Sangha R, Baxter GS, Marshall K, Clayton JK,** In vitro characterization of prostanoid FP- DP- IP- and TP- receptors on the non-pregnant human myometrium, *Br J Pharmacol* 107:215, 1992.

52. **Swanson ML, Lei ZM, Swanson PH, Rao CV, Narumiya S, Hirata M,** The expression of thromboxane A_2 synthase and thromboxane A_2 receptor gene in human uterus, *Biol Reprod* 47:105, 1992.

53. **Zhu HH, Huang JR, Mazella J, Elias J, Tseng L,** Progestin stimulates the biosynthesis of fibronectin and accumulation of fibronectin mRNA in human endometrial cells, *Hum Reprod* 7:141, 1992.

54. **Lessey BA, Damjanovich L, Coutifaris C, Castelbaum A, Albedla SM, Buck CA,** Integrin adhesion molecules in the human endometrium. Correlation with the normal and abnormal menstrual cycles, *J Clin Invest* 90:188, 1992.

55. **Grosskinsky CM, Yowell CW, Sun J, Parise LV, Lessey BA,** Modulation of integrin expression in endometrial stromal cells in vitro, *J Clin Endocrinol Metab* 81:2047, 1996.

56. **Helftenbein G, Misseyanni A, Hagen G, Peter W, Slater EP, Wiehle RD, Suske G, Beato M,** Expression of the uteroglobin promoter in epithelial cell lines from endometrium, In: Bulletti C, Gurpide E, eds. *The Primate Endometrium,* The New York Academy of Sciences, New York, 1991, p 69.

57. **Makrigiannakis A, Margioris A, Markogiannakis E, Stournaras C, Gravanis A,** Steroid hormones regulate the release of immunoreactive ß-endorphin from the Ishikawa human endometrial cell line, *J Clin Endocrinol Metab* 75:584, 1992.

58. **Economos K, MacDonald PC, Casey ML,** Endothelin-1 gene expression and protein biosynthesis in human endometrium: potential modulator of endometrial blood flow, *J Clin Endocrinol Metab* 74:14, 1992.

59. **Kubota T, Kamada S, Hirata Y, Eguchi S, Imai T, Marumo F, Aso T,** Synthesis and release of endothelin-1 by human decidual cells, *J Clin Endocrinol Metab* 75:1230, 1992.

60. **Reynolds LP, Killilea SD, Redmer DA,** Angiogenesis in the female reproductive system, *FASEB J* 6:886, 1992.

61. **Shifren JL, Tseng JF, Zaloudek CJ, Ryan IP, Meng YG, Ferrara N, Jaffe RB, Taylor RN,** Ovarian steroid regulation of vascular endothelial growth factor in the human endometrium: implications for angiogenesis during the menstrual cycle and in the pathogenesis of endometriosis, *J Clin Endocrinol Metab* 81:3112, 1996.

62. **Lessey BA, Killiam AP, Metzger DA, Haney AF, Greene GL, McCarty KS,** Immunohistochemical analysis of uterine estrogen and progesterone receptors throughout the menstrual cycle, *J Clin Endocrinol Metab* 67:334, 1988.

63. **Snijders MPML, de Goeij AFPM, Debets-Te Baerts MJC, Rousch MJM, Koudstaal J, Bosman FT,** Immunocytochemical analysis of oestrogen receptors and progesterone receptors in the human uterus throughout the menstrual cycle and after the menopause, *J Reprod Fertil* 94:363, 1992.

64. **Horie K, Takakura K, Imai K, Liao S, Mori T,** Immunohistochemical localization of androgen receptor in the human endometrium, decidua, placenta and pathological conditions of the endometrium, *Hum Reprod* 7:1461, 1992.

65. **Moy E, Kimzey LM, Nelson LM, Blithe DL,** Glycoprotein hormone alpha-subunit functions synergistically with progesterone to stimulate differentiation of cultured human endometrial stromal cells to decidualized cells: a novel role for free alpha-subunit in reproduction, *Endocrinology* 137:1332, 1996.

66. **Blithe DL, Richards RG, Sklarulis MC,** Free alpha molecules from pregnancy stimulate secretion of prolactin from human decidual cells: a novel function for free alpha in pregnancy, *Endocrinology* 129:2257, 1992.

67. **Handwerger S, Richards RG, Markoff E,** The physiology of decidual prolactin and other decidual protein hormones, *Trends Endocrinol Metab* 3:91, 1992.

68. **Handwerger S, Harman I, Golander A, Handwerger DA,** Prolactin release from perifused human decidual explants: effects of decidual prolactin-releasing factor (PRL-RF) and prolactin release-inhibitory factor (PRL-IF), *Placenta* 13:55, 1992.

69. **Riddick DH, Kusmik WF,** Decidua: a possible source of amniotic fluid prolactin, *Am J Obstet Gynecol* 127:187, 1977.

70. **Pihoker C, Pheeney R, Handwerger S,** Lipocortin 1 inhibits the synthesis and release of prolactin from human decidual cells, *Endocrinology* 128:1123, 1991.

71. **Mora S, Diehl T, Stewart EA,** Prolactin is an autocrine growth regulator for human myometrial and leiomyoma cells, *J Soc Gynecol Invest* 2:396, 1995.

72. **Taylor CM, McLaughlin B, Weiss JB, Maroudas NG,** Concentrations of endothelial-cell-stimulating angiogenesis factor, a major component of human uterine angiogenesis factor, in human and bovine embryonic tissues and decidua, *J Reprod Fertil* 94:445, 1992.

73. **Petraglia F, Tabanelli S, Galassi MC, Garuti GC, Mancini AC, Genazzani AR, Gurpide E,** Human decidua and in vitro decidualized endometrial stromal cells at term contain immunoreactive corticotropin-releasing factor (CRF) and CRF messenger ribonucleic acid, *J Clin Endocrinol Metab* 74:1427, 1992.

74. **Poisner AM, Thrailkill K, Poisner R, Handwerger S,** Cyclic AMP and protein kinase C as second messengers for prorenin release from human decidual cells, *Placenta* 12:263, 1991.

75. **Chao H-S, Poisner A, Poisner R, Handwerger S,** Endothelins stimulate the synthesis and release of prorenin from human decidual cells, *J Clin Endocrinol Metab* 76:615, 1993.

76. **Giudice LC, Dsupin BA, Irwin JC,** Steroid and peptide regulation of insulin-like growth factor-binding proteins secreted by human endometrial cells is dependent on stromal differentiation, *J Clin Endocrinol Metab* 75:1235, 1992.

77. **Tseng L, Gao J-G, Chen R, Zhu HH, Mazella J, Powell DR,** Effect of progestin, antiprogestin, and relaxin on the accumulation of prolactin and insulin-like growth factor-binding protein-1 messenger ribonucleic acid in human endometrial cells, *Biol Reprod* 47:441, 1992.

78. **Thrailkill KM, Clemmons DR, Busby Jr WH, Handwerger S,** Differential regulation of insulin-like growth factor binding protein secretion from human decidual cells by IGF-I, insulin, and relaxin, *J Clin Invest* 86:878, 1990.

79. **Pekonen F, Nyman T, Lahteenmaki P, Haukkamaa M, Rutanen E-M,** Intrauterine progestin induces continuous insulin-like growth factor-binding protein-1 production in the human endometrium, *J Clin Endocrinol Metab* 75:660, 1992.

80. **Kauma S, Matt D, Strom S, Eirman D, Turner T,** Interleukin-1ß, human leukocyte antigen HLA-DRa, and transforming growth factor-ß expression in endometrium, placenta, and placental membranes, *Am J Obstet Gynecol* 163:1430, 1990.

81. **Graham CH, Lysiak JJ, McCrae KR, Lal PK,** Localization of transforming growth factor-beta at the human fetal-maternal interface: role in trophoblast growth and differentiation, *Biol Reprod* 46:561, 1992.

82. **Graham CH, McCrae KR, Lala PK,** Molecular mechanisms of controlling trophoblast invasion of the uterus, *Tropohoblast Res* 7:237, 1993.

83. **Heinonen PK, Saarikoski S, Pystynen P,** Reproductive performance of women with uterine anomalies, *Acta Obstet Gynecol Scand* 61:157, 1982.

84. **Rock JA, Schlaff WD,** The obstetrical consequences of uterovaginal anomalies, *Fertil Steril* 43:681, 1985.

85. **Golan A, Langer R, Bukovsky I, Caspi E,** Congenital anomalies of the müllerian system, *Fertil Steril* 51:747, 1989.

86. **Acién P,** Reproductive performance of women with uterine malformations, *Hum Reprod* 8:122, 1993.

87. **Acién P,** Incidence of Müllerian defects in fertile and infertile women, *Hum Reprod* 12:1372, 1997.

88. **The American Society for Reproductive Medicine,** Classifications of adnexal adhesions, distal tubal occlusion, tubal occlusion secondary to tubal ligation, tubal pregnancies, müllerian anomalies and intrauterine adhesions, *Fertil Steril* 49:944, 1988.

89. **Creatsas G, Cardamakis E, Hassan E, Deligeoroglou E, Salakos N, Aravantinos D,** Congenital uterine anomalies with obstructed cervix, hemivagina, or both during adolescence: report of 22 cases, *J Gynecol Surg* 10:159, 1994.

90. **Andrews MC, Jones Jr HW,** Impaired reproductive performance of the unicornuate uterus: intrauterine growth retardation, infertility, and recurrent abortion in five cases, *Am J Obstet Gynecol* 144:173, 1982.

91. **Heinonen P,** Unicornuate uterus and rudimentary horn, *Fertil Steril* 68:224, 1997.

92. **Raga F, Bauset C, Remohi J, Bonilla-Musoles F, Simón C, Pellicer A,** Reproductive impact of congenital Müllerian anomalies, *Hum Reprod* 12:2277, 1997.

93. **Fedele L, Bianchi S, Agnoli B, Tozzi L, Vignali M,** Urinary tract anomalies associated with unicornuate uterus, *J Urol* 155:847, 1996.

94. **Daly DC, Maier D, Soto-Albors C,** Hysteroscopic metroplasty: six years experience, *Obstet Gynecol* 73:201, 1989.

95. **Fedele L, Bianchi S,** Hysteroscopic metroplasty for septate uterus, *Obstet Gynecol Clin North Am* 22:473089, 1995.

96. **Rock JA, Schlaff WD, Zacur HA, Jones Jr HW,** The clinical management of congenital absence of the uterine cervix, *Int J Gynaecol Obstet* 22:231, 1984.

97. **Kaufman RH, Adan E, Binder GL, Gerthoffer E,** Upper genital tract changes and pregnancy outcome in offspring exposed in utero to diethylstilbestrol, *Am J Obstet Gynecol* 137:299, 1980.

98. **Pellerito JS, McCarthy SM, Doyle MB, Glickman MG, DeCherney AH,** Diagnosis of uterine anomalies: relative accuracy of MR imaging, endovaginal sonography, and hysterosalpingography, *Genitourin Radiol* 183:795, 1992.

99. **Barbieri RL, Andersen J,** Uterine leiomyomas: the somatic mutation theory, *Seminars Reprod Endocrinol* 10:301, 1992.

100. **Andersen J, Barbieri RL,** Abnormal gene expression in uterine leiomyomas, *J Soc Gynecol Invest* 2:663, 1995.

101. **Parker WH, Fu YS, Berek JS,** Uterine sarcoma in patients operated on for presumed leiomyoma and rapidly growing leiomyoma, *Obstet Gynecol* 83:414, 1994.

102. **Cramer SF, Patel D,** The frequency of uterine leiomyomas, *Am J Clin Pathol* 94:435, 1990.

103. **Cramer DW,** Epidemiology of myomas, *Seminars Reprod Endocrinol* 10:320, 1992.

104. **Marshall LM, Spiegelman D, Barbieri RL, Goldman MB, Manson JE, Colditz GA, Willett WC, Hunter DJ,** Variation in the incidence of uterine leiomyoma among premenopausal women by age and race, *Obstet Gynecol* 90:967, 1997.

105. **Marshall LM, Spiegelman D, Goldman MB, Manson JE, Colditz GA, Barbieri RL, Stampfer MJ, Hunter DJ,** A prospective study of reproductive factors and oral contraceptive use in relation to the risk of uterine leiomyomata, *Fertil Steril* 70:432, 1998.

106. **Parazzini F, Negri E, La Vecchia C, Fedele L, Rabaiotti M, Luchini L,** Oral contraceptive use and risk of uterine fibroids, *Obstet Gynecol* 79:430, 1992.

107. **Samadi AR, Lee NC, Flanders D, Boring III JR, Parris EB,** Risk factors for self-reported uterine fibroids: a case-control study, *Am J Public Health* 86:858, 1996.

108. **Otubu JA, Buttram VC, Besch NF, Besch PK,** Unconjugated steroids in leiomyomas and tumor-bearing myometrium, *Am J Obstet Gynecol* 143:130, 1982.

109. **Rein MS, Friedman AJ, Stuart JM, MacLaughlin DT,** Fibroid and myometrial steroid receptors in women treated with the gonadotropin-releasing hormone agonist leuprolide acetate, *Fertil Steril* 53:1018, 1990.

110. **Brandon DD, Erickson TE, Keenan EJ, Strawn EY, Novy MJ, Burry KA, Warner C, Clinton CM,** Estrogen receptor gene expression in human uterine leiomyomata, *J Clin Endocrinol Metab* 80:1876, 1995.

111. **Bulun SE, Simpson ER, Word RA,** Expression of the *CYP 19* gene and its product aromatase cytochrome P450 in human uterine leiomyoma tissues and cells in culture, *J Clin Endocrinol Metab* 78:736, 1994.

112. **Andersen J, DyReyes VM, Barbieri RL, Coachman DM, Miksicek RJ,** Leiomyoma primary cultures have elevated transcriptional response to estrogen compared with autologous myometrial cultures, *J Soc Gynecol Invest* 2:542, 1995.

113. **Deligdish L, Loewenthal M,** Endometrial changes associated with myomata of the uterus, *J Clin Pathol* 23:676, 1970.

114. **Kawaguchi K, Fujii S, Konishi I, Nanbu Y, Nonogaki H, Mori T,** Mitotic activity in uterine leiomyomas during the menstrual cycle, *Am J Obstet Gynecol* 160:637, 1989.

115. **Tiltman AJ,** The effect of progestins on the mitotic activity of uterine fibromyomas, *Int J Gynecol* 4:89, 1985.

116. **Brandon DD, Bethea CL, Strawn EY, Novy MJ, Burry KA, Harrington MS, Erickson TE, Warner C, Keenan EJ, Clinton GM,** Progesterone receptor messenger ribonucleic acid and protein are overexpressed in human uterine leiomyomas, *Am J Obstet Gynecol* 169:78, 1993.

117. **Viville B, Charnock-Jones DS, Sharkey AM, Wetzka B, Smith SK,** Distribution of the A and B forms of the progesterone receptor messenger ribonucleic acid and protein in uterine leiomyomata and adjacent myometrium, *Hum Reprod* 12:815, 1997.

118. **Murphy AA, Morales AJ, Kettel LM, Yen SS,** Regression of uterine leiomyomata to the antiprogesterone RU486: dose-response effect, *Fertil Steril* 64:187, 1995.

119. **Matsuo H, Maruo T, Samoto T,** Increased expression of Bcl-2 protein in human uterine leiomyoma and its up-regulation by progesterone, *J Clin Endocrinol Metab* 82:193, 1997.

120. **Andersen J,** Growth factors and cytokines in uterine leiomyomas, *Seminars Reprod Endocrinol* 14:269, 1996.

121. **Lumsden MA, West CP, Bramley T, Rumgay L, Baird DT,** The binding of epidermal growth factor to the human uterus and leiomyomata in women rendered hypoestrogenic by continuous administration of an LHRH agonist, *Br J Obstet Gynaecol* 95:1299, 1988.

122. **Harrison-Woolrych ML, Charnock-Jones DS, Smith SK,** Quantification of messenger ribonucleic acid for epidermal growth factor in human myometrium and leiomyomata using reverse transcriptase polymerase chain reaction, *J Clin Endocrinol Metab* 78:1179, 1994.

123. **Gloudemans T, Prinsen I, Van Unmik JAM, Lips CJ, Den Otter W, Sussenbach JS,** Insulin-like growth factor gene expression in human smooth muscle tumors, *Cancer Res* 50:6689, 1990.

124. **Giudice LC, Irwin JC, Dsupin BA, Pannier EM, Jin IH, Vu TH, Hoffman AR,** Insulin-like growth factor (IGF), IGF binding protein (IGFBP), and IGF receptor gene expression and IGFBP synthesis in human uterine leiomyomata, *Hum Reprod* 8:1796, 1993.

125. **Vollenhoven BJ, Herington AC, Healy DL,** Messenger ribonucleic acid expression of the insulin-like growth factors and their binding proteins in uterine fibroids and myometrium, *J Clin Endocrinol Metab* 76:1106, 1993.

126. **Weir EC, Goad DL, Daifotis AG, Burtis WJ, Dreyer BE, Nowak RA,** Relative overexpression of the parathyroid hormone-related protein gene in human leiomyomas, *J Clin Endocrinol Metab* 78:784, 1994.

127. **Schmid CH, Beham A, Kratochvil P,** Haematopoiesis in a degenerating uterine leiomyomata, *Arch Gynecol Obstet* 248:81, 1990.

128. **Stewart EA, Nowak RA,** Leiomyoma-related bleeding: a classic hypothesis updated for the molecular era, *Hum Reprod Update* 2:296, 1996.

129. **Buttram VC, Reiter RC,** Uterine leiomyomata: etiology, symptomatology and management, *Fertil Steril* 36:433, 1981.

130. **Verkauf BS,** Myomectomy for fertility enhancement and preservation, *Fertil Steril* 58:1, 1992.

131. **Zawin M, McCarthy S, Scoutt LM, Comite F,** High-field MRI and US evaluation of the pelvis in women with leiomyomas, *Mag Reson Imaging* 8:371, 1990.

132. **Fedele L, Bianchi S, Dorta M, Brioschi D, Zanottie F, Vercellini P,** Transvaginal ultrasonography versus hysteroscopy in the diagnosis of uterine submucous myomas, *Obstet Gynecol* 77:745, 1991.

133. **Malone LJ,** Myomectomy: recurrence after removal of solitary and multiple myomas, *Obstet Gynecol* 34:200, 1969.

134. **Candiani GB, Fedele L, Parazzini F, Villa L,** Risk of recurrence after myomectomy, *Br J Obstet Gynaecol* 98:385, 1991.

135. **Fedele L, Parazzini F, Luchini L, Mezzopane R, Tozzi L, Villa L,** Recurrence of fibroids after myomectomy: a transvaginal ultrasonographic study, *Hum Reprod* 10:1795, 1995.

136. **Vergani P, Ghidini A, Strobelt N, Roneaglia N, Locatelli A, Lapinski R, Mangioni C,** Do uterine leiomyomas influence pregnancy outcome? *Am J Perinatol* 11:356, 1994.

137. **Rossi G, Diamond MP,** Myomas, reproductive function, and pregnancy, *Seminars Reprod Endocrinol* 10:332, 1992.

138. **Katz VL, Dotters DJ, Droegemueller W,** Complications of uterine leiomyomas in pregnancy, *Obstet Gynecol* 73:593, 1989.

139. **Rice JP, Kay HH, Mahony BS,** The clinical significance of uterine leiomyomas in pregnancy, *Am J Obstet Gynecol* 160:1212, 1989.

140. **Stewart EA, Friedman AJ,** Steroidal treatment of myomas: preoperative and long-term medical therapy, *Seminars Reprod Endocrinol* 10:344, 1992.

141. **Hales HA, Peterson CM, Jones KP, Quinn JD,** Leiomyomatosis peritonealis disseminata treated with a gonadotropin-releasing hormone agonist, *Am J Obstet Gynecol* 167:515, 1992.

142. **Hirata JD, Moghissi KS, Ginsburg KA,** Pregnancy after medical therapy of adenomyosis with a gonadotropin-releasing hormone agonist, *Fertil Steril* 59:444, 1993.

143. **Nelson JR, Corson SL,** Long-term management of adenomyosis with a gonadotropin-releasing hormone agonist: a case report, *Fertil Steril* 59:441, 1993.

144. **Friedman AJ, Lobel SM, Rein MS, Barbieri RL,** Efficacy and safety considerations in women with uterine leiomyomas treated with gonadotropin-releasing hormone agonists: the estrogen threshold hypothesis, *Am J Obstet Gynecol* 163:1114, 1990.

145. **Letterie GS, Stevenson D, Shah A,** Recurrent anaphylaxis to a depot form of GnRH analogue, *Obstet Gynecol* 78:943, 1991.

146. **Friedman AJ,** Vaginal hemorrhage associated with degenerating submucous leiomyomata during leuprolide acetate treatment, *Fertil Steril* 52:152, 1989.

147. **Schwartz LB, Diamond MP, Schwartz PE,** Leiomyosarcomas: clinical presentation, *Am J Obstet Gynecol* 168:180, 1993.

148. **Har-Toov J, Brenner SH, Jaffa A, Yavetz H, Peyser MR, Lessing JB,** Pregnancy during long-term gonadotropin-releasing hormone agonist therapy associated with clinical pseudomenopause, *Fertil Steril* 59:446, 1993.

149. **Friedman AJ, Daly M, Juneau-Norcross M, Gleason R, Rein MS, LeBoff M,** Long-term medical therapy for leiomyomata uteri: a prospective, randomized study of leuprolide acetate depot plus either oestrogen-progestin or progestin 'add-back' for 2 years, *Hum Reprod* 9:1618, 1994.

150. **Palomba S, Affinito P, Tommaselli GA, Nappl C,** A clinical trial of the effects of tibolone administered with gonadotropin-releasing hormone analogues for the treatment of uterine leiomyomata, *Fertil Steril* 70:111, 1998.

151. **Felberbaum RE, Germer U, Ludwig M, Riethmuller-Winzen H, Heise S, Buttge I, Bauer O, Reissmann T, Engel J, Diedrich K,** Treatment of uterine fibroids with a slow-release formulation of the gonadotropin releasing hormone antagonist Cetrorelix, *Hum Reprod* 13:1660, 1998.

152. **Sadler TW,** In: *Langman's Medical Embryology,* 7th ed, Williams & Wilkins, Baltimore, 1995, p 296.

5 Neuroendocrinology

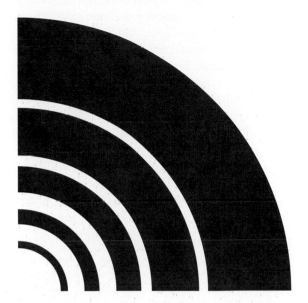

There are two major sites of action within the brain which are important in the regulation of reproductive function, the hypothalamus and the pituitary gland. In the past, the pituitary gland was viewed as the master gland. Then a new concept emerged in which the pituitary was relegated to a subordinate role as part of an orchestra, with the hypothalamus as the conductor, responding to both peripheral and central nervous system messages and exerting its influence by means of neurotransmitters transported to the pituitary by a portal vessel network. Regardless of which site was dominant, the conventional thesis was that the central nervous system-pituitary complex determined and directed the chronology of developmental events within a responsive ovary. However, developments over the past two decades indicate that the complex sequence of events known as the menstrual cycle is controlled by the sex steroids and peptides produced within the very follicle destined to ovulate. The hypothalamus and its direction, and the pituitary, are essential for the operation of the entire mechanism, but the endocrine function that leads to ovulation is brought about by endocrine feedback on the anterior pituitary.

A full understanding of this feature of reproductive biology will benefit the clinician who faces problems in gynecologic endocrinology. With this understanding, the clinician can comprehend the hitherto mysterious, but significant, effects of stress, diet, exercise, and other diverse influences on the pituitary-gonadal axis. Furthermore, we will be prepared to make advantageous use of the numerous neuropharmacologic agents that are the dividends of neuroendocrine research. To these ends, this chapter offers a clinically oriented review of the current status of reproductive neuroendocrinology.

Hypothalamic-Hypophyseal Portal Circulation

The hypothalamus is at the base of the brain just above the junction of the optic nerves. In order to influence the anterior pituitary gland, the brain requires a means of transmission or connection. A direct nervous connection does not exist. The blood supply of the anterior pituitary, however, originates in the capillaries that richly lace the median eminence area of the hypothalamus. The superior hypophyseal arteries form a dense network of capillaries within the median eminence, which then drain into the portal vessels that descend along the pituitary stalk to the anterior pituitary. The direction of the blood flow in this hypophyseal portal circulation is from the brain to the pituitary. Section of the neural stalk which interrupts this portal circulation leads to inactivity and atrophy of the gonads, along with a decrease in adrenal and thyroid activity to basal levels. With regeneration of the portal vessels, anterior pituitary function is restored. Thus, the anterior pituitary gland is under the influence of the hypothalamus by means of neurohormones released into this portal circulation. There also exists retrograde flow so that pituitary hormones can be delivered directly to the hypothalamus, creating the opportunity for pituitary feedback on the hypothalamus. An additional blood supply is provided by short vessels which originate in the posterior pituitary that in turn receives its arterial supply from the inferior hypophyseal arteries.

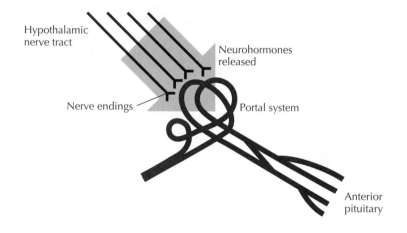

The Neurohormone Concept

A considerable body of evidence indicates that influence of the pituitary by the hypothalamus is achieved by materials secreted in the cells of the hypothalamus and transported to the pituitary by the portal vessel system. Indeed, pituitary cell proliferation and gene expression are controlled by hypothalamic peptides and their receptors. In addition to the stalk section experiments cited above, transplantation of the pituitary to ectopic sites (e.g., under the kidney capsule) results in failure of gonadal function. With retransplantation to an anatomic site under the median eminence, followed by regeneration of the portal system, normal pituitary function is regained. This retrieval of gonadotropic function is not accomplished if the pituitary is transplanted to other sites in the brain. Hence, there is something very special about the blood draining the basal hypothalamus. An exception to this overall pattern of positive influence is the control of prolactin secretion. Stalk secretion and transplantation cause release of prolactin from the anterior pituitary, implying a negative hypothalamic control. Furthermore, cultures of anterior pituitary tissue release prolactin in the absence of hypothalamic tissue or extracts.

Neuroendocrine agents originating in the hypothalamus have positive stimulatory effects on growth hormone, thyroid-stimulating hormone (TSH), adrenocorticotropin hormone (ACTH), as well as the gonadotropins, and represent the individual neurohormones of the hypothalamus. The neurohormone that controls gonadotropins is called gonadotropin-releasing hormone (GnRH). The neurohormone that controls prolactin is called prolactin-inhibiting hormone and is dopamine. Human corticotropin-releasing hormone (CRH) is a 41 amino acid peptide that besides being the principal regulator of ACTH secretion, also activates the sympathetic nervous system. As we

Gonadotropin releasing hormone—
a decapeptide

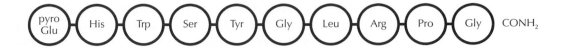

shall see, CRH can suppress gonadotropin secretion, an action partly mediated by endorphin inhibition of GnRH.

In addition to their effects on the pituitary, behavioral effects within the brain have been demonstrated for several of the releasing hormones. Thyrotropin-releasing hormone (TRH) antagonizes the sedative action of a number of drugs and also has a direct antidepressant effect in humans. GnRH evokes mating behavior in male and female animals.[1]

Initially, it was believed that there were two separate releasing hormones, one for follicle-stimulating hormone (FSH) and another for luteinizing hormone (LH). It is now apparent that there is a single neurohormone (GnRH) for both gonadotropins. GnRH is a small peptide with 10 amino acids with some variation in the amino acid sequence among various mammals. Purified or synthesized GnRH stimulates both FSH and LH secretion. The divergent patterns of FSH and LH in response to a single GnRH are due to the modulating influences of the endocrine environment, specifically the feedback effects of steroids on the anterior pituitary gland.

The classic neurotransmitters are secreted at the nerve terminal. Brain peptides require gene transcription, translation, and posttranslational processing, all within the neuronal cell body, the final product being transported down the axon to the terminal for secretion. Small neuroendocrine peptides share common large precursor polypeptides, called polyproteins or polyfunctional peptides. These proteins can serve as precursors for more than one biologically active peptide.

The gene that encodes for the 92 amino acid precursor protein for GnRH is located on the short arm of chromosome 8.[2] The precursor protein for GnRH contains (in the following order) a 23 amino acid signal sequence, the GnRH decapeptide, a 3 amino acid proteolytic processing site, and a 56 amino acid sequence called GAP (GnRH-associated peptide).[3] GAP is a potent inhibitor of prolactin secretion as well as a stimulator of gonadotropins; however, a physiologic role for GAP has not been established. Its primary role may be to provide appropriate conformational support for GnRH.

It is now apparent that GnRH has autocrine/paracrine functions throughout the body. It is present in both neural and nonneural tissues, and receptors are present in many extrapituitary tissues (such as the ovarian follicle and the placenta). Although GnRH is identical in all mammals, other nonmammalian forms exist, indicating that the GnRH molecule has existed for at least 500 million years.[4, 5] The central sequence, Tyr-Gly-Leu-Arg, is the nonconserved segment of GnRH, the segment with the most variability in other species. Accordingly, substitutions in this segment are well tolerated.

A second form of GnRH, known as GnRH-II, has been known to exist in many other species. GnRH-II consists of the following sequence: pGln-His-Trp-Ser-His-Gly-Trp-Tyr-Pro-Gly. Prompted by its existence in other species, a search for its presence in humans was ultimately successful. A gene encoding GnRH-II is located on the human chromosome 20p13, obviously distinct from the GnRH-I gene on 8p21-p11.2.[6] Both genes produce a peptide with a signal sequence, a GnRH decapeptide, a proteolytic site, and a GAP. Human GnRH-II expression is highest outside the brain. An analysis of the evolution of GnRH indicates 3 major forms: GnRH localized to the hypothalamus (GnRH-I), forms in midbrain nuclei and outside the brain (GnRH-II), and forms in several fish species (GnRH-III); thus indicating appearance of the various forms before the emergence of vertebrates.[6]

Perhaps the notion that the pituitary is a master gland should not be discarded. Although it is highly regulated by input from other sites, its function is essential for sustaining life. Pituitary development and activity are under the control of the hypothalamus (with input from other central nervous sytem sites), and pituitary response is finely tuned by hormonal messages from tissues that are the targets of the pituitary trophic hormones. In addition, the pituitary has its own autocrine/paracrine system for enhancement and suppression of growth and function. But the pituitary gland is the focus for all of this activity, and this central, coordinating role is critical for normal life.

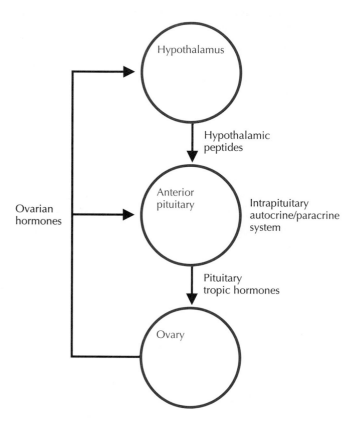

Prolactin Secretion

Prolactin gene expression occurs in the lactotrophs of the anterior pituitary gland, in decidualized endometrium, and the myometrium. The prolactin secreted in these various sites is identical, but there are differences in mRNA indicating differences in prolactin gene regulation.

Transcription of the prolactin gene is regulated by a transcription factor (a protein named Pit-1) that binds to the 5' promoter region and that is also necessary for growth hormone and TSH.[7] In addition, prolactin gene transcription is regulated by the interaction of estrogen and glucocorticoid receptors with 5' flanking sequences. Mutations in the sequences of these flanking regions or in the gene for the Pit-1 protein can result in the failure to secrete prolactin. The Pit-1 gene is also involved in differentiation and growth of anterior pituitary cells, and therefore mutations in this gene can lead not only to absent secretion of growth hormone, prolactin, and TSH, but also an absence of their trophic cells in the pituitary; the result is significant hypopituitarism.[8] Molecular studies indicate that Pit-1 participates in mediating both stimulatory and inhibitory hormone signals for prolactin gene transcription. However, alterations in Pit-1 gene expression are not involved in pituitary tumor formation.[9]

The main function of prolactin in mammals is lactogenesis, while in fish prolactin is important for osmoregulation. The prolactin gene from the Chinook salmon contains coding sequences that are similar to those in mammals, and it is regulated similarly in the pituitary.[10] Pit-1, the pituitary specific transcription factor, therefore, appears to be highly conserved among species.

Prolactin gene expression is further regulated by other species-specific factors. Prolactin gene transcription is stimulated by estrogen and mediated by estrogen receptor binding to estrogen responsive elements. This activation by estrogen requires interaction with Pit-1, in a manner not yet determined. Proximal promoter sequences are also activated by peptide hormones binding to cell surface receptors; e.g., TRH and growth factors. In addition, various agents that control cyclic AMP and calcium channels can stimulate or inhibit prolactin promoter activity.

Pituitary secretion of prolactin is chiefly under the inhibitory control of hypothalamic dopamine released into the portal circulation. The action of dopamine in the pituitary is mediated by receptors that are coupled to the inhibition of adenylate cyclase activity. There are 5 forms of the dopamine receptor, divided into 2 functional groups, D_1 and D_2.[11] The D_2 type is the predominant receptor in the anterior pituitary gland. The structure and function of the dopamine receptors are of the G protein system as described in Chapter 2. Binding of dopamine to the receptor leads to suppression of adenylate cylase and cyclic AMP maintenance of prolactin gene transcription and prolactin secretion. Other mechanisms are also activated, including suppression of intracellular calcium levels. Pit-1 binding sites are involved in this dopamine response. In addition to direct inhibition of prolactin gene expression, dopamine binding to the D_2 receptor also inhibits lactotroph development and growth. These multiple effects of dopamine explain the ability of dopamine agonists to suppress prolactin secretion and the growth of prolactin-secreting pituitary adenomas. No activating or inactivating mutations of the dopamine receptors have been reported.

The secretion of prolactin is inhibited and stimulated by the association and dissociation of dopamine from its receptors.[12] Several factors exert a stimulatory effect on prolactin secretion (prolactin-releasing factors), especially TRH, vasoactive intestinal peptide (VIP), epidermal growth factor, and perhaps GnRH. These factors interact with each other, affecting the overall lactotroph responsiveness.

The Hypothalamus and GnRH Secretion

The hypothalamus is the part of the diencephalon at the base of the brain that forms the floor of the third ventricle and part of its lateral walls. Within the hypothalamus are peptidergic neural cells that secrete the releasing and inhibiting hormones. These cells share the characteristics of both neurons and endocrine gland cells. They respond to signals in the bloodstream, as well as to neurotransmitters within the brain, in a process known as neurosecretion. In neurosecretion, a neurohormone or neurotransmitter is synthesized on the ribosomes in the cytoplasm of the neuron, packaged into a granule in the Golgi apparatus, and then transported by active axonal flow to the neuronal terminal for secretion into a blood vessel or across a synapse.

The cells that produce GnRH originate from the olfactory area. By migration during embryogenesis, the cells move along cranial nerves connecting the nose and the forebrain to their primary location, where eventually 1000–3000 GnRH-producing cells can be found in the arcuate nucleus of the hypothalamus.[13] The GnRH neurons appear in the medial olfactory placode (a thickened plate of ectoderm from which a sense organ develops) and enter the brain with the nervus terminalis, a cranial nerve that projects from the nose to the septal-preoptic nuclei in the brain.[14] This amazing journey accounts for Kallmann's syndrome, an association between an absence of GnRH and a defect in smell (a failure of both olfactory axonal and GnRH neuronal migration from the olfactory placode). Three modes of transmission have been documented: X linked, autosomal dominant, and autosomal recessive.[15] The 5–7-fold increased frequency in males indicates that X-linked transmission is the most common. The mutations responsible for this syndrome result in the failure to produce a protein (homologous to members of the fibronectin family) responsible for cell adhesion and protease inhibition, functions necessary for neuronal migration.[16, 17] Like

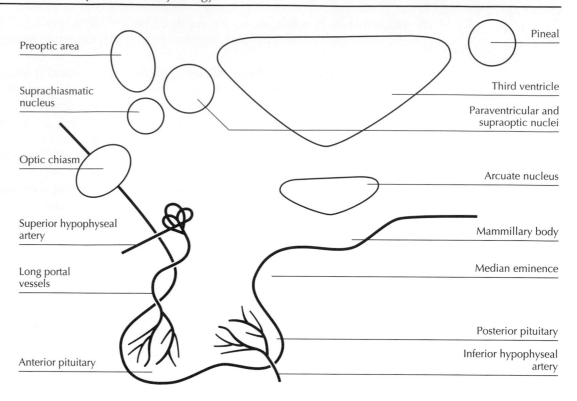

olfactory epithelial cells in the nasal cavity, GnRH neurons have cilia.[18] The olfactory origin and the structural similarity of GnRH neurons and nasal epithelial cells suggest an evolution from reproduction controlled by pheromones.

Pheromones are airborne chemicals released by one individual that can affect other members of the same species. Odorless compounds obtained from the axillae of women in the late follicular phase of their cycles accelerated the LH surge and shorted the cycles of recipient women, and compounds from the luteal phase had the opposite effects.[19] This may be one mechanism by which women who are together much of the time often exhibit a synchrony in menstrual cycle timing.[20, 21]

In primates, the primary network of GnRH cell bodies is located within the medial basal hypothalamus.[22–24] Most of these cell bodies can be seen within the arcuate nucleus where GnRH is synthesized in GnRH neurons. The GnRH neurons exist in a complex network and are connected to each other and to many other neurons. This physical arrangement allows multiple interactions with neurotransmitters, hormones, and growth factors to modulate GnRH release. The delivery of GnRH to the portal circulation is via an axonal pathway, the GnRH tubero-infundibular tract.

Fibers, identified with immunocytochemical techniques using antibodies to GnRH, can also be visualized in the posterior hypothalamus, descending into the posterior pituitary, and in the anterior hypothalamic area projecting to sites within the limbic system.[22] Using hybridization techniques, messenger RNA for GnRH has been localized to the same sites previously identified by immunoreactivity. However, lesions that interrupt GnRH neurons projecting to regions other than the median eminence do not affect gonadotropin release. Only lesions of the arcuate nucleus in the monkey lead to gonadal atrophy and amenorrhea.[25] Therefore, the arcuate nucleus can be viewed with the median eminence as a unit, the key locus within the hypothalamus for GnRH secretion into the portal circulation. The other GnRH neurons may be important for a variety of behavioral responses.

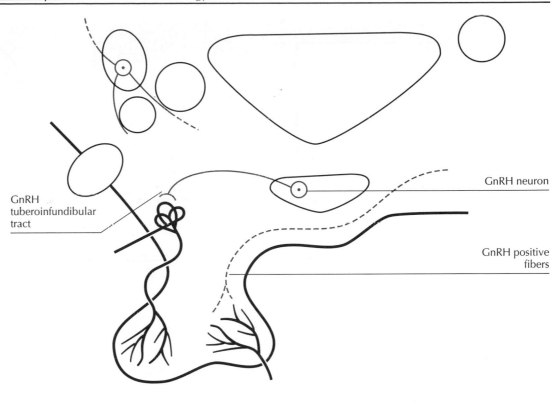

GnRH
tuberoinfundibular
tract

GnRH neuron

GnRH positive
fibers

GnRH Secretion

The half-life of GnRH is only 2–4 minutes. Because of this rapid degradation, combined with the enormous dilution upon entry into the peripheral circulation, biologically effective amounts of GnRH do not escape the portal system. Therefore, control of the reproductive cycle depends on constant release of GnRH. This function, in turn, depends upon the complex and coordinated interrelationships among this releasing hormone, other neurohormones, the pituitary gonadotropins, and the gonadal steroids. The interplay among these substances is governed by feedback effects, both positive stimulatory and negative inhibitory. ***The long feedback loop*** refers to the feedback effects of circulating levels of target gland hormones, and this occurs both in the hypothalamus and the pituitary. ***The short feedback loop*** indicates a negative feedback of pituitary hormones on their own secretion, presumably via inhibitory effects on releasing hormones in the hypothalamus. ***Ultrashort feedback*** refers to inhibition by the releasing hormone on its own synthesis. These signals as well as signals from higher centers in the central nervous system may modify GnRH secretion through an array of neurotransmitters, primarily dopamine, norepinephrine, and endorphin but also serotonin and melatonin. GnRH neurons lack estradiol receptors; therefore, steroid hormone regulation is believed to be mediated through this collection of neurotransmitters.

Dopamine and norepinephrine are synthesized in the nerve terminals by decarboxylation of dihydroxyphenylalanine (DOPA), which in turn is synthesized by hydroxylation of tyrosine. Dopamine is the immediate precursor of norepinephrine, but dopamine itself functions as a key neurotransmitter in the hypothalamus and the pituitary.

A most useful concept is to view the arcuate nucleus as the central site of action, releasing GnRH into the portal circulation in pulsatile fashion. In a classic series of experiments, it was demonstrated that normal gonadotropin secretion requires pulsatile GnRH discharge within a critical range in frequency and amplitude.[26] Even pituitary hormone gene transcription is sensitive to the pulsatile nature of GnRH release.[27]

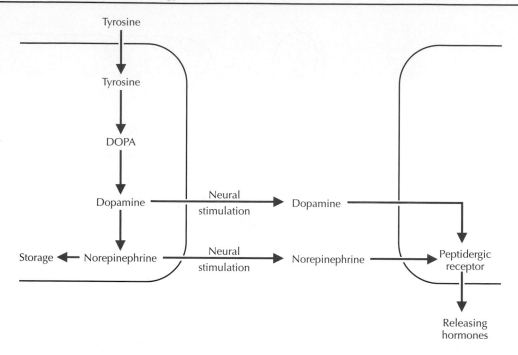

Experimental manipulations have indicated that the critical range of GnRH pulsatile secretion is rather narrow. The administration (to monkeys) of 1 mg GnRH per minute for 6 minutes every hour (1 pulse per hour) produces a portal blood concentration about equal to the peak concentration of GnRH in human portal blood, about 2 ng/mL. Increasing the frequency to 2 and 5 pulses per hour extinguishes gonadotropin secretion. A similar decline in gonadotropin secretion is obtained by increasing the dose of GnRH. Decreasing the pulse frequency decreases LH secretion but increases FSH secretion.

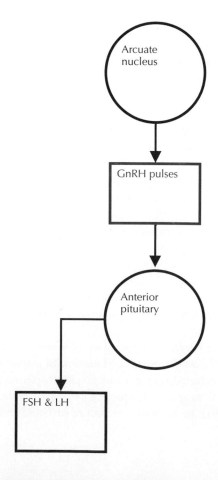

Like GnRH, gonadotropins are also secreted in pulsatile fashion, and indeed, the pulsatile pattern of gonadotropin release reflects the pulsatile GnRH pattern.[28, 29] GnRH and gonadotropin secretion are always pulsatile in nature, but an augmentation of the pulsatile pattern of gonadotropin secretion occurs just before puberty with nighttime increases in LH. After puberty, enhanced pulsatile secretion is maintained throughout the 24-hour period, but it varies in both amplitude and frequency. In puberty, arcuate activity begins with a low frequency of GnRH release and proceeds through a cycle of acceleration of frequency, characterized by passage from relative inactivity, to nocturnal activation, to the full adult pattern. The progressive changes in FSH and LH reflect this activation of GnRH pulsatile secretion. Ovarian steroid release is also pulsatile, coordinated with LH pulses, the major stimulator of ovarian steroidogenesis.[30]

Timing of GnRH Pulses

The measurement of LH pulses is utilized as an indication of GnRH pulsatile secretion (the long half-life of FSH precludes its use for this purpose).[31] The characteristics of LH pulses (and presumably of GnRH pulses) during the menstrual cycle are as follows:[32]

LH pulse mean amplitude:

Early follicular phase	6.5 IU/L.
Midfollicular phase	5.0 IU/L.
Late follicular phase	7.2 IU/L.
Early luteal phase	15.0 IU/L.
Midluteal phase	12.2 IU/L.
Late luteal phase	8.0 IU/L.

LH pulse mean frequency:

Early follicular phase	90 minutes.
Late follicular phase	60–70 minutes.
Early luteal phase	100 minutes.
Late luteal phase	200 minutes

Pulsatile secretion is more frequent but lower in amplitude during the follicular phase compared to the luteal phase. It should be emphasized that these numbers are not inviolate. There is considerable variability between and within individuals and a wide normal range exists.[33] Despite the handicap of the long half-life, it has been ascertained that FSH secretion is correlated with LH secretion.

The anterior pituitary gland also appears to have a pulsatile pattern of its own. Although pulses of significant amplitude are linked to GnRH, small amplitude pulses of high frequency represent spontaneous secretion (at least as demonstrated in isolated pituitary glands in vitro).[34] It is not known whether this has any importance physiologically, and at the present time, the pituitary secretory pattern is thought to reflect GnRH.

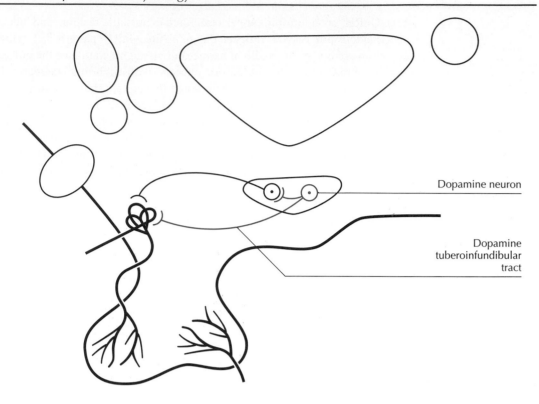

Dopamine neuron

Dopamine
tuberoinfundibular
tract

Control of GnRH Pulses

Normal menstrual cycles require the maintenance of the pulsatile release of GnRH within a critical range of frequency and amplitude. Pulsatile, rhythmic activity is an intrinsic property of GnRH neurons, and the effect of various hormones and neurotransmitters must be viewed as modulating actions.[35]

The Dopamine Tract. Cell bodies for dopamine synthesis can be found in the arcuate and periventricular nuclei. The dopamine tuberoinfundibular tract arises within the medial basal hypothalamus and projects to the median eminence.

The administration of dopamine by intravenous infusion to men and women is associated with a suppression of circulating prolactin and gonadotropin levels.[36] Dopamine does not exert a direct effect on gonadotropin secretion by the anterior pituitary; thus, this effect is mediated through GnRH release in the hypothalamus. Dopamine is directly secreted into the portal blood, thus behaving like a neurohormone. Therefore, dopamine may directly suppress arcuate GnRH activity, and also be transported via the portal system to directly and specifically suppress pituitary prolactin secretion. The hypothalamic tuberoinfundibular dopamine pathway is not the only dopamine pathway in the CNS, and it is only one of two major dopamine pathways in the hypothalamus. But it is this pathway that directly participates in the regulation of prolactin secretion.

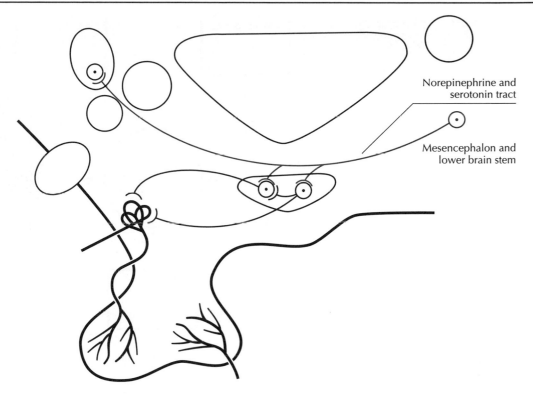

Norepinephrine and serotonin tract

Mesencephalon and lower brain stem

The Norepinephrine Tract. Most of the cell bodies that synthesize norepinephrine are located in the mesencephalon and lower brainstem. These cells also synthesize serotonin. Axons for amine transport ascend into the medial forebrain bundle to terminate in various brain structures including the hypothalamus.

Neuropeptide Y. The secretion and gene expression of neuropeptide Y in hypothalamic neurons is regulated by gonadal steroids.[38] Neuropeptide Y stimulates pulsatile release of GnRH and in the pituitary potentiates gonadotropin response to GnRH.[39] It thus may facilitate pulsatile secretion of GnRH and gonadotropins. In the absence of estrogen, neuropeptide Y inhibits gonadotropin secretion. Because undernutrition is associated with an increase in neuropeptide Y (see Chapter 19) and increased amounts have been measured in cerebrospinal fluid of women with anorexia and bulimia nervosa, it has been proposed that neuropeptide Y is at least one link between nutrition and reproductive function.[40, 41]

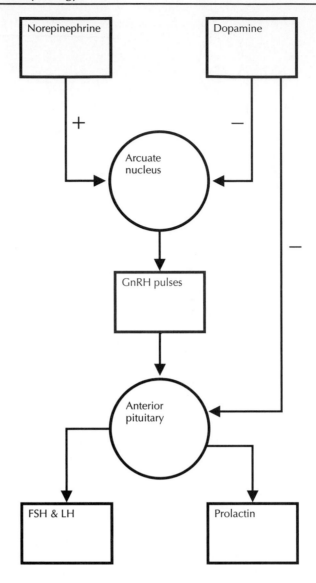

The current concept is that the biogenic catecholamines modulate GnRH pulsatile release.[37] Norepinephrine is thought to exert stimulatory effects on GnRH, while dopamine and serotonin exert inhibitory effects. For an understanding of clinical problems, it is best to view dopamine as an inhibitor of both GnRH and prolactin. Little is known, however, about the role of serotonin. The probable mode of action of catecholamines is to influence the frequency (and perhaps the amplitude) of GnRH discharge. Thus, pharmacologic or psychologic factors that affect pituitary function probably do so by altering catecholamine synthesis or metabolism, and thus the pulsatile release of GnRH.

Pituitary Gonadotropin Secretion

The gene for the α subunit of the gonadotropins is expressed in both the pituitary and placenta. The β-subunit for human chorionic gonadotropin (HCG) is expressed in the placenta but only minimally (and with alterations in structure) in the pituitary, while the LH β-subunit, as expected, is expressed in the pituitary but not significantly in the placenta.[42, 43] Studies of gonadotropin gene expression confirm the relationships established by earlier studies. The sex steroids decrease and castration increases the rate of gonadotropin gene transcription as reflected by the levels of specific messenger RNAs. In addition, the sex steroids can act at the membrane level, affecting the interaction of GnRH with its receptor.[44]

Both LH and FSH are secreted by the same cell, the gonadotrope, localized primarily in the lateral portions of the pituitary gland and responsive to the pulsatile stimulation by GnRH. GnRH is calcium dependent in its mechanism of action and utilizes inositol 1,4,5-triphosphate (IP_3) and 1,2-diacylglycerol (1,2-DG) as second messengers to stimulate protein kinase activity (Chapter 2).[45] These responses require a G protein receptor, and are associated with cyclical release of calcium ions from intracellular stores and the opening of cell membrane channels to allow entry of extracellular calcium. Thus, both protein kinase and calmodulin are mediators of GnRH action. The GnRH receptor, a member of the G protein family, is encoded by a gene on chromosome 4q13.–14q21.1.[46] GnRH receptors are regulated by many agents, including GnRH itself, inhibin, activin, and the sex steroids.[47] A decreased gonadotropin response to continued excessive GnRH stimulation is not due to a loss of GnRH receptors alone but includes desensitization and uncoupling of the receptors (discussed in Chapter 2).

Synthesis of gonadotropins takes place on the rough endoplasmic reticulum. The hormones are packaged into secretory granules by the Golgi cisternae of the Golgi apparatus and then stored as secretory granules. Secretion requires migration (activation) of the mature secretory granules to the cell membrane where an alteration in membrane permeability results in extrusion of the secretory granules in response to GnRH. The rate-limiting step in gonadotropin synthesis is the GnRH-dependent availability of the beta-subunits.

Binding of GnRH to its receptor in the pituitary activates multiple messengers and responses. The immediate event is a secretory release of gonadotropins, while delayed responses prepare for the next secretory release. One of these delayed responses is the self-priming action of GnRH that leads to even greater responses to subsequent GnRH pulses due to a complex series of biochemical and biophysical intracellular events. This self-priming action is important to achieve the large surge in secretion at midcycle; it requires estrogen exposure, and it can be augmented by progesterone. This important action of progesterone depends upon estrogen exposure (for an increase in progesterone receptors) and activation of the progesterone receptor by GnRH stimulated phosphorylation. This latter action is an example of cross-talk between peptide and steroid hormone receptors.

Five different types of secretory cells coexist within the anterior pituitary gland: gonadotropes, lactotropes, thyrotropes, somatotropes, and corticotropes. Autocrine and paracrine interactions combine to make anterior pituitary secretion subject to more complicated control than simply reaction to hypothalamic releasing factors and modulation by feedback signals. Substantial experimental evidence exists to indicate stimulatory and inhibitory influences of various substances on the pituitary secretory cells.

The Intrapituitary Autocrine/Paracrine System

Intrapituitary cytokines and growth factors provide an autocrine/paracrine system for regulating pituitary cell development and replication as well as pituitary hormone synthesis and secretion. The pituitary contains the familiar cast of substances encountered in organs throughout the body, including the interleukins, epidermal growth factor, fibroblast growth factors, the insulin-like growth factors, nerve growth factor, activin, inhibin, and many others.[48] As in most tissues, the interaction among these substances is a complex story, but the activin/inhibin mechanism deserves emphasis.

Activin, Inhibin, and Follistatin

Activin and inhibin are peptide members of the transforming growth factor-β family.[49] Inhibin consists of two dissimilar peptides (known as alpha- and beta-subunits) linked by disulfide bonds. Two forms of inhibin (inhibin A and inhibin B) have been purified, each containing an identical alpha-subunit and distinct but related beta-subunits. Thus, there are three subunits for inhibins:

alpha, beta-A, and beta-B. Each subunit is a product of different messenger RNA; therefore, each is derived from its own large precursor molecule.

Inhibin is secreted by granulosa cells, but messenger RNA for the alpha and beta chains has also been found in pituitary gonadotropes.[50] Inhibin selectively inhibits FSH, but not LH, secretion. Indeed, while suppressing FSH synthesis, inhibin may enhance LH activity.[51] Cells actively synthesizing LH respond to inhibin by increasing GnRH receptor number; FSH dominant cells are suppressed by inhibin.[51] Inhibin has little or no effect on growth hormone, ACTH, and prolactin production.

Activin, also derived from granulosa cells, but present as well in the pituitary gonadotropes, contains two subunits that are identical to the beta-subunits of inhibins A and B. Activin augments the secretion of FSH and inhibits prolactin, ACTH, and growth hormone responses.[52–54] Activin increases pituitary response to GnRH, probably by enhancing GnRH receptor formation.[47] The effects of activin are blocked by inhibin and follistatin.[55] The roles for inhibin and activin in regulating the events of the menstrual cycle are discussed in Chapter 6.

The Two Forms of Inhibin

Inhibin-A:	Alpha-Beta$_A$
Inhibin-B:	Alpha-Beta$_B$

The Three Forms of Activin

Activin-A:	Beta$_A$-Beta$_A$
Activin-AB:	Beta$_A$-Beta$_B$
Activin-B:	Beta$_B$-Beta$_B$

Follistatin is a peptide secreted by a variety of pituitary cells, including the gonadotropes.[56] This peptide has also been called FSH-suppressing protein because of its main action: inhibition of FSH synthesis and secretion and the FSH response to GnRH, probably by binding to activin and in that fashion decreasing the activity of activin.[57, 58] Activin stimulates follistatin production, and inhibin prevents this response.

In summary, GnRH stimulates gonadotropin synthesis and secretion, as well as activin, inhibin, and follistatin. Activin enhances and follistatin suppresses GnRH activity. Evidence in vivo and in vitro indicates that gonadotropin response to GnRH requires activin activity.[59] This relationship may contribute to the down-regulation of pituitary gonadotropin secretion by prolonged GnRH stimulation. Increasing GnRH pulsatile frequency first increases FSH production, and then with high frequency or continuous GnRH stimulation, follistatin production is increased.[59]

The Endogenous Opiates

The most fascinating peptide group is the endogenous opioid peptide family.[60] β-Lipotropin is a 91 amino acid molecule which was first isolated from the pituitary in 1964. Its function remained a mystery for more than 10 years until receptors for opioid compounds were identified, and by virtue of their existence, it was postulated that endogenous opioid compounds must exist and serve important physiological roles. Endorphin was a word coined to denote morphine-like action and endogenous origin in the brain.

Opiate production is regulated by gene transcription and the synthesis of precursor peptides and at a posttranslational level where the precursors are processed into the various bioactive smaller peptides.[61] All opiates derive from one of 3 precursor peptides.

Proopiomelanocortin (POMC) — the source of endorphins.
Proenkephalin A and B — the source of several enkephalins.
Prodynorphin — yields dynorphins.

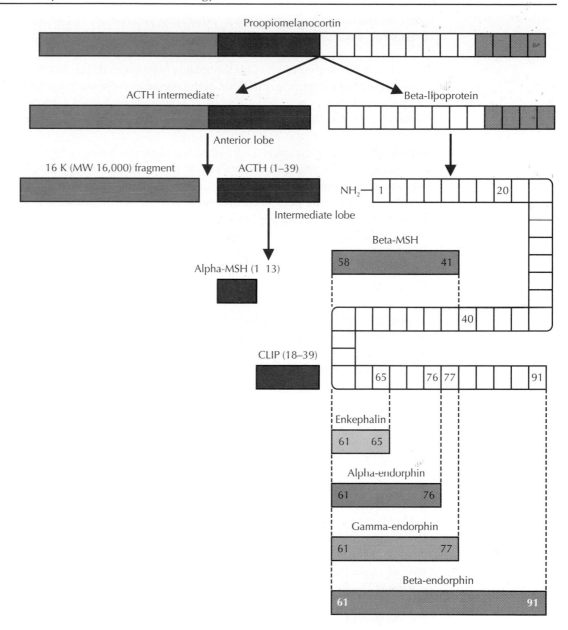

POMC was the first precursor peptide to be identified. It is made in the anterior and intermediate lobes of the pituitary, in the hypothalamus and other areas of the brain, in the sympathetic nervous system, and in other tissues including the gonads, the placenta, the gastrointestinal tract, and the lungs. The highest concentration is in the pituitary gland.

Proopiomelanocortin is split into 2 fragments, an ACTH intermediate fragment and β-lipotropin. β-Lipotropin has no opioid activity but is broken down in a series of steps to β-melanocyte-stimulating hormone (β-MSH), enkephalin, and α-, γ-, and β-endorphins. Melanocyte-stimulating hormone acts in lower animals to stimulate melanin granules within cells, causing darkening of the skin. In humans, there is no known function.

Enkephalin and the α- and γ-endorphins are as active as morphine on a molar basis, while β-endorphin is 5–10 times more potent. In the adult pituitary gland, the major products are ACTH and β-lipotropin, with only small amounts of endorphin. Thus, ACTH and β-lipotropin blood levels show similar courses, and they are major secretion products of the anterior pituitary in response to stress. In the intermediate lobe of the pituitary (which is prominent only during fetal life), ACTH is cleaved to CLIP (corticotropin-like intermediate lobe peptide) and β-MSH. In the placenta and adrenal medulla, POMC processing yields α-MSH-like and β-endorphin peptides. β-Endorphin has also been detected in the ovaries and in the testes.

In the brain, the major products are the opiates, with little ACTH. In the hypothalamus the major products are β-endorphin and α-MSH in the region of the arcuate nucleus and the ventromedial nucleus. The pituitary system is a system for secretion into the circulation while the hypothalamic system allows for distribution via axons to regulate other brain regions and the pituitary gland.

β-Endorphin is appropriately considered a neurotransmitter, a neurohormone, and a neuro-modulator. β-Endorphin influences a variety of hypothalamic functions, including regulation of reproduction, temperature, cardiovascular and respiratory function, as well as extrahypothalamic functions such as pain perception and mood. POMC gene expression in the anterior pituitary is controlled mainly by corticotropin-releasing hormone and influenced by the feedback effects of glucocorticoids. In the hypothalamus, regulation of POMC gene expression is via the sex steroids.[62] In the absence of sex steroids, little, if any, secretion occurs.

Proenkephalin A is produced in the adrenal medulla, the brain, the posterior pituitary, the spinal cord, and the gastrointestinal tract. It yields several enkephalins: methionine-enkephalin, leucine-enkephalin, and other variants. The enkephalins are the most widely distributed endogenous opioid peptides in the brain and are probably mainly involved as inhibitory neurotransmitters in the modulation of the autonomic nervous system. Prodynorphin, found in the brain (concentrated in the hypothalamus) and the gastrointestinal tract, yields dynorphin, an opioid peptide with high analgesic potency and behavioral effects, as well as α-neoendorphin, β-neoendorphin, and leumorphin. The last 13 amino acids of leumorphin constitute another opioid peptide, rimorphin. The prodynorphin products probably function in a fashion similar to endorphin.

It is simpler to say that there are 3 classes of opiates: enkephalins, endorphin, and dynorphin.

Opioid peptides are able to act through different receptors, although specific opiates bind predominantly to one of the various receptor types. Naloxone, used in most human studies, does not bind exclusively to any one receptor type, and thus results with this antagonist are not totally specific. Localization of opioid receptors explains many of the pharmacological actions of the opiates. Opioid receptors are found in the nerve endings of sensory neurons, in the limbic system (site of euphoric emotions), in brainstem centers for reflexes such as respiration, and widely distributed in the brain and the spinal cord.

Opioid Peptides and the Menstrual Cycle

The opioid tone is an important part of menstrual function and cyclicity.[63] Although estradiol alone increases endorphin secretion, the highest levels of endorphin occur with sequential therapy of both estradiol and progesterone (in ovariectomized monkeys). Endogenous endorphin levels, therefore, increase throughout the cycle from nadir levels during menses to highest levels during the luteal phase. Normal cyclicity thus requires sequential periods of high (luteal phase) and low (during menses) hypothalamic opioid activity.

A reduction in LH pulse frequency is linked to increased endorphin release.[64] Naloxone increases both the frequency and the amplitude of LH pulses. ***Thus, the endogenous opiates inhibit gonadotropin secretion by suppressing the hypothalamic release of GnRH.*** Opiates have no effect on the pituitary response to GnRH. The gonadal steroids modify endogenous opioid activity, and the negative feedback of steroids on gonadotropins appears to be mediated by endogenous opiates. Because the fluctuating levels of endogenous opiates in the menstrual cycle are related to the changing levels of estradiol and progesterone, it is attractive to speculate that the sex steroids directly stimulate endogenous opioid receptor activity. There is an absence of opioid effect on postmenopausal and oophorectomized levels of gonadotropins, and the response to opiates is restored with the administration of estrogen, progesterone, or both.[65] Both estrogen and progesterone alone increase endogenous opiates, but estrogen enhances the action of progesterone, which could explain the maximal suppression of GnRH and gonadotropin pulse

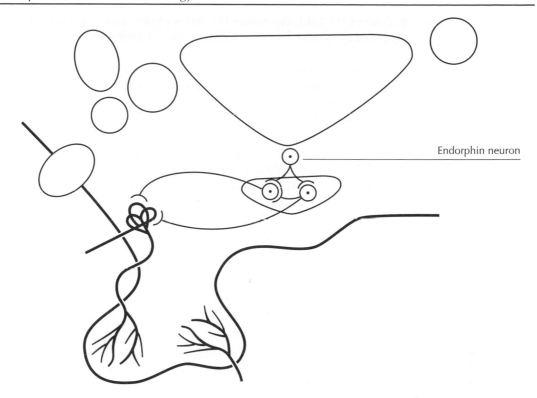

Endorphin neuron

frequency during the luteal phase.[66, 67] In pubertal boys and girls, however, naloxone could not prevent the suppression of LH by estradiol administration, indicating that in this circumstance estradiol may directly inhibit GnRH secretion.[68, 69] Nevertheless, the evidence overall indicates that endogenous opiates exert an inhibiting influence over GnRH secretion.[70]

The inhibiting tone of endogenous opiates is reduced at the time of the ovulatory surge, allowing a release from suppression.[71] This is probably a response to estrogen, specifically an estrogen-induced decrease in opioid receptor binding and opioid release.[72, 73]

Experiments with naloxone administration suggest that the suppression of gonadotropins during pregnancy and the recovery during the postpartum period reflect steroid-induced opioid inhibition, followed by a release from central opioid suppression.

The principal endogenous opiates affecting GnRH release are β-endorphin and dynorphin, and it is probable that the major effect is modulation of the catecholamine pathway, principally norepinephrine. The action does not involve dopamine receptors, acetylcholine receptors, or alpha-adrenergic receptors. On the other hand, endorphin may affect GnRH release directly, without the involvement of any intermediary neuroamine.

Because α-MSH counteracts the effects of β-endorphin, posttranslational processing of POMC can affect hypothalamic-pituitary function by altering the amounts of α-MSH and β-endorphin.[74] This introduces another potential site for neuroendocrine regulation of reproductive function. Gonadal hormones likely have multiple sites for feedback signals.

Clinical Implications

A change in opioid inhibitory tone is not important in the changes of puberty because the responsiveness to naloxone does not develop until after puberty. A change in opioid tone does seem to mediate the hypogonadotropic state seen with elevated prolactin levels, exercise, and other conditions of hypothalamic amenorrhea, while endogenous opioid inhibition does not seem to play a causal role in delayed puberty or hereditary problems such as Kallmann's syndrome.[75, 76] Treatment of patients with hypothalamic amenorrhea (suppressed GnRH pulsatile secretion) with a drug (naltrexone) which blocks opioid receptors restores normal function (ovulation and pregnancy).[77] Thus, the reduced GnRH secretion associated with hypothalamic amenorrhea is mediated by an increase in endogenous opioid inhibitory tone.

Experimental evidence indicates that corticotropin-releasing hormone (CRH) directly inhibits hypothalamic GnRH secretion, both directly and by augmenting endogenous opioid secretion. Women with hypothalamic amenorrhea demonstrate hypercortisolism, suggesting that this could be the pathway by which stress interrupts reproductive function.[78] Mathematical analysis of the associations among FSH, LH, β-endorphin and cortisol pulses support the existence of significant functional coupling between the neuroregulatory systems that control the gonadal and adrenal axes.[79] The CRH gene contains two segments that are similar to estrogen response elements, allowing estrogen enhancement of CRH activity, perhaps explaining the greater vulnerability of the reproductive axis to stress in females.[80]

Cumming concludes that most studies indicate an exercise-induced increase in endogenous opiates, but a significant impact on mood remains to be substantiated.[81] He notes that *runners' high* is more common in California than in Canada (euphoria is hard to come by when running in below freezing temperatures!).

Administration of morphine, enkephalin analogs, and β-endorphin causes release of prolactin. The effect is mediated by inhibition of dopamine secretion in the tuberoinfundibular neurons in the median eminence. Most studies have reported no effect of naloxone on basal, stress-induced, or pregnant levels of prolactin nor on secretion by prolactinomas. Thus a physiological role for endogenous opioid regulation of prolactin does not appear to exist in men and women. However, suppression of GnRH secretion associated with hyperprolactinemia does appear to be mediated by endogenous opiates.[82]

Every pituitary hormone appears to be modulated by opiates. Physiologic effects are important with ACTH, gonadotropins, and possibly vasopressin. Opioid compounds have no direct action on the pituitary, nor do they alter the action of releasing hormones on the pituitary.

POMC-like mRNA is present in the ovary and the placenta.[83] Expression is regulated by gonadotropins in the ovary but not in the placenta. Reasons for endorphin presence in these tissues are not yet apparent. High concentrations of all of the members of the POMC family are found in human ovarian follicular fluid, but only β-endorphin shows significant changes during the menstrual cycle, reaching highest levels just before ovulation.[84]

Catecholestrogens

The enzyme that converts estrogens to catecholestrogens (2-hydroxylase) is richly concentrated in the hypothalamus; hence there are higher concentrations of catecholestrogens than estrone and estradiol in the hypothalamus and pituitary gland. Catecholestrogens have two faces, a catechol side and an estrogen side. Because catecholestrogens have two faces, they have the potential for interacting with both catecholamine and estrogen-mediated systems.[85] To be specific, catecholstrogens can inhibit tyrosine hydroxylase (which would decrease catecholamines) and compete for catechol-*o*-methyltransferase (which would increase catecholamines). Since GnRH, estrogens, and catecholestrogens are located in similar sites, it is possible that catecholestrogens may serve to interact between catecholamines and GnRH secretion. However, these functions remain speculative because a definite role for catecholsteroids has not been established.

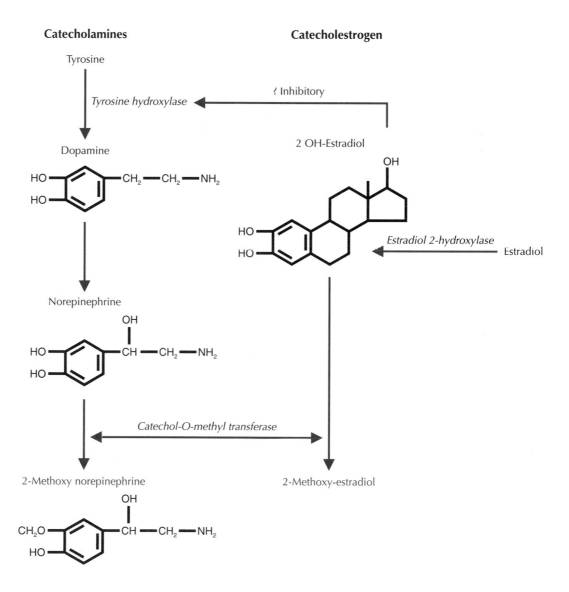

Summary: Control of GnRH Pulses

The key concept is that normal menstrual function requires GnRH pulsatile secretion in a critical range of frequency and amplitude.[29, 31, 86] The normal physiology and pathophysiology of the menstrual cycle, at least in terms of central control, can be explained by mechanisms which affect the pulsatile secretion of GnRH. The pulses of GnRH appear to be directly under the influence of a dual catecholaminergic system: norepinephrine facilitatory and dopamine inhibitory. In turn, the catecholamine system can be influenced by endogenous opioid activity. The feedback effects of steroids may be mediated through this system via catecholsteroid messengers or directly by influencing the various neurotransmitters.

GnRH Agonists and Antagonists

The short half-life of GnRH is due to rapid cleavage of the bonds between amino acids 5-6, 6-7, and 9-10. By altering amino acids at these positions, analogues of GnRH can be synthesized with different properties. Thousands of GnRH analogues have been produced. Substitution of amino acids at the 6 position or replacement of the C-terminal glycine-amide (inhibiting degradation) produces agonists. The GnRH agonists are administered either intramuscularly or subcutaneously or by intranasal absorption. An initial agonistic action (the so-called flare effect) is associated with an increase in the circulating levels of FSH and LH. This response is greatest in the early follicular phase when GnRH and estradiol have combined to create a large reserve pool of gonadotropins. After 1–3 weeks, desensitization and down-regulation of the pituitary produce a hypogonadotropic, hypogonad state. The initial response is due to desensitization, while the sustained response is due to loss of receptors and the uncoupling of the receptor from its effector system. Furthermore, postreceptor mechanisms lead to secretion of biologically inactive gonadotropins, which, however, can still be detected by immunoassay.

Suppression of pituitary secretion of gonadotropins by a GnRH agonist can be utilized for the treatment of endometriosis, uterine leiomyomas, precocious puberty, or the prevention of menstrual bleeding in special clinical situations (e.g., in thrombocytopenic patients). Various tumors contain receptors for GnRH, such as breast, pancreatic, and ovarian, and therefore, there exists a potential for treatment.

GnRH antagonists are synthesized by multiple amino acid substitutions. GnRH antagonists bind to the GnRH receptor and provide competitive inhibition of the naturally occurring GnRH. Thus GnRH antagonists produce an immediate decline in gonadotropin levels with an immediate therapeutic effect. The early products either lacked potency or were associated with undesirable side effects due to histamine release. New analogues continue to be developed and tested, aimed toward the control of fertility.[64] The combination of a GnRH antagonist and testosterone holds promise as a male contraceptive agent.

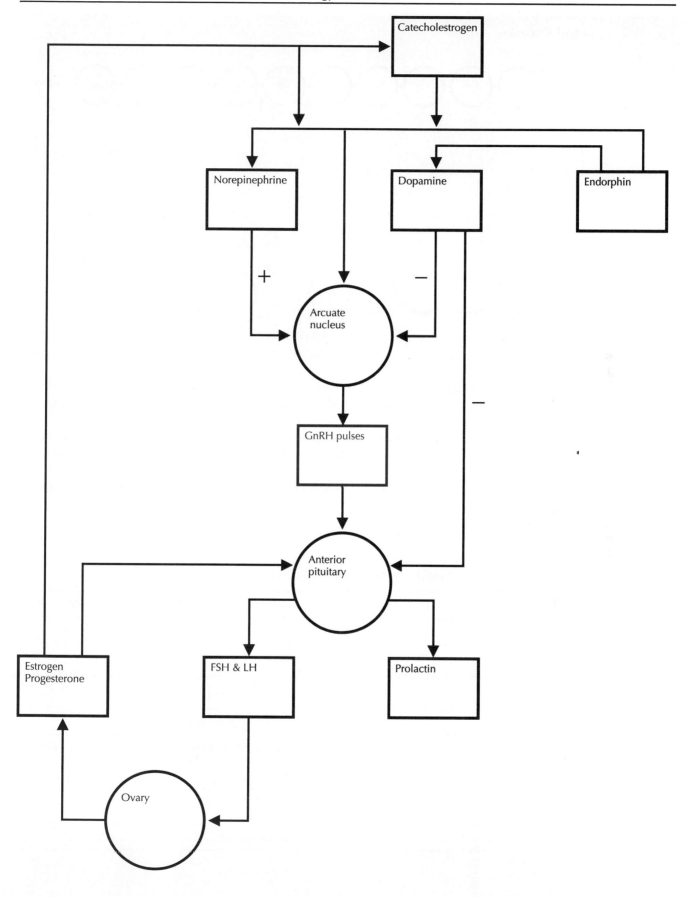

Gonadotropin releasing
hormone

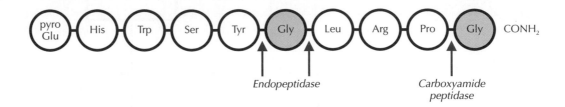

GnRH agonists

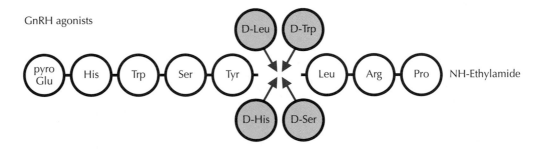

The GnRH analogues cannot escape destruction if administered orally. Higher doses administered subcutaneously can achieve nearly equal effects as observed with intravenous treatment; however, the smaller blood peaks are slower to develop and take longer to return to baseline. Other forms of administration include nasal spray, sustained release implants, and injections of biodegradable microspheres. With the nasal route, absorption enhancers have to be added to increase bioavailability; these agents produce considerable nasal irritation. Goserelin consists of a small biodegradable cylinder which is inserted subcutaneously and monthly using a prepackaged syringe. The depot formulations of GnRH agonists are administered intramuscularly and monthly.

GnRH Agonists in Clinical Use

Position	1	2	3	4	5	6	7	8	9	10
Native GnRH	pGlu	His	Trp	Ser	Tyr	Gly	Leu	Arg	Pro	Gly-NH$_2$
Leuprolide						D-Leu				NH-Ethylamide
Buserelin						D-Ser (tertiary butanol)				NH-Ethylamide
Nafarelin						D-Naphthylalanine (2)				
Histrelin						D-His (tertiary benzyl)				NH-Ethylamide
Goserelin						D-Ser (tertiary butanol)				Aza-Gly
Deslorelin						D-Trp				NH-Ethylamide
Tryptorelin						D-Trp				

Tanycytes

A significant pathway for hypothalamic influence may be via the cerebrospinal fluid (CSF). Tanycytes are specialized ependymal cells whose ciliated cell bodies line the third ventricle over the median eminence. The cells terminate on portal vessels, and they can transport materials from ventricular CSF to the portal system, e.g., substances from the pineal gland, or vasopressin, or oxytocin. Tanycytes change morphologically in response to steroids and exhibit morphological changes during the ovarian cycle.

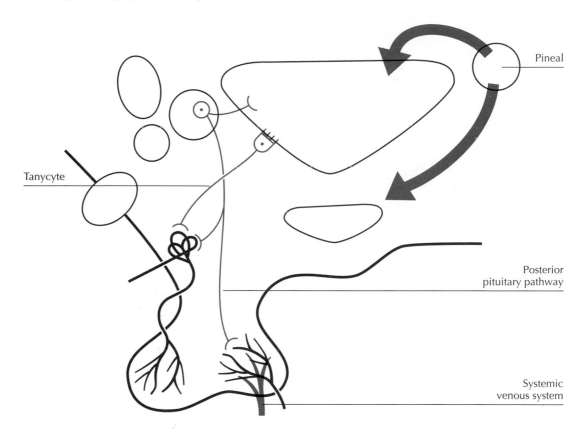

The Posterior Pituitary Pathway

The posterior pituitary is a direct prolongation of the hypothalamus via the pituitary stalk, whereas the anterior pituitary arises from pharyngeal epithelium that migrates into position with the posterior pituitary. Separate neurosecretory cells in both the supraoptic and paraventricular nuclei make vasopressin and oxytocin as parts of large precursor molecules that also contain the transport peptide, neurophysin.[87] Both oxytocin and vasopressin consist of 9 amino acid residues, two of which are half cystines forming a bridge between positions 1 and 6. In the human, vasopressin contains arginine, unlike animals that have lysine vasopressin. The neurophysins are polypeptides with a molecular weight of about 10,000. There are two distinct neurophysins, estrogen-stimulated neurophysin known as neurophysin I, and nicotine-stimulated neurophysin, known as neurophysin II.

The genes for oxytocin and vasopressin are closely linked on chromosome 20, derived from a common ancestor about 400 million years ago.[88] The transcriptional activity of these genes is regulated by endocrine factors, such as the sex steroids and thyroid hormone, through hormone-response elements located upstream. The neurons secrete two large protein molecules, a precursor called pro-pressophysin, which contains vasopressin and its neurophysin, and a precursor called pro-oxyphysin, which contains oxytocin and its neurophysin.[87] Neurophysin I is specifically related to oxytocin, and neurophysin II accompanies vasopressin. Because of this unique packaging, the hormones and their neurophysins are stored together and released at the

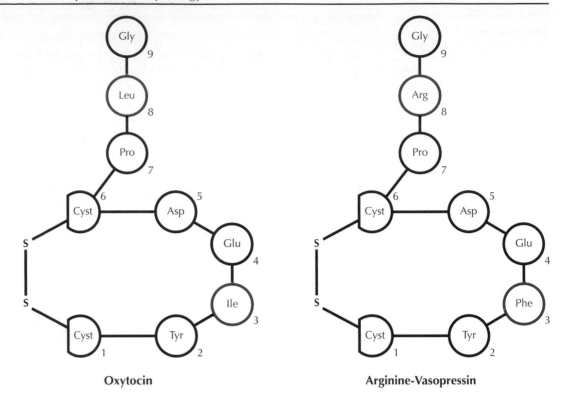

Oxytocin   **Arginine-Vasopressin**

same time into the circulation. The neurophysins are cleaved from their associated neurohormones during axonal transport from the neuronal cell bodies in the supraoptic and paraventricular nuclei to the posterior pituitary. The only known function for the neurophysins is axonal transport for oxytocin and vasopressin.

The posterior pathway is complex and not limited to the transmission of vasopressin and oxytocin to the posterior pituitary. The transportation of vasopressin and oxytocin to the posterior pituitary occurs via nerve tracts which emanate from the supraoptic and paraventricular nuclei and descend through the median eminence to terminate in the posterior pituitary. However, these hormones are also secreted into the cerebrospinal fluid and directly into the portal system. Therefore, vasopressin and oxytocin can reach the anterior pituitary and influence, in the case of vasopressin, ACTH secretion, and in the case of oxytocin, gonadotropin secretion. Vasopressin cooperates with corticotropin-releasing hormone to cause an increased yield of ACTH. Vasopressin and oxytocin-like materials are also found in the ovary, the oviduct, the testis, and the adrenal gland, suggesting that these neurohypophyseal peptides have roles as paracrine or autocrine hormones.[89] The concentrations of these substances in the cerebrospinal fluid exhibit a circadian rhythm (with peak levels occurring during the day), suggesting a different mechanism for CSF secretion compared to posterior pituitary release.[90]

Neurophysin II is called nicotine neurophysin because the administration of nicotine or hemorrhage increases the circulating levels. Neurophysin I is called estrogen neurophysin because estrogen administration increases the levels in the peripheral blood, and peak levels of both neurophysin I and oxytocin are found at the time of the LH surge.[91] Oxytocin neurons and vasopressin neurons have been demonstrated in the rat to contain the estrogen receptor-beta.[92] The rise in estrogen neurophysin begins 10 hours after the rise in estrogen and precedes that of the LH surge, and the elevation of neurophysin lasts longer than the LH surge. Because GnRH and oxytocin are competing substrates for hypothalamic degradation enzymes, it has been hypothesized that oxytocin in the portal blood at the midcycle may inhibit the metabolism of GnRH, thus increasing the amount of GnRH available. Furthermore, oxytocin may have direct actions on the pituitary, ovary, uterus, and fallopian tube during ovulation.

Neurophysin-containing pathways have been traced from the hypothalamic nuclei to various centers in the brainstem and the spinal cord. In addition, behavioral studies suggest a role for vasopressin in learning and memory. Administration of vasopressin has been associated with improvement in memory in brain-damaged human subjects, and enhanced cognitive responses (learning and memory) in both young, normal individuals and depressed patients.

Both oxytocin and vasopressin circulate as the free peptides with a rapid half-life (initial component less than 1 minute, second component of 2–3 minutes). Three major stimuli for vasopressin secretion are changes in osmolality of the blood, alterations in blood volume, and psychogenic stimuli such as pain and fear. The osmoreceptors are located in the hypothalamus; the volume receptors are in the left atrium, aortic arch, and carotid sinus. Angiotensin II also produces a release of vasopressin, suggesting another mechanism for the link between fluid balance and vasopressin. Cortisol may modify the osmotic threshold for the release of vasopressin.

The major functions of vasopressin involve the regulation of osmolality and blood volume. Vasopressin is a powerful vasoconstrictor and antidiuretic hormone. Vasopressin release increases when plasma osmolality rises and is inhibited by water loading (resulting in diuresis). Diabetes insipidus is a condition marked by loss of water because of a lack of vasopressin action in the tubules of the kidney, secondary to a defect in synthesis or secretion of vasopressin. The opposite condition is the continuous and autonomous secretion of vasopressin, the syndrome of inappropriate ADH (antidiuretic hormone) secretion. This syndrome, with its resultant retention of water, is associated with a variety of brain disorders as well as the production of vasopressin and its precursor by malignant tumors.

Oxytocin stimulates muscular contractions in the uterus and myoepithelial contractions in the breast. Thus it is involved in parturition and the letdown of milk. The release of oxytocin is so episodic that it is described as spurts. Ordinarily, there are about 3 spurts every 10 minutes. Oxytocin is released during coitus, probably by the Ferguson reflex (vaginal and cervical stimulation) but also by olfactory, visual, and auditory pathways. Perhaps oxytocin has some role in muscle contractions during orgasm.[93] In the male, release of oxytocin during coitus may contribute to sperm transport during ejaculation.

Using sensitive assays, an increase in maternal levels of oxytocin can be detected prior to parturition, occurring at first only at night.[94, 95] Once labor has begun, oxytocin levels rise significantly, especially during the second stage. Thus, oxytocin may be important for developing the more intense uterine contractions. Extremely high concentrations of oxytocin can be measured in the cord blood at delivery, and release of oxytocin from the fetal pituitary may also be involved in labor. However, this is controversial, and studies in monkeys fail to indicate a role for fetal oxytocin in parturition.[95] Part of the contribution of oxytocin to parturition is the stimulation of prostaglandin synthesis in decidua and myometrium.[96] Cervical dilatation appears to be dependent on oxytocin stimulation of prostaglandin production, probably in the decidua. The greater frequency of labor and delivery at night may be due to greater nocturnal oxytocin secretion.[94] In addition, oxytocin is synthesized in the amnion, chorion, and significantly, in the decidua.[94] This locally produced oxytocin may be a significant stimulus for myometrial and membrane production of prostaglandins.

It is likely that oxytocin action during the initial stages of labor may depend on myometrial sensitivity to oxytocin in addition to the levels of oxytocin in the blood. The concentration of oxytocin receptors in the myometrium is low in the nonpregnant state and increases steadily throughout gestation (an 80 fold increase), and during labor, the concentration doubles. This receptor concentration correlates with the uterine sensitivity to oxytocin.[97] The mechanism for the increase is unknown, but it likely is due to a change in the prostaglandin and hormonal milieu of the uterus. The local production and effects of oxytocin, estrogen, and progesterone combine in a complicated process of autocrine, paracrine, and endocrine actions to result in parturition.

Oxytocin is released in response to suckling, mediated through impulses generated at the nipple and transmitted via the 3rd, 4th, and 5th thoracic nerves to the spinal cord to the hypothalamus. In addition to causing milk ejection, the reflex is responsible for the uterine contractions associated with breastfeeding. Opioid peptides inhibit oxytocin release, and this may be the means by which stress, fear, and anger inhibit milk output in lactating women. Oxytocin is also expressed in many tissues where it exerts autocrine/paracrine actions.

The Brain and Ovulation

Classic studies in a variety of rodents indicated the presence of feedback centers in the hypothalamus that responded to steroids with the release of GnRH. The release of GnRH was the result of the complex, but coordinated, relationships among the neurohormones, the pituitary gonadotropins, and the gonadal steroids designated by the time-honored terms positive and negative feedback.

FSH levels were thought to be largely regulated by a negative inhibitory feedback relationship with estradiol. In the case of LH, there existed both a negative inhibitory feedback relationship with estradiol and a positive stimulatory feedback with high levels of estradiol. The feedback centers were located in the hypothalamus, and they were called the tonic and cyclic centers. The tonic center controlled the day-to-day basal level of gonadotropins and was responsive to the negative feedback effects of steroids. The cyclic center in the female brain was responsible for the midcycle surge of gonadotropins, a response mediated by the positive feedback of estrogen. Specifically, the midcycle surge of gonadotropins was thought to be due to an outpouring of GnRH in response to the positive feedback action of estradiol on the cyclic center of the hypothalamus.

This classic concept was not inaccurate. The problem was that the concept accurately described events in the rodent, but the mechanism is different in the primate.

In the primate, the "center" for the midcycle surge of gonadotropins has moved from the hypothalamus to the pituitary. Experiments in the monkey have demonstrated that GnRH, originating in the hypothalamus, plays a permissive and supportive role. Its pulsatile secretion is an important prerequisite for normal pituitary function,[86] but the feedback responses regulating gonadotropin levels are controlled by ovarian steroid feedback on the anterior pituitary cells.

The present concept is derived from experiments in which the medial basal hypothalamus (MBH) is either destroyed[26] or the hypothalamus is surgically separated from the pituitary.[98] In a typical (and now classic) experiment, lesion of the MBH by radiofrequency waves was followed by loss of LH levels as the source of GnRH was eliminated.[25] Administration of GnRH in a pulsatile fashion by an intravenous pump restored LH secretion. The administration of estradiol was then

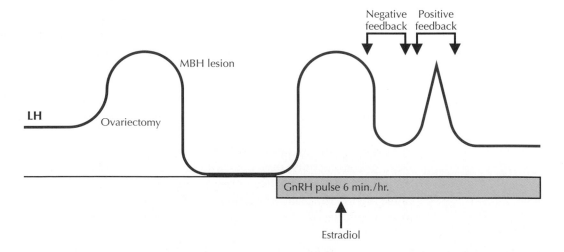

able to produce both negative and positive feedback responses, clearly actions that must be directly on the anterior pituitary because the hypothalamus was absent and GnRH was being administered in a steady and unchanging frequency and dose.

Administration of GnRH intravenously as a bolus produces an increase in blood levels of LH and FSH within 5 minutes, reaching a peak in about 20–25 minutes for LH and 45 minutes for FSH. Levels return to pretreatment values after several hours. When administered by constant infusion at submaximal doses, there is first a rapid rise with a peak at 30 minutes, followed by a plateau or fall between 45 and 90 minutes, then a second and sustained increase at 225–240 minutes. This biphasic response suggests the presence of two functional pools of pituitary gonadotropins.[99] The readily releasable pool (secretion) produces the initial response, and the later response is dependent upon a second, reserve pool of stored gonadotropins.

There are three principal positive actions of GnRH on gonadotropin elaboration.

1. Synthesis and storage (the reserve pool) of gonadotropins.

2. Activation, movement of gonadotropins from the reserve pool to a pool ready for direct secretion, a self-priming action.

3. Immediate release (direct secretion) of gonadotropins.

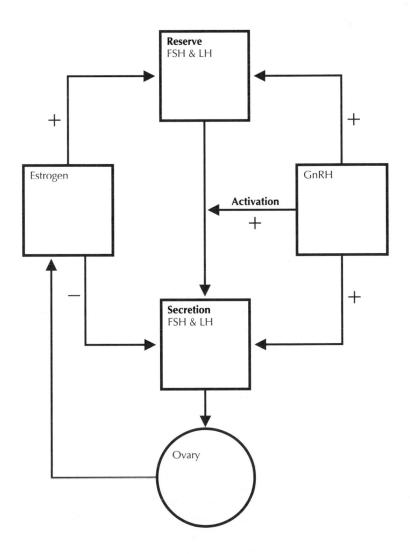

Secretion, synthesis, and storage change during the cycle. At the beginning of the cycle, when estrogen levels are low, both secretion and storage levels are low. With increasing levels of estradiol, a greater increase occurs in storage, with little change in secretion. Thus, in the early follicular phase, estrogen has a positive effect on the synthesis and storage response, building up a supply of gonadotropins in order to meet the requirements of the midcycle surge. Premature release of gonadotropins is prevented by a negative (inhibitory) action of estradiol on the pituitary secretory response to GnRH.

As the midcycle approaches, subsequent responses to GnRH are greater than initial responses, indicating that each response not only induces release of gonadotropins but also activates the storage pool for the next response. This sensitizing or priming action of GnRH also involves an increase in the number of its own receptors and requires the presence of estrogen.[100, 101] Estrogen itself is capable of increasing the number of GnRH receptors.[51, 102] The rise in estrogen at midcycle prepares the gonadotrope to further respond to GnRH.

Because the midcycle surge of LH can be produced in the experimental monkey in the absence of a hypothalamus, and in the face of unchanging GnRH, the ovulatory surge of LH is now believed to be a response to positive feedback action of estradiol on the anterior pituitary. When the estradiol level in the circulation reaches a critical concentration and this concentration is maintained for a critical time period, the inhibitory action on LH secretion changes to a stimulatory action. The mechanism of this steroid action is not known with certainty, but experimental evidence suggests that the positive feedback action involves many mechanisms, including an increase in GnRH receptor concentration, and an increase in pituitary sensitivity to GnRH. The negative feedback of estrogen operates through an uncertain, but different, system.[103–105]

What a logical mechanism! The midcycle surge must occur at the right time of the cycle to ovulate a ready and waiting mature follicle. What better way to achieve this extreme degree of coordination and timing than by the follicle itself, through the feedback effects of the sex steroids originating in the follicle destined to ovulate.

GnRH is increased in the peripheral blood of women and the portal blood of monkeys at midcycle. While this increase may not be absolutely necessary (as demonstrated in the monkey experiments), studies do indicate that activity is occurring in both the hypothalamus and the pituitary.[104, 106, 107] Therefore, although the system can operate with only an unwavering, permissive action of GnRH, fine tuning probably takes place by means of simultaneous effects on GnRH pulsatile secretion and pituitary response to GnRH. This is supported by gonadotropin gene expression studies, indicating steroid effects at both the hypothalamus and the pituitary. The upstream region of the LH β-subunit gene (in the rat) binds the estrogen receptor, providing a means for direct steroid hormone modulation in the pituitary.[108] The human GnRH gene contains a hormone responsive element that binds estrogen and its receptor.[109] However, studies have failed to detect the presence of estrogen receptors in GnRH neurons,[110–112] and this hormone responsive element may be regulated by other substances, or other estrogen responsive neurons may synapse with GnRH cell bodies.[113] Another possibility is that GnRH neurons contain estrogen receptor-beta, and the previous immunoreactive studies have been directed to estrogen receptor-alpha. Nevertheless, in vivo studies in the sheep have demonstrated that estradiol has both negative and positive feedback effects on hypothalamic GnRH secretion, and that a GnRH surge is involved in the preovulatory LH surge.[114–116] Certainly, the presence of GnRH is essential; the administration of a GnRH antagonist to women at midcycle prevents the LH surge.[117]

Influencing the hypothalamic frequency of GnRH secretion can in turn influence pituitary response to GnRH. Faster or slower frequencies of GnRH pulses result in lower GnRH receptor numbers in the pituitary.[118] Thus, a critical peak frequency is necessary for peak numbers of GnRH receptors and the peak midcycle response. Here is a method for the fine tuning at both the hypothalamus (pulse frequency) and the pituitary (receptor number). Indeed, turning off the surge may involve down-regulation because of excessive GnRH. Studies in sheep indicate that a surge of GnRH at the time of the LH surge is associated with a switch from episodic secretion to continuous secretion into the portal circulation, producing the high exposure known to result in down-regulation.[119]

Another aspect of gonadotropin secretion is clinically important. A disparity exists between the quantity of LH measured during the midcycle surge as determined by immunoassay and bioassay. More LH is secreted at midcycle in a molecular form with greater biological activity.[120] There is a well-established relationship between the activity and half-life of glycoprotein hormones and molecular composition (see Chapter 2, under "Heterogeneity" of tropic hormones). The estrogen influence on gonadotropin synthesis is an additional method for maximizing the biologic effects of the midcycle surge. The bioactivity is also very dependent upon pulsatile stimulation by GnRH.

The midcycle surge of FSH has an important clinical purpose. A normal corpus luteum requires the induction of an adequate number of LH receptors on granulosa cells, a specific action of FSH. In addition, FSH accomplishes important intrafollicular changes necessary for the physical expulsion of the ovum. The midcycle surge of FSH, therefore, plays a critical role in ensuring ovulation and a normal corpus luteum. Emerging progesterone secretion, just prior to vulation, is the key.

Progesterone, at low levels and in the presence of estrogen, augments the pituitary secretion of LH and is responsible for the FSH surge in response to GnRH.[121–124] As the rising levels of LH produce the morphologic change of luteinization in the ovulating follicle, the granulosa layer begins to secrete progesterone directly into the bloodstream. The process of luteinization is inhibited by the presence of the oocyte, and therefore progesterone secretion is relatively suppressed, ensuring that only low levels of progesterone reach the brain.

After ovulation, rapid and full luteinization is accompanied by a marked increase in progesterone levels, which, in the presence of estrogen, exercise a profound negative feedback action to suppress gonadotropin secretion. This action of progesterone takes place in two locations.[125–127] First, there definitely is a central action to decrease GnRH.[128] Progesterone fails to block estradiol-induced gonadotropin discharges in monkeys with hypothalamic lesions if pulsatile GnRH replacement is provided. Therefore, high levels of progesterone inhibit ovulation at the hypothalamic level. In addition, progesterone can also block estrogen-induced responses to GnRH at the pituitary level. In contrast, the facilitatory action of low levels of progesterone is exerted only at the pituitary on the response to GnRH.

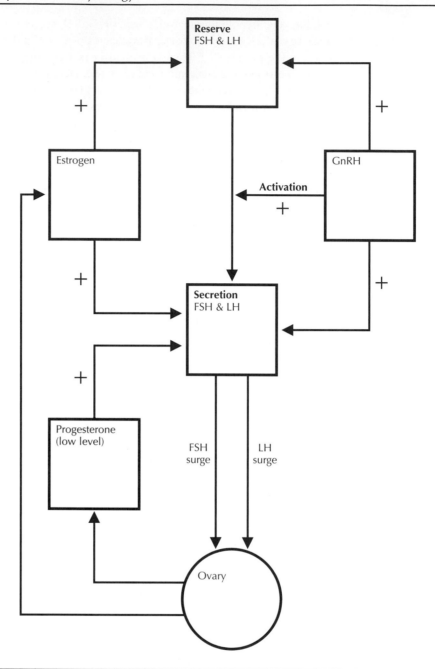

Summary: Key Points

1. Pulsatile GnRH secretion must be within a critical range for frequency and concentration (amplitude). This is absolutely necessary for normal reproductive function.

2. GnRH has only positive actions on the anterior pituitary: synthesis and storage, activation, and secretion of gonadotropins. The gonadotropins are secreted in a pulsatile fashion in response to the similar pulsatile release of GnRH.

3. Low levels of estrogen enhance FSH and LH synthesis and storage, have little effect on LH secretion, and inhibit FSH secretion.

4. High levels of estrogen induce the LH surge at midcycle, and high steady levels of estrogen lead to sustained elevated LH secretion.

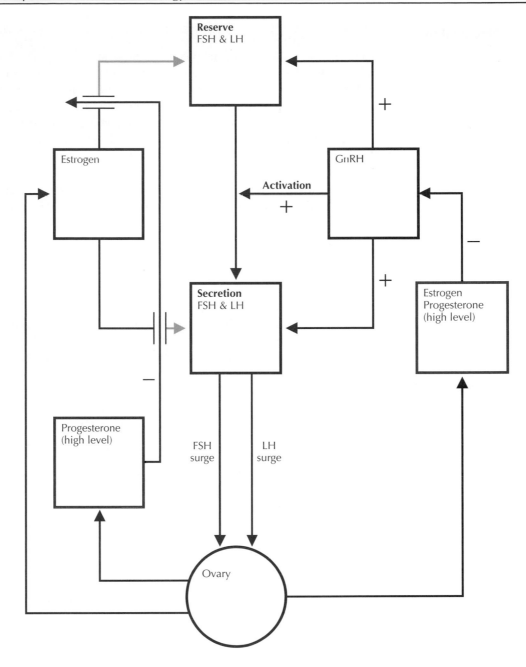

5. Low levels of progesterone acting at the level of the pituitary gland enhance the LH response to GnRH and are responsible for the FSH surge at midcycle.

6. High levels of progesterone inhibit pituitary secretion of gonadotropins by inhibiting GnRH pulses at the level of the hypothalamus. In addition, high levels of progesterone antagonize pituitary response to GnRH by interfering with estrogen action.

The Pineal Gland

Although no physiologic role has been firmly established in the human, the reproductive functions of the hypothalamus may also be under inhibitory control of the brain via the pineal gland. The pineal arises as an outgrowth of the roof of the third ventricle, but soon after birth it loses all afferent and efferent neural connections with the brain. Instead the parenchymal cells receive a new and unusual sympathetic innervation which allows the pineal gland t be an active neuroendocrine organ that responds to photic and hormonal stimuli and exhibits circadian rhythms.[129–131]

The neural pathway begins in the retina and passes through the suprachiasmatic and paraventricular nuclei in the hypothalamus to the inferior accessory optic tracts and the medial forebrain bundle to the upper spinal cord. Preganglionic fibers terminate at the superior cervical ganglion, and postganglionic sympathetic nerves terminate directly on pineal cells. Interruption of this pathway gives the same effect as darkness, which is an increase in pineal biosynthetic activity.

Hydroxyindole-*o*-methyltransferase (HIOMT), an enzyme essential for melatonin synthesis, is found mainly in pineal parenchymal cells, and its products are essentially unique to the pineal. Norepinephrine stimulates tryptophan entry into the pineal cell and also adenylate cyclase activity in the membrane. The resulting increase in cyclic AMP leads to *N*-acetyltransferase activity, the rate-limiting step in melatonin synthesis. Tryptophan is converted by the combined action of *N*-acetyltransferase and HIOMT into melatonin. Thus, melatonin synthesis is controlled by norepinephrine stimulation of adenylate cyclase, and the norepinephrine is liberated by sympathetic stimulation due to the absence of light. HIOMT is also found in the retina where melatonin may serve to regulate the pigment in retinal cells, and in the intestine. However, pinealectomy completely eliminaes detectable levels of melatonin in the circulation. Calcification of the pineal gland is common. It is frequently present in young children, and almost all elderly people have pineal calcification.

The association of hyperplastic pineal tumors with decreased gonadal function, and destructive tumors with precocious puberty, suggested that the pineal is the source of gonadal inhibiting substances. However, pineal mechanisms cannot be absolutely essential for gonadal function. Normal reproductive function returns to the pinealectomized rat several weeks after pinealectomy; blind women have normal fertility, and pinealectomy in a primate did not affect pubertal development.[132]

DARKNESS ⟶ INCREASED MELATONIN ⟶ DECREASED GnRH

A rat in constant light develops a small pineal with decreased HIOMT and melatonin, while the ovarian weight increases. A rat in constant dark has the opposite result, increased pineal size, HIOMT, and melatonin, with decreased ovarian weight and pituitary function. A rhythm is established in pineal HIOMT activity by the presence or absence of light. Short days and long nights result in gonadal atrophy, and this is the major mechanism governing seasonal breeding.[133] In humans, melatonin secretion increases after darkness and peaks in the middle of the night, and then decreases. This rhythm is endogenous, originating in the suprachiasmatic nucleus. Light does not cause the rhythm, but influences its timing.

Possible roles in humans may be to give circadian rhythmicity to other functions such as temperature and sleep. In all vertebrates tested so far, there is a daily and seasonal rhythm in melatonin secretion: high values during the dark and low during light, greater secretion in the winter compared to the summer. Desynchronization with travel across time zones may contribute to the symptom complex known as jet lag. Melatonin ingestion improves both the duration and quality of slee, but the optimal timing of administration is unknown.[131]

The pineal, therefore, serves as an interface between the environment and hypothalamic-pituitary function. In order to correctly interpret day length, animals require a daily rhythm in melatonin secretion. This coordination of temporal, environmental information is especially important in seasonal breeders. This pineal rhythm appears to require the suprachiasmatic nucleus, perhaps the site at which pineal function and light changes are coordinated.

Melatonin is synthesized and secreted by the pineal gland and circulates in the blood like a classical hormone. It affects distant target organs, especially the neuroendocrine centers of the central nervous system. Whether melatonin is secreted primarily into the CSF or blood is still debated, but most evidence favors blood. Melatonin may reach the hypothalamus from the CSF by way of tanycyte transport.

The gonadal changes associated with melatonin are mediated via the hypothalamus and suggest a general suppressive effect on GnRH pulsatile secretion and reproductive function.[134] In humans, melatonin blood levels are highest in the first year of life (with highest levels at night), then decrease with age, eventually releasing, some claim, the suppression of GnRH prior to puberty.[133] This hypothesis is challenged by the association of blindness in human females with an age of menarche that is earlier than normal.[135] Furthermore, pinealectomy in monkeys does not affect puberty.[132]

Pineal activity can be viewed as the net balance between hormone and neuron mediated influences. The pineal contains receptors for the active sex hormones, estradiol, testosterone, dihydrotestosterone, progesterone, and prolactin. Furthermore, the pineal converts testosterone and progesterone to the active 5α-reduced metabolites, and androgens are aromatized to estrogens. The pineal also appears to be unique in that a catecholamine neurotransmitter (norepinephrine), interacting with cell membrane receptors, stimulates cellular synthesis of estrogen and androgen receptors. In general, however, the sympathetic activity producing the circadian rhythm takes precedence over hormonal effects.

Despite a variety of suggestive leads, there is no definitive evidence for a role of the pineal in humans. Nevertheless the important relationship between light exposure and circadian rhythms continues to focus attention on the pineal gland as a coordinator.[136] There is a seasonal distribution in human conception in northern countries with a decrease in ovarian activity and conception rates during the dark winter months.[137, 138] In addition, the pineal can disrupt normal gonadal function. A male with delayed puberty due to hypogonadotropism has been described, who had an enlarged, hyperfunctional pineal gland.[139] Over time, his melatonin levels spontaneously decreased, and normal pituitary-gonadal function developed. Elevated nocturnal levels of melatonin have been reported in patients with hypothalmic amenorrhea and women with anorexia nervosa.[134]

A possible influence of the pineal gland may be the synchronization of menstrual cycles noted among women who spend time together. A significant increase in synchronization of cycles among roommates and among closest friends occurred in the first 4 months of residency in a dormitory of a women's college.[20] A similar increase in synchrony has been observed in women coworkers in occupations characterized by levels of interdependency that were equal to or greater than the levels of encountered job stress.[21] However, efforts to replicate these results have not always been successful.[140]

Melatonin is available in 1 and 5 mg doses that produce blood levels that are 10 to 100 times higher than normal nighttime peaks.[131] The effects include increased sleepiness and decreased alertness. No data are available regarding long-term consequences on reproductive function.

A number of other indoles (also derivatives of tryptophan) have been identified in the pineal gland. Biologic roles for these indoles remain elusive, but one in particular has been extensively investigated. Arginine vasotocin differs from oxytocin by a single amino acid in position 8 and from vasopressin by a single amino acid in position 3. In general, arginine vasotocin has an inhibitory action on the gonads and pituitary secretion of prolactin and LH. Nevertheless a precise role continues to be evasive.

Gonadotropin Secretion Through Fetal Life, Childhood, and Puberty

We have often considered the endocrine events during puberty as an awakening, a beginning. However, endocrinologically, puberty is not a beginning, but just another stage in a development that began at conception. The development of the anterior pituitary in the human starts between the 4th and 5th weeks of fetal life, and by the 12th week of gestation the vascular connection between the hypothalamus and the pituitary is functional. Gonadotropin production has been documented throughout fetal life, during childhood, and into adult life.[141] Remarkable levels of FSH and LH, similar to postmenopausal levels, can be measured in the fetus. GnRH is detectable in the hypothalamus by 10 weeks of gestation, and by 10–13 weeks when the vascular connection is complete, FSH and LH are being produced in the pituitary. The peak pituitary concentrations of FSH and LH occur at about 20–23 weeks of intrauterine life, and peak circulating levels occur at 28 weeks.

The increasing production rate of gonadotropins until midgestation reflects the growing ability of the hypothalamic-pituitary axis to perform at full capacity. Beginning at midgestation, there is an increasing sensitivity to inhibition by steroids and a resultant decrease in gonadotropin secretion. Full sensitivity to steroids is not reached until late in infancy. The rise in gonadotropins after birth reflects loss of the high levels of placental steroids. Thus, in the first year of life there is considerable follicular activity in the ovaries in contrast to later in childhood when gonadotropin secretion is suppressed. Furthermore, the postnatal rise in gonadotropins is even greater in infants born prematurely.

Testicular function in the fetus can be correlated with the fetal hormone patterns. Initial testosterone production and sexual differentiation are in response to the fetal levels of HCG, whereas further testosterone production and masculine differentiation appear to be maintained by the fetal pituitary gonadotropins. Decreased testosterone levels in late gestation probably reflect the decrease in gonadotropin levels. The fetal generation of Leydig cells somehow avoids down-regulation and responds to high levels of HCG and LH by increased steroidogenesis and cell multiplication. This generation of cells is replaced by the adult generation which becomes functional at puberty and responds to high levels of HCG and LH with down-regulation and decreased steroidogenesis.

There is a sex difference in fetal gonadotropin levels. There are higher pituitary and circulating FSH and pituitary LH levels in female fetuses. The lower male levels are probably due to testicular testosterone and inhibin production. In infancy, the postnatal FSH rise is more marked and more sustained in females, while LH values are not as high. This early activity is accompanied by inhibin levels comparable to the low range observed during the follicular phase of the menstrual cycle.[142] After the postnatal rise, gonadotropin levels reach a nadir during early childhood (by about 6 months of age in males and 1–2 years in females) and then rise slightly between 4 and 10 years. This childhood period is characterized by low levels of gonadotropins in the pituitary and in the blood, little response of the pituitary to GnRH, and maximal hypothalamic suppression.

The precise signal that initiates the events of puberty is unknown.[143] In girls, the first steroids to rise in the blood are dehydroepiandrosterone (DHA) and its sulfate (DHAS) beginning at 6–8 years of age, shortly before FSH begins to increase. Estrogen levels, as well as LH, do not begin to rise until 10–12 years of age. If the onset of puberty is triggered by the first hormone to increase in the circulation, then a role for adrenal steroids must be considered. However, there is no evidence to suggest that the adrenal steroids are necessary for the proper timing of puberty, and adrenarche appears to be independent, not controlled by the same mechanism that turns on the gonads.[144] Neither is there a definite relationship demonstrated between melatonin secretion and

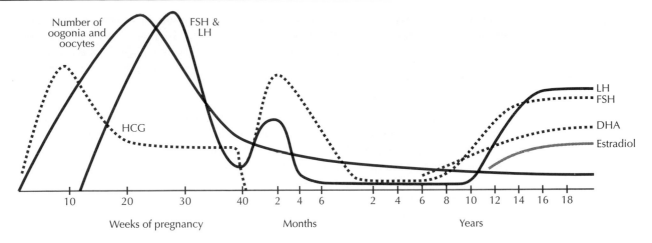

puberty. Because the studies have focused on the amount of melatonin secreted rather than the rhythm of secretion, this question remains open.

Prior to puberty, gonadotropin levels are low but still associated with pulses (although quite irregular).[145] The clinical onset of puberty is preceded by an increase in pulse frequency, amplitude, and regularity, especially during the night.[145-149] At the time of appearance of secondary sex characteristics, the mean LH levels are 2 to 4 times higher during sleep than during wakefulness. This pattern is not present before or after puberty and is an early sign of changes taking place in the hypothalamus, where there is increasing coordination of GnRH neurons with increasing GnRH pulsatile secretion. This pattern can be detected in individuals who develop increasing and decreasing degrees of hypothalamic suppression (such as in individuals with worsening and improving anorexia nervosa). FSH levels plateau by midpuberty, while LH and estradiol levels continue to rise until late puberty. Biologically active LH has been found to rise proportionately more than immunoreactive LH with the onset of puberty.

The rise of gonadotropins at puberty appears to be independent of the gonads in that the same response can be observed in patients with gonadal dysgenesis (who lack functional steroid-producing gonadal tissue). Adolescent girls with Turner syndrome (45,X) also demonstrate augmented gonadotropin secretion during sleep.[150] Thus, maturation at puberty must involve changes in the hypothalamus that are independent of ovarian steroids.

The maturational change in the hypothalamus is followed by an orderly and predictable sequence of events. Increased GnRH secretion leads to increased pituitary responsiveness to GnRH (a combination of steroid influence on the pituitary and a frequency effect of GnRH pulses on GnRH receptor numbers), leading to increasing production and secretion of gonadotropins. Increased gonadotropins are responsible for follicular growth and development in the ovary and increased sex steroid levels. The rising estrogen contributes to achieving an adult pattern of pulsatile GnRH secretion, finally leading to cyclic menstrual patterns.

The trend toward lowering of the menarcheal age and the period of acceleration of growth has halted. In a 10-year prospective study of middle class contemporary American girls, the mean age of menarche was 12.83 with a range of 9.14–17.70 years.[151] The age of onset of puberty is variable and influenced by genetic factors, socioeconomic conditions, and general health. The earlier menarche today compared to the past is undoubtedly due to improved nutrition and better health. It has been suggested that initiation of growth and menarche occur at a particular body weight (48 kg) and percent of body fat (17%).[152] It is thought that this relationship reflects a required stage of metabolism. Although this hypothesis of a critical weight is a helpful concept, the extreme variability in onset of menarche indicates that there is no particular age or size at which an individual girl should be expected to experience menarche.

In the female, the typical sequence of events is growth initiation, thelarche, pubarche, and finally menarche. This generally begins sometime between 8 and 14 years of age. The length of time involved in this evolution is usually 2–4 years. During this time span, puberty is said to occur. Individual variation in the order of appearance of this sequence is great. For example, growth of pubic hair and breast development are not always correlated.

Puberty is due to the reactivation of the hypothalamic-pituitary axis, once fully active during fetal life but suppressed during childhood. If the systems are potentially responsive, what holds function in check until puberty? The hypothalamic-pituitary-gonadal system is operative prior to puberty but is extremely sensitive to steroids and therefore suppressed. The changes at puberty are due to a gradually increasing gonadotropin secretion that takes place because of a decrease in the sensitivity of the hypothalamic centers to the negative-inhibitory action of gonadal steroids. This can be pictured as a slowly rising set point of decreased sensitivity, resulting in increasing GnRH pulsatile secretion, leading to increasing gonadotropin production and ovarian stimulation, and finally to increasing estrogen levels. The reason that FSH is the first gonadotropin to rise at puberty is that arcuate activity begins with a low frequency of GnRH pulses. This is associated with a rise in FSH and little change in LH. With acceleration of frequency, FSH and LH reach adult levels. In addition, there is a qualitative change as a greater increase occurs in the bioactive forms of the gonadotropins.

Negative feedback of steroids, however, cannot be the sole explanation for the low gonadotropin levels in children. Agonadal children show the same decline in gonadotropins from age 2 to 6 as do normal children.[153] This indicates an intrinsic CNS inhibitory mechanism independent of gonadal steroids. Therefore, the restraint of puberty can be viewed as the result of two forces:

1. A CNS inhibitory force, a mechanism suppressing GnRH pulsatile secretion.

2. A very sensitive negative feedback of gonadal steroids (6–15 times more sensitive before puberty).

Because agonadal children show a rise in gonadotropins at pubertal age following suppression to a nadir during childhood, the dominant mechanism must be a CNS inhibitory force. The initial maturational change in the hypothalamus would then be a decrease in this inhibitory influence. A search for this mechanism continues. Some have argued that, rather than a chronic state of inhibition prior to puberty, the GnRH neurons exist in an unrestrained but uncoordinated pattern of activity that prevents adequate secretion.

The development of the positive feedback response to estrogen occurs later. This explains the well-known finding of anovulation in the first months (as long as 18 months) of menstruation. There are frequent exceptions, however, and ovulation can occur even at the time of menarche.

Don't think of puberty as being turned on by a controlling center in the brain but rather as a functional confluence of all factors. This is more a concept than an actual locus of action.

The overall result of this change in the hypothalamus is the development of secondary sex characteristics, attainment of adult set point levels, and the ability to reproduce. Neoplastic and vascular disorders that alter hypothalamic sensitivity can reverse the prepubertal threshold restraint and lead to precocious puberty.

References

1. **Kendrick KM, Dixson AF,** Luteinizing hormone releasing hormone enhances proceptivity in a primate, *Neuroendocrinology* 41:449, 1985.

2. **Hayflick JS, Adelman JP, Seeburg PH,** The complete nucleotide sequence of the human gonadotropin-releasing hormone gene, *Nucleic Acids Res* 17:6403, 1989.

3. **Nikolics K, Mason AJ, Szonyi E, Ramachandran J, Seeburg PH,** A prolactin-inhibiting factor within the precursor for human gonadotropin-releasing hormone, *Nature* 316:511, 1985.

4. **Sherwood NM, Lovejoy DA, Coe IR,** Origin of mammalian gonadotropin-releasing hormones, *Endocr Rev* 14:241, 1993.

5. **King JA, Millar RP,** Evolutionary aspects of gonadotropin-releasing-hormone and its receptor, *Cell Mol Neurobiol* 15:5, 1995.

6. **White RB, Eisen JA, Kasten TL, Fernald RD,** Second gene for gonadotropin releasing hormone in humans, *Proc Natl Acad Sci USA* 95:305, 1998.

7. **Elsholtz HP,** Molecular biology of prolactin: cell-specific and endocrine regulators of the prolactin gene, *Seminars Reprod Endocrinol* 10:183, 1992.

8. **Radovick S, Nations M, Du Y, Berg LA, Weintraub BD, Wondisford FE,** A mutation in the POU-homeodomain of Pit-1 responsible for combined pituitary hormone deficiency, *Science* 257:1115, 1992.

9. **Pellegrini I, Barlier A, Gunz G, Figarella-Branger D, Enjalbert A, Grisoli F, Jaquet P,** Pit-1 gene expression in the human pituitary and pituitary adenomas, *J Clin Endocrinol Metab* 79:189, 1994.

10. **Xiong F, Chin RA, Hew CL,** A gene encoding chinook salmon (Oncorhynchus tschawytscha) prolactin: gene structure and potential cis-acting regulatory elements, *Mol Marine Biol Biotechnol* 1:155, 1992.

11. **Melmed S,** The structure and function of pituitary dopamine receptors, *Endocrinologist* 7:385, 1997.

12. **Martinez de la Escalera G, Weiner RI,** Dissociation of dopamine from its receptor as a signal in the pleiotropic hypothalamic regulation of prolactin secretion, *Endocr Rev* 13:241, 1992.

13. **Schwanzel-Fukuda M, Pfaff DW,** Origin of luteinizing hormone-releasing hormone neurons, *Nature* 338:161, 1989.

14. **Ronnekleiv OK, Resko JA,** Ontogeny of gonadotropin-releasing hormone-containing neurons in early fetal development of rhesus macaques, *Endocrinology* 126:498, 1990.

15. **Waldstreicher J, Seminara SB, Jameson JL, Geyer A, Nachtigall LB, Boepple PA, Holmes LB, Crowley Jr WF,** The genetic and clinical heterogeneity of gonadotropin-releasing hormone deficiency in the human, *J Clin Endocrinol Metab* 81:4388, 1996.

16. **Bick D, Franco B, Sherin RJ, Heye B, Pike L, Crawford J, Maddalena A, Incerti B, Pragliola A, Meitinger T, Ballabio A,** Brief report: intragenic deletion of the KALIG-1 gene in Kallmann's syndrome, *New Engl J Med* 326:1752, 1992.

17. **Hardelin J-P, Levilliers J, Young J, Pholsena M, Legouis R, Kirk J, Boulooux P, Petit C, Schaison G,** Xp22.3 deletions in isolated familial Kallmann's syndrome, *J Clin Endocrinol Metab* 76:827, 1993.

18. **Jennes L, Stumpf WE, Sheedy ME,** Ultrastructural characterization of gonadotropin-releasing hormone (GnRH)-producing neurons, *J Comp Neurol* 232:543, 1985.

19. **Stern K, McClintock MK,** Regulation of ovulation by human pheromones, *Nature* 392:177, 1998.

20. **McClintock MK,** Menstrual synchrony and suppression, *Nature* 229:244, 1971.

21. **Matteo S,** The effect of job stress and job interdependency on menstrual cycle length, regularity and synchrony, *Psychoneuroendocrinology* 12:467, 1987.

22. **Silverman AJ, Antunes JL, Abrams G, Nilaver G, Thau R, Robinson JA, Ferin M, Krey LC,** The luteinizing hormone-releasing pathways in the rhesus (maccaca mulatta) and pigtailed (maccaca nemestrina) monkeys: new observations using thick unembedded sections, *J Comp Neurol* 211:309, 1982.

23. **Silverman AJ, Jhamandas J, Renaud LP,** Localization of luteinizing hormone-releasing hormone (LHRH) neurons that project to the median eminence, *J Neurosci* 7:2312, 1987.

24. **Goldsmith PC, Thind KK, Song T, Kim EJ, Boggan JE,** Location of the neuroendocrine gonadotropin-releasing hormone neurons in the monkey hypothalamus by retrograde tracing and immunostaining, *J Neuroendocrinol* 2:157, 1990.

25. **Nakai Y, Plant TM, Hess DL, Keogh EJ, Knobil E,** On the sites of the negative and positive feedback actions of estradiol in the control of gonadotropin secretion in the rhesus monkey, *Endocrinology* 102:1008, 1978.

26. **Knobil E,** The neuroendocrine control of the menstrual cycle, *Recent Prog Horm Res* 36:53, 1980.

27. **Haisenleder DJ, Dalkin AC, Ortolano GA, Marshall JC, Shupnik MA,** A pulsatile gonadotropin-releasing hormone stimulus is required to increase transcription of the gonadotropin subunit genes: evidence for differential regulation of transcription by pulse frequency in vivo, *Endocrinology* 128:509, 1991.

28. **Van Vugt DA, Diefenbach WP, Ferin M,** Gonadotropin-releasing hormone pulses in third ventricular cerebrospinal fluid of ovariectomized rhesus monkeys: correlation with luteinizing hormone pulses, *Endocrinology* 117:1550, 1985.

29. **Gross KM, Matsumoto AM, Southworth MB, Bremner WJ,** Evidence for decreased luteinizing hormone-releasing hormone frequency in men with selective elevations of follicle-stimulating hormone, *J Clin Endocrinol Metab* 60:197, 1985.

30. **Backstrom CT, McNeilly AL, Leask RM, Baird DT,** Pulsatile secretion of LH, FSH, prolactin, oestradiol and progesterone during the human menstrual cycle, *Clin Endocrinol* 16:29, 1982.

31. **Reame N, Sauder SE, Kelch RP, Marshall JC,** Pulsatile gonadotropin secretion during the human menstrual cycle: evidence for altered frequency of gonadotropin-releasing hormone secretion, *J Clin Endocrinol Metab* 59:328, 1984.

32. **Filicori M, Santoro N, Merriam GR, Crowley Jr WF,** Characterization of the physiological pattern of episodic gonadotropin secretion throughout the human menstrual cycle, *J Clin Endocrinol Metab* 62:1136, 1986.

33. **Veldhuis JD, Evans WS, Johnson ML, Wills MR, Rogol AD,** Physiological properties of the luteinizing hormone pulse signal: impact of intensive and extended venous sampling paradigms on its characterization in healthy men and women, *J Clin Endocrinol Metab* 62:881, 1986.

34. **Gambacciani M, Liu JH, Swartz WH, Tueros VS, Yen SSC,** Intrinsic pulsatility of luteinizing hormone release from the human pituitary in vitro, *Neuroendocrinology* 45:402, 1987.

35. **Stojilkovic SS, Krsmanovic LZ, Spergel DJ, Catt KJ,** GnRH neurons: intrinsic pulsatility and receptor-mediated regulation, *Trends Endocrinol Metab* 5:201, 1994.

36. **Andersen AN, Hagen C, Lange P, Boesgaard S, Djursing H, Eldrup E, Micic S,** Dopaminergic regulation of gonadotropin levels and pulsatility in normal women, *Fertil Steril* 47:391, 1987.

37. **Herbison AE,** Noradrenergic regulation of cyclic GnRH secretion, *Rev Reprod* 2:1, 1997.

38. **Sahu A, Phelps CP, White JD, Crowley WR, Kalra SP, Kalra PS,** Steroidal regulation of hypothalamic neuropeptide Y release and gene expression, *Endocrinology* 130:3331, 1992.

39. **Pau KF, Berria M, Hess DL, Spies HG,** Hypothalamic site-dependent effects of neuropeptide Y on gonadotropin-releasing hormone secretion in rhesus macaques, *J Neuroendocrinol* 7:63, 1995.

40. **Kaye WH, Berrettini W, Gwirtsman H, George DT,** Altered cerebrospinal fluid neuropeptide Y and peptide YY immunoreactivity in anorexia and bulimia nervosa, *Arch Gen Psychiatry* 47:548, 1990.

41. **McShane TM, May T, Miner JL, Keisler DH,** Central actions of neuropeptide-Y may provide a neuromodulatory link between nutrition and reproduction, *Biol Reprod* 46:1151, 1992.

42. **Birken S, Maydelman Y, Gawinowicz MA, Pound A, Liu Y, Hartree AS,** Isolation and characterization of human pituitary chorionic gonadotropin, *Endocrinology* 137:1402, 1996.

43. **Patton PE, Hess DL, Cook DM, Loriaux DL, Braunstein GD,** Human chorionic gonadotropin production by the pituitary gland in a premenopausal women, *Am J Obstet Gynecol* 178:1138, 1998.

44. **Ravindra R, Aronstam RS,** Progesterone, testosterone, and estradiol-17β inhibit gonadotropin-releasing hormone stimulation of G protein GTPase activity in plasma membranes from rat anterior pituitary lobe, *Acta Endocrinol* 126:345, 1992.

45. **Tse A, Hille B,** GnRH-induced Ca²⁺ oscillations and rhythmnic hyperpolarizations of pituitary gonadotropes, *Science* 255:462, 1992.

46. **Sealfon SC, Weinstein H, Millar RP,** Molecular mechanisms of ligand interaction with the gonadotropin-releasing hormone receptor, *Endocr Rev* 18:180, 1997.

47. **Kaiser UB, Conn PM, Chin WW,** Studies of gonadotropin-releasing hormone (GnRH) action using GnRH receptor-expressing pituitary cell lines, *Endocr Rev* 18:46, 1997.

48. **Ray D, Melmed S,** Pituitary cytokine and growth factor expression and action, *Endocr Rev* 18:206, 1997.

49. **Massague J,** The TGF-β family of growth and differentiation factors, *Cell* 49:437, 1987.

50. **Roberts V, Meunier H, Vaughan J, Rivier J, Rivier C, Vale W, Sawchenko P,** Production and regulation of inhibin subunits in pituitary gonadotropes, *Endocrinology* 124:552, 1989.

51. **Bauer-Dantoin AC, Wess J, Jameson JL,** Roles of estrogen, progesterone, and gonadotropin-releasing hormone (GnRH) in the control of pituitary GnRH receptor gene expression at the time of the preovulatory gonadotropin surges, *Endocrinology* 136:1014, 1995.

52. **Kitaoka M, Kojima I, Ogata E,** Activin-A: a modulator of multiple types of anterior pituitary cells, *Biochem Biophys Res Commun* 157:48, 1988.

53. **Billestrup N, Gonzalez-Manchon C, Potter E, Vale W,** Inhibition of somatotroph growth and growth hormone biosynthesis by activin in vitro, *Mol Endocrinol* 4:356, 1990.

54. **Corrigan AZ, Bilezikjian LM, Carroll RS, Bald LN, Schmelzer CH, Fendly BM, Mason AJ, Chin WW, Schwall RH, Vale W,** Evidence for an autocrine role of activin B within rat anterior piuitary cultures, *Endocrinology* 128:1682, 1991.

55. **Bilezikjian LM, Corrigan AZ, Blount AL, Vale WW,** Pituitary follistatin and inhibin subunit messenger ribonucleic acid levels are differentially regulated by local and hormonal factors, *Endocrinology* 137:4277, 1996.

56. **Kaiser UB, Lee BL, Carroll RS, Unabia G, Chin WW, Childs GV,** Follistatin gene expression in the pituitary: localization in gonadotrophs and folliculostellate cells in diestrous rats, *Endocrinology* 130:3048, 1992.

57. **Kogawa K, Nakamura T, Sugiono K, Takio K, Titani K, Sugino H,** Activin-binding protein is present in pituitary, *Endocrinology* 128:1434, 1991.

58. **Besecke LM, Guendner MJ, Sluss PA, Polak AG, Woodruff TK, Jameson JL, Bauer-Dantoin AC, Weiss J,** Pituitary follistatin regulates activin-mediated production of follicle-stimulating hormone during the rat estrous cycle, *Endocrinology* 138:2841, 1997.

59. **Besecke LM, Guendner MJ, Schneyer AL, Bauer-Dantoin AC, Jameson JL, Weiss J,** Gonadotropin-releasing hormone regulates follicle-stimulating hormone-β gene expression through an activin/follistatin autocrine or paracrine loop, *Endocrinology* 137:3667, 1996.

60. **Howlett TA, Rees LH,** Endogenous opioid peptides and hypothalamo-pituitary function, *Ann Rev Physiol* 48:527, 1986.

61. **Bacchinetti F, Petraglia F, Genazzani AR,** Localization and expression of the three opioid systems, *Seminars Reprod Endocrinol* 5:103, 1987.

62. **Micevych PE, Eckersell CB, Brecha N, Holland KL,** Estrogen modulation of opioid and cholecystokinin systems in the limbic-hypothalamic circuit, *Brain Res Bull* 44:335, 1997.

63. **Gindoff PR, Ferin M,** Brain opioid peptides and menstrual cyclicity, *Seminars Reprod Endocrinol* 5:125, 1987.

64. **Rabinovici J, Rothman P, Monroe SE, Nerenberg C, Jaffe RB,** Endocrine effects and pharmacokinetic characteristics of a potent new gonadotropin-releasing hormone antagonist (Ganirelix) with minimal histamine-releasing properties: studies in postmenopausal women, *J Clin Endocrinol Metab* 75:1220, 1992.

65. **Shoupe D, Montz FJ, Lobo RA,** The effects of estrogen and progestin on endogenous opioid activity in oophorectomized women, *J Clin Endocrinol Metab* 60:178, 1985.

66. **Casper RF, Alapin-Rubilovitz S,** Progestins increase endogenous opioid peptide activity in postmenopausal women, *J Clin Endocrinol Metab* 60:34, 1985.

67. **Marunicic M, Casper RF,** The effect of luteal phase estrogen antagonism on luteinizing hormone pulsatility and luteal function in women, *J Clin Endocrinol Metab* 64:148, 1987.

68. **Kletter GB, Padmanaghan V, Beitins IZ, Marshall JC, Kelch RP, Foster CM,** Acute effects of estradiol infusion and naloxone on luteinizing hormone secretion in pubertal boys, *J Clin Endocrinol Metab* 82:4010, 1997.

69. **Cemeroglu AP, Kletter GB, Guo W, Brown MB, Kelch RP, Marshall JC, Padmanabhan V, Foster CM,** In pubertal girls, naloxone fails to reverse the suppression of luteinizing hormone secretion by estradiol, *J Clin Endocrinol Metab* 83:3501, 1998.

70. **Goodman RL, Parfitt DB, Evans NP, Dahl GE, Karsch FJ,** Endogenous opioid peptides control the amplitude and shape of gonadotropin-releasing hormone pulses in the ewe, *Endocrinology* 136:2412, 1995.

71. **Mateo AR, Hammer RP,** Dynamic pattern of medial preoptic mu-opiate receptor regulation by gonadal steroid hormones, *Neuroendocrinology* 55:51, 1992.

72. **Weiland NG, Wise PM,** Estrogen and progesterone regulate oopiate receptor densities in multiple brain regions, *Endocrinology* 126:804, 1990.

73. **Petersen SL, Keller ML, Carder SA, McCrone S,** Differential effects of estrogen and progesterone on levels of POMC mRNA levels in the arcuate nucleus: relationship to the timing of LH surge release, *J Neuroendocrinol* 5:643, 1993.

74. **Shalts E, Feng Y-J, Ferin M, Wardlaw SL,** α-Melanocyte-stimulating hormone antagonizes the neuroendocrine effects of corticotropin-releasing factor and interleukin-1 in the primate, *Endocrinology* 131:132, 1992.

75. **Petraglia F, D'Ambrogio G, Comitini G, Facchinetti F, Volpe A, Genazzani AR,** Impairment of opioid control of luteinizing hormone secretion in menstrual disorders, *Fertil Steril* 43:534, 1985.

76. **Khoury SA, Reame NE, Kelch RP, Marshall JC,** Diurnal patterns of pulsatile luteinizing hormone secretion in hypothalamic amenorrhea: reproducibility and responses to opiate blockade and α_2-adrenergic agonist, *J Clin Endocrinol Metab* 64:755, 1987.

77. **Wildt L, Leyendecker G, Sir-Petermann T, Waibel-Treber S,** Treatment with naltrexone in hypothalamic ovarian failure: induction of ovulation and pregnancy, *Hum Reprod* 8:350, 1993.

78. **Suh BY, Liu JH, Berga SL, Quigley ME, Laughlin GA, Yen SSC,** Hypercortisolism in patients with functional hypothalamic amenorrhea, *J Clin Endocrinol Metab* 66:733, 1988.

79. **Veldhuis JD, Johnson ML, Seneta E, Iranmanesh A,** Temporal coupling among luteinizing hormone, follicle stimulating hormone, β-endorphin and cortisol pulse episodes in vivo, *Acta Endocrinol* 126:193, 1992.

80. **Vamvakopoulos NC, Chrousos GP,** Evidence of direct estrogenic regulation of human corticotropin-releasing hormone gene expression. Potential implications for the sexual dimorphism of the stress response and immune/inflammatory reaction, *J Clin Invest* 92:1896, 1993.

81. **Cumming DC, Wheeler GD,** Opioids in exercise physiology, *Seminars Reprod Endocrinol* 5:171, 1987.

82. **Sarkar DK, Yen SSC,** Hyperprolactinemia decreases the luteinizing hormone-releasing hormone concentration in pituitary portal plasma: a possible role for β-endorphin as a mediator, *Endocrinology* 116:2080, 1985.

83. **Chen CC, Chang C, Krieger DT, Bardin CW,** Expression and regulation of proopiomelanocortin-like gene in the ovary and placenta: comparison with the testis, *Endocrinology* 118:2382, 1986.

84. **Petraglia F, Di Meo G, Storchi R, Segre A, Facchinetti F, Szalay S, Volpe A, Genazzani AR,** Proopiomelanocortin-related peptides and methionine enkephalin in human follicular fluid: changes during the menstrual cycle, *Am J Obstet Gynecol* 157:142, 1987.

85. **Fishman J, Norton B,** Brain catecholestrogens: formation and possible functions, *Adv Biosci* 15:123, 1975.

86. **Mais V, Kazer RR, Cetel NS, Rivier J, Vale W, Yen SSC,** The dependency of folliculogenesis and corpus luteum function on pulsatile gonadotropin secretion in cycling women using a gonadotropin-releasing hormone antagonist as a probe, *J Clin Endocrinol Metab* 62:1250, 1986.

87. **Brownstein MJ, Russel JT, Gainer H,** Synthesis, transport, and release of posterior pituitary hormones, *Science* 207:373, 1980.

88. **Mohr E, Meyerhof W, Richter D,** The hypothalamic hormone oxytocin: From gene expression to signal transduction, *Rev Physiol Biochem Pharmacol* 121:31, 1992.

89. **Kasson BG, Adashi EY, Hsueh AJW,** Arginine vasopressin in the testis: an intragonadal peptide control system, *Endocr Rev* 7:156, 1986.

90. **Perlow MJ, Reppert SM, Artman HA, Fisher DA, Seif SM, Robinson AG,** Oxytocin, vasopressin and estrogen-stimulated neurophysin: daily patterns of concentration in cerebrospinal fluid, *Science* 216:1416, 1983.

91. **Amico JA, Seif SM, Robinson AG,** Elevation of oxytocin and the oxytocin-associated neurophysin in the plasma of normal women during midcycle, *J Clin Endocrinol Metab* 53:1229, 1981.

92. **Hrabovszky E, Kallo I, Hajszan T, Shughrue PJ, Merchenthaler I, Liposits Z,** Expression of estrogen receptor-beta messenger ribonucleic acid in oxytocin and vasopressin neurons of the rat supraoptic and paraventricular nuclei, *Endocrinology* 139:2600, 1998.

93. **Carmichael MS, Humbert R, Dixen J, Palmisano G, Greenleaf W, Davidson JM,** Plasma oxytocin increases in the human sexual response, *J Clin Endocrinol Metab* 64:27, 1987.

94. **Hirst JJ, Chibbart R, Mitchell BF,** Role of oxytocin in the regulation of uterine activity during pregnancy and in the initiation of labor, *Seminars Reprod Endocrinol* 11:219, 1993.

95. **Hirst JJ, Haluska GJ, Cook MJ, Novy MJ,** Plasma oxytocin and nocturnal uterine activity: maternal but not fetal concentrations increase progressively during late pregnancy and delivery in Rhesus monkeys, *Am J Obstet Gynecol* 169:415, 1993.

96. **Wilson T, Liggins GC, Whittaker DJ,** Oxytocin stimulates the release of arachidonic acid and prostaglandin $F_{2\alpha}$ from human decidual cells, *Prostaglandins* 35:771, 1988.

97. **Zeeman GG, Khan-Dawood FS, Dawood MY,** Oxytocin and its receptor in pregnancy and parturition: current concepts and clinical implications, *Obstet Gynecol* 89:873, 1997.

98. **Ferin M, Rosenblatt H, Carmel PW, Antunes JL, Vande Wiele RL,** Estrogen-induced gonadotropin surges in female rhesus monkeys after pituitary stalk section, *Endocrinology* 104:50, 1979.

99. **Yen SSC, Lein A,** The apparent paradox of the negative and positive feedback control system on gonadotropin secretion, *Am J Obstet Gynecol* 126:942, 1976.

100. **Hoff JD, Lasley BL, Yen SSC,** The functional relationship between priming and releasing actions of luteinizing hormone-releasing hormone, *J Clin Endocrinol Metab* 49:8, 1979.

101. **Urban RJ, Veldhuis JD, Dufau ML,** Estrogen regulates the gonadotropin-releasing hormone-stimulated secretion of biologically active luteinizing hormone, *J Clin Endocrinol Metab* 72:660, 1991.

102. **Gregg DW, Nett TM,** Direct effects of estradiol-17β on the number of gonadotropin-releasing hormone receptors in ovine pituitary, *Biol Reprod* 40:288, 1989.

103. **Adams TE, Norman RL, Spies HG,** Gonadotropin-releasing hormone receptor binding and pituitary responsiveness in estradiol-primed monkeys, *Science* 213:1388, 1981.

104. **Menon M, Peegel H, Katta V,** Estradiol potentiation of gonadotropin-releasing hormone responsiveness in the anterior pituitary is mediated by an increase in gonadotropin-releasing hormone receptors, *Am J Obstet Gynecol* 151:534, 1985.

105. **Herbison AE,** Multimodal influence of estrogen upon gonadotropin-releasing hormone neurons, *Endocr Rev* 19:302, 1998.

106. **Xia L, Van Vugt D, Alston EJ, Luckhaus J, Ferin M,** A surge of gonadotropin-releasing hormone accompanies the estradiol-induced gonadotropin surge in the Rhesus monkey, *Endocrinology* 131:2812, 1992.

107. **Woller MJ, Terasawa E,** Changes in pulsatile release of neuropeptide-Y and luteinizing hormone (LH)-releasing hormone during the progesterone-induced LH surge in rhesus monkeys, *Endocrinology* 135:1679, 1994.

108. **Shupnik MA, Weinmann CM, Notides AC, Chin WW,** An upstream region of the rat luteinizing hormone β gene binds estrogen receptor and confers estrogen responsiveness, *J Biol Chem* 264:80, 1989.

109. **Radovick S, Ticknor CM, Nakayama Y, Notides AC, Rahman A, Weintraub BD, Cutler Jr GB, Wondisford FE,** Evidence for direct estrogen regulation of the human gonadotropin-releasing hormone gene, *J Clin Invest* 88:1649, 1991.

110. **Shivers BD, Harlan RE, Morrell JI, Pfaff DW,** Absence of estradiol concentration in cell nuclei of LHRH-immunoreactive neurons, *Nature* 304:345, 1983.

111. **Herbison AE, Horvath TL, Naftolin F, Leranth C,** Distribution of estrogen receptor-immunoreactive cells in monkey hypothalamus: relationship to neurons containing luteinizing hormone-releasing hormone and tyrosine hydroxylase, *Neuroendocrinology* 61:1, 1995.

112. **Sullivan K, Witkin JW, Ferin M, Silverman AJ,** GnRH neurons in the rhesus macaque are not immunoreactive for the estrogen receptor, *Brain Res* 685:198, 1995.

113. **Goldsmith PC, Boggan JE, Thind KK,** Estrogen and progesterone receptor expression in neuroendocrine and related neurons of the pubertal female monkey hypothalamus, *Neuroendocrinology* 65:325, 1997.

114. **Evans NP, Dahl GE, Mauger D, Karsch FJ,** Estradiol induces qualitative and quantitative changes in the pattern of gonadotropin-releasing hormone secretion during the pre-surge period in the ewe, *Endocrinology* 136:1603, 1995.

115. **Evans NP, Dahl GE, Mauger DT, Padmanabhan V, Thrun LA, Karsch FJ,** Does estradiol induce the preovulatory gonadotropin-releasing hormone (GnRH) surge in the ewe by inducing a progressive change in the mode of operation of the GnRH neurosecretory system? *Endocrinology* 136:5511, 1995.

116. **Bowen JM, Dahl GE, Evans NP, Thrun LA, Wang Y, Brown MB, Karsch FJ,** Importance of the gonadotropin-releasing hormone (GnRH) surge for induction of the preovulatory luteinizing hormone surge of the ewe: dose-response relationship and excess of GnRH, *Endocrinology* 139:588, 1998.

117. **Leroy I, d'Acremont MF, Brailly-Tabard S, Frydman R, de Mouzon J, Bouchard P,** A single injection of a gonadotropin-releasing hormone (GnRH) antagonist (Cetrorelix) postpones the luteinizing hormone (LH) surge: further evidence for the role of GnRH during the LH surge, *Fertil Steril* 62:461, 1994.

118. **Katt JA, Duncan JA, Herbon L, Barkan A, Marshall JC,** The frequency of gonadotropin-releasing hormone stimulation determines the number of pituitary gonadotropin-releasing hormone receptors, *Endocrinology* 116:2113, 1985.

119. **Moenter SM, Brand RC, Karsch FJ,** Dynamics of gonadotropin-releasing hormone (GnRH) secretion during the GnRH surge: insights into the mechanism of GnRH surge induction, *Endocrinology* 130:2978, 1992.

120. **Marut EL, Williams RF, Cowan BD, Lynch A, Lerner SP, Hodgen GD,** Pulsatile pituitary gonadotropin secretion during maturation of the dominant follicle in monkeys: estrogen positive feedback enhances the biological activity of LH, *Endocrinology* 109:2270, 1981.

121. **Liu JH, Yen SSC,** Induction of midcycle gonadotropin surge by ovarian steroids in women: a critical evaluation, *J Clin Endocrinol Metab* 57:797, 1983.

122. **Collins RL, Hodgen GD,** Blockade of the spontaneous midcycle gonadotropin surge in monkeys by RU 486: a progesterone antagonist or agonist? *J Clin Endocrinol Metab* 63:1270, 1986.

123. **Turgeon JL, Waring DW,** The timing of progesterone-induced ribonucleic acid and protein synthesis for augmentation of luteinizing hormone secretion, *Endocrinology* 129:3234, 1991.

124. **Waring DW, Turgeon JL,** A pathway for luteinizing hormone releasing-hormone self-potentiation: cross-talk with the progesterone receptor, *Endocrinology* 130:3275, 1992.

125. **Wildt L, Hutchison JS, Marshall G, Pohl CR, Knobil E,** On the site of action of progesterone in the blockade of the estradiol-induced gonadotropin discharge in the rhesus monkey, *Endocrinology* 109:1293, 1981.

126. **Batra SK, Miller WL,** Progesterone decreases the responsiveness of ovine pituitary cultures to luteinizing hormone-releasing hormone, *Endocrinology* 117:1436, 1985.

127. **Araki S, Chikazawa K, Motoyama M, Ljima K, Abe N, Tamada T,** Reduction in pituitary desensitization and prolongation of gonadotropin release by estrogen during continuous administration of gonadotropin-releasing hormone in women: its antagonism by progesterone, *J Clin Endocrinol Metab* 60:590, 1985.

128. **Kasa-Vuvu JZ, Dahl GE, Evans NP, Thrun LA, Moenter SM, Padmanaghan V, Karsch FJ,** Progesterone blocks the estradiol-induced gonadotropin discharge in the ewe by inhibiting the surge of gonadotropin-releasing hormone, *Endocrinology* 131:208, 1992.

129. **Tamarkin L, Baird CJ, Almeida OFX,** Melatonin: a coordinating signal for mammalian reproduction?, *Science* 227:714, 1985.

130. **Reiter RJ,** Pineal melatonin: cell biology of its synthesis and of its physiological interactions, *Endocr Rev* 12:151, 1991.

131. **Brzezinski A,** Melatonin in humans, *New Engl J Med* 336:186, 1997.

132. **Plant TM, Zorub DS,** Pinealectomy in agonadal infantile male rhesus monkeys (Macaca mulatta) does not interrupt initiation of the prepubertal hiatus in gonadotropin secretion, *Endocrinology* 118:227, 1986.

133. **Silman R,** Melatonin and the human gonadotrophin-releasing hormone pulse generator, *J Endocrinol* 128:7, 1991.

134. **Berga S, Mortola J, Yen SSC,** Amplification of nocturnal melatonin secretion in women with functional hypothalamic amenorrhea, *J Clin Endocrinol Metab* 66:242, 1988.

135. **Zacharias L, Wurtman RJ,** Blindness: its relation to age of menarche, *Science* 144:1154, 1964.

136. **Sack RL, Lewy AJ, Blood ML, Keith LD, Nakagawa H,** Circadian rhythm abnormalities in totally blind people: incidence and clinical significance, *J Clin Endocrinol Metab* 75:127, 1992.

137. **Kauppila A, Kivela A, Pakarinen A, Vakkuri O,** Inverse seasonal relationship between melatonin and ovarian activity in humans in a region with a strong seasonal contrast in luminosity, *J Clin Endocrinol Metab* 65:823, 1987.

138. **Rojansky N, Brzezinski A, Schenker JG,** Seasonality in human reproduction: an update, *Hum Reprod* 7:735, 1992.

139. **Puig-Domingo M, Webb SM, Serrano J, Peinado M-A, Corcoy R, Ruscalleda J, Reiter RJ, de Leiva A,** Brief report: melatonin-related hypogoandotropic hypogonadism, *New Engl J Med* 327:1356, 1992.

140. **Wilson HC, Kiefhaber SH, Gravel V,** Two studies of menstrual synchrony: negative results, *Psychoneuroendocrinology* 16:353, 1991.

141. **Huhtaniemi IT, Warren DW,** Ontogeny of pituitary-gonadal interactions: current advances and controversies, *Trends Endocrinol Metab* 1:356, 1990.

142. **Burger HG, Famada Y, Bangah ML, McCloud PI, Warne GL,** Serum gonadotropin, sex steroid, and immunoreactive inhibin levels in the first two years of life, *J Clin Endocrinol Metab* 72:682, 1991.

143. **Reiter EO, Grumbach MM,** Neuroendocrine control mechanisms and the onset of puberty, *Ann Rev Physiol* 44:595, 1982.

144. **Sklar CA, Kaplan SL, Grumbach MM,** Evidence for dissociation between adrenarche and gonadarche: studies in patients with idiopathic precocious puberty, gonadal dysgenesis, isolated gonadotroph deficiency, and constitutionally delayed growth and adolescence, *J Clin Endocrinol Metab* 51:548, 1980.

145. **Dunkel L, Alfthan H, Stenman U-H, Selstam G, Rosberg S, Albertsson-Wikland K,** Developmental changes in 24-hour profiles of luteinizing hormone and follicle-stimulating hormone from prepuberty to midstages of puberty in boys, *J Clin Endocrinol Metab* 74:890, 1992.

146. **Oerter KE, Urarte MM, Rose SR, Barnes KM, Cutler GB,** Gonadotropin secretory dynamics during puberty in normal girls and boys, *J Clin Endocrinol Metab* 71:1251, 1990.

147. **Apter D, Butzow TL, Laughlin GA, Yen SSC,** Gonadotropin-releasing hormone pulse generator activity during pubertal transition in girls: pulsatile and diurnal patterns of circulating gonadotropins, *J Clin Endocrinol Metab* 76:940, 1993.

148. **Cemeroglu AP, Foster CM, Warner R, Kletter GB, Marshall JC, Kelch RP,** Comparison of the neuroendocrine control of pubertal maturation in girls and boys with spontaneous puberty and in hypogonadal girls, *J Clin Endocrinol Metab* 81:4352, 1996.

149. **Clark PA, Iranmanesh A, Veldhuis JD, Rogol AD,** Comparison of pulsatile luteinizing hormone secretion between prepubertal children and young adults: evidence for a mass/amplitutde-dependent difference without gender or day/night contrasts, *J Clin Endocrinol Metab* 82:2950, 1997.

150. **Boyar RM, Ramsey J, Chapman J, Fevere M, Madden J, Marks JF,** Luteinizing hormone and follicle-stimulating hormone secretory dynamics in Turner's syndrome, *J Clin Endocrinol Metab* 47:1078, 1978.

151. **Zacharias L, Rand WM, Wurtman RJ,** A prospective study of sexual development and growth in American girls: the statistics of menarche, *Obstet Gynecol Survey* 31:325, 1976.

152. **Frisch RE,** Body fat, menarche, and reproductive ability, *Seminars Reprod Endocrinol* 3:45, 1985.

153. **Ross JL, Loriaux DL, Cutler GB,** Developmental changes in neuroendocrine regulation of gonadotropin secretion in gonadal dysgenesis, *J Clin Endocrinol Metab* 57:288, 1983.

6 Regulation of the Menstrual Cycle

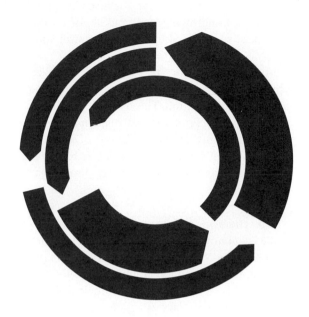

Many superstitious beliefs have surrounded menstruation throughout recorded history. Indeed, attitudes and ideas about this aspect of female physiology have changed slowly. Hopefully, the scientific progress of the last few decades, which has revealed the dynamic relationships between the pituitary and gonadal hormones and the cyclic nature of the normal reproductive process, will yield a new understanding. The hormone changes, correlated with the morphologic and autocrine/paracrine events in the ovary, make the coordination of this system one of the most remarkable events in biology.

The diagnosis and management of abnormal menstrual function must be based on an understanding of the physiologic mechanisms involved in the regulation of the normal cycle. To understand the normal menstrual cycle, it is helpful to divide the cycle into 3 phases: the follicular phase, ovulation, and the luteal phase. We will examine each of these phases, concentrating on the changes in ovarian and pituitary hormones, what governs the pattern of hormone changes, and the effects of these hormones on the ovary, pituitary, and hypothalamus in regulating the menstrual cycle.

The Follicular Phase

During the follicular phase an orderly sequence of events takes place that ensures the proper number of follicles is ready for ovulation. In the human ovary the end result of this follicular development is (usually) one surviving mature follicle. This process, which occurs over the space of 10–14 days, features a series of sequential actions of hormones and autocrine/paracrine peptides on the follicle, leading the follicle destined to ovulate through a period of initial growth from a primordial follicle through the stages of the preantral, antral, and preovulatory follicle.

The Primordial Follicle

The primordial germ cells originate in the endoderm of the yolk sac, allantois, and hindgut of the embryo, and by 5–6 weeks of gestation, they have migrated to the genital ridge. A rapid mitotic multiplication of germ cells begins at 6–8 weeks of pregnancy, and by 16–20 weeks, the maximum number of oocytes is reached: a total of 6–7 million in both ovaries.[1] The primordial follicle is nongrowing and consists of an oocyte, arrested in the diplotene stage of meiotic prophase, surrounded by a single layer of spindle-shaped granulosa cells.

Until their numbers are exhausted, follicles begin to grow and undergo atresia under all physiologic circumstances. Growth and atresia are not interrupted by pregnancy, ovulation, or periods of anovulation. This dynamic process continues at all ages, including infancy and around the menopause. From the maximum number at 16–20 weeks of pregnancy, the number of oocytes will irretrievably decrease. The rate of decrease is proportional to the total number present; thus, the most rapid decrease occurs before birth, resulting in a decline from 6–7 million to 2 million at birth and to 300,000 at puberty. From this large reservoir, about 400 follicles will ovulate during a woman's reproductive years.

The mechanism for determining which follicles and how many will start growing during any one cycle is unknown. The number of follicles that starts growing each cycle appears to be dependent upon the size of the residual pool of inactive primordial follicles.[2, 3] Reducing the size of the pool (e.g., unilateral oophorectomy) causes the remaining follicles to redistribute their availability over time. It is possible that the follicle which is singled out to play the leading role in a particular cycle is the beneficiary of a timely match of follicle "readiness" (perhaps prepared by autocrine/paracrine actions in its microenvironment) and appropriate tropic hormone stimulation. The first follicle able to respond to stimulation may achieve an early lead that it never relinquishes. Nevertheless, each cohort of follicles that begins growth is engaged in a serious competition that ends with only one follicle succeeding.

Rescue From Atresia (Apoptosis)

The follicle destined to ovulate is recruited in the first few days of the cycle.[4] The early growth of follicles occurs over the timespan of several menstrual cycles, but the ovulatory follicle is one of a cohort recruited at the time of the luteal-follicular transition.[5, 6] The total duration of time to achieve preovulatory status is approximately 85 days. The majority of this time (until a late stage) involves responses that are independent of hormonal regulation.[7] Eventually, this cohort of follicles reaches a stage where, unless recruited (rescued) by follicle-stimulating hormone (FSH), the next step is atresia. Thus, follicles are continuously available (2–5 mm in size) for a response to FSH. An increase in FSH is the critical feature in rescuing a cohort of follicles from atresia, the usual fate of most follicles, eventually allowing a dominant follicle to emerge and pursue a path to ovulation. In addition, maintenance of this increase in FSH for a critical duration of time is essential.[8] Without the appearance and persistence of an increase in the circulating FSH level, the cohort is doomed to the process of apoptosis, programmed physiologic cell death to eliminate superfluous cells.[9] "Apoptosis" is derived from Greek and means falling off, like leaves from a tree.

The first visible signs of follicular development are an increase in the size of the oocyte and the granulosa cells becoming cuboidal rather than squamous in shape. These changes may be better viewed as a process of maturation rather than growth. At this same time, small gap junctions develop between the granulosa cells and the oocyte. Gap junctions are channels that when open permit the exchange of nutrients, ions, and regulatory molecules. Thus, the gap junctions serve as the pathway for nutritional, metabolite, and signal interchange between the granulosa cells and

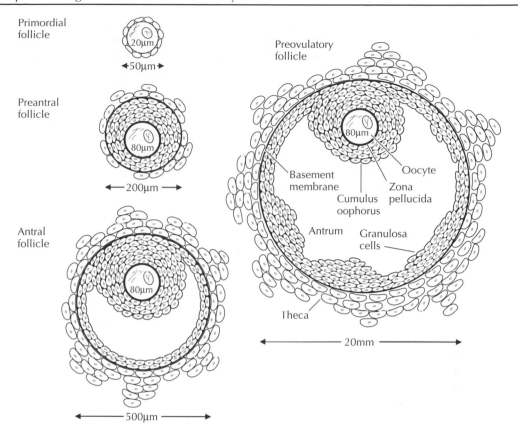

the oocyte. The process of follicular growth is influenced by factors derived from the oocyte. Mice that are genetically deficient in growth differentiation factor-9 (GDF-9), a peptide synthesized only in the oocyte after the primordial follicle becomes a preantral follicle, are infertile because follicular development cannot proceed beyond the primordial follicle stage.[10]

With multiplication of the cuboidal granulosa cells (to approximately 15 cells), the primordial follicle becomes a primary follicle. The granulosa layer is separated from the stromal cells by a basement membrane called the basal lamina. The surrounding stromal cells differentiate into concentric layers designated the theca interna (closest to the basal lamina) and the theca externa (the outer portion). The theca layers appear when granulosa proliferation produces 3–6 layers of granulosa cells.[6]

The belief that the initiation of follicular growth is independent of gonadotropin stimulation is supported by the persistence of this initial growth in gonadotropin-deficient mutant mice and in anencephalic fetuses.[11, 12] In the vast majority of instances this growth is limited and rapidly followed by atresia. In studies of human ovarian follicles, expression of the gene for the FSH receptor could not be detected until after primordial follicles began to growth.[13]

The general pattern of limited growth and quick atresia is interrupted at the beginning of the menstrual cycle when a group of follicles (after approximately 60 days of development) responds to a hormonal change and is propelled to grow. In young women, this cohort numbers 3–11 per ovary.[14]The decline in luteal phase steroidogenesis and inhibin A secretion allows a rise in FSH, beginning a few days before menses.[15, 16] The timing of this important event was based on data derived from the immunoassay of FSH. Using a sensitive measurement of FSH bioactivity, it has been suggested that increasing bioactivity of FSH begins in the mid- to late luteal phase.[17]

Follicular Growth and Development Based on Nonprimate and Primate Data. *The following discussion of events, which mark the growth and development of the ovarian follicle from the preantral stage to ovulation, is based on a formulation that assigns a key role to estradiol functioning as a classic hormone to transmit messages to the brain and as a local regulator within the follicle. This description has been challenged. The belief that the follicular estrogen concentration plays a paramount role within the follicle is based upon evidence (estrogens augment FSH action) derived from rodent experiments. There is no similar evidence derived from primate studies. We will first describe the traditional conventional view regarding ovarian follicular growth and development derived from 10–15 years of scientific pursuit; and then we will consider the differences in primates.* **Local autocrine/paracrine peptides probably have replaced steroid hormones as the principal regulators within primate ovarian follicles.**

The Preantral Follicle

Once growth is accelerated, the follicle progresses to the preantral stage as the oocyte enlarges and is surrounded by a membrane, the zona pellucida. The granulosa cells undergo a multilayer proliferation as the thecal layer continues to organize from the surrounding stroma. This growth is dependent upon gonadotropins and is correlated with increasing production of estrogen. Molecular studies indicate that all of the granulosa cells in mature follicles are derived from as few as 3 precursor cells.[18]

The granulosa cells of the preantral follicle have the ability to synthesize all 3 classes of steroids; however, significantly more estrogens than either androgens or progestins are produced. An aromatase enzyme system acts to convert androgens to estrogens and is a factor limiting ovarian estrogen production. Aromatization is induced or activated through the action of FSH. The binding of FSH to its receptor and activation of the adenylate cyclase mediated signal is followed by expression of multiple mRNAs which encode proteins responsible for cell proliferation, differentiation, and function. Thus, FSH both initiates steroidogenesis (estrogen production) in granulosa cells and stimulates granulosa cell growth.[19]

Specific receptors for FSH are not detected on granulosa cells until the preantral stage,[13] and the preantral follicle requires the presence of FSH in order to aromatize androgens and generate its own estrogenic microenvironment.[20] Estrogen production is, therefore, limited by FSH receptor content. The administration of FSH will raise and lower the concentration of its own receptor on granulosa cells (up- and down-regulation) both in vivo and in vitro.[21] This action of FSH is modulated by growth factors.[22] FSH receptors quickly reach a concentration of approximately 1500 receptors per granulosa cell.[23]

FSH operates through the G protein, adenylate cyclase system (described in Chapter 2), which is subject to down-regulation and modulation by many factors, including a calcium-calmodulin intermediary. Although steroidogenesis in the ovarian follicle is mainly regulated by the gonadotropins, multiple signaling pathways are involved that respond to many factors besides the gonadotropins. Besides the adenylate cyclase enzyme system, these pathways include ion gate channels, tyrosine kinase receptors, and the phospholipase system of second messengers. These pathways are regulated by a multitude of factors, including growth factors, nitric oxide, prostaglandins, and peptides such as gonadotropin-releasing hormone (GnRH), angiotensin II, tissue necrosis factor-α, and vasoactive intestinal peptide. The binding of luteinizing hormone (LH) to its receptor in the ovary is also followed by activation of the adenylate cyclase-cyclic AMP pathway via the G protein mechanism.

FSH combines synergistically with estrogen to exert (at least in the nonprimate) a mitogenic action on granulosa cells to stimulate their proliferation. Together, FSH and estrogen promote a rapid accumulation of FSH receptors, reflecting in part the increase in the number of granulosa cells. The early appearance of estrogen within the follicle allows the follicle to respond to relatively low concentrations of FSH, an autocrine function for estrogen within the follicle. As growth proceeds, the granulosa cells differentiate into several subgroups of different cell populations. This appears to be determined by the position of the cells relative to the oocyte.

There is a system of communication that exists within follicles. Not every cell has to contain receptors for the gonadotropins. Cells with receptors can transfer a signal (by gap junctions), which causes protein kinase activation in cells that lack receptors.[24] Thus, hormone-initiated action can be transmitted throughout the follicle despite the fact that only a subpopulation of cells binds the hormone. This system of communication promotes a coordinated and synchronous performance throughout the follicle, a system that continues to operate in the corpus luteum.

The role of androgens in early follicular development is complex. Specific androgen receptors are present in the granulosa cells.[25] The androgens serve not only as substrate for FSH-induced aromatization but, in low concentrations, can further enhance aromatase activity. When exposed to an androgen-rich environment, preantral granulosa cells favor the conversion of androgens to more potent 5α-reduced androgens rather than to estrogens.[26] These androgens cannot be converted to estrogen and, in fact, inhibit aromatase activity.[27] They also inhibit FSH induction of LH receptor formation, another essential step in follicular development.[28]

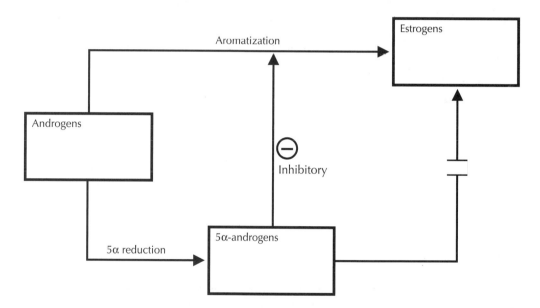

The fate of the preantral follicle is in delicate balance. At low concentrations, androgens enhance their own aromatization and contribute to estrogen production. At higher levels, the limited capacity of aromatization is overwhelmed, and the follicle becomes androgenic and ultimately atretic.[29] Follicles will progress in development only if emerging when FSH is elevated and LH is low. Those follicles arising at the end of the luteal phase or early in the subsequent cycle would be favored by an environment in which aromatization in the granulosa cell can prevail. ***The success of a follicle depends upon its ability to convert an androgen-dominated microenvironment to an estrogen-dominated microenvironment.***[30]

Summary of Events in the Preantral Follicle

1. Initial follicular development occurs independently of hormone influence.

2. FSH stimulation propels follicles to the preantral stage.

3. FSH-induced aromatization of androgen in the granulosa results in the production of estrogen.

4. Together, FSH and estrogen increase the FSH receptor content of the follicle.

The Antral Follicle

Under the synergistic influence of estrogen and FSH there is an increase in the production of follicular fluid that accumulates in the intercellular spaces of the granulosa, eventually coalescing to form a cavity, as the follicle makes its gradual transition to the antral stage. The accumulation of follicular fluid provides a means whereby the oocyte and surrounding granulosa cells can be nurtured in a specific endocrine environment. The granulosa cells surrounding the oocyte are now designated the cumulus oophorus. The differentiation of the cumulus cells is believed to be a response to signals originating in the oocyte.[31]

In the presence of FSH, estrogen becomes the dominant substance in the follicular fluid. Conversely, in the absence of FSH, androgens predominate.[32, 33] LH is not normally present in follicular fluid until the midcycle. If LH is prematurely elevated in plasma and antral fluid, mitotic activity in the granulosa decreases, degenerative changes ensue, and intrafollicular androgen levels rise. Therefore, the dominance of estrogen and FSH is essential for sustained accumulation of granulosa cells and continued follicular growth. Antral follicles with the greatest rates of granulosa proliferation contain the highest estrogen concentrations and the lowest androgen:estrogen ratios, and are the most likely to house a healthy oocyte.[34] An androgenic milieu antagonizes estrogen-induced granulosa proliferation and, if sustained, promotes degenerative changes in the oocyte.

The steroids present in follicular fluid can be found in concentrations several orders of magnitude higher than those in plasma and reflect the functional capacity of the surrounding granulosa and theca cells. The synthesis of steroid hormones is functionally compartmentalized within the follicle—the two-cell system.[23, 29, 33, 35, 36]

The Two-Cell, Two-Gonadotropin System

The aromatase activity of the granulosa far exceeds that observed in the theca. In human preantral and antral follicles, LH receptors are present only on the theca cells and FSH receptors only on the granulosa cells.[37, 38] Thecal interstitial cells, located in the theca interna, have approximately 20,000 LH receptors in their cell membranes. In response to LH, thecal tissue is stimulated to produce androgens that can then be converted, through FSH-induced aromatization, to estrogens in the granulosa cells.

The interaction between the granulosa and theca compartments, with resulting accelerated estrogen production, is not fully functional until later in antral development. Like preantral granulosa cells, the granulosa of small antral follicles exhibits an in vitro tendency to convert significant amounts of androgen to the more potent 5α-reduced form. In contrast, granulosa cells isolated from large antral follicles readily and preferentially metabolize androgens to estrogens. The conversion from an androgen microenvironment to an estrogen microenvironment (a conversion essential for further growth and development) is dependent upon a growing sensitivity to FSH brought about by the action of FSH and the enhancing influence of estrogen.

As the follicle develops, theca cells begin to express the genes for LH receptors, P450scc, and 3β-hydroxysteroid dehydrogenase.[39] The separately regulated (by LH) entry of cholesterol into mitochondria, utilizing internalization of LDL-cholesterol, is essential for steroidogenesis. ***Therefore, ovarian steroidogenesis is LH-dependent to a significant degree.*** Human ovarian granulosa cells, after luteinization and vascularization that occur following ovulation, can use HDL-cholesterol in a system that differs from the LDL-cholesterol pathway. The lipoproteins are not internalized, but rather, the cholesteryl esters are extracted from the lipoproteins at the cell surface and then transferred into the cell.[40]

As the follicle emerges, the theca cells are characterized by their expression of P450c17, the enzyme step which is rate-limiting for the conversion of 21-carbon substrate to androgens.[41] Granulosa cells do not express this enzyme and thus are dependent upon androgens from the theca in order to make estrogen. Increasing expression of the aromatization system (P450arom) is a

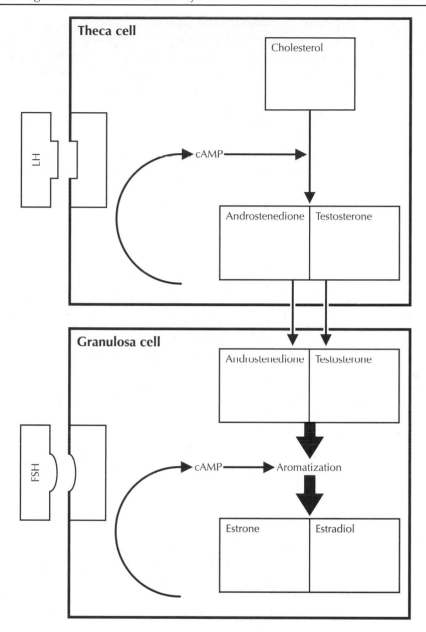

marker of increasing maturity of granulosa cells. The presence of P450c17 only in thecal cells and P450arom only in granulosa cells is impressive evidence confirming the two-cell, two-gonadotropin explanation for estrogen production.[42]

The importance of the two-cell, two-gonadotropin system in the primate is supported by the response of women with a deficiency in gonadotropins to treatment with recombinant (pure) FSH.[43–45] Follicles developed (confirming the essential role of FSH, and the lesser role for LH, in recruitment and initial growth), but estradiol production was limited. Some aromatization occurred, perhaps using androgens originating in the adrenal glands, producing early follicular phase estradiol levels, but the usual robust steroidogenesis was impossible without the presence of LH to provide thecal production of androgen substrate. This same response has been observed in experiments that use a GnRH antagonist to produce LH-deficient monkeys and then the administration of recombinant, pure human FSH.[46, 47] These results indicate that only FSH is required for folliculogenesis, and that in the primate, autocrine/paracrine peptides have replaced estrogen in the important intraovarian role of modulating gonadotropin response.

Selection of the Dominant Follicle

The successful conversion to an estrogen dominant follicle marks the "selection" of a follicle destined to ovulate, the process whereby, with rare exception, only a single follicle succeeds.[48] This selection process is to a significant degree the result of two estrogen actions: 1) a local interaction between estrogen and FSH within the follicle (in the nonprimate model), and 2) the effect of estrogen on pituitary secretion of FSH. While estrogen exerts a positive influence on FSH action within the maturing follicle, its negative feedback relationship with FSH at the hypothalamic-pituitary level serves to withdraw gonadotropin support from the other less developed follicles. The fall in FSH leads to a decline in FSH-dependent aromatase activity, limiting estrogen production in the less mature follicles. Even if a lesser follicle succeeds in achieving an estrogen microenvironment, decreasing FSH support would interrupt granulosa proliferation and function, promote a conversion to an androgenic microenvironment, and thereby induce irreversible atretic change. Indeed, the first event in the process of atresia is a reduction in FSH receptors in the granulosa layer.

The loss of oocytes (and follicles) through atresia is a response to changes in many factors. Certainly gonadotropin stimulation and withdrawal are important, but ovarian steroids and autocrine/paracrine factors are also involved. The consequence of these unfavorable changes, atresia, is a process called *apoptosis*, programmed cell death. This process is heralded by alterations in mRNAs required for cell proteins which maintain follicle integrity.[49] This type of "natural death" is a physiologic process, in contrast to the pathologic cell death of necrosis.

Once cells have entered the process of apoptosis, their response to FSH is modulated by local growth factors. Tumor necrosis factor (TNF), produced in the granulosa cells, inhibits FSH stimulation of estradiol secretion, except in the dominant follicle.[50] An inverse relationship exists between TNF expression and gonadotropin stimulation of granulosa cells. Thus, as the successful follicle increases its response to gonadotropins, its TNF production decreases. Those follicles with a failing response to gonadotropins increase their TNF production, hastening their demise.

An asymmetry in ovarian estrogen production, an expression of the emerging dominant follicle, can be detected in ovarian venous effluent on day 5 of the cycle, corresponding with the gradual fall of FSH levels observed at the midfollicular phase and preceding the increase in diameter that marks the physical emergence of the dominant follicle.[51] This is a crucial time in the cycle. Exogenous estrogen, administered even after selection of the dominant follicle, disrupts preovulatory development and induces atresia by reducing FSH levels below the sustaining level. Because the lesser follicles have entered the process of atresia, loss of the dominant follicle during this period of time requires beginning over, with recruitment of another set of preantral follicles.[52]

The negative feedback of estrogen on FSH serves to inhibit the development of all but the dominant follicle. The selected follicle remains dependent upon FSH and must complete its preovulatory development in the face of declining plasma levels of FSH. The dominant follicle, therefore, must escape the consequences of FSH suppression induced by its own accelerating estrogen production. The dominant follicle has two significant advantages, a greater content of FSH receptors acquired because of a rate of granulosa proliferation that surpasses that of its cohorts and enhancement of FSH action because of its high intrafollicular estrogen concentration (the nonprimate model) or because of local autocrine/paracrine peptides (as will be described below in the primate model). Thus, the dominant follicle is more sensitive to FSH, and as long as a critical duration of FSH exposure was initially present, the dominant follicle continues to develop.[8] As a result, the stimulus for aromatization, FSH, can be maintained, while at the same time it is being withdrawn from among the less developed follicles. A wave of atresia among the lesser follicles, therefore, is seen to parallel the rise in estrogen.

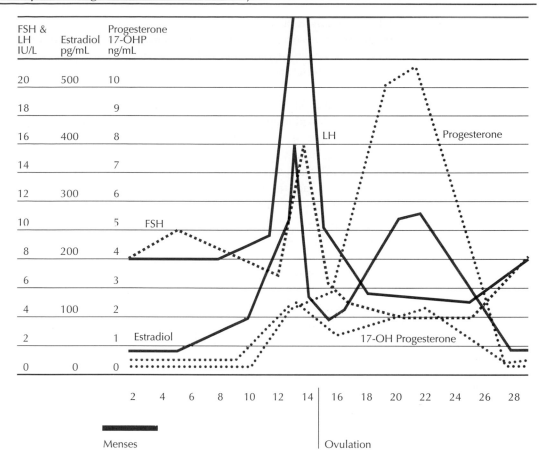

The accumulation of a greater mass of granulosa cells is accompanied by advanced development of the thecal vasculature. By day 9, thecal vascularity in the dominant follicle is twice that of other antral follicles. [53] This allows a preferential delivery of gonadotropins to the follicle, permitting the dominant follicle to retain FSH responsiveness and sustain continued development and function despite waning gonadotropin levels. The monkey ovary expresses a potent growth factor (vascular endothelial growth factor) that induces angiogenesis, and this expression is observed at the two development points when proliferation of capillaries is important: the emerging dominant follicle and the early corpus luteum.[54, 55]

In order to respond to the ovulatory surge and to become a successful corpus luteum, the granulosa cells must acquire LH receptors. FSH induces LH receptor development on the granulosa cells of the large antral follicles. Here again either estrogen (the nonprimate), or local autocrine/paracrine peptides (primate), serves as the chief coordinator.

In the nonprimate model, with increasing concentrations of estrogen within the follicle, FSH changes its focus of action, from up-regulating its own receptor to generation of the LH receptors.[56] The combination of a capacity for continued response despite declining levels of FSH and a high local estrogen environment in the dominant follicle provides optimal conditions for LH receptor development. LH can induce the formation of its own receptor in FSH-primed granulosa cells, but the primary mechanism utilizes FSH stimulation and estrogen enhancement.[57, 58] The role for estrogen goes beyond synergism and enhancement; it is obligatory. Inhibition of estrogen synthesis prevents FSH-stimulated increases in LH receptors.[59]

Although prolactin is always present in follicular fluid, there is no evidence to suggest that prolactin is important during normal ovulatory cycles in the primate.

The Feedback System

Through its own estrogen and peptide production, the dominant follicle assumes control of its own destiny. By altering gonadotropin secretion through feedback mechanisms it optimizes its own environment to the detriment of the lesser follicles.

As reviewed in Chapter 5, gonadotropin-releasing hormone (GnRH) plays an obligatory role in the control of gonadotropin secretion, but the pattern of gonadotropin secretion observed in the menstrual cycle is the result of feedback modulation of steroids and peptides originating in the dominant follicle, acting directly on the hypothalamus and anterior pituitary.[4] In addition, an increase in GnRH accompanies the LH surge, indicating that estrogen positive feedback operates at both pituitary and hypothalamic sites.[60] Estrogen exerts its inhibitory effects in both the hypothalamus and the anterior pituitary, decreasing both GnRH pulsatile secretion and GnRH pituitary response.[61] Progesterone also operates in two sites. Its inhibitory action is at the hypothalamic level, and, like estrogen, its positive action is directly on the pituitary.[62]

The secretion of FSH is very sensitive to the negative inhibitory effects of estrogen even at low levels. At higher levels, estrogen combines with inhibin for a suppression of FSH that is profound and sustained. In contrast, the influence of estrogen on LH release varies with concentration and duration of exposure. At low levels, estrogen imposes a negative feedback relationship with LH. At higher levels, however, estrogen is capable of exerting a positive stimulatory feedback effect on LH release.

The transition from suppression to stimulation of LH release occurs as estradiol rises during the midfollicular phase. There are two critical features in this mechanism: 1) the concentration of estradiol and 2) the length of time during which the estradiol elevation is sustained. In women, the estradiol concentration necessary to achieve a positive feedback is more than 200 pg/mL, and this concentration must be sustained for approximately 50 hours.[63] This level of estrogen essentially never occurs until the dominant follicle has reached a diameter of 15 mm.[64] The estrogen stimulus must be sustained beyond the initiation of the LH surge until after the surge actually begins. Otherwise, the LH surge is abbreviated or fails to occur at all.

Within the well-established monthly pattern, the gonadotropins are secreted in a pulsatile fashion with a frequency and magnitude that vary with the phase of the cycle. The pulsatile pattern is directly due to a similar pulsatile secretion of GnRH, but amplitude and frequency modulation (mean values below) is probably the consequence of steroid feedback on both hypothalamus and anterior pituitary.[65–67] *Pulsatile secretion is more frequent but smaller in amplitude during the follicular phase compared to the luteal phase, with a slight increase in frequency observed as the follicular phase progresses to ovulation.*

LH Pulse Frequency:

Early follicular phase	— 90 minutes.
Late follicular phase	— 60–70 minutes.
Early luteal phase	— 100 minutes.
Late luteal phase	— 200 minutes.

LH Pulse Amplitude:

Early follicular phase	— 6.5 IU/L.
Midfollicular phase	— 5.0 IU/L.
Late follicular phase	— 7.2 IU/L.
Early luteal phase	— 15.0 IU/L.
Midluteal phase	— 12.2 IU/L.
Late luteal phase	— 8.0 IU/L.

The pulsatile pattern of FSH is not easily discerned because of its relatively longer half-life compared to LH, but the experimental data indicate that FSH and LH are secreted simultaneously and that GnRH stimulates the secretion of both gonadotropins. Even as late as only 36–48 hours before menses, gonadotropin secretion is still characterized by infrequent LH pulses and low FSH levels typical of the late luteal phase.[66] During the transition from the previous luteal phase to the next follicular phase, GnRH and the gonadotropins are released from the inhibitory effects of estradiol, progesterone, and inhibin. A progressive and fairly rapid increase in GnRH pulse secretion is associated with a preferential secretion of FSH compared to LH. The frequency of GnRH and LH pulses increases 4.5-fold during this period of time, accompanied by a 3.5-fold increase in the circulating levels of FSH, and a lesser 2-fold increase in LH levels.[68]

The GnRH pulse frequency changes in the luteal phase correlate with duration of exposure to progesterone, while pulse amplitude changes appear to be influenced by changes in progesterone levels.[65] Both estradiol and progesterone are required to achieve the low, suppressed secretory pattern of GnRH during the luteal phase.[69] The studies suggest that steroids influence the hypothalamic release of GnRH for frequency changes and the pituitary for action on amplitude of the gonadotropin pulses. The inhibitory action of luteal phase steroids appears to be mediated by an increase in hypothalamic endogenous opioid peptides. Both estrogen and progesterone can increase endogenous opiates, and administration of clomiphene (an estrogen antagonist) during the luteal phase increases the LH pulse frequency with no effect on amplitude.[70] Thus, estrogen appears to enhance the stimulatory action of progesterone in the luteal phase on endogenous opioid peptides, creating relatively high levels of endogenous opiates during the luteal phase.

Plasma endorphin begins to rise in the 2 days before the LH peak, coinciding with the midcycle gonadotropin surge.[71] The maximal level is reached just after the LH peak, coinciding with ovulation. Levels then gradually decline until the nadir is reached during menses and the early follicular phase. Monkeys have their highest beta-endorphin levels in the hypophyseal portal blood at midcycle.[72] Normal cyclicity requires sequential periods of high (midcycle and luteal phase) and low (during menses) hypothalamic opioid activity.

There is another important action of estrogen. A disparity exists between the patterns of FSH and LH secretion as determined by immunoassay and bioassay, indicating that more biologically active gonadotropins are secreted at midcycle than at other times in the cycle.[73, 74] This quality, bioactivity vs immunoreactivity, is determined by the molecular structure of the gonadotropin molecule, a concept referred to in Chapter 2 as heterogeneity of the tropic hormones. There is a well-established relationship between the activity and half-life of glycoprotein hormones and their sialic acid content. The feedback effects of estrogen include modulation of sialylation and the size and activity of the gonadotropins subsequently released, as well as an augmentation of GnRH-stimulated secretory release of biologically active gonadotropin. It certainly makes sense to intensify the gonadotropin effect at midcycle. The positive feedback action of estrogen, therefore, both increase the quantity and the quality (the bioactivity) of FSH and LH.

There is a diurnal rhythm in FSH and LH secretion.[75] In contrast to the nocturnal rise seen with ACTH, thyroid-stimulating hormone (TSH), growth hormone, and prolactin, FSH and LH exhibit nocturnal decline, probably mediated by endogenous opiates. This diurnal rhythm for LH is present only in the early follicular phase, while FSH maintains a circadian rhythm throughout the menstrual cycle (and thus it is not influenced by steroid hormone feedback) and even in the postmenopausal period of life.

Inhibin, Activin, Follistatin
This family of peptides is synthesized by granulosa cells in response to FSH and secreted into the follicular fluid and ovarian venous effluent.[76–79] The expression of these peptides is not limited to the ovary; they are present in many tissues throughout the body serving as autocrine/paracrine regulators. Inhibin is an important inhibitor of FSH secretion. Activin stimulates FSH release in the pituitary and augments FSH action in the ovary. Follistatin suppresses FSH activity, probably by binding activin.

Inhibin consists of two dissimilar peptides (known as alpha- and beta-subunits) linked by disulfide bonds. Two forms of inhibin (inhibin A and inhibin B) have been purified, each containing an identical alpha-subunit and distinct but related beta-subunits. Thus, there are three subunits for inhibins: alpha, beta-A, and beta-B. Each subunit is a product of different messenger RNA, each derived from its own precursor molecule. Initial efforts to understand the role of inhibin in physiology were hampered by imprecise assays and the fact that multiple forms are present in the circulation, including free subunits.

The 2 Forms of Inhibin:
    Inhibin A: **Alpha-Beta$_A$**
    Inhibin B: **Alpha-Beta$_B$**

FSH stimulates the secretion of inhibin from granulosa cells and, in turn, is suppressed by inhibin — a reciprocal relationship.[80, 81] Refinements in assay techniques have revealed that inhibin B is the form of inhibin predominantly secreted by granulosa cells in the follicular phase of the cycle.[82, 83] The secretion of inhibin is further regulated by local autocrine/paracrine control. GnRH and epidermal growth factor diminish FSH stimulation of inhibin secretion, whereas insulin-like growth factor-I enhances inhibin production. The inhibitory effects of GnRH and epidermal growth factor are consistent with their known ability to decrease FSH-stimulated estrogen production and LH receptor formation. The action of GnRH lends some support for an endogenous ovarian GnRH-like substance (which is found in follicular fluid) and which is involved in inhibin production.

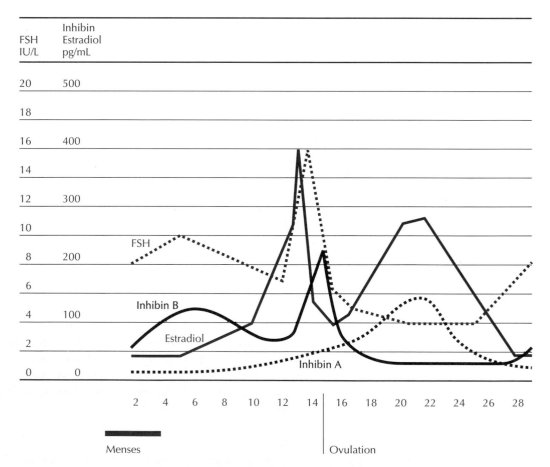

The secretion of inhibin B into the circulation further amplifies the withdrawal of FSH from other follicles, another mechanism by which an emerging follicle secures dominance. Inhibin B rises slowly but steadily, in a pulsatile fashion (60–70 min periodicity) reaching peak levels in the early and midfollicular phases, and then decreasing in the late follicular phase before ovulation to reach a nadir in the midluteal phase.[16, 82, 84, 85] An inhibin B peak the day after ovulation is probably the result of release from the ruptured follicle. This relationship of inhibin B and FSH is supported by the demonstration that Inhibin B levels are lower and FSH levels are higher in the follicular phase in women 45–49 years old compared to younger women.[84, 86]

With the appearance of LH receptors on the granulosa cells of the dominant follicle and the subsequent development of the follicle into a corpus luteum, inhibin expression comes under the control of LH, and expression changes from inhibin B to inhibin A.[87] The circulating levels of inhibin A rise in the late follicular phase to reach a peak level at the midluteal phase.[16, 88] Inhibin A, therefore, contributes to the suppression of FSH to nadir levels during the luteal phase, and to the changes at the luteal-follicular transition.

Inhibin has multiple, diverse inhibitory effects on gonadotropin secretion. Inhibin can block the synthesis and secretion of FSH, prevent the up-regulation of GnRH receptors by GnRH, reduce the number of GnRH receptors present, and, at high concentrations, promote the intracellular degradation of gonadotropins.

Activin is a peptide that is related to inhibin but has an opposite action (the stimulation of FSH release and GnRH receptor number).[83, 89, 90] This peptide contains two subunits that are identical to the beta-subunits of inhibins A and B. Thus, when each of the beta-subunits of the inhibins is combined with an alpha-subunit, the resulting molecule, inhibin A or B, inhibits the release of FSH. If the beta-subunits are paired together, the molecule stimulates the release of FSH. Each activin subunit is encoded by a distinct gene. The structure of the activin genes is homologous to that of transforming growth factor-β, indicating that these products all come from the same gene family.[91] Another important member of this family is the antimüllerian hormone, as well as a protein active during insect embryogenesis, and a protein active in frog embryos.

The 3 Forms of Activin:

Activin A:	**Beta$_A$-Beta$_A$**
Activin AB:	**Beta$_A$-Beta$_B$**
Activin B:	**Beta$_B$-Beta$_B$**

Activin is present in many cell types, regulating growth and differentiation. In the ovarian follicle, activin increases FSH binding in granulosa cells (by regulating receptor numbers) and augments FSH stimulation of aromatization and inhibin production.[78] Considerable evidence derived from human cells exists to indicate that inhibin and activin act directly on thecal cells to regulate androgen synthesis.[92–94] Inhibin enhances the stimulatory action of LH and/or IGF-I, while activin suppresses this action. Inhibin in increasing doses can overcome the inhibitory action of activin. Prior to ovulation, activin suppresses granulosa progesterone production, perhaps preventing premature luteinization. There is a repertoire of cell transmembrane kinase receptors for activin, with differing binding affinities and domain structures.[95] This receptor heterogeneity allows the many different responses elicited by a single peptide. Both activin A and inhibin A have been demonstrated to be very potent in stimulating in vitro maturation of oocytes that subsequently yield a high rate of fertilization.[96]

In the male, activin inhibits and inhibin facilitates LH stimulation of androgen biosynthesis in Leydig cells. In addition, activin stimulates and inhibin decreases spermatogonial proliferation; inhibin is produced in the Sertoli cell, the locus that has the principal role in modulating spermatogenesis. Thus, activin and inhibin play similar autocrine/paracrine roles in both the male and female gonads.

The anterior pituitary expresses the inhibin/activin subunits, and locally produced activin B augments FSH secretion. Activin A has been demonstrated to directly stimulate the synthesis of GnRH receptors in pituitary cells.[90] Follistatin is a peptide secreted by a variety of pituitary cells, including the gonadotropes.[97] This peptide has also been called FSH-suppressing protein because of its main action: inhibition of FSH synthesis and secretion and the FSH response to GnRH, probably by binding to activin and in that fashion decreasing the activity of activin.[98, 99] Activin stimulates follistatin production, and inhibin prevents this response. Follistatin is also expressed by granulosa cells in response to FSH, and, therefore, follistatin, like inhibin and activin, functions locally in the follicle and in the pituitary.[100] Circulating levels of activin increase in the late luteal phase to peak at menses; however, activin A is highly bound in the circulation, and it is not certain it has an endocrine role.[101] Nevertheless, the timing is right for activin to contribute to the rise in FSH during the luteal-follicular transition.

In summary, the pituitary secretion of FSH can be significantly regulated by the balance of activin and inhibin, with follistatin playing a role by inhibiting activin and enhancing inhibin activity. Within the ovarian follicle, activin and inhibin influence growth and development by modulating thecal and granulosal responses to the gonadotropins.

The inhibin-activin family of peptides (also including antimüllerian hormone and transforming growth factor-β) inhibits cell growth and can be considered as a class of tumor-suppressor proteins. Mice have been generated that are deficient in the inhibin alpha-subunit gene.[79] The mice that are homozygous and lack inhibin are susceptible to the development of gonadal stromal tumors which appear after normal sexual differentiation and development. Thus, the alpha-inhibin gene is a specific tumor-suppressor gene for the gonads. A contributing factor to this tumor development could be the high FSH levels associated with the deficiency in inhibin.

Growth Factors

Growth factors are polypeptides that modulate cell proliferation and differentiation, operating through binding to specific cell membrane receptors. They are not classic endocrine substances; they act locally and function in paracrine and autocrine modes. There are multiple growth factors, and most cells contain multiple receptors for the various growth factors.

Insulin-Like Growth Factors. The insulin-like growth factors (also called somatomedins) are peptides that have structural and functional similarity to insulin and mediate growth hormone action.[102] Insulin-like growth factor-I (IGF-I) and insulin-like growth factor-II (IGF-II) are single chain polypeptides containing 3 disulfide bonds. IGF-I is encoded on the long arm of chromosome 12 and IGF-II on the short arm of chromosome 11 (which also contains the insulin gene). The genes are subject to a variety of promoters, and thus differential regulation can govern ultimate actions.

IGF-I mediates the growth promoting actions of growth hormone. The majority of circulating IGF-I is derived from growth hormone dependent synthesis in the liver. However, IGF-I is synthesized in many tissues where production can be regulated in conjunction with growth hormone or ***independently*** by other factors.

IGF-II has little growth hormone dependence. It is believed to be important in fetal growth and development. Both IGFs induce the expression of cellular genes responsible for cellular proliferation and differentiation.

Insulin-like Growth Factor Binding Proteins. There are 6 known nonglycosylated peptides that function as IGF binding proteins, IGFBP-1 to IGFBP-6.[103] These binding proteins serve to carry the IGFs in serum, prolong half-lives, and regulate tissue effects of the IGFs. The regulating action appears to be due to binding and sequestering of the IGFs, preventing their access to the cell membrane surface receptors, and, thus, not permitting the synergistic actions that result when gonadotropins and growth factors are combined. The IGFBPs may also exert direct actions on cellular functions, independently of growth factor functions. IGFBP-1 is the principal BP in amniotic fluid; IGFBP-3 is the main BP in serum and its synthesis, primarily in the liver, is dependent on growth hormone. Circulating levels of IGFBP-3 reflect the total IGF concentration (IGF-I plus IGF-II) and carry at least 90% of the circulating IGFs. These BPs do not bind insulin. The BPs change with age (decreasing levels of IGFBP-3) and during pregnancy (decreasing IGFBP-3 due to a circulating protease unique to pregnancy).

The IGF Receptors. The Type I receptor preferentially binds IGF-1 and can be called the IGF-I receptor. The Type II receptor in a similar fashion can be called the IGF-II receptor. IGF-I also binds to the insulin receptor but with low affinity. Insulin binds to the IGF-I receptor with moderate affinity. The IGF-I receptor and the insulin receptor are similar in structure: tetramers composed of two α-subunits and two β-subunits linked by disulfide bonds. The intracellular component of the β-subunit is a tyrosine kinase that is activated by autophosphorylation. The IGF-II receptor does not bind insulin. It is a single chain glycoprotein, with 90% of its structure extending extracellularly. This receptor functions as a receptor coupled to a G protein. The physiologic effects of IGF-I are mediated by its own receptor, but IGF-II can exert its actions via both receptors. Indeed, the IGF-I receptor binds IGF-I and IGF-II with equal affinity. In human cells, the IGF-I receptor and IGF-II receptor are present in theca and granulosa cells and in luteinized granulosa cells. Ovarian stromal tissue contains IGF-I receptors.

Early Follicular Phase

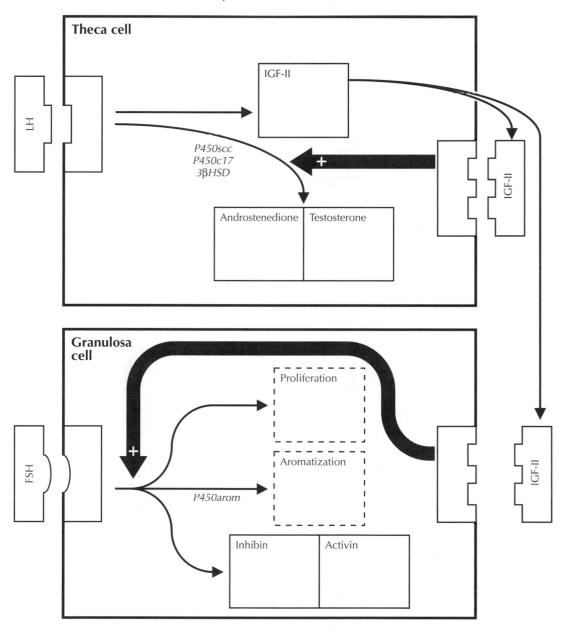

The Ovarian Actions of IGFs. IGF-I has been demonstrated to stimulate the following events in ovarian theca and granulosa cells: DNA synthesis, steroidogenesis, aromatase activity, LH receptor synthesis, and inhibin secretion. IGF-II stimulates granulosa mitosis. In human ovarian cells, IGF-I, in synergy with FSH, stimulates protein synthesis and steroidogenesis. After LH receptors appear, IGF-I enhances LH-induced progesterone synthesis and stimulates proliferation of granulosa-luteal cells. IGF-I, in synergy with FSH, is very active in stimulating aromatase activity in preovulatory follicles. Thus, IGF-I can be involved in both estradiol and progesterone synthesis.

Preovulatory Follicle

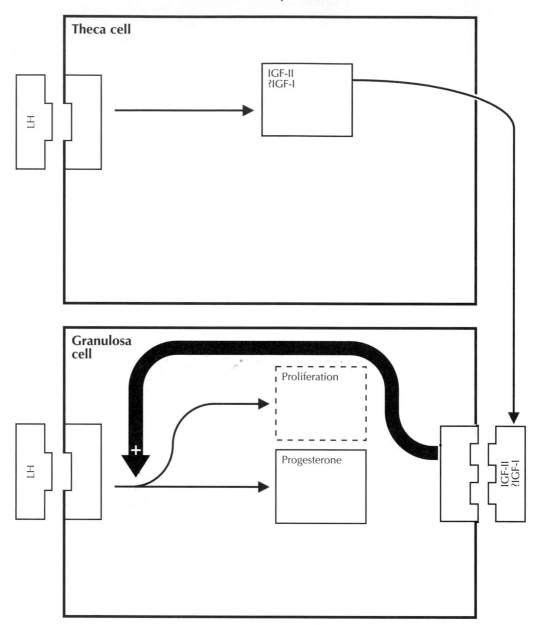

In animal experiments, the synthesis of IGF-I by granulosa cells is dependent upon FSH but enhanced by estradiol. Growth hormone also acts synergistically with FSH and estradiol to increase IGF synthesis. The story becomes confused when various growth factors and regulators are studied, because of their various stimulating and inhibiting effects. In the rat, the granulosa cell is the major site for IGF-I gene expression, which is active only prior to ovulation. It is not detected in atretic follicles or in corpora lutea. Again in the rat, IGF-II gene expression appears to be limited to the theca and interstitial cells. However, the site of IGF expression is different in primates.

In studies with human ovarian tissue, IGF-II is highly expressed in both thecal cells and granulosa cells; however, the level is highest in the granulosa and increases with growth of the follicle.[104, 105] IGF-II is also synthesized by luteinized granulosa and appears to function locally in an autocrine fashion.[106] These findings indicate that IGF-II is the primary IGF in the human ovary. Nevertheless, IGF-I is still a significant product of human thecal cells.[107]

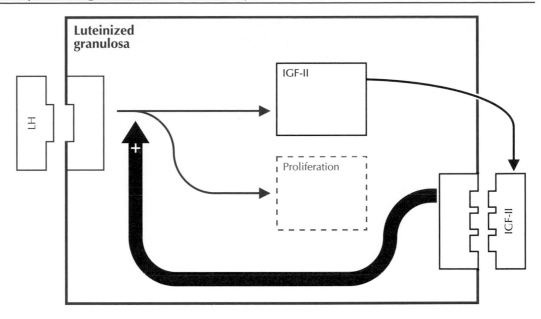

Human thecal cells express mRNA transcripts which encode receptors for both IGF-I and insulin.[108] Because insulin and IGF-II can both activate the receptor for IGF-I, this pathway provides a method for the exertion of a paracrine influence on granulosa cells and autocrine activity in the theca (augmenting LH stimulation of androgen production). In vitro studies confirm that IGF-II is capable of stimulating steroidogenesis and proliferation in human theca and granulosa cells.[109–111] These actions are augmented by growth hormone, which increases IGF production and, thus, indirectly enhances gonadotropin stimulation of ovarian follicles.[112]

This primate scenario is supported by finding higher levels of IGF-II, but not IGF-I, in the follicular fluid of developing follicles, with the highest levels present in dominant follicles.[113] The IGF levels in follicular fluid correlate with estradiol levels and undergo a further short increase after the LH surge. There are no menstrual cycle changes in the circulating levels of IGF-I, IGF-II, IGFBP-1, or IGFBP-3; high levels in the dominant follicle are not associated with an increase in circulating levels.[114]

The 6 IGF binding proteins are synthesized in different amounts in various follicular tissues in response to gonadotropins, insulin, and IGF-I. In the rat, IGFBP-3 is made in the theca, stimulated by growth hormone, and inhibited by FSH and estradiol.[115] In the rat, low concentrations of FSH stimulate the expression of IGFBPs, while FSH at high concentrations inhibits IGFBP synthesis. It is proposed that this biphasic response allows an increase in IGF-I facilitation of mitosis during FSH-induced follicular growth, while IGF-I availability is limited during periods of low FSH when follicular steroidogenesis is the major effort.[116]

In studies with human tissue, IGFBP-1 inhibits IGF-1 mediated steroidogenesis and proliferation of luteinized granulosa cells. The synthesis of IGFBPs by human granulosa is inhibited by FSH, IGF-I, and IGF-II.[117, 118] These findings fit with the overall idea that the BPs counteract the synergistic results of gonadotropins and growth factors. In general, IGFBP-1 expression is found in granulosa cells of growing follicles; IGFBP-3 in theca cells and the granulosa of the dominant follicle; IGFBP-2, -4, and -5 in thecal and granulosa of antral and atretic follicles; and IGFBP-6 has not been found in the ovary.[104] The predominant binding protein in preovulatory follicles is IGFBP-2 in the granulosa and IGFBP-3 in the theca, that increase progressively in the follicle that emerges as the dominant follicle, and then decrease in the late follicular phase.[105, 119, 120] This suggests that –1, -2, and -3 play a role in growing follicles, -2, -4, and -5 in atretic and failing follicles. IGFBP expression in polycystic ovaries is similar to that seen in atretic follicles. The decrease in IGFBP-3 that occurs in dominant follicles should allow an increase in IGF levels and activity. The increase in IGFBP-2 in failing follicles probably correlates with sequestering of IGF, depriving the follicle of an important force in gonadotropin augmentation.

Circulating levels of IGFBP-1 decrease in response to insulin, and thus circulating levels are decreased in women with anovulation and polycystic ovaries who have elevated levels of insulin.[121] These patients also have increased circulating levels of IGF-I, probably a consequence of LH-stimulated synthesis and secretion in theca cells. The level of IGFBP-1 in follicular fluid from polycystic ovaries is decreased; thus this BP is not playing a role inhibiting the action of IGF-I in polycystic ovaries. The levels of IGFBPs -2 and -4 in the follicular fluid from follicles in anovulatory patients are increased (as in atretic follicles).[104, 122] Even though these changes may play a role in anovulatory pathophysiology, they are consistent with failure in development and thus may not be etiologic factors.

IGF activity may also be modulated by the proteases that regulate the activity of the IGF binding proteins.[123] Estrogen-dominant follicular fluid contains very low levels of IGFBP-4, in contrast to the high levels present in androgen-dominant follicular fluid. The low level of IGFBP-4 in estrogen-dominant follicular fluid is associated with the presence of an IGFBP-4 specific protease. This protease would decrease IGFBP activity and enhance IGF activity, another mechanism for ensuring the success of the dominant follicle.

In addition to ovarian activities, IGF-I and its receptor and binding proteins operate in the pituitary gland. In the rat, the hyperplasia of various pituitary cell types appears to be mediated by estrogen regulation of the IGF-I system.[124] This mechanism is of special interest when considering the development of pituitary tumors, such as the prolactin secreting pituitary adenoma.

The insulin-like growth factor story is at once complex, fascinating, and compelling. However, its contribution may be facilitatory and not essential. Laron-type dwarfism is characterized by a deficiency in IGF-I due to an abnormality in the growth hormone receptor. Despite low levels of IGF-I and high levels of IGFBP, a woman with Laron-type dwarfism responded to exogenous gonadotropin stimulation with the production of multiple, mature follicles with good estrogen production and fertilizable oocytes.[125] Another explanation for this observation is that IGF-II, rather than IGF-I, is the important factor in the human dominant follicle. This possibility is supported by evidence indicating that IGF-II is the most abundant IGF in human ovarian follicles.[104, 105] Another possibility is that the Laron-type dwarf is deficient only in growth hormone-dependent IGF-I, and ovarian IGFs are not totally dependent on growth hormone.

Summary of Insulin-Like Growth Factor Action in the Ovary

1. IGF-II stimulates granulosa cell proliferation, aromatase activity, and progesterone synthesis.

2. IGF-II is produced in thecal cells, granulosa cells, and luteinized granulosa cells. In the pig and rat, the primary IGF is IGF-I.

3. Gonadotropins stimulate IGF production, and in animal experiments, this stimulation is enhanced by estradiol and growth hormone.

4. IGF-I receptors are present in theca and granulosa cells, and only IGF-II receptors are present in luteinized granulosa. IGF-II activates both IGF-I and IGF-II receptors.

5. The most abundant IGF in human follicles is IGF-II.

6. FSH inhibits binding protein synthesis, and thus maximizes growth factor availability.

Epidermal Growth Factor. Epidermal growth factor is a mitogen for a variety of cells, and its action is potentiated by other growth factors. Granulosa cells, in particular, respond to this growth factor in a variety of ways related to gonadotropin stimulation, including proliferation. Epidermal growth factor suppresses the up-regulation of FSH on its own receptor.[22]

Transforming Growth Factor. TGF-α is a structural analog of epidermal growth factor and can bind to the epidermal growth factor receptor. TGF-β utilizes a receptor distinct from the epidermal growth factor receptor. These factors are thought to be autocrine growth regulators. Inhibin and activin are derived from the same gene family. TGF-β, secreted by theca cells, enhances FSH induction of LH receptors on granulosa cells, an action which is opposite that of epidermal growth factor.[126] While this action can be viewed as a positive impact on granulosa cells, in the theca, TGF-β has a negative action, inhibiting androgen production.[127]

Fibroblast Growth Factor. This factor is a mitogen for a variety of cells and is present in all steroid-producing tissues. Important roles in the ovarian follicle include stimulation of mitosis in granulosa cells, stimulation of angiogenesis, stimulation of plasminogen activator, inhibition of FSH up-regulation of its own receptor, and inhibition of FSH-induced LH receptor expression and estrogen production.[22, 128] These actions are opposite of those of transforming growth factor-β.

Platelet-Derived Growth Factor. This growth factor modifies cyclic AMP pathways responding to FSH, especially those involved in granulosa cell differentiation. Both platelet-derived growth factor and epidermal growth factor may also modify prostaglandin production within the follicle.

Angiogenic Growth Factors. Vascularization of the follicle is influenced by peptides into the follicular fluid, especially vascular endothelial growth factor (VEGF), a cytokine produced in granulosa cells in response to LH.[129, 130] Luteal cells respond to HCG with greater VEGF output, a probable mechanism contributing to the increased vascular permeability associated with ovarian hyperstimulation that can occur with exogenous gonadotropin administration (Chapter 30).[131]

The Interleukin-1 System. Leukocytes are a prominent component of the ovarian follicle and a major source of interleukins. Interleukin-1 is a member of the cytokine family of immuno-mediators. The human ovary contains the complete interleukin-1 system (ligand and receptor). In the rat, interleukin-1 stimulates ovarian prostaglandin synthesis and perhaps plays a role in ovulation.[132]

Tumor Necrosis Factor-α (TNF-α). TNF-α is also a product of leukocytes (macrophages). It very likely is a key player in the process of apoptosis, a feature of follicular atresia as well as luteolysis of the corpus luteum.

Other Peptides. The follicular fluid is a veritable protein soup! It is composed of exudates from plasma and secretions from follicular cells. A variety of hormones can be found in the follicular fluid, as well as enzymes and peptides, which play important roles in follicular growth and development, ovulation, and modulation of hormonal responses.

Follicular fluid contains ***prorenin,*** the inactive precursor of renin, in a concentration that is about 12 times higher than plasma levels.[133] It appears that LH stimulates its synthesis in the follicle, and there is a midcycle peak in prorenin plasma levels. The circulating levels of prorenin also increase (10-fold) during the early stages of pregnancy, the result of ovarian stimulation by the rise in human chorionic gonadotropin (HCG). These increases in prorenin from the ovary are not responsible for any significant changes in the plasma levels of the active form, renin. Possible roles for this ovarian prorenin-renin-angiotensin system include stimulation of steroidogenesis to provide androgen substrate for estrogen production, regulation of calcium and prostaglandin metabolism, and stimulation of angiogenesis. This system may affect vascular and tissue functions both within and outside the ovary.

Members of the proopiomelanocortin family are found in human follicular fluid.[134] Follicular levels of *ACTH* and *β-lipotropin* remain constant throughout the cycle, but *β-endorphin* levels peak just before ovulation. In addition, enkephalin is present in relatively unchanging concentrations. The corticotropin-releasing hormone (CRH) system is present in thecal cells, but not in granulosa cells, complete with CRH, the CRH receptor, and CRH-binding protein.[135] CRH inhibits LH-stimulated androgen production in thecal cells, apparently by suppressing P450c17 gene expression.[136]

Antimüllerian hormone is produced by granulosa cells and may play a role in oocyte maturation (it inhibits oocyte meiosis) and follicular development.[137, 138] Antimüllerian hormone directly inhibits proliferation of granulosa and luteal cells, as well as epidermal growth factor-stimulated proliferation.

Follicular fluid prevents resumption of meiosis until the preovulatory LH surge either overcomes or removes this inhibition. This action is attributed to *oocyte maturation inhibitor (OMI)*. *Pregnancy-associated plasma protein A,* found in the placenta, is also present in follicular fluid. It may inhibit proteolytic activity within the follicle before ovulation. *Endothelin-1* is a peptide, produced in vascular endothelial cells, which may be the substance previously known as luteinization inhibitor; endothelin gene expression is induced by the hypoxia associated with the avascular granulosa, and it inhibits LH-induced progesterone production.[139] It is uncertain whether *GnRH-like peptides* have a follicular role or represent sequestered GnRH. *Oxytocin* is found in preovulatory follicles and the corpus luteum. Growth hormone-binding protein is present in follicular fluid and similar in characteristics to the same binding protein in serum.

Summary of Events in the Antral Follicle

1. Follicular phase estrogen production is explained by the two-ell, two-gonadotropin mechanism.

2. Selection of the dominant follicle is established during days 5–7, and consequently, peripheral levels of estradiol begin to rise significantly by cycle day 7.

3. Estradiol levels, derived from the dominant follicle, increase steadily and, through negative feedback effects, exert a progressively greater suppressive influence on FSH release.

4. While directing a decline in FSH levels, the midfollicular rise in estradiol exerts a positive feedback influence on LH secretion.

5. The positive action of estrogen also includes modification of the gonadotropin molecule, increasing the quality (the bioactivity) as well as the quantity of FSH and LH at midcycle.

6. LH levels rise steadily during the late follicular phase, stimulating androgen production in the theca.

7. A unique responsiveness to FSH allows the dominant follicle to utilize the androgen as substrate and further accelerate estrogen production.

8. FSH induces the appearance of LH receptors on granulosa cells.

9. Follicular response to the gonadotropins is modulated by a variety of growth factors and autocrine/paracrine peptides.

10. Inhibin B, secreted by the granulosa cells in response to FSH, directly suppresses pituitary FSH secretion.

11. Activin, originating in both pituitary and granulosa, augments FSH secretion and action.

Follicular Growth and Development in the Primate Ovary

Concern that the story for ovarian follicular growth and development might be different in the primate originated with the failure to find estrogen receptors in any of the significant ovarian compartments in the monkey: follicles, stromal tissue, interstitial tissue, or corpora lutea.[140] The importance of this finding in the monkey has been challenged by the discovery that human granulosa cells contain only mRNA for estrogen receptor-beta.[141] However, in further monkey experiments, no reduction in total number or size of follicles resulted when estradiol production was effectively suppressed by treatment with an inhibitor of the aromatase enzyme system or with an inhibitor of 3β-hydroxysteroid dehydrogenase.[142, 143] Oocyte development was not altered, although the subsequent fertilization rate was reduced by this treatment. Another argument against a major role for estrogen in follicular growth and development is the successful stimulation with gonadotropins of normal follicular growth and development in women with 17α-hydroxylase deficiency (an inherited disorder that prevents the production of androgens and estrogens).[144, 145]

A reduced role for estrogen is further supported by the response of women with a deficiency in gonadotropins to treatment with recombinant (pure) FSH.[43–45] Some aromatization occurred, perhaps using androgens originating in the adrenal glands, producing early follicular phase estradiol levels, but the usual robust steroidogenesis was impossible without the presence of LH to provide thecal production of androgen substrate. Nevertheless, oocytes were retrieved, and with in vitro fertilization, pregnancy was achieved. This same response was observed in experiments that used a GnRH antagonist to produce LH-deficient monkeys and then the administration of recombinant, pure human FSH.[46, 47]

These results indicate that only FSH is required for folliculogenesis, and that in the primate, autocrine/paracrine peptides have replaced estrogen in the important role of modulating gonadotropin response. Consider the following actions that have been documented in primate ovaries:

1. *Inhibin and activin regulate androgen synthesis in human theca cells. Inhibin enhances and activin suppresses the stimulatory action of LH and/or IGF-I, and inhibin can overcome the inhibitory action of activin on theca cells.[92-94]*

2. *In immature granulosa cells, activin augments all FSH activities, especially aromatase activity (estrogen production).[78, 146]*

3. *In luteinizing granulosa cells, activin has direct mitogenic activity and suppresses steroidogenesis in response to LH, while inhibin has no effect on LH-dependent aromatase in mature granulosa cells.[146, 147]*

4. *In the follicular phase, granulosa production of inhibin is under the control of FSH, but during the late follicular phase a change occurs, culminating in LH control of luteal synthesis of inhibin.[148, 149]*

5. *As the follicle grows, activin production decreases and inhibin production increases.[150, 151] In addition, follistatin levels increase in follicular fluid with increasing growth of the follicle, a mechanism for decreasing activin activity.[152]*

Early Follicular Phase

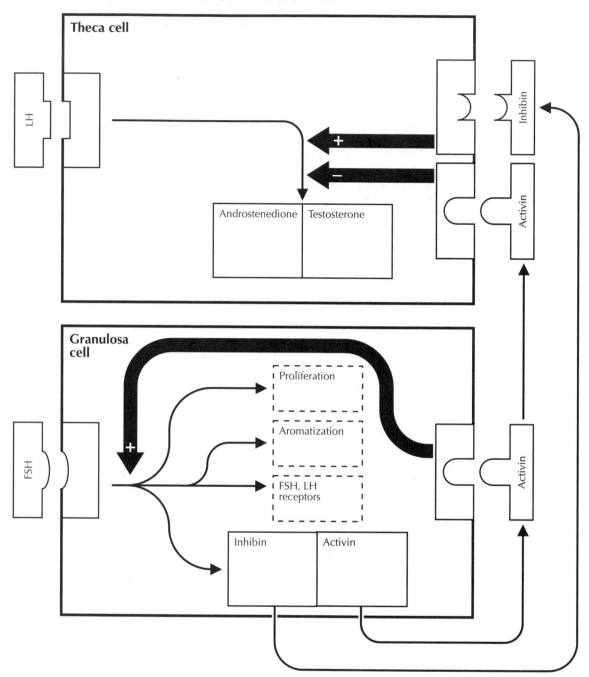

These actions may come together as follows. In the early follicular phase, activin produced by granulosa in immature follicles enhances the action of FSH on aromatase activity and FSH and LH receptor formation, while simultaneously suppressing thecal androgen synthesis. In the late follicular phase, increased production of inhibin by the granulosa (and decreased activin) promotes androgen synthesis in the theca in response to LH and IGF-II to provide substrate for even greater estrogen production in the granulosa. In the mature granulosa of the dominant preovulatory follicle, activin serves to prevent premature luteinization and progesterone production.

The successful follicle is the one that acquires the highest level of aromatase activity and LH receptors in response to FSH. The successful follicle is characterized by the highest estrogen (for central feedback action) and the greatest inhibin production (for both local and central actions).

Late Follicular Phase

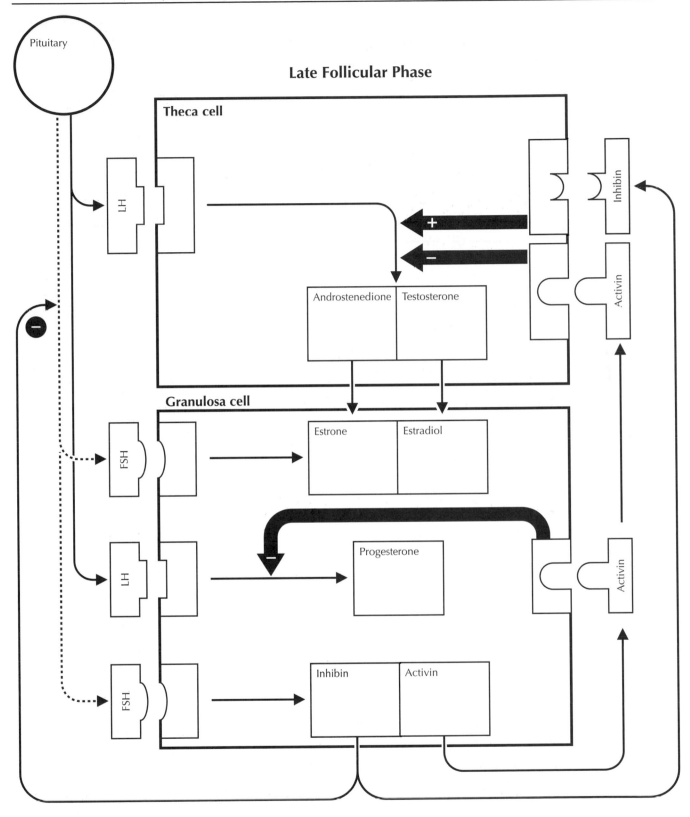

This accomplishment occurs in synchrony with the appropriate activin expression. The highest level of gene activity encoding activin B is found in immature antral follicles and the lowest level in preovulatory follicles. Thus the activin proteins (which enhance FSH activity) are produced in greatest amounts early in follicular development to enhance follicle receptivity to FSH. It is not certain which form of inhibin plays a key role, but as with circulating levels of inhibin, inhibin B is the predominant inhibin in the follicular fluid of growing follicles.[153]

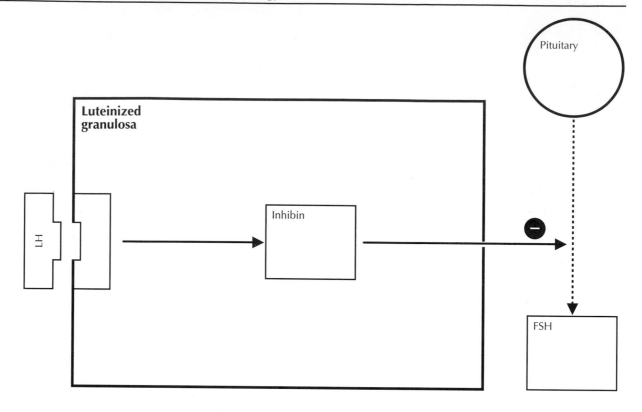

The right concentration of androgens in granulosa cells promotes aromatase activity and inhibin production and, in turn, inhibin promotes LH stimulation of thecal androgen synthesis. With development of the follicle, inhibin expression comes under control of LH. A key to successful ovulation and luteal function is conversion of the inhibin production to LH responsiveness to maintain FSH suppression centrally and enhancement of LH action locally.

A lesser role is assigned to the insulin-like growth factors in view of the successful production of multiple, estrogen-producing follicles which yielded fertilizable oocytes in a woman with IGF-I deficiency treated with gonadotropins.[125] The growth factors assume an important, but perhaps not essential, role as facilitating agents. However, the successful pregnancy in a woman with IGF-I deficiency may indicate the greater importance of IGF-II. In addition, the IGFs in the ovary may not be growth hormone-dependent, and therefore IGF-I and/or IGF-II may also be important in primate ovarian follicles.

Summary of Events in the Primate Ovarian Follicle

1. *FSH stimulates inhibin and activin production by granulosa cells.*

2. *Activin augments FSH activities: FSH receptor expression, aromatization, inhibin/ activin production, and LH receptor expression.*

3. *Inhibin enhances LH stimulation of androgen synthesis in the theca to provide substrate for aromatization to estrogen in the granulosa.*

4. *Inhibin B is secreted by the granulosa cells into the circulation, where it acts in a classic endocrine fashion to suppress FSH secretion by the pituitary gland.*

5. *With the appearance of LH receptors, inhibin production is maintained as it comes under control of LH.*

6. *All functions are modulated by a host of growth factors, and IGF-II may be especially important.*

The Preovulatory Follicle

Granulosa cells in the preovulatory follicle enlarge and acquire lipid inclusions while the theca becomes vacuolated and richly vascular, giving the preovulatory follicle a hyperemic appearance. The oocyte proceeds in meiosis, approaching completion of its reduction division.

Approaching maturity, the preovulatory follicle produces increasing amounts of estrogen. During the late follicular phase, estrogens rise slowly at first, then rapidly, reaching a peak approximately 24–36 hours prior to ovulation.[154] The onset of the LH surge occurs when the peak levels of estradiol are achieved.[155] In providing the ovulatory stimulus to the selected follicle, the LH surge seals the fate of the remaining follicles, with their lower estrogen and FSH content, by further increasing androgen superiority.

Acting through its own receptors, LH promotes luteinization of the granulosa in the dominant follicle, resulting in the production of progesterone. The LH receptor, once expressed, inhibits further cell growth and focuses the cell's energy on steroidogenesis (actions enhanced by IGF).[156] An increase in progesterone can be detected in the venous effluent of the ovary bearing the preovulatory follicle as early as day 10 of the cycle.[51] This small but significant increase in the production of progesterone in the preovulatory period has immense physiologic importance. Prior to the emergence of this follicular progesterone, the circulating level of progesterone was derived from the adrenal gland.[157]

Progesterone receptors begin to appear in the granulosa cells of the dominant follicle in the periovulatory period.[140] The traditional view has been that progesterone receptors are expressed in response to estrogen through an estrogen-receptor mediated mechanism. This is not the case with the primate ovarian follicle. Experimental data in the monkey provide excellent evidence that LH stimulates progesterone receptor expression in granulosa cells.[158] In vitro data with human cells suggest that the preovulatory progesterone and progesterone receptor expression directly inhibit granulosa cell mitosis, probably explainingthe limitation of granulosa cell proliferation as these cells gain LH receptors.[159]

Progesterone affects the positive feedback response to estrogen in both a time and dose dependent manner. When introduced after adequate estrogen priming, progesterone facilitates the positive feedback response, in a direct action on the pituitary, and in the presence of subthreshold levels of estradiol can induce a characteristic LH surge.[160, 161] Hence, the surprising onset of ovulation occasionally observed in an anovulatory, amenorrheic woman administered a prgestin challenge. When administered before the estrogen stimulus, or in high doses (achieving a blood level greater than 2 ng/mL), progesterone blocks the midcycle LH surge. Appropriately low levels of progesterone derived from the maturing follicle contribute to the precise synchronization of the midcycle surge.

In addition to its facilitatory action on LH, progesterone at midcycle is significantly responsible for the FSH surge.[161] This action of progesterone can be viewed as a further step in ensuring completion of FSH action on the follicle, especially making sure that a full complement of LH receptors is in place in the granulosa layer. In certain experimental situations, incremental estradiol alone can elicit simultaneous surges of LH and FSH, suggesting that progesterone certainly enhances the effect of estradiol but may not be obligatory.[162] Nevertheless, blockade of midcycle progesterone synthesis or activity in the monkey impaired the ovulatory process and luteinization.[163] These actions of estrogen and progesterone require the presence and continuous action of GnRH.

The preovulatory period is associated with a rise in plasma levels of 17α-hydroxyprogesterone. This steroid does not appear to have a role in cycle regulation, and its appearance in the blood simply represents the secretion of an intermediate product. As such, however, it signas the LH stimulation of P450scc and P450c17, important enzyme activity for the production of theca androgens, the substrate for granulosa estrogen. After ovulation, some theca cells become luteinized as part of the corpus luteum and lose the ability to express P450c17. Other luteinized theca cells retain P450c17 activity and are believed to continue to produce androgens for aromatization to estrogens.

When the lesser follicles fail to achieve full maturity and undergo atresia, the theca cells return to their origin as a component of stromal tissue, retaining, however, an ability to respond to LH with P450 activity and steroid production. Because the products of thecal tissue are androgens, the increase in stromal tissue in the late follicular phase is associated with a rise in androgen levels in the peripheral plasma at midcycle. There is a 15% increase in androstenedione and a 20% increase in testosterone.[164] This response is enhanced by the rise in inhibin, known to augment LH stimulation of androgen production in thecal cells.

Androgen production at this stage in the cycle may serve two purposes: 1) a local role within the ovary to enhance the process of atresia, and 2) a systemic effect to stimulate libido.

Intraovarian androgens accelerate granulosa cell death and follicular atresia. The specific mechanism for this action is unclear, although it is attractive to suspect an interference with estrogen and the autocrine/paracrine factors in enhancing FSH activity. Therefore, androgens may play a regulatory role in ensuring that only a dominant follicle reaches the point of ovulation.

It is well known that libido can be stimulated by androgens. If the midcycle rise in androgens affects libido, then an increase in sexual activity should coincide with this rise. Early studies failed to demonstrate a consistent pattern in coital frequency in women because of the effect of male partner initiation. If only sexual behavior initiated by women is studied, a peak in female-initiated sexual activity is seen during the ovulatory phase of the cycle.[165] The coital frequency of married couples has also been noted to increase at the time of ovulation.[166] Therefore, the midcycle rise in androgens may serve to increase sexual activity at the time most likely to achieve pregnancy.

Summary of Events in the Preovulatory Follicle

1. Estrogen production becomes sufficient to achieve and maintain peripheral threshold concentrations of estradiol that are required in order to induce the LH surge.

2. Acting through its receptors, LH initiates luteinization and progesterone production in the granulosa layer.

3. The preovulatory rise in progesterone facilitates the positive feedback action of estrogen and may be required to induce the midcycle FSH peak.

4. A midcycle increase in local and peripheral androgens occurs, derived from the thecal tissue of lesser, unsuccessful follicles.

Ovulation

The preovulatory follicle, through the elaboration of estradiol, provides its own ovulatory stimulus. Considerable variation in timing exists from cycle to cycle, even in the same woman. A reasonable and accurate estimate places ovulation approximately 10–12 hours after the LH peak and 24–36 hours after peak estradiol levels are attained.[154, 167] The onset of the LH surge appears to be the most reliable indicator of impending ovulation, occurring 34–36 hours prior to follicle rupture.[168] A threshold of LH concentration must be maintained for 14–27 hours in order for full maturation of the oocyte to occur.[169] Usually the LH surge lasts 48–50 hours.[168]

Because of the careful timing involved in in vitro fertilization programs, we have available some interesting data.[170] The LH surge tends to occur at approximately 3 A.M., beginning between

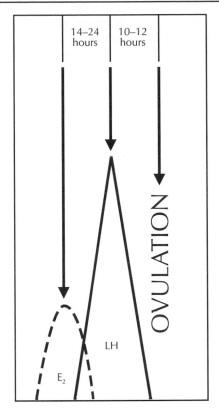

midnight and 8:00 A.M. in over two-thirds of women.[64] Ovulation occurs primarily in the morning during Spring, and primarily in the evening during Autumn and Winter. From July to February in the Northern Hemisphere, about 90% of women ovulate between 4 and 7 P.M.; during Spring, 50% of women ovulate between midnight and 11 A.M.

The gonadotropin surge stimulates a large collection of events that ultimately leads to ovulation, the physical release of the oocyte and its cumulus mass of granulosa cells.[171] This is not an explosive event; therefore, a complex series of changes must occur which cause the final maturation of the oocyte and the decomposition of the collagenous layer of the follicular wall.[172]

The LH surge initiates the continuation of meiosis in the oocyte (meiosis is not completed until after the sperm has entered and the second polar body is released), luteinization of granulosa cells, expansion of the cumulus, and the synthesis of prostaglandins and other eicosanoids essential for follicle rupture. Premature oocyte maturation and luteinization are prevented by local factors. LH-induced cyclic AMP activity overcomes the local inhibitory action of oocyte maturation inhibitor (OMI) and luteinization inhibitor (LI). LI may be endothelin-1, a product of vascular endothelial cells.[139] OMI originates from the granulosa cells, and its activity depends upon an intact cumulus oophorous. Activin also suppresses progesterone production by luteal cells, providing yet another means of preventing premature luteinization.[173, 174]

There is abundant evidence that the oocyte exerts control over granulosa functions.[31] The cumulus oophorus differs from other granulosa cells, lacking in LH receptors and progesterone production; FSH-induced LH receptor expression is suppressed in the contiguous granulosa cells by the oocyte. The oocyte enables cumulus cells to respond to the gonadotropin-induced physical and biochemical changes just before ovulation. The local factors that prevent premature oocyte maturation and luteinization are probably under control of the oocyte.

With the LH surge, levels of progesterone in the follicle continue to rise up to the time of ovulation. The progressive rise in progesterone may act to terminate the LH surge as a negative feedback effect is exerted at higher concentrations. In addition to its central effects, progesterone increases the distensibility of the follicle wall. A change in the elastic properties of the follicular wall is necessary to explain the rapid increase in follicular fluid volume, which occurs just prior to ovulation, unaccompanied by any significant change in intrafollicular pressure. The escape of the ovum is associated with degenerative changes of the collagen in the follicular wall so that just prior to ovulation the follicular wall becomes thin and stretched. FSH, LH, and progesterone stimulate the activity of proteolytic enzymes, resulting in digestion of collagen in the follicular wall and increasing its distensibility. The gonadotropin surge also releases histamine, and histamine alone can induce ovulation in some experimental models.

The proteolytic enzymes are activated in an orderly sequence.[175] The granulosa and theca cells produce plasminogen activator in response to the gonadotropin surge. Plasminogen is activated by either of two plasminogen activators: tissue-type plasminogen activator and urokinase-type plasminogen activator. These activators are encoded by separate genes and are also regulated by inhibitors.

Plasminogen activators produced by granulosa cells activate plasminogen in the follicular fluid to produce plasmin. Plasmin, in turn, generates active collagenase to disrupt the follicular wall. In rat models, plasminogen activator synthesis is triggered by LH stimulation (as well as growth factors and FSH), while plasminogen inhibitor synthesis is decreased.[176] Thus, before and after ovulation, the inhibitor activity is high, while just at ovulation, activator activity is high and the inhibitors are at a nadir. The molecular regulation of these factors is necessary for the coordination that leads to ovulation. Plasminogen activator synthesis in granulosa cells is expressed only at the right preovulatory stage in response to LH. The inhibitor system, which is very active in the thecal and interstitial cells, prevents inappropriate activation of plasminogen and disruption of growing follicles. The inhibitor system has been demonstrated to be present in human granulosa cells and preovulatory follicular fluid and to be responsive to paracrine substances, epidermal growth factor and interleukin-1β.[177–179] Movement of the follicle destined to ovulate to the surface of the ovary is important in that the exposed surface of the follicle is now prone to rupture because it is separated from cells rich in the plasminogen inhibitor system. Ovulation is the result of proteolytic digestion of the follicular apex, a site called the stigma.

In the rat, the gene that encodes for plasminogen activator contains a promoter region which has several sequences for known transcription factors, such as the cyclic AMP-responsive element (CRE). The activation of this CRE (which involves the CRE binding protein) requires FSH stimulation. Thus, both gonadotropins appear to be involved in this process.

Prostaglandins of the E and F series and other eicosanoids (especially HETEs, hydroxy-eicosatetraenoic acid methyl esters) increase markedly in the preovulatory follicular fluid, reaching a peak concentration at ovulation.[180, 181] Prostaglandin synthesis is stimulated by interleukin-1β, implicating this cytokine in ovulation.[182] Inhibition of the synthesis of these products from arachidonic acid blocks follicle rupture without affecting the other LH-induced processes of luteinization and oocyte maturation.[183, 184] Prostaglandins may act to free proteolytic enzymes within the follicular wall, and the HETEs may promote angiogenesis and hyperemia (an inflammatory-like response).[181, 185] Prostaglandins may also contract smooth muscle cells that have been identified in the ovary, thereby aiding the extrusion of the oocyte-cumulus cell mass. ***This role of prostaglandins is so well demonstrated that infertility patients should be advised to avoid the use of drugs that inhibit prostaglandin synthesis.[186, 187]***

A large number of leukocytes enter the follicle prior to ovulation. Neutrophils are a prominent feature in the theca compartment of both healthy and atretic antral follicles.[188] The accumulation of leukocytes is mediated by chemotactic mechanisms of the interleukin system.[189] These immune cells probably contribute to the cellular changes associated with ovulation, corpus luteum function, and apoptosis.

Estradiol levels plunge as LH reaches its peak. This may be a consequence of LH down-regulation of its own receptors on the follicle. Thecal tissue derived from healthy antral follicles exhibits marked suppression of steroidogenesis when exposed to high levels of LH whereas exposure over

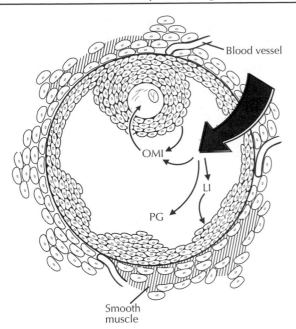

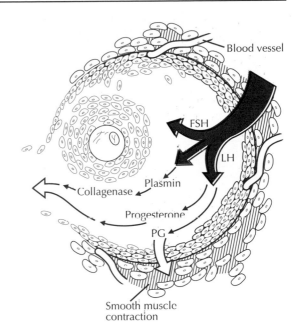

a low range stimulates steroid production. The low midcycle levels of progesterone exert an inhibitory action on further granulosa cell multiplication, and the drop in estrogen may also reflect this local follicular role for progesterone. Finally, estrogen can exert an inhibitory effect on P450c17, a direct action on the gene that is not receptor-mediated.

The granulosa cells that are attached to the basement membrane and enclose the follicle become luteal cells. The cumulus granulosa cells attach to the oocyte. In the mouse, the cumulus cells are metabolically linked to the oocyte and respond to the FSH surge by secreting hyaluronic acid that disperses the cumulus cells prior to ovulation. This hyaluronic acid response depends upon maintenance of the link with the oocyte, indicating the secretion of a supporting factor. The oocyte further secretes factors that promote granulosa cell proliferation and maintain the structural organization of the follicle.[190] Proliferation of the cumulus cells is suppressed by FSH, while FSH stimulates mural granulosa cell proliferation, supported by the oocyte factor or factors.

The FSH peak, partially and perhaps totally dependent on the preovulatory rise of progesterone, has several functions. Plasminogen activator production is sensitive to FSH as well as LH. Expansion and dispersion of the cumulus cells allows the oocyte-cumulus cell mass to become free-floating in the antral fluid just before follicle rupture. The process involves the deposition of a hyaluronic acid matrix, the synthesis of which is stimulated by FSH. Finally, an adequate FSH peak ensures an adequate complement of LH receptors on the granulosa layer. It should be noted that a shortened or inadequate luteal phase is observed in cycles when FSH levels are low or selectively suppressed at any point during the follicular phase.

The mechanism that shuts off the LH surge is unknown. Within hours after the rise in LH, there is a precipitous drop in the plasma estrogens. The decrease in LH may be due to a loss of the positive stimulating action of estradiol or to an increasing negative feedback of progesterone. The abrupt fall in LH levels may also reflect a depletion in pituitary LH content due to down-regulation of GnRH receptors, either by alterations in GnRH pulse frequency or by changes in steroid levels.[191, 192] LH may further be controlled by "short" negative feedback of LH upon the hypothalamus. Direct LH suppression of hypothalamic-releasing hormone production has been demonstrated. However, in the sheep, the LH surge ends before the GnRH signal begins to decline.[193] Another possibility has been suggested, a so-called gonadotropin surge-inhibiting factor (GnSIF) originating in the ovary.[194, 195] GnSIF is produced in granulosa cells under the control of FSH and reaches a peak level in the circulation in the midfollicular phase. Its major role is believed to be prevention of premature luteinization. It is likely that a combination of all of these influences cause the rapid decline in gonadotropin secretion.

The many contributions of progesterone to ovulation are highlighted by the results of experiments in the monkey. Suppression of steroidogenesis at midcycle prevented ovulation, but not resumption of oocyte meiosis.[163] The administration of a progestin agonist to this experimental model restored ovulation.

An adequate gonadotropin surge does not ensure ovulation. The follicle must be at the appropriate stage of maturity in order for it to respond to the ovulating stimulus. In the normal cycle, gonadotropin release and final maturation of the follicle coincide because the timing of the gonadotropin surge is controlled by the level of estradiol, which in turn is a function of follicular growth and maturation. Therefore, gonadotropin release and morphological maturity are usually coordinated and coupled in time. In the majority of human cycles, the requisite feedback relationships in this system allow only one follicle to reach the point of ovulation. Nonidentical multiple births may, in part, reflect the random statistical chance of more than one follicle fulfilling all the requirements for ovulation.

Summary of the Ovulatory Events

1. The LH surge stimulates continuation of reduction division in the oocyte, luteinization of the granulosa, and synthesis of progesterone and prostaglandins within the follicle.

2. Progesterone enhances the activity of proteolytic enzymes responsible, together with prostaglandins, for digestion and rupture of the follicular wall.

3. The progesterone-influenced midcycle rise in FSH serves to free the oocyte from follicular attachments, to convert plasminogen to the proteolytic enzyme, plasmin, and to ensure that sufficient LH receptors are present to allow an adequate normal luteal phase.

Luteal Phase

Before rupture of the follicle and release of the ovum, the granulosa cells begin to increase in size and assume a characteristic vacuolated appearance associated with the accumulation of a yellow pigment, lutein, which lends its name to the process of luteinization and the anatomical subunit, the corpus luteum. During the first 3 days after ovulation, the granulosa cells continue to enlarge. In addition, theca lutein cells may differentiate from the surrounding theca and stroma to become part of the corpus luteum. Dissolution of the basal lamina and rapid vascularization and luteinization make it difficult to distinguish the origin of specific cells.

Capillaries begin to penetrate into the granulosa layer after the cessation of the LH surge, reach the central cavity, and often fill it with blood.[196] Angiogenesis is an important feature of the luteinization process, a response to LH mediated by growth factors produced in luteinized granulosa cells, such as vascular endothelial growth factor (VEGF).[129, 130] By day 8 or 9 after ovulation, a peak of vascularization is reached, associated with peak levels of progesterone and estradiol in the blood. The corpus luteum has one of the highest blood flows per unit mass in the body. On occasion, this ingrowth of vessels and bleeding will result in unchecked hemorrhage and an acute surgical emergency that can present at any time during the luteal phase. Indeed, this is a significant clinical risk in women who are anticoagulated; such women should receive medication to prevent ovulation.

Normal luteal function requires optimal preovulatory follicular development. Suppression of FSH during the follicular phase is associated with lower preovulatory estradiol levels, depressed

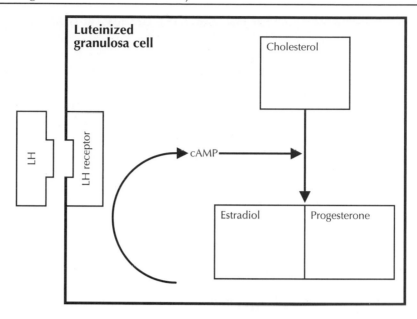

midluteal progesterone production, and a decrease in luteal cell mass.[197] Experimental evidence supports the contention that the accumulation of LH receptors during the follicular phase predetermines the extent of luteinization and the subsequent functional capacity of the corpus luteum. The successful conversion of the avascular granulosa of the follicular phase to the vascularized luteal tissue is also of importance. Because steroid production is dependent upon low-density lipoprotein (LDL) transport of cholesterol, the vascularization of the granulosa layer is essential to allow LDL-cholesterol to reach the luteal cells to provide sufficient substrate for progesterone production. One of the important jobs for LH is to regulate LDL receptor binding, internalization, and postreceptor processing; the induction of LDL receptor expression occurs in granulosa cells during the early stages of luteinization in response to the midcycle LH surge.[198, 199] This mechanism supplies cholesterol to the mitochondria for utilization as the basic building block in steroidogenesis.

The lifespan and steroidogenic capacity of the corpus luteum are dependent on continued tonic LH secretion. Studies in hypophysectomized women have demonstrated that normal corpus luteum function requires the continuous presence of small amounts of LH.[200] The dependence of the corpus luteum on LH is further supported by the prompt luteolysis that follows the administration of GnRH agonists or antagonists or withdrawal of GnRH when ovulation has been induced by the administration of pulsatile GnRH.[201, 202] There is no evidence that other luteotropic hormones, such as prolactin, play a role in primates during the menstrual cycle.[203]

The corpus luteum is not homogeneous. Besides the luteal cells, also present are endothelial cells, leukocytes, and fibroblasts. The nonsteroidogenic cells form the bulk (70–85%) of the total cell population. The leukocyte immune cells produce several cytokines, including interleukin-1β and tumor necrosis factor-α.[204] The many different leukocytes in the corpus luteum are also a rich resource for cytolytic enzymes, prostaglandins, and growth factors involved in angiogenesis, steroidogenesis, and luteolysis.

The corpus luteum is one of the best examples of communication and cross talk in biology. For example, endothelial cells contribute vasoactive compounds, and, in turn, steroidogenic cells contribute factors that influence angiogenesis. The harmonious function of this system is in inverse proportion to its complexity.

Endothelial cells constitute about 50% of the cells in a mature corpus luteum.[205] As elsewhere in the body, endothelial cells participate in immune reactions and endocrine functions. The endothelial cells are a source of endothelin-1, expressed in response to changes in blood flow, blood pressure, and oxygen tension. Studies have now indicated that endothelin-1 may be a mediator of luteolysis.[206, 207]

Even the luteal cell population is not homogeneous, being composed of at least two distinct cell types, large and small cells.[208] Some believe that the large cells are derived from granulosa cells and the small cells from thecal cells. The small cells are the most abundant. Despite the fact that greater steroidogenesis takes place in the large cells, it is the small cells that contain LH and HCG receptors.[209, 210] The absence of LH/HCG receptors on the large cells, presumably derived from granulosa cells that acquire LH receptors in the late follicular phase, requires explanation. Perhaps large cells are functioning at a maximal level with receptors totally occupied and functional, or because of intercellular communication through gap junctions, the large cells do not require direct gonadotropin support. Thus, the large cells can be functioning at a high level, under the control of regulating factors that originate in the small cells in response to gonadotropins. In addition, the overall function is influenced by autocrine/paracrine signals from endothelial and immune cells.

Large luteal cells produce peptides (oxytocin, relaxin, inhibin, and other growth factors) and are more active in steroidogenesis, with greater aromatase activity and more progesterone synthesis than small cells.[211] Human granulosa cells (already luteinizing when recovered from in vitro fertilization patients) contain minimal amounts of P450c17 mRNA. This is consistent with the two-cell explanation, which assigns androgen production (and P450c17) to the cells derived from thecal cells. With luteinization, expression of P450scc and 3β-hydroxysteroid dehydrogenase markedly increases as expected, to account for the increasing production of progesterone, and the continued expression of mRNAs for these enzymes requires LH.[212] The aromatase system (P450arom), of course, continues to be active in luteinized granulosa cells.

Progesterone levels normally rise sharply after ovulation, reaching a peak approximately 8 days after the LH surge. Progesterone acts both locally and centrally to suppress new follicular growth. If progesterone concentrations are monitored in ovarian venous effluents following luteectomy in the monkey, ovulation in the subsequent cycle uniformly occurs on the side opposite the higher progesterone level and contralateral to the previous corpus luteum.[213] If circulating progesterone levels are maintained after luteectomy, the subsequent ovulation again occurs in the ovary having a lower progesterone concentration in its venous effluent.[214] Under normal circumstances (i.e., regular, 28-day cycles), a woman may ovulate from alternate sides.[51, 215] However, short-term ultrasonographic studies have failed to substantiate this pattern.

Initiation of new follicular growth during the luteal phase is further inhibited by the low levels of gonadotropins due to the negative feedback actions of estrogen, progesterone, and inhibin A. With the appearance of LH receptors on the granulosa cells of the dominant follicle and the subsequent development of the follicle into a corpus luteum, inhibin expression comes under the control of LH, and expression changes from inhibin B to inhibin A.[87, 209, 216] The circulating levels of inhibin A rise in the late follicular phase to reach a peak level at the midluteal phase.[16, 88] Inhibin A, therefore, contributes to the suppression of FSH to nadir levels during the luteal phase, and to the changes at the luteal-follicular transition.

The secretion of progesterone and estradiol during the luteal phase is episodic, and the changes correlate closely with LH pulses.[65, 217] Because of this episodic secretion, relatively low midluteal progesterone levels, which some believe are indicative of an inadequate luteal phase, can be found in the course of totally normal luteal phases.

In the normal cycle the time period from the LH midcycle surge to menses is consistently close to 14 days. For practical purposes, luteal phases lasting between 11 and 17 days can be considered normal.[218] The incidence of short luteal phases is about 5–6%. It is well known that significant variability in cycle length among women is due to the varying number of days required for

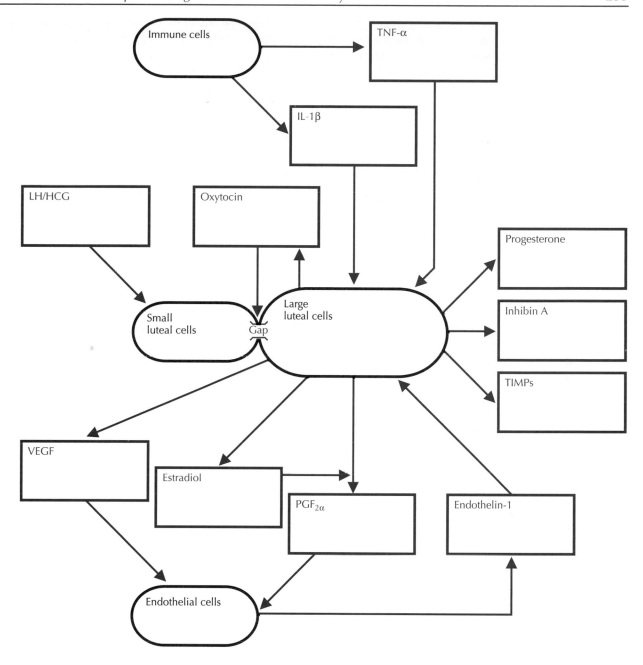

follicular growth and maturation in the follicular phase. The luteal phase cannot be extended indefinitely even with progressively increasing LH exposure, indicating that the demise of the corpus luteum is due to an active luteolytic mechanism.

The corpus luteum rapidly declines 9–11 days after ovulation, and the mechanism of the degeneration remains unknown. In certain nonprimate mammalian species, a luteolytic factor originating in the uterus (prostaglandin $F_{2\alpha}$) regulates the lifespan of the corpus luteum. No definite luteolytic factor has been identified in the primate menstrual cycle, and removal of the uterus in the primate does not affect the ovarian cycle; however, the morphological regression of luteal cells may be induced by the estradiol produced by the corpus luteum. There is evidence to support a role for estrogen in the decline of the corpus luteum.[219] The premature elevation of circulating estradiol levels in the early luteal phase results in a prompt fall in progesterone concentrations. Direct injections of estradiol into the ovary bearing the corpus luteum induce luteolysis while similar treatment of the contralateral ovary produces no effect.[220]

There is another possible role for the estrogen produced by the corpus luteum. In view of the known estrogen requirement for the synthesis of progesterone receptors in endometrium, luteal phase estrogen may be necessary to allow the progesterone-induced changes in the endometrium after ovulation. Inadequate progesterone receptor content due to inadequate estrogen priming of the endometrium is an additional possible mechanism for infertility or early miscarriage, another form of luteal phase deficiency.

Auletta postulated that prostaglandin $F_{2\alpha}$ produced within the ovary bearing the corpus luteum or within the corpus luteum serves as the luteolytic agent, and the production of the prostaglandin is initiated by the luteal estrogen.[220] Experiments using inhibitors of prostaglandin synthesis have not been helpful because luteal tissue also produces members of the prostaglandin family that have stimulating effects (such as PGE and prostacyclin).[221]

Experimental evidence indicates that the luteolytic effect of prostaglandin $F_{2\alpha}$ is mediated by endothelin-1.[206, 207] Prostaglandin $F_{2\alpha}$ stimulates the synthesis of endothelin, and endothelin-1 inhibits luteal steroidogenesis. In addition, endothelin-1 stimulates the release of tumor necrosis factor-α, a growth factor known to induce apoptosis.[222]

A newly appreciated characteristic of the corpus luteum has emerged, the importance of cellular interactions that require cell-to-cell contact. Gap junctions are a prominent feature of luteal cells, just as they are in the follicle before ovulation. When the various cell types of the corpus luteum are studied together, the performance is different compared with studies of single cell types, greater steroidogenesis more closely approximating the total function of the corpus luteum.[223] It is believed that communication and exchange of signals takes place through the gap junction structures, explaining how the small cells respond to LH and HCG, but the large cells are the main site of steroidogenesis. Regulation of the gap junction system is influenced by oxytocin, a paracrine role for oxytocin in the corpus luteum.[224]

When ovulation is induced by the administration of GnRH, normal luteal phase demise occurs despite no change in treatment, arguing against a change in LH as the luteolytic mechanism. In addition, LH receptor binding affinity does not change throughout the luteal phase; thus the decline in steroidogenesis must reflect deactivation of the system (producing a refractoriness of the corpus luteum to LH), perhaps through the uncoupling of the G protein adenylate cyclase system. This is supported by studies in the monkey in which alteration in LH pulse frequency or amplitude did not provoke luteolysis.[225]

The process of luteolysis involves proteolytic enzymes, especially the matrix metalloproteinases (MMPs). These enzymes are held under inhibitory control by tissue inhibitors of metalloproteinases (TIMPs) secreted by the steroidogenic luteal cells, and because TIMP levels do not change in luteal tissue, luteolysis is believed to involve a direct increase in MMP expression. An important part of the rescue mission for human chorionic gonadotropin (HCG) is to prevent this increase in MMP expression.[226] Others have indicated that HCG can increase TIMP production, and this, too, would inhibit MMP activity and luteolysis.[227] In addition, the human ovary contains the complete interleukin-1 system, providing another resource for cytolytic enzymes.

The survival of the corpus luteum is prolonged by the emergence of a new stimulus of rapidly increasing intensity, HCG. This new stimulus first appears at the peak of corpus luteum development (9–13 days after ovulation), just in time to prevent luteal regression.[228] HCG serves to maintain the vital steroidogenesis of the corpus luteum until approximately the 9th or 10th week of gestation, by which time placental steroidogenesis is well established. In some pregnancies placental steroidogenesis will be sufficiently established by the 7th week of gestation.

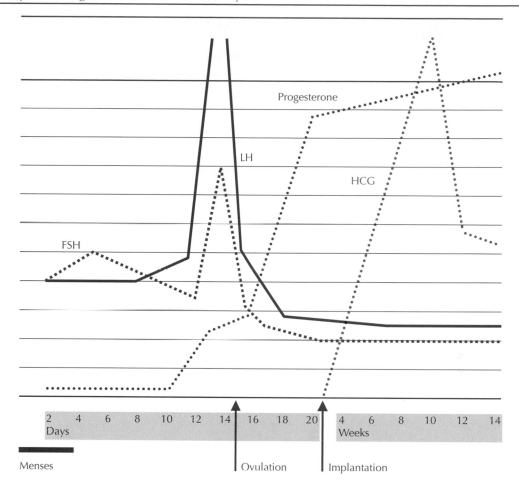

Unlike the biphasic pattern demonstrated by the circulating level of progesterone (a decrease after ovulation and then a new higher peak at the midluteal phase), the mRNA levels for the two major enzymes involved in progesterone synthesis (cholesterol side-chain cleavage and 3β-hydroxy-steroid dehydrogenase) are maximal at ovulation and decline throughout the luteal phase.[229] This suggests that the lifespan of the corpus luteum is established at the time of ovulation, and luteal regression is inevitable unless the corpus luteum is rescued by the HCG of pregnancy. Therefore, primates have developed a system that requires rescue of the corpus luteum in contrast to lower animals that use a mechanism that actively causes the demise of the corpus luteum (luteolysis).

Summary of Events in the Luteal Phase

1. Normal luteal function requires optimal preovulatory follicular development (especially adequate FSH stimulation) and continued tonic LH support.

2. Progesterone acts both centrally and within the ovary to suppress new follicular growth.

3. Regression of the corpus luteum may involve the luteolytic action of its own estrogen production, mediated by an alteration in local prostaglandin and endothelin-1 concentrations.

4. In early pregnancy, HCG rescues the corpus luteum, maintaining luteal function until placental steroidogenesis is well established.

The Luteal-Follicular Transition

The interval extending from the late luteal decline of estradiol and progesterone production to the selection of the dominant follicle is a critical and decisive time, marked by the appearance of menses, but less apparent and very important are the hormone changes that initiate the next cycle. The critical factors include GnRH, FSH, LH, estradiol, progesterone, and inhibin.

Given the important role for FSH-mediated actions on the granulosa cells, it is appropriate that the recruitment of a new ovulating follicle is directed by a selective increase in FSH that begins approximately 2 days before the onset of menses.[230-232] Using a sensitive FSH bioassay, an increase in FSH bioactivity can be measured beginning as early as the midluteal phase.[17] There are at least two influential changes that result in this important increase in FSH: a decrease in luteal steroids and inhibin and a change in GnRH pulsatile secretion.

Inhibin B, originating in the granulosa cells of the corpus luteum and now under the regulation of LH, reaches a nadir in the circulation at the midluteal period. Inhibin A reaches a peak in the luteal phase, and, thus, may help to suppress FSH secretion by the pituitary to the lowest levels reached during a menstrual cycle.[16] The process of luteolysis, whatever the mechanism, with the resulting demise of the corpus luteum, affects inhibin A secretion as well as steroidogenesis. The administration of inhibin A to monkeys effectively suppresses circulating FSH.[233] Thus, an important suppressing influence on FSH secretion is removed from the anterior pituitary during the last days of the luteal phase. The selective action of inhibin on FSH (and not LH) is partly responsible for the greater rise in FSH seen during the luteal-follicular transition, compared to the change in LH. The administration of recombinant (pure) FSH to gonadotropin-deficient women has demonstrated that the early growth of follicles requires FSH, and that LH is not essential during this period of the cycle.[43, 44]

Inhibin B levels begin to rise shortly after the increase in FSH (a consequence of FSH stimulation of granulosa cell secretion of inhibin) and reach peak levels about 4 days after the maximal increase in FSH.[16, 82] Thus, suppression of FSH secretion during the follicular phase is an action exerted by Inhibin B, whereas escape of FSH inhibition during the luteal-follicular transition is partly a response to decreasing inhibin A secretion by the corpus luteum.

Circulating levels of activin increase in the late luteal phase to peak at menses; however, activin A is highly bound in the circulation, and it is not certain it has an endocrine role.[101] Nevertheless, the timing is right for activin to contribute to the rise in FSH during the luteal-follicular transition. Activin enhances and follistatin suppresses GnRH activity. Evidence in vivo and in vitro indicates that gonadotropin response to GnRH requires activin activity.[234]

The selective rise in FSH is also significantly influenced by a change in GnRH pulsatile secretion, previously strongly suppressed by the high estradiol and progesterone levels of the luteal phase.[69] A progressive and rapid increase in GnRH pulses (as assessed by the measurement of LH pulses) occurs during the luteal-follicular transition.[68] From the midluteal peak to menses, there is a 4.5-fold increase in LH pulse frequency (and presumably GnRH) from approximately 3 pulses/24 hours to 14 pulses/24 hours.[68] During this time period, the mean level of LH increases approximately 2-fold, from approximately a mean of 4.8 IU/L to 8 IU/L. The increase in FSH is, as noted, greater than that of LH. FSH pulse frequency increases 3.5-fold from the midluteal period to the time of menses, and FSH levels increase from a mean of approximately 4 IU/L to 15 IU/L.

An increase in GnRH pulse frequency from a low level of secretion has been associated with an initial selective increase in FSH in several experimental models, including the ovariectomized monkey with destruction of the hypothalamus. Treatment of hypogonadal women with pulsatile GnRH results first in predominance of FSH secretion (over LH). This experimental response and the changes during the luteal-follicular transition are similar to that observed during puberty, a predominance of FSH secretion as GnRH pulsatile secretion begins to increase.

The Luteal-Follicular Transition

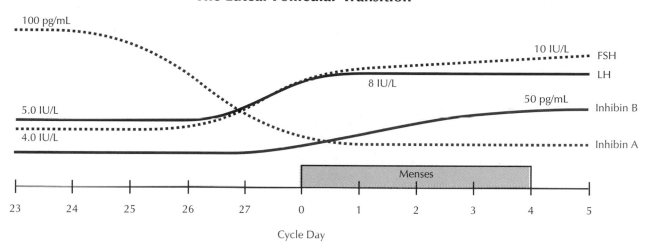

The pituitary response to GnRH is also a factor. Estradiol suppresses FSH secretion by virtue of its classic negative feedback relationship at the pituitary level. The decrease in estradiol in the late luteal phase restores the capability of the pituitary to respond with an increase in FSH secretion.[235]

Summary of Events in the Luteal-Follicular Transition

1. The demise of the corpus luteum results in a nadir in the circulating levels of estradiol, progesterone, and inhibin.

2. The decrease in inhibin A removes a suppressing influence on FSH secretion in the pituitary.

3. The decrease in estradiol and progesterone allows a progressive and rapid increase in the frequency of GnRH pulsatile secretion and a removal of the pituitary from negative feedback suppression.

4. The removal of inhibin A and estradiol and increasing GnRH pulses combine to allow greater secretion of FSH compared with LH, with an increase in the frequency of the episodic secretion.

5. The increase in FSH is instrumental in rescuing a approximately 60-day-old group of ready follicles from atresia, allowing a dominant follicle to begin its emergence.

The Normal Menstrual Cycle

Menstrual cycle length is determined by the rate and quality of follicular growth and development, and it is normal for the cycle to vary in individual women. Our best information comes from two longitudinal studies (with very similar results): the study of Vollman of more than 30,000 cycles recorded by 650 women and the study of Treloar of more that 25,000 woman-years in a little over 2700 women.[236, 237] The observations of Vollman and Treloar documented a normal evolution in length and variation in menstrual cycles.

Menarche is followed by approximately 5–7 years of increasing regularity as cycles shorten to reach the usual reproductive age pattern. In the 40s, cycles begin to lengthen again. The highest incidence of anovulatory cycles is under age 20 and over age 40.[236, 238] At age 25, over 40% of cycles are between 25 and 28 days in length; from 25 to 35, over 60% are between 25 and 28 days. The perfect 28-day cycle is indeed the most common mode, but it totaled only 12.4% of Vollman's

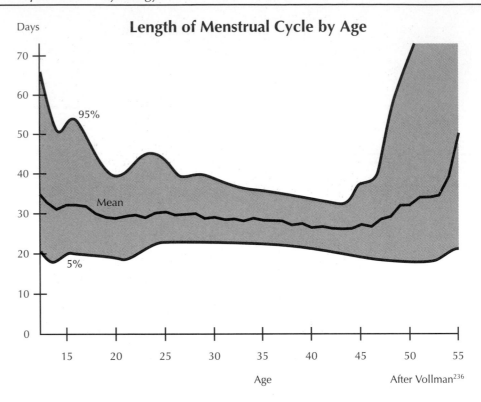

Length of Menstrual Cycle by Age

Days

After Vollman[236]

cycles. Overall, approximately 15% of reproductive age cycles are 28 days in length. Only 0.5% of women experience a cycle less than 21 days long, and only 0.9% a cycle greater than 35 days.[239] Most women have cycles that last from 24 to 35 days, but at least 20% of women experience irregular cycles.

The duration of the follicular phase is the major determinant of cycle length. Sherman and Korenman predicted in 1975 that a factor other than estrogen is the key — inhibin.[240] Cycle lengths are the shortest (with the least variability) in the late 30s, a time when subtle but real increases in FSH and decreases in inhibin are occurring.[86, 218, 241–244] This can be pictured as accelerated follicular growth (because of the changes in FSH and inhibin B). At the same time, fewer follicles grow per cycle as a woman ages.[245] Approximately 2–4 years (6–8 years according to Trelolar) prior to menopause, the cycles lengthen again. In the last 10–15 years before menopause, there is an acceleration of follicular loss.[3] This accelerated loss begins when the total number of follicles reaches approximately 25,000, a number reached in normal women at age 37–38.[246] Eventually menopause occurs because the supply of follicles is depleted.[247]

The changes in the later reproductive years reflect either lesser follicular competence as the better primordial follicles respond early in life, leaving the lesser follicles for later, or the fact that the total follicular pool is reduced in number (or both factors). Arguing in favor of a role for a reduced follicular pool is the observation that follicular fluid obtained from preovulatory follicles of older women contains amounts of inhibin A and B that are similar to that measured in follicular fluid from young women.[248]

References

1. **Baker TG,** A quantitative and cytological study of germ cells in human ovaries, *Proc Roy Soc Lond* 158:417, 1963.

2. **Peters H, Byskov AG, Himelstein-Graw R, Faber M,** Follicular growth: the basic event in the mouse and human ovary, *J Reprod Fertil* 45:559, 1975.

3. **Gougeon A, Echochard R, Thalabard JC,** Age-related changes of the population of human ovarian follicles: increase in the disappearance rate of non-growing and early-growing follicles in aging women, *Biol Reprod* 50:653, 1994.

4. **Mais V, Kazer RR, Cetel NS, Rivier J, Vale W, Yen SSC,** The dependency of folliculogenesis and corpus luteum function on pulsatile gonadotropin secretion in cycling women using a gonadotropin-releasing hormone antagonist as a probe, *J Clin Endocrinol Metab* 62:1250, 1986.

5. **Gougeon A,** Dynamics of follicular growth in the human: a model from preliminary results, *Hum Reprod* 1:81, 1986.

6. **Gougeon A,** Regulation of ovarian follicular development in primates: facts and hypotheses, *Endocr Rev* 17:121, 1996.

7. **Oktay K, Newton H, Mullan J, Gosden RG,** Development of human primordial follicles to antral stages in *SCID/hpg* mice stimulated with follicle stimulating hormone, *Hum Reprod* 13:1133, 1998.

8. **Schipper I, Hop WCJ, Fauser BCJM,** The follicle-stimulating hormone (FSH) threshold/window concept examined by different interventions with exogenous FSH during the follicular phase of the normal menstrual cycle: duration, rather than magnitude, of FSH increase affects follicle development, *J Clin Endocrinol Metab* 83:1292, 1998.

9. **Hsueh AJW, Eisenhauer K, Chun SY, Hsu SY, Billig H,** Gonadal cell apoptosis, *Recent Prog Horm Res* 51:433, 1996.

10. **Dong J, Albertini DF, Nishimori K, Kumar TR, Lu N, Matzuk MM,** Growth differentiation factor-9 is required during early ovarian folliculogenesis, *Nature* 383:531, 1996.

11. **Halpin DMG, Jones A, Fink G, Charlton HM,** Postnatal ovarian follicle development in hypogonadal (hpg) and normal mice and associated changes in the hypothalamic-pituitary axis, *J Reprod Fertil* 77:287, 1986.

12. **Baker TC, Scrimgeour JB,** Development of the gonad in normal and anencephalic human fetuses, *J Reprod Fertil* 60:193, 1980.

13. **Oktay K, Briggs DA, Gosden RG,** Ontogeny of follicle-stimulating hormone receptor gene expression in isolated human ovarian follicles, *J Clin Endocrinol Metab* 82:3748, 1997.

14. **Pache TD, Wladimiroff JW, de Jong FH, Hop WC, Fauser BCJM,** Growth patterns of non dominant ovarian follicles during the normal menstrual cycle, *Fertil Steril* 54:638, 1990.

15. **Vermesh M, Kletzky OA,** Longitudinal evaluation of the luteal phase and its transition into the follicular phase, *J Clin Endocrinol Metab* 65:653, 1987.

16. **Welt CK, Martin KM, Taylor AE, Lambert-Messerlian GM, Crowley Jr WF, Smith JA, Schoenfeld DA, Hall JE,** Frequency modulation of follicle-stimulating hormone (FSH) during the luteal-follicular transition: evidence for FSH control of inhibin B in normal women, *J Clin Endocrinol Metab* 82:2645, 1997.

17. **Christin-Maitre S, Taylor AE, Khoury RH, Hall JE, Martin KA, Smith PC, Albanese C, Jameson JL, Crowley Jr WF, Sluss PM,** Homologous *in vitro* bioassay for follicle-stimulating hormone (FSH) reveals increased FSH biological signal during the mid- to late luteal phase of the human menstrual cycle, *J Clin Endocrinol Metab* 81:2080, 1996.

18. **Van Deerlin PG, Cekleniak N, Coutifaris C, Boyd J, Strauss III JF,** Evidence for the oligoclonal origin of the granulosa cell population of the mature human follicle, *J Clin Endocrinol Metab* 82:3019, 1997.

19. **Yong EL, Baird DT, Hillier SG,** Mediation of gonadotropin-stimulated growth and differentiation of human granulosa cells by adenosine-3',5'-monophosphate: one molecule, two messages, *Clin Endocrinol* 37:51, 1992.

20. **McNatty KP, Makris A, DeGrazia C, Osathanondh R, Ryan KJ,** The production of progesterone, androgens, and estrogens by granulosa cells, thecal tissue, and stromal tissue from human ovaries in vitro, *J Clin Endocrinol Metab* 49:687, 1979.

21. **LaPolt PS, Tilly JL, Aihara T, Nishimori K, Hsueh AJ,** Gonadotropin-induced up- and down-regulation of ovarian follicle-stimulating hormone (FSH) receptor gene expression in immature rats: effects of pregnant mare's serum gonadotropin, human chorionic gonadotropin, and recombinant FSH, *Endocrinology* 130:1289, 1992.

22. **Tilly JL, LaPolt PS, Hsueh AJ,** Hormonal regulation of follicle-stimulating hormone receptor messenger ribonucleic acid levels in cultured rat granulosa cells, *Endocrinology* 130:1296, 1992.

23. **Erickson GF,** An analysis of follicle development and ovum maturation, *Seminars Reprod Endocrinol* 4:233, 1986.

24. **Fletcher WH, Greenan JRT,** Receptor mediated action without receptor occupancy, *Endocrinology* 116:1660, 1985.

25. **Hild-Petito S, West NB, Brenner RM, Stouffer RL,** Localization of androgen receptor in the follicle and corpus luteum of the primate ovary during the menstrual cycle, *Biol Reprod* 44:561, 1991.

26. **McNatty KP, Makris A, Reinhold VN, DeGrazia C, Osathanondh R, Ryan KJ,** Metabolism of androstenedione by human ovarian tissues in vitro with particular reference to reductase and aromatase activity, *Steroids* 34:429, 1979.

27. **Hillier SG, Van Den Boogard AMJ, Reichert LE, Van Hall EV,** Intraovarian sex steroid hormone interactions and the regulation of follicular maturation: aromatization of androgens by human granulosa cells in vitro, *J Clin Endocrinol Metab* 50:640, 1980.

28. **Jia X-C, Kessel B, Welsh Jr TH, Hsueh AJW,** Androgen inhibition of follicle-stimulating hormone-stimulated luteinizing hormone receptor formation in cultured rat granulosa cells, *Endocrinology* 117:13, 1985.

29. **Erickson GF, Magoffin DA, Dyer CA, Hofeditz C,** The ovarian androgen producing cells: a review of structure/function relationships, *Endocr Rev* 6:371, 1985.

30. **Chabab A, Hedon B, Arnal F, Diafouka F, Bressot N, Flandre O, Cristol P,** Follicular steroids in relation to oocyte development and human ovarian stimulation protocols, *Hum Reprod* 1:449, 1986.

31. **Eppig JJ, Chesnel F, Hirao Y, O'Brien MJ, Pendola FL, Watanabe S, Wigglesworth K,** Oocyte control of granulosa cell development: how and why, *Hum Reprod* 12 Natl Suppl, *JBFS* 2:127, 1997.

32. **McNatty KP, Smith DM, Makris A, Osathanondh R, Ryan KJ,** The microenvironment of the human antral follicle; inter-relationships among the steroid levels in antral fluid, the population of granulosa cells, and the status of the oocyte in vivo and in vitro, *J Clin Endocrinol Metab* 49:851, 1979.

33. **McNatty KP, Markris A, DeGraziak C, Osathanondh R, Ryan KJ,** Steroidogenesis by recombined follicular cells from the human ovary in vitro, *J Clin Endocrinol Metab* 51:1286, 1980.

34. **Andersen CY,** Characteristics of human follicular fluid associated with sucessful conception after *in vitro* fertilization, *J Clin Endocrinol Metab* 77:1227, 1993.

35. **McNatty KP, Smith DM, Makris A, DeGrazia C, Tulchinsky D, Osathanondh R, Schiff I, Ryan KJ,** The intraovarian sites of androgen and estrogen formation in women with normal and hyperandrogenic ovaries as judged by in vitro experiments, *J Clin Endocrinol Metab* 50:755, 1980.

36. **Hillier SG,** Paracrine control of follicular estrogen synthesis, *Seminars Reprod Endocrinol* 9:332, 1991.

37. **Kobayashi M, Nakano R, Ooshima A,** Immunohistochemical localization of pituitary gonadotropins and gonadal steroids confirms the two cells two gonadotropins hypothesis of steroidogenesis in the human ovary, *J Endocrinol* 126:483, 1990.

38. **Yamoto M, Shima K, Nakano R,** Gonadotropin receptors in human ovarian follicles and corpora lutea throughout the menstrual cycle, *Hor Res* 37(Suppl 1):5, 1992.

39. **Magoffin DA,** Regulation of differentiated functions in ovarian theca cells, *Seminars Reprod Endocrinol* 9:321, 1991.

40. **Azhar S, Tsai L, Medicherla S, Chandrasekher Y, Giudice L, Reaven E,** Human granulosa cells use high density lipoprotein cholesterol for steroidogenesis, *J Clin Endocrinol Metab* 83:983, 1998.

41. **Sasano H, Okamoto M, Mason JI, Simpson ER, Mendelson CR, Sasano N, Silverberg SG,** Immunolocalization of aromatase, 17α-hydroxylase and side-chain-cleavage cytochromes P-450 in the human ovary, *J Reprod Fertil* 85:163, 1989.

42. **Sasano H,** Functional pathology of human ovarian steroidogenesis: normal cycling ovary and steroid-producing neoplasms, *Endocr Pathol* 5:81, 1994.

43. **Schoot DC, Coelingh-Bennink HJT, Mannaerts BMJL, Lamberts SWJ, Bouchard P, Fauser BCJM,** Human recombinant follicle-stimulating hormone induces growth of preovulatory follicles without concomitant increase in androgen and estrogen biosynthesis in a woman with isolated gonadotropin deficiency, *J Clin Endocrinol Metab* 74:1471, 1992.

44. **Shoham Z, Mannaerts B, Insler V, Coelingh-Bennink H,** Induction of follicular growth using recombinant human follicle-stimulating hormone in two volunteer women with hypogonadotropic hypogonadism, *Fertil Steril* 59:738, 1993.

45. **Ben-Chetrit A, Gotlieb L, Wong PY, Casper RF,** Ovarian response to recombinant human follicle-stimulating hormone in luteinizing hormone-depleted women: examination of the two cell, two gonadotropin theory, *Fertil Steril* 65:711, 1996.

46. **Karnitis VJ, Townson DH, Friedman CI, Danforth DR,** Recombinant human follicle-stimulating hormone stimulates multiple follicular growth, but minimal estrogen production in gonadotropin-releasing hormone antagonist-treated monkeys: examining the role of luteinizing hormone in follicular development and steroidogenesis, *J Clin Endocrinol Metab* 79:91, 1994.

47. **Zelinski-Wooten MB, Hutchison JS, Hess DL, Wolf DP, Stouffer RL,** Follicle stimulating hormone alone supports follicle growth and oocyte development in gonadotropin-releasing hormone antagonist-treated monkeys, *Hum Reprod* 10:1658, 1995.

48. **Goodman AL, Hodgen GD,** The ovarian triad of the primate menstrual cycle, *Recent Prog Hor Res* 39:1, 1983.

49. **Tilly JL, Kowalski KI, Schomberg DW, Hsueh AJ,** Apoptosis in atretic ovarian follicles is associated with selected decreases in messenger ribonucleic acid transcripts for gonadotropin receptors and cytochrome P450 aromatase, *Endocrinology* 131:1670, 1992.

50. **Montgomery Rice V, Limback SD, Roby KF, Terranova PF,** Differential responses of granulosa cells from small and large follicles to follicle stimulating hormone (FSH) during the menstrual cycle and acyclicity: effects of tumour necrosis factor-α, *Hum Reprod* 13:1285, 1998.

51. **Chikasawa K, Araki S, Tameda T,** Morphological and endocrinological studies on follicular development during the human menstrual cycle, *J Clin Endocrinol Metab* 62:305, 1986.

52. **Clark JR, Dierschke DJ, Wolf RC,** Hormonal regulation of ovarian folliculogenesis in rhesus monkeys. III. Atresia of the preovulatory follicle induced by exogenous steroids and subsequent follicular development, *Biol Reprod* 25:3320, 1981.

53. **Zeleznik AJ, Schuler HM, Reichert LE,** Gonadotropin-binding sites in the rhesus monkey ovary: role of the vasculature in the selective distribution of human chorionic gonadotropin to the preovulatory follicle, *Endocrinology* 109:356, 1981.

54. **Ravindranath N, Little-Ihrig L, Phillips HS, Ferrara N, Zeleznik AJ,** Vascular endothelial growth factor messenger ribonucleic acid expression in the primate ovary, *Endocrinology* 131:254, 1992.

55. **Suzuki T, Sasano H, Takaya R, Fukaya T, Yajima A, Nagura H,** Cyclic changes of vasculature and vascular phenotypes in normal human ovaries, *Hum Reprod* 13:953, 1998.

56. **Richards JS, Jahnsen T, Hedin L, Lifka J, Ratoosh SL, Durica JM, Goldring NB,** Ovarian follicular development: from physiology to molecular biology, *Recent Prog Horm Res* 43:231, 1987.

57. **Jia X-C, Hsueh AJW,** Homologous regulation of hormone receptors: luteinizing hormone increases its own receptors in cultured rat granulosa cells, *Endocrinology* 115:2433, 1984.

58. **Kessel B, Liu YX, Jia X-C, Hsueh AJW,** Autocrine role of estrogens in the augmentation of luteinizing hormone receptor formation in cultured rat granulosa cells, *Biol Reprod* 32:1038, 1985.

59. **Knecht M, Brodie AMH, Catt KJ,** Aromatase inhibitors prevent granulosa cell differentiation: an obligatory role for estrogens in luteinizing hormone receptor expression, *Endocrinology* 117:1156, 1985.

60. **Xia L, Van Vugt D, Alston EJ, Luckhaus J, Ferin M,** A surge of gonadotropin-releasing hormone accompanies the estradiol-induced gonadotropin surge in the Rhesus monkey, *Endocrinology* 131:2812, 1992.

61. **Chappel SC, Resko JA, Norman RL, Spies HG,** Studies on rhesus monkeys on the site where estrogen inhibits gonadotropins: delivery of 17β-estradiol to the hypothalamus and pituitary gland, *J Clin Endocrinol Metab* 52:1, 1981.

62. **Wildt L, Hutchison JS, Marshall G, Pohl CR, Knobil E,** On the site of action of progesterone in the blockade of the estradiol-induced gonadotropin discharge in the rhesus monkey, *Endocrinology* 109:1293, 1981.

63. **Young JR, Jaffe RB,** Strength-duration characteristics of estrogen effects on gonadotropin response to gonadotropin-releasing hormone in women. II. Effects of varying concentrations of estradiol, *J Clin Endocrinol Metab* 42:432, 1976.

64. **Cahill DJ, Wardle PG, Harlow CR, Hull MGR,** Onset of the preovulatory luteinizing hormone surge: diurnal timing and critical follicular prerequisites, *Fertil Steril* 70:56, 1998.

65. **Filicori M, Santoro N, Merriam GR, Crowley Jr WF,** Characterization of the physiological pattern of episodic gonadotropin secretion throughout the human menstrual cycle, *J Clin Endocrinol Metab* 62:1136, 1986.

66. **Rossmanith WG, Laughlin GA, Mortola JF, Johnson ML, Veldhuis JD, Yen SSC,** Pulsatile cosecretion of estradiol and progesterone by the midluteal phase corpus luteum: temporal link to luteinizing hormone pulses, *J Clin Endocrinol Metab* 70:990, 1990.

67. **Evans WS, Sollenberger MJ, Booth Jr RA, Rogol AD, Urban RJ, Carlsen EC, Johnson ML, Veldhuis JD,** Contemporary aspects of discrete peak-detection algorithms. II. The paradigm of the luteinizing hormone pulse signal in women, *Endocr Rev* 13:81, 1992.

68. **Hall JE, Schoenfeld DA, Martin KA, Crowley Jr WF,** Hypothalamic gonadotropin-releasing hormone secretion and follicle-stimulating hormone dynamics during the luteal-follicular transition, *J Clin Endocrinol Metab* 74:600, 1992.

69. **Nippold TB, Reame NE, Kelch RP, Marshall JC,** The roles of estradiol and progesterone in decreasing luteinizing hormone pulse frequency in the luteal phase of the menstrual cycle, *J Clin Endocrinol Metab* 69:67, 1989.

70. **Marunicic M, Casper RF,** The effect of luteal phase estrogen antagonism on luteinizing hormone pulsatility and luteal function in women, *J Clin Endocrinol Metab* 64:148, 1987.

71. **Laatikainen T, Raisanen I, Tulenheimo A, Salminen K,** Plasma β-endorphin and the menstrual cycle, *Fertil Steril* 44:206, 1985.

72. **Wehrenberg WB, Wardlaw SL, Frantz AG, Ferin M,** β-Endorphin in hypophyseal portal blood: variations throughout the menstrual cycle, *Endocrinology* 111:879, 1982.

73. **Urban RJ, Veldhuis JD, Dufau ML,** Estrogen regulates the gonadotropin-releasing hormone-stimulated secretion of biologically active luteinizing hormone, *J Clin Endocrinol Metab* 72:660, 1991.

74. **Zambrano E, Olivares A, Mendez JP, Guerrero L, Díaz-Cueto L, Veldhuis JD, Ulloa-Aguirre A,** Dynamics of basal and gonadotropin-releasing hormone-releasable serum follicle-stimulating hormone charge isoform distribution throughout the human menstrual cycle, *J Clin Endocrinol Metab* 80:1647, 1995.

75. **Mortola JF, Laughlin GA, Yen SSC,** A circadian rhythm of serum follicle-stimulating hormone in women, *J Clin Endocrinol Metab* 75:861, 1992.

76. **Rivier C, Rivier J, Vale W,** Inhibin-mediated feedback control of follicle-stimulating hormone secretion in the female rat, *Science* 234:205, 1986.

77. **Bicsak TA, Tucker EM, Cappel S, Vaughan J, Rivier J, Vale W, Hsueh AJW,** Hormonal regulation of granulosa cell inhibin biosynthesis, *Endocrinology* 119:2711, 1986.

78. **Xiao S, Robertson DM, Findlay JK,** Effects of activin and follicle-stimulating hormone (FSH)-suppressing protein/ follistatin on FSH receptors and differentiation of cultured rat granulosa cells, *Endocrinology* 131:1009, 1992.

79. **Matzuk MM, Finegold MJ, Su J-GJ, Hsueh AJW, Bradley A,** α-Inhibin is a tumour-suppressor gene with gonadal specificity in mice, *Nature* 360:313, 1992.

80. **McLachlan RI, Robertson DM, Healy DL, Burger HG, De Kretser DM,** Circulating immunoreactive inhibin levels during the normal human menstrual cycle, *J Clin Endocrinol Metab* 65:954, 1987.

81. **Buckler HM, Healy DL, Burger HG,** Purified FSH stimulates inhibin production from the human ovary, *J Endocrinol* 122:279, 1989.

82. **Groome NP, Illingworth PG, O'Brien M, Pai R, Rodger FE, Mather JP, McNeilly AS,** Measusrement of dimeric inhibin B throughout the human menstrual cycle, *J Clin Endocrinol Metab* 81:1401, 1996.

83. **Lockwood GM, Muttukrishna S, Ledger WL,** Inhibins and activins in human ovulation, conception and pregnancy, *Hum Reprod Update* 4:284, 1998.

84. **Klein NA, Illingworth PJ, Groome NP, McNeilly AS, Battaglia DE, Soules MR,** Decreased inhibin B secretion is associated with the monotropic FSH rise in older, ovulatory women: a study of serum and follicular fluid leavels of dimeric inhibin A and B in spontaneous menstrual cycles, *J Clin Endocrinol Metab* 81:2742, 1996.

85. **Lockwood GM, Muttukrishna S, Groome NP, Matthews DR, Ledger WL,** Mid-follicular phase pulses of inhibin B arc absent in polycystic ovarian syndrome and are initiated by successful laparoscopic ovarian diathermy: a possible mechanism regulating emergence of the dominant follicle, *J Clin Endocrinol Metab* 83:1730, 1998.

86. **Hofmann GE, Danforth DR, Seifer DB,** Inhibin-B: the physiologic basis of the clomiphene citrate challenge test for ovarian reserve screening, *Fertil Steril* 69:474, 1998.

87. **McLachlin RI, Cohen NL, Vale WE, Rivier JE, Burger HG, Bremmer WJ, Soules MR,** The importance of luteinizing hormone in the control of inhibin and progesterone secretion by the human corpus luteum, *J Clin Endocrinol Metab* 68:1078, 1989.

88. **Schipper I, de Jong FH, Fauser BCJM,** Lack of correlation between maximum early follicular phase serum follicle stimulating hormone concentrations and menstrual cycle characteristics in women under the age of 35 years, *Hum Reprod* 13:1442, 1998.

89. **Ling N, Ying S, Ueno N, Shimasaki S, Esch F, Hotta M, Guillemin R,** Pituitary FSH is released by a heterodimer of the β-subunits from the two forms of inhibin, *Nature* 321:779, 1986.

90. **Braden TD, Conn PM,** Activin-A stimulates the synthesis of gonadotropin-releasing hormone receptors, *Endocrinology* 130:2101, 1992.

91. **Mason AJ, Hayflick JS, Ling N, Esch F, Ueno N, Ying SY, Guillemin R, Niall H, Seeburg PH,** Complementary DNA sequences of ovarian follicular fluid inhibin show precursor structure and homology with transforming growth factor-β, *Nature* 318:659, 1985.

92. **Hillier SG, Yong EL, Illingworth PJ, Baird DT, Schwall RH, Mason AJ,** Effect of recombinant inhibin on androgen synthesis in cultured human thecal cells, *Mol Cell Endocrinol* 75:R1, 1991.

93. **Hillier SG, Yong EL, Illingworth PJ, Baird DT, Schwall RH, Mason AJ,** Effect of recombinant activin on androgen synthesis in cultured human thecal cells, *J Clin Endocrinol Metab* 72:1206, 1991.

94. **Sawetawan C, Carr BR, McGee E, Bird IM, Hong TL, Rainey WE,** Inhibin and activin differentially regulate androgen production and 17α-hydroxylasc expression in human ovarian thecal-like cells, *J Endocrinol* 148:213, 1996.

95. **Attisano L, Wrana JL, Cheifetz S, Massague J,** Novel activin receptors: distinct genes and alternative mRNA splicing generate a repertoire of serine/threonine kinase receptors, *Cell* 68:97, 1992.

96. **Alak BM, Smith GD, Woodruff TK, Stouffer RL, Wolf DP,** Enhancement of primate oocyte maturation and fertilization in vitro by inhibin A and activin A, *Fertil Steril* 66:646, 1996.

97. **Kaiser UB, Lee BL, Carroll RS, Unabia G, Chin WW, Childs GV,** Follistatin gene expression in the pituitary: localization in gonadotrophs and folliculostellate cells in diestrous rats, *Endocrinology* 130:3048, 1992.

98. **Kogawa K, Nakamura T, Sugiono K, Takio K, Titani K, Sugino H,** Activin-binding protein is present in pituitary, *Endocrinology* 128:1434, 1991.

99. **Besecke LM, Guendner MJ, Sluss PA, Polak AG, Woodruff TK, Jameson JL, Bauer-Dantoin AC, Weiss J,** Pituitary follistatin regulates activin-mediated production of follicle-stimulating hormone during the rat estrous cycle, *Endocrinology* 138:2841, 1997.

100. **Robertson DM,** Follistatin/activin-binding protein, *Trends Endocrinol Metab* 3:65, 1992.

101. **Muttukrishna S, Fowler PA, George L, Groome NP, Knight PG,** Changes in peripheral serum levels of total activin A during the human menstrual cycle and pregnancy, *J Clin Endocrinol Metab* 81:3328, 1996.

102. **Giudice LC,** Insulin-like growth factors and ovarian follicular development, *Endocr Rev* 13:641, 1992.

103. **Shimasaki S, Ling N,** Identification and molecular characterization of insulin-like growth factor binding proteins (IGFBP-1, -2, -3, -4, -5, and -6), *Prog Growth Factor Res* 3:243, 1992.

104. **El-Roeiy A, Chen X, Roberts VJ, LeRoith D, Roberts Jr CT, Yen SSC,** Expression of insulin-like growth factor-I (IGF-I) and IGF-II and the IGF-I, IGF-II, and insulin receptor genes and localization of the gene products in the human ovary, *J Clin Endocrinol Metab* 77:1411, 1993.

105. **Voutilainen R, Franks S, Mason HD, Martikainen H,** Expression of insulin-like growth factor (IGF), IGF-binding protein, and IGF receptor messenger ribonucleic acids in normal and polycystic ovaries, *J Clin Endocrinol Metab* 81:1003, 1996.

106. **Hernandez ER, Hurwitz A, Vera A, Pellicer A, Adashi EY, LeRoith D, Roberts Jr CT,** Expression of the genes encoding the insulin-like growth factors and their receptors in the human ovary, *J Clin Endocrinol Metab* 74:419, 1992.

107. **Mason HD, Cwyfan-Hughes SC, Heinrich G, Franks S, Holly JMP,** Insulin-like growth factor (IGF) I and II, IGF-binding proteins, and IGF-binding protein proteases are produced by theca and stroma of normal and polycystic human ovaries, *J Clin Endocrinol Metab* 81:276, 1996.

108. **Bergh C, Carlsson B, Olsson J-H, Selleskog U, Hillensjo T,** Regulation of androgen production in cultured human thecal cells by insulin-like growth factor I and insulin, *Fertil Steril* 59:323, 1993.

109. **Nahum R, Thong KJ, Hillier SG,** Metabolic regulation of androgen production by human thecal cells in vitro, *Hum Reprod* 10:75, 1995.

110. **Mason HD, Willis DS, Holly JMP, Franks S,** Insulin preincubation enhances insulin-like growth factor-II (IGF-II) action on steroidogenesis in human granulosa cells, *J Clin Endocrinol Metab* 78:1265, 1994.

111. **DiBlasio AM, Viganó P, Ferrari A,** Insulin-like growth factor-II stimulates human granulosa-luteal cell proliferation *in vitro*, *Fertil Steril* 61:483, 1994.

112. **Barreca A, Artini PG, Del Monte P, Ponzani P, Pasquini P, Cariola G, Volpe A, Genazzani AR, Giordano G, Minuto F,** In vivo and in vitro effect of growth hormone on estradiol secretion by human granulosa cells, *J Clin Endocrinol Metab* 77:61, 1993.

113. **Thierry van Dessel HJHM, Chandrasekher YA, Yap OWS, Lee PDK, Hintz RL, Faessen GHJ, Braat DD, Fauser BC, Giudice LC,** Serum and follicular fluid levels of insulin-like growth factor (IGF)-I, IGF-II, and IGF binding proteins-1 and -3 during the normal menstrual cycle, *J Clin Endocrinol Metab* 81:1224, 1995.

114. **Thierry van Dessel HJHM, Chandrasekher Y, Stephanie Yap OW, Lee PDK, Hintz RL, Faessen GHJ, Braat DDM, Fauser BCJM, Giudice LC,** Serum and follicular fluid levels of insulin-like growth factor I (IGF-I), IGF-II, and IGF-binding protein-1 and -3 during the normal menstrual cycle, *J Clin Endocrinol Metab* 81:1224, 1996.

115. **Ricciarelli E, Hernandez ER, Tedeschi C, Botero LF, Kokia E, Rohan RM, Rosenfeld RG, Albiston AL, Herington AC, Adashi EY,** Rat ovarian insulin-like growth factor binding protein-3: a growth hormone-dependent theca-interstitial cell-derived antigonadotropin, *Endocrinology* 130:3092, 1992.

116. **Adashi EY, Resnick CE, Hurwitz A, Riciarelli E, Hernandez ER, Rosenfeld RG,** Ovarian granulosa cell-derived insulin-like growth factor binding proteins: modulatory role of follicle-stimulating hormone, *Endocrinology* 128:754, 1991.

117. **Grimes RW, Samaras SE, Barber JA, Shimasaki S, Ling N, Hammond JM,** Gonadotropin and cyclic-AMP modulation of insulin-like growth factor-binding protein production in ovarian granulosa cells, *Am J Physiol* 262:E497, 1992.

118. **Dor J, Costritsci N, Pariente C, Rabinovici J, Mashiach S, Lunenfeld B, Kaneti H, Seppala M, Roistinen R, Karasik A,** Insulin-like growth factor-I and follicle-stimulating hormone suppress insulin-like growth factor binding protein-1 secretion by human granulosa-luteal cells, *J Clin Endocrinol Metab* 75:969, 1992.

119. **San Roman GA, Magoffin DA,** Insulin-like growth factor-binding proteins in healthy and atretic follicles during natural menstrual cycles, *J Clin Endocrinol Metab* 76:625, 1992.

120. **Amato G, Izzo A, Tucker A, Bellastella A,** Insulin-like growth factor binding protein-3 reduction in follicular fluid in spontaneous and stimulated cycles, *Fertil Steril* 70:141, 1998.

121. **Cataldo NA, Giudice LC,** Follicular fluid insulin-like growth factor binding protein profiles in polycystic ovary syndrome, *J Clin Endocrinol Metab* 74:695, 1992.

122. **Cataldo NA, Giudice LC,** Insulin-like growth factor binding protein profiles in human ovarian follicular fluid correlate with follicular functional status, *J Clin Endocrinol Metab* 74:821, 1992.

123. **Chandrasekher YA, van Dessel HJHM, Fauser BCJM, Giudice LC,** Estrogen- but not androgen-dominant human ovarian follicular fluid contains an insulin-like growth factor binding protein-4 protease, *J Clin Endocrinol Metab* 80:2734, 1995.

124. **Michels KM, Lee W-H, Seltzer A, Saavedra JM, Bondy CA,** Up-regulation of pituitary [^{125}I]insulin-like growth factor-I (IGF-I) binding and IGF binding protein-2 and IGF-I gene expression by estrogen, *Endocrinology* 132:23, 1993.

125. **Dor J, Ben-Shlomo I, Lunenfeld B, Pariente C, Levran D, Karasik A, Seppala M, Mashiach S,** Insulin-like growth factor-I (IGF-I) may not be essential for ovarian follicular development: evidence from IGF-I deficiency, *J Clin Endocrinol Metab* 74:539, 1992.

126. **Dodson WC, Schomberg DW,** The effect of transforming growth factor on follicle-stimulating hormone-induced differentiation of cultured rat granulosa cells, *Endocrinology* 120:512, 1987.

127. **Hernandez ER, Hurwitz A, Payne DW, Dharmarajan AM, Purchio AF, Adashi EY,** Transforming growth factor-beta inhibits ovarian androgen production: gene expression, cellular localization, mechanisms(s), and site(s) of action, *Endocrinology* 127:2804, 1990.

128. **Oury F, Faucher C, Rives I, Bensaid M, Bouche G, Darbon J-M,** Regulation of cyclic adenosine 3',5'-monophosphate-dependent protein kinase activity and regulatory subunit RIIB content by basic fibroblast growth factor (bFGF) during granulosa cell differentiation: possible implication of protein kinase C in bFGF action, *Biol Reprod* 47:202, 1992.

129. **Christenson LK, Stouffer RL,** Follicle-stimulating hormone and luteinizing hormone/chorionic gonadotropin stimulation of vascular endothelial factor production by macaque granulosa cells from pre- and periovulatory follicles, *J Clin Endocrinol Metab* 82:2135, 1997.

130. **Anasti JN, Kalantaridou SN, Kimzey LM, George M, Nelson LM,** Human follicle fluid vascular endothelial growth factor concentrations are correlated with luteinization in spontaneously developing follicles, *Hum Reprod* 13:1144, 1998.

131. **Lee A, Christenson LK, Patton PE, Burry KA, Stouffer RL,** Vascular endothelial growth factor production by human luteinized granulosa cells *in vitro*, *Hum Reprod* 12:2756, 1997.

132. **Kokia E, Hurwitz A, Ricciarelli E, Tedeschi C, Resnick CE, Mitchell MD, Adashi EY,** Interleukin-1 stimulates ovarian prostaglandin biosynthesis: evidence for heterologous contact-independent cell-cell interaction, *Endocrinology* 130:3095, 1992.

133. **Itskovitz J, Sealey JE,** Ovarian renin-renin-angiotensin system, *Obstet Gynecol Survey* 42:545, 1987.

134. **Petraglia F, Di Meo G, Storchi R, Segre A, Facchinetti F, Szalay S, Volpe A, Genazzani AR,** Proopiomelanocortin-related peptides and methionine enkephalin in human follicular fluid: changes during the menstrual cycle, *Am J Obstet Gynecol* 157:142, 1987.

135. **Asakura H, Zwain IH, Yen SSC,** Expression of genes encoding corticotropin-releasing factor (CRF), type 1 CRF receptor, and CRF-binding protein and localization of the gene products in the human ovary, *J Clin Endocrinol Metab* 82:2720, 1997.

136. **Erden HF, Zwain IH, Asakura H, Yen SSC,** Corticotropin-releasing factor inhibits luteinizing hormone-stimulated P450c17 gene expression and androgen production by isolated thecal cells of human ovarian follicles, *J Clin Endocrinol Metab* 83:448, 1998.

137. **Kim JH, Seibel MM, MacLaughlin DT, Donahoe PK, Ransil BJ, Hametz PA, Richards CJ,** The inhibitory effects of müllerian-inhibiting substance on epidermal growth factor induced proliferation and progesterone production of human granulosa-luteal cells, *J Clin Endocrinol Metab* 75:911, 1992.

138. **Seifer DB, MacLaughlin DT, Penzias AS, Behrman HR, Asmundson L, Donahoe PK, Haning Jr RV, Flynn SD,** Gonadotropin-releasing hormone agonist-induced differences in granulosa cell cycle kinetics are associated with alterations in follicular fluid Müllerian-inhibiting substance and androgen content, *J Clin Endocrinol Metab* 76:711, 1993.

139. **Tedeschi C, Hazum E, Kokia E, Ricciarelli E, Adashi EY, Payne DW,** Endothelin-1 as a luteinization inhibitor: inhibition of rat granulosa cell progesterone accumulation via selective modulation of key steroidogenic steps affecting both progesterone formation and degradation, *Endocrinology* 131:2476, 1992.

140. **Hild-Petito S, Stouffer RL, Brenner RM,** Immunocytochemical localization of estradiol and progesterone receptors in the monkey ovary throughout the menstrual cycle, *Endocrinology* 123:2896, 1988.

141. **Enmark E, Pelto-Huikko M, Grandien K, Lagercrantz S, Lagercrantz J, Fried G, Nordenskjöld M, Gustafsson J-Å,** Human estrogen receptor β-gene structure, chromosomal localization, and expression pattern, *J Clin Endocrinol Metab* 82:4258, 1997.

142. **Zelinski-Wooten MB, Hess DL, Baughman WL, Molskness TA, Wolf DP, Stouffer RL,** Adminstration of an aromatase inhibitor during the late follicular phase of gonadotropin-treated cycles in Rhesus monkeys: effects on follicle development, oocyte maturational, and subsequent luteal function, *J Clin Endocrinol Metab* 76:988, 1993.

143. **Zelinski-Wooten MB, Hess DL, Wolf DP, Stouffer RL,** Steroid reduction during ovarian stimulation impairs ooctye fertilization, but not folliculogenesis, in rhesus monkeys, *Fertil Steril* 61:1147, 1994.

144. **Rabinovici J, Blankstein J, Goldman B, Rudak E, Dor Y, Pariente C, Geier A, Lunenfeld B, Mashiach S,** In vitro fertilization and primary embryonic cleavage are possible in 17-hydroxylase deficiency despite extremely low intrafollicular 17β-estradiol, *J Clin Endocrinol Metab* 68:693, 1989.

145. **Pellicer A, Miro F, Sampaio M, Gomez E, Bonilla-Maroles FM,** In vitro fertilization as a diagnostic and therapeutic tool in a patient with partial 17,20-desmolase deficiency, *Fertil Steril* 55:970, 1991.

146. **Miro F, Hillier SG,** Relative effects of activin and inhibin on steroid hormone synthesis in primate granulosa cells, *J Clin Endocrinol Metab* 75:1556, 1992.

147. **Rabinovici J, Spencer SJ, Doldi N, Goldsmith PC, Schwall R, Jaffe RB,** Activin-A as an intraovarian modulator: actions, localization and regulation of the intact dimer in human ovarian cells, *J Clin Invest* 89:1528, 1992.

148. **Hillier SG, Wickings EJ, Illingworth PI, Yong EL, Reichert Jr LE, Baird DT, McNeilly AS,** Control of immunoactive inhibin production by human granulosa cells, *Clin Endocrinol* 35:71, 1991.

149. **Brannian JD, Stouffer RL, Molskness TA, Chandrasekher YA, Sarkissian A, Dahl KD,** Inhibin production by Macaque granulosa cells from pre- and periovulatory follicles: regulation by gonadotropins and prostaglandin E₂, *Biol Reprod* 46:451, 1992.

150. **Marrs RP, Lobo R, Campeau JD, Nakamura RM, Brown J, Ujita EL, diZerega GS,** Correlation of human follicular fluid inhibin activity with spontaneous and induced follicle maturation, *J Clin Endocrinol Metab* 58:704, 1984.

151. **Schwall RH, Mason AJ, Wilcox JN, Bassett SG, Zeleznik AJ,** Localization of inhibin/activin subunit mRNAs within the primate ovary, *Mol Endocrinol* 4:75, 1990.

152. **Sugawara M, DePaolo L, Nakatani A, DiMarzo S, Ling N,** Radioimmunoassay of follistatin: application for *in vitro* fertilization procedures, *J Clin Endocrinol Metab* 71:1672, 1990.

153. **Magoffin DA, Jakimiuk AJ,** Inhibin A, inhibin B and activin A in the follicular fluid of regularly cycling women, *Hum Reprod* 12:1714, 1997.

154. **Pauerstein CJ, Eddy CA, Croxatto HD, Hess R, Siler-Khodr TM, Croxatto HB,** Temporal relationships of estrogen, progesterone, and luteinizing hormone levels to ovulation in women and infrahuman primates, *Am J Obstet Gynecol* 130:876, 1978.

155. **Fritz MA, McLachlan RI, Cohen NL, Dahl KD, Bremmer WJ, Soules MR,** Onset and characteristics of the midcycle surge in bioactive and immunoactive luteinizing hormone secretion in normal women: influence of physiological variations in periovulatory ovarian steroid hormone secretion, *J Clin Endocrinol Metab* 75:489, 1992.

156. **Yong EL, Baird DT, Yates R, Reicert Jr LE, Hillier SG,** Hormonal regulation of the growth and steroidogenic function of human granulosa cells, *J Clin Endocrinol Metab* 74:842, 1992.

157. **Judd S, Terry A, Petrucco M, White G,** The source of pulsatile secretion of progesterone during the human follicular phase, *J Clin Endocrinol Metab* 74:299, 1992.

158. **Chandrasekher AY, Brenner RM, Molskness TA, Yu Q, Stouffer RL,** Titrating luteinizing hormone surge requirements for ovulatory changes in primate follicles. II. Progesterone receptor expression in luteinizing granulosa cells, *J Clin Endocrinol Metab* 73:584, 1991.

159. **Chaffkin LM, Luciano AA, Peluso JJ,** Progesterone as an autocrine/paracrine regulator of human granulosa cell proliferation, *J Clin Endocrinol Metab* 75:1404, 1992.

160. **Collins RL, Hodgen GD,** Blockade of the spontaneous midcycle gonadotropin surge in monkeys by RU 486: a progesterone antagonist or agonist? *J Clin Endocrinol Metab* 63:1270, 1986.

161. **Couzinet B, Brailly S, Bouchard P, Schaison G,** Progesterone stimulates luteinizing hormone secretion by acting directly on the pituitary, *J Clin Endocrinol Metab* 74:374, 1992.

162. **Liu JH, Yen SSC,** Induction of midcycle gonadotropin surge by ovarian steroids in women: a critical evaluation, *J Clin Endocrinol Metab* 57:797, 1983.

163. **Hibbert ML, Hess DL, Stouffer RL, Wolf DP, Zelinski-Wooten MB,** Midcycle administration of a progesterone synthesis inhibitor prevents ovulation in primates, *Proc Natl Acad Sci USA* 93:1897, 1996.

164. **Judd LH, Yen SSC,** Serum androstenedione and testosterone levels during the menstrual cycle, *J Clin Endocrinol Metab* 38:475, 1973.

165. **Adams DB, Gold AR,** Rise in female-initiated sexual activity at ovulation and its suppression by oral contraceptives, *New Engl J Med* 229:1145, 1978.

166. **Hedricks C, Piccinino LJ, Udry JR, Chimbira THK,** Peak coital rate coincides with onset of luteinizing hormone surge, *Fertil Steril* 48:234, 1987.

167. **World Health Organization Task Force Investigators,** Temporal relationships between ovulation and defined changes in the concentration of plasma estradiol-17β, luteinizing hormone, follicle stimulating hormone, and progesterone, *Am J Obstet Gynecol* 138:383, 1980.

168. **Hoff JD, Quigley ME, Yen SSC,** Hormonal dynamics at midcycle: a reevaluation, *J Clin Endocrinol Metab* 57:792, 1983.

169. **Zelinski-Wooten MB, Hutchison JS, Chandrasekher YA, Wolf DP, Stouffer RL,** Administration of human luteinizing hormone (hLH) to Macaques after follicular development: further titration of LH surge requirements for ovulatory changes in primate follicles, *J Clin Endocrinol Metab* 75:502, 1992.

170. **Testart J, Frydman R, Roger M,** Seasonal influence of diurnal rhythms in the onset of the plasma luteinizing hormone surge in women, *J Clin Endocrinol Metab* 55:374, 1982.

171. **Yoshimura Y, Wallach EE,** Studies on the mechanism(s) of mammalian ovulation, *Fertil Steril* 47:22, 1987.

172. **Gordts S, Campo R, Rombauts L, Brosens I,** Endoscopic visualization of the process of fimbrial ovum retrieval in the human, *Hum Reprod* 13:1425, 1998.

173. **Brannian JD, Woodruff TK, Mather JP, Stouffer RL,** Activin-A inhibits progesterone production by Macaque luteal cells in culture, *J Clin Endocrinol Metab* 75:756, 1992.

174. **Li W, Ho Yeun B, Leung PCK,** Inhibition of progestin accumulation by activin-A in human granulosa cells, *J Clin Endocrinol Metab* 75:285, 1992.

175. **Yoshimura Y, Santulli R, Atlas SJ, Fujii S, Wallach EE,** The effects of proteolytic enzymes on in vitro ovulation in the rabbit, *Am J Obstet Gynecol* 157:468, 1987.

176. **Peng X-R, Leonardsson G, Ohlsson M, Hsueh AJW, Ny T,** Gonadotropin induced transient and cell-specific expression of tissue-type plasminogen activator and plasminogen activator inhibitor type 1 leads to a controlled and directed proteolysis during ovulation, *Fibriolysis* 6(Suppl 14):151, 1992.

177. **Jones PBC, Vernon MW, Muse KN, Curry TE,** Plasminogen activator inhibitor in human preovulatory follicular fluid, *J Clin Endocrinol Metab* 68:1039, 1989.

178. **Piquette GN, Crabtree ME, El-Danasouri I, Milki A, Polan ML,** Regulation of plasminogen activator inhibitor-1 and -2 messenger ribonucleic acid levels in human cumulus and granulosa-luteal cells, *J Clin Endocrinol Metab* 76:518, 1993.

179. **Piquette GN, Simon C, El Danasouri I, Frances A, Polan ML,** Gene regulation on interleukin-1 beta, interleukin-1 receptor type I, and plasminogen activator inhibitor-1 and -2 in human granulosa-luteal cells, *Fertil Steril* 62:760, 1994.

180. **Lumsden MA, Kelly RW, Templeton AA, Van Look PFA, Swanston IA, Baird DT,** Changes in the concentrations of prostaglandins in preovulatory human follicles after administration of hCG, *J Reprod Fertil* 77:119, 1986.

181. **Espey LL, Tanaka N, Adams RF, Okamura H,** Ovarian hydroxyeicodatetraenoic acids compared with prostanoids and steroids during ovulation in rats, *Am J Physiol* 260:E163, 1991.

182. **Watanabe H, Nagai K, Yamaguchi M, Ikenoue T, Mori N,** Interleukin-1 beta stimulates prostaglandin E2 and F2 alpha synthesis in human ovarian granulosa cells in culture, *Prostagland Leukotrienes Essential Fatty Acids* 49:963, 1993.

183. **O'Grady JP, Caldwell BV, Auletta FJ, Speroff L,** The effects of an inhibitor of prostaglandin synthesis (indomethacin) on ovulation, pregnancy, and pseudopregnancy in the rabbit, *Prostaglandins* 1:97, 1972.

184. **Killick S, Elstein M,** Pharmacologic production of luteinized unruptured follicles by prostaglandin synthetase inhibitors, *Fertil Steril* 47:773, 1987.

185. **Miyazaki T, Katz E, Dharmarajan AM, Wallach EE, Atlas SJ,** Do prostaglandins lead to ovulation in the rabbit by stimulating proteolytic enzyme activity? *Fertil Steril* 55:1182, 1991.

186. **Priddy AR, Killick SR, Elstein M, Morris J, Sullivan M, Patel L, Elder M,** The effect of prostaglandin synthetase inhibitors on human preovulatory follicular fluid prostaglandin, thromboxane, and leukotriene concentrations, *J Clin Endocrinol Metab* 71:235, 1990.

187. **Smith G, Roberts R, Hall C, Nuki G,** Reversible ovulatory failure associated with the development of luteinized unruptured follicles in women with inflammatory arthritis, *Br J Rheumatol* 35:458, 1996.

188. **Chang RJ, Gougeon A, Erickson GF,** Evidence for a neutrophil–interleukin-8 system in human folliculogenesis, *Am J Obstet Gynecol* 178:650, 1998.

189. **Brännström M, Mikuni M, Hedin L,** Intra-ovarian events during follicular development and ovulation, *Hum Reprod* 12, Natl Suppl *JBFS* 2:51, 1997.

190. **Vanderhyden BC, Telfer EE, Eppig JJ,** Mouse oocytes promote proliferation of granulosa cells from preantral and antral follicles in vitro, *Biol Reprod* 46:1196, 1992.

191. **Katt JA, Duncan JA, Herbon L, Barkan A, Marshall JC,** The frequency of gonadotropin-releasing hormone stimulation determines the number of pituitary gonadotropin-releasing hormone receptors, *Endocrinology* 116:2113, 1985.

192. **Adams JM, Taylor AE, Schoenfeld DA, Crowley Jr WF, Hall JE,** The midcycle gonadotropin surge in normal women occurs in the face of an unchanging gonadotropin-releasing hormone pulse frequency, *J Clin Endocrinol Metab* 79:858, 1994.

193. **Caraty A, Antoine C, Delaleu B, Locatelli A, Bouchard P, Gautron JP, Evans NP, Karsch FJ, Padmanabhan V,** Nature and bioactivity of gonadotropin-releasing hormone (GnRH) secreted during the GnRH surge, *Endocrinology* 136:3452, 1995.

194. **de Koning J,** Gonadotrophin surge-inhibiting/attenuating factor governs luteinizing hormone secretion during the ovarian cycle: physiology and pathology, *Hum Reprod* 10:2854, 1995.

195. **Fowler PA, Templeton A,** The nature and function of putative gonadotropin surge-attenuating/inhibiting factor (GnSAF/IF), *Endocr Rev* 17:103, 1996.

196. **McClure N, Macpherson AM, Healy DL, Wreford N, Rogers PAW,** An immunohistochemical study of the vascularizaiton of the human Graafian follicle, *Hum Reprod* 9:1401, 1994.

197. **Smith SK, Lenton EA, Cooke ID,** Plasma gonadotrophin and ovarian steroid concentrations in women with menstrual cycles with short luteal phase, *J Reprod Fertil* 75:363, 1985.

198. **Golos TG, Soto EA, Tureck RW, Strauss III JF,** Human chorionic gonadotropin and 8-bromo-adenosine 3',5'-monophosphate stimulate [^{125}I]low density lipoprotein uptake and metabolism by luteinized human granulosa cells in culture, J Clin Endocrinol Metab 61:633, 1985, *J Clin Endocrinol Metab* 61:633, 1985.

199. **Brannian JD, Shiigi SM, Stouffer RL,** Gonadotropin surge increases fluorescent-tagged low-density lipoprotein uptake by Macaque granulosa cells from preovulatory follicles, *Biol Reprod* 47:355, 1992.

200. **Vande Wiele RL, Bogumil J, Dyrenfurth I, Ferin M, Jewelewicz R, Warren M, Rizkallah T, Mikhail G,** Mechanisms regulating the menstrual cycle in women, *Recent Prog Horm Res* 26:63, 1970.

201. **Hutchison JS, Zeleznik AJ,** The rhesus monkey corpus luteum is dependent on pituitary gonadotropin secretion throughout the luteal phase of the menstrual cycle, *Endocrinology* 115:1780, 1984.

202. **Fraser HM, Lunn SF, Morris KD, Deghenghi R,** Initiation of high dose gonadotrophin-releasing hormone antagonist treatment during the late follicular phase in the macaque abolishes luteal function irrespective of effects upon the luteinizing hormone surge, *Hum Reprod* 12:430, 1997.

203. **Richardson DW, Goldsmith LT, Pohl CR, Schallenberger E, Knobil E,** The role of prolactin in the regulation of the primate corpus luteum, *J Clin Endocrinol Metab* 60:501, 1985.

204. **Castro A, Castro O, Troncoso JL, Kohen P, Simón C, Vega M, Devoto L,** Luteal leukocytes are modulators of the steroidogenic process of human mid-luteal cells, *Hum Reprod* 13:1584, 1998.

205. **Lei ZM, Chegini N, Rao CV,** Quantitative cell composition of human bovine corpora lutea from various reproductive states, *Biol Reprod* 44:1148, 1991.

206. **Girsh E, Milvae RA, Wang W, Meidan R,** Effect of endothelin-1 on bovine luteal cell function: role in prostaglandin F2α-induced antisteroidogenic action, *Endocrinology* 137:1306, 1996.

207. **Girsh E, Wang W, Mamluk R, Arditi F, Friedman A, Milvae RA, Meidan R,** Regulation of endothelin-1 expression in the bovine corpus luteum: elevation by prostaglandin F2α, *Endocrinology* 137:5191, 1996.

208. **Retamales I, Carrasco I, Troncoso JL, Las Heras J, Devoto L, Vega M,** Morpho-functional study of human luteal cell subpopulations, *Hum Reprod* 9:591, 1994.

209. **Brannian JD, Stouffer RL,** Progesterone production by monkey luteal cell subpopulations at different stages of the menstrual cycle: changes in agonist responsiveness, *Biol Reprod* 44:141, 1991.

210. **Sanders SL, Stouffer RL, Brannian JD,** Androgen production by monkey luteal cell subpopulations at different stages of the menstrual cycle, *J Clin Endocrinol Metab* 81:591, 1996.

211. **Maas S, Jarry H, Teichmann A, Rath W, Kuhn W, Wuttke W,** Paracrine actions of oxytocin, prostaglandin F2α, and estradiol within the human corpus luteum, *J Clin Endocrinol Metab* 74:306, 1992.

212. **Ravindranath N, Little-Ihrig L, Benyo DF, Zeleznik AJ,** Role of luteinizing hormone in the expression of cholesterol side-chain cleavage cytochrome P450 and 3-hydroxysteroid dehydrogenase 5-4 isomerase messenger ribonucleic acids in the primate corpus luteum, *Endocrinology* 131:2065, 1992.

213. **diZerega GS, Lynch A, Hodgen GD,** Initiation of asymmetrical ovarian estradiol secretion in the primate ovarian cycle after luteectomy, *Endocrinology* 108:1233, 1981.

214. **diZerega GS, Hodgen GD,** The interovarian progesterone gradient: a spatial and temporal regulator of folliculogenesis in the primate ovarian cycle, *J Clin Endocrinol Metab* 54:495, 1982.

215. **Gougeon A, Lefevre B,** Histological evidence of alternating ovulation in women, *J Reprod Fertil* 70:7, 1984.

216. **Brannian JD, Stouffer RL,** Cellular approaches to understanding the function and regulation of the primate corpus luteum, *Seminars Reprod Endocrinol* 9:341, 1991.

217. **Filicori M, Butler JP, Crowley WF,** Neuroendocrine regulation of the corpus luteum in the human: evidence for pulsatile progesterone secretion, *J Clin Invest* 73:1638, 1984.

218. **Lenton EA, Landgren B, Sexton L, Harper R,** Normal variation in the length of the follicular phase of the menstrual cycle: effect of chronological age, *Br J Obstet Gynaecol* 91:681, 1984.

219. **Gore BZ, Caldwell B, Speroff L,** Estrogen-induced human luteolysis, *J Clin Endocrinol Metab* 36:615, 1973.

220. **Auletta FJ, Flint APF,** Mechanisms controlling corpus luteum function in sheep, cows, nonhuman primates, and women especially in relation to the time of luteolysis, *Endocr Rev* 9:88, 1988.

221. **Zelinski-Wooten MB, Stouffer RL,** Intraluteal infusions of prostaglandins of the E, D, I, and A series prevent PGF2α-induced but not spontaneous luteal regression in rhesus monkeys, *Biol Reprod* 43:507, 1990.

222. **Shikone T, Yamoto M, Kokawa K, Yamashita K, Nishimori K, Nakano R,** Apoptosis of human corpora lutea during cyclic luteal regression and early pregancy, *J Clin Endocrinol Metab* 81:2376, 1996.

223. **Grazul-Bilska AT, Redmer DA, Reynolds LP,** Effects of luteinizing hormone and prostaglandin F2α on gap junctional intercellular communication of ovine luteal cells throughout the estrous cycle, *Endocrine* 5:225, 1996.

224. **Khan-Dawood FS,** Oxytocin in intercellular communication in the corpus luteum, *Seminars Reprod Endocrinol* 15:395, 1998.

225. **Zeleznik AJ, Little-Ihrig LL,** Effect of reduced luteinizing hormone concentrations on corpus luteum function during the menstrual cycle of rhesus monkeys, *Endocrinology* 125:2237, 1990.

226. **Duncan WC, McNeilly AS, Illingworth PJ,** The effect of luteal "rescue" on the expression and localization of matrix metalloproteinases and their tissue inhibitors in the human corpus luteum, *J Clin Endocrinol Metab* 83:2470, 1998.

227. **O'Sullivan MJB, Stamouli A, Thomas EJ, Richardson MC,** Gonadotrophin regulation of production of tissue inhibitor of metalloproteinases-1 by luteinized human granulosa cells: a potential mechanism for luteal rescue, *Mol Hum Reprod* 3:405, 1997.

228. **Catt KJ, Dufau ML, Vaitukaitis JL,** Appearance of hCG in pregnancy plasma following the initiation of implantation of the blastocyst, *J Clin Endocrinol Metab* 40:537, 1975.

229. **Bassett SG, Little-Ihrig LL, Mason JI, Zeleznik AJ,** Expression of messenger ribonucleic acids that encode for 3-hydroxysteroid dehydrogenase and cholesterol side-chain cleavage enzyme throughout the luteal phase of the Macaque menstrual cycle, *J Clin Endocrinol Metab* 72:362, 1991.

230. **Roseff SJ, Bangah ML, Kettel LM, Vale W, Rivier J, Burger HG, Yen SSC,** Dynamic changes in circulating inhibin levels during the luteal-follicular transition of the human menstrual cycle, *J Clin Endocrinol Metab* 69:1033, 1989.

231. **Jia X-C, Kessel B, Yen SSC, Tucker EM, Hsueh AJW,** Serum bioactive follicle-stimulating hormone during the human menstrual cycle and in hyper- and hypogonadotropic states: application of a sensitive granulosa cell aromatase bioassay, *J Clin Endocrinol Metab* 62:1243, 1986.

232. **Schneyer AL, Sluss PM, Whitcomb RW, Hall JE, Crowley Jr WF, Freaman RG,** Development of a radioligand receptor assay for measuring follitropin in serum: application to premature ovarian failure, *Clin Chem* 37:508, 1991.

233. **Molskness TA, Woodruff TK, Hess DL, Dahl KD, Stouffer RL,** Recombinant human inhibin-A administered early in the menstrual cycle alters concurrent pituitary and follicular, plus subsequent luteal, function in Rhesus monkeys, *J Clin Endocrinol Metab* 81:4002, 1996.

234. **Besecke LM, Guendner MJ, Schneyer AL, Bauer-Dantoin AC, Jameson JL, Weiss J,** Gonadotropin-releasing hormone regulates follicle-stimulating hormone-β gene expression through an activin/follistatin autocrine or paracrine loop, *Endocrinology* 137:3667, 1996.

235. **Le Nestour E, Marraoui J, Lahlou N, Roger M, de Ziegler D, Bouchard PH,** Role of estradiol in the rise in follicle-stimulating hormone levels during the luteal-follicular transition, *J Clin Endocrinol Metab* 77:439, 1993.

236. **Vollman RF,** The menstrual cycle, In: Friedman E, ed. *Major Problems in Obstetrics and Gynecology,* W.B. Saunders Co., Philadelphia, 1977.

237. **Treloar AE, Boynton RE, Borghild GB, Brown BW,** Variation of the human menstrual cycle through reproductive life, *Int J Fertil* 12:77, 1967.

238. **Collett ME, Wertenberger GE, Fiske VM,** The effect of age upon the pattern of the menstrual cycle, *Fertil Steril* 5:437, 1954.

239. **Munster K, Schmidt L, Helm P,** Length and variation in the menstrual cycle — a cross-sectional study from a Danish county, *Br J Obstet Gynaecol* 99:422, 1992.

240. **Sherman BM, Korenman SG,** Hormonal characteristics of the human menstrual cycle throughout reproductive life, *J Clin Invest* 55:699, 1975.

241. **Lee SJ, Lenton EA, Sexton L, Cooke ID,** The effect of age on the cyclical patterns of plasma LH, FSH, oestradiol and progesterone in women with regular menstrual cycles, *Hum Reprod* 3:851, 1988.

242. **Hughes EG, Robertson DM, Handelsman DJ, Hayward S, Healy DL, de Kretser DM,** Inhibin and estradiol responses to ovarian hyperstimulation: effects of age and predictive value for in vitro fertilization outcome, *J Clin Endocrinol Metab* 70:358, 1990.

243. **Metcalf MG, Livesay JH,** Gonadotropin excretion in fertile women: effect of age and the onset of the menopausal transition, *J Endocrinol* 105:357, 1985.

244. **Klein NA, Battaglia DE, Fujimoto VY, Davis GS, Bremmer WJ, Soules MR,** Reproductive aging: accelerated ovarian follicular devlopment associated with a monotropic follicle-stimulating hormone rise in normal older women, *J Clin Endocrinol Metab* 81:1038, 1996.

245. **Cha KY, Koo JJ, Ko JJ, Choi DH, Han SY, Yoon TK,** Pregnancy after IVF of human follicular oocytes collected from nonstimulated cycles, their culture in vitro and their transfer in a donor oocyte program, *Fertil Steril* 55:109, 1991.

246. **Faddy MJ, Gosden RG, Gougeon A, Richardson SJ, Nelson JF,** Accelerated disappearance of ovarian follicles in mid-life: implications for forecasting menopause, *Hum Reprod* 7:1342, 1992.

247. **Richardson SJ, Senikas V, Nelson JF,** Follicular depletion during the menopausal transition — evidence for accelerated loss and ultimate exhaustion, *J Clin Endocrinol Metab* 65:1231, 1987.

248. **Klein NA, Battaglia DE, Miller PB, Branigan EF, Giudice LC, Soules MR,** Ovarian follicular development and the follicular fluid hormones and growth factors in normal women of advanced reproductive age, *J Clin Endocrinol Metab* 81:1946, 1996.

7 Sperm and Egg Transport, Fertilization, and Implantation

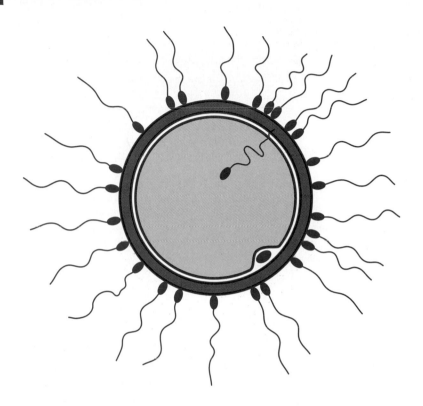

Among his many accomplishments, Galileo Galilei gave to science, in 1609, two important instruments, the telescope and the microscope.[1] Antonj van Leeuwenhoek of Delft, Holland, was fascinated by Galileo's microscope. Leeuwenhoek was a draper and had no medical or scientific training, yet he became a Fellow of the Royal Society of London to which he submitted 375 scientific papers. In 1677, Leewenhoek described (fairly accurately) the "little animals of the sperm." It was another 198 years before Wilhelm August Oscar Hertwig, in Germany, demonstrated the union of sperm and egg, fertilization, in the sea urchin.

The coming together of sperm and egg is one of the essentials of reproduction; however, the remote site of this event and the enclosed origins of the participants made fertilization a difficult subject for study. This changed with the advent of in vitro fertilization. Greater understanding of sperm and egg development and union is one of the major benefits of the clinical application of the assisted reproductive technologies. This chapter examines the mechanisms involved in sperm and egg transport, fertilization, and implantation.

Sperm Transport

The evolution of scrotal mammals and the adoption of internal fertilization are associated with sperm maturation that occurs outside of the testes. This includes epididymal maturation and capacitation in the female before fertilization. The need for capacitation (the final step required to acquire the ability to fertilize) may be an evolutionary consequence of the development of a storage system for inactive sperm in the caudal epididymis.[2]

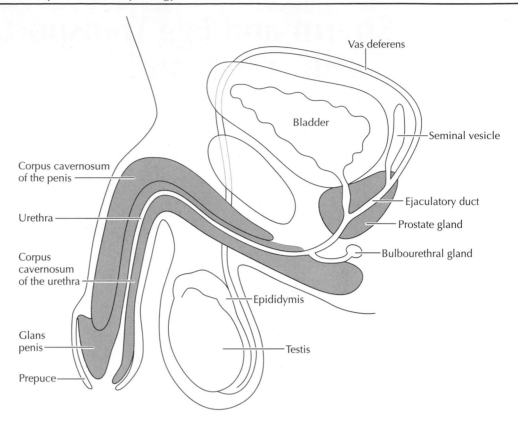

The sperm reach the caudal epididymis approximately 72 days after the initiation of spermatogenesis. At this time, the head of the sperm contains a membrane-bound nucleus capped by the acrosome, a large vesicle of proteolytic enzymes. The inner acrosomal membrane is closely apposed to the nuclear membrane, and the outer acrosomal membrane is next to the surface plasma membrane. The flagellum is a complex structure of microtubules and fibers, surrounded at the proximal end by mitochondria. Motility and the ability to fertilize are acquired gradually as the sperm pass into the epididymis.

The caudal epididymis stores sperm available for ejaculation. The ability to store functional sperm provides a capacity for repetitive fertile ejaculations. Preservation of optimal sperm function during this period of storage requires adequate testosterone levels in the circulation and maintenance of the normal scrotal temperature.[3] The importance of temperature is emphasized by the correlation of reduced numbers of sperm associated with episodes of body fever. The epididymis is limited to a storage role because sperm that have never passed through the epididymis and that have been obtained from the vasa efferentia in men with a congenital absence of the vas deferens can fertilize the human oocyte in vitro and result in pregnancy with live birth.[4] Indeed, the injection of one sperm directly into an oocyte (intracytoplasmic sperm injection) with sperm obtained by testicular biopsy (in men with congenital absence of epididymides) is very successful in achieving fertilization and pregnancy.[5] However, the use of sperm from men with sperm abnormalities, and especially the use of immature germ cells for intracytoplasmic injection should be pursued with some caution. The outcome in subsequent generations must be assessed and appropriate genetic screening must be developed to avoid the transmission of subtle but important genetic alterations.

Semen forms a gel almost immediately following ejaculation but then is liquefied in 20–30 minutes by enzymes derived from the prostate gland. The alkaline pH of semen provides protection for the sperm from the acid environment of the vagina. This protection is transient, and most sperm left in the vagina are immobilized within 2 hours. The more fortunate sperm, by their own motility, gain entrance into the tongues of cervical mucus that layer over the ectocervix. These are the sperm that enter the uterus; the seminal plasma is left behind in the vagina. This entry is rapid, and sperm have been found in mucus within 90 seconds of ejaculation.[6] The

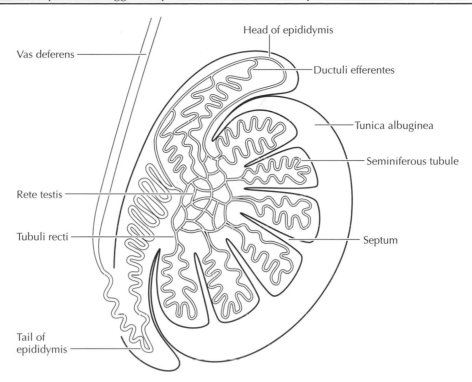

destruction of all sperm in the vagina 5 minutes after ejaculation does not interfere with fertilization in the rabbit, further attesting to the rapidity of transport.[7]

Contractions of the female reproductive tract occur during coitus, and these contractions may be important for entry of sperm into the cervical mucus and further transport. Presumably successful entry is the result of combined female and male forces (the flagellar activity of the sperm). The success of therapeutic insemination, however, indicates that coitus and female orgasm are not essential for sperm transport.

The sperm swim and migrate through pores in the mucus microstructure that are smaller than the sperm head; therefore, the sperm must actively push their way through the mucus.[8] One cause of infertility, presumably, is impaired sperm movement that prevents this transport through the mucus. This movement is probably also influenced by the interaction between the mucus and the surface properties of the sperm head; for example, sperm antibodies on the sperm head inhibit sperm movement in the mucus.[9] Abnormal morphology of the sperm head is often associated with impaired flagellar function; however, abnormal head morphology alone can be a cause of poor mucus penetration.[10, 11] It is generally believed that the cervical mucus has a filtering action; abnormal and less "capable" sperm have difficulty getting through.[12]

Uterine contractions and sperm motility propel the sperm upward, and in the human, sperm can be found in the tube 5 minutes after insemination.[13] It is possible that the first sperm to enter the tube are at a disadvantage. In the rabbit these early sperm have only poor motility, and there is frequent disruption of the head membranes.[14] The sperm in this vanguard are unlikely to achieve fertilization. Other sperm that have colonized the cervical mucus and the cervical crypts then make their way more slowly to the ampulla of the tube in order to meet the egg. The number of sperm in the cervical mucus is relatively constant for 24 hours after coitus, and after 48 hours there are relatively few remaining in the mucus.[15] Although the isthmic region of the tube functions as a sperm reservoir in many species, this does not appear to be the case in human fallopian tubes.[16]

Human sperm have been found in the fallopian tube as long as 80 hours after intercourse, and these sperm can still perform normally with zona-free hamster oocytes.[17] In animals, the fertilizable lifespan is usually one-half the motile lifespan.

Number of sperm (millions)

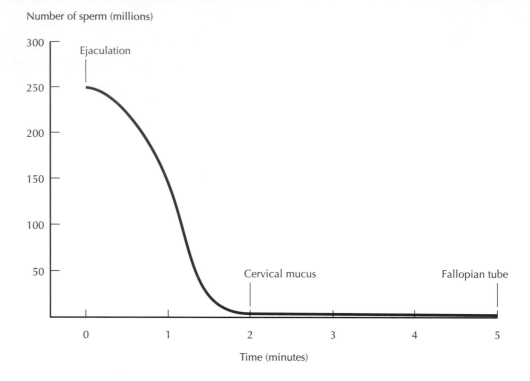

Time (minutes)

The ***attrition in sperm numbers*** from vagina to tube is substantial.[18] Of an average of 200 to 300 million sperm deposited in the vagina, at most only a few hundred, and often less, achieve proximity to the egg.[16] Greater numbers are observed in the tubal ampulla at the time of ovulation. The major loss occurs in the vagina, with expulsion of semen from the introitus playing an important role. Other causes for loss are digestion of sperm by vaginal enzymes and phagocytosis of sperm along the reproductive tract. There are also reports of sperm burrowing into or being engulfed by endometrial cells. Sperm are not stored in the fallopian tube, and indeed, many sperm continue past the oocyte to be lost into the peritoneal cavity. However, the cervix does serve as a reservoir providing a supply of sperm for up to 72 hours.

Within the fallopian tube ampulla, sperm display a new pattern of movement that has been called ***hyperactivated motility***.[19] This motility may be influenced by an interaction with the tubal epithelium that results in greater speed and better direction as well as prevention of attachment and entrapment.

Structure of the Cervical Mucus

The cervical mucus is a complex structure that is not homogeneous.[20] The mucus is secreted in granular form, and a networked structure of the mucus is formed in the cervical canal. Thus, not all areas of the cervical mucus are equally penetrable by the sperm. It is proposed, based upon animal studies, that the outward flow of the cervical mucus establishes a linear alignment of parallel strands that direct the sperm upward. Pressurization of the mucus by contractions of the uterus further aid this alignment and may contribute to the speed of sperm transport. Responding to the midcycle estrogen peak, cervical mucus production, water content, and space between its large glycoproteins reach a maximum in the immediate preovulatory period. The process of capacitation is initiated, and perhaps completed, during the sperm's passage through the cervix.

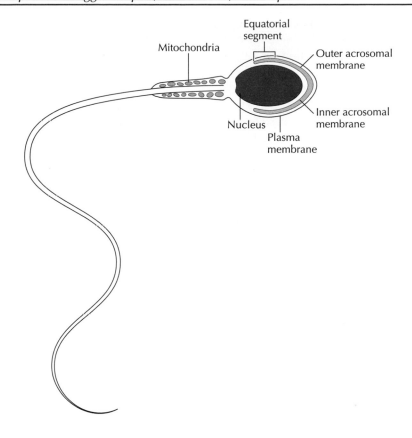

Capacitation

The discovery, in 1951, that rabbit and rat spermatozoa must spend some hours in the female tract before acquiring the capacity to penetrate ova stimulated intensive research efforts to delineate the environmental conditions required for this change in the sperm to occur.[21, 22] The process by which the sperm were transformed was called ***capacitation, the cellular changes that ejaculated spermatozoa must undergo in order to fertilize***.[23] Attention was focused on the hormonal and time requirements and the potential for in vitro capacitation. Capacitation is characterized by 3 accomplishments:

1. The ability to undergo the acrosome reaction.

2. The ability to bind to the zona pellucida.

3. The acquisition of hypermotility.

Capacitation changes the surface characteristics of sperm, as exemplified by removal of seminal plasma factors that coat the surface of the sperm, modification of their surface charge, and restriction of receptor mobility. This is associated with modifications of sperm cell membrane sterols, lipids, and glycoproteins that cause decreased stability of the plasma membrane and the membrane lying immediately under it, the outer acrosomal membrane. The membranes undergo further, more striking, modifications when capacitated sperm reach the vicinity of an oocyte or when they are incubated in follicular fluid. There is a breakdown and merging of the plasma membrane and the outer acrosomal membrane, ***the acrosome reaction***.[24] This allows egress of the enzyme contents of the acrosome, the caplike structure that covers the sperm nucleus. These enzymes, which include hyaluronidase, a neuraminidase-like factor, cumulus-dispersing enzyme, and a protease called acrosin, are all thought to play roles in sperm penetration of the egg investments. The changes in the sperm head membranes also prepare the sperm for fusion with the egg membrane. It is the inner acrosomal membrane that fuses with the oocyte plasma membrane. The acrosome reaction can be induced by zona pellucida proteins of the oocyte and by human follicular fluid in vitro.[25, 26] In addition, capacitation endows the sperm with hyper-motility, and the increased velocity of the sperm is a very critical factor in achieving zona penetration.[19]

The events that constitute the process of capacitation are regulated by the redox status of the sperm cell.[27, 28] Redox reactions induce tyrosine phosphorylation, an absolute requirement for capacitation. These reactions are dependent on a critical increase in intracellular calcium concentrations due to an influx of extracellular calcium, believed to be induced by progesterone.

Although capacitation classically has been defined as a change sperm undergo in the female reproductive tract, it is apparent that sperm of some species, including the human, can acquire the ability to fertilize after a short incubation in defined media and without residence in the female reproductive tract. Therefore, success with assisted reproductive technologies is possible. In vitro capacitation requires a culture medium that is a balanced salt solution containing energy substrates such as lactate, pyruvate, and glucose and a protein such as albumin, or a biologic fluid such as serum or follicular fluid. Sperm-washing procedures probably remove factors that coat the surface of the sperm, one of the initial steps in capacitation. The removal of cholesterol from the sperm membrane is believed to prepare the sperm membrane for the acrosome reaction.[29] The loss of cholesterol regulates the expression of sperm cell membrane surface lectins that are involved in sperm surface receptors for the zona pellucida.[30] The time required for in vitro capacitation is approximately 2 hours.[31]

The final dash to the oocyte is aided by the increased motility due to the state of hyperactivity. This change in motility can be measured by an increase in velocity and flagellar beat amplitude. Perhaps the increase in thrust gained by this hyperactivity is necessary for avoiding attachment to tubal epithelium and achieving penetration of the cumulus and zona pellucida.

Key Steps in Sperm Transport

1. *Approximately 72 days are required to produce spermatozoa, a time period followed by storage in the epididymis prior to ejaculation.*

2. *Sperm enter the cervical mucus and then the fallopian tubes within minutes, but only a few hundred sperm or less reach the oocyte. The cervix serves as a reservoir of sperm for up to 72 hours.*

3. *Capacitation, a process initiated during the sperm's passage through the cervix or during in vitro incubation in an appropriate medium, is characterized by the acquired ability of sperm to undergo the acrosome reaction to bind to the zona pellucida and to acquire hyperactivated motility.*

4. *The acrosome reaction is due to the modification and breakdown, followed by a merger, of the sperm cell membrane and the outer acrosomal membrane, allowing the release of enzymes and changes in the inner acrosomal membrane, necessary for fusion with the oocyte cell membrane.*

Egg Transport

The oocyte, at the time of ovulation, is surrounded by granulosa cells (the **cumulus oophorus**) that attach the oocyte to the wall of the follicle. The **zona pellucida**, a noncellular porous layer of glycoproteins secreted by the oocyte, separates the oocyte from the granulosa cells. The granulosa cells communicate metabolically with the oocyte by means of **gap junctions** between the oocyte plasma membrane and the cumulus cells. In response to the midcycle surge in luteinizing hormone (LH), maturation of the oocyte proceeds with the resumption of meiosis as the oocyte completes the first meiotic division, enters into the second meiotic division, and arrests in the second metaphase. Just before ovulation, the cumulus cells retract their cellular contacts from the oocyte. The disruption of the gap junctions induces maturation and migration of the cortical granules to the outer cortex of the oocyte.[32] Prior to ovulation, the oocyte and its cumulus mass of cells prepare to leave their long residence in the ovary by becoming detached from the follicular wall.

Egg transport encompasses the period of time from ovulation to the entry of the morula into the uterus. The egg can be fertilized only during the early stages of its sojourn in the fallopian tube. Within 2–3 minutes of ovulation, the cumulus and oocyte are in the ampulla of the fallopian tube.

In rats and mice the ovary and distal portion of the tube are covered by a common fluid-filled sac. Ovulated eggs are carried by fluid currents to the fimbriated end of the tube. In contrast, in primates, including humans, the ovulated eggs adhere with their cumulus mass of follicular cells to the surface of the ovary. The fimbriated end of the tube sweeps over the ovary in order to pick up the egg. Entry into the tube is facilitated by muscular movements that bring the fimbriae into contact with the surface of the ovary. Variations in this pattern surely exist, as evidenced by women who achieve pregnancy despite having only one ovary and a single tube located on the contralateral side. Furthermore, eggs deposited in the cul-de-sac by transvaginal injection are picked up by the tubes.[33]

Although there can be a small negative pressure in the tube in association with muscle contractions, oocyte pickup is not dependent on a suction effect secondary to this negative pressure. Ligation of the tube just proximal to the fimbriae does not interfere with pickup.[34]

The fallopian tubes are lined by an epithelium that undergoes cyclic changes comparable to the endometrium, in response to the hormonal changes of the menstrual cycle.[35] The epithelium is composed of nonciliated cells and ciliated cells. The nonciliated cells are characterized by major secretory activity during the follicular phase of the cycle, culminating in the release of cytoplasmic components during the passage of the egg, perhaps providing important metabolic factors for transport and implantation.

Some have described a menstrual cycle variation in ciliated cells in the tube, but most have not.[35] The apparent variation is probably due to differential changes in response to cyclic hormone levels. The cilia on the surface of the fimbriae (where they are present in greater concentrations) display adhesive sites, and these seem to have prime responsibility for the initial movement of the egg into the tube. This movement is dependent on the presence of follicular cumulus cells surrounding the egg, because removal of these cells prior to egg pickup prevents effective egg transport.

In the ampulla of the tube the many cilia beat synchronously in the direction of the uterus. In women and monkeys, this unidirectional beat is also found in the isthmus of the tube. The specific contribution of the cilia to egg transport in the ampulla and isthmus is an unresolved question. Most investigators have credited muscular contractions of the tubes as the primary force for moving the egg.[36] However, interference with muscle contractility in the rabbit did not block egg transport.[37] Reversing a segment of the ampulla of the tube so that the cilia in this segment beat toward the ovary interferes with pregnancy in the rabbit without blocking fertilization. The fertilized ova are arrested when they come in contact with the transposed area.[38] This suggests that ciliary beating is crucial for egg transport. There are *fertile* women who suffer from Kartagener's syndrome in which there is a congenital absence of dynein arms (a protein structure associated with motility) in all bodily cilia, and thus the cilia do not beat. However, motility of cilia in the tube may be disordered and not totally absent.[39]

Transvaginal endoscopic observation of actual ovum and cumulus oophorous pickup in a woman revealed that the process is relatively slow (more than 15 minutes), the fimbriae on the ovulating side are distinguished by being erect (probably due to engorged blood vessels and suggesting a local ovarian influence), and the only observable active mechanism involved ciliary movement.[40]

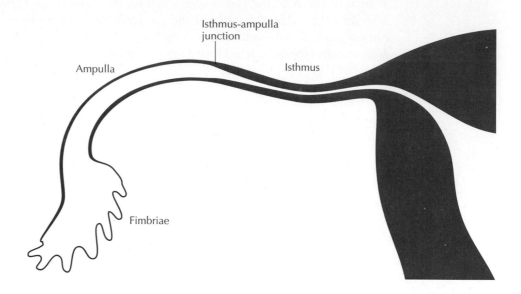

It is probable, therefore, that in normal circumstances, smooth muscle contractions and the flow of secretory fluid in response to ciliary activity work together to accomplish egg transport.

In most species, transport of the ovum (the fertilized oocyte) through the tube requires approximately 3 days.[41] The time spent within the various parts of the tube varies from one species to another. Transport through the ampulla is rapid in the rabbit, whereas in women the egg spends about 80 hours in the tube, 90% of which is in the ampulla.

Attempts to modify tubal function as a method for understanding its physiology have involved three major pharmacologic approaches: 1) altering levels of steroid hormones, 2) interference with or supplementation of adrenergic stimuli, and 3) treatment with prostaglandins. Although there is abundant literature on the effects of estrogen and progesterone on tubal function, it is clouded by the use of different hormones, different doses, and different timing of injections. Because of these variations, it is difficult to obtain a coherent picture and to relate the experimental results to the in vivo situation. In general, pharmacologic doses of estrogen favor retention of eggs in the tube. This "tube-locking" effect of estrogen can be partially reversed by treatment with progesterone.

The isthmus of the tube has an extensive adrenergic innervation. Surgical denervation of the tube, however, does not disrupt ovum transport. Prostaglandins (PG) of the E series relax tubal muscle, whereas those of the F series stimulate muscle activity of the tube. Although $PGF_{2\alpha}$ stimulates human oviductal motility in vivo, it does not cause acceleration of ovum transport.

Is there an essential anatomical segment of the tube? Excision of the ampullary-isthmic junction in rabbits does not prevent fertility.[42] This is equally true if small segments of the ampulla are removed, and pregnancy can occur even if the entire isthmus and uterotubal junction are excised. Although the fimbriae are thought to play a crucial role in fertility, spontaneous pregnancies have been reported following sterilization by fimbriectomy or following surgical repair of tubes whose fimbriated ends had been excised.[43, 44] The fallopian tube appears to readily adapt to anatomical changes and restrictions.

In most species, a period of residence in the tube appears to be a prerequisite for full development. Rabbit eggs can be fertilized in the uterus, but they do not develop unless transferred to the tubes

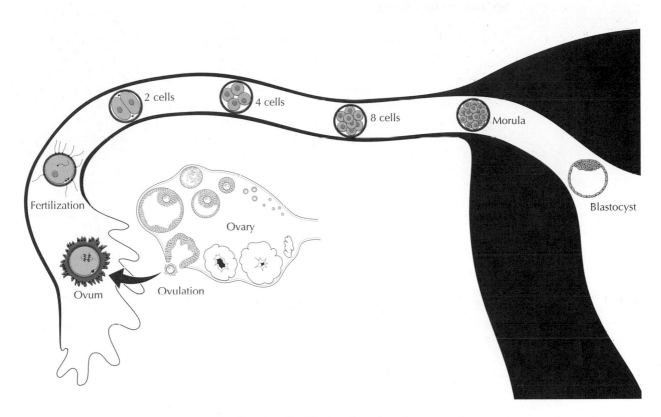

within 3 hours of fertilization.[45] This implies that there may be a component in uterine fluid during the first 48 hours following ovulation that is toxic to the egg.[45] Indirect evidence of an inhospitable environment is also provided by studies indicating that there must be synchrony between development of the endometrium and the egg for successful pregnancy to occur.[46, 47] If the endometrium is in a reduced or advanced stage of development compared with the egg, fertility is compromised. In addition, the blastocyst must undergo cleavage and development in order to gain the capability to implant in the uterus. ***Thus, it is conceptually useful to view the fallopian tube not as an active transport mechanism, but as a structure that provides an important holding action. This functional behavior is coordinated by the changing estrogen and progesterone levels after ovulation, although local embryonic signals may also be involved.***

Successful pregnancies have occurred in the human following the Estes procedure, in which the ovary is transposed to the uterine cornua.[48] Eggs are ovulated directly into the uterus, completely bypassing the tube. Moreover, when fertilized donor eggs are transferred to women who are receiving hormone supplementation, there are several days during the treatment cycle when the blastocysts will implant. This crucial difference between animal and human physiology is of more than academic importance. There has been speculation about the use of drugs that could accelerate tubal transport as a means of providing contraception by ensuring that the egg would reach the uterus when it was in an unreceptive state. Although this may work in animals, it is of doubtful value in the human because perfect synchrony is not required.

Animal and human reproduction also differ in the occurrence of ectopic pregnancy. Ectopic pregnancies are rare in animals, and in rodents, they are not induced even if the uterotubal junction is occluded immediately following fertilization. The embryos reach the blastocyst stage and then degenerate.

Key Steps in Egg Transport

1. *After ovulation, the oocyte and its surrounding cumulus are in the ampulla of the fallopian tube within 2–3 minutes.*

2. *Tubal transport depends on smooth muscle contractions and ciliary-induced flow of secretory fluid.*

3. *The fallopian tube provides an important holding action to allow time for the endometrium to become receptive and the blastocyst to become capable of implantation, a time period of approximately 80 hours, 90% of which is in the ampulla.*

Oocyte Maturation

Oocyte maturation is regulated by the sex hormones, and in nonmammalian species a nongenomic action of progesterone causes an increase in intracellular calcium concentrations. In human oocytes, an influx of extracellular calcium occurs in response to estradiol, followed by secondary rises in calcium ions from intracellular stores, characterized by wavelike oscillations.[49] This is a nongenomic response to estradiol at the cell surface, and the transient increases in intracellular calcium improve the quality of the oocyte and contribute to the capability for fertilization.

Calcium oscillations are a property common to mammalian oocytes and are also an early reaction to the fertilizing spermatozoan.[50] Neither the presence of estradiol nor the calcium oscillations are required for oocytes to resume meiosis. However, improved fertilization following estradiol-induced calcium increases indicates an important role for intrafollicular estradiol in overall oocyte maturation.

Fertilization

The fertilizable life of the human oocyte is unknown, but most estimates range between 12 and 24 hours. However, immature human eggs recovered for in vitro fertilization can be fertilized even after 36 hours of incubation. Equally uncertain is knowledge of the fertilizable lifespan of human sperm. The most common estimate is 48–72 hours, although motility can be maintained after the sperm have lost the ability to fertilize. The extreme intervals that have achieved pregnancy documented after a single act of coitus are 6 days prior to and 3 days after ovulation.[51] The great majority of pregnancies occur when coitus takes place within the 3-day interval just prior to ovulation.[52]

Contact of sperm with the egg, which occurs in the ampulla of the tube, may not be random; there is some evidence for sperm-egg communication that attracts sperm to the oocyte.[53, 54] This chemotactic responsiveness of sperm requires the changes that take place in the capacitation process.[55] Thus, this may be a system to select a sperm that is fully capable of fertilization.

The cumulus oophorus undergoes a preovulatory expansion that may have two important roles. The ampullary space of the human fallopian tube is relatively large (compared with the oocyte), and the expanded cumulus may serve to increase the chances of an encounter with one of the few spermatozoa that have reached the far section of the tube. In addition, this change may facilitate sperm passage through the cumulus. Sperm pass through the cumulus without the release of acrosomal enzymes.[56] It has been suggested, based upon *in vitro* experiments, that the cumulus is essential for full development of the fertilizing ability of sperm; however, removal of the cumulus does not prevent sperm penetration and fertilization.

Despite the evolution from external to internal fertilization over a period of about 100 million years, many of the mechanisms have remained the same.[57, 58] The acellular zona pellucida that surrounds the egg at ovulation and remains in place until implantation has two major functions in the fertilization process:

1. The zona pellucida contains ligands for sperm, which are, with some exceptions, relatively species-specific.

2. The zona pellucida undergoes the *zona reaction* in which the zona becomes impervious to other sperm once the fertilizing sperm penetrates, and thus it provides a bar to polyploidy.[59]

Penetration through the zona is rapid and mediated by acrosin, a trypsinlike proteinase that is bound to the inner acrosomal membrane of the sperm.[60, 61] The pivotal role assigned to acrosin has been disputed. For example, manipulations that increase the resistance of the zona to acrosin do not interfere with sperm penetration, and thus sperm motility may be the critical factor. The zona pellucida is a porous structure due to the many glycoproteins assembled into long, interconnecting filaments. Nevertheless, a preponderance of evidence favors tenacious binding of capacitated spermatozoa to the zona pellucida as a requirement for penetration, although it is clear that penetration requires active motility not only of the tail but of the head as well. Indeed, the sperm head undergoes rapid lateral oscillations of the head about a fulcrum at the head-tail junction, suggesting a scythelike action on the zona.[2]

The acrosome is a lysosomelike organelle in the anterior region of the sperm head, lying just beneath the plasma membrane like a cap over the nucleus. The lower part of the two arms is called the equatorial segment. The acrosome contains many enzymes that are exposed by *the acrosome reaction, the loss of the acrosome immediately before fertilization. This reaction is one of exocytosis, the fusion of an intracellular storage vesicle with the inner surface of the cell membrane, followed by release of the vesicle contents.* This reaction requires an influx of calcium ions, the efflux of hydrogen ion, an increase in pH, and fusion of the plasma membrane with the outer acrosomal membrane, leading to the exposure and escape of the enzymes contained on the inner acrosomal membrane. Binding to the zona pellucida is required to permit a component of the zona to induce the acrosomal reaction. This component is believed to be a glycoprotein sperm receptor, which thus serves dual functions: binding of sperm and induction of the acrosomal reaction.

The initial contact between the sperm and the oocyte is a receptor-mediated process. The zona pellucida is composed of glycoproteins secreted by the oocyte, known as ZP1, ZP2, and ZP3, with ZP3 being the most abundant.[62] ZP3 is the primary ligand for sperm and ZP2 binding occurs after the acrosome reaction, participating in the zona reaction to prevent polyspermy. Structural alteration of these glycoproteins leads to a loss of activity; inactivation of these ligands after fertilization is probably accomplished by one or more cortical granule enzymes. The ZP3 gene is expressed only in growing oocytes. DNA sequence similarities of the ZP3 gene in various mammals indicates that this gene has been evolutionarily conserved and that the sperm-ligand interaction is a common mechanism among mammals.[63] Mice with a disrupted ZP3 gene produce oocytes lacking a zona pellucida and are unable to become pregnant.[64, 65] A vaccine against zona pellucida proteins from pigs is used to control reproduction in female elephants and deer.

The initial binding of the sperm to the zona requires recognition on the part of the sperm of the carbohydrate component of the species-specific glycoprotein ligand molecule.[66] Once binding is accomplished, the acrosome reaction is triggered by the peptide chain component of the receptor glycoprotein. At least one receptor on the sperm head is a tyrosine kinase, activated by binding to the ZP3 glycoprotein and an initiator of the acrosome reaction.[67, 68] This interaction is analogous to the general principle of behavior for hormone-receptor binding and activity. In the case of sperm and oocyte, recognition of the oocyte zona ligand involves an enzyme on the surface of the sperm that becomes exposed during capacitation. Formation of the ZP3-enzyme

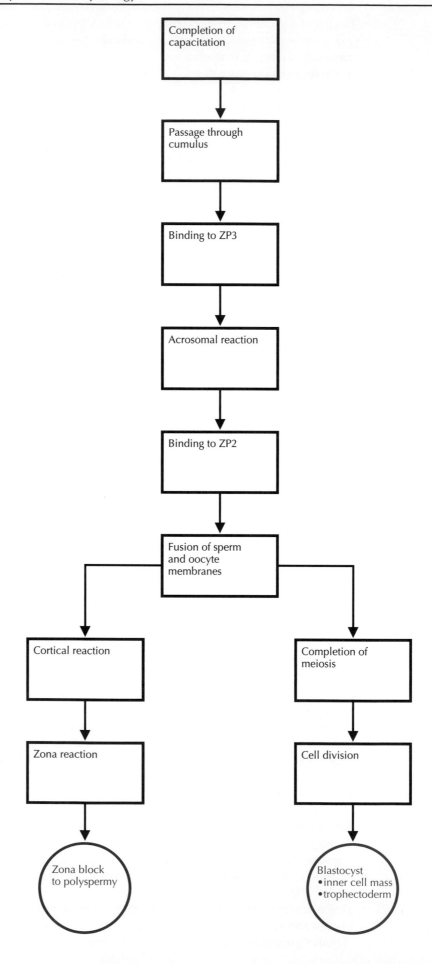

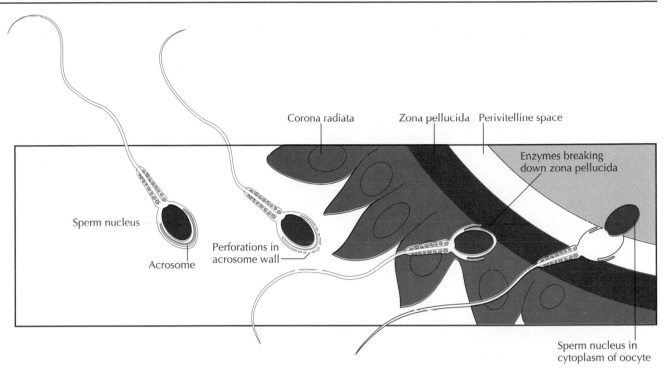

Corona radiata   Zona pellucida   Perivitelline space

Enzymes breaking down zona pellucida

Sperm nucleus

Acrosome

Perforations in acrosome wall

Sperm nucleus in cytoplasm of oocyte

complex, therefore, not only produces binding but also induces the acrosome reaction. The G protein signaling system is also present on sperm heads, and activation at this point in time opens calcium channels to increase intracellular levels of calcium ions, a requirement for the acrosome reaction.[69, 70] Thus, the initial sperm-zona interaction depends on binding of acrosome-intact spermatozoa, followed by a process mediated by the enzymes released by the zona-induced acrosome reaction. Protein kinase C activation is an important step in the acrosomal reaction, leading to phosphorylation of sperm proteins involved in the process.[71]

Spermatozoa enter the perivitelline space at an angle. The oocyte is a spherical cell covered with microvilli. The sperm head is like a flat dish, and the thickness of the head is a little less than the distance between the oocyte microvilli.[72] The region of the equatorial segment of the sperm head, the distal portion of the acrosome, makes initial contact with the vitelline membrane (the egg plasma membrane or oolemma). At first, the egg membrane engulfs the sperm head, and, subsequently, there is fusion of egg and sperm membranes. This fusion is mediated by specific proteins. Two membrane proteins from the sperm head have been sequenced; one (PH-20) is involved in binding to the zona pellucida, and the other (PH-30, also called fertilin) is involved in fusion with the oocyte.[73, 74] PH-20, with hyaluronidase activity, is also active in dispelling the cumulus.[75] The cell membrane of the unfertilized oocyte contains integrin adhesion/fusion molecules that recognize peptides such as fibronectin, laminin, and collagen.[76] Fibronectin appears on the spermatozoa, but it is disputed whether it appears with caudal maturation or after capacitation. Vitronectin is a sperm protein that is activated after capacitation and the acrosome reaction and may be the key peptide interacting with oocyte cell membrane integrins.[77] These steps in the fusion process will occur only with sperm that have undergone the acrosome reaction.

Fusion of the sperm and oocyte membrane is followed by the cortical reaction and metabolic activation of the oocyte. An increase in intracellular free calcium in a periodic, oscillatory pattern always precedes the cortical reaction and oocyte activation at fertilization, and this is believed to be the mechanism by which the spermatozoon triggers these developmental events.[50, 78] A soluble sperm protein, called *oscillin*, has been identified in the equatorial segment of the sperm head that may be the signaling agent for the critical calcium oscillations.[79, 80]

The initiation of the block to penetration of the zona (and the vitellus) by other sperm is mediated by the *cortical reaction,* another example of exocytosis with the release of materials from the *cortical granules*, lysosomelike organelles that are found just below the egg surface.[81] As with other lysosomelike organelles, these materials include various hydrolytic enzymes. Changes brought about by these enzymes lead to the ***zona reaction, the hardening of the extracellular layer by cross-linking of structural proteins, and inactivation of ligands for sperm receptors***.[82] Thus, the zona block to polyspermy is accomplished. The initial change in this zona block is a rapid depolarization of the oocyte membrane associated with a release of calcium ions from calmodulin. The increase in intracellular calcium acts as a signal or trigger to activate protein synthesis in the oocyte. The depolarization of the membrane initiates only a transient block to sperm entry. The permanent block is a consequence of the cortical reaction and release of enzymes, also apparently triggered by the increase in calcium.

Approximately 3 hours after insemination, meiosis is completed.[83] The second polar body is released and leaves the egg with a haploid complement of chromosomes. The addition of chromosomes from the sperm restores the diploid number to the now fertilized egg. The chromatin material of the sperm head decondenses, and the male pronucleus is formed. The male and the female pronuclei migrate toward each other, and as they move into close proximity the limiting membranes break down, and a spindle is formed on which the chromosomes become arranged. Thus, the stage is set for the first cell division.

Embryonic genome activity in the human begins early; DNA synthesis activity can be detected 9–10 hours after insemination.[84] Human gene expression (transcription) begins between the 4- and 8-cell stages of preimplantation cleavage, 2–3 days after fertilization.[85] Early embryonic signals may be derived from a store of maternal messenger RNAs, termed the "maternal legacy."[86] An arrest of development in this pre-blastocyst cleavage stage is well recognized.

The clinician is interested not only in how normal fertilization takes place but also in the occurrence of abnormal events that can interfere with pregnancy. It is worthwhile, therefore, to consider the failures that occur in association with in vivo fertilization. Studies in the nonhuman primate have involved monkeys and baboons. A surgical method was used to flush the uterus of regularly cycling rhesus monkeys, and 9 preimplantation embryos and 2 unfertilized eggs were recovered from 22 flushes. Two of the 9 embryos were morphologically abnormal and probably would not have implanted.[87] Hendrickx and Kraemer used a similar technique in the baboon and recovered 23 embryos, of which 10 were morphologically abnormal.[88] This suggests that, in nonhuman primates, some ovulated eggs are not fertilized and that many early embryos are abnormal and, in all likelihood, will be aborted. Similar findings have been reported in the human in the classic study of Hertig et al.[89] They examined 34 early embryos recovered by flushing and examination of reproductive organs removed at surgery. Ten of these embryos were morphologically abnormal, including 4 of the 8 preimplantation embryos. Because the 4 preimplantation losses would not have been recognized clinically, there would have been 6 losses recorded in the remaining 30 pregnancies.

By using sensitive pregnancy tests, it has been suggested that the total rate of pregnancy loss after implantation is approximately 30%.[90] When the loss of fertilized oocytes before implantation is included, approximately 46% of all pregnancies end before the pregnancy is clinically perceived.[91]

In the postimplantation period, if only clinically diagnosed pregnancies are considered, the generally accepted figure for spontaneous miscarriage in the first trimester is 15%. Approximately 50–60% of these abortuses have chromosome abnormalities.[92] This suggests that a minimum of 7.5% of all human conceptions are chromosomally abnormal. The fact that only 1 in 200 newborns has a chromosome abnormality attests to the powerful selection mechanisms operating in early human gestation. In each ovulatory cycle, only 30% of normally fertile couples can achieve a pregnancy. Once conception is achieved, only 30% survive to birth.[52]

Key Steps in Fertilization

1. *Sperm penetration of the zona pellucida depends on a combination of sperm motility, an acrosomal proteinase, and binding of sperm head receptors to zona ligands.*

2. *Binding of sperm head receptors and zona ligands produces an enzyme complex that induces the acrosome reaction, releasing enzymes essential for the fusion of the sperm and oocyte membranes.*

3. *Fusion of the sperm and oocyte membranes triggers the cortical reaction, the release of substances from the cortical granules, organelles just below the egg cell membrane.*

4. *The cortical reaction leads to the enzyme-induced zona reaction, the hardening of the zona and the inactivation of ligands for sperm receptors, producing an obstacle to polyspermy.*

5. *Cell division begins promptly after fertilization; human gene expression begins between the 4- and 8-cell stages.*

Implantation and Placentation

A normal pregnancy is, of course, impossible without successful implantation and placentation. Because there are differences among the various species, we will focus on the physical and biochemical events that are relevant in human reproduction.[93] Shortly after the 8-cell morula enters the uterine cavity about 4 days after the gonadotropin surge and 3 days after ovulation, a blastocyst (a preimplantation embryo of varying cell number, from 30 to 200) is formed. Implantation (the embedding of the blastocyst in the endometrial stroma) begins with the loss of the zona pellucida (hatching) about 1–3 days after the morula enters the uterine cavity.

Preparation for Implantation

The change from proliferative to secretory endometrium, described in detail in Chapter 4, is an essential part of achieving the receptive conditions required for implantation. The primary endocrine requirement is the presence of progesterone; in the monkey, implantation and pregnancy can be achieved in the absence of luteal phase estrogen.[94] This change is the histologic expression of many biochemical and molecular events. The endometrium is 10–14 mm thick at the time of implantation in the midluteal phase. By this time, secretory activity has reached a peak, and the endometrial cells are rich in glycogen and lipids. Understanding the dynamic endocrine behavior of the endometrium (Chapter 4) increases the appreciation for its active participation in the implantation process. The window of endometrial receptivity is restricted to days 16–22 of a 28-day normal cycle, and days 16–19 of cycles stimulated by exogenous gonadotropins.[47, 95–97] Endometrial receptivity is heralded by formation of ***pinopodes***, surface epithelial microvilli that exhibit a cystic change, appearing and regressing during the window of receptivity.[98] The pinopodes may serve to absorb fluid from the uterine cavity forcing the blastocyst to be in contact with the endometrial epithelium.

Even before the blastocyst adheres to the surface epithelium, but after hatching from the zona pellucida, a dialogue between the mother and the early embryo has begun. Early pregnancy factor (EPF) can be detected in the maternal circulation within 1–2 days after fertilization.[99] EPF prior to implantation is apparently produced by the ovary in response to a signal from the embryo. After implantation, EPF is no longer secreted by the ovary but is derived from the embryo. EPF has immunosuppressive properties and is associated with cell proliferation and growth.

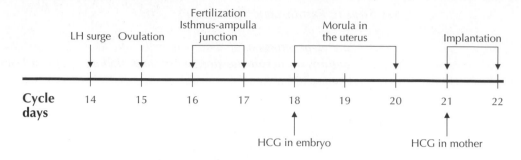

Blastocysts grown in culture produce and secrete human chorionic gonadotropin (HCG), beginning days 7–8 after fertilization.[100] Messenger RNA for HCG can be found in 6- to 8-cell human embryos.[101] Because the 8- to 12-cell stage is achieved about 3 days after fertilization, it is believed that the human embryo begins to produce HCG before implantation when it can be detected in the mother (about 6–7 days after ovulation). The embryo is capable, therefore, of preimplantation signaling, and higher levels of estradiol and progesterone can be measured in the maternal circulation even before maternal HCG is detectable, presumably because of stimulation of the corpus luteum by HCG delivered directly from the uterine cavity to the ovary.[102] Function of the corpus luteum is crucial during the first 7–9 weeks of pregnancy, and luteectomy early in pregnancy can precipitate abortion.[103] Similarly, early pregnancy loss in primates can be induced by injections of anti-HCG serum.[104] Another substance secreted very early by the preimplantation embryo is platelet-activating factor, perhaps part of the immunosuppressive activity required to induce maternal tolerance of the embryo. It is not surprising that various growth factors are produced by the early embryo.[105]

In rodents and rabbits, implantation can be interrupted by injection of prostaglandin inhibitors.[106, 107] Indomethacin prevents the increase in endometrial vascular permeability normally seen just prior to implantation. Additional evidence for a role by prostaglandins in the earliest stages of implantation is the finding of increased concentrations at implantation sites, similar to any inflammatory response.[108] The blastocysts of mice, rabbits, sheep, and cows produce prostaglandins, and prostaglandin E_2 release from human blastocysts and embryos has been demonstrated.[109] The secretory endometrial epithelial cells are also a source of prostaglandin E_2 (but not prostaglandin $F_{2\alpha}$), and its synthesis may be stimulated by the tissue response that accompanies implantation. However, decidual synthesis of prostaglandins is significantly reduced compared with proliferative and secretory endometrium, apparently a direct effect of progesterone activity and perhaps a requirement in order to maintain the pregnancy.[108] Nevertheless, prostaglandin E_2 synthesis is increased at the implantation site, perhaps in response to blastocyst factors, e.g., platelet-activating factor, and correlates with an increase in vascular permeability.[108, 110] In the rabbit, platelet-activating factor also induces the production of early pregnancy factor (discussed above).[111]

As discussed in Chapter 4, the many cytokines, peptides, and lipids secreted by the endometrium are interrelated through the stimulating and inhibiting actions of estrogen and progesterone, as well as the autocrine/paracrine activities of these substances on each other. The response to implantation certainly involves the many members of the growth factor and cytokine families.

Implantation

Implantation is defined as the process by which an embryo attaches to the uterine wall and penetrates first the epithelium and then the circulatory system of the mother to form the placenta. It is a process that is limited in both time and space. Implantation begins 2–3 days after the fertilized egg enters the uterus on day 18 or 19 of the cycle.[97] Thus, implantation occurs 5–7 days after fertilization. The implantation site in the human uterus is usually in the upper, posterior wall in the midsagittal plane. Implantation consists of 3 stages: apposition, adhesion, and invasion (also called migration to denote its benign nature).

Apposition and Adhesion

The human blastocyst remains in the uterine secretions for approximately 1 to 3 days and then hatches from its zona pellucida in preparation for attachment. Implantation is marked initially by apposition of the blastocyst to the uterine epithelium, usually about 2–4 days after the morula enters the uterine cavity. A prerequisite for this contact is a loss of the zona pellucida, which, in vitro, can be ruptured by contractions and expansions of the blastocyst. In vivo, this activity is less critical, because the zona can be lysed by components of the uterine fluid. Nevertheless, blastocyst movement and escape from the zona pellucida appear to involve cytoplasmic projections (this leads to penetrations of the zona by the trophectoderm prior to zona hatching).[112] By this time, the blastocyst has differentiated into an inner cell mass (embryo) and trophectoderm (placenta), both essential for implantation.

The endometrial production of at least 3 cytokines appears to be involved in implantation.[113] These are colony-stimulating factor-1 (CSF-1), leukemia-inhibitory factor (LIF), and interleukin-1 (IL-1). CSF-1 expression and receptors for CSF-1 are found in both the human endometrium (peaking in decidua) and the preimplantation embryo. Mice with an inactivating mutation in the CSF-1 gene are infertile because of low rates of implantation and fetal viability.[114] LIF displays the same pattern of expression as CSF-1, and mice with an LIF gene mutation have a failure of blastocyst implantation.[115, 116] Blocking the interleukin-1 receptor in mice also prevents implantation.[113] However, the role of interleukin-1 is less clear because mice that are deficient in the interleukin receptor have normal reproduction.[117] Perhaps the first maternal change in the implantation process, increased permeability of the capillaries near the adherent blastocyst, is due to a blastocyst-directed change in heparin-binding epidermal growth factor (HB-EGF) expression in the surface epithelium.[118] In addition, the blastocyst contains receptors for epidermal growth factor that respond to HB-EGF and promote growth and zona hatching.

The adhesion process further involves a whole collection of adhesion molecules, including integrins and selectins. The decidualized endometrium and the early embryo express extracellular matrix components, especially laminin and fibronectin, which mediate cell adhesion via the adhesion molecules.[119] Cells are fixed and supported by the extracellular matrix utilizing components such as laminin and fibronectin with attachments to these components via cell surface receptors, especially the integrins. An increase in specific isoforms of laminin in decidua at the time of implantation suggests an important interaction with the invading trophoblast.[120] Thus implantation starts with adhesion due to binding with endometrial integrins, followed by invasion (migration) of the trophoblast by proteinase degradation of the extracellular matrix.

Integrins are members of a family of transmembrane cell surface receptors for collagen, fibronectin, and laminin. Integrins are utilized in cell-cell and cell-matrix interactions, contributing to cell migration, cell differentiation, and tissue structure. A cyclic change in integrin expression in the endometrial epithelial cells indicates peak expression at the time of implantation.[121] It has been suggested that a lack of integrin expression during the implantation window can be a cause of infertility.[122] The blastocyst also expresses integrins in a time sequence and at a site (outgrowing trophoblast cells) that are appropriate for key activity during implantation.[123]

The process of tissue disruption is accompanied by an increase in lymphocytes, another source for cytokines and growth factors in addition to trophoblast and endometrial cells. The distinction between cytokines and growth factors is not always clear, but T lymphocytes and macrophages are significant secretors of cytokines.

In general, cytokines, growth factors, and their receptors have been identified in virtually all tissues associated with implantation. The cataloging is lengthy and often confusing.[113, 124] It is helpful to simply view these various substances as the biochemical tools by which the physical process of trophoblast adhesion and invasion is accomplished.

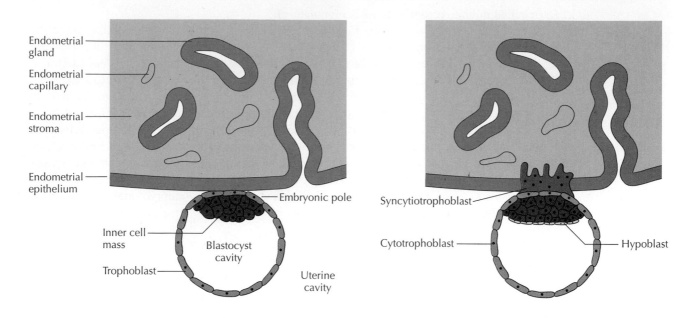

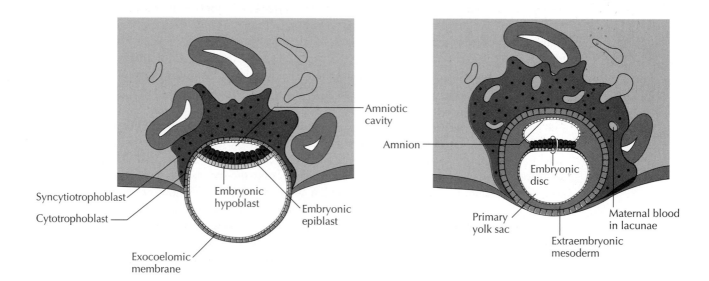

Even if the hormonal milieu and protein composition of the uterine fluid are hospitable to the implantation, it may not occur if the embryo is not at the proper stage of development. It has been inferred from this information that there must be developmental maturation of the surface of the embryo before it is able to achieve attachment and implantation.

Reports on changes in the surface charge of preimplantation embryos differ in their findings, and it is unlikely that changes in surface charge are solely responsible for adherence of the blastocyst to the surface of epithelial cells. Binding of the lectin concanavalin A to the blastocyst changes during the preimplantation period, an indication that the surface glycoproteins of the blastocyst are in transition.[125] It is reasonable to assume that these changes in configuration on the surface occur in order to enhance the ability of the early embryo to adhere to the maternal surface.

As the blastocyst comes into close contact with the endometrium, the microvilli on the surface flatten and interdigitate with those on the luminal surface of the epithelial cells. A stage is reached where the cell membranes are in very close contact and junctional complexes are formed. The early embryo can no longer be dislodged from the surface of the epithelial cells by flushing the uterus with physiologic solutions.

Invasion and Placentation

In the second week after ovulation, the placenta is formed.[119] By this time, the trophoblasts at the implantation site have formed masses of cytotrophoblasts and syncytiotrophoblasts, and invasion of maternal blood vessels has begun. The walls of the spiral arteries are destroyed, as sinusoidal sacs are formed lined with endovascular trophoblast.

Three types of interactions between the implanting trophoblast and the uterine epithelium have been described.[126] In the first, trophoblast cells intrude between uterine epithelial cells on their path to the basement membrane. In the second type of interaction, the epithelial cells lift off the basement membrane, an action that allows the trophoblast to insinuate itself underneath the epithelium. Last, fusion of trophoblast with individual uterine epithelial cells has been identified by electron microscopy in the rabbit.[127] This latter method of gaining entry into the epithelial layer raises interesting questions about the immunologic consequences of mixing embryonic and maternal cytoplasm.

Trophoblast has the ability to phagocytose a variety of cells, but, in vivo, this activity seems largely confined to removal of dead endometrial cells, or cells that have been sloughed from the uterine wall. Similarly, despite the invasive nature of the trophoblast, destruction of maternal cells by enzymes secreted by the embryo does not seem to play a major role in implantation; there is virtually no necrosis. The early embryo does secrete a variety of enzymes (e.g., collagenase and plasminogen activators), and these are important for digesting the intercellular matrix that holds the epithelial cells together. Studies in vitro have demonstrated the presence of plasminogen activator in mouse embryos and in human trophoblast, and its activity is important in the attachment and early outgrowth stages of implantation.[128, 129] Urokinase and proteases, trophoblastic enzymes that convert plasminogen to plasmin, are inhibited by HCG, indicating regulation of this process by the embryo.[130]

The trophoblast at a somewhat later stage of implantation can digest, in vitro, a complex matrix composed of glycoproteins, elastin, and collagen, all of which are components of the normal intercellular matrix.[131, 132] Additional studies in vitro have shown that cells move away from trophoblast in a process called "contact inhibition."[133] Trophoblast then spreads to fill the spaces vacated by the cocultured cells. Once the intracellular matrix has been lysed, this movement of epithelial cells away from trophoblast would allow space for the implanting embryo to move through the epithelial layer. Trophoblast movement is aided by the fact that only parts of its surface are adhesive, and the major portion of the surface is nonadhesive to other cells.

The highly proliferative phase of trophoblastic tissue during early embryogenesis is regulated by the many growth factors and cytokines produced in both fetal and maternal tissues. Invasion of the early trophoblast requires the expression of integrins, stimulated by insulin-like growth factor-II and inhibited by transforming growth factor-β.[134]

Actively migrating trophoblast cells have a different integrin profile than nonmigrating cells, specifically cell surface receptors that preferentially bind laminin.[119, 135] The controlling mechanism (not yet known) for this change in integrin expression must be a key regulator of trophoblast invasion. The specific nature of integrin expression can determine binding to matrix components, a requirement for migration.

Integrin cell surface binding for the matrix components can be also regulated by activating and inactivating the integrins. This would allow trophoblast cells to alternate between adhesive and nonadhesive states, thus achieving directional cell migration.[136] The role of integrin cell surface receptors is not simply to bind to a structural component. Binding activates cellular signaling pathways (similar to the classic endocrine tropic hormone-cell membrane receptor pathway) that activate enzymes that ultimately produce adhesion as well as cellular gene transcription.[119]

The uterine spiral arterioles are invaded by cytotrophoblasts, and the maternal endothelium is replaced by cytotrophoblast tissue as far as the first third of the myometrium. The maternal

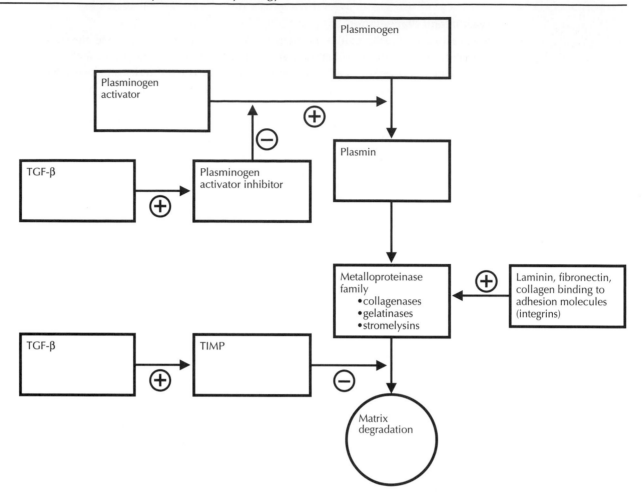

vascular invasion by trophoblast cells and replacement of vascular endothelium with endovascular trophoblast may utilize a different class of surface molecules, the selectin family.[119] The selectins have been demonstrated to be present in decidual vascular endothelial cells, but only at the site of implantation. The selectins are responsive to inflammatory mediators, including cytokines. As the trophoblast cells replace maternal endothelium, the receptor profile for adhesion peptides of the trophoblast changes to resemble endothelial cells.[137] It has been long recognized that this invasion process is limited in pregnancies with preeclampsia. The relative failure in this process in preeclampsia is characterized by insufficient conversion to endothelial adhesion receptors.[138]

The matrix metalloproteinases, significantly involved in the process of menstruation (Chapter 4), are also key players in matrix degradation during trophoblast invasion. The metalloproteinases include collagenases, gelatinases, and the stromelysins. Integrin-mediated adhesion can activate this family of proteolytic enzymes, which then accomplish the degradation of matrix proteins that is necessary in order for trophoblast migration to take place. Production of the metalloproteinases is regulated by the combined actions of plasminogen activators, cytokines, and tissue inhibitors (TIMP).

Further penetration and survival depend on factors that are capable of suppressing the maternal immune response to paternal antigens. The endometrial tissue makes a significant contribution to growth factor activity and immune suppression by synthesizing proteins in response to the blastocyst even before implantation.[139, 140] One of the great mysteries associated with implantation is the mechanism by which the mother rejects a genetically abnormal embryo or fetus. It is possible that the abnormal embryo cannot produce a signal in early pregnancy that can be recognized by the mother.

The embryonic signals will be effective only in a proper hormone milieu. Much of the knowledge concerning the hormone requirements for implantation in animals has been gained from studies of animals with delayed implantation. In a number of species, preimplantation embryos normally lie dormant in the uterus for periods of time, which may extend for as long as 15 months before implantation is initiated. In other species, delayed implantation can be imposed by postpartum suckling or by performing ovariectomy on day 3 of pregnancy. This produces a marked decrease in synthesis of DNA and protein by the blastocyst. The embryo can be maintained at the blastocyst stage by injecting the mother with progesterone. Using this model, hormonal requirements for implantation have been determined. In mice, there is a requirement for estrogen and progesterone. In other species, including the primate, the nidatory stimulus of estrogen is not required, and progesterone alone is sufficient.[94]

Although it is known that the hormone milieu of delayed implantation renders the embryo quiescent, it is not known whether this represents a direct effect on the embryo or whether there is a metabolic inhibitor present in uterine secretions that acts upon the embryo. Removal of the embryo from the uterus to culture dishes allows rapid resumption of normal metabolism, suggesting that there has, in fact, been a release from the inhibitory effects of a uterine product.

Limitation of Invasion

Invasion of the endometrial stromal compartment, breaching of the basement membrane, and penetration of maternal blood vessels are mediated by serine proteases and metalloproteinases. The serine proteases are plasminogen activators that provide plasmin for proteolytic degradation of the extracellular matrix. Plasmin activates the metalloproteinase family. Trophoblast cells contain plasminogen activator receptors. Binding of plasminogen activator to this receptor is believed to be a method by which plasmin proteolysis is exerted in a controlled and limited site.[141]

Many components of the inflammatory response play roles in the process of implantation. Cytokine secretion from the lymphocyte infiltrate in the endometrium activates cellular lysis of trophoblast, perhaps an important process in limiting invasion.[142] The decidua at the time of implantation contains a large number of natural killer cells (large granular lymphocytes). It has been proposed that an interaction between these cells and a human leukocyte antigen uniquely present in invading trophoblast limits invasion by producing appropriate cytokines.[143]

Invasion by the trophoblast is limited by the formation of the decidual cell layer in the uterus. Fibroblast-like cells in the stroma are transformed into glycogen and lipid-rich cells. In the human, decidual cells surround blood vessels late in the nonpregnant cycle, but extensive decidualization does not occur until pregnancy is established. Ovarian steroids govern decidualization, and in the human a combination of estrogen and progesterone is critical.

Histamine may initiate the decidual response.[144] Antihistamines given systemically or directly into the uterus prevent the decidual response in rats. This was disputed when other workers found that systemic antihistamines were not effective in preventing the decidual response. However, there are two different receptors for histamines, H1 and H2. These are not blocked by the same agents, and early experiments demonstrating a lack of effect of antihistamines may have utilized only a block to one receptor. Blockage of both receptors in rats is followed by a decrease in the number of implantation sites.[145] Mast cells in the uterus are a major source of histamine, but it is possible that the embryo can also synthesize histamine.[146]

More recently, limitation of trophoblastic invasion is attributed to the balance of promoting and restraining growth factors, cytokines, and enzymes. Plasminogen activator inhibitor-1 (PAI-1) is a major product of decidual cells, inhibiting excessive bleeding during menses and restraining trophoblast invasion in early pregnancy.[147] PAI-1 binds plasminogen activator with a high affinity and is regulated by cytokines and growth factors. The metalloproteinases that degrade the extracellular matrix components, such as collagens, gelatins, fibronectin, and laminin, are restrained by tissue inhibitors of metalloproteinases (TIMP). In addition, metalloproteinase degradation can be suppressed by inhibiting trophoblast production of these enzymes and by preventing conversion from an inactive to an active form.[148] Decidual TGF-β is a key growth factor involved in limitation of trophoblast invasion by inducing the expression of both TIMP and PAI-1. In addition, TGF-β can inhibit integrin expression and influence cytotrophoblasts to differentiate into non-invasive syncytiotrophoblasts.[134, 149] Even human chorionic gonadotropin (HCG) may exert a governing force by inhibiting protease activity.[130, 150]

Key Steps in Implantation

1. *The early embryo enters the uterine cavity as an 8-cell morula and becomes a 30 to 200-cell blastocyst before implantation.*

2. *Implantation begins with hatching from the zona pellucida about 1–3 days after the morula entered the uterine cavity.*

3. *The endometrium is prepared for implantation by the complex activity of cytokines, growth factors, and lipids modulated by the sex hormones, especially progesterone. The endometrium is receptive for implantation for only a few days.*

4. *The process of implantation begins with apposition and adhesion of the blastocyst to the uterine epithelium, about 2–4 days after the morula enters the uterine cavity. This process is mediated by cytokines and involves adhesion molecules (integrins) that interact with extracellular components, especially laminin and fibronectin.*

5. *Trophoblastic invasion rapidly follows adhesion of the blastocyst, mediated by proteinase degradation of the extracellular matrix. The placenta is formed in the second week after ovulation. Limitation of trophoblastic invasion is due to a restraint imposed by proteinase inhibitors, especially plasminogen activator inhibitor and tissue inhibitors of metalloproteinases.*

Unanswered Questions

Why is gamete production so wasteful? Billions of sperm are produced, but only a few are ever successful in fertilizing an egg. Does it relate to early forms of reproduction; e.g., those in fish, where the sperm are released into the sea and large numbers are needed to ensure that a few reach the egg? Does the overpopulation of sperm allow selection processes to take place, ensuring that the more abnormal sperm are filtered out before the tube is reached? In the human female, approximately 400 ova are ovulated during a woman's life, yet the ovaries contain millions of eggs at birth.

What is the purpose of capacitation? Is it needed to overcome the protective mechanisms that have been built into the sperm, specifically those that prevent premature release of acrosomal enzymes? Penetration by sperm of the egg is desirable, but invasion of other maternal cells might trigger immunologic reactions against sperm. Capacitation does free the sperm from some inhibitors, thus allowing the hypermotility that may be needed for zona penetration.

Why are there so many abnormal embryos? Current estimates are that 50% of embryos in young women and 70% in older women do not survive to term. Why is there a high rate of embryo loss, and, specifically, why is there a high selection against abnormal embryos? Is it because of intrinsic programming defects within the embryo or an inability of the embryo to produce a signal recognized by the mother, or does the maternal organism in some way recognize abnormality and react against it?

Why has embryo transfer in the human following in vitro fertilization resulted in a low number of takes? Can the uterine environment be manipulated in such a way as to increase successful implantation of in vitro fertilization eggs?

References

1. **Medvei VC,** *The History of Clinical Endocrinology,* The Parthenon Publishing Group, New York, 1993.

2. **Bedford JM,** The contraceptive potential of fertilization: a physiological perspective, *Hum Reprod* 9:842, 1994.

3. **Foldesy RG, Bedford JM,** Biology of the scrotum. I. Temperature and androgens as determinants of the sperm storage capacity of the rat cauda epididymis, *Biol Reprod* 26:673, 1982.

4. **Silber SJ, Ord T, Balmaceda J, Patrizio P, Asch RH,** Congenital absence of the vas deferens. The fertilizing capacity of human epididymal sperm, *New Engl J Med* 323:1788, 1990.

5. **Devroey P, Liu J, Nagy Z, Tournaye H, Silber S, Van Steirteghem AC,** Normal fertilization of human oocytes after testicular sperm extraction and intracytoplasmic sperm injection, *Fertil Steril* 62:639, 1994.

6. **Sobrero AJ, MacLeod J,** The immediate postcoital test, *Fertil Steril* 13:184, 1962.

7. **Bedford JM,** The rate of sperm passage into the cervix after coitus in the rabbit, *J Reprod Fertil* 25:211, 1971.

8. **Yudin AI, Hanson FW, Katz DF,** Human cervical mucus and its interaction with sperm: fine structural view, *Biol Reprod* 40:661, 1989.

9. **Wang C, Baker HWG, Jennings MG, Burger HG, Lutjen P,** Interaction between human cervical mucus and sperm surface antibodies, *Fertil Steril* 44:484, 1985.

10. **Morales P, Katz DF, Overstreet JW, Samuels SJ, Chang RJ,** The relationship between the motility and morphology of spermatozoa in human semen, *J Androl* 9:241, 1988.

11. **Katz D, Morales P, Samuels SJ, Overstreet JW,** Mechanisms of filtration of morphologically abnormal human sperm by cervical mucus, *Fertil Steril* 54:513, 1990.

12. **Krzanowska H,** The passage of abnormal spermatozoa through the uterotubal junction of the mouse, *J Reprod Fertil* 38:81, 1974.

13. **Settlage DSF, Motoshima M, Tredway DR,** Sperm transport from the external cervical os to the fallopian tubes in women: a time and quantitation study, *Fertil Steril* 24:655, 1973.

14. **Overstreet JW, Cooper GW,** Sperm transport in the reproductive tract of the female rabbit. I. Rapid transit phase and transport, *Biol Reprod* 19:101, 1978.

15. **Perloff WH, Steinberger E,** In vivo survival of spermatozoa in cervical mucus, *Am J Obstet Gynecol* 88:439, 1964.

16. **Williams M, Hill CJ, Scudamore I, Dunphy B, Cooke ID, Barratt CLR,** Sperm numbers and distribution within the human fallopian tube around ovulation, *Hum Reprod* 8:2019, 1993.

17. **Gould JE, Overstreet JW, Hanson FW,** Assessment of human sperm function after recovery from the female reproductive tract, *Biol Reprod* 31:888, 1984.

18. **Barratt CLR, Cooke ID,** Sperm transport in the human female reproductive trace—a dynamic interaction, *Int J Androl* 14:394, 1991.

19. **Katz DF, Drobnis EZ, Overstreet JW,** Factors regulating mammalian sperm migration through the female reproductive tract and oocyte vestments, *Gamete Res* 22:443, 1989.

20. **Overstreet JW, Katz DF, Yudin AI,** Cervical mucus and sperm transport in reproduction, *Seminars Perinatol* 15:149, 1991.

21. **Chang MC,** Fertilizing capacity of spermatozoa deposited into the fallopian tubes, *Nature* 168:697, 1951.

22. **Austin CR,** Observations on the penetration of the sperm into the mammalian egg, *Aust J Sci Res (Ser B)* 4:581, 1951.

23. **Zaneveld LJD, De Jonge CJ, Anderson RA, Mack SR,** Human sperm capacitation and the acrosome reaction, *Hum Reprod* 6:1265, 1991.

24. **Yanagimachi R,** Capacitation and the acrosome reaction, In: Asch R, Balmaceda JP, Johnston I, eds. *Gamete Physiology,* Serono Symposia, Norewell, Massachusetts, 1990, p 31.

25. **Cross NL, Morales P, Overstreet JW, Hanson FW,** Induction of acrosome reactions by the human zona pellucida, *Biol Reprod* 38:235, 1988.

26. **Suarez SS, Wolf DP, Meizel S,** Induction of the acrosome reaction in human spermatozoa by a fraction of human follicular fluid, *Gamete Res* 14:107, 1986.

27. **Aitken RJ,** Molecular mechanisms regulating human sperm function, *Mol Hum Reprod* 3:169, 1997.

28. **de Lamirande E, Leclerc P, Gagnon C,** Capacitation as a regulatory event that primes spermatozoa for the acrosome reaction and fertilization, *Mol Hum Reprod* 3:175, 1997.

29. **Ravnik SE, Zarutskie PW, Muller CH,** Purification and characterization of a human follicular fluid lipid transfer protein that stimulates human sperm capacitation, *Biol Reprod* 47:1126, 1992.

30. **Benoff S, Hurley I, Cooper GW, Mandel FS, Rosenfeld DL, Hershag A,** Head-specific mannose-ligand receptor expression in human spermatozoa is dependent on capacitation-associated membrane cholesterol loss, *Hum Reprod* 8:2141, 1993.

31. **Overstreet JW, Gould JE, Katz DF,** In vitro capacitation of human spermatozoa after passage through a column of cervical mucus, *Fertil Steril* 34:604, 1980.

32. **Ducibella T,** Mammalian egg cortical granules and the cortical reaction, In: Wassarman PM, ed. *Elements of Mammalian Fertilization,* CRC Press, Boca Raton, Florida, 1991, p 206.

33. **Sharma V, Mason B, Riddle A, Campbell S,** Peritoneal oocyte and sperm transfer, Fifth World Congress on In Vitro Fertilization and Embryo Transfer, Norfolk, Virginia 1987.

34. **Clewe TH, Mastroianni L,** Mechanisms of ovum pickup: I. Functional capacity of rabbit oviducts ligated near the fimbriae, *Fertil Steril* 9:13, 1958.

35. **Crow J, Amso NN, Lewin J, Shaw RW,** Morphology and ultrastructure of Fallopian tube epithelium at different stages of the menstrual cycle and menopause, *Hum Reprod* 9:2224, 1994.

36. **Tao A,** How the myosalpinx works in gamete and embryo transfer, *Arch Biol Med Exp* 24:361, 1991.

37. **Halbert SA, Tam PY, Blandau RJ,** Egg transport in the rabbit oviduct: the roles of cilia and muscle, *Science* 191:1052, 1976.

38. **Eddy CA, Flores JJ, Archer DR, Pauerstein CJ,** The role of cilia in infertility: an evaluation by selective microsurgical modification of the rabbit oviduct, *Am J Obstet Gynecol* 132:814, 1978.

39. **Halbert SA, Patton DL, Zarutskie PW, Soules MR,** Fuction and structure of cilia in the Fallopian tube of an infertile woman with Kartagener's syndrome, *Hum Reprod* 12:55, 1997.

40. **Gordts S, Campo R, Rombauts L, Brosens I,** Endoscopic visualization of the process of fimbrial ovum retrieval in the human, *Hum Reprod* 13:1425, 1998.

41. **Croxatto HB, Ortiz MS,** Egg transport in the fallopian tube, *Gynecol Invest* 6:215, 1975.

42. **Pauerstein CJ, Eddy CA,** The role of the oviduct in reproduction; our knowledge and our ignorance, *J Reprod Fertil* 55:223, 1979.

43. **Tompkins P,** Letter to the editor, *Fertil Steril* 31:696, 1979.

44. **Novy MJ,** Reversal of Kroener fimbriectomy sterilization, *Am J Obstet Gynecol* 137:198, 1980.

45. **Glass RH,** Fate of rabbit eggs fertilized in the uterus, *J Reprod Fertil* 31:139, 1972.

46. **Adams CE,** Consequences of accelerated ovum transport, including a re-evaluation of Estes' operation, *J Reprod Fertil* 55:239, 1979.

47. **Rosenwaks Z,** Donor eggs: their application in modern reproductive technologies, *Fertil Steril* 47:895, 1987.

48. **Ikle FA,** Pregnancy after implantation of the ovary into the uterus, *Gynaecologia* 151:95, 1961.

49. **Tesarik J, Mendoza C,** Nongenomic effects of 17β-estradiol on maturing human oocytes: relationship to oocyte developmental potential, *J Clin Endocrinol Metab* 80:1438, 1995.

50. **Taylor CT, Lawrence YM, Kingand CR, Biljan MM, Cuthbertson KSR,** Oscillations in intracellular free calcium induced by spermatozoa in human oocytes at fertilization, *Hum Reprod* 8:2174, 1993.

51. **France JT, Graham FM, Gosling L, Hair P, Knox BS,** Characteristics of natural conception cycles occurring in a prospective study of sex preselection: fertility awareness symptoms, hormone levels, sperm survival, and pregnancy outcome, *Int J Fertil* 37:244, 1992.

52. **Wilcox AJ, Weinberg CR, Baird DD,** Timing of sexual intercourse in relation to ovulation — effects in the probability of conception, survival of the pregnancy, and sex of the baby, *New Engl J Med* 333:1517, 1995.

53. **Ralt D, Goldenberg M, Fetterolf P, Thompson D, Dor J, Mashiach S, Garbers DL, Eisenbach M,** Sperm attraction to a follicular factor(s) correlates with human egg fertilizability, *Proc Natl Acad Sci USA* 88:2840, 1991.

54. **Eisenbach M, Ralt D,** Precontact mammalian sperm-egg communication and role in fertilization, *Am J Physiol* 262:1095, 1992.

55. **Cohen-Dayag A, Tur-Kaspa I, Dor J, Mashiach S, Eisenbach M,** Sperm capacitation in humans is transient and correlates with chemotactic responsiveness to follicular factors, *Proc Natl Acad Sci USA* 92:11039, 1995.

56. **Talbot P,** Sperm penetration through oocyte investments in mammals, *Am J Anat* 174:331, 1985.

57. **Dietl JA, Rauth G,** Molecular aspects of mammalian fertilization, *Hum Reprod* 4:869, 1989.

58. **Wassarman PM,** Gamete interactions during mammalian fertilization, *Theriogenology* 41:31, 1994.

59. **Hartmann JF, Gwatkin RBL,** Alteration of sites on the mammalian sperm surface following capacitation, *Nature* 234:479, 1971.

60. **Zaneveld LJD, Polakoski KL, Williams WL,** Properties of a proteolytic enzyme from rabbit sperm acrosomes, *Biol Reprod* 6:30, 1972.

61. **Jones R,** Identification and functions of mammalian sperm-egg recognition molecules during fertilization, *J Reprod Fertil* 42(Suppl):89, 1990.

62. **Shabanowitz RB, O'Rand MG,** Characterization of the human zona pellucida from fertilized and unfertilized eggs, *J Reprod Fertil* 82:151, 1988.

63. **Dean J,** Biology of mammalian fertilization: role of the zona pellucida, *J Clin Invest* 89:1055, 1992.

64. **Rankin T, Dean J,** The molecular genetics of the zona pellucida: mouse mutations and infertility, *Mol Hum Reprod* 2:889, 1996.

65. **Liu C, Litscher ES, Mortillo S, Sakai Y, Kinloch RA, Stewart CL, Wassarman PM,** Targeted disruption of the ZP3 gene results in production of eggs lacking a zona pellucida and infertility in female mice, *Proc Natl Acad Sci USA* 93:5431, 1996.

66. **Wassarman PM,** Mouse gamete adhesion molecules, *Biol Reprod* 46:86, 1992.

67. **Leyton L, LeGuen P, Bunch D, Saling PM,** Regulation of mouse gamete interaction by a sperm tyrosine kinase, *Proc Natl Acad Sci USA* 89:11692, 1992.

68. **Burks DJ, Carballada R, Moore HD, Saling PM,** Interaction of a tyrosine kinase from human sperm with the zona pellucida at fertilization, *Science* 269:83, 1995.

69. **Florman HM, Tombes RM, First NL, Babcock DF,** An adhesion-associated agonist from the zona pellucida activates G protein-promoted elevations of internal Ca^{2+} and pH that mediate mammalian sperm acrosomal exocytosis, *Dev Biol* 135:133, 1989.

70. **Ward CR, Storey BT, Kopf GS,** Selective activation of G_{i1} and G_{i2} in mouse sperm by the zona pellucida, the egg's extracellular matrix, *J Biol Chem* 269:13254, 1994.

71. **O'Toole CMB, Roldan ERS, Fraser LR,** Protein kinase C activation during progesterone-stimulated acrosomal exocytosis in human spermatozoa, *Mol Hum Reprod* 2:921, 1996.

72. **Green DPL,** Mammalian fertilization as a biological machine: a working model for adhesion and fusion of sperm and oocyte, *Hum Reprod* 8:91, 1993.

73. **Lathrop WF, Carmichael EP, Myles DG, Primakoff P,** cDNA cloning reveals the molecular structure of a sperm surface protein, PH-20, involved in sperm-egg adhesion and the wide distribution of its gene among mammals, *J Cell Biol* 111:1939, 1990.

74. **Blobel CP, Wolfsberg TG, Turck CW, Myles DG, Primakoff P, White J,** A potential fusion peptide and an integrin ligand domain in a protein active in sperm-egg fusion, *Nature* 356:248, 1992.

75. **Lin Y, Mahan K, Lathrop WF, Myles DG, Primakoff P,** A hyaluronidase activity of the sperm plasma membrane protein PH-20 enables sperm to penetrate the cumulus cell layer surrounding the egg, *J Cell Biol* 125:1157, 1994.

76. **Fusi FM, Vignali M, Gailit J, Bronson Ra,** Mammalian oocytes exhibit specific recognition of the RGD (rg-Gly-Asp) tripeptide and express oolemmal integrins, *Mol Reprod Dev* 36:212, 1993.

77. **Fusi FM, Bernocchi N, Ferrari A, Bronson RA,** Is vitronectin the velcro that binds the gametes together? *Mol Hum Reprod* 2:859, 1996.

78. **Swann K,** Soluble sperm factors and Ca^{2+} release in eggs at fertilization, *Rev Reprod* 1:33, 1996.

79. **Sousa M, Mendoza C, Barros A, Tesarik J,** Calcium responses of human oocytes after intracytoplasmic injection of leukocytes, spermatocytes and round spermatids, *Mol Hum Reprod* 2:853, 1996.

80. **Parrington J, Swann K, Shevchenko VI, Sesay AK, Lai FA,** Calcium oscillations in mammalian eggs triggered by a soluble sperm protein, *Nature* 379:364, 1996.

81. **Barros C, Yanagimachi R,** Induction of zona reaction in golden hamster eggs by cortical granule material, *Nature* 233:2368, 1971.

82. **Sathananthan AH, Trounson AO,** Ultrastructure of cortical granule release and zona interaction in monospermic and polyspermic human ova fertilized *in vitro*, *Gamete Res* 6:225, 1982.

83. **Lopata A, Sathananthan AH, McBain JC, Johnston WIH, Speirs AL,** The ultrastructure of preovulatory human eggs fertilized in vitro, *Fertil Steril* 33:12, 1980.

84. **Balakier H, MacLusky NJ, Casper RF,** Characterization of the first cell cycle in human zygotes: Implications for cryopreservation, *Fertil Steril* 59:359, 1993.

85. **Braude P, Bolton V, Moore S,** Human gene expression first occurs between the four and eight cell stages of preimplantation development, *Nature* 332:459, 1988.

86. **Artley JK, Braude PR,** Biochemistry of the preimplantation embryo, *Assist Reprod Rev* 3:13, 1993.

87. **Hurst PR, Jefferies K, Eckstein P, Wheeler AG,** Recovery of uterine embryos in rhesus monkeys, *Biol Reprod* 15:429, 1976.

88. **Hendrickx AG, Kraemer DC,** Preimplantation stages of baboon embryos, *Anat Rec* 162:111, 1968.

89. **Hertig AT, Rock J, Adams EC, Menkin MC,** Thirty-four fertilized ova, good, bad and indifferent from 210 women of known fertility, *Pediatrics* 23:202, 1959.

90. **Wilcox AJ, Weiberg CR, O'Connor JF, Baird DD, Schlatterer JP, Canfield RE, Armstrong EG, Nisula BC,** Incidence of early loss of pregnancy, *New Engl J Med* 319:189, 1988.

91. **Little AB,** There's many a slip 'twixt' implantation and the crib (editorial), *New Engl J Med* 319:241, 1988.

92. **Ohno M, Maeda T, Matsunobu A,** A cytogenetic study of spontaneous abortions with direct analysis of chorionic villi, *Obstet Gynecol* 77:394, 1991.

93. **Tabibzadeh S, Babaknia A,** The signals and molecular pathways involved in implantation, a symbiotic interaction between blastocyst and endometrium involving adhesion and tissue invasion, *Mol Hum Reprod* 1:1579, 1995.

94. **Ghosh D, De P, Sengupta J,** Luteal phase ovarian oestrogen is not essential for implantation and maintenance of pregnancy from surrogate embryo transfer in the rhesus monkey, *Hum Reprod* 9:629, 1994.

95. **Psychoyos A,** Uterine receptivity for nidation, *Ann NY Acad Sci* 476:36, 1986.

96. **Formigli L, Formigli G, Roccio C,** Donation of fertilized uterine ova to infertile women, *Fertil Steril* 47:162, 1987.

97. **Navot RW, Scott RT, Doresch K, Veeck LL, Liu HC, Rosenwaks Z,** The window of embryo transfer and the efficiency of human conception *in vitro*, *Fertil Steril* 55:114, 1991.

98. **Martel D, Frydman R, Glissant M, Maggioni C, Roche D, Psychoyos A,** Scanning electron microscopy of postovulatory human endometrium in spontaneous cycles and cycles stimulated by hormone treatment, *J Endocrinol* 114:319, 1987.

99. **Morton H, Rolfe BE, Cavanagh AC,** Early pregnancy factor, *Seminars Reprod Endocrinol* 10:72, 1992.

100. **Lopata A, Hay D,** The surplus human embryo: its potential for growth, blastulation, hatching, and human chorionic gonadotropin production in culture, *Fertil Steril* 51:984, 1989.

101. **Bonduelle M, Dodd R, Liebaers I, Steirteghem A, Williamson R, Akhurst R,** Chorionic gonadotropin-β mRNA, a trophoblast marker, is expressed in human 8-cell embryos derived from tripronucleate zygotes, *Hum Reprod* 3:909, 1988.

102. **Stewart DR, Overstreet JW, Nakajima ST, Lasley BL,** Enhanced ovarian steroid secretion before implantation in early human pregnancy, *J Clin Endocrinol Metab* 76:1470, 1993.

103. **Csapo AL, Pulkkinen MO, Wiest WG,** Effects of luteectomy and progesterone replacement in early pregnant patients, *Am J Obstet Gynecol* 115:759, 1973.

104. **Stevens VC,** Potential control of fertility in women by immunization with HCG, *Res Reprod* 7:1, 1975.

105. **Hemmings R, Langlais J, Falcone T, Granger L, Miron P, Guyda H,** Human embryos produce transforming growth factor α activity and insulin-like growth factor II, *Fertil Steril* 58:101, 1992.

106. **Hoffman LH, Davenport GR, Brash AR,** Endometrial prostaglandins and phospholipase activity related to implantation in rabbits: effects of dexamethasone, *Biol Reprod* 38:544, 1984.

107. **Kennedy TG,** Interactions of eicosanoids and other factors in blastocyst implantation, In: Hiller K, ed. *Eicosanoids and Reproduction*, MTP Press, Lancaster, 1987, p 73.

108. **van der Weiden RMF, Helmerhorst FM, Keirse MJNC,** Influence of prostaglandins and platelet activating factor on implantation, *Hum Reprod* 6:436, 1991.

109. **Holmes PV, Sjogren A, Hamberger L,** Prostaglandin-E2 released by pre-implantation human conceptuses, *J Reprod Immunol* 17:79, 1989.

110. **Harper MJK,** Platelet-activating factor: a paracrine factor in preimplantation stages of reproduction? *Biol Reprod* 40:907, 1989.

111. **Sueoka K, Dharmarajan AM, Miyazaki T, Atlas SJ, Wallach E,** Platelet activating factor-induced early pregnancy factor activity from the perfused rabbit ovary and oviduct, *Am J Obstet Gynecol* 159:1580, 1988.

112. **Gonzales DS, Jones JM, Pinyopummintr T, Carnevale EM, Ginther OJ, Shapiro SS, Bavister BD,** Trophectoderm projections: a potential means for locomotion, attachment and implantation of bovine, equine and human blastocysts, *Hum Reprod* 11:2739, 1996.

113. **Simón C, Gimeno MJ, Mercader A, Francés A, Velasco JG, Remohi J, Polan ML, Pellicer A,** Cytokines–adhesion molecules-invasive proteinases. The missing paracrine/autocrine link in embryonic implantation? *Mol Hum Reprod* 2:405, 1996.

114. **Pollard JW, Hunt JS, Wiktor-Jedrzecjczak W, Stanley ER,** A pregnancy defect in the osteopetrotic (op/op) mouse demonstrates the requirement for CSF-1 in female fertility, *Dev Biol* 148:273, 1991.

115. **Stewart CL, Kaspar P, Brunet LJ, Bhatt H, Gadi I, Kontgen F, Abbondanzo SJ,** Blastocyst implantation depends on maternal expression of leukaemia inhibitory factor, *Nature* 359:76, 1992.

116. **Cullinan EB, Abbondanzo SJ, Anderson PS, Pollard JW, A LB, Stewart CL,** Leukemia inhibitory factor (LIF) and LIF receptor expression in human endometrium suggests a potential autocrine/paracrine function in regulating embryo implantation, *Proc Natl Acad Sci USA* 93:3115, 1996.

117. **Abbondanzo SJ, Cullinan EB, McIntyre K, Labow MA, Stewart CL,** Reproduction in mice lacking a functional type 1 IL-1 receptor, *Endocrinology* 137:3598, 1996.

118. **Das SK, Wang X-N, Paria BC, Damm D, Abraham JA, Klagsbrun M, Andrews GK, Dey SK,** Heparin-binding EGF-like growth factor gene is induced in the mouse uterus temporarily by the blastocyst solely at the site of its apposition: a possible ligand for interaction with blastocyst EGF-receptor in implantation, *Development* 120:1071, 1994.

119. **Burrows TD, King A, Loke YW,** Trophoblast migration during human placental implantation, *Hum Reprod Update* 2:307, 1996.

120. **Church HJ, Vicovac LM, Williams DL, Hey NA, Aplin JD,** Laminins 2 and 4 expressed by human decidual cells, *Lab Invest* 74:21, 1996.

121. **Lessey BA, Castelbaum AJ, Buck CA, Lei Y, Yowell CW, Sun J,** Further characterization of endometrial integrins during the menstrual cycle and in pregancy, *Fertil Steril* 62:497, 1994.

122. **Klentzeris LD, Bulmer JN, Trejdosiewicz LK, Morrison L, Cooke ID,** Beta-1 integrin cell adhesion molecules in the endometrium of fertile and infertile women, *Hum Reprod* 8:1223, 1994.

123. **Sutherland AE, Calarco PG, Damsky CH,** Developmental regulation of integrin expression at the time of implantation in the mouse embryo, *Development* 119:1175, 1993.

124. **Chard T,** Cytokines in implantation, *Hum Reprod Update* 1:385, 1995.

125. **Sobel JS, Nebel L,** Changes in concanavalin A agglutinability during development of the inner cell mass and trophoblast of mouse blastocyst in vitro, *J Reprod Fertil* 52:239, 1978.

126. **Schlafke S, Enders AC,** Cellular basis of interaction between trophoblast and uterus at implantation, *Biol Reprod* 12:41, 1975.

127. **Larsen JF,** Electron microscopy of the implantation site in the rabbit, *Am J Anat* 109:319, 1961.

128. **Strickland S, Reich E, Sherman MI,** Plasminogen activator in early embryogenesis: enzyme production by trophoblast and parietal endoderm, *Cell* 9:231, 1976.

129. **Queenan JT, Kao LC, Arboleda CE, Ulloa-Aguirre A, Golos TG, Cines DB, Strauss JF,** Regulation of urokinase-type plasminogen activator production by cultured human cytotrophoblasts, *J Biol Chem* 262:10903, 1987.

130. **Milwidsky A, Finci-Yeheskel Z, Yagel S, Mayer M,** Gonadotropin-mediated inhibition of proteolytic enzymes produced by human trophoblast in culture, *J Clin Endocrinol Metab* 76:1101, 1993.

131. **Glass RH, Aggeler J, Spindle A, Pedersen RA, Werb Z,** Degradation of extracellular matrix by mouse trophoblast outgrowths: a model for implantation, *J Cell Biol* 96:1108, 1983.

132. **Moll UM, Lane BL,** Proteolytic activity of first trimester human placenta: localization of interstitial collagenase in villous and extravillous trophoblast, *Histochemistry* 94:555, 1990.

133. **Glass RH, Spindle AI, Pedersen RA,** Mouse embryo attachment to substratum and the interaction of trophoblast with cultured cells, *J Exp Zool* 203:327, 1979.

134. **Irving JA, Lala PV,** Functional role of cell surface integrins on human trophoblast cell migration: regulation by TGF-β, IGF-II and IGFBP-1, *Exp Cell Res* 217:419, 1995.

135. **Damsky CH, Librach C, Lim K-H, Fitzgerald ML, McMaster MT, Janatpour M, Zhou Y, Logan SK, Fisher SJ,** Integrin switching regulates normal trophoblast invasion, *Development* 120:3657, 1994.

136. **Diamond MS, Springer TA,** The dynamic regulation of integrin adhesiveness, *Curr Biol* 4:506, 1994.

137. **Zhou Y, Fisher SJ, Janatpour M, Genbacev O, Dejana E, Wheelock M, Damsky CH,** Human cytotrophoblasts adopt a vascular phenotype as they differentiate. A strategy for successful endovascular invasion? *J Clin Invest* 99:2139, 1997.

138. **Zhou Y, Damsky CH, Fisher SJ,** Preeclampsia is associated with failure of cytotrophoblasts to mimic a vascular adhesion phenotype: one cause of defective endovascular invasion in this syndrome? *J Clin Invest* 99:2152, 1997.

139. **Clark DA, Slapsys RM, Croy BA, Kreck J, Rossant J,** Local active suppression by suppressor cells in the decidua: a review, *Am J Reprod Immunol* 6:78, 1984.

140. **Salmonsen LA, Doughton BW, Findlay JF,** The effect of the preimplantation blastocyst in vivo and in vitro on protein synthesis and secretion by cultured epithelial cells from sheep endometrium, *Endocrinology* 119:622, 1986.

141. **Roldan A, Cubellis MV, Masucci MT, Behrendt N, Lund LR, Dano K, Appella E, Blasi F,** Cloning and expression of the receptor for human urokinase plasminogen activator, a central molecule in cell surface, plasmin dependent proteolysis, *EMBO J* 9:467, 1990.

142. **King A, Loke YW,** Trophoblast and JEG choriocarcinoma cells are sensitive to lysis by IL-2 stimulated decidual LGL, *Cell Immunol* 129:435, 1990.

143. **Loke YW, King A,** Recent developments in the human maternal-fetal immune interaction, *Curr Opin Immunol* 3:762, 1991.

144. **Shelesnyak MC,** Inhibition of decidual cell formation in the pseudopregnant rat by histamine antagonists, *Am J Physiol* 170:522, 1952.

145. **Brandon JM, Wallis RM,** Effect of mepyramine, a histamine H1-, and burimamide, a histamine H2- receptor antagonist, on ovum implantation in the rat, *J Reprod Fertil* 50:251, 1977.

146. **Dey SK, Johnson DC, Santos JG,** Is histamine production by the blastocyst required for implantation in the rabbit? *Biol Reprod* 21:1169, 1979.

147. **Schatz F, Aigner S, Papp C, Toth-Pal E, Hauskenecht V, Lockwood CJ,** Plasminogen activator activity during decidualization of human endometrial stromal cells is regulated by plasminogen activator inhibitor 1, *J Clin Encrinol Metab* 80:1504, 1995.

148. **McDonnell S, Wright JH, Gaire M, Matrisian LM,** Expression and regulation of stromelysin and matrilysin by growth factors and oncogenes, *Biochem Soc Trans* 22:55, 1994.

149. **Graham CH, Lysiak JJ, McCrae KR, Lal PK,** Localization of transforming growth factor-beta at the human fetal-maternal interface: role in trophoblast growth and differentiation, *Biol Reprod* 46:561, 1992.

150. **Yagel S, Geva TE, Solomon H, Shimonovitz S, Finci-Yeheskel Z, Mayer M, Milwidsky A,** High levels of chorionic gonadotropin retard first trimester trophoblast invasion *in vitro* by decreasing urokinase plasminogen activator and collagenase activities, *J Clin Endocrinol Metab* 77:1506, 1993.

8 The Endocrinology of Pregnancy

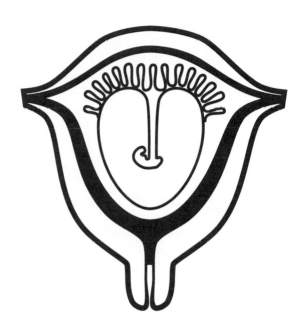

Who is in charge of pregnancy, the mother or her fetus? From the vantage point of an outsider looking in, it seems as if the mother is in charge. But from the fetal point of view, it is overwhelmingly logical that the maternal adaptations of pregnancy are controlled by the fetus. For the fetus, one of the crucial aspects of intrauterine life is its dependency on the effective exchange of nutritive and metabolic products with the mother. It is not surprising that mechanisms exist by which a growing fetus can influence or control the exchange process and, hence, its environment. The methods by which a fetus can influence its own growth and development involve a variety of messages transmitted, in many cases, by hormones. Hormonal messengers from the conceptus can affect metabolic processes, uteroplacental blood flow, and cellular differentiation. Furthermore, a fetus may signal its desire and readiness to leave the uterus by hormonal initiation of parturition. This chapter will review the mechanisms by which the fetus establishes influence over important events during pregnancy. The important process of lactation is discussed in Chapter 16.

Steroid Hormones in Pregnancy

Steroidogenesis in the fetoplacental unit does not follow the conventional mechanisms of hormone production within a single organ. Rather, the final products result from critical interactions and interdependence of separate organ systems that individually do not possess the necessary enzymatic capabilities. It is helpful to view the process as consisting of a fetal compartment, a placental compartment (specifically the syncytiotrophoblast), and a maternal compartment. Separately, the fetal and placental compartments lack certain steroidogenic activities. Together, however, they are complementary and form a complete unit that utilizes the maternal compartment as a source of basic building materials and as a resource for clearance of steroids.

Maternal Plasma Progesterone

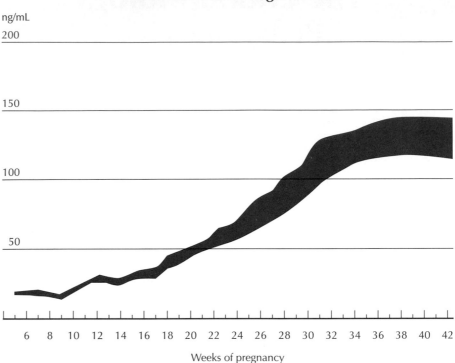

ng/mL

Weeks of pregnancy

Progesterone

In its key location as a way station between mother and fetus, the placenta can utilize precursors from either mother or fetus to circumvent its own deficiencies in enzyme activity. The placenta converts little, if any, acetate to cholesterol or its precursors. Cholesterol, as well as pregnenolone, is obtained from the maternal bloodstream for progesterone synthesis. The fetal contribution is negligible because progesterone levels remain high after fetal demise. Thus, the massive amount of progesterone produced in pregnancy depends on placental-maternal cooperation, although some have argued that the fetal liver is an important source of cholesterol (discussed below).

Progesterone is largely produced by the corpus luteum until about 10 weeks of gestation. Indeed, until approximately the 7th week, the pregnancy is dependent upon the presence of the corpus luteum.[1] Exogenous support for an early pregnancy (until 10 weeks) requires 100 mg of progesterone daily, associated with a maternal circulating level of approximately 10 ng/mL.[2] Despite this requirement, patients pregnant after ovarian stimulation with one of the techniques of assisted reproductive technology have concluded a successful pregnancy after experiencing extremely low progesterone levels.[3, 4] Thus, individual variation is great, and very low circulating levels of progesterone can be encountered occasionally in women who experience normal pregnancies. The predictive value, therefore, of progesterone measurements is limited.

After a transition period of shared function between the 7th week and 10th week during which there is a slight decline in circulating maternal progesterone levels, the placenta emerges as the major source of progesterone synthesis and maternal circulating levels progressively increase.[2, 5, 6] At term, progesterone levels range from 100 to 200 ng/mL, and the placenta produces about 250 mg per day. Most of the progesterone produced in the placenta enters the maternal circulation.

In contrast to estrogen, progesterone production by the placenta is largely independent of the quantity of precursor available, the uteroplacental perfusion, fetal well being, or even the presence of a live fetus. This is because the fetus contributes essentially no precursor. The majority of placental progesterone is derived from maternal cholesterol that is readily available. At term a small portion (3%) is derived from maternal pregnenolone.

The cholesterol utilized for progesterone synthesis enters the trophoblast from the maternal bloodstream as low-density lipoprotein (LDL)-cholesterol, by means of the process of endocytosis (internalization, as described in Chapter 2) involving the LDL cell membrane receptors, a process enhanced in pregnancy by estrogen.[7, 8] Hydrolysis of the protein component of LDL may yield amino acids for the fetus, and essential fatty acids may be derived from hydrolysis of the cholesteryl esters. Unlike steroidogenesis elsewhere, it is not clear whether placental progesterone production requires the control of tropic hormones. Although some evidence suggests tropic hormone support is not necessary, other evidence indicates that a small amount of human chorionic gonadotropin (HCG) must be present.[9, 10]

There is evidence in the baboon that estrogen (estradiol) regulates progesterone production in the placenta.[11] The fetoplacental units in human and baboon pregnancies are virtually identical. Estradiol increases LDL-cholesterol uptake in baboon trophoblastic tissue by increasing LDL receptor gene transcription, and in human syncytiotrophoblast, estradiol increases progesterone production by means of an increase in LDL uptake.[11, 12] Estrogen also stimulates cholesterol production in the human fetal liver to provide circulating LDL-cholesterol substrate for steroido-

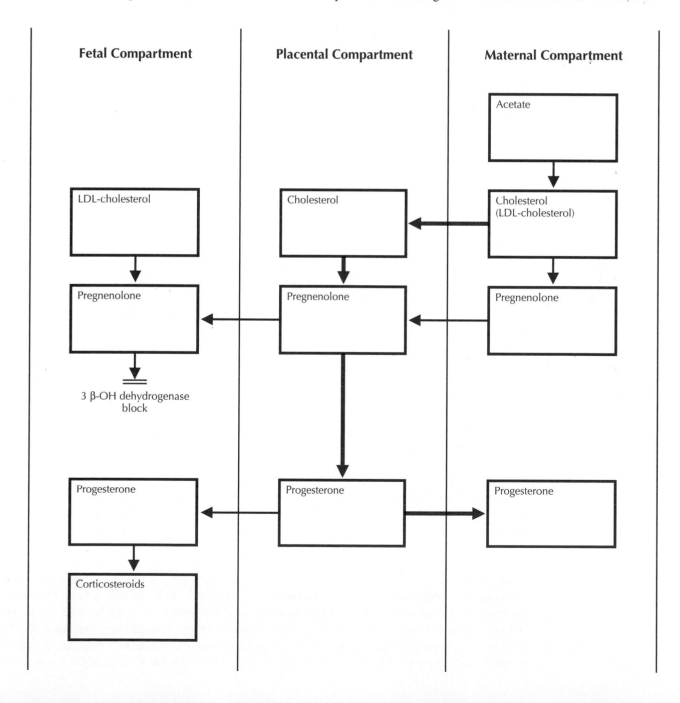

genesis.[13] In addition, estrogen increases placental P450scc enzyme activity that converts cholesterol to pregnenolone, the immediate precursor for progesterone. Because estrogen production ultimately depends on the fetal adrenal gland for precursors, the influence of estrogen on progesterone production would be another example of fetal direction and control in the endocrinology of pregnancy. The proponents of this interaction and dependence of progesterone production on fetal precursors argue that the lack of impact of conditions of estrogen deficiency (e.g., anencephaly, fetal demise) on progesterone production is due to the fact that active, unbound estrogen remains within a critical, effective range, and what is lost reflects the degree of excess production in pregnancy.[11]

The human decidua and fetal membranes also synthesize and metabolize progesterone.[14] In this case, neither cholesterol nor LDL-cholesterol are significant substrates; pregnenolone sulfate may be the most important precursor. This local steroidogenesis may play a role in regulating parturition.

Amniotic fluid progesterone concentration is maximal between 10 and 20 weeks, and then decreases gradually. Myometrial levels are about 3 times higher than maternal plasma levels in early pregnancy, remain high, and are about equal to the maternal plasma concentration at term.

In early pregnancy, the levels of 17α-hydroxyprogesterone rise, marking the activity of the corpus luteum. By the 10th week of gestation, this compound has returned to baseline levels, indicating that the placenta has little 17α-hydroxylase activity. However, beginning about the 32nd week there is a second, more gradual rise in 17α-hydroxyprogesterone due to placental utilization of fetal precursors.

There are two active metabolites of progesterone, that increase significantly during pregnancy. There is about a 10-fold increase of the 5α-reduced metabolite, 5α-pregnane-3,20-dione.[15] This compound contributes to the resistance in pregnancy against the vasopressor action of angiotensin II. The circulating level, however, is the same in normal and hypertensive pregnancies. The concentration of deoxycorticosterone (DOC) at term is 1200 times the nonpregnant levels. Some of this is due to the 3–4-fold increase in cortisol-binding globulin during pregnancy, but a significant amount is due to 21-hydroxylation of circulating progesterone in the kidney.[16] This activity is significant during pregnancy because the rate is proportional to the plasma concentration of progesterone. The fetal kidney is also active in 21-hydroxylation of the progesterone secreted by the placenta into the fetal circulation. At the present time, there is no known physiologic role for DOC during pregnancy.

Progesterone has a role in parturition as will be discussed later in this chapter. It has been suggested that progesterone is important in suppressing the maternal immunological response to fetal antigens, thereby preventing maternal rejection of the trophoblast. Progesterone prepares and maintains the endometrium to allow implantation. The human corpus luteum makes significant amounts of estradiol, but it is progesterone and not estrogen that is required for successful implantation.[17] Because implantation normally occurs about 5–6 days after ovulation, and human chorionic gonadotropin (HCG) must appear by the 10th day after ovulation to rescue the corpus luteum, the blastocyst must successfully implant and secrete HCG within a narrow window of time. In the first 5–6 weeks of pregnancy, HCG stimulation of the corpus luteum results in the daily secretion of about 25 mg of progesterone and 0.5 mg of estradiol. Although estrogen levels begin to increase at 4–5 weeks due to placental secretion, progesterone production by the placenta does not significantly increase until about 10–11 weeks after ovulation.

Progesterone serves as the substrate for fetal adrenal gland production of glucocorticoids and mineralocorticoids; however, cortisol synthesis is also derived from low-density lipoprotein cholesterol (LDL-cholesterol) obtained from the fetal circulation and synthesized in the fetal liver.[13, 18] The fetal zone in the adrenal gland is extremely active, but produces steroids with a 3β-hydroxy-Δ^5 configuration like pregnenolone and dehydroepiandrosterone, rather than 3-keto-Δ^4 products such as progesterone. The fetus, therefore, lacks significant activity of the 3β-hydroxysteroid dehydrogenase, Δ^{4-5} isomerase system. Thus, the fetus must borrow progesterone from the placenta to circumvent this lack in order to synthesize the biologically important corticosteroids. In return, the fetus supplies what the placenta lacks: 19-carbon compounds to serve as precursors for estrogens.

Steroid levels have been compared in maternal blood, fetal blood, and amniotic fluid obtained at fetoscopy in women undergoing termination of pregnancy at 16–20 weeks gestation.[19] Cortisol, corticosterone, and aldosterone are definitely secreted by the fetal adrenal gland independently of the mother. The fetal arterial-venous differences confirm that placental progesterone is a source for fetal adrenal cortisol and aldosterone.

Estrogens

Estrogen production in pregnancy is under the control of the fetus and is a fundamental signaling method by which the fetus directs important physiologic processes that affect fetal well-being. Estrogen influences progesterone production, uteroplacental blood flow, mammary gland development, and fetal adrenal gland function.[11]

The basic precursors of estrogens are 19-carbon androgens. However, there is a virtual absence of 17α-hydroxylation and 17–20 desmolase (lyase) activity (P450c17) in the human placenta. As a result, 21-carbon products (progesterone and pregnenolone) cannot be converted to 19-carbon steroids (androstenedione and dehydroepiandrosterone). Like progesterone, estrogen produced by the placental aromatase (P450arom) enzyme system must derive precursors from outside the placenta.[20]

The androgen compounds utilized for estrogen synthesis in human pregnancy are, in the early months of gestation, derived from the maternal bloodstream. By the 20th week of pregnancy, the vast majority of estrogen excreted in the maternal urine is derived from fetal androgens. In particular, approximately 90% of estriol excretion can be accounted for by dehydroepiandrosterone sulfate (DHAS) production by the fetal adrenal gland.[20, 21] The high output of DHAS by the fetal zone is due to low 3β-hydroxysteroid dehydrogenase gene expression.[22] Removed into cell culture conditions, this gene becomes active in response to adrenocorticotropic hormone (ACTH).

The fetal endocrine compartment is characterized by rapid and extensive conjugation of steroids with sulfate. This is a protective mechanism, blocking the biologic effects of potent steroids present in such great quantities. In order to utilize fetal precursors, the placenta must be extremely efficient in cleaving the sulfate conjugates brought to it via the fetal bloodstream. Indeed, the sulfatase activity in the placenta is rapid and quantitatively very significant. It is recognized that a deficiency in placental sulfatase is associated with low estrogen excretion, giving clinical importance to this metabolic step. This syndrome will be discussed in greater detail later in this chapter.

The fetal adrenal provides DHAS as precursor for placental production of estrone and estradiol. However, the placenta lacks 16α-hydroxylation ability, and estriol with its 16α-hydroxyl group must be derived from an immediate fetal precursor. The fetal adrenal, with the aid of 16α-hydroxylation in the fetal liver, provides the 16α-hydroxydehydroepiandrosterone sulfate for placental estriol formation. After birth, neonatal hepatic 16α-hydroxylation activity rapidly disappears. The maternal contribution of DHAS to total estrogen synthesis must be negligible because, in the absence of normal fetal adrenal glands (as in an anencephalic infant), maternal estrogen levels and excretion are extremely low. The fetal adrenals secrete more than 200 mg of DHAS daily, about 10 times more than the mother.[23] Estriol is the estrogen produced in greatest quantity during pregnancy; estrone and estradiol are derived equally from fetal and maternal precursors.[21]

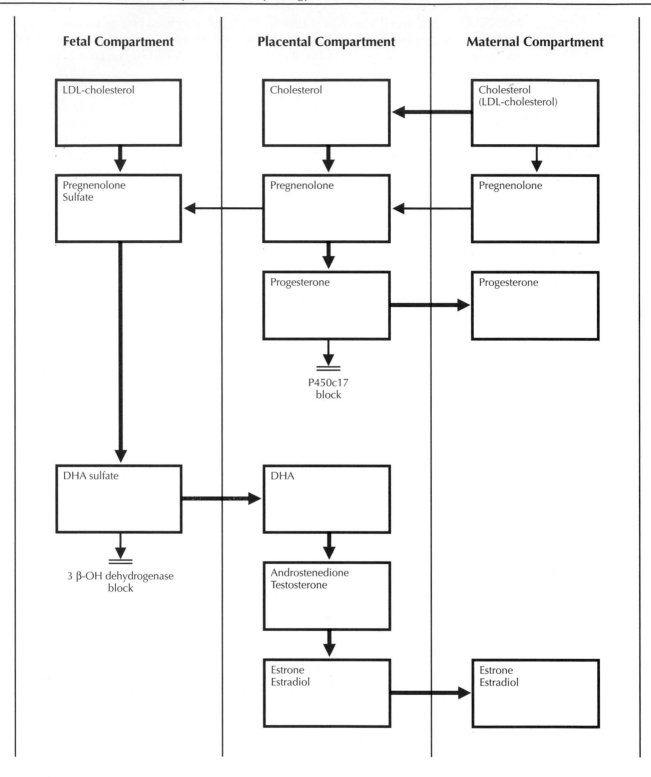

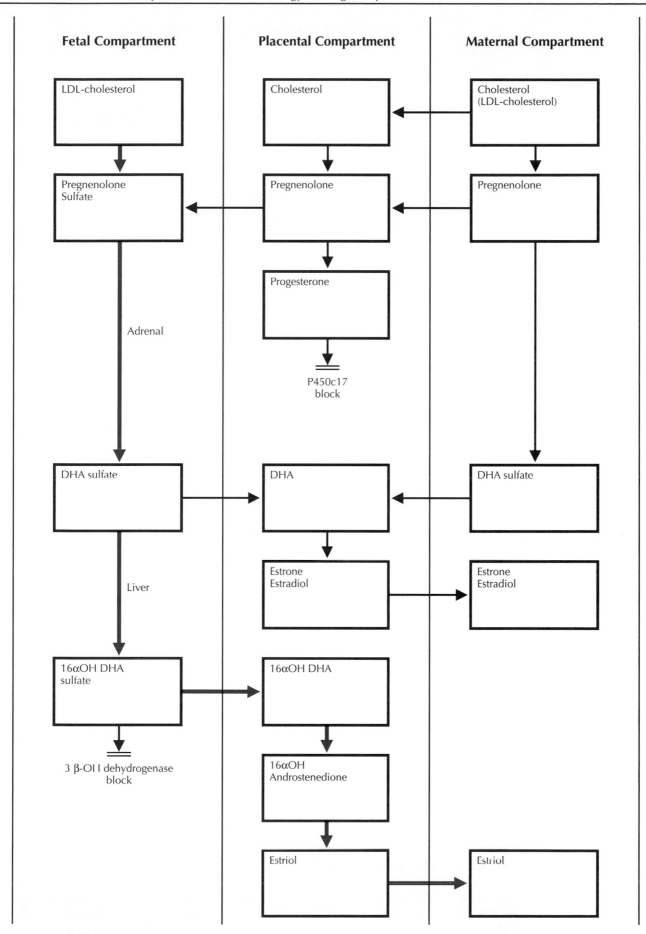

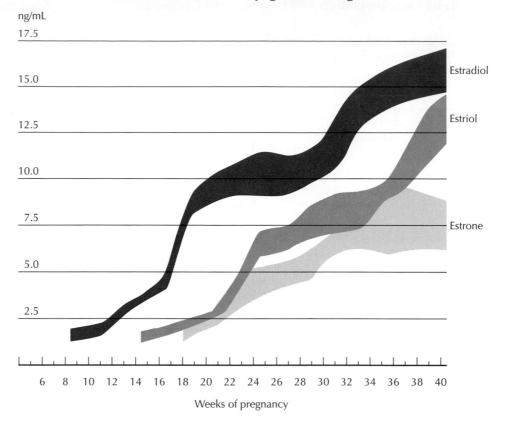

Maternal Plasma Unconjugated Estrogens

ng/mL

Estradiol

Estriol

Estrone

Weeks of pregnancy

The profiles of the unconjugated compounds in the maternal compartment for the 3 major estrogens in pregnancy are:

1. A rise in estrone begins at 6–10 weeks, and individual values range from 2 to 30 ng/mL at term.[24] This wide range in normal values precludes the use of estrone measurements in clinical applications.

2. A rise in estradiol begins in weeks 6–8 when placental function becomes apparent.[2, 25, 26] Individual estradiol values vary between 6 and 40 ng/mL at 36 weeks of gestation and then undergo an accelerated rate of increase.[24] At term, an equal amount of estradiol arises from maternal DHAS and fetal DHAS, and its importance in fetal monitoring is negligible.

3. Estriol is first detectable at 9 weeks when the fetal adrenal gland secretion of precursor begins. Estriol concentrations plateau at 31–35 weeks and then increase again at 35–36 weeks.[27]

During pregnancy, estrone and estradiol excretion is increased about 100 times over nonpregnant levels. However, the increase in maternal estriol excretion is about a thousand-fold. The traditional view that estriol is a weak estrogen metabolite is not accurate. A weak estrogen provided in high concentrations can produce a biologic response equivalent to that of estradiol.[28] Because of its high production rate and concentration, estriol is an important hormone in pregnancy. The maternal level of estradiol is higher than in the fetus; in contrast, the estriol level in the fetus is greater than in the mother.

The maternal cardiovascular adaptations to pregnancy that are so necessary to serve the fetus are appropriately under the influence of the fetus and significantly regulated by estrogen.[29] Blood volume is increased by estrogen stimulation of the maternal and trophoblastic renin-angiotensin systems, and uteroplacental blood flow, that is so critical for the fetus, is influenced by the vasodilatory effects of estrogen.

The enzyme responsible for estrogen synthesis is the cytochrome P450 aromatase enzyme (P450arom), the product of the CYP19 gene.[30] The CYP19 gene is regulated in various tissues by tissue-specific promoters. The placenta, with its huge capacity for estrogen synthesis, uses a powerful, unique promoter that allows specific regulation. An autosomal recessive disorder due to mutations in the P450arom gene is associated with a failure to convert androgen precursors to estrogen by placental aromatase.[31] Consequently, a female fetus and the mother can undergo virilization. Nevertheless, growth and development of the fetus are not impaired, and this disorder raises the question: how much, if any, estrogen is essential in human pregnancy? Is this another example of backup mechanisms operating to achieve the goal?

Normally, placental aromatization is so efficient that little androgen presented to the placenta escapes.[32] For this reason, fetuses are well protected against masculinization, and even in the presence of an androgen-secreting tumor, extremely large amounts of aromatizable androgens or the secretion of nonaromatizable androgens are required to produce unwanted virilization.

The estrogens presented to the maternal bloodstream are rapidly metabolized by the maternal liver prior to excretion into the maternal urine as a variety of more than 20 products. The bulk of these maternal urinary estrogens is composed of glucosiduronates conjugated at the 16-position. Significant amounts of the 3-glucosiduronate and the 3-sulfate-16-glucosiduronate are also excreted. Only approximately 8–10% of the maternal blood estriol is unconjugated.

The Fetal Adrenal Cortex

The fetal adrenal cortex is differentiated by 8–9 weeks gestational age into a thick inner fetal zone and a thin outer definitive zone, the source of cortisol and the forerunner of the adult cortex.[33] Early in pregnancy, adrenal growth and development are remarkable, and the gland achieves a size equal to or larger than that of the kidney by the end of the first trimester. After 20–24 weeks, the adrenal glands slowly decrease in size until a second spurt in growth begins at about 34–35 weeks. The gland remains proportionately larger than the adult adrenal glands. After delivery, the fetal zone (about 80% of the bulk of the gland) rapidly involutes to be replaced by simultaneous expansion of the adrenal cortex composed of the zona glomerulosa, the zona fasciculata, and the zona reticularis. Thus, the specific steroidogenic characteristics of the fetus are associated with a specific adrenal morphology that is dependent on specific factors present during intrauterine life.

Fetal dehydroepiandrosterone (DHA) and DHAS production rises steadily concomitant with the increase in the size of the fetal zone and adrenal weight.[34] DHA and DHAS are the major secretory products of the fetal zone because 3β-hydroxysteroid dehydrogenase-isomerase activity and the expression of this enzyme's gene are suppressed.[22] The well-known increase in maternal estrogen levels is significantly influenced by the increased availability of fetal DHAS as a precursor. Indeed, the accelerated rise in maternal estrogen levels near term can be explained, in part, by an increase in fetal DHAS. The stimulus for the substantial adrenal growth and steroid production has been a puzzle.

Early in pregnancy, the adrenal gland can grow and function without ACTH, perhaps in response to HCG.[33] After 15–20 weeks, fetal ACTH is required. However, during the last 12–14 weeks of pregnancy when fetal ACTH levels are declining, the adrenal quadruples in size.[35] Because pituitary prolactin is the only fetal pituitary hormone to increase throughout pregnancy, paralleling fetal adrenal gland size changes, it was proposed that fetal prolactin is the critical tropic substance. In experimental preparations, however, only ACTH exerts a steroidogenic effect. There is no fetal adrenal response to prolactin, HCG, growth hormone, melanocyte-stimulating hormone (MSH), or thyrotropin-releasing hormone (TRH).[36, 37] Furthermore, in patients treated with bromocriptine, fetal blood prolactin levels are suppressed, but DHAS levels are unchanged.[38] Nevertheless, interest in prolactin persists because both ACTH and prolactin can stimulate steroidogenesis in vivo in the fetal baboon.[39]

There is no question that, in the second half of pregnancy, ACTH is essential for the morphologic development and the steroidogenic mechanism of the fetal adrenal gland.[40, 41] ACTH activates adenylate cyclase, leading to steroidogenesis. Soon the supply of cholesterol becomes rate limiting. Further ACTH action results in an increase in LDL receptors, leading to an increased uptake of circulating LDL-cholesterol, largely derived from the fetal liver.[18] With internalization of LDL-cholesterol, hydrolysis by lysosomal enzymes of the cholesteryl ester makes cholesterol available for steroidogenesis. For this reason, fetal plasma levels of LDL are low, and after birth newborn levels of LDL rise as the fetal adrenal involutes. In the presence of low levels of LDL-cholesterol, the fetal adrenal is capable of synthesizing cholesterol de novo.[42] Thus, near term, both de novo synthesis and utilization of LDL-cholesterol are necessary to sustain the high rates of DHAS and estrogen formation. In addition, ACTH increases adrenal response by increasing the expression of its own receptor.[43]

The tropic support of the fetal adrenal gland by ACTH from the fetal pituitary is protected by placental estrogen. The placenta prevents maternal cortisol from reaching the fetus by converting cortisol to cortisone. This 11β-hydroxysteroid dehydrogenase activity is stimulated by placental estrogen.[44] Regulation of this enzyme by estrogen thus influences fetal ACTH secretion. With increasing estrogen levels in late gestation, even greater 11β-hydroxysteroid dehydrogenase activity would result in even less maternal cortisol reaching the fetal circulation. Thus, it is proposed that, in late gestation, fetal ACTH secretion increases, the fetal adrenal gland undergoes greater maturation, and fetal cortisol synthesis from endogenous cholesterol increases.[45] A relative deficiency in 11β-hydroxysteroid dehydrogenase type 1 (the placental isoform) is correlated with low birth weight, which in turn is correlated with insulin resistance, abnormal lipids, and hypertension in adult life.[46, 47] This enzyme is abundantly expressed in syncytiotrophoblast at the interface between fetal tissue and maternal blood.[48] Expression of the second isoform, type 2 11β-hydroxysteroid dehydrogenase, is found in the liver and the distal nephron of the kidney where enzyme activity excludes glucocorticoids from mineralocorticoid receptors. Fetal hypoxemia down-regulates fetal renal expression of the type 2 enzyme, potentially affecting glucocorticoid availability.[49]

It has been suggested that rising fetal cortisol secretion competes with progesterone for the glucocorticoid receptor in the placenta, thus blocking the inhibitory action of progesterone on corticotropin-releasing hormone (CRH) synthesis, leading to an increase in CRH.[50] Placental production of CRH and the size of the fetal adrenal gland are closely correlated in several primates, both reaching a peak in humans at the time of parturition. The increase in CRH would augment fetal ACTH secretion, producing adrenal growth and even more fetal cortisol in a positive feedback relationship, as well as more DHAS to serve as precursor for the increase in estrogen that occurs prior to parturition. Another possibility is CRH direct stimulation of DHAS by the fetal adrenal gland, as has been demonstrated in vitro.[51]

Adrenal gland steroidogenesis involves autocrine and paracrine regulation by various growth factors.[33] Fetal adrenal cells produce inhibin, and the α-subunit (present only in inhibin) is preferentially increased by ACTH.[52, 53] In the fetal adrenal, the beta-subunit is not expressed; thus, inhibin A and activin A are the principal forms. Inhibin consists of two dissimilar peptides, alpha- and beta-subunits, linked by disulfide bonds. Inhibin A and inhibin B each contain an identical alpha-subunit, but distinct beta-subunits. Activin contains two subunits that are identical to the beta-subunits of the inhibins.

The Two Forms of Inhibin (Heterodimers)

Inhibin-A:	Alpha-Beta$_A$
Inhibin-B:	Alpha-Beta$_B$

The Three Forms of Activin (Homodimers)

Activin-A: $Beta_A$-$Beta_A$
Activin-AB: $Beta_A$-$Beta_B$
Activin-B: $Beta_B$-$Beta_B$

Activin enhances ACTH-stimulated steroidogenesis while inhibiting mitogenesis in human fetal zone adrenal cells.[53] This effect on steroidogenic activity is not present in adult adrenal cells. In vitro, activin enhances a shift in fetal adrenal cells from ACTH stimulation of DHAS production to cortisol production. This shift is analogous to the shift that occurs after birth. Perhaps activin plays this role in the remodeling of the fetal zone in the newborn. A specific action for inhibin in fetal adrenal cells has not been described.

We should not expect the fetal adrenal gland to be an exception to the ubiquitous presence and actions of all growth factors.[33] Basic fibroblast growth factor has potent mitogenic activity mediating the growth response of the fetal adrenal cortex to ACTH. Evidence indicates that the epidermal growth factor receptor is activated in the fetal adrenal, but the ligand using this receptor is probably transforming growth factor-α. Like activin, transforming growth factor-β inhibits fetal zone cellular proliferation, and in addition, suppresses steroidogenesis.

The insulin-like growth factors (IGF-I and IGF-II) are important in mediating the tropic effects of ACTH, particularly increasing adrenal responsiveness to ACTH in the second half of pregnancy.[54] IGF-II production in the fetal adrenal is very significant and is stimulated by ACTH. IGF-II is believed to be important in prenatal growth.[55] The abundance of IGF-II in the fetal adrenal gland implicates this growth factor as a mediator of ACTH-induced growth.[56] Both IGF-I and IGF-II are equally mitogenic in a cell culture system of fetal adrenal cells and enhance the proliferation stimulated by basic fibroblast growth factor and epidermal growth factor.[56] However, only transcription of IGF-II is stimulated by ACTH. IGF-II augments ACTH-stimulated steroidogenesis in the fetal adrenal, specifically by increasing the expression of P450c17.[54] Thus, the growth-promoting and steroidogenic effects of ACTH are mediated by various growth factors, with a principal role played by IGF-II. In this regard, the fetal adrenal differs from the adult adrenal where IGF-I is predominant; however, IGF-II is able to modulate responsiveness to ACTH in the fetal adrenal by activating the IGF-I receptor.

Steroidogenic factor-1 (SF-1) and DAX-1 (named for the location of its gene on the X chromosome) are nuclear receptors for which specific ligands have not been identified ("orphan receptors"). SF-1 influences the expression of genes that encode steroidogenic enzymes, and when genetic expression of SF-1 is disrupted in mice, gonads and adrenal glands fail to develop.[57, 58] Mutations in the DAX-1 gene result in adrenal hypoplasia, and DAX-1 is believed to work with SF-1 in regulating development and function of steroid producing tissues.[59]

The unique features of the fetal adrenal gland can be ascribed to its high-estrogen environment. Tissue culture studies have demonstrated that hormonal peptides of pituitary or placental origin are not the factors that are responsible for the behavior of the fetal adrenal gland.[60–62] Estrogens at high concentration inhibit 3β-hydroxysteroid dehydrogenase-isomerase activity in the fetal adrenal gland and, in the presence of ACTH in conjunction with IGF-II, enhance the secretion of dehydroepiandrosterone (DHA).[63] Estradiol concentrations of 10–100 ng/mL are required to inhibit cortisol secretion.[64] The total estrogen concentrations in the fetus are easily in this range. A study of the kinetics of 3β-hydroxysteroid dehydrogenase activity in human adrenal microsomes reveals that all steroids are inhibitory, and most notably, estrone and estradiol at levels found in fetal life cause almost total inhibition.[65] In a study utilizing a human adrenocortical cell line, estradiol in high concentrations inhibited 3β-hydroxysteroid dehydrogenase and the mechanism appeared to be independent of the estrogen receptor.[66] The hyperplasia of the fetal adrenal may be the result of the high ACTH levels due to the relatively low cortisol levels, a consequence of the enzyme inhibition.

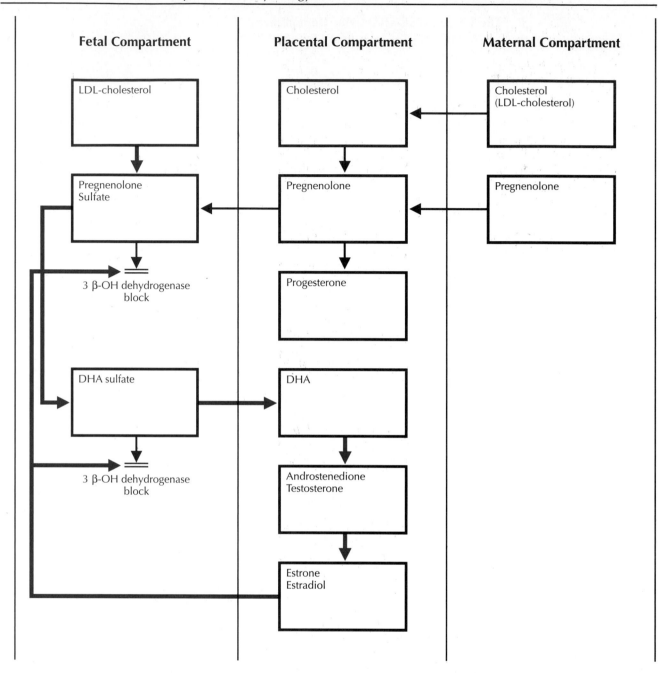

The development of the adrenal gland during human fetal life and during the neonatal period is paralleled in the baboon.[67] The adrenal cortex of the fetal baboon is characterized by the same deficiency in 3β-hydroxysteroid dehydrogenase as that seen in the human, with the same diversion of steroidogenesis into production of DHAS. Treatment of the neonatal baboon with estrogens and progesterone did not halt the regression of the fetal zone and DHAS production, arguing against the hypothesis that the fetal zone is dependent on an estrogen-induced deficiency in 3β-hydroxysteroid dehydrogenase. Treatment of the pregnant baboon with estradiol reduced production of DHAS.[68] It continues to be uncertain, however, whether the internal microenvironment of the adrenal gland can be affected by the exogenous administration of steroids. In the monkey, epidermal growth factor can increase the 3β-hydroxysteroid dehydrogenase content in the fetal adrenal gland, but it is not clear how this action is regulated.[69]

This explanation (estrogen regulation of 3β-hydroxysteroid dehydrogenase) is further challenged by in vitro studies of human fetal zone cells indicating that estradiol and IGF-II combine to direct steroidogenesis to DHAS in a mechanism not due to inhibition of 3β-hydroxysteroid dehydrogenase.[63]

Nevertheless, it is an attractive and useful hypothesis to view the principal mission of the fetal adrenal as providing DHAS as the basic precursor for placental estrogen production. Estrogen, in turn, feeds back to the adrenal to direct steroidogenesis along the Δ^5 pathway to provide even more of its precursor, DHAS. Thus far, this is the only known function for DHAS. With birth and loss of exposure to estrogen, the fetal adrenal gland quickly changes to the adult type of gland.

Measurement of Estrogen in Pregnancy

Because pregnancy is characterized by a great increase in maternal estrogen levels, and estrogen production is dependent on fetal and placental steroidogenic cooperation, the amount of estrogen present in the maternal blood or urine reflects both fetal and placental enzymatic capability and, hence, well-being. Attention focused on estriol because 90% of maternal estriol is derived from fetal precursors. The end product to be assayed in the maternal blood or urine is influenced by a multitude of factors. Availability of precursor from the fetal adrenal gland is a prime requisite as well as the ability of the placenta to perform its conversion steps. Maternal metabolism of the product as well as the efficiency of maternal renal excretion of the product can modify the daily amount of estrogen in the urine. Blood flow to any of the key organs in the fetus, placenta, and mother becomes important.[70, 71] Fetal hypoxemia due to reduced uteroplacental blood flow is associated with a marked increase in adrenal androgen production in response to an increase in fetal ACTH and, in response to the availability of androgen precursors, an increase in maternal estrogen levels.[72] The response to acute stress is in contrast to the effect of chronic uteroplacental insufficiency which is associated with a reduction in fetal androgens and maternal estrogens. In addition, drugs or diseases can affect any level in the cascade of events leading up to the assay of estrogen.

For years, measurement of estrogen in a 24-hour urine collection was the standard hormonal method of assessing fetal well-being. This was replaced by radioimmunoassay of unconjugated estriol in the plasma.[73] Because of its short half-life (5–10 minutes) in the maternal circulation, unconjugated estriol has less variation than urinary or total blood estriol. However, assessment of maternal estriol levels has been superseded by various biophysical fetal monitoring techniques such as nonstress testing, stress testing, and measurement of fetal breathing and activity. Modern screening for fetal aneuploidy (discussed later in the chapter) utilizes 3 markers in the maternal circulation: alpha fetoprotein, human chorionic gonadotropin, and unconjugated estriol.

Amniotic Fluid Estrogen Measurements

Amniotic fluid estriol is correlated with the fetal estrogen pattern rather than the maternal. Most of the estriol in the amniotic fluid is present as 16-glucosiduronate or as 3-sulfate-16-glucosiduronate. A small amount exists as 3-sulfate. Very little unconjugated estriol is present in the amniotic fluid because free estriol is rapidly transferred across the placenta and membranes. Estriol sulfate is low in concentration because the placenta and fetal membranes hydrolyze the sulfated conjugates, and the free estriol is then passed out of the fluid. Because the membranes and the placenta have no glucuronidase activity, the glucosiduronate conjugates are removed slowly from the fetus. The glucosiduronates therefore predominate in the fetal urine and the amniotic fluid. Because of the slow changes in glucosiduronates, measurements of amniotic fluid estriol have wide variations in both normal and abnormal pregnancies. An important clinical use for amniotic fluid estrogen measurements has not emerged.

Estetrol

Estetrol (15α-hydroxyestriol) is formed from a fetal precursor, and is very dependent upon 15α-hydroxylation activity in the fetal liver. The capacity for 15α-hydroxylation of estrogens increases during fetal life, reaching a maximum at term. This activity then declines during infancy and is low, absent, or undetectable in adults. There is no clinical use for maternal blood or urine estetrol measurements during pregnancy. The clinical use of maternal blood and urine estetrol measurements is of no advantage over the usual estriol assessment.

Placental Sulfatase Deficiency

There is an X-linked metabolic disease characterized by a placental sulfatase deficiency in the syncytiotrophoblast, and postnatally, ichthyosis, occurring in about 1 in 2000–3000 newborn males.[74] Patients with the placental sulfatase disorder are unable to hydrolyze DHAS or 16α-hydroxy-DHAS, and, therefore, the placenta cannot form normal amounts of estrogen. A deficiency in placental sulfatase is usually discovered when patients go beyond term and are found to have extremely low estriol levels and no evidence of fetal distress. The patients usually fail to go into labor and require delivery by cesarean section. Most striking is the failure of cervical softening and dilatation; thus, cervical dystocia occurs that is resistant to oxytocin stimulation. There are many case reports of this deficiency, almost all detected by finding low estriol levels. It has been suggested that mothers who are carriers of this disorder are at increased risk for intrauterine growth retardation and perinatal complications even if the fetus is not affected.[75] However, a careful analysis of unexplained low estriol levels concluded that this is a rare occurrence (about 3 per 10,000 pregnancies), and that perinatal complications in pregnancies at risk for placental sulfatase deficiency are not increased (other than a higher cesarean section rate).[76] All newborn children, with a few exceptions, have been male. The steroid sulfatase X-linked recessive ichthyosis locus (the steroid sulfatase gene) has been mapped to the distal short arm portion of the X chromosome. There are no known geographic or racial factors that affect the gene frequency.

The characteristic steroid findings are as follows: extremely low estriol and estetrol levels in the mother with extremely high amniotic fluid DHAS and normal amniotic fluid DHA and androstenedione. The normal DHA and androstenedione with a high DHAS rule out congenital adrenal hyperplasia. The small amount of estriol that is present in these patients probably arises from 16α-hydroxylation of DHAS in the maternal liver, thus providing 16α-hydroxylated DHA to the placenta for aromatization to estriol. Maternal estrone and estradiol are also low but not as markedly reduced because of their utilization of maternal precursors. Measurement in maternal urine of steroids derived from fetal sulfated compounds is a simple and reliable means of prenatal diagnosis. Demonstration of a high level of DHAS in the amniotic fluid is reliable. To establish the diagnosis with certainty, a decrease in sulfatase activity should be demonstrated in an in vitro incubation of placental tissue. The clinician should keep in mind that fresh tissue is needed for this procedure because freezing lowers enzyme activity. Alternatively, steroid sulfatase activity can be assayed in leukocytes.

It is now recognized that steroid sulfatase deficiency is present in other tissues and can persist after birth. These children develop ichthyosis beginning between birth and 6 months of age, characterized by hyperkeratosis (producing scales on the neck, trunk, and palms) and associated with mild corneal opacities, pyloric stenosis, and cryptorchidism. The skin fibroblasts have a low activity of steroid sulfatase, and scale formation that occurs early in the first year of life is thought to be due to an alteration in the cholesterol:cholesteryl ester ratio (due to the accumulation of cholesterol sulfate). This inherited disorder, thus, represents a single entity: placental sulfatase deficiency and X-linked ichthyosis, both reflecting a deficiency of microsomal sulfatase. A family history of scaling in males (as well as repeated postdate pregnancies and cesarean sections) should prompt a consideration for prenatal diagnosis. Because the clinical use of estriol measurements has declined, there is no effective method to identify the presence of this problem in women with normal obstetrical histories. However, a low maternal level of unconjugated estriol can be encountered with multiple marker screening (discussed later in this chapter). Furthermore, consideration should be given to antenatal screening by estriol measurement in pregnancies in which a male fetus is present and there is a previous history of a growth-retarded or stillborn male. However, perinatal outcome is good even when placental sulfatase deficiency is not known to be present and only a very small number of affected boys have serious manifestations of the disorder; therefore, it is difficult to justify the need for antenatal diagnosis.[76]

The Differential Diagnosis of an Extremely Low Estriol

1. **Impending or present fetal demise.**
2. **Adrenal hypofunction.**
3. **Placental sulfatase deficiency.**
4. **Placental aromatase deficiency.**
5. **Drug-related effects.**

Protein Hormones of Pregnancy

The placental villus is composed of trophoblast, mesenchymal cells, and fetal blood vessels. The two main trophoblastic layers consist of the cytotrophoblast, separate mononuclear cells prominent early in pregnancy and sparse late in pregnancy, and the syncytiotrophoblast, a continuous multinuclear layer on the surface of the villi. The cytotrophoblast is the basic placental stem cell from which the syncytiotrophoblasts arise by differentiation. The syncytiotrophoblast is, therefore, the functional cell of the placenta, the major site of hormone and protein production. Control of this important cellular differentiation is still not understood; however, the process is influenced by HCG and, undoubtedly, a variety of growth factors.[77] The protein hormone system is complicated because individual peptides can have multiple functions.[78] The surface of the syncytiotrophoblast is in direct contact with the maternal blood in the intervillous space. This may be a reason why placental proteins are secreted preferentially into the mother.

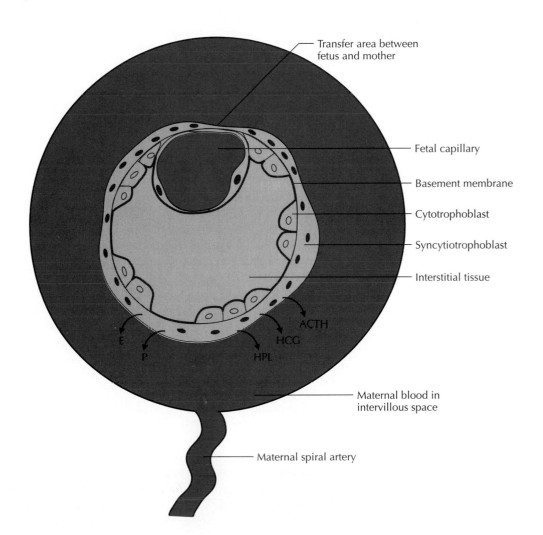

Proteins Associated with Pregnancy

Fetal Compartment	Placental Compartment	Maternal Compartment
Alpha-fetoprotein	Hypothalamic-like hormones 　GnRH 　CRH 　TRH 　Somatostatin 　GHRH	Decidual proteins 　Prolactin 　Relaxin 　IGFBP-1 　Interleukin-1 　Colony stimulating factor-1 　Progesterone-associated 　endometrial protein
	Pituitary-like hormones 　HCG 　HPL 　HGH 　HCT 　ACTH 　Oxytocin	Corpus luteum proteins 　Relaxin 　Prorenin
	Growth factors 　IGF-I 　IGF-II 　Epidermal growth factor 　Platelet-derived growth factor 　Fibroblast growth factor 　Transforming growth factor-α 　Transforming growth factor-β 　Inhibin 　Activin 　Follistatin	
	Cytokines 　Interleukins 　Interferons 　Tissue necrosis factor-α 　Colony stimulating factor-1	
	Other 　Opiates 　Prorenin 　Pregnancy-specific 　β_1-glycoprotein 　Pregnancy-associated 　plasma protein A	

Hypothalamic-like Releasing Hormones

The human placenta contains many releasing and inhibiting hormones, including gonadotropin-releasing hormone (GnRH), corticotropin-releasing hormone (CRH), thyrotropin-releasing hormone (TRH) and somatostatin.[79] Because of the presence of hypothalamic-like releasing hormones in an organ that produces tropic hormones, we are motivated to construct a system of regulation analogous to the hypothalamic-pituitary axis. However, as we shall see, this proves to be very difficult.

Immunoreactive GnRH can be localized in the cytotrophoblast and syncytiotrophoblast. Evidence indicates that placental GnRH regulates placental steroidogenesis and release of prostaglandins as well as HCG.[79–83] In some studies, the highest amount of GnRH was present early in pregnancy when the number of cytotrophoblasts is greatest and HCG secretion reaches its peak; however, others report relatively constant levels throughout pregnancy.[84, 85] The placental receptors for GnRH have a lower affinity than that of GnRH receptors in the pituitary, ovary, and testis.[86, 87] This reflects the situation in which the binding site is in close proximity to the site of secretion for the regulatory hormone. A higher affinity is not necessary because of the large amount of GnRH available in the placenta, and the low affinity receptors avoid response to the low levels of circulating GnRH. GnRH receptors, present in both cytotrophoblasts and syncytiotrophoblasts, are produced in a pattern that parallels the curve of HCG secretion, further evidence that placental GnRH and its receptor regulate HCG secretion.[88] GnRH release is increased by estrogen, activin A, insulin, and prostaglandins, and inhibited by progesterone, endogenous opiates, inhibin, and follistatin.[78]

CRH, identical in structure to hypothalamic CRH, is produced in the trophoblast, the fetal membranes, and the decidua.[78] Its production is regulated by steroids, decreased by progesterone and, in contrast to the usual negative feedback action in the hypothalamus, increased by glucocorticoids.[89] These interactions are consistent with the increase in fetal and maternal ACTH and cortisol associated with the last weeks of pregnancy and labor. Placental CRH is further regulated (as in the hypothalamus) by an array of substances such as vasopressin, norepinephrine, angiotensin-II, prostaglandins, neuropeptide Y, and oxytocin. CRH release is stimulated by activin and interleukin, and inhibited by inhibin and nitric oxide. The progressive increase in maternal CRH levels during pregnancy is due to the secretion of intrauterine CRH into the maternal circulation. The highest levels are found at labor and delivery. A binding protein for CRH exists in the human circulation, and it is produced in placenta, membranes and decidua.[90] Maternal levels of this binding protein are not different in pregnancy until a slight increase at 35 weeks, followed by a major decrease until term. Maternal CRH levels are elevated in women with pregnancies under stress; e.g., with preeclampsia and preterm labor.[78] The increase in placental CRH may be a response to the activation of fetal pituitary ACTH and adrenal cortisol secretion in th presence of hypoxemia.

Trophoblast, amnion, chorion, and decidua also produce a peptide similar to CRH, named urocortin, that binds to CRH receptors and CRH-binding protein.[91] Little is yet known about this peptide.

Human Chorionic Gonadotropin (HCG)

Human chorionic gonadotropin is a glycoprotein, a peptide framework to which carbohydrate side chains are attached.[92] Alterations in the carbohydrate component (about one-third of the molecular weight) change the biologic properties. For example, the long half-life of HCG is approximately 24 hours as compared with 2 hours for luteinizing hormone (LH), a 12-fold difference, which is due mainly to the greater sialic acid content of HCG. As with the other glycoproteins, follicle-stimulating hormone (FSH), LH, and thyroid-stimulating hormone (TSH), HCG consists of two subunits, noncovalently linked by disulfide bonds, called alpha (α) and beta (β).[93] The α-subunit in these glycoprotein hormones is identical, consisting of 92 amino acids. Unique biological activity as well as specificity in radioimmunoassays is attributed to the molecular and carbohydrate differences in the β-subunits (see "Heterogeneity" in Chapter 2).

β-HCG is the largest β-subunit, containing a larger carbohydrate moiety and 145 amino acid residues, including a unique carboxyl terminal tailpiece of 24 amino acid groups. It is this unique part of the HCG structure that allows the production of highly specific antibodies and the utilization of highly specific immunologic assays. The extended sequence in the carboxyl-terminal region of β-HCG contains 4 sites for glycosylation, the reason why HCG is glycosylated to a greater extent than LH, a difference that is responsible for the longer circulating half-life for HCG.

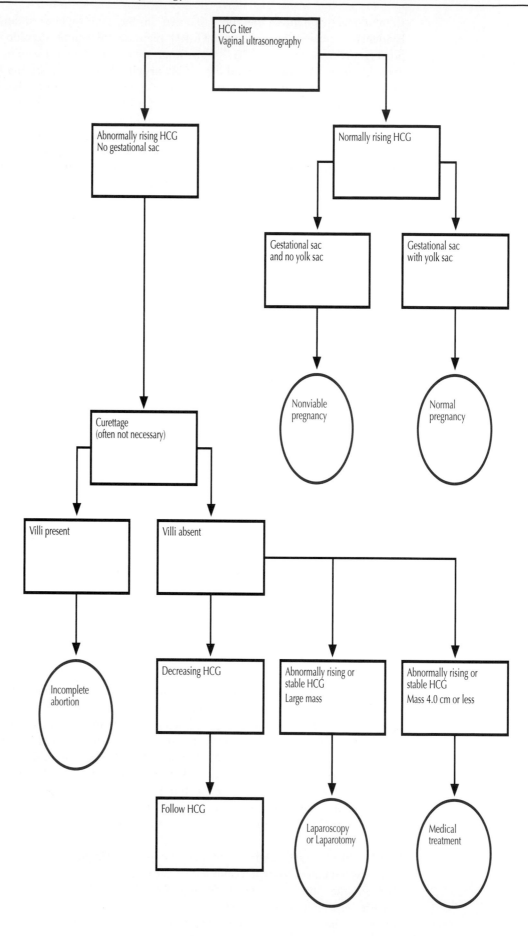

All human tissues appear to make HCG, but the placenta is different in having the ability to glycosylate the protein, thus reducing its rate of metabolism and giving it biologic activity through a long half-life. The carbohydrate components of the glycoproteins are composed of fructose, galactose, mannose, galactosamine, glucosamine, and sialic acid. Although the other sugars are necessary for hormonal function, sialic acid is the critical determinant of biologic half-life. Removal of sialic acid residues in HCG, FSH, and LH leads to very rapid elimination from the circulation.

These differences in structure are associated with a different promoter and transcriptional site that is located upstream in the HCG β-subunit gene compared with the transcriptional site in the LH β-subunit gene. The HCG β-subunit promoter does not contain steroid hormone response elements, allowing HCG secretion to escape feedback regulation by the sex steroids, in contrast to FSH and LH.

Genes for tropic hormones contain promoter and enhancer or inhibitor regions located in the 5' flanking regions upstream from the transcription site. These sites respond to second messengers (cyclic AMP) as well as steroids and other yet unknown regulators. The protein cores of the two glycoprotein subunits are the products of distinct genes.[94] Using recombinant DNA technology, it has been demonstrated that there is a single human gene for the expression of the α-subunit. The gene for the α-subunit shared by FSH, LH, HCG, and TSH is located on chromosome 6p21.1–23. A single promoter site subject to multiple signals and hormones regulates transcription of the α-gene in both placenta and pituitary. The α-subunit gene is expressed in several different cell types, but the β-subunit genes are restricted in cell type. The TSH β-gene is expressed only in thyrotrophs regulated by thyroid hormone; the FSH β-gene is expressed in gonadotrophs regulated by GnRH, activin, inhibin, and gonadal steroids; the LH β-gene, also expressed in gonadotrophs, is regulated by GnRH and is unaffected by activin and inhibin.[95]

The α-subunit gene requires the activation of distinct regulatory elements in thyrotroph and gonadotroph cells, as well as in the placenta. It is the activation of these cell-specific elements that produces tissue specificity for α-gene expression. In gonadotrophs, the GnRH-signaling pathway for α-gene transcription utilizes phosphorylase stimulation of diacyl glycerol (DAG) and inositol triphosphate (IP_3) that lead to a release of intracellular calcium stores. GnRH also stimulates the influx of calcium at the cell membrane. DAG, IP_3, and calcium work together to stimulate protein kinase C activity. Protein kinase regulation of the α-promoter is a principal part of the overall mechanism. This pituitary process is influenced by multiple factors including growth factors and gonadal steroids. In the placenta, the mechanism also utilizes specific regulatory elements, but the primary signal is mediated by the cyclic AMP-protein kinase A pathway.

The genes that encode for the β-subunits of LH, HCG, and TSH are located in a cluster on chromosome 19q13.3. There are 6 genes for the β-subunit of HCG, and only one for β-LH.[96] Transcription for the 6 HCG genes, each with different promoter activity, varies, and it is not certain why HCG requires multigenic expression (perhaps this is necessary to reach the extremely high level of production in early pregnancy). It is thought that β-HCG evolved relatively recently from β-LH, and the unique amino acid terminal extension of β-HCG arose by a read-through mutation of the translation stop codon in the β-LH gene; the DNA sequences of the β-HCG genes and the β-LH gene are 96% identical.[96] Only primates and horses have been demonstrated to have genes for the β-subunit of chorionic gonadotropin. In contrast to human chorionic gonadotropin, equine chorionic gonadotropin exerts both LH and FSH activities in many mammalian species because it contains peptide sequences in its β-subunit that are homologous to those in the pituitary gonadotropins of other species. The equine β-chorionic gonadotropin gene is identical to the equine β-LH gene, and although the primate β-HCG gene evolved from the same ancestral β-LH gene, the horse chorionic gonadotropin gene evolved in a different way. The β-LH gene is not expressed in the placenta.

The placenta-specific expression of β-HCG is due to several differences in DNA sequences between the β-HCG and β-LH genes.[95] The cyclic AMP-mediated enhancement of the β-HCG promoter is influenced by several regulatory proteins. The study of the β-subunit genes has been hampered by difficulties in maintaining glycoprotein-producing cell lines. The availability of choriocarcinoma cell lines, however, has allowed greater investigation of the β-HCG genes.

The genetic complexity for the transcription of β-HCG raises the possibility for mutations of these genes as causes of reproductive problems. A search for β-HCG gene deletions in women with recurrent miscarriage or unexplained infertility and for duplications in women with gestational trophoblastic neoplasia found only normal gene structures.[97]

HCG production and secretion are the result of complex interactions among the sex steroids, cytokines, GnRH, and growth factors. GnRH is synthesized by placental cells; GnRH receptors are present on placental cells, and GnRH stimulates the secretion of HCG and the steroid hormones in in vitro studies of placental cells.[98–100] Similar responses can be demonstrated with other peptides, such as interleukin-1β.[101] Similar to opiate action in the hypothalamus, the endorphins are a major inhibiting influence on HCG secretion.[102] Also similar to the pituitary secretion of gonadotropins, inhibin restrains and activin enhances the GnRH-HCG system, with a positive influence of estrogen and a negative impact by progesterone.[103, 104] Follistatin, by binding activin, prevents the stimulatory activity of activin. Other growth factors, specifically IGF-I, IGF-II, TGF-α, and EGF, also influence HCG secretion.

Although a relatively clear story can be constructed into a working concept regarding the autocrine/paracrine interactions in the regulation of the menstrual cycle (Chapter 6), placental function is more complex, and a simple presentation of the many interactions cannot be produced. For example, epidermal growth factor stimulates HCG secretion, but also stimulates inhibin secretion in placental cells, and inhibin suppresses GnRH stimulation of HCG.[105] Inhibin secretion in the placenta is further stimulated by prostaglandins.[106]

Can the cytotrophoblast-syncytiotrophoblast relationship be compared with the hypothalamic-pituitary axis? It does appear that hypothalamic-like peptides (CRH, GnRH) originate in the cytotrophoblast and influence the syncytiotrophoblast to secrete pituitary-like hormones (HCG, HPL, ACTH). Unraveling the interaction is made more difficult by the incredible complexity of the syncytiotrophoblast, a tissue that produces and responds to steroid and peptide hormones, growth factors, and neuropeptides. The best we can say is that locally produced hormones, growth factors, and peptides work together to regulate placental function.

To this day, the only definitely known function for HCG is support of the corpus luteum, taking over for LH on about the 8th day after ovulation, one day after implantation, when β-HCG first can be detected in maternal blood. HCG has been detected at the 8-cell stage in the embryo using molecular biology techniques.[107] Continued survival of the corpus luteum is totally dependent on HCG, and, in turn, survival of the pregnancy is dependent upon steroids from the corpus luteum until the 7th week of pregnancy.[1] From the 7th week to the 10th week, the corpus luteum is gradually replaced by the placenta, and by the 10th week, removal of the corpus luteum will not be followed by steroid withdrawal abortion.

It is very probable, but not conclusively proven, that HCG stimulates steroidogenesis in the early fetal testes, so that androgen production will ensue, and masculine differentiation can be accomplished.[108] It is also possible that the function of the inner fetal zone of the adrenal cortex depends on HCG for steroidogenesis early in pregnancy. The β-HCG gene is expressed in fetal kidney and fetal adrenal, suggesting that HCG may affect the development and function of these organs.[109]

HCG gene expression is present in both cytotrophoblast and syncytiotrophoblast, but it is synthesized mainly in the syncytiotrophoblast.[110] The maternal circulating HCG concentration is approximately 100 IU/L at the time of the expected but missed menses. A maximal level of about

100,000 IU/L in the maternal circulation is reached at 8–10 weeks of gestation. Why does the corpus luteum involute at the time that HCG is reaching its highest levels? One possibility is that a specific inhibitory agent becomes active at this time. Another is down-regulation of receptors by the high levels of HCG. In early pregnancy, down-regulation may be avoided because HCG is secreted in an episodic fashion.[111] For unknown reasons, the fetal testes escape desensitization; no receptor down-regulation takes place.[108]

HCG levels decrease to about 10,000–20,000 IU/L by 18–20 weeks and remain at that level to term. It is not certain why HCG levels are decreased in the second half of pregnancy. Advancing gestation is associated with increasing amounts of "nicked" HCG molecules in the maternal circulation.[112] These molecules are missing a peptide linkage on the beta-subunit, and therefore, they dissociate into free α- and β-subunits. At any one point in time, the maternal circulation contains HCG, nicked HCG, free subunits, and fragments of HCG. In addition, the carbohydrate content of HCG varies throughout pregnancy, with more glycosylation present in early pregnancy. Overall, there are about 20–30 isoforms in the maternal blood, and the production of normal molecules is maximal in early gestation when the biologic actions of HCG are so important.[113] A major route of clearance for HCG is renal metabolism in which a final reduced fragment of the β-subunit is produced, known as the β-core fragment.

In the complex process of HCG regulation, several inhibiting factors have been identified, including inhibin and progesterone. The decline in HCG occurs at the time of increasing placental progesterone production, and a direct inhibition by this steroid could explain the lower levels of HCG after the 10th week of gestation.[114]

HCG levels close to term are higher in women bearing female fetuses. This is true of serum levels, placental content, urinary levels, and amniotic fluid concentrations. The mechanism and purpose of this difference are not known.

There are two clinical conditions in which blood HCG titers are very helpful: trophoblastic disease and ectopic pregnancies. Early pregnancy is characterized by the sequential appearance of HCG, followed by β-HCG and then α-HCG. The ratio of β-HCG to whole HCG remains constant after early pregnancy. Trophoblastic disease is distinguished by very high β-HCG levels (3–100 times higher than normal pregnancy). Ectopic production of alpha- and beta-HCG by nontrophoblastic tumors is rare. Previous studies with polyclonal antisera suggesting ectopic production were not accurate. The production of whole HCG in such tumors may not occur.

In the United States, hydatidiform moles occur in approximately 1 in 600 induced abortions and 1 in 1000–2000 pregnancies. About 20% of patients with hydatidiform moles will develop malignant complications. Following molar pregnancies, the HCG titer should fall to a non-detectable level by 16 weeks in patients without persistent disease. Patients with trophoblastic disease show an abnormal curve (a titer greater than 500 IU/L) frequently by 3 weeks and usually by 6 weeks.[115, 116] A diagnosis of gestational trophoblastic disease is made when the β-HCG plateaus or rises over a 2-week period, or a continued elevation is present 16 weeks after evacuation. In the United States, the rare occurrence of this disease mandates consultation with a certified subspecialist in gynecologic oncology. Following treatment, HCG should be measured monthly for at least a year, then twice yearly for 5 years. In order to avoid missing the diagnosis of nonmolar trophoblastic disease, abnormal bleeding after any pregnancy should be evaluated with an HCG measurement, and all patients with elevated HCG levels and early pregnancy losses should be followed with serial HCG testing.

In order to avoid unnecessary treatment (prophylactic chemotherapy) of the 80–85% of patients who undergo spontaneous remission, there is a need to identify those at high risk for persistent trophoblastic disease. A radioimmunoassay for the free beta-subunit of HCG may serve this need in that persistent trophoblastic disease is associated with excessive production of the free beta-subunit.[117, 118]

Virtually all ectopic pregnancies are associated with detectable HCG. The HCG level increases at different rates in normal and ectopic pregnancies, and the quantitative measurement of HCG combined with pelvic ultrasonography has had an enormous impact on the diagnosis and management of ectopic pregnancy. This important clinical problem is discussed fully in Chapter 32. The contributions of HCG measurement can be summarized as follows:

1. The quantitative measurement of HCG can assess pregnancy viability. A normal rate of rise usually indicates a normal pregnancy.

2. When the HCG titer exceeds 1000–1500 IU/L, vaginal ultrasonography should identify the presence of an intrauterine gestation.

3. Declining HCG levels are consistent with effective treatment, and persistent or rising levels indicate the presence of viable trophoblastic tissue.

With the use of modern sensitive assays, it is now appreciated that virtually all normal human tissues produce the intact HCG molecule. HCG can be detected in the blood of normal men and women, where it is secreted in a pulsatile fashion in parallel with LH, and apparently the source of this circulating HCG is the pituitary gland.[119–122] The concentration of this pituitary HCG normally reaches the sensitivity of the usual modern assay only in a rare postmenopausal woman with high LH levels. HCG produced in sites other than the placenta has little or no carbohydrate, and, therefore, it has a very short half-life and is rapidly cleared from the circulation. Significant levels of free α-subunit are also present in the circulation of healthy individuals; however, the levels of the β-subunit are extremely low.

Human Placental Lactogen (HPL)

Human placental lactogen (sometimes called human chorionic somatomammotropin), also secreted by the syncytiotrophoblast, is a single-chain polypeptide of 191 amino acids held together by two disulfide bonds. It is very similar in structure to human growth hormone (HGH), but has only 3% of HGH somatotropin activity. The growth hormone-HPL gene family consists of 5 genes on chromosome 17q22–q24. Two genes encode for HGH and 3 for HPL; however, only 2 of the HPL genes are abundantly active in the placenta, each producing the same HPL hormone.[123] The third HPL gene does generate a protein in the placenta, but its activity is limited.[124]

Although HPL has about 50% of the lactogenic activity of sheep prolactin in certain bioassays, its lactogenic contribution in human pregnancy is uncertain. Its half-life is short, about 15 minutes; hence its appeal as an index of placental problems. The level of HPL in the maternal circulation is correlated with fetal and placental weight, steadily increasing until plateauing in the last 4 weeks of pregnancy (5–7 mg/mL). There is no circadian variation, and only minute amounts of HPL enter the fetal circulation. Very high maternal levels are found in association with multiple gestations; levels up to 40 mg/mL have been found with quadruplets and quintuplets. An abnormally low level is anything less than 4 mg/mL in the last trimester.

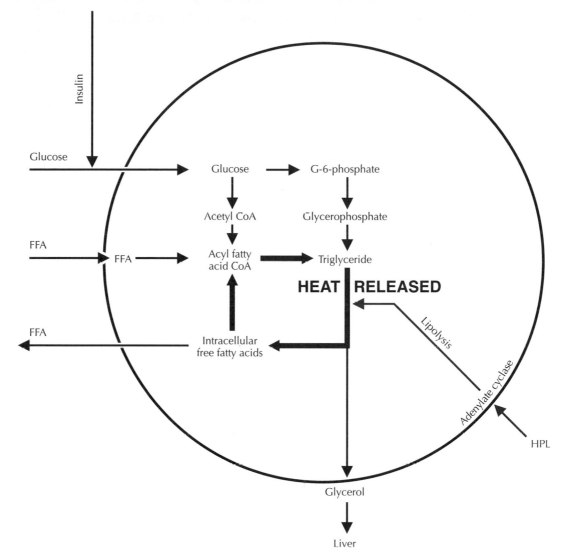

Physiologic Function

Although similar in structure to growth hormone, neither growth hormone-releasing hormone nor somatostatin influence placental HPL secretion. One would expect the regulatory mechanism to involve placental growth factors and cytokines, as is the case with other placental steroids and peptides.

In the mother, HPL stimulates insulin secretion and IGF-I production and induces insulin resistance and carbohydrate intolerance. Experimentally, the maternal level of HPL can be altered by changing the circulating level (chronically, not acutely) of glucose. HPL is elevated with hypoglycemia and depressed with hyperglycemia. This information and studies in fasted pregnant women have led to the following formulation for the physiologic function of HPL.[125–131]

The metabolic role of HPL is to mobilize lipids as free fatty acids. In the fed state, there is abundant glucose available, leading to increased insulin levels, lipogenesis, and glucose utilization. This is associated with decreased gluconeogenesis and a decrease in the circulating free fatty acid levels, because the free fatty acids are utilized in the process of lipogenesis to deposit storage packets of triglycerides (see Chapter 19, Obesity).

HPL Changes in the Fed State

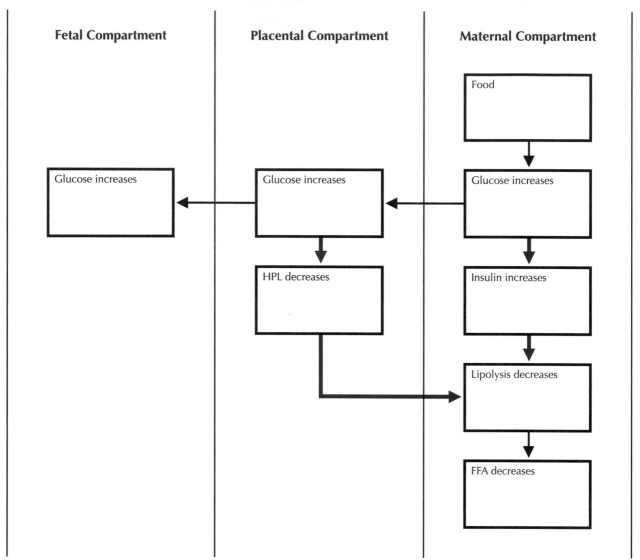

Pregnancy has been likened to a state of "accelerated starvation," characterized by a relative hypoglycemia in the fasting state.[128] This state is due to two major influences:

1. Glucose provides the major, although not the entire, fuel requirement for the fetus. A difference in gradient causes a constant transfer of glucose from the mother to the fetus.

2. Placental hormones, specifically estrogen and progesterone, and especially HPL, interfere with the action of maternal insulin. In the second half of pregnancy when HPL levels rise approximately 10-fold, HPL is a major force in the diabetogenic effects of pregnancy. The latter is characterized by increased levels of insulin associated with decreased cellular response (peripheral insulin resistance and hyperinsulinemia).

As glucose decreases in the fasting state, HPL levels rise. This stimulates lipolysis leading to an increase in circulating free fatty acids. Thus, a different fuel is provided for the mother so that glucose and amino acids can be conserved for the fetus. With sustained fasting, maternal fat is utilized for fuel to such an extent that maternal ketone levels rise. There is limited transport of free fatty acids across the placenta. Therefore, when glucose becomes scarce for the fetus, fetal tissues utilize the ketones that do cross the placenta. Thus, decreased glucose levels lead to

HPL Changes in the Fasting State

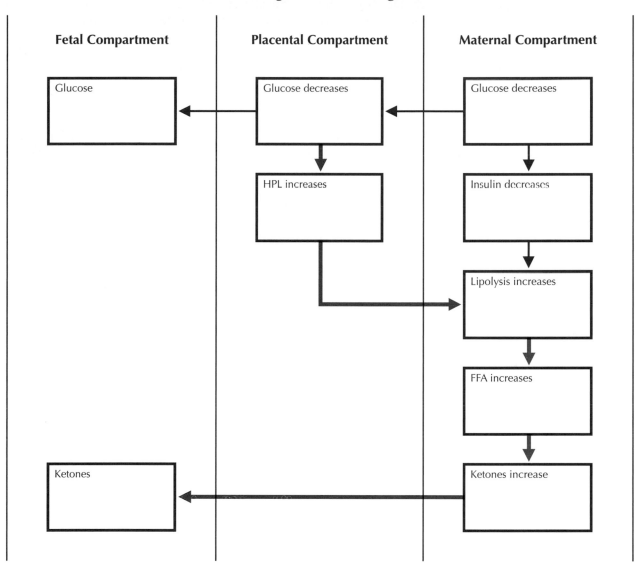

decreased insulin and increased HPL, increasing lipolysis and ketone levels. HPL also may enhance the fetal uptake of ketones and amino acids. The mechanism for the insulin antagonism by HPL may be the HPL-stimulated increase in free fatty acid levels, which, in turn, directly interfere with insulin-directed entry of glucose into cells. These interactions significantly involve growth factors, particularly insulin-like growth factor, at the cellular level.

This mechanism can be viewed as an important means to provide fuel for the fetus between maternal meals. However, with a sustained state of inadequate glucose intake, the subsequent ketosis may impair fetal brain development and function. Pregnancy is not the time to severely restrict caloric intake. Indeed, impaired fetal growth and development are now recognized to correlate with adverse cardiovascular risk factors and disease in adult life.[47, 132]

The lipid, lipoprotein, and apolipoprotein changes during pregnancy are positively correlated with changes in estradiol, progesterone, and HPL.[133] The lipolytic activity of HPL is an important factor because HPL is also linked to the maternal blood levels of cholesterol, triglycerides, phospholipids, and insulin-like growth factor-I.

When glucose is abundant, as in pregnant women with diabetes mellitus, the flow of nutritional substrates (in this case, glucose and amino acids) is in the direction of the fetus. The subsequent hyperinsulinemia in the fetus becomes a strong stimulus to growth, perhaps compounded by maternal hyperinsulinemia caused by obesity as well as the hyperinsulinemia due to the peripheral resistance produced by the hormones of pregnancy.[134] Fetal undernutrition lowers fetal IGF-I levels, and this is associated with a high prevalence of insulin resistance later as adults.[135] In vitro studies indicate that HPL, despite its lower levels in the fetus, directly affects fetal tissue metabolism, including synergistic actions with insulin, especially on glycogen synthesis in the liver. The failure of fetal growth hormone to affect fetal growth (e.g., normal growth in anencephalics) further indicates that HPL may be the fetal growth hormone.

HPL Clinical Uses

Blood levels of HPL are related to placental function. Although some studies indicated that HPL was valuable in screening patients for potential fetal complications, others id not support the use of HPL measurements. Even though utilization of the HPL assay can have an impact on perinatal care, fetal heart rate-monitoring techniques are more reliably predictive and sensitive for assessing fetal well-being. Furthermore, totally uneventful pregnancies have been reported, despite undetectable HPL.[136, 137]

Previous suggestions that a low or declining level of HPL and a high level of HCG are characteristic of trophoblastic disease were not accurate. Because of the rapid clearance of HPL (half-life of about 20 minutes), aborting molar pregnancies are likely to have low levels of HPL, whereas the level of HCG is still high. However, intact molar pregnancies can have elevated levels of both HPL and HCG.[138]

Human Chorionic Thyrotropin (HCT)

The human placenta contains two thyrotropic substances. One is called human chorionic thyrotropin (HCT), similar in size and action to pituitary TSH. Te content in the normal placenta is very small, and it is unlikely that it has any physiologic importance. HCT differs from the other glycoproteins in that it does not appear to share the common α-subunit. Antiserum generated to α-HCG does not neutralize the biologic activities of HCT, but it does neutralize that of HCG and pituitary TSH.

Rarely, patients with trophoblastic disease have hyperthyroidism. Studies have indicated that HCG has intrinsic thyrotropic activity, suggesting that HCG is the second placental thyrotropic substance.[139–141] It has been calculated that HCG contains approximately 1/4000th of the thyrotropicactivity of human TSH. In conditions with very elevated HCG levels, the thyrotropic activity can be sufficient to produce hyperthyroidism, and this can even be encountered in normal pregnancy.[142] There is a correlation between elevated thyroid function and hyperemesis gravidarum. These clinical manifestations in normal pregnancies may be linked to a specific subpopulation of HCG molecules with greater thyrotropic bioactivity (beause highly purified, standard HCG has only trivial TSH-like activity).[143] Specifically, HCG with reduced sialic acid content is increased in pregnant patients with hyperemesis and hyperthyroidism.[144] The thyroid hormone changes in pregnancy and the role of HCG as a thyroid stimulator are discussed in Chapter 20.

Human Chorionic Adrenocorticotropin

The rise in maternal free cortisol that takes place throughout pregnancy is due to ACTH and corticotropin-releasing hormone (CRH) production ad secretion into the maternal circulation by the placenta.[145–147] The placental content of ACTH is higher than can be aunted for by the contribution of sequestered blood. In addition, cortisol levels in pregnant women are resist to dexamethasone suppression, suggesting that there is a component of maternal ACTH and CRH that does not originate in the maternal pituitary gland. The placental production of ACTH in the syncytiotrophoblast (and the increase in maternal ACTH levels) is probably due to stimulation by the locally produced CRH in the cytotrophoblast.[148] Placental pro-opiomelanocortin (POMC) gene expression and ACTH content are present throughout pregnancy and increase in the weeks before term.[149] One can speculate that placental ACTH and CRH raise maternal adrenal activity in order to provide the basic building blocks (cholesterol and pregnenolone) for placental steroidogenesis. There is no passage of ACTH between the fetal and maternal opartments.

The maternal ACTH response to the administration of CRH during pregnancy is blunted, indicating a high level of endogenous CRH and ACTH activity. Vasopressin stimulates ACTH secretion in the pituitary, both directly and indirectly by potentiating the action of CRH. In contrast to the blunted response to CRH during pregnancy, the ACTII response to vasopressin is increased.[150] This is further evidence that placental CRH produces a state of chronic stimulation for the maternal pituitary-adrenal axis. Thus, in contrast to nonpregnant women, CRH levels in maternal plasma are relatively high, rising in the second trimester to peak values at term.[151, 152] In contrast to the hypothalamic-pituitary axis, placental CRH and ACTII are not suppressed by glucocorticoids, and, therefore, maternal ACTH levels are little affected by corticosteroid administration to the mother. Oxytocin is a potent stimulator of CRH and ACTH placental production, a logical mechanism to meet the stress of labor and delivery. The fall in CRH-binding protein near term further increases the cortisol availability during labor and delivery.

Both maternal and fetal levels of CRH are further elevated in pathologic states such as premature labor, hypertension, fetal asphyxia, and intrauterine growth retardation.[153] Because CRH also stimulates prostaglandin synthesis in the placenta and fetal membranes, it is implicated in the premature labor that accompanies pathologic conditions.[154]

Growth Hormone, Growth Hormone-Releasing Hormone, and Somatostatin

Growth hormone-releasing hormone (GHRH) and somatostatin are found in the placenta, and somatostatin is present indecidua.[78, 155] The amount of somatostatin decreases ith increasing gestation. Pregnancy GHRH and somatostatin do not contribute to maternal circulating levels of these peptides. One of the two growth hormone genes on chromosome 17 is expressed only in the syncytiotrophoblast of the placenta.[124] The placental growth hormone is not identical to pituitary growth hormone, and after 15–20 weeks of pregnancy, placental growth hormone gradually replaces pituitary growth hormone in the aternal circulation.[124, 156] Indeed, by term, maternal pituitary growth hormone is undetectable. Placental growth hormone is not present in fetal blood. The changes in maternal levels of insulin-like growth factors and insulin-like growth factor binding proteins reflect regulation by this placental growth hormone.[157] Maternal IGF-I levels in the circulation increase uring pregnancy in a pattern similar to that of placental growth hormone. Placental growth hormone is not regulated by placental GHRH, but responds inversely to maternal glucose levels, protecting glucose availability for the fetus.[124] Placental growth hormone can also stimulate gluconeogenesis and lipolysis in maternal organs. It is believed, therefore, that placental growth hormone influences fetal growth by affecting maternal metabolism.

Alpha-Fetoprotein

Alpha-fetoprotein (AFP) is a relatively unique glycoprotein (590 amino acids and 4% carbohydrate) derived largely from fetal liver and partially from the yolk sac until it degenerates at about 12 weeks. In early pregnancy (5–12 weeks), amniotic fluid AFP is mainly from yolk sac origin, whereas maternal circulating AFP is mainly from the fetal liver.[158] Its function is unknown, but it is comparable in size to albumin and contains 39% sequence homology; it may serve as a protein carrier of steroid hormones in fetal blood. AFP may also be a modulator of cell proliferation, synergizing with various growth factors.[159]

Peak levels of AFP in the fetal blood are reached at the end of the first trimester; then levels decrease gradually until a rapid decrease begins at 32 weeks. Maternal blood levels are much lower than fetal levels, rising until week 32 (probably because of the great increase in trophoblast villous surface area during this time period) and then declining. Because AFP is highly concentrated in the fetal central nervous system, abnormal direct contact of CNS with the amniotic fluid (as with neural tube defects) results in elevated amniotic fluid and maternal blood levels. Other fetal abnormalities, such as intestinal obstruction, omphalocele, and congenital nephrosis, are also associated with high levels of AFP in the amniotic fluid. Besides indicating a variety of fetal anomalies, elevated maternal AFP levels are also present with multiple pregnancies and associated with an increased risk of spontaneous miscarriage, stillbirth, preterm birth, preeclampsia, neonatal death, and low birth weight (probably reflecting an increase in villous surface area in response to an adverse intrauterine environment).[160, 161]

Multiple Marker Screening

Down syndrome is a very common genetic cause of abnormal development. The majority of cases are due to trisomy 21, an extra chromosome usually due to nondisjunction in maternal meiosis. A low maternal level of AFP is associated with trisomy 21. However, there is extensive overlap between normal and affected pregnancies responsible for a significant false-positive rate. Several placental products are secreted in increased amounts in pregnancies with trisomy 21, including HCG and HPL, whereas the maternal circulating level of unconjugated estriol is lower in affected pregnancies. The free β-subunit of HCG usually circulates in low concentrations, but in the presence of a fetus with Down syndrome, the levels are high. With trisomy 18, all markers are decreased. Modern screening for fetal aneuploidy combines three markers: AFP, HCG, or β-HCG, and unconjugated estriol.[162–164] This protocol will detect 85% of open neural tube defects and 80% of Down syndrome. However, Down syndrome represents only about 50% of the chromosomal abnormalities that can be detected.

The multiple marker screening protocol measures AFP, HCG, and unconjugated estriol in maternal serum at 16–18 weeks gestation, the optimal time for neural tube defect detection. Using the patient's age and the laboratory results, patients are provided a statistical estimation of risks for both neural tube defects and Down syndrome. Corrections are applied for race and weight. A pattern similar to that of Down syndrome has also been reported to be associated with hydropic fetal Turner syndrome.[165] A comparison trial concluded that a combination of AFP and the free β-subunit of HCG is more accurate and less expensive than the utilization of the 3 markers, AFP, HCG, and unconjugated estriol.[166]

The most critical factor for correct risk assessment is accurate gestational dating. A two-week error in dating can change the calculated risk for Down syndrome ten-fold. Therefore, ultrasound confirmation of gestational dating is essential. In addition, ultrasonography will indicate fetal number and assess the fetus for anomalies.

The multiple marker protocol is for screening a low-risk population regardless of age, and amniocentesis is necessary for final diagnosis. Genetic amniocentesis is still recommended for older women; however, although multiple marker screening does not detect all chromosomal abnormalities, some have argued that the detection rate is so high that screening as an option should be offered even to older women.[163, 167]

The detection of a very low unconjugated estriol level in the second trimester is associated with an increased risk of early fetal demise.[168] In addition, a low estriol can be a marker for placental sulfatase deficiency.

Relaxin

Relaxin is a peptide hormone produced by the corpus luteum of pregnancy, which is not detected in men or nonpregnant women. It is composed of two short peptide chains (24 and 29 amino acids, respectively) linked by disulfide bridges. While it has been argued that the human corpus luteum is the sole source of relaxin in pregnancy, it has also been identified in human placenta, decidua, and chorion.[169–171] The maternal serum concentration rises during the first trimester when the corpus luteum is dominant and declines in the second trimester.[172] This suggests a role in maintaining early pregnancy, but its function is not really known. In animals, relaxin softens the cervix (ripening), inhibits uterine contractions, and relaxes the pubic symphysis. The animal cervical changes are comparable to those seen with human labor, and in in vitro studies of human cervical stromal cells, relaxin induces changes consistent with clinical ripening.[173, 174] To examine the contribution of the corpus luteum, normally pregnant women were compared with women pregnant with donated oocytes (and therefore without corpora lutea).[175] Relaxin was undetectable in the women without functioning ovaries, confirming that its major source is the corpus luteum. No effect on prolactin secretion was observed, but it did appear that relaxin enhanced growth hormone secretion by the pituitary. Obviously, relaxin is not necessary for the maintenance of pregnancy and labor because the rest of pregnancy and the outcomes did not differ between those women with circulating levels of relaxin and those with undetectable levels. However, recombinant relaxin is being tested for ripening of the cervix.

Prolactin

Following ovulation, the endometrium becomes a secretory organ and remains so throughout pregnancy. Decidualized endometrium secretes renin, which may be involved in the regulation of water and electroytes in the amniotic fluid, and relaxin, which may influence prostaglandin production in the membranes. One of the best studied special endocrine functions of the decidual endometrium is the secretion of prolactin. Prolactin is synthesized by endometrium during a normal menstrual cycle, but this synthesis is not initiated until histologic decidualization begins about day 23.[176, 177] The control of prolactin secretion by decidual tissue has not been definitively established. Some argue that once decidualization is established, prolactin secretion continues in the absence of either progesterone or estradiol, although there is evidence for an inhibitory feedback by decidual proteins (perhaps prolactin itself).[176, 178] Others indicate that endometrial prolactin production requires the combined effects of progestin and estrogen hormones plus the presence of other placental and decidual factors, including relaxin, IGF-I, and specific stimulatory and inhibitory proteins.[179]

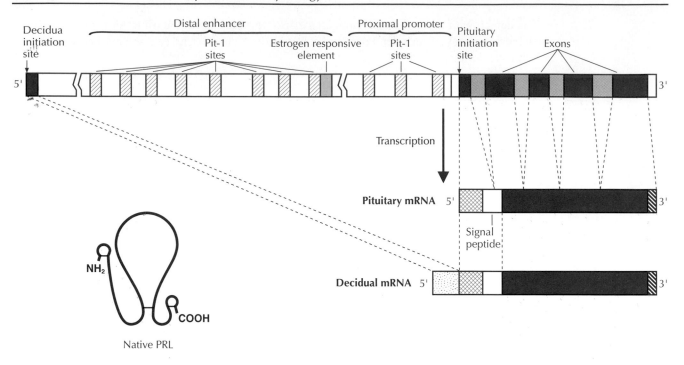

During pregnancy, prolactin secretion is limited to the fetal pituitary, the maternal pituitary, and the uterus. Neither trophoblast nor fetal membranes synthesize prolactin, but both the myometrium and endometrium can produce prolactin. The endometrium requires the presence of progesterone to initiate prolactin, whereas progesterone suppresses prolactin synthesis in the myometrium. Prolactin derived from the decidua is the source of prolactin found in the amniotic fluid.[180] The prolactin in the fetal circulation is derived from the fetal pituitary. Decidual prolactin is transcribed by a gene with an additional exon compared with the pituitary, accounting for a different system of regulation.[181]

During pregnancy, prolactin levels rise from the normal level of 10–25 ng/mL to high concentrations, beginning about 8 weeks and reaching a peak of 200–400 ng/mL at term.[182, 183] The increase in prolactin parallels the increase in estrogen beginning at 7–8 weeks gestation, and the mechanism for increasing prolactin secretion (discussed in Chapter 5) is believed to be estrogen suppression of the hypothalamic prolactin inhibiting factor, dopamine, and direct stimulation of prolactin gene transcription in the pituitary.[184, 185] There is marked variability in maternal prolactin levels in pregnancy, with a diurnal variation similar to that found in nonpregnant persons.

Amniotic fluid concentrations of prolactin parallel maternal serum concentrations until the 10th week of pregnancy, rise markedly until the 20th week, and then undergo a decrease until delivery. The maternal and fetal blood levels of prolactin are derived from the respective pituitary glands, and, therefore, dopamine agonist suppression of pituitary secretion of prolactin throughout pregnancy produces minimal maternal and fetal blood levels, yet there is normal fetal growth and development, and amniotic fluid levels are unchanged.[186] Fortunately, decidual secretion of prolactin is unaffected by dopamine agonist treatment because decidual prolactin is important for fluid and electrolyte regulation of the amniotic fluid. This decidual prolactin is transported across the membranes in a process that requires the intact state of amnion and chorion with adherent decidua. The prolactin receptor is expressed in fetal and maternal tissues in the following descending order of intensity: chorionic cytotrophoblast, decidua, amnion, and syncytiotrophoblast.[187] This molecular expression is consistent with local actions.

No clinical significance can be attached to maternal and fetal blood levels of prolactin in abnormal pregnancies. Decidual and amniotic fluid prolactin levels are lower, however, in hypertensive pregnancies and in patients with polyhydramnios.[188, 189] Prolactin receptors are present in the chorion laeve, and their concentration is lower in patients with polyhydramnios.[190] Prolactin reduces the permeability of the human amnion in the fetal to maternal direction. This receptor-mediated action takes place on the epithelium lining the fetal surface.[191] There is also evidence that prolactin derived from the fetal pituitary contributes to the regulation of fetal water and electrolyte balance by acting as an antidiuretic hormone.[192]

The increase in maternal levels of prolactin represents maternal pituitary secretion in response to estrogen as the fetus prepares the mother for breastfeeding. The mechanisms for pituitary secretion of prolactin are discussed in Chapters 2, 5, and 16.

Cytokines and Growth Factors

The placenta synthesizes many proteins that are part of the normal composition of cells throughout the body. Local placental cytokine production is believed to be important for embryonic growth, and in the maternal immune response essential for survival of the pregnancy.[193] Interleukin-1β is produced in the decidualized endometrium during pregnancy, and colony-stimulating factor-1 (CSF-1) is produced by both decidua and placenta. CSF-1 gene expression in response to interleukin-1β has been localized to mesenchymal fibroblasts from the core of placental villi.[194] Thus, a system of communication is present between maternal decidual and fetal tissue to provide growth factor support for the placenta which would include fetal hematopoiesis, a known response to CSF-1. The placenta also produces interleukin-6, and both interleukins stimulate HCG release by activation of the interleukin-6 receptor.[195] Thus, the interleukin-1 influence on HCG secretion is mediated by the interleukin-6 system. Both trophoblast derived interleukin-1 and tumor necrosis factor-α (TNF-α) synergistically release interleukin-6 and activate the interleukin-6 system to secrete HCG.[196] Interferons and their receptors are present in virtually all cells, and thus, it is not surprising that they are found in the tissues of pregnancy.

The insulin-like growth factors, IGF-I and IGF-II, are involved in prenatal and postnatal growth and development. These growth factors do not cross the placenta into the fetal circulation; however, they may be involved in placental growth.[197] The maternal levels of IGF-I are significantly regulated by growth hormone-dependent liver synthesis. The fetus can influence maternal IGF-I levels by means of the placental secretion of HPL. An increase in maternal IGF-I levels during pregnancy with a rapid decrease after delivery indicates a significant placental influence. There is no major change in maternal IGF-II levels throughout pregnancy.

The 6 IGF binding proteins transport IGFs in the circulation, protect IGFs against metabolism and clearance, and, importantly, affect the biologic activity of IGFs by modulating IGF availability at the cellular level. Pregnancy is marked by a rise in maternal levels of insulin-like growth factor binding protein-1 (IGFBP-1), beginning at the end of the first trimester and reaching a peak at term.[198] IGFBP-1 is now recognized to be the same as placental protein-12, a decidual protein. Thus, IGFBP-1 originates in the decidua, regulated by progesterone, as well as in the liver. The prominence of IGFBP-1 in the pregnant state is in contrast to the nonpregnant state when IGFBP-3 is the main circulating IGFBP. During pregnancy, the levels of IGFBP-3 and IGFBP-2 decrease, apparently due to the activity of a pregnancy-associated serum protease (IGFBP-3 protease).[198] These changes would promote the bioavailability of IGF-I in maternal tissues, and this may be important in enhancing nutrient transfer from the mother to the placenta. There is evidence to indicate that the mother can alter IGFBP-3 proteolytic activity according to her nutritional state; thus increased proteolysis would decrease IGFBP-3 levels increasing the bioavailability of maternal IGF-I.[199]

How these changes interact to regulate growth and development of different organs and tissues is a new area of research activity. For example, in the pregnant ewe and fetal lamb, glucose and other nutritional factors regulate the gene expression and, therefore, the circulating levels of IGF binding proteins.[200] Fasting and feeding increased and decreased, respectively, the IGFBP concentrations, perhaps partly a response to insulin levels and the effect of insulin on liver synthesis of IGFBPs. These changes are consistent with IGF and IGFBP involvement in the responses to nutrition and stress. Because IGFBP-1 appears to be the principal binding protein in pregnancy, attention is focused on the changes in IGF-I and IGFBP-1. IGF-I, produced in the placenta, regulates transfer of nutrients across the placenta to the fetus and, thus, enhances fetal growth; IGFBP-1, produced in the decidua, interferes with IGF-I action and inhibits fetal growth.[201] Thus, newborn birth weight correlates directly with maternal levels of IGF-I and inversely with levels of IGFBP-1.

Intrauterine growth retardation is associated with reduced fetal blood levels of IGF-I and IGFBP-3 and increased levels of IGFBP-1 and IGFBP-2.[202] In view of the strong relationship between the IGF system and fetal nutrition, it is logical that fetal glucose availability and insulin are the principal regulating agents. In experimental animals, an increase in fetal insulin or glucose elevates IGF-I levels, whereas nutritional restriction causes an increase in IGFBP-1 and IGFBP-2, and a decrease in IGFBP-3.[203] Insulin is believed to influence growth by promoting cellular uptake of nutrients and by increasing IGF-I production. The fetal blood levels of IGF-II parallel those of IGF-I, and IGF-II promotes fetal growth by means of the IGF-I receptor. IGF-II appears to be important early in embryonic growth, and then after organ development is complete, IGF-I becomes the dominant factor.

Epidermal growth factor (EGF) is present in both cytotrophoblast and syncytiotrophoblast, but more intensely in syncytiotrophoblast, and probably is involved in the differentiation of cytotrophoblast into syncytiotrophoblast. EGF is well known as a mitogen. Other growth factors isolated from human placenta include platelet-derived growth factor, nerve growth factor, fibroblast growth factor, and transforming growth factors. These factors are probably all involved in the proliferation and growth associated with pregnancy.

Inhibin, Activin, and Follistatin

The placenta produces inhibin, which is responsible for the marked increase in maternal inhibin levels throughout pregnancy.[204, 205] Inhibin A is the principal bioactive inhibin secreted during pregnancy, rising in the maternal circulation at the time of the emergence of placental function, peaking at 8 weeks gestation, and then decreasing before increasing again in the third trimester to reach a level at term that is 100 times greater than that during the normal menstrual cycle.[206–208] Undoubtedly, the high levels of inhibin and estrogen during pregnancy account for the profound suppression of maternal gonadotropins. Trophoblastic inhibin synthesis is inhibited by activin A and stimulated by HCG, GnRH, epidermal growth factor, transforming growth factor-α, and PGE_2 and $PGF_{2\alpha}$, the major placental prostaglandins.[205] Activin A, the major trophoblastic activin product, also increases in the maternal circulation, with elevated but stable levels from 8 to 24 weeks, and then increasing to reach a level at term that is 100 times greater than that during the normal menstrual cycle.[209]

Similar to their action in the ovarian follicle, inhibin and activin are regulators within the placenta for the production of GnRH, HCG, and steroids; as expected, activin is stimulatory, and inhibin is inhibitory.[103] GnRH and the subunits for inhibin and activin can be found in the same placental cells, in both cytotrophoblast and syncytiotrophoblast, but not in all cells.[210] The maternal levels of inhibin B are very low throughout pregnancy; however, inhibin B is significantly expressed in the amnion where it is believed to influence prostaglandin synthesis.[211] Trophoblast synthesis and release of inhibin and activin are part of the complex placental story, involving many hormones and locally produced factors. The placental and decidual appearance of inhibin and activin occurs early in pregnancy in time for possible roles in embryogenesis and local immune responses. The measurement of inhibin A has promise as a screening test for Down syndrome.[212, 213]

Follistatin is an activin-binding protein expressed in placenta, membranes, and decidua.[214]

Because follistatin binds activin, it antagonizes the stimulatory effects of activin on placental steroid and peptide production.

Endogenous Opiates

Fetal and maternal endogenous opiates originate from the pituitary glands and are secreted in parallel with ACTH, in response to corticotropin-releasing hormone, which is, in part, derived from the placenta.[215] There is reason to believe that in pregnancy the intermediate lobe of the maternal pituitary gland is a major source of elevated circulating endorphin levels. However, the syncytiotrophoblast in response to CRH produces all of the products of proopiomelanocortin (POMC) metabolism, including β-endorphin, enkephalins, and dynorphins. The placenta and membranes are richly endowed with G protein opioid receptors.[216] The presence of CRH in the placenta and placental opiate production in response to CRH and oxytocin indicate an interaction similar to that in the hypothalamic-pituitary axis.[217]

It is not certain whether maternal blood levels of endogenous opiates increase with advancing gestation.[78] However, a marked increase in maternal values is reached during labor, coinciding with full cervical dilatation. The maternal levels also correlate with the degree of pain perception and use of analgesia. On the fetal side, hypoxia is a potent stimulus for endorphin release.

There are many hypotheses surrounding the function of endogenous opiates in pregnancy. These include roles related to stress; inhibition of oxytocin, vasopressin and gonadotropins; the promotion of prolactin secretion; and, of course, a natural analgesic agent during labor and delivery.

The Renin-Angiotensin System

The circulating levels of prorenin, the inactive precursor of renin, increase (10-fold) during early pregnancy, the result of ovarian stimulation by HCG.[218, 219] This increase in prorenin from the ovary is not associated with any significant change in the blood levels of the active form, renin. Possible roles for this ovarian prorenin-renin-angiotensin system include the following: stimulation of steroidogenesis to provide androgen substrate for estrogen production, regulation of calcium and prostaglandin metabolism, and stimulation of angiogenesis. This system may affect vascular and tissue functions both in and outside the ovary. Prorenin also originates in chorionic tissues and is highly concentrated in the amniotic fluid. The highest biologic levels of prorenin are found in gestational sacs in early pregnancy; its possible roles in embryonic growth and development remain speculative.[219] Renin and angiotensinogen (the renin substrate) are expressed by the following fetal tissues: chorion, amnion, and placenta.[220] This system responds to a variety of factors, affecting vascular resistance and blood volume.[221] Maternal renin activity is increased four-fold by midgestation, partly a response to an estrogen-induced increase in angiotensinogen, but largely a compensatory response to maintain blood pressure in the presence of vasodilatation.[222] There is little evidence that fetal or uterine prorenin or renin contribute to the maternal circulation.

Atrial Natriuretic Peptide

Atrial natriuretic peptide (ANP) is derived from human atrial tissue and the placenta.[223] It is a potent natriuretic, diuretic, and smooth muscle-relaxant peptide that circulates as a hormone. Maternal ANP increases in the third trimester and during labor, and cord levels on the arterial side suggest that ANP is a circulating hormone in the fetus.[224] In the mother, ANP release is stimulated by atrial stretch, and this is another mechanism for regulating the volume and electrolyte changes associated with pregnancy and delivery.[225]

Other Proteins

The mother responds to a pregnancy even before implantation. Remarkably, early pregnancy factor (EPF) can be detected in the maternal circulation within 1–2 days after coitus results in a pregnancy.[226] It remains throughout pregnancy, but interestingly, disappears before parturition. EPF prior to implantation is apparently produced by the ovary in response to a signal from the embryo. After implantation, EPF is no longer secreted by the ovary but now is derived from the embryo. EPF is a protein associated with cell proliferation and growth and, therefore, is present in many nonpregnant tissues such as neoplasms. EPF has immunosuppressive properties and is abundant in platelets. We are just beginning to learn about this fetal and maternal protein. Neuropeptide Y, a peptide extensively distributed in the brain, is found in trophoblast, membranes, and decidua, with higher but nonchanging maternal blood levels during pregnancy.[78]

Pregnancy-specific γ_1-glycoprotein (PSG) was previously known as Schwangerschaftsprotein 1. The physiologic function of PSG produced by the placenta is unknown, but it has been used as a test for pregnancy and a marker for malignancies, including choriocarcinoma. Molecular studies have revealed that PSG consists of a family of closely related glycoproteins encoded by genes on chromosome 19.[227] The PSG family is closely related to the carcinoembryonic antigen (CEA) proteins. Pregnancy-associated plasma protein-A (PAPP-A) is a placental protein that is similar to a macroglobulin in the serum and still in search of specific functions. Progesterone-associated endometrial protein, previously called placental protein 14, is now recognized to originate in secretory endometrium and decidua. No role for this protein has been described thus far.

Prostaglandins

Prostaglandin Biosynthesis

The family of prostaglandins with the greatest biologic activity is that having two double bonds, derived from arachidonic acid.[228, 229] Arachidonic acid can be obtained from two sources, directly from the diet (from meats) or by formation from its precursor linoleic acid, which is found in vegetables. In the plasma, 1–2% of the total free fatty acid content is free arachidonic acid. The majority of arachidonic acid is covalently bound in esterified form as a significant proportion of the fatty acids in phospholipids and in esterified cholesterol. Arachidonic acid is only a minor fatty acid in the triglycerides packaged in adipose tissue.

The rate-limiting step in the formation of the prostaglandin family is the release of free arachidonic acid. A variety of hydrolases may be involved in arachidonic acid release, but phospholipase A_2 activation is an important initiator of prostaglandin synthesis because of the abundance of arachidonate in the 2 position of phospholipids. In addition, phospholipase C activity can provide arachidonic acid. Types of stimuli that activate such lipases include burns, infusions of hypertonic and hypotonic solutions, thrombi and small particles, endotoxin, snake venom, mechanical stretching, catecholamines, bradykinin, angiotensin, and the sex steroids.

"Eicosanoids" refer to all the 20-carbon derivatives, whereas "prostanoids" indicate only those containing a structural ring. After the release of arachidonic acid, the synthetic path can go in two different directions: the lipoxygenase pathway or the cyclooxygenase (prostaglandin endoperoxide H synthase) pathway, depending upon the local cellular context. There are 3 lipoxygenase enzymes that lead to active compounds. Arachidonic acid is first converted to hydroperoxyeicosatetraenoic acids (HPETEs), and then to hydroxyeicosatetraenoic acids (HETEs), lipoxins,

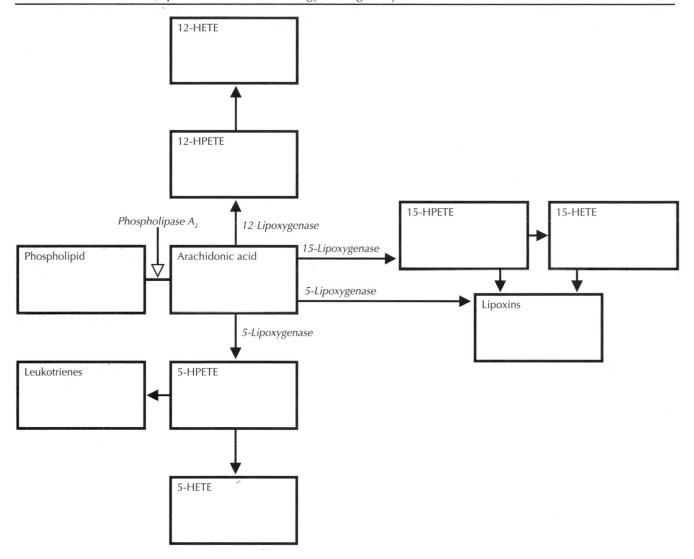

or leukotrienes. The leukotrienes are formed by 5-lipoxygenase oxygenation of arachidonic acid at C-5, forming an unstable intermediate, LTA_4.[230] LTB_4 is formed by hydration and LTC_4 by the addition of glutathione. The remaining leukotrienes are metabolites of LTC_4. The previously known slow reacting substance of anaphylaxis consists of a mixture of LTC_4, LTD_4, and LTE_4. The leukotrienes are involved in the defense reactions of white cells and participate in hypersensitivity and inflammatory responses. LTB_4 acts primarily on leukocytes (stimulation of leukocyte emigration from the bloodstream), whereas LTC_4, LTD_4, and LTE_4 affect smooth muscle cells (bronchoconstriction in the lungs and reduced contractility in the heart). All leukotrienes increase microvascular permeability. Thus, the leukotrienes are major agonists, synthesized in response to antigens provoking asthma and airway obstruction. Leukotrienes are 100–1000 times more potent than histamine in the pulmonary airway. Asthma can now be treated with a specific leukotriene receptor antagonist.

The 12-lipoxygenase pathway leads to 12-hydroxyeicosatetraenoic acid (12-HETE). Little is known about 12-HETE other than its function as a leukostatic agent. The lipoxins (LXA and LXB), products of the 5- and 15-lipoxygenase pathways, inhibit natural killer cell cytotoxicity and are vasodilators.[230]

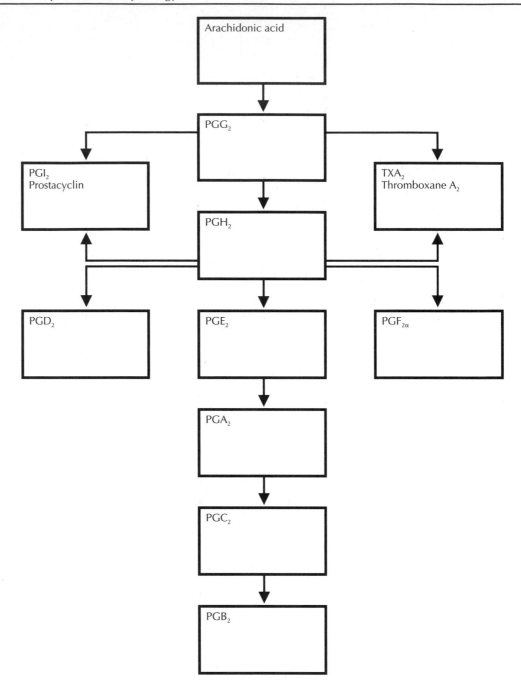

The cyclooxygenase pathway leads to the prostaglandins. The first true prostaglandin (PG) compounds formed are PGG_2 and PGH_2 (half-life of about 5 minutes), the mothers of all other prostaglandins. The numerical subscript refers to the number of double bonds. This number depends on which of the three precursor fatty acids has been utilized. Besides arachidonic acid, the other two precursor fatty acids are linoleic acid, which gives rise to the PG_1 series, and pentanoic acid, the PG_3 series. The latter two series are of less importance in physiology, hence, the significance of the arachidonic acid family. The prostaglandins of original and continuing relevance to reproduction are PGE_2 and $PGF_{2\alpha}$ and possibly PGD_2. The α in $PGF_{2\alpha}$ indicates the α steric configuration of the hydroxyl group at the C-9 position. The A, B, and C prostaglandins either have little biologic activity or do not exist in significant concentrations in biologic tissues. In the original work, the prostaglandin more soluble in ether was named PGE, and the one more soluble in phosphate (spelled with an F in Swedish) buffer was named PGF. Later, naming became alphabetical.

The cyclooxygenase enzyme (prostaglandin synthase) exists in two forms, COX-1 and COX-2, products of separate genes.[231–233] Prostacyclin is produced by COX-1, the constitutive form of the enzyme found in virtually all tissues, whereas COX-2 is induced in responses to inflammatory stimuli. COX-2 is expressed only after stimulation by various growth factors, cytokines, and endotoxins, and, therefore, it is called the inducible form. Thus selective inhibition of COX-2 would be therapeutically advantageous, possibly avoiding the side effects associated with inhibition of COX-1.

Thromboxane and Prostacyclin

Thromboxanes are not true prostaglandins because of the absence of the pentane ring, but prostacyclin (PGI_2) is a legitimate prostaglandin. Thromboxane (TX) (half-life about 30 seconds) and PGI_2 (half-life about 2–3 minutes) can be viewed as opponents, each having powerful biologic activity that counters or balances the other. TXA_2 is the most powerful vasoconstrictor known, whereas PGI_2 is a potent vasodilator. These two agents also have opposing effects on platelet function. Platelets, lungs, and the spleen predominately synthesize TXA_2, while the heart, stomach, and blood vessels throughout the body synthesize PGI_2. The lungs are a major source of prostacyclin. Normal pulmonary endothelium makes prostacyclin while TXA_2 appears in response to pathologic stimuli.[234] The pulmonary release of prostacyclin may contribute to the body's defense against platelet aggregation.

Let's take a closer look at platelets. The primary function of platelets is the preservation of the vascular system. Blood platelets stick to foreign surfaces or other tissues, a process called adhesion. They also stick to each other and form clumps; this process is called aggregation. Because platelets synthesize TXA_2, a potent stimulator of platelet aggregation, the natural tendency of platelets is to clump and plug defects and damaged spots. The endothelium, on the other hand, produces PGI_2 and its constant presence inhibits platelet aggregation and adherence, keeping blood vessels free of platelets and ultimately clots. Thus, prostacyclin has a defensive role in the body. It is 4 to 8 times more potent a vasodilator than the E prostaglandins, and it prevents the adherence of platelets to healthy vascular endothelium. However, when the endothelium is damaged, platelets gather, beginning the process of thrombus formation. Even in this abnormal situation, prostacyclin strives to fulfill its protective role because increased PGI_2 can be measured in injured endothelium, thrombosed vessels, and in the vascular tissues of hypertensive animals.

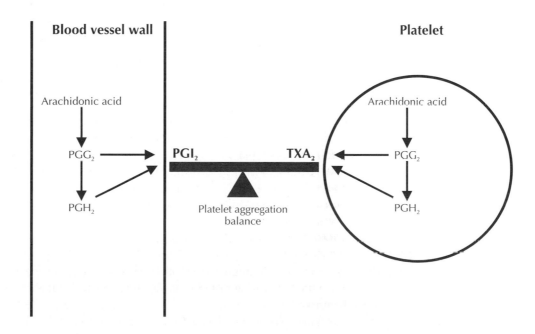

It is believed that endothelial production of prostacyclin plays an important role in the impressive vasodilatation that is associated with pregnancy. The placenta is a major source of thromboxane, and preeclampsia may, in part, reflect an imbalance between the vasodilator, prostacyclin, and the vasoconstrictor, thromboxane.[235]

Conditions associated with vascular disease can be understood through the prostacyclin-thromboxane mechanism.[236] For example, atheromatous plaques and nicotine inhibit prostacyclin synthesis. Increasing the cholesterol content of human platelets increases the sensitivity to stimuli that cause platelet aggregation due to increased thromboxane production. The well-known association between low-density and high-density lipoproteins (LDL-cholesterol and HDL-cholesterol) and cardiovascular disease may also be partly explained in terms of PGI_2. LDL from men and postmenopausal women inhibits and HDL stimulates prostacyclin production.[237] Platelets from diabetics and from class A diabetic pregnant women make more TXA_2 than platelets from normal pregnant women. Smokers who use oral contraceptives have increased platelet aggregation and an inhibition of prostacyclin formation.[238] Incidentally, onion and garlic inhibit platelet aggregation and TXA_2 synthesis.[239] Perhaps the perfect contraceptive pill is a combination of progestin, estrogen, and some onion or garlic.

In some areas of the world, there is a low incidence of cardiovascular disease. This can be directly attributed to diet and the protective action of prostacyclin.[240] The diet of Eskimos and Japanese has a high content of pentanoic acid and low levels of linoleic and arachidonic acids. Pentanoic acid is the precursor of prostaglandin products with 3 double bonds, and, as it happens, PGI_3 is an active agent while TXA_3 is either not formed, or it is inactive. The fat content of most common fish is 8–12% pentanoic acid, and more than 20% in the more exotic (and expensive) seafoods such as scallops, oysters, and caviar.

Metabolism

Prostaglandin metabolism is initiated by 15-hydroxyprostaglandin dehydrogenase. The metabolism of prostaglandins occurs primarily in the lungs, kidneys, and liver. The lungs are important in the metabolism of E and F prostaglandins. Indeed, there is an active transport mechanism that specifically carries E and F prostaglandins from the circulation into the lungs. Nearly all active prostaglandins in the circulation are metabolized during one passage through the lungs. Therefore, members of the prostaglandin family have a short half-life, and in most instances, exert autocrine/paracrine actions at the site of their synthesis. Because of the rapid half-lives, studies are often performed by measuring the inactive end products, for example 6-keto-$PGF_{1\alpha}$, the metabolite of prostacyclin, and TXB_2, the metabolite of thromboxane A_2.

Prostaglandin Inhibition

A review of prostaglandin biochemistry is not complete without a look at the inhibition of the biosynthetic cascade of products. Corticosteroids were thought to inhibit the prostaglandin family by stabilizing membranes and preventing the release of phospholipase. It is now proposed that corticosteroids induce the synthesis of proteins called lipocortins (or annexins) which block the action of phospholipase.[241] Thus far, corticosteroids and some local anesthetic agents are the only substances known to work at this step. Because corticosteroids reduce the availability of arachidonic acid for both the lipoxygenase and cyclooxygenase pathways, they are very effective anti-inflammatory agents and antihypersensitivity agents, especially for the treatment of asthma.

Aspirin is an irreversible inhibitor, selectively acetylating the cyclooxygenase involved in prostaglandin synthesis. The other inhibiting agents, nonsteroidal anti-inflammatory agents such as indomethacin and naproxen, are reversible agents, forming a reversible bond with the active site of the enzyme. Acetaminophen inhibits cyclooxygenase in the central nervous system, accounting for its analgesic and antipyretic properties, but has no anti-inflammatory properties

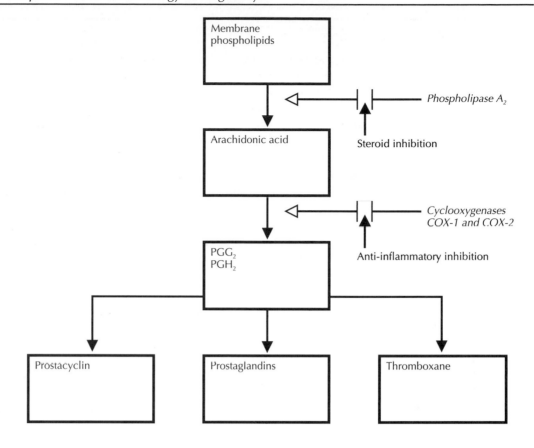

nor does it affect platelets. However, acetaminophen does reduce prostacyclin synthesis; the reason for this preferential effect is unknown.[242] The analgesic, antipyretic, and anti-inflammatory actions of these agents are mediated by inhibition of the cyclooxygenase enzymes, COX-1 and COX-2. Aspirin, indomethacin, and ibuprofen are more potent inhibitors of COX-1 than COX-2.[243] Diclofenac, acetaminophen, and naproxen inhibit both enzymes equally. The side effects associated with each agent are a reflection of the degree of selectivity towards the two enzymes; inhibition of COX-1, the constitutive form, being associated with significant side effects, and inhibition of COX-2, the inducible form, being therapeutic. Part of the anti-inflammatory activity of glucocorticoids is due to inhibition of COX-2 formation. The well-known gastric ulcerogenic side effect of anti-inflammatory drugs is due to the fact that PGE_2 protects the gastric mucosa by inhibiting gastric acid secretion, and COX-1 is the predominant enzyme in the gastric mucosa.

Because of the irreversible nature of the inhibition by aspirin, aspirin exerts a long lasting effect on platelets, maintaining inhibition in the platelet for its lifespan (8–10 days). Prostacyclin synthesis in the endothelium recovers more quickly because the endothelial cells can resynthesize new cyclooxygenase. Platelets, lacking nuclei, cannot produce new enzyme, probably exclusively COX-1. The sensitivity of the platelets to aspirin may explain the puzzling results in the early studies in which aspirin was given to prevent subsequent morbidity and mortality following thrombotic events. It takes only a little aspirin to effectively inhibit thromboxane synthesis in platelets. Going beyond this dose will not only inhibit thromboxane synthesis in platelets, but also the protective prostacyclin production in blood vessel walls. Some suggest that a dose of 3.5 mg/kg (about half an aspirin tablet) given at 3-day intervals effectively induces maximal inhibition of platelet aggregation without affecting prostacyclin production by the vessel walls.[244] Others indicate that the dose which effectively and selectively inhibits platelet cyclooxygenase is 20–40 mg daily.[245, 246] The major handicap with the use of inhibitors of PG synthesis is that they strike blindly and with variable effect from tissue to tissue. Obviously, drugs that selectively inhibit TXA_2 synthesis would be superior to aspirin in terms of antithrombotic effects.

The Endocrinology of Parturition

Perhaps the best example of the interplay among fetus, placenta, and mother is the initiation and maintenance of parturition. Hormonal changes in the uteroplacental environment are the principal governing factors accounting for the eventual development of uterine contractions. The sequence of events has been repeatedly reviewed in detail, where references to the original work are available.[247–249]

Extensive work in the sheep has implicated the fetal pituitary-adrenal axis in normal parturition. The sequence of events in the sheep begins about 10 days prior to labor with elevation of fetal cortisol in response to fetal pituitary ACTH, in turn a response to increased release of hypothalamic CRH. Fetal adrenalectomy or hypophysectomy prolongs pregnancy, whereas infusion of ACTH or glucocorticoids into the sheep fetus stimulates premature labor. Maternal stimulation of the fetal adrenal is not a factor because in sheep (and in women) there is little or no placental transfer of maternal ACTH into the fetal circulation. Thus, parturition in the ewe is initiated by a signal in the fetal brain activating ACTH secretion.

Increased cortisol secretion by the fetal adrenal gland starts a chain of events associated with labor. The sequence of events continues in the sheep with a decline in progesterone. This change is brought about by the induction of 17α-hydroxylase, 17,20-lyase enzyme activity (P450c17) in the sheep placenta. The up-regulation of P450c17 may be mediated by PGE_2. COX-2 activity is stimulated by cortisol, while at the same time, cortisol inhibits the activity of 15-hydroxy-prostaglandin dehydrogenase. Thus, an increase in PGE_2 correlates with the increasing activity of P450c17.

Glucocorticoid treatment of sheep placental tissue specifically increases the rate of production of 17α,20α-dihydroxypregn-4-en-3-one. This dihydroxyprogesterone compound also has been identified in sheep placental tissue obtained after spontaneous labor. Thus, direct synthesis of progesterone does not decline, but increased metabolism to a 17α-hydroxylated product results in less available progesterone. Progesterone withdrawal is associated with a decrease in the resting potential of myometrium; i.e., an increased response to electric and oxytocic stimuli. Conduction of action potential through the muscle is increased, and the myometrial excitability is increased.

Changes in Sheep Pregnancy

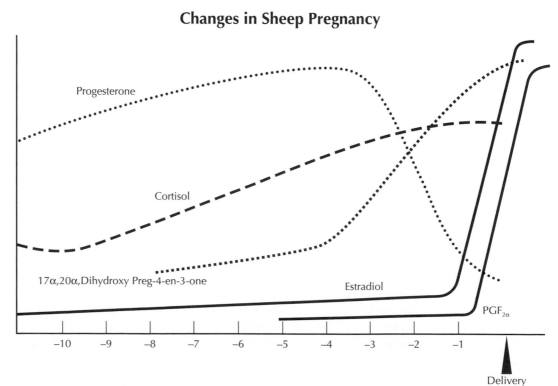

Dihydroxyprogesterone also serves as a precursor for the rise in estrogen levels, which occurs a few days prior to parturition. Estrogens enhance rhythmic contractions, as well as increasing vascularity and permeability, and the oxytocin response. Thus, progesterone withdrawal and estrogen increase lead to an enhancement of conduction and excitation.

The final event in the ewe is a rise in $PGF_{2\alpha}$ production hours before the onset of uterine activity. A cause-and-effect relationship between the rise in estrogen and the appearance of $PGF_{2\alpha}$ has been demonstrated in sheep. These events indicate that the decline in progesterone, the rise in estrogen, and the increase in $PGF_{2\alpha}$ are all secondary to direct induction of a placental enzyme by fetal cortisol.

Human Parturition

The steroid events in human pregnancy are not identical to events in the ewe. In addition, there is a more extended time scale. Steroid changes in the sheep occur over the course of several days, while in human pregnancy the changes begin at approximately 34–36 weeks and occur over the last 5 weeks of pregnancy. However, if the time course is expressed as a percentage of gestational length, the percentages in sheep and primates are impressively comparable.

Cortisol rises dramatically in amniotic fluid, beginning at 34–36 weeks, and correlates with pulmonary maturation. Cord blood cortisol concentrations are high in infants born vaginally or by cesarean section following spontaneous onset of labor. In contrast, cord blood cortisol levels are lower in infants born without spontaneous labor, whether delivery is vaginal (induced labor) or by cesarean section (elective repeat section). In keeping with the extended time scale of events, administration of glucocorticoids is not followed acutely by the onset of labor in pregnant women (unless the pregnancy is past due).

It is unlikely that the cortisol increments in the fetus represent changes due to increased adrenal activity in the mother in response to stress. Although maternal cortisol crosses the placenta readily, it is largely (85%) metabolized to cortisone in the process. This, in fact, may be the mechanism by which suppression of the fetal adrenal gland by maternal steroids is avoided. In contrast to the maternal liver, the fetal liver has a limited capacity for transforming the biologically inactive cortisone to the active cortisol. On the other hand, the fetal lung does possess the capability of changing cortisone to cortisol, and this may be an important source of cortisol for the lung. Cortisol itself induces this conversion in lung tissue. Increased fetal adrenal activity is followed by changes in steroid levels as well as important developmental accomplishments (e.g., increased pulmonary surfactant production and the accumulation of liver glycogen). In human parturition an important contribution of the fetal adrenal, in addition to cortisol, is its effect on placental estrogen production. The common theme in human pregnancies associated with failure to begin labor on time is decreased estrogen production; e.g., anencephaly and placental sulfatase deficiency.[250] In contrast, mothers bearing fetuses who cannot form normal amounts of cortisol, such as those with congenital adrenal hyperplasia, deliver on time.[251]

Progesterone maintenance of uterine quiescence and increased myometrial excitability associated with progesterone withdrawal are firmly established as mechanisms of parturition in lower species. In primates, the role of progesterone is less clear, largely because of the inability to demonstrate a definite decline in peripheral blood levels of progesterone prior to parturition.[252] Nevertheless, pharmacologic treatment with progesterone or synthetic progestational agents has some effect in preventing premature labor, although not labor at term.[253, 254] There is also reason to believe that progesterone concentration is regulated locally, especially in the fetal membranes and the decidua, and progesterone withdrawal can be accomplished by a combination of binding and metabolism.[255] Interruption of exposure to progesterone (e.g., with the antiprogesterone, RU486) leads to uterine contractions.[256] Furthermore, inhibition of progesterone production in the second trimester of human or the third trimester of monkey pregnancies is followed by a decrease in maternal, fetal and amniotic fluid progesterone concentrations and preterm labor and

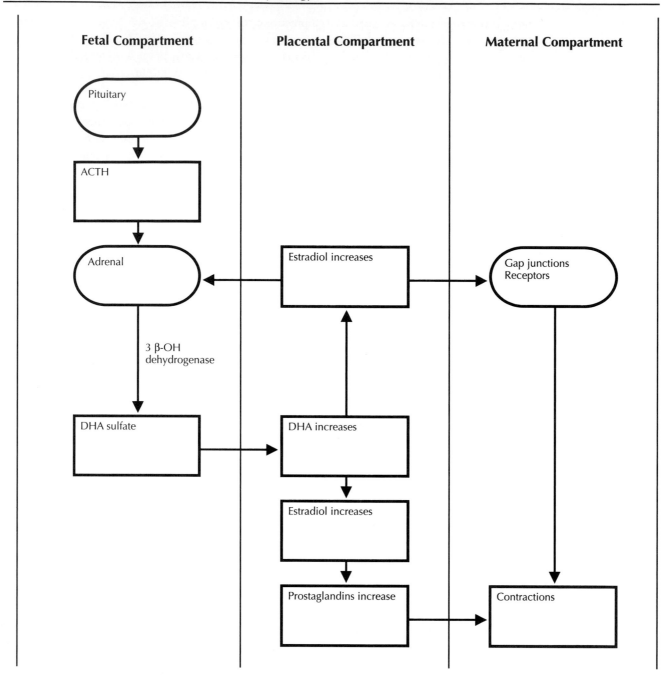

delivery.[257, 258] Perhaps multiple mechanisms exist, which affect in a subtle fashion the local concentration and actions of progesterone, as well as the production of progesterone in fetal membranes.[259]

An increase in estrogen levels in maternal blood begins at 34–35 weeks of gestation, but a late increase just before parturition (as in the sheep) has not been observed in human pregnancy. Perhaps a critical concentration is the signal in human pregnancy rather than a triggering increase. Or the changes are taking place at a local level and are not reflected in the maternal circulation.[260] Although it has not been definitely demonstrated, increased or elevated estrogen levels, as well as a local decrease in progesterone production, are thought to play a key role in increasing prostaglandin production.

Evidence for a role of prostaglandin in parturition includes the following:

1. Prostaglandin levels in maternal blood and amniotic fluid increase in association with labor.

2. Arachidonic acid levels in the amniotic fluid also rise in labor, and arachidonate injected into the amniotic sac initiates parturition.

3. Patients taking high doses of aspirin have a highly significant increase in the average length of gestation, incidence of postmaturity, and duration of labor.

4. Indomethacin prevents the normal onset of labor in monkeys and stops premature labor in human pregnancies.

5. Stimuli known to cause the release of prostaglandins (cervical manipulation, stripping of membranes, and rupture of membranes) augment or induce uterine contractions.

6. The process of cervical ripening and softening is mediated by prostaglandins.

7. Prostaglandins induce labor.

The precursor fatty acid for prostaglandin production in part may be derived from storage pools in the fetal membranes, the decidua, or both.[241] Phospholipase A_2 has been demonstrated in both human chorioamnion and uterine decidua. Although the precise mechanism for initiating prostaglandin synthesis, presumably by activation of the enzyme phospholipase A_2, remains unknown, the availability of arachidonic acid for prostaglandin production during parturition follow the stimulation of hydrolysis of phosphatidylethanolamine and phosphatidylinositol in decidual, amnion, and chorion laeve tissues.[261–263] Microsomes from amnion, chorion laeve, and decidua vera tissues contain lipases that hydrolyze fatty acids esterified in the 2 position. Specific phospholipase activity (phospholipase A_2 acting on phosphatidylethanolamine and phospholipase C acting on phosphatidylinositol) combined with a diacylglycerol lipase that also has a specificity for arachidonic acid provides a mechanism for the release of arachidonic acid. The activity of these enzymes in fetal membranes and decidua vera tissue increases with increasing length of gestation.

The key may be the increasing formation of estrogen (both estradiol and estriol) in the maternal circulation as well as in the amniotic fluid or, more importantly, locally within the uterus. The marked rise in estrogen near term may affect the activity of the lipase enzymes, leading to the liberation of arachidonic acid. The activity of these phospholipases is increased by increasing concentrations of calcium, and, therefore, the regulation of intracellular calcium is an important mechanism. Nevertheless, a role for local progesterone withdrawal in the activation of prostaglandin production cannot be discounted.[258]

The human fetal membranes and decidua are incredibly active. Human chorion and decidua produce estrogen utilizing a variety of substrates, especially estrone sulfate and dehydroepiandrosterone sulfate (DHAS), and this activity is increased around the time of parturition.[264, 265] In addition, the human fetal membranes synthesize and metabolize progesterone.[14] The membranes contain a 17,20-hydroxysteroid dehydrogenase system. One active site converts 20α-dihydroxyprogesterone to progesterone, while another active site on this enzyme converts estrone to estradiol. Thus, this enzyme can play an important role in altering the estrogen:progesterone ratio. The membranes and the decidua contain distinct cell populations with different biochemical activities (which change with labor).[266] Steroidogenic and prostaglandin interactions among these cells could produce the changes necessary for parturition without affecting the concentrations of circulating hormones. In addition, relaxin derived from decidua and/or chorion may exert a paracrine action on amnion prostaglandin production.[171] Throughout most of pregnancy, the amnion and chorion may exert an inhibitory influence over the myometrium by suppressing calcium channel activity.[267] Finally, the fetus may take a very direct role in this scenario by secreting substances into the amniotic fluid, which interact with the fetal membranes to signal the initiation of parturition.

The following observations support an important role for placental corticotropin-releasing hormone (CRH):

1. CRH is produced in trophoblast, the fetal membranes, and decidua.[78]

2. During pregnancy, CRH levels in the amniotic fluid and the maternal circulation progressively increase, and although amniotic fluid levels do not further increase with labor, the highest maternal levels are found at labor and delivery.

3. Levels of the CRH-binding protein (also produced in trophoblast, membranes, and decidua) are decreased in the amniotic fluid and maternal circulation prior to labor.[266, 268] This decrease in the CRH-binding protein would allow an increase in CRH activity.

4. CRH stimulates prostaglandin release in fetal membranes, decidua, and myometrium.[90, 269]

5. Increased CRH and decreased CRH-binding protein have been measured in women with preterm labor and in women with threatened preterm labor who subsequently deliver within 24 hours.[270–272]

6. Cortisol, in the presence of progesterone, stimulates (probably by blocking progesterone inhibition) trophoblastic CRH synthesis.[50, 273]

These observations are consistent with a key mechanism involving CRH activity in the initial triggering events of parturition. Although in the sheep the CRH signal begins in the fetal brain, in women, it appears to begin in the uterus. Progesterone is the only major inhibiting factor for CRH production in placental tissues. It has been hypothesized that rising fetal cortisol secretion competes with progesterone for the glucocorticoid receptor in the placenta, thus blocking the inhibitory action of progesterone on CRH synthesis, leading to an increase in CRH.[50] The increase in CRH would augment fetal ACTH secretion, producing more fetal cortisol as well as more DHAS to serve as precursor for the increase in estrogen that occurs prior to parturition; this indicates the important role of the fetal brain in the overall process. The competitive inhibition of progesterone would in effect be a mechanism of progesterone withdrawal. This sequence of events could be started by an increase in CRH or a decrease in CRH-binding protein, or both. On the other hand, consistent with the sheep studies, the initiating step in this sequence of events could be an increase in fetal ACTH secretion; e.g., in response to relative hypoxemia. Regardless of the specific triggering event, it is increasingly clear that the fetus plays a pivotal, if not controlling, role in parturition.

The Role of Prostaglandins

With labor, the arachidonic acid pathway in the fetal membranes shifts toward the cyclooxygenase direction with a large increase in the production of PGE_2 due to the induction of COX-2 activity. This COX-2 activity is a response to the increase in cortisol that in turn is a response to CRH. In addition, CRH can directly stimulate prostaglandin production in the membranes.

Specific protein inhibitors of prostaglandin synthase have been demonstrated in placenta, amnion, and chorion, and these proteins cannot be found in tissue from patients who have established labor.[241, 274] The link between infection and the onset of labor (especially preterm labor) may be due to the conversion by bacterial medium (with factors such as the interleukins)

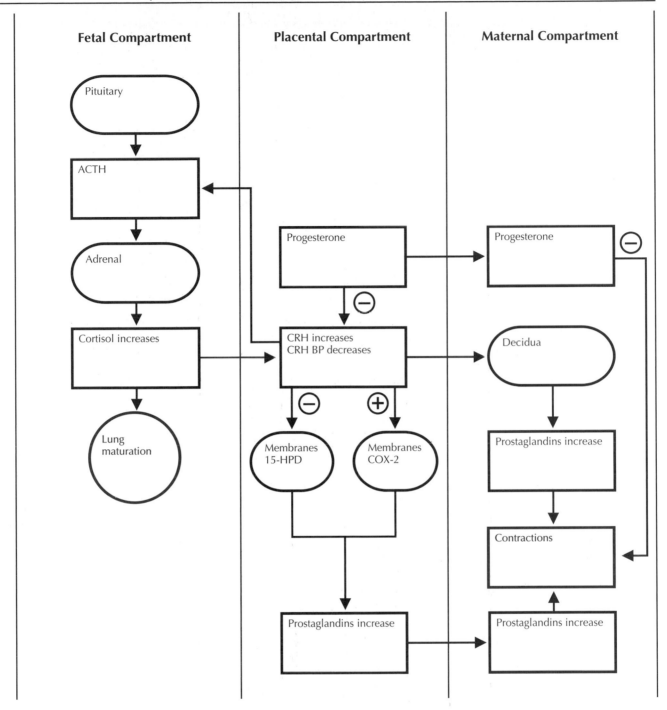

Fetal Compartment   **Placental Compartment**   **Maternal Compartment**

of arachidonic metabolism in the membranes and decidua to a condition associated with labor marked by the production of PGE_2.[241, 275, 276] In this case, prostaglandin production may be a consequence of inflammatory induction of the second cyclooxygenase enzyme, COX-2.[277]

Undoubtedly, prostaglandin production during pregnancy reflects the usual complex interaction of a host of autocrine/paracrine factors. Platelet-activating factor, epidermal growth factor, and transforming growth factor-α stimulate prostaglandin production by the fetal membranes apparently by regulating intracellular calcium concentrations.[278, 279] Secretory products of the fetal membranes themselves are active stimulators of membrane prostaglandin production, including renin derived from chorion prorenin.[280] Decidual $PGF_{2\alpha}$ production is enhanced by bradykinin, epidermal growth factor and transforming growth factor-α, and these responses are further increased by interleukin-1β.[281, 282] Prostaglandin production by amnion, chorion, and decidual cells is stimulated by corticotropin-releasing hormone and modulated by progesterone.[89] The ubiquitous substances, activin and inhibin, are involved here as well. Amnion and chorion produce the activin and inhibin subunits, and activin stimulates prostaglandin PGE_2 release from amnion cells.[211]

During labor the maternal circulating levels of PGE_2, $PGF_{2\alpha}$, and the $PGF_{2\alpha}$-metabolite are increased, a change which can be directly attributed to uterine production in that the gradient across the uterus for these substances is also increased. This increase in production of prostaglandins within the uterus must be the key factor, because the concentration and affinity of prostaglandin receptors do not change at parturition.[283] Meanwhile, prostacyclin and its metabolite are not increased. Prostacyclin is produced (at least in vitro) by a variety of tissues involved in pregnancy: endometrium, myometrium, placenta, amnion, chorion, and decidua. Prostacyclin and thromboxane are probably more important in the vascular responses of mother and fetus, and in all likelihood do not play a role in initiating or maintaining uterine contractions.[284]

Decidua produces both PGE_2 and $PGF_{2\alpha}$, but the amnion and chorion produce primarily PGE_2.[285] The inducible cyclooxygenase, COX-2, is expressed at a high level at term in the amnion and chorion.[286] As in sheep, prostaglandin synthesis in membranes and decidua is probably stimulated by cortisol; glucocorticoid receptors are present in the same cells that contain cyclooxygenase.[287]

There is evidence for the transfer of prostaglandin E_2 across the membranes to the decidua and possibly the myometrium.[288] The paradox of PGE_2 production in the amnion being matched not by a PGE-metabolite in the maternal circulation, but by a $PGF_{2\alpha}$-metabolite, is explained by transfer across the membranes and conversion of PGE_2 to $PGF_{2\alpha}$ in the decidua.[289] However, continued study of this issue strongly indicates that prostaglandins produced on one side of the membranes do not contribute to the prostaglandins on the other side, arguing that uterine contractions must be primarily influenced by decidual or myometrial prostaglandins.[290] On the other hand, there is reason to believe that the myometrial exposure to prostaglandins is governed by the activity of a catabolic enzyme in the chorion.

At term, prostaglandin synthesis occurs mainly in the amnion and decidua, and throughout pregnancy the chorion forms a barrier preventing passage of bioactive prostaglandins to the myometrium because of a large capacity to catabolize prostaglandins via 15-hydroxyprostaglandin dehydrogenase.[291] The activity of this enzyme is decreased in the presence of labor, including preterm labor, and after premature rupture of membranes or when infection is present.[292] Thus, a combination of increased biosynthesis and a decrease in chorionic 15-hydroxyprostaglandin dehydrogenase achieve the increase in prostaglandins associated with parturition, probably mediated by the local changes in estrogen and progesterone bioavailability and activity, with a key role also played by CRH and cortisol. Cortisol decreases and progesterone increases 15-hydroxyprostaglandin dehydrogenase in placental tissues.[330]

Oxytocin and Myometrial Responses

Using sensitive assays, an increase in maternal levels of oxytocin can be detected prior to parturition, occurring at first only at night.[293, 294] Once labor has begun, oxytocin levels rise significantly, especially during the second stage. Thus, oxytocin may be important for developing the later, more intense uterine contractions. Extremely high concentrations of oxytocin can be measured in the cord blood at delivery, and release of oxytocin from the fetal pituitary may also be involved in labor. However, this is controversial, and studies in monkeys fail to indicate a role for fetal oxytocin in parturition.[294] Part of the contribution of oxytocin to parturition is the stimulation of prostaglandin synthesis in decidua and myometrium.[295] Cervical dilatation appears to be dependent on oxytocin stimulation of prostaglandin production, probably in the decidua. The greater frequency of labor and delivery at night may be due to greater nocturnal oxytocin secretion.[293] In addition, oxytocin is synthesized in the amnion, chorion, and significantly, in the decidua.[293, 296, 297] This locally produced oxytocin may be a significant stimulus for myometrial and membrane production of prostaglandins.

It is likely that oxytocin action during the initial stages of labor may depend on myometrial sensitivity to oxytocin in addition to the levels of oxytocin in the blood. The concentration of

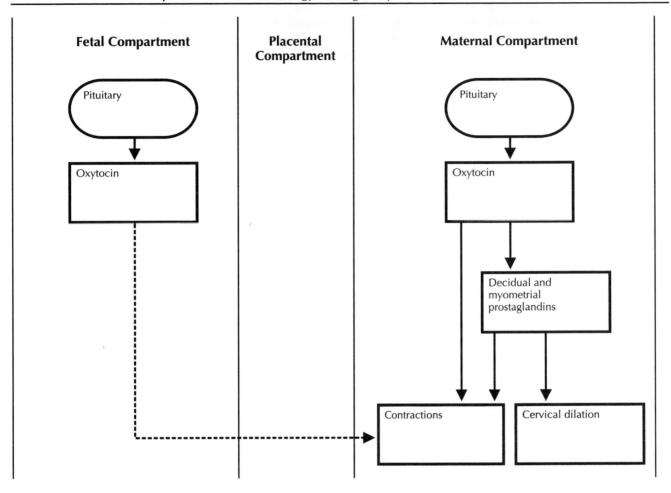

oxytocin receptors in the myometrium is low in the nonpregnant state and increases steadily throughout gestation (an 80-fold increase), and during labor, the concentration doubles. This receptor concentration correlates with the uterine sensitivity to oxytocin.[298] The mechanism for the increase is unknown, but it likely is due to a change in the prostaglandin and hormonal milieu of the uterus. The local production and effects of oxytocin, estrogen, and progesterone combine in a complicated process of autocrine, paracrine, and endocrine actions to result in parturition. In mice lacking the prostaglandin F receptor, the sequence of progesterone withdrawal, appearance of oxytocin receptors, and parturition fails to occur, indicating a key role for prostaglandin initiation of luteolysis in mice as a requisite for labor and delivery.[299] Mice lacking oxytocin, however, undergo normal parturition, but fail to nurse their offspring.[300]

Animal studies have implicated the formation of low-resistance pathways in the myometrium, called *gap junctions,* as an important action of steroids and prostaglandins during labor.[301] In the gap junction, a pore forms, which allows communication from cytoplasm to cytoplasm between two cells. The pore is a cylinder-shaped channel formed of 6 special proteins called *connexins.* Either substances or electrical current (ions) can follow this pathway without leakage into extracellular space. Thus, gap junctions provide a means of communication between myometrial cells, allowing enhancement of electrical conductivity and synchronization of activity. Gap junction formation is related to the estrogen/progesterone ratio (estrogen is stimulatory and progesterone is inhibitory) and to the presence of the stimulating prostaglandins, PGE_2 and $PGF_{2\alpha}$. Therefore it is not surprising that the number of gap junctions increases in the final weeks of pregnancy, especially just before labor. The modulation of the number and the permeability of gap junctions is another contributing factor in the control of uterine contractility.

The final contraction of uterine muscle results from increased free calcium concentrations in the myofibril, the result of prostaglandin action, an action opposed to that of progesterone which promotes calcium binding in the sarcoplasmic reticulum.[302] Thus, prostaglandins and oxytocin increase while progesterone decreases intracellular calcium levels. The intracellular calcium concentration is affected by cellular entry and exit of calcium as well as binding in the sarcoplasmic reticulum. It is the intracellular concentration of calcium which determines the rate of myosin phosphorylation and the contractile state of the myometrium. Tocolytic therapy (the use of beta-adrenergic agents) stimulates adenylate cyclase activity, which increases the levels of cellular cyclic AMP, which, in turn, decreases intracellular calcium concentration as well as inhibiting actin-myosin interaction by modulating kinase phosphorylation.

Ducsay and colleagues propose that the coordination of this complex relationship of physiologic, endocrine, and molecular mechanisms is expressed in rhythms.[67] Both mother and fetus experience 24-hour rhythms in hormone secretions, and uterine activity is correlated with day and night (photoperiod regulation). The coordination and enhancement of this rhythmicity play a role in parturition. Improved detection and measurement of this activity could contribute to better prevention and treatment of preterm labor.

Concluding Thought

Imagine yourself as a fetus within a pregnant uterus. Your growth, development, and survival require keeping the uterus quiescent for most of pregnancy. This is accomplished by maintaining progesterone inhibitory dominance of the myometrium. When ready to begin extrauterine life or when your environment becomes inhospitable, you are able to prepare or "activate" the parturition mechanisms by means of hormonal and autocrine/paracrine messengers. Ultimately, uterine contractions and cervical ripening are stimulated, and amazingly, even if you are incapable of initiating these events, the sequence will eventually begin, and delivery will ensue. The extraordinary experience and wonder of labor and birth, as perceived by parents and birth assistants, are matched by your ability and the complexity of the systems you influence.

Treatment of Labor With Prostaglandin Inhibition

The key role for prostaglandins in parturition raises the potential for treatment of premature labor with inhibitors of prostaglandin synthesis. The concern has been that such treatment would result in intrauterine closure of the ductus arteriosus and pulmonary hypertension. Clinical studies, however, indicate that use of the nonsteroidal anti-inflammatory agents for short periods of time (3 days) yields good results and does not result in this complication.[303] Beyond 34 weeks, the fetus is more sensitive to this pulmonary action, and treatment should be limited to pregnancies less than 32 weeks and with caution from 32–34 weeks. Perhaps it is the treatment of choice for the inhibition of labor during a maternal transport. If the drug is failing, it should not be maintained because increased blood loss can occur at delivery. Because indomethacin inhibits the synthesis of all members of the prostaglandin family, including the vasodilating prostacyclin, it should be used with caution in hypertensive patients.[304] Sulindac is just as effective as a tocolytic but does not affect urine output and amniotic fluid, and it has a lesser impact on the fetal ductus arteriosus.[305, 306]

Treatment of pregnant women with indomethacin reduces the amniotic fluid volume due to a decrease in fetal urine output. This is reversible with a decrease in dose. This treatment has been used for polyhydramnios with good response and no effect on the newborn despite treatment for 2 to 11 weeks.[307]

Induction of Labor and Cervical Ripening

Pharmacologically and physiologically, prostaglandins have two direct actions associated with labor: ripening of the cervix and myometrial stimulation. Successful parturition requires organized changes in both the upper uterus and in the cervix. The cervical changes are in response to the estrogen/progesterone ratio and the local release of prostaglandins. Whether relaxin plays a role in human parturition is not established; however, recombinant relaxin is being tested for cervical ripening.

Ripening of the cervix is the result of a change that includes an increase in hyaluronic acid and water and a decrease in dermatan sulfate and chondroitin sulfate (these compounds hold the collagen fibers in a rigid structure). How prostaglandins operate in this change is unknown, but enzyme activation must be involved. For ripening of the cervix, PGE_2 is very effective, while $PGF_{2\alpha}$ has little effect. The purpose of pharmacologically achieving ripening of the cervix is to increase the success rate with induction of labor and lower the proportion of cesarean sections. Intravaginal prostaglandin E_2 administered as tablets, suppositories, and mixed in gels has been very effective for cervical ripening. The commercial formulation currently available in the U.S. consists of 0.5 mg PGE_2 dissolved in a triacetin viscous gel base, also containing a colloid silicone dioxide, provided in a prefilled syringe for application.[308] A synthetic PGE_1 analogue, misoprostol, is also safe and effective when used intravaginally for cervical ripening and labor induction.[309]

A major clinical application for the induction of labor in the United States is the use of intravaginal PGE_2 in cases of fetal demise and anencephalic fetuses. Based on our own experience, certain precautions have been developed. The patient should be well hydrated with an electrolyte solution to counteract the induced vasodilatation and decreased peripheral resistance. If satisfactory uterine activity is established, the next application should be withheld. And, finally, because there is a synergistic effect when oxytocin is used shortly after prostaglandin administration, there should be a minimum of 6 hours between the last prostaglandin dose and beginning oxytocin augmentation.

Prostaglandins are used to induce term labor. Intravenous prostaglandins are not an acceptable method due to the side effects achieved by the high dosage necessary to reach the uterus. The intravaginal and oral administration of PGE_2 is as effective as intravenous oxytocin, even including patients with previous cesarean sections.[310, 311] The intravaginal administration of misoprostol, the synthetic prostaglandin E_1 analogue, is safe, effective, and relatively inexpensive.[312] These methods, plus intracervical administration, are in routine use in many parts of the world.

Induced Abortion

Prostaglandins are effective for postcoital contraception and first trimester abortion but impractical because of the high incidence of side effects, including an unacceptable rate of incomplete abortions. For midtrimester abortions, intra-amniotic prostaglandin, intramuscular methyl esters, and vaginal PGE suppositories are available. The major clinical problems have been the efficacy in accomplishing complete expulsion and the high level of systemic side effects. Overall, there is a higher risk of hemorrhage, fever, infection, antibiotic administration, readmission to the hospital, and more operative procedures when compared with saline abortions. The surgical procedure, D&E (dilatation and evacuation) is safer and less expensive than medical methods, and it is better tolerated by patients.

The combination of prostaglandin's oxytocic action with the antiprogesterone effect of RU486 (mifepristone) has proved to be a safe and effective medical treatment for the induction of therapeutic abortion prior to 9 weeks gestation.[313–315] An orally active methyl ester of prostaglandin E_1 is only 20% effective as an abortifacient when administered by itself. Combining the prostaglandin with RU486 achieves greater than 95% efficacy, safely and inexpensively.

Prostaglandins and Postpartum Hemorrhage

When routine methods of management for postpartum hemorrhage caused by uterine atony have failed, an analogue of prostaglandin $F_{2\alpha}$ has been used with excellent results (80–90% successful).[316] Prostin 15 M is (15-S)-15-methyl prostaglandin $F_{2\alpha}$-tromethamine. The dose is 0.25-0.5 mg, repeated up to 4 times and given with equal efficacy either intramuscularly or directly into the myometrium. It can also be used after the replacement of an inverted uterus. Failures are usually associated with infections or magnesium sulfate therapy. It should not be used in patients with severe hypertension or symptomatic asthma. Diarrhea is a frequent side effect.

Prostaglandins and the Fetal Circulation

The predominant effect of prostaglandins on the fetal and maternal cardiovascular system is to maintain the ductus arteriosus, renal, mesenteric, uterine, placental, and probably the cerebral and coronary arteries in a relaxed or dilated state. The importance of the ductus arteriosus can be appreciated by considering that 59% of the cardiac output flows through this connection between the pulmonary artery and the descending aorta.

Control of ductal patency and closure is mediated through prostaglandins. The arterial concentration of oxygen is the key to the caliber of the ductus. With increasing gestational age, the ductus becomes increasingly responsive to increased oxygen. In this area, too, attention has turned to PGI_2 and TXA_2.

Fetal lamb ductus homogenates produce mainly PGI_2 when incubated with arachidonic acid. PGE_2 and $PGF_{2\alpha}$ are formed in small amounts and TXA_2 not at all. Although PGE_2 is less abundant than PGI_2 in the ductus, it is a more potent vasodilator of the ductus and is more responsive to oxygen (decreasing vasodilatation with increasing oxygen).[317] Thus, PGE_2 appears to be the most important prostaglandin in the ductus from a functional point of view, while PGI_2, the major product in the main pulmonary artery, appears to be the major factor in maintaining vasodilatation in the pulmonary bed. The ductus is dilated maximally in utero by production of prostaglandins, and a positive vasoconstrictor process is required to close it. The source of the vasoconstrictor is probably the lung. With increasing maturation, the lung shifts to TXA_2 formation. This fits with the association of ductal patency with prematurity. With the onset of pulmonary ventilation at birth leading to vascular changes that deliver blood to the duct directly from the lungs, TXA_2 can now serve as the vasoconstrictor stimulus. The major drawback to this hypothesis is the failure of inhibitors to affect the constriction response to oxygen.

Administration of vasodilating prostaglandins can maintain patency after birth, while preparing an infant for surgery to correct a congenital lesion causing pulmonary hypertension. Infants with persistent ductus patency may be spared thoracotomy by treatment with an inhibitor of prostaglandin synthesis. The use of indomethacin to close a persistent ductus in the premature infant is successful about 40% of the time.[317] An important factor is early diagnosis and treatment because with increasing postnatal age the ductus becomes less sensitive to prostaglandin inhibitors, probably because of more efficient clearance of the drug.[318] The highest incidence of successful indomethacin ductus closure has been with infants less than 30 weeks gestation and less than 10 days old.

This aspect of the use of prostaglandin inhibitors is of concern in considering the use of agents to inhibit premature labor. The drug half-life in the fetus and newborn is prolonged because the metabolic pathways are limited, and there is reduced drug clearance because of immature renal function. In utero constriction of the ductus can cause congestive heart failure and fetal pulmonary hypertension.[319] Prolonged ductus constriction leads to subendocardial ischemia and fibrotic lesions in the tricuspid valve muscles. Infants with persistent pulmonary hypertension have hypoxemia, cardiomegaly, and right to left shunting through the foramen ovale or the ductus. Infants of mothers given either indomethacin or salicylates chronically have been reported to have this syndrome. Duration of exposure and dosage are critical. It takes occlusion of the ductus for more than 2 weeks to produce fetal pulmonary hypertension and cardiac hypertrophy. This side effect is rare in pregnancies less than 27 weeks gestation; the ductus arteriosus usually begins to respond at 27–30 weeks, and after 30 weeks, this is an important side effect which can be minimized if long-term use is avoided.[320]

Prostaglandins and Fetal Breathing

Prior to parturition, fetal breathing is very shallow. It is proposed that placental PGE_2 suppresses breathing by acting in the fetal brain.[321] Occlusion of the umbilical cord is rapidly followed by a loss of this PGE_2 influence and the onset of air breathing. The administration of indomethacin to fetal sheep increases, while infusion of PGE suppresses, fetal breathing movements. This may be the explanation for the decrease in fetal breathing movements observed during human labor (associated with an increase in prostaglandin levels).

Fetal Lung Maturation

The pulmonary alveoli are lined with a surface-active phospholipid-protein complex called pulmonary surfactant, which is synthesized in the type II pneumocyte of mature lungs. It is this surfactant that decreases surface tension, thereby facilitating lung expansion and preventing atelectasis. In full-term fetuses, surfactant is present at birth in sufficient amounts to permit adequate lung expansion and normal breathing. In premature fetuses, however, surfactant is present in lesser amounts, and when insufficient, postnatal lung expansion and ventilation are frequently impaired, resulting in progressive atelectasis, the clinical syndrome of respiratory distress.

Phosphatidylcholine (lecithin) has been identified as the most active and most abundant lipid of the surfactant complex. The second most active and abundant material is phosphatidylglycerol (PG), which significantly enhances surfactant function. Both are present in only small concentrations until the last 5 weeks of pregnancy. Beginning at 20–22 weeks of pregnancy, a less stable and less active lecithin, palmitoylmyristoyl lecithin, is formed. Hence, a premature infant does not always develop respiratory distress syndrome; however, in addition to being less active, synthesis of this lecithin is decreased by stress and acidosis, making the premature infant more susceptible to respiratory distress. At about the 35th week of gestation, there is a sudden surge of dipalmitoyl lecithin, the major surfactant lecithin, which is stable and very active. Because secretion by the fetal lungs contributes to the formation of amniotic fluid and the sphingomyelin concentration of amniotic fluid changes relatively little throughout pregnancy, assessment of the lecithin/sphingomyelin (L/S) ratio in amniotic fluid at approximately 34–36 weeks of pregnancy can determine the amount of dipalmitoyl lecithin available and thus the degree to which the lungs will adapt to newborn life.

Gluck and colleagues were the first to demonstrate that the L/S ratio correlates with pulmonary maturity of the fetal lung.[322] In normal development, sphingomyelin concentrations are greater than those of lecithin until about gestational week 26. Prior to 34 weeks, the L/S ratio is approximately 1:1. At 34–36 weeks, with the sudden increase in lecithin, the ratio rises acutely. In general, a ratio of 2.0 or greater indicates pulmonary maturity and that respiratory distress syndrome will not develop in the newborn. Respiratory distress syndrome associated with a ratio greater than 2.0 usually follows a difficult delivery with a low 5-minute Apgar score, suggesting that severe acidosis can inhibit surfactant production. A ratio in the transitional range (1.0–1.9) indicates that respiratory distress syndrome may develop but that the fetal lung has entered the period of lecithin production, and a repeat amniocentesis in 1 or 2 weeks usually reveals a mature L/S ratio. The rise from low to high ratios may actually occur within 3–4 days.

An increase in the surfactant content of phosphatidylglycerol at 34–36 weeks marks the final maturation of the fetal lung. When the L/S ratio is greater than 2.0 and PG is present, the incidence of respiratory distress syndrome is virtually zero. The assessment of PG is especially helpful when the amniotic fluid is contaminated because the analysis is not affected by meconium, blood, or vaginal secretions.

Abnormalities of pregnancy may affect the rate of maturation of the fetal lung, resulting either in an early mature L/S ratio or a delayed rise in the ratio. Accelerated maturation of the ratio is associated with hypertension, advanced diabetes, hemoglobinopathies, heroin addiction, and poor maternal nutrition. Delayed maturation is seen with diabetes (without hypertension) and Rh sensitization. In general, accelerated maturation is associated with reductions in uteroplacental blood flow (and presumably increased fetal stress). With vigorous and effective control of maternal diabetes, the risk of respiratory distress syndrome in the newborns is not significantly different from infants born to nondiabetics.

Since Liggins observed survival of premature lambs following the administration of cortisol to the fetus, it has become recognized that fetal cortisol is the principal requisite for surfactant biosynthesis. This is true despite the fact that no increase in fetal cortisol can be demonstrated to correlate with the increases in fetal lung maturation. For that reason, fetal lung maturation can be best viewed as the result of not only cortisol, but the synergistic action of cortisol, prolactin, thyroxine, estrogens, prostaglandins, growth factors, and perhaps other yet unidentified agents.[323] Insulin directly inhibits surfactant protein expression in fetal lung tissue, which explains the increase in respiratory distress syndrome associated with hyperglycemia in pregnancy (although this effect can be overcome by the stress associated with advanced diabetes).[324]

Corticosteroid therapy of pregnant women threatened with preterm delivery reduces neonatal mortality, respiratory distress syndrome, and intraventricular hemorrhage.[325] In general, maximal benefit in terms of enhanced fetal pulmonic maturity has been demonstrated with glucocorticoid administration at 24–32 weeks of gestational age, with some benefit between 32–34 weeks, and no benefit beyond 34 weeks. The optimal effect requires that 48 hours elapse after initiation of therapy, and this benefit is lost after 7 days; however, it is recommended that treatment be limited to 2 doses. The effect of antenatal corticosteroid treatment is additive to that of postnatal surfactant. Although every case of respiratory distress syndrome and subsequent chronic lung disease cannot be prevented, a significant impact can be achieved on infant mortality, and the incidence and severity of respiratory distress syndrome. Additional treatment with thyrotropin-releasing hormone (TRH) was initially believed to be beneficial; however, clinical trials indicate that TRH does not further reduce the incidence of chronic lung disease in glucocorticoid-treated very low birth weight infants.[326, 327]

The Postpartum Period

The immediate postpartum period is a time of rapid readjustment to the nonpregnant endocrine state. About 10–15% of women become clinically depressed during this time, and an endocrine mechanism has been suggested.[328] The clinician should always have a high index of suspicion for thyroid dysfunction because of the 5–10% incidence of postpartum thyroiditis in the 3–6 months after delivery. Because of the relative hypercortisolism in the last trimester of pregnancy, it has been suggested that persistent suppression of hypothalamic CRH secretion (and thus the pituitary-adrenal axis) in the postpartum period is a characteristic finding in women with postpartum depression, and that this suppression also contributes to a greater vulnerability to autoimmune diseases, like thyroiditis.[329]

References

1. **Csapo AL, Pulkkinen MO, Wiest WG,** Effects of luteectomy and progesterone replacement in early pregnant patients, *Am J Obstet Gynecol* 115:759, 1973.

2. **Schneider MA, Davies MC, Honour JW,** The timing of placental competence in pregnancy after oocyte donation, *Fertil Steril* 59:1059, 1993.

3. **Azuma K, Calderon I, Besanko M, Maclachlan V, Healy D,** Is the luteo-placental shift a myth? Analysis of low progesterone levels in sucessful ART pregnancies, *J Clin Endocrinol Metab* 77:195, 1993.

4. **Sultan KM, Davis OK, Liu H-C, Rosenwaks Z,** Viable term pregnancy despite "subluteal" serum progesterone levels in the first trimester, *Fertil Steril* 60:363, 1993.

5. **Mishell DR, Thorneycroft IH, Nagata Y, Murata T, Nakamura RM,** Serum gonadotropin and steroid patterns in early human gestation, *Am J Obstet Gynecol* 117:631, 1973.

6. **Tulchinsky D, Hobel CJ,** Plasma human and chorionic gonadotropin, estrogen, estradiol, estriol, progesterone and 17α-hydroxyprogesterone in human pregnancy, *Am J Obstet Gynecol* 117:884, 1973.

7. **Parker CR, Illingworth DR, Bissonnette J, Carr BR,** Endocrine changes during pregnancy in a patient with homozygous familial hypobetalipoproteinemia, *New Engl J Med* 314:557, 1986.

8. **Albrecht ED, Pepe GJ,** Placental steroid hormone biosynthesis in primate pregnancy, *Endocr Rev* 11:124, 1990.

9. **Begum-Hasan J, Murphy BEP,** In vitro stimulation of placental progesterone production by 19-nortestosterone and C19 steroids in early human pregnancy, *J Clin Endocrinol Metab* 75:838, 1992.

10. **Bhattacharyya S, Chaudhary J, Das C,** Antibodies to hCG inhibit progesterone production from human syncytiotrophoblast cells, *Placenta* 13:135, 1992.

11. **Pepe GJ, Albrecht ED,** Actions of placental and fetal adrenal steroid hormones in primate pregnancy, *Endocr Rev* 16:608, 1995.

12. **Grimes RW, Pepe GJ, Albrecht ED,** Regulation of human placental trophoblast low-density lipoprotein uptake *in vitro* by estrogen, *J Clin Endocrinol Metab* 81:2675, 1996.

13. **Carr BR, Simpson ER,** Cholesterol synthesis by human fetal hepatocytes: effect of lipoproteins, *Am J Obstet Gynecol* 150:551, 1984.

14. **Mitchell BF, Challis JRG, Lukash L,** Progesterone synthesis by human amnion, chorion, and decidua at term, *Am J Obstet Gynecol* 157:349, 1987.

15. **Parker CR, Everett RB, Quirk JG, Whalley PJ, Gant NF,** Hormone production during pregnancy in the primigravid patient: I. Plasma levels of progesterone and 5-pregnane-3,20-dione throughout pregnancy of normal women and women who developed pregnancy-induced hypertension, *Am J Obstet Gynecol* 135:778, 1979.

16. **Parker CR, Everett RB, Whalley PJ, Quirk JG, Gant NF, MacDonald PC,** Hormone production during pregnancy in the primigravid patient: II. Plasma levels of deoxycorticosterone throughout pregnancy of normal women and women who developed pregnancy-induced hypertension, *Am J Obstet Gynecol* 138:626, 1980.

17. **Rothchild I,** Role of progesterone in initiating and maintaining pregnancy, In: Bardin CW, Milgrom E, Mauvais-Jarvis P, eds. *Progesterone and Progestins,* Raven Press, New York, 1983, p 219.

18. **Carr BR, Simpson ER,** Lipoprotein utilization and cholesterol synthesis by the human fetal adrenal gland, *Endocr Rev* 2:306, 1981.

19. **Partsch C-J, Sippell WG, Mackenzie IZ, Aynsley-Green A,** The steroid hormonal milieu of the undisturbed human fetus and mother at 16-20 weeks gestation, *J Clin Endocrinol Metab* 73:969, 1991.

20. **Siiteri PK, MacDonald PC,** The utilization of circulating dehydroisoandrosterone sulfate for estrogen synthesis during human pregnancy, *Steroids* 2:713, 1963.

21. **Siiteri PK, MacDonald PC,** Placental estrogen biosynthesis during human pregnancy, *J Clin Endocrinol Metab* 26:751, 1966.

22. **Voutilainen R, Ilvesmaki V, Miettinen PJ,** Low expression of 3β-hydroxy-5-ene steroid dehydrogenase gene in human fetal adrenals in vivo; adrenocorticotropin and protein dinase C-dependent regulation in adrenocortical cultures, *J Clin Endocrinol Metab* 72:761, 1991.

23. **Madden JD, Gant NF, MacDonald PC,** Study of the kinetics of conversion of maternal plasma dehydroisoandrosterone sulfate to 16-hydroxydehydroisoandrosterone sulfate, estradiol, and estriol, *Am J Obstet Gynecol* 132:392, 1978.

24. **Buster JE, Abraham GE,** The applications of steroid hormone radioimmunoassays to clinical obstetrics, *Obstet Gynecol* 46:489, 1975.

25. **Devroey P, Camus M, Palermo G, Smitz J, Van Waesberghe L, Wsanto A, et al,** Placental production of estradiol and progesterone after oocyte donation in patients with primary ovarian failure, *Am J Obstet Gynecol* 162:66, 1990.

26. **Salat-Baroux J, Cornet D, Alvarez S, Antoine JM, Mandelbaum J, Plachot M,** Hormonal secretions in singleton pregnancies arising from the implantation of fresh or frozen embryos after oocyte donation in women with ovarian failure, *Fertil Steril* 57:150, 1992.

27. **Buster JE, Sakakini Jr J, Killam AP, Scragg WH,** Serum unconjugated estriol levels in the third trimester and their relationship to gestational age, *Am J Obstet Gynecol* 125:672, 1975.

28. **Katzenellenbogen BS,** Biology and receptor interactions of estriol and estriol derivatives in vitro and in vivo, *J Steriod Biochem* 20:1033, 1984.

29. **Longo LD,** Maternal blood volume and cardiac output during pregnancy: an hypothesis of endocrinologic control, *Am J Physiol* 245:R720, 1983.

30. **Simpson ER, Mahendroo MS, Means GD, Kilgore MW, Hinshelwood MM, Graham-Lorence S, Amarneh B, Ito Y, Fisher CR, Michael MD, Mendelson CR, Bulun SE,** Aromatase cytochrome P450, the enzyme responsible for estrogen biosynthesis, *Endocr Rev* 15:342, 1994.

31. **Morishima A, Grumbach MM, Simpson ER, Fisher C, Qin K,** Aromatase deficiency in male and female siblings caused by a novel mutation and the physiological role of estrogens, *J Clin Endocrinol Metab* 80:3689, 1995.

32. **MacDonald PC, Siiteri PK,** Origin of estrogen in women pregnant with an anencephalic fetus, *J Clin Invest* 44:465, 1965.

33. **Mesiano S, Jaffe RB,** Developmental and functional biology of the primate fetal adrenal cortex, *Endocr Rev* 18:378, 1997.

34. **Parker Jr CR, Leveno K, Car BR, Hauth J, MacDonald PC,** Umbilical cord plasma levels of dehydroepiandrosterone sulfate during human gestation, *J Clin Endocrinol Metab* 54:1216, 1982.

35. **Winters AJ, Oliver C, Colston C, MacDonald PC, Porter JC,** Plasma ACTH levels in the human fetus and neonate as related to age and parturition, *J Clin Endocrinol Metab* 39:2690, 1974.

36. **Walsh SW, Norman RL, Novy MJ,** In utero regulation of rhesus monkey fetal adrenals: effects of dexamethasone, adrenocorticotropin, thyrotropin-releasing hormone, prolactin, human chorionic gonadotropin, and α-melanocyte-stimulating hormone on fetal and maternal plasma steroids, *Endocrinology* 104:1805, 1979.

37. **Abu-Hakima M, Branchaud CL, Goodyer CG, Murphy BEP,** The effects of human chorionic gonadotropin on growth and steroidogenesis of the human fetal adrenal gland in vitro, *Am J Obstet Gynecol* 156:681, 1987.

38. **del Pozo E, Bigazzi M, Calaf J,** Induced human gestational hypoprolactinemia: lack of action on fetal adrenal androgen synthesis, *J Clin Endocrinol Metab* 51:936, 1980.

39. **Walker ML, Pepe GJ, Albrecht ED,** Regulation of baboon fetal adrenal androgen formation by pituitary peptides at mid- and late gestation, *Endocrinology* 122:546, 1988.

40. **McNulty WP, Novy MJ, Walsh SW,** Fetal and postnatal development of the adrenal glands in Macaca mulatta, *Biol Reprod* 25:1079, 1981.

41. **Pepe GJ, Albrecht ED,** Regulation of the primate fetal adrenal cortex, *Endocr Rev* 11:151, 1990.

42. **Mason JI, Rainey WE,** Steroidogenesis in the human fetal adrenal: a role for cholesterol synthesized de novo, *J Clin Endocrinol Metab* 64:140, 1987.

43. **Mesiano S, Fujimioto VY, Nelson LR, Lee JY, Voytek CC, Jaffe RB,** Localization and regulation of corticotropin receptor expression in the midgestation human fetal adrenal cortex: implications for *in utero* homeostasis, *J Clin Endocrinol Metab* 81:340, 1996.

44. **Baggia S, Albrecht ED, Pepe GJ,** Regulation of 11 beta-hydroxysteroid dehydrogenase activity in the baboon placenta by estrogen, *Endocrinology* 126:2742, 1990.

45. **Pepe GJ, Davies WA, Albrecht ED,** Activation of the baboon fetal pituitary-adrenocortical axis at midgestation by estrogen: enhancement of fetal pituitary proopiomelanocortin messenger ribonucleic acid expression, *Endocrinology* 135:2581, 1994.

46. **Edwards CR, Benediktsson R, Lindsay RS, Seckl JR,** Dysfunction of placental glucocorticoid barrier: link between fetal environment and adult hypertension? *Lancet* 341:355, 1993.

47. **Fall CHD, Osmond C, Barker DJP, Clark PMS, Hales CN, Stirling Y, Meade TW,** Fetal and infant growth and cardiovascular risk factors in women, *Br Med J* 310:428, 1995.

48. **Brown RW, Chapman KE, Kotelevtsev Y, Yau JLW, Lindsay RS, Brett L, Leckie C, Murad P, Lyons V, Mullins JJ, Edwards CRW, Seckl JR,** Cloning and production of antisera to human placental 11β-hydroxysteroid dehydrogenase type 2, *Biochem J* 313:1007, 1996.

49. **Yang K, Shearman K, Asano H, Richardson BS,** Effects of hypoxemia on 11β-hydroxysteroid dehydrogenase types 1 and 2 gene expression in preterm fetal sheep, *J Soc Gynecol Invest* 4:124, 1997.

50. **Karalis K, Goodwin G, Majzoub JA,** Cortisol blockade of progesterone: a possible molecular mechanism involved in the initiation of human labor, *Nature Med* 2:556, 1996.

51. **Smith R, Mesiano S, Chan E-C, Brown S, Jaffe RB,** Corticotropin-releasing hormone directly and preferentially stimulates dehydroepiandrosterone sulfate secretion by human fetal adrenal cortical cells, *J Clin Endocrinol Metab* 83:2916, 1998.

52. **Voutilainen R, Eramaa M, Ritvos O,** Hormonally regulated inhibin gene expression in human fetal and adult adrenals, *J Clin Endocrinol Metab* 73:1026, 1991.

53. **Spencer SJ, Rabinovici J, Mesiano S, Goldsmith PC, Jaffe RB,** Activin and inhibin in the human adrenal gland. Regulation and differential effects in fetal and adult cells, *J Clin Invest* 90:1420, 1992.

54. **Mesiano S, Katz SL, Lee JY, Jaffe RB,** Insulin-like growth factors augment steroid production and expression of steroidogenic enzymes in human fetal adrenal cortical cells: implications for adrenal androgen regulation, *J Clin Endocrinol Metab* 82:1390, 1997.

55. **D'Ercole AJ,** Somatomedins/insulin-like growth factors and fetal growth, *J Dev Physiol* 9:481, 1987.

56. **Mesiano S, Mellon SH, Jaffe RB,** Mitogenic action, regulation, and localization of insulin-like growth factors in the human fetal adrenal gland, *J Clin Endocrinol Metab* 76:968, 1993.

57. **Luo X, Ikeda Y, Parker KL,** A cell-specific nuclear receptor is essential for adrenal and gonadal development and sexual differentiation, *Cell* 77:481, 1994.

58. **Parker KL, Schimmer BP,** Steroidogenic factor 1: a key determinant of endocrine development and function, *Endocr Rev* 18:361, 1997.

59. **Burris TP, Guo W, McCabe ER,** The gene responsible for adrenal hypoplasia congenita, DAX-1, encodes a nuclear hormone receptor that defines a new class within the superfamily, *Recent Prog Horm Res* 51:241, 1996.

60. **Fujieda K, Faiman C, Reyes FI, Winter JSD,** The control of steroidogenesis by human fetal adrenal cells in tissue culture: I. Responses to adrenocorticotropin, *J Clin Endocrinol Metab* 53:34, 1981.

61. **Fujieda K, Faiman C, Reyes FI, Thliveris J, Winter JSD,** The control of steroidogenesis by human fetal adrenal cells in tissue culture: II. Comparison of morphology and steroid production in cells of the fetal and definitive zones, *J Clin Endocrinol Metab* 53:401, 1981.

62. **Fujieda K, Faiman C, Reyes FI, Winter JSD,** The control of steroidogenesis by human fetal adrenal cells in tissue culture: III. The effects of various hormonal peptides, *J Clin Endocrinol Metab* 53:690, 1981.

63. **Mesiano S, Jaffe RB,** Interaction of insulin-like growth factor-II and estradiol directs steroidogenesis in the human fetal adrenal toward dehydroepiandrosterone sulfate production, *J Clin Endocrinol Metab* 77:754, 1993.

64. **Fujieda K, Faiman C, Reyes FI, Winter JSD,** The control of steroidogenesis by human fetal adrenal cells in tissue culture: IV. The effects of exposure to placental steroids, *J Clin Endocrinol Metab* 54:89, 1982.

65. **Byrne GC, Perry YS, Winter JSD,** Steroid inhibitory effects upon human adrenal 3β-hydroxysteroid dehydrogenase activity, *J Clin Endocrinol Metab* 62:413, 1986.

66. **Gell JS, Oh J, Rainey WE, Carr BR,** Effect of estradiol on DHEAS production in the human adrenocortical cell line, H295R, *J Soc Gynecol Invest* 5:144, 1998.

67. **Ducsay CA, Hess DL, McClellan MC, Novy MJ,** Endocrine and morphological maturation of the fetal and neonatal adrenal cortex in baboons, *J Clin Endocrinol Metab* 73:385, 1991.

68. **Albrecht ED, Pepe GJ,** Suppression of maternal adrenal dehydroepiandrosteorne (DHA) and DHA sulphate (DHAS) by estrogen during baboon pregnancy, *J Soc Gynecol Invest* 2:P375A, 1995.

69. **Coulter CL, Read LC, Carr BR, Tarantal AF, Barry S, Syne DM,** A role for epidermal growth factor in the morphological and functional maturation of the adrenal gland in the fetal rhesus monkey in vivo, *J Clin Endocrinol Metab* 81:1254, 1996.

70. **Fritz MA, Stanczyk FZ, Novy MJ,** Relationship of uteroplacental blood flow to the placental clearance of maternal dehydroepiandrosterone through estradiol formation in the pregnant baboon, *J Clin Endocrinol Metab* 61:1023, 1985.

71. **Fritz MA, Stanczyk FZ, Novy MJ,** Maternal estradiol response to alterations in uteroplacental blood flow, *Am J Obstet Gynecol* 155:1317, 1986.

72. **Shepherd RW, Stanczyk FZ, Bethea CL, Novy MJ,** Fetal and maternal endocrine responses to reduced uteroplacental blood flow, *J Clin Endocrinol Metab* 75:301, 1992.

73. **Distler W, Gabbe SG, Freeman RK, Mestman JH, Goebelsmann U,** Estriol in pregnancy: V. Unconjugated and total plasma estriol in the management of pregnant diabetic patients, *Am J Obstet Gynecol* 130:424, 1978.

74. **Bradshaw KD, Carr BR,** Placental sulfatase deficiency: maternal and fetal expression of steroid sulfatase deficiency and X-linked ichthyosis, *Obstet Gynecol Survey* 41:401, 1986.

75. **Rizk DEE, Johansen KA,** Maternal steroid sulfatase deficiency — cause of high-risk pregnancy? *Am J Obstet Gynecol* 171:566, 1994.

76. **Bradley LA, Canick JA, Palomaki GE, Haddow JE,** Undetectable maternal serum unconjugated estriol levels in the second trimester: risk of perinatal complications associated with placental sulfatase deficiency, *Am J Obstet Gynecol* 176:531, 1997.

77. **Shi QJ, Lei ZM, Rao CV, Lin J,** Novel role of human chorionic gonadotropin in differentiation of human cytotrophoblasts, *Endocrinology* 132:1387, 1993.

78. **Petraglia F, Florio P, Nappi C, Genazzani AR,** Peptide signaling in human placenta and membranes: autocrine, paracrine, and endocrine mechanisms, *Endocr Rev* 17:156, 1996.

79. **Siler-Khodr TM, Khodr GS,** Production and activity of placental releasing hormones, In: Novy MJ, Resko JA, eds. *Fetal Endocrinology,* Academic Press, New York, 1981, p 183.

80. **Siler-Khodr TM, Kuehl TJ, Vickery BH,** Effects of a gonadotropin-releasing antagonist on hormone levels in the pregnant baboon and on fetal outcome, *Fertil Steril* 41:448, 1984.

81. **Siler-Khodr TM, Khodr GS, Harper MJK, Rhode J, Vickery BH, Nestor Jr JJ,** Differential inhibition of human placental prostaglandin release in vitro by a GnRH antagonist, *Prostaglandins* 31:1003, 1986.

82. **Siler-Khoder TM, Khodr GS, Rhode J, Vickery BH, Nestor Jr JJ,** Gestational age-related inhibition of placental hCG, alpha hCG and steroid hormone release in vitro by a GnRH antagonist, *Placenta* 8:1, 1987.

83. **Belisle S, Guevin J-F, Bellabarba D, Lehoux J-G,** Luteinizing hormone-releasing hormone binds to enriched placental membranes and stimulates in vitro the synthesis of bioactive human chorionic gonadotropin, *J Clin Endocrinol Metab* 59:119, 1984.

84. **Miyake A, Sakumoto T, Anono T, Kawamura Y, Maeda T, Kurachi K,** Changes in luteinizing hormone-releasing hormone in human placenta throughout pregnancy, *Obstet Gynecol* 60:444, 1982.

85. **Kelly AC, Rodgers A, Dong K-W, Barrezueta NX, Blum M, Roberts JL,** Gonadotropin-releasing hormone and chorionic gonadotropin gene expression in human placental development, *DNA Cell Biol* 10:411, 1991.

86. **Iwashita M, Evans MI, Catt KJ,** Characterization of a gonadotropin-releasing hormone receptor site in term placenta and chorionic villi, *J Clin Endocrinol Metab* 62:127, 1986.

87. **Bramley TA, Mcphie CA, Menzies GS,** Human placental gonadotropin-releasing hormone (GnRH) binding sites. I. characterization, properties and ligand specificity, *Placenta* 13:555, 1992.

88. **Lin L-S, Roberts VJ, Yen S,** Expression of human gonadotropin-releasing hormone receptor gene in the placenta and its functional relationship to human chorionic gonadotropin secretion, *J Clin Endocrinol Metab* 80:580, 1995.

89. **Jones SA, Brooks AN, Challis JRG,** Steroids modulate corticotropin-releasing hormone production in human fetal membranes and placenta, *J Clin Endocrinol Metab* 68:825, 1989.

90. **Challis JRG, Matthews SG, Van Meir C, Ramirez MM,** Current topic: the placental corticotrophin-releasing hormone-adrenocorticotrophin axis, *Placenta* 16:481, 1995.

91. **Petraglia F, Florio P, Gallo R, Simoncini T, Saviozzi M, Di Blasio AM, Vaughan J, Vale W,** Human placenta and fetal membranes express human urocortin mRNA and peptide, *J Clin Endocrinol Metab* 81:3807, 1996.

92. **Ren S-G, Braunstein GD,** Human chorionic gonadotropin, *Seminars Reprod Endocrinol* 10:95, 1992.

93. **Lapthorn AJ, Harris DC, Littlejohn A, Lustbader JW, Canfield RE, Machin KJ, Mogan FJ, Isaacs NW,** Crystal structure of human chorionic gonadotropin, *Nature* 369:455, 1994.

94. **Gharib SD, Wierman ME, Shupnik MA, Chin WW,** Molecular biology of the pituitary gonadotropins, *Endocr Rev* 11:177, 1990.

95. **Albanese C, Colin IM, Crowley WF, Ito M, Pestell RG, Weiss J, Jameson JL,** The gonadotropin genes: evolution of distinct mechanisms for hormonal control, *Recent Prog Hormone Res* 51:23, 1996.

96. **Jameson JL, Hollenberg AN,** Regulation of chorionic gonadotropin gene expression, *Endocr Rev* 14:203, 1993.

97. **Layman LC, Edwards JL, Osborne WE, Peak DB, Gallup DG, Tho SPT, Reindollar RH, Roach DJ, McDonough PG, Lanclos KD,** Human chorionic gonadotrophin-β gene sequences in women with disorders of HCG production, *Mol Hum Reprod* 3:315, 1997.

98. **Tan L, Rousseau P,** The chemical identity of the immunoreactive LHRH-like peptide biosynthesized in the placenta, *Biochem Biophys Res Commun* 109:1061, 1982.

99. **Merz WE, Dorner M,** Studies on structure-function relationships of human choriogonadotropins with C-teminally shortened alpha subunits. I. Receptor binding and immunologic properties, *Biochem Biophys Acta* 844:62, 1985.

100. **Siler-Khodr TM, Khodr GS, Valenzuelea G, Rhode J,** Gonadotropin-releasing hormone effects on placental hormones during gestation. II. Progesterone, estrogen, estradiol and estriol, *Biol Reprod* 34:255, 1986.

101. **Steele GL, Currie WD, Leung E, Ho Yuen B, Leung PCK,** Rapid stimulation of human chorionic goandotropin secretion by interleukin-1 from perifused first trimester trophoblast, *J Clin Endocrinol Metab* 75:783, 1992.

102. **Barnea ER, Ashkenazy R, Tal Y, Kol S, Sarne Y,** Effect of β-endorphin on human chorionic gonadotrophin secretion by placental explants, *Hum Reprod* 6:1327, 1991.

103. **Petraglia F, Vaughn J, Vale W,** Inhibin and activin modulate the release of gonadotropin-releasing hormone, human chorionic gonadotropin, and progesterone from cultured placental cells, *Proc Natl Acad Sci USA* 86:5114, 1989.

104. **Petraglia F, Vaughan J, Vale W,** Steroid hormones modulate the release of immunoreactive gonadotropin-releasing hormone from cultured human placental cells, *J Clin Endocrinol Metab* 70:1173, 1990.

105. **Qu J, Brulet C, Thomas K,** Effect of epidermal growth factor on inhibin secretion in human placental cell culture, *Endocrinology* 131:2173, 1992.

106. **Qu J, Thomas K,** Prostaglandins stimulate the secretion of inhibin from human placental cells, *J Clin Endocrinol Metab* 77:556, 1993.

107. **Bonduelle M, Dodd R, Liebaers I, Steirteghem A, Williamson R, Akhurst R,** Chorionic gonadotropin-β mRNA, a trophoblast marker, is expressed in human 8-cell embryos derived from tripronucleate zygotes, *Hum Reprod* 3:909, 1988.

108. **Rabinovici J, Jaffe RB,** Development and regulation of growth and differentiated function of human and subhuman primate fetal gonads, *Endocr Rev* 11:532, 1990.

109. **Rothman PA, Chao VA, Taylor MR, Kuhn RW, Jaffe RB, Taylor RN,** Extraplacental human fetal tissues express mRNA transcripts encoding the human chorionic gonadotropin-β subunit protein, *Mol Reprod Dev* 33:1, 1992.

110. **Hoshina M, Boothby M, Boime I,** Cytological localization of chorionic gonadotropin α and placental lactogen mRNA during development of human placenta, *J Cell Biol* 93:19098, 1982.

111. **Nakajima ST, McAuliffe T, Gibson M,** The 24-hour pattern of the levels of serum progesterone and immunoreactive human chorionic gonadotropin in normal early pregnancy, *J Clin Endocrinol Metab* 71:345, 1990.

112. **Cole LA, Kardan A, Andrade-Gordon P, Gawinowicz MA, Morris JC, Bergert ER, O'Connor J, Birken S,** The heterogeneity of hCG: III. The occurrence, biological and immunological activities of nicked hCG, *Endocrinology* 129:1559, 1991.

113. **Wide L, Lee J-Y, Rasmussen C,** A change in the isoforms of human chorionic gonadotropin occurs around the 13th week of gestation, *J Clin Endocrinol Metab* 78:1419, 1994.

114. **Maruo T, Matsuo H, Ohtani T, Hoshina M, Mochizuchi M,** Differential modulation of chorionic gonadotropin (CG) subunit messenger ribonucleic acid level and CG secretion by progesterone in normal placenta and choriocarcinoma cultured in vitro, *Endocrinology* 119:858, 1986.

115. **Schlaerth JB, Morrow CP, Kletzky OA, Nalick RH, D'Ablaing GA,** Prognostic characteristics of serum human chorionic gonadotropin titer regression following molar pregnancy, *Obstet Gynecol* 58:478, 1981.

116. **Yedema KA, Verheijen RH, Kenemans P, Schijf CP, Borm GF, Segers MJ, Thomas CM,** Identification of patients with persistent trophoblastic disease by means of a normal human chorionic gonadotropin regression curve, *Am J Obstet Gynecol* 168:787, 1993.

117. **Khazaeli MB, Hedayat MM, Hatach KD, To ACW, Soong S-J, Shingleton HM, Boots LR, LoBuglio AF,** Radioimmunoassay of free β-subunit of human chorionic gonadotropin as a prognostic test for persistent trophoblastic disease in molar pregnancy, *Am J Obstet Gynecol* 155:320, 1986.

118. **Khazaeli MB, Buchina ES, Pattillo RA, Soong S-J, Hatch KD,** Radioimmunoassay of free β-subunit of human chorionic gonadotropin in diagnosis of high-risk and low-risk gestational trophoblastic disease, *Am J Obstet Gynecol* 160:444, 1989.

119. **Odell WD, Griffin J,** Pulsatile secretion of human chorionic gonadotropin in normal adults, *New Engl J Med* 317:1688, 1987.

120. **Odell WD, Griffin J,** Pulsatile secretion of chorionic gonadotropin during the normal menstrual cycle, *J Clin Endocrinol Metab* 69:528, 1989.

121. **Birken S, Maydelman Y, Gawinowicz MA, Pound A, Liu Y, Hartree AS,** Isolation and characterization of human pituitary chorionic gonadotropin, *Endocrinology* 137:1402, 1996.

122. **Patton PE, Hess DL, Cook DM, Loriaux DL, Braunstein GD,** Human chorionic gonadotropin production by the pituitary gland in a premenopausal women, *Am J Obstet Gynecol* 178:1138, 1998.

123. **Walker WH, Fitzpatrick SL, Barrera-Saldana HA, Resendes-Perez D, Saunders GF,** The human placental lactogen genes: structure, function, evolution and transcriptional regulation, *Endocr Rev* 12:316, 1991.

124. **Alsat E, Guibourdenche J, Luton D, Frankenne F, Evain-Brion D,** Human placental growth hormone, *Am J Obstet Gynecol* 177:1526, 1997.

125. **Grumbach MM, Kaplan SL, Vinik A,** HCS, In: Berson SA, Yalow RS, eds. *Peptide Hormones,* Vol. 2B, North-Holland, Amsterdam, 1973, p 797.

126. **Spellacy WN, Buhi WC, Schram JC, Birk SA, McCreary SA,** Control of human chorionic somatomammotropin levels during pregnancy, *Obstet Gynecol* 37:567, 1971.

127. **Felig P, Lynch V,** Starvation in human pregnancy: hypoglycemia, hypoinsulinemia, and hyperketonemia, *Science* 170:990, 1970.

128. **Felig P,** Maternal and fetal fluid homeostasis in human pregnancy, *Am J Clin Nutr* 26:998, 1973.

129. **Felig P, Kim YJ, Lynch V, Hendler R,** Amino acid metabolism during starvation in human pregnancy, *J Clin Invest* 51:1195, 1972.

130. **Kim YJ, Felig P,** Plasma chorionic somatomammotropin levels during starvation in mid-pregnancy, *J Clin Endocrinol Metab* 32:864, 1971.

131. **Handwerger S,** Clinical counterpoint: the physiology of placental lactogen in human pregnancy, *Endocr Rev* 12:329, 1991.

132. **Barker DJP, Martyn CN, Osmond C, Hales CN, Fall CHD,** Growth in utero and serum cholesterol concentrations in adult life, *Br Med J* 307:1524, 1993.

133. **Desoye G, Schweditsch MO, Pfeiffer KP, Zechner R, Kostner GM,** Correlation of hormones with lipid and lipoprotein levels during normal pregnancy and postpartum, *J Clin Endocrinol Metab* 64:704, 1987.

134. **Kalkhoff RK,** Impact of maternal fuels and nutritional state on fetal growth, *Diabetes* 40 (Suppl 2):61, 1991.

135. **Barker DJP, Hales CN, Fall CHD, Osmond C, Phipps K, Clark PMS,** Type 2 non-insulin-dependent-diabetes mellitus, hypertension and hyperlipidaemia (syndrome X): relation to reduced fetal growth, *Diabetologia* 36:620, 1993.

136. **Nielsen PV, Pedersen H, Kampmann E,** Absence of human placental lactogen in an otherwise uneventful pregnancy, *Am J Obstet Gynecol* 135:322, 1979.

137. **Sideri M, de Virgiliis G, Guidobono F, Borgese N, Sereni LP, Nicolini U, Remotti G,** Immunologically undetectable human placental lactogen in a normal pregnancy. Case report, *Br J Obstet Gynaecol* 90:771, 1983.

138. **Dawood MY, Teoh ES,** Serum human chorionic somatomammotropin in unaborted hydatidiform mole, *Obstet Gynecol* 47:183, 1976.

139. **Pekonen F, Althan H, Stenman U, Ylikorkala O,** Human chorionic gonadotropin (hCG) and thyroid function in early human pregnancy: circadian variation and evidence for intrinsic thyrotropic activity of hCG, *J Clin Endocrinol Metab* 66:853, 1988.

140. **Kimura M, Amino N, Tamaki H, Mitsuda N, Miyai K, Tanizawa O,** Physiologic thyroid activation in normal early pregnancy is induced by circulating hCG, *Obstet Gynecol* 75:775, 1990.

141. **Ballabio M, Poshyachinda M, Ekins RP,** Pregnancy-induced changes in thyroid function: role of human chorionic gonadotropin as putative regulator of maternal thyroid, *J Clin Endocrinol Metab* 73:824, 1991.

142. **Kimura M, Amino N, Tamaki H, Ito E, Mitsuda N, Miyai K, Tanizawa O,** Gestational thyrotoxicosis and hyperemesis gravidarum: possible role of hCG with higher stimulating activity, *Clin Endocrinol* 38:345, 1993.

143. **Yamazaki K, Sato K, Shizume K, Kanaji Y, Ito Y, Obara T, Nakagawa T, Koizumi T, Nishimura R,** Potent thyrotropic activity of human chorionic gonadotropin variants in terms of ^{125}I incorporation and *de novo* synthesized thyroid hormone release in human thyroid follicles, *J Clin Endocrinol Metab* 80:473, 1995.

144. **Tsuruta E, Tada H, Tamaki H, Kashiwai T, Asahio K, Takeoka K, Mitsuda N, Amino N,** Pathogenic role of asialo human chorionic gonadotropin in gestational thyrotoxicosis, *J Clin Endocrinol Metab* 80:350, 1995.

145. **Rees LH, Buarke CW, Chard T, Evans SW, Letchorth AT,** Possible placental origin of ACTH in normal human pregnancy, *Nature* 254:620, 1975.

146. **Goland RS, Wardlaw SL, Blum M, Tropper PJ, Stark RI,** Biologically active corticotropin-releasing hormone in maternal and fetal plasma during pregnancy, *Am J Obstet Gynecol* 159:884, 1988.

147. **Goland R, Conwell I, Warren W, Wardlaw S,** Placental CRH and pituitary-adrenal function during pregnancy, *Neuroendocrinology* 56:749, 1992.

148. **Petraglia F, Sawchenko PE, Rivier J, Vale W,** Evidence for local stimulation of ACTH secretion by corticotropin-releasing factor in human placenta, *Nature* 328:717, 1987.

149. **Cooper ES, Greer IA, Brooks AN,** Placental proopio-melanocortin gene expression, adrenocorticotropin tissue concentrations, and immunostaining increase throughout gestation and are unaffected by prostaglandins, antiprogestins, or labor, *J Clin Endocrinol Metab* 81:4462, 1996.

150. **Goland RS, Wardlaw SL, MacCarter G, Warren WB, Stark RI,** Adrenocorticotropin and cortisol responses to vasopressin during pregnancy, *J Clin Endocrinol Metab* 73:257, 1991.

151. **Laatikainen T, Virtanen T, Raiosanen I, Salminen K,** Immunoreactive corticotropin releasing factor and corticotropin in plasma during pregnancy, labor and puerperium, *Neuropeptides* 10:343, 1987.

152. **Goland RS, Jozak S, Conwell I,** Placental corticotropin-releasing hormone and the hypercortisolism of pregnancy, *Am J Obstet Gynecol* 171:1287, 1994.

153. **Wolfe CDA, Patel SP, Linton EA, Campbell EA, Anderson J, Dornhorst A, Lowry PJ, Jones MT,** Plasma corticotrophin-releasing factor (CRH) in abnormal pregnancy, *Br J Obstet Gynaecol* 95:1003, 1988.

154. **Jones SA, Challis JRG,** Local stimulation of prostaglandin production by corticotropin-releasing hormone in human fetal membranes and placenta, *Biochem Biophys Res Commun* 159:192, 1989.

155. **Frankenne F, Closset J, Gomez F, Scippo ML, Smal J, Hennen G,** The physiology of growth hormones (GHs) in pregnant women and partial characterization of the placental GH variant, *J Clin Endocrinol Metab* 66:1171, 1988.

156. **Daughaday WH, Trivedi B, Winn HN, Yan H,** Hypersomatotropism in pregnant women, as measured by a human liver radioreceptor assay, *J Clin Endocrinol Metab* 70:215, 1990.

157. **Mirlesse V, Grankenne F, Alsat E, Poncelet M, Hennen G, Evain-Brion D,** Placental growth hormone levels in normal pregnancy and in pregnancies with intrauterine growth retardation, *Pediatr Res* 34:439, 1993.

158. **Jauniaux E, Gulbis B, Jurkovic D, Schaaps JP, Campbell S, Meuris S,** Protein and steroid levels in embryonic cavities in early human pregnancy, *Hum Reprod* 8:782, 1993.

159. **Keel BA, Eddy KB, Cho S, Gangrade BK, May JV,** Purified human alpha fetoprotein inhibits growth factor-stimulated estradiol production by porcine granulosa cells in monolayer culture, *Endocrinology* 130:3715, 1992.

160. **Williams MA, Hickok DE, Zingheim RW, Luthy DA, Kimelman J, Nyberg DA, Mahony BS,** Elevated maternal serum α-fetoprotein levels and midtrimester placental abnormalities in relation to subsequent adverse pregnancy outcomes, *Am J Obstet Gynecol* 167:1032, 1992.

161. **Waller DK, Lustig LS, Cunningham GC, Feuchtbaum LB, Hook EB,** The association between maternal serum alpha-fetoprotein and preterm birth, small for gestational age infants, preeclampsia, and placental complications, *Obstet Gynecol* 88:816, 1996.

162. **Phillips OP, Elias S, Shulman LP, Andersen RN, Morgan CD, Simpson JL,** Maternal serum screening for fetal Down syndrome in women less than 35 years of age using alpha-fetoprotein, hCG, and unconjugated estriol: a prospective 2-year study, *Obstet Gynecol* 80:353, 1992.

163. **Haddow JE, Palomaki GE, Knoght GJ, Williams J, Pulkkinen A, Canick JA, Saller Jr DN, Bowers GB,** Prenatal screening for Down's syndrome with use of maternal serum markers, *New Engl J Med* 327:588, 1992.

164. **Kellner LH, Weiner Z, Weiss RR, Neuer M, Martin GM, Mueenuddin M, Bombard A,** Triple marker (α-fetoprotein, unconjugated estriol, human chorionic gonadotropin) versus α-fetoprotein plus free-β subunit in second-trimester maternal serum screening for fetal Down syndrome: a prospective comparison study, *Am J Obstet Gynecol* 173:1306, 1995.

165. **Saller DN, Canick JA, Schwartz S, Blitzer MG,** Multiple-marker screening in pregnancies with hydropic and nonhydropic Turner syndrome, *Am J Obstet Gynecol* 167:1021, 1992.

166. **Extermann P, Bischof P, Marguerat P, Mermillod B,** Second-trimester maternal serum screening for Down's syndrome: free β-human chorionic gonadotrophin (HCG) and α-fetoprotein, with or without unconjugated oestriol, compared with total HCG, α-fetoprotein and unconjugated oestriol, *Hum Reprod* 13:220, 1998.

167. **Kellner LH, Weiss RR, Weiner Z, Neuer M, Martin GM, Schulman H, Lipper S,** The advantages of using triple-marker screening for chromosomal abnormalities, *Am J Obstet Gynecol* 172:831, 1995.

168. **Schleifer RA, Bradley LA, Richards DS, Ponting NR,** Pregnancy outcome for women with very low levels of maternal serum unconjugated estriol on second-trimester screening, *Am J Obstet Gynecol* 173:1152, 1995.

169. **Weiss G, O'Byrne EM, Hochman J, Steinetz BG, Goldsmith L, Flitcraft JG,** Distribution of relaxin in women during pregnancy, *Obstet Gynecol* 52:569, 1978.

170. **Fields PA, Larkin LH,** Purification and immunohistochemical localization of relaxin in the human term placenta, *J Clin Endocrinol Metab* 52:79, 1981.

171. **Lopez Bernal A, Bryant-Greenwood GD, Hansell DJ, Hicks BR, Greenwood FC, Turnbull AC,** Effect of relaxin on prostaglandin E production by human amnion: changes in relation to the onset of labour, *Br J Obstet Gynaecol* 94:1045, 1987.

172. **Quagliarello J, Steinetz BG, Weiss G,** Relaxin secretion in early pregnancy, *Obstet Gynecol* 53:62, 1979.

173. **MacLennan AH, Katz M, Creasy R,** The morphologic characteristics of cervical ripening induced by the hormones relaxin and prostaglandin F2 in a rabbit model, *Am J Obstet Gynecol* 152:691, 1985.

174. **Hwang JJ, Macinga D, Rorke EA,** Relaxin modulates human cervical stromal cell activity, *J Clin Endocrinol Metab* 81:3379, 1996.

175. **Emmi AM, Skurnick J, Goldsmith LT, Gagliardi CL, Schmidt CL, Kleinberg D, Weiss G,** Ovarian control of pituitary hormone secretion in early human pregnancy, *J Clin Endocrinol Metab* 72:1359, 1991.

176. **Daly DC, Kuslis S, Riddick DH,** Evidence of short-loop inhibition of decidual prolactin synthesis by decidual proteins, Part II, *Am J Obstet Gynecol* 155:363, 1986.

177. **Maslar IA, Ansbacher R,** Effects of progesterone on decidual prolactin production by organ cultures of human endometrium, *Endocrinology* 118:2102, 1986.

178. **Daly DC, Kuslis S, Riddick DH,** Evidence of short-loop inhibition of decidual prolactin synthesis by decidual proteins, Part I, *Am J Obstet Gynecol* 155:358, 1986.

179. **Handwerger S, Brar A,** Placental lactogen, placental growth hormone, and decidual prolactin, *Seminars Reprod Endocrinol* 10:106, 1992.

180. **McCoshen JA, Barc J,** Prolactin bioactivity following decidual synthesis and transport by amniochorion, *Am J Obstet Gynecol* 153:217, 1985.

181. **Gellersen B, DiMattia G, Friesen HG, Bohnet H,** Prolactin (PRL) mRNA from human decidua differs from pituitary PRL mRNA but resembles IM-9-P3 lymphoblast PRL transcript, *Mol Cell Endocrinol* 64:127, 1989.

182. **Tyson JE, Hwang P, Guyda H, Friesen HG,** Studies of prolactin secretion in human pregnancy, *Am J Obstet Gynecol* 113:14, 1972.

183. **Kletzky OA, Marrs RP, Howard WF, McCormick W, Mishell Jr DR,** Prolactin synthesis and release during pregnancy and puerperium, *Am J Obstet Gynecol* 136:545, 1980.

184. **Tyson JE, Friesen HG,** Factors influencing the secretion of human prolactin and growth hormone in menstrual and gestational women, *Am J Obstet Gynecol* 116:377, 1973.

185. **Barberia JM, Abu-Fadil S, Kletzky OA, Nakamura RM, Mishell Jr DR,** Serum prolactin patterns in early human gestation, *Am J Obstet Gynecol* 121:1107, 1975.

186. **Ho Yuen B, Cannon W, Lewis J, Sy L, Wooley S,** A possible role for prolactin in the control of human chorionic gonadotropin and estrogen secretion by the fetoplacental unit, *Am J Obstet Gynecol* 136:286, 1980.

187. **Maaskant RA, Bogic LV, Gilger S, Kelly PA, Bryant-Greenwood GD,** The human prolactin receptor in the fetal membranes, decidua, and placenta, *J Clin Endocrinol Metab* 81:396, 1996.

188. **Luciano AA, Varner MW,** Decidual, amniotic fluid, maternal, and fetal prolactin in normal and abnormal pregnancies, *Obstet Gynecol* 63:384, 1984.

189. **Golander A, Kopel R, Lasebik N, Frenkel Y, Spirer Z,** Decreased prolactin secretion by decidual tissue of pre-eclampsia in vitro, *Acta Endocrinol* 108:111, 1985.

190. **Healy DL, Herington AC, O'Herlihy C,** Chronic polyhydramnios is a syndrome with a lactogen receptor defect in the chorion laeva, *Br J Obstet Gynaecol* 92:461, 1985.

191. **Raabe MA, McCoshen JA,** Epithelial regulation of prolactin effect on amnionic permeability, *Am J Obstet Gynecol* 154:130, 1986.

192. **Pullano JG, Cohen-Addad N, Apuzzio JJ, Ganesh VL, Josimovich JB,** Water and salt conservation in the human fetus and newborn. I. Evidence for a role of fetal prolactin, *J Clin Endocrinol Metab* 69:1180, 1989.

193. **Ben-Rafael Z, Orvieto R,** Cytokines — involvement in reproduction, *Fertil Steril* 58:1093, 1992.

194. **Harty JR, Kauma SW,** Interleukin-1 stimulates colony-stimulating factor-1 production in placental villous core mesenchymal cells, *J Clin Endocrinol Metab* 75:947, 1992.

195. **Masuhiro K, Matsuzaki N, Nishino E, Taniguchi T, Kameda T, Li Y, Saji F, Tanizawa O,** Trophoblast-derived interleukin-1 (IL-1) stimulates the release of human chorionic gonadotropin by activating IL-6 and IL-6-receptor system in first trimester human trophoblasts, *J Clin Endocrinol Metab* 72:594, 1991.

196. **Li Y, Matsuzaki N, Masuhiro K, Kameda T, Tamiguchi T, Saji F, Yone K, Tanizawa O,** Trophoblast-derived tumor necrosis factor induces release of human chorionic gonadotropin using interleukin-6 (IL-6) and Il-6-receptor-dependent system in the normal human trophoblasts, *J Clin Endocrinol Metab* 74:184, 1992.

197. **Pekonen F, Suikkari A-M, Makinen T, Rutanen E-M,** Different insulin-like growth factor binding species in human placenta and decidua, *J Clin Endocrinol Metab* 67:1250, 1988.

198. **Giudice LC, Farrell EM, Pham H, Lamson G, Rosenfeld RG,** Insulin-like growth factor binding proteins in maternal serum throughout gestation and in the puerperium: effects of a pregnancy-associated serum protease activity, *J Clin Endocrinol Metab* 71:806, 1990.

199. **Langford KS, Nicolaides KH, Jones J, Abbas A, McGregor AM, Miell JP,** Serum insulin-like growth factor-binding protein-3 (IGFBP-3) levels and IGFBP-3 protease activity in normal, abnormal, and multiple human pregnancy, *J Clin Endocrinol Metab* 80:21, 1995.

200. **Osborn BH, Fowlkes J, Han VKM, Fremark M,** Nutritional regulation of insulin-like growth factor-binding protein gene expression in the ovine fetus and pregnant ewe, *Endocrinology* 131:1743, 1992.

201. **Iwashita M, Kobayashi M, A M, Nakayama S, Mimuro T, Takeda Y, Sakamoto S,** Feto-maternal interactions of IGF-I and its binding proteins in fetal growth, *Early Hum Dev* 29:187, 1992.

202. **Lassarre C, Hardouin S, Daffos F, Forestier F, Frankenne F, Binoux M,** Serum insulin-like growth factors and insulin-like growth factor binding proteins in the human fetus. Relationships with growth in normal subjects and in subjects with intrauterine growth retardation, *Pediatr Res* 29:219, 1991.

203. **Gluckman PD,** The endocrine regulation of fetal growth in late gestation: the role of insulin-like growth factors, *J Clin Endocrinol Metab* 80:1047, 1995.

204. **Abe Y, Hasegawa Y, Miyamoto K, Yamaguchi M, Andoh A, Ibuki Y,** High concentrations of plasma immunoreactive inhibin during normal pregnancy in women, *J Clin Endocrinol Metab* 71:133, 1990.

205. **Qu J, Ying S-Y, Thomas K,** Inhibin production and secretion in human placental cells cultured in vitro, *Obstet Gynecol* 79:705, 1992.

206. **Muttukrishna S, George L, Fowler PA, Groome NP, Knight PG,** Measurement of serum concentrations of dimeric inhibin during human pregnancy, *Clin Endocrinol* 42:391, 1994.

207. **Qu J, Thomas K,** Inhibin and activin production in human placenta, *Endocr Rev* 16:485, 1995.

208. **Illingworth PJ, Groome NP, Duncan WC, Grant V, Tovanabutra S, Baird DT, McNeilly AS,** Measurement of circulating inhibin forms during the establishment of pregnancy, *J Clin Endocrinol Metab* 81:1471, 1996.

209. **Muttukrishna S, Fowler PA, George L, Groome NP, Knight PG,** Changes in peripheral serum levels of total activin A during the human menstrual cycle and pregnancy, *J Clin Endocrinol Metab* 81:3328, 1996.

210. **Petraglia F, Woodruff TK, Botticelli G, Botticelli A, Genazzani AR, Mayo KE, Vale W,** Gonadotropin-releasing hormone, inhibin, and activin in human placenta: evidence for a common cellular localization, *J Clin Endocrinol Metab* 74:1184, 1992.

211. **Petraglia F, Anceschi MM, Calza L, Garuti GC, Fusaro P, Giardino L, Genazzani AR, Vale W,** Inhibin and activin in human fetal membranes: evidence for a local effect on prostaglandin release, *J Clin Endocrinol Metab* 77:542, 1993.

212. **Cuckle HS, Holding S, Jones R, Wallace EM, Groome NP,** Maternal serum dimeric inhibin A in second-trimester Down's syndrome pregnancies, *Prenat Diagn* 15:385, 1995.

213. **Aitken DA, Wallace EM, Crossley JA, Swanston IA, van Pareren Y, van Maarle M, Groome NP, Macri JN, Connor JM,** Dimeric inhibin A as a marker for Down's syndrome in early pregnancy, *New Engl J Med* 334:1231, 1996.

214. **Petraglia F, Gallinelli A, Grande A, Florio P, Ferrari S, Genazzani AR, Ling N, DePaolo V,** Local production and action of follistatin in human placenta, *J Clin Endocrinol Metab* 78:205, 1994.

215. **Hung TT,** The role of endogenous opioids in pregnancy and anesthesia, *Seminars Reprod Endocrinol* 5:161, 1987.

216. **Xie G-X, Miyajima A, Goldstein A,** Expression cloning of cDNA encoding a seven-helix receptor from human placenta with affinity for opioid ligands, *Proc Natl Acad Sci USA* 89:4124, 1992.

217. **Margioris AN, Grino M, Protos P, Gold PW, Chrousos GP,** Corticotropin-releasing hormone and oxytocin stimulate the release of placental proopiomelanocortin peptides, *J Clin Endocrinol Metab* 66:922, 1988.

218. **Derkx FHM, Alberda AT, De Jong FH, Zeilmaker FH, Makovitz JW, Schalekamp MADH,** Source of plasma prorenin in early and late pregnancy: observations in a patient with primary ovarian failure, *J Clin Endocrinol Metab* 65:349, 1987.

219. **Itskovitz J, Rubattu S, Levron J, Sealey JE,** Highest concentrations of prorenin and human chorionic gonadotropin in gestational sacs during early human pregnancy, *J Clin Endocrinol Metab* 75:906, 1992.

220. **Lenz T, Sealey JE, August P, James GD, Laragh JH,** Tissue levels of active and total renin, angiotensinogen, human chorionic gonadotrophin, estradiol, and progesterone in human placentas from different methods of delivery, *J Clin Endocrinol Metab* 69:31, 1989.

221. **Myatt L,** Control of vascular resistance in the human placenta, *Placenta* 13:329, 1992.

222. **August P, Mueller FB, Sealey JE, Edersheim TG,** Role of renin-angiotensin system in blood pressure regulation in pregnancy, *Lancet* 345:896, 1995.

223. **Lim AT, Gude NM,** Atrial natriuretic factor production by the human placenta, *J Clin Endocrinol Metab* 80:3091, 1995.

224. **Yamaji T, Hirai N, Ishibashi M, Takaku F, Yanaihara T, Nakayama T,** Atrial natriuretic peptide in umbilical cord blood: evidence for a circulating hormone in human fetus, *J Clin Endocrinol Metab* 63:1414, 1986.

225. **Pouta AM, rasanen JP, Airaksinen KE, Vuolteenaho OJ, Laatikainen TJ,** Changes in maternal heart dimensions and plasma atrial natriuretic peptide levels in the early puerperium of normal and preeclamptic pregnancies, *Br J Obstet Gynaecol* 103:988, 1996.

226. **Morton H, Rolfe BE, Cavanagh AC,** Early pregnancy factor, *Seminars Reprod Endocrinol* 10:72, 1992.

227. **Chou JY, Plouzek CA,** Pregnancy-specific 1-glycoprotein, *Seminars Reprod Endocrinol* 10:116, 1992.

228. **Ramwell PW, Foegh M, Loeb R, Leovey EMK,** Synthesis and metabolism of prostaglandins, prostacyclin, and thromboxanes: the arachidonic acid cascade, *Seminars Perinatol* 4:3, 1980.

229. **Smith WL, Marnett LJ, DeWitt DL,** Prostaglandin and thromboxane biosynthesis, *Pharmacol Ther* 49:153, 1991.

230. **Samuelsson B, Dahlen S-E, Lindgren JA, Rouzer CA, Serhan CN,** Leukotrienes and lipoxins: structures, biosynthesis, and biological effects, *Science* 237:1171, 1987.

231. **Funk CD, Funk LB, Kennedy ME, Pong AS, FitzGerald GA,** Human platelet/erythroleukemia cell prostaglandin G/H synthase: cDNA cloning, expression and gene chromosomal assignment, *FASEB J* 5:2304, 1991.

232. **Jones DA, Carlton DP, McIntyre TM, Zimmerman GA, Prescott SM,** Molecular cloning of human prostaglandin endoperoxide synthase type II and demonstration of expression in response to cytokines, *J Biol Chem* 268:9049, 1993.

233. **Williams CS, Du Bois RN,** Prostaglandin endoperoxide synthase: why two isoforms? *Am J Physiol* 270:393, 1996.

234. **Gryglewski RJ, Korbut R, Oetkiewicz A, Splawinski J, Wojtaszek B, Swies J,** Lungs as a generator of prostacyclin — hypothesis on physiological significance, *Arch Pharmacol* 304:45, 1979.

235. **Walsh SW,** Preeclampsia: an imbalance in placental prostacyclin and thromboxane production, *Am J Obstet Gynecol* 152:335, 1985.

236. **Moncada S, Vance JR,** Arachidonic acid metabolites and the interactions between platelets and blood vessel walls, *New Engl J Med* 300:1142, 1979.

237. **Beitz J, Muller G, Forster W,** Effect of HDL and LDL from pre and post menopausal women on prostacylcin synthesis, *Prostaglandins* 30:179, 1985.

238. **Mileikowsky GN, Nadler JL, Huey F, Francis R, Roy S,** Evidence that smoking alters prostacyclin formation and platelet aggregation in women who use oral contraceptives, *Am J Obstet Gynecol* 159:1547, 1988.

239. **Makheja A, Vanderhoek JY, Bailey JM,** Inhibition of platelet aggregation and thromboxane synthesis by onion and garlic, *Lancet* 1:781, 1979.

240. **Fischer S, Weber PC,** The prostacyclin/thromboxane balance is favourably shifted in Greenland Eskimos, *Prostaglandins* 32:235, 1986.

241. **Olson DM, Zakart T,** Intrauterine tissue prostaglandin synthesis: regulatory mechanisms, *Seminars Reprod Endocrinol* 11:234, 1993.

242. **Green K, Drvota V, Vesterqvist O,** Pronounced reduction of *in vivo* prostacyclin synthesis in humans by acetaminophen (paracetamol), *Prostaglandins* 37:311, 1989.

243. **Mitchell JA, Akarasereenont P, Thiemermann C, Flower RJ, Vane JR,** Selectivity of nonsteroidal antiinflammatory drugs as inhibitors of constitutive and inducible cyclooxygenase, *Proc Natl Acad Sci USA* 90:11693, 1993.

244. **Masotti G, Poggesi L, Galanti G, Abbate R, Neri S, Neri GG,** Differential inhibition of prostacyclin production and platelet aggregation by aspirin, *Lancet* 2:1213, 1979.

245. **Bochner F, Lloyd J,** Is there an optimal dose and formulation of aspirin to prevent arterial thrombo-embolism in man? *Clin Sci* 71:625, 1987.

246. **FitzGerald DJ, Mayo G, Catella F, Entman SS, FitzGerald GA,** Increased thromboxane biosynthesis in normal pregnancy is mainly derived from platelets, *Am J Obstet Gynecol* 157:325, 1987.

247. **Mitchell MD,** Mechanisms of human parturition: role of prostaglandins and related compounds, *Adv Prostglandin Thromboxane Leukotriene Res* 15:613, 1985.

248. **Casey ML, MacDonald PC,** The initiation of labor in women: regulation of phospholipid and arachidonic acid metabolism and of prostaglandin production, *Seminars Perinatol* 10:270, 1986.

249. **Challis JRG, Gibb W,** Control of parturition, *Prenatal Neonatal Med* 1:283, 1996.

250. **Honnebier WJ, Swaab DF,** The influence of anencephaly upon intrauterine growth of fetus and placenta and upon gestation length, *J Obstet Gynaecol Br Common* 80:577, 1973.

251. **Price HV, Cone BA, Keogh M,** Length of gestation in congenital adrenal hyperplasia, *J Obstet Gynaecol Br Common* 78:430, 1971.

252. **Walsh SW, Stanczyk FZ, Novy MJ,** Daily hormonal changes in the maternal, fetal and amniotic fluid compartments before parturition in a primate species, *J Clin Endocrinol Metab* 58:629, 1984.

253. **Femini M, Borenstein R, Dreazen E, Apelman Z, Mogilner BM, Kessler I, Lancet M,** Pevention of premature labor by 17α-hydroxyprogesterone caproate, *Am J Obstet Gynecol* 151:574, 1985.

254. **Erny R, Pigne A, Prouvost C, Gamerre M, Malet C, Serment H, Barrat J,** The effects of oral administration of progesterone for premature labor, *Am J Obstet Gynecol* 154:525, 1986.

255. **Khan-Dawood FS,** In vitro conversion of pregnenolone to progesterone in human term placenta and fetal membranes before and after onset of labor, *Am J Obstet Gynecol* 157:1333, 1987.

256. **Haluska GJ, Stanczyk FZ, Cook MJ, Novy MJ,** Temporal changes in uterine activity and prostaglandin response to RU 486 in rhesus macaques in late gestation, *Am J Obstet Gynecol* 157:1487, 1987.

257. **Selinger M, MacKenzie IZ, Gillmet MD, Phipps SL, Ferguson J,** Progesterone inhibition in mid-trimester termination of pregnancy: physiological and clinical effects, *Br J Obstet Gynaecol* 94:1218, 1987.

258. **Haluska GJ, Cook MJ, Novy MJ,** Inhibition and augmentation of progesterone production during pregnancy: effects on parturition in rhesus monkeys, *Am J Obstet Gynecol* 176:682, 1997.

259. **Mitchell BF, Wong S,** Changes in 17β,20α-hydroxysteroid dehydrogenase activity supporting an increase in the estrogen/progesterone ratio of human fetal membranes at parturition, *Am J Obstet Gynecol* 168:1377, 1993.

260. **Davidson BJ, Murray RD, Challis JRG, Valenzuela GJ,** Estrogen, progesterone, prolactin, prostaglandin E_2, prostaglandin $F_{2\alpha}$, 13,14-dihydro-15-keto-prostaglandin $F_{2\alpha}$, and 6-keto-prostaglandin $F_{1\alpha}$ gradients across the uterus in women in labor and not in labor, *Am J Obstet Gynecol* 157:54, 1987.

261. **Okazaki T, Sagawa N, Okita JR, Bleasdale JE, MacDonald PC, Johnston JM,** Diacylglycerol metabolism and arachidonic acid release in human fetal membranes and decidua vera, *J Biol Chem* 256:7316, 1981.

262. **Okazaki T, Sagawa N, Bleasdale JE, Okita JR, MacDonald PC, Johnston JM,** Initiation of human parturition: XIII. Phospholipase C, phospholipase A2, and diacylglycerol lipase activities in fetal membranes and decidua vera tissues from early and late gestation, *Biol Reprod* 25:103, 1981.

263. **DiRenzo GC, Johnston JM, Okazaki T, Okita JR, MacDonald PC, Bleasdale JE,** Phosphatidylinositol specific phospholipase C in fetal membranes and uterine decidua, *J Clin Invest* 67:847, 1981.

264. **Romano WM, Lukash LA, Challis JRG, Mitchell BF,** Substrate utilization for estrogen synthesis by human fetal membranes and decidua, *Am J Obstet Gynecol* 155:11700, 1986.

265. **Chibbar R, Hobkirk R, Mitchell BF,** Sulfohydrolase activity for estrone sulfate and dehydroepiandrosterone sulfate in human fetal membranes and decidua around the time of parturition, *J Clin Endocrinol Metab* 62:90, 1986.

266. **Challis JRG, Vaughan M,** Steroid synthetic and prostaglandin metabolizing activity is present in different cell populations from human fetal membranes and decidua, *Am J Obstet Gynecol* 157:1474, 1987.

267. **Collins PL, Moore JJ, Idriss E, Kulp TM,** Human fetal membranes inhibit calcium L-channel activated uterine contractions, *Am J Obstet Gynecol* 175:1173, 1996.

268. **Florio P, Woods RJ, Genazzani AR, Lowry PJ, Petraglia F,** Changes in amniotic fluid immunoreactive corticotropin-releasing factor (CRF) and CRF-binding protein levels in pregnant women at term and during labor, *J Clin Endocrinol Metab* 82:835, 1997.

269. **Bendetto C, Petraglia F, Marozio L, Florio P, Genazzani AR, Massobrio M,** CRH increases prostaglandin $F_{2\alpha}$ in human myometrium *in vitro*, *Am J Obstet Gynecol* 171:126, 1994.

270. **McLean M, Bisit A, Davies J, Woods R, Lowry PJ, Smith R,** A placental clock controlling the length of human pregnancy, *Nature Med* 1:460, 1995.

271. **Berkowitz GS, Lapinski RH, Lockwood CJ, Florio P, Blackmore-Prince C, Petraglia F,** Corticotropin-releasing factor and its binding protein: maternal serum levels in term and preterm deliveries, *Am J Obstet Gynecol* 174:1477, 1996.

272. **Korebrits C, Ramirez MM, Watson L, Brinkman E, Bocking AD, Challis JRG,** Maternal corticotropin-releasing hormone is increased with impending preterm birth, *J Clin Endocrinol Metab* 83:1585, 1998.

273. **Marinoni E, Korebrits C, Di Iorio R, Cosmi EV, Challis JRG,** Effect of betamethasone in vivo on placental corticotropin-releasing hormone in human pregnancy, *Am J Obstet Gynecol* 178:770, 1998.

274. **Mortimer G, Hunter IC, Stimson WH, Govan ADT,** A role for amniotic epithelium in control of human parturition, *Lancet* 1:1074, 1985.

275. **Bennett PR, Rose MP, Myatt L, Elder MG,** Preterm labor: stimulation of arachidonic acid metabolism in human amnion cells by bacterial productions, *Am J Obstet Gynecol* 156:649, 1987.

276. **Romero R, Avila C, Brekus CA, Morotti R,** The role of systemic and intrauterine infection in preterm parturition, *Ann NY Acad Sci* 622:355, 1991.

277. **Silver RM, Edwin SS, Trautman MS, Simmons DL, Branch DW, Dudley DJ, Mitchell MD,** Bacterial lipopolysaccharide-mediated fetal death. Production of a newly recognized form of inducible cyclooxygenase (COX-2) in murine decidua in response to lipopolysaccharide, *J Clin Invest* 95:725, 1995.

278. **Morris C, Khan H, Sullivan MHF, Elder MG,** Effects of platelet-activating factor on prostaglandin E2 production by intact fetal membranes, *Am J Obstet Gynecol* 166:1228, 1992.

279. **Tahara M, Tasaka K, Masumoto N, Adachi K, Adachi H, Ikebuchi Y, Kurachi H, Miyake A,** Expression of messenger ribonucleic acid for epidermal growth factor (EGF), transforming growth factor-alpha (TGF alpha), and EGF receptor in human amnion cells: possible role of TGF alpha in prostaglandin E_2 synthesis and cell proliferation, *J Clin Endocrinol Metab* 80:138, 1995.

280. **Lundin-Schiller S, Mitchell MD,** Renin increases human amnion cell prostaglandin E2 biosynthesis, *J Clin Endocrinol Metab* 73:436, 1991.

281. **Mitchell MD,** The regulation of decidual prostaglandin biosynthesis by growth factors, phorbol esters, and calcium, *Biol Reprod* 44:871, 1991.

282. **Schrey MP, Monaghan H, Holt JR,** Interaction of paracrine factors during labour: interleukin-1β causes amplification of decidua cell prostaglandin $F_{2\alpha}$ production in response to bradykinin and epidermal growth factor, *Prostaglandins Leukotrienes Essential Fatty Acids* 45:137, 1992.

283. **Giannopoulis G, Jackson K, Kredentser J, Tulchinsky D,** Prostaglandin E_2 and $F_{2\alpha}$ receptors in human myometrium during the menstrual cycle and in pregnancy and labor, *Am J Obstet Gynecol* 153:904, 1985.

284. **Shellhaas CS, Coffman T, Dargie PJ, Killam AP, Kay HH,** Intravillous eicosanoid compartmentalization and regulation of placental blood flow, *J Soc Gynecol Invest* 4:58, 1997.

285. **Okazaki T, Casey ML, Okita JR, MacDonald PC, Johnston JM,** Initiation of human parturition: XII. Biosynthesis and metabolism of prostaglandins in human fetal membranes and uterine decidua vera, *Am J Obstet Gynecol* 139:373, 1981.

286. **Gibb W, Sun M,** Localization of prostaglandin H synthase type 2 protein and mRNA in term human fetal membranes and decidua, *J Endocrinol* 150:497, 1996.

287. **Sun M, Ramirez M, Challis JR, Gibb W,** Immunohistochemical localization of the glucocorticoid receptor in human fetal membranes and decidua at term and preterm delivery, *J Endocrinol* 149:243, 1996.

288. **Nakla S, Skinner K, Mitchell BF, Challis JRG,** Changes in prostaglandin transfer across human fetal membranes obtained after spontaneous labor, *Am J Obstet Gynecol* 155:1337, 1986.

289. **Niesert S, Christopherson W, Korte K, Mitchell MD, MacDonald PC, Casey ML,** Prostaglandin E_2 9-ketoreductase activity in human decidua vera tissue, *Am J Obstet Gynecol* 155:1348, 1986.

290. **Mitchell BF, Rogers K, Wong S,** The dynamics of prostaglandin metabolism in human fetal membranes and decidua around the time of parturition, *J Clin Endocrinol Metab* 77:759, 1993.

291. **Sangha RK, Walton JC, Ensor CM, Tai H-H, Challis JRG,** Immunohistochemical localization, messenger ribonucleic acid abundance, and activity of 15-hydroxyprostaglandin dehydrogenase in placenta and fetal membranes during term and preterm labor, *J Clin Endocrinol Metab* 78:982, 1994.

292. **van Meir CA, Matthews SG, Keirse MJNC, Ramirez MM, Bocking A, Challis JRG,** 15-Hydroxyprostaglandin dehydrogenase: implications in preterm labor with and without ascending infection, *J Clin Endocrinol Metab* 82:969, 1997.

293. **Hirst JJ, Chibbart R, Mitchell BF,** Role of oxytocin in the regulation of uterine activity during pregnancy and in the initiation of labor, *Seminars Reprod Endocrinol* 11:219, 1993.

294. **Hirst JJ, Haluska GJ, Cook MJ, Novy MJ,** Plasma oxytocin and nocturnal uterine activity: maternal but not fetal concentrations increase progressively during late pregnancy and delivery in Rhesus monkeys, *Am J Obstet Gynecol* 169:415, 1993.

295. **Wilson T, Liggins GC, Whittaker DJ,** Oxytocin stimulates the release of arachidonic acid and prostaglandin $F_{2\alpha}$ from human decidual cells, *Prostaglandins* 35:771, 1988.

296. **Chibbar R, Miller FD, Mitchell BF,** Synthesis of oxytocin in amnion, chorion, and decidua may influence the timing of human parturition, *J Clin Invest* 91:185, 1993.

297. **Chibbar R, Wong S, Miller FD, Mitchell BF,** Estrogens stimulate oxytocin gene expression in human chorio-decidua, *J Clin Endocrinol Metab* 80:567, 1995.

298. **Zeeman GG, Khan-Dawood FS, Dawood MY,** Oxytocin and its receptor in pregnancy and parturition: current concepts and clinical implications, *Obstet Gynecol* 89:873, 1997.

299. **Sugimoto Y, Yamasaki A, Segi E, Tsuboi K, Aze Y, Nishimura T, Oida H, Yoshida N, Tanaka T, Katsuyama M, Hasumoto K, Murata T, Hirata M, Ushikubi F, Negishi M, Ichikawa A, Narumiya S,** Failure of parturition in mice lacking the prostaglandin F receptor, *Science* 277:681, 1997.

300. **Nishimori K, Young LJ, Guo Q, Wang Z, Insel TR, Matzuk MM,** Oxytocin is required for nursing but is not essential for parturition or reproductive behavior, *Proc Natl Acad Sci USA* 93:11699, 1996.

301. **Burghardt RC, Barhoumi R, Dookwah H,** Endocrine regulation of myometrial gap junctions and their role in parturition, *Seminars Reprod Endocrinol* 11:250, 1993.

302. **Carsten ME, Miller JD,** A new look at uterine muscle contraction, *Am J Obstet Gynecol* 157:1303, 1987.

303. **Van den Veyyer IB, Moise Jr KJ,** Prostaglandin synthetase inhibitors in pregnancy, *Obstet Gynecol Survey* 48:493, 1993.

304. **Sorensen TK, Easterling TR, Carlson KL, Brateng DA, Benedetti TJ,** The maternal hemodynamic effect of indomethacin in normal pregnancy, *Obstet Gynecol* 79:661, 1992.

305. **Carlan SJ, O'Brien WF, O'Leary TD, Mastrogiannis D,** Randomized comparative trial of indomethacin and sulindac for the treatment of refractory preterm labor, *Obstet Gynecol* 79:223, 1992.

306. **Rasanen J, Jouppila P,** Fetal cardiac function and ductus arteriosus during indomethacin and sulindac therapy for threatened preterm labor: a randomized study, *Am J Obstet Gynecol* 173:20, 1995.

307. **Cabrol D, Landesman R, Muller J, Uzan M, Sureau C, Saxena BB,** Treatment of polyhydramnios with prostaglandin synthetase inhibitor (indomethacin), *Am J Obstet Gynecol* 157:422, 1987.

308. **Bernstein P,** Prostaglandin E_2 gel for cervical ripening and labor induction: a multicentre placebo-controlled trial, *Can Med Assoc J* 145:1249, 1991.

309. **Sanchez-Ramos L, Kaunitz AM, Wears RL, Delke I, Gaudier FL,** Misoprostol for cervical ripening and labor induction: a meta-analysis, *Obstet Gynecol* 89:633, 1997.

310. **Ray DA, Garite TJ,** Prostaglandin E_2 for induction of labor in patients with premature rupture of membranes at term, *Am J Obstet Gynecol* 166:836, 1992.

311. **Sanchez-Ramos L, Kaunitz AM, Del Valle GO, Delke I, Schroeder PA, Briones DK,** Labor induction with the prostaglandin E_1 methyl analogue misoprostol versus oxytocin: a randomized trial, *Obstet Gynecol* 81:332, 1993.

312. **Sanchez-Ramos L, Chen A, Kaunitz AM, Gaudier FL, Delke I,** Labor induction with intravaginal misoprostol in term premature rupture of membranes: a randomized study, *Obstet Gynecol* 89:909, 1997.

313. **Peyron R, Aubeny E, Targosz V, Silvestre L, Renault M, Elkik F, Leclerc P, Ulmann A, Baulieu EE,** Early termination of pregnancy with mifepristone (RU 486) and the orally active prostaglandin misoprostol, *New Engl J Med* 328:1509, 1993.

314. **El-Rafaey HJ, Rajasekar D, Abdalla M, Calder L, Templeton A,** Induction of abortion with mifepristone (RU 486) and oral or vaginal misoprostol, *New Engl J Med* 332:983, 1995.

315. **Webster D, Penney GC, Templeton A,** A comparison of 600 and 200 mg mifepristone prior to second trimester abortion with the prostaglandin misoprostol, *Br J Obstet Gynaecol* 103:706, 1996.

316. **O'Leary JA,** Prostaglandins and postpartum hemorrhage, *Seminars Reprod Endocrinol* 3:247, 1985.

317. **Coceani F, Olley PM, Lock JE,** Prostaglandins, ductus arteriosus, pulmonary circulation: current concepts and clinical potential, *Eur J Clin Pharmacol* 18:75, 1980.

318. **Brash AR, Hickey DE, Graham TP, Stahlman MT, Oates JA, Cotton RB,** Pharmacokinetics of indomethacin in the neonate: relation of plasma indomethacin levels to response of the ductus arteriosus, *New Engl J Med* 305:67, 1981.

319. **Rudolph AM,** The effects of nonsteroidal antiinflammatory compounds on fetal circulation and pulmonary function, *Obstet Gynecol* 58:635, 1981.

320. **Vermillion ST, Scardo JA, Lashus AG, Wiles HB,** The effect of indomethacin tocolysis on fetal ductus arteriosus constriction with advancing gestational age, *Am J Obstet Gynecol* 177:256, 1997.

321. **Thorburn GD,** The placenta, PGE_2 and parturition, *Early Hum Dev* 29:63, 1992.

322. **Gluck L, Kulovich MV, Borer RC, Brenner PH, Anderson GG, Spellacy WN,** Diagnosis of respiratory distress syndrome by amniocentesis, *Am J Obstet Gynecol* 109:440, 1971.

323. **Mendelson CR, Boggaram V,** Hormonal control of the surfactant system in the fetal lung, *Ann Rev Physiol* 53:415, 1991.

324. **Dekowski SA, Snyder JM,** Insulin regulation of messenger ribonucleic acid for the surfactant-associated proteins in human fetal lung in vitro, *Endocrinology* 131:669, 1992.

325. **National Institutes of Health Consensus Development Conference Statement,** Effect of corticosteroids for fetal maturation on perinatal outcomes, February 28-March 2, 1994, *Am J Obstet Gynecol* 173:246, 1995.

326. **Ballard RA, Ballard PL, Creasy RK, Padbury J, Polk DH, Bracken M, Moya FR, Gross I, and the TRH Study Group,** Respiratory disease in very-low-birthweight infants after prenatal thyrotropin-releasing hormone and glucocorticoids, *Lancet* 339:510, 1992.

327. **ACTOBAT Study Group,** Australian collaborative trial of antenatal thyrotropin-releasing hormone (ACTOBAT) for prevention of neonatal respiratory disease, *Lancet* 345:877, 1995.

328. **Wisner KL, Stowe ZN,** Psychobiology of postpartum mood disorders, *Seminars Reprod Endocrinol* 15:77, 1997.

329. **Magiakou M-A, Mastorakos G, Rabin D, Dubbert B, Gold PW, Chrousos GP,** Hypothalamic corticotropin-releasing hormone suppression during the postpartum period: implications for the increase in psychiatric manifestations at this time, *J Clin Endocrinol Metab* 81:1912, 1996.

330. **Patel FA, Clifton VL, Chwalisz K, Challis JRG,** Steroid regulation of prostaglandin dehydrogenase activity and expression in human term placenta and chorio-decidua in relation to labor, *J Clin Endocrinol Metab* 84:291, 1999.

Part II

Clinical Endocrinology

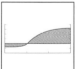

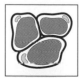

9 Normal and Abnormal Sexual Development

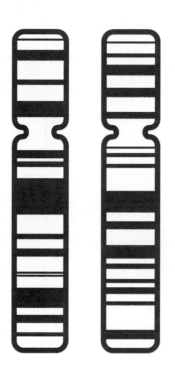

Abnormalities of sexual differentiation are seen infrequently in an individual clinician's practice. There are, however, few practitioners who have not been challenged at least once by a newborn with ambiguous genitalia or by a young woman with primary amenorrhea on a genetic basis. The categorization of the various syndromes in this area has been confusing, requiring constant reference to multiple textbooks, and dependence upon memory of eponym-laden, seemingly endless lists of syndromes. Happily, this "catalogue" state of affairs has changed; major advances in reproductive science have yielded clarification and consolidation. As a result, an informed basis for clinical practice has emerged and is readily applicable.

This chapter will present classification of the major problems and our clinical approach to diagnosis. Normal sexual differentiation will be considered in order to provide a basis of understanding for the various types of abnormal development. This is followed by a section on the diagnosis and management of ambiguous genitalia. Some subjects are discussed in other chapters, but brief descriptions will be repeated here in order to present a complete picture. It will be seen that analysis of phenotypic ambiguity follows a fundamental, pervasive theme: too little androgen effect in males, too much androgen effect in females. Whereas androgen biologic "availability" may be excessive in females because of abnormally high levels of intake or production, reduced androgen effects in males can be the result of defects in synthesis, peripheral and target organ conversion, abnormalities in androgen receptor or receptor-DNA interactions, as well as defective gonadal development and function.

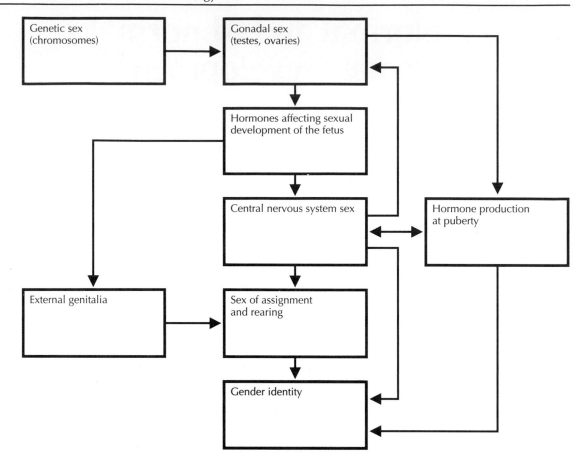

Normal Sexual Differentiation

The gender identity of a person (whether an individual identifies as a male or a female) is the end result of genetic, hormonal, and morphologic sex as influenced by the environment of the individual. It includes all behavior with any sexual connotation, such as body gestures and mannerisms, habits of speech, recreational preferences, and content of dreams. Sexual expression, both homosexual and heterosexual, can be regarded as the result of all influences on the individual, both prenatal and postnatal. Specifically, gender identity is the result of the following determinants: genetic sex, gonadal sex, the internal genitalia, the external genitalia, the secondary sexual characteristics that appear at puberty, and the role assigned by society in response to all of these developmental manifestations of sex.

Prenatally, sexual differentiation follows a specific sequence of events. First is the establishment of the genetic sex. Second, under the control of the genetic sex the gonads differentiate, determining the hormonal environment of the embryo, the differentiation of internal duct systems, and the formation of the external genitalia. It has become apparent that the embryonic brain is also sexually differentiated, perhaps via a control mechanism very similar to that which determines the sexual development of the external genitalia. The inductive influences of hormones on the central nervous system may have an effect on the patterns of hormone secretion and sexual behavior in the adult.[1-6]

Gonadal Differentiation

In human embryos, the gonads begin development during the 5th week of gestation as protuberances overlying the mesonephric ducts. The migration of primordial germ cells into these gonadal ridges occurs between weeks 4 and 6 of gestation. Although germ cells do not induce gonadal development, if the germ cells fail to arrive, gonads do not develop and only the fibrous streak

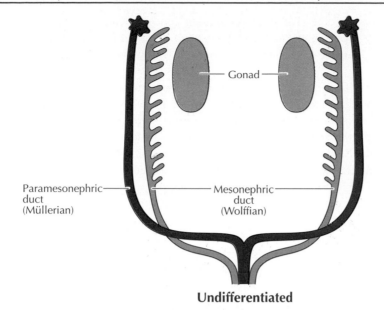

Undifferentiated

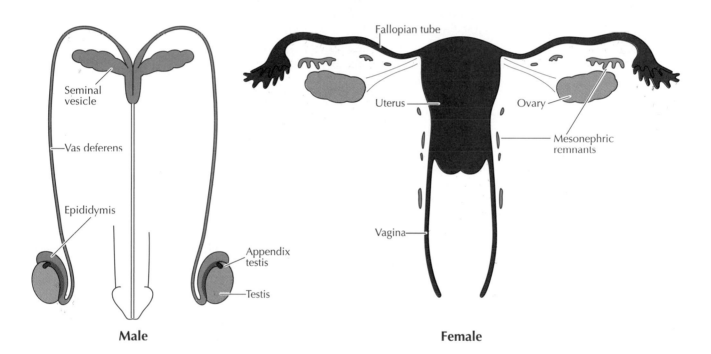

Male

Female

of gonadal agenesis will exist (Chapter 3). At 6 weeks of gestation (4 weeks after ovulation) the gonads are indifferent but bipotential, possessing both cortical and medullary areas, and are capable of differentiation into either testes or ovaries. They are composed of germ cells, special epithelia (potential granulosa/Sertoli cells), mesenchyme (potential theca/Leydig cells), and the mesonephric duct system. Wolffian and müllerian ducts exist side by side; external genitalia are undifferentiated.[7] Subsequent sexual differentiation requires direction by various genes, with a single gene determinant on the Y chromosome (testes determining factor — TDF) necessary for testicular differentiation, beginning at 6–7 weeks gestation.[8]

The distal ends of the short arms of the X and Y chromosomes are called the pseudoautosomal regions because during meiosis the homologous distal short arms of the X and Y chromosomes pair, and interchange of genetic material occurs as in autosomes. The genes in the pseudoautosomal regions are doubly present in both sexes, and therefore escape X inactivation. Gene deletions in this area of the X chromosome (Xp22.3) are associated with various conditions, known as contiguous gene syndromes: short stature, mental retardation, X-linked ichthyosis,

Kallmann's syndrome. The testes-determing gene is located on the distal short arm of the Y, immediately adjacent to the pseudoautosomal region. Loss of the TDF gene causes gonadal dysgenesis. Transfer of the TDF gene to the X results in an XX male.

Since the identification of the Y chromosome's importance to male differentiation over 4 decades ago, three proteins have been suggested as the Y-encoded, gene expressed, testes determining factor. The first was the H-Y histocompatibility antigen and the second, ZFY (a zinc finger protein). Both were abandoned because of inconsistencies of expression in various cell types (in XX males and XY females), as well as absent expression in indisputable males with testes. More recently, SRY (Sex determining Region Y) has been isolated, almost certainly the true sex-determining region on the short arm of the Y chromosome, the only gene on the Y chromosome required for sex determination.[9]

SRY is a single copy gene located in the smallest Y chromosome region capable of sex reversal. It is expressed in the genital ridge only during the appropriate time of embryonic development when testicular cords form; it is deleted or mutated in cases of human XY females, and present in 46,XX males, and it can sex-reverse XX mice into males.[10–12] The 204 amino acid protein product contains an 80 amino acid domain with a motif shared by a recognized family of transcription factors (the high mobility group) that bind to DNA and regulate gene transcription. Investigations of the DNA binding properties of the SRY high mobility group (HMG) box in the promoter regions of P450 aromatase (conversion of testosterone to estradiol which is down-regulated in the male embryo) and anti-müllerian hormone (responsible for regression of the müllerian ducts) support the hypothesis that SRY directly controls male development through sequence-specific regulation of target genes.[13]

SRY participation in morphogenesis leading to a testis from the bipotential genital ridge is a model "genetic switch" between alternative inherent programs. Whereas testes formation is an active event, female sex determination is the default pathway occurring if SRY is absent or deficient. Genes other than SRY are also required for proper gonadogenesis.[14, 15] In the human, autosomal genes are essential for gonadal development. These autosomal genes regulate migration of the germ cells and coding of the steroidogenic enzymes. The formation of the testicle precedes any other sexual development in time, and a functionally active testis controls subsequent sexual development, therefore SRY presumably controls these autosomal genes. Thus, testicular hormones activate or repress genes to direct development away from an otherwise predetermined course of female differentiation.

Steroidogenic factor-1 (SF-1) and DAX-1 (named for the location of its gene on the X chromosome) are nuclear receptors for which specific ligands have not been identified ("orphan receptors"). SF-1 influences the expression of genes that encode steroidogenic enzymes, and when genetic expression of SF-1 is disrupted in mice, gonads and adrenal glands fail to develop.[16, 17] SF-1 is also believed to be involved in the production of anti-müllerian hormone.[18] Mutations in the DAX-1 gene result in adrenal hypoplasia, and DAX-1 is believed to work with SF-1 in regulating development and function of steroid-producing tissues.[19]

The *WT1* gene is named after the Wilms' tumor nephroblastoma because it is one of the genes on chromosome 11 deleted in patients with this tumor. Mutant mice lacking *WT1* fail to develop kidneys and gonads. *WT1* mutations, however, could not be detected in 25 patients with a congenital absence of the uterus and vagina, indicating that *WT1* may be necessary for normal renal and gonadal development, but not for early müllerian duct development.[20]

Testicular differentiation begins at 6–7 weeks; first with Sertoli cells that aggregate to form spermatogenic cords, then seminiferous tubules, followed by Leydig cell formation a week later. Human chorionic gonadotropin (HCG) stimulation produces Leydig cell hypertrophy, and peak fetal testosterone levels are seen at 15–18 weeks.[14] It is very probable, but not conclusively proven, that HCG stimulates steroidogenesis in the early fetal testes, so that androgen production will ensue and masculine differentiation can be accomplished.[21]

In an XX individual, without the active influence of a Y chromosome, the bipotential gonad develops into an ovary about 2 weeks later than testicular development. The cortical zone develops and contains the germ cells, while the medullary portion regresses with its remnant being the rete ovarii, a compressed nest of tubules and Leydig cells in the hilus of the ovary. The germ cells proliferate by mitosis, reaching a peak of 5–7 million by 20 weeks. By 20 weeks, the fetal ovary achieves mature compartmentalization with primordial follicles containing oocytes, initial evidence of follicle maturation and atresia, and an incipient stroma. Degeneration (atresia) begins even earlier, and by birth, approximately 1–2 million germ cells remain. These have become surrounded by a layer of follicular cells, forming primordial follicles with oocytes that have entered the first meiotic division. Meiosis is arrested in the prophase of the first meiotic division until reactivation of follicular growth that may not occur until years later. Excessively rapid atresia (germ cell attrition) in gonadal dysgenesis (45,X) accounts for the streak gonad seen in these cases.[22] A complete 46,XX chromosomal complement is necessary for normal ovarian development.[23] The second X chromosome, therefore, contains elements essential for ovarian development and maintenance.

Duct System Differentiation

Caspar Wolff described the mesonephros in 1759 in his doctoral dissertation when he was 26 years old.[24] The paired structures of the mesonephros of the early vertebrate embryo were named wolffian bodies by the 19th century embryologist, Rathke, in recognition of Wolff's initial discovery and description. Johannes Müller, a German physiologist with a prodigious academic output, described the embryology of the genitalia in 1830. The paramesonephric ducts received his name, not because of his original contributions, but because of his ability to synthesize current knowledge in his effective writings. His physiology text was a standard in many European countries.

Renal development goes through 3 stages: pronephric, mesonephric, and metanephric. The mesonephric ducts remain for development as internal genitalia. At this stage the mesonephric ducts are called the wolffian ducts. The paired paramesonephric ducts are the müllerian ducts. The wolffian and müllerian ducts are discrete primordia which temporarily coexist in all embryos during the ambisexual period of development (up to 8 weeks). Thereafter, one type of duct system persists normally and gives rise to special ducts and glands, whereas the other disappears during the 3rd fetal month, except for nonfunctional vestiges.

Hormonal control of mammalian somatic sex differentiation was established by the classic experiments of Alfred Jost.[25] In Jost's landmark studies, the active role of male determining factors was defined as the directing feature of sex differentiation. This principle applies not only to the internal ducts but to the gonad, external genitalia, and perhaps even the brain. The critical factors in determining which of the duct structures stabilize or regress are the secretions from the testes: testosterone and anti-müllerian hormone (AMH), also known as müllerian inhibiting substance or müllerian inhibiting factor.

AMH is a member of the transforming growth factor-β family of glycoprotein differentiation factors that includes inhibin and activin.[26, 27] The gene for AMH has been mapped to the short arm of chromosome 19, and the AMH receptor gene is on chromosome 12. AMH is synthesized by Sertoli cells (activated by SRY) soon after testicular differentiation and is responsible for the ipsilateral regression of the müllerian ducts by 8 weeks, before the emergence of testosterone and stimulation of the wolffian ducts.[28] Despite its presence in serum up to puberty, lack of regression of the uterus and tubes is the only consistent expression of AMH gene mutations. Knockout mice for AMH develop normal testes and ovaries.[29] In the absence of AMH, the fetus will develop fallopian tubes, uterus, and upper vagina from the paramesonephric ducts (the müllerian ducts). *This development requires the prior appearance of the mesonephric ducts, and for this reason, abnormalities in the renal system are associated with abnormalities in development of the tubes, uterus, and upper vagina.*

AMH has extra müllerian functions. AMH exerts an inhibitory effect on oocyte meiosis, plays a role in the descent of the testes, and inhibits surfactant accumulation in the lungs.[30] Proteolytic cleavage of AMH produces fragments which have the ability to inhibit growth of various tumors (a potential therapeutic application). Testicular descent occurs in stages. Transabdominal movement of the testes is the result of rapid gubernacular growth, apparently under AMH control. Movement through the inguinal canal is mediated by androgens.

AMH, secreted by the Sertoli cells, is detectable in the serum of males during infancy, childhood, adolescence, and adulthood (with a decline to barely detectable levels after puberty). In contrast, AMH, secreted by granulosa cells, is not measurable until puberty in females. This difference allows serum measurement to be a sensitive marker for the presence of testicular tissue in intersex anomalies.[31] After puberty, testosterone, with an added contribution from meiotic germ cells, suppresses AMH secretion in males, and, therefore, individuals with the androgen insensitivity syndrome (androgen receptor defects) have very high AMH levels after puberty.[32] The failure of testosterone to suppress AMH secretion during fetal and newborn life is explained by the absence of the androgen receptor in Sertoli cells until later in life.

Testosterone is secreted by the fetal testes soon after Leydig cell formation (at 8 weeks) and rapidly rises to peak concentrations at 15–18 weeks. This testosterone secretion stimulates development of the wolffian duct system into epididymis, vas deferens, and seminal vesicles. Testosterone levels in the male fetus correlate with Leydig cell development, overall gonadal weight, 3β-hydroxysteroid dehydrogenase activity, and chorionic gonadotropin (HCG) concentrations. As HCG declines (approximately 20 weeks) the fetal pituitary luteinizing hormone (LH) assumes control of Leydig cell testosterone secretion; anencephalics and other forms of congenital hypopituitarism display diminished androgen effects on internal and external genitalia.

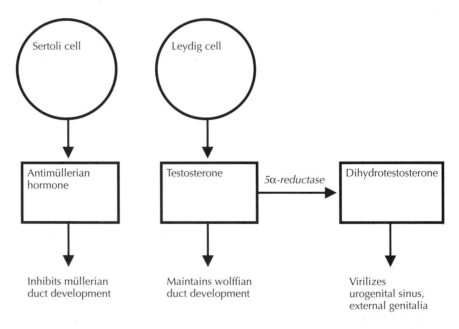

The wolffian ducts receive testosterone signals directly from nearby Leydig cells as well as the general fetal circulation. This local paracrine effect is essential to the stimulation of ipsilateral differentiation into the epididymis, vas deferens, and seminal vesicles. Duct system differentiation will proceed, therefore, according to the nature of the adjacent gonad. The wolffian ducts do not form dihydrotestosterone, so the direct high concentration is crucial for normal development.[33] Because of this local paracrine action, wolffian development cannot be stimulated in females exposed to adrenal or exogenous androgens.

The internal genitalia possess the intrinsic tendency to feminize. In the absence of a Y chromosome and a functional testis, the lack of AMH allows retention of the müllerian system and development of fallopian tubes, uterus, and upper vagina. In the absence of testosterone, the wolffian system regresses. In the presence of a normal ovary or the absence of any gonad, müllerian duct development takes place. These classic roles for the presence and absence of testosterone are undisputed; however, estrogen may make a contribution in this process. Knockout mice for the estrogen receptor-α have a marked retention of wolffian tubules, indicating that estrogen plays a role in the degeneration of the wolffian system.[34]

External Genitalia Differentiation

In the bipotential state (6th gestational week), the external genitalia consist of a genital tubercle, a urogenital sinus, and two lateral labioscrotal swellings. Unlike the internal genitalia where both duct systems initially coexist, the external genitalia are neutral primordia able to develop into either male or female structures depending on gonadal steroid hormone signals. Normally, this differentiation is under the active influence of androgen from the Leydig cells of the testis. The genital tubercle forms the penis, labioscrotal folds fuse to form a scrotum, and folds of the urogenital sinus form the penile urethra. The testis begins androgen secretion by 8–9 weeks; masculinization of the external genitalia is manifest 1 week later and is completed by 14 weeks. To achieve this morphologic change, external genitalia target tissue cells must convert testosterone to dihydrotestosterone (DHT) by the intracellular enzyme 5α-reductase. In the male, DHT mediates the following androgen events: temporal hairline recession, growth of facial and body hair, development of acne, and development of the external genitalia and prostate.

Bipotential Stage

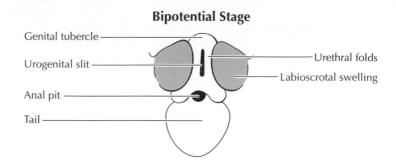

Female   **Male**

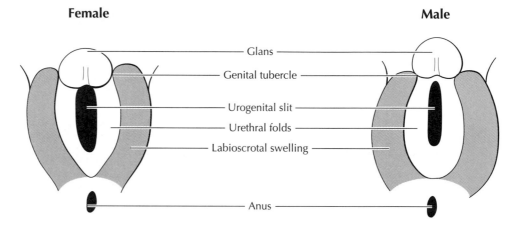

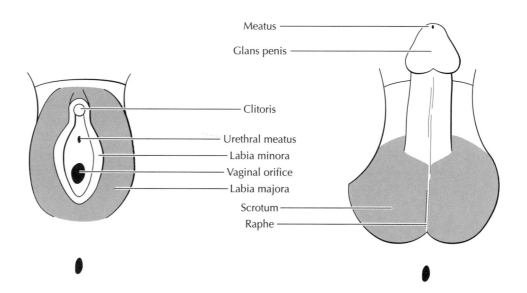

In the absence of this androgen effect (the absence of a Y chromosome, the presence of an ovary, the absence of a gonad, abnormalities in androgen receptor or postreceptor events, or defects of the 5α-reductase enzyme), the folds of the urogenital sinus remain open, forming the labia minora, the labioscrotal folds form the labia majora, the genital tubercle forms the clitoris, and the urogenital sinus differentiates into the vagina and the urethra. Thus, the lower vagina is formed as part of the external genitalia.

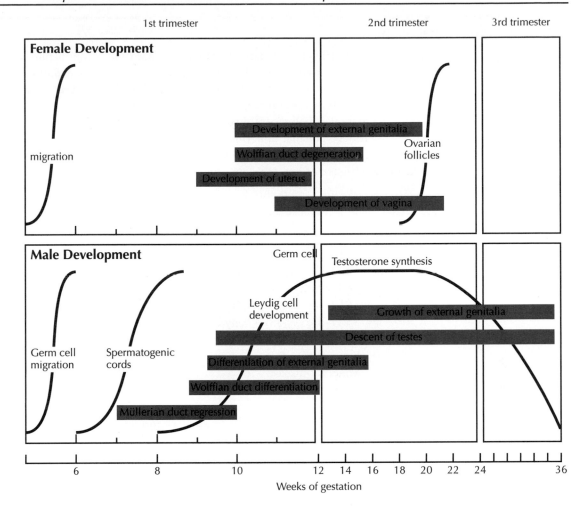

Exposure to androgens at critical time periods leads to variable masculinization. Androgen exposure at 9–14 weeks superimposes variable external ambiguity on the basic female phenotype (clitoral hypertrophy, hypospadias, scrotalization of nonfused labia). By the same token, incompletely masculinized genitalia will result if sufficient local androgen concentration or activity is not achieved by the 12th week in the male. Because of shared common tissue origin, male-female external genital structural ambiguities reflect abnormal androgen impact: males too little, females too much.

Central Nervous System Differentiation

At the same time the presence or absence of androgens is playing a critical role in genitalia development, the neuroendocrine mechanism of the central nervous system is also being influenced. Androgens present in sufficient amounts during the appropriate critical stage of development may program the central nervous system (CNS) to induce the potential for male sexual behavior.[3, 5, 6, 35–37] Experimental and analytical evidence suggests that a behavioral effect can be traced to this early androgen influence. Inappropriate fetal hormonal programming may contribute, therefore, to the spectrum of psychosexual behavior seen in humans. In addition, gender role is heavily influenced by assignment of sex of rearing followed by social interaction based upon genital appearance and the development of secondary sexual characteristics.

Abnormal Sexual Differentiation

The standard classification of individuals with intersexuality (hermaphroditism) proceeds according to gonadal morphology. In this terminology, a **true hermaphrodite** possesses both ovarian and testicular tissue. A **male pseudohermaphrodite** has testes, but external and sometimes internal genitalia take on female phenotypic aspects. A **female pseudohermaphrodite** has ovaries, but genital development displays masculine characteristics. These classifications are modified to reflect gonadal abnormalities due to abnormal sex chromosome constitution or abnormalities of phenotype attributable to an inappropriate fetal hormone environment. Hypospadias in the absence of any other deformity is not included in this classification.

Disorders of Fetal Endocrinology

Masculinized females (female pseudohermaphroditism)
Congenital adrenal hyperplasia
21-Hydroxylase (P450c21) deficiency
11β-Hydroxylase (P450c11β) deficiency
3β-Hydroxysteroid dehydrogenase deficiency
Elevated androgens in the maternal circulation
Drug intake
Maternal disease
Aromatase (P450arom) deficiency

Incompletely masculinized males (male pseudohermaphroditism)
Androgen insensitivity syndromes
5α-Reductase deficiency
Testosterone biosynthesis defects
3β-Hydroxysteroid dehydrogenase deficiency
17α-Hydroxylase (P450c17) deficiency
17β-Hydroxysteroid dehydrogenase deficiency
Gonadotropin resistant testes
Anti-müllerian hormone deficiency

Disorders of Gonadal Development

Male pseudohermaphroditism
Primary gonadal defect — Swyer syndrome
Anorchia

True hermaphroditism

Gonadal dysgenesis
Turner syndrome
Mosaicism
Normal karyotype — Noonan syndrome

Masculinized Females

Masculinized females possess ovaries and are female by genetic sex (XX), but the external genitalia are not those of a normal female. Of all infants with ambiguous genitalia, 40–45% have adrenal hyperplasia. Rarer causes of female pseudohermaphroditism are excess maternal androgen caused by drug ingestion, tumor secretion, or possibly aromatase deficiency.

Congenital Adrenal Hyperplasia (the Adrenogenital Syndrome)

Congenital adrenal hyperplasia in females is characterized by masculinized external genitalia, and is diagnosed by demonstrating excessive androgen production by the adrenal cortex, caused by either tumor or hyperplasia.[38–40] The syndrome may appear in utero or develop postnatally.

Depending on the time of onset, quantity available, and duration of exposure, the presence of excessive androgens is manifested by varying degrees of fusion of the labioscrotal folds, clitoral enlargement, and anatomical changes of the urethra and vagina. Generally, the urethra and vagina share a urogenital sinus formed by the fusion of labial folds. This sinus opens at the base of the clitoris, which is usually enlarged. The degree of urogenital sinus deformity is related to the timing in prenatal development of the onset of masculinizing androgen effect. Because there is no anomalous secretion of anti-müllerian hormone in females with congenital adrenal hyperplasia, the fallopian tubes, uterus, and upper vagina develop normally. Since wolffian duct development and maintenance depend on high local androgen levels provided by the male gonad, the excessive androgens of adrenal hyperplasia origin cannot stimulate this process, and no wolffian development is retained. The external genitalia on the other hand can be substantially altered by adrenal hyperplasia. After the 10th week, when the vagina and urethra have separated, the emerging excess androgen effect may be limited to clitoral hypertrophy. High androgen levels earlier than the 12th week of fetal age, however, can cause progressive fusion of the labia, formation of a urogenital sinus, and even variable closure of the urethra along the phallus (hypospadias). The absence of palpable testes may be the only clinical marker suggesting female pseudohermaphroditism.

Excessive adrenal activity does not affect internal genitalia differentiation. This is because the internal genitalia are completely formed by the 10th week of gestation, whereas the adrenal cortex does not reach a level of significant function until 10–12 weeks.

Because the female external genitalia phenotype is not completed until 20 weeks of fetal age, early androgen excess (10–12 weeks gestation) may fully masculinize, whereas late (18–20 weeks gestation) androgen may create limited ambiguity of the basically female appearance of the urogenital sinus and genital folds. The size of the clitoris depends on the quantity rather than timing of androgen excess. Cases of incorrect sex assignment in the female are due to the similarity between these external genitalia and hypospadias and bilateral cryptorchidism in a male infant.

If untreated, the female with adrenal hyperplasia will develop signs of progressive virilization postnatally. Pubic hair will appear by age 2–4, followed by axillary hair, then body hair and beard. Bone age is advanced by age 2, and because of early epiphyseal closure, height in childhood is achieved at the expense of shortened stature in adulthood. Progressive masculinization continues with the development of the male habitus, acne, deepened voice, and primary amenorrhea and infertility.

In addition to sexual changes, patients can present with metabolic disorders such as salt-wasting, hypertension, or rarely, hypoglycemia. An electrolyte imbalance of the salt-losing type is usually apparent within a few days of birth and occurs in approximately two-thirds of patients with virilizing adrenal hyperplasia. A salt-losing crisis usually begins 5–15 days after birth. Beginning with a refusal to feed, failure to thrive, apathy, and vomiting, the infant goes on to an Addisonian-like crisis with hyponatremia, hyperkalemia, and acidosis. Rapid diagnosis and treatment are necessary to save these infants. Less frequent is hypertension, which occurs in approximately 5% of patients with virilizing adrenal hyperplasia.

Virilizing adrenal hyperplasia is the result of an inherited abnormality of steroid biosynthesis that results in an inability to synthesize glucocorticoids. The hypothalamic-pituitary axis reacts to the low level of cortisol by elevated ACTH secretion in a homeostatic response to achieve normal levels of cortisol production. This stimulation induces a hyperplastic adrenal cortex that produces androgens as well as corticoid precursors in abnormal quantities. Therefore, one can see a well-compensated infant who has achieved normal cortisol levels but at the expense of extensive masculinization. In summary, the clinical picture resulting from a specific enzyme deficiency is due to the effects of both the inadequate production of cortisol/aldosterone and excess accumulation of precursors, with diversion into biosynthetic pathways yielding androgens.

The most common enzymatic defects are the 21-hydroxylase (P450c21), the 11β-hydroxylase (P450c11), and the 3β-hydroxysteroid dehydrogenase types. Very rarely, blocked synthesis of cortisol can be due to a defect in P450c17.

Enzyme Defect in Adrenal Only: Deficient 21-Hydroxylase (P450c21). The 21-hydroxylase block is the most common form of congenital adrenal hyperplasia (95% of cases), the most frequent cause of sexual ambiguity, and the most frequent endocrine cause of neonatal death. With severe uncompensated blocks of this type, salt-wasting and shock accompany significant virilization. In less severe variations, when sufficient cortisol can be produced, virilization due to excess androgen is still present in utero, at birth, or later in life. Three different clinical forms are recognized representing the spectrum of severity: the salt-wasting, the simple virilizing, and the nonclassical (previously known as the late-onset, attenuated, or acquired adrenal hyperplasia). The first and second are associated with female pseudohermaphroditism at birth, while the third usually becomes apparent at adolescence or beyond and causes hirsutism, menstrual irregularities, and infertility.

Developments in molecular biology and genetics have greatly expanded our understanding of this condition.[41]

1. The disorder is inherited as a monogenic autosomal recessive trait.

2. Two 21-hydroxylase genes exist, designated CYP21A and CYP21B, located on chromosome 6, in tandem duplication with the genes encoding the fourth component of complement. Only CYP21B is active in adrenal steroidogenesis; CYP21A is not involved (a pseudogene, also known as CYP21P, because it is inactive).

3. A variety of mutations affecting CYP21B lead to 21-hydroxylase deficiency, but 85% are gene conversions. Most patients are compound heterozygotes, having a different genetic lesion on each copy of chromosome 6, one from each parent. The severity of the condition is determined by the activity of the least affected allele.

The 21-hydroxylase genes are located in the midst of the human leukocyte antigen (HLA) complex on the short arm of chromosome 6. By combined HLA genotyping and ACTH stimulation testing (see 17-OHP nomogram in Chapter 13) of families that contained patients with nonclassical and classical disease, a concept of variations in 21-hydroxylase activity evolved.[42, 43] Salt-wasting, simple virilizing, and nonclassical clinical manifestations, respectively, are due to the most, less, and the least deficiency of 21-hydroxylase. Some family members exhibit abnormal responses to ACTH, and, although some of these have clinical evidence of androgen excess, others are entirely normal and represent a "cryptic" form of 21-hydroxylase deficiency. Finally, heterozygotes for either the mild or severe deficiency exhibit the mildest enzyme deficiency and are clinically asymptomatic.

Enzyme Defect in Adrenal Only: Deficient 11β-Hydroxylase (P450c11). The final step in cortisol synthesis is blocked in this condition. In classic 11β-hydroxylase deficiency, 11-deoxycortisol is not converted to cortisol. Accumulated precursors are shunted into androgen biosynthesis with virilization similar to that seen with 21-hydroxylase deficiency. However, a parallel defect also exists so that deoxycorticosterone (DOC) is not converted to corticosterone. This pathway is used in the zona glomerulosa to synthesize aldosterone, and the degree to which aldosterone levels are affected lends clinical heterogeneity to the classic presentation of 11β-hydroxylase deficiency (virilization, hypertension, volume overload). About 5–8% of cases of

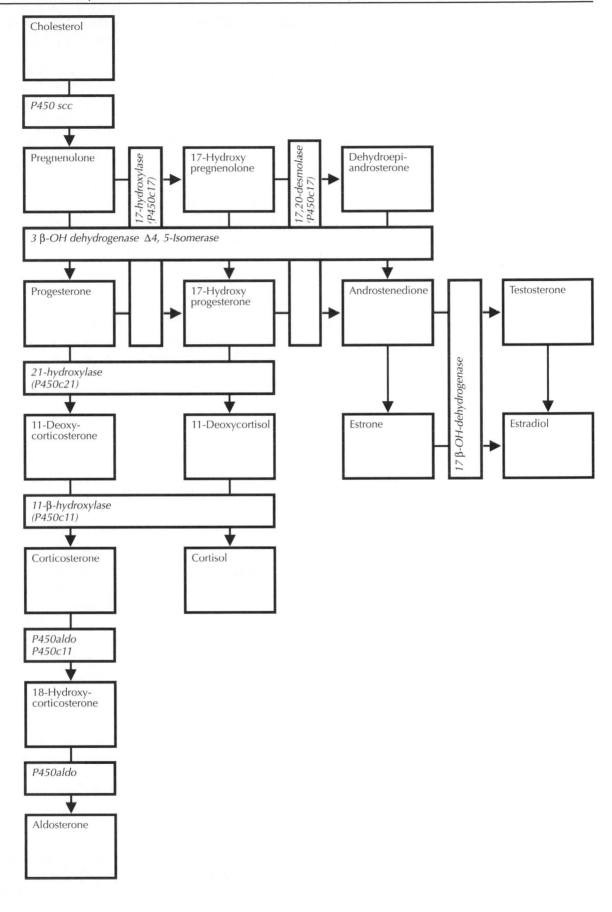

congenital adrenal hyperplasia are due to 11β-hydroxylase deficiency, about 1 in 100,000 births, with a higher incidence in Jewish people who originated in Morocco.[44]

Usually as a result of 11β-hydroxylase deficiency, metabolically active precursors of corticosterone and cortisol add to excess androgen synthesis as further liabilities of ACTH-induced hyperplasia. Hypertension and hypokalemic alkalosis are induced by elevated deoxycorticosterone with reduced renin and aldosterone. Virilization is caused by androgens of the "deoxy" type (dehydroepiandrosterone, dehydroepiandrosterone sulfate, and androstenedione). The diagnosis is confirmed by high plasma deoxycorticosterone and compound S (11-deoxycortisol) levels.

About two-thirds of untreated patients with 11β-hydroxylase deficiency become hypertensive, usually of mild to moderate degree (150/90 mm Hg) and only after several years of life. A mild nonclassic form of 11β-hydroxylase deficiency, as in 21-hydroxylase defects, has also been documented; it is characterized by mild biochemical abnormalities, and the patients are only slightly virilized and rarely hypertensive.

Contrary to 21-hydroxylase deficiency, the 11β-hydroxylase deficiency locus is remote from the HLA complex. The gene for the enzyme is on the long arm of chromosome 8, and the deficiency is inherited in autosomal recessive fashion.[45] Actually there are two isozymes with 11β-hydroxylase activity, encoded by two genes on chromosome 8.[44] One, CYP11B1 or P450c11, is the enzyme classically referred to as 11β-hydroxylase and regulated by ACTH. The other, CYP11B2 or P450c18 (or P450aldo), has been called aldosterone synthase and is regulated by angiotensin II. P450c18 has strong 11β-hydroxylase activity, but also hydroxylates and oxidizes at the C-18 position. Deficiency in 11β-hydroxylase results from mutations in P450c11 (CYP11B1).[44]

Enzyme Defects in Adrenal and Ovary: Deficient 3β-Hydroxysteroid Dehydrogenase.
Lack of this essential step in the formation of all biologically active steroids affects both the adrenal cortex and the ovary and is also inherited in autosomal recessive fashion. Thus, there is decreased synthesis of glucocorticoids, mineralocorticoids, androgens, and estrogens. These infants are severely ill at birth and rarely survive. The external genitalia ambiguity results from the massive increase in dehydroepiandrosterone that is androgenic when available in excess, and also can be utilized to form more potent androgens in peripheral tissues. Thus, females may be slightly virilized and males incompletely masculinized with a variable degree of hypospadias. The spectrum of clinical phenotypes also includes both salt wasting and non-salt wasting forms. The degree of the enzyme defect cannot be extrapolated from the degree of external genitalia ambiguity. As in 21-hydroxylase deficiency, milder nonclassic cases may occur with mild hirsutism and elevated dehydroepiandrosterone and dehydroepiandrosterone sulfate being the only distinguishing features. Some argue that late-onset 3β-hydroxysteroid dehydrogenase deficiency is encountered more frequently than 21-hydroxylase deficiency.[46] However, although an exaggerated 17α-hydroxypregnenolone response to ACTH stimulation is common in women with hyperandrogenism, the response is consistent with adrenal hyperactivity and not an enzyme deficiency.[47] Furthermore, molecular studies fail to find mutations in the genes for the two 3β-hydroxysteroid dehydrogenase enzymes in patients with apparent mild to moderate 3β-hydroxysteroid dehydrogenase deficiency.[48, 49]

Enzyme Defect in Adrenal and Ovary: Deficient 17α-Hydroxylase (P450c17).
With block of the 17α-hydroxylase enzyme (P450c17), synthesis of cortisol, androgens, and estrogens is curtailed. Only the non-17-hydroxylated corticoids, deoxycorticosterone and corticosterone, are formed.[50] The molecular basis for this enzyme deficiency is due to a variety of mutations which result in multiple base deletions and duplications in the CYP17 gene on chromosome 10q24–25.[51, 52] The resulting syndrome is composed of hypertension (due to hypernatremia and hypervolemia), hypokalemia, infantile female external genitalia, which do not mature at puberty, and primary amenorrhea with elevated follicle-stimulating hormone (FSH) and luteinizing hormone (LH). Genital ambiguity is a problem only in male infants.

Epidemiology

Only the 21-hydroxylase deficiency has been studied extensively, in part because it is not only the most frequent cause of genital ambiguity and congenital adrenal hyperplasia but also because of the high prevalence of the nonclassical, late onset forms of the disease. Within families, the clinical picture is uniform, the type of syndrome (simple, salt-wasting, hypertensive) is usually, but not always, the same in affected siblings. The genetic defect in virilizing adrenal hyperplasia is an autosomal recessive gene. The ratio in offspring of unaffected parents is one affected to three nonaffected individuals. Treated patients have a 1:100 to 1:200 chance of producing an affected infant. Males and females are at equal risk. The classic form is a relatively common inborn error of metabolism. One out of every 100 Caucasians is likely to be a genetic carrier of the classic type, and neonatal screening tests indicate an incidence of 1 in 14,000 births. The highest frequency for congenital adrenal hyperplasia is in Alaskan Yupik Eskimos.

For the nonclassical types, frequency rates established by the usual methodology (neonatal screening, case surveys) are likely to markedly underestimate what may be one of the most common autosomal recessive disorders in humans. Extrapolations from ACTH testing suggest the following frequency:[53]

	Nonclassical Disease	Heterozygous Carrier
Eastern European Jews	1 in 30	1 in 3
Hispanics	1 in 40	1 in 4
Slavs	1 in 50	1 in 5
Italians	1 in 333	1 in 9
Others	1 in 1000	1 in 14

Prenatal Diagnosis

The diagnosis of congenital adrenal hyperplasia due to 21-hydroxylase deficiency can be obtained prenatally by demonstrating elevated levels of 17-hydroxyprogesterone (17-OHP), 21-deoxycortisol, and androstenedione in the amniotic fluid. 17-OHP may be elevated only in the salt-losing form of adrenal hyperplasia, but androstenedione is usually increased with all forms. The 11β-hydroxylase deficiency is associated with elevated levels of 11-deoxycortisol in amniotic fluid and tetrahydro-11-deoxycortisol in maternal urine.[54] Because amniotic fluid steroids may be within the normal range with less severe deficiencies, hormonal measurements have been replaced by molecular genetic diagnosis.

Prenatal diagnosis of the 21-hydroxylase deficiency by chorion villus biopsy utilizing DNA probes offers the timely options of termination or in utero therapy.[55] With chorion villus biopsy, diagnosis can be made and therapy instituted before the critical period of fetal genital differentiation with avoidance of genital ambiguity in affected female fetuses. In addition, masculinization of the fetal brain can be avoided which might have an impact on gender identity and adult sexual behavior.[2, 4, 5] Despite the fact that prenatal diagnosis is not 100% accurate, prenatal treatment beginning at 4–5 weeks gestation has been administered with dexamethasone in fetuses at risk for 21-hydroxylase deficiency.[56–60] Using multiple daily doses of dexamethasone (total no greater than 1.5 mg/day), complete prevention has been achieved in some newborns and diminished virilization in others. No congenital malformations or low birth weight or height have resulted from pregnancy-long cortisol derivative therapy. However, this treatment is associated with significant maternal side effects, such as severe striae with permanent scarring,

Prenatal Treatment and Diagnosis of 21-Hydroxylase Deficiency

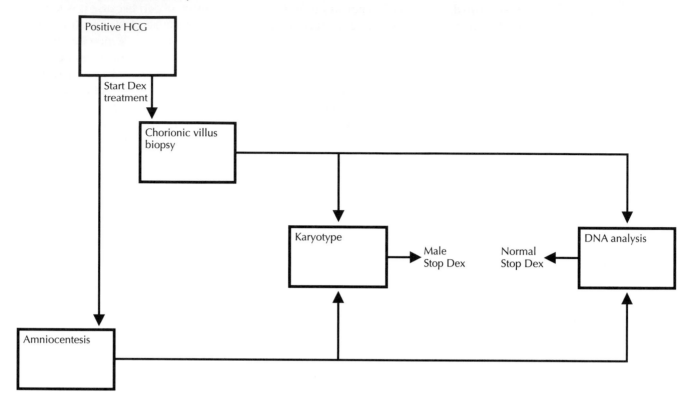

hyperglycemia, hypertension, gastrointestinal symptoms, and emotional lability.[61] A reduction in dosage during the second half of pregnancy is recommended; dosage can be titered by maintaining the maternal serum estriol levels in the normal range.

Given that only one in four siblings is at risk and one-half will be males (who do not suffer genital ambiguity from the excess androgen associated with 21-hydroxylase deficiency) then only 1 of 8 fetuses requires treatment. Therefore 7 of 8 fetuses will be exposed to very high glucocorticoid doses unnecessarily. Until the long-term effects and safety of this therapy are established, treatment should be governed by appropriate research-type institutional protocols.

Diagnosis of Adrenal Hyperplasia

For years the demonstration of a metabolic defect and its location depended upon the study of urinary steroid excretion. Today, the immunoassay of blood 17-hydroxyprogesterone (17-OHP) has become the primary assessment for the diagnosis and management of congenital adrenal hyperplasia. With the 21-hydroxylase and 11β-hydroxylase deficiencies, the 17-OHP level will be 50–400-fold above normal. In addition, plasma renin activity is measured to assess the degree of mineralocorticoid deficiency.

During delivery of normal infants, the concentration of 17-OHP is elevated in cord blood (1000–3000 ng/dL), but it rapidly decreases to 100–200 ng/dL after 24 hours. A delay in measurement gains accuracy. In contrast to 17-ketosteroids in the urine where the delay must be several days, with 17-OHP the delay need be only a day or two. In affected infants, 17-OHP ranges from 3000 to 40,000 ng/dL. Measurement of 17-OHP is the basis for the newborn screening programs currently in place in many countries and some states in the U.S. In Texas, the screening program detected classic congenital adrenal hyperplasia in 1 in 16,000 births, with a ratio of salt-wasting to simple virilizing of 2.7:1.[62]

In adults, 17-OHP must be measured first thing in the morning to avoid later elevations due to the diurnal pattern of ACTH secretion. The baseline 17-OHP level should be less than 200 ng/dL. Levels greater than 200 ng/dL, but less than 800 ng/dL, require ACTH testing (discussed in Chapter 13). Levels over 800 ng/dL are virtually diagnostic of the 21-hydroxylase deficiency. The dehydroepiandrosterone sulfate level is usually normal. The hallmarks of nonclassical adrenal hyperplasia are elevated levels of 17-OHP and a dramatic increase after ACTH stimulation. The elevated levels of 17-OHP are often not impressive (e.g., overlapping with those found in women with polycystic ovaries due to anovulation), and a simple ACTH stimulation test must be utilized. *To distinguish the 21-hydroxylase deficiency from other disorders, all of the following in addition to 17-OHP should be measured at zero and 60 minutes after ACTH stimulation: pregnenolone, 17-hydroxypregnenolone, dehydroepiandrosterone, 11-deoxycortisol, cortisol, and testosterone.*

Of course, in patients with 3β-hydroxysteroid dehydrogenase or 17-hydroxylase blocks, the 17-OHP level will not be elevated. With the 3β-hydroxysteroid dehydrogenase block, the blood levels of DHA and DHA sulfate (DHAS) will be markedly increased. In the 11β-hydroxylase deficiency, in addition to elevated 17-OHP, elevation of 11-deoxycortisol is diagnostic. In this deficiency, plasma renin activity will be low, whereas in 21-hydroxylase and 3β-hydroxysteroid dehydrogenase deficiencies plasma renin activity is elevated in the salt losing forms.

Treatment

Treatment of adrenal hyperplasia is to supply the deficient hormone, cortisol. This decreases ACTH secretion and lowers production of androgenic precursors. The addition of salt-retaining hormone to glucocorticoid therapy has improved the control of the disease. When the plasma renin activity is normalized, ACTH and androgen levels are further decreased, and a decrease in the glucocorticoid dose is also possible. Therefore, the modern management of hormonal control requires the measurement of the blood levels of 17-OHP, androstenedione, testosterone, and plasma renin activity.[38, 39] The drugs of choice are hydrocortisone (cortisol), approximately 10 mg per day, and 9-fluorohydrocortisone, approximately 100 mg/day. This method of treatment and monitoring applies to all forms of adrenal hyperplasia. The standard dose of cortisol is 12–18 mg/m^2 or 3.5–5 mg/m^2 of prednisone, but larger doses given on alternate days (14 mg/m^2 of prednisone, about 20 mg) can maintain adrenal androgen suppression and perhaps achieve better growth and pubertal development, despite higher levels of 17-hydroxyprogesterone.[63] The 17-OHP level should be maintained in the range of 500 to 4000 ng/dL, thereby avoiding both overtreatment and undertreatment. Minor stresses will cause brief elevations of adrenal androgens but usually do not require readjustment of dosage. With major stress, such as surgery, additional hormonal support is necessary.

The surgical treatment of the anatomical abnormalities should be carried out in the first few years of life, when the patient is still too young to remember the procedure and too young to have developed psychological problems centered about the abnormal external genitalia. If clitoridectomy is necessary, the clitoral recession procedure, conserving the glans and its innervation, should be employed. It is important to know that women who undergo total clitoral amputations have no subsequent impairment of erotic responsiveness or capacity for orgasm. Significant vaginal reconstruction, if necessary, is best accomplished after puberty when mature compliance is possible.

Normal reproduction is possible with replacement therapy of the cortisol deficiency. Unfortunately, poor compliance with therapy and less than satisfactory surgical reconstruction of the vagina result in decreased fertility and sexuality.[2] Greater attention to these factors is needed to improve the sexual experience and fertility of these women. Many cases come to cesarean section because normal anatomy of the perineum may be obscured by scar tissue from earlier plastic surgery; therefore, greater blood loss and the risk of a hematoma with a vaginal delivery are significant factors. A masculine pelvis is not expected since the adult form and size of the inlet of the pelvis are assumed largely during the growth spurt in puberty. However, a small pelvis might be anticipated if the bone age is up to age 13–14 when treatment is initiated. Fertility in women with nonclassical adrenal hyperplasia is only slightly reduced, dependent upon the degree of hormonal dysfunction (which is promptly corrected with glucocorticoid therapy).[64] Consistent with the belief that androgens can program sexual behavior during fetal development, women with congenital adrenal hyperplasia report a decrease in heterosexual activity and an increase in homosexual activity.[2, 4]

The maintenance steroid dose usually does not need to be changed during pregnancy. The dosage of steroids used in the treatment of this syndrome replaces the approximate amount normally produced and, therefore, is a physiologic dose. At these low doses, teratogenic effects would be unlikely, and none have been noted. The need for additional steroids during the stress of labor and delivery is obvious and is usually met by the administration of cortisone acetate intramuscularly and cortisol intravenously. Infection and impaired wound healing have not been problems. Aside from the liability associated with genetic transmission of this syndrome, the children born to patients with adrenal hyperplasia have been normal. The newborn should be closely observed for adrenal insufficiency due to steroid crossover and suppression of the fetal adrenal in utero.

Treatment Problems

Overtreatment causes Cushing's syndrome and poor growth; undertreatment is associated with short stature, hirsutism, and infertility. In some cases, undertreatment and increased androgen secretion lead to premature pubertal maturation that may require treatment with a gonadotropin-releasing hormone (GnRH) agonist. The adult height achieved by most patients is less than normal, testimony to overtreatment and undertreatment (which both compromise growth). Mineralocorticoid therapy should be maximized (maintaining the plasma renin activity at its lower limit of normal) to eliminate hypovolemia as a stimulus for ACTH secretion, via the angiotensin II pathway.

Because it is now recognized that estrogen is the primary regulator of bone response in both males and females,[65] low-dose hydrocortisone and fludrocortisone treatment was combined with flutamide (an antiandrogen) and testolactone (an inhibitor of androgen to estrogen aromatization). In a preliminary study, normalization of growth was achieved.[66]

Masculinization Due to Elevated Androgens in the Maternal Circulation

Masculinization of the female fetus, although in most cases due to fetal virilizing adrenal hyperplasia, can be produced by an androgen-secreting maternal tumor or can be due to the intake of exogenous androgenic substances, such as progestins and danazol. When not caused by an error in the metabolism of the fetal adrenal gland, virilization is not progressive, blood steroids are not elevated, and no hormonal therapy is needed. Subsequent development will be normal. Therefore, surgical correction of abnormalities in the external genitalia is the only indicated treatment.

The occurrence of an androgen-secreting tumor in a mother during pregnancy is rarely seen. On the other hand, the iatrogenic cause of masculinization is a well known story. The majority of these cases resulted from antenatal maternal treatment of threatened or recurrent miscarriage with various progestin compounds. In view of the lack of evidence for positive results with such therapy, progestin compounds, other than progesterone, are no longer administered to pregnant women.

Aromatase (P450arom) Deficiency

P450arom is encoded by the CYP19 gene on chromosome 15p21.1. A deficiency in this enzyme is very uncommon, and only rare mutations in P450arom have been reported.[65, 67–69] An individual with this deficiency will be first affected by the failure to achieve normal levels of aromatization within the placenta. A placental deficiency in aromatase activity would allow an accumulation of the fetal androgen precursors utilized in placental estrogen synthesis. This condition is associated with virilization of the mother during the second half of pregnancy, low estrogen levels in the mother, and a female newborn with masculinization. Accurate prenatal diagnosis requires a loading test with DHA and DHAS. A patient with a placental sulfatase deficiency will increase her estrogen levels in response to DHA and not to DHAS. A patient with an aromatase deficiency will respond to neither steroid. Pubertal development is prevented because the ovary cannot aromatize androgens in order to produce estrogen; a patient can present with primary amenorrhea (hypergonadotropic hypogonadism) and mild virilization.

Incompletely Masculinized Males

Incompletely masculinized males are male by genetic sex (XY) and possess testicles, but the external genitalia are not normally male. Male pseudohermaphrodites may arise in one of four ways:

1. Defective responses in androgen dependent tissues — Androgen Insensitivity Syndromes.

2. Abnormal androgen synthesis.

3. Gonadotropin resistant testes.

4. Absent or defective anti-müllerian hormone.

Syndromes of Androgen Insensitivity

Factors that influence the response to androgens in specific target cells include the following:

1. The intracellular concentration of androgen.

2. The relative binding affinity of these steroids to their nuclear androgen receptors.

3. The binding capacity of the receptor.

4. The nuclear content of androgen receptors.

5. The cellular concentrations of catabolic and/or synthetic enzymes (e.g., 5α-reductase, aromatase, 17β-hydroxysteroid dehydrogenase).

6. The adequacy of the nuclear (chromatin) acceptor site.

7. The adequacy of regulatory molecules (adapter proteins) controlling chromatin "read" of the androgen message.

8. RNA processing and translation.

9. The quality of the protein gene product.

Defects in androgenization of targets theoretically can occur as a result of failure in any of these steps. Three major clinical conditions are worthy of detailed review.

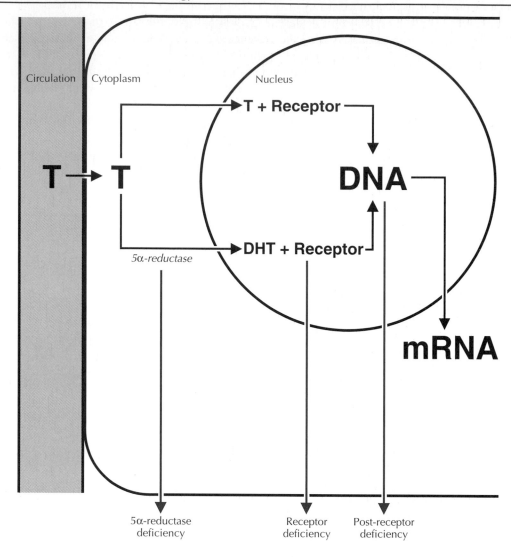

Complete Androgen Insensitivity — Testicular Feminization

Complete androgen insensitivity was first described in detail by Morris at Yale, who provided the descriptive term, testicular feminization.[70] The phenotype of this condition (also discussed in Chapter 11) is female, despite the normal male karyotype, 46,XY. There is a congenital insensitivity to androgens, transmitted by means of a maternal X-linked recessive gene responsible for the androgen intracellular receptor.[71] Therefore, androgen induction of wolffian duct development does not occur. However, anti-müllerian hormone activity is present, and the individual does not have müllerian development (a natural experiment that indicates the presence of an anti-müllerian hormone). Frequently the testes have descended to the inguinal ring because AMH mediates the transabdominal descent of the testes. The vagina is short (derived from the urogenital sinus only) and ends blindly. The uterus and tubes are absent. The testes are normally developed but abnormally positioned. Testosterone production is normal or slightly increased. There is no problem of sex assignment because there is no trace of androgen activity. The diagnosis is likely when an individual presents following breast development at puberty, with primary amenorrhea, absent pubic and axillary hair, a short vagina, and an absent cervix and uterus. Males with enzyme defects that prevent testosterone synthesis will have a female phenotype, but breast development does not occur. Individuals with complete androgen insensitivity have augmented breast development because of a total absence of androgen influence. Androgen insensitivity accounts for about 10% of all cases of primary amenorrhea, third most common after gonadal dysgenesis and congenital absence of the vagina. The hormone profile in these individuals is typical: high LH, normal to slightly elevated male testosterone levels, high

Androgen Insensitivity Syndromes

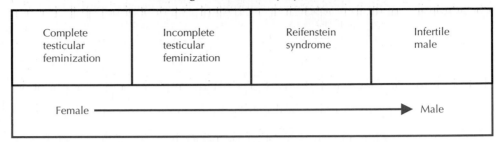

Phenotypic Spectrum

estradiol (for men), and normal to elevated FSH. Individuals with complete androgen insensitivity perform less well in tests of visual-spatial ability, suggesting that androgens exert an organizing effect in the brain during development.[72]

An absent uterus in a normal appearing female is encountered in only two conditions: androgen insensitivity and müllerian agenesis (the Mayer-Rokitansky-Kuster-Hauser syndrome). The latter is easily diagnosed because of the presence of pubic and axillary hair and a normal 46,XX karyotype (discussed in Chapter 11).

The "complete" form indicates that there is no androgen response; therefore, normal external female development occurs, and these infants should be reared as females. The testes (azoospermic with hyperplastic Leydig cells) may be present in the inguinal canals. Children with inguinal hernias and/or inguinal masses should be suspected of testicular feminization. There is no virilization at puberty because of the lack of androgen response. In contrast to dysgenetic gonads with a Y chromosome, the occurrence of gonadal tumors is relatively late, rarely before age 25, and the overall incidence is less, about 5–10%.[73–76] Therefore, gonadectomy should be performed at approximately age 16–18, to allow endogenous hormonal changes and a smooth transition through puberty.

Because of the importance of prophylactic gonadectomy, detection of this syndrome demands careful investigation for other affected family members. This syndrome follows an X-limited recessive pattern of inheritance. Apparent sisters of affected individuals have a 1 in 3 chance of being XY. Female offspring of a normal sister of an affected individual have a 1 in 6 chance of being XY. About a third of the patients have negative family histories and presumably represent new mutations.

In the past, conventional wisdom warned against unthinking and "needless" disclosure of the gonadal and chromosomal sex to a patient with complete androgen insensitivity. This attitude has changed as, more and more, patients desire and appreciate a full understanding of themselves. Although infertile, these patients are certainly completely female in their gender identity, and this should be reinforced rather than challenged. We now strongly advocate combining a truthful education with appropriate psychological counseling of patient and parents. A good resource is the international support group, A^L^I^A^S, that is headquartered in the United Kingdom (2 Shirburn Avenue, Mansfield, Nottinghamshire, NG18 2BY, UK); http//www.medhelp.org/www/ais/.

Incomplete Androgen Insensitivity

A spectrum of disorders, all due to an X-linked recessive trait, are known as incomplete forms of testicular feminization. Incomplete androgen insensitivity is one-tenth as common as the complete syndrome.[76] The clinical presentation ranges from almost complete failure of virilization to essentially complete phenotypic masculinization. Between these poles exist examples of mild clitoromegaly and slight labial fusion to significant genital ambiguity. Reifenstein's syndrome is now applied to all the intermediate forms that were initially given individual names (such as Lubs syndrome). Males have been described whose only indication of androgen insensitivity was azoospermic or severe oligospermic infertility. Indeed, the incidence may approach 40% or more of men with infertility due to azoospermia or severe oligospermia. However, the defect in androgen receptor function may be so subtle that some affected men are fertile.[77] The undervirilized fertile male syndrome is another manifestation of this androgen receptor disorder. The diversity of presentation represents variable manifestations of the same mutant gene. The biochemical abnormality depends upon the degree of function of the androgen receptor or postreceptor events.

Molecular analysis of the androgen receptor gene in individuals with androgen insensitivity has demonstrated a spectrum of disorders in which both the complete and partial forms result from androgen receptor gene mutations.[71] The gene encoding the androgen receptor is localized to the q11–12 region (the long arm) of the X chromosome.[78, 79] About 200 unique mutations have been identified.[80]

Two types of defective androgen receptor function are recognized: abnormalities of androgen binding and abnormalities of DNA binding. The molecular defects responsible for these deficiencies have been identified and characterized. These include major structural abnormalities of the androgen receptor gene in which complete deletion of the gene or deletions of the exons encoding the androgen binding domain or the DNA binding domain each result in the clinical picture of complete androgen insensitivity.[81-84] In addition, point mutations that result in a defective receptor or alter receptor mRNA and cause reduced receptor protein production also result in complete androgen insensitivity.[85] On the other hand, single base mutations that change a single amino acid yield subjects displaying either complete or partial androgen insensitivity.[86] Alterations in receptor function, therefore, range from complete loss to subtle qualitative changes in the stimulation and transcription of androgen dependent target genes. Less understandable, however, is the poor correlation between receptor levels (and androgen binding affinity) with the degree of masculinization seen in partial androgen insensitivity. Nevertheless, the same mode of inheritance, despite differences in androgen receptor functioning, indicates that all forms originate in changes in the structural gene responsible for the androgen receptor.

Some men with partial androgen insensitivity can respond to androgen treatment with enhanced virilization. For example, a man with Reifenstein syndrome due to a mutation in the DNA-binding domain of the androgen receptor responded to high-dose testosterone administration with normal virilization.[87] However, there is no test or measurement that will predict response, and only a few of these patients are able to respond to androgen therapy.

Sex assignment may be a problem when ambiguous genitalia exist because of a partial response of the receptor. If sex assignment is female, early gonadectomy is performed to avoid neoplasia. In Reifenstein syndrome, the phallus may be large enough to allow a male sex assignment at birth, despite the perineal hypospadias. After puberty, however, the inadequate androgen receptor function becomes evident. The receptor function is inadequate to respond to the surge of androgen at puberty; without androgen effect, estrogen activity prevails, and feminization with gynecomastia occurs. These individuals are infertile and cannot react to exogenous androgen. The karyotype is male XY, distinguishing it from other feminizing syndromes of puberty in phenotypic males (e.g., Klinefelter's syndrome).

The endocrine profiles of both the complete and incomplete forms are similar: normal to elevated FSH levels, mildly elevated LH (due to absence of negative androgen feedback), and high blood levels of testosterone and estradiol (increased testicular response to LH and increased peripheral conversion).

The Androgen Insensitivity Syndromes[76]

	5α-reductase	Complete	Incomplete	Reifenstein	Infertile
Inheritance	Autosomal recessive	X-linked recessive	X-linked recessive	X-linked recessive	X-linked recessive
Spermatogenesis	Decreased	Absent	Absent	Absent	Decreased
Müllerian	Absent	Absent	Absent	Absent	Absent
Wolffian	Male	Absent	Male	Male	Male
External	Female	Female	Female clitoromegaly	Male hypospadias	Male
Breasts	Male	Female	Female	Gynecomastia	Gynecomastia

5α-Reductase Deficiency

This form of familial incomplete male (46,XY) pseudohermaphroditism is due to an autosomal recessive trait that leads to a deficiency of the 5α-reductase enzyme (and, in some individuals, enzyme that is present but unstable) and is characterized by severe perineal hypospadias and underdevelopment of the vagina.[88] In the past it was known as pseudovaginal perineoscrotal hypospadias (PPH). It differs from the incomplete forms of testicular feminization because, at puberty, masculinization occurs (the breasts remain male). Normal testicular function occurs, and there is no lack of response to endogenous or exogenous androgen. At birth, however, the external genitalia are similar to that of incomplete androgen insensitivity; i.e., hypospadias, varying failure of fusion of labioscrotal folds and a urogenital opening, or separate urethral and vaginal openings. The cleft in the scrotum appears to be a vagina (there are no müllerian ducts), and these patients have been reared as girls with an enlarged clitoris. At birth, steroid levels are normal, ruling out adrenal disorders.

Diagnosis can be established by demonstrating an elevated T:DHT ratio based upon the blood levels of testosterone and dihydrotestosterone, especially after HCG stimulation. The karyotype is XY, and, as with other incompletely masculinized males, the sex assignment is female if the phallus is inadequate. Gonadectomy is necessary to avoid not only neoplasia but the virilization that is certain to appear at puberty. On the other hand, early correction of cryptorchidism and hypospadias can preserve fertility and allow a male life. The deficiency is believed to be due to the homozygous state, manifest clinically only in males. Homozygous 46,XX females have reduced body hair, and although menarche may be delayed, fertility is normal.[89]

At least 3 "types" of enzyme deficiency have been described in affected families:

1. Abnormally low concentration of enzyme.

2. Reduced enzyme activity due to enzyme instability.

3. Normal enzyme concentration but defective affinity for testosterone and/or essential cofactors leading to reduced enzyme activity.

Two 5α reductase genes have been cloned.[90] One isoenzyme (5α-reductase-1) is encoded on chromosome 5; mutations in the other isoenzyme (5α-reductase-2) encoded on chromosome 2 are responsible for male pseudohermaphroditism due to 5α-reductase deficiency. Because this deficiency in females does not affect fertility, this contributes to the high incidence of the disorder. The relatively easy switch of individuals reared as girls to boys at puberty suggests that the other 5α-reductase gene is operative in the brain.

Study of this syndrome points out important lessons in intersexuality.[91] In this condition, the wolffian duct virilizes in a normal male fashion, but the urogenital sinus and genital tubercle persist as female structures. The failure is due to inadequate DHT formation intracellularly in these external genitalia tissues at the time the normal male fetus virilizes. In the 5α-reductase deficiencies, the seminal vesicles, ejaculatory ducts, epididymis, and vas deferens, which are all testosterone-dependent, are present, whereas the DHT-dependent structures, external genitalia, urethra, and prostate, do not develop along male lines. Affected men have less facial and body hair, less temporal hairline recession, and no problems with acne. However, spermatogenesis, muscle mass, male libido, and deepening of the voice do occur in these men. DHT presence is a requirement only in the fetus, as indicated by the significant genital virilization these patients undergo at puberty and thereafter.[92] These individuals require surgical correction of hypospadias and cryptorchidism. Whereas the conversion from male to female role is exceedingly traumatic psychologically, the reversal of sex identity (female to male) some of these patients have undergone at puberty was apparently uncomplicated.[35] In one such case, a "double-life" was conducted. Although functioning in all public respects as a female, one 5α-reductase individual conducted numerous and prolonged heterosexual affairs, which were quite satisfactory, albeit clandestine. He had known of his male sexual identity since puberty but delayed medical assistance for fear that exposure would bring shame and guilt to his religiously devoted elderly "old world" mother. He decided to keep his secret until his mother died. He finally sought diagnostic help at age 65, however, because his mother at age 93 continued to enjoy good health.

Abnormal Androgen Synthesis

Defective male development may stem from a secretory failure of the testes during the critical period of sex differentiation. In addition to the obvious specific and often familial defects in enzymatic steps leading to testosterone biosynthesis, a variety of other intrinsically testicular problems can lead to male pseudohermaphroditism. In all, the following conditions account for 4% of male pseudohermaphroditism:

1. Aberrations in testicular organogenesis (dysgenetic testes).

2. Gonadotropin resistant testes (LH receptor mutations).

3. Congenital lipoid adrenal hyperplasia.

4. Defective synthesis, secretion, or response to anti-müllerian hormone.

Defects in testosterone synthesis can be at any one of the 3 required enzymatic reactions that lead from cholesterol to testosterone: 3β-hydroxysteroid dehydrogenase, P450c17, and 17β-hydroxysteroid dehydrogenase. These defects are inherited as autosomal recessive traits, and the phenotypes range from partial to complete male pseudohermaphroditism.

Patients with male pseudohermaphroditism who are considered variants of testicular feminization upon partial virilization at puberty may actually have a defect in androgen synthesis. The diagnosis is made by demonstrating elevated blood levels of androstenedione and estrogens, while the blood level of testosterone is low or low-normal. When the enzyme involves a reaction that is active in the adrenal gland (all but the 17β-hydroxysteroid dehydrogenase), the adrenal blocks are usually severe with adrenal failure and death in the newborn period.

The male pseudohermaphrodite due to deficient testicular 17β-hydroxysteroid dehydrogenase activity because of mutations in the encoding gene has male internal genitalia and no müllerian structures. The characteristic clinical findings in these patients are external female genitalia at birth with testes usually located in the inguinal canal. Raised as females, these individuals can undergo virilization at puberty because of an increase in testosterone levels. This increase in pubertal testosterone is derived by conversion of elevated circulating levels of androstenedione (in response to the increase in LH at puberty) by unaffected 17β-hydroxysteroid dehydrogenase isoenzymes.[93] In individuals being raised as girls, early gonadectomy is required to avoid virilization at puberty and testicular neoplasia.

Gonadotropin Resistant Testes

Male pseudohermaphrodites, due to agenesis or abnormal differentiation of Leydig cells, are characterized by reduced responsiveness to LH/HCG. All these cases can be termed "gonadotropin resistant testes." In general, the characteristics of the syndrome include basically female but ambiguous genitalia, male cryptorchid testes with degenerated Leydig cells (Leydig cell hypoplasia or agenesis), no müllerian ducts but present vas deferens and epididymis, elevated gonadotropins (FSH rises further after gonadectomy, indicating the presence of inhibin).[94]

Molecular studies have revealed that these XY gonadotropin resistant individuals with varying degrees of masculinization (from total feminization to nearly normal male genitalia) reflect the amount of Leydig cell function allowed by mutations in the LH receptor.[95, 96] These mutations are inherited by recessive transmission, and, therefore, heterozygous parents have no characteristic affected phenotypes.[97]

Congenital Lipoid Adrenal Hyperplasia

Most of the cholesterol used for steroid synthesis is derived from the mobilization and transport of intracellular stores.[98, 99] Indeed, the rate-limiting step in steroidogenesis is the transfer of cholesterol from the outer mitochondrial membrane to the inner mitochondrial membrane where fully active P450scc waits for substrate. The rate-limiting transfer of hydrophobic cholesterol through the aqueous space between the outer and inner mitochondrial membranes is mediated by protein activation stimulated by tropic hormones. Long-term, chronic steroidogenesis requires gene transcription and protein synthesis, but short-term, acute responses occur independently of new RNA synthesis, although protein synthesis is still necessary, specifically the proteins that regulate cholesterol transfer across the mitochondrial membrane.

Several proteins have been characterized and proposed as regulators of acute intracellular cholesterol transfer. Sterol carrier protein 2 (SCP2) is able to bind and transfer cholesterol between compartments within a cell. Another candidate is a small molecule, steroidogenesis activator polypeptide (SAP), and still another is peripheral benzodiazepine receptor (PBR), which affects cholesterol flux through a pore structure. But the most studied and favored protein as a regulator of acute cholesterol transfer is ***steroidogenic acute regulator (StAR) protein***.[100, 101] StAR messenger RNA and protein are induced concomitantly with acute steroidogenesis in response to cyclic AMP stimulation; StAR increases steroid production; and StAR is imported and localized in the mitochondria. But most impressively, congenital lipoid adrenal hyperplasia (an autosomal recessive disorder) has been demonstrated to be a failure in adrenal and gonadal steroidogenesis due to a mutation in the StAR gene, which results in premature stop codons.[102, 103] With this mutation, a low level of steroidogenesis is possible, even permitting feminization at puberty, but continuing tropic hormonal stimulation results in an accumulation of intracellular lipid deposits that destroy steroidogenic capability.[104]

StAR mediates the transport of cholesterol into mitochondria in adrenal and gonadal steroidogenesis, but not in the placenta and brain. It is synthesized in a precursor form as a 285-amino acid protein that has a 25-residue sequence cleaved from the NH$_2$-terminal after transport into mitochondria.[105] The mutant forms of StAR undergo premature truncation that prevents this proteolytic cleavage. Mutations of the StAR gene, located on chromosome 8p11.2, are the only inherited disorder of steroidogenesis not caused by a defect in one of the steroidogenic enzymes. The absence of StAR expression in placenta and brain indicates the presence of different mechanisms for cholesterol transport in those tissues.

Abnormal Anti-Müllerian Hormone

Hernia Uterine Inguinale (Uterine Hernia Syndrome)

Individuals with this syndrome appear to be normal males, but relatively well-differentiated müllerian duct structures are found, usually a uterus and tubes in an inguinal hernia sac. This is due to a failure of AMH function either as a result of failure of Sertoli cell secretion of this polypeptide or an inability of the müllerian ducts to respond to AMH. Therefore, this syndrome is due to mutations in either the gene for AMH or its receptor. The mutation is inherited as a recessive trait, either X-linked or autosomal. Fertility is usually preserved.

Disorders of Gonadal Development

The proper development and eventual function of the gonad depend on the presence of germ cells, the appropriate sex chromosome constitution, and appropriate gonadal ridge somatic cells. Errors in meiotic division can cause aneuploidy and abnormal sex chromosomes. These occur by nondisjunction, anaphase lag, translocation, breakage, rearrangements, or deletions. Mitosis can also be marred by nondisjunction and anaphase lag leading to mosaicism. Two or more different cell lines can persist and appear in different tissues. Finally, abnormal gonadogenesis may occur as a result of structural or disease related catastrophes leading to loss of fetal gonadal function.

Bilateral Dysgenesis of the Testes (Swyer Syndrome)

Affected individuals have an XY karyotype but normal (infantile) female external and internal genitalia.[106] There are fibrous bands in place of the gonads yielding primary amenorrhea and lack of secondary sexual development at puberty. It is a matter of prudent practice to avoid the possibility of virilization or neoplasm; therefore, removal of these band areas is advocated as soon as the diagnosis is made. Presumably, testes failed to develop or were eliminated (testicular regression) before internal or external genital differentiation.[107] At least one cause of this syndrome is a mutation in the SRY gene.[108] Estrogen and progestin sequential therapy supports female secondary sex development.

Anorchia

Affected XY individuals have infantile unambiguous male external genitalia, and male wolffian ducts and lack müllerian ducts. There are, however, no detectable testes. Early testis function did occur (wolffian presence, AMH function) but was not sustained in sufficient amounts or duration to develop a normal size phallus. It is frequently called "the disappearing testis syndrome." Sex of assignment depends on the extent of external genitalia development.

True Hermaphroditism

Hermaphroditus, the Greek god with bisexual attributes, was the son-daughter of Hermes, the god of athletics, secrets, and occult philosophy, and Aphrodite, the goddess of love. The bisexual theme was immortalized in countless statues by the Greeks and Romans, depicting a normal woman with normal male external genitalia (not a combination commonly encountered in real life). Pliny (23–79 AD) was the first to apply the term hermaphrodite to humans, presenting a description in his massive work, *Historia Naturalis.*

Abnormal sexual differentiation can occur as a result of a mixture of gonadal sex (true hermaphroditism) or complete uncertainty of gonadal sex (gonadal dysgenesis with some virilization).[109, 110] A true hermaphrodite possesses both ovarian and testicular tissue. Both types may be contained in one gonad (ovotestis) or less often, one side may be an ovary, the other a testis. The internal structures correspond to the adjacent gonad. In the majority, external genitalia are ambiguous with sufficient male character to allow male sex assignment. However, three-fourths develop gynecomastia and half menstruate after puberty. Sixty percent are genetic females (XX), few are XY, the rest are mosaics with at least one cell line XX. 46,XX individuals without SRY may have a mutation of an autosomal gene that permits testicular determination in the absence of the testes determining factor.[111]

Gonadal Dysgenesis

Gonadal dysgenesis with bilateral rudimentary streak gonads due to an abnormality in or absence of one of the X chromosomes in all cell lines is called Turner syndrome. Approximately 60% of Turner patients have the total loss of one X chromosome; the remainder have either a structural abnormality in one of the X chromosomes or mosaicism with an abnormal X. Henry Hughbert Turner, born in 1892, became chief of endocrinology and associate dean of the University of Oklahoma school of medicine. He was president of the Endocrine Society in 1968, and died in 1970. Turner's clinical description of this syndrome was presented to the annual meeting of the Association for the Study of Internal Secretions in 1938.[112]

In the absence of gonadal development, these individuals are phenotypic females. The well-known characteristics are short stature (142–147 cm, 56–58 inches), sexual infantilism, and streak gonads. The streak gonad is composed of white fibrous stromal tissue, 2–3 cm long and about 0.5 cm wide, containing no ova or follicular derivatives. Other congenital problems in this syndrome are a webbed neck, a high arched palate, cubitus valgus, a broad shield-like chest with widely spaced nipples, a low hairline on the neck, short fourth metacarpal bones, disproportionately short legs, and renal abnormalities (horseshoe kidney, unilateral pelvic kidney, rotational abnormalities, and partial or complete duplication of the collecting system). Autoimmune disorders are common, such as Hashimoto's thyroiditis, Addison's disease, alopecia, and vitiligo. Hypothyroidism is present in about 10% of young patients and may reach 50% later in life. Mild insulin resistance and hearing loss are also common. Patients with Turner syndrome are very prone to keloid formation. One-third of patients with Turner syndrome have cardiovascular abnormalities, including bicuspid aortic valves, coarctation of the aorta, mitral valve prolapse, and aortic aneurysms. Often the diagnosis is not made until puberty when amenorrhea and lack of sexual development become apparent. At birth, however, lymphedema (due to hypoplasia of superficial vessels) of the extremities may indicate the condition. It is important to assess the aorta, aortic root, and aortic valve with ultrasonography at least in infancy and again during the teens. Patients with Turner syndrome have normal intelligence; however, there may be difficulty with mathematical ability, visual-motor coordination, and spatial-temporal processing, problems that remain throughout life.

Almost all (99%) of conceptuses with only one X chromosome abort. The remaining 1% account for an incidence of Turner syndrome between 1 in 2500 and 1 in 5000 liveborn girls. [113]

Because of the high incidence of assorted abnormalities in patients with Turner syndrome, the following evaluations should be performed, some only once at the time of diagnosis, and others annually as part of on-going surveillance: thyroid function testing (annually) and antibodies (at least once), intravenous pyelogram or renal ultrasonography (once if normal), echocardiography, audiometry, and annual evaluation of the lipid profile and glucose metabolism.

Spontaneous puberty has been reported in 10–20% and spontaneous menstruation in 2–5% of girls with Turner syndrome.[114] Rare pregnancies have been reported in those who have had spontaneous menstruation.[115] The presence of menstrual function and reproduction in a patient with Turner phenotype may be due to an undetected mosaic complement, such as a 46,XX line in addition to 45,X. When pregnancy does occur in an X deficient subject, the infant has a 30% chance of congenital anomalies, including Down syndrome, spina bifida, and congenital heart disease.

A large variety of mosaic patterns is seen with gonadal dysgenesis. From analysis of the various combinations, it is apparent that short stature is related to loss of regions on the short arm of one X chromosome. Distal long arm deletions of one of the X chromosomes are associated with

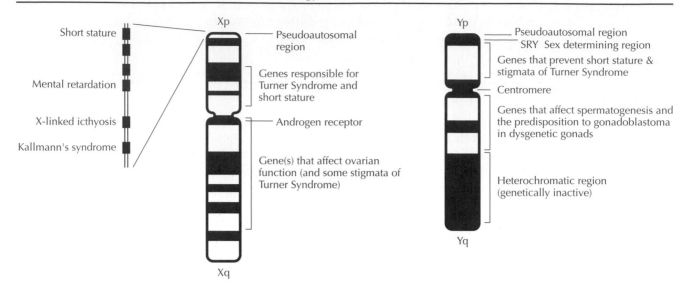

amenorrhea (usually secondary after some ovarian function) and streak gonads, but the patients are not always growth compromised nor do they display other Turner somatic malformations. Long arm deletions near the centromere are associated with primary amenorrhea. Thus, loss of material from the short arms of the X chromosome leads to short stature and the other stigmata of Turner syndrome. This suggests that normal ovarian development requires two loci, one on the long arm and one on the short arm; loss of either results in gonadal failure. Thyroid autoimmunity is common in Turner syndrome, but Hashimoto's thyroiditis may be specific to 46,XXqi cases. It should be emphasized that any of the Turner syndrome characteristics can be seen with any karyotype.

Just as X chromosome monosomy, with deletion of the second X chromosome, results in Turner's phenotype, the same will apply to loss of the Y chromosome. The 45,X karyotype derived from leukocyte culture does not guarantee that a mosaic does not exist with a gonadal line containing XY. For this reason, annual pelvic examinations and appropriate screening are required to detect incipient signs of gonadal neoplasia as an adnexal mass. If a presumed 45,X patient develops breasts or sexual hair without exogenous therapy, a gonadoblastoma or dysgerminoma should be considered and ruled out. Heterosexual signs require scrutiny in all 45,X individuals. ***Expert consultation should be obtained to pursue further analysis with X- and Y-specific DNA probes.*** Why not screen all patients with some form of gonadal dysgenesis with molecular techniques? For example, 3–4% of 45,X patients had Y-derived DNA detected by polymerase chain reaction analysis.[116] In one series of 40 Turner syndrome patients, one patient had identifiable Y chromosome material using polymerase chain reaction of the gene from the SRY region of the Y chromosome.[117] In 3 of 18 patients (none of whom had evidence of Y chromosomal material by cytogenetic analysis), Y chromosomal segments from the SRY region were detected by polymerase chain amplification and Southern blot analysis.[118] Therefore the prevalence of undetected Y material is low.[119] Furthermore, is it necessary to know of the presence of silent Y mosaicism?

The problem is that we do not know if there is any clinical significance to Y-derived material detected only by molecular techniques. Another shortcoming of this approach is that polymerase chain reaction and in situ hybridization identify only those DNA sequences that correspond to the probes used in the analysis. There may be a sequence from a Y chromosome that does not correspond to the selected probes. A totally reliable method awaits identification of the gene responsible for tumor formation or the complete mapping of the Y chromosome sequences. Until then, ***the recommendation is to seek Y chromosomal material in patients with virilization or when a chromosomal fragment of uncertain origin is identified on the karyotype.***

The term "gonadal dysgenesis" is frequently used to describe all subjects with female genitalia, normal müllerian structures and streak gonads (with either 46,XX or 46,XY karyotypes). Not all possess the spectrum of Turner phenotype anomalies, and some show none of these characteristics. The latter groups are referred to as "pure gonadal dysgenesis." Ovarian development and subsequent internal and external genitalia development proceed normally. However, at variable times thereafter, the gonads undergo accelerated germ cell loss, and premature degeneration of the ovaries ensues. A similar morphologic consequence of premature ovarian degeneration exists in 46,XX gonadal dysgenesis. In these instances, a mutation in an autosomal gene is considered the likely etiologic factor, inherited in autosomal recessive fashion.[75] Perrault syndrome is the combination of XX gonadal dysgenesis and neurosensory deafness.

Subjects with 46,XY karyotype can also have gonadal dysgenesis; most, but not all, with the pure gonadal dysgenesis form are without Turner stigmata.[120] The 46,XY gonadal dysgenesis patients are diagnosed in early adolescence with delayed pubertal development. As expected they show elevated gonadotropins, normal female levels of androgen, and low levels of estrogens, female external genitalia, a uterus, and fallopian tubes. Minimal breast enlargement reflects peripheral aromatization of androgens. Menstrual function suggests tumor development in the streak gonad. These streaks often display ovarian stroma but no follicles. Their propensity to tumor development is significant, a 20–30% incidence. Patients with mosaic patterns in the karyotype have a reduced risk of tumor, but it still amounts to 15–20%. The most common tumor is the often bilateral gonadoblastoma, but dysgerminomas and even the more threatening embryonal carcinoma are also seen. Intraabdominal testes should be removed as early in life as possible because of the known risk of tumor development. If well visualized, streak gonads can be removed by laparoscopy.[121–123] The uterus and tubes should be retained for the possibility of pregnancy with donor oocytes.

The etiology of this defect is thought to be a short arm Y chromosome deletion involving SRY, a mutation in other genes that leads to inhibition of SRY function, or a XXqi mutation of SRY.[12] There is evidence to suggest that some cases of 46,XY gonadal dysgenesis are due to impaired function of a gene on the X chromosome that is necessary for normal SRY function.[124, 125] The absence of Turner stigmata in these patients suggests the preservation of a nearby gene that protects XY individuals from developing Turner features.[126] In 46,XY partial gonadal dysgenesis individuals there is some testicular development, and therefore, they present as newborns with ambiguous genitalia.[127] The degree of external masculinization and the relative proportions of müllerian and wolffian duct structures present correlate with the extent of testes differentiation.

Curiously, to date analysis of a large number of 46,XY gonadal dysgenesis patients has not demonstrated mutations of the coding region of the SRY gene. The association of this form of gonadal dysgenesis with duplications of the short arm of the X chromosome, and various inherited syndromes of multiple congenital anomalies, indicate the role of several genes other than SRY in testes development. There are several reports of 46,XY male pseudohermaphroditism because of mutations in the LH receptor gene.[128, 129] The 46,XX sisters of these individuals present with primary amenorrhea and a normal female phenotype.

Males who have a 46,XX karyotype usually have SRY present, probably by translocation from the Y to an X chromosome.[126] Some subjects, however, lack SRY, indicating that more than one genetic defect yields 46,XX maleness.

Multiple X females (47,XXX) have normal development and reproductive function, although mental retardation may be more frequent. Secondary amenorrhea and/or eunuchoidism can be seen.

Mixed Gonadal Dysgenesis

Mosaicism involving the Y chromosome can be associated with abnormalities of sex differentiation. Of the variety of karyotypes possible from loss of the Y by nondisjunction, 45,X/46,XY is the most common. A wide variety of phenotypes is displayed by these individuals from newborns with ambiguous genitalia to normal fertile males or normal female phenotype with bilateral streak gonads. Most have short stature, and one-third have other Turner stigmata.

In the "typical" mixed gonadal dysgenesis case presenting with abnormal sex differentiation, the usual gonadal pattern is a streak gonad on one side and a dysgenetic or normal appearing testis on the other side of the abdomen. Müllerian and wolffian duct development correlates with the character of the ipsilateral gonad. All possible permutations combining streaks, and dysgenetic and apparently normal testes have been encountered. The diversity of presentation is presumed to reflect the relative proportion of 45,X and 46,XY cells in the gonadal ridge. The incidence of gonadal tumors is 25%.

Surgical Removal of Gonadal Tissue

There is no debate that gonadal tissue having any Y chromosome component in phenotypic females requires removal as soon as the diagnosis is made to avoid the risk of malignant gonadal tumors. There is one exception to this rule. Because gonadal tumors occur relatively late in patients with complete androgen insensitivity, surgery is delayed until after puberty. An accomplished laparoscopist can attempt this procedure, with the option of laparotomy if the gonads prove to be inaccessible. Streak gonads have been removed in this fashion, as well as the testes in androgen insensitivity.[121–123] With androgen insensitivity, the gonads can be close to the external iliac artery and herniated into the inguinal canals. The procedure is more difficult, and care must be taken to extract the gonad from the inguinal canal to secure complete excision. It may also be necessary to make a small abdominal incision or a culdotomy to extract the gonad in order to avoid morcellation. Preoperative magnetic resonance imaging can be helpful in order to accurately localize gonadal tissue and select the correct operative approach.

The uterus and tubes should be preserved for the possibility of pregnancy with donor oocytes.

Hormone Treatment of Patients Without Ovaries

When ovaries are absent in individuals being reared as females, either because of surgery or streak gonads, hormonal treatment will be necessary at puberty and thereafter. Estrogen will initiate and sustain maturation and function of secondary sexual characteristics, and promote the achievement of the full height potential. The adolescent increase in bone density is a very important determinant of an individual's later risk for osteoporosis. This alone is sufficient reason for treatment.[130] Very small amounts of estrogen will promote growth and development. Early treatment with estrogen, however, can reduce overall growth.[131] Start at about age 12–14 with unopposed estrogen (0.3 mg conjugated estrogens or 0.5 mg estradiol daily). After 6 months to 1 year, move to a sequential program with 0.625 mg conjugated estrogens or 1.0 mg estradiol daily and 5 mg medroxyprogesterone acetate or an equivalent progestin for the first 14 days each month (if a uterus is present). Although not proven by appropriate studies, most clinicians believe an increase in estrogen dose to 1.25 mg conjugated estrogens or 2.0 mg estradiol is warranted (along with adequate calcium intake) to maximize bone and breast responses. Adequacy of treatment can be assessed by following bone age changes, although this is unnecessary in most cases. In patients with genetic shortness in stature (e.g., Turner syndrome), estrogen treatment is not started until bone age is greater than 12 to avoid epiphysial closure and to allow a longer period of time for long bone growth. Clinicians should strive for good compliance with life-long hormone therapy in order to protect against osteoporosis and cardiovascular disease. Patients can receive helpful education and support from the Turner's Syndrome Society of the United States, 1313 SE Fifth St., Suite 327, Minneapolis, MN 55414, http://www.turner-syndrome-us.org

Stimulation of Growth

Short stature occurs in virtually all patients with a 45,X karyotype and nearly all patients with Turner syndrome who have other karyotypes.[132] This growth impairment begins in utero, is apparent throughout childhood, and results in a short adult height (a mean of 143 cm, about 4 feet 8 inches).[133] This attenuation of growth is partly due to insufficient growth hormone secretion due to the deficiency in sex steroids and also to an end organ resistance to insulin-like growth factor-I.[134] Anabolic steroids have been used to stimulate growth, especially in patients with Turner syndrome. Short-term growth can be stimulated by anabolic steroids; however, the effect on final adult height is equivocal because epiphyseal maturation is also enhanced. Furthermore, virilizing side effects are a drawback. The combination of low doses of an anabolic steroid (e.g., oxandrolone) and recombinant growth hormone under the direction of a pediatric endocrinologist offers the best prospect. Treatment with growth hormone (50 µg/kg/day) yields significant growth acceleration that can be sustained for at least 6 years, achieving an adult height as much as 10 cm over the initial predicted height, and most patients can achieve a height that is greater than 150 cm (about 4 feet 11 inches).[131, 135] The future may see effective use of growth hormone-releasing hormone for this purpose. It is worth noting that adolescents with Turner syndrome either treated with growth hormone or not do not lose bone mineral density prior to estrogen treatment; hence, it is unnecessary to begin estrogen treatment at an early age (when it might counteract the goal of growth hormone therapy: achieving maximal height).[132, 136]

Now that the success of growth hormone treatment is recognized and accepted, an argument can be made for chromosomal screening by molecular analysis of all growth-retarded girls. In a screening of 375 mildly growth-retarded girls, 18 cases of Turner syndrome were identified; 14 of whom had none of the typical clinical features.[137]

The Possibility of Pregnancy

In women who have variants of gonadal dysgenesis and who menstruate, pregnancy can occur. However, there is a 30% incidence of congenital anomalies in the offspring, including spina bifida and Down syndrome. Sex chromosome abnormalities are frequent in the children born to mosaic mothers.[115] Prenatal diagnosis by amniocentesis or chorionic villus biopsy is highly advised. Assisted reproductive technology with donated oocytes yields excellent results in women with streak gonads (see Chapter 31). There is an important consideration in regards to those patients who become pregnant. ***Fatal aortic events (aneurysm, dissection, or rupture) can occur during pregnancy in patients with gonadal dysgenesis. A cardiology consultation with an echocardiogram is strongly advised for these women prior to pregnancy.***

Noonan Syndrome

Both affected males and females with Noonan syndrome have apparently normal chromosome complements and normal gonadal function. The phenotypic appearance of the female is that of a patient with Turner syndrome: short stature, webbed neck, shield chest, and cardiac malformations.[138] The cardiac lesions, however, are different. Pulmonic stenosis is most frequent in Noonan syndrome as opposed to aortic coarctation in Turner syndrome. In the past these patients have been referred to as male Turner's or Turner's with normal chromosomes. Noonan's are fertile and transmit the trait as an autosomal dominant with variable expression.

Diagnosis of Ambiguous Genitalia

Ambiguous external genitalia in a newborn infant represents not only a major diagnostic challenge, but a social and medical emergency. The physician is involved in a pressure-filled situation because of the necessity for making such an influential decision as the sex of sexual rearing. Rapid and organized evaluation must be initiated to assign the appropriate gender, identify a possible life-threatening medical condition, and begin necessary medical, surgical, and psychological interventions.[139] Input from a team of experts in endocrinology, genetics, neonatology, psychology, surgery, and urology is essential. Nevertheless, the primary clinician should be the sole contact with the family. Diagnostic procedures may delay the decision, but it is well recognized that a period of delay is far better than later reversal of the sex assignment. Naming of the child should be delayed until a gender is firmly assigned. Parental education and guidance are essential in this anxiety-ridden situation.

The most important point to remember when confronted with a newborn infant with ambiguous genitalia, or an apparently male infant with bilateral cryptorchidism, is that the prime diagnosis until ruled out is congenital adrenal hyperplasia. The reason is clear: adrenal hyperplasia is the only condition that is life threatening. Signs of adrenal failure such as vomiting, diarrhea, dehydration, and shock may develop rapidly. Furthermore, most infants with ambiguous genitalia are virilized females, and most of these have congenital adrenal hyperplasia.

The history of a previously affected relative may aid in the diagnosis of testicular feminization or any of its variants. Similarly, the history of a sibling with genital ambiguity or the history of a previous neonatal death in a sibling strongly suggest the possibility of adrenal hyperplasia. A history of maternal exposure to androgenic compounds may be difficult to elicit. The mother may be unaware of the nature of her medications, and the obstetrician should be consulted to determine if medication was used for threatened or recurrent miscarriage or endometriosis.

Although the appearance of the external genitalia in intersex infants may be similar regardless of etiology, and a definitive diagnosis unachievable by physical examination alone, certain useful clues can be discerned.

Are gonads palpable? Palpation of the genital and inguinal regions is the most important part of the physical examination. Gonads in the inguinal regions or in scrotal folds are almost certainly testes. Ovaries are not found in scrotal folds or in the inguinal regions. The testicles, however, may be intraabdominal. If testicles are not palpable, the infant should be considered to have congenital adrenal hyperplasia until demonstrated otherwise.

What is the phallus length and diameter? Measured from the pubic ramus to the tip of the glans, a stretched penile length of less than 2.5 cm is 2.5 standard deviations below the mean for infants at 40 weeks of gestational age (2.0 cm for 36 weeks and 1.5 cm for 32 weeks).[139] The normal newborn clitoris measures less than 1 cm long; a normal newborn penis measures 2.8–4.2 cm in length.

What is the position of the urethral meatus? The urethral meatus can range from a mild hypospadias to an opening in the perineal area into a urogenital sinus. Hypospadias is almost always accompanied by chordee, which is a ventral curvature of the phallus resulting from a shortened urethra.

To what degree are the labioscrotal folds fused? The findings can range from unfused labia majora of a normal female through labia with variable degrees of posterior fusion, a bifid scrotum, to a fully fused normal appearing male scrotum. The distance from the anus to the edge of the vagina divided by the distance from the anus to the base of the clitoris is a ratio which is less than 0.5 in normal females. A ratio greater than 0.5 indicates some degree of labioscrotal fusion.

Is there a vagina, vaginal pouch, or urogenital sinus? Does the rectal examination suggest a midline structure that might be a uterus? A uterus can be palpable, especially shortly after birth when the uterus is a little enlarged in response to maternal estrogen.

Further important physical signs include evidence of hyperpigmentation due to the melanocyte stimulation associated with high levels of ACTH in adrenal hyperplasia, dehydration, hypotension, hypertension, and the manifestations of Turner syndrome such as webbed neck, low hairline, edema of hands and feet, and cardiac and renal anomalies. Careful examination of the phallus may differentiate between a clitoris and a penis. The penis has a midline ventral frenulum, while the clitoris has two folds which extend from the lateral aspects of the clitoris to the labia minora.

All patients with ambiguous genitalia require pelvic ultrasonography (to detect a uterus and ovaries or undescended testes) and a retrograde injection of contrast media into the urogenital orifice to outline the urethra and/or vaginal anatomy, the existence of a urogenital sinus, and the presence of a cervix.[140] Magnetic resonance imaging of the newborn pelvis can supplant both of these procedures.[141]

Rapid testing of blood leukocytes for karyotype analysis, serum electrolytes, serum androgens (androstenedione, testosterone, dehydroepiandrosterone, dehydroepiandrosterone sulfate), 17-hydroxyprogesterone, 11-deoxycorticosterone, and 11-deoxycortisol is an essential laboratory component in the evaluation of intersex. In selected circumstances, ACTH testing and genital skin biopsy provide specific amplifying information. Currently, there is no rapid test using DNA probes for diagnosing the etiology of ambiguous genitalia.

Differential Diagnosis

The presence or absence of palpable gonads, the presence or absence of a uterus, and the karyotype places the patient in one of four categories: female pseudohermaphroditism, male pseudohermaphroditism, true hermaphroditism, or gonadal dysgenesis.

Clinical signs of adrenal failure indicate that the newborn has some form of adrenal enzyme defect regardless of the steroid pattern. The diagnosis is certain if such an infant is hyperkalemic and hyponatremic (due to aldosterone deficiency) or hypertensive and hypokalemic (secondary to elevated deoxycorticosterone).

In the absence of maternal androgen excess, the diagnosis of genetic females with excess androgen (female pseudohermaphroditism) must distinguish 3 forms of congenital virilizing adrenal hyperplasia. The diagnosis of 21-hydroxylase deficiency is confirmed by finding an elevated level of 17-hydroxyprogesterone in the serum. Elevated levels of 11-deoxycorticosterone and 11-deoxycortisol are found in 11β-hydroxylase deficiency, while the precursors to cortisol and androgen, 17-hydroxypregnenolone and dehydroepiandrosterone, are high in the 3β-hydroxysteroid dehydrogenase deficiency. Marginal basal aberrations can be accentuated by an ACTH stimulation test.

Male pseudohermaphroditism (genetic males with too little androgen) can be the result of one of the relatively rare enzyme disorders. Four derive from enzymatic errors in the biosynthesis of testosterone. P450c17 deficient patients display elevated progesterone, whereas individuals with 3β-hydroxysteroid dehydrogenase deficiency have elevated DHA and 17-hydroxypregnenolone levels. Again, ACTH testing can be useful in amplifying compensated defects. A testosterone biosynthetic error which leads to deficient masculinization involves an enzyme not required for glucocorticoid or mineralocorticoid synthesis. Thus no evidence of adrenal insufficiency with electrolyte disturbance is seen in 17β-hydroxysteroid dehydrogenase deficiency. Using HCG stimulation testing, elevated androstenedione and DHA are abnormally high. In Leydig cell hypoplasia, HCG stimulation reveals very low circulating testosterone and its precursors, but no adrenal defects, confirming a specific cellular defect in the testes.

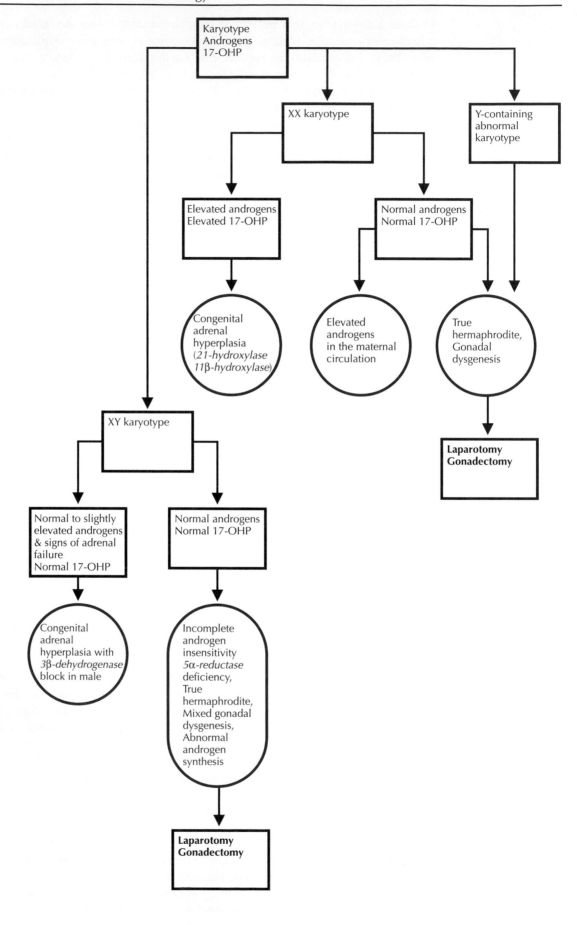

HCG stimulation tests and cultures of genital skin fibroblasts are useful in the laboratory differentiation of 5α-reductase deficiency and partial androgen insensitivity in the newborn. An elevated ratio of testosterone to dihydrotestosterone after HCG stimulation suggests 5α-reductase deficiency that can be confirmed in culture. On the other hand, patients with androgen insensitivity will have normal ACTH and HCG stimulation tests and abnormal androgen binding or androgen receptor gene mutations in cultured cells.

Although laparotomy is not necessary for assignment of sex, it may be the only way to arrive at a definitive diagnosis. Laparotomy is indicated in the following situations (laparoscopic evaluation is inadequate because gonads may be small and hidden in the inguinal canal).

1. The XX infant with ambiguous genitalia, normal androgens, in apparent good health, and no history of maternal androgen exposure. This is either a true hermaphrodite or a variant of mixed gonadal dysgenesis, and gonadectomy is indicated.

2. The XY patient with ambiguous genitalia, without palpable gonads, and normal androgens. The possibilities are incompletely masculinized males (variants of testicular feminization), a true hermaphrodite, mixed gonadal dysgenesis, and 5α-reductase deficiency. Sex of rearing will be female, and gonadectomy is necessary to avoid virilization at puberty and the propensity to develop gonadal neoplasia.

Only laparotomy, gonadal biopsy, and/or gonadectomy confirm the diagnosis of true hermaphroditism in individuals with ambiguous genitalia and 46,XY or 45X/46,XY karyotypes. It should be emphasized that evaluations for mutations in the SRY gene are powerful research tools, but these tests are not currently available for clinical determinations.[142]

Assignment of Sex of Rearing

In a newborn who presents a problem of correct sex assignment, it is better to delay than to reverse the sex assignment at a later date. Generally, the decision can be made within a few days, at most a few weeks. In dealing with the parents, terms with unfortunate connotations, such as hermaphrodite, should be avoided. An easy way to explain ambiguous genital development to parents is to indicate that the genitals are unfinished, rather than abnormal from a sexual point of view.

Despite the wealth of knowledge derived from the world of molecular biology, the decision regarding sex of rearing remains a clinical judgment. When all the information is in place, gender assignment will rest on:

1. Future fertility,

2. The projected appearance of genitalia after puberty,

3. Penile adequacy for coital function.

The future fertility in all masculinized females is unaffected. With proper treatment, reproduction is possible, since the internal genitalia and gonads are those of a normal female. Therefore, all masculinized females should be reared as females.

The only other category of patients with ambiguous genitalia with reproductive capability consists of males with 1) isolated hypospadias, 2) the male with repaired isolated cryptorchidism, and 3) the male with the uterine hernia syndrome.

All other patients with ambiguous genitalia will be sterile. Except for salt-wasting adrenal hyperplasia, the physician's prime concern is not with physical survival, but to enable the patient to grow into a psychologically normal, healthy, and well-adjusted adult. The sex of assignment depends upon only one judgment: can the phallus ultimately develop into a penis adequate for intercourse. The success of a penis is dependent upon erectile tissue, and the genitalia should not only be serviceable but also erotically sensitive. Technically, the construction of female genitalia is easier, and therefore the physician must be convinced that a functional penis is possible.[143, 144]

All decisions regarding sex of rearing and the overall treatment program should be made early in life. If a case has been neglected, sex reassignments must be made according to the gender identity in which a child has developed. Reassignment of sex can probably be made safely up to age 18 months.

Socialization and hormone therapy are important for gender identity and sexual function. Future gender role and identity can be in accord with assigned sex if 4 conditions are met:

1. The parents are comfortable in their ability to raise their child and their resolution of any doubts or uncertainty about the sex of the child. In this acceptance and adaptation, the parents must have participated in and agreed to the sex reassignment decision. Ambiguous names should be discouraged to ensure normal gender identity.

2. Genital reconstruction should take place as early as possible, certainly well before 18 months. Thereafter, sex reassignment is difficult and adjustment impaired.

3. Properly timed hormonal and/or additional surgical interventions must be provided at puberty.

4. The patient should be informed about his or her condition as deemed age-appropriate.

Sex Testing in Athletics

Gender verification tests were introduced into competitive sports in the 1960s because of the concern that individuals might masquerade as the opposite sex to gain a competitive advantage. Sex testing can be based on chromosomal or other histological assays, hormone measurements, or anatomical criteria. Such testing could identify 3 potential groups of problem athletes: transsexuals who have undergone sex change operations, impersonators, and individuals with intersex conditions. Neither sex changed individuals nor masqueraders have been a problem in athletic events. However, sex testing creates the possibility of public exposure and embarrassment for intersex individuals. In addition, sex testing has the potential for revealing to an unaffected individual an underlying diagnosis in a shocking, difficult manner. For all of these reasons, it is argued that physical examination alone should suffice, and any individual with a female phenotype should be allowed to compete as a woman.[145] Even individuals with mild disorders would be able to pass the physical examination requirement. Gender testing of athletes is unnecessary and fraught with potential harm. Gender testing was eliminated in 1992 by the International Amateur Athletic Federation, but it is still required in the Olympic Games.

References

1. **Money J, Schwartz M, Lewis VG,** Adult heterosexual status and fetal hormonal masculinization and demasculinization: 46,XX congenital virilizing adrenal hyperplasia and 46,XY androgen-insensitivity syndrome compared, *Psychoneuroendocrinology* 9:405, 1984.

2. **Mulaikal RM, Migeon CJ, Rock JA,** Fertility rates in female patients with congenital adrenal hyperplasia due to 21-hydroxylase deficiency, *New Engl J Med* 316:178, 1987.

3. **Dittmann RW, Kappes ME, Kappes MH,** Sexual behavior in adolescent and adult females with congenital adrenal hyperplasia, *Psychoneuroendocrinology* 17:153, 1992.

4. **Kuhnle U, Bollinger M, Schwarz HP, Knorr D,** Partnership and sexuality in adult female patients with congenital adrenal hyperplasia. First results of a cross-sectional quality-of-life evaluation, *J Steroid Biochem Mol Biol* 45:123, 1993.

5. **Meyer-Bahlburg HF, Gruen RS, New MI, Bell JJ, Morishima A, Shimshi M, Bueno Y, Vargas I, Baker SW,** Gender change from female to male in classical congenital adrenal hyperplasia, *Horm Behav* 30:319, 1996.

6. **Rubinow DR, Schmidt PJ,** Androgens, brain, and behavior, *Am J Psychiatr* 153:974, 1996.

7. **Van Wagenen G, Simpson ME,** *Embryology of the Ovary and Testis, Homo Sapiens and Mucaca Mulatta,* Yale University Press, New Haven, Connecticut, 1965.

8. **Sinclair AH, Berta P, Palmer MS, Hawkins JR, Griffiths BL, Smith JJ, Foster JW, Frischauf A-M, Lovell-Badge R, Goodfellow PN,** A gene from the human sex-determining region encodes a protein with homology to a conserved DNA-binding motif, *Nature* 346:240, 1990.

9. **Berta P, Hawkins JR, Sinclair AH, Taylor A, Griffiths BL, Goodfellow PN, Fellows M,** Genetic evidence equating SRY and the testes-determining factor, *Nature* 348:448, 1990.

10. **Jager RJ, Anvret M, Hall K, Scherer G,** A human XY female with a frame shift mutation in the candidate testis-determining gene SRY, *Nature* 348:452, 1990.

11. **Moore CCD, Grumbach MM,** Sex determination and gonadogenesis: a transcription cascade of sex chromosome and autosome genes, *Seminars Perinatol* 16:266, 1992.

12. **Muller J, Schwartz M, Skakkebaek NE,** Analysis of the sex-determining region of the Y chromosome (SRY) in sex reversed patients: point-mutation in SRY causing sex-reversion in a 46,XY female, *J Clin Endocrinol Metab* 75:331, 1992.

13. **Haqq CM, King C-Y, Donahoe PK, Weiss MA,** SRY recognizes conserved DNA sites in sex-specific promoters, *Proc Natl Acad Sci USA* 90:1097, 1993.

14. **Wilson JD, Griffin JE, George FW, Leshin M,** The role of gonadal steroids in sexual differentiation, *Recent Prog Hor Res* 37:1, 1981.

15. **Harley VR, Goodfellow PN,** The biochemical role of SRY in sex determination, *Mol Reprod Dev* 39:184, 1994.

16. **Luo X, Ikeda Y, Parker KL,** A cell-specific nuclear receptor is essential for adrenal and gonadal development and sexual differentiation, *Cell* 77:481, 1994.

17. **Parker KL, Schimmer BP,** Steroidogenic factor 1: a key determinant of endocrine development and function, *Endocr Rev* 18:361, 1997.

18. **Shen W-H, Moore CCD, Ikeda Y, Parker KL, Ingraham HA,** Nuclear receptor steroidogenic factor 1 regulates the müllerian inhibiting substance gene: a link to the sex determination cascade, *Cell* 77:651, 1994.

19. **Burris TP, Guo W, McCabe ER,** The gene responsible for adrenal hypoplasia congenita, DAX-1, encodes a nuclear hormone receptor that defines a new class within the superfamily, *Recent Prog Horm Res* 51:241, 1996.

20. **van Lingen BL, Reindollar RH, Davis AJ, Gray MR,** Further evidence that the *WT1* gene does not have a role in the development of the derivatives of the müllerian duct, *Am J Obstet Gynecol* 179:597, 1998.

21. **Rabinovici J, Jaffe RB,** Development and regulation of growth and differentiated function of human and subhuman primate fetal gonads, *Endocr Rev* 11:532, 1990.

22. **Singh RP, Carr DH,** The antomy and histology of XO human embryos and fetuses, *Anat Rec* 155:369, 1966.

23. **Krauss CM, Turksoy RN, Atkins L, McGlaughlin C, Brown LG, Page DC,** Familial premature ovarian failure due to an interstitial deletion of the long arm of the X chromosome, *New Engl J Med* 317:125, 1987.

24. **Speert H,** *Obstetric & Gynecologic Milestones Illustrated,* The Parthenon Publishing Group, New York, 1996.

25. **Jost A, Vigier B, Prepin J, Perchellet JP,** Studies on sex differentiation in mammals, *Recent Prog Hormone Res* 29:1, 1973.

26. **Picard JY, Josso N,** Purification of testicular anti müllerian hormone allowing direct visualization of the pure glycoprotein and determination of yield and purification factor, *Mol Cell Endocrinol* 34:23, 1984.

27. **Pepinsky RB, Sinclair LK, Chow EP, Mattaliano RJ, Manganaro TF, Donahoe PK, Cate RL,** Proteolytic processing of müllerian inhibiting substance produces a transforming growth factor-beta-like fragment, *J Biol Chem* 263:18961, 1988.

28. **Taguchi O, Cunha GR, Lawrence WD, Robboy SJ,** Timing and irreversibility of müllerian duct inhibition in the embryonic reproductive tract of the human male, *Dev Biol* 106:394, 1984.

29. **Behringer RR, Finegold MJ, Cate RL,** Müllerian-inhibiting substance function during mammalian sexual development, *Cell* 79:415, 1994.

30. **Lee MM, Donahoe PK,** Müllerian inhibiting substance: a gonadal hormone with multiple functions, *Endocr Rev* 14:152, 1993.

31. **Gustafson ML, Lee MM, Asmundson L, MacLaughlin DT, Donahoe PK,** Müllerian inhibiting substance in the diagnosis and management of intersex and gonadal abnormalities, *J Pediatr Surg* 28:439, 1993.

32. **Rey R, Mébarki F, Forest MG, Mowszowicz I, Cate RL, Morel Y, Chaussain JL, Josso N,** Anti-müllerian hormone in children with androgen insensitivity, *J Clin Endocrinol Metab* 79:960, 1994.

33. **Siiteri PK, Wilson JD,** Testosterone formation and metabolism during male sexual differentiation in the human embryo, *J Clin Endocrinol Metab* 38:113, 1974.

34. **Rosenfeld CS, Bagegni A, Lubahn DB,** Estrogen receptor-α knockout mice reveal a role for estrogen in mammalian female sexual development (Abstract OR20-3), The Endocrine Society, Annual Meeting, 1998.

35. **Imperato-McGinley J, Peterson RE, Gaultier T, Sturla E,** Androgens and the evolution of male gender identity among male pseudohermaphrodites with 5α-reductase deficiency, *New Engl J Med* 300:1233, 1979.

36. **LeVay S,** A difference in hypothalamic structure between heterosexual and homosexual men, *Science* 253:1034, 1991.

37. **Hofman MA, Swaab DF,** Sexual dimorphism of the human brain: myth and reality, *Exp Clin Endocrinol* 98:161, 1991.

38. **White PC, New MI, Dupont B,** Congenital adrenal hyperplasia, *New Engl J Med* 316:1519, 1987.

39. **White PC, New MI, Dupont B,** Congenital adrenal hyperplasia, *New Engl J Med* 316:1580, 1987.

40. **New MI,** Female pseudohermaphroditism, *Seminars Perinatol* 16:289, 1992.

41. **Speiser PW, Dupont J, Zhu D, Serrat J, Buegeleisen M, Tusie-Luna MT, Lesser M, New MI, White PC,** Disease expression and molecular genotype in congenital adrenal hyperplasia due to 21-hydroxylase deficiency, *J Clin Invest* 90:584, 1992.

42. **Kohn B, Levine LS, Pollack MS, Pang S, Lorenzen F, Levy DJ, Lerner AJ, Gian FR, Dupont B, New MI,** Late-onset steroid 21-hydroxylase deficiency: a variant of classical congenital adrenal hyperplasia, *J Clin Endocrinol Metab* 55:817, 1982.

43. **Spenser PW, New MI,** Genotype and hormonal phenotype in nonclassical 21-OH deficiency, *J Clin Endocrinol Metab* 64:86, 1987.

44. **White PC, Curnow KM, Pascoe L,** Disorders of steroid 11 β-hydroxylase isozymes, *Endocr Rev* 15:421, 1994.

45. **Chua CH, Szabo P, Vitek A, Grzeschik K-H, John M, White PC,** Cloning of cDNA encoding steroid 11 beta-hydroxylase (P450c11), *Proc Natl Acad Sci USA* 84:7193, 1987.

46. **Schram P, Zerah M, Mani P, Jewelewicz R, Jaffe S, New MI,** Nonclassical 3β-hydroxysteroid dehydrogenase deficiency: a review of our experience with 25 female patients, *Fertil Steril* 58:129, 1992.

47. **Azziz R, Bradley Jr EL, Potter HD, Boots LR,** 3β-Hydroxysteroid dehydrogenase deficiency in hyperandrogenism, *Am J Obstet Gynecol* 168:889, 1993.

48. **Zerah M, Rheame E, Mani P, Schram P, Simard J, Labrie F, New MI,** No evidence of mutations in the genes for type I and type II 3β-hydroxysteorid dehydrogenase (3β-HSD) in nonclassic 3β-HSD deficiency, *J Clin Endocrinol Metab* 79:1811, 1994.

49. **Chang YT, Zhang L, Alkaddour HS, Mason JL, Lin K, Yang X, Garibaldi LR, Bourdony CJ, Dolan LM, Donaldson DL, et al,** Absence of molecular defect in the type II 3β-hydroxysteroid dehydrogenase (3β-HSD) gene in premature pubarche children and hirsute female patients with moderately decreased adrenal 3β-HSD activity, *Pediatr Res* 37:820, 1995.

50. **Biglieri EG, Herron MA, Brust N,** 17-Hydroxylation deficiency in man, *J Clin Invest* 45:1946, 1966.

51. **Yanase T, Sanders D, Shibata A, Matsui N, Simpson ER, Waterman MR,** Combined 17α-hydroxylase/17,20-lyase deficiency due to a 7-basepair duplication in the N-terminal region of the cytochrome P450c17 (CYP17) gene, *J Clin Endocrinol Metab* 70:1325, 1990.

52. **Fardella CE, W HD, Homoki J, Miller WL,** Point mutation of Arg440 to His in cytochrome P450c17 causes severe 17α-hydroxylase deficiency, *J Clin Endocrinol Metab* 79:160, 1994.

53. **Sherman SL, Aston CE, Morton NE, Speiser PW, New MI,** A segregation and linkage study of classical and nonclassical 21-hydroxylase deficiency, *Am J Hum Genet* 42:830, 1988.

54. **Rosler A, Weshler N, Leiberman E, Hochberg Z, Weidenfeld J, Sack J, Chemke J,** 11β-hydroxylase deficiency congenital adrenal hyperplasia: update of prenatal diagnosis, *J Clin Endocrinol Metab* 66:830, 1988.

55. **Reindollar RH, Lewis JB, White PC, Fernhoff PM, McDonough PG, Whitney III JB,** Prenatal diagnosis of 21-hydroxylase deficiency by the complementary deoxyribonucleic acid probe for cytochrome P-450C-21OH, *Am J Obstet Gynecol* 158:545, 1988.

56. **Petersen KE, Damkjaer-Nielsen M, Buus O, Couillin P,** Congenital adrenal hyperplasia. Prenatal treatment, *Pediatr Res* 20:1201, 1986.

57. **Forest MG, Betull H, David M,** Antenatal treatment of congenital adrenal hyperplasia due to 21 hydroxylase deficiency: a multicenter study, *Ann Endocrinol (Paris)* 48:31, 1987.

58. **Speiser PW, Laforgia N, Kato K, Pareira J, Khan R, Yang SY, Whorwood C, White PC, Elias S, Schriock E, Schriock E, Simpson JL, Taslimi M, Najjar J, May S, Mills G, Crawford C, New MI,** First trimester prenatal treatment and molecular genetic diagnosis of congenital adrenal hyperplasia (21-hydroxylase deficiency), *J Clin Endocrinol Metab* 70:838, 1990.

59. **Karaviti L, Mercado AB, Mercado MB, Speiser PW, Buegeleisen M, Crawford C, Antonian L, White PC, New MI,** Prenatal diagnosis/treatment in families at risk for infants with steroid 21-hydroxylase deficiency (congenital adrenal hyperplasia), *J Steroid Biochem Mol Biol* 41:445, 1992.

60. **Mercado AB, Wilson RC, Cheng KC, Wei J-Q, New MI,** Prenatal treatment and diagnosis of congenital adrenal hyperplasia owing to steroid 21-hydroxylase deficiency, *J Clin Endocrinol Metab* 80:2014, 1995.

61. **Pang S, Clark AT, Freeman LC, Dolan LM, Immken L, Mueller OT, Stiff D, Shulman DI,** Maternal side effects of prenatal dexamethasone therapy for fetal congenital adrenal hyperplasia, *J Clin Endocrinol Metab* 75:249, 1992.

62. **Therrell Jr BL, Berenbaum SA, Manter-Kapanke V, Simmank J, Korman K, Prentice L, Gonzalez J, Gunn S,** Results of screening 1.9 million Texas newborns for 21-hydroxylase-deficient congenital adrenal hyperplasia, *Pediatrics* 101:583, 1998.

63. **Linder B, Feuillan P, Chrousos GP,** Alternate day prednisone therapy in congenital adrenal hyperplasia: adrenal androgen suppression and normal growth, *J Clin Endocrinol Metab* 69:191, 1989.

64. **Feldman S, Billaud L, Thalabard J-C, Raux-Demay M-C, Mowszowicz I, Kuttenn F, Mauvais-Jarvis P,** Fertility in women with late-onset adrenal hyperplasia due to 21-hydroxylase deficiency, *J Clin Endocrinol Metab* 74:635, 1992.

65. **Morishima A, Grumbach MM, Simpson ER, Fisher C, Qin K,** Aromatase deficiency in male and female siblings caused by a novel mutation and the physiological role of estrogens, *J Clin Endocrinol Metab* 80:3689, 1995.

66. **Laue L, Merke DP, Jones JV, Barnes KM, Hill S, Cutler Jr GB,** A preliminary study of flutamide, testolactone, and reduced hydrocortisone dose in the treatment of congenital adrenal hyperplasia, *J Clin Endocrinol Metab* 81:3535, 1996.

67. **Shozu M, Akasofu K, Harada T, Kubota Y,** A new cause of female pseudohermaphroditism: placental aromatase deficiency, *J Clin Endocrinol Metab* 72:560, 1991.

68. **Conte FA, Grumbach MM, Ito Y, Fisher CR, Simpson ER,** A syndrome of female pseudohermaphrodism, hypergonadotropic hypogonadism, and multicystic ovaries associated with missense mutations in the gene encoding aromatase (P450arom), *J Clin Endocrinol Metab* 78:1287, 1994.

69. **Mullis PE, Yoshimura N, Kuhlmann B, Lippuner K, Jaeger P, Harada H,** Aromatase deficiency in a female who is compound heterozygote for two new point mutations in the P450arom gene: impact of estrogens on hypergonadotropic hypogonadism, multicystic ovaries, and bone densitometry in childhood, *J Clin Endocrinol Metab* 82:1739, 1997.

70. **Morris JM, Mahesh BV,** The syndrome of testicular feminization in male pseudohermaphrodites, *Am J Obstet Gynecol* 65:1192, 1953.

71. **Quigley CA, De Bellis A, Marschke KB, El-Awady MK, Wilson EM, French FS,** Androgen receptor defects: historical, clinical, and molecular perspectives, *Endocr Rev* 16:271, 1995.

72. **Imperato-McGinley J, Pichardo M, Gautier T, Voyer D, Bryden MP,** Cognitive abilities in androgen-insensitive subjects: comparison with control males and females from the same kindred, *Clin Endocrinol* 34:341, 1991.

73. **Manuel M, Katayama KP, Jones Jr HW,** The age of occurrence of gonadal tumors in intersex patients with a Y chromosome, *Am J Obstet Gynecol* 124:293, 1976.

74. **Rutgers JL, Scully RE,** The androgen insensitivity syndrome (testicular feminization): a clinicopathologic study of 43 cases, *Int J Gynecol Path* 10:126, 1991.

75. **Simpson JL,** Genetics of sexual differentiation, In: Rock JA, Carpenter SE, eds. *Pediatic and Adolescent Gynecology,* Raven Press, New York, 1992, p 1.

76. **Griffin JE,** Androgen resistance — the clinical and molecular spectrum, *New Engl J Med* 326:611, 1992.

77. **Grino PB, Griffin JE, Cushard Jr WG, Wilson JD,** A mutation of the androgen receptor associated with partial androgen resistance, familial gynecomastia, and fertility, *J Clin Endocrinol Metab* 66:754, 1988.

78. **Lubahn DB, Joseph DR, Sullivan PM, Willard HF, French FS, Wilson EM,** Cloning of human androgen receptor complementary DNA and localization to the X chromosome, *Science* 240:327, 1988.

79. **Lubahn DB, Brown TR, Simental JA, Higgs HN, Migeon CJ, Wilson EM, French FS,** Sequence of intron/exon junctions of the coding region of the human androgen receptor gene and identification of a point mutation in a family with complete androgen insensitivity, *Proc Natl Acad Sci USA* 86:9534, 1989.

80. **Gottlieb B, Trifiro M, Lumbroso R, Pinsky L,** The androgen receptor gene mutations database, *Nucleic Acids Res* 25:158, 1997.

81. **Brown TR, Lubahn DB, Wilson EM, Joseph DR, French FS, Migeon CJ,** Deletion of the steroid binding domain of the human androgen receptor gene in one family with complete androgen insensitivity syndrome: evidence for further heterogeneity in this syndrome, *Proc Natl Acad Sci USA* 85:8151, 1988.

82. **Trifero M, Gottlieb B, Pinsky L,** The 56/58 K Da androgen binding protein in male genital skin fibroblasts with a deleted androgen receptor gene, *Mol Cell Endocrinol* 75:37, 1991.

83. **Quigley CA, Evans BA, Simental JA, Marschke KB, Sar M, Lubahn DB, Davies P, Hughes IA, Wilson EM, French FS,** Complete androgen insensitivity due to deletion of exon C of the androgen receptor gene highlights the functional importance of the second zinc finger of the androgen receptor in vivo, *Mol Endocrinol* 6:1103, 1992.

84. **Brinkman AO, Jenster G, Kuiper GGJM, Ris C, van Laar JH, van der Korput JAGM, Degenhart HJ, Trifiro MA, Pinsky L, Romalo G, Schweikert HU, Veldscholte J, Mulder E, Trapman J,** The human androgen receptor: structure/function relationship in normal and pathological situations, *J Steroid Biochem Mol Biol* 41:361, 1992.

85. **Marcelli M, Tilley WD, Wilson CM, Wilson JD, Griffin JE, McPhaul MJ,** A single nucleotide substitution introduces a premature termination codon into the androgen receptor gene of a patient with receptor negative androgen resistance, *J Clin Invest* 85:1522, 1990.

86. **Zoppi S, Marcelli M, Deslypere J-P, Griffin JE, Wilson JD, McPhaul MJ,** Amino acid substitutions in the DNA-binding domain of the human androgen receptor are a frequent cause of receptor binding positive androgen resistance, *Mol Endocrinol* 6:409, 1992.

87. **Weidemann W, Peters B, romalo G, Spindler K-D, Schweikert H-U,** Response to androgen treatment in a patient with partial androgen insensitivity and a mutation in the deoxyribonucleic acid-binding domain of the androgen receptor, *J Clin Endocrinol Metab* 83:1173, 1998.

88. **Peterson RE, Imperato-McGinley J, T G, Sturia E,** Male pseudohermaphroditism due to steroid 5α-reductase deficiency, *Am J Med* 62:170, 1977.

89. **Katz MD, Cai L-Q, Zhu Y-S, Herrera C, DeFillo-Ricart M, Shackleton CHL, Imperato-McGinley J,** The biochemical and phenotypic characterization of females homozygous for 5α-reductase-2 deficiency, *J Clin Endocrinol Metab* 80:3160, 1995.

90. **Thigpen AE, Davis DL, Gautier T, Imperato-McGinley J, Russell DW,** Brief report: The molecular basis of steroid 5α-reductase deficiency in a large Dominican kindred, *New Engl J Med* 327:1216, 1992.

91. **Fratianni CM, Imperato-McGinley J,** The syndrome of 5α-reductase-2 deficiency, *Endocrinologist* 4:301, 1994.

92. **Wilson JD, George FW, Griffin JE,** The hormonal control of sexual development, *Science* 211:1278, 1981.

93. **Andersson S, Geissler WM, Wu L, Davis DL, Grumbach MM, New MI, Schwarz HP, Blethen SL, Mendonca BB, Bloise W, Witchel SF, Cutler Jr GB, Griffin JE, Wilson JD, Russell DW,** Molecular genetics and pathophysiology of 17β-hydroxysteorid dehydrogenase 3 deficiency, *J Clin Endocrinol Metab* 81:130, 1996.

94. **Perez-Palacios G, Scaglia HE, Kofman-Alfaro S,** Inherited male pseudohermaphroditism due to gonadotropin unresponsiveness, *Acta Endocrinol* 98:148, 1981.

95. **Kremer H, Kraaij R, Toledo SPA, Post M, Fridman JB, Hayashida CY, van Reen M, Milgrom E, Ropers H, Mariman E, et al,** Male pseudohermaphroditism due to a homozygous missense mutation of the luteinizing hormone receptor gene, *Nat Genet* 9:160, 1995.

96. **Laue L, Wu SM, Kudo M, Hsueh AJ, Cutler Jr GB, Griffin JE, Wilson JD, Brain C, Berry AC, Grant DB, et al,** A nonsense mutation of the human luteinizing hormone receptor gene in Leydig cell hypoplasia, *Hum Mol Genet* 4:1429, 1995.

97. **Misrahi M, Meduri G, Pissard S, Bouvattier C, Beau I, Loosfelt H, Jolivet A, Rappaport R, Milgrom E, Bougneres P,** Comparison of immunocytochemical and molecular features with the phenotype in a case of incomplete male pseudohermaphroditism associated with a mutation of the luteinizing hormone receptor, *J Clin Endocrinol Metab* 82:2159, 1997.

98. **Liscum L, Dahl NK,** Intracellular cholesterol transport, *J Lipid Res* 33:1239, 1992.

99. **Reaven E, Tsai L, Azhar S,** Cholesterol uptake by the 'selective' pathway of ovarian granulsoa cells: early intracellular events, *J Lipid Res* 36:1602, 1995.

100. **Clark BJ, Wells J, King SR, Stocco DM,** The purification, cloning, and expression of a novel LH-induced mitochondrial protein in MA-10 mouse Leydig tumor cells: characterization of the steroidogenic acute regulatory protein (StAR), *J Biol Chem* 269:28314, 1994.

101. **Clark BJ, Soo SC, Caron KM, Ikeda Y, Parker KL, Stocco DM,** Hormonal and developmental regulation of the steroidogenic acute regulatory (StAR) protein, *Mol Endocrinol* 9:1346, 1995.

102. **Lin D, Sugawara T, Strauss III JF, Clark BJ, Stocco DM, Saenger P, Rogol A, Miller WL,** Role of steroidogenic acute regulatory protein in adrenal and gonadal steroidogenesis, *Science* 267:1828, 1995.

103. **Tee M, Lin D, Sugaware T, Holt JA, Guiguen Y, Buckingham B, Strauss III JF, Miller WL,** T-A transversion 11 bp from a splice acceptor site in the human gene for steroidogenic acute regulatory protein causes congenital lipoid adrenal hyperplasia, *Hum Mol Genet* 4:2299, 1995.

104. **Bose H, Pescovitz OH, Miller WL,** Spontaneous feminization in a 46,XX female patient with congenital lipoid adrenal hyperplasia due to a homozygous frameshift mutation in the steroidogenic acute regulatory protein, *J Clin Endocrinol Metab* 82:1511, 1997.

105. **Sugawara T, Holt JA, Driscoll D, Strauss III JF, Lin D, Miller WL, Patterson D, Clancy KP, Hart IM, Clark BJ, Stocco DM,** Human steroidogenic acute regulatory protein: functional activity in COS-1 cells, tissue-specific expression, and mapping of the gene to 8p11.2 and a pseudogene to chromosome 13, *Proc Natl Acad Sci USA* 92:4778, 1995.

106. **Swyer GIM,** Male pseudohermaphroditism: a hitherto undescribed form, *Br Med J* ii:709, 1955.

107. **Coulam CB,** Testicular regression syndrome, *Obstet Gynecol* 53:44, 1979.

108. **Hines RS, Tho SPT, Zhang YY, Plouffe Jr L, Hansen KA, Khan I, McDonough PG,** Paternal somatic and germ-line mosaicism for a sex-determining region on Y (SRY) missense mutation leading to recurrent 46,XY sex reversal, *Fertil Steril* 67:675, 1997.

109. **Simpson JL,** True hermaphroditism: etiology and phenotypic considerations, *Birth Defects* 14:9, 1978.

110. **Krob G, Braun A, Kuhnle U,** True hermaphroditism: geographical distribution, clinical findings, chromosomes and gonadal histology, *Eur J Pediatr* 153:2, 1994.

111. **Berkovitz GD, Fechner PY, Marcantonio SM, Bland G, Stetten G, Goodfellow PN, Smith KD, Migeon CJ,** The role of the sex-determining region of the Y chromosome (SRY) in the etiology of 46,XX true hermaphroditism, *Hum Genet* 88:411, 1992.

112. **Turner HH,** A syndrome of infantilism, congenital webbed neck, and cubitus valgus, *Endocrinology* 28:566, 1938.

113. **Gravholt C, Juul S, Naeraa R, Hansen J,** Prenatal and postnatal prevalence of Turner's syndrome: a registry study, *Br Med J* 312:16, 1996.

114. **Pasquino AM, Passeri F, Pucarelli I, Segni M, Municchi G,** Spontaneous pubertal development in Turner's syndrome. Italian Study Group for Turner's Syndrome, *J Clin Endocrinol Metab* 82:1810, 1997.

115. **Kaneko N, Kawagoe S, Hiroi M,** Turner's syndrome — review of the literature with reference to a successful pregnancy outcome, *Gynecol Obstet Invest* 29:81, 1990.

116. **Chu CE, Conner JM, Donaldson MDC, Kelnar CJH, Smail PJ, Greene SA,** Detection of Y mosaicism in patients with Turner's syndrome, *J Med Genet* 32:578, 1995.

117. **Medlej R, Lobaccaro JM, Berta P, Belon C, Leheup B, Toublanc JE, Weill J, Chevalier C, Dumas R, Sultan C,** Screening for Y-derived sex determining gene SRY in 40 patients with Turner syndrome, *J Clin Endocrinol Metab* 75:1289, 1992.

118. **Kocova M, Siegel SF, Wenger SL, Lee PA, Trucco M,** Detection of Y chromosome sequences in Turner's syndrome by Southern blot analysis of amplified DNA, *Lancet* 342:140, 1993.

119. **Binder G, Koch A, Wajs E, Ranke MB,** Nested polymerase chain reaction study of 53 cases with Turner's syndrome: is cytogenetically undetected Y mosaicism common? *J Clin Endocrinol Metab* 80:3532, 1995.

120. **Berkovitz GD, Fechner PY, Zacur HW, Rock JA, Snyder HM, Migeon CJ, Perlman EJ,** Clinical and pathologic spectrum of 46,XY gonadal dysgenesis: its relevance to the understanding of sex differentiation, *Medicine* 70:375, 1991.

121. **Droesch K, Droesch J, Chumas J, Bronson R,** Laparoscopic gonadectomy for gonadal dysgenesis, *Fertil Steril* 53:360, 1990.

122. **Shalev E, Zabari A, Romano S, Luboshitzky R,** Laparoscopic gonadectomy in 46XY female patient, *Fertil Steril* 57:459, 1992.

123. **Gililland J, Cummings D, Hibbert ML, Crain T, Rozanski T,** Laparoscopic orchiectomy in a patient with complete androgen insensitivity, *J Laparoendoscopic Surg* 3:51, 1993.

124. **Fechner PY, Marcantonio SM, Ogata T, Rosales TO, Smith KD, Goodfellow PN, Migeon CJ, Berkovitz GD,** Report of a kindred with X-linked (or autosomal dominant sex-linked) 46,XY partial gonadal dysgenesis, *J Clin Endocrinol Metab* 76:1248, 1993.

125. **Bardoni B, Zanaria E, Guioli S, Foridia G, Worley KC, Tonini G, Ferrante E, Chiumello G, McCabe ERB, Fraccaro M, Zuffardi O, Camerino G,** A dosage sensitive locus at chromosome Xp21 is involved in male to female sex reversal, *Nature Genet* 7:497, 1994.

126. **Fisher EMC, Beer-Romero P, Brown LG, Ridley A, McNeil JA, Lawrence JB, Willard HF, Bieber FR, Page DC,** Homologous ribosomal protein genes on the human X and Y chromosome: escape from X inactivation and possible implications for Turner syndrome, *Cell* 63:1205, 1990.

127. **Fechner PY, Marcantonio SM, Jaswaney V, Stetten G, Goodfellow PN, Migeon CJ, Smith KD, Berkovitz GD,** The role of the sex-determining region Y gene in the etiology of 46,XX maleness, *J Clin Endocrinol Metab* 76:690, 1993.

128. **Toledo SPA, Brunner HG, Kraaij R, Post M, Dahia PLM, Hayashida CY, Kremer H, Themmen APN,** An inactivating mutation of the luteinizing hormone receptor causes amenorrhea in a 46,XX female, *J Clin Endocrinol Metab* 81:3850, 1996.

129. **Stavrou SS, Zhu Y-S, Cai L-Q, Katz MD, Herrera C, Defillo-Ricart M, Imperato-McGinley J,** A novel mutation of the human luteinizing hormone receptor in 46XY and 46XX sisters, *J Clin Endocrinol Metab* 83:2091, 1998.

130. **Neely EK, Marcus R, Rosenfeld RG, Bachrach LK,** Turner syndrome adolescents receiving growth hormone are not osteopenic, *J Clin Endocrinol Metab* 75:861, 1993.

131. **Nilsson KO, Albertsson-Wikland K, Alm J, Aronson S, Gustafsson J, Hagenäs L, Häger A, Ivarsson SA, Karlberg J, Kriström B, Marcus C, Moell C, Ritzén M, Tuvemo T, Wattsgård C, Westgren U, Westphal O, Åman J,** Improved final height in girls with Turner's syndrome treated with growth hormone and oxandrolone, *J Clin Endocrinol Metab* 81:635, 1996.

132. **Park E, Bailey JD, Cowell CA,** Growth and maturation of patients with Turner's syndrome, *Pediatr Res* 17:1, 1983.

133. **Lyon AL, Preece MA, Grant DB,** Growth curve for girls with Turner syndrome, *Arch Dis Child* 60:932, 1985.

134. **Zadik Z, Landau H, Chen M, Altman Y, Lieberman E,** Assessment of growth hormone (GH) axis in Turner's syndrome using 24-hour integrated concentrations of GH, insulin-like growth factor-I, plasma GH-binding activity, GH binding to IM9 cells, and GH response to pharmacological stimulation, *J Clin Endocrinol Metab* 75:412, 1992.

135. **Rosenfeld RG, Attie KM, Frane J, Brasel JA, Burstein S, Cara JF, Chernausek S, Gotlin RW, Kuntze J, Lippe BM, Mahoney CP, Moore WV, Saenger P, Johanson AJ,** Growth hormone therapy of Turner's syndrome: beneficial effect on adult height, *J Pediatr* 132:319, 1998.

136. **Shaw NJ, Rehan VK, Husain S, Marshall T, Smith CS,** Bone mineral density in Turner's syndrome—a longitudinal study, *Clin Endocrinol* 47:367, 1997.

137. **Gicquel C, Gaston V, Cabrol S, Le Bouc Y,** Assessment of Turner's syndrome by molecular analysis of the X chromosome in growth-retarded girls, *J Clin Endocrnol Metab* 83:1472, 1998.

138. **Allanson JE, Hall JG, Hughes HE, Preus M, Witt RD,** Noonan syndrome: the changing phenotype, *Am J Med Genet* 21:507, 1985.

139. **Myers-Seifer CH, Charest NJ,** Diagnosis and management of patients with ambiguous genitalia, *Seminars Perinatol* 16:332, 1992.

140. **Siegel MJ,** Pediatric gynecologic sonography, *Radiology* 179:593, 1991.

141. **Hricak H, Chang YCF, Thurnher S,** Vagina: evaluation with MR imaging. Part I: Normal anatomy and congenital anomalies, *Radiology* 169:169, 1988.

142. **Hawkins JR, Taylor A, Goodfellow PN, Migeon CJ, Smith KD, Berkovitz GD,** Evidence for increased prevalence of SRY mutations in XY females with complete rather than partial gonadal dysgenesis, *Am J Hum Genet* 51:979, 1992.

143. **Coran AG, Porley TZ,** Surgical management of ambiguous genitalia in the infant and child, *J Pediatr Surg* 26:812, 1991.

144. **Donahoe PK, Powell DM, Lee MK,** Clinical management of intersex abnormalities, *Curr Prob Surg* 28:515, 1992.

145. **Ljungqvist A, Simpson JL,** Medical examination for health of all athletes replacing the need for gender verification in international sports: the International Amateur Athletic Federation plan, *JAMA* 267:850, 1992.

10　Abnormal Puberty and Growth Problems

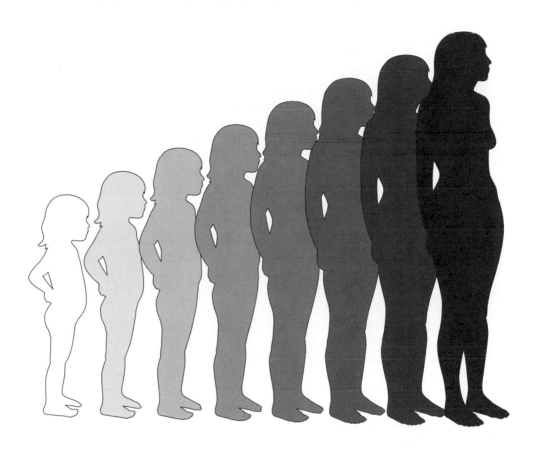

I n many societies throughout history, puberty has been a time of celebration. The changes of puberty announce the acquisition of fertility. However, it is precisely these psychological, social, and cultural forces that make this a stressful, difficult transition for many individuals. Unfortunately, the earlier age of puberty in modern times has made it difficult to cope with an earlier sexuality. Early teenage pregnancies are a relatively new problem (previously they were a biological impossibility). This change in modern life, probably due to improved nutrition and living conditions, makes it all the more important to understand puberty.

The ability to diagnose and manage disorders of female pubescence requires a thorough understanding of the physical and hormonal events that mark the evolution of the child into a sexually mature adult capable of reproduction. Abnormalities in this process of developmental endocrinology either lead to premature, attenuated, or retarded (delayed) puberty. This chapter reviews the important landmarks and mechanisms of normal female maturation as well as the abnormalities which lead to precocious or delayed puberty.

The Physiology of Puberty

The Period of Infancy and Childhood

The hypothalamus, anterior pituitary gland, and gonads of the fetus, neonate, the prepubertal infant and child are all capable of secreting hormones in adult concentrations. Even during fetal life, serum concentrations of follicle-stimulating hormone (FSH) and luteinizing hormone (LH) reach adult levels at midgestation but fall thereafter as the high level of pregnancy steroid hormones exerts inhibitory feedback.[1] Separation of the newborn from its sources of maternal and placental estrogen and progesterone releases newborn FSH and LH from this negative feedback. A prompt rise in gonadotropin secretion follows (along with an increase in inhibin B levels) that, in female neonates, may occasionally reach levels greater than those in the normal adult menstrual cycle.[2, 3] As a result, transient estradiol secretion equivalent to the level of the midfollicular phase of the menstrual cycle is induced and is associated with waves of ovarian follicle maturation and atresia. Full negative feedback is rapidly attained; ovarian steroids and gonadotropins decline and remain at very low levels until 6–8 years of age. During this period, the hypothalamic-pituitary system controlling gonadotropins (the "gonadostat") is highly sensitive to negative feedback of estrogen (estradiol concentration in these years remains low at 10 pg/mL). Studies on gonadal dysgenesis and other hypogonadal infants indicate that the "gonadostat" is 6–15 times more sensitive to negative feedback at this period than in the adult.[4] Therefore, gonadotropin secretion is in part restrained by even extraordinarily low levels of estrogen.

This reduction in the infant's gonadotropins is not entirely due to exquisite sensitivity to negative feedback. Low levels of FSH and LH even exist in hypogonadal children (with gonadal dysgenesis) between the ages of 5 and 11 years and are similar to the low levels in normal infants of this age.[5] Because gonadotropin-releasing hormone (GnRH) infusion stimulates moderate LH and FSH secretion in these agonadal subjects, a central nonsteroidal suppressor of endogenous GnRH and gonadotropin synthesis appears to be operative.[6]

Although peptide hormone concentrations are low throughout infancy and the prepubertal child, FSH and LH display evidence of pulsatile secretion.[7–9] As noted, pituitary gonadotropins react with small but significant responses to exogenously administered GnRH, which although quantitatively less than those achieved in puberty are nevertheless capable of inducing the immature gonad to respond with modest steroid secretion. Immaturity of the various endocrine components is not the rate-limiting factor in the onset of puberty.

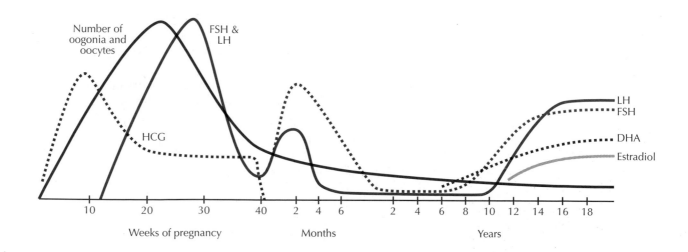

The Prepubertal Period

As puberty approaches, three critical changes in the low endocrine homeostatic function of childhood emerge:

1. Adrenarche.

2. Decreasing repression of the "gonadostat."

3. Gradual amplification of the peptide-peptide and peptide-steroid interactions leading to "gonadarche."

Adrenarche

The growth of pubic and axillary hair is due to an increased production of adrenal androgens at puberty. Thus, this phase of puberty is often referred to as adrenarche (or pubarche). ***Premature adrenarche*** by itself is occasionally seen; i.e., pubic and axillary hair without any other sign of sexual development. ***Premature thelarche*** (breast development) without other signs of puberty is very rare, but does occur. Increased adrenal cortical function, expressed by a rise in circulating dehydroepiandrosterone (DHA), dehydroepiandrosterone sulfate (DHAS), and androstenedione associated with increased adrenal 17α-hydroxylase and 17,20-lyase activity (the P450c17 enzyme), occurs progressively in late childhood from about age 6–7 to adolescence (13–15 years of age).[10] This steroid secretion is associated with an increase in size and differentiation of the inner zone (zona reticularis) of the cortex. Generally, the beginning of adrenarche precedes by 2 years the linear growth spurt, the rise in estrogens and gonadotropins of early puberty, and menarche at midpuberty. Because of this temporal relationship, activation of adrenal androgen secretion has been suggested as a possible initiating event in the ontogeny of the pubertal transition.

Considerable evidence, however, supports a *dissociation* of the control mechanisms that initiate adrenarche and those governing GnRH-pituitary-ovarian maturation ("gonadarche").[11] Premature adrenarche (precocious appearance of pubic and axillary hair before age 8 years) is not associated with a parallel abnormal advancement of gonadarche.[12] In hypergonadotropic hypogonadism (gonadal dysgenesis) or in hypogonadotropic states such as Kallmann's syndrome, adrenarche occurs despite the absence of gonadarche. When adrenarche is absent, as in children with cortisol-treated Addison's disease (hypoadrenalism), gonadarche still occurs. Finally, in true precocious puberty occurring before 6 years of age, gonadarche precedes adrenarche.

Plasma levels of adrenal androgens change without corresponding changes in cortisol and ACTH during fetal life, puberty, and aging. Furthermore, in other circumstances such as chronic disease, surgical stress, recovery from secondary adrenal insufficiency, and anorexia nervosa, changes in ACTH-induced cortisol secretion are not accompanied by corresponding changes in plasma adrenal androgen levels.[13] Thus, adrenarche does not appear to be under direct control of gonadotropins or ACTH.

A pituitary adrenal androgen stimulating factor formed by cleavage of a high molecular weight precursor, proopiomelanocortin (POMC), which also contains ACTH and β-lipotropin, acting on an ACTH prepared and maintained adrenal, has been suggested as the agent stimulating adrenarche. A large glycoprotein has been identified that also displayed adrenal androgen stimulating activity.[14] However, in a study confirming the dissociation between plasma adrenal androgens and cortisol in children and adolescents with Cushing's disease and ectopic ACTH producing tumors, all known proopiomelanocortin-related peptides, including ACTH, β-endorphin, and β-lipotropin did not have a determinative role in the initiation of adrenarche.[15] Studies fail to demonstrate a relationship between melatonin secretion and adrenarche.[16]

A study of the kinetics of the 3β-hydroxysteroid dehydrogenase enzyme in human adrenal microsomes suggests that the changes in adrenal secretion from fetal life to adulthood can be explained by local steroid inhibition of key enzymes within the adrenal, acting to a variable degree in different layers of the cortex and at different stages of development.[17] Puberty is associated with the emerging prominence of a zona reticularis (the source of DHA and DHAS) that is relatively deficient in 3β-hydroxysteroid dehydrogenase activity, a state that is maintained during adult life.[18, 19] The factors that regulate and suppress this enzyme activity remain unknown. Another hypothesis suggests that serine phosphorylation of P450c17 is necessary for 17,20-lyase activity, and that this phosphorylation, stimulated by a yet unknown mechanism, is responsible for the initiation of adrenarche.[20] It is fair to say that the factors controlling adrenarche remain obscure.

Decreasing Repression of the "Gonadostat"

Regardless of its relation to adrenarche, factors which induce gonadarche in late prepuberty involve derepression of the central nervous system (CNS)-pituitary gonadostat, progressive responsiveness of the anterior pituitary to exogenous (and presumably endogenous) GnRH, and follicle reactivity to FSH and LH.

For approximately 8 years, from early infancy to the prepubertal period, LH and FSH are suppressed to very low levels. The mechanisms for this restraint on gonadotropin secretion are a highly sensitive negative feedback of low level gonadal estrogen on hypothalamic and pituitary sites, and an intrinsic central inhibitory influence on GnRH that reduces basal gonadotropin concentrations even in agonadal children. Gonadal dysgenesis patients display marked elevations of gonadotropins for the first 2–3 years of life. Thereafter, a striking decline in concentrations of FSH and LH occurs, reaching a nadir at 6–8 years. By age 10–11 (at the time puberty would have occurred), however, gonadotropins are elevated once again to the postmenopausal range. The overall pattern of basal gonadotropin secretion in agonadal children is qualitatively similar to that observed in normal females.

Whereas negative feedback inhibition may play the more important role in early childhood, the central intrinsic inhibitor becomes functionally dominant in midchildhood and persists up to prepuberty. Suppression of, or damage to, the neural source of this inhibition has been postulated in the pathogenesis of the precocious puberty secondary to hypothalamic lesions that compress or destroy posterior hypothalamic areas.[21] Thus, normal pubertal timing of gonadarche, with the reactivation of gonadotropin synthesis and secretion, results from the combined reduction in intrinsic suppression of GnRH and decreased sensitivity to the negative feedback of estrogen.[22]

It has been suggested that the reversal of central intrinsic suppression is due to a reduction in melatonin secretion by the pineal gland. In lower animals affected by photoperiodicity, pineal melatonin appears to inhibit hypothalamic-pituitary gland secretion. While melatonin may play a role in the altered timing of puberty associated with pineal tumors and in the pathophysiology of central precocious puberty, there is no evidence that it is important in the physiologic onset of normal puberty in humans.[23] In two large studies of circadian rhythms of serum melatonin from infancy to adulthood (1–18 years) the decline in the nocturnal surge of melatonin, thought to have been exclusively related to the pubertal conversion, was observed to begin in infancy and progressively decline through pubescence.[24, 25] Pinealectomy in agonadal primates does not prevent the inhibition of FSH and LH seen during transition from infancy to childhood nor the return of gonadotropins with the advent of puberty.[26]

The fascinating search for the factor(s) involved in the derepression of the "gonadostat" so crucial to the timing of puberty continues. POMC-related peptides do not appear to change during the transitional period.[27] The ontogeny of the GnRH gene and its expression, so elegantly demonstrated in rodents, is yet to be extended to the primate.

Alteration and Amplification of GnRH-Gonadotropin and Gonadotropin-Ovarian Steroid Interactions

FSH and LH levels increase during the progress through the stages of puberty. Rhythmic pulses of GnRH given to immature rhesus monkeys will initiate activity of the pituitary-gonadal apparatus, supporting the primacy of endogenous GnRH in the establishment and maintenance of puberty. Similar effects have been demonstrated in prepubertal girls.[28] Normal pubertal maturation in girls is also accompanied by changes in the pattern of gonadotropin responses to the hypothalamic-releasing hormone GnRH. FSH responses to GnRH are initially pronounced but decrease steadily throughout the onset of puberty. In contrast, LH responses are low in prepubertal girls and increase strikingly during puberty.[29] This is the basis of the observation that in general FSH rises initially and plateaus in midpuberty while LH tends to rise more slowly and reaches adult levels in late puberty. The increased amplitude and frequency of pulsatile GnRH are believed to provoke progressively enhanced responses of FSH and LH secretion. GnRH acts as a self-primer on the gonadotrope cells of the anterior pituitary by inducing cell surface receptors specific for GnRH and necessary for its action (up-regulation). Thus, gonadotrope cells increase their capacity to respond to GnRH first by synthesis and later by secretion of gonadotropins. As gonadotropin secretion appears, ovarian follicle steroid synthesis is stimulated and estrogen secretion rises.

Elsewhere (Chapters 5 and 6), the evidence for the dichotomous effects of estrogen feedback on the anterior pituitary has been reviewed. Suffice to say, by midpuberty estrogen enhances LH secretory responses to GnRH (positive feedback) while combining with inhibin to maintain relative inhibition (negative feedback) of FSH response.

The amplification of peptide-steroid interactions during pubescence is not restricted to the GnRH impact on gonadotropin or steroid feedback on the pituitary and hypothalamus. As the pubertal transition advances there is a disproportionate rise of biologically potent LH beyond the increase seen in immunologic LH. This marked increase in the bioactive to immunoreactive ratio is due to molecular alterations in the glycosylation pattern of LH, as reviewed in Chapter 2 under "Heterogeneity."[30]

Prior to puberty, gonadotropin levels are low but still associated with pulses.[9] The onset of augmented GnRH pulses first occurs during sleep. There is sleep-associated release of LH in both sexes, a consequence of LH responses to endogenous GnRH. The early stages of puberty are associated with a marked nocturnal augmentation of FSH and LH pulses (both amplitude and frequency, but especially frequency); this difference between nighttime and daytime switches by late puberty with an increase in daytime and a decrease in sleep pulsatility.[8, 31–33] It should be noted that day-night differences exist before puberty, but the differences become more marked with the onset of puberty. This change is not abrupt with the onset of puberty. Very sensitive assays can detect an increase in FSH and LH (both day and night) in the months preceding the beginning of breast development.[31]

Sleep-related LH pulses also are seen in children with idiopathic precocious puberty, in anorexia nervosa patients during intermediate stages of exacerbation and recovery, and also in agonadal patients during the pubertal age period when their gonadotropins are returning from mid-childhood reductions.[34] GnRH pulses appear and are maintained independent of steroid feedback.

Puberty

The cascade of events initiated by the release of pulsatile GnRH from prepubertal feedback and central negative inhibition results in increased levels of gonadotropins and steroids with appearance of secondary sexual characteristics and eventual adult function (menarche and, later, ovulation). Between the ages of 10 and 16 the endocrine sequence observed includes, first, increased pulsatile patterns of LH during sleep, followed by similar pulses of less amplitude occurring throughout the 24-hour day. Episodic peaks of estradiol result and menarche appears.

By mid to late puberty, maturation of the positive feedback relationship between estradiol and LH is established, leading to ovulatory cycles.

Timing of Puberty

Although the major determinant of the timing of puberty is genetic, other factors appear to influence the time of initiation and the rate of progression of puberty: geographic location, exposure to light, general health and nutrition, and psychologic factors. For example, children with a family history of early puberty start early.[35] Children closer to the equator, at lower altitudes, those in urban areas, and mildly obese children start earlier than those in Northern latitudes, at higher elevations above sea level, in rural areas, and normal weight children, respectively. There is a fairly good correlation between the times of menarche of mothers and daughters and between sisters.[35] There is a correlation between age of onset and duration of puberty; the earlier the onset, the longer the duration.[36]

The decline in the age of menarche displayed by children in developed countries undoubtedly reflects improved nutritional status and healthier living conditions. Frisch argued that a critical body weight (47.8 kg) must be reached by a girl to achieve menarche.[37] Possibly more important than total weight is the shift in body composition to a greater percent fat (from 16.0 to 23.5%), which in turn is influenced by the nutritional state.[38] Indeed, moderately obese girls (20–30% over normal weight) have earlier menarche than normal weight girls.[39] Conversely, anorectics and intense exercisers (low weight or low percent fat component of weight) have delayed menarche or secondary amenorrhea. That other factors are involved is indicated by the delayed menarche experienced by morbidly obese girls (greater than 30% overweight), diabetics, and intense exercisers of normal weight. Intriguingly, blind girls experience earlier menarche.[40] Furthermore, girls with idiopathic central precocious puberty may undergo menarche at a total body fat of 19%, and girls with no signs of puberty may have measured total body fat of 27%.[41]

It is reasonable to hypothesize that central mechanisms bring about maturation of the hypothalamic-pituitary-ovarian axis, which in turn stimulates growth to the critical weight as well as the increases in body fat composition. However, not all auxologic studies have found a relationship between the onset of puberty and either body fat mass or body fat distribution.[42] Nevertheless, the identification of leptin (discussed in Chapter 19) has revitalized the importance of a relationship between body fat and reproductive function.

Leptin is a peptide secreted in adipose tissue that circulates in the blood bound to a family of proteins, and acts on the central nervous system neurons that regulate eating behavior and energy balance. Several observations support a role for leptin in reproductive physiology.

1. Leptin administration accelerates the onset of puberty in rodents.[43]

2. Leptin levels increase at puberty in boys.[44]

3. Low leptin levels are present in athletes and in patients with anorexia, or delayed puberty.[45]

4. Mice lacking leptin undergo normal sexual development, but remain prepubertal and never ovulate, but fertility is restored with leptin administration.[43]

Leptin levels increase during childhood until the onset of puberty, suggesting that a threshold level of leptin (and, therefore, a critical amount of adipose tissue, the source of leptin) is necessary for puberty to begin.[46] The higher the level of leptin, the earlier the age of menarche.[47] Girls with idiopathic precocious puberty have higher levels of leptin.[48] These relationships support the existence of communication between the central nervous system and body fat in the process of puberty, with leptin serving as the messenger.

After puberty, leptin levels in boys return to the prepubertal range (apparent suppression by testosterone). In girls, leptin levels are higher than in boys and decrease with increasing Tanner stages of puberty.[49] Thus with puberty, there is increasing sensitivity to leptin. Or, in another way to look at this relationship, a decrease in leptin during puberty may allow greater food intake for growth by lowering the satiety signal.

Stages of Pubertal Development

On the average, the pubertal sequence of accelerated growth, breast development, adrenarche, and menarche requires a period of 4.5 years (range 1.5 to 6 years). The largest body of data was accumulated in healthy European girls; current North American standards are approximately 6 months earlier for each stage.[50–56] Secondary sex characteristics develop earlier in black girls than in white girls.

In the early 1990s, the American Academy of Pediatrics performed a cross-sectional study of pubertal development in American girls seen in pediatric office practices.[57] Although this study was handicapped by deriving data from office practices rather than a randomized population sampling, it is the largest study available, containing 17,077 girls (9.6% black Americans and 90.4% white). The important findings are as follows:

	Black Americans	White Americans
Breast and/or pubic hair at age 7:	27.2%	6.7%
at age 8:	48.3%	14.7%
Menarche at age 11:	27.9%	13.4%
at age 12:	62.1%	35.2%
Mean age for thelarche:	8.87 years	9.96 years
Mean age for adrenarche:	8.78 years	10.51 years
Mean age for menarche:	12.16 years	12.88 years

The data from the American Academy of Pediatrics study indicates that a substantial number of girls display development 6 months to one year earlier than previously documented, although the age of menarche has remained stable. On average, black American girls begin puberty between ages 8 and 9, and white American girls by age 10.

In general, the first sign of puberty is an acceleration of growth followed by breast budding (thelarche). Breast development follows a well-recognized sequence of events. Breast budding is a change distinguished by enlargement and elevation of the nipples and areolae. This is followed by elevation of the breast by the building of the breast mound. Just prior to the formation of the final adult contours, the areolae form secondary mounds.

Although the sequence may be reversed, adrenarche usually appears after the breast bud with axillary hair growth 2 years later. In approximately 20% of children, pubic hair growth is the first sign of puberty. Menarche is a late event, occurring after the peak of growth has passed.

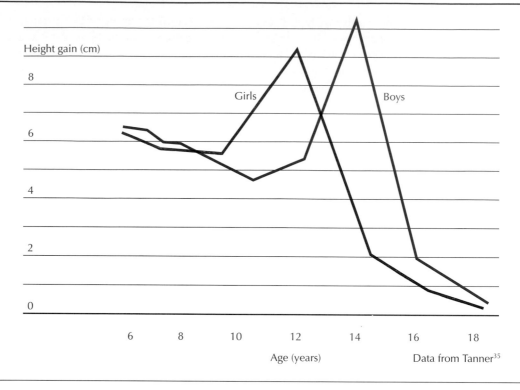

Growth

An adolescent girl's growth spurt occurs 2 years earlier (at 11–12 years) than that of a boy, and in 1 year, her rate of growth doubles, yielding a height increment of between 6 and 11 cm (2.4–4.3 inches).[58] The average girl reaches this growth peak about 2 years after breast budding and 1 year prior to menarche. Evidence suggests that growth acceleration is due to estrogen and concomitant increases in growth hormone production and secondary stimulation of insulin-like growth factor-I (IGF-I) levels.[59] Adrenal androgens are not involved because cortisol-repleted Addisonian patients display normal pubertal growth patterns.

In a remarkable study of African pygmies, it was discovered that the short stature of adult pygmies is due primarily to a failure of growth to accelerate during puberty, and that the principal factor responsible for normal pubertal growth is insulin-like growth factor-I (IGF-I).[60] Growth hormone exerts its action through a locally produced mediator, insulin-like growth factor-I. In addition, growth hormone can directly stimulate epiphyseal cartilage growth. Normal growth at puberty requires the concerted action of growth hormone, insulin-like growth factor-I, and sex steroids. The increase in circulating insulin-like growth factor-I at puberty correlates with sexual development and results from the interaction between sex steroids and growth hormone. Specifically, the increase in sex steroids in turn increases the secretion of growth hormone, which stimulates the production of insulin-like growth factor-I.[61] However, studies also indicate that the sex steroids can have a direct effect on bone growth independent of growth hormone.[62] Thus, Laron-type dwarfs (who have a genetic defect in the growth hormone receptor and cannot stimulate IGF-I secretion) can undergo a growth spurt at puberty in response to the sex steroids. However, normal pubertal growth velocities require the combined action of the sex steroids and growth hormone. The sex steroid hormones also limit the ultimate height attained by stimulating epiphyseal fusion. The principal sex steroid involved in pubertal growth is probably estrogen in both boys and girls, with aromatization of androgens being the source of estrogen in boys.[63]

The most abundant hormone produced by the pituitary gland is growth hormone, which is secreted not as a single substance but as one predominant form and one smaller variant.[64] Growth hormone is encoded by 5 genes located on chromosome 17q22-q24. One gene is for the predominant form in the pituitary; 3 of the genes are expressed in the placenta. The pituitary gene is regulated by growth hormone-releasing hormone, thyroid hormone, and glucocorticoids.

Besides the stimulation of IGF-I in cartilage, growth hormone also stimulates IGF-I production in a variety of tissues throughout the body, especially in the liver (the main source of circulating IGF-I).

The hepatic production of insulin-like growth factor binding protein-1 (IGFBP-1) is regulated by insulin. The circulating levels of IGFBP-1 decrease throughout puberty, in response to the relative hyperinsulinemia that accompanies puberty in response to increasing insulin resistance.[65] This change would allow greater metabolic activity of IGF-I, an important mediator of growth.

Like the gonadotropins, growth hormone is secreted in pulsatile fashion, and during puberty, the amplitude of the pulses increases, especially during sleep. Your grandmother was right when she said: sleep and you'll grow. The age at which an increase in pulse amplitude first occurs corresponds to the age of most rapid growth. The growth response to growth hormone is correlated with the increases in pulse amplitude, not a change in baseline levels.[66, 67] Slower growing children display fewer and smaller pulses of growth hormone. The pulsatile pattern of growth hormone secretion is regulated by stimulation from growth hormone-releasing hormone and inhibition from somatropin release-inhibiting hormone, both released into the hypothalmic-pituitary portal circulation from hypothalamic nuclei. This mechanism is influenced at multiple levels by estrogens and androgens. Prior to puberty, the sex steroid hormones are not involved with growth hormone secretion, beyond a low maintenance effect on secretion. At puberty, however, the dynamics of growth hormone secretion are critically dependent on the gonadal sex steroid hormones. Growth hormone secretion must be very sensitive to the stimulatory effect of estrogens because growth hormone levels increase before any signs of sexual development appear.

The amounts of estrogen required to stimulate long-bone cortical growth are incredibly small. Doses of 100 nanograms of estradiol per kilogram body weight per day increase the amplitude of growth hormone pulsatile secretion and produce maximal growth in agonadal recipients. These doses are insufficient to cause breast budding, vaginal cornification, or an increase in sex hormone-binding globulin.[68, 69] These low dose effects are consistent with the observation that girls attain peak height velocity early in puberty at a serum estradiol concentration of 20 pg/mL which is one-sixth the mean level of adult women. Furthermore, at low doses, estrogen stimulates growth hormone-induced IGF-I secretion, while high doses suppress IGF-I levels.

Estrogen is a critical hormone in both males and females. Males with mutations in the estrogen receptor alpha or who have aromatase deficiencies grow slowly and have markedly reduced bone densities.[70, 71] Analysis of the decline in testosterone and estrogen circulating levels with aging indicates that the amount of bioavailable estrogen circulating in the blood is the most consistent predictor of bone density in men and women.[72] And most impressively, a man with an aromatase deficiency, treated with estrogen, demonstrated that both androgens and estrogens are necessary in order to for males to reach optimal bone mass.[73]

Osteoporosis and vertebral fractures are less common in black than in white women. Vertebral bone density increases rapidly and significantly during adolescence, and the increase is greater in black girls, providing one explanation for the racial difference in osteoporosis.[74] The pubertal increase in bone density ranges from 10% to 20%, an accumulation which provides 10–20 years of protection against the normal age-related loss of skeletal mass. Calcium supplementation during adolescence results in a significant increase in bone density and skeletal mass, providing even greater protection against future osteoporosis.[75] Optimal growth has both immediate and long-term consequences. Adolescents with abnormal menstrual function (suppressed estrogen levels) should not be ignored, but properly evaluated and treated. The influence of the sex steroid levels on bone mass is underscored by the fact that almost all of the bone mass in the hip and the vertebral bodies will be accumulated in young women by late adolescence (age 18), and the years immediately following menarche (11–14) are especially important.[76, 77]

Menarche

As mentioned previously, environmental factors are important in the onset of puberty. Improved living standards and nutrition in the mother antenatally, and in children postnatally, have played a significant role in producing taller, heavier children with earlier maturation. Studies of identical twins and nonidentical twins indicate that the age at menarche is chiefly controlled by genetic factors when the environment is optimal. In affluent cultures, the trend toward lowering of the menarcheal age and puberty halted around 1960.[51] In the 1700s, the mean age of voice change in the Boys' Bach Choir in Leipzig was 18, now it is 13.5 years. Recent studies have indicated a very slight upward trend in the age of menarche, perhaps a response to some environmental deterioration.[78]

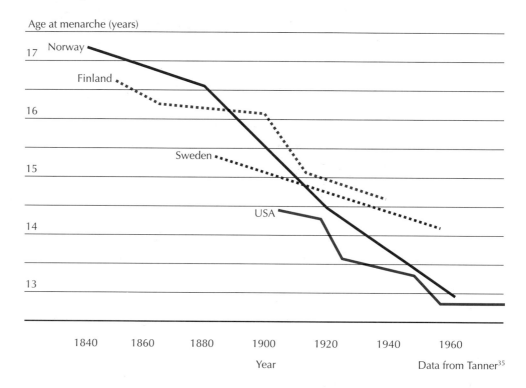

The relationship between menarche and the growth spurt is relatively fixed: menarche occurs after the peak in growth velocity has passed. Hence slower growth, totaling no more than 6 cm (2.4 inches) is noted after initiation of menses.

The normal age range of menarche in U.S. girls is 9.1–17.7 years with a median of 12.8.[51, 52] The final endocrine hallmark of puberty is the development of positive estrogen feedback on the pituitary and hypothalamus. This feedback stimulates the midcycle surge of LH required for ovulation. Thus, the menses following menarche are usually anovulatory, irregular, and occasionally heavy. Anovulation lasts as long as 12–18 months after menarche, but there are reports of pregnancy before menarche. Ovulation increases in frequency as puberty progresses, but it is common for 25–50% of adolescents to still be anovulatory 4 years after menarche.[53, 54]

Summary of Pubertal Events

The onset of puberty is an evolving sequence of maturational steps. The hypothalamic-pituitary-gonadal system differentiates and functions during fetal life and early infancy. Thereafter, it is suppressed to low activity levels during childhood by a combination of hypersensitivity of the "gonadostat" to estrogen negative feedback and an intrinsic CNS inhibitor. All the components located below GnRH (below the CNS) are competent to respond at all ages (as will be seen in the pathogenesis of precocious puberty). After a decade of functional GnRH insufficiency (between

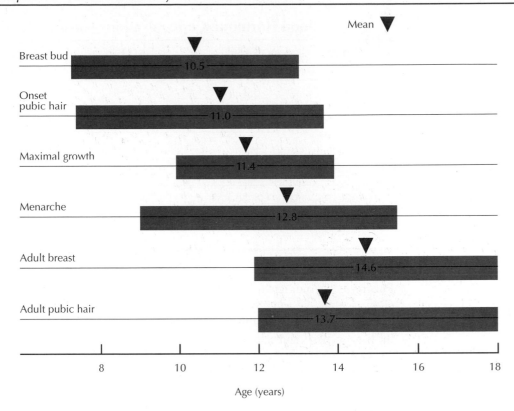

Age (years)

late infancy and the onset of puberty), GnRH secretion is resumed and gonadarche (the reactivation of the CNS-pituitary-ovarian apparatus) appears. Prolongation of intrinsic CNS suppression or disability in any of the components of the gonadarche cascade leads to delayed or absent pubescence.

1. FSH and then LH levels rise moderately before the age of 10 and are followed by a rise in estradiol. An increase in LH pulses is first seen only in sleep but gradually extends throughout the day. In the adult, they occur at roughly 1.5–2 hourly intervals.

2. As gonadal estrogen increases (gonadarche), breast development, female fat distribution, and vaginal and uterine growth occur. Skeletal growth rapidly increases as a result of initial gonadal secretion of low levels of estrogen, which increases the secretion of growth hormone, which in turn stimulates the production of IGF-I.

3. Adrenal androgen (adrenarche) and, to a lesser degree, gonadal androgen secretion cause pubic and axillary hair growth. Adrenarche plays little, if any, part in skeletal growth. While temporarily related to gonadarche, adrenarche is an independent, functionally unrelated biological event.

4. At midpuberty, sufficient gonadal estrogen secretion proliferates the endometrium, and the first menses (menarche) occurs.

5. Postmenarcheal cycles are initially anovulatory. Sustained, predictable positive LH surge responses to estradiol with ovulation are late pubertal events.

Blood Hormone Concentrations During Female Puberty [79–85]

Tanner Stage	FSH IU/L	LH IU/L	Estradiol pg/mL	DHA ng/dL
Stage 1	0.9–5.1	1.8–9.2	<10	19–302
Stage 2	1.4–7.0	2.0–16.6	7–37	45–1904
Stage 3	2.4–7.7	5.6–13.6	9–59	125–1730
Stage 4	1.5–11.2	7–14.4	10–156	153–1321
Adult: follicular	3–20	5–25	30–100	162–1620

Precocious Puberty

Puberty is the biologic transition between immature and adult reproductive function. Its timing, endocrine milieu, and physical expressions have been characterized sufficiently to set clinically reasonable time limits for the normal appearance of female maturity and to allow recognition of the pathogenesis and pathophysiology of most of the causes of premature or delayed pubescence.

If one accepts the mean ±2.5 standard deviations as encompassing the normal range, then pubertal changes before the age of 8 are regarded as precocious. However, the most recent cross-sectional study (by the American Academy of Pediatrics) indicates that a substantial number of normal girls begin pubertal development before age 8.[57] Certainly, thelarche and adrenarche before age 6 deserves evaluation. From age 6 to age 8, the clinician's response will be influenced by the anxiety and distress in patient and parents, and the clinical presentation. Increased growth is often the first change in precocious puberty. This is usually followed by breast development and growth of pubic hair. On occasion, adrenarche, thelarche, and linear growth occur simultaneously. Menarche, however, can be the first sign.

Traditionally, precocious puberty has been divided into two classifications:

1. **GnRH-Dependent Precocious Puberty.** Complete, isosexual, central (or specifically GnRH- and gonadotropin-dependent) precocity — also known as *true precocious puberty.* These terms all refer to early activation of the hypothalamic-pituitary-gonadal axis.

2. **GnRH-Independent Precocious Puberty.** Incomplete, isosexual or heterosexual, peripheral or *precocious pseudopuberty.* Sexual maturation in these instances may be due to extra pituitary secretion of human chorionic gonadotropin (HCG) or sex steroid secretion independent of hypothalamic-pituitary gonadotropin stimulation. Thus, this mechanism is GnRH-independent.

In clinical practice, these classifications are of little practical use. Precocity occurs in girls 5 times more frequently than boys, and almost three-quarters of precocity in girls is idiopathic. Nevertheless, in the face of any precocious development, the clinician is obligated to rule out a serious disease process in central or peripheral sites. In girls over 4 years old a specific etiology is rarely found. In younger girls, a CNS lesion is usually present.

A classification of sexual precocity is presented to provide a guide to the possible conditions and the relative incidences encountered. It should be noted that a GnRH-dependent cause is found in up to 80% of girls, with a lesser occurrence in boys. Ovarian tumors, adrenal disease, and the McCune-Albright syndrome make up the majority of noncentral precocity in girls.

Classification and Relative Occurrence of Precocious Puberty[86–88]

	Female	Male
GnRH-Dependent (True Precocity)		
Idiopathic	74.0%	41.0%
CNS problem	7.0%	26.0%
GnRH-Independent (Precocious Pseudopuberty)		
Ovarian (cyst or tumor)	11.0%	—
Testicular	—	10.0%
McCune-Albright syndrome	5.0%	1.0%
Adrenal feminizing	1.0%	0.0%
Adrenal masculinizing	1.0%	22.0%
Ectopic gonadotropin production	0.5%	0.5%

Particular attention should be given to the following possibilities: drug ingestion, cerebral problems such as cranial trauma or encephalitis, retarded growth with symptoms of hypothyroidism, and a pelvic or abdominal mass. A left hand-wrist film (for use with atlases) should be obtained for bone age. Determination of thyroid function is indicated, and blood levels of gonadotropins and steroids should be measured. CT or MRI imaging of the brain is indicated in patients with precocious puberty, even in the face of a normal overall evaluation, including normal routine skull x-rays. Other procedures should be dictated by the clinical findings. Virilization, of course, demands a full adrenal evaluation.

Sexual development does not require ovulatory capability. Evaluation of a patient's possible fertility, for example, with basal body temperatures or progesterone assays, is an unnecessary procedure. More importantly, complete sexual precocity with potential fertility and adult levels of gonadotropins does not rule out the possibility of a serious disease process (e.g., a CNS tumor). While it is true that the most common form of sexual precocity in females is idiopathic or constitutional precocity (true sexual precocity), this must be a diagnosis by exclusion with prolonged follow-up in an effort to detect slowly developing lesions of the brain, ovary, or adrenal gland.

GnRH-Dependent Precocious Puberty (Precocious Development Due to Stimulation of Gonadotropin Secretion, True Precocious Puberty)

The signs of *constitutional* sexual precocity are due to premature maturation of the hypothalamic-pituitary-ovarian axis, resulting in production of gonadotropins and sex steroids. These patients experience an increase in growth that is associated with pubertal levels of insulin-like growth factor-I. Constitutional precocity runs in families and usually occurs very close to the "borderline" age of 8 years. On the other hand, *idiopathic* precocious puberty does not run in families and occurs much earlier in childhood. It must be reemphasized that these benign diagnoses should be made only by exclusion and deserve long-term follow-up, because cerebral abnormalities may not become apparent until adulthood.

Clinical presentation of true precocity may not follow the usual progression of breast and pubic hair growth, acceleration of growth rate and then menses. It is not unusual for adrenarche or menarche to be the first sign (or an adult body odor) with others following. This progression is variable, usually slower in idiopathic cases, but telescoped in precocity due to central disease.

Sexual precocity is consistent with normal reproductive life and it is not associated with premature menopause. The most serious effect of precocity is the resultant adult short stature. Because the skeleton is very sensitive to even the lowest levels of estrogen, these children are transiently tall for their age, but as a result of early epiphyseal fusion, eventually short stature results. Fifty percent are less than 5 feet tall (152 cm).

Intellectual and psychosocial development are also commensurate with chronologic age rather than stage of puberty. Expectations of emotional, social, sexual, and intellectual competence corresponding to their pubertal state leave these youngsters and their families with potentially serious difficulties on all levels of social and emotional function.

A number of CNS problems, including abnormal skull development due to rickets, can cause true precocious development. Various tumors can induce precocity, including hamartomas in the hypothalamus (the most common lesion in very young girls), craniopharyngioma, astrocytoma, glioma, neurofibroma, ependymoma, and suprasellar teratoma — all usually near the hypothalamus. Pineal tumors, for unknown reasons, have been seen only in male precocious puberty. Nontumorous causes include encephalitis, meningitis, hydrocephalus, and von Recklinghausen's disease. An injury to the skull may stimulate sexual development.[89] The mechanism is unknown, and a latent period of 1–2 months is usually seen. A hamartoma is a hyperplastic congenital malformation in the floor of the third ventricle that usually produces precocity in the first few years of life; magnetic resonance imaging is the most sensitive method for the detection of small tumors like a hamartoma. Patients with true precocious puberty and known CNS lesions or a history of cranial irradiation should be evaluated for growth hormone deficiency because of the recognized association of these defects.[62]

There is no unifying pathophysiologic mechanism linking this diverse spectrum of etiologies for central precocity. Increased intracerebral pressure and a predilection for posterior hypothalamic lesions have suggested numerous theories. The finding that transforming growth factor-α (TGF-α) accumulates in areas of brain injury as a result of trauma-induced activation of gene expression in glial cells presents an intriguing model in that TGF-α stimulates GnRH release.[90] Hamartomas can produce gonadotropin-releasing hormone pulses, just as the normal hypothalamic tissue from which they are derived.

Ectopic gonadotropin production is a rare cause of sexual precocity accounting for less than 0.5% of cases. The most common tumors producing human chorionic gonadotropin (HCG) are chorioepithelioma and dysgerminoma of the ovary, and liver hepatoblastoma.[91, 92] Tumor spread may be present at the time of pubertal development; pelvic and abdominal masses accompanied by ascites are usually detectable.

True sexual precocity occurs in a small number of children with long-standing hypothyroidism. There is evidence to support the possibility that high levels of thyroid-stimulating hormone (TSH) can stimulate the FSH receptor.[93] In addition to short stature (but not bone age acceleration), galactorrhea may be present. The sella turcica is frequently enlarged, but with thyroid replacement pubertal development will stop and even regress. The sella films will return to normal. Although reported cases have been severe and, therefore, clinically obvious, laboratory evaluation of thyroid function is indicated in all cases of sexual precocity.

GnRH-Independent Precocious Puberty (Development Due to Availability of Sex Steroids, Precocious Pseudopuberty)

Eleven percent of girls with precocious puberty have an ovarian tumor. The tumor is usually an estrogen-producing neoplasm or cyst. Five percent of granulosa cell tumors and 1% of theca cell tumors occur before puberty. However, gonadoblastomas, teratomas, lipoid cell tumors, cystadenomas and even ovarian cancers have been reported as causes of precocity. Bleeding is irregular and menorrhagic — clearly anovulatory. A pelvic mass is readily palpable in 80% of cases. The palpation of a pelvic or abdominal mass demands surgical exploration. Increasing use has been made of pelvic ultrasonography and whole body (abdominal) imaging for the work-up of precocious puberty. In addition to estrogen and androgens, these tumors can secrete HCG.

A feminizing adrenal tumor is very rare (1% of cases) and is associated with increased blood levels of DHAS.

Drug ingestion should be suspected in all cases of precocity, especially when there is dark pigmentation of the nipples and breast areolae, an effect of certain synthetic estrogens such as stilbestrol. Common sources are oral contraceptives, anabolic steroids, and hair or facial creams.

McCune-Albright syndrome (polyostotic fibrous dysplasia) accounts for 5% of female precocity and consists of multiple disseminated cystic bone lesions that easily fracture, cafe au lait skin spots of various sizes and shapes, and sexual precocity. In addition, this syndrome can be associated with ovarian cysts, growth hormone- and prolactin-secreting adenomas, hyperthyroidism, adrenal hypercortisolism, and osteomalacia. Premature menarche may be the first sign of the syndrome. Skeletal abnormalities may become evident following the onset of puberty. The combination of multiple bone fractures, cafe au lait patches, and premature development should lead to the diagnosis. But remember that the manifestations of this syndrome can be varied and sometimes subtle. A technetium-99 bone scan may be necessary to demonstrate the areas of bony fibrous dysplasia.

Sexual precocity in McCune-Albright syndrome is now demonstrated to be the result of autonomous early production of estrogen by the ovaries.[94] FSH and LH levels are low, respond poorly to GnRH stimulation, and there is an absence of nocturnal gonadotropin pulsations (all unlike central precocity). In addition, Cushing's disease, acromegaly, hyperparathyroidism, and hyperthyroidism have been reported in this syndrome. The protean manifestations of this disorder suggested that the pathophysiology results from a basic defect in cellular regulation at the level of the G protein-cAMP-kinase function in affected tissues.[95] A mutation in the alpha-subunit ($G_S\alpha$) of the G protein that stimulates cAMP formation (as described in Chapter 2) has been identified in all affected tissues in patients with McCune-Albright syndrome. This mutation attenuates GTPase activity that is necessary to terminate adenylate cyclase activation; thus, affected tissues have autonomous activity. Somatic mosaicism of the alpha-subunit accounts for the fact that this mutation is not lethal and for the variation in site and activity throughout the body. This mutation can also occur in nonendocrine tissues in patients with McCune-Albright syndrome, thus explaining the occurrence of hepatitis, intestinal polyps, and cardiac arrhythmias. It is possible that this mechanism is responsible for childhood diseases other than McCune-Albright syndrome. For this reason, it has been suggested that this genetic disorder should be called inherited $G_S\alpha$ deficiency.[96] Eventual fertility is unimpaired, and adult height is usually normal. These positive factors must be considered in the choice of management of the syndrome. In keeping with the autonomous nature of the gonadal activity, treatment with a GnRH agonist fails to suppress gonadal hormone secretion or reverse the sexual precocity.[97]

Familial male precocious puberty is inherited in an autosomal dominant fashion and is caused by mutations in the LH receptor gene that lead to activation.[98] Thus far, no effects in females of activating mutations of either the LH receptor gene or the FSH receptor gene have been reported.

Yet another example of precocity due to GnRH-independent gonadal secretion of estrogen is by autonomous benign ovarian follicular or luteal cysts.[99] These children demonstrate an absence of gonadotropin pulsations, variable responses to GnRH, and a lack of suppression of puberty by a long-acting GnRH agonist. The cysts may enlarge and involute and then recur so that signs of sexual precocity and vaginal bleeding remit and exacerbate.[100] The cysts are unusually large and therefore palpable. GnRH testing is useful in differentiating the autonomous (nonreactive) cyst from those secondary to the FSH and LH stimulation of central true precocity (reactive).

It is now understood that nearly every cause of peripheral precocious puberty may *secondarily activate* the hypothalamic-pituitary-gonadal axis with development and superimposition of a central GnRH-dependent true precocity process. Presumably the central mechanism controlling the onset of puberty can be activated once a critical threshold of somatic development has been achieved by the premature production of estrogen *regardless* of source of secretion. This explains the previously paradoxical observations of continuing progressive puberty despite effective treatment of specific causative disease as well as the variable effectiveness of GnRH agonist therapy in McCune-Albright and the syndrome of recurrent ovarian cyst formation. GnRH testing to determine the level of activation will dictate the need for additional GnRH agonist suppression, inhibition of steroidogenesis, or peripheral aromatase inhibition therapy in these cases.

Laboratory Findings in Disorders Producing Precocious Puberty

	Gonadal Size	Basal FSH/LH	Estradiol or Testosterone	DHAS	GnRH Response
Idiopathic	Increased	Increased	Increased	Increased	Pubertal
Cerebral	Increased	Increased	Increased	Increased	Pubertal
Gonadal	Unilat. incr.	Decreased	Increased	Increased	Flat
Albright	Increased	Decreased	Increased	Increased	Flat
Adrenal	Small	Decreased	Increased	Increased	Flat

Special Cases of Precocious Development

Special cases of precocious development include the isolated appearance of one sexual characteristic: premature adrenarche or pubarche (pubic hair), premature thelarche (breast development), or premature isolated menarche. These cases present a special dilemma for the concerned clinician. Are they benign, self-limited variants of normal sexual development that do not require treatment or the first sign of a potentially accelerating process in which early exhaustive diagnosis and long-term therapy may be necessary?

Typically linear growth and skeletal maturation are not advanced, and baseline hormone levels are normal for age and sexual development. However, there is a spectrum of conditions of premature sexual maturation defined by idiopathic central precocious puberty at one end and isolated premature thelarche or premature adrenarche at the other. Between these poles are examples of mixed atypical problems with variable tendencies for stability or progression. Guidelines are emerging that address the issues of when sophisticated diagnostic testing (ACTH stimulation, GnRH testing, ultrasonography, bone assessments) is indicated.

Premature Thelarche

Premature thelarche usually occurs in the first few years of life and is usually self-limited, requiring no therapy. Follow-up has revealed that these children experience normal puberty and growth and, eventually, normal reproduction.[101] The breast growth may regress after a few months, wax and wane for years, or last until puberty. Premature thelarche can be unilateral.

Premature Menarche

Isolated premature menarche without other evidence of maturation is an exceedingly rare presentation of precocity; infection, the presence of a foreign body, abuse and trauma, and local neoplasms should be considered. Normal growth, development, and fertility are not affected.[102]

Premature Adrenarche

Premature adrenarche, the appearance of pubic hair before age 8 in girls, is the consequence of an early modest increase in the adrenal androgens, androstenedione, dehydroepiandrosterone and dehydroepiandrosterone sulfate. Normal levels according to stage of puberty are available in the literature.[103] An adrenal enzyme deficit should be excluded by appropriate laboratory testing, but it is rarely discovered in a prepubertal child who presents only with early growth of pubic hair.[104, 105] Thus, an ACTH stimulation test is not necessary; a measurement of the circulating early morning level of 17-hydroxyprogesterone will suffice. Treatment is not necessary because the transient acceleration in growth and bone maturation has no major influence on puberty or final height.[106, 107] Surveillance of these patients should be continued because, although not certain, it has been suggested that they have an increased incidence of anovulation, hirsutism, and hyperinsulinemia.[108–110] Sparse hair growth on the vulva does not represent precocious pubarche.

An ACTH stimulation test should be performed in patients who have an advanced bone age and circulating androgen levels that are greater than those seen in the early stages of puberty. ACTH testing of all children with premature adrenarche will yield results in some that are consistent with mild errors of steroidogenesis. However, even if present, these mild enzyme changes do not require treatment, and hence, exact diagnosis is not necessary. Treatment is indicated only for unequivocal cases of 21-hydroxylase deficiency, in whom baseline 17-hydroxyprogesterone levels will be diagnostic.

Tanner Staging

	Breast	**Pubic Hair**
Stage 1 (prepubertal)	Elevation of papilla only	No pubic hair
Stage 2	Elevation of breast and papilla as small mound, areola diameter enlarged. Median age: 9.8 years	Sparse, long, pigmented hair chiefly along labia majora. Median age: 10.5 years
Stage 3	Further enlargement without separation of breast and areola. Median age: 11.2 years	Dark, coarse, curled hair sparsely spread over mons. Median age: 11.4 years
Stage 4	Secondary mound of areola and papilla above the breast. Median age: 12.1 years	Adult-type hair, abundant but limited to the mons. Median age: 12.0 years
Stage 5	Recession of areola to contour of breast. Median age: 14.6 years	Adult-type spread in quantity and distribution. Median age: 13.7 years

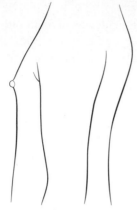

1 Prepubertal

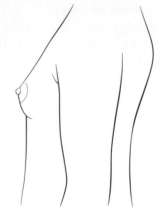

2 Breast bud

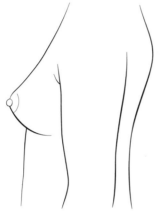

3 Breast elevation

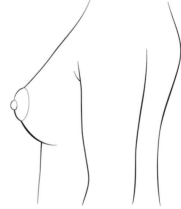

4 Areolar mound

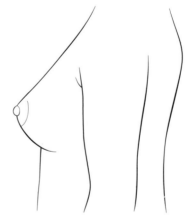

5 Adult contour

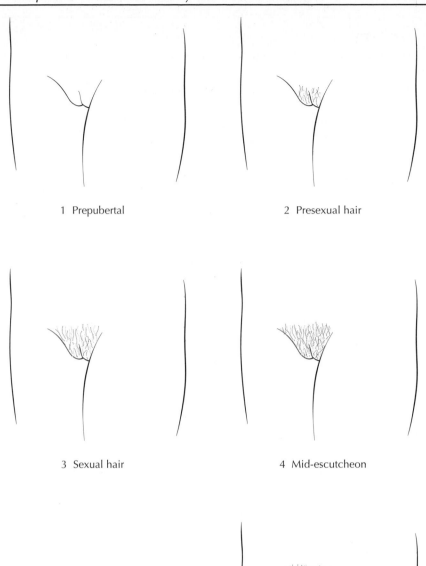

1 Prepubertal

2 Presexual hair

3 Sexual hair

4 Mid-escutcheon

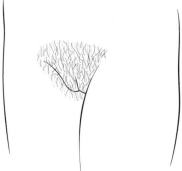

5 Female escutcheon

Diagnosis of Precocious Puberty

The cause of precocious development may be obvious by findings in the history or physical examination. Familial occurrence helps to exclude certain disease processes (tumors). Clinically, the nature of precocity dictates certain diagnostic priorities.

1. **Rule out life-threatening disease.** This includes neoplasms of the CNS, ovary, and adrenal.

2. **Define the velocity of the process.** Is it progressing or stabilized? Management decisions hinge on this determination. Isolated, nonendocrine causes of vaginal bleeding (trauma, foreign body, vaginitis, genital neoplasm) must be excluded.

Differential Diagnostic Steps

Physical Diagnosis:
Record of growth, Tanner stages, height and weight percentiles.
External genitalia changes.
Abdominal, pelvic, neurologic examination.
Signs of androgenization.
Special findings: McCune-Albright, hypothyroidism.

Laboratory Diagnosis:
Bone age.
Head CT scan or MRI, ultrasonography of abdomen and pelvis.
FSH, LH, HCG assay.
Thyroid function tests (TSH and free T_4).
Steroids (serum DHAS, testosterone, estradiol, progesterone, 17-hydroxyprogesterone).
GnRH testing.

If the full signs of sexual precocity are present, and basal or GnRH-stimulated gonadotropins are in the pubertal range, a pituitary source of gonadotropins is suspected. A simplified GnRH test can be used as follows:[111]

GnRH, 100 µg, administered subcutaneously;
Serum LH level 40 minutes after injection should be less than 8 IU/L.

Any abnormality on neurologic exam or imaging points toward central (CNS in origin) precocious puberty. If these are all normal, idiopathic sexual precocity is the most likely diagnosis. It should be emphasized that basal serum gonadotropins may be in the prepubertal range in the early stages of idiopathic or central precocious puberty; with time and progression of sexual development these will rise to the pubertal range. However, an ectopic source of HCG should be considered if serum gonadotropins are suppressed while estradiol is markedly elevated; a situation easily confirmed by an immunoassay specific for the β-subunit of HCG. The rare feminizing adrenal tumor may be present if the laboratory picture is more one of elevated adrenal androgens with only slightly elevated serum estradiol and suppressed serum gonadotropins. Abdominal and pelvic ultrasonography or magnetic resonance imaging (MRI) is indicated.

When signs of sexual precocity are associated with accelerated growth and skeletal maturation, in the absence of virilization, the etiology may be an ovarian tumor or cyst. A pelvic mass is usually palpable. In this situation, serum FSH and LH are suppressed, while serum estradiol is usually elevated. An elevated serum progesterone suggests an ovarian luteoma. Pelvic ultrasound or imaging can help to confirm the presence of an ovarian mass. Laparotomy is indicated to confirm the diagnosis and carry out surgical resection.

Adrenal hyperplasia or a virilizing adrenal or ovarian tumor must be considered if signs of sexual precocity are accompanied by virilization. With elevation of serum 17-hydroxyprogesterone (17-OHP) and adrenal androgens, the diagnosis of 21-hydroxylase deficient adrenal hyperplasia is established, whereas an elevation of serum 11-deoxycortisol leads to the diagnosis of 11β-hydroxylase deficient adrenal hyperplasia. If these two serum hormones are normal, while serum DHAS or androstenedione is elevated, an adrenal tumor or a virilizing ovarian tumor is suspect. Ultrasound examination and abdominal imaging can be utilized to further localize the tumor.

Breast development usually correlates with a bone age of 11 and menarche with a bone age of 13. If breast and genital development, pubic hair growth, and vaginal bleeding are seen in a short child with a *delayed* bone age, primary hypothyroidism is the most likely diagnosis. This can be confirmed by finding a low serum T_4 and elevated TSH concentration. Serum FSH and LH levels may be in the pubertal range, but these will decrease following thyroid treatment. Galactorrhea may be present along with elevated serum prolactin concentrations. These return to normal with thyroid treatment.

Treatment of Precocious Development

The objectives of management and treatment of precocious puberty include:

1. Diagnose and treat intracranial disease.

2. Arrest maturation until normal pubertal age.

3. Attenuate and diminish established precocious characteristics.

4. Maximize eventual adult height.

5. Avoidance of abuse, reduction of emotional problems, and contraception if necessary.

A number of therapies have been used to achieve these goals. These have included medroxyprogesterone acetate, cyproterone acetate, and danazol. In addition to undesireable side effects, bone maturation and growth were not regularly or sufficiently controlled. Major progress has been made with the use of GnRH analogues for the treatment of true precocious puberty.

The short half-life of GnRH is due to rapid cleavage of bonds between amino acids 5-6, 6-7, and 9-10. Substitution of amino acids at position 6 and replacement of the C-terminal glycine amide has produced effective GnRH agonists. Agents can be chosen that are administered subcutaneously, intranasally daily, or in long-acting depot forms.

After an initial short-term "flare" stimulation of gonadotropin release, desensitization and down-regulation follow, yielding profound reduction in gonadotropins, steroid production, and biologic effects. Substantial regression of pubertal characteristics, amenorrhea, and reduction in growth velocity are rapidly achieved and maintained within the first year of treatment.[112] Final bone height is increased but is dependent upon the stage at which medication is begun, the bone age at which the drug is stopped, and the adequacy of the dose regimen.[113, 114] Even individuals with advanced bone ages will achieve greater growth because suppression of gonadal steroids will delay epiphyseal fusion and prolong the duration of growth. Treatment is more effective if begun before bone age exceeds 12 years.[115] With idiopathic GnRH-dependent precocious puberty, height predictions are more accurate using the Bayley-Pinneau tables for average girls, despite advanced bone ages in patients. Some patients will demonstrate a marked slowing of growth with GnRH agonist treatment, and in these patients, the addition of growth hormone will produce an excellent growth response.[116]

GnRH Agonists in Clinical Use

Position	1	2	3	4	5	6	7	8	9	10
Native GnRH	pGlu	His	Trp	Ser	Tyr	Gly	Leu	Arg	Pro	Gly-NH$_2$
Leuprolide						D-Leu				NH-Ethylamide
Buserelin						D-Ser (tertiary butanol)				NH-Ethylamide
Nafarelin						D-Naphthylalanine (2)				
Histrelin						D-His (tertiary benzyl)				NH-Ethylamide
Goserelin						D-Ser (tertiary butanol)				Aza-Gly
Deslorelin						D-Trp				NH-Ethylamide
Tryptorelin						D-Trp				

The dose of GnRH agonist treatment can be monitored by measuring estradiol levels. Because estradiol is the hormone that triggers growth and development, the objective is to maintain an estradiol less than 10 pg/mL, a prepubertal range.[117] Because many commercial estradiol assays lack sensitivity in this range, it may be necessary to confirm adequate suppression by demonstrating a lack of gonadotropin response to the administration of GnRH. In general, children require higher doses of GnRH agonists to achieve suppression compared to adults. Even with treatment, adrenarche will probably continue, true to its independent control system.

Sustained release pellets (goserelin) or sustained release injections (leuprolide) allow once a month dosing.[118] Treatment is maintained until the epiphyses are fused or until appropriate pubertal and chronological ages are matched. Discontinuation of therapy is followed by prompt reactivation of the pubertal process and the development of regular ovulatory function in a pattern similar to that of normal adolescents.[119] GnRH agonist treatment is also recommended for GnRH-secreting hamartomas of the hypothalamus.[120, 121] The progress of the tumor can be monitored by imaging, and risky surgery can be avoided.

GnRH agonist treatment is not effective for noncentral forms of precocious puberty such as McCune-Albright syndrome, GnRH-independent sexual precocity, or congenital adrenal hyperplasia. However, should patients with McCune-Albright syndrome or congenital adrenal hyperplasia mature their hypothalamic-pituitary-gonadal axis and develop true sexual precocity, then supplementary GnRH agonist therapy is helpful.[122, 123] Primary treatment in these cases is directed toward suppression of gonadal steroidogenesis. Medroxyprogesterone acetate can be utilized in depot form to suppress LH secretion, or testolactone, an aromatase inhibitor, can be administered.

If a specific etiology for precocious puberty is identified, treatment is aimed at curing the underlying disorder. Neurosurgical excision of hypothalamic, pituitary, cerebral, or pineal tumors must be individualized in each patient. If these tumors are small and do not extend around or into vital brain structures, their removal may be successful. If complete surgical excision is not possible, radiation therapy should be considered. Although many tumors are said not to be radiosensitive, this may be the only treatment available, although new chemotherapy protocols are of benefit with some tumors. The tumors that secrete ectopic HCG, such as chorioepitheliomas, teratomas, hepatomas, should be managed in a manner consistent with current specific treatment protocols for HCG-secreting neoplasms.

If an ovarian or adrenal tumor is identified, surgical excision is the treatment of choice. In the case of an ovarian cyst, it may be difficult to know whether the cyst is an autonomous source of estrogens or whether its growth is secondary to gonadotropin stimulation. GnRH testing is useful in resolving this question. If multiple bilateral cysts are discovered, these are usually secondary to central gonadotropin secretion. If the cyst is solitary and the contralateral ovary appears immature, then cyst resection is justified. With primary hypothyroidism, thyroid replacement will prevent further progression of sexual precocity. If adrenal hyperplasia is identified, treatment with appropriate doses of glucocorticoids (and mineralocorticoids if salt-wasting is present) will also prevent further progression of pubertal development. If these patients have a bone age of 11–12 years, glucocorticoid therapy may result in onset of true sexual precocity.

Careful consideration must be given to the management of psychosocial problems in all children with precocious puberty. As mentioned previously, these children have intellectual, behavioral and psychosexual maturation in keeping with their chronological age, not their physical or pubertal age. They do not have early heterosexual activity or abnormal sexual libido. Unfortunately, parents, teachers, and peers may have unrealistic expectations of their intellectual and athletic abilities, and these children may even inappropriately be labeled as retarded. Careful explanation of these considerations must be given to parents. The children should be counseled that their secondary sexual characteristics are normal albeit early. If the child is bright, advancement in school may be possible with special tutoring and this may prove beneficial. Children with precocious puberty may place a stress on the marital or family relationship, and in these situations formal psychological counseling can be useful.

Prognosis

The prognosis for precocious puberty depends on the underlying cause. With primary hypothyroidism, the prognosis is excellent. Children with adrenal hyperplasia tend to be short as adults. Removal of benign ovarian tumors and adrenal tumors carries a good prognosis, while malignant carcinomas often have metastatic disease at the time of presentation, with consequent poor prognosis. Approximately 20% of granulosa cell tumors are malignant, and the prognosis is guarded for recurrences as late as 25 years after removal. Approximately 25% of ovarian Sertoli-Leydig cell tumors are malignant.

With CNS causes of sexual precocity, the prognosis again depends on the exact etiology. If tumors of the CNS are completely resectable, the prognosis is good; however, this tends to be the exception rather than the rule. Some tumors, though, such as hamartomas, are slow growing and may only be discovered during a routine autopsy following death due to other causes. Other tumors, such as craniopharyngiomas, are developmental remnants rather than true neoplasms, and with partial resection and radiation therapy patients may go into remission for many years. With other conditions, such as congenital cysts, hydrocephalus, encephalitis, McCune-Albright syndrome, and neurofibromatosis, the prognosis is related to associated neurologic deficits.

Psychometric testing indicates that girls with precocious puberty have higher verbal IQ scores. Behavioral testing demonstrates that a majority of girls do not have problems; a minority may show a tendency toward social difficulties related to apparent age and physical maturation, such as depression, social withdrawal, moodiness, aggression and hyperactivity. However, with the exception of short stature as an adult, the prognosis for idiopathic sexual precocity remains good if the children enter adult life without psychosexual scars. The mean height in adult women is approximately 152 cm (5 feet). Even with prompt GnRH agonist treatment final adult height is likely to be somewhat compromised because some stimulation to epiphyseal closure will already have occurred before treatment is initiated. One can consider adding growth hormone to patients who appear to be falling short of their predicted height, however the expense of growth hormone is a factor (discussed in Chapter 9). Most women have normal menstrual cycles and fertility, and they do not have premature menopause.[124]

Delayed Puberty

Since there is such a wide variation in normal development it is difficult to define the patient with abnormally delayed sexual maturation. Nearly all U.S. white girls and all U.S. black girls have entered puberty by age 13.[52] However, some evaluation is needed whenever a patient and parents are concerned enough to seek a clinician's advice. Patients who have not developed signs of puberty by age 17 are very likely to have a specific problem and not physiological delay of puberty.

Delayed puberty is a rare condition in girls, and a genetic problem or hypothalamic-pituitary disorder must be suspected. In addition, anatomic abnormalities of the target organ (uterus and endometrium) or outflow tract are unique but important elements to consider in amenorrheic but otherwise normal pubertal adolescents.

The history and physical examination are very useful in the diagnostic work-up of delayed puberty. Special note should be taken of past general health, height and weight records, and the height and pubertal milestone experience of older siblings and parents, and relevant behavior such as extreme exercise or abnormal eating habits. Physiological delayed puberty tends to be familial. On physical examination, in addition to body measurements and Tanner staging of any secondary sexual characteristics present, a search for signs of hypothyroidism, gonadal dysgenesis, hypopituitarism, or chronic illness should be made. Persistent deciduous teeth are typical of hypothyroidism. The absence of pubic hair in a patient with a uterus and vagina indicates hypopituitarism. The absence of pubic hair in a patient with a vaginal pouch indicates that the patient has androgen insensitivity syndrome.

The failure of growth in stature suggests several possibilities. Isolated growth hormone deficiency is associated with somewhat delayed sexual maturity. Menarche may eventually occur, albeit delayed, but with bone age still several years below chronologic age. More global pituitary hormone deficiency will result in total pubertal delay. Finally, gonadal dysgenesis (45,X) will be associated with decreased height and sexual infantilism with normal to slightly reduced bone age and hypergonadotropism.

Neurologic examination is important; evidence of intracranial disease, restricted visual fields, or absent sense of smell are key findings. Anatomic defects of the müllerian ducts must be sought, especially when a disparity between normal puberty and absent menses is encountered.

As will be seen in the discussion of the work-up, the diverse etiologic possibilities for delayed puberty are best classified by the level of gonadotropin encountered. The distribution of diagnostic frequencies in the three categories — hypergonadotropic hypogonadism, hypogonadotropic hypogonadism and eugonadism — are depicted below, representing the findings in 326 patients.[125]

Relative Frequency of Delayed Pubertal Abnormalities[125]

Hypergonadotropic Hypogonadism		**43.0%**
Ovarian failure, abnormal karyotype		26.0%
Ovarian failure, normal karyotype		17.0%
46, XX	15.0%	
46, XY	2.0%	
Hypogonadotropic Hypogonadism		**31.0%**
Reversible		18.0%
Physiologic delay	10.0%	
Weight loss/anorexia	3.0%	
Primary hypothyroidism	1.0%	
Congenital adrenal hyperplasia	1.0%	
Cushing's syndrome	0.5%	
Prolactinomas	1.5%	
Irreversible		13.0%
GnRH deficiency	7.0%	
Hypopituitarism	2.0%	
Congenital CNS defects	0.5%	
Other pituitary adenomas	0.5%	
Craniopharyngioma	1.0%	
Malignant pituitary tumor	0.5%	
Eugonadism		**26.0%**
Müllerian agenesis		14.0%
Vaginal septum		3.0%
Imperforate hymen		0.5%
Androgen insensitivity syndrome		1.0%
Inappropriate positive feedback		7.0%

Laboratory Assessments of Delayed Puberty

Laboratory work-up of delayed puberty usually includes x-rays for bone age, skull imaging (if hypogonadotropic), gonadotropin and prolactin levels, appropriate adrenal and gonadal steroid measurements, and assessment of thyroid function. In addition, general laboratory screening for systemic disorders is worthwhile. Evaluation according to the program outlined in Chapter 11 will lead to the proper diagnosis. Patients with elevated gonadotropins require a karyotype. Measurements of serum IGF-I, IGFBP-3, and IGFBP-2 can distinguish between delayed puberty and growth hormone deficiency; normal levels according to age, body mass index, and stage of puberty are available in the literature.[126, 127]

Hypergonadotropic Hypogonadism

If gonadotropins are increased into the postmenopausal range (hypergonadotropic hypogonadism), then some type of gonadal deficiency usually is the basis of delayed maturation. The most common disorder of this type is gonadal dysgenesis. In the 45,X patient, the typical phenotypic stigmata of Turner syndrome will be displayed. However, these may be minimal or absent in sex chromosome mosaicism or structural deletions of the X chromosome. A Y-bearing cell line requires gonadal excision as prophylaxis against the risk of gonadal malignancy. Intersex patients (Chapter 9) can present with delayed puberty.

A hypergonadotropic 46,XX individual presents interesting possibilities. If hypertension, sexual infantilism, and an elevated serum progesterone are found, 17α-hydroxylase deficiency in steroid synthesis is likely. Acquired ovarian damage from torsion or inflammation should be ruled out. In sickle cell disease, approximately 20% of patients have delayed puberty and hypergonadotropism Finally, the 46,XX patient may have pure gonadal dysgenesis (gonadal streaks) or the resistant ovary syndrome. See the discussion in Chapter 11 under "Premature Ovarian Failure."

Hypogonadotropic Hypogonadism

Decreased secretion of LH (less than 6 IU/L), associated with depressed FSH, is seen in hypothalamic amenorrhea, amenorrhea and anosmia — Kallmann's syndrome, pituitary (tumor) disorders, hyperprolactinemia, or nonpathologic constitutional (physiologic) delay in development. Physiological delayed puberty can be regarded as a physiologic variant in development. The typical patient with physiological delay is short with appropriate bone maturation delay. Physiological delay accounts for only 10% of cases with delayed puberty, emphasizing the need to seek another diagnosis. As previously noted, physiological delay is frequently seen in a familial pattern with the expectation of a late but otherwise normal growth pattern and adult reproductive function.

Poor nutrition (anorexia nervosa, malabsorption, chronic illness, regional ileitis, renal disease) can lead to hypogonadotropic delayed growth and development. Exercise and/or stress-induced amenorrhea can also delay puberty. Unfortunately, illegal drug use (especially marijuana) must be considered.

In the presence of normal olfaction and normal prolactin levels, exclusion of pituitary, parapituitary, or hypothalamic tumor by specialized neuroradiologic procedures is necessary. If tumor or vascular malformation is not found, the diagnosis is (by exclusion) physiological delayed puberty.

Craniopharyngioma. This tumor is the most common neoplasm associated with delayed puberty. Craniopharyngioma is a tumor of Rathke's pouch, originating from the pituitary stalk with suprasellar extension. The peak incidence is between ages 6 and 14.[128] Imaging reveals an abnormal sella and calcifications in 70% of cases. Treatment consists of a combination of surgery and irradiation.

Eugonadism

Müllerian tube segmental discontinuities, müllerian agenesis, or androgen insensitivity syndrome will present as delayed menarche despite normal development of an adult female phenotype (Chapter 11). Müllerian agenesis accounts for one-seventh of cases of prolonged primary amenorrhea. Other obstructive anomalies of the müllerian ducts are less frequently seen. Anovulation and polycystic ovaries, and androgen-producing adrenal disease, can present as primary amenorrhea. Virilization raises the possibility of adrenal hyperplasia or an intersex problem.

Treatment of Sexual Infantilism (Delayed Puberty)

The first priority in therapy is removal or correction of primary etiology when possible. In this regard, thyroid therapy for hypothyroidism, growth hormone for isolated growth hormone deficiency, and treatment of ileitis are examples of specific therapy. In XY individuals, properly timed gonadectomy followed by sex hormone treatment is required. In physiological delay, reassurance that the anticipated development will occur is the only management step needed, especially when there is a family history of delayed puberty. Early hormone treatment is worthwhile in order to minimize psychological stress.

In hypogonadism, hormonal therapy will initiate and sustain maturation and function of secondary sexual characteristics and promote the achievement of full height potential. The importance of the adolescent increase in bone density should not be underrated. This is sufficient reason to recommend hormone treatment.

Hormone treatment should conform to what we have learned about the early stages of puberty. Very small amounts of estrogen will promote growth and development. Start with unopposed estrogen, 0.3 mg conjugated estrogens or 0.5 mg estradiol daily. After 6 months to 1 year, move to a sequential program with 0.625 mg conjugated estrogens or 1.0 mg estradiol daily and 5 mg medroxyprogesterone acetate or an equivalent progestin for the first 14 days each month. Patients with physiological delay of puberty will continue development on their own when bone age has advanced to 13 years.

Monthly menstruation is an important experience for adolescents. Regular and visible bleeding serves to reinforce the young patient's identification with the feminine gender role. However, remember that the doses used for this therapy will not protect against pregnancy in the event the hypothalamic-pituitary-ovarian axis is activated. In a sexually active patient, it would be wiser to use oral contraception to provide the missing estrogen.

Treatment with pulsatile GnRH is both a logical and effective means of inducing a physiologic puberty.[129] However, this treatment regimen is not practical. Although its expense is an important consideration, the technical aspects associated with the parenteral administration of GnRH pulses make this method too cumbersome and difficult.

Growth Problems in Normal Adolescents

Perhaps the worst thing about an adolescent growth problem is that it makes the individual "different." It is probably true that more than anyone else the adolescent does not like to be different. Therefore, excessive or insufficient growth is not a problem to be dismissed lightly, and psychologic support and reassurance are key features in the management of such problems. A willingness to listen to problems, together with an adult-to-adult attitude, will place the adolescent-clinician relationship at the proper level of mutual respect.

The basic and essential laboratory procedure is a left hand-wrist x-ray for bone age. The Bayley-Pinneau tables predict future adult height, utilizing the bone age and present height.[130] To use the tables, one needs a measurement of height, the patient's age, and an x-ray of the left hand and wrist for bone age. All of the hand epiphyses and those of the distal end of the arm are used to determine the skeletal age. The Bayley-Pinneau tables begin at the end of this chapter.

To predict a patient's adult height, use the tables as follows. Go down the left column to the patient's present height, follow this horizontal row to the column under the bone age which is given by 6-month intervals across the top. The number at the intersection represents the predicted adult height. The predicted height can be easily extrapolated if figures do not fall at the 1-inch or 6-month intervals used on the tables.

It is important to use the table suitable for the rate of maturing. If the bone age is within 1 year of the chronologic age, use the table for average girls; if the bone age is accelerated 1 year or more, use the table for accelerated girls; if the bone age is retarded 1 year or more, use the table for retarded girls. Girls with idiopathic central precocious puberty are an exception to this recommendation. With idiopathic GnRH-dependent precocious puberty, despite advanced bone age, height predictions are more accurate using the Bayley-Pinneau tables for average girls.[115]

The tables are for use with bone age films of the hand and wrist only in conjunction with the Greulich-Pyle Atlas. Use with bone age determined by any other method is less accurate.

Short Stature

Thorough medical history and physical examination will eliminate the usual disorders associated with short stature: malnutrition, chronic urinary tract disease, chronic infectious disease, hypothyroidism, mental illness, panhypopituitarism, and gonadal dysgenesis. In the history, the heights and weights of parents, siblings, and relatives should be obtained along with timing of growth in the family, dietary history, daily activities, and sleep habits. Normal history and examination in an individual with a bone age only 1 year behind the chronologic age suggest a constitutional pattern that does not require treatment.

Endocrine disease is an uncommon basis for impairment of growth. Congenital hypothyroidism is the most frequent problem of this type, followed by hypopituitarism, hypothyroidism with onset during childhood, and excess cortisol.

It is unlikely that a patient with congenital hypothyroidism will present undiagnosed and untreated as an adolescent. However, juvenile hypothyroidism must be suspected in an adolescent with obesity and short stature and normal early childhood development. Similarly, an adolescent with hypopituitarism due to a slow growing pituitary tumor may present with a failure to develop secondary sexual characteristics and a failure to grow. Cortisol excess may be due to Cushing's disease (rare in childhood) or to therapy with corticosteroids. Excess endogenous or exogenous corticosteroids suppress skeletal maturation and growth. Moderate overdosage of cortisol; e.g., when treating children with adrenal hyperplasia, can suppress growth.

Treatment of Short Stature. Support and observation are indicated if the physician concludes that an adolescent suffers from a delay of normal growth and no disease process is present. Reassurance is essential if the bone age is more than 1 year below the chronologic age, but the family history reveals a consistent pattern of retarded but eventual normal growth. It is helpful to point out the x-ray, indicating that the individual has 1 year or more of unused potential in which to catch up with her friends.

Hormone treatment can be considered when continued failure to grow is evident in the absence of disease. Presently the use of growth hormone is limited to use in growth hormone deficiency. The increment in height achieved with growth hormone treatment of short, but normal, children is too small (about 2.5 cm) to warrant such treatment.[131] Illicit sources of growth hormone have been administered by parents and young people eager to "grow" to achieve greater athletic prowess. This dangerous practice all too often leads to growth but of fragile bones unsupported by the sought-after muscular capacities.

Anabolic-androgenic steroids are illegally utilized by both adolescent males and females to increase athletic performance and even in an effort to look better.[132] Response to these agents ranges from increased strength and libido (virilization and menstrual dysfunction in women) to liver diseases, impotence, and oligospermia. Excessive androgen use by adolescents can prevent individuals from reaching their genetic height potential. Although not well studied, most experts believe that there are significant psychological and behavioral effects (such as enhanced aggression), as well as psychological dependence. In addition, adolescents who use anabolic steroids are more likely to use other drugs and to share needles (a major risk factor for human immunodeficiency virus infection).[133]

Fortunately, it is rare to see a female adolescent complaining of short stature. More commonly it is an adolescent boy who is sensitive to reduced growth, and in whom the use of testosterone may be indicated. In cases of gonadal failure, estrogen can be used in a female to stimulate epiphyseal growth, bringing the bone age to match the chronologic age. Conjugated estrogens (0.3 mg) or estradiol (0.5 mg) administered daily are effective in hypogonadal individuals (this is a much smaller dose than previously used). Patients should be observed at monthly intervals to document the pattern of growth and development. Hormone treatment may be discontinued when the bone age matches the chronologic age.

Tall Stature

This is rarely a problem in boys. Basketball has provided a ready outlet, and fortunately participation in sports is now appealing to girls as well. But girls who are the daughters of very tall parents may come for help. The Bayley-Pinneau tables are accurate in predicting the height of tall girls. A predicted height greater than 6 feet probably deserves treatment.

A hand-wrist x-ray for bone age is necessary. The degree of development of secondary sexual characteristics is important, because the more mature a girl is, the less effective treatment is in influencing her eventual height.

Treatment of Tall Stature. It is difficult to make a decision for treatment, and parental participation in the decision is essential. In a case where some success can be achieved, the patient is relatively young and may find it hard to know what to think about the future problem.

Because the adolescent growth spurt precedes menarche, treatment must begin before menarche in order to be optimally successful.[134] This would be as early as 8 or 9 years, and certainly before the age of 12. However, treatment begun after menarche may still achieve up to an inch of growth reduction.[135, 136] Once begun, treatment must continue until epiphyses are fused. If treatment is stopped earlier, further growth will occur.[137] The parents and patient must be informed of possible problems with menorrhagia, breast symptoms, and water retention.

A simple regimen that provides high doses of estrogen is to use oral contraceptives; a 50 μg ethinyl estradiol oral contraceptive provides 10 times the estrogen usually administered to postmenopausal women. Hand-wrist films should be taken every 6 months until epiphyseal closure is demonstrated. In view of the sensitivity of growth physiology to low levels of estrogen, it is not certain that these high doses are necessary. Although 10-year follow-up of a large number of women treated with high doses of estrogens did not detect any adverse consequences on reproductive function,[138] it would be reasonable to consider the usual replacement dose (0.625–1.25 mg conjugated estrogens or 1–2 mg estradiol), especially if the high doses elicit unpleasant symptoms.

References

1. **Kaplan SL, Grumbach MM, Aubert ML,** The ontogenesis of pituitary hormones and hypothalamic factors in the human fetus: maturation of central nervous system regulation of anterior pituitary function, *Recent Prog Hor Res* 32:161, 1976.

2. **Burger HG, Famada Y, Bangah ML, McCloud PI, Warne GL,** Serum gonadotropin, sex steroid, and immunoreactive inhibin levels in the first two years of life, *J Clin Endocrinol Metab* 72:682, 1991.

3. **Andersson A-M, Toppari J, Haavisto A-M, Petersen JH, Simell T, Simell O, Skakkebæk NE,** Longitudinal reproductive hormone profiles in infants: peak of inhibin B levels in infant boys exceeds levels in adult men, *J Clin Endocrinol Metab* 83:675, 1998.

4. **Winter JSD, Faiman C,** The development of cyclic pituitary-gonadal function in adolescent females, *J Clin Endocrinol Metab* 37:714, 1973.

5. **Conte FA, Grumbach MM, Kaplan SL, Reiter EO,** Correlation of LHRF induced LH and FSH release from infancy to 19 years with the changing pattern of gonadotropin secretion in agonadal patients: relation to restraint of puberty, *J Clin Endocrinol Metab* 50:165, 1980.

6. **Roth JC, Kelch RP, Kaplan SL, Grumbach MM,** FSH and LH response to luteinizing hormone-releasing factor in prepubertal and pubertal children, adult males and patients with hypogonadotropic and hypergonadotropic hypogonadism, *J Clin Endocrinol Metab* 37:680, 1973.

7. **Jakacki RI, Kelch RP, Sander SE, Lloyd JS, Hopwood NJ, Marshall JC,** Pulsatile secretion of luteinizing hormone in children, *J Clin Endocrinol Metab* 53:453, 1982.

8. **Oerter KE, Urarte MM, Rose SR, Barnes KM, Cutler GB,** Gonadotropin secretory dynamics during puberty in normal girls and boys, *J Clin Endocrinol Metab* 71:1251, 1990.

9. **Dunkel L, Alfthan H, Stenman U-H, Selstam G, Rosberg S, Albertsson-Wikland K,** Developmental changes in 24-hour profiles of luteinizing hormone and follicle-stimulating hormone from prepuberty to midstages of puberty in boys, *J Clin Endocrinol Metab* 74:890, 1992.

10. **Sizonenko PC, Paunier L, Carmignac D,** Hormonal changes during puberty: IV. Longitudinal study of adrenal androgen secretion, *Horm Res* 7:288, 1976.

11. **Counts DR, Pescovitz OH, Barnes KM, Hench KD, Chrousos GP, Sherins RJ, Comite F, Loriaux DL, Cutler Jr GB,** Dissociation of adrenarche and gonadarche in precocious puberty and in isolated hypogonadotropic hypogonadism, *J Clin Endocrinol Metab* 64:1174, 1987.

12. **Sklar CA, Kaplan SL, Grumbach MM,** Evidence for dissociation between adrenarche and gonadarche: studies in patients with idiopathic precocious puberty, gonadal dysgenesis, isolated gonadotroph deficiency, and constitutionally delayed growth and adolescence, *J Clin Endocrinol Metab* 51:548, 1980.

13. **Zumoff B, Walsh BT, Katz JL,** Subnormal plasma dehydroisoandrosterone to cortisol ratio in anorexia nervosa: a second hormonal parameter of ontogenetic regression, *J Clin Endocrinol Metab* 56:668, 1983.

14. **Parker LN, Lifrak AT, Odell WD,** A 60,000 molecular weight glycoprotein stimulates adrenal androgen secretion, *Endocrinology* 113:2092, 1983.

15. **Hauffa BP, Kaplan SL, Grumbach MM,** Dissociation between plasma adrenal androgens and cortisol in Cushing's disease and ectopic ACTH producing tumor: relation to adrenarche, *Lancet* i:1373, 1984.

16. **Cavallo A,** Melatonin secretion during adrenarche in normal human puberty and in pubertal disorders, *J Pineal Res* 12:71, 1992.

17. **Byrne GC, Perry YS, Winter JSD,** Steroid inhibitory effects upon human adrenal 3β-hydroxysteroid dehydrogenase activity, *J Clin Endocrinol Metab* 62:413, 1986.

18. **Endoh A, Kristiansen SB, Casson PR, Buster JE, Hornsby PJ,** The zona reticularis is the site of biosynthesis of dehydroepiandrosterone and dehydroepiandrosterone sulfate in the adult human adrenal cortex resulting from its low expression of 3β-hydroxysteroid dehydrogenase, *J Clin Endocrinol Metab* 81:3558, 1996.

19. **Gell JS, Carr BR, Sasano H, Atkins B, Margraf L, Mason JI, Rainey WE,** Adrenarche results from development of a 3β-hydroxysteroid dehydrogenase-deficient adrenal reticularis, *J Clin Endocrinol Metab* 83:3695, 1998.

20. **Zhang L, Rodriguez H, Ohno S, Miller WL,** Serine phosphorylation of human P450c17 increases 17,20-lyase activity: implications for adrenarche and the polycystic ovary syndrome, *Proc Natl Acad Sci USA* 92:10619, 1995.

21. **Terasawa E, Noonan JJ, Nass TE, Loose MD,** Posterior hypothalamic lesions advance the onset of puberty in the female rhesus monkey, *Endocrinology* 115:224, 1984.

22. **Foster DL, Ryan KD,** Endocrine mechanisms governing transition into adulthood: a marked decrease in inhibitory feedback action of estradiol on tonic secretion of LH in the lamb during puberty, *Endocrinology* 105:896, 1979.

23. **Waldhauser F, Boepple PA,** The pubertal growth spurt in eight patients with true precocious puberty and growth hormone deficiency: evidence for a direct role of sex steroids, *J Clin Endocrinol Metab* 71:975, 1990.

24. **Attanasio A, Borrelli P, Gupta D,** Circadian rhythms in serum melatonin from infancy to adolescence, *J Clin Endocrinol Metab* 61:388, 1985.

25. **Cavallo A, Richards GE, Smith ER,** Relation between nocturnal melatonin profile and hormonal markers of puberty in humans, *Horm Res* 37:185, 1992.

26. **Plant TM, Zorub DS,** Pinealectomy in agonadal infantile male rhesus monkeys (Macaca mulatta) does not interrupt initiation of the prepubertal hiatus in gonadotropin secretion, *Endocrinology* 118:227, 1986.

27. **Genazzani AR, Fachinetti F, Petraglia F, Pintor C, Corda R,** Hyperendorphinemia in obese children and adolescents, *J Clin Endocrinol Metab* 62:36, 1986.

28. **Marshall JC, Kelch RP,** Low dose pulsatile GnRH in anorexia nervosa: a model of human pubertal development, *J Clin Endocrinol Metab* 49:712, 1979.

29. **Job JC, Garnier PE, Chaussain JL, Milhaud G,** Elevation of serum gonadotropins (LH and FSH) after releasing hormone (LH-RH) injection in normal children and in patients with disorders of puberty, *J Clin Endocrinol Metab* 35:473, 1972.

30. **Burstein S, Schaff-Blass E, Blass J, Rosenfield R,** Changing ratio of bioactive to immunoactive LH through puberty, *J Clin Endocrinol Metab* 61:508, 1985.

31. **Apter D, Butzow TL, Laughlin GA, Yen SSC,** Gonadotropin-releasing hormone pulse generator activity during pubertal transition in girls: pulsatile and diurnal patterns of circulating gonadotropins, *J Clin Endocrinol Metab* 76:940, 1993.

32. **Cemeroglu AP, Foster CM, Warner R, Kletter GB, Marshall JC, Kelch RP,** Comparison of the neuroendocrine control of pubertal maturation in girls and boys with spontaneous puberty and in hypogonadal girls, *J Clin Endocrinol Metab* 81:4352, 1996.

33. **Clark PA, Iranmanesh A, Veldhuis JD, Rogol AD,** Comparison of pulsatile luteinizing hormone secretion between prepubertal children and young adults: evidence for a mass/amplitutde-dependent difference without gender or day/night contrasts, *J Clin Endocrinol Metab* 82:2950, 1997.

34. **Kapen S, Boyar RM, Hellman L, Weltzman ED,** 24-Hour patterns of LH secretion in humans: ontogenic and sexual consideration, *Prog Brain Res* 42:103, 1975.

35. **Tanner JM,** *Growth at Adolescence,* 2nd ed, Blackwell Scientific Publications, Oxford, 1962.

36. **Marti-Henneberg C, Vizmanos B,** The duration of puberty in girls is related to the timing of its onset, *J Pediatr* 131:618, 1997.

37. **Frisch RE, Revelle R,** Menstrual cycles: fatness as a determinant of minimum weight-for-height for their maintenance or onset, *Science* 185:949, 1974.

38. **Maclure M, Travis LB, Willett W, MacMahon B,** A prospective cohort study of nutrient intake and age at menarche, *Am J Clin Nutr* 54:649, 1991.

39. **Zacharias L, Wurtman RJ, Schatzott M,** Sexual maturation in contemporary American girls, *Am J Obstet Gynecol* 108:833, 1970.

40. **Zacharias L, Wurtman RJ,** Blindness: its relation to age of menarche, *Science* 144:1154, 1964.

41. **Crawford JD, Osler DC,** Body composition at menarche: the Frisch Revelle hypothesis revisited, *Pediatrics* 56:449, 1975.

42. **de Ridder CM, Thijssen JHH, Bruning PF, Van den Brande JL, Zonderland ML, Erich WBM,** Body fat mass, body fat distribution, and pubertal development: a longitudinal study of physical and hormonal sexual maturation of girls, *J Clin Endocrinol Metab* 75:442, 1992.

43. **Chehab FF, Mounzih K, Lu R, Lim ME,** Early onset of reproductive function in normal female mice treated with leptin, *Science* 275:88, 1997.

44. **Mantzoros CS, Flier JS, Rogol AD,** A longitudinal assessment of hormonal and physical alterations during normal puberty in boys. V. Rising leptin levels may signal the onset of puberty, *J Clin Endocrinol Metab* 82:1066, 1997.

45. **Hanaoka I, Hosoda K, Ogawa Y, Masuzaki H, Miyawaki T, Natsui K, Hiraoka J, Matsuoka N, Yasuno A, Satoh H, Matsuda J, Shintani M, Azuma Y, Kou T, Nishimura H, Yoshimasa Y, Nishi S, Nakao K,** Decreased plasma leptin levels in anorexia nervosa, P2-539, The Endocrine Society Annual Meeting, 1997.

46. **Garcia-Mayor RV, Andrade MA, Rios M, Lage M, Dieguex C, Casanueva FF,** Serum leptin levels in normal children: relationship to age, gender, body mass index, pituitary-gonadal hormones, and pubertal stage, *J Clin Endocrinol Metab* 82:2849, 1997.

47. **Matkovic V, Ilich JZ, Skugor M, Badenhop NE, Goel P, Clairmont A, Klisovic D, Nahhas RW, Landoll JD,** Leptin is inversely related to age at menarche in human females, *J Clin Endocrinol Metab* 82:1066, 1997.

48. **Palmert MR, Radovick S, Boepple PA,** Leptin levels in children with central precocious puberty, *J Clin Endocrinol Metab* 83:2260, 1998.

49. **Hassink SG, Sheslow DV, de Lancey E, Opentanova I, Considine RV, Caro JF,** Serum leptin in children with obesity: relationship to gender and development, *Pediatrics* 98:201, 1996.

50. **Marshall WA, Tanner JM,** Variations in the pattern of pubertal changes in girls, *Arch Dis Child* 44:291, 1969.

51. **Zacharias L, Rand WM, Wurtman RJ,** A prospective study of sexual development and growth in American girls: the statistics of menarche, *Obstet Gynecol Survey* 31:325, 1976.

52. **Harlan WR, Harlan EA, Grillo GP,** Secondary sex characteristics of girls 12 to 17 years of age: the U.S. Health Examination Survey, *J Pediatr* 96:1074, 1980.

53. **Read G, Wilson D, Hughes I, Griffiths K,** The use of salivary progesterone assays in the assessment of ovarian function in postmenarcheal girls, *J Endocrinol* 102:265, 1984.

54. **Vuorento T, Huhtaniemi I,** Daily levels of salivary progesterone during menstrual cycle in adolescent girls, *Fertil Steril* 58:685, 1992.

55. **Lee PA,** Normal ages of pubertal events among American males and females, *J Adolesc Health Care* 1:26, 1980.

56. **Beller FK, Borsos A, Kieback D, Csoknyay J, Lampe L,** Geschlechtsentwicklung: die entwicklung der sekundaren geschlechtsmerkmale — die Tannerstadien 25 jahre spater, *Zentralbl Gynakol* 113:499, 1991.

57. **Herman-Giddens ME, Slora EJ, Wasserman RC, Bourdony CJ, Bhapkar MV, Koch GG, Hasemeier CM,** Secondary sexual characteristics and menses in young girls seen in office practice: a study from the Pediatric Research Office Settings Network, *Pediatrics* 99:505, 1997.

58. **Fried RI, Smith EE,** Postmenarcheal growth patterns, *J Pediatr* 61:562, 1962.

59. **Harris DA, Van Vliet G, Egli LA, Grumbach MM, Kaplan SL, Styne DM, Vainsel M,** Somatomedin-C in normal puberty and in true precocious puberty before and after treatment with a potent luteinizing hormone-releasing hormone agonist, *J Clin Endocrinol Metab* 61:152, 1985.

60. **Merimee TJ, Zapf J, Hewlett B, Cavalli-Sforza LL,** Insulin-like growth factors in pygmies, *New Engl J Med* 316:906, 1987.

61. **Mansfield MJ, Rudlin CR, Crigler Jr JF, Karol KA, Crawfod JD, Boepple PA, Crowley Jr WF,** Changes in growth and serum growth hormone and plasma somatomedin-C levels during suppression of gonadal sex steroid secretion in girls with central precocious puberty, *J Clin Endocrinol Metab* 66:3, 1988.

62. **Attie KM, Ramierez NR, Conte FA, Kaplan SL, Grumbach MM,** The pubertal growth spurt in eight patients with true precocious puberty and growth hormone deficiency: evidence for a direct role of sex steroids, *J Clin Endocrinol Metab* 71:975, 1990.

63. **Veldhuis JD, Metzger DL, Martha Jr PM, Mauras N, Kerrigan JR, Keenan B, Rogol AD, Pincus SM,** Estrogen and testosterone, but not a non-aromatizable androgen, direct network integration of the hypothalamo-somatorope (GH-IGF-I axis in the human: evidence from pubertal pathophysiology and sex-steroid hormone replacement, *J Clin Endocrinol Metab* 82:3414, 1997.

64. **Kerrigan JR, Rogol AD,** The impact of gonadal steroid hormone action on growth hormone secretion during childhood and adolescence, *Endocr Rev* 13:281, 1992.

65. **Travers SH, Labarta JI, Gargosky SE, Rosenfeld RG, Jeffers BW, Eckel RH,** Insulin-like growth factor binding protein-I levels are strongly associated with insulin sensitivity and obesity in early pubertal children, *J Clin Endocrinol Metab* 83:1935, 1998.

66. **Hindmarsh PC, Matthews DR, Stratton I, Pringle PJ, Brook CDG,** Rate of change (modulation) of serum growth hormone concentrations is a more important factor in determining growth rate than duration of exposure, *Clin Endocrinol* 36:165, 1992.

67. **Bridges NA, Hindmarsh PC, Matthews DR, Brook CGD,** The effect of changing gonadotropin-releasing hormone pulse frequency on puberty, *J Clin Endocrinol Metab* 79:841, 1994.

68. **Ross JL, Long LM, Skerda M, Cassorla F, Kurtz D, Loriaux DL, Cutler Jr GG,** Effect of low doses of estradiol on 6-month growth rates and predicted height in patients with Turner syndrome, *J Pediatr* 109:950, 1986.

69. **Bohnet HG,** New aspects of oestrogen/gestagen-induced growth and endocrine changes in individuals with Turner syndrome, *Eur J Pediatr* 145:275, 1986.

70. **Smith EP, Boyd J, Frank GR, Takahashi H, Cohen RM, Specker B, Williams TC, Lubahn DB, Korach KS,** Estrogen resistance caused by a mutation in the estrogen-receptor gene in a man, *New Engl J Med* 331:1056, 1994.

71. **Carani C, Qin K, Simoni M, Faustini-Fustini M, Serpente S, Boyd J, Korach KS, Simpson ER,** Effect of testosterone and estradiol in a man with aromatase deficiency, *New Engl J Med* 337:91, 1997.

72. **Khosla S, Melton III LJ, Atkinson EJ, O'Fallon WM, Klee GG, Riggs BL,** Relationship of serum sex steroid levels and bone turnover markers with bone mineral density in men and women: a key role for bioavailable estrogen, *J Clin Endocrinol Metab* 83:2266, 1998.

73. **Bilezikian JP, Morishima A, Bell J, Grumbach MM,** Increased bone mass as a result of estrogen therapy in a man with aromatase deficiency, *New Engl J Med* 339:599, 1998.

74. **Gilsanz V, Roe TF, Mora S, Costin G, Goodman WG,** Changes in vertebral bone density in black girls and white girls during childhood and puberty, *New Engl J Med* 325:1597, 1991.

75. **Lloyd T, Andon MB, Rollings N, Martel JK, Landis JR, Demers LM, Eggli DF, Kiesselhorst K, Kulin HE,** Calcium supplementation and bone mineral density in adolescent girlls, *JAMA* 270:841, 1993.

76. **Theitz G, Buch B, Rizzoli R, Slosman D, Clavien H, Sizonko PC, Bonjour JPH,** Longitudinal monitoring of bone mass accumulation in healthy adolescents: evidence for a marked reduction after 16 years of age at the levels of lumbar spine and femoral neck in female subjects, *J Clin Endocrinol Metab* 75:1060, 1992.

77. **Matkovic V, Jelic T, Wardlaw GM, Ilich J, Goel PK, Wright JK, Andon MB, Smith KT, Heaney RP,** Timing of peak bone mass in caucasian females and its implication for the prevention of osteoporosis: inference from a cross-sectional model, *J Clin Invest* 93:799, 1994.

78. **Dann TC, Koberts DF,** Menarcheal age in University of Warwick young women, *J Biosoc Sci* 25:531, 1993.

79. **Sizonenko PC, Paunier L,** Hormonal changes in puberty III: correlation of plasma dehydroepiandrosterone, testosterone, FSH and LH with stage of puberty and bone age in normal boys and girls and in patients with Addison's disease or hypogonadism or premature or late adrenarche, *J Clin Endocrinol Metab* 41:894, 1975.

80. **Hung W, August GP, Glasgow AM,** *Pediatric Endocrinology,* Medical Examination Publishing Co., Garden City, 1978.

81. **Jenner MR, Kelch RP, Kaplan SL, Grumbach MM,** Hormonal changes in puberty. IV. Plasma estradiol, LH and FSH in prepubertal children, pubertal females, and in precocious puberty, premature thelarche, hypogonadism and in a child with a feminizing ovarian tumor, *J Clin Endocrinol Metab* 34:521, 1972.

82. **Raiti S, Johanson A, Light C, Migeon CJ, Blizzard RM,** Measurement of immunologically reactive follicle stimulating hormone in serum of normal male children and adults, *Metabolism* 18:234, 1969.

83. **Johanson J, Guyda H, Light C, Migeon CG, Blizzard RM,** Serum luteinizing hormone by radioimmunoassay in normal children, *J Pediatr* 74:416, 1969.

84. **Frasier SD, Gafford F, Horton R,** Plasma androgens and adolescence, *J Clin Endocrinol Metab* 29:1404, 1969.

85. **Lee PA, Migeon CJ,** Puberty in boys: correlation of plasma levels of gonadotropins (LH, FSH), androgens (testosterone, androstenedione, dehydroepiandrosterone and its sulfate), estrogens (estrone and estradiol) and progestins (progesterone and 17-hydroxyprogesterone), *J Clin Endocrinol Metab* 41:556, 1975.

86. **Jolly H,** *Sexual precocity,* Charles C. Thomas, Springfield, Illinois, 1955.

87. **Wilkins L,** *The Diagnosis and Treatment of Endocrine Disorders in Childhood and Adolescence,* 3rd ed, Charles C. Thomas, Springfield, Illinois, 1965.

88. **Stein DT,** New developments in the diagnosis and treatment of sexual precocity, *Am J Med Sci* 303:53, 1992.

89. **Maxwell M, Karacostas D, Ellenbogen RG, Brzezinski A, Zervas NT, Black PM,** Precocious puberty following head injury, *J Neurosurg* 73:123, 1990.

90. **Junier MP, Ma YJ, Costa ME, Hoffman G, Hill DF, Ojeda SR,** Transforming growth factor-β contributes to the mechanism by which hypothalamic injury induces precocious puberty, *Proc Natl Acad Sci USA* 88:9743, 1991.

91. **Pomariede R, Finidori J, Cernichow P, Pfister A, Hirsch JF, Rappaport R,** Germinoma in a boy with precocious puberty: evidence of HCG secretion by the tumoral cells, *Child Brain* 11:298, 1984.

92. **Navarro C, Corretser JM, Sancho A, Rovira J, Morales L,** Paraneoplastic precocious puberty. Report of a new case with hepatoblastoma and review of the literature, *Cancer* 56:1725, 1985.

93. **Anasti JN, Flack MR, Froehlich J, Nelson LM, Nisula BC,** A potential novel mechanism for precocious puberty in juvenile hypothyroidism, *J Clin Endocrinol Metab* 80:276, 1995.

94. **Lee PA, Van Dop C, Migeon CJ,** McCune-Albright syndrome: long-term follow-up, *JAMA* 256:290, 1986.

95. **Schwindenger WF, Francomano CA, Levine MA,** Identification of a mutation in the gene encoding the alpha subunit of the stimulatory G protein adenyl cyclase in McCune-Albright syndrome, *Proc Natl Acad Sci USA* 89:5152, 1992.

96. **Miric A, Vechio JD, Levine MA,** Heterogeneous mutations in the gene encoding the α-subunit of the stimulatory G protein of adenyl cyclase in Albright hereditary osteodystrophy, *J Clin Endocrinol Metab* 76:1560, 1993.

97. **Comite F, Shawker TH, Pescovitz OH, Loriaux DL, Cutler Jr GB,** Cyclical ovarian function resistant to treatment with an analogue of luteinizing hormone releasing hormone in McCune-Albright syndrome, *New Engl J Med* 311:1032, 1984.

98. **Yano K, Saji M, Hidaka A, Moriya N, Okuno A, Kohn LD, Cutler GB,** A new constitutively activating point mutation in the luteinizing hormone/choriogonadotropin receptor gene in cases of male-limited precocious puberty, *J Clin Endocrinol Metab* 80:1162, 1995.

99. **Lightner ES, Kelch RP,** Treatment of precocious pseudopuberty associated with ovarian cysts, *Am J Dis Child* 138:126, 1984.

100. **Millar DM, Blake JM, Stringer DA, Hara H, Babiak C,** Prepubertal ovarian cyst formation: 5 years' experience, *Obstet Gynecol* 81:434, 1993.

101. **Van Winter JT, Noller KL, Zimmerman D, Melton LJ,** Natural history of premature thelarche in Olmsted County, Minnesota 1940 to 1984, *J Pediatr* 116:278, 1990.

102. **Murram D, Dewhurst J, Grant DB,** Premature menarche: a follow-up study, *Arch Dis Child* 58:142, 1983.

103. **Lashansky G, Saenger P, Fishman K, Gautier T, Mayes D, Berg G, DiMartino-Nardi J, Reiter E,** Normative data for adrenal steroidogenesis in a healthy pediatric population: age and sex-related changes after ACTH stimulation, *J Clin Endocrinol Metab* 73:674, 1991.

104. **Saenger P, Rester EO,** Premature adrenarche: a normal variant of puberty, *J Clin Endocrinol Metab* 74:236, 1992.

105. **Morris AH, Reiter EO, Geffner ME, Lippe BM, Itami RM, Mayes DM,** Absence of nonclassical congenital adrenal hyperplasia in patients with precocious adrenarche, *J Clin Endocrinol Metab* 69:709, 1989.

106. **Ibáñez L, Virdis R, Potau N, Zampolli M, Ghizzoni L, Albisu MA, Carrascosa A, Bernasconi S, Vicens-Calvet E,** Natural history of premature pubarche: an auxological study, *J Clin Endocrinol Metab* 74:254, 1992.

107. **Pere A, Perheentupa J, Peter M, Voutilainen R,** Follow-up of growth and steroids in premature adrenarche, *Eur J Pediatr* 154:346, 1995.

108. **Ibáñez L, Potau N, Virdis R, Zampolli M, Terzi C, Gussinye M, Carrascosa A, Vicens-Calvet E,** Postpubertal outcome in girls diagnosed of premature pubarche during childhood: increased frequency of functional ovarian hyperandrogenism, *J Clin Endocrinol Metab* 76:1599, 1993.

109. **Ibáñez L, Potau N, Georgopoulos N, Prat N, Gussinye M, Carrascosa A,** Growth hormone, insulin-like growth factor-I axis, and insulin secretion in hyperandrogenic adolescents, *Fertil Steril* 64:1113, 1995.

110. **Ibáñez L, Potau N, Zampolli M, Riqué S, Saenger P, Carrascosa A,** Hyperinsulincmia and decreased insulin-like growth factor-binding protein-1 are common features in prepubertal and pubertal girsl with a history of premature pubarche, *J Clin Endocrinol Metab* 82:2283, 1997.

111. **Eckert KL, Wilson DM, Bachrach LK, Anhalt H, Habiby RL, Olney RC, Hintz RL, Neely EK,** A single-sample, subcutaneous gonadotropin-releasing hormone test for central precocious puberty, *Pediatrics* 97:517, 1996.

112. **Wheeler MD, Styne DM,** The treatment of precocious puberty, *Endocrinol Metab Clin North Am* 20:183, 1991.

113. **Manasco PK, Pescovitz OH, Hill SC, Jones JM, Barnes KM, Hench KD, Loriaux DL, Cutler C,** Six-year results of luteinizing hormone releasing hormone (LHRH) agonist treatment in children with LHRH-dependent precocious puberty, *J Pediatr* 115:105, 1989.

114. **Cook JS, Doty KL, Conn PM, Hansen JR,** Assessment of depot leuprolide acetate dose adequacy for central precocious puberty, *J Clin Endocrinol Metab* 74:1206, 1992.

115. **Kauli R, Galatzer A, Kornreich L, Lazar L, Pertzelan A, Laron Z,** Final height of girls with central precocious puberty, untreated versus treated with cyproterone acetate or GnRH analogue. A comparative study with re-evaluation of predictions by the Bayley-Pinneau method, *Horm Res* 47:54, 1997.

116. **Pasquino AM, Municchi G, Pucarelli I, Segni M, Mancini MA, Troiani S,** Combined treatment with gonadotropin-releasing hormone analog and growth hormone in central precocious puberty, *J Clin Endocrinol Metab* 81:948, 1996.

117. **Klein KO, Baron J, Barnes KM, Pescovitz OH, Cutler Jr GB,** Use of an ultrasensitive recombinant cell bioassay to determine estrogen levels in girls with precocious puberty treated with a luteinizing hormone-releasing hormone agonist, *J Clin Endocrinol Metab* 83:2387, 1998.

118. **Parker KL, Baine-Bailon RG, Lee PA,** Depot leuprolide acetate dosage for sexual precocity, *J Clin Endocrinol Metab* 73:50, 1991.

119. **Jay N, Mansfield MJ, Blizzard RM, Crowley Jr WF, Schoenfeld D, Rhubin L, Boepple PA,** Ovulation and menstrual function of adolescent girls with central precocious puberty after therapy with gonadotropin-releasing hormone agonists, *J Clin Endocrinol Metab* 75:890, 1992.

120. **Mahachoklertwattana P, Kaplan S, Grumbach MM,** The luteinizing hormone-releasing hormone-secreting hypothalamic hamartoma is a congenital malformation: natural history, *J Clin Endocrinol Metab* 77:118, 1993.

121. **Stewart L, Steinbok P, Daaboul J,** Role of surgical resection in the treatment of hypothalamic hamartomas causing precocious pubert. Report of six cases, *J Neurosurg* 88:340, 1998.

122. **Mansfield MJ, Beardsworth DE, Loughlin JS, Crawford JD, Bode HH, Rivier J, Vale W, Kushner DC, Crigler Jr JF, Crowley Jr WF,** Long-term treatment of central precocious puberty with a long-acting analogue of luteinizing hormone-releasing hormone. effects on somatic growth and skeletal maturation, *New Engl J Med* 309:1286, 1983.

123. **Pescovitz OH, Comite F, Cassorla F, Dwyer AJ, Poth MA, Sperling MA, Hench K, McNemar A, Skerda M, Loriaux DL, Cutler Jr GB,** True precocious puberty complicating congenital adrenal hyperplasia: treatment with a luteinizing hormone-releasing hormone analog, *J Clin Endocrinol Metab* 58:857, 1984.

124. **Murran D, Dewhurst J, Grant DB,** Precocious puberty: a follow-up study, *Arch Dis Child* 59:77, 1984.

125. **Reindollar RH, Tho SPT, McDonough PG,** Delayed puberty: an updated study of 326 patients, *Trans Am Gynecol Obstet Soc* 8:146, 1989.

126. **Smith WJ, Nam TJ, Underwood LE, Busby WH, Clenicker A, Clemmons DR,** Use of IGFBP-2, IGFBP-3, and IGF-I for assessing growth hormone status in short children, *J Clin Endocrinol Metab* 77:1294, 1993.

127. **Juul A, Bang P, Hertel NT, Main K, Dalgaard P, Jørgensen K, Müller J, Hall K, Skakkebæk NE,** Serum insulin-like growth factor-I in 1030 healthy children, adolescents, and adults: relation to age, sex, stage of puberty, testicular size, and body mass index, *J Clin Endocrinol Metab* 78:744, 1994.

128. **Stanhope R, Pringle PJ, Brook CGD, Adams J, Jacobs HS,** Induction of puberty by pulsatile gonadotropin releasing hormone, *Lancet* ii:552, 1987.

129. **Thomsett JJ, Conte FA, Kaplan SL, Grumbach MM,** Endocrine and neurologic outcome in childhood craniopharyngioma: review of effect of treatment in 42 patients, *J Pediatr* 97:728, 1980.

130. **Bayley N, Pinneau SR,** Tables for predicting adult height from skeletal age: revised for use with the Greulich-Pyle hand standards, *J Pediatr* 40:423, 1952.

131. **Hindmarsh PC, Brook CGD,** Final height of short normal children treated with growth hormone, *Lancet* 348:13, 1996.

132. **Rogol AD, Yesalis III CE,** Clinical review 31: anabolic-androgenic steroids and athletes: what are the issues? *J Clin Endocrinol Metab* 74:465, 1992.

133. **DuRant RH, Rickert VI, Ashworth CS, Newman C, Slavens G,** Use of multiple drugs among adolescents who use anabolic steroids, *New Engl J Med* 328:922, 1993.

134. **Drop SLS, de Waal WJ, de Muinck Keizer-Schrama SMPF,** Sex steroid treatment of constitutionally tall stature, *Endocr Rev* 19:540, 1998.

135. **Schoen EJ, Solomon IL, Warner D, Wingerd J,** Estrogen treatment of tall girls, *Am J Dis Child* 125:71, 1973.

136. **Norman H, Wettenhall B, Cahill C, Roche AF,** Tall girls: a survey of 15 years of management and treatment, *Adolesc Med* 86:602, 1975.

137. **de Waal WJ, Greyn-Fokker MH, Stijnen T, van Gurp EAFJ, Toolens AMP, de Muinck Keizer-Schrama SMPF, Aarsen RSR, Drop SLS,** Accuracy of final height prediction and effect of growth-reductive therapy in 362 constitutionally tall children, *J Clin Endocrinol Metab* 81:1206, 1996.

138. **de Waal WJ, Torn M, de Muinck Keizer-Schrama SM, Aarsen RS, Drop SL,** Long term sequelae of sex steroid treatment in the management of constitutionally tall stature, *Arch Dis Child* 73:311, 1995.

Bayley-Pinneau Table for Average Girls
(J Pediatr 40:423, 1952)

To predict height, find vertical column corresponding to skeletal age and horizontal row for the present height. The number at the intersection is the predicted height in inches. If figures do not fall at the whole inch or 6-month intervals, the predicted height must be extrapolated.

Skeletal Age		6/0	6/6	7/0	7/6	8/0	8/6	9/0	9/6	10/0	10/6	11/0	11/6	12/0
Height in inches	37	51.4												
	38	52.8	51.5											
	39	54.2	52.8	51.5										
	40	55.6	54.2	52.8	51.8									
	41	56.9	55.6	54.2	53.1	51.9								
	42	58.3	56.9	55.5	54.4	53.2	51.9							
	43	59.7	58.3	56.8	55.7	54.4	53.1	52.0						
	44	61.1	59.6	58.1	57.0	55.7	54.3	53.2	52.1	51.0				
	45	62.5	61.0	59.4	58.3	57.0	55.6	54.4	53.3	52.2				
	46	63.9	62.3	60.8	59.6	58.2	56.8	55.6	54.5	53.4	52.0			
	47	65.8	63.7	62.1	60.9	59.5	58.0	56.8	55.7	54.5	53.2	51.9	51.4	51.0
	48	66.7	65.0	63.4	62.2	60.8	59.3	58.0	56.9	55.7	54.3	53.0	52.5	52.1
	49	68.1	66.4	64.7	63.5	62.0	60.5	59.3	58.1	56.8	55.4	54.1	53.6	53.1
	50	69.4	67.8	66.1	64.8	63.3	61.7	60.5	59.2	58.0	56.6	55.2	54.7	54.2
	51	70.8	69.1	67.4	66.1	64.6	63.0	61.7	60.4	59.2	57.7	56.3	55.8	55.3
	52	72.2	70.5	68.7	67.4	65.8	64.2	62.9	61.6	60.3	58.8	57.4	56.9	56.4
	53	73.6	71.8	70.0	68.7	67.1	65.4	64.1	62.8	61.5	60.0	58.5	58.0	57.5
	54		73.2	71.3	69.9	68.4	66.7	65.3	64.0	62.6	61.1	59.6	59.1	58.6
	55		74.5	72.7	71.2	69.6	67.9	66.5	65.2	63.8	62.2	60.7	60.2	59.7
	56			74.0	72.5	70.9	69.1	67.7	66.4	65.0	63.3	61.8	61.3	60.7
	57				73.8	72.2	70.4	68.9	67.5	66.1	64.5	62.9	62.4	61.8
	58					73.4	71.6	70.1	68.7	67.3	65.6	64.0	63.5	62.9
	59					74.7	72.8	71.3	69.9	68.4	66.7	65.1	64.6	64.0
	60						74.1	72.6	71.1	69.6	67.9	66.2	65.6	65.1
	61							73.8	72.3	70.8	69.0	67.3	66.7	66.2
	62								73.5	71.9	70.1	68.4	67.8	67.2
	63								74.6	73.1	71.3	69.5	68.9	68.3
	64									74.2	72.4	70.6	70.0	69.4
	65										73.5	71.7	71.1	70.5
	66										74.7	72.9	72.2	71.6
	67											74.0	73.3	72.7
	68												74.4	73.8
	69													74.8
	70													
	71													
	72													
	73													
	74													

12/6	13/0	13/6	14/0	14/6	15/0	15/6	16/0	16/6	17/0	17/6	18/0	
												37
												38
												39
												40
												41
												42
												43
												44
												45
												46
												47
51.0												48
52.1	51.1											49
53.1	52.2	51.3	51.0									50
54.2	53.2	52.4	52.0	51.7	51.5	51.4	51.2	51.2	51.1	51.0	51.0	51
55.3	54.3	53.4	53.1	52.7	52.5	52.4	52.2	52.2	52.1	52.0	52.0	52
56.3	55.3	54.4	54.1	53.8	53.5	53.4	53.2	53.2	53.1	53.0	53.0	53
57.4	56.4	55.4	55.1	54.8	54.5	54.4	54.2	54.2	54.1	54.0	54.0	54
58.4	57.4	56.5	56.1	55.8	55.6	55.4	55.2	55.2	55.1	55.0	55.0	55
59.5	58.5	57.5	57.1	56.8	56.6	56.4	56.2	56.2	56.1	56.0	56.0	56
60.6	59.5	58.5	58.2	57.8	57.6	57.4	57.2	57.2	57.1	57.0	57.0	57
61.6	60.5	59.5	59.2	58.8	58.6	58.4	58.2	58.2	58.1	58.0	58.0	58
62.7	61.6	60.6	60.2	59.8	59.6	59.4	59.2	59.2	59.1	59.0	59.0	59
63.8	62.6	61.6	61.2	60.9	60.6	60.4	60.2	60.2	60.1	60.0	60.0	60
64.8	63.7	62.6	62.2	61.9	61.6	61.4	61.2	61.2	61.1	61.0	61.0	61
65.9	64.7	63.7	63.3	62.9	62.6	62.4	62.2	62.2	62.1	62.0	62.0	62
67.0	65.8	64.7	64.3	63.9	63.6	63.4	63.3	63.2	63.1	63.0	63.0	63
68.0	66.8	65.7	65.3	64.9	64.6	64.4	64.3	64.2	64.1	64.0	64.0	64
69.1	67.8	66.7	66.3	65.9	65.7	65.5	65.3	65.2	65.1	65.0	65.0	65
70.1	68.9	67.8	67.3	66.9	66.7	66.5	66.3	66.2	66.1	66.0	66.0	66
71.2	69.9	68.8	68.4	68.0	67.7	67.5	67.3	67.2	67.1	67.0	67.0	67
72.3	71.0	69.8	69.4	69.0	68.7	68.5	68.3	68.2	68.1	68.0	68.0	68
73.3	72.0	70.8	70.4	70.0	69.7	69.5	69.3	69.2	69.1	69.0	69.0	69
74.4	73.1	71.9	71.4	71.0	70.7	70.5	70.3	70.2	70.1	70.0	70.0	70
	74.1	72.9	72.4	72.0	71.7	71.5	71.3	71.2	71.1	71.0	71.0	71
		73.9	73.5	73.0	72.7	72.5	72.3	72.2	72.1	72.0	72.0	72
		74.9	74.5	74.0	73.7	73.5	73.3	73.2	73.1	73.0	73.0	73
					74.7	74.5	74.3	74.2	74.1	74.0	74.0	74

Bayley-Pinneau Table for Accelerated Girls

To predict height, find vertical column corresponding to skeletal age and horizontal row for the present height. The number at the intersection is the predicted height in inches. If figures do not fall at the whole inch or 6-month intervals, the predicted height must be extrapolated.

Skeletal Age		7/0	7/6	8/0	8/6	9/0	9/6	10/0	10/6	11/0	11/6	12/0
Height in inches	37	52.0										
	38	53.4	51.9									
	39	54.8	53.3	52.0								
	40	56.2	54.6	53.3	51.9							
	41	57.6	56.0	54.7	53.2	51.9						
	42	59.0	57.4	56.0	54.5	53.2	51.9					
	43	60.4	58.7	57.3	55.8	54.4	53.2	51.9				
	44	61.8	60.1	58.7	57.1	55.7	54.4	53.1	51.4			
	45	63.2	61.5	60.0	58.4	57.0	55.6	54.3	52.6	54.0		
	46	64.6	62.8	61.3	59.7	58.2	56.9	55.6	53.7	52.1	51.6	51.1
	47	66.0	64.2	62.7	61.0	59.5	58.1	56.8	54.9	53.2	52.7	52.2
	48	67.4	65.6	64.0	62.3	60.8	59.3	58.0	56.1	54.4	53.9	53.3
	49	68.8	66.9	65.3	63.6	62.0	60.6	59.2	57.2	55.5	55.0	54.4
	50	70.2	68.3	66.7	64.9	63.3	61.8	60.4	58.4	56.6	56.1	55.5
	51	71.6	69.7	68.0	66.1	64.6	63.0	61.6	59.6	57.8	57.2	56.6
	52	73.0	71.0	69.3	67.4	65.8	64.3	62.8	60.7	58.9	58.4	57.7
	53	74.4	72.4	70.7	68.7	67.1	65.5	64.0	61.9	60.0	59.5	58.8
	54		73.8	72.0	70.0	68.4	66.7	65.2	63.1	61.2	60.6	59.9
	55			73.3	71.3	69.6	68.0	66.4	64.3	62.3	61.7	61.0
	56			74.7	72.6	70.9	69.2	67.6	65.4	63.4	62.8	62.2
	57				73.9	72.2	70.5	68.8	66.6	64.6	64.0	63.3
	58					73.4	71.7	70.0	67.8	65.7	65.1	64.4
	59					74.7	72.9	71.3	68.9	66.8	66.2	65.5
	60						74.2	72.5	70.1	68.0	67.3	66.6
	61							73.7	71.3	69.1	68.5	67.7
	62							74.9	72.4	70.2	69.6	68.8
	63								73.6	71.3	70.7	69.9
	64								74.8	72.5	71.8	71.0
	65									73.6	72.9	72.1
	66									74.7	74.1	73.3
	67											74.4
	68											
	69											
	70											
	71											
	72											
	73											
	74											

12/6	13/0	13/6	14/0	14/6	15/0	15/6	16/0	16/6	17/0	17/6	
											37
											38
											39
											40
											41
											42
											43
											44
											45
											46
											47
51.9											48
53.0	51.9	50.9									49
54.1	52.9	51.9	51.4	51.0							50
55.2	54.0	53.0	52.5	52.0	51.7	51.5	51.4	51.3	51.1	51.0	51
56.3	55.0	54.0	53.5	53.1	52.7	52.5	52.4	52.3	52.1	52.0	52
57.4	56.1	55.0	54.5	54.1	53.8	53.5	53.4	53.3	53.1	53.0	53
58.4	57.1	56.1	55.6	55.1	54.8	54.5	54.4	54.3	54.1	54.0	54
59.5	58.2	57.1	56.6	56.1	55.8	55.5	55.4	55.3	55.1	55.0	55
60.6	59.3	58.2	57.6	57.1	56.8	56.5	56.4	56.3	56.1	56.0	56
61.7	60.3	59.2	58.6	58.2	57.8	57.6	57.4	57.3	57.1	57.0	57
62.8	61.4	60.2	59.7	59.2	58.8	58.6	58.4	58.3	58.1	58.0	58
63.9	62.4	61.3	60.7	60.2	59.8	59.6	59.4	59.3	59.1	59.0	59
64.9	63.5	62.3	61.7	61.2	60.9	60.6	60.4	60.3	60.1	60.0	60
66.0	64.6	63.3	62.8	62.2	61.9	61.6	61.4	61.3	61.1	61.0	61
67.1	65.6	64.4	63.8	63.3	62.9	62.6	62.4	62.3	62.1	62.0	62
68.2	66.7	65.4	64.8	64.3	63.9	63.6	63.4	63.3	63.1	63.0	63
69.3	67.7	66.5	65.8	65.3	64.9	64.6	64.4	64.3	64.1	64.0	64
70.3	68.8	67.5	66.9	66.3	65.9	65.7	65.5	65.3	65.1	65.0	65
71.4	69.8	68.5	67.9	67.3	66.9	66.7	66.5	66.3	66.1	66.0	66
72.5	70.9	69.6	68.9	68.4	68.0	67.7	67.5	67.3	67.1	67.0	67
73.6	72.0	70.6	70.0	69.4	69.0	68.7	68.5	68.3	68.1	68.0	68
74.7	73.0	71.7	71.0	70.4	70.0	69.7	69.5	69.3	69.1	69.0	69
	74.1	72.7	72.0	71.4	71.0	70.7	70.5	70.3	70.1	70.0	70
		73.7	73.0	72.4	72.0	71.7	71.5	71.4	71.1	71.0	71
		74.8	74.1	73.5	73.0	72.7	72.5	72.4	72.1	72.0	72
				74.5	74.0	73.7	73.5	73.4	73.1	73.0	73
						74.4	74.5	74.4	74.1	74.0	74

Bayley-Pinneau Table for Retarded Girls

To predict height, find vertical column corresponding to skeletal age and horizontal row for the present height. The number at the intersection is the predicted height in inches. If figures do not fall at the whole inch or 6-month intervals, the predicted height must be extrapolated.

Skeletal Age		6/0	6/6	7/0	7/6	8/0	8/6	9/0	9/6	10/0	10/6	11/0	11/6
Height in inches	38	51.8											
	39	53.2	51.9										
	40	54.6	53.3	51.9									
	41	55.9	54.6	53.2	52.0								
	42	57.3	55.9	54.5	53.3	52.2	51.0						
	43	58.7	57.3	55.8	54.6	53.5	52.2	51.1					
	44	60.0	58.6	57.1	55.8	54.7	53.5	52.3	51.3				
	45	61.4	59.9	58.4	57.1	56.0	54.7	53.5	52.4	51.5			
	46	62.8	61.3	59.7	58.4	57.2	55.9	54.7	53.6	52.6	51.3		
	47	64.1	62.6	61.0	59.6	58.5	57.1	55.9	54.8	53.8	52.5	51.2	
	48	65.5	63.9	62.3	60.9	59.7	58.3	57.1	55.9	54.9	63.6	52.3	51.8
	49	66.9	65.2	63.6	62.2	60.9	59.5	58.3	57.1	56.1	54.7	53.4	52.9
	50	68.2	66.6	64.9	63.5	62.2	60.8	59.5	58.3	57.2	55.8	54.5	54.0
	51	69.6	67.9	66.2	64.7	63.4	62.0	60.6	59.4	58.4	56.9	55.6	55.1
	52	70.9	69.2	67.5	66.0	64.7	63.2	61.8	60.6	59.5	58.0	56.6	56.2
	53	72.3	70.6	68.8	67.3	65.9	64.4	63.0	61.8	60.6	59.2	57.7	57.2
	54	73.7	71.9	70.1	68.5	67.2	65.6	64.2	62.9	61.8	60.3	58.8	58.3
	55		73.2	71.4	69.8	68.4	66.8	65.4	64.1	62.9	61.4	59.9	59.4
	56		74.6	72.7	71.1	69.7	68.0	66.6	65.3	64.1	62.5	61.0	60.5
	57			74.0	72.3	70.9	69.3	67.8	66.4	65.2	63.6	62.1	61.6
	58				73.6	72.1	70.5	69.0	67.6	66.4	64.7	63.2	62.6
	59				74.9	73.4	71.7	70.2	68.8	67.5	65.8	64.3	63.7
	60					74.6	72.9	71.3	69.9	68.7	67.0	65.4	64.8
	61						74.1	72.5	71.1	69.8	68.1	66.4	65.9
	62							73.7	72.3	70.9	69.2	67.5	67.0
	63							74.7	73.4	72.1	70.3	68.6	68.0
	64								74.6	73.2	71.4	69.7	69.1
	65									74.4	72.5	70.8	70.2
	66										73.7	71.9	71.3
	67										74.8	73.0	72.4
	68											74.1	73.4
	69												74.5
	70												
	71												
	72												
	73												
	74												

12/0	12/6	13/0	13/6	14/0	14/6	15/0	15/6	16/0	16/6	17/0	
											38
											39
											40
											41
											42
											43
											44
											45
											46
											47
51.5											48
52.6	51.6										49
53.6	52.7	51.9	51.2								50
54.7	53.7	52.9	52.2	51.9	51.6	51.3	51.2	51.1	51.1	51.0	51
55.8	54.8	53.9	53.2	52.9	52.6	52.3	52.2	52.1	52.1	52.0	52
56.9	55.8	55.0	54.2	53.9	53.6	53.3	53.2	53.1	53.1	53.0	53
57.9	56.9	56.0	55.3	54.9	54.6	54.3	54.2	54.1	54.1	54.0	54
59.0	58.0	57.1	56.3	56.0	55.6	55.3	55.2	55.1	55.1	55.0	55
60.1	59.0	58.1	57.3	57.0	56.6	56.3	56.2	56.1	56.1	56.0	56
61.2	60.1	59.1	58.3	58.0	57.6	57.3	57.2	57.1	57.1	57.0	57
62.2	61.1	60.2	59.4	59.0	58.6	58.3	58.2	58.1	58.1	58.0	58
63.3	62.2	61.2	60.4	60.0	59.7	59.4	59.2	59.1	59.1	59.0	59
64.4	63.2	62.2	61.4	61.0	60.7	60.4	60.2	60.1	60.1	60.0	60
65.5	64.3	63.3	62.4	62.1	61.7	61.4	61.2	61.1	61.1	61.0	61
66.5	65.3	64.3	63.5	63.1	62.7	62.4	62.2	62.1	62.1	62.0	62
67.6	66.4	65.3	64.5	64.1	63.7	63.4	63.3	63.1	63.1	63.0	63
68.7	67.4	66.4	65.5	65.1	64.7	64.4	64.3	64.1	64.1	64.0	64
69.7	68.5	67.4	66.5	66.1	65.7	65.4	65.3	65.1	65.1	65.0	65
70.8	69.5	68.5	67.6	67.1	66.7	66.4	66.3	66.1	66.1	66.0	66
71.9	70.6	69.5	68.6	68.2	67.7	67.4	67.3	67.1	67.1	67.0	67
73.0	71.7	70.5	69.6	69.2	68.8	68.4	68.3	68.1	68.1	68.0	68
74.0	72.7	71.6	70.6	70.2	69.8	69.4	69.3	69.1	69.1	69.0	69
	73.8	72.6	71.6	71.2	70.8	70.4	70.3	70.1	70.1	70.0	70
	74.8	73.6	72.7	72.2	71.8	71.4	71.3	71.1	71.1	71.0	71
		74.7	73.7	73.3	72.8	72.4	72.3	72.1	72.1	72.0	72
			74.7	74.3	73.8	73.4	73.3	73.1	73.1	73.0	73
					74.8	74.4	74.3	74.1	74.1	74.0	74

11   Amenorrhea

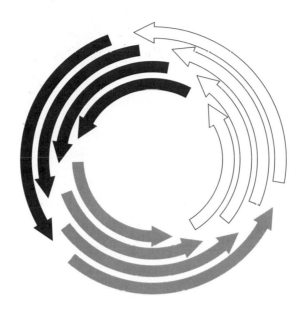

Few problems in gynecologic endocrinology are as challenging or taxing to the clinician as amenorrhea. The clinician must be concerned with an array of potential diseases and disorders involving, in many instances, unfamiliar organ systems, some carrying morbid and even lethal consequences for the patient. Not infrequently, the otherwise confident and experienced clinician dismisses the problem as too complex for a busy practice and refers the patient to a "specialist" in the field. In doing so, the nonavailability of sophisticated laboratory techniques is often cited as necessitating the costly and frequently inconvenient transfer of the patient.

The intent of this chapter is to provide a simple mechanism for the differential diagnosis of amenorrhea of all types and chronology, using procedures available to all clinicians. Strict adherence to this design will unerringly pinpoint the organ system locus of disorder leading to the presenting symptom of amenorrhea. Once this is accomplished, the detailed evidence confirming the diagnosis can be sought and the assistance of appropriate specialists (neurosurgeon, internist, endocrinologist, psychiatrist) confidently chosen. In the end, the patient receives the most reliable diagnosis and therapy at minimum cost and optimum convenience. The majority of patients with amenorrhea have relatively simple problems that can be managed easily by the patients' primary care clinicians. This happy outcome is also consistent with the modern health care emphasis on cost-effectiveness.

The "workup" to be described is not new. With minor modifications, it has been continuously and successfully applied for several decades. Before presenting the diagnostic workup in detail, it is necessary to provide a definition of amenorrhea, designating the appropriate selection of patients. In addition, a brief review of the physiologic mechanisms by which a menstrual flow is produced is presented to clarify the logic of the various steps in the diagnostic procedures.

Definition of Amenorrhea

Any patient fulfilling the following criteria should be evaluated as having the clinical problem of amenorrhea:

1. No period by age 14 in the absence of growth or development of secondary sexual characteristics.

2. No period by age 16 regardless of the presence of normal growth and development with the appearance of secondary sexual characteristics.

3. In a woman who has been menstruating, the absence of periods for a length of time equivalent to a total of at least 3 of the previous cycle intervals or 6 months of amenorrhea.

Having affirmed the traditional criteria, let us now point out that strict adherence to these criteria can result in improper management of individual cases. There is no reason to defer the evaluation of a young girl who presents with the obvious stigmata of Turner syndrome. Similarly, the 14-year-old girl with an absent vagina who is otherwise completely normal should not be told to return in 2 years. A patient deserves a considerate evaluation whenever her anxieties, or those of her parents, bring her to a clinician. Finally, the possibility of pregnancy should always be considered.

Another tradition has been to categorize amenorrhea as primary or secondary in nature. Although these stipulations are inherent in the classic definitions noted above, experience has shown that premature categorization of this sort leads to diagnostic omission in certain instances, and frequently, unnecessary and expensive diagnostic procedures. Because the prescribed workup to be detailed here applies comprehensively to all forms of amenorrhea, the classic definitions are not retained.

Basic Principles in Menstrual Function

The clinical demonstration of menstrual function depends on visible external evidence of the menstrual discharge. This requires an intact outflow tract that connects the internal genital source of flow with the outside. As such, the outflow tract requires patency and continuity of the vaginal orifice, the vaginal canal, and the endocervix with the uterine cavity. The presence of a menstrual flow depends on the existence and development of the endometrium lining the uterine cavity. This tissue is stimulated and regulated by the proper quantity and sequence of the steroid hormones, estrogen and progesterone. The secretion of these hormones originates in the ovary, but more specifically, in the evolving spectrum of follicle development, ovulation, and corpus luteum function. This essential maturation of the follicular apparatus is guided by the stimuli provided by the sequence and magnitude of the gonadotropins, follicle-stimulating hormone (FSH) and luteinizing hormone (LH), originating in the anterior pituitary. The secretion of these hormones is in turn dependent on gonadotropin-releasing hormone (GnRH), the specific peptide-releasing hormone produced in the basal hypothalamus and blood borne via the portal vessels of the stalk to receptive cells within the anterior pituitary. The entire system is regulated by a complex mechanism that integrates biophysical and biochemical information composed of interactive levels of hormonal signals, autocrine/paracrine factors, and target cell reactions.

At 6–8 weeks of gestation, the first signs of ovarian differentiation are reflected in the rapid mitotic multiplication of germ cells, reaching 6–7 million oogonia by 16–20 weeks.[1, 2] This represents the maximal oogonal content of the gonad. From this point in time germ cell content will irretrievably decrease until, some 50 years later, the store of oocytes will be finally exhausted. Chromosomal anomalies can accelerate germ cell loss. Individuals with Turner syndrome (45,X) experience normal migration and mitosis of germ cells, but the oogonia do not

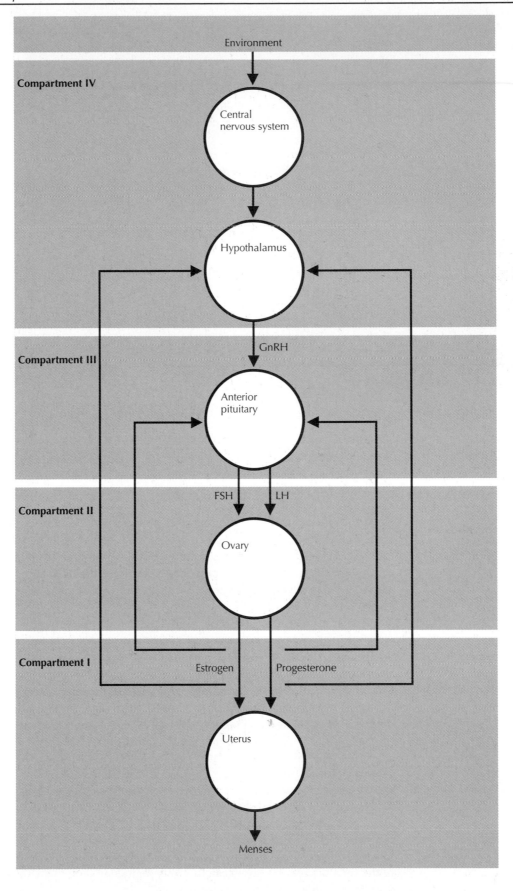

undergo meiosis, and rapid loss of oocytes leaves the gonad without follicles by birth, and it appears as a fibrous streak.

The basic principles underlying the physiology of menstrual function permit formulation of several discrete compartmental systems on which proper menstruation depends. It is useful to employ a diagnostic evaluation that segregates causes of amenorrhea into the following compartments:

Compartment I:
Disorders of the outflow tract or uterine target organ.

Compartment II:
Disorders of the ovary.

Compartment III:
Disorders of the anterior pituitary.

Compartment IV:
Disorders of central nervous system (hypothalamic) factors.

Evaluation of Amenorrhea

A careful history and physical examination should seek the following: evidence for psychological dysfunction or emotional stress, family history of apparent genetic anomalies, signs of a physical problem with a focus on nutritional status, abnormal growth and development, the presence of a normal reproductive tract, and evidence for CNS disease. A patient with amenorrhea is then exposed to a combined therapeutic and laboratory dissection according to the depicted flow diagrams. Because a significant number of patients with amenorrhea also have galactorrhea (nonpuerperal breast secretion), and there are similarities in the evaluation of these two conditions, the workup as described is appropriate for patients who have amenorrhea, galactorrhea, or both. Galactorrhea is an important clinical physical sign, whether it is spontaneous or present only with careful expression by the examiner, unilateral or bilateral, persistent or intermittent. ***Hormonal secretions usually come from multiple duct openings in contrast to pathologic discharge that usually comes from a single duct.*** Galactorrhea is considered in greater detail in Chapter 16.

Amenorrhea and galactorrhea need be the sole pertinent initial items of information. Although additional data are undoubtedly available at this time, derived from history and physical examination and evaluation of other endocrine glands such as the thyroid and adrenal, these items should not be utilized for diagnostic purposes until the entire workup is completed. Experience has shown that premature diagnostic bias at this point, while frequently accurate, not uncommonly leads to erroneous judgments as well as inappropriate, costly, and useless testing.

Step 1

The initial step in the workup of the amenorrheic patient after excluding pregnancy begins with a measurement of thyroid-stimulating hormone (TSH), a prolactin level, and a progestational challenge. The initial step in the patient presenting with galactorrhea, regardless of menstrual history, also includes TSH and prolactin measurements but adds a coned-down, lateral x-ray view of the sella turcica. The x-ray can be safely omitted in those patients who have galactorrhea, but also have regular, ovulatory menstrual cycles.

Only a few patients presenting with amenorrhea and/or galactorrhea will have hypothyroidism that is not clinically apparent. Although it seems rather extravagant to measure TSH in such a

large number of patients for such a small return, because treatment for hypothyroidism is so simple and is rewarded by such a prompt return of ovulatory cycles, and, if galactorrhea is present, by a disappearance of the breast secretions (a slower process that can take several months), TSH measurement is warranted.

The duration of the hypothyroidism is important with regard to the mechanism of the galactorrhea; the longer the duration the higher the incidence of galactorrhea and the higher the prolactin levels.[3] This is thought to be associated with declining hypothalamic content of dopamine with on-going hypothyroidism. This would lead to an unopposed thyrotropin-releasing hormone (TRH) stimulatory effect on the pituitary cells that secrete prolactin. In our experience, prolactin levels associated with primary hypothyroidism have always been less than 100 ng/mL.

Constant stimulation by hypothalamic-releasing hormones can result in hypertrophy or hyperplasia of the pituitary. The imaging picture of a tumor (distortion, expansion, or erosion of the sella turcica) can be seen, therefore, with primary hypothyroidism and in patients with elevated GnRH and gonadotropin secretion due to premature ovarian failure.[4,5] Appropriate treatment is followed by rapid normalization of the initial image. Patients with primary hypothyroidism and hyperprolactinemia can present with either primary or secondary amenorrhea.[6]

The purpose of the progestational challenge is to assess the level of endogenous estrogen and the competence of the outflow tract. A course of a progestational agent totally devoid of estrogenic activity is administered. There are 3 choices: parenteral progesterone in oil (200 mg), the oral administration of micronized progesterone (300 mg), or orally active medroxyprogesterone acetate, 10 mg daily for 5 days. The use of an orally active agent avoids an unpleasant intramuscular injection (although this might be necessary when compliance is a concern). The dose of micronized progesterone is relatively high and should be administered at bedtime to avoid side effects. Other hormonal preparations, such as oral contraceptives, are not appropriate because they do not exert a purely progestational effect.

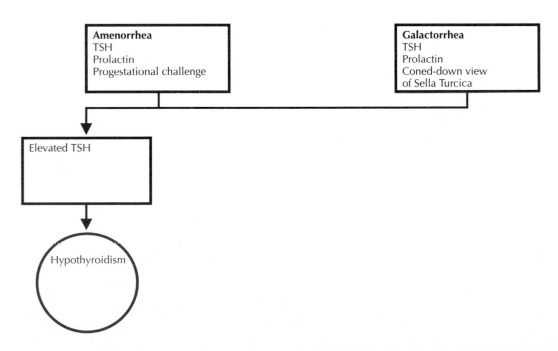

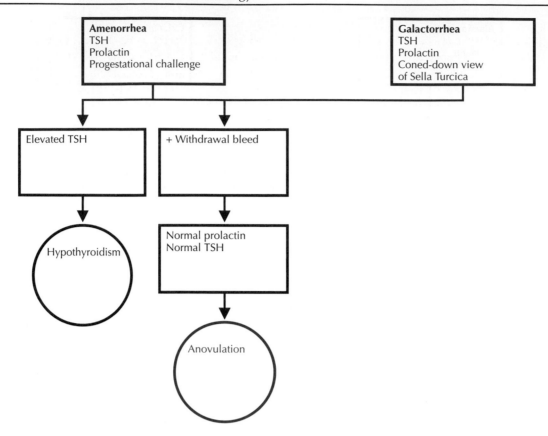

Within 2–7 days after the conclusion of progestational medication, the patient will either bleed or not bleed. If the patient bleeds, a diagnosis of anovulation has been reliably and securely established. The presence of a functional outflow tract and a uterus lined by reactive endometrium sufficiently prepared by endogenous estrogen is confirmed. With this demonstration of the presence of estrogen, minimal function of the ovary, pituitary, and CNS is established. In the absence of galactorrhea, with a normal prolactin level, and a normal TSH, further evaluation is unnecessary.

How much bleeding constitutes a positive withdrawal response? The appearance of only a few blood spots following progestational medication implies marginal levels of endogenous estrogen. Such patients should be followed closely and periodically reevaluated, because the marginally positive response may progress to a clearly negative response, placing the patient in a new diagnostic category. Bleeding in any amount beyond a few spots is considered a positive withdrawal response.

There are two rare situations associated with a negative withdrawal response, despite the presence of adequate levels of endogenous estrogen. In both situations, the endometrium is decidualized, and, therefore, it will not be shed following the withdrawal of exogenous progestin. The first condition finds the endometrium decidualized in response to high androgen levels, e.g., due to the anovulatory state (with polycystic ovaries). In the second unusual clinical situation, the endometrium is decidualized by high progesterone levels associated with a specific adrenal enzyme deficiency.

All anovulatory patients require therapeutic management, and with this minimal evaluation, therapy can be planned immediately. Because of the short latent period in the progression from normal endometrial tissue to atypia to cancer, clinicians are sensitive to the issue of endometrial cancer. But all too often, the clinician believes that this is a problem limited to older age. The critical feature is the duration of exposure to constant, unopposed estrogen. Therefore, even young women, anovulatory for relatively long periods of time, can develop endometrial cancer. If there is any concern, evaluation of the endometrium (with aspiration curettage) is in order. On the other hand, the latent phase for breast cancer is long, perhaps as long as 20 years. Women who are anovulatory when they are young may have an increased risk of breast cancer when they are postmenopausal.[7] This could reflect exposure to unopposed estrogen, or it could be the consequence of infertility and the absence of the protection against breast cancer that pregnancy early in the reproductive years confers. However, some studies have not observed a link between anovulation and the risk of breast cancer (discussed with full references in Chapter 16).

Minimal therapy of anovulatory women requires the monthly administration of a progestational agent. An easily remembered program is to prescribe 10 mg medroxyprogesterone acetate daily for the first 10 days of each month. Experience with the endometrium in estrogen therapy programs has established the importance of a time period of at least 10 days to provide adequate protection against the growth-promoting effects of constant estrogen. When reliable contraception is essential, the use of low-dose oral contraceptive pills in the usual cyclic fashion is appropriate. Attempts to demonstrate a relationship between pill use and subsequent postpill amenorrhea have not been successful. Anovulation with amenorrhea or oligomenorrhea should not be viewed as a contraindication to the use of oral contraception.

If, at any time, an anovulatory patient fails to have withdrawal bleeding on a monthly progestin program, this is a sign (providing the patient is not pregnant) that she has moved to the negative withdrawal bleed category, and the remainder of the workup must be pursued. The progestational challenge will occasionally trigger an ovulation in an anovulatory patient. The tip-off will be a later withdrawal bleed, 14 days after the progestational challenge!

In the absence of galactorrhea and if the serum prolactin level is normal (less than 20 ng/mL in most laboratories), further evaluation for a pituitary tumor is unnecessary provided the patient has undergone a withdrawal bleed. Random single samples for prolactin are sufficient, because variations in the amplitude of the spikes of secretion and the sleep-related and food-related increases appear to be attenuated in both functional and tumor hyperprolactinemic states. If the prolactin is elevated, imaging evaluation of the sella turcica is essential (as discussed below). At this point in the workup, the following statement is a useful clinical rule of thumb: *A positive withdrawal bleeding response to progestational medication, the absence of galactorrhea, and a normal prolactin level together effectively rule out the presence of a significant pituitary tumor.*

Ectopic production of prolactin is rarely encountered. Increased prolactin secretion should draw attention to the pituitary gland. However, to be complete, we should mention case reports with ectopic secretion associated with pituitary tissue in the pharynx, bronchogenic carcinoma, renal cell carcinoma, a gonadoblastoma, and women with amenorrhea and hyperprolactinemia due to a prolactinoma in the wall of an ovarian dermoid cyst or teratoma.[8–12]

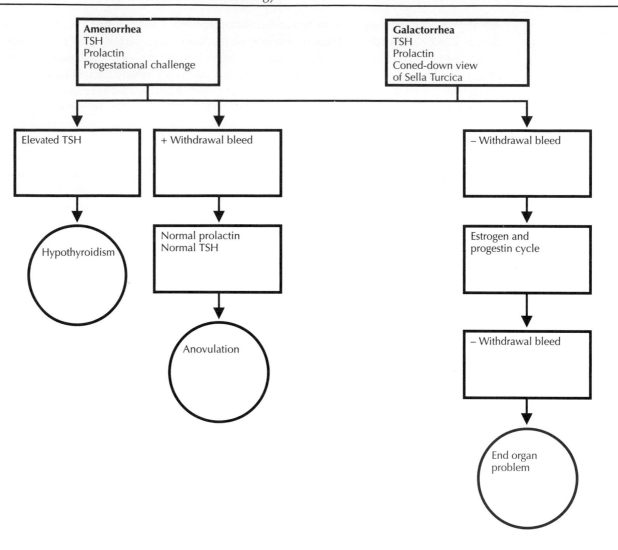

Step 2

If the course of progestational medication does not produce withdrawal flow, either the target organ outflow tract is inoperative or preliminary estrogen proliferation of the endometrium has not occurred. Step 2 is designed to clarify this situation. Orally active estrogen is administered in quantity and duration certain to stimulate endometrial proliferation and withdrawal bleeding provided that a completely reactive uterus and patent outflow tract exist. An appropriate dose is 1.25 mg conjugated estrogens or 2 mg estradiol daily for 21 days. The terminal addition of an orally active progestational agent (medroxyprogesterone acetate 10 mg daily for the last 5 days) is necessary to achieve withdrawal. In this way the capacity of Compartment I is challenged by exogenous estrogen. In the absence of withdrawal flow, a validating second course of estrogen is a wise precaution.

As a result of the pharmacologic test of Step 2, the patient with amenorrhea will either bleed or not bleed. If there is no withdrawal flow, the diagnosis of a defect in the Compartment I systems (endometrium, outflow tract) can be made with confidence. If withdrawal bleeding does occur, one can assume that Compartment I systems have normal functional abilities if properly stimulated by estrogen.

From a practical point of view, in a patient with normal external and internal genitalia by pelvic examination, and in the absence of a history of infection or trauma (such as curettage), an abnormality of the outflow tract is unlikely. Outflow tract problems include either destruction of the endometrium, generally the result of an overzealous curettage or the result of an infection, or primary amenorrhea resulting from the discontinuity or disruption of the müllerian tube. ***Abnormalities in the systems of Compartment I are not commonly encountered, and in the absence of a reason to suspect a problem, Step 2 can be omitted.***

Step 3

With the elucidation of the amenorrheic patient's inability to provide adequate stimulatory amounts of estrogen, the physiologic mechanisms responsible for the elaboration of this steroid must be tested. In order to produce estrogen, ovaries containing a normal follicular apparatus and sufficient pituitary gonadotropins to stimulate that apparatus are required. Step 3 is designed to determine which of these two crucial components (gonadotropins or follicular activity) is functioning improperly.

This step involves an assay of the level of gonadotropins in the patient. Because Step 2 involved administration of exogenous estrogen, endogenous gonadotropin levels may be artificially and temporarily altered from their true baseline concentrations. Hence, a delay of 2 weeks following Step 2 must ensue before doing Step 3, the gonadotropin assay. One should keep in mind that the midcycle surge of LH is approximately 3 times the baseline level. Therefore, if the patient does not bleed 2 weeks after the blood sample was obtained, a high level can be safely interpreted as abnormal.

Step 3 is designed to determine whether the lack of estrogen is due to a fault in the follicle (Compartment II) or in the CNS-pituitary axis (Compartments III and IV). The result of the gonadotropin assay in the amenorrheic woman who does not bleed following a progestational agent will be abnormally high, abnormally low, or in the normal range.

Clinical State	Serum FSH	Serum LH
Normal adult female	5–20 IU/L, with the ovulatory midcycle peak about 2 times the base level	5–20 IU/L, with the ovulatory midcycle peak about 3 times the base level
Hypogonadotropic state: Prepubertal, hypothalamic, or pituitary dysfunction	Less than 5 IU/L	Less than 5 IU/L
Hypergonadotropic state: Postmenopausal, castrate, or ovarian failure	Greater than 20 IU/L	Greater than 40 IU/L

High Gonadotropins

The clinical implications of elevated gonadotropins are very significant, and, therefore, repeated measurements, several months apart, are worthwhile to document a more than transient state. The association between castrate or postmenopausal levels of gonadotropins and absent ovarian follicles due to accelerated atresia is very reliable, but not totally reliable. There are rare situations in which high gonadotropins can be accompanied by ovaries that contain follicles.

1. On rare occasions, tumors can produce gonadotropins. This situation is usually associated with lung cancer and is so infrequent that, with a normal history and physical examination, routine chest x-ray is not warranted in amenorrheic patients.

2. There have been a handful of reports of a single gonadotropin deficiency. The importance of measuring both FSH and LH can be appreciated because a high level of one and a baseline or undetectable level of the other would reveal this rare condition. The rare cases of a true single gonadotropin deficiency are probably due to homozygous mutations in the gonadotropin genes. A case of hypogonadism due to an LH β-subunit mutation and a woman with primary amenorrhea due to a mutation in the FSH β-subunit have been reported.[13, 14] The mutated β-subunit genes produce alterations in the β-subunits that yield no immunoreactivity or bioactivity. Hence, hypogonadism will be associated with one high and one low gonadotropin level. Heterozygote carriers have a problem of relative infertility. Treatment with exogenous gonadotropins will achieve pregnancy in these rare patients. When a high FSH and a normal or low LH are encountered, an elevated level of α-subunit and the presence of a pituitary mass indicate a gonadotroph adenoma.

3. Elevated gonadotropins can be due to a gonadotropin-secreting pituitary adenoma. However, gonadotropin-secreting adenomas are *NOT* associated with hypogonadism (amenorrhea), and, therefore, are hard to diagnose.[15–17] There is no specific symptom or symptom complex associated with hypersecretion of gonadotropins. Thus, these tumors are usually diagnosed because of tumor growth that results in headaches and visual disturbances. Previously it was believed that these tumors were very rare and more common in men. This belief was due to the difficulty in recognizing these adenomas, especially in women. However, tumors of the pituitary are relatively common, and most are not nonsecreting, but, in fact, they arise from gonadotroph cells, and they are active.[18] In addition to secreting FSH and, rarely, LH, these tumors secrete high levels of the α-subunit of the glycopeptide hormones, and sometimes only the α-subunit. Patients suspected of having a pituitary tumor, the nature of which is uncertain or puzzling, should have their gonadotropin and α-subunit levels measured.

4. During the perimenopausal period, it is normal for FSH levels to begin to rise even before bleeding has ceased.[19] This is true whether the perimenopausal period is premature at age 25–35 or at the usual time. This increase in FSH is associated with a decrease in inhibin. During the perimenopausal period, the remaining follicles may be viewed as the least sensitive of all follicles because they have remained in place and failed to respond to gonadotropins for many years. The rise in FSH prior to menopause is due to the declining inhibin production by either the less competent ovarian follicles or because the cohort of follicles is reduced in number. Attention must be paid to this situation because a period of elevated levels of FSH can be followed by a pregnancy. An elevated FSH level is not an absolute indicator of infertility. It is not unusual to encounter a pregnancy in a woman after a diagnosis of premature ovarian failure.[20]

5. In the resistant or insensitive ovary syndrome, the patient with amenorrhea and normal growth and development has elevated gonadotropins, despite the presence of ovarian follicles. In this condition, the ovarian follicles are unresponsive to stimulation compared with premature depletion of follicles in the most common type of premature ovarian failure. This syndrome may be due to absent or defective gonadotropin receptors on the follicles or a postreceptor-signaling defect.[21] Molecular biology studies of patients with premature ovarian failure are discovering rare cases of point mutations; e.g., mutations in the gonadotropin receptor genes that prevent ovarian response.[22, 23] We anticipate that more and more such cases will be identified. In addition, translocations between regions on X and Y chromosomes that share sequence homology have been reported in patients with secondary amenorrhea and ovarian failure.[24] It is also possible that this is a subtle form of autoimmune ovarian failure. In these cases, laparotomy is the only definitive way to evaluate the ovaries, because follicles are contained deep within the ovary, yielding only to a full thickness biopsy.[25] Because this condition is very rare, and the chance of achieving pregnancy is probably impossible, even with large doses of exogenous gonadotropins, laparotomy is *NOT* recommended for every patient with amenorrhea and high gonadotropins.

6. Secondary amenorrhea caused by premature ovarian failure can be due to autoimmune disease.[26] The ovaries contain normal-appearing primordial follicles, but developing follicles are surrounded by nests of lymphocytes and plasma cells with lymphocytic infiltration of the thecal layer of cells. The exact mechanism of resistance to gonadotropins is not known. Antibodies blocking FSH and LH receptors cannot be demonstrated in immunoglobulin G from women with premature ovarian failure.[27] Most commonly, evidence of abnormal thyroid function is detected, and, therefore, complete thyroid testing (with antibodies) is necessary in all patients with premature ovarian failure. The extensive polyglandular syndrome (autoimmune polyglandular syndrome) that includes hypoparathyroidism, adrenal insufficiency, thyroiditis, and moniliasis, is rare; at least one gene mutation has been identified in this autosomal recessive disorder.[28] In patients with adrenal insufficiency and ovarian failure, antibodies have been detected directed against P450scc, the cholesterol side-chain cleavage enzyme essential for steroidogenesis.[29] It is believed that antibodies can be directed against any of the vital enzymes involved in steroidogenesis. Other rare conditions associated with premature ovarian failure include myasthenia gravis, idiopathic thrombocytopenic purpura, rheumatoid arthritis, vitiligo, and autoimmune hemolytic anemia. Classically, premature ovarian failure precedes adrenal failure, and, thus, a case can be made for continuing adrenal surveillance.[30] Frequently, various endocrine disorders will be present among family members. Very rare pregnancies have been reported in women with ovarian failure and autoimmune disease. Ovulation has been restored temporarily with corticosteroid treatment, and at least one patient had a temporary spontaneous return of menstrual ovarian activity.[31] Because pregnancy is extremely unlikely, consideration should be given to donor oocytes. However, an impressive pregnancy rate has been reported by one group combining suppression with a GnRH agonist, corticosteroid treatment, and induction of ovulation with high doses of exogenous gonadotropins.[32]

7. Galactosemia is a rare inherited autosomal recessive disorder of galactose metabolism due to a deficiency of galactose-1-phosphate uridyl transferase.[33] The problem in patients with galactosemia is primarily gonadal; fewer oogonia may be the result of a direct toxic effect of galactose metabolites on germ cell migration to the genital ridge.[34] Premature ovarian failure is common and usually irreversible.

8. The final rare clinical situation associated with high gonadotropins despite the presence of ovarian follicles is that associated with specific enzymatic deficiencies. The 17-hydroxylase deficiency (P450c17) is present in both ovaries and the adrenal gland. A patient with a deficiency of 17-hydroxylase is readily detectable because she would present with absent secondary sexual development (sex steroids cannot be produced due to the enzyme block in the adrenal glands and the ovaries), and hypertension, hypokalemia, and high blood levels of progesterone. A deficiency in the aromatase enzymes is another rare cause of hypergonadotropic amenorrhea and a failure of pubertal development.

The Need for Chromosome Evaluation

All patients under the age of 30 who have been assigned the diagnosis of ovarian failure on the basis of elevated gonadotropins must have a karyotype determination. The presence of mosaicism with a Y chromosome requires excision of the gonadal areas because the presence of any testicular component within the gonad carries with it a significant chance of malignant tumor formation. These are highly malignant secondary tumors from germ cells: gonadoblastomas, dysgerminomas, yolk sac tumors, and choriocarcinoma. Approximately 30% of patients with a Y chromosome will not develop signs of virilization. Therefore, even the normal-appearing adult woman with elevated gonadotropin levels must be karyotyped. Even if the karyotype is normal, as an added precaution all patients with ovarian failure should have an annual pelvic examination. Such preventive care is also indicated because these patients will be receiving hormone therapy. Over the age of 30, amenorrhea with high gonadotropins is best labeled premature menopause. Genetic evaluation is unnecessary because it is essentially unheard of to have a gonadal tumor appear in these patients after the age of 30. Most of these tumors appear before age 20, but a significant number are detected from age 20 to 30.[35, 36]

The clinician and patient should give consideration to whether it is worth obtaining an expensive karyotype to seek identification of chromosomal abnormalities that have clinical implications for other family members. Deletions of the X chromosome can be responsible for premature ovarian failure.[37] Accurate diagnosis of these deletions is not essential for decision making regarding the patient; however, the presence of such abnormalities within a family is associated with infertility due to premature ovarian failure. Having this information can influence the family planning decisions of family members. We recommend that women with premature ovarian failure who are less than 63 inches tall (160 cm) be karyotyped because of the close conjunction of the genes responsible for stature and normal ovarian function. *Because an individual with a mosaic karyotype (e.g., XX/XO) can experience normal pubertal development, menses, and even pregnancy before the onset of a premature menopause, it is appropriate to consider obtaining a karyotype, regardless of menstrual pattern, in an adolescent or young woman less than 60 inches tall.* Spontaneous puberty has been reported in 10–20% and spontaneous menstruation in 2–5% of girls with Turner syndrome.[38]

Premature Ovarian Failure: A Clinical Dilemma

Patients with repeatedly elevated gonadotropin levels can be reliably diagnosed as having ovarian failure and can be considered sterile. In the past this was a diagnosis made with great confidence, and careful explanation was given to the patient indicating that future pregnancy was impossible. However, as many as 10–20% of patients presenting with secondary amenorrhea and elevated gonadotropins (with normal karyotypes), several months later, have demonstrated resumption of normal function.[20, 39, 40] Often, this has been associated with the use of estrogen therapy, suggesting that the estrogen may activate receptor formation on follicles, and the high gonadotropins may, thus, stimulate follicular growth and development. On the other hand, spontaneous recovery of ovarian function may be the reason for apparent success with treatment. In some patients, return of normal ovarian function with pregnancy has occurred in the absence of any

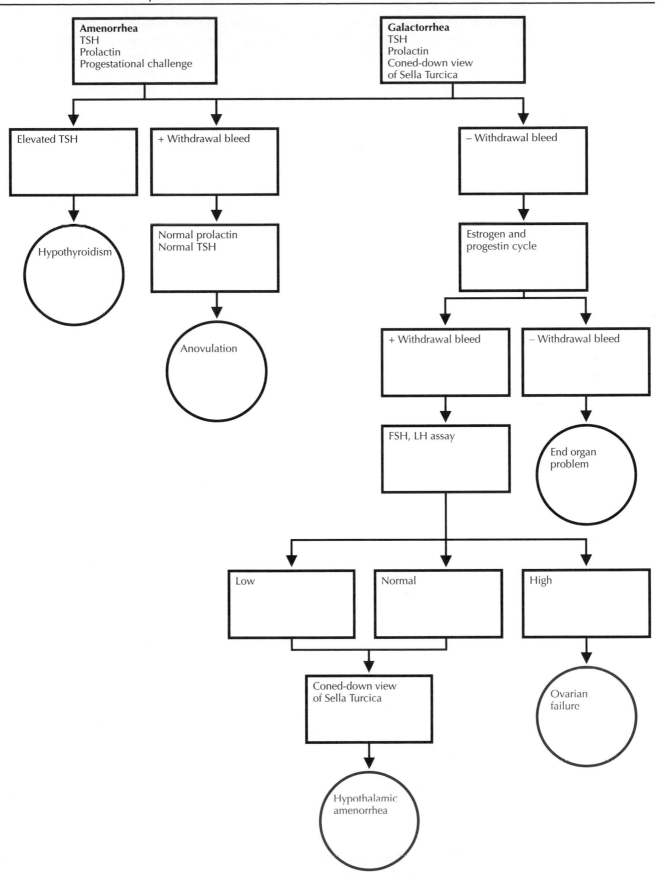

treatment. Indeed, careful study of estrogen treatment in women with hypergonadotropic amenorrhea could detect no impact on ovarian folliculogenesis.[41] Although resumption of normal function is extremely rare, it is now necessary to tell patients who fit into this category that there is a very remote possibility of future pregnancy (but it should be emphasized this is very unlikely). In addition the feasibility of pregnancy with the transfer of a fertilized donated ovum should be presented as a possible option (Chapter 31).

A number of cases of ovarian failure have been reported with autoimmune disorders. Indirect immunofluorescence has been used for the detection of ovarian antibodies, but the results have been variable and of little clinical meaning. Comparing several methodologies currently available, only a small number of women with premature ovarian failure test positively, results are inconsistent, and a need or indication for ovarian antibody testing cannot be established.[42] The search for antibodies to gonadotropin receptors has been equally unrewarding.[27]

A reasonable empiric approach is to perform a few selected blood tests for autoimmune disease. These tests should also be obtained periodically (perhaps every few years) as part of the long-term surveillance against associated autoimmune disorders.

> Calcium
> Phosphorus
> Fasting glucose
> A.M. cortisol
> Free T_4
> TSH
> Thyroid antibodies, if thyroid function is abnormal
> Complete blood count and sedimentation rate
> Total protein, albumin:globulin ratio
> Rheumatoid factor
> Antinuclear antibody

Testing for adrenocorticotropic hormone (ACTH) reserve (with corticotropin stimulation or metyrapone) is not necessary if clinical appearance and other laboratory tests are normal. Periodic surveillance for adrenal failure is in order because ovarian failure usually precedes adrenal failure. It is not worthwhile to seek the presence of antiovarian antibodies in serum or antibodies to the gonadotropins; there is no correlation between the clinical state and the results from such testing.[30]

Other than hypothyroidism, it is uncommon to encounter other disorders associated with premature ovarian failure. In a series of 119 patients with premature ovarian failure and normal karyotypes, recruited by the National Institute of Child Health and Human Development in Bethesda, 10 new cases of hypothyroidism and 3 new cases of diabetes mellitus were discovered; there were no new cases of adrenal insufficiency, hypoparathyroidism, or pernicious anemia.[43]

It has been suggested that blood gonadotropins and estradiol should be measured weekly on 4 occasions.[20] If FSH is not higher than LH (an FSH:LH ratio less than 1.0), and if estradiol is greater than 50 pg/mL, induction of ovulation can be considered. Prior to treatment with exogenous gonadotropins, no advantage has been demonstrated to first bringing the elevated gonadotropins down to normal range with administration of a GnRH agonist.[44] The experience with this approach has been unrewarding, and we do not recommend it.

The clinician needs to compare the choice of a full-thickness ovarian biopsy with empirical treatment. In our view, empirical treatment appears to outweigh the cost and risk of laparotomy, since only a very rare woman with hypergonadotropic amenorrhea can be expected to conceive. In other words, even if there is some gonadotropic and estradiol evidence of follicular activity, the response to exogenous gonadotropin stimulation has been very disappointing. We believe that ovarian biopsy is not indicated or necessary.

Transvaginal ultrasonography can identify ovarian follicular activity in many of these patients. However, the meaning of this finding is uncertain. Are patients with ovarian follicles present on ultrasonography more likely to respond to treatment and achieve pregnancy? In time, clinical studies should provide us with an answer.

This clinical problem requires scientific study. Ovarian failure may be the consequence of more than one abnormal condition. One recognized example is ovarian failure due to an accelerated rate of follicular atresia leading to the premature depletion of the follicular supply. Other cases may be due to a failure in the gonadotropin receptor mechanism. Unsuccessful binding can be due to defective receptors, blockage of receptors (e.g., by autoantibodies), or to genetic mutations that direct the production of gonadotropins of altered structure which are incapable of binding. Molecular studies of these patients should bring important clinical clarification in the coming years.

Normal Gonadotropins

Why is it that hypoestrogenic (negative progestational withdrawal) patients will frequently have normal circulating levels of FSH and LH as measured by immunoassay? If normal gonadotropins were truly present in the circulation, follicular growth should be maintained and estrogen levels would be adequate to provide a positive withdrawal bleed. The answer to this paradox lies in the heterogeneity of the glycoprotein hormones (as discussed in Chapter 2).

The molecules of gonadotropins produced by these amenorrheic patients have increased amounts of sialic acid in the carbohydrate portion. Therefore, the molecules are qualitatively altered and biologically inactive. The antibodies in the immunoassay, however, are able to recognize a sufficient portion of the molecule to return a normal answer. Another very rare possibility is an inherited disorder of gonadotropin synthesis leading to the production of immunologically active but biologically inactive hormones.[45]

The significant clinical point is the following: FSH and LH levels in the normal range in a patient with a negative progestational withdrawal test are consistent with pituitary-CNS failure. Indeed, this is the most commonly encountered clinical situation. Extremely low or nondetectable gonadotropins are seldom found, usually only with large pituitary tumors or in patients with anorexia nervosa. Further evaluation, therefore, is in order and follows the recommendations for low gonadotropins.

Low Gonadotropins

If the gonadotropin assay is abnormally low, or in the normal range, one final localization is required to distinguish between a pituitary (Compartment III) or CNS-hypothalamic (Compartment IV) cause for the amenorrhea. This is achieved by imaging evaluation of the sella turcica for signs of abnormal change.

Imaging of the Sella Turcica

The diagnostic modality of choice is either thin-section coronal computed tomography (CT scan) with intravenous contrast enhancement or magnetic resonance imaging (MRI) with gadolinium enhancement. CT scanning (capable of high-resolution 1.5 mm cuts) is able to evaluate the contents of the sella turcica as well as the suprasellar area; however, total accuracy is not achieved.[46] Magnetic resonance imaging is even more sensitive than the CT scan, but it is also more expensive, and it requires a lengthy period of time to obtain the images. MRI provides highly accurate assessments without biologic hazard, and it is better for evaluation of extrasellar extensions and the empty sella turcica.[47] Most neuroradiologists and neurosurgeons prefer MRI,

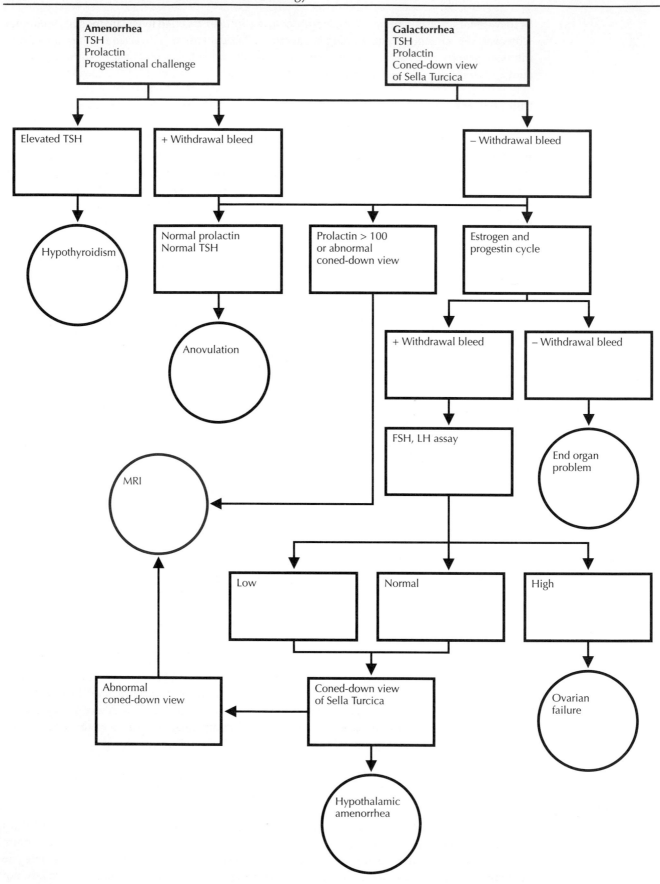

as do we. The intention of this workup is to be conscious of cost and to isolate those few patients who require sophisticated but expensive imaging.

There has been growing conservatism in the management of small pituitary tumors because of an appreciation that the majority of these tumors never change.[48–50] We have adopted the conservative approach of close surveillance, recommending dopamine agonist treatment for those prolactin-secreting tumors that display rapid growth, or those tumors that are already large, and reserving surgery only for those tumors that are unresponsive to medical therapy. This means that small tumors (microadenomas are less than 10 mm in diameter) need not be treated at all. Hence, the initial x-ray evaluation for amenorrheic patients with or without galactorrhea is the coned-down lateral view of the sella turcica. This will detect the presence of a large tumor, although an incredibly rare suprasellar extension might escape this method. The coned-down lateral view of the sella is also a good screen for other lesions, such as a craniopharyngioma. Combining this screening technique with the prolactin assay, we are able to select those few patients who require more sensitive sellar imaging. If the prolactin level is greater than 100 ng/mL, or if the coned-down view of the sella turcica is abnormal, we recommend CT scan evaluation or MRI. *A double floor of the sella is often seen on the coned-down view and, in the absence of enlargement and/ or demineralization, is interpreted as a normal variation rather than asymmetrical depression of the sellar floor by a tumor.*

The presence of visual problems and/or headaches should also encourage CT scan or MRI evaluation. Headaches are definitely correlated with the presence of a pituitary adenoma.[51] Although they are usually bifrontal, retro-orbital, or bitemporal, no locations or features are specific for pituitary tumors.

The prolactin level of 100 ng/mL for determining a more aggressive approach has been empirically chosen. Both in our own experience, and that of others, large tumors are most frequently associated with prolactin levels greater than 100 ng/mL. *Large masses associated with prolactin levels less than 100 ng/mL are more likely to be tumors other than prolactin-secreting adenomas, causing stalk compression and interruption of the normal dopamine regulation of prolactin secretion. These tumors will be associated with abnormal changes present in the coned-down view of the sella turcica.*

If imaging rules out an empty sella syndrome, or a suprasellar problem, treatment is dictated by the patient's desires, the size of the tumor, and the rapidity of growth of the tumor.

The above approach to the problem of pituitary tumors implies that patients with prolactin levels less than 100 ng/mL and with normal coned-down views of the sella turcica can be offered a choice between treatment and surveillance. An annual prolactin level and a periodic coned-down view (at first annually, and then at increasing intervals) are indicated for continued observation to detect an emerging and slow-growing tumor. Dopamine agonist therapy is recommended for patients wishing to achieve pregnancy and for those patients who have galactorrhea to the point of discomfort. Thus far, long-term therapy with a dopamine agonist has not been proven to be successful in producing a complete reversal of the problem (with either permanent suppression of elevated prolactin levels or elimination of small tumors). Thus, a very strong argument can be made for a "need not to know" the presence of a pituitary microadenoma. If treatment and management are not changed, it is not necessary to document the presence of a microadenoma.

Reasons Why the Diagnosis of Microadenoma Is Not Necessary

1. *Microadenomas are very common.*

2. *Microadenomas very rarely grow during pregnancy.*

3. *Microadenomas very rarely progress to a macroadenoma (10 mm or more in diameter).*

4. *There is a significant recurrence rate after surgery.*

5. *The natural course is unaffected by dopamine agonist treatment.*

6. *There is no contraindication to hormone therapy or oral contraception.*

7. *It is better to avoid the problem of the pituitary incidentaloma.*

Contemporary reviews point out the short comings of the coned-down view of the sella turcica, citing the limitation of excluding only macroadenomas.[52] Indeed, reviews of our text have faulted this chapter for being less than the state-of-the-art, emphasizing that where we use the coned-down view, MRI should be uniformly obtained. We would argue that the state-of-the-art approach is to use the MRI when necessary, to avoid the compulsion to document the presence of a microadenoma for the reasons stated above, to be cost-effective. This takes strength of conviction when your radiologist reports that a coned-down view of the sella turcica is not sufficient.

The Pituitary Incidentaloma

The percentage of pituitary glands found to contain unsuspected adenomas, all microadenomas, ranged from 9% to 27% in autopsy series.[53-57] Therefore, many individuals, probably 10%,[58] have silent pituitary masses that are endocrinologically inactive and have no adverse effects on well-being. These lesions are being found incidentally because of the increased use of CT scanning and MRI. Silent microadenomas (less than 10 mm diameter) do not grow, and even macroadenomas (10 mm or more diameter) grow slowly and only rarely.[49, 50] This benign course argues against immediate intervention in patients who have no evidence of hormonal disturbances; long-term surveillance is appropriate.[59] Imaging reassessment of a microadenoma should be obtained at 1, 2, and 5 years, and if there is no change, no further studies are necessary. Imaging reassessment of a macroadenoma should be obtained at 0.5, 1, 2, and 5 years. Growth, of course, requires treatment. Although it is reasonable to screen hormonal function in the presence of a macroadenoma, the value of hormonal screening in a normal individual with a microadenoma is debatable. Minimal hormonal screening includes prolactin, TSH, IGF-I, and a 24-hour urinary cortisol or the overnight dexamethasone suppression test (Chapter 13).

Evaluation of the Abnormal Sella Turcica and/or High Prolactin

The high incidence of pituitary tumors in patients with amenorrhea has prompted a search for a reliable method of diagnosing the condition. Expectations for the utilization of endocrine testing to discriminate between disorders of the hypothalamus and the anterior pituitary have not been realized. These endocrine maneuvers include GnRH stimulation, TRH stimulation, and other steps to alter prolactin, growth hormone, and ACTH secretion. TRH stimulation of the prolactin response is the most consistently abnormal response (a blunter response of prolactin), but some patients with tumors respond normally. Variability in response to all maneuvers is the rule.

Frankly, the endocrine maneuvers yield no more useful information than the two major screening procedures, the blood prolactin and the coned-down view of the sella turcica. Visual field examination is not useful in screening for pituitary tumors because abnormalities are seen only with large tumors that are evident by prolactin, x-ray evaluation, and/or visual symptoms and headaches.

If the coned-down view is abnormal and/or the prolactin level is over 100 ng/mL, further evaluation and treatment require consultation with expert endocrine resources. These patients are rare, and accumulated experience that can provide the necessary clinical judgment can be found only with the referral resource. On the other hand, our workup easily deals with the vast majority of patients, and the few who require a multidisciplinary team approach are readily identified.

Hypogonadotropic Hypogonadism

Patients with amenorrhea and without galactorrhea who have reached this point in the workup and have normal imaging studies are classified as ***hypothalamic amenorrhea.*** The mechanism of the amenorrhea is suppression of pulsatile GnRH secretion below its critical range. This is a diagnosis by exclusion because we can identify probable causes (e.g., anorexia and weight loss) but we cannot test, manipulate, or measure the hypothalamus to prove our diagnosis.

Specific Disorders Within Compartments

With only modest effort, expense, and time, the problem of amenorrhea has been dissected into compartments of dysfunction which positively correlate with specific organ systems. At this point, with the specific anatomic locus of the defect defined, the clinician can now undertake steps to elucidate the specific disorder leading to amenorrhea. Congenital abnormalities are limited to amenorrhea that presents in the pubertal period of life. In a collection of 262 patients with secondary amenorrhea of adult onset, the following diagnostic frequencies were most often observed:[60]

Compartment I	
Asherman's syndrome	7.0%
Compartment II	
Abnormal chromosomes	0.5%
Normal chromosomes	10.0%
Compartment III	
Prolactin tumors	7.5%
Compartment IV	
Anovulation	28.0%
Weight loss/anorexia	10.0%
Hypothalamic suppression	10.0%
Hypothyroidism	1.0%

Compartment I: Disorders of the Outflow Tract or Uterus

Asherman's Syndrome

Secondary amenorrhea follows destruction of the endometrium (Asherman's syndrome).[61] This condition generally is the result of an overzealous postpartum curettage resulting in intrauterine scarification. A typical pattern of multiple synechiae is seen on a hysterogram. Diagnosis by hysteroscopy is more accurate and will detect minimal adhesions that are not apparent on a hysterogram. In the presence of normal ovarian function, the basal body temperature will be biphasic. The adhesions may partially or completely obliterate the endometrial cavity, the internal cervical os, the cervical canal, or combinations of these areas. Surprisingly, despite stenosis or atresia of the internal os, hematometra does not inevitably occur. The endometrium, perhaps in response to a buildup of pressure, becomes refractory, and simple cervical dilatation cures the problem. Asherman's syndrome also can occur following uterine surgery, including cesarean section, myomectomy, or metroplasty. Very severe adhesions have been noted following postpartum curettage and postpartum hypogonadism; e.g., in Sheehan's syndrome.

Patients with Asherman's syndrome can present with other problems besides amenorrhea, including miscarriages, dysmenorrhea, or hypomenorrhea. They can even have normal menses. Infertility can be present with mild adhesions, an association not readily explainable. Patients with repeated miscarriages, infertility, or pregnancy wastage should have investigation of the endometrial cavity by hysterogram or hysteroscopy.

Impairment of the endometrium resulting in amenorrhea can be caused by tuberculosis, a condition that is rare in the United States. Diagnosis is made by culture of the menstrual discharge or tissue obtained by endometrial biopsy. Uterine schistosomiasis is another rare cause of end organ failure, and eggs of the parasite may be found in urine, feces, rectal scrapings, menstrual discharge, or endometrium. We have seen the syndrome following intrauterine device (IUD)-related infections and severe, generalized pelvic infections.

Asherman's syndrome in the past was treated with a dilatation and curettage to break up the synechiae and, if necessary, an on-the-table hysterogram to ensure a free uterine cavity. Hysteroscopy with direct lysis of adhesions by cutting, cautery, or laser yields better results than the "blind" dilatation and curettage. Following operation, a method should be utilized to prevent the sides of the uterine cavity from adhering. Previously an IUD was used for this purpose; however, a pediatric Foley catheter appears to be a better option. The bag is filled with 3 mL fluid, and the catheter is removed after 7 days. A broad-spectrum antibiotic is started preoperatively and maintained for 10 days. An inhibitor of prostaglandin synthesis can be used if uterine cramping is a problem. The patient is treated for 2 months with high stimulatory doses of estrogen (e.g., conjugated estrogens 2.5 mg daily 3 of 4 weeks with medroxyprogesterone acetate 10 mg daily added during the 3rd week). When the initial attempt fails to re-establish menstrual flow, repeated attempts are worthwhile. Persistent treatment with repeated procedures may be necessary to regain reproductive potential. Approximately 70–80% of patients with this condition have achieved a successful pregnancy. Pregnancy is frequently complicated, however, by premature labor, placenta accreta, placenta previa, and/or postpartum hemorrhage.

Müllerian Anomalies

In primary amenorrheas, discontinuity by segmental disruptions of the müllerian tube should be ruled out. Thus, imperforate hymen, obliteration of the vaginal orifice, and lapses in continuity of the vaginal canal must be ruled out by direct observation. The cervix or the entire uterus may be absent. Far less common, the uterus may be present, but the cavity absent, or, in the presence of a cavity, the endometrium may be congenitally lacking. With the exception of the latter abnormalities, the clinical problem of amenorrhea due to obstruction is compounded by the painful distension of hematocolpos, hematometra, or hematoperitoneum. In all instances, an effort must be made to incise and drain from below at the points of closure of the müllerian tube. Even in complicated circumstances reestablishment of müllerian duct continuity usually can be achieved surgically. The unfortunate consequences of operative extirpation of painful masses from above with damage to bladder, ureter, and rectum, as well as irretrievable loss of distended but otherwise healthy reproductive organs, are rare but well remembered.

Knowing what to expect prior to attempting surgical correction is a great advantage. Imaging (MRI) can be utilized to accurately delineate the anatomical abnormality.[62, 63] A correct preoperative diagnosis will certainly facilitate the planning and execution of surgery.

Müllerian Agenesis

Lack of müllerian development *(Mayer-Rokitansky-Kuster-Hauser syndrome)* is the diagnosis for the individual with primary amenorrhea and no apparent vagina.[64] This is a relatively common cause (about 1 in 4000 female births) of primary amenorrhea, more frequent than congenital androgen insensitivity and second only to gonadal dysgenesis. These patients have an absence or hypoplasia of the internal vagina, and usually an absence of the uterus and fallopian tubes. However, rarely, the uterus may be normal, but lacking a conduit to the introitus, or there may only be rudimentary, bicornuate cords present. If a partial endometrial cavity is present, cyclic abdominal pain may be a complaint. Because of the similarity to some types of male pseudohermaphroditism, it is worthwhile to demonstrate the normal female karyotype. Because the ovaries are not müllerian structures, ovarian function is normal and can be documented with basal body temperatures or peripheral levels of progesterone. Growth and development are normal.

The exact cause of müllerian agenesis is unknown; however, likely causes are mutations of the gene for antimüllerian hormone or the gene for the antimüllerian hormone receptor. The underlying mechanism would be unwanted exposure to antimüllerian hormone activity. Thus far, no activating mutations have been reported, in contrast to inactivating mutations that cause persistence of müllerian structures.[65] Although usually sporadic, occasional occurrence may be noted within a family. A mutation has been identified in galactose-1-phosphate uridyl transferase in daughters with müllerian agenesis and their mothers.[66] This is different from classic galactosemia; however, it is postulated that increased intrauterine exposure to galactose because of this error in galactose metabolism can be a biologic basis for müllerian agenesis. High-galactose feeding of pregnant mice delays vaginal opening in female offspring. In this group of patients with müllerian agenesis, oocyte depletion (and premature ovarian failure) may be more common.

Further evaluation should include radiologic studies. Approximately one-third of patients have urinary tract abnormalities, and 12% or more have skeletal anomalies, most involving the spine, although absent digits and syndactyly (webbing or fusion of fingers or toes) can occur. Renal tract abnormalities include ectopic kidney, renal agenesis, horseshoe kidney, and abnormal collecting ducts. When the presence of a uterine structure is suspected on examination, ultrasound can be utilized to depict the size and symmetry of the structure. When the anatomic picture on ultrasonography is not certain, MRI is indicated.[67, 68] Laparoscopic visualization of the pelvis is not necessary. MRI is more accurate than ultrasonography and less expensive and invasive than laparoscopy. Extirpation of the müllerian remnants is certainly not necessary unless they are causing a problem such as uterine fibroid growth, hematometra, endometriosis, or symptomatic herniation into the inguinal canal.

Because of the difficulties and complications experienced in surgical series, we favor, when possible, an alternative to the surgical construction of an artificial vagina. Instead, we encourage the use of progressive dilatation as initially described by Frank[69] and later by Wabrek et al.[70] Beginning first in a posterior direction, and then after 2 weeks changing upward to the usual line of the vaginal axis, pressure with commercially available vaginal dilators is performed for 20 min daily to the point of modest discomfort. Utilizing increasingly larger dilators, a functional vagina can be created in several months.[71] Plastic syringe covers can be used instead of the expensive commercial glass dilators. An easier and very effective technique is to hold the dilator in place with a tight garment, maintaining pressure by sitting on a racing bicycle seat (mounted on a special stool or even on a bicycle).[72]

In patients who are unwilling or unable to undergo the dilatation program, the Vecchietti operation applies a traction device either transabdominally or by laparoscopy.[73] Postoperative traction creates a functional vagina in 7–9 days.

Operative treatment should be reserved for those women in whom the Frank method is unacceptable, or fails, or when a well-formed uterus is present and fertility might be preserved. The symptoms of retained menstruation should identify these patients. One recommendation is to perform an initial laparotomy to evaluate the cervical canal; if the cervix is atretic, the uterus should be removed.[74] If it is the relatively simple problem of an imperforate hymen or a transverse vaginal septum, surgery is indicated. Most have recommended against trying to preserve fertility in the presence of complete vaginal agenesis. The morbidity subsequent to this surgery argues for removal of the müllerian structures at the time of construction of a neovagina.

Patients with a transverse vaginal septum, which is a failure of canalization of the distal third of the vagina, usually present with symptoms of obstruction and urinary frequency. A transverse septum can be differentiated from an imperforate hymen by a lack of distension at the introitus with Valsalva's maneuver. A transverse vaginal septum can be accompanied by abnormalities of the upper reproductive tract; e.g., absent segments or atresia of the fallopian tubes or unilateral absence of the fallopian tube and ovary.[75]

Distal obstruction of the genital tract is the only condition in this category that can be considered an emergency. Delay in surgical treatment can lead to infertility due to inflammatory changes and endometriosis. Definitive surgery should be accomplished as soon as possible. Diagnostic needling should be avoided because a hematocolpos can be converted into a pyocolpos.

Reassurance and support are necessary to carry a patient through these procedures. Problems with body image and sexual enjoyment can be avoided, and, although infertile, a full and normal life as a woman can be achieved. Furthermore, genetic offspring can be achieved by collection of oocytes from the genetic mother, fertilization by the genetic father, and placement into a surrogate carrier.[76] An analysis of 34 surrogacy live births resulting from oocytes retrieved from 58 women with congenital absence of the uterus and vagina could find no indication of inheritance in a dominant fashion, making surrogate pregnancy a reasonable option for patients with this disorder.[77]

Androgen Insensitivity (Testicular Feminization)

Complete androgen insensitivity (testicular feminization) is the likely diagnosis when a blind vaginal canal is encountered and the uterus is absent (also discussed in Chapter 9). This is the third most common cause of primary amenorrhea after gonadal dysgenesis and müllerian agenesis. The patient with testicular feminization is a male pseudohermaphrodite. The adjective male refers to the gonadal sex; thus, the individual has testes and an XY karyotype. Pseudohermaphrodite means that the genitalia are opposite of the gonads; thus, the individual is phenotypically female but with absent or meager pubic and axillary hair.

Differences between Müllerian Agenesis and Testicular Feminization

	Müllerian Agenesis	Testicular Feminization
Karyotype	46,XX	46,XY
Heredity	Not known	Maternal X-linked recessive; 25% risk of affected child, 25% risk of carrier
Sexual hair	Normal female	Absent to sparse
Testosterone level	Normal female	Normal to slightly elevated male
Other anomalies	Frequent	Rare
Gonadal neoplasia	Normal incidence	5% incidence of malignant tumors

The male pseudohermaphrodite is a genetic and gonadal male with failure of virilization. Failures in male development can be considered a spectrum with incomplete forms of androgen insensitivity being represented by some androgen response. Transmission of this disorder is by means of an X-linked recessive gene that is responsible for the androgen intracellular receptor (see Chapter 9 for a discussion of the androgen receptor defect). Clinically, the diagnosis should be considered in:

1. A female child with inguinal hernias because the testes are frequently partially descended.

2. A patient with primary amenorrhea and an absent uterus.

3. A patient with absent body hair.

These patients appear normal at birth except for the possible presence of an inguinal hernia, and most patients are not seen by a physician until puberty. Growth and development are normal, although overall height is usually greater than average, and there may be an eunuchoidal tendency (long arms, big hands, and big feet). The breasts, although large, are abnormal; actual glandular tissue is not abundant, nipples are small, and the areolae are pale. More than 50% have an inguinal hernia, the labia minora are usually underdeveloped, and the blind vagina is less deep than normal. Rudimentary fallopian tubes are composed of fibromuscular tissue with only occasional epithelial lining. Horseshoe kidneys have been reported.

The testes may be intra-abdominal, but often are in a hernia. They are similar to any cryptorchid testis except that they may be nodular. After puberty, the testis displays immature tubular development, and tubules are lined by immature germ cells and Sertoli cells. There is no spermatogenesis. The incidence of neoplasia in these gonads is high. In 50 reported cases, there were 11 malignancies, 15 adenomas, and 10 benign cysts: a 22% incidence of malignancy and a 52% incidence of neoplasia.[78] More recent series indicate a lower overall incidence of gonadal tumors, about 5–10%.[35, 79–81] Therefore, once full development is attained after puberty, the gonads should be removed at approximately age 16–18, and the patient should receive hormone therapy. ***This is the only exception to the rule that gonads with a Y chromosome should be removed as soon as a diagnosis is made.*** There are two reasons: first, the development achieved with hormone treatment does not seem to match the smooth pubertal changes due to endogenous hormones, and second, gonadal tumors in these patients have not been encountered prior to puberty. Removal of gonadal tissue can be accomplished by a skilled operator through the laparoscope, reserving the option of laparotomy if the gonads are inaccessible.[82]

When testicular feminization was first studied, it was found that the urinary 17-ketosteroids were normal, and it was suggested that there might be a resistance to androgen action rather than an absence of androgens — a congenital androgen insensitivity. Indeed, the plasma levels of testosterone are in the normal to high male range, and the plasma clearance and metabolism of testosterone are normal. Thus, these patients produce testosterone, but they do not respond to androgens, either their own or those given locally or systemically. Therefore, the critical steps in sexual differentiation, which require androgens, fail to take place, and development is totally female. Because antimüllerian hormone is present, development of the müllerian duct is inhibited, hence the absence of uterus, tubes, and upper vagina.

This syndrome is marked by a unique combination:

1. Normal female phenotype.

2. Normal male karyotype, 46,XY.

3. Normal or slightly elevated male blood testosterone levels and a high LH.

Cases of **incomplete androgen insensitivity** (one-tenth as common as the complete syndrome) represent individuals with some androgen effect. These individuals may have clitoral enlargement, or a phallus may even be present. Axillary hair and pubic hair develop along with breast growth. Gonadectomy should not be deferred in such cases because it will obviate unwanted further virilization. Patients with a deficit in testicular 17β-hydroxysteroid dehydrogenase activity will have impaired testosterone production and present clinically as incomplete androgen insensitivity. Because treatment (gonadectomy) is the same, precise diagnosis is not essential.

In the past, conventional wisdom warned against unthinking and "needless" disclosure of the gonadal and chromosomal sex to a patient with complete androgen insensitivity. This attitude has changed as, more and more, patients desire and appreciate a full understanding of themselves. Although infertile, these patients are certainly completely female in their gender identity, and this should be reinforced rather than challenged. We now strongly advocate combining a truthful education with appropriate psychological counseling of patient and parents. A good resource is the international support group, A^{L}I^{A}S, that is headquartered in the United Kingdom (2 Shirburn Avenue, Mansfield, Nottinghamshire, NG18 2BY, UK); http://www.medhelp.org/www/ais/.

Compartment II: Disorders of the Ovary

Problems in gonadal development can present with either primary or secondary amenorrhea. From 30 to 40% of primary amenorrhea cases have gonadal streaks due to abnormal development: gonadal dysgenesis. These patients can be grouped according to the following karyotypes:

        50% — 45,X
        25% — Mosaics
        25% — 46,XX

Women with gonadal dysgenesis can also present with secondary amenorrhea. The karyotypes associated with this presentation are, in order of decreasing frequency:

        46,XX (most common).
        Mosaics (e.g., 45,X/46,XX).
        Deletions in X short and long arms.
        47,XXX
        45,X

Both X chromosomes must be present and active in oocytes to avoid the accelerated loss of follicles. The finding of a normal karyotype in patients with ovarian failure, the most common situation, is most perplexing, suggesting subtle reasons for loss of activity, probably due to specific gene alterations. There is reason to believe that specific genes confined to a portion of the X chromosome are necessary for normal ovarian function.[83]

Gonadal dysgenesis associated with a normal karyotype is also linked to neurosensory deafness (Perrault syndrome). Auditory evaluation should be considered in all 46,XX gonadal dysgenesis cases.

Pure gonadal dysgenesis indicates the presence of bilateral streak gonads, regardless of karyotype. Mixed gonadal dysgenesis indicates testicular tissue on one side and a streak gonad on the other.

Turner Syndrome

Turner syndrome (an abnormality in or an absence of one of the X chromosomes) is a well known and thoroughly studied entity. (See Chapter 9 for a full discussion.) The characteristics of short stature, webbed neck, shield chest, and increased carrying angle at the elbow, combined with hypergonadotropic hypoestrogenic amenorrhea, make a diagnosis possible on the most superficial evaluation. Due to a lack of ovarian follicles, there is no gonadal sex hormone production at puberty, and thus patients present with primary amenorrhea. However, special attention must be given to the less common variations of this syndrome. Autoimmune disorders, cardiovascular abnormalities, and various renal anomalies must be ruled out. A karyotype should be performed on all patients with elevated gonadotropins, despite the appearance of a typical case of Turner syndrome. The presence of a pure syndrome, 45,X chromosome single-cell line, should be confirmed. This expensive test cannot be viewed just as a step toward academic perfection. Forty percent of individuals who appear to have Turner syndrome are mosaics or have structural aberrations in the X or Y chromosome.

Mosaicism

The presence of mosaicism (multiple cell lines of varying sex chromosome composition) must be ruled out for a very important reason. The presence of a Y chromosome in the karyotype requires excision of the gonadal areas because the presence of any medullary (testicular) component within the gonad is a predisposing factor to tumor formation and to heterosexual development (virilization). Only in the patient with the complete form of androgen insensitivity can laparotomy be deferred until after puberty, because the individual is resistant to androgens and gonadal tumors occur late. In all other patients with a Y chromosome, gonadectomy should be performed as soon as the diagnosis is made to avoid virilization and early tumor formation. One should be aware that approximately 30% of patients with a Y chromosome will not develop signs of virilization. Therefore, even the normal-appearing adult patient with elevated serum levels of gonadotropins must be karyotyped to detect a silent Y chromosome so that prophylactic gonadectomy can be performed before neoplastic changes occur. The fully stained and banded karyotype continues to be the best method to detect the presence of testicular tissue or other mosaic combinations. When standard cytogenetic analysis is uncertain, expert consultation should be obtained to pursue further analysis with X- and Y-specific DNA probes.[84] Probing for Y chromosomal material is also indicated when virilization occurs, despite no apparent Y on the karyotype and when a chromosomal fragment of uncertain origin is identified (discussed in chapter 9).

The impact of mosaicism, even in the absence of a Y-containing line, is significant. With an XX component (e.g., XX/XO), functional cortical (ovarian) tissue can be found within the gonad, leading to a variety of responses, including some degree of female development, and, on occasion, even menses and reproduction. These individuals may appear normal, attaining normal stature before premature menopause is experienced. More commonly, these patients are short. Most patients with missing sex chromosome material are less than 63 inches (160 cm) in height. The menopause is early, because the functioning follicles undergo an accelerated rate of atresia.

This complex array of gonadal dysgenesis variations, from the typical pure form to an otherwise normal-appearing and functioning woman with premature menopause, is the result of a variety of mosaicism, which produces a complex mixture of cortical and medullary gonadal tissue. The clinical importance of this information justifies obtaining karyotypes in all cases of elevated gonadotropins in women under age 30. Although more uncommon, even autosomal abnormalities can be associated with hypergonadotropic ovarian failure; e.g., a 28-year-old woman with secondary amenorrhea and elevated gonadotropins has been reported with trisomy 18 mosaicism.[85] All patients with absent ovarian function and quantitative alterations in the sex chromosomes are categorized as having **gonadal dysgenesis** (Chapter 9).

XY Gonadal Dysgenesis

A female patient with an XY karyotype who has a palpable müllerian system, normal female testosterone levels, and lack of sexual development has **Swyer's syndrome.** Tumor transformation in the gonadal ridge can occur at any age, and extirpation of the gonadal streaks should be performed as soon as the diagnosis is made.

Gonadal Agenesis

No complicated clinical problems accompany the gonadal failure due to agenesis. Without precise information, only conjecture about the causes of absent development can be made. Thus, viral and metabolic influences in early gestation or undiscovered genetic mutations are suspected. Nevertheless, the final result is irretrievable — hypergonadotropic hypogonadism. In the absence of gonadal function, development is female. Surgical removal of the gonadal streaks is necessary to avoid the possibility of neoplasia.

The Resistant Ovary Syndrome

There is a rare patient with amenorrhea and normal growth and development who has elevated gonadotropins despite the presence of unstimulated ovarian follicles, and there is no evidence of autoimmune disease. Laparotomy is necessary to arrive at a correct diagnosis by obtaining adequate histological evaluation of the ovaries. This can demonstrate not only the presence of follicles but the absence of the lymphocytic infiltration seen with autoimmune disease. Because of the rarity of this condition and the very low chance of achieving pregnancy even with high doses of exogenous gonadotropins, we do not believe it is worthwhile to perform a laparotomy for the purpose of ovarian biopsy on every patient with amenorrhea, high gonadotropins, and a normal karyotype. These patients are excellent candidates for oocyte donation.

Premature Ovarian Failure

Premature ovarian failure (the early depletion of ovarian follicles) is surprisingly common. Approximately 1% of women will experience ovarian failure before the age of 40, and in women with primary amenorrhea, the prevalence ranges from 10% to 28%.[26, 86] The etiology of premature ovarian failure is unknown in most cases. It is useful to explain to the patient that it is probably a genetic disorder with an increased rate of follicle disappearance. Often, specific sex chromosome anomalies can be identified.[87] The most common abnormalities are 45,X and 47,XXY, followed by mosaicism and specific structural abnormalities on the sex chromosomes. Searching for 45,X/46,XX mosaicism using fluorescence in situ hybridization, a higher percentage of cells containing a single X chromosome can be detected in women who present with premature ovarian failure.[88] The cause of ovarian failure is most likely accelerated follicular atresia because even 45,X (Turner syndrome) patients begin with a full complement of germ cells. In addition, premature ovarian failure can be due to an autoimmune process, or perhaps to destruction of follicles by infections, such as mumps oophoritis, or a physical insult, such as irradiation or chemotherapy.

The problem can present at varying ages, depending on the number of follicles left. It is useful to view the various presentations as representing a stage in the process of perimenopausal change, no matter what the chronological age of the patient. If loss of follicles has been rapid, then primary amenorrhea and lack of sexual development will be present. If loss of follicles takes place during or after puberty, then the extent of adult phenotypic development and the time of onset of secondary amenorrhea will vary accordingly.

In view of the many case reports documenting resumption of normal function in patients with normal karyotypes (10–20% of these patients), we cannot be certain that these patients will be sterile forever. On the other hand, laparotomy and full-thickness ovarian biopsy surely are not necessary for all of these patients. We believe that a minimal approach, with a survey for autoimmune disease (recognizing that there is no practical clinical method to accurately diagnose autoimmune ovarian failure) and an assessment of ovarian-pituitary activity, is sufficient. As with other hypogonadal patients, hormone therapy is recommended. However, because of spontaneous ovulations, an oral contraceptive is a better treatment regimen choice if pregnancy is not desired. The best prospect for pregnancy is with donated oocytes; however, it should be noted that pregnancy rates are reduced when using a sibling's donated oocytes.[89]

Molecular Explanations for Ovarian Failure

A group of patients with ovarian failure and normal chromosomes has been identified in Finland, displaying a recessive inheritance pattern.[90] A point mutation was detected in the FSH receptor gene and demonstrated to be the cause of ovarian failure in this population.[22] This mutation accounted for 29% of 75 Finnish women with ovarian failure. Ovarian follicles were present in these women, as detected by ultrasonography, although the ovaries were small in volume.[23] Finland is known to harbor an increased number of inherited conditions. A search for this same mutation in American and Brazilian women could not detect a single case in women presenting with premature ovarian failure.[91, 92]

As more women with premature ovarian failure undergo genetic studies, we anticipate the identification of multiple subgroups, each with a different biologic basis for the ovarian failure, results that would be consistent with a heterogeneous condition with multiple causes. For example, a case of hypergonadotropic primary amenorrhea has been reported due to a point mutation in the LH receptor gene; FSH and LH were only slightly elevated and multiple ovarian follicles were present with development and steroidogenesis up to an early antral stage.[93] The almost normal gonadotropin levels were probably due to inhibition by inhibin, because inhibin secretion by granulosa cells is FSH-dependent and not influenced by LH. This patient had two siblings who were 46,XY male pseudohermaphrodites due to Leydig cell hypoplasia because of the same LH receptor gene mutation. In another example, translocations between regions on X and Y chromosomes that share sequence homology have been reported in patients with secondary amenorrhea and ovarian failure.[24] Sequences on the long arm of the X chromosome (Xq27-28) share homology with sequences on the long arm of the Y chromosome (Yq11.22) allowing errors in the process of crossing-over. In addition, less than complete mutations (so-called premutations) of the site that transmits the fragile X syndrome have been reported to occur at a greater frequency in women with premature ovarian failure.[94]

The Effect of Radiation and Chemotherapy

The effect of radiation is dependent upon age and the x-ray dose.[95, 96] Steroid levels begin to fall and gonadotropins rise within 2 weeks after irradiation to the ovaries. The higher number of oocytes in younger age is responsible for the resistance to total castration in young women exposed to intense radiation. Function can resume after many years of amenorrhea. On the other hand, the damage may not appear until later in the form of premature ovarian failure. If pregnancy does occur, the risk of congenital abnormalities is no greater than normal. When the irradiation field excludes the pelvis, there is no risk of premature ovarian failure.[97] For this reason, elective transposition by laparoscopy of the ovaries out of the pelvis prior to irradiation provides a good prospect for future fertility.[98] Gonads are not in danger in the kitchen; microwave ovens utilize wavelengths with low tissue-penetrating power.

The following table indicates the risk of sterilization according to dose.[99]

Ovarian Dose	Sterilization Effect
60 rads	No effect
150 rads	Some risk over age 40
250–500 rads	Ages 15–40: 60% sterilized
500–800 rads	Ages 15–40: 60–70% sterilized
over 800 rads	100% permanently sterilized

Alkylating agents are very toxic to the gonads. As with radiation, there is an inverse relationship between the dose required for ovarian failure and age at the start of therapy.[100] Other chemotherapeutic agents have the potential for ovarian damage, but they have been less well studied. The effect of combination chemotherapies is similar to those of the alkylating agents. Approximately two-thirds of premenopausal women with breast cancer and treated with cyclophosphamide, methotrexate, and fluorouracil lose ovarian function.[101] Resumption of menses and pregnancy can occur, but there is no way to predict which patient will reacquire ovulatory function. As with radiotherapy, damage may present late with premature ovarian failure.[102]

Is it possible that maintenance of ovarian follicles in a "dormant" state by suppressing FSH secretion can prevent ovarian failure? In a monkey model, gonadotroph suppression by treatment with a GnRH agonist during radiation did not protect against loss of ovarian follicles.[103] In contrast, GnRH agonist treatment of monkeys did protect the ovarian follicles against damage by cyclophosphamide.[104]

The harvesting and cryopreservation of oocytes prior to irradiation and/or chemotherapy will, in our opinion, ultimately prove to be best means of preserving fertility for these patients.

Compartment III: Disorders of the Anterior Pituitary

A consideration of the disorders of the hypothalamic-pituitary axis must first focus on the problem of the pituitary tumor. Fortunately, malignant tumors are almost never encountered. Through 1997, there were approximately 40 reported cases of prolactin cell metastatic carcinomas (mostly in men) and through 1989, no more than 40 cases of primary pituitary cancer in the world literature,[105–111] but growth of a benign tumor can cause problems because it expands in a confined space. The tumor grows upward, compressing the optic chiasm and producing the classic findings of bitemporal hemianopsia. With small tumors, however, abnormal visual fields are rarely encountered. In contrast, other tumors of this region (e.g., craniopharyngioma, usually marked by calcifications on x-ray) may be associated with the early development of blurring of vision and visual field defects because of their close proximity to the optic chiasm. Besides craniopharyngioma, other very rare tumors include meningiomas, gliomas, metastatic tumors, and chordomas. Increased melatonin secretion, probably from a cystic pineal lesion, has been reported as a cause of delayed puberty.[112] ***Hypogonadism and delayed puberty deserve brain evaluation by MRI.***

Sometimes, the suspicion of a pituitary tumor is increased because of clinical signs of acromegaly caused by excessive secretion of growth hormone, or Cushing's disease due to excessive secretion of ACTH. Rarely, a TSH-secreting tumor (less than 1–3% of pituitary tumors) will cause secondary hyperthyroidism.[113, 114] Amenorrhea and/or galactorrhea may precede the eventual full clinical expression of a tumor that secretes ACTH or growth hormone. If clinical criteria suggest Cushing's disease, ACTH levels and the 24-hour urinary levels of free cortisol should be measured, and the rapid suppression test (Chapter 13) should be utilized. If acromegaly is suspected, growth hormone should be measured during an oral glucose tolerance test (lack of suppression of growth hormone levels is diagnostic), and the circulating level of IGF-I should be measured. However, the 2 most common tumors are prolactin-secreting adenomas and clinically nonfunctioning tumors. Though usually a problem in adult life, prolactin-secreting tumors can be seen in preadolescent and adolescent children, and, thus, can be a cause of failure of growth and development or of primary amenorrhea.[115]

Because acromegaly can initially present with an elevated prolactin level and amenorrhea, the circulating level of IGF-I should be measured in all patients with a macroadenoma (>10 mm diameter).

The majority of clinically nonfunctioning (null) adenomas (30–40% of all pituitary tumors) are of gonadotroph origin and actively secrete FSH, free α-subunit, and rarely, LH (all of which do not exert clinical effects, and, therefore, patients with these tumors usually present with symptoms due to mass effects).[17] The α-subunit can be used as a tumor marker; however, in postmenopausal women (the age at which most gonadotroph adenomas present) the situation can be confusing because increased free α-subunit secretion accompanies increased secretion of gonadotropins. One premenopausal woman with a gonadotroph adenoma has been reported, distinguished by multiple ovarian cysts, high estradiol levels, and endometrial hyperplasia.[116] In contrast to patients with normal pituitary glands, patients with pituitary adenomas usually fail to down-regulate gonadotropin secretion in response to GnRH agonist treatment, and repeated GnRH agonist administration is associated with persistent elevations in either FSH or α-subunit. Most patients with these tumors, however, have reduced secretion of gonadotropins (and amenorrhea) because of tumor compression of the pituitary stalk and interference with the delivery of hypothalamic GnRH. For this reason, these patients often present with modest elevations of prolactin (due to the inability of dopamine to reach the anterior pituitary). ***Elevated gonadotropins in the presence of a pituitary microadenoma in a woman with amenorrhea are not a consequence of secretion by the tumor; another explanation must be pursued.***

Not all intrasellar masses are neoplastic. Cysts, tuberculosis, sarcoidosis, and fat deposits have been reported as causes of pituitary compression leading to hypogonadotropic amenorrhea. Lymphocytic hypophysitis is a rare autoimmune infiltration of the pituitary that can mimic a pituitary tumor, often occurring during pregnancy or in the first 6 months postpartum.[117] In the initial phase of hypophysitis, hyperprolactinemia is common, followed by hypopituitarism. Transsphenoidal surgery is both diagnostic and therapeutic for this potentially lethal condition.

Nearby lesions, such as internal carotid artery aneurysms and obstruction of the aqueduct of Sylvius, can also cause amenorrhea. Pituitary insufficiency can be secondary to ischemia and infarction and appear as a late sequela to obstetrical hemorrhage — the well known Sheehan's syndrome. These problems, as well as genetic disorders such as Laurence-Moon-Biedl and Prader-Willi syndromes, are so rarely encountered that consultation with textbooks and colleagues is necessary. In a large transsphenoidal surgical series, 91% of sellar and parasellar masses were pituitary adenomas.[118] Diabetes insipidus is not associated with pituitary adenomas, but commonly accompanies masses not of pituitary origin.

Treatment of Nonfunctioning Adenomas

If imaging discovers a microadenoma (less than 10 mm in diameter) in an asymptomatic patient, no treatment is necessary. These tumors are often incidental findings. A follow-up imaging is recommended in a year or two to be sure there is no growth. If a macroadenoma (greater than 10 mm in diameter) is present and symptomatic, surgery is necessary; these tumors are commonly not detected until the onset of symptoms (headaches and visual disturbances). Because of their large size and the high risk of recurrence, adjunctive irradiation is recommended if residual tumor and elevated gonadotropins and α-subunit are present after surgery. Follow-up imaging is obtained every 6 months for 1 year, and then yearly for 3–5 years. The radiation dose is high (4500 rads), and the incidence of hypopituitarism may reach 50% over a 10-year period.[17] Ongoing surveillance of adrenal and thyroid function is necessary. With careful imaging follow-up after surgery, postoperative irradiation can be avoided in some patients.[119] Although a response to dopamine agonist therapy has been reported, in general, results are not satisfactory.[15, 120] The response to the somatostatin analogue, octreotide, has also been disappointing.[121] Nevertheless, because good tumor size reduction occasionally occurs, the option of medical treatment should be considered.

Pituitary Prolactin-Secreting Adenomas

Prolactin-secreting adenomas are the most common pituitary tumors, and they account for 50% of all pituitary adenomas identified at autopsy. Classically, pituitary adenomas have been grouped according to their staining ability as eosinophilic, basophilic, or chromophobic. This classification is misleading and of no clinical usefulness. Pituitary adenomas should be classified according to their function; e.g., prolactin-secreting adenoma.

With the utilization of the serum prolactin assay and the increased sensitivity of the new imaging techniques, the association of amenorrhea and small pituitary tumors has become recognized as a relatively common problem. This is not a new phenomenon, rather it reflects more sensitive diagnostic techniques. Attempts to link the problem to oral contraceptive use have proved negative.[122]

The exact incidence of this clinical problem is unknown. In autopsy series the percentage of pituitary glands found to contain microadenomas ranged from 9% to 27%.[53–57] The age distribution ranged from 2 to 86, with the greatest incidence in the 6th decade of life. The sex distribution was equal. However, clinical manifestations, mainly a disruption of the reproductive mechanism, occur more commonly in women and are probably due to estrogen-induced activity of the pituitary lactotrophs.

A high prolactin level is encountered in about one-third of women with no obvious cause of amenorrhea.[123] Only one-third of women with high prolactin levels will have galactorrhea, probably because the low estrogen environment associated with the amenorrhea prevents a normal response to prolactin. Another possible explanation again focuses on the heterogeneity of peptide hormones. Prolactin circulates in various forms with structural modifications, which are the result of glycosylation, phosphorylation, deletions, and additions. The various forms are associated with varying bioactivity (manifested by galactorrhea) and immunoreactivity (recognition by immunoassay). The predominant variant is little prolactin (80–85%), which also has more biological activity than the larger sized variants. Therefore, it is not surprising that big prolactins compose the major form of circulating prolactin in women with normal menses and minimal galactorrhea.[124] This is not always the case, however, because a high blood level (350–400 ng/mL) of prolactin composed predominantly of high molecular weight prolactin has been reported in a woman with oligomenorrhea and galactorrhea but with no evidence of a pituitary tumor.[125] These high levels of relatively inactive prolactin in the absence of a tumor may be due to the creation of macromolecules of prolactin by antiprolactin autoantibodies.[126] Explanations for clinically illogical situations can be found in the variable molecular heterogeneity of the peptide hormones. At any one point in time, the bioactivity and the immunoreactivity of prolactin represent the cumulative effect of the circulating family of structural variants.

Very high prolactin levels (greater than 1000 ng/mL) are associated with invasive tumors. These very rare tumors do not yield themselves to surgery, but, fortunately, they can usually be effectively treated and controlled with a dopamine agonist.

Approximately one-third of women with galactorrhea have normal menses.[127, 128] As the prolactin concentration increases, a woman can progress sequentially from normal ovulation to an inadequate luteal phase to intermittent anovulation to total anovulation to complete suppression and amenorrhea.

Probably as many as one-third of patients with secondary amenorrhea will have a pituitary adenoma, and if galactorrhea is also present, half will have an abnormal sella turcica.[123] The clinical symptoms do not always correlate with the prolactin level, and patients with normal prolactin levels can have pituitary tumors.[128] The highest prolactin levels, however, are associated with amenorrhea, with or without galactorrhea.

The amenorrhea associated with elevated prolactin levels is due to prolactin inhibition of the pulsatile secretion of GnRH. The pituitary glands in these patients respond normally to GnRH, or in augmented fashion (perhaps due to increased stores of gonadotropins), thus indicating that the mechanism of the amenorrhea is a decrease in GnRH.[129, 130] Short-term administration of an opioid antagonist suggests that this inhibition is mediated by increased opioid activity.[131] However, chronic administration of naltrexone (a long-acting opioid antagonist) does not restore menstrual function.[132] Nevertheless, treatment that lowers the circulating levels of prolactin restores ovarian responsiveness and menstrual function. This is true whether the treatment consists of removal of a prolactin-secreting tumor or suppression of prolactin secretion. Interestingly, postmenopausal women with elevated levels of prolactin do not experience vasomotor symptoms (hot flushes) until prolactin levels are restored to normal.[133]

The increased ability to detect pituitary tumors has been accompanied by the development of a surgical technique that effectively removes the small tumors with a high margin of safety. Utilizing the operating microscope, the transsphenoidal technique approaches via a sublabial incision (under the upper lip), with dissection under the nasal mucosa, removal of the nasal septum to expose the sphenoidal sinus, and resection of the floor of the sphenoid sinus to expose the sella turcica. Tumor tissue is usually distinguishable from the yellow-orange, firm tissue of the normal anterior pituitary. However, because pituitary adenomas do not have a capsule, the borderline between tumor and normal tissue is often vague. The ideal time for excision is when the adenoma is a small nodule. When enlarged, it becomes more difficult to distinguish normal from pathological tissue. Once the adenoma grows beyond the sella, total removal is essentially impossible.

The development of transsphenoidal surgery was paralleled by the availability and clinical application of the drug, bromocriptine, which specifically suppresses prolactin secretion. Initially, appropriate decisions between the surgical approach and medical treatment were difficult to make. With increasing experience, clinical perspective has been achieved, and reasonable judgments are now possible. Let us first consider results with surgery, and then examine dopamine agonist treatment.

Results With Surgery

Transsphenoidal neurosurgery achieves immediate resolution of hyperprolactinemia with resumption of cyclic menses in approximately 30% of patients with macroadenomas and 70% of patients with microadenomas. Besides an inability to achieve a complete cure, surgery may be followed by recurrence of tumor (long-term cure rate is about 50% overall, ranging from as high as 70% for microadenomas to as low as 10% for macroadenomas), depending upon the skill and experience of the neurosurgeon and the size of the tumor, and a still unknown but significant percentage (perhaps as high as 10–30% after surgery for macroadenomas) of development of panhypopituitarism.[134, 135] Other complications of surgery include cerebrospinal fluid leaks, an occasional case of meningitis, and the frequent postoperative problem of diabetes insipidus. The diabetes insipidus is usually a transient problem, rarely lasting as long as 6 months, but it can be permanent. There is a mortality rate of less than 1%. Although initial follow-up reports of the results of transsphenoidal adenomectomy were discouraging (high recurrence rates), other authors have argued that surgical techniques improved with time, and recurrent hyperprolactinemia is relatively low.[136] The best results are in patients with prolactin levels in the 150–500 ng/mL range; the higher the prolactin the lower the cure rate. In the largest series (409 women) with long-term follow-up, the recurrence rate was 26% when postoperative prolactin levels were 20 ng/mL or less.[137] The higher the postoperative prolactin level, the lower the cure rate. Overall, approximately 50% of both microadenomas and macroadenomas were cured by surgery. There were no deaths, but adrenal hormone replacement (hypopituitarism) was necessary in 4%. Importantly, pregnancy (achieved by 88% within 1 year in those desiring conception) did not cause exacerbation or recurrence in a single patient.

There are 3 possible explanations for the recurrence or persistence of hyperprolactinemia after surgery.

1. The prolactin-producing tumor looks like the surrounding normal pituitary, and it is difficult to resect completely.

2. The tumor may be multifocal in origin.

3. There may be a continuing abnormality of the hypothalamus giving rise to chronic stimulation of the lactotrophs. In other words, this is a problem of recurrent hyperplasia, not adenomas. However, molecular biology studies indicate that pituitary tumors are monoclonal.[138] If dysfunction were the etiologic factor, one would expect the tumors to be polyclonal.

When persistent or recurrent tumors are treated with repeat surgery, only about one-third are cured and the complication rate is high.[139] Irradiation after surgery has many problems, including the possibility of stroke and other brain tumors.[140, 141]

We recommend the following management for those patients who have had surgery:

1. If cyclic menses return: periodic evaluation for the problem of anovulation.

2. If amenorrhea or oligomenorrhea and hyperprolactinemia persist or recur: prolactin levels every 6 months and imaging yearly for 2 years, and then a coned-down view every few years. If tumor growth becomes evident, control of growth should be achieved with dopamine agonist treatment. In addition, a dopamine agonist can be used to induce ovulation if pregnancy is desired. If the reason for surgery was lack of response or side effects with bromocriptine, one of the other dopamine agonists should be used.

Results With Radiation

Results with radiation therapy are less satisfactory than with surgery. In addition, response is very slow; prolactin concentrations may take several years to fall. After radiation, panhypopituitarism can occur as long as 10 years after treatment.[142] Patients who have been treated with radiation should be followed for a long time, and any symptoms suggestive of pituitary failure require investigation. It is not yet known whether focusing the delivery of radiation (stereotactic radiotherapy) can avoid the problem of hypopituitarism, presumably by sparing the hypothalamus from radiation. Furthermore, it is believed that focused irradiation is better for small tumors or small amounts of residual tumor after surgery. Irradiation should be reserved as adjunctive therapy for controlling postoperative persistence or regrowth of large tumors and shrinking large tumors that are unresponsive to medical treatment. Overall, a small number of irradiated women return to normal hormonal function.[137]

Dopamine Agonist Treatment

Bromocriptine is a lysergic acid derivative with a bromine substitute at position 2.[143] It is available as the methane-sulfonate (mesylate) in 2.5 mg tablets. It is a dopamine agonist, binding to dopamine receptors and, therefore, directly mimicking dopamine inhibition of pituitary prolactin secretion. Prolactin-secreting tumors do not have inactivating mutations in the dopamine receptor gene; thus, dopamine agonists can bind and exert inhibiting activity.[144] Absorption from the gastrointestinal tract is rapid but not complete; 28% is absorbed and 94% metabolized in the first pass through the liver. Bromocriptine is metabolized into at least 30 excretory products. Excretion is mainly biliary, and more than 90% appears in the feces over 5 days after a single dose of 2.5 mg. A small part, 6–7%, is excreted unchanged or as metabolites in the urine.

The oral dose that suppresses prolactin is 10 times lower than that which improves the symptoms of Parkinson's disease. For some patients, one pill a day (or half a pill bid) will be effective. On the other hand, an occasional patient will require 7.5 mg or 10 mg daily in order to suppress adenoma secretion of prolactin.

Bromocriptine is also available in a long-acting form (depot-bromocriptine) for intramuscular injection and as a slow-release oral form. Depot-bromocriptine is administered in a dose of 50–75 mg monthly; the dose of the oral slow-release formulation is 5–15 mg daily. These forms are equally effective as the standard oral preparation and are associated with the same side effect severity and prevalence.[145] The response to the intramuscular form appears to be more rapid, and thus this preparation would offer an advantage in cases with large tumors with visual field impairment.[146, 147]

Approximately 10% of patients cannot tolerate oral bromocriptine. Nausea, headache, and faintness are the usual initial problems. The faintness is due to orthostatic hypotension, which can be attributed to relaxation of smooth muscle in the splanchnic and renal beds, as well as inhibition of transmitter release at noradrenergic nerve endings and central inhibition of sympathetic activity. Neuropsychiatric symptoms, occasionally with hallucinations, occur in less than 1% of patients. This may be due to hydrolysis of the lysergic acid part of the molecule. Other side effects include dizziness, fatigue, nasal congestion, vomiting, and abdominal cramps.

Side effects can be minimized by slowly building tolerance toward the usual dose, 2.5 mg bid. Treatment should be started with an initial dose of 2.5 mg given at bedtime. It may help to take the tablet with a glass of milk and snack. The peak level is achieved 2 hours after ingestion, and the biological half-life is about 3 hours. If intolerance occurs with this initial dose, then the tablet should be cut in half, and an even slower program should be followed. Usually a week after the initial dose, the second 2.5 mg dose can be added at breakfast or lunch. Patients who are extremely sensitive to the drug should be instructed to divide the tablets and to devise their own schedule of increasing dosage in order to achieve tolerance. A very small percentage of patients cannot tolerate any dosage.

Vaginal administration of bromocriptine is an excellent method to avoid side effects. One 2.5 mg tablet is inserted high into the vagina at bedtime. This dose will provide excellent clinical results and few side effects.[148, 149] In contrast to oral bromocriptine which is not absorbed completely and that which is absorbed is largely metabolized in the first pass through the liver, vaginal absorption is nearly complete, and avoidance of the liver first-pass effect (with longer maintenance of systemic levels) allows achievement of therapeutic results at a lower dose.

There are two bromocriptine treatment methods to follow in those patients seeking pregnancy. The first is simply daily administration of 2.5 mg bid until the patient is pregnant as judged by the basal body temperature chart. In the second method, bromocriptine is administered during the follicular phase, and the drug is stopped when a basal body temperature rise indicates that ovulation has occurred, thus avoiding high drug levels early in pregnancy. The drug is resumed at menses when it is apparent the patient is not pregnant. No comparative study has been performed to tell us whether the follicular phase only method is as effective as the daily method. Furthermore, there has been no evidence that bromocriptine ingestion during early pregnancy is harmful to the fetus.[150, 151]

Results of Treatment. In 22 clinical trials, 80% of patients with amenorrhea/galactorrhea, associated with hyperprolactinemia but no demonstrable tumors, had menses restored.[152] The average treatment time to the initiation of menses was 5.7 weeks. Complete cessation of galactorrhea occurred in 50–60% of patients in an average time of 12.7 weeks, and a 75% reduction of breast secretions was achieved in 6.4 weeks. *It is important to advise patients that the cessation of galactorrhea is a slower and less certain response than restoration of ovulation and menses.* Amenorrhea recurred in 41% of the patients within an average of 4.4 weeks of discontinuing treatment; galactorrhea recurred in 69% at an average of 6.0 weeks. Approximately 5% of patients terminated treatment because of adverse reactions.

Regression of Tumors With Bromocriptine. There is no question that macroadenomas will regress with bromocriptine treatment.[120, 143, 153] In some, there is prompt shrinkage with low-dose treatment (5–7.5 mg daily); in others, prolonged treatment is required with higher doses. If a prolactin adenoma fails to shrink with 10 mg daily, further increases in dose are not useful. Visual improvement may be noted within several days. Reduction in tumor size can take place in several days to 6 weeks, but in some cases it is not observed until 6 months or more. In most cases, rapid shrinkage occurs during the first 3 months of therapy, followed by slower reduction.[154] Very high prolactin levels, greater than 2000–3000 ng/mL, are probably the result of invasion of the cavernous sinuses with release directly into the bloodstream. Levels greater than 1000 ng/mL are associated with locally invasive tumors. Even these cases show remarkable resolution with bromocriptine treatment. Indeed, surgical results with invasive tumors are so poor that long-term control with a dopamine agonist is recommended. Although tumor shrinkage is always preceded by a decrease in prolactin levels, the overall response cannot be predicted by the basal prolactin level, the absolute or relative fall in prolactin, or even the attainment of normal prolactin levels. Visual impairment improves rapidly, but maximal effects may take several months. However, a prolactin level nonresponder will be a tumor size nonresponder.

The response of macroadenomas to bromocriptine is impressive, and a most compelling reason in favor of its use is that it has been successful when previous surgery or radiation has failed.[120] The problem, however, is that it probably must be taken indefinitely, because there is yet to be a convincing report of complete disappearance and resolution of tumor that can be attributed to drug therapy and not spontaneous resolution. Light and electron microscopic, immuno-histochemical, and morphometric analyses all indicate that bromocriptine causes not only a reduction in the size of individual cells but also necrosis of the cells with replacement fibrosis.[154] Nevertheless, prolactin levels generally return to an elevated state after discontinuation of the drug. There are cases of improvement in sellar imaging; however, the occurrence of spontaneous regression of prolactin-secreting tumors makes it impossible to attribute "cures" to bromo-criptine. Recurrence of hyperprolactinemia has been observed following as many as 4–8 years of treatment.

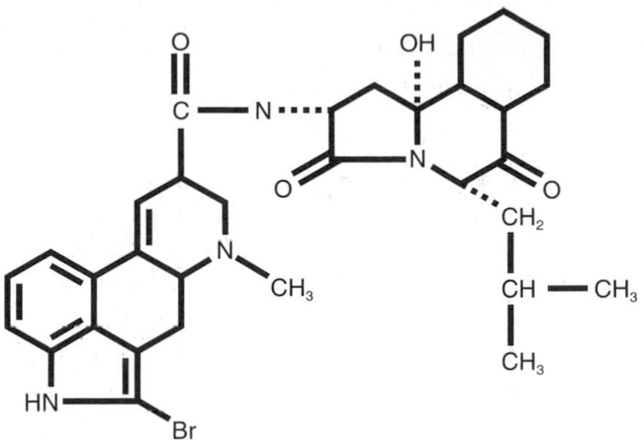

Bromocriptine

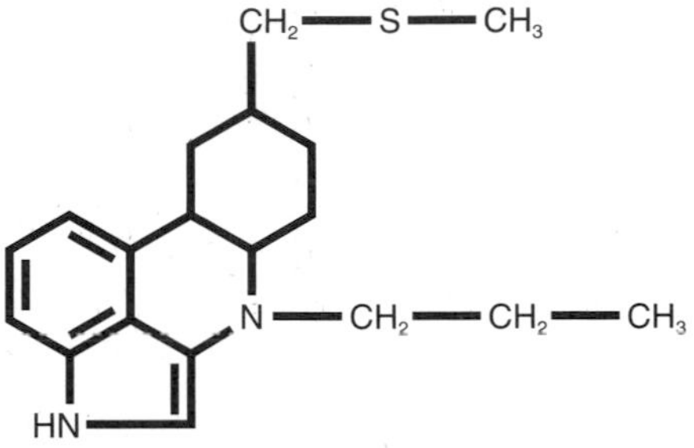

Pergolide

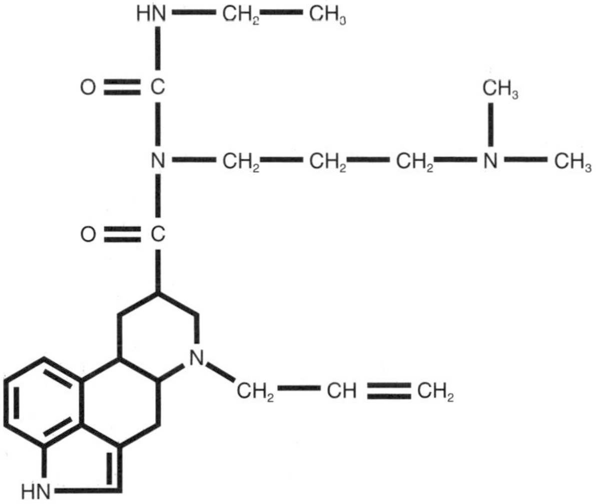

Cabergoline

Other Dopamine Agonists

Other ergoline derivatives with dopaminergic activity are available throughout the world. Pergolide is more potent, longer-lasting, and better tolerated by some patients than bromocriptine. Pergolide is given in a single daily dose of 50–150 mg, and it may be effective in bromocriptine-resistant patients.[155] Others are lysuride, terguride, metergoline, and cabergoline. Quinagolide (CV 205-502) is a nonergot long-acting dopamine agonist given in a daily bedtime dse of 75–300 mg. Because quinagolide has a higher affinity for the dopamine receptor, tumors resistant to bromocriptine have responded to this drug.[156] Side effects are reduced with quinagolide, and it appears to have antidepressive properties.[157] Side effects and intolerance with one of these drugs is often solved by using another. *A patient who fails to respond to one dopamine agonist may respond to another.*

Cabergoline. Cabergoline is also an ergot-derived dopamine agonist.[158] Patients resistant to both bromocriptine and quinagolide have been reported to respond to cabergoline.[159] Cabergoline can be administered orally at doses of 0.5 to 3.0 mg only once weekly, although it can be given twice weekly if necessary, with minimal dopamine agonist side effects (headache being the most common complaint).[160–163] *The low rate of side effects and the once weekly dosage make cabergoline an attractive choice for initial treatment, replacing bromocriptine.* The only reservation (a small one) is a more limited experience documenting fetal safety for patients being treated for infertility.[164] Cabergoline can also be administered vaginally for the rare patient who cannot tolerate it orally.[165]

Summary: Therapy of Pituitary Prolactin-Secreting Adenomas

Macroadenomas

Currently dopamine agonist treatment is advocated for the treatment of macroadenomas, utilizing as low a dose as possible. Shrinkage of a tumor may require 5–10 mg bromocriptine daily, but once shrinkage has occurred, the daily dose should be progressively reduced until the lowest maintenance dose is achieved. The serum prolactin level can be utilized as a marker, checking levels every 3 months until stable. In many (but not all) patients, control of tumor growth correlates with maintenance of a baseline prolactin level and can be achieved in some patients with as little as one-quarter of a tablet (0.625 mg) daily.[166] Withdrawal of the drug is usually associated with regrowth or reexpansion of the tumor, and, therefore, treatment must be long-term if not indefinite. If there is a good response in prolactin levels, and if present, visual field defects, the MRI should be repeated after 1 year of treatment to establish size reduction of the tumor. Some patients will prefer surgery rather than long-term medical treatment, and it is certainly a legitimate option. In view of better results claimed in more recent times, this choice should be presented to the patient. Transsphenoidal surgery is recommended when suprasellar extension or visual impairment persists after dopamine agonist treatment of a macroadenoma. For some patients, side effects with dopamine agonist treatment and difficulty with medication compliance make surgery a reasonable alternative. Because tumor recurrence is high, radiotherapy should be considered.[167] All patients receiving radiotherapy require ongoing surveillance for the development of hypopituitarism. Surgery should be considered as a debulking procedure for very large tumors with or without invasion prior to long-term dopamine agonist therapy.

Short-term treatment (several weeks) with a dopamine agonist can make surgery easier because of a reduction in size (although not all neurosurgeons agree); however, long-term treatment (3 months or more) is associated with fibrosis, which makes complete surgical removal more difficult and more likely to be associated with the sacrifice of other pituitary hormonal function.[168] Even though prolactin levels usually increase when dopamine agonist treatment is discontinued after several years, many tumors (70–80%) do not regrow.[169] Pregnancy should be deferred until repeat imaging confirms shrinkage of the macroadenoma.

Approximately 10% of macroadenomas do not shrink with dopamine agonist therapy. *The failure of a tumor to shrink significantly in size despite a normalization of prolactin levels is consistent with a nonfunctioning tumor that is interrupting the supply of dopamine to the pituitary by stalk compression. Early surgery is indicated.* A tumor that continues to grow despite dopamine agonist treatment may be a rare carcinoma.

Microadenomas

The treatment of microadenomas should be directed to alleviating one of two problems: infertility or breast discomfort. Treatment with a dopamine agonist is the method of choice. Again, some patients, deliberately and understandably, choose the surgical approach in hopes of achieving a cure and avoiding the worry and annoyance of continuing surveillance.

The major therapeutic dilemma can be expressed by the following question: should chronic dopamine agonist treatment be utilized to retrieve ovarian function in those patients with hypoestrogenic amenorrhea, or should estrogen treatment be offered? Until a clear-cut benefit is demonstrated by clinical studies, we cannot advocate widespread dopamine agonist therapy for those patients not interested in becoming pregnant. This conservative approach is supported by documentation of a benign clinical course with spontaneous resolution in many patients.[170–172] Patients with hypoestrogenic amenorrhea are encouraged to be on an estrogen therapy program to maintain the health of their bones and the vascular system. Low-dose oral contraception is recommended for those patients who require contraception. *Estrogen-induced tumor expansion or growth has not been a problem in both our experience and in that of others.*[173, 174]

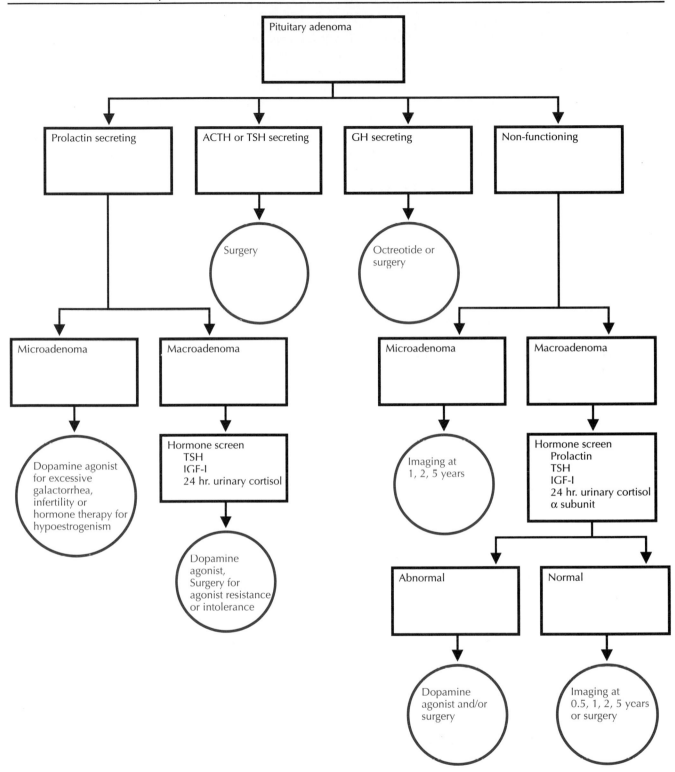

Long-Term Follow-Up

Because these tumors can grow slowly, it is appropriate in the absence of symptoms to evaluate patients with microadenomas annually for 2 years. The evaluation consists of a measurement of the prolactin level and a coned-down view of the sella turcica. If the course is unchanged, annual evaluation can be limited to measurement of the prolactin level. More sophisticated sellar imaging is reserved for patients with a change in the coned-down x-ray view, an increasing prolactin, or the development of headaches and/or visual complaints. It should be noted that progressively increasing prolactin levels have been observed *without* associated tumor growth of a microadenoma.[175] The rare microadenoma that grows deserves treatment. Patients with macroadenomas deserve an initial period of follow-up after treatment every 6 months, and if the adenoma appears to be clinically stable, prolactin levels should be measured annually. CT scanning or MRI is reserved for situations suggestive of tumor expansion. If clinician and patient need reassurance regarding tumor size, imaging intervals can be prolonged if the tumor is stable; e.g., at 1 year, 2 years, 4 years, 8 years. Tumor expansion and recurrent tumors after surgery or radiotherapy deserve a trial of treatment with a dopamine agonist.

Patients who have been on dopamine agonist treatment for 5–10 years with successful tumor size reduction can have a gradual reduction, and then stopping of treatment, followed by monitoring of prolactin levels every 3 months. If a normal prolactin level is maintained, we recommend an imaging study 1 year later. Of course, tumor reexpansion requires resumption of treatment with the gradual program that should always be used when starting therapy.

Pregnancy and Prolactin Adenomas

Approximately 80% of hyperprolactinemic women achieve pregnancy with dopamine agonist treatment.[176] ***Breastfeeding, if desired, can be experienced normally without fear of stimulating tumor growth.*** There is no increase in the normal rates of spontaneous miscarriages, ectopic pregnancies, and complications of pregnancy.

Interestingly, some women resume cyclic menses after pregnancy. This spontaneous improvement may be due to tumor infarction brought about by the expansion and shrinkage during and after pregnancy, or there may be a correction of a hypothalamic dysfunction followed by a disappearance of the associated pituitary hyperplasia.

A very small percentage (less than 2%) of women with hyperprolactinemia and microadenomas will develop signs or symptoms suggestive of tumor growth during pregnancy.[176] Approximately 5% of these patients will develop asymptomatic tumor enlargement (determined by radiologic techniques), and essentially none will ever require surgical intervention. The risk is higher with macroadenomas, approximately 15%. Headaches usually precede visual disturbances, and both may occur in any trimester. There is no characteristic headache; they are variable in intensity, location, and character. Bitemporal hemianopsia is the classic visual field finding, but other defects can occur. It has been argued in the past that a desire for pregnancy was a reason for the surgical approach. This argument hinged on the risk of tumor enlargement during pregnancy due to the well known stimulatory effects of estrogen on the pituitary lactotrophs. As noted above, however, experience has indicated that very few patients develop problems. In a series of 65 consecutive pregnant women with untreated pituitary adenomas, not one with a microadenoma developed visual loss; however, 6 of 8 women with macroadenomas did develop some visual field loss.[177]

It is impossible to identify which patient is at risk for symptomatic expansion during pregnancy. Other than a very large tumor, the size is not critical because both microadenomas and macroadenomas can undergo uneventful pregnancies. There is no increase in miscarriages, or perinatal mortality or morbidity. It is virtually unheard of to develop a problem that results in perinatal damage or serious maternal sequelae. Nevertheless, an occasional serious event can occur; e.g., hemorrhage of the tumor with diabetes insipidus and the potential for permanent visual impairment or life-threatening sequelae.[178]

Surveillance during pregnancy at first consisted of monthly visual field and prolactin measurements. With experience, this proved to be unnecessary. The patient and the clinician can be guided by the development of symptoms. Assessment of visual fields, prolactin, and the sella turcica by imaging can await the onset of headaches or visual disturbances. Even macroprolactinomas with suprasellar extension can be followed closely; discontinuation of a dopamine agonist after conception is usually not associated with tumor growth during the pregnancy.[179] With repeated pregnancies, tumor regression often occurs with the development of an empty sella.

Definite evidence of tumor expansion, as well as the symptoms of headaches and visual changes, promptly regresses with dopamine agonist treatment.[120] Termination of pregnancy or neurosurgery, therefore, should rarely, if ever, be necessary. Although bromocriptine treatment profoundly lowers both maternal and fetal blood levels of prolactin, no adverse effects on the pregnancy or the newborn have been noted.[150, 176, 180–182] Fortunately, amniotic fluid prolactin (and its presumed action on regulation of amniotic fluid water and electrolytes) is derived from decidual tissue, and its secretion is controlled by estrogen and progesterone, not dopamine. Therefore, dopamine agonist treatment does not affect amniotic fluid levels of prolactin.

The Empty Sella Syndrome

A patient may have an abnormal sella turcica, but rather than a tumor, she may have the empty sella syndrome. In this condition, there is a congenital incompleteness of the sellar diaphragm that allows an extension of the subarachnoid space into the pituitary fossa. The pituitary gland is separated from the hypothalamus and is flattened. The sella floor may be demineralized due to pressure from the cerebrospinal fluid, and the x-ray picture on coned-down views will be similar to a tumor. The empty sella syndrome can also occur secondary to surgery, radiotherapy, or infarction of a pituitary tumor.

An empty sella is found in approximately 5% of autopsies, and approximately 85% are in women, previously thought to be concentrated in middle-aged and obese women.[183] A closer look at the sella turcica, brought about by our pursuit of elevated prolactin levels, has revealed an incidence of empty sellas in 4–16% of patients who present with amenorrhea/galactorrhea.[123, 128] Galactorrhea and elevated prolactin levels can be seen with an empty sella, and there may be a coexisting prolactin-secreting adenoma. This suggests that the empty sella in these patients may have arisen because of tumor infarction.

This condition is benign; it does not progress to pituitary failure. The chief hazard to the patient is inadvertent treatment for a pituitary tumor. Even though enlargement of the sella turcica with a normal shape is more likely associated with an empty sella than a tumor, all patients should have examination by imaging for confirmation.

Because of the possibility of a coexisting adenoma, patients with elevated prolactin levels or galactorrhea and an empty sella should undergo annual surveillance (prolactin assay and coned-down view) for a few years to detect tumor growth. It is totally safe and appropriate to offer hormone treatment or induction of ovulation.

Sheehan's Syndrome

Acute infarction and necrosis of the pituitary gland due to postpartum hemorrhage and shock is known as Sheehan's syndrome.[184] The symptoms of hypopituitarism are usually seen early in the postpartum period, especially failure of lactation and loss of pubic and axillary hair. Deficiencies in growth hormone and gonadotropins are most common, followed by ACTH, and last, by TSH in frequency.[185] Diabetes insipidus is not usually present. This can be a life-threatening condition, but fortunately, because of good obstetrical care, this syndrome is never encountered by most of us.

Compartment IV: Central Nervous System Disorders

Hypothalamic Amenorrhea

Patients with hypothalamic amenorrhea (hypogonadotropic hypogonadism) have a deficiency in GnRH pulsatile secretion. Hypothalamic problems are usually diagnosed by exclusion of pituitary lesions and are the most common category of hypogonadotropic amenorrhea, a functional suppression of reproduction, often a psychobiologic response to life events.[186] Frequently, there is an association with a stressful situation, such as in business or in school. There is also a higher proportion of underweight women and a higher occurrence of previous menstrual irregularity. Indeed, many women with hypothalamic amenorrhea display the endocrine and metabolic characteristics associated with eating disorders and athletics, suggesting the presence of a subclinical eating disorder.[187] Nevertheless, the clinician is obliged to go through the process of exclusion prior to prescribing hormone therapy or attempting induction of ovulation to achieve pregnancy.

The degree of GnRH suppression determines how these patients present clinically. Mild suppression can be associated with a marginal effect on reproduction, specifically an inadequate luteal phase. Moderate suppression of GnRH secretion can yield anovulation with menstrual irregularity, and profound suppression is manifested by hypothalamic amenorrhea.

Patients with hypothalamic amenorrhea are categorized by low or normal gonadotropins, normal prolactin levels, a normal imaging evaluation of the sella turcica, and a failure to demonstrate withdrawal bleeding. A good practice is to evaluate such patients annually. This annual surveillance should include a prolactin assay and the coned-down view of the sella turcica. The x-ray is necessary only every 2–3 years after several years with no change. In the only long-term follow-up of a large group of women with secondary amenorrhea, it was noted that amenorrhea associated with psychological stress or weight loss demonstrated a spontaneous recovery after 6 years in 72% of the women.[188] This still leaves a significant percentage of women who require ongoing surveillance. In patients with eating disorders, the return of menstrual function is associated with a gain in body weight, an obvious marker for clinical improvement in the underlying condition.[189]

Experimental evidence in the monkey indicates that corticotropin-releasing hormone (CRH) inhibits gonadotropin secretion, probably by augmenting endogenous opioid secretion.[190] This is the probable pathway by which stress interrupts reproductive function. Women with hypothalamic amenorrhea have reduced secretion of FSH, LH, and prolactin, but increased secretion of cortisol.[191–193] There is also evidence to indicate that some patients with hypothalamic amenorrhea have dopaminergic inhibition of GnRH pulse frequency.[194] The suppression of GnRH pulsatile secretion may be the result of increases in both endogenous opioids and dopamine. Thus far, abnormalities in the genes for GnRH and the beta-subunits for FSH and LH have not been detected in patients with hypothalamic amenorrhea.[195, 196]

Even though a patient may not be currently interested in pursuing pregnancy, it is important to assure these patients that, at the appropriate time, treatment for the induction of ovulation will be available and that fertility can be achieved. Concern with potential fertility is often an unspoken fear, especially in the younger patients, even teenagers. On the other hand, induction of ovulation should be performed only for the purpose of producing a pregnancy. There is no evidence that cyclic hormone administration or induction of ovulation will stimulate the return of normal function.

Weight Loss, Anorexia, Bulimia

St. Wilgefortis was the 7th daughter of the King of Portugal, living around the year 1000.[197] When confronted with an arranged marriage (she had made a vow of virginity to become a nun), she turned to intense prayer. The intensity of the prayer was marked by anorexia and the growth of body hair. Confronted with this new appearance, the King of Sicily changed his mind about the marriage, and Wilgefortis's father had her crucified. Around 1200, the legend of Wilgefortis spread throughout Europe.

St. Wilgefortis became a symbol, a woman who liberated herself of female problems, and she became a protectress of women with sexual problems, including problems associated with childbirth. Indeed, women who wished to rid themselves of their husbands prayed to her, because she had successfully resisted both a father and a potential husband. In England, rather than St. Wilgefortis, she was known as St. Uncumber because women believed she could uncumber them of their husbands.

Thus emerged the medieval dark ages explanation (with ascendancy to sainthood) of a girl's response (anorexia nervosa) to her fears of marriage and sexuality. Our understanding of the reason for this extraordinary behavior continues today to focus on an inability to cope with the onset of adult sexuality, with a return to the prepubertal state. Both anorexia nervosa and bulimia nervosa (binge eating) are distinguished by a morbid fear of fatness.

Obesity can be associated with amenorrhea, but amenorrhea in an obese patient is usually due to anovulation, and a hypogonadotropic state is not encountered unless the patient also has a severe emotional disorder. Conversely, acute weight loss, in some unknown way, can lead to the hypogonadotropic state. Again, the clinician must pursue the presence of a pituitary tumor, and the diagnosis of hypothalamic amenorrhea is made by exclusion.

Clinically a spectrum is encountered that ranges from a limited period of amenorrhea associated with a crash diet, to the severely ill patient with the life-threatening attrition of anorexia nervosa. It is a common experience for a clinician to be the first to recognize anorexia nervosa in a patient presenting with the complaint of amenorrhea. It is also not infrequent that a clinician will evaluate and manage an infertility problem due to hypogonadotropism and not be aware of a developing case of anorexia. Because the mortality rate associated with this syndrome is significant (5–15%), it warrants close attention.[198, 199]

Diagnosis of Anorexia Nervosa

1. Onset between ages 10 and 30.
2. Weight loss of 25% or weight 15% below normal for age and height.
3. Special attitudes:
   —Denial,
   —Distorted body image,
   —Unusual hoarding or handling of food.
4. At least one of the following:
   —Lanugo,
   —Bradycardia,
   —Overactivity,
   —Episodes of overeating (bulimia),
   —Vomiting, which may be self-induced.
5. Amenorrhea.
6. No known medical illness.
7. No other psychiatric disorder.
8. Other characteristics:
   —Constipation,
   —Low blood pressure,
   —Hypercarotenemia,
   —Diabetes insipidus.

Anorexia nervosa has been recognized to occur frequently in young white middle to upper class females under age 25, but it is now apparent that this problem occurs at all socioeconomic levels in about 1% of young women.[200] The families of anorectics are success-achievement-appearance oriented. Serious problems may be present within the family, but the parents make every effort to maintain an apparent marital harmony, glossing over or denying conflicts. In one psychiatric interpretation, each parent, in secret dissatisfaction with the other, expects affection from their "perfect" child. Anorexia begins when the role of the perfect child becomes too difficult. The pattern usually starts with a voluntary diet to control weight. This brings a sense of power and accomplishment, soon followed by a fear that weight cannot be controlled if discipline is allowed to relax. A reasonable view is to consider anorexia as a mechanism that identifies a generally disturbed family.[201] The symptom pattern is the expression of the various psychological, familial, and cultural factors involved.

At puberty, the normal weight gain may be interpreted as excessive, and this can trip the teenager over into true anorexia nervosa. Excessive physical activity can be the earliest sign of incipient anorexia nervosa. The children are characteristically overachievers and strivers. They seldom give any trouble, but are judgmental and demand that others live up to their rigid value system, often resulting in social isolation. Patients with eating disorders usually demonstrate delayed psychosexual development marked by sexual experiences occurring at a later age.[202]

The cultural value our society places on thinness definitely plays a role in eating disorders. Both occupational and recreational environments that stress thinness put women at greater risk for anorexia nervosa and bulimia. But basically, an eating disorder is a method being utilized to solve a psychological dilemma.

Besides amenorrhea, constipation is a common symptom, often severe and accompanied by abdominal pain. The preoccupation with food may manifest itself by large intakes of lettuce, raw vegetables, and low-calorie foods. Hypotension, hypothermia, rough dry skin, soft lanugo-type hair on the back and buttocks, bradycardia, and edema are the most commonly encountered signs. Long-term diuretic and laxative abuse may produce significant hypokalemia. An elevation of the serum carotene is not always associated with a large intake of yellow vegetables, suggesting that a defect in vitamin A utilization is present. The yellowish coloration of the skin is usually seen on the palms. Hypercarotenemia should be regarded as a metabolic marker, but not every woman with hypercarotenemia will be amenorrheic or anovulatory.[203]

Bulimia is a syndrome marked by episodic and secretive binge eating followed by self-induced vomiting, fasting, or the use of laxatives and diuretics.[198, 204] It appears to be a growing problem among young women; however, careful study indicates that although bulimic behaviors may be relatively common, clinically significant bulimia is not (approximately 1.0% of female students and 0.1% of male students in a college sample), and the overall prevalence of eating disorders may be declining.[205–207] Bulimic behavior is frequently seen in patients with anorexia nervosa (about half), but not in all. Patients with bulimia have a high incidence of depressive symptoms, and a problem with shoplifting (usually food). Little is known about the long-term outcome. There is a growing tendency to divide patients with anorexia nervosa into bulimic anorectics and dieters. Bulimic anorectics are older, less isolated socially, and have a higher incidence of family problems. Body weight in a "pure" bulimic fluctuates, but it does not fall to the low levels seen in anorectics.

The serious case of anorexia nervosa is seen more often by an internist. However, the borderline anorectic frequently presents to a gynecologist, pediatrician, or family physician as a teenager who has low body weight, amenorrhea, and hyperactivity (excellent grades and many extracurricular activities). The amenorrhea can precede, follow, or appear coincidentally with the weight loss.

The various problems associated with anorexia represent dysfunction of the body mechanisms regulated by the hypothalamus: appetite, thirst and water conservation, temperature, sleep, autonomic balance, and endocrine secretion.[208] Endocrine studies can be summarized as follows: FSH and LH levels are low, cortisol levels are elevated, prolactin levels are normal, TSH and thyroxine (T_4) levels are normal, but the 3,5,3'-triiodothyronine (T_3) level is low, and reverse T_3 is high. Indeed, many of the symptoms can be explained by relative hypothyroidism (constipation, cold intolerance, bradycardia, hypotension, dry skin, low metabolic rates, hypercarotenemia). There appears to be a compensation to the state of undernourishment, with diversion from formation of the active T_3 to the inactive metabolite, reverse T_3. With weight gain, all of the metabolic changes revert to normal. Even though normal gonadotropin secretion may be restored with weight gain, 30% of patients remain amenorrheic, a good sign of ongoing psychological conflict.[206]

The central origin for the amenorrhea is suggested by the demonstration that the response to GnRH is regained at approximately 15% below the ideal weight, and this return to normal responsiveness occurs before the resumption of menses.[209] Patients with anorexia nervosa have persistent low levels of gonadotropins similar to prepubertal children. With weight gain, sleep-associated episodic secretion of LH appears, similar to the early pubertal child. With full recovery, the 24-hour pattern is similar to that of an adult, marked by fluctuating peaks. This sequence of changes with increasing and decreasing weight is explained by increasing and decreasing pulsatile secretion of GnRH. Neuropeptide Y may be a link between the control of food intake and GnRH secretion.[210] Neuropeptide Y cell bodies are located in the arcuate nucleus of the hypothalamus. This peptide both stimulates feeding behavior and inhibits gonadotropin secretion (presumably by suppressing GnRH pulses, although a direct action on the pituitary is also possible). In response to food deprivation, the endogenous levels of neuropeptide Y increase, and elevated concentrations of neuropeptide Y can be measured in the cerebrospinal fluid of anorexic women. This is consistent with the known actions of leptin, as discussed with full references in Chapter 19.

This is one of the rare conditions in which gonadotropins may be undetectable (large pituitary tumors and genetic deficiencies are the others). If necessary, a high plasma cortisol can differentiate this condition from pituitary insufficiency. However, extensive laboratory testing in these patients is not necessary. Adherence to our scheme for the evaluation of amenorrhea is indicated to rule out other pathological processes. Further endocrine assessment, however, is not essential for patient management.

A careful and gentle revelation to the patient of the relationship between the amenorrhea and the low body weight is often all that is necessary to stimulate the patient to return to normal weight and normal menstrual function. Occasionally, it is necessary to see the patient frequently and become involved in a program of daily calorie counting (a minimum intake of 2600 calories) in order to break the patient's established eating habits. If progress is slow, hormone therapy should be initiated. In an adult weighing less than 100 pounds, continued weight loss requires psychiatric consultation. Some would argue that any patient with an eating disorder requires psychiatric intervention.

Going away to school or the development of a relationship with a male friend often are turning points for young women with mild to moderate anorexia. A failure to respond to these life changes is relatively ominous, predicting a severe problem with a protracted course.

It is disappointing that despite the impressive studies on anorexia, there is no specific or new therapy available. This only serves to emphasize the need for early recognition to allow psychologic intervention before the syndrome is entrenched in its full severity.[211] The use of serotonin antagonists or uptake blockers is restricted to patients who, as is frequently the case, have the comorbidity of clinical depression.[212] Clinicians (and parents) should pay particular attention to weight and diet in young women with amenorrhea. Even in amenorrheic adolescents of normal or above-normal body weights, disordered eating patterns (fasting and purging) are often present, a sign of an underlying stressful disorder.[213]

Exercise and Amenorrhea

Soranus of Ephesus in the 1st century AD observed in his famous treatise, "On the Diseases of Women," that amenorrhea is frequently observed in the youthful, the aged, the pregnant, in singers, and in those who take much exercise. Late in the 20th century, there was a new awareness that competitive female athletes, as well as women engaged in strenuous recreational exercise and women engaged in other forms of demanding activity, such as ballet and modern dance, have a significant incidence of menstrual irregularity and amenorrhea, in the pattern called hypothalamic suppression. The extent of this problem has perhaps been underestimated because of a lack of attention to anovulatory cycles. As many as two-thirds of runners who have menstrual periods have short luteal phases or are anovulatory.[214] When training starts before menarche, menarche can be delayed by as much as 3 years, and the subsequent incidence of menstrual irregularity is higher. In some individuals, secondary amenorrhea is associated with delayed menarche even though training did not begin until after menarche. It is suggested that some girls with these characteristics may be socially influenced to pursue athletic training. Contrary to the female situation, exercise has little effect on the timing of puberty in boys. Although changes in testicular function can be demonstrated in males, the changes are more subtle and less meaningful clinically.[215]

There appear to be two major influences: a critical level of body fat and the effect of stress itself. Young women who weigh less than 115 pounds and lose more than 10 pounds while exercising are the women most likely to develop the problem,[216] an association that supports the critical weight concept of Frisch.[217]

The critical weight hypothesis states that the onset and regularity of menstrual function necessitate maintaining weight above a critical level, and, therefore, above a critical amount of body fat. In dealing with patients, it is helpful to use the nomogram derived from Frisch, which is based on the calculation of the amount of total body water as a percentage of body weight. This relates to the percentage of body fat and, therefore, is an index of fatness. The 10th percentile at age 16 is equivalent to about 22% body fat, the minimal weight for height necessary for sustaining menstruation, and the 10th percentile at age 13 is equivalent to 17% body fat, the minimum for initiating menarche. A loss of body weight in the range of 10–15% of normal weight for height

A Fatness Index Nomogram
modified from Frisch

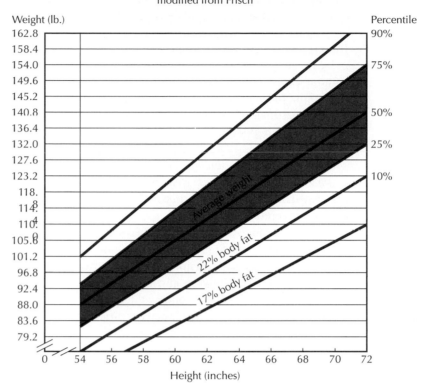

Weight (lb.)

Height (inches)

represents a loss of approximately one-third of the body fat, which will result in a drop below the 22% line and may result in abnormal menstrual function.[218]

Although the nomogram is useful to show these relationships to patients, individual variation is such that the nomogram cannot be utilized to predict without fail the return of menses for an individual patient. Indeed, the accuracy of the nomogram has been challenged.[219] The fat criteria were derived from the indirect estimation of body fat from predicted total body water, with a regression equation that employs height and weight. There is no question that the most reliable and accurate method for estimating body fatness is hydrostatic weighing of body density, although dual-energy x-ray absorptiometry (DEXA) is also excellent. But one can hardly maintain a small pool for this purpose in a clinical office. Granted that the nomogram, and specifically the 22% body fat criterion, are not absolutely accurate; nevertheless, the concept is useful, and the nomogram remains helpful to illustrate the concept to patients.

The competitive female athlete has about 50% less body fat than the noncompetitor, very much under the 10th percentile for secondary amenorrhea (the 22% body fat line). This change in body fat can occur with no discernible change in total body weight, because fat is converted to lean muscle mass.[220] A critical look at the critical weight hypothesis argues that there is not a cause-and-effect relationship between body fat and menstrual function, only a correlation.[221, 222] For this reason, considerable variation is seen with many examples of normal and abnormal menstrual function at all levels of body fat content. On the other hand, the correlation does exist, and body fat content and body weight are useful guides to the relationship between menstrual function and the energy balance of the body. Indeed, the leptin story (Chapter 19) has restored credibility to the critical weight hypothesis. It has always been a mystery how total body fat could talk with the brain. A mystery no longer! Fat talks to the brain via leptin, and the leptin system affects reproduction.

In addition to the role of body fat, stress and energy expenditure appear to play an independent role. Warren has pointed out that dancers will have a return of menses during intervals of rest, despite no change in body weight or percent body fat.[223] High-energy output and stress, therefore, can act independently, as well as additively, to low body fat in suppressing reproductive function. It is not surprising that a woman with low body weight who is engaged in competitive activity (athletic or aesthetic) is highly susceptible to anovulation and amenorrhea.

Running in the dark is even more risky. Studies indicate that ovarian activity can be affected independently by strenuous activity and seasonal variation.[224] Decreased ovarian activity in autumn could be related to a greater dark photoperiod with increased pineal secretion of melatonin. Indeed, the conception rate of women living in northern Scandinavia is higher during the summer than in the winter. The practical conclusion is that serious runners can expect to encounter more problems with menstrual function in autumn and winter.

This menstrual disruption is similar to the hypothalamic dysfunction which is more marked in the classic cases of anorexia nervosa. Acute exercise decreases gonadotropins and increases prolactin, growth hormone, testosterone, ACTH, the adrenal steroids, and endorphins as a result of both enhanced secretion and reduced clearance.[225] The prolactin increase is in contrast to the absence of prolactin changes in undernourished women. The prolactin increases are variable, small in amplitude, and exceedingly short in duration. Thus, it is unlikely that the prolactin increase is responsible for the suppression of the menstrual cycle. Most importantly, insignificant differences occur in prolactin when amenorrheic runners are compared with eumenorrheic runners or nonrunners.[226] In addition, women athletes have elevated daytime melatonin levels, and amenorrheic athletes have an exaggerated nocturnal secretion of melatonin.[227] The nocturnal increase in melatonin is also seen in women with hypothalamic amenorrhea and appears to reflect suppression of GnRH pulsatile secretion.[228] Another contrast to undernourished women is found in the thyroid axis. Athletes have relatively low T_4 levels, but amenorrheic athletes have an overall suppression of all circulating thyroid hormones, including reverse T_3.[229]

It has been suggested that a suboptimal amount of body fat adversely affects estrogen metabolism, specifically leading to an increased conversion of biologically active estrogens to relatively inactive catecholestrogens.[230] The conversion of estradiol to its catecholestrogens rapidly yields 2-hydroxyestrone and 4-hydroxyestrone, relatively inactive metabolites, that are metabolized further by methylation to 2-methoxyestrogen and 4-methoxyestrogen. These products, and, thus, this metabolic pathway, are increased by physical exercise.[231, 232] The extent of 2-hydroxylation correlates inversely with body fat, increasing with decreasing adiposity.[220, 233] This could be a mechanism that interferes with the important feedback and local roles for estradiol in pituitary-ovarian interactions.

Among runners, there is frequent talk about the runner's "high," the feeling of euphoria and exhilaration after competition or an extensive workout. It is still not clear whether this is a psychologic reaction or whether it is due to an increase in endogenous opiates. The site of GnRH secretion, the arcuate nucleus area in the hypothalamus, is rich in opioid receptors and endorphin production. There is considerable evidence indicating that endogenous opiates inhibit gonadotropin secretion by suppressing hypothalamic GnRH. Women studied during a period of endurance conditioning demonstrated a steadily increasing endorphin output after exercise.[234–237] This link of endorphins to the menstrual suppression associated with exercise is very plausible. Naltrexone, a long-acting opioid receptor blocker, restores menstrual function when administered long-term to women with amenorrhea associated with weight loss; this indicates a key role of endorphins in stress-related hypothalamic amenorrhea.[238] The measurement of circulating β-endorphin levels may not reflect central mechanisms; both eumenorrheic and amenorrheic athletes have exercise-induced increases in the blood levels of β-endorphin.[237]

Corticotropin-releasing hormone (CRH) directly inhibits hypothalamic GnRH secretion, probably by augmenting endogenous opioid secretion.[239, 240] Women with hypothalamic amenorrhea (including exercisers and women with eating disorders) demonstrate hypercortisolism (due to increased CRH and ACTH), suggesting that this is the pathway by which stress interrupts reproductive function.[192, 241, 242] Indeed, amenorrheic athletes who have cortisol levels that return to normal range regain menstrual function within 6 months, in contrast to athletes who maintain elevated cortisol levels and continue to be amenorrheic.[243]

Amenorrheic athletes are in a state of negative energy balance, further distinguished by elevated levels of insulin-like growth factor binding protein-1 (IGFBP-1), increased insulin sensitivity, decreased insulin levels, and increased growth hormone levels.[244] The increase in IGFBP-1 can limit IGF activity in the hypothalamus and thus provide another mechanism for suppression of GnRH secretion.

Λ unifying hypothesis focuses on energy balance.[222] When available energy is excessively diverted, as in exercise, or when insufficient, as with eating disorders, reproduction is suspended in order to support essential metabolism for survival. Thus reproduction is not directly affected by the level of body fat, rather body fat is a marker of the metabolic energy state. From a teleologic point of view, there is sense to these relationships; the responses that assist the body to withstand stress also inhibit menstrual function because a stressful period is not the ideal time for reproduction.

The effect of leptin on reproduction can be viewed as an additional role in maintaining responses to stress. Weight loss is known to be associated with an increased adrenal response and a decrease in thyroid function; these endocrine changes, along with suppression of the estrous cycle, occur in fasted mice and are reversed by treatment with leptin.[245]

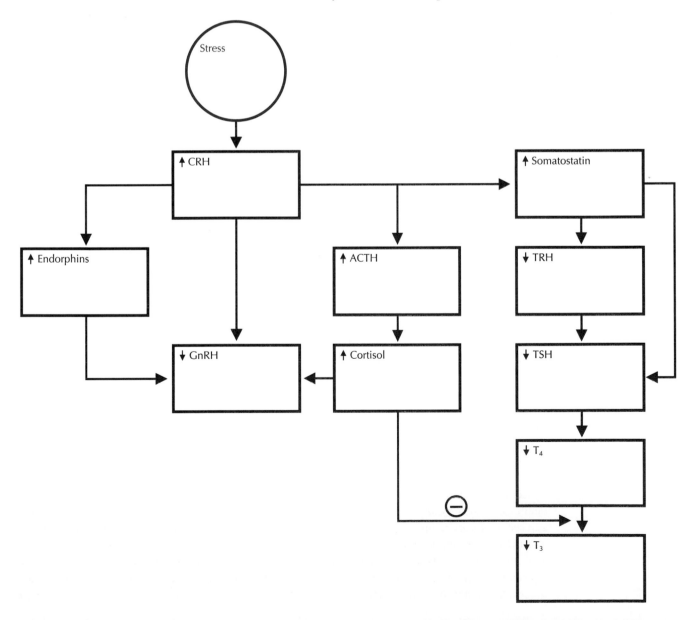

The puzzle is why CRH is elevated in stress amenorrhea (especially that associated with weight loss) in contrast to fasting in normal and obese individuals. One possibility is that the decrease in leptin and increase in NPY associated with stress-related weight loss is the expected response, but it is inadequate to suppress the stress-induced increase in CRH. The blunted patterns in amenorrheic athletes support this. The increase in CRH and resulting hypercortisolism further increases metabolism and weight loss.

Athletes with cyclic menses demonstrate a normal diurnal rhythm in leptin levels. However, amenorrheic athletes do not have a diurnal pattern.[246] Both cycling athletes and amenorrheic athletes have low leptin levels (3-fold reduction) that correlate with reduced body fat, but the levels are further lowered by hypoinsulinemia and hypercortisolemia. In addition, amenorrheic athletes have a blunted leptin response to the increase in insulin following meals. An increase in menstrual irregularity and amenorrhea is correlated with a decrease in body fat below 15% of body weight and leptin levels that are less than 3 ng/ml.[247]

Because of the high levels of leptin present in overweight people, the purpose of leptin function may be limited to an effect at low levels. A low circulating level of leptin may serve as a signal that fat stores are not sufficient for growth and reproduction. Thus low levels would ordinarily stimulate hyperphagia, reduce energy expenditure, and suppress gonadotropin secretion and reproduction. The high levels of leptin and the apparent resistance to leptin action associated with excess body weight and fat would then reflect not resistance, but a lack of physiologic effect.

In regards to reproduction, the final pathway is suppression of GnRH, a response to multiple inputs indicating the availability of metabolic fuel.[248] Even in runners with regular menstrual patterns, LH pulsatile frequency and amplitude are significantly reduced.[249, 250] A central inhibition of GnRH can be discerned even before there is perceptible evidence of menstrual irregularity. The clinical presentation (inadequate luteal phase, anovulation, or amenorrhea) will depend on the degree of GnRH suppression. Insufficient estrogen secretion at a critical time during growth can impede the growth spurt and yield short stature.

The characteristics of women in the subculture of exercise and amenorrhea strikingly remind one of anorexia nervosa: significant physical exercise, a necessity for control of the body, striving for artistic and technical proficiency, and the consequent preoccupation with the body, combined with the stressful pressures of performing and competition.[251, 252] Individuals in this lifestyle are prone to develop what can be called the anorectic reaction.[253] Fries has described four stages of dieting behavior that can form a continuum:[254]

1. Dieting for cosmetic reasons.

2. Dieting due to neurotic fixation on food intake and weight.

3. The anorectic reaction.

4. True anorexia nervosa.

There are several important distinctions between the anorectic reaction and true anorexia nervosa. Psychologically, the patient with true anorexia nervosa has a misperception of reality and a lack of insight into the disease and her problem. She does not consider herself underweight and displays an impressive lack of concern over her dreadful physical condition and appearance. The clinician–patient relationship is difficult with no visible emotional involvement and a great deal of mistrust. Patients with the anorectic reaction have the capability for self-criticism. They can see the problem and describe it with insight and an absence of denial. The exercising woman and the competing athlete or dancer can develop an anorectic reaction. The anorectic reaction develops consciously and voluntarily, just as in anorexia nervosa, as the exercising woman deliberately makes an effort to decrease body weight. A clinician may be the first to be aware of the problem having encountered the patient because of the presenting complaint of either amenorrhea or now uncontrolled weight loss. Early recognition, concentrated counseling, and confidential support can intercept and prevent a progressive problem. The high prevalence of eating disorders among female athletes indicates that the threat of progression should not be underrated.[252] It is estimated that the prevalence (in the general population, not just athletes) of the early or partial disorder is twice that of the full syndrome, and progression from pathologic dieting to the full syndrome can occur in some individuals in as short a time period as 1–2 years.[255]

Prognosis is excellent with early recognition, and simple weight gain may reverse the state of amenorrhea. The degree of reversibility is unknown, although general experience indicates that the majority of women regain ovulation when stress and exercise diminish or cease.[256, 257] However, these patients are often unwilling to give up their routines of exercise, and a sensitive clinician can perceive that the exercise is an important means for coping with daily life. Hormone therapy is, therefore, encouraged for these hypoestrogenic patients to provide protection against the loss of bone and cardiovascular changes. However, in patients with an eating disorder, restoration of normal hormonal levels is not sufficient to return bone density to normal; resumption of an adequate diet and weight gain are essential.[258–260] When pregnancy is desired, a reduction in the amount of exercise and a gain in weight should be recommended, or induction of ovulation must be pursued.

Eating Disorders and Pregnancy

It has been estimated that a typical pregnancy requires approximately 300 extra calories per day above that needed in the nonpregnant state.[261] With sufficient caloric intake, weight gain during pregnancy averages 10–12 kg (22–26 lb). Women who are underweight prior to pregnancy need to increase their energy intake and gain 12–15 kg (26–33 lb). Imagine the reaction of a patient with an eating disorder when confronted with these facts. This is fuel for the fire (the morbid fear of fatness).

Prior to the 1970s, obstetricians vigorously advised their patients to limit weight gain during pregnancy. This sadly misplaced advice can be traced to the false belief that excessive weight gain caused preeclampsia, made labor more difficult, and had a permanently detrimental impact on a woman's figure. More appropriate recommendations emerged in the 1970s, based upon a growing body of information derived from scientific studies. These studies documented the importance of prepregnancy weight as well as weight gain during pregnancy as two very important determinants for infant birth weight.

The critical issue is the relationship between the diet of the mother and the well-being of the fetus. There are three classic studies of acute famine in Leningrad, Holland, and Wuppertal during the worst days of World War II.[262–264] The mean birth weight during the siege of Leningrad declined 550 g to 2,789 g. During the Dutch famine, mean birth weight decreased by 300 g; there was no decrease in the birth weight of infants conceived during the famine whose mothers received adequate rations during the third trimester. In Wuppertal, mean birth weight was depressed by 170–227 g. These differences were proportional to the level of official rations, the conditions being the worst in Leningrad.

Studies of restriction of calories during pregnancy have indicated a ready achievement of lesser maternal weight gain, at the expense of lighter birth weights.[265] Women who gain less than 20 pounds compared with those who gain more than 20 pounds are 2.3 times more likely to deliver infants of low birth weight and 1.5 times more likely to have a fetal death.[266] These studies finally led to the abandonment of caloric limitation.

In general, studies of dietary supplementation have indicated increases in mean birth weights.[266] The Special Supplemental Food Program for Women, Infants, and Children (WIC) was begun in the U.S. in 1973. A review of this program found a significant impact on decreasing preterm labor and delivery, an increase in mean birth weight, and a reduction in late fetal death.[267] These improvements are attributed to an improved maternal physiologic status, not upgraded health care. The head circumferences of infants of mothers who participated in WIC were significantly larger, presumably reflecting accelerated brain growth.

Gradually it came to be appreciated that there is a linear relationship between birth weight and maternal weight gain at all levels of prepregnancy weight.[268–273] However, as prepregnancy weight increases, the importance of maternal weight gain diminishes.[274] Thus, in underweight women, the importance of each factor, prepregnancy weight and the weight gain during pregnancy, is magnified.

Now that the many circumstances that influence infant birth weight are better recognized, a modern look at this subject is especially helpful. After adjusting for maternal age, race, parity, weight gain, socioeconomic status, cigarette consumption, and gestational age, there continues to be a statistically significant linear relationship between prepregnancy body mass and birth weight, as well as between prenatal weight gain and birth weight.[275, 276] Furthermore, the fetal death rate increases exponentially as birth weight decreases at each gestational age.[277] Most importantly, a low prepregnancy weight can be overcome; weight gain during pregnancy (beginning in the first trimester) in underweight women can bring an infant into the normal range for birth weight.[278]

Low birth weight in an infant can be directly attributed mainly to two influencing factors: prematurity and fetal growth retardation. Underweight status before pregnancy and inadequate weight gain during the second half of pregnancy each separately increase the risk of preterm birth.[279] In patients with eating disorders, the outcome of pregnancy is significantly influenced by both preterm delivery and intrauterine growth retardation.

In view of the well-recognized correlation between maternal weight (prepregnancy weight and pregnancy weight gain) and infant size, it is certainly logical to expect a problem with pregnancy outcome in patients with eating disorders. Older reports were anecdotal in nature and usually failed to provide birth weights, because our awareness of the importance of body weight to pregnancy outcome is a relatively recent development.[280–286]

More recent reports have documented problems with intrauterine growth retardation and preterm labor. The average weight gain in 7 pregnancies in patients with anorexia nervosa was 8 kg; all infants demonstrated intrauterine growth retardation in the third trimester, followed by accelerated growth after birth.[287] A review of 23 pregnancies in 74 women treated for anorexia or bulimia documented the importance of the severity of the disorder.[288] Women in remission gained more weight and had higher birth weights and 5-minute Apgar scores. Women with active disease had worsening symptoms and psychological problems during pregnancy. The smallest birth weights were born to those with anorexia and bulimia. All the women who were ill at conception continued to be ill. Nine of the 10 women who successfully breastfed for 6 months were in remission. The rate of preterm labor and delivery in patients with eating disorders is twice the normal incidence, and in a study of 50 Danish anorectic women, the perinatal mortality rate was 6 times the normal rate.[289] In an Australian review of 14 consecutive women who failed to respond to clomiphene, all the women had a history of an eating or exercise disorder, and one-third of the eventual live births weighed less than 2500 g.[290] There is a suggestion in retrospective data that the risk of spontaneous miscarriage is increased in pregnant women who are actively bulimic.[291]

Some patients with eating disorders do well during pregnancy; however, even during pregnancy, many patients continue their abnormal eating behavior, and characteristically minimize or lie about their eating behaviors to clinicians, family, and friends.[292] After the pregnancy, rapid deterioration usually takes place.[293] In contrast, normal women are more accepting of their body size and weight gain during pregnancy, and dieting is unusual.[294] Ultimately, the impact on weight is the key. There is no evidence that psychological distress independently influences fetal growth.[295]

Expert help during the pregnancy is highly recommended. Some useful warning signs are the following:

1. Unusual concern regarding body shape.

2. Aversion to being weighed.

3. Lack of weight gain.

Approximately 25% of patients with amenorrhea are underweight due to self-imposed dietary restriction.[296] Because underweight women frequently are anovulatory, it is not surprising that they represent a significant population in whom ovulation is induced. Comparing the outcome of pregnancy in underweight women after spontaneous and induced ovulation, it is apparent that inadequate weight has serious consequences.[297] Underweight women who undergo induction of ovulation often fail to gain weight adequately during pregnancy despite care and counseling. As expected, intrauterine growth retardation and preterm labor are significant problems.

The seriousness of the problem is heightened because of its presence at conception and during the first trimester. A study of adolescent pregnancy concluded that inadequate weight gain before 24 weeks gestation was associated with a significantly increased risk of having a small for gestational age infant, *even when later weight gains brought the cumulative weight gain within normal adult standards.*[298] Later inadequate weight gain was associated with an increased risk of preterm delivery. These results suggest that prevention of preterm delivery and intrauterine growth retardation requires an effort encompassing the entire pregnancy, best beginning prior to conception. A rise in weight of more than 6 kg by the 28th week of pregnancy has predictive value, indicating with a high degree of probability that the rest of pregnancy will progress normally.[299]

In summary, dietary restriction decreases birth weight and can have as great an impact as a serious famine. The impact on perinatal morbidity and mortality has been poorly assessed, but there is reason to believe that preterm labor is increased and that children with intrauterine growth retardation have more problems later in life. Although the impact of the eating disorder on parenting after the delivery has not been well studied, there is evidence that the children of parents with eating disorders are not adequately nourished.[300–302] Mealtimes for these children are often filled with conflict, interfering with the important communication between parent and infant that usually takes place during feeding.[303] The critical factor affecting the parental-infant interaction is the mother's preoccupation with her own body and shape.

Because intrauterine growth retardation before the third trimester is associated with significant long-term morbidity, clinicians treating amenorrhea associated with weight loss should consider solving the dietary problem before subjecting a fetus to a struggle during intrauterine life. Patients with an active eating disorder should wait for remission before getting pregnant. These messages, therefore, especially apply to two groups of physicians: obstetricians and reproductive endocrinologists.

When encountering a patient who is pregnant and has an eating disorder, the obstetrician should seek expert consultation in order to achieve and maintain remission of the disorder during the pregnancy. Careful monitoring of maternal weight gain and fetal growth is essential. Consideration should be given to special dietary supplementation, especially when delayed fetal growth is demonstrated. Full exploitation of the pregnancy is warranted to provide motivation for effective resolution of this psychodynamic disorder.

The best results can be achieved with stabilization of the disorder prior to pregnancy. The reproductive endocrinologist should hesitate before embarking on a program of ovulation induction. The reward of pregnancy should be offered as an inducement to reach a normal prepregnancy weight. Patients with an eating disorder who are considering pregnancy must be made aware of the potential adverse impact on fetal growth and development. The persistence of amenorrhea is not a good sign. Persistent amenorrhea is associated with longer duration of the eating disorder and more affective disorders.[189]

The timing of psychiatric intervention is important. The prospect of pregnancy should stimulate a preconceptual effort by the patient's physicians. At no other time will the patient's physicians have such a strong ally, the motivating force behind the desire for pregnancy.

Inherited Genetic Defects

Specific inherited defects that cause hypogonadotropic hypogonadism have not been commonly recognized; however, with the increasing sophistication of molecular biology, this may change.[304] No mutations of the α-subunit have been reported. Deficient secretion of GnRH is a consequence of Kallmann's syndrome and the inherited disorder of adrenal hypoplasia. A case of hypogonadism due to an LH β-subunit mutation and women with primary amenorrhea and delayed puberty due to a mutation in the FSH β-subunit have been reported.[13, 14, 305] The mutated β-subunit genes produce alterations in the β-subunits that yield no immunoreactivity or bioactivity. Hence, hypogonadism will be associated with one high and one low gonadotropin level. Treatment with exogenous gonadotropins will achieve pregnancy in these rare patients; transmission is autosomal recessive. *When a high FSH and a normal or low LH are encountered, an elevated level of α-subunit and the presence of a pituitary mass indicate a gonadotroph adenoma.*

Amenorrhea and Anosmia, Kallmann's Syndrome

A rare condition in females is the syndrome of congenital hypogonadotropic hypogonadism due to deficient secretion of GnRH, associated with anosmia or hyposmia, known as Kallmann's syndrome. There is a chronology of eponyms assigning credit for original descriptions of this syndrome, but with all due respect to the physicians who first recognized this association, it is far easier to remember it in a descriptive way, as a syndrome of amenorrhea and anosmia.[306–309] In the female, this problem is characterized by primary amenorrhea, infantile sexual development, low gonadotropins, a normal female karyotype, and the inability to perceive odors; e.g., coffee grounds or perfume. Often the affected individuals are not aware of their olfactory defect. The gonads can respond to gonadotropins, therefore induction of ovulation with exogenous gonadotropins is successful. However, clomiphene is ineffective.

Kallmann's syndrome is associated with a specific anatomic defect. Magnetic resonance imaging (as well as postmortem examination) demonstrates hypoplastic or absent olfactory sulci in the rhinencephalon.[310] This defect is a consequence of the failure of both olfactory axonal and GnRH neuronal migration from the olfactory placode in the nose. The cells that produce GnRH originate in the olfactory area and migrate during embryogenesis along fibers of the cranial nerve I complex (the terminal nerve) that connect the nose and the forebrain.[311]

Three modes of transmission have been documented: X-linked, autosomal dominant, and autosomal recessive.[312] The 5–7-fold increased frequency in males indicates that X-linked transmission is the most common. X-linked Kallmann's syndrome can be associated with other disorders due to deletions or translocations of contiguous genes on the distal short arm of the X chromosome (such as X-linked short stature or ichthyosis and sulfatase deficiency).

The X-linked mutations (there is no consistent mutation) responsible for this syndrome involve a single gene (KAL) on the short arm of the X chromosome (at Xp22.3) that encodes a protein responsible for functions necessary for neuronal migration.[313–315] This protein has been named anosmin-1.[316] The syndrome of anosmia and amenorrhea associated with X-linked mutations results from the failure of this nerve complex to penetrate the forebrain, preventing the successful migration of GnRH neurons. Other neurologic abnormalities (mirror movements, hearing loss, cerebellar ataxia) can be present, suggesting more widespread neurologic defects. Renal and bone abnormalities, hearing deficit, color blindness, and cleft lip and palate (the most common associated abnormality) also occur in affected individuals, probably reflecting the fact that the gene is expressed in tissues other than the hypothalamus.[317] The syndrome occurs as an inherited or sporadic defect.

Molecular Explanations for Hypogonadotropic Amenorrhea

It is possible that patients with hypothalamic amenorrhea due to isolated deficiency of GnRH secretion (and no other abnormalities) have a defect similar to that of Kallmann's syndrome. With a lesser penetrance, only the GnRH migratory defect is expressed. In some individuals with amenorrhea and a normal sense of smell, family members can be identified with anosmia. Some patients with GnRH deficiency, but without anosmia, have an autosomal mode of transmission; however, a defect in the GnRH gene has not been commonly detected and X-linked mutations are uncommon.[195, 312]

A brother and sister have been described with hypogonadotropic hypogonadism due to mutations of the GnRH receptor gene.[318] The parents and one sister were heterozygotes and normal; thus, the mutations were transmitted as an autosomal recessive trait. Screening 46 men and women with hypogonadotropic hypogonadism revealed the existence of an autosomally inherited GnRH gene receptor mutation in one of the 14 families with an affected female.[319] This mutation produces an interference in signal transduction resulting in resistance to GnRH stimulation. Thus this infrequent mutation causes hypogonadotropic amenorrhea that is not readily treated with GnRH, but response to exogenous gonadotropins is unimpaired. ***Because most individuals with hypogonadotropic amenorrhea respond to GnRH, this genetic defect is not common, and worth pursuing only in patients who have family members with similar presentations.*** This approach is supported by the failure to detect GnRH receptor gene deletions or rearrangements in patients with idiopathic hypogonadotropic hypogonadism.[320]

Adrenal Hypoplasia

Adrenal hypoplasia is an X-linked inherited disorder that results in adrenal insufficiency, and in survivors, hypogonadotropic hypogonadism.[321] This condition is caused by mutations in the DAX-1 gene, a gene that encodes a protein that is similar in structure to receptors that have no identified ligands (orphan receptors). These rare patients have both deficient secretion of GnRH and impaired response to GnRH.

Postpill Amenorrhea

In the past, it was assumed that secondary amenorrhea reflected persistent suppressive effects of oral contraceptive medication or the use of the intramuscular depot form of medroxyprogesterone acetate (Depo-Provera). It is now recognized that the fertility rate is normal following discontinuance of either of these forms of contraception (Chapter 22), and attempts to identify a cause-effect relationship in case-control studies have failed. Therefore, amenorrhea following the use of steroids for contraception requires investigation as described in order to avoid missing a significant problem. This investigation should be pursued if a patient is amenorrheic 6 months after discontinuing oral contraception or 12 months after the last injection of Depo-Provera.

Hormone Therapy

The patient who is hypoestrogenic and who is not a candidate for induction of ovulation deserves hormone therapy. This includes patients appropriately evaluated and diagnosed as having gonadal failure, patients with hypothalamic amenorrhea, and postgonadectomy patients. The long-term impact of the hypoestrogenic state in terms of cardiovascular disease has long been recognized. To some degree, the beneficial impact of exercise on the lipoprotein profile is reversed by estrogen deficiency; however, athletes have high, exercise-induced levels of HDL-cholesterol, which should be cardioprotective.[322, 323]

We want to emphasize that the bone density in women is dependent on normal reproductive age levels of estrogen and progesterone. Even the most strenuous of exercise does not balance the consequences of hypoestrogenism on the bones, especially in adolescents.[324–327] The degree of bone loss is influenced by the specific athletic activity; e.g., gymnasts have a higher bone density than runners despite similar menstrual patterns and body fat.[328] In one study, ballet dancers were able to maintain bone density at weight-bearing sites, despite oligomenorrhea and reduced body weight, whereas another study found reduced bone mass in weight-bearing bones.[208, 329] It makes sense that different exercises have different osteogenic effects according to the mechanical forces generated. In addition, the effect of bone loss is greater in the spine because trabecular bone is more sensitive to the loss of estrogen. Whether specific individuals and activities are threatened with osteoporosis-related fractures later in life requires follow-up data that are not available at this point in time.

In the absence of estrogen, the normal response of bone to stress (to become stronger) is impaired.[330] The same arguments that apply to hormone treatment in older women (Chapters 17 and 18) can be convincingly used to encourage these younger women to replace the estrogen they are lacking. The amenorrheic exerciser should be made aware that the hypoestrogenic state is associated with a greater risk of stress fractures.[331–336] Indeed, the loss of bone in amenorrheic athletes, with some exceptions as noted above, occurs at all skeletal sites that are weight bearing and subject to stress fractures.[337] Ballet dancers with delayed menarche are more prone to scoliosis as well as stress fractures.[335] It is not certain, however, whether this greater risk of stress fractures is influenced solely by bone density changes in that some studies fail to correlate fractures with reductions in bone density.[338] It should be noted that bone loss in amenorrheic women shows the same pattern over time as seen in postmenopausal women.[339] The loss is most rapid in the first few years, emphasizing the need for early treatment. The bone density increase in response to estrogen-progestin treatment of women with exercise-induced amenorrhea is impressive and worth achieving.[340] Long-term estrogen treatment of women with Turner syndrome effectively maintains bone density.[341]

It is worth emphasizing the importance of bone mineralization early in life. The subsequent risk of fracture from osteoporosis will depend upon bone mass at the time of menopause and the rate of bone loss following menopause. There is only a relatively narrow window of opportunity for acquiring bone mass. Almost all of the bone mass in the hip and the vertebral bodies will be accumulated by late adolescence (age 18), and the years following menarche (11–14) are especially important.[342, 343] The importance of a normal diet and normal hormonal support during adolescence cannot be overrated.

In patients with eating disorders, bone density correlates with body weight.[344] The response to hormone therapy will be impaired as long as an abnormal weight is maintained.[260] The failure to respond to estrogen treatment with an increase in bone density may be due to the adverse bone effects of the hypercortisolism associated with stress disorders. Furthermore, because the pubertal gain in bone density is so significant, individuals who fail to experience this adolescent increase may continue to have a deficit in bone mass despite hormone treatment. Reduced menstrual function for any reason early in life (even beyond adolescence) may leave a residual deficit in bone density that cannot be totally retrieved with resumption of menses or with hormone treatment.[345, 346] Interventions that improve diet and reduce overtraining can restore hormonal function, and even improve athletic performance (presumably because of better energy balance).[347]

Several reports have indicated that patients with hyperprolactinemia are at risk for osteoporosis. At first this appeared not to be related to estrogen status, suggesting an independent effect of prolactin. Results have been confusing for several reasons. Controls in various studies were matched in different fashions; e.g., only for age, ignoring height and weight. Photon absorptiometry, the method of study in some reports, has a reduced sensitivity and significant variation when used to assess the axial skeleton. And finally, the estrogen status of the hyperprolactinemic patients was not always carefully quantified. It is now recognized that the bone density changes observed in hyperprolactinemic amenorrheic women are due to the hypoestrogenic state.[348–350]

The standard program for estrogen therapy should be used. A good schedule is the following: 0.625 mg conjugated estrogens or 1 mg estradiol daily with 5 mg medroxyprogesterone acetate for two weeks every month. If the progestational agent is responsible for side effects, patients do well upon changing to 0.7 mg norethindrone. In a few individuals, the estrogen dosage may have to be increased in order to achieve menstrual bleeding. Whether a flow-provoking dose of estrogen is necessary for optimal protection of the bones has not been addressed in a clinical study. In patients who have not undergone pubertal development, a lower dose regimen should be used initially, as outlined in Chapter 10. *Periodic measurements of bone density are worthwhile to assess adequacy of hormonal treatment and to provide evidence of lifestyle and dieting changes.*

Menstruation generally occurs 3 days after the last day of progestin medication. Bleeding that occurs at any time other than the usual expected time may be a sign that endogenous function has returned. The hormone treatment program should be discontinued and the patient monitored for the resumption of ovulation.

The importance of monthly menstruation to a young woman cannot be overemphasized. Regular and visible menstrual bleeding is often a gratifying experience in the young patient with gonadal dysgenesis and serves to reinforce her identification with the feminine gender role. On the other hand, serious exercisers (such as athletes and dancers) may want to avoid menstrual bleeding. One can provide hormone therapy to these women utilizing the daily combination approach: 0.625 mg conjugated estrogens and 2.5 mg medroxyprogesterone acetate or equivalent preparations given together every day without a break.

If for some reason, a hypoestrogenic woman refuses hormone treatment, supplemental calcium (1000–1500 mg daily) should be strongly encouraged. High calcium intake when combined with a high level of exercise is more effective in protecting the vertebral bone density than either exercise or calcium alone.[351] Even patients receiving hormone therapy should be cautioned to maintain a normal intake of calcium and vitamin D, and this usually requires supplementing the teenage diet.

Patients with hypothalamic amenorrhea must be cautioned that hormone therapy will not protect against pregnancy in the event that normal function unknowingly returns. In the patient who desires effective contraception, it is reasonable to utilize a low-dose oral contraceptive to provide the missing estrogen.[352] This is an excellent option in patients with premature ovarian failure because a spontaneous resumption of ovarian function can occur without warning. Athletes and others interested in avoiding menstruation can take oral contraceptives every day without a pill-free interval.

It is not enough to provide hormone therapy when disturbed menstrual function is secondary to psychobiologic stress responses. Appropriate support and counseling are necessary to help patients develop coping mechanisms other than extreme dieting and exercise. All available skills and resources should be utilized to promote healthy attitudes and healthy behaviors. The presence of amenorrhea in athletes and recreational exercisers should be regarded as a sign of negative energy balance, a condition requiring appropriate interventions.

References

1. **Baker TG,** A quantitative and cytological study of germ cells in human ovaries, *Proc Roy Soc Lond* 158:417, 1963.

2. **Gondos B, Bhiraleus P, Hobel C,** Ultrastructural observations on germ cells in human fetal ovaries, *Am J Obstet Gynecol* 110:644, 1971.

3. **Contreras P, Generini G, Michelson H, Pumarino H, Campino C,** Hyperprolactinemia and galactorrhea: spontaneous versus iatrogenic hypothyroidism, *J Clin Endocrinol Metab* 53:1036, 1981.

4. **Danziger J, Wallace S, Handel S, Samaan NG,** The sella turcica in primary end organ failure, *Radiology* 131:111, 1979.

5. **Sarlis NJ, Brucker-Davis F, Doppman JL, Skarulis MC,** MRI-demonstrable regression of a pituitary mass in a case of primary hypothyroidism after a week of actue thyroid hormone therapy, *J Clin Endocrinol Metab* 82:808, 1997.

6. **Poretsky L, Garber J, Kleefield J,** Primary amenorrhea and pseudoprolactinoma in a patient with primary hypothyroidism, *Am J Med* 81:180, 1986.

7. **Coulam CB, Annegers JF,** Breast cancer and chronic anovulation syndrome, *Surg Forum* 33:474, 1982.

8. **Lloyd RV, Chandler WF, Kovacs K, Ryan N,** Ectopic pituitary adenomas with normal anterior pituitary glands, *Am J Surg Path* 10:546, 1986.

9. **Stanisic TH, Donova J,** Prolactin secreting renal cell carcinoma, *J Urol* 136:85, 1986.

10. **Hoffman WH, Gala RR, Kovacs K, Subramanian MG,** Ectopic prolactin secretion from a gonadoblastoma, *Cancer* 60:2690, 1987.

11. **Kallenberg GA, Pesce CM, Norman B, Ratner RE, Silvergerg SG,** Ectopic hyperprolactinemia resulting from an ovariana teratoma, *JAMA* 263:2472, 1990.

12. **Palmer PE, Bogojavlensky S, Bhan AK, Scully RE,** Prolactinoma in wall of ovarian dermoid cyst with hyperprolactinemia, *Obstet Gynecol* 75:540, 1990.

13. **Weiss J, Axelrod L, Whitcomb RW, Harris PE, Crowley WF, Jameson JL,** Hypogonadism caused by a single amino acid substitution in the β-subunit of luteinizing hormone, *New Engl J Med* 326:179, 1992.

14. **Matthews CH, Borgato S, Beck-Peccoz P, Adams M, Tone Y, Gambino G, Casagrande S, Tedeschini G, Benedetti A, Chatterjee VKK,** Primary amenorrhoea and infertility due to a mutation in the β-subunit of follicle-stimulating hormone, *Nature Genetics* 5:83, 1993.

15. **Comtois R, Bouchard J, Robert F,** Hypersecretion of gonadotropins by a pituitary adenoma: pituitary dynamic studies and treatment with bromocriptine in one patient, *Fertil Steril* 52:569, 1989.

16. **Katznelson L, Alexander JM, Bikkal HA, Jameson JL, Hsu DW, Klibanski A,** Imbalanced follicle-stimulating hormone - subunit hormone biosynthesis in human pituitary adenomas, *J Clin Endocrinol Metab* 74:1343, 1992.

17. **Katznelson L, Alexander JM, Klibanski A,** Clinically nonfunctioning pituitary adenomas, *J Clin Endocrinol Metab* 76:1089, 1993.

18. **Daneshdoost L, Gennarelli TA, Bashey HM, Savino PJ, Sergott RC, Bosley TM, Snyder P,** Recognition of gonadotroph adenomas in women, *New Engl J Med* 324:589, 1991.

19. **Buckler HM, Evans A, Mamlora H, Burger HG, Anderson DC,** Gonadotropin, steroid and inhibin levels in women with incipient ovarian failure during anovulatory and ovulatory 'rebound' cycles, *J Clin Endocrinol Metab* 72:116, 1991.

20. **Rebar RW, Connolly HV,** Clinical features of young women with hypergonadotropic amenorrhea, *Fertil Steril* 53:804, 1990.

21. **Talbert LM, Raj MHG, Hammond MG, Greer T,** Endocrine and immunologic studies in a patient with resistant ovary syndrome, *Fertil Steril* 42:741, 1984.

22. **Aittomäki K, Dieguez Lucena JL, Pakarinen P, Sistonen P, Tapanainein J, Gromoll J, Kaskikari R, Sankila EM, Lehvaslaiho H, Engel AB, et al,** Mutation in the follicle-stimulating hormone receptor gene causes hereditary hypergonadotropic ovarian failure, *Cell* 82:959, 1995.

23. **Aittomäki K, Herva R, Stenman U-H, Juntunen K, Ylöstalo P, Hovatta O, de la Chapelle A,** Clinical features of primary ovarian failure caused by a point mutation in the follicle-stimulating hormone receptor gene, *J Clin Endocrinol Metab* 81:3722, 1996.

24. **Delon B, Lallaoui H, Abel-Lablanche C, Geneix A, Bellec V, Benkhalifa M,** Fluorescent in-situ hybridization and sequence-tagged sites for delineation of an X:Y translocation in a patient with secondary amenorrhea, *Mol Hum Reprod* 3:439, 1997.

25. **Sutton C,** The limitations of laparoscopic ovarian biopsy, *J Obstet Gynaecol Br Commonwlth* 81:317, 1974.

26. **Alper MM, Garner PR,** Premature ovarian failure: its relationship to autoimmune disease, *Obstet Gynecol* 66:27, 1985.

27. **Anasti JN, Flack MR, Froehlich J, Nelson LM,** The use of human recombinant gonadotropin receptors to search for immunoglobulin G-mediated premature ovarian failure, *J Clin Endocrinol Metab* 80:824, 1995.

28. **Consortium, Autoimmune Polyendocrinopathy-Candidiasis-Ectodermal Dystrophy,** An autoimmune disease, APECED, caused by mutations in a novel gene featuring two PHD-type zinc-finger domains, *Nat Genet* 17:399, 1997.

29. **Winqvist O, Gebre-Medhin G, Fustafsson J, Ritzén EM, Lundkvist Ö, Karlsson FA, Kämpe O,** Identification of the main gonadal autoantigens in patients with adrenal insufficiency and associated ovarian failure, *J Clin Endocrinol Metab* 80:1717, 1995.

30. **Hoek A, Schoemaker J, Drexhage HA,** Premature ovarian failure and ovarian autoimmunity, *Endocr Rev* 18:107, 1997.

31. **Cowchock FS, McCabe JL, Montgomery BB,** Pregnancy after corticosteroid administration in premature ovarian failure (polyglandular endocrinopathy syndrome), *Am J Obstet Gynecol* 158:118, 1988.

32. **Blumenfeld Z, Halachmi S, Peretz BA, Shmuel Z, Golan D, Makler A, Brandes JM,** Premature ovarian failure — the prognostic application of autoimmunity on conception after ovulation induction, *Fertil Steril* 59:750, 1993.

33. **Levy HL, Driscoll SG, Porensky RS, Wender DF,** Ovarian failure in galactosemia, *New Engl J Med* 310:50, 1984.

34. **Robinson ACR, Dockeray CJ, Cullen MJ, Sweeney EC,** Hypergonadotrophic hypogonadism in classical galactosaemia: evidence for defective oogenesis: case report, *Br J Obstet Gynaecol* 91:199, 1984.

35. **Manuel M, Katayama KP, Jones Jr HW,** The age of occurrence of gonadal tumors in intersex patients with a Y chromosome, *Am J Obstet Gynecol* 124:293, 1976.

36. **Troche V, Hernandez E,** Neoplasia arising in dysgenetic gonads, *Obstet Gynecol Survey* 41:74, 1986.

37. **Bione S, Sala C, Manzini C, Arrigo G, Zuffardi O, Banfi S, Borsani G, Jonveaux P, Philippe C, Zuccotti M, Ballabio A, Toniolo D,** A human homologue of the Drosophila melanogaster diaphenous gene is disrupted in a patient with premature ovarian failure: evidence for conserved function in oogenesis and implications for human sterility, *Am J Hum Genet* 62:533, 1998.

38. **Pasquino AM, Passeri F, Pucarelli I, Segni M, Municchi G,** Spontaneous pubertal development in Turner's syndrome. Italian Study Group for Turner's Syndrome, *J Clin Endocrinol Metab* 82:1810, 1997.

39. **Aiman J, Smentek C,** Premature ovarian failure, *Obstet Gynecol* 66:9, 1985.

40. **Nelson LM, Anasti JN, Kimzey LM, Defensor RA, Lipetz KJ, White BJ, Shawker TH, Merino MJ,** Development of luteinized graafian follicles in patients with karyotypically normal spontaneous premature ovarian failure, *J Clin Endocrinol Metab* 79:1470, 1994.

41. **Taylor AE, Adams JM, Mulder JE, Martin KA, Sluss PM, Crowley Jr WF,** A randomized, controlled trial of estradiol replacement therapy in women with hypergonadotropic amenorrhea, *J Clin Endocrinol Metab* 81:3615, 1996.

42. **Wheatcroft NJ, Salt C, Milford-Ward A, Cooke ID, Weetman AP,** Identification of ovarian antibodies by immunofluorescence, enzyme-linked immunosorbent assay or immunoblotting in premature ovarian failure, *Hum Reprod* 12:2617, 1997.

43. **Kim TJ, Anasti JN, Flack MR, Kimzey LM, Defensor RA, Nelson LM,** Routine endocrine screening for patients with karyotypically normal spontaneous premature ovarian failure, *Obstet Gynecol* 89:777, 1997.

44. **Nelson LM, Kimzey LM, Merriam GR,** Gonadotropin suppression for the treatment of karyotypically normal spontaneous premature ovarian failure: a controlled trial, *Fertil Steril* 57:50, 1992.

45. **Axelrod L, Neer RM, Kliman B,** Hypogonadism in a male with immunologically active, biologically inactive luteinizing hormone: an exception to a venerable rule, *J Clin Endocrinol Metab* 48:279, 1979.

46. **Teasdale E, Teasdale G, Mohsen F, MacPherson P,** High-resolution computed tomography in pituitary microadenoma: is seeing believing? *Clin Radiol* 37:227, 1986.

47. **Stein AL, Levenick MN, Kletzky OA,** Computed tomography versus magnetic resonance imaging for the evaluation of suspected pituitary adenomas, *Obstet Gynecol* 73:996, 1989.

48. **Schlechte J, Dolan K, Sherman B, Chapler F, Luciano A,** The natural history of untreated hyperprolactinemia: a prospective analysis, *J Clin Endocrinol Metab* 68:412, 1989.

49. **Reincke M, Allolio B, Saeger W, Menzel J, Winkelmann W,** The 'incidentaloma' of the pituitary gland, *JAMA* 263:2772, 1990.

50. **Donovan LE, Corenblum B,** The natural history of the pituitary incidentaloma, *Arch Intern Med* 155:181, 1995.

51. **Strebel PM, Zacur HA, Gold EB,** Headache, hyperprolactinemia, and prolactinomas, *Obstet Gynecol* 68:195, 1986.

52. **Yazigi RA, Quintero CH, Salameh WA,** Prolactin disorders, *Fertil Steril* 67:215, 1997.

53. **Costello RT,** Subclinical adenoma of the pituitary gland, *Am J Pathol* 12:191, 1936.

54. **Kraus HE,** Neoplastic diseases of the human hypophysis, *Arch Pathol* 39:343, 1945.

55. **McCormick WF, Halmi NS,** Absence of chromophobe adenomas from a large series of pituitary tumors, *Arch Pathol* 92:231, 1971.

56. **Sheline GE,** Untreated and recurrent chromophobe adenomas of the pituitary, *Radiology* 112:768, 1971.

57. **Burrow GN, Wortzman G, Rewcastle NB, Holgate RC, Kovacs K,** Microadenomas of the pituitary and abnormal sellar tomograms in an unselected autopsy series, *New Engl J Med* 304:156, 1981.

58. **Hall WA, Luciano MG, Doppman JL, Patronas NJ, Oldfield EH,** Pituitary magnetic resonance imaging in normal human volunteers: occult adenomas in the general population, *Ann Intern Med* 120:817, 1994.

59. **Molitch ME,** Evaluation and treatment of the patient with a pituitary incidentaloma, *J Clin Endocrinol Metab* 80:3, 1995.

60. **Reindollar RH, Novak M, Tho SPT, McDonough PG,** Adult-onset amenorrhea: a study of 262 patients, *Am J Obstet Gynecol* 155:531, 1986.

61. **Schenker JG, Margalioth EJ,** Intrauterine adhesions: an updated appraisal, *Fertil Steril* 37:593, 1982.

62. **Markham SM, Parmley TH, Murphy AA, Huggins GR, Rock JA,** Cervical agenesis combined with vaginal agenesis diagnosed by magnetic resonance imaging, *Fertil Steril* 48:143, 1987.

63. **Reinhold C, Hricak H, Forstner R, Ascher SM, Bret PM, Meyer WR, Semelka RC,** Primary amenorrhea: evaluation with MR imaging, *Radiology* 203:383, 1997.

64. **Griffin JE, Edwards C, Ladden JD, Harrod MJ, Wilson JD,** Congenital absence of the vagina, *Ann Intern Med* 85:224, 1976.

65. **Imbeaud S, Faure E, Lamarre I, Matéi MG, di Clemente N, Tizard R, Carre-Eusebe D, Belville C, Tragethon L, Tonkin C, et al,** Insensitivity to anti-mullerian hormone due to a mutation in the human anti-mullerian hormone receptor, *Nat Genet* 11:382, 1995.

66. **Cramer DW, Goldstein DP, Fraer C, Reichardt JKV,** Vaginal agenesis (Mayer-Rokitansky-Kuster-Hauser syndrome) associated with the N314D mutation of galactose-1-phosphate uridyl transferase (GALT), *Mol Hum Reprod* 2:145, 1996.

67. **Letterie GS, Wilson J, Miyazawa K,** Magnetic resonance imaging of müllerian tract abnormalities, *Fertil Steril* 50:365, 1988.

68. **Fedele L, Dorta M, Brioschi D, Giudici MN, Candiani GB,** Magnetic resonance imaging in Mayer-Rokitansky-Kuster-Hauser Syndrome, *Obstet Gynecol* 76:593, 1990.

69. **Frank RT,** Formation of artificial vagina without operation, *Am J Obstet Gynecol* 35:1053, 1938.

70. **Wabrek AJ, Millard PR, Wilson Jr WB, Pion RJ,** Creation of a neovagina by the Frank nonoperative method, *Obstet Gynecol* 37:408, 1971.

71. **Costa EMF, Mendonca BB, Inácio M, Arnhold IJP, Silva FAQ, Lodovici O,** Mangement of ambiguous genitalia in pseudohermaphrodites: new perspectives on vaginal dilation, *Fertil Steril* 67:229, 1997.

72. **Ingram J,** The bicycle seat stool in the treatment of vaginal agenesis and stenosis: a preliminary report, *Am J Obstet Gynecol* 140:867, 1981.

73. **Veronikis DK, McClure GB, Nichols DH,** The Vecchietti opertion for construction of a neovagina: indications, instrumentation, and techniques, *Obstet Gynecol* 90:301, 1997.

74. **Bates GW, Wiser WL,** A technique for uterine conservation in adolescents with vaginal agenesis and a functional uterus, *Obstet Gynecol* 66:290, 1985.

75. **Polasek PM, Erickson LD, Stanhope CR,** Transverse vaginal septum associated with tubal atresia, *Mayo Clin Proc* 70:965, 1995.

76. **Batzer FR, Corson SL, Gocial B, Daly DC, Go K, English ME,** Genetic offspring in patients with vaginal agenesis: specific medical and legal issues, *Am J Obstet Gynecol* 167:1288, 1992.

77. **Petrozza JC, Gray MR, Davis AJ, Reindollar RH,** Congenital absence of the uterus and vagina is not commonly transmitted as a dominant genetic trait: outcomes of surrogate pregnancies, *Fertil Steril* 67:387, 1997.

78. **Morris JM, Mahesh VB,** Further observations on the syndrome "testicular feminization," *Am J Obstet Gynecol* 87:731, 1963.

79. **Rutgers JL, Scully RE,** The androgen insensitivity syndrome (testicular feminization): a clinicopathologic study of 43 cases, *Int J Gynecol Path* 10:126, 1991.

80. **Simpson JL,** Genetics of sexual differentiation, In: Rock JA, Carpenter SE, eds. *Pediatic and Adolescent Gynecology,* Raven Press, New York, 1992, p 1.

81. **Griffin JE,** Androgen resistance — the clinical and molecular spectrum, *New Engl J Med* 326:611, 1992.

82. **Gililland J, Cummings D, Hibbert ML, Crain T, Rozanski T,** Laparoscopic orchiectomy in a patient with complete androgen insensitivity, *J Laparoendoscopic Surg* 3:51, 1993.

83. **Powell CM, Taggart RT, Drumheller TC, Wangsa D, Qian C, Nelson LM, White BJ,** Molecular and cytogenetic studies of an X:autosome translocation in a patient with premature ovarian failure and review of the literature, *Am J Med Genet* 52:19, 1994.

84. **Medlej R, Lobaccaro JM, Berta P, Belon C, Leheup B, Toublanc JE, Weill J, Chevalier C, Dumas R, Sultan C,** Screening for Y-derived sex determining gene SRY in 40 patients with Turner syndrome, *J Clin Endocrinol Metab* 75:1289, 1992.

85. **Uehara S, Obara Y, Obara T, Funato T, Yaegashi N, Fukaya T, Yajima A,** Trisomy 18 mosaicism associated with secondary amenorrhea: ratios of mosaicism in different samples and complications, *Clin Genet* 49:91, 1996.

86. **Coulam CB, Adamsen SC, Annegers JF,** Incidence of premature ovarian failure, *Obstet Gynecol* 67:604, 1986.

87. **Dewald GW, Spurbeck JL,** Sex chromosome anomalies associated with premature gonadal failure, *Seminars Reprod Endocrinol* 1:79, 1983.

88. **Devi AS, Metzger DA, Luciano AA, Benn PA,** 45, X/46,XX mosaicism in patients with idiopathic premature ovarian failure, *Fertil Steril* 70:89, 1998.

89. **Sung L, Bustillo M, Mukherjee T, Booth G, Karstaedt A, Copperman AB,** Sisters of women with premature ovarian failure may not be ideal ovum donors, *Fertil Steril* 67:912, 1997.

90. **Aittomäki K,** The genetics of XX gonadal dysgenesis, *Am J Hum Genet* 54:844, 1994.

91. **Layman LC, Amde S, Cohen DP, Jin M, Xie J,** The Finnish follicle-stimulating hormone receptor gene mutation is rare in North American women with 46,XX ovarian failure, *Fertil Steril* 69:300, 1998.

92. **Beatriz da Fonte Kohek M, Cidade Batista M, Russell AJ, Vass K, Ricardo Giacaglia L, Bilharinho Mendonca B, Caludia Latronico A,** No evidence of the inactivating mutation (C566T) in the follicle-stimulating hormone receptor gene in Brazilian women with premature ovarian failure, *Fertil Steril* 70:565, 1998.

93. **Toledo SPA, Brunner HG, Kraaij R, Post M, Dahia PLM, Hayashida CY, Kremer H, Themmen APN,** An inactivating mutation of the luteinizing hormone receptor causes amenorrhea in a 46,XX female, *J Clin Endocrinol Metab* 81:3850, 1996.

94. **Conway GS, Payne NP, Webb J, Murray A, Jacobs PA,** Fragile X premutation screening in women with premature ovarian failure, *Hum Reprod* 13:1184, 1998.

95. **Gradishar WJ, Schilsky RL,** Ovarian function following radiation and chemotherapy, *Seminars Oncol* 16:425, 1989.

96. **Wallace WH, Shalet S, MCrowne EC, Morris-Jones PH, Gattamanen HR,** Ovarian failure following abdominal irradiation in childhood: natural history and prognosis, *Clin Oncol* 1:75, 1989.

97. **Madsen BL, Giudice L, Donaldson SS,** Radiation-induced premature menopause: a misconception, *Int J Radiat Oncol Biol Phys* 32:1461, 1995.

98. **Morice P, Thiam-Ba R, Castaigne D, Haie-Meder C, Gerbaulet A, Pautier P, Duvillard P, Michel G,** Fertility results after ovarian transposition for pelvic malignancies treated by external irradiation or brachytherapy, *Hum Reprod* 13:660, 1998.

99. **Asch P,** The influence of radiation on fertility in man, *Br J Radiol* 53:271, 1980.

100. **Byrne J, Mulvihill JJ, Myers MH, Connelly RR, Naughton MD, Krauss MR, Steinhorn SC, Hassinger DD, Austin DF, Bragg K, et al,** Effects of treatment on fertility in long-term survivors of childhood cancer, *New Engl J Med* 317:1315, 1987.

101. **Bines J, Oleske DM, Cobleigh MA,** Ovarian function in premenopausal women treated with adjuvant chemotherapy for breast cancer, *J Clin Oncol* 14:1718, 1996.

102. **Clark ST, Radford JA, Crowther D, Swindell R, Shalet SM,** Gonadal function following chemotherapy for Hodgkin's disease: a comparative study of MVPP and a seven-drug hybrid regimen, *J Clin Oncol* 13:134, 1995.

103. **Ataya K, Pydyn E, Ramahi-Ataya A, Orton CG,** Is radiation-induced ovarian failure in rhesus monkeys preventable by luteinizing hormone-releasing hormone agonists? Preliminary observations, *J Clin Endocrinol Metab* 80:790, 1995.

104. **Ataya K, Rao LV, Lawrence E, Kimmel R,** Luteinizing hormone-releasing hormone agonist inhibits cyclophosphamide-induced ovarian follicular depletion in Rhesus monkeys, *Biol Reprod* 52:365, 1995.

105. **Schelthauer BW, Randall RV, Laws Jr ER, Kovacs KT, Horvath E, Whitaker MD,** Prolactin cell carcinoma of the pituitary, *Cancer* 55:598, 1985.

106. **Mountcastle RB, Roof BS, Mayflied RK, Mordes DB, Sagel J, Biggs PJ, Rawe SE,** Case report: pituitary adenocarcinoma in an acromegalic patient. Response to bromocriptine and pituitary testing: a review of the literature on 36 cases of pituitary carcinoma, *Am J Med Sci* 298:109, 1989.

107. **Walker JD, Grossman A, Anderson JV, Ur E, Trainer PJ, Benn J, Lowy C, Sonksen PH, Plowman PN, Lowe DG, Doniach I, Wass JAH, Besser GM,** Malignant prolactinoma with extracranial metastases: A report of three cases, *Clin Endocrinol* 38:411, 1993.

108. **Long MA, Colquhoun IR,** Case report: multiple intra-cranial metastases from a prolactin-secreting pituitary tumor, *Clin Radiol* 49:356, 1994.

109. **Saeger W, Bosse U, Pfingst E, Schierke G, Kulinna H, Atkins D, Gullotta F,** Prolactin producing hypophyseal carcinoma. Case report of an extremely rare metastatic tumor, *Pathologe* 16:354, 1995.

110. **Saeger W, Lübke D,** Pituitary carcinomas, *Endocr Pathol* 7:21, 1996.

111. **Hurel SJ, Harris PE, McNicol AM, Foster S, Kelly WF, Baylis PH,** Metastatic prolactinoma: effect of ostretotide, cabergoline, carboplatin and etoposide; immunocytochemical analysis of proto-oncogene expression, *J Clin Endocrinol Metab* 82:2962, 1997.

112. **Walker AB, English J, Arendt J, MacFarlane IA,** Hypogonadotrophic hypogonadism and primary amenorrhoea associated with increased melatonin secretion from a cystic pineal lesion, *Clin Endocrinol* 45:353, 1996.

113. **Mindermann T, Wilson CB,** Thyrotropin-producing pituitary adenomas, *J Neurosurg* 79:521, 1993.

114. **Losa M, Giovanelli M, Persani L, Mortini P, Faglia G, Beck-Peccoz P,** Criteria of cure and follow-up of central hyperthyroidism due to thyrotropin-secreting pituitary adenomas, *J Clin Endocrinol Metab* 81:3084, 1996.

115. **Colao A, Loche S, Cappa M, Di Sarno A, Luisa Landi M, Sarnacchiaro F, Facciolli G, Lombardi G,** Prolactinomas in children and adolescents. Clinical presentation and long-term follow-up, *J Clin Endocrinol Metab* 83:2777, 1998.

116. **Djerassi A, Coutifaris C, West VA, Asa SL, Kapoor SC, Pavlou SN, Snyder PJ,** Gonadotroph adenoma in a premenopausal woman secreting follicle-stimulating hormone and causing ovarian hyperstimulation, *J Clin Endocrinol Metab* 80:591, 1995.

117. **Ezzat S, Josse RG,** Autoimmune hypophysitis, *Trends Endocrinol Metab* 8:74, 1997.

118. **Freda PU, Wardlaw SL, Post KD,** Unusual causes of sellar/parasellar masses in a large transsphenoidal surgical series, *J Clin Endocrinol Metab* 81:3455, 1996.

119. **Bradley KM, Adams CBT, Potter CPS, Wheeler DW, Anslow PJ, Burke CW,** An audit of selected patients with non-functioning pituitary adenoma treated by transsphenoidal surgery without irradiation, *Clin Endocrinol* 41:655, 1994.

120. **Bevan JS, Webster J, Burke CW, Scanlon MF,** Dopamine agonists and pituitary tumor shrinkage, *Endocr Rev* 13:220, 1992.

121. **Lamberts SWJ, Van Der Lely A-J, De Herder WW, Hofland LJ,** Octreotide, *New Engl J Med* 334:246, 1996.

122. **Pituitary Adenoma Study Group,** Pituitary adenomas and oral contraceptives: a multicenter case-control study, *Fertil Steril* 39:753, 1983.

123. **Schlechte J, Sherman B, Halmi N, Van Gilder J, Chapler FK, Dolan K, Granner D, Duello T, Harris C,** Prolactin-secreting pituitary tumors, *Endocr Rev* 1:295, 1980.

124. **Jackson RD, Wortsman J, Malarkey WB,** Characterization of a large molecular weight prolactin in women with idiopathic hyperprolactinemia and normal menses, *J Clin Endocrinol Metab* 61:258, 1985.

125. **Jackson RD, Wortsman J, Malarkey WB,** Macroprolactinemia presenting like a pituitary tumor, *Am J Med* 78:346, 1985.

126. **Hattori N, Ishihara T, Ikekubo K, Moridera K, Hino M, Kurahachi H,** Autoantibody to human prolactin in patients with idiopathic hyperprolactinemia, *J Clin Endocrinol Metab* 75:1226, 1992.

127. **Kleinberg DL, Noel CL, Frantz AG,** Galactorrhea: a study of 235 cases including 48 with pituitary tumors, *New Engl J Med* 296:589, 1977.

128. **Speroff L, Levin RM, Haning Jr RV, Kase NG,** A practical approach for the evaluation of women with abnormal polytomography or elevated prolactin levels, *Am J Obstet Gynecol* 135:896, 1979.

129. **Monroe SE, Levine L, Chang RJ, Keye Jr WR, Yamamoto M, Jaffe RB,** Prolactin-secreting pituitary adenomas: V. Increased gonadotropin responsivity in hyperprolactinemic women with pituitary adenomas, *J Clin Endocrinol Metab* 52:1171, 1981.

130. **Sauder SE, Frager M, Case GD, Kelch RP, Marshall JC,** Abnormal patterns of pulsatile luteinizing hormone secretion in women with hyperprolactinemia and amenorrhea: responses to bromocriptine, *J Clin Endocrinol Metab* 59:941, 1984.

131. **Cook CB, Nippoldt TB, Kletter GB, Kelch RP, Marshall JC,** Naloxone increases the frequency of pulsatile luteinizing hormone secretion in women with hyperprolactinemia, *J Clin Endocrinol Metab* 73:1099, 1991.

132. **Matera C, Freda PU, Ferin M, Wardlaw SL,** Effect of chronic opioid antagonism on the hypothalamic-pituitary-ovarian axis in hyperprolactinemic women, *J Clin Endocrinol Metab* 80:540, 1995.

133. **Maor Y, Berezin M,** Hyperprolactinemia in postmenopausal women, *Fertil Steril* 67:693, 1997.

134. **Schlechte JA, Sherman BM, Chapler FK, Van Gilder J,** Long term follow-up of women with surgically treated prolactin-secreting pituitary tumors, *J Clin Endocrinol Metab* 62:1296, 1986.

135. **Parl FF, Cruz VE, Cobb CA, Bradley CA, Aleshire SL,** Late recurrence of surgically removed prolactinomas, *Cancer* 57:422, 1986.

136. **Thomson JA, Davies DL, McLaren EH, Teasdale GM,** Ten year follow up of microprolactinoma treated by transsphenoidal surgery, *Br Med J* 309:1409, 1994.

137. **Feigenbaum SL, Downey DE, Wilson CB, Jaffe RB,** Transsphenoidal pituitary resection for preoperative diagnosis of prolactin-secreting pituitary adenoma in women: long term follow-up, *J Clin Endocrinol Metab* 81:1711, 1996.

138. **Herman V, Fagin J, Gonsky R, Kovacs K, Melmed S,** Clonal origin of pituitary adenomas, *J Clin Endocrinol Metab* 71:1427, 1990.

139. **Laws ER, Fode NC, Redmond MJ,** Transsphenoidal surgery following unsuccessful prior therapy: an assessment of benefits and risks in 158 patients, *J Neurosurg* 63:823, 1985.

140. **Bowen J, Paulsen CA,** Stroke after pituitary irradiation, *Stroke* 23:908, 1992.

141. **Tsang RW, Laperriere NJ, Simpson WJ, Brierley J, Panazrella T, Smyth HS,** Glioma arising after radiation therapy for pituitary adenoma, *Cancer* 72:2227, 1993.

142. **Snyder PJ, Fowble BF, Schatz NJ, Savino PJ, Gennarelli TA,** Hypopituitarism following radiation theratpy of pituitary adenomas, *Am J Med* 81:457, 1986.

143. **Vance ML, Evans WS, Thorner MO,** Bromocriptine, *Ann Intern Med* 100:78, 1984.

144. **Friedman E, Adams EF, Höög A, Gejman PV, Carson E, Larsson C, De Marco L, Werner S, Fahlbusch R, Nordenskjöld M,** Normal structural dopamine type 2 receptor gene in prolactin-secreting and other pituitary tumors, *J Clin Endocrinol Metab* 78:568, 1994.

145. **Merola B, Colao A, Caruso E, Sarnacchiaro F, Briganti F, Lancranjan I, Lombardi G, Schettini G,** Oral and injectable long-lasting bromocriptine preparations in hyperprolactinemia: comparison of their prolactin lowering activity, tolerability, and safety, *Gynecol Endocrinol* 5:267, 1991.

146. **Beckers A, Petrossians P, Abs R, Flandroy P, Stadnik T, de Longueville M, Lancranjan I, Stevenaert A,** Treatment of macroprolactinomas with the long-acting and repeatable form of bromocriptine: a report on 29 cases, *J Clin Endocrinol Metab* 75:275, 1992.

147. **Brue T, Lancranjan I, Louvet J-P, Dewailly D, Roger P, Jaquet P,** A long-acting repeatable form of bromocriptine as long-term treatment of prolactin-secreting macroadenomas: a multicenter study, *Fertil Steril* 57:74, 1992.

148. **Katz E, Schran HF, Adashi EY,** Successful treatment of a prolactin-producing pituitary macroadenoma with intravaginal bromocriptine mesylate: a novel approach to intolerance of oral therapy, *Obstet Gynecol* 73:517, 1989.

149. **Ginsburg J, Hardiman P, Thomas M,** Vaginal bromocriptine — clinical and biochemical effects, *Gynecol Endocrinol* 6:119, 1992.

150. **Turkalj I, Braun P, Krupp P,** Surveillance of bromocriptine in pregnancy, *JAMA* 247:1589, 1982.

151. **Weil C,** The safety of bromocriptine in long-term use: a review of the literature, *Curr Med Res Opin* 10:25, 1986.

152. **Cuellar FG,** Bromocriptine mesylate (Parlodel) in the management of amenorrhea/galactorrhea associated with hyperprolactinemia, *Obstet Gynecol* 55:278, 1980.

153. **Sieck JO, Niles NL, Jinkins JR, Al-Mefty O, Elo-Akkad S, Woodhouse N,** Extrasellar prolactinomas: successful management of 24 patients using bromocriptine, *Horm Res* 23:167, 1986.

154. **Mori H, Mori S, Saitoh Y, Arita N, Aono T, Uozumi T, Mogami H, Matsumoto K,** Effects of bromocriptine on prolactin-secreting pituitary adenomas, *Cancer* 56:230, 1985.

155. **Lamberts SWJ, Quik RFP,** A comparison of the efficacy and safety of pergolide and bromocriptine in the treatment of hyperprolactinemia, *J Clin Endocrinol Metab* 72:635, 1991.

156. **Brue T, Pellegrini I, Gunz G, Morange I, Dewailly D, Brownell J, Enjalbert A, Jaquet P,** Effects of the dopamine agonist CV 205-502 in human prolactinomas resistant to bromocriptine, *J Clin Endocrinol Metab* 74:577, 1992.

157. **Lappohn RE, van de Wiel HBM, Brownell J,** The effect of two dopaminergic drugs on menstrual function and psychological state in hyperprolactinemia, *Fertil Steril* 58:321, 1992.

158. **Rains CP, Bryson HM, Fitton A,** Cabergoline. A review of its pharmacological properties and therapeutic potential in the treatment of hyperprolactinemia and inhibition of lactation, *Drugs* 49:255, 1995.

159. **Colao A, Di Sarno A, Sarnacchiaro F, Ferone D, Di Renzo G, Merola B, Annunziato L, Lombardi G,** Prolactinomas resistant to standard dopamine agonists respond to chronic cabergoline treatment, *J Clin Endocrinol Metab* 82:876, 1997.

160. **Ciccarelli E, Giusti M, Miola C, Potenzoni F, Sghedoni D, Camanni F, Giordano G,** Effectiveness and tolerability of long term treatment with cabergoline, a new long-lasting ergoline derivative in hyperprolactinemic patients, *J Clin Endocrinol Metab* 69:725, 1989.

161. **Webster J, Piscitelli G, Polli A, Ferrari CI, Ismail I, Scanlon MF, for the Cabergoline Comparative Study Group,** A comparison of cabergoline and bromocriptine in the treatment of hyperprolactinemic amenorrhea, *New Engl J Med* 331:904, 1994.

162. **Biller BMK, Molitch ME, Vance ML, Cannistraro KB, Davis KR, Simons JA, Schoenfelder JR, Klibanski A,** Treatment of prolactin-secreting macroadenomas with the once-weekly dopamine agonist cabergoline, *J Clin Endocrinol Metab* 81:2338, 1996.

163. **Colao A, Di Sarno A, Landi ML, Cirillo S, Sarnacchiaro F, Gacciolli G, Pivonello R, Cataldi M, Merola B, Annuziato L, Lombardi G,** Long-term and low-dose treatment with cabergoline induces macroprolactinoma shrinkage, *J Clin Endocrinol Metab* 82:3574, 1997.

164. **Robert E, Musatti L, Piscitelli G, Ferrari CI,** Pregnancy outcome after treatment with the ergot drivative, cabergoline, *Reprod Toxicol* 10:333, 1996.

165. **Motta T, deVincentiis S, Marchinin M, Colombo N, D'Alberton A,** Vaginal cabergoline in the treatment of hyperprolactinemic patients intolerant to oral dopaminergics, *Fertil Steril* 65:440, 1996.

166. **Liuzzi A, Dallabonzana D, Oppizzi G, Verde GG, Cozzi R, Chiodini P, Luccarelli G,** Low doses of dopamine agonists in the long-term treatment of macroprolactinomas, *New Engl J Med* 313:656, 1985.

167. **Tsagarakis S, Grossman A, Plowman PN, Jones AE, Touzel R, Rees LH, Wass JA, Besser GM,** Megavoltage pituitary irradiation in the management of prolactomas: long-term follow-up, *Clin Endocrinol* 34:399, 1991.

168. **Bevan JS, Adams CBT, Burke CW, Morton KE, Molyneux AJ, Moore RA, Esiri MM,** Factors in the outcome of transsphenoidal surgery for prolactinoma and non-functioning pituitary tumour, including pre-operative bromocriptine therapy, *Clin Endocrinol* 26:541, 1987.

169. **Johnston DG, Hall K, Kendall-Taylor P, Patrick D, Watson MJ, Cook DB,** Effect of dopamine agonist withdrawal after long-term therapy in prolactinomas. Studies with high-definition computerized tomography, *Lancet* 2:187, 1984.

170. **Martin TL, Kim M, Malarkey WB,** The natural history of idiopathic hyperprolactinemia, *J Clin Endocrinol Metab* 60:855, 1985.

171. **Sluijmer AV, Lappohn RE,** Clinical history and outcome of 59 patients with idiopathic hyperprolactinemia, *Fertil Steril* 58:72, 1992.

172. **Jeffcoate WJ, Pound N, Sturrock NDC, Lambourne J,** Long-term follow-up of patients with hyperprolactinaemia, *Clin Endocrinol* 45:299, 1996.

173. **Corenblum B, Donovan L,** The safety of physiological estrogen plus progestin replacement therapy and oral contraceptive therapy in women with pathological hyperprolactinemia, *Fertil Steril* 59:671, 1993.

174. **Testa G, Vegetti W, Motta T, Alagna F, Bianchedi D, Carlucci C, Bianchi M, Parazzini F, Crosignani PG,** Two-year treatment with oral contraceptives in hyperprolactinemic patients, *Contraception* 58:69, 1998.

175. **Sisam DA, Sheehan JP, Schumacher OP,** Lack of demonstrable tumor growth in progressive hyperprolactinemia, *Am J Med* 80:279, 1986.

176. **Molitch ME,** Pregnancy and the hyperprolactinemic woman, *New Engl J Med* 312:1362, 1985.

177. **Kupersmith MJ, Rosenberg C, Kleinberg D,** Visual loss in pregnant women with pituitary adenomas, *Ann Intern Med* 121:473, 1994.

178. **Freeman R, Wezenter B, Silverstein M, Kuo D, Weiss KL, Kantrowitz AB, Schubart UK,** Pregnancy-associated subacute hemorrhage into a prolactinoma resulting in diabetes insipidus, *Fertil Steril* 58:427, 1992.

179. **Ahmed M, Al-Dossary E, Woodhouse NJY,** Macroprolactinomas with suprasellar extension: effect of bromocriptine withdrawal during one or more pregnancies, *Fertil Steril* 58:492, 1992.

180. **De Wit W, Coelingh Bennink HJT, Gerards LJ,** Prophylactic bromocriptine treatment during pregnancy in women with macroprolactinomas: report of 13 pregnancies, *Br J Obstet Gynaecol* 91:1059, 1984.

181. **Ruiz-Velasco V, Tolis G,** Pregnancy in hyperprolactinemic women, *Fertil Steril* 41:793, 1984.

182. **Holmgren U, Bergstrand G, Hagenfeldt K, Werner S,** Women with prolactinoma-effect of pregnancy and lactation on serum prolactin and on tumour growth, *Acta Endocrinol* 111:452, 1986.

183. **Hodgson SF, Randall RV, Holman CB, MacCarty CS,** Empty sella syndrome, *Med Clin North Am* 56:897, 1972.

184. **Sheehan HL, Murdoch R,** Postpartum necrosis of the anterior pituitary: pathological and clinical aspects, *J Obstet Gynaecol Br Emp* 45:456, 1938.

185. **Veldhuis JH, Hammond JM,** Endocrine function after spontaneous infarction of the human pituitary: report, review, and reappraisal, *Endocr Rev* 1:100, 1980.

186. **Berga SL,** Behaviorally induced reproductive compromise in women and men, *Seminars Reprod Endocrinol* 15:47, 1997.

187. **Laughlin GA, Dominguez CE, Yen SSC,** Nutritional and endocrine-metabolic aberrations in women with functional hypothalamic amenorrhea, *J Clin Endocrinol Metab* 83:25, 1998.

188. **Hirvonen E,** Etiology, clinical features and prognosis in secondary amenorrhea, *Int J Fertil* 22:69, 1977.

189. **Copeland PM, Sacks NR, Herzog DB,** Longitudinal follow-up of amenorrhea in eating disorders, *Psychosom Med* 57:121, 1995.

190. **Olster DH, Ferin M,** Corticotropin-releasing hormone inhibits gonadotropin secretion in the ovariectomized Rhesus monkey, *J Clin Endocrinol Metab* 65:262, 1987.

191. **Berga SL, Mortola JF, Suh GB, Laughlin G, Pham P, Yen SSC,** Neuroendocrine aberrations in women with functional hypothalamic amenorrhea, *J Clin Endocrinol Metab* 68:301, 1989.

192. **Biller BMK, Federoff HJ, Koenig JI, Klibanski A,** Abnormal cortisol secretion and responses to corticotropin-releasing hormone in women with hypothalamic amenorrhea, *J Clin Endocrinol Metab* 70:311, 1990.

193. **Berga SL, Daniels TL, Giles DE,** Women with functional hypothalamic amenorrhea but not other forms of anovulation display amplified cortisol concentrations, *Fertil Steril* 67:1024, 1997.

194. **Berga SL, Loucks AB, Rossmanith WG, Kettel LM, Laughlin GA, Yen SSC,** Acceleration of luteinizing hormone pulse frequency in functional hypothalamic amenorrhea by dopaminergic blockade, *J Clin Endocrinol Metab* 72:151, 1991.

195. **Weiss J, Adams E, Whitcomb RW, Crowley Jr WF, Jameson JL,** Normal sequence of the gonadotropin-releasing hormone gene in patients with idiopathic hypogonadotropic hypogonadism, *Biol Reprod* 45:743, 1991.

196. **Layman LC, Wilson JT, Huey LO, Lanclos KD, Plouffe Jr L, McDonough PG,** Gonadotropin-releasing hormone, follicle-stimulating hormone beta, luteinizing hormone beta gene structure in idiopathic hypogonadotropic hypogonadism, *Fertil Steril* 57:42, 1992.

197. **Lacey JH,** Anorexia nervosa and a bearded female saint, *Br Med J* 285:1816, 1982.

198. **Garner DM,** Pathogenesis of anorexia nervosa, *Lancet* 341:1631, 1993.

199. **Sullivan PF,** Mortality in anorexia nervosa, *Am J Psychiatr* 152:1073, 1995.

200. **Halmi KA,** Eating disorder research in the past decade, *Ann N Y Acad Sci* 789:67, 1996.

201. **North C, Gowers S, Byram V,** Family functioning in adolescent anorexia nervosa, *Br J Psychiatr* 167:673, 1995.

202. **Schmidt U, Evans K, Tiller J, Treasure J,** Puberty, sexual milestones and abuse: how are they related in eating disorder patients? *Psychol Med* 25:413, 1995.

203. **Martin-Du Pan RC, Herrmann W, Chardon F,** Hypercarotinémie, aménorrhée, et régime végétarien, *J Gynécol Obstet Biol Reprod* 19:290, 1990.

204. **Herzog DB, Copeland PM,** Eating disorders, *New Engl J Med* 313:295, 1985.

205. **Schotte DE, Stunkard AJ,** Bulimia vs bulimic behaviors on a college campus, *JAMA* 258:1213, 1987.

206. **Kins MB,** Eating disorders in a general practice population. Prevalence, characteristics and follow-up at 12 to 18 months, *Psychiatr Med* (Suppl)14:1, 1989.

207. **Heatherton TF, Nichols P, Mahamedi F, Keel P,** Body weight, dieting, and eating disorder symptoms among college students, 1982 to 1992, *Am J Psychiatr* 152:1623, 1995.

208. **Warren MP, Vande Wiele RL,** Clinical and metabolic features of anorexia nervosa, *Am J Obstet Gynecol* 117:435, 1973.

209. **Warren MP, Jewelewicz R, Dyrenfurth I, Ans R, Khalaf S, Vande Wiele RL,** The significance of weight loss in the evaluation of pituitary response to LH-RH in women with secondary amenorrhea, *J Clin Endocrinol Metab* 40:601, 1975.

210. **McShane TM, May T, Miner JL, Keisler DH,** Central actions of neuropeptide-Y may provide a neuromodulatory link between nutrition and reproduction, *Biol Reprod* 46:1151, 1992.

211. **Beumont PJV, Russell JD, Touyz SW,** Treatment of anorexia nervosa, *Lancet* 341:1635, 1993.

212. **Crow SJ, Mitchell JE,** Rational therapy of eating disorders, *Drugs* 48:372, 1994.

213. **Selzer R, Caust J, Hibbert M, Bowes G, Patton G,** The association between secondary amenorrhea and common eating disordered weight control practices in an adolescent population, *J Adolesc Health* 19:56, 1996.

214. **Prior JC,** Luteal phase defects and anovulation: adaptive alterations occurring with conditioning exercise, *Seminars Reprod Endocrinol* 3:27, 1985.

215. **Cumming DC, Wheeler GD,** Exercise-associated changes in reproduction: a problem common to women and men, In: Frisch RE, ed. *Adipose Tissue and Reproduction,* Vol. 14, Prog Reprod Biol Med, 1990, p 125.

216. **Speroff L, Redwine DB,** Exercise and menstrual function, *Physician Sport Med* 8:42, 1980.

217. **Frisch RE,** Body fat, menarche, and reproductive ability, *Seminars Reprod Endocrinol* 3:45, 1985.

218. **Falsetti L, Pasinetti E, Mazzani MD, Gastaldi A,** Weight loss and menstrual cycle: clinical and endocrinological evaluation, *Gynecol Endocrinol* 6:49, 1992.

219. **Loucks AB, Horvath SM, Freedson PS,** Menstrual status and validation of body fat prediction in athletes, *Hum Biol* 56:383, 1984.

220. **Frisch RE, Snow RC, Johnson LA, Gerard B, Barbieri R, Rosen B,** Magnetic resonance imaging of overall and regional body fat, estrogen metabolism, and ovulation of athletes compared to controls, *J Clin Endocrinol Metab* 77:471, 1993.

221. **Bronson FH, Manning JM,** The energetic regulation of ovulation: a realistic role for body fat, *Biol Reprod* 44:945, 1991.

222. **Wade GN, Schneider JE, Li H-Y,** Control of fertility by metabolic cues, *Am J Physiol* 270(Endocrinol Metab 33):E1, 1996.

223. **Warren MP,** Effect of exercise and physical training on menarche, *Seminars Reprod Endocrinol* 3:17, 1985.

224. **Ronkainen H, Pakarinen A, Kirkinen P, Kauppila A,** Physical exercise-induced changes and season-associated differences in the pituitary-ovarian function of runners and joggers, *J Clin Endocrinol Metab* 60:416, 1985.

225. **Cumming DC, Rebar RW,** Hormonal changes with acute exercise and with training in women, *Seminars Reprod Endocrinol* 3:55, 1985.

226. **Chang FE, Richards SR, Kim MH, Malarkey WB,** Twenty-four hour prolactin profiles and prolactin responses to dopamine in long distance runners, *J Clin Endocrinol Metab* 59:631, 1984.

227. **Laughlin GA, Loucks AB, Yen SSC,** Marked augmentation of nocturnal melatonin secretion in amenorrheic athletes, but not in cycling athletes: unaltered by opioidergic or dopaminergic blockade, *J Clin Endocrinol Metab* 73:1321, 1991.

228. **Berga S, Mortola J, Yen SSC,** Amplification of nocturnal melatonin secretion in women with functional hypothalamic amenorrhea, *J Clin Endocrinol Metab* 66:242, 1988.

229. **Loucks AB, Laughlin GA, Mortola JF, Girton L, Nelson JC, Yen SSC,** Hypothalamic-pituitary-thyroidal function in eumenorrheic and amenorrheic athletes, *J Clin Endocrinol Metab* 75:514, 1992.

230. **Fishman J, Boyar RM, Hellman L,** Influence of body weight on estradiol metabolism in young women, *J Clin Endocrinol Metab* 41:989, 1975.

231. **Snow RC, Barbieri RL, Frisch RE,** Estrogen 2-hydroxylase oxidation and menstrual function among elite oarswomen, *J Clin Endocrinol Metab* 69:369, 1989.

232. **De Crée C, Van Kranenburg G, Geurten P, Fujimori Y, Keizer HA,** 4-Hydroxycatecholestrogen metabolism responses to exercise and training: possible implications for menstrual cycle irregularities and breast cancer, *Fertil Steril* 67:505, 1997.

233. **Frisch RE, Snow R, Gerard E, Johnson L, Kennedy D, Barbieri R, Rosen BR,** Magnetic resonance imaging of body fat of athletes compared with controls, and the oxidative metabolism of estradiol, *Metabolism* 41:191, 1992.

234. **Howlett TA, Tomlin S, Hgahfoong L, Rees LH, Bullen BA, Skrinar GS, McArthur JW,** Release of beta-endorphin and met-enkephalin during exercise in normal women: response to training, *Br Med J* 288:1950, 1984.

235. **Russell JB, Mitchell DE, Musey PI, Collins DC,** The role of beta-endorphins and catechol estrogens on the hypothalamic-pituitary axis in female athletes, *Fertil Steril* 42:690, 1984.

236. **Laatikainen T, Virtanen T, Apter D,** Plasma immunoreactive beta-endorphin in exercise-associated amenorrhea, *Am J Obstet Gynecol* 154:94, 1986.

237. **Harber VJ, Sutton JR, MacDougall JD, Woolever CA, Bhavnani BR,** Plasma concentrations of β-endorphin in trained eumenorrheic and amenorrheic women, *Fertil Steril* 67:648, 1997.

238. **Genazzani AD, Petraglia F, Gastaldi M, Volpogni C, Gamba O, Genazzani AR,** Naltrexone treatment restores menstrual cycles in patients with weight loss-related amenorrhea, *Fertil Steril* 64:951, 1995.

239. **Gindoff PR, Ferin M,** Endogenous peptides modulate the effect of corticotropin-releasing factor on gonadotropin release in the primate, *Endocrinology* 121:837, 1987.

240. **Barbarino A, de Marinis L, Tofani A, Della Casa S, D'Amico C, Mancini A, Corsello SM, Sciuto R, Barini A,** Corticotropin-releasing hormone inhibiton of gonadotropin release and the effect of opioid blockade, *J Clin Endocrinol Metab* 68:523, 1989.

241. **Chrousos GP, Gold PW,** The concepts of stress and stress system disorders: overview of physical and behavioral homeostasis, *JAMA* 267:1244, 1992.

242. **Dorn LD, Chrousos GP,** The neurobiology of stress: understanding regulation of affect during female biological transitions, *Seminars Reprod Endocrinol* 15:19, 1997.

243. **Ding JH, Sheckter C, Drinkwater B, Soules M, Bremmer W,** High serum cortisol levels in exercise-associated amenorrhea, *Ann Intern Med* 108:530, 1988.

244. **Laughlin GA, Yen SSC,** Nutritional and endocrine-metabolic aberrations in amenorrheic athletes, *J Clin Endocrinol Metab* 81:4301, 1996.

245. **Ahima RS, Prabakren D, Mantzoros C, Ou D, Lowell B, Maratzoros-Flier E, Flier J,** Role of leptin in the neuroendocrine response to fasting, *Nature* 382:250, 1996.

246. **Laughlin GA, Yen SSC,** Hypoleptinemia in women athletes: absence of a diurnal rhythm with amenorrhea, *J Clin Endocrinol Metab* 82:318, 1997.

247. **Tataranni PA, Monroe MB, Dueck CA, Traub SA, Nicolson M, Manore MM, Matt KS, Ravussin E,** Adiposity, plasma leptin concentration and reproductive function in active and sedentary females, *Int J Obes Relat Metab Disord* 21:818, 1997.

248. **Veldhuis JD, Evans WS, Demers LM, Thorner MO, Wakat D, Rogol AD,** Altered neuroendocrine regulation of gonadotropin secretion in women distance runners, *J Clin Endocrinol Metab* 61:557, 1985.

249. **Cumming DC, Vickovic MM, Wall SR, Fluker MR,** Defects in pulsatile LH release in normally menstruating runners, *J Clin Endocrinol Metab* 60:810, 1985.

250. **Loucks AB, Mortola JF, Girton L, Yen SSC,** Alterations in the hypothalamic-pituitary-ovarian and the hypothalamic-pituitary-adrenal axes in athletic women, *J Clin Endocrinol Metab* 68:402, 1989.

251. **Smith NJ,** Excessive weight loss and food aversion in athletes simulating anorexia nervosa, *Pediatrics* 66:139, 1980.

252. **Tofler IR, Stryer BK, Micheli LJ, Herman LR,** Physical and emotional problems of elite female gymnasts, *New Engl J Med* 335:281, 1996.

253. **Gadpaille WJ, Sanborne CF, Wagner WW,** Athletic amenorrhea, major affective disorders and eating disorders, *Am J Psychiatr* 144:939, 1987.

254. **Fries H,** Secondary amenorrhea, self-induced weight reduction and anorexia nervosa, *Acta Psychiatr Scand* Suppl 248, 1974.

255. **Shisslak CM, Crago M, Estes LS,** The spectrum of eating disturbances, *Int J Eating Disorders* 18:209, 1995.

256. **Bullen BA, Skriinar GS, Beitins IZ, von Mering G, Turnbull BA, McArthur JW,** Induction of menstrual disorders by strenuous exercise in untrained women, *New Engl J Med* 312:1349, 1985.

257. **Stager JM, Ritchie-Flanagan RB, Robertshaw D,** Reversibility of amenorrhea in athletes, *New Engl J Med* 310:51, 1984.

258. **Carmichael KA, Carmichael DH,** Bone metabolism and osteopenia in eating disorders, *Medicine* 74:254, 1995.

259. **Iketani T, Kiriike N, Nakanishi S, Nakasuji T,** Effects of weight gain and resumption of menses on reduced bone density in patients with anorexia nervosa, *Biol Psychiatr* 37:521, 1995.

260. **Klibanski A, Biller BMK, Schoenfeld DA, Herzog DB, Saxe VC,** The effects of estrogen administration on trabecular bone loss in young women with anorexia nervosa, *J Clin Endocrinol Metab* 80:898, 1995.

261. **Hytten FE, Chamberlain G,** eds, *Clinical Physiology in Obstetrics,* Blackwell Oxford, 1980.

262. **Antonov AN,** Children born during the siege of Leningrad in 1942, *J Pediatr* 30:250, 1947.

263. **Smith CA,** The effect of wartime starvation in Holland upon pregnancy and its product, *Am J Obstet Gynecol* 53:599, 1947.

264. **Dean RFA,** (Medical Research Councl Special Report Series, Her Majesty's Stationery Office), The size of the baby at birth and the yield of breast milk, 1951, Report No. 275, 1951.

265. **Campbell DM, MacGillivray I,** The effect of a low calorie diet or a thiazide diuretic on the incidence of pre-eclampsia and on birthweight, *Br J Obstet Gynaecol* 82:572, 1975.

266. **Rush D,** Effects of changes in protein and calorie intake during pregnancy on the growth of the human fetus, In: Calmers I, Enkin M, Keirse MJNC, eds. *Effective Care in Pregnancy and Childbirth,* Oxford University Press, Oxford, 1989, p 255.

267. **Taffel SM,** (Public Health Service, U.S. Government Printing Office), Maternal weight gain and the outcome of pregnancy: United States, 1980, National Center for Health Statistics, Series 21-No.44, DHHS (PHS), 1986.

268. **Peckham CH, Christianson RE,** The relationship between prepregnancy weight and certain obstetric factors, *Am J Obstet Gynecol* 111:1, 1971.

269. **Simpson JW, Lawless RW, Mitchell CA,** Responsiblity of the obstetrician to the fetus. II. Influence of prepregnancy weight gain on birthweight, *Obstet Gynecol* 45:481, 1975.

270. **Harrison GG, Udall JN, Morrow G,** Maternal obesity, weight gain in pregnancy, and infant birth weight, *Am J Obstet Gynecol* 136:411, 1980.

271. **Gormican A, Valentine J, Satter E,** Relationships of maternal weight gain, prepregnancy weight, and infant birth weight, *J Am Diet Assoc* 77:662, 1980.

272. **Arbuckle TE, Sherman GJ,** Comparison of the risk factors for pre-term delivery and intrauterine growth retardation, *Paediatr Perinat Epidemiol* 3:115, 1989.

273. **Johnson AA, Knight EM, Edwards CH, Oyemade UJ, Cole OJ, Westney OE, Westney LS, Laryea H, Jones S,** Dietary intakes, anthropometric measurements and pregnancy outcomes, *J Nutr* 124:936S, 1994.

274. **Winikoff B, Debrovner CH,** Anthropometric determinants of birth weight, *Obstet Gynecol* 58:678, 1981.

275. **Abrams BF, Laros RK,** Prepregnancy weight, weight gain, and birth weight, *Am J Obstet Gynecol* 154:503, 1986.

276. **Seidman DS, Ever-Hadani P, Gale R,** The effect of maternal weight gain in pregnancy on birth weight, *Obstet Gynecol* 74:240, 1989.

277. **Myers SA, Ferguson R,** A population study of the relationship between fetal death and altered fetal growth, *Obstet Gynecol* 74:325, 1989.

278. **Bruce L, Tchabo JG,** Nutrition intervention program in a prenatal clinic, *Obstet Gynecol* 74:310, 1989.

279. **Siega-Riz AM, Adair LS, Hobel CJ,** Maternal underweight status and inadequate rate of weight gain during the third trimester of pregnancy increases the risk of preterm delivery, *J Nutr* 126:146, 1996.

280. **Kay DWK, Leigh D,** The natural history, treatment and prognosis of anorexia based on a study of 38 patients, *J Ment Sci* 100:411, 1954.

281. **Beck JC, Brockner-Mortensen K,** Observation on the prognosis in anorexia nervosa, *Acta Med Scand* 149:409, 1954.

282. **Dally P, Sargant W,** Treatment and outcome of anorexia nervosa, *Br Med J* 2:793, 1966.

283. **Farquharson RF, Hyland H,** Anorexia nervosa: the course of 15 patients treated from 20 to 30 years previously, *J Can Med Assoc* 94:411, 1969.

284. **Theander S,** Anorexia nervosa: a psychiatric investigation of 94 female patients, *Acta Psychiatr Scand* 214(Suppl):1, 1970.

285. **Hart T, Kase N, Kimball CP,** Induction of ovulation and pregnancy in patients with anorexia nervosa, *Am J Obstet Gynecol* 108:880, 1970.

286. **Willi J, Hagemann R,** Langzeitverlaufe von anorexia nervosa, *Schweiz Med Wochenschr* 106:1459, 1976.

287. **Treasure JL, Russell GFM,** Intrauterine growth and neonatal weight gain in babies of women with anorexia nervosa, *Br Med J* 296:1036, 1988.

288. **Stewart DE, Rasking J, Garfinkel PE, MacDonald OL, Robinson GE,** Anorexia nervosa, bulimia, and pregnancy, *Am J Obstet Gynecol* 157:1194, 1987.

289. **Brinch M, Isager T, Telstrup K,** Anorexia nervosa and motherhood: reproduction pattern and mothering behaviour of 50 women, *Acta Psychiatr Scand* 77:611, 1988.

290. **Abraham S, Mira M, Llewellyn-Jones D,** Should ovulation be induced in women recovering from an eating disorder or who are compulsive exercisers? *Fertil Steril* 53:566, 1990.

291. **Mitchell JE, Seim HC, Glotter D, Soll EA, Pyle RL,** A retrospective study of pregnancy in bulimia nervosa, *Int J Eating Dis* 10:209, 1991.

292. **Hollifield J, Hobdy J,** The course of pregnancy complicated by bulimia, *Psychotherapy* 27:249, 1990.

293. **Lacey JH, Smith G,** Bulimia nervosa. The impact of pregnancy on mother and baby, *Br J Psychiatr* 150:777, 1987.

294. **Davies K, Wardle J,** Body image and dieting in pregnancy, *J Psychosom Res* 38:787, 1994.

295. **Hedegaard M, Henriksen TB, Sabroe S, Secher NJ,** The relationship between psychological distress during pregnancy and birth weight for gestational age, *Acta Obstet Gynecol Scand* 75:32, 1996.

296. **Knuth UA, Hull MGR, Jacobs HS,** Amenorrhoea and loss of weight, *Br J Obstet Gynaecol* 84:801, 1977.

297. **van der Spuy ZM, Steer PJ, McCusker M, Steele SJ, Jacobs HS,** Outcome of pregnancy in underweight women after spontaneous and induced ovulation, *Br Med J* 296:962, 1988.

298. **Hediger ML, Scholl TO, Belsky DH, Ances IG, Salmon RW,** Patterns of weight gain in adolescent pregnancy: effects on birth weight and preterm delivery, *Obstet Gynecol* 74:6, 1989.

299. **Lauckner A, Lauckner W,** Significance of initial weight and weight development for the course and outcome of pregnancy, *Zentralbl Gynakol* 110:1018, 1988.

300. **Stein A, Fairburn CG,** Children of mothers with bulimia nervosa, *Br Med J* 299:777, 1989.

301. **van Wezel-Meijler G, Wit JM,** The offspring of mothers with anorexia nervosa: a high risk group for undernutrition and stunting? *Eur J Paediat* 149:130, 1989.

302. **Woodside DB, Shekter-Wolfson LF,** Parenting by parents with anorexia nervosa and bulimia nervosa, *Int J Eating Dis* 9:303, 1990.

303. **Stein A, Woolley H, Cooper SD, Fairburn CG,** An observational study of mothers with eating disorders and their infants, *J Child Psychol Psychiatr* 35:733, 1994.

304. **Jameson JL,** Inherited disorders of the gonadotropin hormones, *Mol Cellular Endocrinol* 125:143, 1996.

305. **Layman LC, Lee E-J, Peak DB, Namnoum AB, Vu KV, van Lingen BL, Gray MR, McDonough PG, Reindollar RH, Jameson JL,** Delayed puberty and hypogonadism caused by mutations in the follicle-stimulating hormone β-subunit gene, *New Engl J Med* 337:607, 1997.

306. **Maestre de San Juan A,** Falta total de los nervious olfaatorios con anosmia en un individuo en quien existia una atrofia congenita de los testiculos y meiembro viril, *Siglo Medico* 131:211, 1856.

307. **Kallmann FJ, Schoenfeld WA, Barrera SE,** The genetic aspects of primary eunuchoidism, *Am J Ment Defic* 48:203, 1944.

308. **De Morsier G, Gauthier G,** La dysplasie olfacto genitale, *Pathol Biol* 11:1267, 1963.

309. **Tagatz G, Fialkow PJ, Smith D, Spadoni L,** Hypogonadotropic hypogonadism associated with anosmia in the female, *New Engl J Med* 282:1326, 1970.

310. **Knorr JR, Ragland RL, Brown RS, Gelber N,** Kallmann's syndrome: MR findings, *Am J Neuroradiol* 14:845, 1993.

311. **Quinton, R, Hasan W, Grant W, Thrasivoulou C, Quiney RE, Besser GM, Bouloux PG,** Gonadotropin-releasing hormone immunoreactivity in the nasal epithelia of adults with Kallmann's syndrome and isolated hypogonadotropic hypogonadism and in the early midtrimester human fetus, *J Clin Endocrinol Metab* 82:309, 1997.

312. **Waldstreicher J, Seminara SB, Jameson JL, Geyer A, Nachtigall LB, Boepple PA, Holmes LB, Crowley Jr WF,** The genetic and clinical heterogeneity of gonadotropin-releasing hormone deficiency in the human, *J Clin Endocrinol Metab* 81:4388, 1996.

313. **Bick D, Franco B, Sherin RJ, Heye B, Pike L, Crawford J, Maddalena A, Incerti B, Pragliola A, Meitinger T, Ballabio A,** Brief report: intragenic deletion of the KALIG-1 gene in Kallmann's syndrome, *New Engl J Med* 326:1752, 1992.

314. **Hardelin J-P, Levilliers J, Young J, Pholsena M, Legouis R, Kirk J, Bouloux P, Petit C, Schaison G,** Xp22.3 deletions in isolated familial Kallmann's syndrome, *J Clin Endocrinol Metab* 76:827, 1993.

315. **Maya-Nuñez G, Zenteno JC-A, A, Kofman-Alfaro S, Mendez JP,** A recurrent missense mutation in the KAL gene in patients with X-linked Kallmann's syndrome, *J Clin Endocrinol Metab* 83:1650, 1998.

316. **Soussi-Yanicostas N, Hardelin J-P, del Mar Arroyo-Jimenez M, Ardovin O, Legouis R, Levilliers J, Traincard F, Betton JM, Cabanie L, Petit C,** Initial characterizationof anosmin-1, a putative extracellular matrix protein synthesized by definite neuronal cell populations in the central nervous system, *J Cell Sci* 109:1749, 1996.

317. **Franco B, Guioli S, Pragliola A, Incerti B, Bardoni B, Tonlorenzi R, Carrozzo R, Maestrini E, Pieretti M, Taillon-Miller P, Brown CJ, Willard HF, Lawrence C, Persico MG, Camerino G, Ballabio A,** A gene detected in Kallmann syndrome shares homology with neural cell adhesion and axonal pathfinding molecules, *Nature* 353:529, 1991.

318. **de Roux N, Young J, Misrahi M, Genet R, Chanson P, Schaison G, Milgrom E,** A family with hypogonadotropic hypogonadism and mutations in the gonadotropin-releasing hormone receptor, *New Engl J Med* 337:1597, 1997.

319. **Layman LC, Cohen DP, Jin M, Xie J, Li Z, Reindollar RH, Bolbolan S, Bick DP, Sherins RR, Duck LW, Musgrove LC, Sellers JC, Neill JD,** Mutations in gonadotropin-releasing hormone receptor gene cause hypogonadotropic hypogonadism, *Nature Genet* 18:14, 1998.

320. **Layman LC, Peak DB, Xie J, Sohn SH, Reindollar RH, Gray MR,** Mutation analysis of the gonadotropin-releasing hormone receptor gene in idiopathic hypogonadotropic hypogonadism, *Fertil Steril* 68:1079, 1997.

321. **Habiby RL, Boepple P, Nachtigall L, Sluss PM, Crowly Jr WF, Jameson JL,** Adrenal hypoplasia congenita with hypogonadotropic hypogonadism: evidence that DAX-1 mutations lead to combined hypothalamic and pituitary defects in gonadotropin production, *J Clin Invest* 98:1055, 1996.

322. **Lamon-Fava S, Fisher EC, Nelson ME, Evans WJ, Millar JS, Ordovas JM, Schaefer EJ,** Effect of exercise and menstrual cycle status on plasma lipids, low density lipoprotein particle size, and apolipoproteins, *J Clin Endocrinol Metab* 68:17, 1989.

323. **Friday KE, Drinkwater BL, Bruemmer B, Chesnut III C, Chait A,** Elevated plasma low-density lipoprotein and high-density lipoprotein cholesterol levels in amenorrheic athletes: effects of endogenous hormone status and nutrient intake, *J Clin Endocrinol Metab* 77:1605, 1993.

324. **Drinkwater BL, Nilson K, Chesnut CH, Bremmer WJ, Shainholtz S, Southworth MB,** Bone mineral content of amenorrheic and eumenorrheic athletes, *New Engl J Med* 311:277, 1984.

325. **Drinkwater BL, Nilson K, Ott S, Chesnut III CH,** Bone mineral density after resumption of menses in amenorrheic athletes, *JAMA* 256:380, 1986.

326. **Myerson M, Gutin B, Warren MP, Wang J, Lichtman S, Pierson Jr RN,** Total bone density in amenorrheic runners, *Obstet Gynecol* 79:9730, 1992.

327. **Baer JT, Taper LJ, Gwazdauskas GF, Walberg JL, Novascone M-A, Ritchey SJ, Thye FW,** Diet, hormonal, and metabolic factors affecting bone mineral density in adolescent amenorrheic and eumenorrheic female runners, *J Sports Med Phys Fitness* 32:51, 1992.

328. **Robinson TL, Snow-Harter C, Taaffe DR, Gillis D, Shaw J, Marcus R,** Gymnasts exhibit higher bone mass than runners despite similar prevalence of amenorrhea and oligomenorrhea, *J Bone Min Res* 10:26, 1995.

329. **Young N, Formica C, Szmukler G, Seeman E,** Bone density at weight-bearing and nonweight-bearing sites in ballet dancers: the effects of exercise, hypogonadism, and body weight, *J Clin Endocrinol Metab* 78:449, 1994.

330. **Warren MP, Brooks-Gunn J, Fox RP, Lancelot C, Newman D, Hamilton WG,** Lack of bone accretion and amenorrhea: evidence for a relative osteopenia in weight-bearing bones, *J Clin Endocrinol Metab* 72:847, 1991.

331. **Lindberg JS, Fears WB, Hunt MM, Powell MR, Boll D, Wade CE,** Exercise-induced amenorrhea and bone density, *Ann Intern Med* 101:647, 1984.

332. **Marcus R, Cann C, Madvig P, Minkoff J, Goddard M, Bayer M, Martin M, Gaudiani L, Haskell W, Genant H,** Menstrual function and bone mass in elite women distance runners, *Ann Intern Med* 102:158, 1985.

333. **Lloyd T, Triantafyllou SJ, Baker ER, Houts PS, Whiteside JA, Kalenak A, Stumpf PG,** Women athletes with menstrual irregularity have increased musculoskeletal injuries, *Med Sci Sports Exerc* 18:374, 1986.

334. **Barrow GW, Subrata S,** Menstrual irregularity and stress fractures in collegiate female distance runners, *Am J Sports Med* 16:209, 1988.

335. **Warren MP, Brooks-Gunn J, Hamilton LH, Warren LF, Hamilton WG,** Scoliosis and fractures in young ballet dancers, *New Engl J Med* 314:1348, 1986.

336. **Myburgh KH, Hutchins J, Fataar AB, Hough SF, Noakes TD,** Low bone density is an etiologic factor for stress fractures in athletes, *Ann Intern Med* 113:754, 1990.

337. **Rencken ML, Chesnut III CH, Drinkwater BL,** Bone density at multiple skeletal sites in amenorrheic athletes, *JAMA* 276:238, 1996.

338. **Carbon R, Sambrook PN, Deakin V, Fricker P, Eisman JA, Kelly P, Maguire K, Yeates MG,** Bone density of elite female athletes with stress fractures, *Med J Aust* 153:373, 1990.

339. **Cann CE, Martin MC, Jaffe RB,** Duration of amenorrhea affects rate of bone loss in women runners: implications of therapy, *Med Sci Sports Exerc* 17:214, 1985.

340. **Cumming DC,** Exercise-associated amenorrhea, low bone density, and estrogen replacement therapy, *Arch Intern Med* 156:2193, 1996.

341. **Sylvén L, Hagenfeldt K, Ringertz H,** Bone mineral density in middle-aged women with Turner's syndrome, *Eur J Endocrinol* 132:47, 1995.

342. **Theitz G, Buch B, Rizzoli R, Slosman D, Clavien H, Sizonko PC, Bonjour JPH,** Longitudinal monitoring of bone mass accumulation in healthy adolescents: evidence for a marked reduction after 16 years of age at the levels of lumbar spine and femoral neck in female subjects, *J Clin Endocrinol Metab* 75:1060, 1992.

343. **Matkovic V, Jelic T, Wardlaw GM, Ilich J, Goel PK, Wright JK, Andon MB, Smith KT, Heaney RP,** Timing of peak bone mass in caucasian females and its implication for the prevention of osteoporosis: inference from a cross-sectional model, *J Clin Invest* 93:799, 1994.

344. **Bachrach LK, Katzman DK, Litt IF, Guido D, Marcus R,** Recovery from osteopenia in adolescent girls with anorexia nervosa, *J Clin Endocrinol Metab* 72:602, 1991.

345. **Drinkwater BL, Bruemmer B, Chesnut III CH,** Menstrual history as a determinant of current bone density in young athletes, *JAMA* 263:545, 1990.

346. **Jonnavithula S, Warren MP, Fox RP, Lazaro MI,** Bone density is compromised in amenorrheic women despite return of menses: a 2-year study, *Obstet Gynecol* 81:669, 1993.

347. **Dueck CA, Matt KS, Manore MM, Skinner JS,** Treatment of athletic amenorrhea with a diet and training intervention program, *Int J Sport Nutr* 6:24, 1996.

348. **Klibanski A, Biller BMK, Rosenthal DI, Schoenfeld DA, Saxe V,** Effects of prolactin and estrogen deficiency in amenorrheic bone loss, *J Clin Endocrinol Metab* 67:124, 1988.

349. **Schlechte J, Walkner L, Kathol M,** A longitudinal analysis of premenopausal bone loss in healthy women and women with hyperprolactinemia, *J Clin Endocrinol Metab* 75:698, 1992.

350. **Biller BMK, Baum HBA, Rosenthal DI, Saxe VC, Charpie MP, Klibanski A,** Progressive trabecular osteopenia in women with hyperprolactinemic amenorrhea, *J Clin Endocrinol Metab* 75:692, 1992.

351. **Kanders BS, Lindsay R,** The effect of physical activity and calcium intake on the bone density of young women age 24-35, *Med Sci Sports Exerc* 17:284, 1985.

352. **Hergenroeder AC, Smith EO, Shypailo R, Jones LA, Klish WJ, Ellis K,** Bone mineral changes in young women with hypothalamic amenorrhea treated with oral contraceptives, medroxyprogesterone, or placebo over 12 months, *Am J Obstet Gynecol* 176:1017, 1997.

12 Anovulation and The Polycystic Ovary

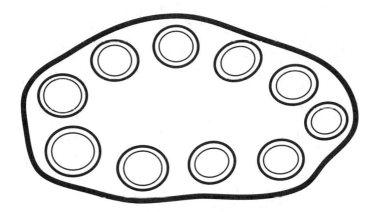

Anovulation is a very common problem that presents in a variety of clinical manifestations, including amenorrhea, irregular menses, and hirsutism. Serious consequences of chronic anovulation are infertility and a greater risk for developing carcinoma of the endometrium and perhaps the breast. There is a new appreciation for the role of hyperinsulinemia in this condition and for the clinical effect of hyperinsulinemia and hyperandrogenism on the risks of developing cardiovascular disease and diabetes mellitus. The clinician must recognize the clinical impact of anovulation and undertake therapeutic management of all anovulatory patients to avoid these unwanted consequences. We cannot overemphasize the importance of a new attitude toward this common female problem. Concern for anovulation and the polycystic ovary is a legitimate component of modern preventive health care.

Normal ovulation requires coordination of the menstrual system at all levels: the central hypothalamic-pituitary axis, the feedback signals, and local responses within the ovary. The loss of ovulation can be due to any one of an assortment of factors operating at each of these levels. The end result is a dysfunctional state: anovulation and the polycystic ovary. In this chapter, we will discuss the variety of mechanisms by which dysfunction of the ovulatory cycle can occur and how the clinical expressions of the resulting abnormal menstrual function are produced.

Pathogenesis of Anovulation

Just before and during menses, escape from the negative feedback of estrogen, progesterone, and inhibin results in increased follicle-stimulating hormone (FSH) secretion by the anterior pituitary. This initial increase in FSH is essential for follicular growth and steroidogenesis. With continued growth of the follicle, autocrine/paracrine factors produced within the follicle maintain follicular sensitivity to FSH, allowing conversion from a microenvironment dominated by androgens to one dominated by estrogen, a change necessary for a complete and successful follicular lifespan. Continuing and combined action of FSH and activin leads to the appearance of luteinizing hormone (LH) receptors on the granulosa cells, a prerequisite for ovulation and luteinization. Ovulation is triggered by the rapid rise in circulating levels of estradiol. A positive feedback response at the level of the anterior pituitary (and perhaps at the hypothalamus as well) results in the midcycle surge of LH necessary for expulsion of the egg and formation of the corpus luteum. A rise in progesterone follows ovulation along with a second rise in estradiol, producing the 14-day luteal phase characterized by low FSH and LH levels. The demise of the corpus luteum, concomitant with a fall in hormone levels, allows FSH to increase again, thus initiating a new cycle.

In the early follicular phase, activin produced by granulosa in immature follicles enhances the action of FSH on aromatase activity and FSH and LH receptor formation, while simultaneously suppressing thecal androgen synthesis. In the late follicular phase, increased production of inhibin by the granulosa (and decreased activin) promotes androgen synthesis in the theca in response to LH and insulin-like growth factor-II (IGF-II) to provide substrate for even greater estrogen production in the granulosa. Refinements in assay techniques have revealed that inhibin B is the form of inhibin predominantly secreted by granulosa cells in the follicular phase of the cycle.[1] In the mature granulosa, activin serves to prevent premature luteinization and progesterone production.

The successful follicle is the one that acquires the highest level of aromatase activity and LH receptors in response to FSH. The successful follicle is characterized by the highest estrogen (for central feedback action) and the greatest inhibin production (for both local and central actions. This accomplishment occurs in synchrony with the appropriate activin and growth factor expression. The activin proteins (which enhance FSH activity) are produced in greatest amounts early in follicular development to enhance follicle receptivity to FSH.

The right concentration of androgens in granulosa cells promotes aromatase activity and inhibin production, and, in turn, inhibin promotes LH stimulation of thecal androgen synthesis. LH stimulation of androgen production in thecal cells is further enhanced by the autocrine activity of insulin-like growth factor. Evidence indicates that the endogenous insulin-like growth factor in the human ovarian follicle is IGF-II in both the granulosa and the thecal cells.[2] Studies indicating activity of IGF-I with human ovarian tissue can be explained by the fact that both IGF-I and IGF-II activities can be mediated by the type I IGF receptor, which is structurally similar to the insulin receptor. With development of the follicle, inhibin expression comes under control of LH. A key to successful ovulation and luteal function is conversion of the inhibin production to LH responsiveness, to maintain FSH suppression centrally and enhancement of LH action locally.

This recycling mechanism is regulated by substances functioning as classic hormones (FSH, LH, estradiol, and inhibin) transmitting messages between the ovary and the hypothalamic-pituitary axis, and autocrine/paracrine factors (IGF-II, inhibin, and activin, among others), which coordinate sequential activities within the follicle destined to ovulate. The negative feedback relationship between corpus luteum products (estradiol, progesterone, and inhibin) and FSH results in the critical initial rise in FSH during menses, and the positive feedback relationship between estradiol and LH is the ovulatory stimulus. Within the ovary, IGF-II, inhibin, and activin modify follicular receptor responses necessary for growth and function. Dysfunction in the cycle can be due to an abnormality in one of the various roles for any one of these substances or an inability to respond to signals.

Central Defects

The hypothalamic-pituitary axis may be unable to respond, even if given adequate and appropriately timed feedback signals. A pituitary tumor represents an obvious example of a central defect in menstrual function and is discussed in Chapter 11, Amenorrhea.

Although difficult to demonstrate definitively, malfunction within the hypothalamus is both a likely, as well as a favorite, explanation for ovulatory failure. Normal pituitary ovulatory response to the follicle's steroid signals requires the presence of gonadotropin-releasing hormone (GnRH) pulsatile secretion within a critical range. The teenager between menarche and the onset of ovulation cannot generate a normal cycle until full GnRH pulsatile secretion is achieved. Increasing intensity of GnRH suppression is associated with increasing dysfunction and a changing clinical presentation. A variety of problems, such as stress and anxiety, borderline anorexia nervosa, and acute weight loss after a crash diet, is associated with an inhibition of normal GnRH pulsatile secretion. The mechanism for this suppression of GnRH is excessive hypothalamic activity of corticotropin-releasing hormone (CRH), a response to stress.[3] These patients present more commonly with amenorrhea, as discussed in Chapter 11. However if GnRH is only partially suppressed, homeostatic pituitary-ovarian function is maintained, and the patients will be anovulatory.[4–6]

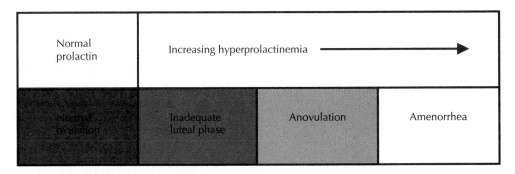

At least one specific clinical syndrome of central anovulatory dysfunction has been recognized: hyperprolactinemia. Increasing levels of prolactin can cause a woman to progress through a spectrum, beginning with an inadequate luteal phase to anovulation to the amenorrhea associated with complete GnRH suppression. *A search for galactorrhea and measurement of the prolactin level are important screening procedures for all women who are not ovulating normally.* The presence of galactorrhea or elevated prolactin levels dictates a choice of dopamine agonist treatment for the induction of ovulation. Indeed, even in women with normal prolactin levels, long-term treatment with a dopamine agonist can reduce androgen levels and restore menstrual function, either through a direct central dopaminergic effect or because of further suppression of normal prolactin levels.[7]

Anovulatory women with polycystic ovaries have a higher LH (and presumably GnRH) pulse frequency and amplitude when compared to the normal midfollicular phase.[8] Central opioid tone appears to be suppressed because there is no difference in response to naloxone.[9] The enhanced pulsatile secretion of GnRH can be attributed to a reduction in hypothalamic opioid inhibition because of the chronic absence of progesterone.[10] Interaction at the dopamine-endorphin sites may be altered because pretreatment with a dopamine precursor leads to a naloxone-induced increase in LH in anovulatory women compared with controls.

Abnormal Feedback Signals

Abnormal cycles can be due to failures within the system or due to the introduction of confounding factors. In order to achieve the appropriate changes within the cycle, estradiol levels must rise and fall in synchrony with morphologic events. Therefore, two possible signal failures may occur: 1) estradiol levels may not fall low enough to allow sufficient FSH response for the initial growth stimulus, and 2) levels of estradiol may be inadequate to produce the positive stimulatory effects necessary to induce the ovulatory surge of LH.

Loss of FSH Stimulation

In order to achieve recycling, a nadir in blood sex steroid levels must occur so that the initial event in the cycle, the rise in FSH, can take place. Sustained estrogen at such a key moment would not permit FSH stimulation of follicular growth and maturation, and recycling would be thwarted. The necessary decline in blood estrogen requires reduction of secretion, appropriate clearance and metabolism, and the absence of a significant contribution of estrogen to the circulation by extragonadal sources.

Persistent Estrogen Secretion. The most common clinical example of anovulation associated with continued secretion of sex steroids is pregnancy. Persistent and elevated secretion of estrogen can be encountered rarely with an ovarian or adrenal tumor. In such a case, anovulation or amenorrhea may bring the patient to a clinician's attention.

Abnormal Estrogen Clearance and Metabolism. The clearance and metabolism of estrogen can be impaired by other pathologic conditions, such as thyroid or hepatic disease. It is for this reason that a careful history and physical examination are important elements in the differential diagnosis of anovulation. Both hyperthyroidism and hypothyroidism can cause persistent anovulation by altering not only metabolic clearance but also the peripheral conversion rates among the various steroids. *The subtle presence of hypothyroidism, which may be associated with elevated prolactin levels, demands screening of anovulatory and amenorrheic women with a thyroid-stimulating hormone (TSH) level.*

Extraglandular Estrogen Production. Extragonadal contribution to the blood estrogen level can reach significant proportions. Although the adrenal gland does not secrete appreciable amounts of estrogen into the circulation, it indirectly contributes to the total estrogen level. This is accomplished by the extragonadal peripheral conversion of C-19 androgenic precursors, mainly androstenedione, to estrogen. In this manner, psychological or physical stress may increase the adrenal contribution of estrogenic precursor, and subsequent conversion to estrogen may sustain the blood level of estrogen at a time when a decline is necessary for successful recycling of the menstrual cycle. Adipose tissue is capable of converting androstenedione to estrogen; hence, the percent conversion increases with increasing body weight.[11] This is at least one mechanism for the well-known association between obesity and anovulation.

Loss of LH Stimulation

A failure in gonadal production of estrogen need not be absolute. Obviously, the patient with gonadal dysgenesis and ovarian failure will present with amenorrhea and infertility because of a total lack of estrogen secretion. More commonly, the clinician is concerned with the patient who has gonadotropin and estrogen production but does not ovulate. The failure to achieve a critical midcycle level of estradiol necessary to trigger the gonadotropin surge may be due to a relative deficiency in steroid production. The perimenopausal woman undergoes a terminal period of anovulation, which may represent steroidogenic refractoriness within the remaining elderly follicles. This inadequacy may be due to intrinsic follicular weaknesses or impairment in the follicular-gonadotropin interaction. In any case, the end result is the same—a failure to achieve critical signal levels of estradiol at the appropriate time in midcycle.

Local Ovarian Conditions

An understanding of the critical balances within the follicle indicates possible points of failure that may lead to anovulation. Local autocrine/paracrine factors prevent atresia despite declining FSH levels by enhancing the action of FSH in increasing the number of FSH receptors within the follicle, thus increasing follicular sensitivity to FSH. In addition, these factors enhance the induction of LH receptors by FSH, making it possible for the follicle to respond to the LH surge at midcycle. A follicle can fail to grow and ovulate because of inadequate expression or impaired function of any of the following local ovarian activities (described in detail in Chapter 6):

1. Selection of the dominant follicle is established during days 5–7, and consequently, peripheral levels of estradiol begin to rise significantly by cycle day 7.

2. Derived from the dominant follicle, estradiol levels increase steadily and, through negative feedback effects, exert a progressively greater suppressive influence on FSH release.

3. Insulin-like growth factor-II (IGF-II) is produced in theca cells in response to gonadotropin stimulation, and this response is enhanced by estradiol and growth hormone. In an autocrine action, IGF-II increases LH stimulation of androgen production in thecal cells.

4. IGF-II stimulates granulosa cell proliferation, aromatase activity, and progesterone synthesis.

5. FSH inhibits IGF binding protein synthesis and thus maximizes growth factor availability.

6. FSH stimulates inhibin and activin production by granulosa cells.

7. Activin augments FSH activities: FSH receptor expression, aromatization, inhibin/activin production, and LH receptor expression.

8. Inhibin enhances LH stimulation of androgen synthesis in the theca to provide substrate for aromatization to estrogen in the granulosa.

9. While directing a decline in FSH levels, the midfollicular rise in estradiol exerts a positive feedback influence on LH secretion. LH levels rise steadily during the late follicular phase, stimulating androgen production in the theca.

10. The positive action of estrogen also includes modification of the gonadotropin molecule, increasing the quality (the bioactivity) as well as the quantity of LH at midcycle.

11. Inhibin and, less importantly, follistatin, secreted by the granulosa cells in response to FSH, directly suppress pituitary FSH secretion.

12. FSH induces the appearance of LH receptors on granulosa cells.

The factors that control follicular growth and development are now understood in terms of the two-cell explanation described in Chapter 2 and Chapter 6. A very precise coordination is necessary between morphologic development and hormone stimulation. Perturbations may arise from an infectious process, from the presence of endometriosis, or by abnormal qualitative or quantitative changes in tropic hormone receptors (ovarian insensitivity), or the necessary biologic effects may be blocked by an improper molecular constitution of the gonadotropins (heterogeneity of the glycopeptide hormones).

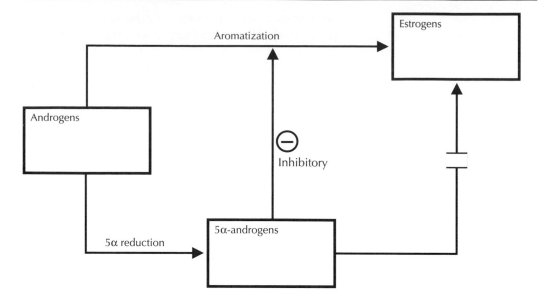

A Critical Role for the Concentration of Androgens in the Ovarian Follicle

Serving as substrate for FSH-induced aromatization, the androgens in low concentrations enhance aromatase activity and estrogen production. At higher concentrations, the granulosa cells favor the conversion of androgens to more potent 5α-reduced androgens, that cannot be converted to estrogen and, in addition, are capable of inhibiting aromatase activity and FSH induction of LH receptors (Chapter 6). Thus, raising the local androgen concentration above a critical level inhibits the emergence of a dominant follicle and leads to follicular atresia. Although this action in the normal cycle may be important in ensuring that only one follicle reaches the point of ovulation, an excessive concentration of androgens (no matter what the source) can prevent normal cycling and cause chronic anovulation.

Excess Body Weight

The frequency of obesity in women with anovulation and polycystic ovaries has been reported to be from 35% to 60%.[12–15] Obesity is associated with three alterations that interfere with normal ovulation, and weight loss improves all three:

1. Increased peripheral aromatization of androgens to estrogens.

2. Decreased levels of sex hormone-binding globulin (SHBG), resulting in increased levels of free estradiol and testosterone.

3. Increased insulin levels that can stimulate ovarian stromal tissue production of androgens.

Precise Etiology

The normal ovulatory function of the menstrual system relies on a dynamic coordination of complex actions. Abnormal function may represent discordance at all of the levels reviewed in the above paragraphs. Thus, a minor deficiency in the estradiol signal will be associated with a subnormal central response and an impaired or inappropriate degree of follicular growth and function. Dysfunction is sustained by the internal feedback mechanisms within the system, and anovulation can become a persistent problem.

It is usually impossible to reduce the issue of etiology to a single factor of abnormal menstrual function, except in severe states such as pituitary tumors, anorexia nervosa, gonadal dysgenesis, and perhaps hyperprolactinemia and obesity. Not only is it often impossible, but it is usually unnecessary to define the precise etiology. Regardless of the nature of the initial cause of the problem, the final clinical statement of the dysfunction is predictable, and easily diagnosed and managed. In patients who have abnormal or absent menstrual function, but are otherwise medically normal, the diagnosis will fall into one of three categories:

1. Ovarian Failure. Hypergonadotropic hypogonadism, the inability of the ovary to respond to any gonadotropic stimulation, usually due to the absence of follicular tissue on a genetic basis (discussed in Chapter 11).

2. Central Failure. Hypogonadotropic hypogonadism, hypothalamic or pituitary suppression as expressed in abnormal low or normal serum gonadotropins (discussed in Chapter 11).

3. Anovulatory Dysfunction. The patient who has asynchronous gonadotropin and estrogen production and does not ovulate presents with a variety of clinical manifestations. The associated clinical signs and symptoms depend on the level of gonadal function preserved and are represented by the following principal problems:

> Amenorrhea (Chapter 11).
> Hirsutism (Chapter 13).
> Dysfunctional uterine bleeding (Chapter 15).
> Endometrial hyperplasia and cancer (Chapter 18).
> Breast disease (Chapter 16).
> Infertility and induction of ovulation (Chapter 30).
> The polycystic ovary (this chapter).

The Polycystic Ovary

In 1935, Irving F. Stein and Michael L. Leventhal first described a symptom complex associated with anovulation.[16] Both gynecologists were born in Chicago, both were graduates of Rush Medical College, and both spent their entire professional careers at Michael Reese Hospital.[17] Stein and Leventhal described 7 patients (4 of whom were obese) with amenorrhea, hirsutism, and enlarged, polycystic ovaries. They reported the results of bilateral wedge resection, removing one-half to three-fourths of each ovary; all 7 patients resumed regular menses, and 2 became pregnant. Stein and Leventhal developed the wedge resection after they observed that several of their amenorrheic patients menstruated after ovarian biopsies. They reasoned that the thickened tunic was preventing follicles from reaching the surface of the ovary.

Acceptance of this syndrome as a singular clinical entity led to a rather rigid approach to this problem for many years. Only those women qualified who had a history of oligomenorrhea, hirsutism, and obesity, together with a demonstration of enlarged, polycystic ovaries, a clinical state now recognized to be characteristic of extreme cases. It is far more useful clinically to avoid the use of eponyms and even the term polycystic ovary syndrome or disease. It is better to consider this problem as one of persistent anovulation with a spectrum of etiologies and clinical manifestations, that now includes insulin resistance and hyperinsulinemia, as well as hyperandrogenism. Of course, specific conditions must be pursued and excluded, such as adrenal hyperplasia, Cushing's syndrome, hyperprolactinemia, and androgen-producing tumors.

A question that has puzzled gynecologists and endocrinologists for many years is what causes polycystic ovaries. There is an answer that is appealing in its logic and clinical applicability. ***The characteristic polycystic ovary emerges when a state of anovulation persists for any length of time.*** Whether diagnosis is by ultrasonography or by the traditional clinical and biochemical criteria, a cross section of anovulatory women at any one point of time will reveal that

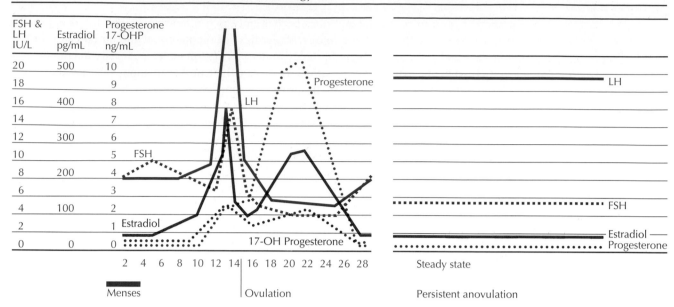

approximately 75% will have polycystic ovaries.[15, 18] Because there are many causes of anovulation, there are many causes of polycystic ovaries. A similar clinical picture and ovarian condition can reflect any of the dysfunctional states discussed above. In other words, the polycystic ovary is the result of a functional derangement, not a specific central or local defect.

Insistence on a specific endocrine or clinical criterion for the diagnosis of the polycystic ovary syndrome results in the inclusion of a collection of patients that represents a focused segment isolated from the broad clinical spectrum in which these patients really belong. This especially applies to the use of ultrasonography to make the diagnosis of the polycystic ovary syndrome (the presence of an increased number of ovarian follicles, often in a necklace-like pattern, and an increase in ovarian volume, largely due to an increase in stroma). From 8% to 25% of normal women will demonstrate ultrasonographic findings typical of polycystic ovaries![19–22] Even 14% of women on oral contraceptives have been found to have this ultrasonographic picture.[20] Ultrasonography as a diagnostic tool for this condition is unnecessary, and we vigorously discourage its use for this purpose. Magnetic resonance studies further confirm the unreliability of the imaging finding presumed to be diagnostic of this condition.[23]

It is argued that normally ovulating women with polycystic ovaries on ultrasonography have underlying metabolic abnormalities.[14, 19] However, the great majority of ovulatory women with polycystic ovaries on ultrasonography are endocrinologically normal, and only occasionally is an androgen level minimally elevated.[24] We are not convinced that such subtle changes are of clinical importance. Even if this argument were correct and a basic disorder is present, but homeostatic adjustments allow the maintenance of normal physiologic mechanisms and there are no clinical consequences, it is hard to justify medical interventions.

In contrast to the characteristic picture of fluctuating hormone levels in the normal cycle, a "steady state" of gonadotropins and sex steroids can be depicted in association with persistent anovulation. This steady state is only relative, and is being exaggerated in the diagram to present a concept of this clinical problem. In patients with persistent anovulation, the average daily production of estrogen and androgens is both increased and dependent on LH stimulation.[25, 26] This is reflected in higher circulating levels of testosterone, androstenedione, dehydroepiandrosterone (DHA), dehydroepiandrosterone sulfate (DHAS), 17-hydroxyprogesterone (17-OHP), and estrone.[27] The testosterone, androstenedione, and DHA are secreted directly by the ovary, whereas the DHAS, elevated in about 50% of anovulatory women with polycystic ovaries, is almost exclusively an adrenal contribution.[28, 29]

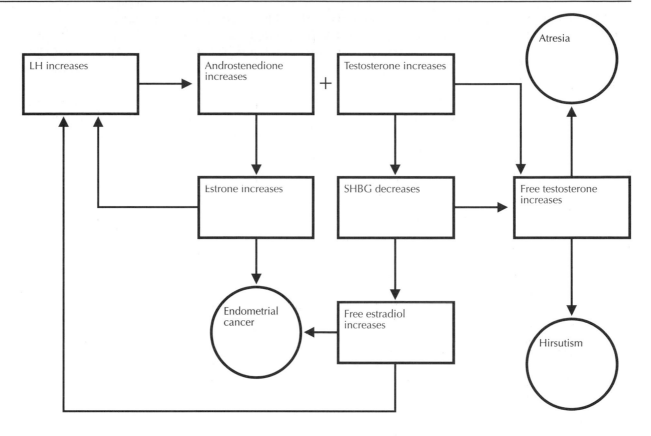

Treatment of women with polycystic ovaries with a GnRH agonist (to produce a hypo-gonadotropic hypogonadal state) is associated with the following helpful observations:[25, 30, 31]

1. The increases in androstenedione and testosterone are almost exclusively from the ovary.

2. The increase in 17-OHP is also from the ovary.

3. Secretion of DHA, DHAS, and cortisol are not influenced by short-term GnRH agonist treatment; however, long-term treatment is associated with a decrease in DHAS in some but not all women with polycystic ovaries.[30, 31] It is suggested that increased adrenal androgen production in some women is secondary to P450c17 17,20 lyase hyperactivity, and in others it is an acquired response due to the anovulatory hormonal steady state.[31, 32]

The ovary does not secrete increased amounts of estrogen, and estradiol levels are equivalent to early follicular phase concentrations.[33] Circulating estrone levels are slightly elevated. The increased total estrogen is due to peripheral conversion of the increased amounts of androstene-dione to estrone. That is not to say that there is no ovarian secretion of estrogen. Both estrone and estradiol continue to be secreted in significant, although low, amounts.[34]

When compared with levels found in normal women, patients with persistent anovulation have higher mean concentrations of LH, but low or low-normal levels of FSH.[35, 36] The elevated LH levels are partly due to an increased sensitivity of the pituitary to releasing hormone stimulation, manifested by an increase in LH pulse amplitude and frequency, but mainly amplitude.[33, 37, 38] This is consistent with the concepts discussed in Chapter 5, linking a high estrogen environment with anterior pituitary secretion of LH and suppression of FSH. It is noteworthy that this high level of LH is characterized by an increased level of LH bioactivity.[26, 37]

The gonadotropin pattern (high LH and low FSH) can also be due to increased frequency of GnRH pulsatile secretion.[38, 39] Central opioid tone appears to be suppressed because there is no difference in response to naloxone.[9] Indeed, the enhanced pulsatile secretion of GnRH can be attributed to a reduction in hypothalamic opioid inhibition because of the chronic absence of progesterone.[10, 40] This is associated with an increase in amplitude and frequency of LH secretion that is correlated with the level of circulating estrogen.[41] It is likely that this increased activity is taking place at both hypothalamic and pituitary sites. This altered state is also associated with a change in the circadian pattern with the highest LH values occurring in late afternoon rather than at night.[33]

The increase in LH pulse frequency and pituitary response to GnRH are characteristic of the anovulatory state, and are independent of obesity.[42] Obesity attenuates the LH response to GnRH, and LH pulse amplitude is relatively normal in overweight women with polycystic ovaries, although the increase in pulse frequency is maintained.[43, 44] The overall LH reduction may be a direct effect of the greater hyperandrogenism in obese women.[45, 46]

The increased pituitary and hypothalamic sensitivity can be attributed to the increased estrone levels,[47] but an important contributing factor is the impact of the decreased SHBG concentration. The levels of sex hormone-binding globulin (SHBG) are controlled by a balance of hormonal influences on its synthesis in the liver; testosterone is inhibitory, estrogen and thyroxine are stimulatory. In anovulatory women with polycystic ovaries, there is an approximately 50% reduction in circulating levels of SHBG, a response to the increased testosterone, and in patients with hyperinsulinemia, due to a direct insulin effect on the liver (discussed later in this chapter). Despite no increase in estradiol secretion, free estradiol levels are increased because of the significant decrease in SHBG. The clinical consequences of uninterrupted estrogen stimulation (endometrial and perhaps breast cancer) as well as the increased LH are the result of the two estrogenic influences, estrone and free estradiol.

The increased LH secretion as expressed by the LH:FSH ratio is positively correlated with the increased free estradiol.[39, 48] The lower FSH levels represent the sensitivity of the FSH negative feedback system to the elevated estrogen, both free estradiol and the estrone formed from peripheral conversion of androstenedione. In addition, the altered pattern of GnRH secretion can contribute to this characteristic LH:FSH ratio.[39] There is no evidence to support a role for inhibin suppression of FSH.[49, 50] In fact, consistent with impaired granulosa cell function, inhibin production in granulosa cells from polycystic ovaries is reduced.[51, 52] However, it is possible that these early findings with inhibin reflect the lack of precision associated with the first immunoassays. A sensitive assay for inhibin B has detected high levels in women with polycystic ovaries, suggesting that multiple small follicles can suppress FSH levels by increasing the circulating levels of inhibin B.[53]

Because the FSH levels are not totally depressed, new follicular growth is continuously stimulated, but not to the point of full maturation and ovulation.[54] Despite the fact that full growth potential is not realized, follicular lifespan may extend several months in the form of multiple follicular cysts, 2–10 mm in diameter (some can be as large as 15 mm). These follicles are surrounded by hyperplastic theca cells, often luteinized in response to the high LH levels. The accumulation of follicular tissue in various stages of development allows an increased and relatively constant production of steroids in response to the gonadotropin stimulation. This condition is self-sustaining. As various follicles undergo atresia, they are immediately replaced by new follicles of similar limited growth potential.

The tissue derived from follicular atresia is also sustained by the steady state and now contributes to the stromal compartment of the ovary. In terms of the two-cell explanation of follicular steroidogenesis, atresia is associated with a degenerating granulosa, leaving the theca cells to contribute to the stromal compartment of the ovary. It is not surprising, therefore, that this functioning stromal tissue secretes significant amounts of androstenedione and testosterone, the usual products of theca cells. In response to the elevated LH levels, the androgen production rate is increased. In turn, in a vicious cycle, the elevated androgen levels compound the problem through the process of extraglandular conversion as well as the suppression of SHBG synthesis, resulting in elevated estrogen levels. In addition, the decrease in SHBG is associated with a two-fold increase in free testosterone.

The elevated androgens contribute to the morphologic effect within the ovary preventing normal follicular development and inducing premature atresia. Indeed, in another aspect of the vicious cycle, the local androgen block is a major obstacle that maintains the steady state of persistent anovulation. When ovarian androgen concentrations are high, they can be converted to 5α-reduced metabolites that inhibit aromatase activity and estrogen production.[55] A sustained reduction in androgen levels following surgical wedge resection of the ovaries precedes the return of ovulatory cycles, indicating that the intraovarian androgen effect is a principal factor in preventing normal cycling.[56–59] The success of wedge resection is directly proportional to the volume of androgen-producing tissue removed. Tissue removal and destruction are the key factors, not the shape and procedure of the "wedge." Indeed, even a unilateral oophorectomy is followed by resumption of ovulation in anovulatory women with polycystic ovaries.[60]

This is further supported by the results of treatment with flutamide, an antiandrogen at the receptor level. In 8 young anovulatory, hirsute women with polycystic ovaries, treatment with flutamide restored ovulation in every subject.[61] In addition, testosterone can have a direct inhibitory action on the hypothalamic-pituitary axis.[62]

In this manner, the classic picture of the polycystic ovary is attained, displaying numerous follicles in the early stages of development and atresia and dense stromal tissue. The loss of recycling has resulted in a hormonal steady state causing persistent anovulation that can be associated with an increase in the production of androgens and the bioavailability of estrogen.

The polycystic ovary is the result of a "vicious cycle," which can be initiated at any one of many entry points. Altered function at any point in the cycle leads to the same result: the polycystic ovary. Recent studies, in an effort to be accurate, have usually included only patients fulfilling strict criteria. Thus, only certain subgroups of a large heterogeneous clinical population have been characterized. ***Don't lose sight of the fact that the polycystic ovary is a sign, not a disease.***

The polycystic ovary is usually enlarged and is characterized by a smooth pearly white capsule. For years, it was erroneously believed that the thick sclerotic capsule acted as a mechanical barrier to ovulation. A more accurate concept is that the polycystic ovary is a consequence of the loss of ovulation and the achievement of the steady state of persistent anovulation. The characteristics of the ovary reflect this dysfunctional state:[63]

1. The surface area is doubled, giving an average volume increase of 2.8 times.

2. The same number of primordial follicles is present, but the number of growing and atretic follicles is doubled. Each ovary may contain 20–100 cystic follicles.

3. The thickness of the tunica (outermost layer) is increased by 50%.

4. A one-third increase in cortical stromal thickness and a 5-fold increase in subcortical stroma are noted. The increased stroma is due both to hyperplasia of thecal cells and to increased formation subsequent to the excessive follicular maturation and atresia.

5. There are 4 times more ovarian hilus cell nests (hyperplasia).

Hyperthecosis refers to patches of luteinized theca-like cells scattered throughout the ovarian stroma. It is characterized by the same histologic findings as seen in polycystic ovaries.[64] The clinical picture of more intense androgenization is a result of greater androgen production. This condition is associated with lower LH levels, which is a possible consequence of the higher testosterone levels blocking estrogen action at the hypothalamic-pituitary level.[45, 46] It seems appropriate to view hyperthecosis as a manifestation of the same process, persistent anovulation, but with greater intensity. A greater degree of insulin resistance is correlated with the degree of hyperthecosis.[46] And in turn, because insulin and IGF-I stimulate proliferation of thecal interstitial cells, hyperinsulinemia may be an important incitement toward hyperthecosis.[65]

The typical histologic changes of the polycystic ovary can be encountered with any size ovary. There is a spectrum of time involved in the development of this condition, and it is useful to view the attainment of large ovaries as a stage of maximal effect of persistent anovulation. Increased size of the ovaries is not a critical feature, nor is it necessary for diagnosis. The key to understanding this clinical problem is an appreciation for the disruption in ovulatory recycling function.

There is no specific pathophysiologic defect. The hypothalamic-pituitary response is entirely appropriate, a response to chronically elevated estrogen feedback. The changes are a functional derangement brought about by accumulated and increased androgen due to a failure of ovulation, whatever the reason. Hence, the polycystic ovary may be associated with extragonadal sources of androgens,[66, 67] or with ovarian androgen-producing tumors,[68, 69] and even with the administration of exogenous androgens to female-to-male transsexuals.[70]

The functional problem can be understood in terms of the two-cell explanation of steroidogenesis (Chapter 6). The follicles are unable to successfully change their microenvironment from androgen dominance to estrogen dominance, the change that is essential for continued follicular growth and development.[71] Measurement of the insulin-like growth factor binding proteins (IGFBPs) in follicular fluid reveals that the profile in polycystic ovaries is the same as that found in atretic follicles, higher levels of IGFBP-2 and -4.[72, 73] This is consistent with limitation of IGF-I and IGF-II activity, reducing the expression of aromatase action and allowing androgenic dominance in the microenvironment. However, there is a striking difference comparing polycystic granulosa cells with granulosa cells from atretic follicles. Granulosa cells from polycystic ovaries are very sensitive to FSH; granulosa cells from atretic follicles are not.[74] Thus, the granulosa cells from the follicles in polycystic ovaries are not apoptotic (atretic), but simply arrested in development, and capable of responding to FSH stimulation.[75, 76]

The functional picture that emerges (arrested granulosa cells and very active theca cells) corresponds to the morphologic histology of underdeveloped granulosa and hyperplastic and luteinized theca. Granulosa cells obtained from the small follicles of polycystic ovaries produce negligible amounts of estradiol but show a dramatic increase in estrogen production when FSH or IGF-I is added and a synergistic action when FSH and IGF-I are added together.[77, 78] In terms of the two-cell explanation, this behavior is consistent with a blockage of FSH response (probably through various growth factors), not an intrinsic steroid synthesis enzyme defect. Successful treatment depends, therefore, on altering the ratio of FSH to androgens; either increasing FSH (with clomiphene) or decreasing androgens (wedge resection) to overcome the androgen block at the granulosa level. This permits development of aromatization to bring about conversion of the microenvironment to estrogen dominance. Because anovulation with polycystic ovaries is a functional derangement, it is not surprising that these patients occasionally may ovulate spontaneously. Indeed, ovulation is unpredictable, and contraception may be necessary.

Genetic Considerations

The familial clustering of anovulation and polycystic ovaries suggests an underlying genetic basis.[79–81] At least one group of patients with this condition has been described inheriting the disorder, possibly by means of an X-linked dominant transmission. There was a two-fold higher incidence of hirsutism and oligomenorrhea with paternal transmission but with marked variability of phenotypic expression.[82] On the other hand, studies of large families suggested inheritance in an autosomal dominant fashion, with premature balding as the phenotype in males.[83, 250] The strong link between hyperinsulinemia and hyperandrogenism also suggests that the stimulatory effect of insulin on ovarian androgen production is influenced by a genetic predisposition or susceptibility. Family members of women with anovulation, hyperandrogenism, and polycystic ovaries have an increased incidence of hyperinsulinemia in females and premature baldness in males.[84] Initial searches for genes that are associated with a susceptibility to anovulation and polycystic ovaries have implicated a locus on the insulin gene and the gene encoding P450scc (*CYP11a*), but not the gene encoding P450c17α (CYP17).[85, 86] ***These studies imply an autosomal dominant mode of inheritance, directing clinicians to counsel families that theoretically 50% of mothers and sisters within a family can manifest this disorder.*** The actual expression is less (perhaps 40%) due to modification by both genetic and environmental factors.

P450c17 Dysregulation

A popular hypothesis in the 1990s explained this ovarian hyperandrogenic state as a consequence of an enzymatic dysregulation, specifically of P450c17, the enzyme responsible for both 17α-hydroxylase and 17,20-lyase activities.[87] Abnormal hyperactivity of this enzyme would account for the altered steroidogenesis in both the ovaries and the adrenal glands. Indeed, the adrenal gland is involved in this clinical problem. Higher circulating levels of DHAS, almost exclusively an adrenal product, testify to adrenal participation. The mechanism and the clinical importance of this involvement will be further discussed in Chapter 13, Hirsutism. It is difficult, if not impossible, to know whether abnormal enzyme activity comes first or is a reflection of the anovulatory dysfunctional state. Indeed, in 92 consecutive women with hirsutism, the steroidogenic response to ACTH stimulation was not consistent with an inherent disorder in P450c17.[88] Testing both ovarian and adrenal responses to stimulation fails to delineate a clear-cut or characteristic disorder of P450c17.[89] Genetic screening of anovulatory women with polycystic ovaries has not detected sequence variations in the promoter or coding regions of the P450c17 gene.[90] In our view, a more straight forward and clinically manageable concept is to consider enzyme changes as secondary to the dysfunctional state.

Insulin Resistance, Hyperinsulinemia, and Hyperandrogenism

The first recognition of an association between glucose intolerance and hyperandrogenism was the famous report of the bearded diabetic woman by Archard and Thiers in 1921.[91] The association between increased insulin resistance and polycystic ovaries is now well recognized. This clinical association of hyperinsulinemia and anovulatory hyperandrogenism is commonly found throughout the world and among different ethnic groups.[92–94] In addition, hyperandrogenism and insulin resistance are often associated with acanthosis nigricans.[95] Acanthosis nigricans is a gray–brown velvety, sometimes verrucous, discoloration of the skin, usually at the neck, groin, axillae, and under the breasts, which is a marker for insulin resistance. Hyperkeratosis and papillomatosis are the histological characteristics of acanthosis nigricans. The presence of acanthosis nigricans in hyperandrogenic women is dependent on the presence and severity of hyperinsulinemia.[96] It is most highly correlated with the magnitude of peripheral insulin resistance and less well with the hyperinsulinemia measured by a glucose tolerance test. The mechanism responsible for the development of acanthosis nigricans is uncertain. Conflicting studies suggest mediation through various growth factor receptors, not just insulin or insulin-like growth factor. Because acanthosis nigricans can be present in normal women, its presence is not an absolute marker for hyperandrogenism and hyperinsulinemia.

Insulin resistance is defined as a reduced glucose response to a given amount of insulin. Resistance to insulin-stimulated glucose uptake is a relatively common phenomenon, sometimes referred to as syndrome X.[97] The majority of patients with noninsulin-dependent diabetes mellitus have peripheral insulin resistance, but not all women who are insulin resistant are hyperandrogenic. The state of chronic hyperinsulinemia represents a compensatory response to the target tissue problem. These relationships involve changes in plasma free fatty acid concentrations. If the insulin levels necessary to suppress free fatty acid levels cannot be achieved, then the increase in free fatty acids leads to increased hepatic glucose production and hyperglycemia.

There are several mechanisms for the state of insulin resistance: peripheral target tissue resistance, decreased hepatic clearance, or increased pancreatic sensitivity.[98] The ***euglycemic clamp technique*** establishes a steady state of hyperinsulinemia with a normal glucose level at which point the glucose infusion rate equals glucose utilization. Adding insulin will measure the glucose uptake rate (the more insulin required, the greater the peripheral resistance, also referred to as a measure of ***insulin sensitivity***). Studies with this technique indicate that hyperandrogenic women with hyperinsulinemia have peripheral insulin resistance and, in addition, a reduction in the insulin clearance rate due to decreased hepatic insulin extraction.[98, 99]

The clinical presentation of patients with insulin resistance (whether they have impaired glucose tolerance or diabetes mellitus) depends on the ability of the pancreas to compensate for the target tissue resistance to insulin. At first, compensation is effective, and the only metabolic abnormality is hyperinsulinemia. In many patients, the beta cells of the pancreas eventually fail to meet the challenge, and declining insulin levels lead to impaired glucose tolerance and type II noninsulin-dependent diabetes mellitus. Indeed, beta cell dysfunction can be detected in women with polycystic ovaries even before the appearance of glucose intolerance.[100]

Hyperinsulinemia leads to hypertension and an increased risk of coronary heart disease; a direct relationship exists between plasma insulin levels and blood pressure.[101] Resistance to insulin is further associated with increased triglycerides and decreased HDL-cholesterol levels, a potent bad combination that promotes coronary heart disease.[102] Although the adverse lipid effect is present in anovulatory women with polycystic ovaries, hypertension is not encountered in these women until later in life, not in their reproductive years.[103–105]

Hyperinsulinemia and polycystic ovaries are also associated with an increased production of plasminogen activator inhibitor type 1 (PAI-1).[105, 106] Increased PAI-1 levels are correlated with an increased risk of coronary heart disease; impaired fibrinolysis may affect vascular tissue changes associated with vascular disease.

There are rare causes of hyperinsulinemia and hyperandrogenism that are congenital in origin. Peripheral insulin resistance associated with hyperandrogenism and acanthosis nigricans, known as "type A syndrome," can be due to mutations of the insulin receptor gene (which leads to decreased numbers of insulin receptors in target tissues).[107] Leprechaunism is a rare syndrome in young girls with a mutation in the insulin receptor gene and perhaps defects in growth factor receptors; it is associated with severe insulin resistance, polycystic ovaries, hyperandrogenism, and acanthosis nigricans.[108] Another subgroup, "type B syndrome," consists of patients with autoantibodies to insulin receptors. This leaves a large collection of women with neither reduced nor abnormal insulin receptors nor autoantibodies, the most common clinical entity encountered, anovulatory women with hyperandrogenism and hyperinsulinemia. Possible mechanisms for the hyperinsulinemia include functional problems in the insulin receptor (which could also be a consequence of insulin receptor gene mutations) and inhibitors, which can interfere with insulin-receptor function after binding.[109] Thus, there are at least 3 categories for peripheral target tissue insulin resistance: decreased insulin receptor numbers, decreased insulin binding, and post receptor failures.

There is experimental evidence to indicate that in women with polycystic ovaries, the peripheral insulin resistance is due to a defect beyond activation of the receptor kinase, specifically leading to reduced tyrosine autophosphorylation of the insulin receptor.[110, 111] The phosphorylation of serine and threonine residues on the insulin receptor reduces signal transmission, and excessive serine phosphorylation (by a mechanism extrinsic to the insulin receptor) has been demonstrated as a possible postreceptor defect in these patients, changing signal transduction.[111] It has been

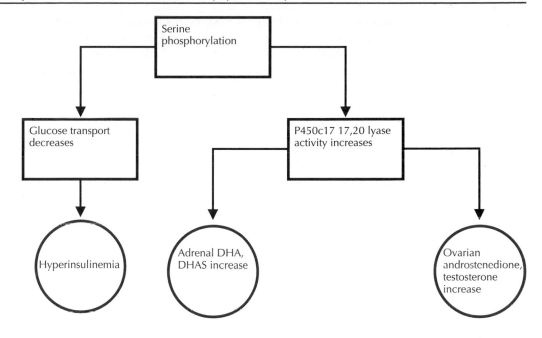

suggested that serine phosphorylation of the beta chain of the insulin receptor and at the same time of the adrenal and ovarian P450c17 enzyme (the origin or cause of serine phosphorylation is uncertain, but presumably it would have a genetic basis) would explain both the hyperinsulinemia and hyperandrogenism (serine phosphorylation increases and dephosphorylation decreases 17,20-lyase activity and androgen production).[32] Stated simply, serine instead of tyrosine phosphorylation is an "off" mechanism for glucose transport, but an "on" mechanism for P450c17 enzyme activity.

This change in phosphorylation would be consistent with no abnormality in the number of receptors or in receptor function; the impaired insulin signal for glucose transport would be due to a postreceptor problem. Indeed, structural defects in the insulin receptor cannot be identified.[112, 113] Of course, different patients with the same clinical presentation may have different reasons for the insulin resistance, a spectrum of etiologies with a common clinical expression. The defect in insulin action is limited to glucose metabolism; other biologic actions of insulin are not impaired.

Because of the tight connection between insulin and leptin levels in mice, and the now well-recognized prevalence of hyperinsulinemia in women with polycystic ovaries, it makes sense to examine leptin levels in these women. Although an initial study reported increased leptin levels in women with polycystic ovaries, the study was criticized for not adjusting for body weight.[114] At least 4 studies, controlling for weight, have detected no differences in leptin levels comparing women with and without polycystic ovaries.[115–118] In women with polycystic ovaries, the relationship between leptin and body weight is maintained. Thus, in contrast to the rodent model, hyperinsulinemia and insulin resistance do not affect leptin levels in these women.

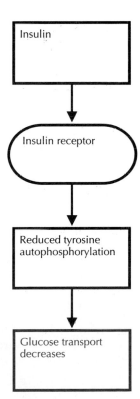

However, a role for leptin in the changes associated with polycystic ovaries should not yet be discounted. There may be subtle differences that have biologic consequences. At least one study demonstrated a correlation between leptin levels and 24-hour insulin levels in women with polycystic ovaries.[115] Furthermore, a drug that lowers insulin resistance, troglitazone, inhibits transcription of the leptin gene and may be especially suited for obese women with polycystic ovaries.[119]

Is the Link Between Hyperinsulinemia and Hyperandrogenism Explained Solely by the Presence of Obesity in Hyperandrogenic Patients?

Overweight, anovulatory women with hyperandrogenism have a characteristic distribution of body fat known as android obesity.[120–122] Android obesity is the result of fat deposited in the abdominal wall and visceral mesenteric locations. This fat is more sensitive to catecholamines, less sensitive to insulin, and more active metabolically. This fat distribution is associated with hyperinsulinemia, impaired glucose tolerance, diabetes mellitus, and an increase in androgen production rates resulting in decreased levels of sex hormone-binding globulin and increased levels of free testosterone and estradiol.[120–122]

Central body (android) obesity is associated with cardiovascular risk factors, including hypertension and unfavorable cholesterol-lipoprotein profiles.[123] The waist:hip ratio is the variable most strongly and inversely associated with the level of HDL_2, the fraction of HDL-cholesterol most consistently linked with protection from cardiovascular disease.[124] A waist:hip ratio greater than 0.85 indicates android fat distribution. The adverse impact of excess weight in adolescence can be explained by the fact that deposition of fat in adolescence is largely central in location.[125, 126] Weight loss in women with lower body obesity is mainly cosmetic, whereas loss of central body weight is more important for general health because an improvement in cardiovascular risk is associated with loss of central body fat.

Hyperinsulinemia and hyperandrogenism, however, are not confined to anovulatory women who are overweight. It is important to note that the combination of increased androgen secretion and insulin resistance has been reported in both obese and nonobese anovulatory women.[42, 127–130] However, insulin levels are higher and LH, SHBG, and IGFBP-1 levels are lower in obese women with polycystic ovaries compared to nonobese women with polycystic ovaries.[42, 131, 132] For this reason, some have suggested that hyperandrogenic women with polycystic ovaries could be divided into two groups: those with obesity, insulin resistance, hyperinsulinemia, and normal or minimally elevated LH levels; and those with elevated LH, no insulin resistance, and normal insulin levels.[133, 134] In our view, these two groups represent the ends of a spectrum, and division of this clinically broad spectrum of patients is artifactual and unhelpful.

Hyperinsulinemia and hyperandrogenism are not explained, therefore, solely by obesity, and specifically, android obesity. *However, the presence of obesity adds the insulin resistance and hyperinsulinemia associated with obesity to that which is specifically unique to the anovulatory, polycystic ovary state.*[42, 135, 136]

Which Comes First, the Hyperinsulinemia or the Hyperandrogenism?

There are studies indicating that androgens can induce hyperinsulinemia. However, most of the evidence supports hyperinsulinemia as the primary factor, especially the experiments in which turning off the ovary with a GnRH agonist does not change the hyperinsulinemia or insulin resistance.[98, 137–139] This indicates that disordered insulin action precedes the increase in androgens. Large doses of insulin were administered to a 16-year-old female with insulin resistance secondary to insulin receptor autoantibodies; the increased insulin levels increased her circulating testosterone levels.[140] With resolution of her insulin resistance, her testosterone levels returned to normal, indicating that the hyperinsulinemia stimulates and increases testosterone and not vice versa. Indeed, there are 6 reasons to believe that hyperinsulinism causes hyperandrogenism:

1. The administration of insulin to women with polycystic ovaries increases circulating androgen levels.[141]

2. The administration of glucose to hyperandrogenic women increases the circulating levels of both insulin and androgens.[142]

3. Weight loss decreases the levels of both insulin and androgens, and increases the levels of IGFBP-1.[143]

4. In vitro, insulin stimulates thecal cell androgen production.[144, 145]

5. The experimental reduction of insulin levels in women reduces androgen levels in women with polycystic ovaries, but not in normal women.[146]

6. After normalization of androgens with GnRH agonist treatment, the hyperinsulin response to glucose tolerance testing remains abnormal in obese women with polycystic ovaries.[139, 147]

Nevertheless, antiandrogen treatment and prolonged androgen suppression can ameliorate the degree of insulin resistance.[148, 149] However, the effect is not great, and may be limited to lean patients with mild hyperinsulinemia.

How Does Hyperinsulinemia Produce Hyperandrogenism?

There is an impressive correlation between the degree of hyperinsulinemia and hyperandrogenism.[127, 129, 130] At higher concentrations, insulin binds to the type I IGF receptors (which are similar in structure to insulin receptors; both IGF and insulin transmit their signals by initiating tyrosine autophosphorylation of their receptors). Thus, when insulin receptors are blocked or deficient in number, it is to be expected that insulin would bind to the type I IGF receptors.[150] In view of the known actions of IGF-I in augmenting the thecal androgen response to LH, activation of IGF-I receptors by insulin would lead to increased androgen production in thecal cells.[151] *It should be noted that evidence indicates that the endogenous insulin-like growth factor in the human ovarian follicle is IGF-II in both the granulosa and the thecal cells.[2] Studies indicating activity of IGF-I with human ovarian tissue can be explained by the fact that both IGF-I and IGF-II activities can be mediated by the type I IGF receptor, which is structurally similar to the insulin receptor.*

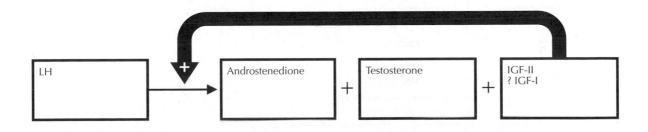

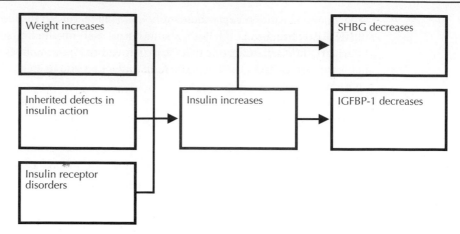

Because the increase in insulin is not always extreme, it has been proposed that insulin activates a signaling system separate from glucose transport, specifically, that insulin operates via inositolphosphoglycan to stimulate steroidogenesis.[152] This pathway would operate by means of insulin binding to its own receptor, not the IGF receptor, a pathway supported by in vitro studies of both granulosa cells and thecal cells.[153–155]

There are two other important actions of insulin which contribute to hyperandrogenism in the presence of hyperinsulinemia: inhibition of hepatic synthesis of sex hormone-binding globulin and inhibition of hepatic production of insulin-like growth factor binding protein-1.

Independently of any effect on sex steroids, increased insulin will inhibit the hepatic synthesis of sex hormone-binding globulin.[156] In vitro studies indicate that both insulin and IGF-I directly inhibit SHBG secretion by human hepatoma cells.[157, 158] This is now known to be the mechanism for the inverse relationship between body weight and the circulating levels of SHBG. Because SHBG is regulated by insulin, decreased SHBG levels in women represent an independent risk factor for noninsulin-dependent diabetes mellitus, regardless of body weight and fat distribution.[159] Of course, a decrease in SHBG allows more androgen and estrogen to be bioavailable.

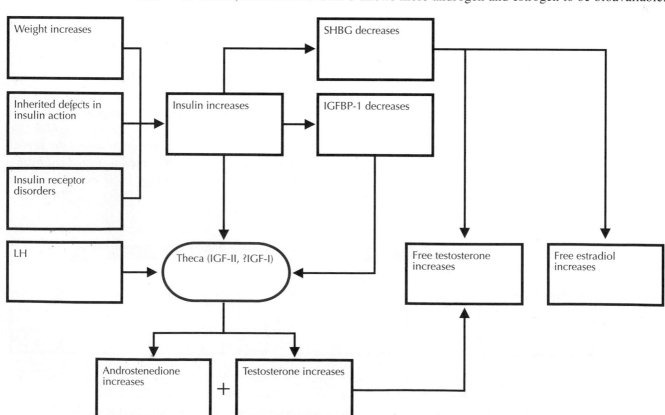

Nutritional intake decreases the circulating levels of insulin-like growth factor binding protein-1 (IGFBP-1) because of the increase in insulin, which then directly inhibits IGFBP-1 production in the liver.[160] Obese individuals with increased insulin levels and women with polycystic ovaries and hyperinsulinemia have lower circulating levels of IGFBP-1.[161] This lower level of IGFBP-1 allows an increase in circulating levels of IGF-I and greater local activity of IGF-I and/or IGF-II in the ovary. In addition, greater IGF-I activity in the endometrium due to reduced levels of IGFBP-1 and direct insulin activation of IGF receptors or its own receptor are possible mechanisms for endometrial growth (and the increased risk for endometrial cancer) in these patients. On the other hand, a greater IGF binding protein capacity in the follicular fluid from polycystic ovaries would yield a reduced bioavailability of IGFs within the follicle.[72, 73] Although these findings (increased circulating IGF availability and decreased follicular IGF availability) at first seem paradoxical, they are compatible with increased thecal androgen production by the IGF pathway and disrupted follicular maturation by the FSH system. It is likely that these characteristics of polycystic ovaries are secondary to increased anovulation, hyperinsulinemia, and increased androgens, rather than indicating a primary, etiologic role.

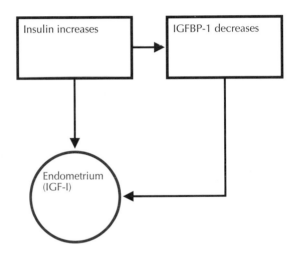

Finally, there is evidence that insulin can increase LH secretion in some anovulatory, overweight women.[162]

Why are not all patients with hyperinsulinemia also hyperandrogenic; e.g., many women with noninsulin-dependent diabetes mellitus? The answer to this question is not known, but a logical speculation is that an ovarian genetic susceptibility is required,[163] although it may be that the existence of long-term anovulation must be present and even precede hyperinsulinemia.

Can Ovarian Hyperandrogenism be Treated with Diabetes Drugs?

There is a variety of pharmacologic agents available to reduce insulin levels. Diazoxide and octreotide, the long-acting analogue of somatostatin, both inhibit insulin secretion, but are accompanied by worsening glucose intolerance.[146, 164] The best approach is to improve peripheral insulin sensitivity, thus achieving reductions in insulin secretion and stability of glucose tolerance. Metformin and troglitazone, oral agents used to treat diabetes mellitus, have been administered to anovulatory women with polycystic ovaries.

Metformin improves insulin sensitivity, but the primary effect is a significant reduction in gluconeogenesis, thus decreasing hepatic glucose production. Metformin treatment (500 mg tid) reduces hyperinsulinemia, basal and stimulated LH levels, free testosterone concentrations, and PAI-1 levels in overweight women with polycystic ovaries.[165–167] A significant number of these anovulatory women ovulate and achieve pregnancy.[168, 169] In a group of obese women with polycystic ovaries, 90% of the women treated with metformin and 50 mg clomiphene ovulated compared with 8% in the group treated with placebo and clomiphene.[170] However, there has been controversy, suggesting that the improvement was the result of the weight loss that often accompanies the use of metformin.[171] In a study designed to control the effect of body weight, the administration of metformin was without effect on insulin resistance in extremely overweight women with polycystic ovaries.[172] In another well-designed study, metformin again had no effect on insulin resistance when body weights remained unchanged, and in this study baseline weights and hyperinsulinemia were only modestly increased.[173] In lean, anovulatory women with hyperinsulinemia, metformin treatment reduced hyperandrogenemia although there was no change in body weight; however, a decrease in the waist to hip ratio accompanied a reduction in the hyperinsulinemia.[174] This study indicates that both obese and nonobese patients with hyperinsulinemia respond to metformin treatment. The reasons for the differences among the studies are not apparent. Perhaps only certain patients will respond to metformin, and, thus, patient selection could influence the reported results.

The thiazolidinediones markedly improve insulin sensitivity and insulin secretion (improved peripheral glucose utilization and β-cell function) without weight changes. Troglitazone (400 mg daily) decreases hyperinsulinemia, and improvements in metabolic abnormalities (decreased androgens, increased SHBG, decreased PAI-1 consistent with improved fibrinolytic capacity, and decreased LH) and a return to ovulation in very obese women have been reported with this agent.[175, 176]

There is little doubt that these drugs can produce significant and beneficial improvements in this condition, although metformin may be effective only when weight loss occurs. However, is short-term use better than our standard methods of the induction of ovulation, and are these drugs safe during pregnancy and lactation? Is long-term use for preventive health care cost-effective and compatible with good drug compliance? How effective are these agents in women who are of normal or only slightly elevated body weight? Are there any unwanted effects associated with long-term use (liver enzyme changes have occurred in rare patients with troglitazone)? Appropriate clinical trials are required to answer these questions.

We believe there will be rapid progress in this area. It is our prediction that during the clinical lifetime of this text, metformin and troglitazone (and perhaps new related drugs) will be increasingly used for anovulatory women resistant to clomiphene treatment and to prevent the cardiovascular and metabolic consequences of hyperinsulinemia.

The Clinical Consequences of Persistent Anovulation

Anovulation is the key feature of this condition and presents as amenorrhea in approximately 50% of cases and with irregular, heavy bleeding (dysfunctional uterine bleeding) in 30%.[12, 177] True virilization is rare, but 70% of anovulatory patients complain of cosmetically disturbing hirsutism. The development of hirsutism depends not only on the concentration of androgens in the blood but on the genetic sensitivity of hair follicles to androgens. Thus, anovulatory, hyperandrogenic women can be free of the clinical sign of hirsutism. Alopecia and acne can also be consequences of hyperandrogenism.[14, 178] Obesity has been classically regarded as an important feature, but in view of the concept of persistent anovulation arising from many causes, its presence is extremely variable (about 35–60% of anovulatory women with polycystic ovaries) and has no diagnostic value.[12–14] However, the greater the body mass index, the higher the testosterone levels, and, therefore, hirsutism is more common in overweight anovulatory women.

How many anovulatory women with polycystic ovaries have hyperinsulinemia? It is impossible to provide an accurate estimate. It does appear that the more aggressively clinicians pursue hyperinsulinemia in these patients the more often it is being demonstrated. Certainly not every anovulatory patient has hyperinsulinemia, not even every overweight, anovulatory patient. However, subtle abnormalities in insulin dynamics may be present early in the course of this condition, and appear more prominently with time.[179] Thus, when anovulation and hyperandrogenism are present, hyperinsulinemia may be an underlying disorder in most, if not all. As an anovulatory woman gains weight, the insulin resistance and hyperinsulinemia associated with obesity are now added to the underlying problem, and the abnormality is now more easily detected.[42, 135, 136]

Although an elevated LH value in the presence of a low or low-normal FSH may be diagnostic, the diagnosis is easily made by the clinical presentation alone. About 20–40% of patients with this condition do not have elevated LH levels with reversal of the LH:FSH ratio.[180–182] We do not routinely measure FSH and LH levels in anovulatory patients. The selection of a specific criterion to make this diagnosis will inevitably fail to include many patients with this clinical problem that covers a broad spectrum of manifestations. This failing also applies to the diagnostic use of ultrasonographic criteria.[22]

The Clinical Consequences of Persistent Anovulation

1. **Infertility.**
2. **Menstrual bleeding problems, ranging from amenorrhea to dysfunctional uterine bleeding.**
3. **Hirsutism, alopecia, and acne.**
4. **An increased risk of endometrial cancer and, perhaps, breast cancer.**
5. **An increased risk of cardiovascular disease**
6. **An increased risk of diabetes mellitus in patients with insulin resistance.**

There are potentially severe clinical consequences of the steady state of hormone secretion. Besides the problems of bleeding, amenorrhea, hirsutism, and infertility, the effect of the unopposed and uninterrupted estrogen is to place the patient at considerable risk for cancer of the endometrium and, perhaps, cancer of the breast.[183–186] The risk of endometrial cancer is increased 3-fold, while chronic anovulation during the reproductive years has been reported to be associated with a 3–4 times increased risk of breast cancer appearing in the postmenopausal years. However, the statistical power of these observational studies on breast cancer was limited by small numbers (all fewer than 15 cases). Others have failed to find a link between anovulation and the risk of breast cancer.[187–189] Women with the most irregular menstrual cycles (and thus presumably anovulatory) in the Nurses' Health Study appeared to have a reduced risk of breast cancer.[190]

If left unattended, patients with persistent anovulation develop clinical problems, and, therefore, appropriate therapeutic management is essential for all anovulatory patients. In a long-term follow-up of women with polycystic ovaries, the problems of android obesity and hyper-insulinemia were observed to persist into the postmenopausal years.[103] Although it is yet to be documented by appropriate epidemiologic studies, it is logical to expect postmenopausal women who have previously been anovulatory, hyperandrogenic, and hyperinsulinemic to experience a reduction in life expectancy because of cardiovascular disease and diabetes mellitus. These women will derive important benefits from an aggressive preventive health care attitude on the part of the clinician that results in amelioration of adverse metabolic risk factors.

Growing support for an inherited basis for this disorder (autosomal dominant) makes it important to consider appropriate family counseling. Sisters and daughters may have a 50% chance of having the same problems as the patient.

The typical patient presents with anovulation and irregular menses or amenorrhea with withdrawal bleeding after a progestational challenge. Documentation of anovulation is usually unnecessary, especially in the presence of menstrual irregularity with periods of amenorrhea. In the patient who has long-standing anovulation, an endometrial biopsy (with extensive sampling) is a wise precaution. The well-known association between this condition and abnormal endometrial changes must be kept in mind. Endometrial cancer can be encountered in young, anovulatory women.[191–193] *The decision to perform an endometrial biopsy should not be influenced by the patient's age. It is the duration of exposure to unopposed estrogen that is critical.*

Therapy of most anovulatory patients can be planned at the first visit. If the patient desires pregnancy, she is a candidate for the medical induction of ovulation (Chapter 30). When pregnancy is achieved, patients with polycystic ovaries appear to have an increased risk of spontaneous miscarriage.[194–196] This increased risk has been attributed to elevated levels of LH that may produce an adverse environment for the oocyte, perhaps even inducing premature maturation and completion of the first meiotic division. For this reason, consideration should be given to pretreatment suppression prior to the induction of ovulation (Chapter 30).

If the patient presents with amenorrhea, an investigation must be pursued as outlined in Chapter 11. The management of significant dysfunctional uterine bleeding is discussed in Chapter 16 and hirsutism in Chapter 13.

For the patient who does not wish to become pregnant and does not complain of hirsutism, but is anovulatory and has irregular bleeding, therapy is directed toward interruption of the steady state effect on the endometrium and breast. The use of medroxyprogesterone acetate (5–10 mg daily for the first 10 days of every month) is favored to ensure complete withdrawal bleeding and to prevent endometrial hyperplasia and atypia. The monthly 10-day duration has been demonstrated to be essential to protect the endometrium from cancer in women on postmenopausal estrogen therapy. Until specific clinical data are available, it seems logical that young, anovulatory women also require at least 10 days of progestational exposure every month. The patient will be aware of the onset of ovulatory cycles because bleeding will occur at a time other than the expected withdrawal bleed. In our opinion, when reliable contraception is essential, the use of low-dose combination oral contraception in the usual cyclic fashion is appropriate.

Besides contraception, there is another argument in favor of continuous suppression with low-dose oral contraceptives rather than periodic progestational interruption. The lipid profile in androgenized women with polycystic ovaries (who are also exposed to relatively lower estrogen levels over time) is similar to the male pattern with higher levels of cholesterol, triglycerides, and LDL-cholesterol, and lower levels of HDL-cholesterol, and this abnormal pattern is independent of body weight.[197–201] Although the elevated androgens associated with polycystic ovaries and anovulation offer some protection against osteoporosis, the adverse impact on the risk for cardiovascular disease is a more important consideration.[202] An adverse lipid profile is a distinguishin feature of these patients even when body mass index, insulin, and age are controlled in case-control studies.[203] Subclinical atherosclerosis can be demonstrated by carotid ultrasonography to be prevalent in premenopausal women with a history of anovulation and polycystic ovaries.[204] In women undergoing coronary angiography, the prevalence of polycystic ovaries is increased, and women with polycystic ovaries have more extensive coronary atherosclerosis.[205] Thus anovulatory women with polycystic ovaries develop risk factors for atherosclerosis and ultimately clinical disease, comparable with that found in older, very overweight, postmenopausal women.

Monthly periodic treatment with a progestational agent has no significant effect on the androgen production by polycystic ovaries. Thus, if contraception is not required and hirsutism is not a complaint, assessment of the lipoprotein profile is a reasonable clinical response, and in the presence of a male pattern, serious consideration should be given to suppression with oral contraceptives. Short-term studies with low-dose oral contraceptives have not revealed an adverse effect on the already abnormal lipid profile.[206] Indeed, one would expect an improvement in the lipid profile to accompany suppression of androgen production. Similarly, interference with androgen actions with an agent like flutamide improves the lipid profile.[207] Long-term suppression of hyperandrogenism should be beneficial; however, epidemiologic data on this important question are not available.

Because older, high-dose oral contraceptives increased insulin resistance, it has been suggested that this treatment should be avoided in anovulatory, overweight women. However, low-dose oral contraceptives have minimal effects on carbohydrate metabolism, and the majority of hyper-

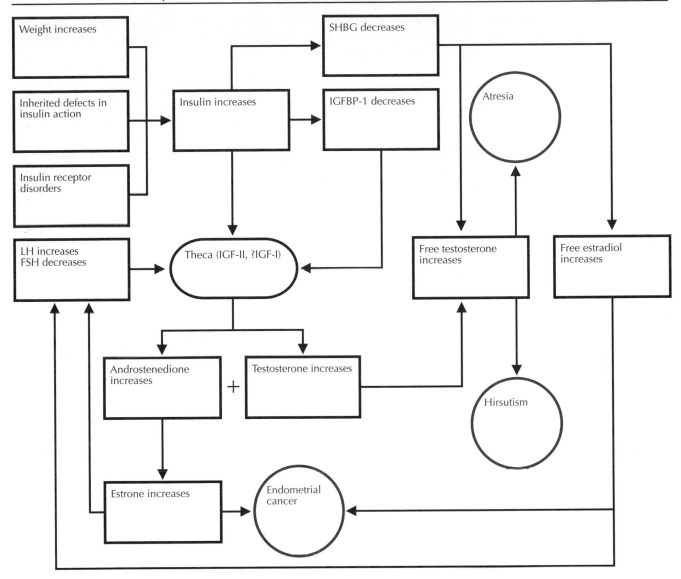

insulinemic, hyperandrogenic women can be expected to respond favorably to treatment with oral contraceptives.[208] Insulin and glucose changes with low-dose (less than 50 μg ethinyl estradiol) oral contraceptives are so minimal, that it is now believed that they are of no clinical significance.[209] Long-term follow-up studies have failed to detect any increase in the incidence of diabetes mellitus or impaired glucose tolerance (even in past and current users of high-dose pills).[210, 211] Furthermore, there is no evidence of an increase in risk of cardiovascular disease among past users of oral contraceptives.[212, 213] In addition, low-dose oral contraceptives have been administered to women with recent gestational diabetes without an adverse impact, and in women with insulin-dependent diabetes mellitus, low-dose oral contraceptives have not produced deterioration of lipid and biochemical markers for cardiovascular disease or increased the development of retinopathy or nephropathy.[214–217] And finally, the administration of a low-dose oral contraceptive to women with extreme obesity and insulin resistance resulted in only a mild deterioration of glucose tolerance.[218]

This experience supports the safety of oral contraceptive treatment for anovulatory, hyperandrogenic, hyperinsulinemic women. Patients resistant to oral contraceptive treatment may require suppression with a GnRH agonist. Because glucocorticoids increase insulin resistance, they should be used with caution in patients with hyperinsulinemia. Spironolactone and flutamide do not affect insulin sensitivity in anovulatory women.[219, 220]

A contributing factor to the abnormal lipid pattern in many of these patients is hyperinsulinemia,[201, 221] and therefore, a major effort must be directed to control of body weight in those patients who are overweight.

Hyperandrogenic and hyperinsulinemic, anovulatory women must be cautioned regarding their increased risk of future diabetes mellitus. Not only are anovulatory, hyperinsulinemic women at greater risk for noninsulin-dependent diabetes, but the age of onset is about 30 years earlier than the general population.[222, 249] Not surprising, these patients are more likely to develop glucose tolerance problems in pregnancy.[223] And patients who have experienced gestational diabetes are more likely to demonstrate the entire metabolic syndrome (hyperandrogenism and hyperinsulinemia) later in life.[224] In a long-term follow-up study, anovulatory women with polycystic ovaries had a 5-fold increased risk of diabetes mellitus compared with age-matched controls.[103] *It is apropriate, and indeed essential, to monitor glucose tolerance with periodic glucose tolerance testing.*

Hyperinsulinemia also contributes to the increased risk of cardiovascular disease both by means of a direct atherogenic action and indirectly by adversely affecting the lipoprotein profile. Insulin resistance may be a more significant factor than androgens in determining the abnormal lipoprotein profile in overweight, anovulatory women.[201] It has also been suggested that the increased insulin stimulation of IGF-I could produce bone changes similar to that seen in acromegaly.[225] Hyperinsulinemia may be a factor contributing to the higher risk of endometrial cancer in these patients by increasing IGF-I activity in the endometrium.[226]

The best therapy for these women is weight loss. Both the hyperinsulinemia and the hyperandrogenism can be reduced with weight loss, which is at least more than 5% of the initial weight.[143, 227–231] Increased PAI-1 levels associated with hyperinsulinemia also improve with weight loss.[230] These metabolic improvements are associated with an impressive rate of resumption of ovulation and pregnancy.[232, 233] In one study, 60 of 67 anovulatory women, who lost from 4 to 15 kg, resumed ovulation.[234] A goal for weight loss that correlates with a good chance of achieving pregnancy (improved menstrual function), a reduction in insulin levels, and a decrease in free testosterone levels is a body mss index of less than 27 (see the nomogram for calculating body mass index in Chapter 19). Insulin resistance is not detected in normal women with a body mass index less than 27.[135] However, it is likely that women with this condition can still manifest some degree of insulin resistance despite weight loss. Nevertheless, the impact of mild or incipient hyperinsulinemia is uncertain, and a major improvement in clinical consequences can be achieved by weight loss, and it should be emphasized, that only a relatively small percentage of weight (5–10%) need be lost to have a beneficial impact upon insulin resistance and cardiovascular hemodynamic function.[235]

The best application of drugs, such as metformin and troglitazone, remains to be determined by data from appropriate clinical trials; however, the mechanism of action and the logic behind this treatment offer impressive potential for preventive health benefits for these women. Clinical (ovulatory) and laboratory responses can be expected within 3 months. *As we have previously noted, we believe these drugs will prove to be an important component of the health care of anovulatory women with polycystic ovaries.*

Although changes are uncommon, liver function must be monitored during troglitazone treatment. The pharmaceutical company's package information should be consulted for the currently recommended monitoring regimen of serum alanine aminotransferase levels. Troglitazone was found to be associated with a 30% decrease in the circulating estrogen and progestin levels in oral contraceptive users in a small number of women who have been studied in clinical trials (pharmaceutical company data), an effect probably secondary to troglitazone's stimulation of hepatic enzyme activity; however, it is by no means certain that this will result in a loss of contraceptive efficacy. Lactic acidosis is a rare complication in patients treated with metformin; however, virtually all cases have occurred in patients with complicated medical problems, such as sepsis, renal insufficiency, and congestive heart failure. Patients who become ill should discontinue metformin treatment, and metformin should not be administered to women who have abnormal renal chemistries.

Treatment with low doses of dehydroepiandrosterone to increase insulin sensitivity is effective in the short-term, but well-designed studies are necessary to demonstrate long-term efficacy and safety.[236]

Overall Goals of Treatment

1. **Reduce the production and circulating levels of androgens.**
2. **Protect the endometrium against the effects of unopposed estrogen.**
3. **Support lifestyle changes to achieve normal body weight.**
4. **Lower the risk for cardiovascular disease.**
5. **Avoid the effects of hyperinsulinemia on the risks of cardiovascular disease and diabetes mellitus.**
6. **Induction of ovulation to achieve pregnancy.**

Who Should Be Tested for Hyperinsulinemia?

Do all anovulatory patients require testing for hyperinsulinemia? Both lean and obese women with polycystic ovaries can be found to have hyperinsulinemia, but not all hyperandrogenic women withpolycystic ovaries (lean and obese) have hyperinsulinemia.[14, 147, 237] However, it is more common and severe in overweight women and androgenic effects are more intense. Furthermore, lean women with hyperinsulinemia do not appear to have the same risk of future diabetes mellitus, although clinical follow-up may in time document an onset later in life of noninsulin-dependent diabetes mellitus compared to an earlier onset in obese women. It has been reported that anovulatory women with polycystic ovaries who have a parent with noninsulin-dependent diabetes mellitus are more likely to have impaired beta cell secretion of insulin in addition to insulin resistance.[238]

Because of the probable inherited susceptibility for anovulation and insulin resistance, consideration should be given to a glucose tolerance and insulin evaluation for family members of already diagnosed patients. Both brothers and sisters of anovulatory, hyperandrogenic women can be insulin resistant.[84]

What about those women who are ovulatory and have no clinical complaints, yet supposedly have an underlying hyperinsulinemic disorder? In our view, if this is real, it is a homeostatic compensatory state, and until appropriate data reveal adverse outcomes in these women, diagnostic and therapeutic interventions are not indicated.

It would be ideal if all patients with android obesity were tested for hyperinsulinemia. The waist:hip ratio is a means of estimating the degree of upper to lower body obesity; the ratio ccurately predicts the amount of intra-abdominal fat (which is greater with android obesity).[239, 240] However, studies have demonstrated that the more easily determined circumference of the waist is a better predictor of central, android abdominal fat.[241, 242] *A waist circumference greater than 100 cm (about 40 inches) in men and 90 cm (about 35 inches) in women is predictive of abnormal endocrinologic and metabolic function and is associated with an increased risk of cardiovascular disease.*[241]

Teenagers who present with persistent anovulation would also be good candidates for hyperinsulinemia testing. During puberty, insulin resistance develops, probably because of the increase in sex steroids and growth hormone, resulting in a secondary increase in insulin and IGF-I.[243, 244] The increase in insulin leads to a decrease in SHBG, which would allow greater sex steroid activity for pubertal developmentThere is reason to believe that some teenagers fail to normalize the hyperinsulinemia associated with the growth hormone increase in early puberty.[179] It would be important to identify these teenagers who are at an increased risk for the development of diabetes mellitus and are destined to struggle with all of the problems associated with anovulation and polycystic ovaries. There is also reason to believe that many cases of premature adrenarche are due to hyperinsulinemia, and these patients go on to develop the full characteristics of anovulation, hyperandrogenism, and polycystic ovaries.[245, 246]

When clinical circumstances are encountered that do not seem to make sense, give consideration to the presence of hyperinsulinemia. We have experienced several examples where hyperinsulinemia proved to be the underlying answer. Several instances involved women in the reproductive age range, with significant hirsutism and very high testosterone levels. Evaluation failed to reveal an ovarian tumor or an adrenal lesion. The demonstration of hyperinsulinemia has avoided unnecessary surgical exploration for a "small tumor." Another example was the onset of hirsutism in elderly women associated with testosterone levels greater than 200 ng/mL and normal imaging evaluations of the ovaries and adrenal glands. Again, hyperinsulinemia was the cause, not a hidden tumor.

Unfortunately, it is not certain what levels of insulin in the fasting state or in response to an oral glucose tolerance test are correlated with clinical outcome. However, in individuals with normal glucose tolerance, the fasting insulin level is strongly correlated with insulin resistance.[247] In most laboratories, the upper limit of normal for a fasting insulin level is 10–20 U/mL. Because there is considerable overlap between normal women and patients with anovulation and polycystic ovaries, it is reasonable to assume that all overweight, anovulatory women with polycystic ovaries are hyperinsulinemic. Nevertheless we recommend the measurement of the ratio of fasting glucose to fasting insulin in order to provide evidence that lends credence and importance to counseling efforts. ***A ratio of less than 4.5 is consistent with insulin resistance.***[248]

Based upon the information reviewed in this chapter, we offer the following recommendations:

All anovulatory women who are hyperandrogenic should be assessed for insulin resistance and glucose tolerance with measurements of:

1. **The fasting glucose:insulin ratio, followed by**
2. **The 2-hour glucose level after a 75 g glucose load:**
normal	less than 140 mg/dL
impaired	140–199 mg/dL
noninsulin-dependent diabetes mellitus	200 mg/dL and higher

Anovulory women who do not exhibit signs of hyperandrogenism should be evaluated for the presence of a metabolic abnormality by measuring the free testosterone level; if elevated, insulin resistance and glucose tolerance should be assessed. *However, a fasting glucose:insulin ratio is about one-third the cost of a free testosterone level. It may be more economical to measure this ratio in all anovulatory women.*

In women who continue to manifest this disorder, periodic surveillance is necessary. The frequency is uncertain, but annual assessment is appropriate in women who continue to be obese.

Conclusion

We are truly entering a new era in our understanding and management of women with polycystic ovaries and hyperandrogenism. In the past we have effectively treated the specific problems of infertility, dysfunctional uterine bleeding, and hirsutism. We now have an opportunity to have an impact on the quality and quantity of life to be experienced by these patients. By creating and supporting a preventive health care attitude in anovulatory women, we can not only correct specific clinical consequences of anovulation, we can reduce major adverse effects on overall health.

References

1. **Groome NP, Illingworth PG, O'Brien M, Pai R, Rodger FE, Mather JP, McNeilly AS,** Measurement of dimeric inhibin B throughout the human menstrual cycle, *J Clin Endocrinol Metab* 81:1401, 1996.

2. **Voutilainen R, Franks S, Mason HD, Martikainen H,** Expression of insulin-like growth factor (IGF), IGF-binding protein, and IGF receptor messenger ribonucleic acids in normal and polycystic ovaries, *J Clin Endocrinol Metab* 81:1003, 1996.

3. **Judd SJ, Wong J, Saloniklis S, Maiden M, Yeap B, Filmer S, Michailov L,** The effect of alprazolam on serum cortisol and luteinizing hormone pulsatility in normal women and in women with stress-related anovulation, *J Clin Endocrinol Metab* 80:818, 1995.

4. **Lundberg U, Hansson U, Andersson K, Eneroth P, Frankenhausen M, Hagenfeld K,** Hirsute women with elevated testosterone: psychological characteristics, steroid hormones and catecholamines, *J Psychosom Obstet Gynecol* 2:86, 1983.

5. **Lobo RA, Granger LR, Paul WL, Goebelsmann U, Mishell Jr DR,** Psychological stress and increases in urinry norepinephrine metabolites, platelet serotonin, and adrenal androgens in women with polycystic ovary syndrome, *Am J Obstet Gynecol* 145:496, 1983.

6. **Orenstein H, Raskind MA, Wyllie D, Raskind WH, Soules MR,** Polysymptomatic complaints and Briquet's syndrome in polycystic ovary disease, *Am J Psychiatr* 143:768, 1986.

7. **Paoletti AM, Cagnacci A, Depau GF, Orrù M, Ajossa S, Melis GB,** The chronic administration of cabergoline normalizes androgen secretion and improves menstrual cyclicity in women with polycystic ovary syndrome, *Fertil Steril* 66:527, 1996.

8. **Burger CW, Korsen T, van Kessel H, van Dop PA, Caron JM, Schoemaker J,** Pulsatile luteinizing hormone patterns in the follicular phase of the menstrual cycle, polycystic ovarian disease (PCOD) and non-PCOD secondary amenorrhea, *J Clin Endocrinol Metab* 61:1126, 1985.

9. **Barnes RB, Lobo RA,** Central opioid activity in polycystic ovary syndrome with and without dopaminergic modulation, *J Clin Endocrinol Metab* 61:779, 1985.

10. **Berga SL, Yen SSC,** Opioidergic regulation of LH pulsatility in women with polycystic ovary syndrome, *Clin Endocrinol* 30:177, 1989.

11. **Siiteri PK, MacDonald PC,** Role of extraglandular estrogen in human endocrinology, In: Geyer SR, Astwood EB, Greep RO, eds. *Handbook of Physiology, Section 7, Endocrinology,* American Physiology Society, Washington, DC, 1973, p 615.

12. **Goldzieher JW, Axelrod LR,** Clinical and biochemical features of polycystic ovarian disease, *Fertil Steril* 14:631, 1963.

13. **Dunaif A, Graf M, Mandeli J, Laumas V, Dobrjansky A,** Characterization of groups of hyperandrogenic women with acanthosis nigricans, impaired glucose tolerance and/or hyperinsulinemia, *J Clin Endocrinol Metab* 65:499, 1987.

14. **Conway GS, Honour JW, Jacobs HS,** Heterogeneity of the polycystic ovary syndrome: clinical endocrine and ultrasound features in 556 patients, *Clin Endocrinol* 30:459, 1989.

15. **Franks S,** Polycystic ovary syndrome, *New Engl J Med* 333:853, 1995.

16. **Stein IF, Leventhal ML,** Amenorrhea associated with bilateral polycystic ovaries, *Am J Obstet Gynecol* 29:181, 1935.

17. **Speert H,** *Obstetric & Gynecologic Milestones Illustrated,* The Parthenon Publishing Group, New York, 1996.

18. **Hull MGR,** Epidemiology of infertility and polycystic ovarian disease: endocrinological and demographic studies, *Gynaecol Endocrinol* 1:235, 1987.

19. **Polson DW, Wadsworth J, Adams J, Franks S,** Polycystic ovaries: a common finding in normal women, *Lancet* ii:870, 1988.

20. **Clayton RN, Ogden V, Hodgkinson J, Worswick L, Rodin DA, Dyer S, Meade TW,** How common are polycystic ovaries in normal women and what is their significance for the fertility of the population? *Clin Endocrinol* 37:127, 1992.

21. **Farquhar CM, Birdsall M, Manning P, Mitchell JM, France JT,** The prevalence of polycystic ovaries on ultrasound scanning in a population of randomly selected women, *Aust NZ Obstet Gynaecol* 34:67, 1994.

22. **van Santbrink EJP, Hop WC, Fauser BCJM,** Classification of normogonadotropic infertility: polycystic ovaries diagnosed by ultrasound vesus endocrine characteristics of polycystic ovary syndrome, *Fertil Steril* 67:452, 1997.

23. **Kimura I, Togashi K, Kawakami S, Nakano Y, Takakura K, Mori T, Konishi J,** Polycystic ovaries: implications of diagnosis with MR imaging, *Radiology* 201:549, 1996.

24. **Carmina E, Wong L, Chang L, Paulson RJ, Sauer MV, Stanczyk FZ, Lobo RA,** Endocrine abnormalities in ovulatory women with polycystic ovaries on ultrasound, *Hum Reprod* 12:905, 1997.

25. **Chang RJ,** Ovarian steroid secretion in polycystic ovarian disease, *Seminars Reprod Endocrinol* 2:244, 1984.

26. **Calogero AE, Macchi M, Montanini V, Mongioi A, Maugeri G, Vicari E, Coniglione F, Sipione C, D'Agata R,** Dynamics of plasma gonadotropin and sex steroid release in polycystic ovarian disease after pituitary-ovarian inhibition with an analog of gonadotropin-releasing hormone, *J Clin Endocrinol Metab* 64:980, 1987.

27. **Laatikainen TJ, Apter DL, Paavonen JA, Wahlstrom TR,** Steroids in ovarian and peripheral venous blood in polycystic ovarian disease, *Clin Endocrinol* 13:125, 1980.

28. **Hoffman DI, Klove K, Lobo RA,** The prevalence and significance of elevated dehydroepiandrosterone sulfate levels in anovulatory women, *Fertil Steril* 42:76, 1984.

29. **Carmina E, Rosato F, Janni A,** Increased DHEAS levels in PCO syndrome: evidence for the existence of two groups of patients, *J Endocrinol Invest* 9:5, 1986.

30. **Gonzalez F, Hatala DA, Speroff L,** Basal and dynamic hormonal responses to gonadotropin releasing hormone agonist treatment in women with polycystic ovaries with high and low dehydroepiandrosterone sulfate levels, *Am J Obstet Gynecol* 165:535, 1991.

31. **Gonzalez F, Chang L, Horab T, Lobo RA,** Evidence for heterogeneous etiologies of adrenal dysfunction in polycystic ovary syndrome, *Fertil Steril* 66:354, 1996.

32. **Zhang L, Rodriguez H, Ohno S, Miller WL,** Serine phosphorylation of human P450c17 increases 17,20-lyase activity: implications for adrenarche and the polycystic ovary syndrome, *Proc Natl Acad Sci USA* 92:10619, 1995.

33. **Venturoli S, Porcu E, Fabbri R, Magrini O, Gammi L, Paradisi R, Forcacci M, Bolzani R, Flamigni C,** Episodic pulsatile secretion of FSH, LH, prolactin, oestradiol, oestrone, and LH circadian variations in polycystic ovary syndrome, *Clin Endocrinol* 28:93, 1988.

34. **Wajchenberg BL, Achando SS, Mathor MM, Czeresnia CE, Neto DG, Kirschner MA,** The source(s) of estrogen production in hirsute women with polycystic ovarian disease as determined by simultaneous adrenal and ovarian venous catheterization, *Fertil Steril* 49:56, 1988.

35. **Kletzky OA, Davajan V, Nakamura RM, Thorneycroft IH, Mishell Jr DR,** Clinical categorization of patients with secondary amenorrhea using progesterone induced uterine bleeding and measurement of serum gonadotropin levels, *Am J Obstet Gynecol* 121:695, 1975.

36. **Rebar RW,** Gonadotropin secretion in polycystic ovary disease, *Seminars Reprod Endocrinol* 2:223, 1984.

37. **Imse V, Holzapfel G, Hinney B, Kuhn W, Wuttke W,** Comparison of luteinizing hormone pulsatility in the serum of women suffering from polycystic ovarian disease using a bioassay and five different immunoassays, *J Clin Endocrinol Metab* 74:1053, 1992.

38. **Hayes FJ, Taylor AE, Martin KA, Hall JE,** Use of a gonadotropin-releasing hormone antagonist as a physiologic probe in polycystic ovary syndrome: assessment of neuroendocrine and androgen dynamics, *J Clin Endocrinol Metab* 83:2343, 1998.

39. **Waldstreicher J, Santoro NF, Hall JE, Filicori M, Crowley Jr WF,** Hyperfunction of the hypothalamic-pituitary axis in women with polycystic ovarian disease: indirect evidence for partial gonadotroph desensitization, *J Clin Endocrinol Metab* 66:165, 1988.

40. **Cheung AP, Lu JKH, Chang RJ,** Pulsatile gonadotrophin secretion in women with polycystic ovary syndrome after gonadotropin-releasing hormone agonist treatment, *Hum Reprod* 12:1156, 1997.

41. **Schoemaker J,** Neuroendocrine control in polycystic ovary-like syndrome, *Gynecol Endocrinol* 5:277, 1991.

42. **Morales AJ, Laughlin GA, Bützow T, Maheshwari H, Baumann G, Yen SSC,** Insulin, somatotropic, and luteinizing hormone axes in lean and obese women with polycystic ovary syndrome: common and distinct features, *J Clin Endocrinol Metab* 81:2854, 1996.

43. **Taylor AE, McCourt B, Martin KA, Anderson EJ, Adams JM, Schoenfeld D, Hall JE,** Determinants of abnormal gonadotropin secretion in clinically defined women with polycystic ovary syndrome, *J Clin Endocrinol Metab* 82:2248, 1997.

44. **Arroyo A, Laughlin GA, Morales AJ, Yen SSC,** Inappropriate gonadotropin secretion in polycystic ovary syndrome: influence of adiposity, *J Clin Endocrinol Metab* 82:3728, 1997.

45. **Nagamani M, Lingold JC, Gomez LG, Barza JR,** Clinical and hormonal studies in hyperthecosis of the ovaries, *Fertil Steril* 36:326, 1981.

46. **Nagamani M, Dinh TV, Kelver ME,** Hyperinsulinemia in hyperthecosis of the ovaries, *Am J Obstet Gynecol* 154:384, 1986.

47. **Chang RJ, Mandel FP, Lu JK, Judd HL,** Enhanced disparity of gonadotropin secretion by estrone in women with polycystic ovarian disease, *J Clin Endocrinol Metab* 54:490, 1982.

48. **Lobo RA, Granger L, Goebelsmann U, Mishell Jr DR,** Elevations in unbound serum estradiol as a possible mechanism for inappropriate gonadotropin secretion in women with PCO, *J Clin Endocrinol Metab* 52:156, 1981.

49. **Buckler HM, McLachlan RI, McLachlan VB, Healy DL, Burger HG,** Serum inhibin levels in polycystic ovary syndrome: basal levels and response to luteinizing hormone-releasing hormone agonist and exogenous gonadotropin administration, *J Clin Endocrinol Metab* 66:798, 1988.

50. **Lambert-Messerlian GM, Hall JE, Sluss PM, Taylor AE, Martin KA, Groome NP, Crowley Jr WF, Schneyer AL,** Relatively low levels of dimeric inhibin circulate in men and women with polycystic ovarian syndrome using a specific two-site enzyme-linked immunosorbent assay, *J Clin Endocrinol Metab* 79:45, 1994.

51. **Yamoto M, Minami S, Nakano R,** Immunohistochemical localization of inhibin subunits in polycystic ovary, *J Clin Endocrinol Metab* 77:859, 1993.

52. **Roberts VJ, Barth S, El-Roeiy A, Yen SSC,** Localization of inhibin/activin subunit and follistatin peptides and mRNAs in ovaries from women with polycystic ovarian syndrome, *J Clin Endocrinol Metab* 79:1434, 1994.

53. **Lockwood GM, Muttukrishna S, Groome NP, Matthews DR, Ledger WL,** Mid-follicular phase pulses of inhibin B are absent in polycystic ovarian syndrome and are initiated by successful laparoscopic ovarian diathermy: a possible mechanism regulating emergence of the dominant follicle, *J Clin Endocrinol Metab* 83:1730, 1998.

54. **Fauser BC,** Observations in favor of normal early follicle development and disturbed dominant follicle selection in polycystic ovary syndrome, *Gynecol Endocrinol* 8:75, 1994.

55. **Agarwal SK, Judd HL, Magoffin DA,** A mechanism for the suppression of estrogen production in polycystic ovary syndrome, *J Clin Endocrinol Metab* 81:3686, 1996.

56. **Judd HL, Rigg LA, Anderson DC, Yen SSC,** The effect of ovarian wedge resection on circulating gonadotropin and ovarian steroid levels in patients with polycystic ovary syndrome, *J Clin Endocrinol Metab* 43:347, 1976.

57. **Mahesh VB, Bratlid D, Lindabeck T,** Hormone levels following wedge resection in polycystic ovary syndrome, *Obstet Gynecol* 51:64, 1978.

58. **Katz M, Carr PJ, Cohen BM, Milhin RP,** Hormonal effects of wedge resection of polycystic ovaries, *Obstet Gynecol* 51:437, 1978.

59. **Casper RF, Greenblatt EM,** Laparoscopic ovarian cautery for induction of ovulation in women with polycystic ovarian disease, *Seminars Reprod Endocrinol* 8:2080, 1990.

60. **Kaaijk EM, Beek JF, Hamerlynck JVTH, van der Veen F,** Unilateral oophorectomy in polycystic ovary syndrome: a treatment option in highly selected cases? *Hum Reprod* 12:2370, 1997.

61. **De Leo V, Lanzetta D, D'Antona D, la Marca A, Morgante G,** Hormonal effects of flutamide in young women with polycystic ovary syndrome, *J Clin Endocrinol Metab* 83:99, 1998.

62. **Serafini P, Silva PD, Paulson RJ, Elkind-Hirsch K, Hernandez M, Lobo RA,** Acute modulation of the hypothalamic-pituitary axis by intravenous testosterone in normal women, *Am J Obstet Gynecol* 155:1288, 1986.

63. **Hughesdon PE,** Morphology and morphogenesis of the Stein-Leventhal ovary and of so-called "hyperthecosis," *Obstet Gynecol Survey* 37:59, 1982.

64. **Judd HL, Scully RE, Herbst AL, Yen SSC, Ingersol FM, Kliman B,** Familial hyperthecosis: comparison of endocrinologic and histologic findings with polycystic ovarian disease, *Am J Obstet Gynecol* 117:979, 1973.

65. **Duleba AJ, Spaczynski RZ, Olive DL,** Insulin and insulin-like growth factor I stimulate the proliferation of human ovarian theca-interstitial cells, *Fertil Steril* 69:335, 1998.

66. **Kase N, Kowal J, Perloff W, Soffer LJ,** In vitro production of androgens by a virilizing adenoma and associated polycystic ovaries, *Acta Endocrinol* 44:15, 1963.

67. **Amerikia H, Savoy-Moore RT, Sundareson AS, Moghissi KS,** The effects of long-term androgen treatment on the ovary, *Fertil Steril* 45:202, 1986.

68. **Zourlas PA, Jones Jr HW,** Stein-Leventhal syndrome with masculinizing ovarian tumors, *Obstet Gynecol* 34:861, 1969.

69. **Dunaif A, Scully RE, Andersen RN, Chapin DS, Crowley Jr WF,** The effects of continuous androgen secretion on the hypothalamic-pituitary axis in women: evidence from a luteinized thecoma of the ovary, *J Clin Endocrinol Metab* 59:389, 1984.

70. **Pache TD, Fauser BCJM,** Polycystic ovaries in female-to-male transsexuals, *Clin Endocrinol* 39:702, 1993.

71. **McNatty KP, Smith DM, Makris A, DeGrazia C, Tulchinsky D, Osathanondh R, Schiff I, Ryan KJ,** The intraovarian sites of androgen and estrogen formation in women with normal and hyperandrogenic ovaries as judged by in vitro experiments, *J Clin Endocrinol Metab* 50:755, 1980.

72. **Cataldo NA, Giudice LC,** Follicular fluid insulin-like growth factor binding protein profiles in polycystic ovary syndrome, *J Clin Endocrinol Metab* 74:695, 1992.

73. **San Roman GA, Magoffin DA,** Insulin-like growth factor binding proteins in ovarian follicles from women with polycystic ovarian disease: cellular source and levels in follicular fluid, *J Clin Endocrinol Metab* 75:1010, 1992.

74. **Erickson GF, Magoffin DA, Garzo VG, Cheung AP, Chang RJ,** Granulosa cells of polycystic ovaries: are they normal or abnormal? *Hum Reprod* 7:293, 1992.

75. **Mason HD, Willis DS, Beard RW, Winston RML, Margara R, Franks S,** Estradiol production by granulosa cells of normal and polycystic ovaries: relationship to menstrual cycle history and concentrations of gonadotropins and sex steroids in follicular fluid, *J Clin Endocrinol Metab* 79:1355, 1994.

76. **Almahbobi G, Anderiesz C, Hutchinson P, McFarlane JR, Wood C, Trounson AO,** Functional integrity of granulosa cells from polycystic ovaries, *Clin Endocrinol* 44:571, 1996.

77. **Erickson GF, Hsueh AJN, Quigley ME, Rebar R, Yen SSC,** Functional studies of aromatase activity in human granulosa cells from normal and polycystic ovaries, *J Clin Endocrinol Metab* 49:514, 1979.

78. **Mason HD, Margara R, Winston RL, Seppala M, Koistinen R, Franks S,** Insulin-like growth factor-I (IGF-I) inhibits production of IGF-binding protein-1 while stimulating estradiol secretion in granulosa cells from normal and polycystic human ovaries, *J Clin Endocrinol Metab* 76:1275, 1993.

79. **Cooper H, Spellacy W, Prem K, Cohen W,** Hereditary factors in the Stein-Leventhal syndrome, *Am J Obst Gynecol* 100:371, 1968.

80. **Ferriman D, Purdie A,** The inheritance of PCO and possible relationship to premature balding, *Clin Endocrinol* 11:291, 1979.

81. **Lunde O, Magnus P, Sandvik L, Hoglo S,** Familial clustering in the polycystic ovarian syndrome, *Gynecol Obstet Invest* 28:23, 1989.

82. **Givens JR,** Familial polycystic ovarian disease, *Endocrinol Metab Clin North Am* 17:1, 1988.

83. **Carey AH, Chan KL, Short F, White DM, Williamson R, Franks S,** Evidence for a single gene effect in polycystic ovaries and male pattern baldness, *Clin Endocrinol* 38:653, 1993.

84. **Norman RJ, Masters S, Hague W,** Hyperinsulinemia is common in family members of women with polycystic ovary syndrome, *Fertil Steril* 66:942, 1996.

85. **Franks S, Gharani N, Waterworth D, Batty S, White D, Williamson R, McCarthy M,** The genetic basis of polycystic ovary syndrome, *Hum Reprod* 12:2641, 1997.

86. **Waterworth DM, Bennett ST, Gharani N, McCarthy MI, Hague S, Batty S, Conway GS, White D, Todd JA, Franks S, Williamson R,** Linkage and association of insulin gene VNTR regulatory polymorphism with polycystic ovary syndrome, *Lancet* 349:986, 1997.

87. **Ehrmann DA, Barnes RB, Rosenfield RL,** Polycystic ovary syndrome as a form of functional ovarian hyperandrogensim due to dysregulation of androgen secretion, *Endocr Rev* 16:322, 1995.

88. **Azziz R, Bradley Jr EL, Potter HD, Boots LR,** Adrenal androgen excess in women: lack of a role for 17-hydroxylase and 17,20-lyase dysregulation, *J Clin Endocrinol Metab* 80:400, 1995.

89. **Sahin Y, Kelestimur F,** 17-hydroxyprogesterone responses to gonadotrophin-releasing hormone agonist buserelin and adrenocorticotrophin in polycystic ovary syndrome: investigation of adrenal and ovarian cytochrome P450c17α dysregulation, *Hum Reprod* 12:910, 1997.

90. **Techatraisak K, Conway GS, Rumsby G,** Frequency of a polymorphism in the regulatory region of the 17α-hydroxylase-17,20-lyase (CYP17) gene in hyperandrogenic states, *Clin Endocrinol* 46:131, 1997.

91. **Archard C, Thiers J,** Le virilisme pilaire et son association a l'insuffisance glycolytique (diabete des femmes a barbe), *Bull Acad Natl Med* 86:51, 1921.

92. **Carmina E, Koyama T, Chang T, Stanczyk FZ, Lobo RA,** Does ethnicity influence the prevalence of adrenal hyperandrogenism and insulin resistance in polycystic ovary syndrome? *Am J Obstet Gynecol* 167:1807, 1992.

93. **Osei K, Schuster DP,** Ethnic differences in secretion, sensitivity, and hepatic extraction of insulin in black and white Americans, *Diabetic Med* 11:755, 1994.

94. **Norman RJ, Mahabeer S, Masters S,** Ethnic differences in insulin and glucose response to glucose between white and Indian women with polycystic ovary syndrome, *Fertil Steril* 63:58, 1995.

95. **Barbieri RL, Ryan KJ,** Hyperandrogenism, insulin resistance and acanthosis nigricans: a common endocrinopathy with distinct pathophysiologic features, *Am J Obstet Gynecol* 147:90, 1983.

96. **Dunaif A, Green G, Phelps RG, Lebwohl M, Futterweit W, Lewy L,** Acanthosis nigricans, insulin action, and hyperandrogenism: clinical, histological, and biochemical findings, *J Clin Endocrinol Metab* 73:590, 1991.

97. **Reavens GM,** Role of insulin resistance in human disease, *Diabetes* 37:1595, 1988.

98. **Poretsky L,** On the paradox of insulin-induced hyperandrogenism in insulin-resistant states, *Endocr Rev* 12:3, 1991.

99. **O'Meara NM, Blackman JD, Ehrman DA, Barnes RB, Jaspan JB, Rosenfeld RL, Polonsky KS,** Defects in beta-cell function in functional ovarian hyperandrogenism, *J Clin Endocrinol Metab* 76:1241, 1993.

100. **Dunaif A, Finegood DT,** β-Cell dysfunction independent of obesity and glucose intolerance in the polycystic ovary syndrome, *J Clin Endocrinol Metab* 81:942, 1996.

101. **Reaven GM, Lithell H, Landsberg L,** Hypertension and associated metabolic abnormalities — the role of insulin resistance and the sympathoadrenal system, *New Engl J Med* 334:374, 1996.

102. **Haffner SM, Valdez RA, Hazuda HP, Mitchell BD, Morales PH, Stern MP,** Prospective analysis of the insulin-resistance syndrome (syndrome X), *Diabetes* 41:715, 1992.

103. **Dahlgren E, Johansson S, Lindstedt G, Knutsson F, Oden A, Janson PO, Mattson L-A, Crona N, Lundberg P-A,** Women with polycystic ovary syndrome wedge resected in 1956 to 1965: a long-term follow-up focusing on natural history and circulating hormones, *Fertil Steril* 57:505, 1992.

104. **Zimmerman S, Phillips RA, Wikenfeld C, Dunaif A, Finegood D, Ardeljan M, Wallenstein S, Gorlin R, Krakoff L,** Polycystic ovary syndrome: lack of hypertension despite insulin resistance, *J Clin Endocrinol Metab* 75:508, 1992.

105. **Sampson M, Kong C, Patel A, Unwin R, Jacobs H,** Ambulatory blood pressure profiles and plasminogen activator inhibitor (PAI-1) activity in lean women with and without polycystic ovary syndrome, *Clin Endocrinol* 45:623, 1996.

106. **Schneider D, Sobel B,** Synergistic augmentation of expression of PAI-1 induced by insulin, VLDL, and fatty acids, *Coronary Artery Dis* 7:813, 1996.

107. **Imano E, Kadowaki H, Kadowaki T, Iwama N, Watarai T, Kawamori R, Kamada T, Taylor SI,** Two patients with insulin resistance due to decreased levels of insulin-receptor mRNA, *Diabetes* 40:548, 1991.

108. **Reddy SSK, Kahn CR,** Epidermal growth factor receptor defects in leprechaunism: a multiple growth factor resistant syndrome, *J Clin Invest* 84:1569, 1989.

109. **Kadowaki T, Kadowaki H, Rechler MM, Serrrano-Rios M, Roth J, Gorden P, Taylor SI,** Five mutant alleles of the insulin receptor gene in patients with genetic forms of insulin resistance, *J Clin Invest* 86:254, 1990.

110. **Ciaraldi TP, El-Roeiy A, Madar Z, Reichart D, Olefsky JM, Yen SSC,** Cellular mechanisms of insulin resistance in polycystic ovarian syndrome, *J Clin Endocrinol Metab* 75:577, 1992.

111. **Dunaif A, Xia J, Book C-B, Schenker E, Tang Z,** Excessive insulin receptor serine phosphorylation in cultured fibroblasts and in skeletal muscle: a potential mechanism for insulin resistance in the polycystic ovary syndrome, *J Clin Invest* 96:801, 1995.

112. **Sorbara LR, Tang Z, Cama Z, Xia J, Schenker E, Kohansi RA, Poretsky L, Koller E, Taylor SI, Dunaif A,** Absence of insulin receptor gene mutations in three women with the polycystic ovary syndrome, *Metabolism* 43:1568, 1994.

113. **Talbot JA, Bricknell EJ, Rajkhowa M, Drook A, O'Rahilly S, Clayton RN,** Molecular scanning of the insulin receptor gene in women with polycystic ovarian syndrome, *J Clin Endcrinol Metab* 81:1979, 1996.

114. **Brzechffa PR, Jakimiuk J, Agarwal SK, Weitsman SR, Buyalos RP, Magoffin DA,** Serum immunoreactive leptin concentrations in women with polycystic ovary syndrome, *J Clin Endocrinol Metab* 81:4166, 1996.

115. **Laughlin GA, Yen SSC,** Serum leptin levels in women with polycystic ovary syndrome: the role of insulin resistance/hyperinsulinemia, *J Clin Endocrinol Metab* 82:1692, 1997.

116. **Mantzoros CS, Dunaif A, Flier JS,** Leptin concentrations in the polycystic ovary syndrome, *J Clin Endocrinol Metab* 82:1687, 1997.

117. **Rouru J, Anttila L, Koskinen P, Penttilä T-A, Irjala K, Huupponen R, Koulu M,** Serum leptin concentrations in women with polycystic ovary syndrome, *J Clin Endocrinol Metab* 82:1697, 1997.

118. **Gennarelli G, Holte J, Wide L, Berne C, Lithell H,** Is there a role for leptin in the endocrine and metabolic aberrations of polycystic ovary syndrome? *Hum Reprod* 13:535, 1998.

119. **Nolan JJ, Olefsky JM, Nyce MR, Considine RV, Caro JF,** Effect of troglitazone on leptin production: studies in vitro and in human subjects, *Diabetes* 45:1276, 1996.

120. **Peiris AN, Sothmann MS, Aiman EJ, Kissebah AH,** The relationship of insulin to sex hormone binding globulin: role of adiposity, *Fertil Steril* 52:69, 1989.

121. **Kirschner MA, Samojlik E, Drejda M, Szmal E, Schneider G, Ertel N,** Androgen-estrogen metabolism in women with upper body versus lower body obesity, *J Clin Endocrinol Metab* 70:473, 1990.

122. **Pasquali R, Casimirri F, Balestra V, Flamia R, Melchionda N, Fabbri R, Barbara L,** The relative contribution of androgens and insulin in determining abdominal fat distribution in premenopausal women, *J Endocrinol Invest* 14:839, 1991.

123. **Lapidus L, Bengtsson C, Larsson B, Pennert K, Rybo E, Sjostrom L,** Distribution of adipose tissue and risk of cardiovascular disease and death: a 12 year follow up of participants in the population study of women in Gothenburg, *Br Med J* 289:1257, 1984.

124. **Ostlund Jr RE, Staten M, Kohrt W, Schultz J, Malley M,** The ratio of waist-to-hip circumference, plasma insulin level, and glucose intolerance as independent predictors for the HDL$_2$ cholesterol level in older adults, *New Engl J Med* 322:229, 1990.

125. **Deutsch MI, Mueller WH, Malina RM,** Androgyny in fat patterning is associated with obesity in adolescents and young adults, *Ann Hum Biol* 12:275, 1985.

126. **Must A, Jacques PF, Dallal GE, Bajema CJ, Dietz WH,** Long-term morbidity and mortality of overweight adolescents: a follow-up of the Harvard Growth Study of 1922 to 1935, *New Engl J Med* 327:1350, 1992.

127. **Chang RJ, Nakamura RM, Judd HL, Kaplan SA,** Insulin resistance in non-obese patients with polycystic ovarian disease, *J Clin Endocrinol Metab* 57:356, 1983.

128. **Jialal I, Naiker P, Reddi K, Moodley J, M JS,** Evidence for insulin resistance in nonobese patients with polycystic ovarian disease, *J Clin Endocrinol Metab* 64:1066, 1987.

129. **Dunaif A, Segal K, Futterweit W, Dobrjansky A,** Profound peripheral resistance independent of obesity in polycystic ovary syndrome, *Diabetes* 38:1165, 1989.

130. **Buyalos RP, Geffner ME, Bersch N, Judd HL, Watanabe RM, Bergman RN, Golde DW,** Insulin and insulin-like growth factor-I responsiveness in polycystic ovarian syndrome, *Fertil Steril* 57:796, 1992.

131. **Anttila L, Ding Y-Q, Ruutiainen K, Erkkola R, Irjala K, Huhtaniemi I,** Clinical features and circulating gonadotropin, insulin, and androgen interactions in women with polycystic ovarian disease, *Fertil Steril* 55:1057, 1991.

132. **Insler V, Shoham Z, Barash A, Koistinen R, Seppälä M, Hen M, Lunenfeld B, Zadik Z,** Polycystic ovaries in non-obese and obese patients: possible pathophysiological mechanism based on new interpretation of facts and findings, *Hum Reprod* 8:379, 1993.

133. **Dale PO, Tanbo T, Vaaler S, Abyholm T,** Body weight, hyperinsulinemia, and gonadotropin levels in the polycystic ovarian syndrome: evidence of two distinct populations, *Fertil Steril* 58:487, 1992.

134. **Homburg R, Pariente C, Lunenfeld B, Jacobs RS,** The role of insulin-like growth factor-I (IGF-I) and IGF binding protein-1 (IGFBP-1) in the pathogenesis of polycystic ovary syndrome, *Hum Reprod* 7:1379, 1992.

135. **Campbell PJ, Gerich JE,** Impact of obesity on insulin action in volunteers with normal glucose tolerance: demonstration of a threshold for the adverse effect of obesity, *J Clin Endocrinol Metab* 70:1114, 1990.

136. **Jahanfar S, Eden JA, Warren P, Seppälä M, Nguyen TV,** A twin study of polycystic ovary syndrome, *Fertil Steril* 63:478, 1995.

137. **Geffner ME, Kaplan SA, Bersch N, Golde DW, Landaw EM, Chang RJ,** Persistence of insulin resistance in polycystic ovarian disease after inhibition of ovarian steroid secretion, *Fertil Steril* 45:327, 1986.

138. **Grainger D, Thornton K, Rossi G, Connoly-Diamond M, DeFronzo R, Sherwin R, Diamond MP,** Influence of basal androgen levels in euandrogenic women on glucose homeostasis, *Fertil Steril* 58:1113, 1992.

139. **Dunaif A, Green G, Futterweit W, Dobrjansky A,** Suppression of hyperandrogenism does not improve peripheral or hepatic insulin resistance in the polycystic ovary syndrome, *J Clin Endocrinol Metab* 70:699, 1990.

140. **DeClue TJ, Shah SC, Marchese M, Malone JI,** Insulin resistance and hyperinsulinemia induce hyperandrogenism in a young type B insulin-resistant female, *J Clin Endocrinol Metab* 72:1308, 1991.

141. **Elkind-Hirsch KE, Valdes CT, McConnell TG, Malinak LR,** Androgen responses to acutely increased endogenous insulin levels in hyperandrogenic and normal cycling women, *Fertil Steril* 55:486, 1991.

142. **Smith S, Ravnikar VA, Barbieri RL,** Androgen and insulin response to an oral glucose challenge in hyperandrogenic women, *Fertil Steril* 48:72, 1987.

143. **Kiddy DS, Hamilton-Fairley D, Seppälä M, Koistinen R, James VHT, Reed MJ, Franks S,** Diet-induced changes in sex hormone binding globulin and free testosterone in women with normal or polycystic ovaries: correlation with serum insulin and insulin-like growth factor-I, *Clin Endocrinol* 31:757, 1989.

144. **Barbieri RL, Makris A, Ryan KJ,** Insulin stimulates androgen accumulation in incubations of human ovarian stroma and theca, *Obstet Gynecol* 64:73S, 1984.

145. **Barbieri RL, Makris A, Randall RW, Daniels G, Kistner RW, Ryan KJ,** Insulin stimulates androgen accumulation in incubations of ovarian stroma obtained from women with hyperandrogenism, *J Clin Endocrinol Metab* 62:904, 1986.

146. **Nestler JC, Barlascini CO, Matt DW, Steingold KA, Plymate SR, Clore JN, Blackard WG,** Suppression of serum insulin by diazoxide reduces serum testosterone levels in obese women with polycystic ovary syndrome, *J Clin Endocrinol Metab* 68:1027, 1989.

147. **Dale PO, Tanbo T, Djoseland O, Jervell J, Abyholm T,** Persistence of hyperinsulinemia in polycystic ovary syndrome after ovarian suppression by gonadotropin-releasing hormone agonist, *Acta Endocrinol* 126:132, 1992.

148. **Elkind-Hirsch KE, Valdes CT, Malinak LR,** Insulin resistance improves in hyperandrogenic women treated with Lupron, *Fertil Steril* 60:634, 1993.

149. **Moghetti P, Tosi F, Castello R, Magnani CM, Negri C, Brun E, Furiani L, Caputo M, Muggeo M,** The insulin resistance in women with hyperandrogenism is partially reversed by antiandrogen treatment: evidence that androgens impair insulin action in women, *J Clin Endocrinol Metab* 81:952, 1996.

150. **Fradkin JE, Eastman RC, Lesniak MA, Roth J,** Specificity spillover at the hormone receptor: exploring its role in human disease, *New Engl J Med* 320:640, 1989.

151. **Bergh C, Carlsson B, Olsson J-H, Selleskog U, Hillensjo T,** Regulation of androgen production in cultured human thecal cells by insulin-like growth factor I and insulin, *Fertil Steril* 59:323, 1993.

152. **Nestler JE,** Role of hyperinsulinemia in the pathogenesis of the polycystic ovary syndrome, and its clinical implications, *Seminars Reprod Endocrinol* 15:111, 1997.

153. **Willis D, Franks S,** Insulin action in human granulosa cells from normal and polycystic ovaries is mediated by the insulin receptor and not the type-I insulin-like growth factor receptor, *J Clin Endocrinol Metab* 80:3788, 1995.

154. **Willis D, Mason H, Gilling-Smith C, Franks S,** Modulation by insulin of follicle-stimulating hormone and luteinizing hormone actions in human granulosa cells of normal and polycystic ovaries, *J Clin Endocrinol Metab* 81:302, 1996.

155. **Nestler JE, Jakubowicz DJ, de Vargas AF, Brik C, Quintero N, Medina F,** Insulin stimulates testosterone biosynthesis by human thecal cells from women with polycystic ovary syndrome by activating its own receptor and using inositolglycan mediators as the signal transduction system, *J Clin Endocrinol Metab* 83:2001, 1998.

156. **Nestler JE, Powers LP, Matt DW, Steingold KA, Plymate SR, Rittmaster RS, Clore JN, Blackard WG,** A direct effect of hyperinsulinemia on serum sex hormone-binding globulin levels in obese women with the polycystic ovary syndrome, *J Clin Endocrinol Metab* 72:83, 1991.

157. **Plymate SR, Matej LA, Jones RE, Friedl KE,** Inhibition of sex hormone binding globulin production in human hepatoma (hep G2) cell line by insulin and prolactin, *J Clin Endocrinol Metab* 67:460, 1988.

158. **Singh A, Hamilton-Fairley D, Koistinen R, Seppälä M, James VHT, Franks S, Reed MJ,** Effect of insulin-like growth factor-I (IGF-I) and insulin on the secretion of sex hormone-binding globulin and IGF-binding protein (IGFBP-1) by human hepatoma cells, *J Endocrinol* 124:R1, 1990.

159. **Haffner SM, Valdez RA, Morales PA, Hazuda HP, Stern MP,** Decreased sex hormone-binding globulin predicts noninsulin-dependent diabetes mellitus in women but not in men, *J Clin Endocrinol Metab* 77:56, 1993.

160. **Conover CA, Lee PDK, Kanaley JA, Clarkson JT, Jensen MD,** Insulin regulation of insulin-like growth factor binding protein-1 in obese and nonobese humans, *J Clin Endocrinol Metab* 74:1355, 1992.

161. **Buyalos RP, Pekonen F, Halme JK, Judd HL, Rutanen EM,** The relationship between circulating androgens, obesity, and hyperinsulinemia in serum insulin-like growth factor binding protein-1 in the polycystic ovary syndrome, *Am J Obstet Gynecol* 172:932, 1995.

162. **Nestler JE,** Role of hyperinsulinemia in the pathogenesis of the polycystic ovary syndrome, and its clinical implications, *Seminars Reprod Endocrinol* 15:111, 1997.

163. **Legro RS, Muhleman D, Comings D, Lobo RA, Kovacs B,** D_3 receptor polymorphisms are associated with hyperandrogenic chronic anovulation and clomiphene citrate failure among female Hispanics, *Fertil Steril* 63:779, 1995.

164. **Prelevic GM, Wurzburger MI, Balint-Peric L, Nesic JS,** Inhibitory effect of sandostatin on secretion of luteinising hormone and ovarian steroids in polycystic ovary syndrome, *Lancet* 336:900, 1990.

165. **Velázquez EM, Mendoza S, Hamer T, Sosa F, Glueck CJ,** Metformin therapy in polycystic ovary syndrome reduces hyperinsulinemia, insulin resistance, hyperandrogenemia, and systolic blood pressure, while facilitating normal menses and pregnancy, *Metabolism* 43:647, 1994.

166. **Nestler JE, Jakubowicz DJ,** Decreases in ovarian cytochrome P450c17 alpha activity and serum free testosterone after reduction of insulin secretion in polycystic ovary syndrome, *New Engl J Med* 335:617, 1996.

167. **Velázquez EM, Mendoza SG, Wang P, Glueck CJ,** Metformin therapy is associated with a decrease in plasma plasminogen activator inhibitor-1, lipoprotein (a), and immunoreactive insulin levels in patients with the polycystic ovary syndrome, *Metabolism* 46:454, 1997.

168. **Velázquez E, Acosta A, Mendoza SG,** Menstrual cyclicity after metformin therapy in polycystic ovary syndrome, *Obstet Gynecol* 90:392, 1997.

169. **Diamanti-Kandarakis E, Kouli C, Tsianateli T, Bergiele A,** Therapeutic effects of metformin on insulin resistance and hyperandrogenism in polycystic ovary syndrome, *Eur J Endocrinol* 138:269, 1998.

170. **Nestler JE, Jakubowicz DJ, Evans WS, Pasquali R,** Effects of metformin on spontaneous and clomiphene-induced ovulation in the polycystic ovary syndrome, *New Engl J Med* 338:1876, 1998.

171. **Crave J-C, Fimbel S, Lejeune H, Cugnardey N, Dechaud H, Pugeat M,** Effects of diet and metformin administration on sex hormone-binding globulin, androgens, and insulin in hirsute and obese women, *J Clin Endocrinol Metab* 80:2057, 1995.

172. **Ehrmann DA, Cavaghan MK, Imperial J, Sturis J, Rosenfield RL, Polonsky KS,** Effects of metformin on insulin secretion, insulin action, and ovarian steroidogenesis in women with polycystic ovary syndrome, *J Clin Endocrinol Metab* 82:524, 1997.

173. **Açbay O, Gündogdu S,** Can metformin reduce insulin resistance in polycystic ovary syndrome? *Fertil Steril* 65:946, 1996.

174. **Nestler JE, Jakubowicz DJ,** Lean women with polycystic ovary syndrome respond to insulin reduction with decreases in ovarian P450c17α activity and serum androgens, *J Clin Endocrinol Metab* 82:4075, 1997.

175. **Dunaif A, Scott D, Finegood D, Quintana B, Whitcomb R,** The insulin-sensitizing agent troglitazone improves metabolic and reproductive abnormalities in the polycystic ovary syndrome, *J Clin Endocrinol Metab* 81:3299, 1996.

176. **Ehrmann DA, Schneider DJ, Sobel BE, Cavaghan MK, Imperial J, Rosenfield RL, Polonsky KS,** Troglitazone improves defects in insulin action, insulin secretion, ovarian steroidogenesis, and fibrinolysis in women with polycystic ovary syndrome, *J Clin Endocrinol Metab* 82:2108, 1997.

177. **Prunty FTG,** Hirsutism, virilism, and apparent virilism, and their gonadal relationships, *J Endocrinol* 38:203, 1967.

178. **Futterweit W, Dunaif A, Yeh HC, Kingsley P,** The prevalence of hyperandrogenism in 109 consecutive female patients with diffuse alopecia, *J Am Acad Dermatol* 19:831, 1988.

179. **Apter D, Butzow T, Laughlin GA, Yen SSC,** Metabolic features of polycystic ovary syndrome are found in adolescent girls with hyperandrogenism, *J Clin Endocrinol Metab* 80:2966, 1995.

180. **Ehrmann DA, Rosenfield RL, Barnes RB, Brigell DF, Sheikh Z,** Detection of functional ovarian hyperandrogensim in women with androgen excess, *New Engl J Med* 327:157, 1992.

181. **Fauser BCJM, Pache TD, Hop WCJ, de Jong FH, Dahl KD,** The significance of a single LH measurement in women with cycle disturbances: discrepancies between immunoreactive and bioactive hormone estimates, *Clin Endocrinol* 37:445, 1992.

182. **Pache TD, de Jong FH, Hop WC, Fauser BCJM,** Association between ovarian changes assessed by transvaginal sonography and clinical and endocrine signs of the polycystic ovary syndrome, *Fertil Steril* 59:544, 1993.

183. **Coulam CB, Annegers JF,** Breast cancer and chronic anovulation syndrome, *Surg Forum* 33:474, 1982.

184. **Coulam CB, Annegers JF, Krans JS,** Chronic anovulation syndrome and associated neoplasia, *Obstet Gynecol* 61:403, 1983.

185. **Ron E, Lunenfeld B, Menczer J, Blumstein T, Katz L, Oelsner G, Serr D,** Cancer incidence in a cohort of infertile women, *Am J Epidemiol* 125:780, 1987.

186. **Escobedo LG, Lee NC, Peterson HB, Wingo PA,** Infertility-associated endometrial cancer risk may be limited to specific subgroups of infertile women, *Obstet Gynecol* 77:124, 1991.

187. **Gammon MD, Thompson WD,** Infertility and breast cancer: a population-based case-control study, *Am J Epidemiol* 132:708, 1990.

188. **Gammon MD, Thompson WD,** Polycystic ovaries and the risk of breast cancer, *Am J Epidemiol* 134:818, 1991.

189. **Anderson KE, Sellers TA, Chen P-L, Rich SS, Hong C-P, Folsom AR,** Association of Stein-Leventhal syndrome with the incidence of postmenopausal breast carcinoma in a large prospective study of women in Iowa, *Cancer* 79:494, 1997.

190. **Garland M, Hunter DJ, Colditz GA, Manson JE, Stampfer MJ, Spiegelman D, Speizer F, Willett WC,** Menstrual cycle characteristics and history of ovulatory infertility in relation to breast cancer risk in a large cohort of US women, *Am J Epidemiol* 147:636, 1998.

191. **Farhi DC, Nosanchuk J, Silverberg SG,** Endometrial adenocarcinoma in women under 25 years of age, *Obstet Gynecol* 68:741, 1986.

192. **Dockerty MB, Lovelady SB, Faust GT,** Carcinoma of the corpus uteri in young women, *Am J Obstet Gynecol* 61:966, 1991.

193. **Gitsch G, Hanzal E, Jensen D, Hacker NF,** Endometrial cancer in premenopausal women 45 years and younger, *Obstet Gynecol* 85:504, 1995.

194. **Sagle M, Bishop K, Ridley N, Alexander FM, Michel M, Bonney RC, Beard RW, Franks S,** Recurrent early miscarriage and polycystic ovaries, *Br Med J* 297:1027, 1988.

195. **Regan L, Owen EJ, Jacobs HS,** Hypersecretion of luteinising hormone, infertility, and miscarriage, *Lancet* 336:1141, 1990.

196. **Tulppala M, Stenman U-H, Cacciatore B, Ylikorkala O,** Polycystic ovaries and levels of gonadotrophins and androgens in recurrent miscarriage: prospective study in 50 women, *Br J Obstet Gynaecol* 100:348, 1993.

197. **Wild RA, Painter PC, Coulson PB, Carruth KB, Ranney GB,** Lipoprotein lipid concentrations and cardiovascular risk in women with polycystic ovary syndrome, *J Clin Endocrinol Metab* 61:946, 1985.

198. **Wild RA, Van Nort JJ, Grubb B, Bachman W, Hartz A, Bartholomew M,** Clinical signs of androgen excess as risk factors for coronary artery disease, *Fertil Steril* 54:255, 1990.

199. **Graf MJ, Richards CJ, Brown V, Meissner L, Dunaif A,** The independent effects of hyperandrogenaemia, hyperinsulinaemia, and obesity on lipid and lipoprotein profiles in women, *Clin Endocrinol* 33:119, 1990.

200. **Conway GS, Agrawal R, Betteridge DJ, Jacobs HS,** Risk factors for coronary artery disease in lean and obese women with polycystic ovary syndrome, *Clin Endocrinol* 37:119, 1992.

201. **Wild RA, Alaupovic P, Parker IJ,** Lipid and apolipoprotein abnormalities in hirsute women. I. The association with insulin resistance, *Am J Obstet Gynecol* 166:1191, 1992.

202. **DiCarlo C, Shoham Z, MacDougall J, Patel A, Hall ML, Jacobs HS,** Polycystic ovaries as a relative protective factor for bone mineral loss in young women with amenorrhea, *Fertil Steril* 57:314, 1992.

203. **Talbott E, Guzick DS, Clerici A, Berga S, Detre K, Weimer K, Kuller L,** Coronary heart disease risk factors in women with polycystic ovary syndrome, *Arterioscler Thromb Vasc Biol* 15:821, 1995.

204. **Guzick DS, Talbott EO, Sutton-Tyrrell K, Herzog HC, Kuller LH, Wolfson Jr SK,** Carotid atherosclerosis in women with polycystic ovary syndrome: initial results from a case-control study, *Am J Obstet Gynecol* 174:1224, 1996.

205. **Birdsall MA, Farquhar CM, White HD,** Association between polycystic ovaries and extent of coronary artery disease in women having cardiac catheterization, *Ann Intern Med* 126:32, 1997.

206. **Korytkowski MT, Mokan M, Horwitz MJ, Berga SL,** Metabolic effects of oral contraceptives in women with polycystic ovary syndrome, *J Clin Endocrinol Metab* 80:3327, 1995.

207. **Diamanti-Kandarakis E, Mitrakou A, Raptis S, Tolis G, Duleba AJ,** The effect of a pure antiandrogen receptor blocker, flutamide, on the lipid profile in the polycystic ovary syndrome, *J Clin Endocrinol Metab* 83:2699, 1998.

208. **Azziz R,** The hyperandrogenic-insulin-resistant acanthosis nigricans syndrome: therapeutic response, *Fertil Steril* 61:570, 1994.

209. **Gaspard UJ, Lefebvre PJ,** Clinical aspects of the relationship between oral contraceptives, abnormalities in carbohydrate metabolism, and the development of cardiovascular disease, *Am J Obstet Gynecol* 163:334, 1990.

210. **Duffy TJ, Ray R,** Oral contraceptive use: Prospective follow-up of women with suspected glucose intolerance, *Contraception* 30:197, 1984.

211. **Hannaford PC, Kay CR,** Oral contraceptives and diabetes mellitus, *Br Med J* 299:315, 1989.

212. **Stampfer MJ, Willett WC, Coldtiz GA, Speizer FE, Hennekens CH,** Past use of oral contraceptives and cardiovascular disease: a meta-analysis in the context of the Nurses' Health Study, *Am J Obstet Gynecol* 163:285, 1990.

213. **Colditz GA, and the Nurses' Health Study Research Group,** Oral contraceptive use and mortality during 12 years of follow-up: the Nurses' Health Study, *Ann Intern Med* 120:821, 1994.

214. Kjos SL, Shoupe D, Douyan S, Friedman RL, Bernstein GS, Mestman JH, Mishell Jr DR, Effect of low-dose oral contraceptives on carbohydrate and lipid metabolism in women with recent gestational diabetes: results of a controlled, randomized, prospective study, *Am J Obstet Gynecol* 163:1822, 1990.

215. Kjos SL, Peters RK, Xiang A, Thomas D, Schaefer U, Buchanan TA, Contraception and the risk of type 2 diabetes in Latino women with prior gestational diabetes, *JAMA* 280:533, 1998.

216. Garg SK, Chase HP, Marshall G, Hoops SL, Holmes DL, Jackson WE, Oral contraceptives and renal and retinal complications in young women with insulin-dependent diabetes mellitus, *JAMA* 271:1099, 1994.

217. Petersen KR, Skouby SO, Sidelmann J, Mølsted-Petersen L, Jespersen J, Effects of contraceptive steroids on cardiovascular risk factors in women with insulin-dependent diabetes mellitus, *Am J Obstet Gynecol* 171:400, 1994.

218. Nader S, Riad-Gabriel MG, Saad M, The effect of a desogestrel-containing oral contraceptive on glucose tolerance and leptin concentrations in hyperandrogenic women, *J Clin Endocrinol Metab* 82:3074, 1997.

219. Ramsay LE, Yeo WW, Jackson PR, Influence of diuretics, calcium antagonists, and alpha-blockers on insulin sensitivity and glucose tolerance in hypertensive patients, *J Cardiovasc Phys* 20S:49, 1992.

220. Diamanti-Kandarakis E, Mitrakou A, Hennes MM, Platanissiotis D, Kaklas N, Spina J, Georgiadou E, Hoffman RG, Kissebah AH, Raptis S, Insulin sensitivity and antiandrogenic therapy in women with polycystic ovary syndrome, *Metabolism* 44:525, 1995.

221. Slowinska-Srzednicka J, Zgliczynski S, Wierzbicki M, Srzednicki M, Stopinska-Gluszak U, Zgliczynski W, Soszynski P, Chotkowska E, Bednarska M, Sadowski Z, The role of hyperinsulinemia in the development of lipid disturbances in non-obese and obese women with the polycystic ovary syndrome, *J Endocrinol Invest* 14:569, 1991.

222. Dunaif A, Hyperandrogenic anovulation (PCOS): a unique disorder of insulin action associated with an increased risk of non-insulin-dependent diabetes mellitus, *Am J Med* 98(Suppl 1A):33S, 1995.

223. Lanzone A, Fulghesu AM, Cucinelli F, Guido M, Pavone V, Caruso A, Mancuso S, Preconceptional and gestational evaluation of insulin secretion in patients with polycystic ovary syndrome, *Hum Reprod* 11:2382, 1996.

224. Holte J, Gennarelli G, Wide L, Lithell H, Berne C, High prevalence of polycystic ovaries and associated clinical, endocrine, and metabolic features in women with previous gestational diabetes mellitus, *J Clin Endocrinol Metab* 83:1143, 1998.

225. Fox R, Wardle PG, Clarke L, Hull MGR, Acromegaloid bone changes in severe polycystic ovarian disease: an effect of hyperinsulinaemia? *Br J Obstet Gynaecol* 98:410, 1991.

226. Giudice LC, Dsupin BA, Jin IH, Vu TH, Hoffman AR, Differential expression of messenger ribonucleic acids encoding insulin-like growth factors and their receptors in human uterine endometrium and decidua, *J Clin Endocrinol Metab* 76:1115, 1993.

227. Pasquali R, Antenucci D, Casimirri F, Venturoli S, Paradisi R, Fabbri R, Balestra V, Melchiondra N, Barbara L, Clinical and hormonal characteristics of obese amenorrheic hyperandrogenic women before and after weight loss, *J Clin Endocrinol Metab* 68:173, 1989.

228. Kiddy DS, Hamilton-Fairley D, Bush A, Short F, Anyaoku V, Reed MJ, Franks S, Improvement in endocrine and ovarian function during dietary treatment of obese women with polycystic ovary syndrome, *Clin Endocrinol* 36:105, 1992.

229. Guzick DS, Wing R, Smith D, Berga S, Winters SJ, Endocrine consequences of weight loss in obese, hyperandrogenic anovulatory women, *Fertil Steril* 61:598, 1994.

230. Andersen P, Selifeflot I, Abdelnoor M, Arnese H, Dale PO, Lovik A, Birkeland K, Increased insulin sensitivity and fibrinolytic capacity after dietary intervention in obese women with polycystic ovary syndrome, *Metabolism* 44:611, 1995.

231. Jakubowicz DJ, Nestler JE, 17α-Hydroxyprogesterone responses to leuprolide and serum androgens in obese women with and without polycystic ovary syndrome after dietary weight loss, *J Clin Endocrinol Metab* 82:556, 1997.

232. Clark AM, Ledger W, Galletly C, Tomlinson L, Blaney F, Wang X, Norman RJ, Weight loss results in significant improvement in pregnancy and ovulation rates in anovulatory obese women, *Hum Reprod* 10:2705, 1995.

233. Hollmann M, Runnebaum B, Gerhard I, Effects of weight loss on the hormonal profile in obese, infertile women, *Hum Reprod* 11:1884, 1996.

234. Clark AM, Thornley B, Tomlinson L, Galletley C, Norman RJ, Weight loss in obese infertile women results in improvement in reproductive outcome for all forms of fertility treatment, *Hum Reprod* 13:1502, 1998.

235. Muscelli E, Camastra S, Catalano C, Galvan AQ, Ciociaro D, Baldi S, Ferrannini E, Metabolic and cardiovascular assessment in moderate obesity: effect of weight loss, *J Clin Endocrinol Metab* 82:2937, 1997.

236. Bates GW, Egerman RS, Umstot ES, Buster JE, Casson PR, Dehydroepiandrosterone attenuates study-induced declines in insulin sensitivity in postmenopausal women, *Ann NY Acad Sci* 774:291, 1995.

237. Ovesen P, Moller J, Ingerslev HJ, Jørgensen JOL, Mengel A, Schmitz O, Alberti KGMM, Moller N, Normal basal and insulin-stimulated fuel metabolism in lean women with the polycystic ovary syndrome, *J Clin Endocrinol Metab* 77:1636, 1993.

238. Ehrmann DA, Sturis J, Byrne MM, Karrison T, Rosenfield RL, Polonsky KS, Insulin secretory defects in polycystic ovary syndrome. Relationship to insulin sensitivity and family history of non-insulin-dependent diabetes mellitus, *J Clin Invest* 96:520, 1995.

239. Ashwell M, Chinn S, Stalley S, Garrow JS, Female fat distribution — a simple classification based on two circumference measurements, *Int J Obesity* 6:143, 1982.

240. Ashwell M, Cole TJ, Dixon AK, Obesity: new insight into the anthropometric classification of fat distribution shown by computed tomography, *Br Med J* 290:1692, 1985.

241. Pouliot MC, Despres JP, Lemieux S, Moorjani S, Bouchard C, Tremblay A, Nadeau A, Lupren PJ, Waist circumference and abdominal sagittal diameter: best simple anthropometric indexes of abdominal visceral adipose tissue accumulation and related cardiovascular risk in men and women, *Am J Cardiol* 73:460, 1994.

242. Lean MEJ, Han TS, Durenberg P, Predicting body composition by densitometry from simple anthropometric measurements, *Am J Clin Nutr* 63:4, 1996.

243. Bloch CA, Clemons P, Sperling MA, Puberty decreased insulin sensitivity, *J Pediatr* 110:481, 1987.

244. Savage MO, Smith CP, Dunger DB, Gale EA, Holly JM, Preece MA, Insulin and growth factors adaptation to normal puberty, *Horm Res* 3:70, 1992.

245. Ibáñez L, Potau N, Virdis R, Zampolli M, Terzi C, Gussinye M, Carrascosa A, Vicens-Calvet E, Postpubertal outcome in girls diagnosed of premature pubarche during childhood: increased frequency of functional ovarian hyperandrogenism, *J Clin Endocrinol Metab* 76:1599, 1993.

246. Ibáñez L, Potau N, Georgopoulos N, Prat N, Gussinye M, Carrascosa A, Growth hormone, insulin-like growth factor-I axis, and insulin secretion in hyperandrogenic adolescents, *Fertil Steril* 64:1113, 1995.

247. **Laakso M,** How good a marker is insulin level for insulin resistance? *Am J Epidemiol* 137:959, 1993.

248. **Legro RS, Finegood D, Dunaif A,** A fasting glucose to insulin ratio is a useful measure of insulin sensitivity in women with polycystic ovary syndrome, *J Clin Endocrinol Metab* 83:2694, 1998.

249. **Legro RS, Kunselman AR, Dodson WC, Dunaif A.** Prevalence and predictors of risk for type 2 diabetes mellitus and impaired glucose tolerance in polycystic ovary syndrome: a prospective, controlled study in 254 affected women, *J Clin Endocrinol Metab* 84:165, 1999.

250. **Govind A, Obhral MS, Clayton RN,** Polycystic ovaries are inherited as an autosomal dominant trait: analysis of 29 polycystic ovary syndrome and 10 control families, *J Clin Endocrinol Metab* 84:38, 1999.

13 Hirsutism

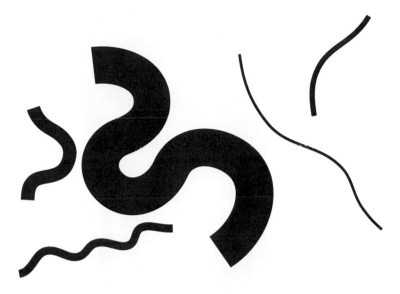

Hirsutism, excessive facial and body hair caused by excess androgen production, is usually associated with anovulatory ovaries and loss of cyclic menstrual function. The more severe states of virilism (clitoromegaly, deepening of the voice, balding, and changes in body habitus) are rarely seen and usually are secondary to adrenal hyperplasia or androgen-producing tumors of adrenal or ovarian origin. Although these are rare, diagnostic evaluation is required.

A concerned and sympathetic approach must be offered to women who complain of hirsutism. The responsible clinician must view hirsutism both as an endocrine problem and as a cosmetic problem. To the affected woman, hair growth over the face, abdomen, or breasts is disturbing on several levels. Is there disease? Is sexuality changing? Is social acceptance altered? Is fertility impaired?

This chapter reviews the biology of hair growth and the endocrine causes that can yield hirsutism. An uncomplicated, effective program for diagnostic evaluation and therapeutic management is presented.

The Biology of Hair Growth[1]

Embryology

Each hair follicle develops at about 8–10 weeks of gestation as a derivative of the epidermis. It is composed initially of a solid column of cells that proliferates from the basal layers of the epidermis and protrudes downward into the dermis. As the column elongates it encounters a cluster of mesodermal cells (the dermal papilla) that it envelops at its bulbous tip (bulb). The solid epithelial column then hollows out to form a hair canal, and the pilosebaceous apparatus (a hair follicle, sebaceous glands, and arrector pili muscles) is laid down.

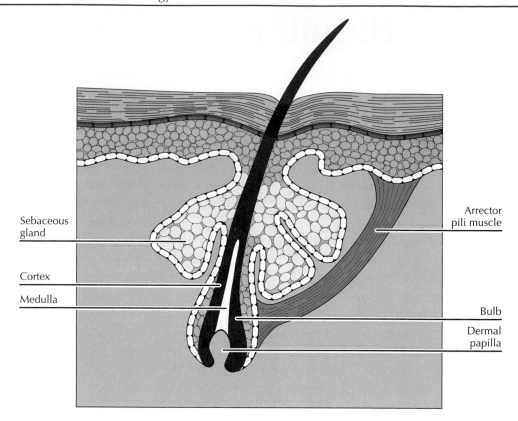

Hair growth begins with proliferation of the epithelial cells at the base of the column in contact with the dermal papilla. The ***lanugo hair*** that covers the fetus is lightly pigmented, thin in diameter, short in length, and fragile in attachment. Important to note is the fact that the total endowment of hair follicles is made at an early gestational stage (by 22 weeks) and no new hair follicles will be produced de novo. The concentration of hair follicles laid down per unit area of facial skin does not differ materially between sexes but does differ between races and ethnic groups (Caucasian > Oriental; Mediterranean > Nordic). In addition, hair growth differences between races probably reflect hair follicle differences in 5α-reductase activity (the production of the active androgen, dihydrotestosterone).[2] The pattern of hair growth is genetically predetermined.

Structure and Growth

Hair does not grow continuously but, rather, in a cyclic fashion with alternating phases of activity and inactivity. The cycles are referred to by the following terms:

> **Anagen — the growing phase.**
> **Catagen — rapid involution phase.**
> **Telogen — quiescent phase.**

In the resting phase (telogen), the hair is short and loosely attached to the base (the bulb) of the epithelial canal. As growth begins (anagen), epithelial matrix cells at the base begin to proliferate and extend downward into the dermis. The epithelial column elongates some 4–6 times from the resting state. Once downward extension is completed, continued rapid growth of the matrix cells pushes upward to the skin surface. The tenuous contact of the previous hair is broken, and that hair is shed. The superficial matrix cells differentiate forming a keratinized column. Growth continues as long as active mitoses persist in the basal matrix cells. When finished (catagen), the column shrinks, the bulb shrivels, and the resting state is reachieved (telogen).

The length of hair is primarily determined by duration of the growth phase (anagen). Scalp hair remains in anagen for 3 years and has only a relatively short resting phase. Elsewhere (forearm) a short anagen and long telogen will lead to short hair of stable nongrowing length. The appearance of continuous growth (or periodic shedding) is determined by the degree to which individual hair follicles act asynchronously with their neighbors. Scalp hair is asynchronous and, therefore, always seems to be growing. The resting phase that some hairs (10–15%) are in is not apparent. If marked synchrony is achieved, then all hairs may undergo telogen at the same time leading to shedding that is called *telogen effluvium*. Occasionally, women will complain of marked hair loss from the scalp, but this time period of shedding is usually limited (6–8 months), and growth resumes when asynchrony is re-established. *However, it is worthwhile to rule out thyroid disease with a TSH measurement.*

Hypertrichosis is a generalized increase in hair of the fetal lanugo type, associated with the use of drugs or malignancy. *Vellus hair* is the downy, unpigmented hair associated with the prepubertal years. *Terminal hair* is the coarse, pigmented hair that grows on various parts of the body during the adult years. Hirsutism implies a vellus to terminal hair transformation.

Factors That Influence Hair Growth

The dermal papilla is the director of the events that control hair growth. Despite major injury to the epithelial component of the follicle (such as freezing, x-rays, or a skin graft), if the dermal papilla survives, the hair follicle will regenerate and regrow hair. Injury to or degeneration of the dermal papilla (such as that achieved with properly performed electrolysis) is the crucial factor in permanent hair loss.

Sexual hair is defined as hair that responds to the sex steroids. Sexual hair grows on the face, lower abdomen, anterior thighs, the chest, the breasts, the pubic area, and in the axillae. Once androgen influences hair follicles in sexual areas and larger, longer, more pigmented hair is induced, these final hair characteristics recur in typical cycles of activity and inactivity, even in the absence of sustaining androgen. Androgenic stimulation of the hair follicle requires the conversion of testosterone to dihydrotestosterone, and therefore the sensitivity of the hair follicle to androgens is determined by the level of 5α-reductase activity. The individual variability in hair response is believed to reflect genetic differences in 5α-reductase activity.

From animal studies and human disease patterns, the following list of hormonal effects can be compiled:

1. Androgens, particularly testosterone, initiate growth, increase the diameter and pigmentation of the keratin column, and probably increase the rate of matrix cell mitoses in all but scalp hair.

2. Estrogens act essentially opposite from androgens, retarding the rate and initiation of growth, and leading to finer, less pigmented and slower growing hair. In the mouse, estrogen arrests hair follicles in the telogen phase of the cycle.[3]

3. Progestins have minimal direct effects on hair.

4. Pregnancy (high estrogen and progesterone) can increase the synchrony of hair growth, leading to periods of growth or shedding.

An important clinical characteristic of hair growth can be understood from studies of the effects of castration. If castration occurs before puberty, the male will not grow a beard. If castration occurs after puberty with beard and sexual hair distribution fully developed, then these hairs continue to grow albeit more slowly and with finer caliber. Androgen stimulates sexual hair follicle conversion from lanugo to terminal adult hair growth patterns, but *once established, these patterns persist despite withdrawal of androgen.*

Sexual and nonsexual hair growth can be affected by endocrine problems. In hypopituitarism, there is marked reduction of hair growth. Acromegaly will be associated with hirsutism in 10–15% of patients. Although the impact of thyroid hormone is not clear, hypothyroid individuals sometimes display scalp alopecia as well as less axillary, pubic, and curiously, lateral eyebrow hair. 5α-Reductase activity is stimulated by insulin-like growth factor-I (IGF-I).[4] Increased IGF-I activity in anovulatory patients with insulin resistance and hyperinsulinemia can intensify the hirsute response in these hyperandrogenic patients.

Hair growth can be influenced by nonhormonal factors, such as local skin temperature, blood flow, and edema. Hair grows faster in the summer than in the winter.[5] Hair growth can be seen in association with central nervous system (CNS) pathology such as encephalitis, cranial trauma, multiple sclerosis, and with certain drugs.

Androgen Production

The production rate of testosterone in the normal female is 0.2 to 0.3 mg/day. Approximately 50% of testosterone is derived from peripheral conversion of androstenedione, whereas the adrenal gland and ovary contribute approximately equal amounts (25%) to the circulating levels of testosterone, except at midcycle when the ovarian contribution increases by 10–15%. Dehydroepiandrosterone sulfate (DHAS) arises almost exclusively from the adrenal gland, while 90% of dehydroepiandrosterone (DHA) is from the adrenal.

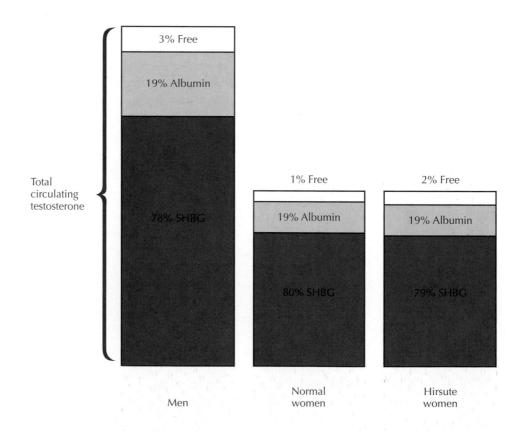

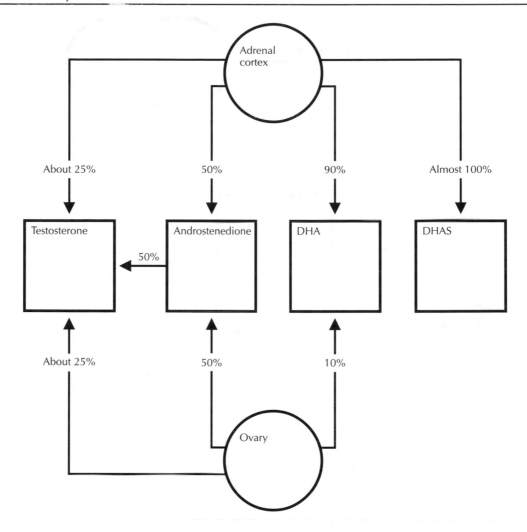

About 80% of circulating testosterone is bound to a beta-globulin known as sex steroid hormone-binding globulin (SHBG). In women, approximately 19% is loosely bound to albumin, leaving about 1% unbound. Androgenicity is dependent mainly on the unbound fraction and partly upon the fraction associated with albumin. DHA, DHAS, and androstenedione are not significantly protein bound, and routine immunoassay reflects their biologically available hormone activity. This is not the case with testosterone because routine assays measure the total testosterone concentration, bound and unbound.

SHBG production in the liver is decreased by androgens. Hence, the binding capacity in men is lower than in normal women, and 2–3% of testosterone circulates in the free, active form in men. SHBG is decreased by insulin, and increased by estrogens and thyroid hormone. Therefore, binding capacity is increased in women with hyperthyroidism, in pregnancy, and by estrogen-containing medication. In a hirsute woman, the SHBG level is depressed by the excess androgen (and, when present, by hyperinsulinemia), and the percent free and active testosterone is elevated as is the metabolic clearance rate of testosterone. The total testosterone concentration, therefore, can be in the normal range in a woman who is hirsute. However, there is little clinical need for a specific assay for the free portion of testosterone. The very presence of hirsutism or masculinization indicates increased androgen effects. One can reliably interpret a normal total testosterone level in these circumstances as being compatible with decreased binding capacity and increased free testosterone.

In hirsute women, only 25% of the circulating testosterone arises from peripheral conversion, and most is due to direct glandular secretion. Indeed, data overwhelmingly indicate that the ovary is the major source of increased testosterone and androstenedione in hirsute women.[6] The most common cause of hirsutism in women is persistent anovulation and excessive androgen production by the ovaries. Adrenal causes are most uncommon.

3α-Androstanediol Glucuronide

Although testosterone is the major circulating androgen, dihydrotestosterone (DHT) is the major nuclear androgen in many sensitive tissues, including hair follicles and the pilosebaceous unit in skin. 3α-Androstanediol is the peripheral tissue metabolite of DHT, and its glucuronide, 3α-androstanediol glucuronide (3α-AG) has been utilized as a marker of target tissue cellular action.[7, 8] There is an excellent correlation between the serum levels of 3α-AG and the clinical manifestations of androgens. Specifically, 3α-AG correlates with the level of 5α-reductase activity (testosterone and androstenedione to dihydrotestosterone) in the skin.

Thus, there are 3 principal laboratory measurements of *potential* clinical use for the evaluation of androgen excess:

1. Testosterone — a measure of ovarian and adrenal activity.

2. DHAS — a measure of adrenal activity.

3. 3α-AG — a measure of peripheral target tissue activity.

Hirsutism is not a disorder of hair; rather, it reflects increased 5α-reductase activity which produces more DHT, leading to the stimulation of hair growth. This enzyme activity is increased by an increased availability of precursor (the circulating level of testosterone, therefore, is a primary factor) or by still unknown local tissue mechanisms. Measurement of 3α-AG has revealed that true idiopathic hirsutism may not exist (or at least it is very rare). In the presence of other laboratory measurements that are normal, increased levels of 3α-AG indicate an increased activity of 5α-reductase in the peripheral compartment.[9] However, 3α-AG also reflects hepatic conjugation activity and the impact of major precursors that are derived from the adrenal gland and not from peripheral sources.[10] Therefore 3α-AG is not solely a measure of cutaneous androgen metabolism.

There are 2 reasons why the measurement of 3α-AG is not part of the routine clinical approach to the problem of hirsutism. First, it is not an absolute measurement. Values in hirsute women overlap the normal range by about 20%. Second, and most importantly, the ultimate diagnosis and therapy of the problem are not affected by this test.

Prostate-Specific Antigen

The prostate-specific antigen (PSA) is a serine protease, produced in the prostate gland, and used as a tumor marker for the diagnosis and management of prostate cancer. PSA has also been detected in female tissues, and using a very sensitive assay, circulating levels of PSA can be measured in women. Because androgens increase the expression of the PSA gene, it is reasonable to expect hyperandrogenic women to have increased circulating levels of PSA. Indeed, circulating levels of PSA are higher in hirsute women and are correlated with 3α-AG levels.[11] These elevated levels do not respond to ovarian and adrenal stimulation or ovarian suppression, indicating a widespread origin.[12] However, at the present time, there is no clinical application for PSA measurements in women.

Evaluation of Hirsutism

Cosmetically disturbing hirsutism is the end result of a number of factors:

1. The number of hair follicles present (Asian women bearing androgen-producing tumors rarely are hirsute because of the low concentration of hair follicles per unit skin area).

2. The degree to which androgen has converted resting vellus hair to terminal adult hair.

3. The ratio of the growth to resting phases in affected hair follicles.

4. The asynchrony of growth cycles in aggregates of hair follicles.

5. The thickness and degree of pigmentation of individual hairs.

The primary factor in hirsutism is an increase in androgen levels (usually testosterone) that produces an initial growth stimulus and then acts to sustain continued growth. Essentially, every woman with hirsutism will have an increased production rate of testosterone and androstenedione.[13]

Anovulatory women who are not hirsute can often be found to have laboratory evidence of increased androgen production.[14] However, the most common complaint voiced by women and associated with increased androgen production is hirsutism. This is followed in order by acne and increased oiliness of the skin, increased libido, clitoromegaly, and, finally, masculinization. Masculinization and virilization are terms reserved for extreme androgen effects (usually, but not always, associated with a tumor) leading to the development of a male hair pattern, clitoromegaly, deepening of the voice, increased muscle mass, and general male-like body habitus. The Ferriman-Gallwey scoring system used to quantify the amount of hirsutism is of little clinical use, and it is reserved for studies of hirsutism, but even for this purpose, it is limited by subjective variability.[15]

Alopecia can be a vexing problem for patient and clinician. In many instances, alopecia is a temporary phenomenon, a response of the scalp hair to some change that has induced a period of synchronous hair growth and loss. This can be a response to acute, stressful events. Telogen effluvium often occurs near the end of a pregnancy or postpartum. With time, usually 6 months to a year, the scalp hair becomes asynchronous again and the hair thickens. In a series of consecutive patients presenting with diffuse alopecia, the majority had no evidence of hirsutism or menstrual dysfunction; however, anovulation with polycystic ovaries was the most common problem, and nearly 40% demonstrated hyperandrogenism.[16] Patients complaining of alopecia deserve evaluation for hyperandrogenism because a significant number of them can be appropriately treated. In addition, a laboratory survey is indicated for thyroid dysfunction or chronic illness. However, because alopecia reflects increased scalp 5α-reductase activity, normal circulating hormone levels should not preclude treatment.[17, 18] Hair loss is also a consequence of aging, beginning in both sexes about the age of 50.[19]

Acne is another sign of increased androgen activity. Up to 60% of women with acne who have normal circulating levels of androgens display evidence of increased 5α-reductase activity in the pilosebaceous unit.[20] These are the women who benefit from antiandrogenic treatment.

Acanthosis nigricans in an overweight patient with hirsutism is a reliable clinical marker of insulin resistance and hyperinsulinemia. This gray–brown velvety discoloration of the skin is usually present at the neck, groin, and axillae; however, the vulva is a very common site in hirsute women.[21] Acanthosis nigricans indicates the need to determine the state of glucose metabolism, as discussed in Chapter 12. Serious consideration should be given to the presence of hyperinsulinemia in hyperandrogenic women.

The most common clinical problem is the hirsute woman with irregular menses, with the onset of hirsutism during teenage years or in the early 20s, and long, gradual worsening of the condition. About 70% of anovulatory women develop hirsutism. The picture is so characteristic that a careful history is often sufficient for the diagnosis.

A good history can reveal some of the rare causes of hirsutism: environmental factors producing chronic irritation or reactive hyperemia of the skin, the use of drugs, changes associated with Cushing's syndrome or acromegaly, or even the presence of pregnancy (indicating the possibility of a luteoma). Hair-stimulating drugs include methyltestosterone, anabolic agents such as Nilevar or Anavar, phenytoin, diazoxide, danazol, cyclosporin, and minoxidil. Hirsutism associated with drugs that are not androgens typically consists of fine hairs distributed diffusely over the trunk and face (hypertrichosis). The 19-nortestosterones in the current low-dosage oral contraceptives rarely (if ever) cause acne or hirsutism. Postmenopausal women being treated with androgens can develop hirsutism despite low doses. Dehydroepiandrosterone, available as a food supplement, increases testosterone levels in women and can cause hirsutism and acne, even at the lowest doses.

Especially important in the history is the rapidity of development. A woman who develops hirsutism after the age of 25 and demonstrates very rapid progression of masculinization over several months usually has an androgen-producing tumor.

Late-onset adrenal hyperplasia caused by an enzymatic deficiency *presenting* in adult life is rare. Classical congenital adrenal hyperplasia that can lead to hirsutism is usually diagnosed and treated prior to puberty. Hirsutism in childhood is usually caused by classical congenital adrenal hyperplasia or androgen-producing tumors. Genetic problems, such as Y-containing mosaics or incomplete androgen sensitivity, will produce signs of androgen stimulation at puberty.

Virilization during pregnancy raises the suspicion of a luteoma, which is not a true tumor but an exaggerated reaction of the ovarian stroma to normal levels of chorionic gonadotropin.[22] The solid luteoma is unilateral in 45% of cases and associated with a normal pregnancy. Theca-lutein cysts (also called ***hyperreactio luteinalis***) seen with trophoblastic disease are virtually always bilateral. Maternal virilization occurs in 30% of pregnancies with theca-lutein cysts. Hyperreactio luteinalis can also be seen with the high human chorionic gonadotropin (HCG) titers associated with multiple gestation. Because a luteoma regresses postpartum, the only risk is masculinization of a female fetus; a risk not reported with theca-lutein cysts.[23, 24] Luteomas cause maternal virilization in 35% of the cases, and in these pregnancies, about 80% of female fetuses will exhibit some signs of masculinization. Subsequent pregnancies are usually normal, but maternal virilization is occasionally recurrent.[25] There have been several rare case reports of recurrent maternal virilization during pregnancy associated with hyperthecosis or polycystic ovaries.[26] These cases should also be regarded as examples of hyperreactio luteinalis.

Androgen-secreting ovarian tumors are very rarely encountered during pregnancy, probably because the excess androgen usually suppresses ovulation.[23, 24] Ultrasonographic evaluation of the pelvis in women experiencing virilization in pregnancy is very helpful. Malignancy is frequently encountered when a solid unilateral ovarian lesion is present.

Hirsutism, therefore, is usually associated with persistent anovulation (Chapter 12). Although anovulatory ovaries are usually the source of excess androgens, a minimal workup is necessary, dedicated to ruling out the adrenal sources and tumors. It should be emphasized that hospitalization for extensive evaluation of hirsutism is required only rarely.

The Diagnostic Workup for Hirsutism

The initial laboratory evaluation of hirsutism consists of assays for the blood levels of testosterone and 17α-hydroxyprogesterone (17-OHP). We no longer consider the measurement of DHAS to be necessary (discussed later). As part of the evaluation for anovulation, prolactin levels and thyroid function should be assessed, careful examination of the breasts for the presence of galactorrhea is important, and an aspiration endometrial biopsy should be considered. A thyroid-stimulating hormone (TSH) screen is also indicated in women complaining of alopecia. In addition, consideration should be directed to the possible presence of hyperinsulinemia. *Patients with intense androgen action may be amenorrheic due to endometrial suppression (with a decidual response) and may not demonstrate withdrawal bleeding after a progestational challenge.*

Cushing's syndrome can present with hirsutism, and later, masculinization. Remember that one of the most common referral diagnoses is Cushing's syndrome, but this is one of the least common final diagnoses. When clinical suspicion is high, a screen for Cushing's syndrome is indicated.

The Screen for Cushing's Syndrome

Cushing's syndrome is the persistent oversecretion of cortisol. It can develop in 5 different ways: pituitary adrenocorticotropic hormone (ACTH) overproduction (Cushing's disease), ectopic ACTH overproduction by tumors, autonomous cortisol secretion by the adrenal or, very rarely, ovarian tumors, or a fifth extremely rare possibility, the secretion of corticotropin-releasing hormone (CRH) by a tumor. A clinician must first make the diagnosis of Cushing's syndrome (excessive cortisol secretion) before determining the etiology.[27]

The most useful measurements in the basal state to detect Cushing's syndrome are the 24-hour urinary free cortisol excretion (10–90 μg) and the late evening plasma cortisol level (less than 15 μg/dL). The urinary excretion of 17-ketosteroids and 17-hydroxysteroids and measurement of morning and afternoon plasma cortisol levels are less reliable because of a significant overlap between normal and abnormal patients.

We prefer to start with the single-dose overnight dexamethasone test. Dexamethasone (1 mg) is given orally at 11 PM, and a plasma cortisol is drawn at 8:00 the next morning. A value less than 5 μg/dL rules out Cushing's syndrome. Cushing's syndrome is unlikely with intermediate values between 5 and 10 μg/dL, whereas a value higher than 10 μg/dL is diagnostic of adrenal hyperfunction. The number of patients with Cushing's syndrome who show a normal suppression in the single-dose overnight test is negligible (less than 1%).[28] Obese patients, however, have a false-positive rate up to 13%.

If the single-dose overnight test is abnormal, establish the diagnosis by measuring the 24-hour urinary free cortisol. The low-dose, 2-day suppression test provides final confirmation. Dexamethasone (0.5 mg every 6 hours) is administered for 2 consecutive days after 2 days of baseline 24-hour urinary 17-hydroxysteroid and free cortisol measurements. Patients with Cushing's will not lower their urinary 17-hydroxysteroids below 2.5 mg/day and the free cortisol below 10 μg on the second day of dexamethasone suppression. Combining the low-dose test with the 24-hour urinary free cortisol should definitely provide the diagnosis of Cushing's syndrome. A 24-hour urinary free cortisol greater than 250 μg is virtually diagnostic of Cushing's syndrome, and a urinary free cortisol greater than 200 μg/day provides 90% diagnostic accuracy.

Pseudo-Cushing's states exist in patients with mild hypercortisolism due to conditions such as alcoholism, response to stress, anorexia and bulimia nervosa, severe obesity, and depression. Although usually not necessary, combining the low-dose dexamethasone suppression test with CRH stimulation is an accurate method to distinguish the real syndrome from the hypercortisolism associated with these other conditions.[29] After two days of low-dose dexamethasone

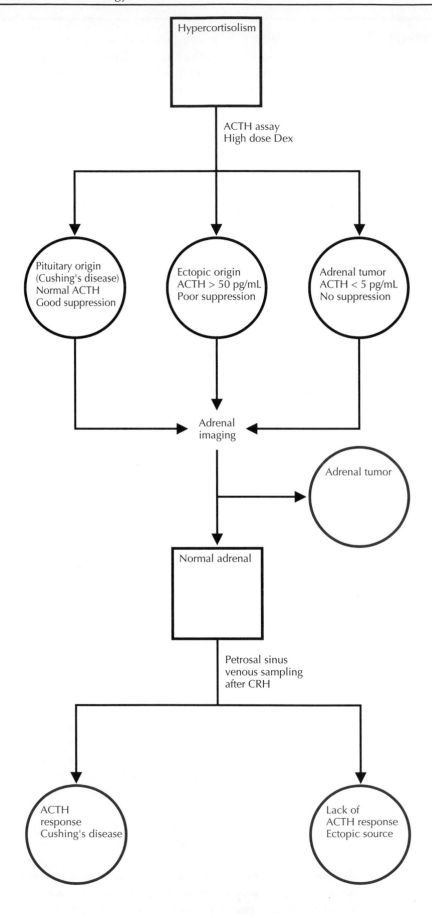

suppression, a single plasma cortisol level is obtained 15 minutes after administering CRH (1 μg/kg) intravenously. A 15-minute cortisol level greater than 1.4 μg/dL requires further evaluation.

The etiology of Cushing's syndrome can be established by combining a high dose dexamethasone suppression test with measurement of the basal state blood ACTH level. Dexamethasone (2 mg every 6 hours) is administered for 2 days, and the urinary 17-hydroxysteroid and cortisol levels on the second day are compared with basal levels. If basal ACTH is less than 5 pg/mL, and the urinary steroids do not decrease by at least 40%, an adrenal tumor is likely. When ACTH is measurable in the blood (more than 20 pg/mL), an ectopic ACTH-producing tumor is unlikely if the urinary steroids decrease by at least 40%. Cushing's disease is present when the blood ACTH level is in the normal range, a chest x-ray is normal, and imaging detects an abnormal sella turcica. A level of plasma ACTH greater than 50 pg/mL suggests ectopic ACTH release; a level less than 5 pg/mL suggests an autonomous cortisol-secreting tumor.

Imaging is very accurate and reliable in detecting adrenal tumors.[30] In addition, imaging reliably predicts which patients have ectopic ACTH-producing tumors by detecting bilateral adrenal enlargement in such patients. CT scanning of the adrenal glands provides better resolution and is preferred over MRI and ultrasonography.

The evaluation of a patient with Cushing's syndrome can yield inconclusive results, and a failure to recognize an occult, ectopic ACTH-secreting neoplasm can lead to unnecessary pituitary or adrenal surgery. Bilateral venous sampling from the inferior petrosal sinus (sampling the blood draining from the pituitary gland) for the measurement of ACTH before and after CRH stimulation is an effective means to achieve accurate diagnosis of a pituitary origin for the ACTH.[31–33] Approximately 15% of patients with ACTH-dependent Cushing's syndrome will have an occult, ectopic source for the ACTH. Most of these ACTH-secreting lesions are in the thorax (usually small-cell lung carcinoma), some in the abdomen.[34] Petrosal sinus sampling is recommended in all patients with ACTH-dependent Cushing's syndrome who do not have an obvious adrenal tumor on imaging.[35]

A very rare cause of Cushing's syndrome is the autonomous production of cortisol by an ovarian tumor.[36] Chest and abdominal imaging is recommended for all atypical presentations.

Assessment of Insulin Secretion

Hyperandrogenism and hyperinsulinemia are commonly associated, as discussed in detail with complete references in Chapter 12. In many patients, a disorder in insulin action precedes the increase in androgens. Hyperinsulinemia can directly augment thecal cell androgen production in the ovary, and in addition, hyperinsulinemia contributes to the hyperandrogenism by inhibiting hepatic synthesis of sex hormone-binding globulin and insulin-like growth factor binding protein-1, actions that increase free testosterone levels and augment IGF-I stimulation of thecal androgen synthesis, respectively.

Weight loss reduces both hyperinsulinemia and hyperandrogenism, and is often followed by a return to ovulatory function. The use of oral agents such as troglitazone and metformin for the treatment of these patients offers great promise. Overweight, hyperandrogenic and hyperinsulinemic, anovulatory women must be counseled regarding their increased risk of future diabetes mellitus and cardiovascular disease.

The mechanism of hyperandrogenism can be attributed to hyperinsulinemia in an occasional case in which the circumstances are hard to understand; for example, the onset of hirsutism in an elderly woman who is found to have hyperthecosis in the ovaries. The appearance of hirsutism in such a case is not due to an ovarian response to hypergonadotropism but, rather, to the development of hyperinsulinemia.

For these reasons, we make the following recommendations:

All anovulatory women who are hyperandrogenic should be assessed for insulin resistance and glucose tolerance with measurements of:

1. **The fasting glucose:insulin ratio, followed by**
2. **The 2-hour glucose level after a 75 g glucose load:**

normal	less than 140 mg/dL
impaired	140–199 mg/dL
noninsulin-dependent diabetes mellitus	200 mg/dL and higher

In women who continue to manifest this disorder, periodic surveillance is necessary. The frequency is uncertain, but annual assessment is appropriate in women who continue to be obese.

Unfortunately, testing for hyperinsulinemia is not straightforward. Clinical guidelines for the interpretation of insulin levels and response to glucose loading have not been established. Because there is considerable overlap between normal women and patients with anovulation and polycystic ovaries, it is reasonable to assume that all overweight, anovulatory women with polycystic ovaries are hyperinsulinemic. Nevertheless, we recommend the measurement of the ratio of fasting glucose to fasting insulin in order to provide evidence that lends credence and importance to counseling efforts. *A ratio of less than 4.5 is consistent with insulin resistance.*[37]

The DHAS Level

DHAS circulates in higher concentration than any other steroid and is derived almost exclusively from the adrenal gland. It is, therefore, a direct measure of adrenal androgen activity, correlating clinically with the urinary 17-ketosteroids.[38] The upper limit of normal in most laboratories is 350 µg/dL, but, because of laboratory variation, attention must be paid to the local range of normal.

A random sample of DHAS is sufficient for the evaluation of hirsutism, needing no corrections for body weight, creatinine excretion, or episodic variation. Variations are minimized because of its high circulating concentration and its long half-life. A slow turnover rate results in a large and stable pool in the blood with insignificant variation. Elevated levels of DHAS contribute to the clinical problem of hirsutism because DHAS serves as a prehormone in hair follicles, providing substrate for the hair follicle synthesis of androgens.[39]

Aging is associated with a decrease in the blood concentration of DHAS. The decrease accelerates after menopause, and DHAS is almost undetectable after age 70.[40] This decline is 4 times greater than the age-related decline in cortisol, which is further support for the contention that cortisol and DHAS secretion are separately controlled.

Both 17-ketosteroids and circulating levels of DHAS are elevated in association with hyperprolactinemia.[41, 42] The levels return to normal with prolactin suppression by dopamine agonist treatment. In addition, increased free testosterone levels associated with decreased SHBG are often found in hyperprolactinemic women.[43, 44] This underscores the need to search for galactorrhea and to obtain a prolactin measurement in all anovulatory women. The androgen changes are probably secondary to the persistent anovulatory state induced by the elevated prolactin, although direct prolactin effects on the adrenal, ovary, or SHBG are possible.

When the DHAS level is normal, adrenal disease is most unlikely, and the diagnosis of excess androgen production by the ovaries is likely. There are only rare cases of adrenal tumors with normal DHAS levels, and further evaluation of such cases would be indicated by the presence of markedly elevated blood levels of testosterone.[45] These rare tumors are responsive to luteinizing hormone (LH), suggesting that they are derived from embryonic rest cells. Nonclassical (late-onset) adrenal hyperplasia commonly is not associated with an increased level of DHAS; the diagnosis of this condition relies on the measurement of 17-OHP for screening.

The clinical problem with DHAS measurements in the evaluation of hirsutism is the frequent finding of a moderately elevated DHAS level in anovulatory patients with polycystic ovaries. This is similar to the moderate elevations of 17-ketosteroids encountered in these patients. If the 17-OHP level is normal, we believe that it is not worthwhile to subject these patients to a search for an adrenal enzyme defect. Clinical experience has established that moderate elevations of DHAS are associated with anovulation; suppression of ovarian function restores the DHAS level to normal.

A DHAS level of 700 µg/dL or greater has been accepted as a marker for abnormal adrenal function. But how often is a DHAS of this level encountered? *DHAS levels of 700 µg/dL or more are confronted so rarely that we must now question the clinical usefulness of measuring DHAS. We cannot identify a single case in our experience in which the DHAS level changed patient management. Even if a DHAS of 700 µg/dL or greater is encountered, we believe that the adrenal secretion of extremely high levels of DHAS will be associated with high levels of testosterone, either by direct secretion or by peripheral conversion of the DHAS. Therefore, in the absence of Cushing's syndrome, we believe that measurement of testosterone will suffice to screen for adrenal abnormalities. An imaging assessment of the adrenal glands whenever a markedly elevated testosterone is encountered will be more cost-effective than measuring DHAS in all hirsute women.*

Nonclassical Adrenal Hyperplasia

Congenital adrenal hyperplasia is due to an enzyme defect leading to excessive androgen production. This severe condition, with its prenatal onset, is inherited in an autosomal recessive fashion (discussed in Chapter 9). A milder form of the disease, appearing later in life, has been designated by a variety of adjectives, including late-onset, partial, nonclassical, attenuated, and acquired adrenal hyperplasia.[46, 47] An asymptomatic form, cryptic adrenal hyperplasia, is revealed only with biochemical testing.

Although each of the enzymatic steps from cholesterol to cortisol can be affected in specific clinical disease, the most common enzymes to be deficient are 21-hydroxylase (p450c21), 11β-hydroxylase (p450c11), and 3β-hydroxysteroid dehydrogenase.

The 21-Hydroxylase Defect

Women with late-onset adrenal hyperplasia due to a 21-hydroxylase deficiency respond to ACTH stimulation in a moderate fashion, between the classical homozygote response and the mild heterozygote reaction (see the 17-OHP nomogram). A 21-hydroxylase deficiency is now recognized to be the most common autosomal recessive disorder, surpassing cystic fibrosis and sickle cell anemia.[48] The clinical presentation is extremely variable, and the symptoms may appear and disappear over time. Therefore, the diagnosis requires laboratory evaluation as discussed under "The 17-OHP Level." The genetic diagnosis for known mutations in the CYP21 gene is discussed in Chapter 9.

There are at least 3 reasons that make it worthwhile to seek the correct diagnosis:

1. Therapy should be accurately applied because it must be long-term.

2. Pregnant couples with this condition require genetic counseling for the prenatal diagnosis and possible treatment of the congenital form of the disease, as well as the assessment of asymptomatic offspring. However, without knowing the father's carrier status, an accurate estimate of risk is impossible. Although the risk of having a child with congenital adrenal hyperplasia is very low, the couple should consider paternal testing for heterozygosity. If the father tests positively, prenatal diagnosis and treatment would be reasonable.

3. Theoretically, these patients might be subject to cortisol deficiency during severe stress; however, to our knowledge this has not been a clinical problem.

Other Enzyme Defects

The 3β-hydroxysteroid (type II) dehydrogenase deficiency exists in both the ovaries and adrenals. This defect precludes significant androgen production; however, this enzyme activity appears to remain intact in peripheral tissues. Therefore, hirsutism seen with this deficiency is probably due to target tissue conversion of the increased secretion of precursors.[49] Unlike 21-hydroxylase deficiency, no genetic markers are currently available; diagnosis requires ACTH stimulation and demonstration of an altered 17α-hydroxypregnenolone to 17-OHP ratio. Some argue that late-onset 3β-hydroxysteroid dehydrogenase deficiency is encountered more frequently than 21-hydroxylase deficiency.[50] However, although an exaggerated 17α-hydroxypregnenolone response to ACTH stimulation is common in women with hyperandrogenism, the response is consistent with adrenal hyperactivity and not an enzyme deficiency.[51] Furthermore, molecular studies fail to find mutations in the genes for the two 3β-hydroxysteroid dehydrogenase enzymes in patients who appear to have mild to moderate deficiencies in 3β-hydroxysteroid dehydrogenase.[52, 53] We believe that this deficiency is so subtle that accurate diagnosis is not essential. Our usual therapeutic approach to hirsutism will be effective. The 11β-hydroxylase deficiency is quite rare, and it is usually diagnosed at a younger age (Chapter 9). It is not worth measuring the 11-deoxycortisol response to ACTH stimulation in adult hirsute women in an effort to detect this rare deficiency.[54]

The 17-OHP Level

From 1 to 5% of women who complain of hirsutism display a biochemical response that is consistent with the less severe form of adrenal hyperplasia of the 21-hydroxylase variety.[55–57] This relative frequency of late-onset adrenal hyperplasia dictates routine 17-OHP screening of women who complain of hirsutism. On the other hand, the routine use of the ACTH stimulation test is not warranted.[55, 58] Heterozygosity for CYP21 mutations does not increase the risk of clinically significant hirsutism.[59]

Besides using the 17-OHP screen to make a cost-effective decision regarding ACTH stimulation, one can be swayed by pertinent clinical findings.[60] A strong family history of androgen excess suggests the presence of an inherited disorder. Hirsutism due to an adrenal enzyme defect usually is more severe and begins at a young age, typically at puberty. Short stature and very high blood levels of androgens also signify a more severe problem. Finally, it is worth considering the following: ***With normal baseline steroid levels, even if a woman has a subtle enzyme defect, the management of the problem does not require its discovery.***

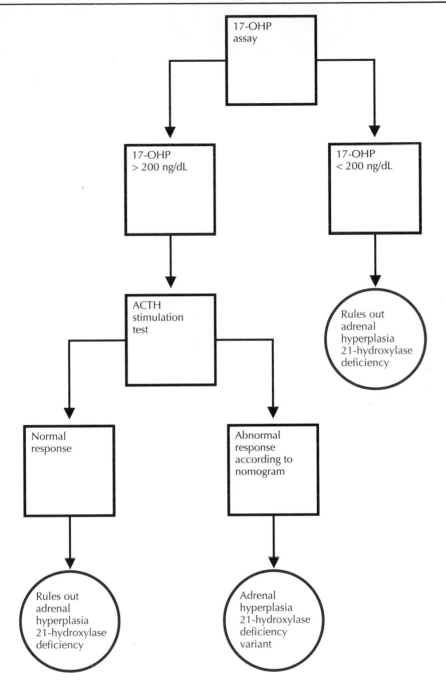

17-OHP must be measured first thing in the morning to avoid later elevations due to the diurnal pattern of ACTH secretion. The baseline 17-OHP level should be less than 200 ng/dL.[58] Levels greater than 200 ng/dL, but less than 800 ng/dL, require ACTH testing. Levels over 800 ng/dL are virtually diagnostic of the 21-hydroxylase deficiency. The DHAS level is usually normal. The hallmarks of late-onset adrenal hyperplasia are elevated levels of 17-OHP and a dramatic increase after ACTH stimulation.[56] However, the elevated baseline levels of 17-OHP are often not impressive (e.g., overlapping with those found in women with polycystic ovaries due to anovulation), and a simple ACTH stimulation test must be utilized.

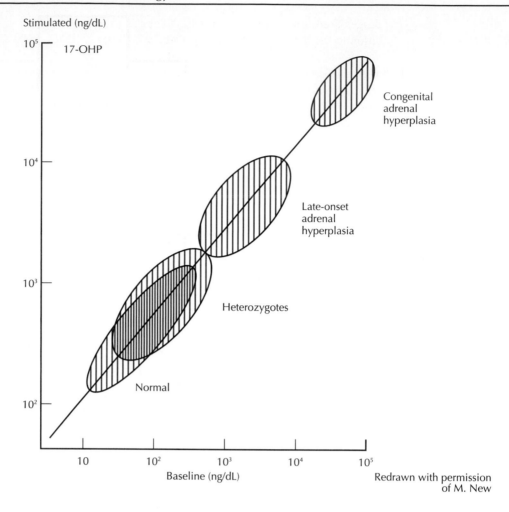

Stimulated (ng/dL)

Redrawn with permission
of M. New

The ACTH Stimulation Test

Synthetic ACTH (Cortrosyn) is administered intravenously in a dose of 250 μg. Blood samples for the measurement of 17-OHP are obtained at time 0 and again at 1 hour. The testing must be performed in the morning (8 AM), but it can be scheduled at any time during the menstrual cycle. The 1 hour value is plotted on the nomogram which predicts the genotype of homozygote and heterozygote forms of the 21-hydroxylase deficiency.[61] Dexamethasone pretreatment the night before is not necessary.[62] Heterozygote carriers for 21-hydroxylase deficiency have ACTH-stimulated levels of 17-OHP up to 1000 ng/dL; patients with late-onset deficiency have stimulated levels above 1200 ng/dL.

For the diagnosis of the 3β-hydroxysteroid dehydrogenase deficiency, the same ACTH stimulation test is utilized, measuring 17-OHP and 17-hydroxypregnenolone. An abnormal 17-hydroxypregnenolone/17-OHP ratio is usually greater than 6.0.[49] This deficiency is also usually marked by a significant elevation of DHAS in the face of normal or mildly elevated testosterone levels. In the 11β-hydroxylase deficiency, the level of 11-deoxycortisol will be increased; it is normal with the 21-hydroxylase defect.

The Adrenal Gland and Anovulation

Adrenal involvement in the syndrome of anovulation and hirsutism has long been recognized. Adrenal suppression, for example, will induce regular menses and ovulation in some patients, and empiric treatment with glucocorticoids has been advocated in the past.

Late-onset adrenal hyperplasia does not explain every anovulatory woman encountered with a moderate elevation in DHAS. The important clinical question is the following: is excessive androgen secretion by the adrenal gland a primary disorder in these women, or is it a secondary reaction to the hormonal milieu associated with anovulation?

One possibility is that the adrenal hyperactivity (as indicated by elevated DHAS levels) is due to an estrogen-induced 3β-hydroxysteroid dehydrogenase insufficiency. Considerable effort has been devoted to demonstrating an estrogen influence on adrenal androgen secretion. Unfortunately there is no clear-cut conclusion, with both positive[63–67] and negative[68–72] results reported.

This picture may be similar to that of the fetal adrenal gland. Studies have demonstrated that the low level of 3β-hydroxysteroid dehydrogenase activity and high secretion of DHAS by the fetal adrenal cortex are due to estrogen.[73, 74] Inconsistent with this explanation is the fact that ACTH levels in adult anovulatory women are not elevated;[75, 76] however, the period of increased ACTH response would exist only until normal cortisol levels are re-achieved (a new set point). Indeed, studies of anovulatory women with elevated levels of DHAS indicate that the increase in adrenal activity is because of a mechanism within the adrenal gland, not because of an increase in pituitary response to CRH and not because of increased adrenal response to ACTH stimulation.[77]

The activity of 3β-hydroxysteroid dehydrogenase is inhibited by both androgens and estrogens in concentrations to be expected within the adrenal gland but difficult to achieve with exogenous administration; changes in adrenal secretion, therefore, can reflect varying action of steroids, especially estrogen, in different layers of the adrenal cortex.[78] The failure to affect adrenal steroidogenesis with the exogenous administration of androgens is consistent with this hypothesis.[79] Thus, it remains attractive to explain adrenal hyperactivity seen in anovulatory women as a secondary reaction induced and maintained by the constant estrogen state associated with persistent anovulation. Indeed, in patients with polycystic ovaries and increased adrenal androgen activity, a correlation can be demonstrated between adrenal sensitivity to ACTH and estrogen levels.[80] This relationship, however, may be the result of mechanisms other than inhibition of 3β-hydroxysteroid dehydrogenase (see discussion of the fetal adrenal gland in Chapter 8).

Suppression of ovarian function by treatment with a GnRH agonist has been utilized in hopes of bringing clarity to this puzzle by assessing adrenal function after elimination of ovarian steroid production. Short-term suppression (3–6 months) has been reported to have no impact on adrenal androgen production.[81, 82] However, these studies did not include women with high levels of DHAS. When anovulatory women with levels of DHAS greater than normal are treated with a gonadotropin-releasing hormone (GnRH) agonist for at least 3 months, in some women, but not all, the elevated DHAS levels are suppressed.[83, 84] Thus, the exact nature of the adrenal-ovarian relationship in these women may vary, consistent with the clinical heterogeneity characteristic of these patients. It has been suggested that increased adrenal androgen production in some women is secondary to P450c17 17,20 lyase hyperactivity, and in others it is an acquired response due to the anovulatory hormonal steady state.[84–86] In those women with P450c17 hyperactivity, the underlying disorder may be hyperinsulinemia.[87]

Regardless of differences in weight, diet, race, and environmental factors, excess adrenal androgen activity is present in one-half to two-thirds of anovulatory women and hyperinsulinemia in approximately 70%.[88] It makes sense that similar growth factor modulation takes place in adrenal steroid-producing cells as in the ovary. Women with polycystic ovaries (both obese and nonobese) and hyperinsulinemia have a greater steroidogenic response to ACTH than anovulatory patients with normal insulin levels.[89]

Insulin and IGF-I receptors are present on adrenal cells. The infusion of insulin into women causes a decrease in DHAS, and hyperinsulinemia inhibits adrenal 17,20 lyase (P450c17) activity, suggesting that insulin decreases the production of this adrenal androgen.[90, 91] It is further suggested that the age-related decline in DHAS may be related to increasing insulin resistance.[92] How do these changes relate to DHAS levels in anovulatory women, levels that range from normal to moderately elevated? A simple inverse relationship between insulin and adrenal androgen levels in anovulatory women does not exist.[93] Furthermore, in a study of 92 consecutive women with hirsutism, the steroidogenic response to ACTH stimulation was not consistent with an inherent disorder of P450c17.[94]

An ovulatory response following the treatment of anovulatory women with dexamethasone can be explained in part by a contribution made to ovarian androgen production by circulating DHAS. A significant percentage of testosterone production by the ovarian follicle can be attributed to circulating DHAS serving as a substrate or prehormone.[95] Thus, dexamethasone suppression cannot separate adrenal and ovarian testosterone secretion in that the two glands are involved in a complex interaction, with DHAS providing at least one mechanism for this interaction.

The inconclusiveness of this situation and the rarity of a true adrenal enzyme deficiency in adult women make a cost-effective argument against routine endocrine testing. Accordingly, we have adopted a 17-OHP level of 200 ng/dL, below which we do not pursue the possibility of a primary adrenal enzyme problem, and we now find little use for DHAS measurements. Mild adrenal enzyme defects can be treated by our usual methods and do not require glucocorticoid administration.

The Testosterone Level

Plasma testosterone levels (normal 20–80 ng/dL) are elevated in the majority of women (70%) with anovulation and hirsutism. Individual variation is great, however, largely because of the changes in the testosterone-binding capacity of the sex hormone-binding globulin in the blood. Because the binding globulin levels are depressed by androgen and insulin, the total testosterone concentration can be in the normal range in a woman who is hirsute even though the percent unbound and active testosterone is elevated. Indeed, the unbound or free testosterone is approximately twice normal (an increase from 1% to 2%) in women with anovulation and polycystic ovaries.[96] Therefore, a normal total testosterone level in hirsute women is still consistent with elevated androgen production rates.

It is not necessary to measure the free testosterone (a technically difficult and expensive assay) because a routine total testosterone assay adequately serves the purpose of screening for testosterone-secreting tumors. Such tumors are associated with testosterone levels that are usually in the male range, and, therefore, the fine discrimination of the free testosterone level is unnecessary.[97, 98] *If the testosterone level exceeds 200 ng/dL, an androgen-producing tumor must be suspected.*

The arbitrary cutoff point has been challenged because variations in secretion can yield misleading values, and not all androgen-producing tumors will be this active, and some women with polycystic ovaries (especially hyperthecosis) will have testosterone levels greater than 200 ng/dL.[99, 100] Nevertheless, the combination of the patient's historical chronology of the development of hirsutism, the pelvic examination, and the 200 ng/dL testosterone level will provide accurate diagnosis in virtually all cases. *A patient with an acute, rapid course of virilizing symptoms requires a full evaluation for the presence of an androgen-producing tumor even if the testosterone concentration is less than the cutoff level.*

Be aware that testosterone levels are significantly elevated during normal pregnancy. Levels are greater than 100 ng/dL in the first trimester and reach 500 to 800 ng/dL by term.[101] This is mainly due to the estrogen-induced increase in sex hormone-binding globulin; however, even the free testosterone level is elevated in the third trimester. Mother and fetus are protected from these high androgen levels by many mechanisms, including binding to sex hormone-binding globulin and placental aromatization of androgens to estrogens.

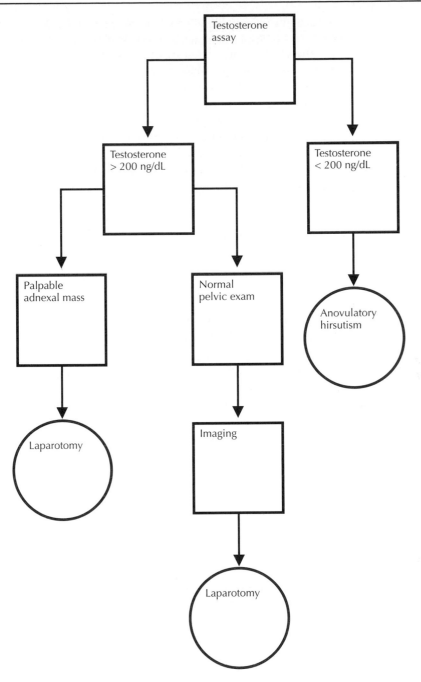

Androgen-Producing Tumors

There are two findings that should stimulate the clinician to suspect the presence of an androgen-producing tumor. One is a history of rapidly progressive masculinization. Hirsutism associated with anovulation is generally slow to develop, usually covering a time period of at least several years. Tumors are associated with a short time course, measured in months. The second finding that should arouse suspicion is a testosterone level greater than 200 ng/dL.

In our view, androgen-producing tumors are one of medicine's vastly overrated problems. First, they are incredibly rare, yet they attract an inordinate amount of attention at our meetings and a disproportionate number of printed pages in texts and journals. Second, there is an endocrine mystique surrounding the functioning tumor. Actually it is a straightforward problem.

Functioning ovarian tumors are almost all palpable, and like any ovarian mass, rapid laparotomy and surgical removal are in order. It is well recognized, however, that very small ovarian tumors (usually in the hilus of the ovary) can secrete testosterone. And occasionally, virilization is encountered with a nonfunctional tumor due to tumor stimulation of androgen secretion in the surrounding stromal tissue.[102]

The only diagnostic dilemma is when to explore the patient in whom a mass is not palpable. Suppression and stimulation tests are known to falsely lead to oophorectomy in the presence of a virilizing adrenal adenoma.[98] In addition, suppression and stimulation methods do not specifically isolate ovarian or adrenal function.[102, 103] Ovarian androgen-producing tumors are responsive to LH and, therefore, will respond to ovarian suppression and stimulation.[104–106]

Selective angiography with venous sampling and measurement of adrenal and ovarian steroids is not without problems. It is technically difficult to achieve bilateral catheterization of the ovaries, steroid secretion is episodic (especially by the adrenal glands), and the technique is not without risk. Selective retrograde catheterization of ovarian and adrenal veins by an expert should be reserved for those few patients who have been imaged with negative findings and yet the clinical history is suggestive of a tumor. Surgical exploration and bivalving of the ovaries may be necessary if the catheterization studies are negative. However, a surgical approach requires the presence of an appropriately rapid appearance of virilizing signs.

In postmenopausal women with hyperandrogenism, it is usually appropriate to be more aggressive surgically; however, keep in mind that hyperinsulinemia in the postmenopausal years can stimulate hyperthecosis, which would simulate the presentation of a tumor.[107] GnRH agonist treatment can avoid surgery in these patients because insulin-induced steroidogenic activity in the ovary is still LH-dependent.

When an androgen-producing tumor is suspected and an adnexal mass is not palpable, imaging of the adrenal glands and ovaries should be obtained. Imaging of the adrenal is a sensitive diagnostic technique for small tumors that produce Cushing's syndrome as well as for virilizing adrenal adenomas.[30, 98] For adrenal imaging, CT scanning provides better resolution and is preferred over MRI and ultrasonography. For ovarian imaging, transvaginal ultrasonography is the method of choice.

The Incidental Adrenal Mass

Adrenal masses will be discovered incidentally in approximately 10% of postmortem examinations, and therefore, it is to be expected that an incidental adrenal mass will be discovered occasionally with abdominal imaging.[108] Bilateral lesions are more serious. Common causes of bilateral lesions are metastatic cancer (most commonly from breast, kidney, or lung), infection (tuberculous and fungal), and adrenal hyperplasia; hence, surgery is rarely indicated. A primary malignancy of the adrenal is usually associated with excess secretion of glucocorticoids and androgens. The size of a lesion is significant.[109] The probability of malignancy roughly parallels the diameter of the lesion. Bilateral lesions less than 3 cm usually are due to metastatic disease. Thus, the current recommendation is to excise unilateral masses if they are of significant size, usually greater than 4 cm in diameter. Fine needle aspiration is also recommended for all unilateral adrenal lesions, after excluding a pheochromocytoma, to rule out metastatic lesions.[108] When following a mass, imaging should be performed at 3, 9, and 18 months. Any mass that is stable after 18 months can be left in place.

Incidental adrenal masses require evaluation for biochemical function. The presence of hypertension raises the suspicion of Cushing's syndrome, hyperaldosteronism, or pheochromocytoma. The evaluation should include a screening test for pheochromocytoma (24-hour urinary catecholamines), electrolyte, aldosterone, and renin activity assessment for aldosteronism, a 24-

hour urinary free cortisol, and a testosterone level. If these tests are normal, subclinical hormone secretion can be present. A relatively high incidence of cortisol-secreting tumors in the presence of normal 24-hour urinary free cortisol excretion indicates the need to perform an overnight dexamethasone suppression test in patients with asymptomatic incidental adrenal masses.[110] There appears to be a high incidence of adrenal masses in patients with adrenal hyperplasia, presumably because of chronic excess ACTH stimulation. These need not be removed surgically, but a laboratory evaluation for adrenal hyperplasia is, therefore, indicated in patients with incidental adrenal masses to avoid unnecessary surgery.[111] Finally, the clonidine suppression test is useful to diagnose a subclinical pheochromocytoma. Adrenal scintigraphy uses radiotracers accumulated by functioning tissue and is recommended when biochemical testing is normal.[109] When uptake in the mass is less than in the contralateral adrenal (a "discordant" pattern), fine-needle aspiration is indicated to rule out a malignant lesion.

Screening Tests for Incidental Adrenal Masses

24-hour urinary catecholamines and free cortisol

Testosterone

Renin activity, aldosterone, and electrolytes

Provocative Tests for Subclinically Active Incidental Adrenal Masses

Dexamethasone overnight suppression test

17-Hydroxyprogesterone response to ACTH

Clonidine suppression test (clonidine, 0.3 mg p.o in a supine position, followed by plasma norepinephrine levels at 0, 2, and 3 hours; a norepinephrine level above 500 pg/mL or 50% greater than the 0-hour level is a positive result)

Summary of Key Recommendations for the Evaluation of Hirsutism

1. **The laboratory evaluation of hirsutism consists of the measurement of the circulating levels of testosterone and 17-OHP. When alopecia is present, a TSH screen for thyroid function is also indicated.**

2. **The single-dose overnight dexamethasone test is used to screen for Cushing's syndrome. Abnormal results are confirmed by measuring the 24-hour urinary free cortisol.**

3. **A clinician should always consider the possibility of hyperinsulinemia and emphasize preventive health interventions (as discussed in Chapter 12).**

4. **Any patient with rapidly progressive virilization must be evaluated for an androgen-secreting tumor regardless of the results of screening laboratory tests.**

5. **Incidentally discovered adrenal masses require evaluation.**

Treatment of Hirsutism

Almost all patients presenting with hirsutism represent excess androgen production in association with the steady state of persistent anovulation. Treatment is directed toward interruption of the steady state. In those patients who wish to become pregnant, ovulation can be induced as discussed in Chapter 30. In patients who do not want to become pregnant, the steady state can be interrupted by suppression of ovarian steroidogenesis by utilizing the potent inhibitory action on LH of progestational agents.

Androgen production in hirsute women is usually an LH-dependent process. Suppression of ovarian steroidogenesis depends upon adequate LH suppression. In addition to the inhibitory action of the progestational component, oral contraceptives provide a further benefit because of the increase in SHBG levels induced by the estrogen component. The increase in SHBG results in a greater androgen-binding capacity with a decrease in free testosterone levels. The progestins in oral contraceptives also inhibit 5α-reductase activity in skin, further contributing to the clinical impact of oral contraceptives on hirsutism.[112]

The low-dose oral contraceptives are effective in treating acne and hirsutism. Suppression of free testosterone levels is comparable with that achieved with higher dosage.[113, 114] The beneficial clinical effect is the same with low-dose preparations containing levonorgestrel, previously recognized to cause acne at high dosage.[114, 115] Formulations with desogestrel, gestodene, and norgestimate are associated with greater increases in sex hormone-binding globulin and significant decreases in free testosterone levels. Comparison studies with oral contraceptives containing these progestins can detect no differences in effects on various androgen measurements among the various products.[116] Theoretically, these products would be more effective in the treatment of acne and hirsutism; however, this is not documented by clinical studies. It is likely that all low-dose formulations through the combined effects of an increase in sex hormone-binding globulin and a decrease in testosterone production produce an overall similar clinical response, especially over time (a year or more).

Even in women being treated with antiandrogens, oral contraceptives are important and useful to provide both cycle control and contraception.

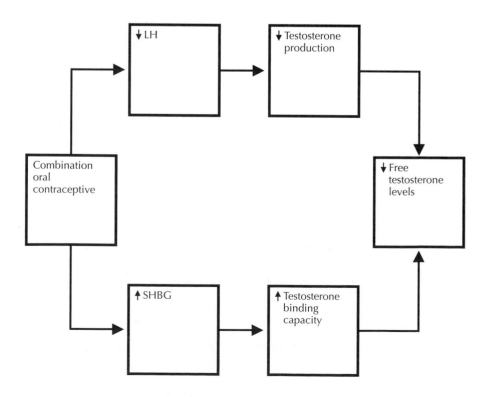

In the patient in whom oral contraceptives are contraindicated or unwanted, good results can be achieved with the use of medroxyprogesterone acetate, either 150 mg intramuscularly every 3 months or 10–20 mg orally per day. The mechanism of action of medroxyprogesterone acetate is slightly different from that of the combination oral contraceptive. Suppression of gonadotropins is less intense; hence, ovarian follicular activity continues. LH suppression is significant, however, and testosterone production is decreased, although to a lesser degree than with combined oral contraceptives. In addition, testosterone clearance from the circulation is increased.[117] This latter effect is due to an induction of liver enzyme activity. Medroxyprogesterone acetate decreases SHBG so that less testosterone is bound; however, suppression of total testosterone production is so great that the actual amount of free testosterone decreases.[118] The overall effect yields a clinical result comparable with that achieved with the combination oral contraceptive.

A noteworthy feature of hirsutism is the slow response to treatment. Because of the hair growth cycle, change takes time. The patient should be cautioned that treatment with hormonal suppression will be necessary for at least 6 months before an observable diminution in hair growth occurs. Combined treatment with electrolysis is not recommended, therefore, until hormonal suppression has been used at least 6 months.

New hair follicles will no longer be stimulated to grow, but hair growth that has been previously established will not disappear with hormone treatment alone. This can be affected temporarily by shaving, tweezing, waxing, or the use of depilatories.[119] Contrary to a common belief, these methods do not stimulate growth or increase the rate of growth of hair. None of these tactics alters the inherent growth of the hair; therefore, they must be reapplied at frequent intervals. Permanent removal of hair can be accomplished only by electrocoagulation of dermal papillae. Patients should be counseled to make sure their electrologists use disposable needles.

Some patients return after a period of treatment expressing disappointment because hair is still present. The effect of the treatment (prevention of new hair growth) may not be apparent unless the previously established hair is removed. The combination of ovarian suppression preventing new hair growth and electrolysis removing the old hair yields the most complete and effective treatment of hirsutism.

How long should treatment be continued? After 1–2 years, it is worthwhile to stop the medication and observe the patient for a return of ovulatory cycles. Even in those patients who continue to be anovulatory, testosterone suppression continues for 6 months to 2 years after discontinuing treatment. Of course, if anovulation is still present, one can expect the eventual return of hirsutism.

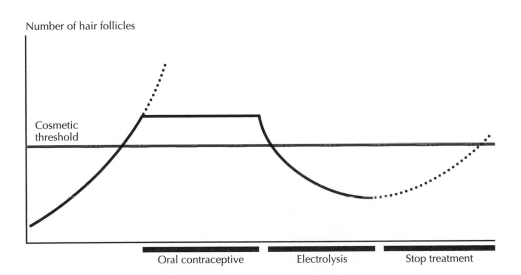

The really resistant patient deserves further consideration. Combination therapy with one of the methods discussed below is worthwhile, preferably an oral contraceptive combined with either spironolactone or finasteride.

In most patients, DHAS levels are suppressed by progestational treatment.[120, 121] The mechanism is not definitely known, but there are several possible explanations. If the original stimulus for the increased DHAS secretion is the steady estrogen state of anovulation, then the change in the endocrine milieu of the adrenal gland brought about by the suppression of ovarian steroidogenesis will restore a normal adrenal secretory pattern. Oral contraceptives may also produce subtle but significant alterations in ACTH secretion or response in the adrenal gland.

The effectiveness of adrenal suppression in inducing ovulatory cycles in some anovulatory patients can be attributed to a lowering of circulating androgen levels due to a decrease in the adrenal contribution as well as a reduction in the amount of DHAS available for conversion to testosterone within the ovarian follicle. The intraovarian androgen level is decreased, therefore lowering the inhibitory action of androgens on follicular growth and development. In terms of ovulation, the frequency of successful response with this type of treatment does not match that of the first drug of choice, clomiphene. In terms of treatment of hirsutism, progestin suppression of ovarian steroidogenesis is more effective and should remain the first therapeutic approach. Adrenal suppression should be reserved for patients with a clearly established diagnosis of an adrenal enzyme deficiency.

In an older woman who has no further desire for fertility, and in the woman for whom continued use of steroid medication is disturbing because of increasing risks with increasing age, serious consideration should be given to a surgical solution. A persistent problem of hirsutism, especially if it is progressive in severity, is a reasonable indication for hysterectomy and bilateral salpingo-oophorectomy. Patients with hyperthecosis respond poorly to suppression and are usually older. Surgical treatment for these patients is often very appropriate. Of course, an estrogen regimen is recommended for these patients postoperatively.

Keep in mind the strong association between hyperandrogenism and hyperinsulinemia as discussed in Chapter 12. Treating the problem of hirsutism by suppression of androgen production and action will not restore glucose metabolism to normal; these patients will continue to demonstrate insulin resistance. In overweight, hyperandrogenic patients, a weight control program is essential to reduce the risks of diabetes mellitus and cardiovascular disease, and consideration should be given to the preventive health benefits expected from long-term treatment with metformin or troglitazone. Nevertheless, hirsutism in hyperandrogenic women with hyperinsulinemia will respond favorably to treatment with oral contraceptives.[122]

Additional Methods of Treatment

Spironolactone

Spironolactone is an aldosterone-antagonist diuretic. In the treatment of hirsutism, spironolactone has multiple actions, inhibiting the ovarian and adrenal biosynthesis of androgens, competing for the androgen receptor in the hair follicle, and directly inhibiting 5α-reductase activity. The inhibition of steroidogenesis is achieved through an effect on the cytochrome p450 system, but the steroid suppressive effects are so variable that the receptor-blocking action is the most important mechanism.[123] It is probably for this reason that cortisol, DHA, and DHAS levels are not significantly changed with spironolactone treatment, even though androstenedione levels are decreased.[124]

The impact of spironolactone treatment on hirsutism is related to dosage, and a better effect is seen with a dose of 200 mg daily.[125–127] After a period of time, one can usually lower the dose of

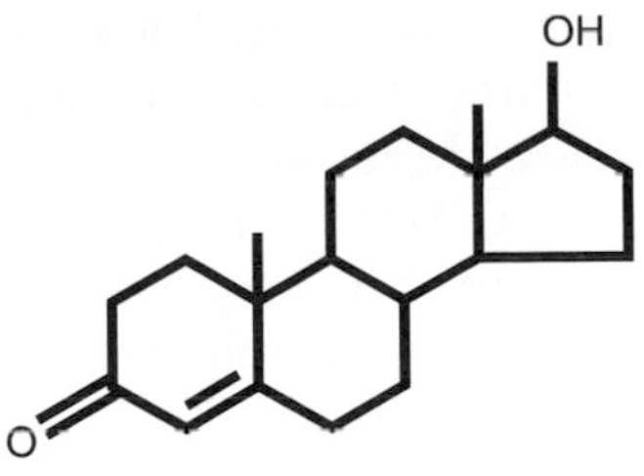

Testosterone

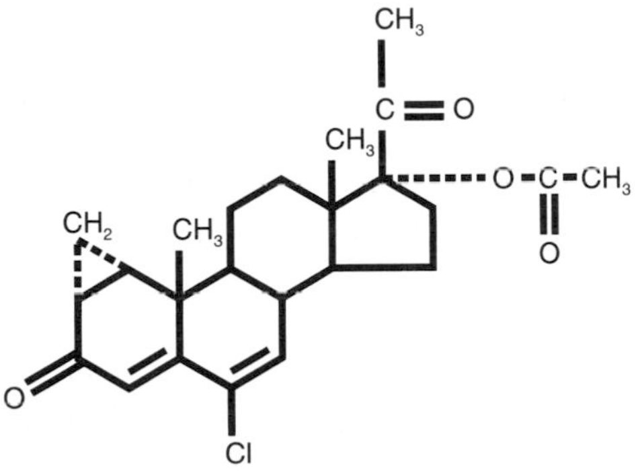

Cyproterone acetate

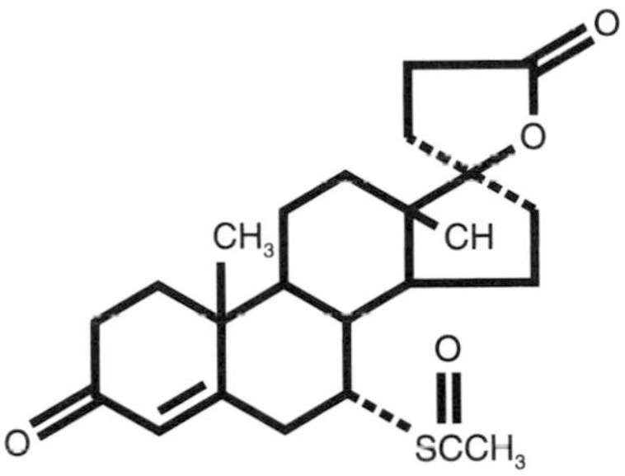

Spironolactone

spironolactone to a maintenance dose of 25–50 mg daily. As with progestational agents, the response is relatively slow, and a maximal effect can be demonstrated only after 6 months of treatment. Side effects are minimal, including diuresis in the first few days of use, occasional complaints of fatigue, ad dysfunctional uterine bleeding. Remember that the anovulatory state requires progestational management in order to avoid abnormal uterine bleeding (and endometrial hyperplasia). Because of the possibility of hyperkalemia, spironolactone should be used with caution in women who are elderly, diabetic, or using drugs that raise the potassium level.

We use spironolactone when patients find oral contraceptives unacceptable or the response is disappointing. Indeed, it makes sense to combine the peripheral tissue action of spironolactone with oral contraceptives to achieve a more dramatic result; however, the results with combined treatment regimens have not been impressively better than single agent therapy.[128, 129] Acne has been effectively treated with the local application of a cream containing 2–5% spironolactone.[130] Systemic absorption does not occur, and there are no side effects.

One word of caution: with inhibition of androgen secretion, ovulation can occur, and effective contraception is important. Theoretically, spironolactone interference with testosterone action could result in the feminization of a male fetus; however, a disrupting effect on the external genitalia has not occurred, despite fetal exposure to high doses.[131] Combined treatment with an oral contraceptive may produce a better clinical effect and, at the same time, prevent menstrual irregularity and provide contraception.

Cyproterone Acetate

Cyproterone is a potent progestational agent that both inhibits gonadotropin secretion and blocks androgen action by binding to the androgen receptor. In many parts of the world, it has been used in an oral contraceptive agent called "Diane" (2 mg cyproterone acetate and 50 μg ethinyl estradiol). "Dianette" or "Diane 35" contains 2 mg cyproterone acetate and 35 μg ethinyl estradiol. In a method for the treatment of hirsutism called the reversed sequential regimen, cyproterone acetate is given in a dose of 50 or 100 mg daily on days 5–14, with 30 or 50 μg of ethinyl estradiol daily on days 5–25.[132] In a comparison of Diane with the high dose (100 mg) cyproterone acetate treatment, the therapeutic effect was greater (but probably not of clinical significance) with the higher dose, and there was a similar incidence of side effects with both treatments.[133] In a comparison of Dianette with higher doses of cyproterone acetate (20 and 100 mg), the clinical response with the 2 mg dose of cyproterone in Dianette was equal to that of the higher doses.[134] The most common reactions include fatigue, edema, loss of libido, weight gain, and mastalgia. Significant improvement in facial hirsutism is seen by the 3rd month of treatment. In comparisons of spironolactone and cyproterone acetate, a monophasic low-dose oral contraceptive combined with spironolactone 100 mg daily was as effective as the reversed sequential regimen of 50 or 100 mg cyproterone and estrogen.[135–137]

Dexamethasone

Dexamethasone suppression of endogenous ACTH secretion is used in women who have an adrenal enzyme deficiency. Dexamethasone is given nightly (to achieve maximal suppression of the central nervous system-adrenal axis that peaks during sleep) in a dose of 0.5 mg. An equivalent dose of prednisone is 5–7.5 mg. If this treatment suppresses the morning plasma cortisol level below 2.0 μg/dL, the dose should be reduced to avoid an inability to react to stress. Fortunately, adrenal androgen secretion is more sensitive to suppression by dexamethasone than is cortisol secretion.[138] Patients with adrenal hyperplasia may require higher doses to normalize the steroid blood levels. With higher doses, alternate day therapy can still accomplish significant adrenal androgen suppression without affecting cortisol secretion.[139] It should be emphasized that moderate elevations of DHAS do not indicate patients who will benefit from dexamethasone treatment.[140] Maximal effectiveness against hirsutism in patients with an adrenal enzyme deficiency may require treatment besides glucocorticoid supplementation.[141, 142] The addition of an oral contraceptive or antiandrogen should be considered.

Treatment With GnRH Agonists

Because ovarian androgen production is LH-dependent, suppression of the pituitary with chronic GnRH agonist treatment improves hirsutism. However, inconsistent results in the literature attest to the fact that sufficient dosage must be administered to achieve effective suppression and clinical response. Therefore, monitoring dosage and response is recommended. A greater dose of GnRH agonist is required to suppress ovarian androgen secretion compared with estradiol secretion.[143] We recommend the use of depot administration of a GnRh agonist with monitoring treatment by measuring testosterone levels (the goal being less than 40 ng/dL). To avoid the problems associated with estrogen deficiency, estrogen-progestin add-back should be initiated after the maintenance dose of a long-acting GnRH agonist has been established. We recommend the daily administration of 0.625 mg conjugated estrogens or 1.0 mg estradiol combined with 2.5 mg medroxyprogesterone acetate or 0.35 mg norethindrone, or, even better, an oral contraceptive.

Although a combination of a GnRH agonist and an oral contraceptive produces a greater reduction in free testosterone levels, improvement of hirsutism is similar, comparing the combination to treatment with only an agonist; however, treatment with an agonist has been reported to be more effective than oral contraceptives alone.[144–146] In one clinical trial, the improved response associated with agonist treatment was observed only in the first 3 months of treatment; by 6 months the combination of oral contraceptives and a GnRH agonist was no more effective than oral contraceptives.[147] The addition of a long-acting agonist to Dianette (2 mg cyproterone acetate and 35 μg ethinyl estradiol) did not significantly improve clinical results.[148] After one year, a comparison of GnRH agonist treatment with the high dose cyproterone acetate regimen indicated equal efficacy, although agonist treatment was followed by a more prolonged remission.[149] These mixed results reflect variability in the severity of the condition and the degree in androgen suppression. The impact of a GnRH agonist-oral contraceptive combination is maximal when testosterone levels are suppressed below 40 ng/dL and in patients who are overweight with severe hirsutism.

This method of treatment is relatively complicated and expensive and should be reserved for the severe case of ovarian hyperandrogenism, which is usually due to significant hyperthecosis and marked hyperinsulinemia (a condition that responds less well to the usual methods of treatment). An alternative that deserves consideration is treatment of the hyperinsulinemia with metformin or troglitazone. Once maximal response has been obtained with one of these more expensive methods, long-term suppression of hair growth can be maintained with an oral contraceptive or an antiandrogen.

Flutamide

Flutamide (Eulexin) is a nonsteroidal antiandrogen at the receptor level.[150] Flutamide directly inhibits hair growth without many side effects (dry skin is the most common); however, hepatotoxicity is possible.[151] Because of the uncommon but severe toxic effect on the liver, a low-dose approach is recommended. A dose of 250 mg daily can have a marked beneficial impact on hirsutism within 6 months.[152] Despite the use of lower doses, however, it is prudent to monitor liver enzymes. In a comparison study, flutamide (250 mg bid) was not more effective than spironolactone (100 mg/day).[153] Treatment with fluta-mide should be combined with a method of contraception; blockage of androgen receptors in a male fetus could interfere with normal male development. In our view, the potential for hepatotoxicity makes flutamide an unsatis-factory choice for treatment of hirsutism.

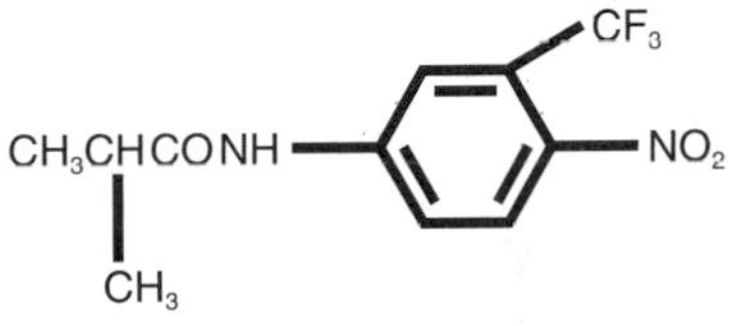

Flutamide

Finasteride

Finasteride inhibits 5α-reductase activity, thus blocking conversion of testosterone into dihydro-testosterone. The 5α-reductase enzyme exists in two forms, type I and II, each encoded by a separate gene, with the type I enzyme found in skin and the type II reductase predominately expressed in reproductive tissues.[154] Finasteride (Proscar), used to treat prostate cancer, effec-tively inhibits both isoenzymes, and, therefore, can be used to treat hirsutism. A dose of 5 mg per day decreases hirsutism without side effects.[155] A lower dose is probably as effective. Finasteride has been available only as a 5 mg unscored tablet, but it can with care be cut into quarters. A smaller dose, 1 mg (Propecia), has now been approved for the treatment of hair loss in men. In a randomized, clinical trial finasteride and spironolactone (100 mg daily) were equally effective.[156] In another randomized clinical trial, spironolactone in a dose of 100 mg daily was more effective than finasteride.[157] The main advan-tage of finasteride is the lack of side effects. Because the development of the urogenital sinus and urogenital tu-bercle into the male external genitalia, urethra, and prostate requires the action of dihydrotestosterone, pa-tients being treated with finasteride should be cautioned regarding this possible risk during pregnancy, and an effective method of contraception must be used.

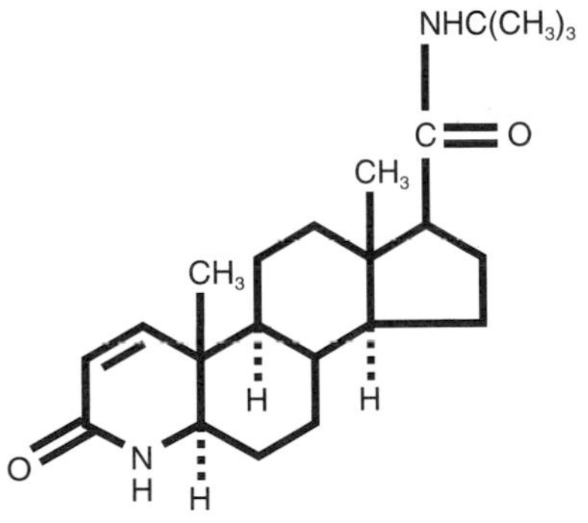

Finasteride

Other Agents

Cimetidine (300 mg qid) has been used to treat hirsutism, but it is the least potent of the androgen receptor blockers, and the clinical response is disappointing.[158] The use of a skin cream containing progesterone is effective, but it must be applied frequently (because of rapid metabolic clearance) and its action is very concentrated at the point of application.[159] Minoxidil in a topical application produces a moderate increase in hair growth in women with alopecia; however, indefinite, on-going treatment is necessary, and a return to the previous hair pattern cannot be achieved.[160] Ketoconazole in a dose of 400 mg daily blocks androgen synthesis by inhibiting the cytochrome P450 system. Although the impact on hirsutism is significant, there is a high incidence of side effects as well as changes in liver enzymes.[161] Ketoconazole, at best, should be a last resort, requiring frequent monitoring of liver function. In addition, chronic treatment with ketoconazole may suppress adrenal corticosteroid production.

End Organ Hypersensitivity (Idiopathic Hirsutism)

There are some patients who present with hirsutism, but ovulate regularly. This category of patients has in the past been labeled idiopathic or familial hirsutism and is more pronounced in certain geographic areas and among certain ethnic groups (especially those from the Mediterranean area). The only satisfactory explanation for this distressing problem is hypersensitivity of the skin's hair apparatus to normal levels of androgens, probably due to increased 5α-reductase activity.[162] Because of this excessive sensitivity, normal levels of androgen stimulate hair growth. Even in these cases, hirsutism responds to ovarian suppression with a combination oral contraceptive. Suppression of normal female androgen levels to subnormal concentrations diminishes the stimulus to the hair follicles, yielding the same stabilizing results seen in other hirsute women. Spironolactone, flutamide, and finasteride are also effective for this group of patients. Clinical response to pharmacologic treatment correlates with the circulating levels of 3α-AG, supporting the diagnosis of a target tissue (hair follicle) locus for this problem.[163] Thus 5α-reductase inhibition with finasteride may be preferred for this condition (although there have been no comparison studies) because it is directed at the source of the complaint, and there is some evidence that a benefit is sustained after finasteride treatment is discontinued.[164] For this same reason, finasteride may be the treatment of choice for women who have normal circulating androgen levels but suffer from alopecia, a problem due to increased scalp 5α-reductase activity. Although hirsutism due to an endocrine disorder requires control, end organ hypersensitivity is treated only for the purpose of cosmetic improvement. Electrolysis is a useful adjunct in this group of patients.

Summary of Recommendations for the Treatment of Hirsutism

1. The initial treatment of choice for anovulatory women with hirsutism is a low-dose (less than 50 μg estrogen) oral contraceptive.

2. Response is relatively slow, and at least 6 months of treatment are required to demonstrate an impact.

3. When patients do not respond well to oral contraceptives, an antiandrogen should be added, preferably (in order) spironolactone or finasteride.

4. There is no overwhelming evidence that one agent is better than another, and choices should be governed by cost and side effects.

5. The addition of a GnRH agonist should be reserved for patients resistant to initial therapy.

6. Finasteride may be more effective for idiopathic hirsutism and androgenic alopecia.

Limitations and Pitfalls

We have outlined a simple, straightforward approach for the evaluation and management of the hirsute woman; however, as in all of medicine, exceptions occur.

1. Occasionally, testosterone levels may be extremely elevated with anovulation, leading to very heavy hair growth and even masculinization. A testosterone level over 200 ng/dL does not absolutely indicate the presence of a tumor.

2. Enlarged ovaries are not necessary for the clinical syndrome of anovulation and excessive androgen production. On the other hand, the presence of enlarged, polycystic ovaries does not ensure the diagnosis of anovulation and excess ovarian production of androgen. They can be associated with adrenal disease or exogenous androgen ingestion.

3. Laparoscopy and ovarian biopsy are not indicated procedures in the evaluation of hirsutism.

4. The association of elevated testosterone production and hirsutism with normal ovulatory cycles should make the clinician suspicious of an adrenal problem.

5. Suppression of elevated androgens by progestin treatment does not rule out the presence of an ovarian tumor. Functional ovarian tumors are gonadotropin-dependent and responsive.

6. Failure of progestin treatment to suppress hair growth and testosterone levels after 6–12 months raises the suspicion of adrenal disease or a very small ovarian tumor.

7. Androgen levels in postmenopausal women are lower. In this age group, a testosterone level greater than 100 ng/dL is suspicious for a tumor.

References

1. **Uno H,** Biology of hair growth, *Seminars Reprod Endocrinol* 4:131, 1986.

2. **Lookingbill DP, Demers LM, Wang C, Leung A, Rittmaster RS, Santen RJ,** Clinical and biochemical parameters of androgen action in normal and healthy caucasian versus Chinese subjects, *J Clin Endocrinol Metab* 72:1242, 1991.

3. **Oh H-S, Smart RC,** An estrogen receptor pathway regulates the telogen-anagen hair follicle transition and influences epidermal cell proliferation, *Proc Natl Acad Sci USA* 93:12525, 1996.

4. **Horton R,** Dihydrotestosterone is a peripheral paracrine hormone, *J Androl* 13:23, 1992.

5. **Randall VA, Ebling FJG,** Seasonal changes in hair growth, *Br J Dermatol* 124:146, 1991.

6. **Chang RJ,** Ovarian steroid secretion in polycystic ovarian disease, *Seminars Reprod Endocrinol* 2:244, 1984.

7. **Serafini P, Lobo R,** Increased 5α-reductase activity in idiopathic hirsutism, *Fertil Steril* 43:74, 1985.

8. **Serafini P, Ablan F, Lobo RA,** 5α-Reductase activity in the genital skin of hirsute women, *J Clin Endocrinol Metab* 60:349, 1985.

9. **Greep N, Hoopes M, Horton R,** Androstanediol glucuronide plasma clearance and production rates in normal and hirsute women, *J Clin Endocrinol Metab* 62:22, 1986.

10. **Rittmaster RS,** Androgen conjugates: physiology and clinical significance, *Endocr Rev* 14:121, 1993.

11. **Melegos DN, Mala HY, Wang C, Stanczyk F, Diamandis EP,** Prostate-specific antigen in female serum, a potential new marker of androgen excess, *J Clin Endocrinol Metab* 82:777, 1997.

12. **Escobar-Morreale H, Serrano-Gotarredona J, Avila S, Villar-Palasí J, Varela C, Sancho J,** The increased circulating prostate-specific antigen concentrations in women with hirsutism do not respond to acute changes in adrenal or ovarian function, *J Clin Endocrinol Metab* 83:2580, 1998.

13. **Bardin CW, Lipsett M,** Testosterone and androstenedione blood production rates in normal women and women with idiopathic hirsutism and polycystic ovaries, *J Clin Invest* 46:891, 1967.

14. **Allen SE, Potter HD, Azziz R,** Prevalence of hyperandrogenemia among nonhirsute oligo-ovulatory women, *Fertil Steril* 67:569, 1997.

15. **Ferriman D, Gallwey JD,** Clinical assessment of body hair growth in women, *J Clin Endocrinol Metab* 21:1440, 1961.

16. **Futterweit W, Dunaif A, Yeh HC, Kingsley P,** The prevalence of hyperandrogenism in 109 consecutive female patients with diffuse alopecia, *J Am Acad Dermatol* 19:831, 1988.

17. **Matteri RK, Stancyzk FZ, Gentzschein EE, Delgado C, Lobo RA,** Androgen sulfate and glucuronide conjugates in nonhirsute and hirsute women with polycystic ovarian syndrome, *Am J Obstet Gynecol* 161:1704, 1989.

18. **Legro RS, Carmina E, Stanczyk FZ, Gentzschein E, Lobo RA,** Alterations in androgen conjugate levels in women and men with alopecia, *Fertil Steril* 62:744, 1994.

19. **Reid RL, Van Vugt DA,** Hair loss in the female, *Obstet Gynecol Survey* 43:1350, 1988.

20. **Carmina E, Lobo RA,** Evidence for increased androsterone metabolism in some normoandrogenic women with acne, *J Clin Endocrinol Metab* 76:1111, 1993.

21. **Grassinger CC, Wild RA, Parker IJ,** Vulvar acanthosis nigricans: a marker for insulin resistance in hirsute women, *Fertil Steril* 59:583, 1993.

22. **Garcia-Buneul R, Berek JS, Woodruff JD,** Luteomas of pregnancy, *Obstet Gynecol* 45:407, 1975.

23. **McClamrock HD, Adashi EY,** Gestational hyperandrogenism, *Fertil Steril* 57:257, 1992.

24. **Manganiello PD, Adams LV, Harris RD, Ornvold K,** Virilization during pregnancy with spontaneous resolution postpartum: a case report and review of the English literature, *Obstet Gynecol Survey* 50:404, 1995.

25. **VanSlooten AJ, Rechner SF, Dodds WG,** Recurrent maternal virilization during pregnancy caused by benign androgen-producing ovarian lesions, *Am J Obstet Gynecol* 167:1342, 1992.

26. **Ben-Chetrit A, Greenblatt EM,** Recurrent maternal virilization during pregnancy associated with polycystic ovarian syndrome: a case report and review of the literature, *Hum Reprod* 10:3057, 1995.

27. **Orth DN,** Cushing's syndrome, *New Engl J Med* 332:791, 1995.

28. **Meikle AW,** A diagnostic approach to Cushing's syndrome, *Endocrinologist* 3:311, 1993.

29. **Yanovski JA,** The dexamethasone-suppressed corticotropin-releasing hormone test in the differential diagnosis of hypercortisolism, *Endocrinologist* 5:169, 1995.

30. **White FE, White MC, Drury PL, Fry IK, Besser GM,** Value of computed tomography of the abdomen and chest in investigation of Cushing's syndrome, *Br Med J* 284:771, 1982.

31. **Findling JW, Kehoe ME, Shaker JL, Raff H,** Routine inferior petrosal sinus sampling in the differential diagnosis of adrenocorticotropin (ACTH)-dependent Cushing's syndrome: early recognition of the occult ectopic ACTH syndrome, *J Clin Endocrinol Metab* 73:408, 1991.

32. **Oldfield EH, Doppman JL, Nieman LK, Chrousos GP, Miller DL, Katz DA, Cutler Jr GB, Loriaux DL,** Petrosal sinus sampling with and without corticotropin-releasing hormone for the differential diagnosis of Cushing's syndrome, *New Engl J Med* 325:897, 1991.

33. **Booth GL, Redelmeier DA, Grossman H, Kovacs K, Smyth HS, Ezzat S,** Improved diagnostic accuracy of inferior petrosal sinus sampling over imaging for localizing pituitary pathology in patients with Cushing's disease, *J Clin Endocrinol Metab* 83:2291, 1998.

34. **Findling JW, Tyrrell JB,** Occult ectopic secretion of corticotropin, *Arch Intern Med* 146:929, 1986.

35. **Yanovski JA, Cutler Jr GB, Doppman JL, Miller DL, Chrousos GP, Oldfield EH, Nieman LK,** The limited ability of inferior petrosal sinus sampling with corticotropin-releasing hormone to distinguish Cushing's disease from pseudo-Cushing states or normal physiology, *J Clin Endocrinol Metab* 77:503, 1993.

36. **Chetkowski RJ, Judd HL, Jagger PI, Nieberg RK, Chang RJ,** Autonomous cortisol secretion by a lipoid cell tumor of the ovary, *JAMA* 254:2628, 1985.

37. **Legro RS, Finegood D, Dunaif A,** A fasting glucose to insulin ratio is a useful measure of insulin sensitivity in women with polycystic ovary syndrome, *J Clin Endocrinol Metab* 83:2694, 1998.

38. **Lobo RA, Paul WL, Goebelsmann U,** Dehydroepiandrosterone sulfate as an indicator of adrenal androgen function, *Obstet Gynecol* 57:69, 1981.

39. **Haning Jr RV, Flood CA, Hackett RJ, Loughlin JS, McClure N, Longcope C,** Metabolic clearance rate of dehydroepiandrosterone sulfate, its metabolism to testosterone, and its intrafollicular metabolism to dehydroepiandrosterone, androstenedione, testosterone, and dihydrotestosterone in vivo, *J Clin Endocrinol Metab* 72:1088, 1991.

40. **Cumming DC, Rebar RW, Hopper BR, Yen SSC,** Evidence for an influence of the ovary on circulating dehydroepiandrosterone sulfate levels, *J Clin Endocrinol Metab* 54:1069, 1982.

41. **Lobo RA, Kletsky OA, Kaptein EM, Goebelsmann U,** Prolactin modulation of dehydroepiandrosterone sulfate secretion, *Am J Obstet Gynecol* 138:632, 1980.

42. **Schiebinger RJ, Chrousos GP, Cutler Jr GB, Loriaux DL,** The effect of serum prolactin on plasma adrenal androgens and the production and metabolic clearance rate of dehydroepiandrosterone sulfate in normal and hyperprolactinemic subjects, *J Clin Endocrinol Metab* 62:202, 1986.

43. **Vermeulen A, Ando S, Verdonck L,** Prolactinomas, testosterone-binding globulin and androgen metabolism, *J Clin Endocrinol Metab* 54:409, 1982.

44. **Glickman SP, Rosenfield RL, Bergenstal RM, Helke J,** Multiple androgenic abnormalities, including elevated free testosterone, in hyperprolactinemic women, *J Clin Endocrinol Metab* 55:251, 1982.

45. **Kamilaris TC, DeBold CR, Manolas KJ, Hoursanidis A, Panageas S, Yiannatos J,** Testosterone-secreting adrenal adenoma in a peripubertal girl, *JAMA* 258:2558, 1987.

46. **White PC, New MI, Dupont B,** Congenital adrenal hyperplasia, *New Engl J Med* 316:1519, 1987.

47. **White PC, New MI, Dupont B,** Congenital adrenal hyperplasia, *New Engl J Med* 316:1580, 1987.

48. **Speiser PW, Dupont B, Rubenstein P, Piazza A, Kastelan A, New MI,** High frequency of non-classical steroid 21-hydroxylase deficiency, *Am J Hum Genet* 37:650, 1985.

49. **Pang S, Lerner AJ, Stoner E, Levine LS, Oberfield SE, Engle I, New MI,** Late-onset adrenal steroid 3β-hydroxysteroid dehydrogenase deficiency. I. A cause of hirsutism in pubertal and postpubertal women, *J Clin Endocrinol Metab* 60:428, 1985.

50. **Schram P, Zerah M, Mani P, Jewelewicz R, Jaffe S, New MI,** Nonclassical 3β-hydroxysteroid dehydrogenase deficiency: a review of our experience with 25 female patients, *Fertil Steril* 58:129, 1992.

51. **Azziz R, Bradley Jr EL, Potter HD, Boots LR,** 3β-Hydroxysteroid dehydrogenase deficiency in hyperandrogenism, *Am J Obstet Gynecol* 168:889, 1993.

52. **Zerah M, Rheame E, Mani P, Schram P, Simard J, Labrie F, New MI,** No evidence of mutations in the genes for type I and type II 3β-hydroxysteroid dehydrogenase (3β-HSD) in nonclassic 3β-HSD deficiency, *J Clin Endocrinol Metab* 79:1811, 1994.

53. **Chang YT, Zhang L, Alkaddour HS, Mason JL, Lin K, Yang X, Garibaldi LR, Bourdony CJ, Dolan LM, Donaldson DL, et al,** Absence of molecular defect in the type II 3β-hydroxysteroid dehydrogenase (3β-HSD) gene in premature pubarche children and hirsute female patients with moderately decreased adrenal 3β-HSD activity, *Pediatr Res* 37:820, 1995.

54. **Azziz R, Boots LR, Parker Jr CR, Bradley E, Zacur HA,** 11β-Hydroxylase deficiency in hyperandrogenism, *Fertil Steril* 55:733, 1991.

55. **Cobin RH, Futterweit W, Fiedler RP, Thornton JC,** Adrenocorticotropic hormone testing in idiopathic hirsutism and polycystic ovarian disease: a test of limited usefulness, *Fertil Steril* 44:224, 1985.

56. **Kuttenn F, Couillin P, Girard F, Billaud L, Vincens M, Boucekkine C, Thalabarad J-C, Maudelonde T, Spritzer P, Mowszowicz I, Boue A, Mauvais-Jarvis P,** Late-onset adrenal hyperplasia in hirsutism, *New Engl J Med* 313:224, 1985.

57. **Benjamin F, Deutsch S, Saperstein H, Seltzer BVL,** Prevalence of and markers for the attenuated form of congenital adrenal hyperplasia and hyperprolactinemia masquarading as polycystic ovarian disease, *Fertil Steril* 46:215, 1986.

58. **Azziz R, Zacur H,** 21-Hydroxylase deficiency in female hyperandrogenism: screening and diagnosis, *J Clin Endocrinol Metab* 69:577, 1989.

59. **Knochenhauer ES, Cortet-Rudelli C, Cunnigham RD, Conway-Myers BA, Dewailly D, Azziz R,** Carriers of 21-hydroxylase deficiency are not at increased risk for hyperandrogenism, *J Clin Endocrinol Metab* 82:479, 1997.

60. **Lobo RA,** The role of the adrenal in polycystic ovary syndrome, *Seminars Reprod Endocrinol* 2:251, 1984.

61. **New MI, Lorenzen F, Lerner AJ, Kohn B, Oberfield SE, Pollack MS, Dupont B, Stoner E, Levy DJ, Pang S, Levine LS,** Genotyping steroid 21-hydroxylase deficiency: hormonal reference data, *J Clin Endocrinol Metab* 57:320, 1983.

62. **Rosenfield RL, Helke J, Lucky AW,** Dexamethasone preparation does not alter corticoid and androgen responses to adrenocorticotropin, *J Clin Endocrinol Metab* 60:585, 1985.

63. **Sobrino L, Kase N, Grunt J,** Changes in adrenocortical function in patients with gonadal dysgenesis after treatment with estrogen, *J Clin Endocrinol Metab* 33:110, 1971.

64. **Abraham G, Maroulis G,** Effect of exogenous estrogen on serum pregnenolone, cortisol and androgens in postmenopausal women, *Obstet Gynecol* 45:271, 1975.

65. **Lucky AW, Marynick SP, Rebar RW, Cutler GB, Glen M, Johnsonbaugh E, Loriaux DL,** Replacement oral ethinyloestradiol therapy for gonadal dysgenesis: growth and adrenal androgen studies, *Acta Endocrinol* 91:519, 1979.

66. **Lobo RA, March CM, Goebelsmann U, Mishell Jr DR,** The modulating role of obesity and of 17β-estradiol (E2) on bound and unbound E2 and adrenal androgens in oophorectomized women, *J Clin Endocrinol Metab* 54:320, 1982.

67. **Lobo RA, Goebelsmann U, Brenner PF, Mishell Jr DR,** The effects of estrogen on adrenal androgens in oophorectomized women, *Am J Obstet Gynecol* 142:471, 1982.

68. **Rosenfield RL, Famg IS,** The effects of prolonged physiologic estradiol therapy on the maturation of hypogonadal teenagers, *J Pediatr* 85:830, 1974.

69. **Anderson D, Yen SSC,** Effects of estrogens on adrenal 3β-hydroxysteroid dehydrogenase in ovariectomized women, *J Clin Endocrinol Metab* 43:561, 1976.

70. **Rose DP, Fern M, Liskowski L, Milbrath JR,** Effect of treatment with estrogen conjugates on endogenous plasma steroids, *Obstet Gynecol* 49:80, 1977.

71. **Steingold K, de Ziegler D, Cedars M, Meldrum DR, Lu JKH, Judd HL, Chang RJ,** Clinical and hormonal effects of chronic gonadotropin-releasing hormone agonist treatment in polycystic ovarian disease, *J Clin Endocrinol Metab* 65:773, 1987.

72. **Tazuke S, Khaw K-T, Barrett-Connor E,** Exogenous estrogen and endogenous sex hormones, *Medicine* 71:44, 1992.

73. **Fujieda K, Faiman C, Reyes FI, Winter JSD,** The control of steroidogenesis by human fetal adrenal cells in tissue culture: IV. The effects of exposure to placental steroids, *J Clin Endocrinol Metab* 54:89, 1982.

74. **Gell JS, Oh J, Rainey WE, Carr BR,** Effect of estradiol on DHEAS production in the human adrenocortical cell line, H295R, *J Soc Gynecol Invest* 5:144, 1998.

75. **Chang RJ, Mandel FP, Wolfren AR, Judd HL,** Circulating levels of plasma adrenocorticotropin in polycystic ovary disease, *J Clin Endocrinol Metab* 54:1265, 1982.

76. **Stewart PM, Penn R, Holder R, Parton A, Ratcliffe JG, London DR,** The hypothalamo-pituitary-adrenal axis across the normal menstrual cycle and in polycystic ovary syndrome, *Clin Endocrinol* 38:387, 1993.

77. **Azziz R, Black V, Hines GA, Fox LM, Boots LR,** Adrenal androgen excess in the polycystic ovary syndrome: sensitivity and responsivity of the hypothalamic-pituitary-adrenal axis, *J Clin Endocrinol Metab* 83:2317, 1998.

78. **Byrne GC, Perry YS, Winter JSD,** Steroid inhibitory effects upon human adrenal 3β-hydroxysteroid dehydrogenase activity, *J Clin Endocrinol Metab* 62:413, 1986.

79. **Futterweit W, Green G, Tarlin N, Dunaif A,** Chronic high-dosage androgen administration to ovulatory women does not alter adrenocortical steroidogenesis, *Fertil Steril* 58:124, 1992.

80. **Ditkoff EC, Fruzzetti FA, Chang L, Stancyzk FZ, Lobo RA,** The impact of estrogen on adrenal androgen sensitivity and secretion in polycystic ovary syndrome, *J Clin Endocrinol Metab* 80:603, 1995.

81. **Dunaif A, Green G, Futterweit W, Dobrjansky A,** Suppression of hyperandrogenism does not improve peripheral or hepatic insulin resistance in the polycystic ovary syndrome, *J Clin Endocrinol Metab* 70:699, 1990.

82. **Wild RA, Alaupovic P, Parker IJ,** Lipid and apolipoprotein abnormalities in hirsute women. I. The association with insulin resistance, *Am J Obstet Gynecol* 166:1191, 1992.

83. **Gonzalez F, Hatala DA, Speroff L,** Basal and dynamic hormonal responses to gonadotropin releasing hormone agonist treatment in women with polycystic ovaries with high and low dehydroepiandrosterone sulfate levels, *Am J Obstet Gynecol* 165:535, 1991.

84. **Gonzalez F, Chang L, Horab T, Lobo RA,** Evidence for heterogeneous etiologies of adrenal dysfunction in polycystic ovary syndrome, *Fertil Steril* 66:354, 1996.

85. **Zhang L, Rodriguez H, Ohno S, Miller WL,** Serine phosphorylation of human P450c17 increases 17,20-lyase activity: implications for adrenarche and the polycystic ovary syndrome, *Proc Natl Acad Sci USA* 92:10619, 1995.

86. **Escobar-Morreale HG, Serrano-Gotarredona J, García-Robles R, Sancho JM, Varela C,** Lack of an ovarian function influence on the increased adrenal androgen secretion present in women with functional ovarian hyperandrogenism, *Fertil Steril* 67:654, 1997.

87. **Moghetti P, Castello R, Negri C, Tosi F, Spiazzi GG, Brun E, balducci R, Toscano V, Muggeo M,** Insulin infusion amplifies 17α-hydroxycorticosteroid intermediates response to ACTH in hyperandrogenic women: apparent relative impairment of 17,20-lyase activity, *J Clin Endocrinol Metab* 81:881, 1996.

88. **Carmina E, Koyama T, Chang T, Stanczyk FZ, Lobo RA,** Does ethnicity influence the prevalence of adrenal hyperandrogenism and insulin resistance in polycystic ovary syndrome? *Am J Obstet Gynecol* 167:1807, 1992.

89. **Lanzone A, Fulghesu AM, Guido M, Fortini A, Caruso A, Mancuso S,** Differential androgen response to adrenocorticotropic hormone stimulation in polycystic ovarian syndrome: relationship with insulin secretion, *Fertil Steril* 58:296, 1992.

90. **Nestler JE, Clore JN, Strauss III JF, Blackard WG,** Effects of hyperinsulinemia on serum testosterone, progesterone, dehydroepiandrosterone sulfate, and cortisol levels in normal women and in a woman with hyperandrogenism, insulin resistance and acanthosis nigricans, *J Clin Endocrinol Metab* 64:180, 1987.

91. **Nestler JE, McClanahan MA, Clore JN, Blackard WG,** Insulin inhibits adrenal 17,20-lyase activity in man, *J Clin Endocrinol Metab* 74:362, 1992.

92. **Liu CH, Laughlin GA, Fischer UG, Yen SSC,** Marked attenuation of ultradian and circadian rhythms of dehydroepiandrosterone in postmenopausal women: evidence for a reduced 17,20-desmolase enzymatic activity, *J Clin Endocrinol Metab* 71:900, 1990.

93. **Alper MM, Garner PR,** Elevated serum dehydroepiandrosterone sulfate levels in patients with insulin resistance, hirsutism, and acanthosis nigricans, *Fertil Steril* 47:255, 1987.

94. **Azziz R, Bradley Jr EL, Potter HD, Boots LR,** Adrenal androgen excess in women: lack of a role for 17-hydroxylase and 17,20-lyase dysregulation, *J Clin Endocrinol Metab* 80:400, 1995.

95. **Haning Jr RV, Hackett RJ, Flood CA, Loughlin JS, Zhao QY, Longcope C,** Plasma dehydroepiandrosterone sulfate serves as a prehormone for 48% of follicular fluid testosterone during treatment with menotropins, *J Clin Endocrinol Metab* 76:1301, 1993.

96. **Easterling Jr WE, Talbert LM, Potter HD,** Serum testosterone levels in the polycystic ovary syndrome, *Am J Obstet Gynecol* 120:385, 1974.

97. **Meldrum DR, Abraham GE,** Peripheral and ovarian venous concentrations of various steroid hormones in virilizing ovarian tumors, *Obstet Gynecol* 53:36, 1979.

98. **Gabrilove JL, Seman AT, Sabet R, Mitty HA, Nicolis GL,** Virilizing adrenal adenoma with studies on the steroid content of the adrenal venous effluent and a review of the literature, *Endocr Rev* 2:462, 1981.

99. **Friedman CI, Schmidt GE, Kim MH, Powell J,** Serum testosterone concentrations in the evaluation of androgen-producing tumors, *Am J Obstet Gynecol* 153:44, 1985.

100. **Surrey ES, de Ziegler D, Gambone JC, Judd HL,** Preoperative localization of androgen-secreting tumors: clinical, endocrinologic, and radiologic evaluation of ten patients, *Am J Obstet Gynecol* 158:1313, 1988.

101. **Bammann BL, Coulam CB, Jiang N-S,** Total and free testosterone during pregnancy, *Am J Obstet Gynecol* 137:293, 1980.

102. **Moltz L, Schwartz U,** Gonadal and adrenal androgen secretion in hirsute females, *Clin Endocrinol Metab* 15:229, 1986.

103. **Brumsted JR, Chapitis J, Riddick D, Gibson M,** Norethindrone inhibition of testosterone secretion by an ovarian Sertoli-Leydig cell tumor, *J Clin Endocrinol Metab* 65:194, 1987.

104. **Kennedy L, Trasub AI, Atkinson AB, Sheridan B,** Short-term administration of gonadotropin-releasing hormone analog to a patient with a testosterone-secreting ovarian tumor, *J Clin Endocrinol Metab* 64:1320, 1987.

105. **Cohen I, Shapira M, Cuperman S, Goldberger S, Siegal A, Altaras M, Beyth Y,** Direct in-vivo detection of atypical hormonal expression of a Sertoli-Leydig cell tumour following stimulation with human chorionic gonadotropin, *Clin Endocrinol* 39:491, 1993.

106. **Pascale M-M, Pugeat M, Roberts M, Rousset H, Déchaud H, Dutrieux-Berger N, Tourniaire J,** Androgen suppressive effect of GnRH agonist in ovarian hyperthecosis and virilizing tumours, *Clin Endocrinol* 41:571, 1994.

107. **Leedman PJ, Bierre AR, Martin FIR,** Virilizing nodular ovarian stromal hyperthecosis, diabetes mellitus and insulin resistance in a postmenopausal woman. Case report, *Br J Obstet Gynaecol* 96:1095, 1989.

108. **Cook DM, Loriaux DL,** The incidental adrenal mass, *Am J Med* 101:88, 1996.

109. **Kloos RT, Gross MD, Francis IR, Korobkin M, Shapiro B,** Incidentally discovered adrenal masses, *Endocr Rev* 16:460, 1995.

110. **Reincke M, Nieke J, Krestin GP, Saeger W, Allolio B, Winkelman W,** Preclinical Cushing's syndrome in adrenal "incidentalomas:" comparison with adrenal Cushing's syndrome, *J Clin Endocrinol Metab* 75:826, 1992.

111. **Jaresch S, Kornely E, Kley H-K, Schlaghecke R,** Adrenal incidentaloma and patients with homozygous or heterozygous congenital adrenal hyperplasia, *J Clin Endocrinol Metab* 74:685, 1992.

112. **Cassidenti DL, Paulson RJ, Serafini P, Stanczyk FZ, Lobo RA,** Effects of sex steroids on skin 5α-reductase activity in vitro, *Obstet Gynecol* 78:103, 1991.

113. **van der Vange N, Blankenstein MA, Kloosterboer HJ, Haspels AA, Thijssen JHH,** Effects of seven low-dose combined oral contraceptives on sex hormone binding globulin, corticosteroid binding globulin, total and free testosterone, *Contraception* 41:345, 1990.

114. **Lemay A, Dewailly SD, Grenier R, Huard J,** Attenuation of mild hyperandrogenic activity in postpubertal acne by a triphasic oral contraceptive containing low doses of ethynyl estradiol and d,l-norgestrel, *J Clin Endocrinol Metab* 71:8, 1990.

115. **Palatsi R, Hirvensalo E, Liukko P, Malmiharju T, Mattila L, Riihiluoma P, Ylöstalo P,** Serum total and unbound testosterone and sex hormone binding globulin (SHBG) in female acne patients treated with two different oral contraceptives, *Acta Derm Venereol* 64:517, 1984.

116. **Coenen CMH, Thomas CMG, Borm GF, Rolland R,** Changes in androgens during treatment with four low-dose contraceptives, *Contraception* 53:171, 1996.

117. **Gordon GG, Southern AL, Tochimoto S, Olivo J, Altman K, Rand J, Lemberger L,** Effect of medroxyprogesterone acetate (Provera) on the metabolism and biological activity of testosterone, *J Clin Endocrinol Metab* 30:449, 1970.

118. **Wortsman J, Khan MS, Rosner W,** Suppression of testosterone-estradiol binding globulin by medroxyprogesterone acetate in polycystic ovary syndrome, *Obstet Gynecol* 67:705, 1986.

119. **Richards RN, Uy M, Meharg G,** Temporary hair removal in patients with hirsutism: a clinical study, *Cutis* 45:199, 1990.

120. **Wild RA, Umstot ES, Andersen RN, Givens JR,** Adrenal function in hirsutism: II. Effect of an oral contraceptive, *J Clin Endocrinol Metab* 54:676, 1982.

121. **Wiebe RH, Morris CV,** Effect of an oral contraceptive on adrenal and ovarian androgenic steroids, *Obstet Gynecol* 63:12, 1984.

122. **Azziz R,** The hyperandrogenic-insulin-resistant acanthosis nigricans syndrome: therapeutic response, *Fertil Steril* 61:570, 1994.

123. **Young RL, Goldzieher JW, Elkind-Hirsch K,** The endocrine effects of spironolactone used as an antiandrogen, *Fertil Steril* 48:223, 1987.

124. **Serafini P, Lobo RA,** The effects of spironolactone on adrenal steroidogenesis in hirsute women, *Fertil Steril* 44:595, 1985.

125. **Lobo RA, Shoupe D, Serafini P, Brinton D, Horton R,** The effects of two doses of spironolactone on serum androgens and anagen hair in hirsute women, *Fertil Steril* 43:200, 1985.

126. **Evans DJ, Burke CW,** Spironolactone in the treatment of idiopathic hirsutism and the polycystic ovary syndrome, *J Roy Soc Med* 79:453, 1986.

127. **Barth JH, Cherry CA, Wojnarowaka F, Dawber RP,** Spironolactone is an effective and well tolerated systemic anti-androgen therapy for hirsute women, *J Clin Endocrinol Metab* 68:966, 1989.

128. **Pittaway DE, Maxson WS, Wentz AC,** Spironolactone in combination drug therapy for unresponsive hirsutism, *Fertil Steril* 43:878, 1985.

129. **Kelestimur F, Sahin Y,** Comparison of Diane 35 and Diane 35 plus spironolactone in the treatment of hirsutism, *Fertil Steril* 69:66, 1998.

130. **Messina M, Manieri C, Rizzi G, Gentile L, Milani P,** Treating acne with antiandrogens: the confirmation of the validity of a percutaneous treatment with spironolactone, *Curr Ther Res Clin Exp* 38:269, 1985.

131. **Groves TD, Corenblum B,** Letter to the Editors: Spironolactone therapy during human pregnancy, *Am J Obstet Gynecol* 172:1655, 1995.

132. **Miller JA, Jacobs HS,** Treatment of hirsutism and acne with cyproterone acetate, *Clin Endocrinol Metab* 15:373, 1986.

133. **Belisle S, Love EJ,** Clinical efficacy and safety of cyproterone acetate in severe hirsutism: results in a multicentered Canadian study, *Fertil Steril* 46:1015, 1986.

134. **Barth JH, Cherry CA, Wojnarowska F, Dawber RPR,** Cyproterone acetate for severe hirsutism: results of a double-blind dose-ranging study, *Clin Endocrinol* 35:5, 1991.

135. **Chapman MG, Dowsett M, Dewhurst CJ, Jeffcoate SL,** Spironolactone in combination with an oral contraceptive: an alternative treatment for hirsutism, *Br J Obstet Gynaecol* 92:983, 1985.

136. **O'Brien RC, Cooper ME, Murray RML, Seeman E, Thomas AK, Jerums G,** Comparison of sequential cyproterone acetate/estrogen versus spironolactone/oral contraceptive in the treatment of hirsutism, *J Clin Endocrinol Metab* 72:1008, 1991.

137. **Erenus M, Yücelten D, Gürbüz O, Durmusoglu F, Pekin S,** Comparison of spironolactone-oral contraceptive versus cyproterone acetate-estrogen regimens in the treatment of hirsutism, *Fertil Steril* 66:216, 1996.

138. **Rittmaster RS, Loriaux DL, Cutler Jr GB,** Sensitivity of cortisol and adrenal androgens to dexamethasone suppression in hirsute women, *J Clin Endocrinol Metab* 61:462, 1985.

139. **Avgerinos PC, Cutler Jr GB, Tsokos GC, Gold PW, Feuillan P, Galucci WT, Pillemer SR, Loriaux DL, Chrousos GP,** Dissociation between cortisol and adrenal androgen secretion in patients receiving alternate day prednisone therapy, *J Clin Endocrinol Metab* 65:24, 1987.

140. **Steinberger E, Smith KD, Rodriguez-Rigau J,** Testosterone, dehydroepiandrosterone, and dehydroepiandrosterone sulfate in hyperandrogenic women, *J Clin Endocrinol Metab* 59:471, 1984.

141. **Carmina E, Lobo RA,** Ovarian suppression reduces clinical and endocrine expression of late-onset congenital adrenal hyperplasia due to 21-hydroxylase deficiency, *Fertil Steril* 62:738, 1994.

142. **Azziz R, Slayden SM,** The 21-hydroxylase-deficient adrenal hyperplasias: more than ACTH oversecretion, *J Soc Gynecol Invest* 3:297, 1996.

143. **Rittmaster RS,** Differential suppression of testosterone and estradiol in hirsute women with the superactive gonadotropin-releasing hormone agonist leuprolide, *J Clin Endocrinol Metab* 67:651, 1988.

144. **Falsetti L, Pasinetti E,** Treatment of moderate and severe hirsutism by gonadotropin releasing hormone agonists in women with polycystic ovary syndrome and idiopathic hirsutism, *Fertil Steril* 61:817, 1994.

145. **Elkind-Hirsch KE, Anania C, Mack M, Malinak R,** Combination gonadotropin-releasing hormone agonist and oral contraceptive therapy improves treatment of hirsute women with ovarian hyperandrogenism, *Fertil Steril* 63:970, 1995.

146. **Azziz R, Ochoa TM, Bradley Jr EL, Potter HD, Boots LR,** Leuprolide and estrogen *versus* oral contraceptive pills for the treatment of hirsutism: a prospective randomized study, *J Clin Endocrinol Metab* 80:3406, 1995.

147. **Carr BR, Breslau NA, Givens C, Byrd W, Barnett-Hamm C, Marshburn PB,** Oral contraceptive pills, gonadotropin-releasing hormone agonists, or use in combination for treatment of hirsutism: a clinical research center study, *J Clin Endocrinol Metab* 80:1169, 1995.

148. **Acién P, Mauri M, Gutierrez M,** Clinical and hormonal effects of the combination gonadotrophin-releasing hormone agonist plus oral contraceptive pills containing ethinyl-oestradiol (EE) and cyproterone acetate (CPA) versus the EE-CPA pill alone on polycystic ovarian disease-related hyperandrogenism, *Hum Reprod* 12:423, 1997.

149. **Carmina E, Lobo RA,** Gonadotrophin-releasing hormone agonist therapy for hirsutism is as effective as high dose cyproterone acetate but results in a longer remission, *Hum Reprod* 12:663, 1997.

150. **Marcondes JAM, Minnani SL, Luthold WW, Wajchenberg BL, Samojlik E, Kirschner MA,** Treatment of hirsutism in women with flutamide, *Fertil Steril* 57:543, 1992.

151. **Wallace C, Lalor EA, Chik CL,** Hepatotoxicity complicating flutamide treatment of hirsutism, *Ann Intern Med* 119:1150, 1993.

152. **Müderis II, Bayram F, Sahin Y, Kelestimur F,** A comparison of two doses of flutamide (250 mg/d and 500 mg/d) in the treatment of hirsutism, *Fertil Steril* 68:644, 1997.

153. **Erenus M, Gürbüz O, Durmusoglu F, Demircay Z, Pekin S,** Comparison of the efficacy of spironolactone versus flutamide in the treatment of hirsutism, *Fertil Steril* 61:613, 1994.

154. **Russell DW, Wilson JD,** Steroid 5α-reductase: two genes/two enzymes, *Ann Rev Biochem* 63:25, 1994.

155. **Tolino A, Petrone A, Sarnacchiaro F, Cirillo D, Ronsini S, Lombardi G, Nappi C,** Finasteride in the treatment of hirsutism: new therapeutic perspectives, *Fertil Steril* 66:61, 1996.

156. **Wong IL, Morris RS, Chang L, Spahn M-A, Stanczyk FZ, Lobo RA,** A prospective randomized trial comparing finasteride to spironolactone in the treatment of hirsute women, *J Clin Endocrinol Metab* 80:233, 1995.

157. **Erenus M, Yücelten D, Durmusoglu F, Gürbüz O,** Comparison of finasteride versus spironolactone in the treatment of idiopathic hirsutism, *Fertil Steril* 68:1000, 1997.

158. **Golditch IM, Price VH,** Treatment of hirsutism with cimetidine, *Obstet Gynecol* 75:911, 1990.

159. **Rowe TC, Mezei M, Hilchie J,** Treatment of hirsutism with liposomal progesterone, *Prostate* 5:346, 1984.

160. **De Villez RL, Jacobs JP, Szpunar CA, Warner ML,** Androgenetic alopecia in the female. Treatment with 2% topical minoxidil solution, *Arch Dermatol* 130:303, 1994.

161. **Venturoli S, Fabbri R, Dal Prato L, Mantovani B, Capelli M, Magrini O, Flamigni C,** Ketoconazole therapy for women with acne and/or hirsutism, *J Clin Endocrinol Metab* 71:335, 1990.

162. **Paulson RJ, Serafini PC, Catalino JA, Lobo RA,** Measurements of 3α-, 17β-androstenediol glucuronide in serum and urine and the correlation with skin 5α-reductase activity, *Fertil Steril* 46:222, 1986.

163. **Kirschner MA, Samojlik E, Szmal E,** Clinical usefulness of plasma androstanediol glucuronide measurements in women with idiopathic hirsutism, *J Clin Endocrinol Metab* 65:597, 1987.

164. **Castello R, Tosi F, Perrone F, Negri C, Muggeo M, Moghetti P,** Outcome of long-term treatment with the 5α-reductase inhibitor finasteride in idiopathic hirsutism: clinical and hormonal effects during a 1-year course of therapy and 1-year follow-up, *Fertil Steril* 66:734, 1996.

14 Menstrual Disorders

	1	2	3	4	5	6
7	8	9	10	11	12	13
14	15	16	17	18	19	20
21	22	23	24	25	26	27
28	29	30	31			

S ince antiquity, the appearance of menses in correlation with lunar phases has inspired names for menses, such as a period or the monthly time. The regularity of this appearance was easily appreciated; more difficult was understanding the purpose of the bleeding. Ancient physicians viewed menstruation as a process of detoxification, and throughout history myths and attitudes toward menstruation have kept alive negative connotations that range from magic to danger and poison.[1]

The health care profession has an obligation to promote menstrual education. This must start with ourselves. We must have an understanding of reproductive physiology in order to impart it to our patients, and we must be sensitive to the need to present a positive attitude regarding sexual and reproductive functions. An educated understanding of these normal events is a powerful mechanism for dealing with perceived discomforts and disorders of menstruation.

Unfortunately, some menstrual disorders are still not well understood (such as the premenstrual syndrome), although others, such as dysmenorrhea, can be physiologically explained in a framework that provides for appropriate pharmacologic treatment. In this chapter we will consider several medical problems that are linked to menstruation and do our best to provide an objective point of view based on physiology.

The Premenstrual Syndrome

The simplest definition of the premenstrual syndrome (PMS) is a commonsense one: the cyclic appearance of one or more of a large constellation of symptoms (over 100) just prior to menses, occurring to such a degree that lifestyle or work is affected, followed by a period of time entirely free of symptoms. The most frequently encountered symptoms include the following: abdominal bloating, anxiety or tension, breast tenderness, crying spells, depression, fatigue, lack of energy, unprovoked anger or irritability, difficulty concentrating, thirst and appetite changes, and variable degrees of edema of the extremities — usually occurring in the last 7 to 10 days of the cycle. The exact collection of symptoms in an individual is irrelevant; the diagnosis is made by prospectively and accurately charting the cyclic nature of the symptoms. However, the symptoms are not to be underrated; the various symptoms of premenstrual syndrome have been recounted time and time again in clinicians' offices in poignant detail, often noting a feeling of being "overwhelmed" or "out of control."

When women's daily moods are prospectively charted, a subgroup emerges in which mood changes demonstrate a cyclic pattern with increasing symptoms during the luteal phase and an elimination of symptoms at or soon after menses. Fewer than 50% of women who complain of premenstrual syndrome can be demonstrated to have a pattern of mood changes with a cyclic pattern.[2]

There are two established guidelines for the diagnosis of PMS. The first is from the American Psychiatric Association (APA) and consists of the criteria for what the APA has designated as the ***premenstrual dysphoric disorder***. According to the American Psychiatric Association, this disorder should be differentiated as more severe than PMS; however, most assuredly, there is a broad spectrum of severity, and this differentiation is not helpful or useful. The APA criteria for diagnosis (which correspond to our simple definition above) are as follows:

A.   Symptoms are temporally related to the menstrual cycle, beginning during the last week of the luteal phase and remitting after the onset of menses.

B.   The diagnosis requires at least 5 of the following, and one of the symptoms must be one of the first 4:

1.   Affective lability; e.g., sudden onset of being sad, tearful, irritable, or angry.
2.   Persistent and marked anger or irritability.
3.   Anxiety or tension.
4.   Depressed mood, feelings of hopelessness.
5.   Decreased interest in usual activities.
6.   Easy fatigability or marked lack of energy.
7.   Subjective sense of difficulty in concentrating.
8.   Changes in appetite, overeating, or food craving.
9.   Hypersomnia or insomnia.
10. Feelings of being overwhelmed or out of control.
11. Physical symptoms, such as breast tenderness, headaches, edema, joint or muscle pain, weight gain.

C.   The symptoms interfere with work or usual activities or relationships.

D.   The symptoms are not an exacerbation of another psychiatric disorder. Thus, PMS is, in part, a diagnosis of exclusion.

The guidelines from the National Institute of Mental Health (NIMH) state that the diagnosis of PMS requires the documentation of at least a 30% increase in severity of symptoms in the 5 days prior to menses compared with the 5 days following menses.[3] Using the NIMH and APA criteria, it is estimated that about 5% of women of reproductive age can be diagnosed with disruptive PMS.[4, 5]

Approximately 40% of women report problems related to their cycles, and about 2–10% report a degree of impact on work or lifestyle.[6] The exact prevalence, however, is difficult to ascertain. The symptoms are variable and difficult to quantitate. A further problem that complicates the evaluation of published studies, as well as dealing with individual cases, is that behavior is usually related to menstruation in a retrospective fashion. This is prone to considerable subjective bias.[7] For example, studies in the literature point out that some women do not actually experience problems in relation to menstruation but believe that they do.[7] It is argued, rather convincingly, that men and women in our culture have been conditioned to expect symptoms in a woman's premenstrual phase and have been taught to expect fluid retention, pain, and emotional reactions. These stereotypic expectations are precisely what are reported when retrospective charting is utilized. Most importantly, carefully constructed studies (prospective with appropriate statistical analyses) show no significant variation associated with the cycle for cognitive, motor, or social behavior.[8]

Is PMS due to an individual pathologic problem or is it due to cultural beliefs, beliefs that lead to the menstrual cycle being associated with a variety of negative reactions, or a combination of both? There is a significant correlation between menstrual symptoms in daughters and mothers, and between sisters, suggesting that these are responses that can be learned.[9, 10] Throughout our recorded history, we find evidence of menstrual taboos. What if our societies and cultures had celebrated menstruation as a time of pleasure (and even public joy) rather than something private (to be hidden) and negative? Would we have PMS today? The answer may lie in the unraveling of the role of our shared beliefs about menstruation in society, rather than the functioning of those beliefs in individuals.

It is generally recognized that R. T. Frank, chief of obstetrics and gynecology at Mt. Sinai Hospital in New York City, first defined premenstrual syndrome in 1931. His description still stands as a graphic and vivid statement. He wrote the following:[11]

> The group of women to whom I refer especially complain of a feeling of indescribable tension from 10 to 7 days preceding menstruation which in most instances continues until the time that the menstrual flow occurs. The patients complain of unrest, irritability, like jumping out of their skin and a desire to find relief by foolish and ill considered actions. Their personal suffering is intense and manifests itself in many reckless and sometimes reprehensible actions. Not only do they realize their own suffering, but they feel conscience-stricken toward their husbands and families, knowing well that they are unbearable in their attitude and reactions. Within an hour or two after the onset of the menstrual flow complete relief from both physical and mental tension occurs.

Frank went on to summarize 15 cases. He reported that he could obtain relief by withdrawing blood from his patients, and, therefore, theorized that the problem was due to an excess of female sex hormones because of inadequate excretion. Accordingly, he used treatments to enhance excretion, such as calcium lactate, caffeine, and laxatives. For severe cases, he produced ovarian failure by irradiation. S. Leon Israel, in the 1930s, was the first to propose the counterargument that the syndrome was due to defective luteinization resulting in a progesterone deficiency and only a relative hyperestrogenic state.[12] The phrase, "premenstrual syndrome," was first used in 1953 by Dalton in a report of 84 cases with Greene,[13]

For many years, we were handicapped by a lack of knowledge as to what the premenstrual syndrome really is, how to establish a diagnosis, and how best to treat the condition. In the last decade, however, a degree of understanding has emerged, and treatment guidelines are now available derived from clinical studies.[14]

But first let's take a brief look backwards into history where we find reason enough to conclude that we are limited in our reactions to menses, limited by what has been provided by our culture throughout history.

Historical Myths

Recorded beliefs, many of them truly ancient, include magical beliefs, superstitions regarding the milk supply from cows, and beliefs about crops and animals.[15] It was thought, almost universally, that the menstrual woman was possessed by an evil spirit.

Pliny, born in 23 AD, consulted approximately 2000 available books by physicians in writing his *Historia Naturalis*. Pliny's treatise was a resource throughout the Dark Ages, and there are still more than 100 copies of it, all 37 volumes. The oft-quoted Pliny, who clearly was unencumbered with the burden of objectivity, wrote almost exhaustively on menstruation.[16]

> Contact with it turns new wine sour, crops touched by it become barren, grafts die, seeds in gardens are dried up, the fruit of trees falls off, the edge of steel and the gleam of ivory are dulled, hives of bees die, even bronze and iron are at once seized by rust, and a horrible smell fills the air; to taste it drives dogs mad and infects their bites with an incurable poison. If a woman strips herself naked while she is menstruating and walks around a field of wheat, the caterpillars, worms, beetles, and other vermin will fall off from the ears of corn. All plants will turn of a yellow complexion on the approach of a woman who has the menstrual discharge upon her. Bees will forsake their hives at her touch, for they have a special aversion to a thief and a menstrous woman, and a glance of her eyes suffices to kill a swarm of bees.

Household articles were not immune. Aristotle said that a menstrous woman could dull a mirror with a look, and the next person to look into it would be bewitched. There were numerous tales of women breaking things at the time of menses — needles snapping, glasses breaking, and clocks stopping. In general, there has been a universal horror of blood throughout early history. It is not surprising, therefore, that this (probably) instinctive horror led to taboos on blood and all that came in contact with it. This led in turn to prohibition and seclusion. Almost universally, menstruating women were isolated and prevented from handling food. Most primitive peoples regarded women as unclean during menstruation and subjected menstruating women to segregation and special rituals. Ultimately, with growing sophistication, this led to a generally negative attitude.

The scientific study of menstruation has been hampered by the overpowering influence of traditions and social and cultural beliefs. We have all, men and women, been conditioned to view menstruation in a negative way. Perhaps, it is time to look at menstruation from another point of view. How many fine novels have been finished in a burst of creativity in the premenstrual period? How many great ideas have been born premenstrually? If PMS reflects socially mediated expectations, the answer may lie in social re-education.

The Social Consequences of PMS

It was a common view in Europe in the 19th and early 20th centuries that menstruation was associated with antisocial behavior.[17] A domestic servant who murdered one of her employer's children in 1845 was acquitted on the grounds of insanity due to obstructed menstruation. In 1851, a woman was acquitted of murdering her baby niece on the grounds of insanity due to disordered menstruation. Acquittals for shoplifting because of suppression of menses date back to 1845. When we consider the fact that PMS (although not known by this specific phrase) has been recognized throughout recorded history, it is not unexpected that it has been used as a defense in the courts before modern times.

Dalton argued that PMS is responsible for an increased incidence of crime, jailing for alcoholism, school misdemeanors, sickness in industry, hospitalization for accidents, and general hospital admissions.[18] However studies on premenstrual symptoms that have appropriate controls and statistical treatment find no significant variation associated with the menstrual cycle for cognitive or motor behavior.[8, 19, 20] Social behavior (including crime and suicide) reveals effects similar to all others seen in self-report studies. When social or psychological expectations are altered, the effect disappears. Today, PMS is accepted by courts in the same manner that factors related to social and psychological stress or physical illness are accepted, and such factors do not absolve the accused of criminal responsibility.

Unfortunately, PMS is still used to explain apparently motiveless and impulsive acts, as well as poor academic performance. In contrast to Dalton's contention that schoolgirls have impaired academic performance during the premenstrual phase, the results of 244 female medical and paramedical students in all examinations taken during one year did not reveal any significant menstrual cycle effects on examination performance.[21]

One of the biggest problems with the studies that have sought to link behavior with menstrual cycles is an underlying assumption that the premenstrual phase is the crucial variable, ignoring the fact that any phase of the cycle is vulnerable to life stresses. In other words, the premenstrual phase must be controlled for all life stresses in order to conclude that that phase of the cycle has an etiologic influence on some life event.

Etiologies and Treatments

Where scientists have failed to provide proof, practitioners have seldom failed to provide theories. The list of biological theories is impressive:

> Low progesterone levels
> High estrogen levels
> Falling estrogen levels
> Changes in estrogen:progesterone ratios
> Increased aldosterone activity
> Increased renin-angiotensin activity
> Increased adrenal activity
> Endogenous endorphin withdrawal
> Subclinical hypoglycemia
> Central changes in catecholamines
> Response to prostaglandins
> Vitamin deficiencies
> Excess prolactin secretion

Studies prior to 1983 did not incorporate appropriate diagnostic criteria and, therefore, suffer from inaccuracy and heterogeneity. Since 1983, efforts to isolate a specific pathophysiologic mechanism have failed to demonstrate differences between women with and without symptoms for all hormone levels throughout the menstrual cycle (including estrogens, progesterone, testosterone, follicle-stimulating hormone, luteinizing hormone, prolactin, and sex hormone-binding globulin) or weight gain and measurements of substances involved in fluid regulation, such as aldosterone.[22] This further includes both the circulating levels as well as the pattern of secretion over the menstrual cycle. In addition, no connection could be demonstrated between PMS and two endogenous metabolites of progesterone, allopregnanolone and pregnanolone.[23] Dynamic testing has revealed no abnormalities in the hypothalamic-pituitary axis and its relationships with the adrenal glands, the thyroid gland, and the ovaries. No differences can be detected in magnesium, zinc, vitamin A, vitamin E, thiamin, or vitamin B_6.[24] Some have argued for a greater change in endorphins, proposing that the luteal phase symptom complex is due to a withdrawal from endogenous opioids (in effect, an autoaddiction and withdrawal), but others have been unable to detect a difference in circulating endorphins in symptomatic patients.[25–27]

Differences have been reported in various biologic factors, but these differences are not always confined to the luteal phases. Some of these factors, besides the endorphins, include the response to thyrotropin-releasing hormone (TRH), melatonin secretion, red blood cell magnesium levels, growth hormone and cortisol responses to tryptophan, cortisol response to corticotropin-releasing hormone, free cortisol secretion, and cortisol secretion patterns. The strongest argument against a luteal phase hormonal change is derived from experiments at the National Institute of Mental Health.[28] These experiments utilized the progesterone antagonist, RU486, in combination with human chorionic gonadotropin (HCG) or placebo to induce bleeding at various times during the cycle. Altering the menstrual cycle had no effect on the timing or severity of the PMS symptoms; thus, the neuroendocrine and endocrine events during the luteal phase should not be involved.

In general, thyroid function is normal in patients with PMS.[29] About 10% of women with PMS have abnormal thyroid function, but this compares with the prevalence rate of subclinical hypothyroidism. Although there are no differences in thyroid-stimulating hormone (TSH) responses to TRH, patients with PMS do demonstrate more abnormal responses, both exaggerated and blunted (which would balance out in group comparisons).[30] However, these abnormal responses occur just as often in the follicular phase as in the luteal phase. Furthermore, there is no evidence of a therapeutic response to thyroxine compared with placebo, even in patients with abnormal responses to TRH.

Various methods of treatment have been proposed, each championing a presumed etiology. All of the following have failed to demonstrate any clear-cut benefits over placebo: oral contraceptives, vitamin B_6, bromocriptine, monamine oxidase inhibitors, and synthetic progestational agents.[14] The use of spironolactone has many advocates, especially for women with a major complaint of bloating; however, appropriate double-blind, placebo-controlled trials have failed to demonstrate a clinical impact (other than on bloatedness) greater than placebo.[31, 32] It has been argued that patients with PMS have a deficiency in fatty acid metabolism, and evening of primrose oil has been advocated for therapy. Evening of primrose oil is extracted from the seed of the evening primrose; it provides linoleic and gamma-linoleic acids (precursors of prostaglandin E). Appropriately blinded and controlled studies failed to find a difference comparing primrose oil with placebo.[33–35] The one positive study used retrospective assessment of symptoms, a method known to be inaccurate.[36] Significant improvement has been noted with the use of prostaglandin synthesis inhibitors, but it is difficult to know if this is influenced by a positive impact on dysmenorrhea.[37]

In the past, there was an enormous amount of publicity given to the use of progesterone treatment by injection or vaginal suppository, long proposed and promoted by Dalton.[18] Four early studies that failed to detect a positive effect of progesterone were criticized for study size and progesterone dosage.[38–41] A very well-designed study attempted to remove a placebo effect by providing no contact with the investigators or any health care providers during the course of the study; both progesterone and placebo failed to achieve an improvement in symptoms.[42] The criticism of study size and progesterone dose was effectively answered in a randomized placebo-controlled, double-blind, clinical crossover trial of 168 women.[43] Progesterone in doses of 400 mg and 800 mg (doses used by Dalton) did not differ from placebo. A later study by this same group utilizing a very large dose (1200 mg daily) also found no difference between progesterone and placebo treatments.[44] Only one study has reported beneficial effects with progesterone, a study of only 23 highly motivated women, and the major effect occurred only in the first month of treatment.[45]

Medical and surgical oophorectomy has been described to have dramatic success. A lasting response to surgical hysterectomy and oophorectomy was reported in women unresponsive to medical therapy.[46, 47] Gonadotropin-releasing hormone (GnRH) agonist treatment can produce hypogonadotropic hypogonadism, in effect, a medical oophorectomy. GnRH agonist treatment has been effective; adding estrogen-progestin to avoid the side effects of the GnRH agonist diminished somewhat the improvement in symptoms. However, the beneficial impact was still considerable.[48–50] While medical and surgical oophorectomy is undoubtedly effective, it is impossible to blind such treatment, and the mechanism is, therefore, uncertain. In the GnRH agonist-steroid add-back study, patients receiving a placebo instead of estrogen-progestin had a return of symptoms (despite continued GnRH agonist treatment), probably in anticipation of a negative reaction to estrogen-progestin. This experience is a strong statement of the power of the placebo response (in this case, a negative response). In general, the response to ovarian suppression with GnRH agonist treatment indicates that the symptoms of PMS represent an abnormal response to normal hormonal changes.[51]

The only randomized trials, double-blinded and placebo-controlled, which have had consistent, excellent results are those with the antidepressants, fluoxetine, clomipramine, sertraline, paroxetine, and alprazolam.[44, 52–58] A dose (20–60 mg daily) of fluoxetine (which inhibits neuronal uptake of serotonin) effectively abolished symptoms without side effects.[52–54] Further studies have established that a 20 mg dose of fluoxetine is as effective as higher doses, achieving a rapid response within 2–3 months and avoiding the side effects associated with the higher doses.[57, 59] For some women, treatment limited to the premenstrual phase can be effective.[60] Alprazolam is a short-acting benzodiazepine with anxiolytic, antidepressant, and smooth muscle relaxant properties. A dose of 0.25 mg bid-tid during the luteal phase is effective, although some women may require an alprazolam daily dose of 2.5 mg.[44, 61, 62] In contrast, lithium has no effect.

Problems and Questions

The problems and questions are many:

1. The clinical symptoms are variable, difficult to quantitate, and enormous in number. The symptoms cover emotions, sexual feelings, mood states, behavioral changes, and somatic complaints. Despite multiple questionnaires, we are still not convinced that there exists a reliable, objective method for observing and measuring symptoms that are experienced internally, rather than manifested via external behavior.[7]

2. The discrepancy between retrospective and prospective accounts regarding cyclic changes is now well documented and recognized.[63] Women use menses as a marker of time, and unpleasant, easily remembered experiences are attributed to an easily recognized signpost. If women in our culture have been conditioned to expect symptoms in the premenstrual phase and have been taught to expect fluid retention, pain, and emotional reactions, that is precisely what will be reported.[63] Our lives are rhythmical. Day alternates with night. There are sleeping and waking, being hungry and being full, the circadian rhythms of our glands, and the ultimate rhythm: the sexual cycle. It is the most natural thing to seek a rhythm for our behavior.

   The Ruble study is now a classic.[64] In this study, 44 undergraduates at Princeton University were deliberately deceived about which phase of the menstrual cycle they were experiencing. A bogus electroencephalogram, complete with electrodes attached to the head, was heralded as a new technique capable of predicting the date of menstruation. Subjects were told they were either premenstrual (due in 1–2 days) or intermenstrual (due in 7–10 days). Only those women who were led to believe that their period would begin in 2 days reported significantly higher symptom ratings on pain, water retention, and eating habit changes. This was interpreted as a realization of stereotypic expectations.

3. Is there a specific syndrome? A syndrome must have a specific pathophysiology; specific signs and symptoms can be documented; and a specific treatment achieves a beneficial response in most patients. One of the basic problems is that we have lumped everything into PMS, including behavioral changes, somatic complaints, and psychological problems, implying the existence of a specific syndrome. Part of the problem is that all the tools of research reflect the way the author of the tool conceptualizes PMS, which, in turn, is based on the background and training of the author.[65]

4. The experimenter expectancy effect has to be properly controlled. Subjects tend to comply with what they think is the experimenter's hypothesis. This has been studied in regard to PMS, and no significant difference in PMS symptomatology can be demonstrated when the purpose of the study is disguised, and, in addition, the responses can be influenced by positive or negative manipulations.[66–68] This relates to findings of negative mood changes when subjects are asked to assess their menstrual distress retrospectively.

5. Studies are complicated by high placebo responses. Clinical studies of premenstrual syndrome typically demonstrate a 30–50% response to placebo and, if a positive effect is anticipated by the subjects, up to 80%. Only well-designed, double-blind, placebo-controlled, randomized trials yield reliable data.

The Placebo Response

The strange sounding word, placebo, comes from the Latin verb meaning "I shall please." Clinicians and patients have been educated to observe a prescription ritual. Most people seem to feel that their complaints are not taken seriously unless they are in possession of a prescription. But the placebo is not so much a pill as a process.[69]

The process begins with patient confidence in the clinician and extends through to the full functioning of the patient's own healing system. Interaction with the clinician provides a better understanding of what's going on (at least some elimination of unfounded fears) and provides some hope. Many of the treatment modalities for PMS, if not all, provide a woman with a greater sense of control over life; thus, minimal interaction, such as focusing on diet or lifestyle, can yield a positive result. In the process of making detailed, prospective observations of one's own life, a patient can experience an increase in self-control, which is in itself a therapeutic process.

Leon Eisenberg has written the following insightful and helpful thoughts on the placebo:[70]

> So emphatically does the phrase "placebo response" discredit the psychosocial aspects of the therapeutic encounter that it may be time to eradicate it from our language. Let us replace it by some such term as "the response to care," "the response to the doctor," or "the healing response" in order to emphasize that it is (a). powerful, (b). no less "real" than drug actions, and (c). embedded in every therapeutic transaction. . . Its mechanisms are some compound of the arousal of hope, the comfort of reassurance, taking an active rather than a passive role in managing the illness experience, and reinterpreting the meaning of the illness. . . It is perverse that "placebo" has almost become an epithet implying charlatanism rather than a descriptor of a fundamental characteristic of medical practice. . . We ought equally to seek an understanding of the healing response rather than disdaining it, as the "hard" scientist does, or being deceived by it, as practitioners often are.

Until PMS is better understood, the placebo response will continue to play an important role in therapy. There is a psychosocial subjective component of medicine that makes the placebo process a legitimate part of every patient–clinician interaction.

Treatment of Premenstrual Syndrome

The first step is to be convinced (both patient and clinician) that the problem is cyclic. The only instrument of diagnosis available at the present time is the menstrual calendar. There is no single calendar that has emerged as superior and acceptable to all; however, several are available in the literature.[71, 72] At least 3 months of prospective recording, aided if possible by other observers (such as family members), are necessary in order to document a recurring problem in the luteal phase of the cycle, interfering with work or lifestyle, and followed by a period entirely free of symptoms. This time period should be used to develop a solid patient–clinician relationship and, in so doing, to provide as much education as possible for the patient.

We offer our perspective on this syndrome, suggesting that it is not a single disorder, but rather a collection of different problems. We believe that PMS has a basic psychophysiologic origin, tied to the menstrual cycle, primarily biologically, but with a psychosociologic overlay. This can be a learned response or it can be a response in vulnerable individuals triggered by normal neuroendocrine and hormonal changes. The hormonal changes of the menstrual cycle are not an etiologic factor, but they can operate to produce in susceptible women mood changes or a destabilization of mood, and specifically involving the serotonergic system.[73] This may be the reason that elimination of menses with drugs or oophorectomy is often effective. The problem presumably lies within the central nervous system with a mechanism that determines susceptibility.

Often, patients present to the clinician totally focused on complaints that occur premenstrually. With exploration of lifestyle, relationships, and interactions, the focus on a premenstrual syndrome can be shifted to the underlying issues that are producing conflict and lack of control. Helping a patient to come to grips with the subtle nature of this problem, the fundamental psychologic response involved, and the need to take charge of one's life represent the type of broad involvement required of a clinician. Without this type of broad involvement, only a short-term response can be achieved with little hope for long-term success.

Any changes that allow individuals to exert greater control over their lives will produce a positive impact. It is for this reason that lifestyle changes are effective in the treatment of PMS. Changes in diet, changes in exercise, changes in work or recreation — all are examples of exerting control over life rather than having life's circumstances control the individual.

If the practitioner is convinced of the cyclic nature of a problem (by a prospective record of at least 3 months duration), try to isolate the specific symptoms and treat with a specific therapy. If fluid retention is perceived by the patient as a principal problem, offer diuretic therapy with spironolactone. If dysmenorrhea is a component of the symptom complex, try one of the inhibitors of prostaglandin synthetase or oral contraceptives. Calcium supplementation (1200 mg daily) was observed in a placebo-controlled, randomized trial to be associated with a 48% reduction in symptom scores (compared with a 30% reduction in the placebo-treated group).[74] These are safe and relatively inexpensive approaches that deserve initial consideration.

A failure to identify a specific disorder with a specific mechanism suggests that premenstrual syndrome represents a variety of psychological manifestations triggered by normal, physiologic hormonal changes. This process can be either physiologic in nature or psychosocial and deeply rooted in our cultural history. For that reason, it makes some sense to completely eliminate endogenous sex steroid variability. This can be achieved with daily oral contraceptives, or medroxyprogesterone acetate, 10–30 mg daily, or depot-medroxyprogesterone acetate, 150 mg every 3 months. On occasion, we have induced beneficial and gratifying results in patients with incapacitating emotional swings. But in view of the vague and subjective nature of this syndrome, any such empiric therapeutic treatment must be pursued in a fully informed fashion. If a patient is willing to undergo an empiric trial, we are willing. In doing so, however, neither partner in this contract should be deceived; we must remember that the placebo response may be the underlying basis for any positive response. But keep in mind that the placebo response is another example of an individual exerting control. In this case, it represents the subtle effort of the body at a subconscious level to exert self-healing.

Last resort treatments, in our view, are the expensive and complicated medical oophorectomy by GnRH agonist combined with estrogen-progestin add-back (in doses used for postmenopausal therapy), and the use of the selective serotonin reuptake inhibitors and alprazolam. Because alprazolam can be abused, and because the clinical effect is not impressive, the serotonin reuptake inhibitors are preferred.[75] Clinical studies have indicated that ovarian suppression with GnRH agonist treatment is more effective for behavioral and physical symptoms and less effective for psychological symptoms.[50, 76] Furthermore, the response is not overwhelming; treatment with a GnRH agonist can be expected to achieve success in 60–70% of women with PMS.[51] These reasons also favor the use of serotonin reuptake inhibitors. Long-term effectiveness of fluoxetine has been documented, with decreased libido being the most common side effect.[77] To minimize side effects, intermittent treatment (7–14 days during the luteal phase) should be assessed first.[60]

The clinical studies with medical oophorectomy or the use of serotonin reuptake inhibitors are very convincing, but this serious medical therapy does not diminish the important contribution to be made by the clinician in an ongoing relationship and interaction with the patient.

Dysmenorrhea

Dysmenorrhea is pain with menstruation, usually cramping in nature and centered in the lower abdomen. Studies on the prevalence of dysmenorrhea are few. In a random sample of 19-year-old women in Gothenburg, Sweden, 72% reported dysmenorrhea, 15% had to limit their daily activity and the severity was unimproved by analgesics, 8% missed school or work at every menses, and 38.2% regularly used medical treatment.[78] Oral contraceptive use and previous vaginal deliveries were associated with less dysmenorrhea. The severity of dysmenorrhea was directly related to the duration and amount of menstrual flow. In a longitudinal American study of 17–19-year-old university students, 13% reported severe pain in more than half of their menstrual periods, and 42% indicated interference with activity at least once.[79] A survey in Turkey reported that 25.6% of adolescents missed school because of dysmenorrhea.[80] In another older but good prevalence study, 45% of surveyed women had moderate or severe dysmenorrhea.[81] Most adolescents experience dysmenorrhea in the first 3 years after menarche. In the U.S., about 60% of menstruating adolescents were reported to have some dysmenorrhea, and 14% regularly missed school.[82] Menstrual problems, including dysmenorrhea, are more common in individuals who smoke.[83, 84] Dysmenorrhea improves in most women after a full-term pregnancy.[85]

Primary dysmenorrhea, a condition associated with ovulatory cycles, is due to myometrial contractions induced by prostaglandins originating in secretory endometrium, while secondary dysmenorrhea is associated with a variety of pathological conditions.[86] Other symptoms associated with menstrual flow, such as headache, nausea and vomiting, backache, and diarrhea, can be explained by entry of the prostaglandins and prostaglandin metabolites into the systemic circulation. There is a 3-fold increase in prostaglandin levels in the endometrium from the follicular phase to the luteal phase, with a further increase during menstruation.[87] Women with primary dysmenorrhea have greater endometrial production of prostaglandins than asymptomatic women. Most of the release of prostaglandins during menstruation occurs during the first 48 hours, which coincides with the greatest intensity of the symptoms.

Prostaglandin $F_{2\alpha}$ ($PGF_{2\alpha}$) is the agent responsible for dysmenorrhea. It always stimulates uterine contractions, whereas the E prostaglandins inhibit contractions in the nonpregnant uterus. Uterine muscle from both normal and dysmenorrheic women is sensitive to $PGF_{2\alpha}$, but the amount of $PGF_{2\alpha}$ produced is the major differentiating factor.

The clinical benefit derived from the pharmacologic use of inhibitors of prostaglandin synthesis depends on a significant decrease in prostaglandin production in the endometrium, as well as shortened and diminished menstrual flow. An additional role may be attributed to decreased prostaglandins from the platelets participating in the clotting of menstrual blood. The explanation for the benefit seen with oral contraceptives is decreased prostaglandin synthesis associated with the atrophic decidualized endometrium. Oral contraception is a good choice for therapy, combining contraception with a beneficial impact on dysmenorrhea, menstrual flow, and menstrual irregularity.[88]

In women who do not desire hormonal contraception, the best therapy is one of the agents that inhibit prostaglandin synthesis. There are several families of nonsteroidal anti-inflammatory agents. The acetic acid group is associated with more side effects, and these agents are not the drugs of choice for dysmenorrhea; indomethacin belongs to this group. The propionic acid derivatives (ibuprofen, naproxen, ketoprofen) and the fenamates (mefenamic acid, meclofenamate, flufenamic acid) are very effective for the treatment of dysmenorrhea.

The findings in 51 clinical trials of prostaglandin synthetase inhibitors indicated that the fenamates are more effective, but not substantially, for relieving pain.[89] The fenamates, in addition to inhibiting prostaglandin synthesis, also have an antagonistic action, competing for prostaglandin-binding sites. Side effects associated with these agents are minimal, but can include blurred vision, headaches, dizziness, and gastrointestinal discomfort. The latter can be reduced by taking the medication with milk or food. All of these agents are more potent than aspirin, because the uterus is relatively insensitive to aspirin. The major contraindications to the use of these agents include gastrointestinal ulcers and hypersensitivity to aspirin and similar agents.

Approximately 80% of dysmenorrheic women are relieved by prostaglandin inhibitors. Improvement is noted in the symptoms associated with menses, specifically cramping, backache, nausea, vomiting, dizziness, leg pain, insomnia, and headache. A trial of up to 6 months is warranted, with necessary changes in dosage and inhibitors, before abandoning this therapy. Initially, it was believed that better relief was achieved if treatment was started 2–3 days before menses in order to lower the tissue level of prostaglandins before breakdown of the endometrium. Fortunately, studies have indicated that treatment is just as effective if begun at the sign of first bleeding, thus decreasing the possibility of taking one of these agents early in pregnancy. Another benefit of prostaglandin inhibition is a reduction in the amount of blood lost with periods. Indeed, the agents may be used to treat idiopathic menorrhagia, or the excess flow associated with an intrauterine device (IUD). Most women do not need to take the medication more than 2–3 days.

If dysmenorrhea is not relieved by one of the nonsteroidal, anti-inflammatory analgesics, laparoscopy should be seriously considered to determine the cause of the symptoms. Conditions associated with dysmenorrhea include müllerian duct anomalies, endometriosis, and pelvic inflammatory disease. *We should especially be aware that endometriosis occurs in adolescents; dysmenorrhea caused by endometriosis in adolescents usually begins 3 or more years after menarche.*

Menstrual Headache

Headaches are very common, but it is rare when the cause of the headache is a serious problem. Most headaches are due to vasodilatation, muscle contraction, or psychologic stress. Menstrual headaches include all headaches related in temporal fashion to menses, beginning before or during menstrual flow.[90] For many women with premenstrual syndrome, headache is part of the constellation of PMS symptoms. Here, we are considering the occurrence of headache as a single, solitary symptom associated with menses.

Migraine headaches have a peak incidence of first occurrence at age 15–19; they are most prevalent in women in their late 30s to early 40s, and rare after menopause.[91, 92] An association with menses is observed by 60% of women with migraine headaches. In 7–14% of women with migraine, headaches occur exclusively with menses. Because menstrual migraine improves in two-thirds of migraineurs with pregnancy, this type of migraine seems to be due to falling levels of estrogen and progesterone, triggering a host of responses such as release of prostaglandins and changes in neurotransmitters.[93, 94]

Classic migraine is associated with a visual aura, including bright lights, zigzag lights, or flashes and sparkles. *Common migraine* is not associated with neurologic auras. Complicated migraine refers to headache associated with dramatic focal neurologic features that are transient; e.g, blindness, unilateral paresthesias, or paresis. With increasing age, the focal neurologic phenomena can occur without headache.

Vascular Headaches

Acute and throbbing headaches are due to abnormal vasodilatation. The vasodilatation associated with migraine headaches is believed to follow a period of vasoconstriction. Migraine headaches are usually, but not always, preceded by prodromal symptoms (which may reflect the period of vasoconstriction). Significant vascular headaches can be precipitated by stress, alcohol, or tyramine and tryptophan rich foods (red wine, chocolate, ripe cheeses). Vascular headaches can accompany other problems, such as systemic viral infections, fever, or hypertension. Common migraine headaches are known as "migraine without aura."[91] Classic migraine is referred to as "migraine with aura." Migraine headaches associated with menstruation are typically migraine without aura.[92]

Tension Headaches

The common tension headache is due to prolonged and excessive muscle contraction. The pain is dull, steady, bilateral, and worsens throughout the day. The headaches frequently occur with worry or emotional stress and commonly last for hours or a couple of days; however, everyday minor hassles are a more important factor in the pathogenesis of tension headaches than major stressful events.

Secondary Headaches

This type of headache is due to underlying organic disease. The pain is usually due to pressure or pulling of structures. Headaches associated with brain tumors are usually accompanied by neurologic abnormalities. Other causes are brain abscesses, subdural hematomas, hypertension, drug use, and concussions. The main cause of inflammatory headaches is meningitis.

Evaluation

The acute onset of severe headache pain deserves attention. The following signs suggest the presence of a serious problem: neck stiffness, altered mental status, focal neurologic abnormalities, visual impairment, and fever. Any patient with meningeal signs requires hospitalization. Keep carbon monoxide exposure and drug withdrawal in mind as etiologic agents.

Chronic headaches should be characterized according to location, quality, and course over time. Head trauma in the past is an important piece of information, raising the suspicion of a subdural hematoma. When the headache is cyclic, with periodic complete resolution, one can comfortably ascribe the headache to a vascular origin. Tension headaches are either variable or relatively constant without relentless progression. Any recurrent or chronic headache that gets worse with time deserves a neurologic evaluation.

Management

Menstrually related migraines are more refractory to the battery of therapy used by neurologists, although oral and subcutaneous sumatriptan has been effective.[91, 92, 95] The nonsteroidal anti-inflammatory agents are also effective, particularly when headaches are associated with dysmenorrhea.

Early studies of menstrual migraine indicated that administration of estrogen could delay the onset of migraine even if menses were not delayed.[96] Progesterone administration delayed menses, but not the onset of headache. Others have claimed effective treatment of menstrual migraine with maintenance of estrogen levels (there is reason to believe that a relatively high estrogen level is necessary; e.g., the use of the 100 μg transdermal patch).[97, 98] Still others have reported success with tamoxifen or danazol treatment. Unfortunately this field suffers from a lack of well-designed, double-blind, placebo-controlled studies, and we must make our judgments based on experience.

We have had personal success (anecdotal to be sure) alleviating headaches by eliminating the menstrual cycle, either with the use of *daily* oral contraceptives (not the progestin-only minipill) or the daily administration of a progestational agent (such as 10 mg medroxyprogesterone acetate). Some menstrual migraineurs have extremely gratifying responses.

If menstrual headaches are a reaction to cyclic changes in circulating levels of the sex steroids, it makes sense to avoid cyclicity and maintain a relatively steady state with daily administration of exogenous hormones. A more expensive approach, but one with documented success, is the utilization of a long-acting GnRH agonist combined with estrogen-progestin add-back therapy.[99] Another option is to use an estrogen transdermal application during the menstrual time period.

The elimination of cyclicity can be applied to postmenopausal women who experience exacerbation or onset of headaches on a sequential hormone regimen. The maintenance of daily, relatively constant hormone levels with the daily, continuous program of combined estrogen-progestin has been effective in our experience.

The run-of-the-mill headache is treated with mild analgesics such as aspirin, acetaminophen, or the nonsteroidal anti-inflammatory agents. A problem of severe headaches on oral contraception requires an immediate response. The conservative reaction is to discontinue the oral contraceptives. On the other hand, the headache can be due to stress or some other reversible condition. We would argue that automatic discontinuation of oral contraception is not necessary with the low-dose preparations. It would be better to evaluate the patient and find out if the patient can continue her contraceptive protection, by discovering an explanation for the headaches. Case-control studies with the old higher dose oral contraceptives indicated that migraine headaches were linked to a risk of stroke. Strokes are essentially no longer seen with low-dose oral contraception. (Chapter 22 with full references) This probably reflects both lower dosage as well as the reluctance of clinicians to prescribe oral contraception to women with severe headaches.

True severe vascular headaches (migraine with aura) represent a contraindication for the use of combined oral contraceptives and their appearance is an indication to discontinue oral contraception. The symptom complex that deserves serious consideration includes headaches that last a long time; dizziness, nausea, or vomiting with headaches; scotomata or blurred vision; episodes of blindness; unilateral, unremitting headaches; and headaches that continue despite medication.

Concern over headaches with oral contraception should be limited to the use of combined oral contraceptives. The progestin-only methods are not associated with problems with headaches. Therefore, the sustained release progestin-only methods are also free of headache concern.

Catemenial Seizures

Catamenial epilepsy in ancient times was attributed to the moon, giving rise to the word, "lunatic."[100] Epileptic seizures increase in frequency during menstruation and decrease during the luteal phase.[101-103] Exacerbation of seizure activity with menses occurs in 50% of epileptic women.[104] In addition, seizure frequency increases at the time of the midcycle peak in estrogen and during anovulatory cycles. In animal experiments, estrogen increases seizure activity, and progesterone is antiepileptic. These observations suggest an antiepileptic effect of progesterone.

Progestational hormones are known to have a sedative effect on the central nervous system. This pharmacologic effect combined with the observations indicating increased seizure activity at times when circulating levels of progesterone are low indicated that treatment with a progestin would have a beneficial impact on seizures. Treatment with orally administered progesterone during the luteal phase has been reported to decrease seizure activity.[105]

Antiepileptic drugs enhance hepatic metabolic activity, and, therefore, doses must be relatively high. Oral medroxyprogesterone acetate is relatively ineffective, probably because it is difficult to achieve high blood levels. Intramuscular injections of depot-medroxyprogesterone acetate can improve seizure control. Depot-medroxyprogesterone acetate, 150 mg im every 1–2 months, can decrease seizure frequency by approximately 50%.[106] In a case report of an 8-year-old girl, 150 mg administered every 2 weeks abolished seizure activity.[104] Intravenous progesterone (producing luteal phase levels) can produce a significant decrease in spike frequency.[107]

In women with a seizure pattern consistently linked to menses, elimination of cyclic hormonal changes can bring impressive relief. The administration of daily oral contraceptives, or intramuscular depot-medroxyprogesterone acetate, or GnRH agonist treatment with estrogen-progestin add-back can be used for this purpose.

Premenstrual Asthma

Approximately 30–40% of women with asthma have an increase in symptoms associated with menstruation.[108–110] Even asthmatics not aware of a link to menstruation demonstrate a menstrual worsening of pulmonary function.[111, 112] The mechanism is not known, but obvious effects of menstrual hormonal changes have been suggested, such as prostaglandin release, changes in the immune system, or a direct impact of declining estrogen and progesterone on bronchial smooth muscle. The administration of estrogen (estradiol 2 mg orally daily) improves symptoms and measurements of pulmonary function.[112] In another report, the administration of intramuscular progesterone ameliorated premenstrual asthma.[113] Once again, the logic is appealing that the elimination of menstrual periods (with the daily administration of oral contraceptives or intramuscular depot-medroxyprogesterone acetate or with a long-acting GnRH agonist together with an estrogen-progestin supplement) can have a beneficial impact on a menstrual condition, in this case premenstrual asthma, a disorder that can even be lethal.

Catamenial Pneumothorax

Very rarely, recurrent pneumothoraces, often due to pulmonary endometriosis, occur at the time of menses.[114] Effective medical treatment requires the long-term suppression of menstruation.[115] The two best therapeutic choices are again the daily administration of oral contraceptives or treatment with a long-acting GnRH agonist supplemented with a daily estrogen-progestin combination.

References

1. **Golub S,** *Periods, from Menarche to Menopause,* Sage Publications, Newbury Park, California, 1992.

2. **Rubinow DR,** The premenstrual syndrome: new views, *JAMA* 168:1908, 1992.

3. **Osofsky JH, Blumenthal SJ,** eds, *Premenstrual Syndrome: Current Findings and Future Directions,* American Psychiatric Press, Washington, D.C., 1985.

4. **Ramacharan S, Love EJ, Fick GH, Goldfien A,** The epidemiology of premenstrual symptoms in a population based sample of 2650 urban women, *J Clin Epidemiol* 45:377, 1992.

5. **Merikangas KR, Foeldenyi M, Angst J,** The Zurich Study. XIX. Patterns of menstrual disturbances in the community: results of the Zurich Cohort Study, *Eur Arch Psychiatry Clin Neurosci* 243:23, 1993.

6. **Logue CM, Moos RH,** Perimenstrual symptoms: prevalence and risk factors, *Psychosom Med* 48:388, 1986.

7. **Rubinow DR, Roy-Byrne P,** Premenstrual syndromes: overview from a methodologic perspective, *Am J Psychiatr* 141:2, 1984.

8. **Sommer B,** The effect of menstruation on cognitive and perceptual-motor behavior: a review, *Psychosom Med* 35:515, 1973.

9. **Freeman EW, Sondheimer SJ, Rickels K,** Effects of medical history factors on symptom severity in women meeting criteria for premenstrual syndrome, *Obstet Gynecol* 72:236, 1988.

10. **Wilson CA, Turner CW, Keye WR,** Firstborn adolescent daughters and mothers with and without premenstrual sydnrome: a comparison, *J Adolesc Health* 12:130, 1991.

11. **Frank RT,** The hormonal causes of premenstrual tension, *Arch Neurol Psychiatr* 26:1052, 1931.

12. **Israel SL,** Premenstrual tension, *JAMA* 110:1721, 1934.

13. **Greene R, Dalton K,** The premenstrual syndrome, *Br Med J* i:1007, 1953.

14. **Parry BL,** Psychobiology of premenstrual dysphoric disorder, *Seminars Reprod Endocrinol* 15:55, 1997.

15. **Crawford R,** Superstitions of menstruation, *Lancet* ii:1331, 1915.

16. **Secundus Plinius C,** *Historia Naturalis,* Carbondale HP, Translator, Southern Illinois Press, 1962.

17. **d'Orban PT,** Medicolegal aspects of the premenstrual syndrome, *Br J Hosp Med,* December, 1983.

18. **Dalton K,** *The Premenstrual Syndrome and Progesterone Therapy,* 2nd edition, Yearbook Medical Publishers, Inc., Chicago, 1984.

19. **Gannon FL,** Evidence for a psychological etiology of menstrual disorders: a critical review, *Psychol Rep* 48:287, 1981.

20. **Morgan M, Rapkin AJ, D'Elia L, Reading A, Goldman L,** Cognitive functioning in premenstrual syndrome, *Obstet Gynecol* 88:961, 1996.

21. **Walsh RM, Budtz-Olsen I, Leader C, Cummins RA,** The menstrual cycle, personality, and academic performance, *Arch Gen Psychiat* 38:219, 1981.

22. **Rubinow DR, Schmidt PJ,** Premenstrual sydnrome: a review of endocrine studies, *Endocrinologist* 2:47, 1992.

23. **Schmidt PJ, Purdy RH, Moore Jr PH, Paul SM, Rubinow DR,** Circulating levels of anxiolytic steroids in the luteal phase in women with premenstrual syndrome and in control subjects, *J Clin Endocrinol Metab* 79:1256, 1994.

24. **Mira M, Stewart PM, Abraham SF,** Vitamin and trace element status in premenstrual syndrome, *Am J Clin Nutr* 47:636, 1988.

25. **Facchinetti F, Martignoni E, Petraglia F, Sances MG, Nappi G, Genazzani AR,** Premenstrual fall of plasma β-endorphin in patients with premenstrual syndrome, *Fertil Steril* 47:570, 1987.

26. **Tulenheimo A, Laatikainen T, Salminen K,** Plasma β-endorphin immunoreactivity in premenstrual tension, *Br J Obstet Gynaecol* 94:26, 1987.

27. **Chuong CJ, Coulam CB, Bergstralh EJ, O'Fallon WM, Steinmetz GI,** Clinical trial of naltrexone in premenstrual syndrome, *Obstet Gynecol* 72:332, 1988.

28. **Schmidt PJ, Nieman LK, Grover GN, Muller KL, Merriam GR, Rubinow DR,** Lack of effect of induced menses on symptoms in women with premenstrual syndrome, *New Engl J Med* 324:1174, 1991.

29. **Korzekwa MI, Lamont JA, Steiner M,** Late luteal phase dysphoric disorder and the thyroid axis revisited, *J Clin Endocrinol Metab* 81:2280, 1996.

30. **Schmidt PJ, Grover GN, Roy-Byrne PP, Rubinow DR,** Thyroid function in women with premenstrual sydnrome, *J Clin Endocrinol Metab* 76:671, 1993.

31. **Vellacott ID, Shroff NE, Pearce MY, Stratford ME, Akbar FA,** A double-blind, placebo-controlled evaluation of spironolactone in the premenstrual syndrome, *Curr Med Res Opin* 10:450, 1987.

32. **Burnet RB, Radden HS, Easterbrook EG, McKinnon RA,** Premenstrual syndrome and spironolactone, *Aust NZ J Obstet Gynaecol* 31:366, 1991.

33. **Khoo SK, Munro C, Battistutta D,** Evening primrose oil and treatment of premenstrual syndrome, *Med J Aust* 153:189, 1990.

34. **Collins A, Cerin A, Coleman G, Landgren B-M,** Essential fatty acids in the treatment of premenstrual syndrome, *Obstet Gynecol* 81:93, 1993.

35. **Budeiri DJ, LiWanPo A, Dornan JC,** Is evening primrose oil of value in the treatment of premenstrual syndrome? *Control Clin Trials* 17:60, 1996.

36. **Puolakka J, Makarainen L, Viinikka L, Ylikorkola O,** Biochemical and clinical effects of treating the premenstrual syndrome with prostaglandin synthesis precursors, *J Reprod Med* 30:149, 1985.

37. **Mira M, McNeil D, Fraser IS, Vizzard J, Abraham S,** Mefenamic acid in the treatment of premenstrual syndrome, *Obstet Gynecol* 68:395, 1986.

38. **Sampson GA,** Premenstrual syndrome: a double-blind controlled trial of progesterone and placebo, *Br J Psychiatr* 135:209, 1979.

39. **Van der Meer YG, Benedek-Jaszmann LJ, Van Loenen AC,** Effects of high-dose progesterone on the premenstrual syndrome: a double-blind cross-over trial, *J Psychosom Obstet Gynecol* 2:220, 1983.

40. **Andersch B, Hahn L,** Progesterone treatment of premenstrual tension — a double blind study, *J Psychosom Res* 29:489, 1985.

41. **Richter MA, Haltvick R, Shapiro SS,** Progesterone treatment of premenstrual syndrome, *Curr Ther Res* 36:840, 1984.

42. **Maddocks S, Hahn P, Moller F, Reid RL,** A double-blind placebo-controlled trial of progesterone vaginal suppositories in the treatment of premenstrual syndrome, *Am J Obstet Gynecol* 154:573, 1986.

43. **Freeman E, Rickels K, Sondheimer SJ, Plansky M,** Ineffectiveness of progesterone suppository treatment for premenstrual syndrome, *JAMA* 264:349, 1990.

44. **Freeman EW, Richels K, Sondheimer SJ, Polansky M,** A double-blind trial of oral progesterone, alprazolam, and placebo in treatment of severe premenstrual syndrome, *JAMA* 274:51, 1995.

45. **Dennerstein L, Spencer-Gardner C, Gotts G, Brown JB, Smith MA, Burrows GD,** Progesterone and the premenstrual syndrome: a double blind cross-over trial, *Br Med J* 290:1617, 1985.

46. **Casson P, Hahn PM, Van Vugt DA, Reid RL,** Lasting response to ovariectomy in severe intractable premenstrual syndrome, *Am J Obstet Gynecol* 162:99, 1990.

47. **Casper RF, Hearn MT,** The effect of hysterectomy and bilateral oophorectomy in women with severe premenstrual syndrome, *Am J Obstet Gynecol* 162:105, 1990.

48. **Mortola JF, Girton L, Fischer U,** Successful treatment of severe premenstrual syndrome by combined use of gonadotropin-releasing hormone agonist and estrogen/progestin, *J Clin Endocrinol Metab* 71:252, 1991.

49. **Hussain SY, Massil JH, Matta WH, Shaw RW, O'Brien PMS,** Buserelin in premenstrual syndrome, *Gynecol Endocrinol* 6:57, 1992.

50. **Brown CS, Ling FW, Andersen RN, Farmer RG, Arheart KL,** Efficacy of depo leuprolide in premenstrual syndrome: effect of symptom severity and type in a controlled trial, *Obstet Gynecol* 84:779, 1994.

51. **Schmidt PJ, Nieman LK, Danaceau MA, Adams LF, Rubinow DR,** Differential behavioral effects of gonadal steroids in women with and in those without premenstrual syndrome, *New Engl J Med* 338:209, 1998.

52. **Stone AB, Pearlstein TB, Brown WA,** Fluoxetine in the treatment of late luteal phase dysphoric disorder, *J Clin Psychiatr* 52:290, 1991.

53. **Wood SH, Mortola JF, Chan Y-F, Moossazadeh F, Yen SSC,** Treatment of premenstrual sydrome with fluoxetine: a double-blind, placebo-controlled, crossover study, *Obstet Gynecol* 80:339, 1992.

54. **Menkes DB, Taghavi E, Mason PA, Spears GFS, Howard RC,** Fluoxetine treatment of severe premenstrual syndrome, *Br Med J* 305:346, 1992.

55. **Sundblad C, Hedberg MA, Eriksson E,** Clomipramine administered during the luteal phase reduces the symptoms of premenstrual syndrome: a placebo-controlled trial, *Neuropsychopharmacology* 9:133, 1993.

56. **Eriksson E, Hedber MA, Andersch B, Sundblad C,** The serotonin reuptake inhibitor paroxetine is superior to the noradrenaline reuptake inhibitor maprotiline in the treatment of premenstrual syndrome: a placebo-controlled trial, *Neuropsychopharmacology* 12:169, 1995.

57. **Steiner M, Steinberg S, Stewart D, Carter D, Berger C, Reid R, Grover D, Streiner D, for the Canadian Fluoxetine/Premenstrual Dysphoria Collaborative Study Group,** Fluoxetine in the treatment of premenstrual dysphoria, *New Engl J Med* 332:1529, 1995.

58. **Yonkers KA, Halbreich U, Freeman E, Brown C, Endicott J, Frank E, Parry B, Pearlstein T, Severino S, Stout A, Stone A, Harrison W, for the Sertraline Premenstrual Dysphoric Collaborative Study Group,** Symptomatic improvement of premenstrual dysphoric disorder with sertraline treatment. A randomized controlled trial, *JAMA* 278:983, 1997.

59. **Pearlstein TB, Stone AB, Lund SA, Scheft H, Zlotnick C, Brown WA,** Comparison of fluoxetine, bupropion, and placebo in the treatment of premenstrual dysphoric disorder, *J Clin Psychopharmacol* 17:261, 1997.

60. **Halbreich U, Smoller JW,** Intermittent luteal phase sertraline treatment of dysphoric premenstrual syndrome, *J Clin Psychiatry* 58:1, 1997.

61. **Smith S, Rinehart JS, Ruddock VE, Schiff I,** Treatment of premenstrual syndrome with alprazolam: results of a double-blind, placebo-controlled, randomized crossover clinical trial, *Obstet Gynecol* 70:37, 1987.

62. **Harrison WM, Endicott J, Nee J,** Treatment of premenstrual dysphoria with alprazolam, *Arch Gen Psychiatr* 47:270, 1990.

63. **Brooks J, Ruble D, Clark A,** College women's attitudes and expectations concerning menstrual-related changes, *Psychosom Med* 39:288, 1977.

64. **Ruble DN,** Premenstrual symptoms: a reinterpretation, *Science* 197:291, 1977.

65. **Halbreich U, Endicott J,** Methodological issues in studies of premenstrual changes, *Psychoneuroendocrinology* 10:15, 1985.

66. **Vila J, Breech HR,** Premenstrual symptomatology: an interaction hypothesis, *Br J Soc Clin Psychol* 19:73, 1980.

67. **AuBuchon PG, Calhoun KS,** Menstrual cycle symptomatology: the role of social expectancy and experimental demand characteristics, *Psychosom Med* 47:35, 1985.

68. **Olasov B, Jackson J,** Effects of expectancies on women's reports of moods during the menstrual cycle, *Psychosom Med* 49:65, 1987.

69. **Cousins N,** *Anatomy of an Illness,* Bantam Books, New York, 1979.

70. **Eisenberg L,** The subjective in medicine, *Perspectives Biol Med* 27:48, 1983.

71. **Reid RL,** Premenstrual syndrome, *Curr Prob Obstet Gynecol Fertil* 8:1, 1985.

72. **Mortola JF, Girton L, Beck L, Yen SS,** Diagnosis of premenstrual syndrome by a simple prospective and reliable instrument: the calendar of premenstrual experiences, *Obstet Gynecol* 76:302, 1990.

73. **Leibenluft E, Fiero PL, Rubinow DR,** Effects of the menstrual cycle on dependent variables in mood disorder research, *Arch Gen Psychiatry* 51:761, 1994.

74. **Thys-Jacobs S, Starkey P, Bernstein D, Tian J, and the Premenstrual Syndrome Study Group,** Calcium carbonate and the premenstrual syndrome: effects on premenstrual and menstrual symptoms, *Am J Obstet Gynecol* 179:444, 1998.

75. **Schmidt PJ, Grover GN, Rubinow DR,** Alprazolam in the treatment of premenstrual syndrome: a double-blind, placebo-controlled trial, *Arch Gen Psychiatry* 50:467, 1993.

76. **West CP, Hillier H,** Ovarian suppression with the gonadotrophin-releasing hormone agonist goserelin (Zoladex) in management of the premenstrual tension syndrome, *Hum Reprod* 9:1058, 1994.

77. **Pearlstein TB, Stone AB,** Long-term fluoxetine treatment of late luteal phase dysphoric disorder, *J Clin Psychiatry* 55:332, 1994.

78. **Andersch B, Milsom I,** An epidemiologic study of young women with dysmenorrhea, *Am J Obstet Gynecol* 144:655, 1982.

79. **Harlow SD, Park M,** A longitudinal study of risk factors for the occurrence, duration and severity of menstrual cramps in a cohort of college women, *Br J Obstet Gynaecol* 103:1134, 1996.

80. **Vicdan K, Kukner S, Dabakoglu T, Ergin T, Keles G, Gokmen O,** Demographic and epidemiologic features of female adolescents in Turkey, *J Adolesc Health* 18:54, 1996.

81. **Coppen A, Kessel N,** Menstruation and personality, *Br J Psychiatr* 109:771, 1963.

82. **Klein JR, Litt IF,** Epidemiology of adolescent dysmenorrhea, *Pediatrics* 68:661, 1981.

83. **Parazzini F, Tozzi L, Mezzopane R, Luchini L, Marchini M, Fedele L,** Cigarette smoking, alcohol consumption, and risk of primary dysmenorrhea, *Epidemiology* 5:469, 1994.

84. **Charlton A, While D,** Smoking and menstrual problems in 16-year-olds, *J Roy Soc Med* 89:193, 1996.

85. **Sundell G, Milsom I, Andersch B,** Factors influencing the prevalence and severity of dysmenorrhea in young women, *Br J Obstet Gynaecol* 97:588, 1990.

86. **Dawood MY**, ed, *Dysmenorrhea,* Williams & Wilkins, Baltimore, 1981.

87. **Eldering JA, Nay MG, Hoberg LM, Longcope C, McCracken JA,** Hormonal regulation of prostaglandin production by Rhesus monkey endometrium, *J Clin Endocrinol Metab* 71:596, 1990.

88. **Robinson JC, Plichter S, Weisman CS, Nathanson CA, Ensminger M,** Dysmenorrhea and use of oral contraceptives in adolescent women attending a family planning clinic, *Am J Obstet Gynecol* 166:578, 1992.

89. **Owens PR,** Prostaglandin synthetase inhibitors in the treatment of primary dysmenorrhea: outcome trials reviewed, *Am J Obstet Gynecol* 148:96, 1984.

90. **Nattero G,** Menstrual headache, *Adv Neurol* 33:215, 1982.

91. **Sheftell FD, Silberstein SD, Rapoport AM, Rossum RW,** Migraine and women: diagnosis, pathophysiology, and treatment, *J Women's Health* 1:5, 1992.

92. **MacGregor EA,** Menstruation, sex hormones, and migraine, *Adv Headache* 15:125, 1997.

93. **Marcus DA,** Interrelationships of neurochemicals, estrogen, and recurring headache, *Pain* 62:129, 1995.

94. **Fioroni L, Martignoni E, Facchinetti F,** Changes of neuroendocrine axes in patients with menstrual migraine, *Cephalagia* 15:297, 1995.

95. **Facchinetti F, Bonellie G, Kangasniemi P, Fascual J, Shuaib A,** The efficacy and safety of subcutaneous sumatriptan in the acute treatment of menstrual migraine, *Obstet Gynecol* 86:911, 1995.

96. **Somerville BW,** Estrogen-withdrawal migraine. II. Attempted prophylaxis by continuous estradiol administration, *Neurology* 25:245, 1975.

97. **de Ligniéres B, Vincens M, Mauvais-Jarvis P, Mas JL, Touboul PJ, Bousser MG,** Prevention of menstrual migraine by percutaneous oestradiol, *Br Med J* 193:1540, 1986.

98. **Granella F, Sances G, Messa G, de Marinis M, Manzoni GC,** Treatment of menstrual migraine, *Cephalalgia* 17(Suppl 20):35, 1997.

99. **Murray SC, Muse KN,** Effective treatment of severe menstrual migraine headaches with gonadotropin-releasing hormne agonist and "add-back" therapy, *Fertil Steril* 67:390, 1997.

100. **Newmark ME, Penry JK,** Catamenial epilepsy: a review, *Epilepsia* 21:281, 1980.

101. **Backstrom T,** Epileptic seizures in women related to plasma estrogen and progesterone during the menstrual cycle, *Acta Neurol Scand* 54:321, 1976.

102. **Mattson RH, Kamer JA, Cramer JA, Caldwell BV,** Seizure frequency and the menstrual cycle: a clinical study, *Epilepsia* 22:242, 1981.

103. **Lundberg PO,** Catamenial epilepsy: a review, *Cephalalgia* 17(Suppl 20):42, 1997.

104. **Zimmerman AW, Holden KR, Reiter EO, Dekaban AS,** Medroxyprogesterone acetate in the treatment of seizures associated with menstruation, *J Pediatr* 83:959, 1973.

105. **Herzog AG,** Progesterone therapy in women with complex partial and secondary generalized seizures, *Neurol* 45:1660, 1995.

106. **Mattson RH, Cramer JA, Caldwell BV, Siconolfi BC,** Treatment of seizures with medroxyprogesterone acetate: preliminary report, *Neurol* 34:1255, 1984.

107. **Backstrom T, Zetterlund B, Blom S, Romano M,** Effects of intravenous progesterone infusions on the epileptic discharge frequency in women with partial epilepsy, *Acta Neurol Scand* 69:240, 1984.

108. **Hanley SP,** Asthma variation with menstruation, *Br J Dis Chest* 75:306, 1981.

109. **Enright T, Lim DT, Devnani R, Mariano R,** Cyclical exacerbations of bronchial asthma, *Ann Allergy* 58:405, 1987.

110. **Skobeloff EM, Spivey WH, Silverman RA, Eskin BA, Harchelroad FP, Alessi TV,** The effect of the menstrual cycle on asthma presentations in the emergency department, *Arch Intern Med* 156:1837, 1996.

111. **Pauli BD, Reid RL, Munt PW, Wigle RD, Forkert L,** Influence of the menstrual cycle on airway function in asthmatic and normal subjects, *Am Rev Respir Dis* 140:358, 1989.

112. **Chandler MHH, Schuldheisz S, Phillips BA, Muse KN,** Premenstrual asthma: the effect of estrogen on symptoms, pulmonary function, and β_2-receptors, *Pharmacotherapy* 17:224, 1997.

113. **Beynon HLC, Garbett ND, Barnes PJ,** Severe premenstrual exacerbations of asthma: effect of intramuscular progesterone, *Lancet* ii:370, 1988.

114. **Lillington GA, Mitchell SP, Wood GA,** Catamenial pneumothorax, *JAMA* 219:1328, 1972.

115. **Dotson RL, Peterson M, Doucette RC, Quinton R, Rawson DY, Parker Jones K,** Medical therapy for recurring catamenial pneumothorax following pleurodesis, *Obstet Gynecol* 82:656, 1993.

15 Dysfunctional Uterine Bleeding

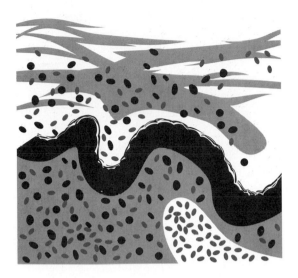

Dysfunctional uterine bleeding is defined as a variety of bleeding manifestations of anovulatory cycles (in the absence of pathology or medical illness). It can be confidently managed without surgical intervention by therapeutic regimens founded on sound physiologic principles. Our formulation is based on knowledge of how the post-ovulatory menstrual function is naturally controlled, and uses pharmacologic application of sex steroids to reverse the abnormal tissue factors that lead to the excessive and prolonged flow typical of anovulatory cycles.

Three major categories of dysfunctional endometrial bleeding are dealt with:

1. Estrogen withdrawal bleeding,

2. Estrogen breakthrough bleeding, and

3. Progestin breakthrough bleeding.

In each instance, the manner in which the endometrium deviates from the norm is characterized, and specific sex steroid therapy is recommended to counter the difficulties each situation presents.

This mode of clinical management has been in regular use for many years, and failure to control vaginal bleeding with this therapy, despite appropriate application and utilization, excludes the diagnosis of dysfunctional uterine bleeding. If this occurs, attention is directed to a pathologic entity within the reproductive tract as the cause of abnormal bleeding.

Heavy but regular menstrual bleeding can be encountered in ovulating women. In the absence of a specific pathologic cause, it is presumed that this reflects subtle disturbances in the endometrial tissue mechanisms discussed in Chapter 4. In essentially all cases, evaluation and treatment are identical to the approach detailed in this chapter.

Length of Menstrual Cycles

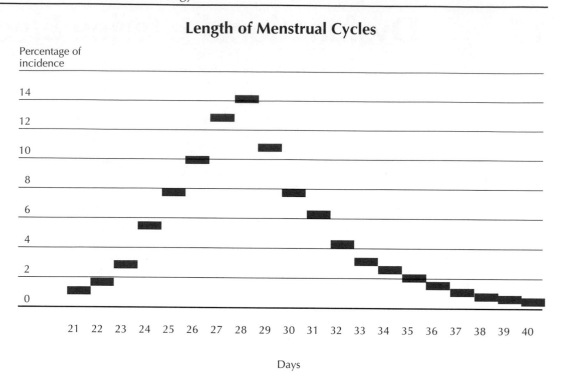

Percentage of incidence

Days

Normal Withdrawal (Menstrual) Bleeding

Of all the types of hormonal-endometrial relationships, the most stable endometrium and the most reproducible menstrual function in terms of quantity and duration occurs with postovulatory estrogen-progesterone withdrawal bleeding. It is so controlling that many women over the years come to expect a certain characteristic flow pattern. Any slight deviations, such as plus or minus 1 day in duration or minor deviation from expected napkin or tampon utilization, are causes for major concern in the patient. So ingrained is the expected flow that considerable clinician reassurance may be required in some instances of minor variability. Although variability of menstrual cycles is a common feature during teenage years and the perimenopausal transition, the characteristics of menstrual bleeding do not undergo appreciable change during the reproductive years.[1]

Menarche is followed by approximately 5–7 years of relatively long cycles at first, and then there is increasing regularity as cycles shorten to reach the usual reproductive age pattern. In the 40s, cycles begin to lengthen again. The highest incidence of anovulatory cycles is under age 20 and over age 40.[2, 3] At age 25, over 40% of cycles are between 25 and 28 days in length; from 25 to 35, over 60% are between 25 and 28 days. Overall, approximately 15% of reproductive age cycles are 28 days in length. Only 0.5% of women experience a cycle less than 21 days long, and only 0.9% a cycle greater than 35 days.[4] Most women have cycles that last from 24 to 35 days, but at least 20% of women experience irregular cycles.[1] When women are in their 40s, anovulation becomes more prevalent, and prior to anovulation, menstrual cycle length increases, beginning 2 to 8 years before menopause.[5]

The usual duration of flow is 4–6 days, but many women flow as little as 2 days, and as much as 7 days. The normal volume of menstrual blood loss is 30 mL.[6] Greater than 80 mL is abnormal. Most of the blood loss occurs during the first 3 days of a period, so excessive flow may exist without prolongation of flow.[7, 8]

Menstrual Period Characteristics

	Normal	Abnormal
Duration of flow	4–6 days	Less than 2; more than 7 days
Volume of flow	30 mL	More than 80 mL
Cycle	24–35 days	

Although the postovulatory phase averages 14 days, greater variability in the proliferative phase produces a distribution in the duration of a menstrual cycle. Based on the normal experience, menstrual bleeding more often than every 24 days or less often than every 35 days deserves evaluation.[1, 5] Flow that lasts 7 or more days also deserves evaluation. A flow that totals more than 80 mL per month usually leads to anemia and should be treated.[9, 10] In general, however, an effort to quantitate menstrual flow beyond historical information is not necessary because evaluation and treatment are responses to a patient's own perceptions regarding duration, amount, and timing of her menstrual bleeding. Although the correlation between a patient's perceptions and actual menstrual blood loss is poor,[11] an individual patient's anxiety and concern deserve consideration and evaluation. Midcycle bleeding can be a consequence of the preovulatory fall in estrogen; however, intermenstrual bleeding is often due to pathology.

The histologic changes in the endometrium of a normal, ovulatory menstrual cycle have been detailed in Chapter 4. An understanding of these events provides the foundation and framework to understand abnormal endometrial bleeding. There are three reasons for the self-limited character of estrogen-progesterone withdrawal bleeding.

1. *It is a universal endometrial event.* Because the onset and conclusion of menses are related to a precise sequence of hormonal events, menstrual changes occur almost simultaneously in all segments of the endometrium.

2. *The endometrial tissue that has responded to an appropriate sequence of estrogen and progesterone is structurally stable, and random breakdown of tissue due to fragility is avoided.* The events leading to ischemic disintegration of the endometrium are orderly and progressive, being related to rhythmic waves of vasoconstriction of increasing duration.

3. *Inherent in the events that start menstrual function following estrogen-progesterone are the factors involved in stopping menstrual flow.* Just as waves of vasoconstriction initiate the ischemic events, prolonged vasoconstriction abetted by the stasis associated with endometrial collapse enables clotting factors to seal off the exposed bleeding sites. Additional and significant effects are obtained by resumed estrogen activity.

The withdrawal of estrogen and progesterone initiates important endometrial events: vasomotor reactions, the process of apoptosis, tissue loss, and, finally, menstruation. The most prominent immediate effect of this hormone withdrawal is a modest shrinking of the tissue height and remarkable spiral arteriole vasomotor responses. The following vascular sequence has been constructed from direct observations of rhesus endometrium.[12, 13] With shrinkage of height, blood flow within the spiral vessels diminishes, venous drainage is decreased, and vasodilatation ensues. Thereafter, the spiral arterioles undergo rhythmic vasoconstriction and relaxation. Each successive spasm is more prolonged and profound, leading eventually to endometrial blanching. Within the 24 hours immediately preceding menstruation, these reactions lead to endometrial ischemia and stasis. White cells migrate through capillary walls, at first remaining adjacent to vessels, but then extending throughout the stroma. During arteriolar vasomotor changes, red blood cells escape into the interstitial space. Thrombin-platelet plugs also appear in superficial vessels. The prostaglandin content ($PGF_{2\alpha}$ and PGE_2) in the secretory endometrium reaches its highest levels at the time of menstruation. The vasoconstriction and myometrial contractions associated with the menstrual events are believed to be significantly mediated by $PGF_{2\alpha}$ from glandular cells and the potent vasoconstrictor, endothelin-1, derived from stromal decidual cells.

In the first half of the secretory phase, acid phosphatase and potent lytic enzymes are confined to lysosomes. Their release is inhibited by progesterone stabilization of the lysosomal membranes. With the waning of estrogen and progesterone levels, the lysosomal membranes are not maintained, and the enzymes are released into the cytoplasm of epithelial, stromal, and endothelial cells, and, eventually, into the intercellular space. These active enzymes will digest their cellular constraints, leading to the release of prostaglandins, extravasation of red blood cells, tissue necrosis, and vascular thrombosis. This process is one of *apoptosis* (programmed cell death, characterized by a specific morphologic pattern that involves cell shrinkage and chromatin condensation culminating in cell fragmentation) mediated by cytokines.[14]

Endometrial tissue breakdown involves a family of enzymes, matrix metalloproteinases, that degrade components (including collagens, gelatins, fibronectin, and laminin) of the extracellular matrix and basement membrane.[15] The metalloproteinases include collagenases that degrade interstitial and basement membrane collagens, gelatinases that further degrade collagens, and stromelysins that degrade fibronectin, laminin, and glycoproteins. The expression of metalloproteinases in human endometrium follows a pattern correlated with the menstrual cycle, indicating a sex steroid response as part of the growth and remodeling of the endometrium, with a marked increase in late secretory and early menstrual endometrium.[16] Progesterone withdrawal from endometrial cells induces matrix metalloproteinase secretion that is followed by the breakdown of cellular membranes and the dissolution of extracellular matrix.[17] Appropriately, this enzyme expression increases in the decidualized endometrium of the late secretory phase, during the time of declining progesterone levels. With the continuing progesterone secretion of early pregnancy, the decidua is maintained and metalloproteinase expression is suppressed, in a mechanism mediated by TFG-β.[18] In a nonpregnant cycle, metalloproteinase expression is suppressed after menses, presumably by increasing estrogen levels. Metalloproteinase activity is restrained by specific tissue inhibitors, designated as TIMP. Thus progesterone withdrawal can lead to endometrial breakdown through a mechanism that is independent of vascular events (specifically ischemia), a mechanism that involves cytokines.[14]

Eventually considerable leakage occurs as a result of diapedesis, and, finally, interstitial hemorrhage occurs due to breaks in superficial arterioles and capillaries. As ischemia and weakening progress, the continuous binding membrane is fragmented, and intercellular blood is extruded into the endometrial cavity. New thrombin-platelet plugs form intravascularly upstream at the shedding surface, limiting blood loss. Increased blood loss is a consequence of reduced platelet numbers and inadequate hemostatic plug formation. Menstrual bleeding is influenced by activation of clotting and fibrinolysis. Fibrinolysis is principally the consequence of the potent enzyme, plasmin, formed from its inactive precursor, plasminogen. Endometrial stromal cell tissue factor (TF) and plasminogen activators and inhibitors are involved in achieving a balance in this process. TF stimulates coagulation, initially binding to factor VII. TF and plasminogen activator inhibitor-1 (PAI-1) expression accompanies decidualization, and the levels of these factors may govern the amount of bleeding.[19] PAI-1, in particular, exerts an important restraining action on fibrinolysis and proteolytic activity.[20]

With further tissue disorganization, the endometrium shrinks even more, and coiled arterioles are buckled. Additional ischemic breakdown ensues with necrosis of cells and defects in vessels adding to the menstrual effluvium. A natural cleavage point exists between basalis and spongiosum, and, once breached, the loose, vascular, edematous stroma of the spongiosum desquamates and collapses. The process is initiated in the fundus and inexorably extends throughout the uterus. In the end, the typical deflated shallow dense menstrual endometrium results. Within 13 hours, the endometrial height shrinks from 4 mm to 1.25 mm.[21] Menstrual flow stops as a result of the combined effects of prolonged vasoconstriction, tissue collapse, vascular stasis, and estrogen-induced "healing." In contrast to postpartum bleeding, myometrial contractions are not important for control of menstrual bleeding. Thrombin generation in the basal endometrium in response to extravasation of blood is essential for hemostasis. Thrombin promotes the generation of fibrin, the activation of platelets and clotting cofactors, and angiogenesis.

Platelets and fibrin play a direct part in the hemostasis achieved in a bleeding menstrual endometrium. Deficiencies in these constituents cause the increased blood loss seen in von Willebrand's disease and in thrombocytopenia. The blood loss at menses in afibrinogenemia indicates the importance of fibrin-generating and fibrinolytic factors in the menstrual process. Intravascular thrombi are observed in the functional layers and are localized to the shedding surface of the tissue. These are known as impeding "plugs" because blood may flow past these only partially occlusive barriers. Therefore, thrombi continue to develop within the menstrual blood, accounting for the platelets and large amounts of fibrin found in this effluent. Fibrinolysis occurs in the endometrial tissue, limiting fibrin deposition in the proximal, still unshed layer. Despite large holes in vessel walls, with blood exposed to collagen surfaces, no occlusive surface thrombus is formed. After early dependence on thrombin plugs to restrain blood loss, later generalized vasoconstrictive hemostasis without thrombin plugs occur. The healing endometrium is pale, collapsed, and disorderly, but no thrombi and no fibrin deposits are seen.

Lockwood assigns a key role to decidual cells in both the process of endometrial bleeding (menstruation) and the process of endometrial hemostasis (implantation and placentation).[22] Implantation requires endometrial hemostasis and the maternal uterus requires resistance to invasion. Inhibition of endometrial hemorrhage can be attributed, to a significant degree, to appropriate changes in critical factors as a consequence of decidualization; e.g., lower plasminogen activator levels, reduced expression of the enzymes that degrade the stromal extracellular matrix (such as the metalloproteinases), increased levels of plasminogen activator inhibitor-1 and tissue factor. Withdrawal of estrogen and progesterone support, however, leads to changes in the opposite directions, consistent with endometrial breakdown.

Traditional Definitions

Oligomenorrhea:	**Intervals greater than 35 days.**
Polymenorrhea:	**Intervals less than 24 days.**
Menorrhagia:	**Regular normal intervals, excessive flow and duration.**
Metrorrhagia:	**Irregular intervals, excessive flow and duration.**

Endometrial Responses to Steroid Hormones: Physiologic and Pharmacologic

Obviously, estrogen and progesterone withdrawal is not the only type of endometrial bleeding provoked by the presence of sex steroids and their effects on the endometrium. There are clinical examples for estrogen withdrawal bleeding and estrogen breakthrough bleeding, as well as for progesterone withdrawal and breakthrough bleeding.

Estrogen Withdrawal Bleeding

This category of uterine bleeding can occur after bilateral oophorectomy, radiation of mature follicles, or administration of estrogen to a castrate and then discontinuation of therapy. Similarly, the bleeding that occurs postcastration can be delayed by concomitant estrogen therapy. Flow will occur on discontinuation of exogenous estrogen. Midcycle bleeding can occur secondary to the decrease in estrogen that immediately precedes ovulation.

Estrogen Breakthrough Bleeding

Here a semiquantitative relationship exists between the amount of estrogen stimulating the endometrium and the type of bleeding that can ensue. Relatively low doses of estrogen yield intermittent spotting that may be prolonged, but is generally light in quantity of flow. On the other hand, high levels of estrogen and sustained availability lead to prolonged periods of amenorrhea followed by acute, often profuse bleeds with excessive loss of blood.

Progesterone Withdrawal Bleeding

Removal of the corpus luteum will lead to endometrial desquamation. Pharmacologically, a similar event can be achieved by administration and discontinuation of progesterone or a nonestrogenic synthetic progestin. Progesterone withdrawal bleeding occurs only if the endometrium is initially proliferated by endogenous or exogenous estrogen. If estrogen therapy is continued as progesterone is withdrawn, the progesterone withdrawal bleeding still occurs. Only if estrogen levels are increased 10–20-fold will progesterone withdrawal bleeding be delayed.[23]

Progesterone Breakthrough Bleeding

Progesterone breakthrough bleeding occurs only in the presence of an unfavorably high ratio of progesterone to estrogen. In the absence of sufficient estrogen, continuous progesterone therapy will yield intermittent bleeding of variable duration, similar to low-dose estrogen breakthrough bleeding noted above. This is the type of bleeding associated with the long-acting progestin-only contraceptive methods, Norplant and Depo-Provera.[24]

Suggestions for Why Anovulatory Bleeding Is Excessive

Most instances of anovulatory bleeding are examples of estrogen withdrawal or estrogen breakthrough bleeding. The heaviest bleeding is secondary to high sustained levels of estrogen associated with polycystic ovaries, obesity, immaturity of the hypothalamic-pituitary-ovarian axis as in postpubertal teenagers, and late anovulation, usually involving women in their late 30s and 40s. In the absence of growth-limiting progesterone and periodic desquamation, the endometrium attains an abnormal height without concomitant structural support. The tissue increasingly displays intense vascularity, back-to-back glandularity, but without an intervening stromal support matrix. This tissue is fragile and will suffer spontaneous superficial breakage and bleeding. As one site heals, another, and yet another new site of breakdown will appear. The typical clinical picture is that of a pale frightened teenager who has bled for weeks. Also frequently encountered is the older woman with prolonged bleeding who is deeply concerned over this experience as a manifestation of cancer.

In these instances, the usual endometrial control mechanisms are missing. This bleeding is not a universal event, but, rather, it involves random portions of the endometrium at variable times and in asynchronous sequences. The fragility of the vascular adenomatous hyperplastic tissue is responsible for this experience, in part because of excessive growth, but mostly because of irregular stimulation in which the structural rigidity of a well-developed stroma or stratum compactum does not occur. Finally, the flow is prolonged and excessive not only because there is a large quantity of tissue available for bleeding, but more importantly, because there is a disorderly, abrupt, random, breakdown of tissue with consequent opening of multiple vascular channels. There is no vasoconstrictive rhythmicity, no tight coiling of spiral vessels, no orderly collapse to induce stasis. The anovulatory tissue can only rely on the "healing" effects of endogenous estrogen to stop local bleeds. However, this is a vicious cycle in that this healing is only temporary. As quickly as it rebuilds, tissue fragility and breakdown recur at other endometrial sites.

Alternate Hypothesis

Another explanation for the control of postovulatory endometrial bleeding and regeneration has been presented.[25] Based on light and scanning electron microscopy of hysterectomy specimens, this thesis favors nonhormone-related regeneration of surface epithelium from basal glands and cornual area residual tissue with restoration of the continuous binding membrane as the critical events in cessation of blood flow. Endometrial regeneration is viewed as a response to tissue loss, not hormonal changes. By this account, estrogen withdrawal or breakthrough bleeding is uncontrolled because there is insufficient stimulus (loss of tissue) for binding surface restoration to occur. Furthermore, curettage is effective in this condition by reachieving sufficient basal glandular denudation (as is seen also in combined estrogen and progestin withdrawal), which stimulates regeneration of surface integrity and, thus, controls blood flow.

Additional studies are needed to clarify the difference of opinion concerning the pathophysiology of dysfunctional uterine bleeding. Our therapeutic approach favored in this book uses hormonal control of endometrial events and rarely finds it necessary to resort to surgery.

Differential Diagnosis

Dysfunctional uterine bleeding is a diagnosis made by exclusion. A very common cause of abnormal uterine bleeding is pregnancy and pregnancy-related problems such as ectopic pregnancy or spontaneous miscarriage. This category of problems should always receive diagnostic consideration because the most common cause of an abrupt departure from a normal menstrual pattern is pregnancy or a complication of pregnancy. Patients may be using medications unknowingly with an impact on the endometrium. For example, the use of ginseng, an herbal root, has been associated with estrogenic activity and abnormal bleeding.[26] Pathology of the menstrual outflow tract includes cancers of the cervix and endometrium, endometrial polyps, leiomyomata uteri, and infections. Although uterine bleeding is a common problem with various contraceptive methods and postmenopausal hormonal therapy, the clinician should always be convinced no pathology is present. Abnormal menstrual cycles are occasionally the first sign of either hypothyroidism or hyperthyroidism.[27] Irregular, serious bleeding is often associated with severe organ disease, such as renal failure and liver failure. Finally, careful examination is worthwhile to discover genital injury or a foreign object.

One should keep in mind that as many as 20% of adolescents with dysfunctional uterine bleeding will have a coagulation defect, although the most common cause is anovulation.[28, 29] In 150 women aged 15–50 in Helsinki who were referred for the evaluation of menorrhagia, an inherited bleeding disorder was diagnosed in 26 of the patients; the most common diagnoses were von Willebrand's disease (13%) and factor XI deficiency (4%).[30] Bleeding secondary to a blood dyscrasia is usually a heavy flow with regular, cyclic menses (menorrhagia), and this same pattern can be seen in patients being treated with anticoagulants.[31] Bleeding disorders are usually associated with menorrhagia since menarche and a history of bleeding with surgery or trauma. Menorrhagia may be the only sign of an inherited bleeding disorder.[32]

The effects of tubal ligation are still not certain. The first well-controlled studies of this issue demonstrated no change in menstrual patterns, volume, or pain.[33, 34] Subsequently, these same authors reported an increase in dysmenorrhea and changes in menstrual bleeding.[35, 36] However, these authors failed to agree in their findings (a change found by one group was not confirmed by the other). Adding to the confusion, the incidence of hysterectomy for bleeding disorders in women after tubal sterilization was reported to be increased by some,[37] but not by others.[38] In a large cohort of women in a group health plan, hospitalization for menstrual disorders was significantly increased; however, the authors believed this reflected bias by patient and physician preference for surgical treatment.[39] In the U.S. prospective long-term follow-up study of sterilization, the increased risk of hysterectomy after sterilization was concentrated in women who were treated for gynecologic disorders before tubal sterilization.[40] These discordant reports do not make patient counseling about the long-term effects of tubal sterilization an easy task. It is possible that extensive electrocoagulation of the fallopian tubes can change ovarian steroid production. Perhaps this is why menstrual changes were detected with longer (4 years) follow-up, while no changes have been noted with the use of rings or clips.[39, 41, 42] However, attempts to relate poststerilization menstrual changes with extent of tissue destruction fail to find a correlation, and an increase in hospitalization for menstrual disorders after unipolar cautery cannot be documented.[39, 42] Still another long-term follow-up study (3-4.5 years) failed to document any significant changes in menstrual cycles.[43] This inconsistency can reflect differences in sterilization techniques, as well as the fact that a surgical solution is more likely to be chosen if continuing fertility is no longer an issue. The best answer for now is that some women experience menstrual changes, but most do not.

Laboratory tests that can be helpful (but not always necessary) are coagulation studies (prothrombin time, partial thromboplastin time, platelet count, bleeding time, and the ristocetin cofactor assay for the von Willebrand factor), complete blood count, quantitative human chorionic gonadotropin (HCG), prolactin, thyroid function tests, liver function tests, and appropriate cervical cultures.

Treatment Program for Anovulatory Bleeding

The immediate objective of medical therapy in anovulatory bleeding is to retrieve the natural controlling influences missing in this tissue: universal, synchronous endometrial events, structural stability, and vasomotor rhythmicity.

Progestin Therapy

Most women will, at sometime during their reproductive years, either fail to ovulate or not sustain adequate corpus luteum function or duration. But this occurs with increased frequency in adolescence and in the decade prior to menopause. The usual clinical presentation is oligomenorrhea with bouts of heavy bleeding. Women correctly seek medical advice promptly because these menstrual aberrations suggest unplanned pregnancy or uterine pathology. Under most circumstances, progestin therapy will suffice to control the abnormality once uterine pathology is ruled out.

Progesterone and progestins are powerful antiestrogens when given in pharmacologic doses. Progestins stimulate 17β-hydroxysteroid dehydrogenase and sulfotransferase activity, which convert estradiol to estrone sulfate (which is rapidly excreted from the cell).[44] Progestins also diminish estrogen effects on target cells by inhibiting the augmentation of estrogen receptors that ordinarily accompanies estrogen action (receptor replenishment inhibition). In addition, progestins suppress estrogen-mediated transcription of oncogenes.[45] These influences account for the antimitotic, antigrowth impact of progestins on the endometrium (prevention and reversal of hyperplasia, limitation of growth postovulation, and the marked atrophy during pregnancy or in response to combined oral contraceptives).

In the treatment of oligomenorrhea, orderly limited withdrawal bleeding can be accomplished by administration of a progestin such as medroxyprogesterone acetate, 5–10 mg daily for at least 10 days every month. Absence of induced bleeding requires workup. In the treatment of dysfunctional menometrorrhagia or polymenorrhea, progestins are prescribed for 10 days to 2 weeks (to induce stabilizing predecidual stromal changes) followed by a withdrawal flow — the so-called "medical curettage." Thereafter, repeat progestin is offered cyclically for at least the first 10 days of each month to ensure therapeutic effect. Failure of progestin to correct irregular bleeding requires diagnostic reevaluation. ***If contraception is desired, the use of an oral contraceptive is a better choice.***

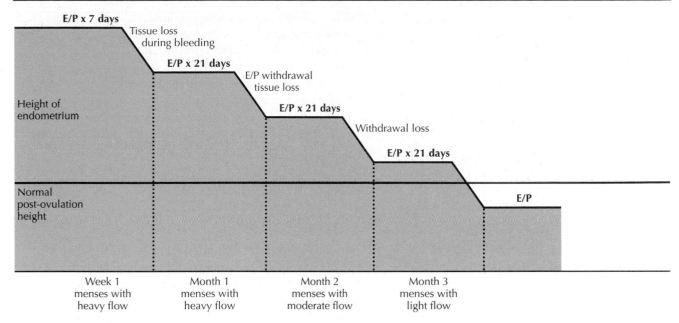

E/P = Estrogen-Progestin combination

Oral Contraceptive Therapy

In young women, anovulatory bleeding may be associated with prolonged endometrial buildup, delayed diagnosis, and heavy blood loss. In these cases, combined progestin-estrogen therapy is used in the form of combined oral contraceptives. Any of the low-dose oral combination monophasic tablets are useful. Whatever formulation is available or chosen, therapy is administered as one pill twice a day for 5–7 days. This therapy is maintained despite cessation of flow within 12–24 hours. If flow does not abate, other diagnostic possibilities (polyps, incomplete abortion, and neoplasia) should be reevaluated.

If flow does diminish rapidly, the remainder of the week of treatment can be given over to the evaluation of causes of anovulation, investigation of hemorrhagic tendencies, and blood replacement or initiation of iron therapy. In addition, the week provides time to prepare the patient for the estrogen-progestin withdrawal flow that will soon be induced. For the moment, therapy has produced the structural rigidity intrinsic to the compact pseudodecidual reaction. Continued random breakdown of formerly fragile tissue is avoided and blood loss stopped. However, a large amount of tissue remains to react to estrogen-progestin withdrawal. The patient must be warned to anticipate a heavy and severely cramping flow 2–4 days after stopping therapy. If not prepared in this way, it is certain that the patient will view the problem as recurrent disease or failure of hormonal therapy.

In successful therapy, on the 5th day of flow or in the usual Sunday start fashion, a low dose combination oral contraceptive medication (one pill a day) is started. This will be repeated for several (usually three) 3-week treatments, punctuated by 1-week withdrawal flow intervals. A decrease in volume and pain with each successive cycle is reassuring. Oral contraceptives reduce menstrual flow by at least 60% in normal uteri.[46] Early application of the estrogen-progestin combination limits growth and allows orderly regression of excessive endometrial height to normal controllable levels. If the estrogen-progestin combination is not applied, abnormal endometrial height and persistent excessive flow will recur.

In the patient not requiring contraception, in whom cyclic estrogen-progestin for 3 months has reduced endometrial tissue to normal height, the oral contraceptive can be discontinued and unopposed endogenous estrogen permitted to reactivate the endometrium. In the absence of spontaneous menses, the recurrence of the anovulatory state is suspected, and a brief preemptive course of an orally active progestin is administered to counter endometrial proliferation. Once pregnancy is ruled out, medroxyprogesterone acetate, 5–10 mg orally daily for at least 10 days, is given monthly. Reasonable flow (progestin withdrawal flow) will occur 2–7 days after the last pill. With this therapy, excessive endometrial buildup is avoided, and an increased risk of endometrial and possibly breast cancer is avoided. If contraception is desired, routine use of oral contraception is warranted and will also be of prophylactic value.

Depot-medroxyprogesterone acetate in the dose used for contraception, 150 mg intramuscularly every 3 months, is a useful option for poorly compliant patients. Breakthrough bleeding is treated with estrogen as discussed below.

Estrogen Therapy

Intermittent vaginal spotting is frequently associated with minimal (low) estrogen stimulation (estrogen breakthrough bleeding). In this circumstance, where minimal endometrium exists, the beneficial effect of progestin treatment is not achieved, because there is insufficient tissue on which the progestin can exert action. A similar circumstance also exists in the younger anovulatory patient in whom prolonged hemorrhagic desquamation leaves little residual tissue.

In these circumstances, when bleeding is acute and heavy, high-dose estrogen therapy is applied by using as much as 25 mg conjugated estrogen intravenously every 4 hours until bleeding abates or for 24 hours.[47] This is the sign that the "healing" events are initiated to a sufficient degree. The mechanism of action for estrogen is believed to be a stimulus to clotting at the capillary level.[48] Progestin treatment (usually an oral contraceptive) is started at the same time. Where bleeding is less, lower oral doses of estrogen (1.25 mg of conjugated estrogens or 2.0 mg estradiol daily for 7–10 days) can be prescribed initially. When bleeding is moderately heavy, a more intensive oral program can be utilized, 1.25 mg conjugated estrogens or 2 mg estradiol every 4 hours for 24 hours, followed by the single daily dose for 7–10 days. All estrogen therapy must be followed by progestin coverage and a withdrawal bleed.

Estrogen therapy is also useful in two examples of problems associated with progestin breakthrough bleeding. These are the breakthrough bleeding episodes occurring with use of oral contraception or with depot forms of progestational agents. In the absence of sufficient endogenous and exogenous estrogen, the endometrium shrinks by pharmacologically induced pseudoatrophy. Furthermore, it is composed almost exclusively of pseudodecidual stroma and blood vessels with minimal glands. Peculiarly, experience indicates that this type of endometrium also leads to the fragility bleeding more typical of pure estrogen stimulation.

The usual clinical story is a patient on long-standing oral contraception who, after experiencing marked diminution or absence of withdrawal flow in the pill-free interval, begins to see breakthrough bleeding while on medication. Conjugated estrogens, 1.25 mg, or estradiol, 2.0 mg daily for 7 days during, and, in addition to, the usual birth control pill administration are effective. This treatment rejuvenates the endometrium and intermenstrual flow stops. Another frequently encountered problem is the progestin breakthrough bleeding experienced with chronic depot administration of progestin (Depo-Provera). This therapy is used not only for contraception, but also in the treatment of endometriosis and the prevention of menses during chemotherapy. In 75% of recipients, continuous therapy is not associated with abnormal menstrual bleeding. In the remainder, breakthrough progestin bleeding occurs. Judicious use of estrogen is the appropriate and effective therapy in these instances.

Bleeding problems are common with Norplant, another example of the effect of persistent progestational influence on the endometrium. Patients who can no longer tolerate prolonged bleeding will benefit from a short course of oral estrogen as above.[49]

The Risk Associated with Estrogen Therapy

There is concern that high doses of estrogen could precipitate a thrombotic event. More than one oral contraceptive per day and multiple doses of oral or intravenous estrogen in a 24-hour period certainly should be regarded as high doses. There are no data available, however, to verify or quantitate any risk associated with this use of hormonal therapy. This treatment must be chosen by clinician and patient after weighing the risk-benefit considerations that surround the uterine bleeding problem. As a matter of clinical judgment and prudent practice, lower doses can be used in patients with lifestyle or medical history consistent with an increased risk of vascular complications. In women with a past episode or a positive family history of idiopathic venous thromboembolism, exposure to high doses of estrogen should be avoided.

The Use of Antiprostaglandins

There seems little doubt that prostaglandins (PG) have important actions on the endometrial vasculature and, presumably, on endometrial hemostasis. The concentrations of PGE_2 and $PGF_{2\alpha}$ increase progressively in human endometrium during the menstrual cycle, and nonsteroidal eicosanoid synthesis inhibitors decrease menstrual blood loss perhaps by also altering the balance between the platelet proaggregating vasoconstrictor thromboxane A_2 (TXA_2) and the anti-aggregating vasodilator prostacyclin (PGI_2).[50] Excessive bleeding in women with menorrhagia can be reduced by approximately 40–50%.[51] In a comparison study of ovulating women with menorrhagia, treatment during menses with a prostaglandin synthetase inhibitor was no more effective than high-dose progestin supplementation during the 7 days preceding menstruation, but both treatments were effective.[52] Occasionally, a woman will demonstrate, for unknown reasons, an anomalous response to this treatment, with an increase in menstrual bleeding.[53] A study of postoperative surgical specimens after mefenamic acid treatment revealed evidence of vasoconstriction and improved platelet aggregation.[54]

Whatever the exact mechanism, prostaglandin synthetase inhibitors diminish menstrual bleeding in normal women as well as in the bleeding secondary to intrauterine device (IUD) use. This approach should be considered as a first line of defense in the absence of pathology in those women who are ovulatory but bleed heavily. Side effects are unusual because treatment is limited, usually beginning with the onset of bleeding and continuing for 3–4 days. This treatment will also relieve the other symptoms of menstrual molimina.

Treatment With a Progestin IUD

The delivery of a progestational agent directly to the endometrium in a local fashion is possible with an intrauterine device which releases progesterone or levonorgestrel.[55, 56] In a comparison trial with a prostaglandin synthase inhibitor and an antifibrinolytic agent, the levonorgestrel-releasing IUD outperformed the medical treatment dramatically.[56] The reduction in menstrual flow reached 96% after 12 months, and some patients even become amenorrheic. In a comparison of the levonorgestrel-releasing IUD with endometrial ablation, symptomatic response and patient satisfaction were relatively comparable; approximately 20% of patients become amenorrheic and another 50% have a less than normal menstrual flow.[57] This is an attractive option in patients with intractable bleeding associated with chronic illnesses (such as renal failure). A progestin-releasing IUD is also a good choice for normally ovulating women who have extremely heavy menstrual bleeding.

Treatment with GnRH Agonists

Treatment with a GnRH agonist can achieve short-term relief from a bleeding problem, for example, in a patient with renal failure or a blood dyscrasia. This choice is a good one for patients who experience menstrual bleeding problems after organ transplantation (especially after liver transplantation) where the toxicity of immunosuppressive drugs makes the use of sex steroids less desirable. However, the expense and long-term side effects make this an unlikely choice for chronic therapy. If long-term GnRH agonist therapy is chosen, after gonadal suppression is achieved (2–4 weeks), we recommend add-back treatment with a daily combination of 0.625 mg conjugated estrogens or 1.0 mg estradiol and 2.5 mg medroxyprogesterone acetate or 0.35 mg norethindrone.

Treatment With Desmopressin

Desmopressin acetate is a synthetic analog of arginine vasopressin. It has been used to treat abnormal uterine bleeding in patients with coagulation disorders, especially in patients with von Willebrand's disease.[58, 59] It can be administered intranasally, but the intravenous route (0.3 µg/kg diluted in 50 mL saline and administered over 15–30 minutes) is more effective. Treatment is followed by a rapid increase in coagulation factor VIII and von Willebrand's factor, which lasts approximately 6 hours. This treatment should be regarded as a last resort for selected patients with coagulation problems. The nasal spray is very effective for patients with von Willebrand's disease type I.[59]

Ablation of the Endometrium

Persistent bleeding despite treatment is both aggravating and concerning. Hysterectomy is an appropriate choice for some of these patients. Others would prefer to avoid a major operation, and still others have conditions that make major surgery a high-risk procedure. Patients and clinicians should consider the option of hysteroscopic endometrial ablation. Ablation of the endometrium can be accomplished with either a laser, a resectoscope with a loop or rolling ball electrode, or radio frequency-induced thermal destruction. A new method employs a uterine balloon to expose the endometrium to an 85°C temperature for 10–15 minutes using the circulation of hot saline.[60] In a comparison with the rolling ball technique, the thermal balloon was as effective and with fewer side effects.[61] In a randomized comparison of medical treatment of menorrhagia compared with hysteroscopic endometrial ablation, overall results were better with surgical management.[62] Nevertheless, for most women, medical management is a better first approach (certainly in terms of cost).

Success with these methods is not 100%. Approximately 90% of women with menorrhagia will have an improvement following an ablation procedure; only 40–50% will become amenorrheic.[63–65] Some women will continue to have menorrhagia. In a randomized trial comparing endometrial resection and hysterectomy, subsequent surgery was required by 22% of the women after endometrial resection compared with 9% in the hysterectomy group.[66] The best results are obtained if the endometrium is first suppressed for 4–6 weeks with either a high dose of a progestin, GnRH agonist treatment, or danazol. Caution must be exercised regarding the possibility of excessive absorption of irrigating fluid with subsequent fluid overload. Despite the advantages of lower risk, fewer complications, and more rapid recovery with endometrial resection, patients treated by hysterectomy tend to be more satisfied with the outcome.[66, 67]

There is concern that obliteration of segments of the uterine cavity can allow isolated, residual endometrium to progress to carcinoma without recognition.[68] Endometrial ablation is not recommended for patients who are considered to be at high risk for endometrial cancer.[69]

Less Appealing Choices

Antifibrinolytic agents (e.g., tranexamine acid) are associated with a large number of side effects. Danazol effectively reduces menstrual blood loss, but treatment requires significant doses maintained for a long time period. The expense and androgenic side effects associated with danazol make it a poor choice.[70]

Hyperplasia Versus Neoplasia

Ferenczy argues that there are two separate and biologically unrelated diseases: endometrial hyperplasia and endometrial neoplasia.[71, 72] He suggests that all hyperplasia without atypia be referred to as *endometrial hyperplasia*, and this is usually not a precursor of carcinoma. He further proposes that lesions with cytologic atypia be referred to as *endometrial intraepithelial neoplasia (EIN).* In these cases, persistence after multiple curettings or high-dose progestin therapy is approximately 75%. EIN would replace the following terms: atypical adenomatous hyperplasia and carcinoma in situ of the endometrium. This lesion is characterized by nuclear atypia of the cells lining the endometrial glands (enlargement, rounding, and pleomorphism of the nuclei with aneuploid DNA content). Invasive carcinoma is distinguished from EIN by stromal invasion.

EIN is best treated surgically! If future pregnancy is desired, daily progestin therapy (30 mg medroxyprogesterone acetate daily) should be followed by repeat endometrial aspiration curettage in 3–4 months. If EIN is still present, the choice is between surgery and high dose progestin (200 mg medroxyprogesterone acetate daily, 500 mg megestrol acetate biweekly, or depot medroxyprogesterone acetate 1000 mg weekly) with repeat biopsy surveillance.

The benign lesions include all of the following traditional interpretations: anovulatory, proliferative, cystic glandular hyperplasia, simple hyperplasia, adenomatous hyperplasia without atypia. These lesions are basically the same (perhaps exaggerations at most) as preovulatory, proliferative endometrium. This hyperplasia regresses spontaneously, after curettage, or with hormonal treatment.[72, 73] *This argument is an important one: benign lesions can be treated hormonally. With one exception, only the presence of cytonuclear atypia should raise immediate and serious concern for progression to cancer. The exception is the patient with an apparently benign lesion that does not respond to progestin therapy. Was the diagnosis accurate? Will clinical data eventually indicate that this type of patient is also at higher risk for progression?*

Summary of Key Points in Therapy of Anovulatory (Dysfunctional) Bleeding

Teenager	Adult
Preliminary:	*Preliminary:*
Pelvic or rectal examination	Pelvic examination
Rule out pregnancy	PAP smear
Appropriate laboratory tests	Rule out pregnancy
	Appropriate laboratory tests
	Endometrial biopsy

1. Intense estrogen-progestin therapy for 7 days.

2. Cyclic low-dose oral contraceptive for 3 months.

3. If contraception is desired, continue oral contraception.

4. If not exposed to pregnancy, medroxyprogesterone acetate, 5–10 mg daily for at least 10 days every month.

If bleeding has been prolonged, if biopsy yields minimal tissue, if the patient is on progestin medication, or if follow-up is uncertain:

Conjugated estrogens (1.25 mg) or estradiol (2.0 mg) daily for 7–10 days, followed by the daily estrogen combined with 10 mg medroxyprogesterone acetate for 7 days. If acute bleeding is moderately heavy, the oral estrogen dose can be administered every 4 hours during the first 24 hours. For very heavy, acute bleeding, conjugated estrogen, 25 mg intravenously every 4 hours until bleeding stops or significantly slows, and then proceed to Step 1 above. If no response in 24 hours, proceed to D and C.

The clinical problem of dysfunctional bleeding is associated with either anovulation and estrogen withdrawal or breakthrough bleeding, or with anovulation caused by exogenous progestin medication and bleeding due to progestational endometrial breakthrough. These categories of bleeding lack the three important characteristics of normal estrogen-progesterone withdrawal bleeding:

1. Universal, simultaneous change in all segments of the endometrium.

2. An orderly progression of events involving a rigid, compact structure.

3. Vasomotor rhythmicity with vasoconstriction, structural collapse, and clotting.

Questioning should be directed by the differential diagnosis of abnormal uterine bleeding. Clues to the diagnosis may be apparent on physical examination, such as hirsutism, acne, galactorrhea, thyroid enlargement, evidence of an eating disorder, bruises, and, of course, abnormalities on examination of the pelvis. Brown, dark colored bleeding is often secondary to obstruction in a müllerian anomaly. Laboratory tests that can be helpful (but not always necessary) are coagulation studies (prothrombin time, partial thromboplastin time, platelet count, bleeding time, and the ristocetin cofactor assay for von Willebrand's factor), quantitative human chorionic gonadotropin (HCG), prolactin, thyroid function tests, liver function tests, and appropriate cervical cultures. However, it is appropriate to move quickly to empirical hormonal therapy because pathology will eventually declare itself.

Office aspiration biopsy of the endometrium should always be performed in patients considered to be at high risk for endometrial hyperplasia and cancer. Texts and review articles continue to emphasize that endometrial biopsy is in order if the patient is older; e.g., greater than 35 or 40 years old. *It is not the age of the patient that is critical; it is the duration of exposure to unopposed estrogen. Women in their 20s and even teenagers can develop endometrial cancer.*[74] The small flexible suction cannulas are preferred for greater patient comfort, and results are comparable with the older, traditional methods.[75-77] Office hysteroscopy is also useful for the direction of biopsies and the detection of polyps and submucous myomas.

Therapy involves an initial choice between intensive estrogen-progestin combination medication or relatively high doses of estrogen. The estrogen-progestin combination will be ineffective unless endometrium of sufficient quantity and responsiveness to allow the formation of pseudo-decidual tissue is present. Therefore, the initial choice of therapy should be estrogen in the following situations:

1.   When bleeding has been heavy for many days and it is likely that the uterine cavity is now lined only by a raw basalis layer.

2.   When the endometrial curet yields minimal tissue.

3.   When the patient has been on progestin medication (oral contraceptives, or intramuscular progestins) and the endometrium is shallow and atrophic.

4.   When follow-up is uncertain, because estrogen therapy will temporarily stop all categories of dysfunctional bleeding.

If estrogen therapy does not significantly abate flow within 24 hours, reevaluation is mandatory, and the need for curettage is likely. It is believed that patients with coagulation disorders respond better if the uterine cavity is first evacuated with a suction curet. Consideration should be given to the empirical administration of fresh frozen plasma to adolescents who present with acute, serious bleeding. It is prudent to combine hysteroscopy with curettage in order to achieve full accuracy in diagnosis and treatment.

Once the acute bleeding episode in an anovulatory patient is under control, the patient should not be forgotten. With persistent anovulation, recurrent hemorrhage is a common pattern, and, more importantly, chronic unopposed estrogen stimulation to the endometrium can eventually lead to atypical tissue changes. It is absolutely necessary that the patient undergo periodic progestational withdrawal either with a routine oral contraceptive regimen or if contraception is not desired, a progestational agent (medroxyprogesterone acetate, 5–10 mg daily for at least 10 days) should be administered every month.

Curettage is *not* the first line of defense, but, rather, the last. The use of appropriate steroids for the clinical management of dysfunctional bleeding is based on a physiologic understanding of the endometrium and its responses to hormones. Adherence to this program will avoid D and C except in a rare case of dysfunctional bleeding and except in those cases in which bleeding is due to a pathologic entity within the reproductive tract where D and C is truly indicated and necessary.

Remember to seek pathology if dysfunctional uterine bleeding is persistent or recurrent after hormonal treatment. If a patient has recurrent bleeding despite repeated medical therapy, submucous myomas or endometrial polyps must be suspected. Thorough curettage can miss such pathology, and further diagnostic study can be helpful. Either hysterosalpingography with slow instillation of dye and careful fluoroscopic examination or hysteroscopy (especially with filling of the uterine cavity with fluid) may reveal a myoma or polyp; hysteroscopy can also direct a more accurate biopsy of the endometrium.[78-80] A pathologic problem such as this should especially be suspected in the puzzling case of the patient who has abnormal bleeding and ovulatory cycles.

Patients who are ovulating but have a heavy menstrual flow (menorrhagia) can be effectively treated with prostaglandin inhibitors, progestins administered daily for the 7 days preceding menses, or oral contraceptives in the routine manner. If contraception is not required, we prefer the use of one of the fenamate prostaglandin inhibitors (which block both synthesis and prostaglandin receptors). Women who have menorrhagia but are ovulating should be evaluated for a coagulation disorder (prothrombin time, partial thromboplastin time, platelet count, bleeding time, and the ristocetin cofactor assay for von Willebrand's factor). The IUD that releases progesterone or a progestin is a good choice for ovulating women with menorrhagia, and it should be also considered in patients with chronic illnesses.

References

1. **Belsey EM, Pinol APY, and Task Force on Long-Acting Systemic Agents for Fertility Regulation,** Menstrual bleeding patterns in untreated women, *Contraception* 55:57, 1997.

2. **Collett ME, Wertenberger GE, Fiske VM,** The effect of age upon the pattern of the menstrual cycle, *Fertil Steril* 5:437, 1954.

3. **Chiazze Jr L, Brayer FT, Macisco Jr JJ, Parker MP, Duffy BJ,** The length and variability of the human menstrual cycle, *JAMA* 203:377, 1968.

4. **Munster K, Schmidt L, Helm P,** Length and variation in the menstrual cycle — a cross-sectional study from a Danish county, *Br J Obstet Gynaecol* 99:422, 1992.

5. **Treloar AE, Boynton RE, Borghild GB, Brown BW,** Variation of the human menstrual cycle through reproductive life, *Int J Fertil* 12:77, 1967.

6. **Hallberg L, Högdahl A, Nilsson L, Rybo G,** Menstrual blood loss — a population study, *Acta Obstet Gynecol Scand* 45:320, 1966.

7. **Rybo G,** Menstrual blood loss in relation to parity and menstrual pattern, *Acta Obstet Gynecol Scand* 7:119, 1966.

8. **Haynes PJ, Hodgson H, Anderson ABM, Turnbull AC,** Measurement of menstrual blood loss in patients complaining of menorrhagia, *Br J Obstet Gynaecol* 84:763, 1977.

9. **Higham JM, O'Brien PMS, Shaw RM,** Assessment of menstrual blood loss using a pictorial chart, *Br J Obstet Gynaecol* 97:734, 1990.

10. **Cohen BJB, Gibor J,** Anemia and menstrual blood loss, *Obstet Gynecol Survey* 35:597, 1980.

11. **Fraser IS, McCarron G, Markham R,** A preliminary study of factors influencing perception of menstrual blood loss volume, *Am J Obstet Gynecol* 149:788, 1984.

12. **Markee JE,** Menstruation in intraocular endometrial transplants in the rhesus monkey, *JAMA* 250:2167, 1946.

13. **Markee JE,** Morphological basis for menstrual bleeding: relation of regression to the initiation of bleeding, *Bull NY Acad Med* 24:253, 1948.

14. **Tabibzadeh S,** The signals and molecular pathways involved in human menstruation, a unique process of tissue destruction and remodelling, *Mol Hum Reprod* 2:77, 1996.

15. **Salamonsen LA,** Matrix metalloproteinases and endometrial remodelling, *Cell Biol Int* 18:1139, 1994.

16. **Rodgers WH, Matrisian LM, Giudice LC, Dsupin B, Cannon P, Svitek C, Gorstein F, Osteen KG,** Patterns of matrix metalloproteinase expression in cycling endometrium imply differential functions and regulation by steroid hormones, *J Clin Invest* 94:946, 1994.

17. **Irwin JC, Kirk D, Gwatkin RBL, Navre M, Cannon P, Giudice LC,** Human endometrial matrix metalloproteinase-2, a putative menstrual proteinase. Hormonal regulation in cultured stromal cells and messenger RNA expression during the menstrual cycle, *J Clin Invest* 97:438, 1996.

18. **Bruner KL, Rodgers WH, Gold LI, Korc M, Hargrove JT, Matrisian LM, Osteen KG,** Transforming growth factor beta mediates the progesterone suppression of an epithelial metalloproteinase by adjacent stroma in the human endometrium, *Proc Natl Acad Sci USA* 92:7362, 1995.

19. **Lockwood C, Krikun G, Papp C, Toth-Pal E, Markiewicz L, Wang EY, Kerenyi T, Zhou X, Hauskenecht V, Papp Z,** The role of progestionally regulated stromal cell tissue factor and type-1 plasminogen activator inhibitor (PAI-1) in endometrial hemostasis and menstruation, *Ann NY Acad Sci* 734:57, 1994.

20. **Schatz F, Aigner S, Papp C, Toth-Pal E, Hauskenecht V, Lockwood CJ,** Plasminogen activator activity during decidualization of human endometrial stromal cells is regulated by plasminogen activator inhibitor 1, *J Clin Encrinol Metab* 80:1504, 1995.

21. **Christiaens GCML, Sixma JJ, Haspels AA,** Hemostasis in menstrual endometrium: a review, *Obstet Gynecol Survey* 37:281, 1982.

22. **Lockwood CJ, Schatz F,** A biological model for the regulation of peri-implantional hemostasis and menstruation, *J Soc Gynecol Invest* 3:159, 1996.

23. **de Ziegler D, Bergeron C, Cornel C, Medalie A, Massai MR, Milgrom E, Frydman R, Bouchard P,** Effects of luteal estradiol on the secretory transformation of human endometrium and plasma gonadotropins, *J Clin Endocrinol Metab* 74:322, 1992.

24. **Belsey EM, Task Force on Long-Acting Systemic Agents for Fertility Regulation,** Vaginal bleeding patterns among women using one natural and eight hormonal methods of contraception, *Contraception* 38:181, 1988.

25. **Ferenczy A,** Studies on the cytodynamics of human endometrial regeneration. I. Scanning electron microscopy, *Am J Obstet Gynecol* 124:64, 1976.

26. **Hopkins MP, Androff L, Benninghoff AS,** Ginseng face cream and unexplained vaginal bleeding, *Am J Obstet Gynecol* 159:1121, 1988.

27. **Wilansky DL, Greisman B,** Early hypothyroidism in patients with menorrhagia, *Am J Obstet Gynecol* 160:673, 1989.

28. **Claessens EA, Cowell CL,** Acute adolescent menorrhagia, *Am J Obstet Gynecol* 139:377, 1981.

29. **Smith YR, Quint EH, Hertzberg RB,** Menorrhagia in adolescents requiring hospitalization, *J Pediatr Adolesc Gynecol* 11:13, 1998.

30. **Kadir RA, Economides DL, Sabin CA, Owens D, Lee CA,** Frequency of inherited bleeding disorders in women with menorrhagia, *Lancet* 351:485, 1998.

31. **van Eijkeren MA, Christiaens GCML, Haspels AA, Sixma JJ,** Measured menstrual blood loss in women with a bleeding disorder or using oral anticoagulant therapy, *Am J Obstet Gynecol* 162:1261, 1990.

32. **Edlund M, Blomback M, von Schoultz B, Andersson O,** On the value of menorrhagia as a predictor for coagulation disorders, *Am J Hematol* 53:234, 1996.

33. **Rulin MC, Turner JH, Dunworth R, Thompson D,** Post tubal sterilization syndrome: a misnomer, *Obstet Gynecol* 151:13, 1985.

34. **DeStefano F, Huezo CM, Peterson HB, Rubin GL, Layde PM, Ory HW,** Menstrual changes after tubal sterilization, *Obstet Gynecol* 62:673, 1983.

35. **Rulin MC, Davidson AR, Philliber SG, Graves WL, Cushman LF,** Changes in menstrual symptoms among sterilized and comparison women: a prospective study, *Obstet Gynecol* 79:749, 1989.

36. **DeStefano F, Perlman J, Peterson HB, Diamond E,** Long-term risk of menstrual disturbances after tubal sterilization, *Am J Obstet Gynecol* 152:835, 1985.

37. **Kjer J, Knudsen L,** Hysterectomy subsequent to laparoscopic sterilization, *Eur J Obstet Gynecol* 35:63, 1990.

38. **Stergachis A, Shy KK, Gouthaus LC, Wagner EH, Hecht JA, G A, Normand EH, Raboud J,** Tubal sterilization and the long-term risk of hysterectomy, *JAMA* 264:2893, 1990.

39. **Shy KK, Stergachis A, Grothaus LG, Wagner EH, Hecth J, Anderson G,** Tubal sterilization and risk of subsequent hospital admission for menstrual disorders, *Am J Obstet Gynecol* 166:1698, 1992.

40. **Hillis SD, Marchbanks PA, Tylor LR, Peterson HB, for the U.S. Collaborative Review of Sterilization Working Group,** Higher hysterectomy risk for sterilized than nonsterilized women: findings from the U.S. Collaborative Review of Sterilization, *Obstet Gynecol* 91:241, 1998.

41. **Thranov I, Hertz JB, Kjer JJ, Andresen A, Micic S, Nielsen J, Hancke S,** Hormonal and menstrual changes after laparoscopic sterilization by Falope-rings or Filshie-clips, *Fertil Steril* 57:751, 1992.

42. **Wilcox LS, Martinez-Schnell B, Peterson HB, Ware JH, Hughes JM,** Menstrual function after tubal sterilization, *Am J Epidemiol* 135:1368, 1992.

43. **Rulin MC, Davidson AR, Philliber SG, Graves WL, Cushman LF,** Long-term effect of tubal sterilization on menstrual indices and pelvic pain, *Obstet Gynecol* 82:118, 1993.

44. **Gurpide E, Gusberg S, Tseng L,** Estradiol binding and metabolism in human endometrial hyperplasia and adenocarcinoma, *J Steroid Biochem* 7:891, 1976.

45. **Kirkland JL, Murthy L, Stancel GM,** Progesterone inhibits the estrogen-induced expression of *c-fos* messenger ribonucleic acid in the uterus, *Endocrinology* 130:3223, 1992.

46. **Nelson L, Rybo G,** Treatment of menorrhagia, *Am J Obstet Gynecol* 110:713, 1971.

47. **DeVore GR, Owens O, Kase N,** Use of intravenous premarin in the treatment of dysfunctional uterine bleeding — a double-blind randomized control study, *Obstet Gynecol* 59:285, 1982.

48. **Livio M, Mannucci PM, Vigano G, Mingardi G, Lombardi R, Mecca G, Remuzzi G,** Conjugated estrogens for the management of bleeding associated with renal failure, *New Engl J Med* 315:731, 1986.

49. **Diaz S, Croxatto HB, Pavez M, Belhadj H, Stern J, Sivin I,** Clinical assessment of treatments for prolonged bleeding in users of Norplant implants, *Contraception* 42:97, 1990.

50. **Fraser IS,** Prostaglandin inhibitors in gynaecology, *Aust NZ J Obstet Gynecol* 25:114, 1985.

51. **Hall P, Maclachlan N, Thorn N, Nudd MWE, Taylor CG, Garrioch DB,** Control of menorrhagia by the cyclo-oxygenase inhibitors naproxen sodium and mefenamic acid, *Br J Obstet Gynaecol* 94:554, 1987.

52. **Cameron IT, Haining R, Lumsden M-A, Thomas VR, Smith SK,** The effects of mefenamic acid and norethisterone on measured menstrual blood loss, *Obstet Gynecol* 76:85, 1990.

53. **Fraser IS, McCarron G,** Randomized trial of 2 hormonal and 2 prostaglandin-inhibiting agents in women with a complaint of menorrhagia, *Aust NZ J Obstet Gynecol* 31:66, 1991.

54. **van Eijkeren MA, Christianes GCML, Geuze JH, Haspels AA, Sixma JJ,** Effects of mefenamic acid on menstrual hemostasis in essental menorrhagia, *Am J Obstet Gynecol* 166:1419, 1992.

55. **Bergqvist A, Rybo G,** Treatment of menorrhagia with intrauterine release of progesterone, *Br J Obstet Gynaecol* 90:255, 1983.

56. **Milsom I, Andersson K, Andersch B, Rybo G,** A comparison of flurbiprogen, tranexamic acid, and a levonorgestrel-releasing intrauterine contraceptive device in the treatment of idiopathic menorrhagia, *Am J Obstet Gynecol* 164:879, 1991.

57. **Crosignani PG, Vercellini P, Mosconi P, Oldani S, Cortesi I, De Giorgi O,** Levonorgestrel-releasing intrauterine device versus hysteroscopic endometrial resection in the treatment of dysfunctional uterine bleeding, *Obstet Gynecol* 90:257, 1997.

58. **Kubrinsky NL, Tulloch H,** Treatment of refractory thrombocytopenic bleeding with desamino-8-D-arginine vasopressin (desmopressin), *J Pediatr* 112:993, 1988.

59. **Rose EH, Aledort LM,** Nasal spray desmopressin (DDAVP) for mild hemophilia A and von Willebrand disease, *Ann Intern Med* 114:563, 1991.

60. **Bustos-Lopez HH, Baggish M, Valle RF, Vadillo-Ortega F, Ibarra V, Nava G,** Assessment of the safety of intrauterine instillation of heated saline for endometrial ablation, *Fertil Steril* 69:155, 1998.

61. **Meyer WR, Walsh BW, Grainger DA, Peacock LM, Loffer FD, Steege JF,** Thermal balloon and rollerball ablation to treat menorrhagia: a multicenter comparison, *Obstet Gynecol* 92:98, 1998.

62. **Cooper KG, Parker DE, Garratt AM, Grant AM,** A randomised comparison of medical and hysteroscopic management in women consulting a gynaecologist for treatment of heavy menstrual loss, *Br J Obstet Gynaecol* 104:1360, 1997.

63. **Townsend DE, Richart RM, Paskowitz RA, Woolfork RE,** Rollerball coagulation of the endometrium, *Obstet Gynecol* 76:310, 1990.

64. **Phipps JH, Lewis BV, Prior MF, Roberts T,** Experimental and clinical studies with radio frequency-induced thermal endometrial ablation for functional menorrhagia, *Obstet Gynecol* 76:876, 1990.

65. **O'Connor H, Magos A,** Endometrial resection for the treatment of menorrhagia, *New Engl J Med* 335:151, 1996.

66. **O'Connor H, Broadbent JAM, Magos AL, McPherson K,** Medical Research Council randomised trial of endometrial resection versus hysterectomy in management of menorrhagia, *Lancet* 349:897, 1997.

67. **Crosignani PG, Vercellini P, Apolone G, De Giorgi O, Cortesi I, Meschia M,** Endometrial resection versus vaginal hysterectomy for menorrhagia: long-term clinical and quality-of-life outcomes, *Am J Obstet Gynecol* 177:95, 1997.

68. **Horowitz IR, Copas PR, Aarono M, Spann CO, McGuire WP,** Endometrial adenocarcinoma following endometrial ablation for postmenopausal bleeding, *Gynecol Oncol* 56:460, 1995.

69. **Valle RF, Baggish MS,** Endometrial carcinoma after endometrial ablation: high-risk factors predicting its occurrence, *Am J Obstet Gynecol* 179:569, 1998.

70. **Higham JM, Shaw RW,** A comparative study of danazol, a regimen of decreasing doses of danazol, and norethindrone in the treatment of objectively proven unexplained menorrhagia, *Am J Obstet Gynecol* 169:1134, 1993.

71. **Ferenczy A, Gelfand MM, Tzipris F,** The cytodynamics of endometrial hyperplasia and carcinoma, a review, *Ann Pathol* 3:189, 1983.

72. **Ferenczy A, Gelfand M,** The biologic significance of cytologic atypia in progestogen-treated endometrial hyperplasia, *Am J Obstet Gynecol* 160:126, 1989.

73. **Kurman RJ, Kaminski PT, Norris HJ,** The behavior of endometrial hyperplasia. A long-term study of "untreated" hyperplasia in 170 patients, *Cancer* 56:402, 1985.

74. **Farhi DC, Nosanchuk J, Silverberg SG,** Endometrial adenocarcinoma in women under 25 years of age, *Obstet Gynecol* 68:741, 1986.

75. **Silver MM, Miles P, Rosa C,** Comparison of Novak and Pipelle endometrial biopsy instruments, *Obstet Gynecol* 78:828, 1991.

76. **Eddowes HA, Read MD, Codling BW,** Pipelle: a more acceptable technique for outpatient endometrial biopsy, *Br J Obstet Gynaecol* 97:961, 1990.

77. **Fothergill DJ, Brown VA, Hill AS,** Histological sampling of the endometrium — A comparison between formal curettage and the Pipelle sampler, *Br J Obstet Gynaecol* 99:779, 1992.

78. **Gimpelson RJ, Rappold HD,** A comparative study between panoramic hysteroscopy with directed biopsies and dilatation and curettage, *Am J Obstet Gynecol* 158:489, 1988.

79. **Loffer DD,** Hysteroscopy with selective endometrial sampling compared with D&C for abnormal uterine bleeding: the value of a negative hysteroscopic view, *Obstet Gynecol* 73:16, 1989.

80. **Fraser IS,** Hysteroscopy and laparoscopy in women with menorrhagia, *Am J Obstet Gynecol* 162:1264, 1992.

16   The Breast

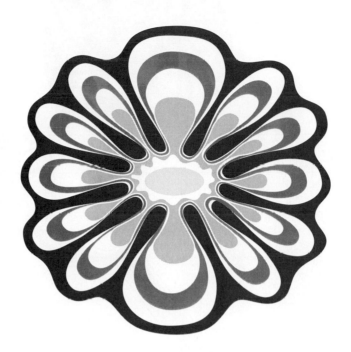

The form, function, and pathology of the human female breast are major concerns of medicine and society. As mammals, we define our biologic class by the function of the breast in nourishing our young. Breast contours occupy our attention. As obstetricians, we seek to enhance or diminish function, and as gynecologists, the appearance of inappropriate lactation (galactorrhea) may signify serious disease. Cancer of the breast is the most prevalent cancer in women.

In this chapter, the factors involved in normal growth and development of the breast will be reviewed, including the physiology of normal lactation. A description of the numerous factors leading to inappropriate lactation will follow, and, finally, the endocrine aspects of breast cancer will be considered.

Growth and Development

The basic component of the breast lobule is the hollow alveolus or milk gland lined by a single layer of milk-secreting epithelial cells, derived from an ingrowth of epidermis into the underlying mesenchyme at 10–12 weeks of gestation. Each alveolus is encased in a crisscrossing mantle of contractile myoepithelial strands. Also surrounding the milk gland is a rich capillary network.

The lumen of the alveolus connects to a collecting intralobular duct by means of a thin nonmuscular duct. Contractile muscle cells line the intralobular ducts that eventually reach the exterior via 15–20 collecting ducts in a radial arrangement, corresponding to the 15–20 distinct mammary lobules in the breast, each of which contains many alveoli.

Growth of this milk-producing system is dependent on numerous hormonal factors that occur in two sequences, first at puberty and then in pregnancy. Although there is considerable overlapping of hormonal influences, the differences in quantities of the stimuli in each circumstance and the availability of entirely unique inciting factors (human placental lactogen and prolactin) during

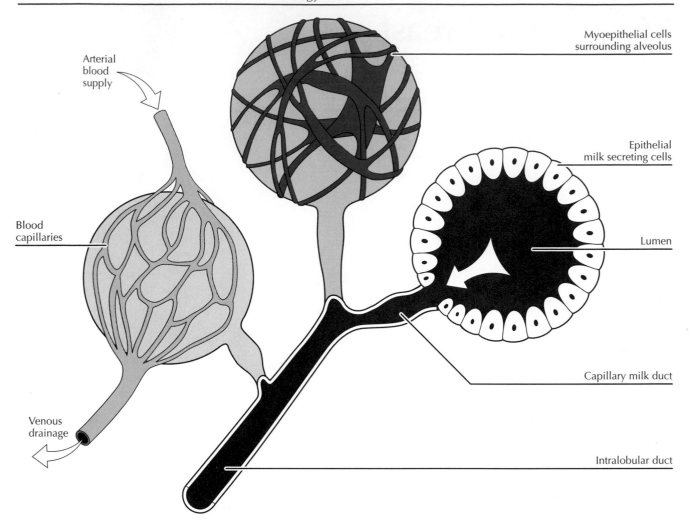

Arterial blood supply

Myoepithelial cells surrounding alveolus

Blood capillaries

Epithelial milk secreting cells

Lumen

Venous drainage

Capillary milk duct

Intralobular duct

pregnancy permit this chronologic distinction. The strength of the hormonal stimulus to breast tissue during pregnancy is responsible for the fact that nearly half of male and female newborns have breast secretions.

The major influence on breast growth at puberty is estrogen. In most girls, the first response to the increasing levels of estrogen is an increase in size and pigmentation of the areola and the formation of a mass of breast tissue just underneath the areola. Breast tissue binds estrogen in a manner similar to the uterus and vagina. The human breast expresses both estrogen receptors, ER-α and ER-β.[1] The development of estrogen receptors in the breast does not occur in the absence of prolactin. The primary effect of estrogen in subprimate mammals is to stimulate growth of the ductal portion of the gland system. Progesterone in these animals influences growth of the alveolar components of the lobule.[2] However, neither hormone alone, or in combination, is capable of yielding optimal breast growth and development. Full differentiation of the gland requires insulin, cortisol, thyroxine, prolactin, and growth hormone.[3] Of course, the ubiquitous growth factors are also involved, but the molecular mechanisms remain to be determined. Nevertheless, experimental evidence in mice indicates that progesterone is the key hormone required for mammary growth and differentiation; estrogen is necessary because the synthesis of progesterone receptors requires the critical presence of estrogen.[2]

The pubertal response is a manifestation of closely synchronized central (hypothalamus-pituitary) and peripheral (ovary-breast) events. For example, gonadotropin-releasing hormone (GnRH) is known to stimulate prolactin release, and this action is potentiated by estrogen.[4] This suggests a paracrine interaction between gonadotrophs and lactotrophs, linked by estrogen, ultimately with an impact on the breast.

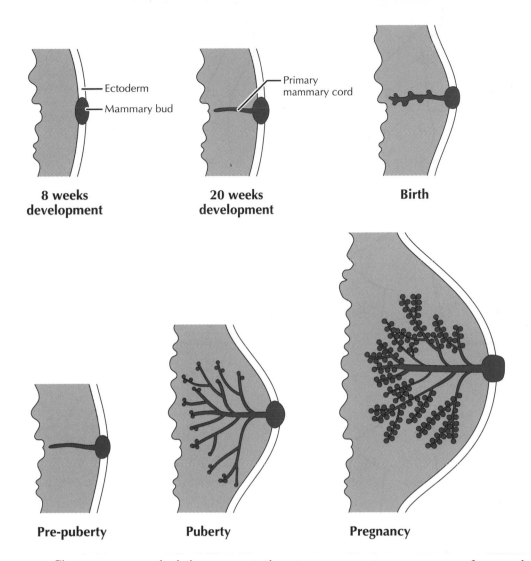

Changes occur routinely in response to the estrogen-progesterone sequence of a normal menstrual cycle. Maximal size of the breast occurs late in the luteal phase. Fluid secretion, mitotic activity, and DNA production of nonglandular tissue and glandular epithelium peak during the luteal phase.[5-7] This accounts for cystic and tender premenstrual changes.

During the normal menstrual cycle, estrogen receptors in mammary gland epithelium decrease in number during the luteal phase, whereas progesterone receptors remain at a high level throughout the cycle.[8] Studies using tissue from reduction mammoplasties or from breast tissue near a benign or malignant lesion have demonstrated a peak in mitotic activity during the luteal phase.[6, 9, 10] Using fine needle biopsy tissue, an immunocytochemical marker of proliferation was higher in the luteal phase than in the proliferative phase.[8] And in this study there was a direct correlation with serum progesterone levels. However, important studies indicate that with increasing duration of exposure, progesterone imposes a limitation on breast cell proliferation.[11-13] Therefore, breast and endometrium epithelial cells may be more similar than initially proposed.

Final differentiation of the alveolar epithelial cell into a mature milk cell is accomplished by the gestational increase in estrogen and progesterone, combined with the presence of prolactin, but only after prior exposure to cortisol and insulin. The complete reaction depends on the availability of minimal quantities of thyroid hormone. Thus, the endocrinologically intact individual in whom estrogen, progesterone, thyroxine, cortisol, insulin, prolactin, and growth hormone are available can have appropriate breast growth and function. During the first trimester of pregnancy, growth and proliferation are maximal, changing to differentiation and secretory activity as pregnancy progresses.

Breast tissue changes with aging. During teenage years the breasts are dense and predominantly glandular. As the years go by, the breasts contain progressively more fat, but after menopause, this process accelerates so that soon into the postmenopausal years, the breast glandular tissue is mostly replaced by fat.

Abnormal Shapes and Sizes

Early differentiation of the mammary gland anlage is under fetal hormonal control. Abnormalities in adult size or shape may reflect the impact of hormones (especially the presence or absence of testosterone) during this early period of development. This prenatal hormonal influence programs the breast development that will occur in response to the increase in hormones at puberty. Occasionally, the breast bud will begin to develop on one side first. Similarly, one breast may grow faster than the other. These inequalities usually disappear by the time development is complete. However, exact equivalence in size may not be attained. Significant asymmetry is correctable only by a plastic surgeon. Likewise hypoplasia and hypertrophy can be treated only by corrective surgery. With one exception, hormone therapy is totally ineffective in producing a permanent change in breast shape or size. Of course in patients with primary amenorrhea due to deficient ovarian function, estrogen treatment will induce significant and gratifying breast growth. Breast size can be increased in current users of oral contraceptives, but there is no lasting effect associated with past use.[14]

Accessory nipples can be found anywhere from the groin to the neck, remnants of the mammary line that extends early in embryonic life (6th week) along the ventral, lateral body wall. They occur in approximately 1% of women and require no therapy.

Pregnancy and Lactation

Prolactin Secretion

In most mammalian species, prolactin is a single chain polypeptide of 199 amino acids, 40% similar in structure to growth hormone and placental lactogen. All three hormones are believed to have originated from a common ancestral protein about 400 million years ago.

Prolactin is encoded by a single gene on the short arm of chromosome 6, producing a molecule that in its major form is maintained in 3 loops by disulfide bonds. Simultaneous measurements of prolactin by both bioassay and immunoassay reveal discrepancies. Chemical studies have revealed structural modifications that include glycosylation, phosphorylation, and variations in binding and charge. This heterogeneity is the result of many influences at many levels: transcription, translation, post translational modification, and peripheral metabolism.[15, 16] Other variations exist. Enzymatic cleavage of the prolactin molecule yields fragments that may be capable of biologic activity. Prolactin that has been glycosylated continues to exert activity; differences in the carbohydrate moieties can produce differences in biologic activity and immunoreactivity. However, the non-glycosylated form of prolactin is the predominant form of prolactin secreted into the circulation.[17] Modification of prolactin also includes phosphorylation, deamidation, and sulfation. Little prolactin probably results from the proteolytic deletion of amino acids. Big prolactin can result from the failure to remove introns; it has little biologic activity and does not cross react with antibodies to the major form of prolactin. The so-called big big variants of prolactin are due to separate molecules of prolactin binding to each other, either noncovalently or by interchain disulfide bonding. Some of the apparently larger forms of prolactin are prolactin molecules complexed to binding proteins.

At any one point of time, the bioactivity (e.g., galactorrhea) and the immunoreactivity (circulating levels by immunoassay) of prolactin represent the cumulative effect of the family of structural variants. Remember, immunoassays do not always reflect the biologic situation (e.g., a normal prolactin level in a woman with galactorrhea). Nevertheless, the routine radioimmunoassay of prolactin is generally clinically reliable, especially at extremely high levels associated with prolactin-secreting pituitary tumors.

The anterior pituitary cells that produce prolactin, growth hormone, and thyroid-stimulating hormone (lactotrophs, somatotrophs, and thyrotrophs) require the presence of Pit-1, a transcription factor, for development. Pit-1 also binds to the prolactin gene in multiple sites in both the promoter region and in an adjacent region, designated as a distal enhancer; Pit-1 binding is a requirement for prolactin promoter activity and gene transcription. Many hormones, neurotransmitters, and growth factors influence the prolactin gene, involved in a level of function beyond that allowed by Pit-1. Fundamental modulation of prolactin secretion is exerted by estrogen, producing both differentiation of lactotrophs and direct stimulation of prolactin production.[18, 19] An estrogen response element is adjacent to one of the Pit-1 binding sites in the distal enhancer region, and estrogen stimulation of the prolactin gene involves interaction with this Pit-1 binding site. Estrogen also influences prolactin production by suppressing dopamine secretion.[20]

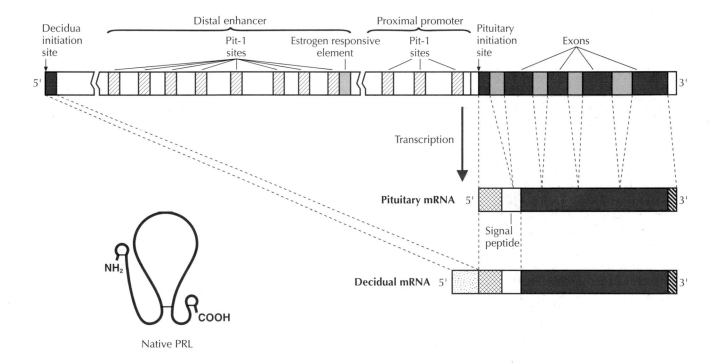

Prolactin is involved in many biochemical events during pregnancy. Surfactant synthesis in the fetal lung is influenced by prolactin, and decidual prolactin modulates prostaglandin-mediated uterine muscle contractility.[21, 22] Prolactin also contributes to the prevention of the immunologic rejection of the conceptus by suppressing the maternal immune response. Prolactin is both produced and processed in breast cells. The mechanisms and purpose for mammary production of prolactin remain to be determined, but prolactin in milk is believed to be derived from local synthesis. Transmission of this prolactin to the newborn may be important for immune functions.

Prolactin Inhibiting Factor

The hypothalamus maintains suppression of pituitary prolactin secretion by delivering a prolactin inhibiting factor (PIF) to the pituitary via the portal circulation. Suckling suppresses the formation of this hypothalamic substance, which is believed to be dopamine (as discussed in Chapter 5).[23] Dopamine is secreted by the basal hypothalamus into the portal system and conducted to the anterior pituitary. Dopamine binds specifically to lactotroph cells and suppresses the secretion of prolactin into the general circulation; in its absence, prolactin is secreted. Dopamine binds to a G protein-coupled receptor (Chapter 2) that exists in a long form and a short form, but only the D_2 (long form) is present on lactotrophs. The molecular mechanism for dopamine's inhibitory action is still not known. There are several other PIFs, but a specific role has been established only for dopamine.

Prolactin Releasing Factor

Prolactin secretion may also be influenced by a positive hypothalamic factor, prolactin-releasing factor (PRF). PRF does exist in various fowl (e.g., pigeon, chicken, duck, turkey, and the tricolored blackbird). While the identity of this material has not been elucidated, or its function substantiated in normal human physiology, it is possible that thyrotropin-releasing hormone (TRH) is a potent stimulant of prolactin secretion in humans. The smallest doses of TRH which are capable of producing an increase in TSH also increase prolactin levels, a finding which supports a physiologic role for TRH in the control of prolactin secretion, at least in response to suckling.[24] TRH stimulation of prolactin release involves calcium mechanisms (both internal release and influx via calcium channels) in response to the TRH receptor, also a member of the G protein family. However, except in hypothyroidism, normal physiologic changes as well as abnormal prolactin secretion are easily explained and understood in terms of variations in the prolactin inhibiting factor, dopamine. A large collection of peptides has been reported to stimulate the release of prolactin in vitro. These include growth factors, angiotensin II, GnRH, vasopressin, and others. But it is unknown whether these peptides participate in the normal physiologic regulation of prolactin secretion.

The Prolactin Receptor

The prolactin receptor is encoded by a gene on chromosome 5p13–14 that is near the gene for the growth hormone receptor. The prolactin receptor belongs to a receptor family that includes many cytokines and some growth factors, supporting a dual role for prolactin as a classic hormone and as a cytokine.[25]

Prolactin receptors exist in more than one form, all containing an extracellular region, a single transmembrane region, and a relatively long cytoplasmic domain. There is evidence for more than one receptor, depending upon the site of action (e.g., decidual and placenta).[26] The amino acid identity between prolactin and growth hormone receptors is approximately 30%, with certain regions having up to 70% homology.[27] Prolactin receptors are expressed in many tissues throughout the body. Because of the various forms and functions of prolactin, it is likely that multiple signal mechanisms are involved, and for that reason, no single second messenger for prolactin's intracellular action has been identified. A protein also exists that functions as a receptor/transporter, translocating prolactin from the blood into the cerebrospinal fluid, the amniotic fluid, and milk.

Amniotic Fluid Prolactin

Amniotic fluid concentrations of prolactin parallel maternal serum concentrations until the 10th week of pregnancy, rise markedly until the 20th week, and then decrease. Maternal prolactin does not pass to the fetus in significant amounts. Indeed, the source of amniotic fluid prolactin is neither the maternal pituitary nor the fetal pituitary. The failure of dopamine agonist treatment to suppress amniotic fluid prolactin levels, and studies with in vitro culture systems, indicate a primary decidual source with transfer via amnion receptors to the amniotic fluid, requiring the intactness of amnion, chorion, and adherent decidua. This decidual synthesis of prolactin is initiated by progesterone, but once decidualization is established, prolactin secretion continues in the absence of both progesterone and estradiol.[28] Various decidual factors regulate prolactin synthesis and release, including relaxin, insulin, and insulin-like growth factor-I (discussed in Chapter 4). Prolactin produced in extrapituitary sites involves an alternative exon upstream of the pituitary start site, generating a slightly larger RNA transcript compared with the pituitary product. However, the amino acid sequence and the chemical and biological properties of decidual prolactin are identical to those of pituitary prolactin. It is hypothesized that amniotic fluid prolactin plays a role in modulating electrolyte economy not unlike its ability to regulate sodium transport and water movement across the gills in fish (allowing the ocean-dwelling salmon and steelhead to return to freshwater streams for reproduction). Thus prolactin would protect the human fetus from dehydration by control of salt and water transport across the amnion. Prolactin reduces the permeability of the human amnion in the fetal to maternal direction by a receptor-mediated action on the epithelium lining the fetal surface.[29]

Lactation

During pregnancy, prolactin levels rise from the normal level of 10–25 ng/mL to high concentrations, beginning about 8 weeks and reaching a peak of 200–400 ng/mL at term.[30, 31] The increase in prolactin parallels the increase in estrogen beginning at 7–8 weeks gestation, and the mechanism for increasing prolactin secretion (discussed in Chapter 5) is believed to be estrogen suppression of the hypothalamic prolactin-inhibiting factor, dopamine, and direct stimulation of prolactin gene transcription in the pituitary.[32, 33] There is marked variability in maternal prolactin levels in pregnancy, with pulsatile secretion and a diurnal variation similar to that found in nonpregnant subjects. The peak level occurs 4–5 hours after the onset of sleep.[34]

Made by the placenta and actively secreted into the maternal circulation from the 6th week of pregnancy, human placental lactogen (HPL) rises progressively reaching a level of approximately 6000 ng/mL at term. HPL, though displaying less activity than prolactin, is produced in such large amounts that it may exert a lactogenic effect.

Although prolactin stimulates significant breast growth, and is available for lactation, only colostrum (composed of desquamated epithelial cells and transudate) is produced during gestation. Full lactation is inhibited by progesterone, which interferes with prolactin action at the alveolar cell prolactin receptor level. Both estrogen and progesterone are necessary for the expression of the lactogenic receptor, but progesterone antagonizes the positive action of prolactin on its own receptor while progesterone and pharmacologic amounts of androgens reduce prolactin binding.[27, 35, 36] In the mouse, inhibition of milk protein production is due to progesterone suppression of prolactin receptor expression.[37] The effective use of high doses of estrogen to suppress postpartum lactation indicates that pharmacologic amounts of estrogen also block prolactin action.

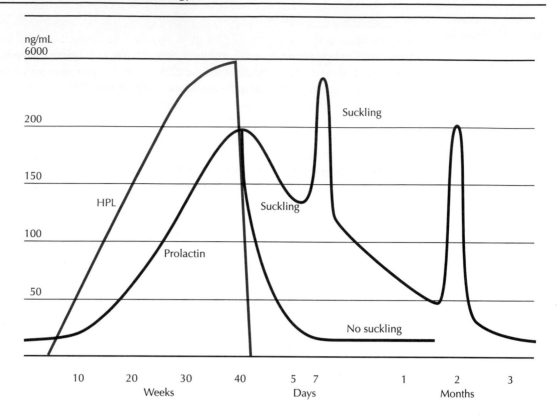

Progesterone can directly suppress milk production. A nuclear peptide (a corepressor) has been identified that binds to specific sites in the promoter region of the casein gene, thus inhibiting transcription.[38] Progesterone stimulates the generation of this corepressor. After delivery, the loss of progesterone leads to a decrease in this inhibitory peptide.

The principal hormone involved in milk biosynthesis is prolactin. Without prolactin, synthesis of the primary protein, casein, will not occur, and true milk secretion will be impossible. The hormonal trigger for initiation of milk production within the alveolar cell and its secretion into the lumen of the gland is the rapid disappearance of estrogen and progesterone from the circulation after delivery. The clearance of prolactin is much slower, requiring 7 days to reach non-pregnant levels in a non-breastfeeding woman. These discordant hormonal events result in removal of the estrogen and progesterone inhibition of prolactin action on the breast. Breast engorgement and milk secretion begin 3–4 days postpartum when steroids have been sufficiently cleared. Maintenance of steroidal inhibition or rapid reduction of prolactin secretion (with a dopamine agonist) are effective in preventing postpartum milk synthesis and secretion. Augmentation of prolactin (by TRH or sulpiride, a dopamine receptor blocker) results in increased milk yield.

In the first postpartum week, prolactin levels in breastfeeding women decline approximately 50% (to about 100 ng/mL). Suckling elicits increases in prolactin, which are important in initiating milk production. Until 2–3 months postpartum, basal levels are approximately 40–50 ng/mL, and there are large (about 10–20-fold) increases after suckling. Throughout breastfeeding, baseline prolactin levels remain elevated, and suckling produces a two-fold increase that is essential for continuing milk production.[39, 40] The pattern or values of prolactin levels does not predict the postpartum duration of amenorrhea or infertility.[41] The failure to lactate within the first 7 days postpartum may be the first sign of Sheehan's syndrome (hypopituitarism following intrapartum infarction of the pituitary gland).

Maintenance of milk production at high levels is dependent on the joint action of both anterior and posterior pituitary factors. By mechanisms to be described in detail shortly, suckling causes the release of both prolactin and oxytocin as well as thyroid-stimulating hormone (TSH).[42, 43]

Prolactin sustains the secretion of casein, fatty acids, lactose, and the volume of secretion, while oxytocin contracts myoepithelial cells and empties the alveolar lumen, thus enhancing further milk secretion and alveolar refilling. The increase in TSH with suckling suggests that thyrotropin-releasing hormone (TRH) may play a role in the prolactin response to suckling. The optimal quantity and quality of milk are dependent upon the availability of thyroid, insulin and the insulin-like growth factors, cortisol, and the dietary intake of nutrients and fluids.

Secretion of calcium into the milk of lactating women approximately doubles the daily loss of calcium.[44] In women who breastfeed for 6 months or more, this is accompanied by significant bone loss even in the presence of a high calcium intake.[45] However, bone density rapidly returns to baseline levels in the 6 months after weaning.[46] The bone loss is due to increased bone resorption, probably secondary to the relatively low estrogen levels associated with lactation. It is possible that recovery is impaired in women with inadequate calcium intake; total calcium intake during lactation should be at least 1500 mg per day. Nevertheless, calcium supplementation has no effect on the calcium content of breast milk or on bone loss in lactating women who have normal diets.[47] Furthermore, studies indicate that any loss of calcium and bone associated with lactation is rapidly restored, and, therefore, there is no impact on the risk of postmenopausal osteoporosis.[48, 49]

Antibodies are present in breast milk and contribute to the health of an infant. Human milk prevents infections in infants both by transmission of immunoglobulins and by modifying the bacterial flora of the infant's gastrointestinal tract. Viruses are transmitted in breast milk, and although the actual risks are unknown, women infected with cytomegalovirus, hepatitis B, or human immunodeficiency virus are advised not to breastfeed. Vitamin A, vitamin B_{12}, and folic acid are significantly reduced in the breast milk of women with poor dietary intake. As a general rule approximately 1% of any drug ingested by the mother appears in breast milk. In a study of Pima Indians, exclusive breastfeeding for at least 2 months was associated with a lower rate of adult onset noninsulin-dependent diabetes mellitus, partly because overfeeding and excess weight gain are more common with bottlefeeding.[50]

Frequent emptying of the lumen is important for maintaining an adequate level of secretion. Indeed, after the 4th postpartum month, suckling appears to be the only stimulant required; however, environmental and emotional states also are important for continued alveolar activity. Vigorous aerobic exercise does not affect the volume or composition of breast milk, and therefore infant weight gain is normal.[51]

The ejection of milk from the breast does not occur as the result of a mechanically induced negative pressure produced by suckling. Tactile sensors concentrated in the areola activate, via thoracic sensory nerve roots 4, 5, and 6, an afferent sensory neural arc that stimulates the paraventricular and supraoptic nuclei of the hypothalamus to synthesize and transport oxytocin to the posterior pituitary. The efferent arc (oxytocin) is blood-borne to the breast alveolus-ductal systems to contract myoepithelial cells and empty the alveolar lumen. Milk contained in major ductal repositories is ejected from openings in the nipple. This rapid release of milk is called "letdown." This important role for oxytocin is evident in knockout mice lacking oxytocin who undergo normal parturition, but fail to nurse their offspring.[52]

In many instances, the activation of oxytocin release leading to letdown does not require initiation by tactile stimuli. The central nervous system can be conditioned to respond to the presence of the infant, or to the sound of the infant's cry, by inducing activation of the efferent arc. These messages are the result of many stimulating and inhibiting neurotransmitters. Suckling, therefore, acts to refill the breast by activating both portions of the pituitary (anterior and posterior) causing the breast to produce new milk and to eject milk. The release of oxytocin is also important for uterine contractions that contribute to involution of the uterus.

The oxytocin effect is a release phenomenon acting on secreted and stored milk. Prolactin must be available in sufficient quantities for continued secretory replacement of ejected milk. This requires the transient increase in prolactin associated with suckling. The amount of milk produced correlates with the amount removed by suckling. The breast can store milk for a maximum of 48 hours before production diminishes.

Breastfeeding by Adopting Mothers

Adopting mothers occasionally request assistance in initiating lactation.[53] Successful breastfeeding can be achieved by approximately half of the women by ingestion of 25 mg chlorpromazine tid together with vigorous nipple stimulation every 1–3 hours. Milk production will not appear for several weeks. This preparation ideally should be practiced for several months.

Cessation of Lactation

Lactation can be terminated by discontinuing suckling. The primary effect of this cessation is loss of milk letdown via the neural evocation of oxytocin. With passage of a few days, the swollen alveoli depress milk formation probably via a local pressure effect (although milk itself may contain inhibitory factors). With resorption of fluid and solute, the swollen engorged breast diminishes in size in a few days. In addition to the loss of milk letdown the absence of suckling reactivates dopamine (PIF) production so that there is less prolactin stimulation of milk secretion. Routine use of a dopamine agonist for suppression of lactation is not recommended because of reports of hypertension, seizure, myocardial infarctions, and strokes associated with its postpartum use.

Contraceptive Effect of Lactation

A moderate contraceptive effect accompanies lactation and produces child-spacing, which is very important in the developing world as a means of limiting family size. The contraceptive effectiveness of lactation, i.e., the length of the interval between births, depends on the level of nutrition of the mother (if low, the longer the contraceptive interval), the intensity of suckling, and the extent to which supplemental food is added to the infant diet. If suckling intensity and/or frequency is diminished, contraceptive effect is reduced. Only amenorrheic women who exclusively breastfeed (full breastfeeding) at regular intervals, including nighttime, during the first 6 months have the contraceptive protection equivalent to that provided by oral contraception (98% efficacy); with menstruation or after 6 months, the chance of ovulation increases.[54, 55] With full or nearly full breastfeeding, approximately 70% of women remain amenorrheic through 6 months and only 37% through one year; nevertheless with exclusive breastfeeding, the contraceptive efficacy at one year is high, at 92%.[55] Fully breastfeeding women commonly have some vaginal bleeding or spotting in the first 8 postpartum weeks, but this bleeding is not due to ovulation.[56]

Supplemental feeding increases the chance of ovulation (and pregnancy) even in amenorrheic women.[57] Total protection is achieved by the exclusively breastfeeding woman for a duration of only 10 weeks.[56] Half of women studied who are not fully breastfeeding ovulate before the 6th week, the time of the traditional postpartum visit; a visit during the 3rd postpartum week is strongly recommended for contraceptive counseling.

Rule of 3's for Postpartum Initiation of Contraception

Full breastfeeding;   **Begin in *3rd postpartum month.***
Partial or no breastfeeding: **Begin in *3rd postpartum week.***

In nonbreastfeeding women, gonadotropin levels remain low during the early puerperium and return to normal concentrations during the 3rd to 5th week when prolactin levels have returned to normal. In an assessment of this important physiologic event (in terms of the need for contraception), the mean delay before first ovulation was found to be approximately 45 days, while no woman ovulated before 25 days after delivery.[54] Of the 22 women, however, 11 ovulated before the 6th postpartum week, underscoring the need to move the traditional postpartum medical visit to the 3rd week after delivery. In women who do receive dopamine agonist treatment at or immediately after delivery, return of ovulation is slightly accelerated, and contraception is required a week earlier, in the 2nd week postpartum.[58, 59]

The mechanism of the contraceptive effect is of interest because a similar interference with normal pituitary-gonadal function is seen with elevated prolactin levels in nonpregnant women, the syndrome of galactorrhea and amenorrhea. Prolactin concentrations are increased in response to the repeated suckling stimulus of breastfeeding. Given sufficient intensity and frequency, prolactin levels will remain elevated. Under these conditions, follicle-stimulating hormone (FSH) concentrations are in the normal range (having risen from extremely low concentrations at delivery to follicular range in the 3 weeks postpartum) and luteinizing hormone (LH) values are in the low normal range. Despite the presence of gonadotropin, the ovary, during lactational hyperprolactinemia, does not display follicular development and does not secrete estrogen.

Earlier experimental evidence suggested that the ovaries might be refractory to gonadotropin stimulation during lactation, and, in addition, the anterior pituitary might be less responsive to GnRH stimulation. Other studies, done later in the course of lactation, indicated, however, that the ovaries as well as the pituitary were responsive to adequate tropic hormone stimulation.[60]

These observations suggest that high concentrations of prolactin can work at both central and ovarian sites to produce lactational amenorrhea and anovulation. Prolactin appears to affect granulosa cell function in vitro by inhibiting the synthesis of progesterone. It also may change the testosterone:dihydrotestosterone ratio, thereby reducing aromatizable substrate and increasing local antiestrogen concentrations. Nevertheless, a direct effect of prolactin on ovarian follicular development does not appear to be a major factor. The central action predominates.

Elevated levels of prolactin inhibit the pulsatile secretion of GnRH.[61, 62] Prolactin excess has short loop positive feedback effects on dopamine. Increased dopamine reduces GnRH by suppressing arcuate nucleus function, perhaps in a mechanism mediated by endogenous opioid activity.[63, 64] However, blockade of dopamine receptors with a dopamine antagonist or the administration of an opioid antagonist in breastfeeding women does not always affect gonadotropin secretion.[65] The exact mechanism for the suppression of GnRH secretion remains to be unraveled. The principle of GnRH suppression by prolactin is reinforced by the demonstration that treatment of amenorrheic, lactating women with pulsatile GnRH fully restores pituitary secretion and normal ovarian cyclic activity.[66]

At weaning, as prolactin concentrations fall to normal, gonadotropin concentrations increase, and estradiol secretion rises. This prompt resumption of ovarian function is also indicated by the occurrence of ovulation within 14–30 days of weaning.

Inappropriate Lactation — Galactorrheic Syndromes

Galactorrhea refers to the mammary secretion of a milky fluid, which is non-physiologic in that it is inappropriate (not immediately related to pregnancy or the needs of a child), persistent, and sometimes excessive. Although usually white or clear, the color may be yellow or even green. In the latter circumstance, local breast disease should be considered. To elicit breast secretion, pressure should be applied to all sections of the breast beginning at the base of the breast and working up toward the nipple. *Hormonally-induced secretions usually come from multiple duct openings in contrast to pathologic discharge that usually comes from a single duct.* A bloody discharge is more typical of cancer. The quantity of secretion is not an important criterion. Any galactorrhea demands evaluation in a nulliparous woman and if at least 12 months have elapsed since the last pregnancy or weaning in a parous woman. Galactorrhea can involve both breasts or just one breast. Amenorrhea does not necessarily accompany galactorrhea, even in the most serious provocative disorders.

Differential Diagnosis of Galactorrhea

The differential diagnosis of galactorrhea is a difficult and complex clinical challenge. The difficulty arises from the multiple factors involved in the control of prolactin release. In most pathophysiologic states the final common pathway leading to galactorrhea is an inappropriate augmentation of prolactin release. The following considerations are important:

1. Increased prolactin release may be a consequence of prolactin elaboration and secretion from pituitary tumors which function independently of the otherwise appropriate restraints exerted by PIF from a normally functioning hypothalamus. This infrequent but potentially dangerous tumor, which has endocrine, neurologic, and ophthalmologic liabilities that can be disabling, makes the differential diagnosis of persistent galactorrhea a major clinical challenge. Beyond producing prolactin, the tumor may also suppress pituitary parenchyma by expansion and compression, interfering with the secretion of other tropic hormones. Other pituitary tumors may be associated with lactotroph hyperplasia and present with the characteristic syndrome of hyperprolactinemia and amenorrhea.

2. A variety of drugs can inhibit hypothalamic PIF.[67] There are nearly 100 phenothiazine derivatives with indirect mammotropic activity. In addition, there are many phenothiazine-like compounds, reserpine derivatives, amphetamines, and an unknown variety of other drugs (opiates, diazepams, butyrophenones, α-methyldopa, and tricyclic antidepressants) that can initiate galactorrhea via hypothalamic suppression. The final action of these compounds is either to deplete dopamine levels or to block dopamine receptors. Chemical features common to many of these drugs are an aromatic ring with a polar substituent as in estrogen and at least two additional rings or structural attributes making spatial arrangements similar to estrogen. Thus, these compounds may act in a manner similar to estrogens to decrease PIF or to act directly on the pituitary. In support of this conclusion, it has been demonstrated that estrogen and phenothiazine derivatives compete for the same receptors in the median eminence. Prolactin is uniformly elevated in patients on therapeutic amounts of phenothiazines, but essentially never as high as 100 ng/mL. Approximately 30–50% will exhibit galactorrhea that should not persist beyond 3–6 months after drug treatment is discontinued.

3. Hypothyroidism (juvenile or adult) can be associated with galactorrhea. With diminished circulating levels of thyroid hormone, hypothalamic TRH is produced in excess and acts as a PRF to release prolactin from the pituitary. Reversal with thyroid hormone is strong circumstantial evidence to support the conclusion that TRH stimulates prolactin.

4. Excessive estrogen (e.g., oral contraceptives) can lead to milk secretion via hypothalamic suppression, causing reduction of PIF and release of pituitary prolactin, and direct stimulation of the pituitary lactotrophs. Galactorrhea developing during oral contraceptive administration may be most noticeable during the days free of medication (when the steroids are cleared from the body and the prolactin interfering action of the estrogen and progestin on the breast wanes). Galactorrhea caused by excessive estrogen disappears within 3–6 months after discontinuing medication. This is now a rare occurrence with the lower dose pills.[68] A longitudinal study of 126

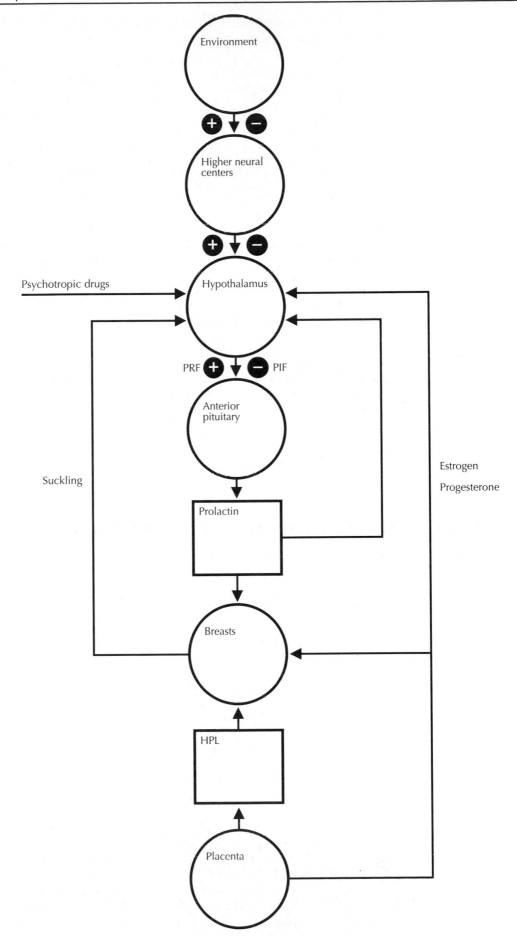

women did demonstrate a 22% increase in prolactin values over mean control levels, but the response to low-dose oral contraceptives was not out of the normal range.[69]

5. Prolonged intensive suckling can also release prolactin, via hypothalamic reduction of PIF. Similarly, thoracotomy scars, cervical spinal lesions, and herpes zoster can induce prolactin release by activating the afferent sensory neural arc, thereby simulating suckling.

6. Stresses can inhibit hypothalamic PIF, thereby inducing prolactin secretion and galactorrhea. Trauma, surgical procedures, and anesthesia can be seen in temporal relation to the onset of galactorrhea.

7. Hypothalamic lesions, stalk lesions, or stalk compression (events that physically reduce production or delivery of PIF to the pituitary) allow release of excess prolactin leading to galactorrhea.

8. Increased prolactin concentrations can result from non-pituitary sources such as lung and renal tumors and even a uterine leiomyoma. Severe renal disease requiring hemodialysis is associated with elevated prolactin levels due to the decreased glomerular filtration rate.

The Clinical Problem of Galactorrhea

A variety of eponymic designations have been applied to variants of the lactation syndromes. These were based on the association of galactorrhea with intrasellar tumor (Forbes, Henneman, Griswold, and Albright, 1951), antecedent pregnancy with inappropriate persistence of galactorrhea (Chiari and Frommel, 1852), and in the absence of previous pregnancy (Argonz and del Castillo, 1953). In all, the association of galactorrhea with eventual amenorrhea was noted.

On the basis of currently available information, categorization of individual cases according to these eponymic guidelines is neither helpful nor does it permit discrimination of patients who have serious intrasellar or suprasellar pathology.

Hyperprolactinemia may be associated with a variety of menstrual cycle disturbances: oligo-ovulation, corpus luteum insufficiency, as well as amenorrhea. About one-third of women with secondary amenorrhea will have elevated prolactin concentrations. Pathologic hyperprolactinemia inhibits the pulsatile secretion of GnRH, and the reduction of circulating prolactin levels restores menstrual function.

Mild hirsutism may accompany ovulatory dysfunction caused by hyperprolactinemia. Whether excess androgen is stimulated by a direct prolactin effect on adrenal cortex synthesis of DHA (dehydroepiandrosterone) and its sulfate (DHAS) or is primarily related to the chronic anovulation of these patients (and hence ovarian androgen secretion) is not settled.

Not all patients with hyperprolactinemia display galactorrhea. The reported incidence is about 33% (Chapter 11). The disparity may not be due entirely to the variable zeal with which the presence of nipple milk secretion is sought during physical examination. The absence of galactorrhea may be due to the usually accompanying hypoestrogenic state. A more attractive explanation focuses on the concept of heterogeneity of tropic hormones (Chapter 2). The immunoassay for prolactin may not discriminate among heterogeneous molecules of prolactin. A high circulating level of prolactin may not represent material capable of interacting with breast prolactin receptors. On the other hand, galactorrhea can be seen in women with normal prolactin serum concentrations. Episodic fluctuations and sleep increments may account for this clinical discordance, or, in this case, bioactive prolactin may be present that is immunoreactively not detectable. Remember that at any one point in time, the bioactivity (galactorrhea) and the

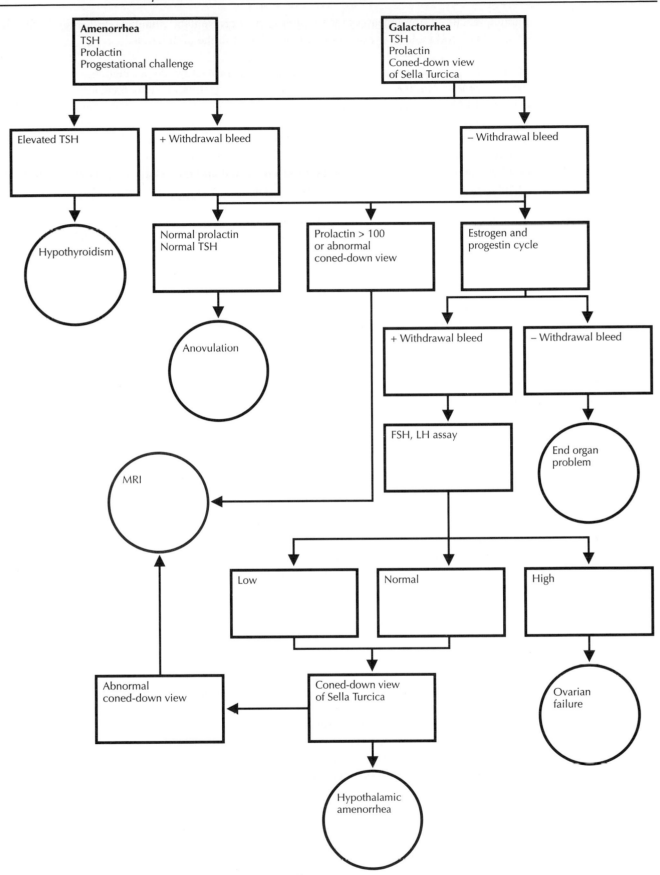

immunoreactivity (immunoassay result) of prolactin represent the cumulative effect of the family of structural and molecular prolactin variants present in the circulation.

In the pathophysiology of male hypogonadism, hyperprolactinemia is much less common, and the incidence of actual galactorrhea quite rare. Hyperprolactinemia in men usually presents with decreased libido and potency.

If galactorrhea has been present for 6 months to 1 year, or hyperprolactinemia is noted in the process of working up menstrual disturbances, infertility, or hirsutism, the probability of a pituitary tumor must be recognized. The workup of hyperprolactinemia is presented in detail in Chapter 11, "Amenorrhea." It is worth reemphasizing the salient clinical issues here.

With the current diagnostic techniques there is no difficulty in discovering and monitoring the size and function of a pituitary prolactin-secreting tumor. With few exceptions the combination of elevation in basal levels of prolactin and radiographic imaging offers complete confidence in diagnosing sellar pathology. The major concern remains in determining management—medical, surgical, or expectant? The considerations that influence management include:

1. Microadenomas, if exclusively prolactin-producing, rarely progress to macro-adenoma size. Most are exceedingly slow-growing or stable.

2. Some tumors regress spontaneously. Medical therapy with dopamine agonists shrinks tumors and can prevent growth, although complete elimination of a tumor by dopamine agonist treatment does not occur, and rapid regrowth usually follows discontinuation of the drug.

3. Transsphenoidal microsurgery is a very safe procedure, but there is a high recurrence rate.

4. The presence of a prolactin-secreting adenoma does not represent a contraindication to pregnancy or the use of exogenous hormones such as oral contraceptives.

As a result of these considerations, many patients can be observed, others treated medically, and, rarely, some treated with surgery, with or without prior medically-induced tumor reduction (see Chapter 11).

Treatment of Galactorrhea

Galactorrhea as an isolated symptom of hypothalamic dysfunction existing in an otherwise healthy woman does not require treatment. Periodic prolactin levels will, if within normal range, confirm the stability of the underlying process. However, some patients find the presence or amount of galactorrhea sexually, cosmetically, and emotionally burdensome. Treatment with combined oral contraceptives, androgens, danazol, and progestins has met with minimal success. Dopamine agonist treatment, therefore, is the therapy of choice. Even with normal prolactin concentrations and normal imaging, treatment with a dopamine agonist can eliminate galactorrhea.

We have adopted a conservative approach of close surveillance for pituitary prolactin-secreting adenomas, recommending surgery only for those tumors that display rapid growth or those tumors that are already large and do not shrink in response to dopamine agonists. If the prolactin level is greater than 100 ng/mL, or if the coned-down view of the sella turcica is abnormal, we recommend magnetic resonance imaging (MRI) evaluation. If the MRI rules out an empty sella syndrome or a suprasellar problem, surgical intervention after preoperative dopamine agonist treatment is then dictated by the patient's desires, the size of the tumor, and the response of the tumor to a dopamine agonist. In patients with prolactin levels less than 100 ng/mL and with normal coned-down views of the sella turcica, an annual prolactin level and periodic coned-down views are indicated for continued observation to detect a growing tumor. Dopamine agonist therapy is recommended for patients wishing to achieve pregnancy, and for those patients who have galactorrhea to the point of discomfort.

The Management of Mastalgia

The cyclic premenstrual occurrence of breast discomfort is a common problem and is occasionally associated with dysplastic, benign histologic changes in the breast. Neither a specific etiology (although the response is probably secondary to the hormonal stimulation of the luteal phase) nor an adverse consequence (such as an increased risk of breast cancer) has been established.[70] Approximately 70% of women report premenstrual breast discomfort in surveys, and interference with activities is recorded in 10–30%.[70]

Medical treatment of mastalgia has historically included a bewildering array of options. Several are of questionable value. Diuretics have little impact, and thyroid hormone treatment is indicated only when hypothyroidism is documented. Steroid hormone treatment has been tried in many combinations, mostly unsupported by controlled studies. An old favorite, with many years of clinical experience testifying to its effectiveness, is testosterone. One must be careful, however, to avoid virilizing doses. A good practice is to start with 5 mg methyltestosterone every other day during the time of discomfort. In recent years, however, these methods have been supplanted by several new approaches.

Danazol in a dose of 100–200 mg/day is effective in relieving discomfort as well as decreasing nodularity of the breast.[71, 72] A daily dose is recommended for a period of 6 months. This treatment may achieve long-term resolution of histologic changes in addition to the clinical improvement. Doses below 400 mg daily do not assure inhibition of ovulation, and a method of effective contraception is necessary because of possible teratogenic effects of the drug. Significant improvement has been noted with vitamin E, 600 units/day of the synthetic tocopherol acetate. No side effects have been noted, and the mechanism of action is unknown. Bromocriptine (2.5 mg/day, which can be administered vaginally if side effects are a problem) and antiestrogens such as tamoxifen (10 or 20 mg daily) are also effective for treating mammary discomfort and benign disease.[72–74]

Clinical observations had suggested that abstinence from methylxanthines leads to resolution of symptoms. Methylxanthines (caffeine, theophylline, and theobromine) are present in coffee, tea, chocolate, and cola drinks. In controlled studies, however, a significant placebo response rate (30–40%) has been observed. Careful assessments of this relationship have failed to demonstrate a link between methylxanthine use and mastalgia, mammographic changes, or atypia (premalignant tissue changes).[75, 76]

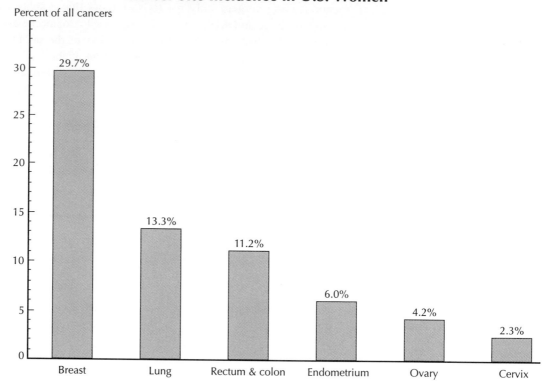

Figure title: **Cancer Site Incidence in U.S. Women**[77]

Percent of all cancers

- Breast: 29.7%
- Lung: 13.3%
- Rectum & colon: 11.2%
- Endometrium: 6.0%
- Ovary: 4.2%
- Cervix: 2.3%

Cancer of the Breast

Scope of the Problem

Currently, female American newborns have a lifetime probability of developing breast cancer of 12.5%, about 1 in 8, double the risk in 1940.[77] The incidence increased over the past 4 decades but plateaued in 1987 (about 180,000 new cases of invasive breast cancer per year). Mortality rates remained disappointingly constant (44,000 deaths per year) until a decline began in 1990. The 5-year survival rate for localized breast cancer (about 60% of breast cancers) has risen from 72% in the 1940s to 97%.[77] This is attributed to earlier diagnosis because of the greater utilization of screening mammography and increased use of chemotherapy, and a continuing decline in mortality should be observed. With regional spread, the 5-year survival rate for breast cancer is 76%; with distant metastases, the rate is 21%. The overall survival rates (all stages combined) are approximately 84% at 5 years after diagnosis, 67% after 10 years, and 56% after 15 years.[77]

The incidence of breast cancer steadily increased until 1990 throughout the world since breast cancer registration began in the 1930s. The increase was almost entirely due to an increasing incidence in women over age 50. This long-term steady increase was present long before the beginning of widespread mammography screening in the 1980s. From 1982 through 1987, there occurred a more rapid increase in the incidence of breast cancer due to the detection by screening mammography of early stage, small tumors; the incidence of larger tumors and metastatic tumors actually decreased slightly.[77] For these reasons, the long-term increase (about 1% per year) cannot be attributed solely to the widespread availability of screening mammography. Because the incidence since 1990 has plateaued, the long-term increase over the past decades is attributed to lifestyle and reproductive changes (diet and exercise; reduced parity and delayed child-bearing).

Cancer Deaths in U.S. Women[77]

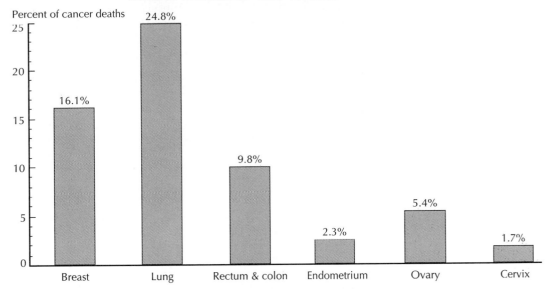

The breast is the leading site of cancer in U.S. women (29.7% of all cancers) and is now, unfortunately, (because smoking is obviously the reason) exceeded by lung cancer as the leading cause of death from cancer in women.[77]

Mortality rate per 100,000 female population[77]

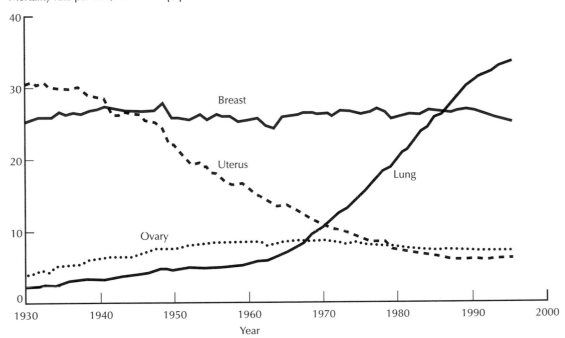

Breast cancer has an increasing frequency with age. Nearly 77% of all breast cancers occur in women over age 50; only 6.5% of all cases occur under age 40, 15% under age 50. A woman at age 70 has almost 16 times the risk as a 40-year-old woman. However, after menopause, although the incidence rate continues to increase, it is less dramatic than the rise before menopause. Over the age of 50, American white women are more likely to develop breast cancer than black American women; under the age of 50, the opposite is true.[77] The 5-year survival rate for women who develop breast cancer under age 45 is 79% compared to 87% for women ages 65 and older.

The Chances of Developing Breast Cancer According to Age[78]

By age 25	1 in 19,608
By age 30	1 in 2,525
By age 35	1 in 622
By age 40	1 in 217
By age 45	1 in 93
By age 50	1 in 50
By age 55	1 in 33
By age 60	1 in 24
By age 65	1 in 17
By age 70	1 in 14
By age 75	1 in 11
By age 80	1 in 10
By age 85	1 in 9
Lifetime	1 in 8

Over the years, breast cancer has continued its deadly impact despite advances in surgical and diagnostic techniques. Classically, the single most useful prognostic information in women with operable breast cancer has been the histologic status of the axillary lymph nodes.[79, 80] The survival rate is higher with axillary lymph nodes negative for disease compared with positive nodes. Because of this recognition for the importance of the axillary nodes, the traditional surgical approach to breast cancer was based on the concept that breast cancer is a disease of stepwise progression. *There has been an important change in concept. Breast cancer is now viewed as a systemic disease, with spread to local and distant sites at the same time. Breast cancer is best viewed as occultly metastatic at the time of presentation.* Therefore, dissemination of tumor cells has occurred by the time of surgery in many patients. However, this is not the story for all patients. Surely, some (if not many) cancers prior to invasion (and perhaps even some small invasive cancers) are not systemic at the time of diagnosis. For this reason, surgery is curative for many early cases of breast cancer.

Because we have been dealing with a disease that has already reached the point of dissemination in many patients, we must move the diagnosis forward several years in order to have an impact on breast cancer mortality. Earlier diagnosis requires that we be aware of what it is that makes a high-risk patient. *However, keep in mind that the great majority of women (85%) who develop breast cancer do not have an identifiable risk factor other than age, and, therefore, every woman must be considered at risk.*

Risk Factors

A constellation of factors influences the risk for breast cancer. These include reproductive experience, ovarian activity, benign breast disease, familial tendency, genetic differences, dietary considerations, and specific endocrine factors.

Reproductive Experience

The risk of breast cancer increases with the increase in age at which a woman bears her first full-term child. A woman pregnant before the age of 18 has about one-third the risk of one who first delivers after the age of 35. To be protective, pregnancy must occur before the age of 30. In fact, women over the age of 30 years at the time of their first birth have a greater risk than women who never become pregnant.[81] Indeed, there is reason to believe that the age at the time of birth of the last child is the most important influence (an increasing risk with increasing age).[82] There is, however, a significant protective effect with increasing parity, present even when adjusted for age at first birth and other risk factors.[83, 84] Delayed childbearing and fewer children in modern times are believed to have contributed significantly to the increased incidence of breast cancer observed over the last decades.

Data from the Nurses' Health Study indicate that a positive family history for breast cancer overwhelms the protective effect of pregnancy, and women with a mother or sister history of breast cancer actually had an increase in risk enhanced by first pregnancy.[85]

Although pregnancy at an early age produces an overall lifetime reduction in risk, there is evidence that the first few years after delivery are associated with a transient increase in risk.[86] This increase may reflect accelerated growth of an already present malignancy by the hormones of pregnancy. A very large case-control study concluded that pregnancy transiently increases the risk (perhaps for up to 3 years) after a woman's first childbirth, and this is followed by a lifetime reduction in risk.[87] And some have found that a concurrent or recent pregnancy (3–4 years previously) adversely affects survival (even after adjustment for size of tumor and number of nodes).[88, 89] It is argued that breast cells which have already begun malignant transformation are adversely affected by the hormones of pregnancy, while normal stem cells become more resistant.

Conflicting results have been reported in over 20 studies examining the risk of breast cancer associated with the number of abortions (especially induced abortions) experienced by individual patients.[90, 91] Concern for an adverse effect has been based on the theoretical suggestion that a full-term pregnancy protects against breast cancer by invoking complete differentiation of breast cells, but abortion increases the risk by allowing breast cell proliferation in the first trimester of pregnancy, but not allowing the full differentiation that occurs in later pregnancy. In these studies there has been a major problem of recall bias; women who develop breast cancer are more likely to truthfully reveal their history of induced abortion than healthy women. In studies that avoided recall bias (e.g., by deriving data from national registries instead of personal interviews), the risk of breast cancer was identical in women with and without induced abortions.[92, 93]

The fact that pregnancy early in life is associated with a reduction in the risk of breast cancer implies that etiologic factors are operating during that period of life. The protection afforded only by the first pregnancy suggests that the first full-term pregnancy has a trigger effect which either produces a permanent change in the factors responsible for breast cancer, or changes the breast tissue and makes it less susceptible to malignant transformation. There is evidence for a lasting impact of a first pregnancy on a woman's hormonal milieu. A small but significant elevation of estriol, a decrease in dehydroepiandrosterone and dehydroepiandrosterone sulfate, and lower prolactin levels all persist for many years after delivery.[94, 95] These changes take on significance when viewed in terms of the endocrine factors considered below.

Lactation may offer a weak to moderate protective effect (20% reduced risk) only for premenopausal breast cancer.[96–99] There is a unique and helpful study of the Chinese Tanka, who are boat people living on the coast of southern China.[100] The women of the Chinese Tanka wear clothing with an opening only on the right side, and they breastfeed only with the right breast. All breast cancers were in postmenopausal women, and the cancers were equally distributed between the two sides, suggesting a protective effect only for premenopausal breast cancer. The Nurses' Health Study could not detect a protective effect of lactation, and a Norwegian prospective study, including a high percentage of women with long durations of breastfeeding, found no benefit on either premenopausal or postmenopausal breast cancer incidence.[101, 102] The impact of lactation, if significant, must be small.

In both cohort and case-control studies, there is good evidence that cosmetic breast augmentation does not increase the risk of breast cancer.[103–105] Specifically, studies have failed to indicate an increased risk of breast cancer in women who have had cosmetic breast implants.[106, 107]

Ovarian Activity

Women who have a premenopausal oophorectomy have a lower risk of breast cancer, and the lowered risk is greater the younger a woman is when ovariectomized. There is a 70% risk reduction in women who have oophorectomy before age 35. There is a small decrease in risk with late menarche and a moderate increase in risk with late natural menopause, indicating that ovarian activity plays a continuing role throughout reproductive life.[108]

Benign Breast Disease

Women with prior benign breast disease form only a small proportion of breast cancer patients, approximately 5%. With obstruction of ducts (probably by stromal fibrosis), ductule-alveolar secretion persists, the secretory material is retained, and cysts form from the dilatation of terminal ducts (duct ectasia) and alveoli. There is good reason to eliminate the phrase "fibrocystic disease of the breast." In a review of over 10,000 breast biopsies in Nashville, Tennessee, 70% of the women were found to not have a lesion associated with an increased risk for cancer.[109] The most important variable on biopsies is the degree and character of the epithelial proliferation. Women with atypical hyperplasia had a relative risk of 5.3, while women with atypia and a family history of breast cancer had a relative risk of 11. In the Nurses' Health Study, biopsies with proliferative disease had a relative risk of breast cancer of 1.6, and with atypical hyperplasia, the relative risk was 3.7.[110] Only 4–10% of benign biopsies have atypical hyperplasia. The point is that we needlessly frighten patients with the use of the phrase fibrocystic disease. For most women, this is not a disease, but a physiologic change brought about by cyclic hormonal activity. ***Let's call this problem FIBROCYSTIC CHANGE OR CONDITION.***

The College of American Pathologists supports this position and has offered this classification.[111]

Classification of Breast Biopsy Tissue According to Risk for Breast Cancer

    No increased risk:
        Adenosis
        Duct ectasia
        Fibroadenoma
        Fibrosis
        Mild hyperplasia (3–4 cells deep)
        Mastitis
        Periductal mastitis
        Squamous metaplasia

    Slightly increased risk (1.5–2.0 times):
        Moderate or florid hyperplasia
        Papilloma

    Risk increased 3–5 times:
        Atypical hyperplasia

Familial Tendency

Most breast cancers are sporadic; i.e., they arise in individuals without a family history of breast cancer. However, female relatives of women with breast cancer have about twice the rate of the general population. There is an excess of bilateral disease among patients with a family history of breast cancer. Relatives of women with bilateral disease have about a 45% lifetime chance of developing breast cancer. In data from the Centers for Disease Control and Prevention (CDC), these relative risks were observed:[112]

Affected mother or sister:	**2.3 relative risk.**
Affected aunt or grandmother:	**1.5 relative risk.**
Affected mother and sister:	**14.0 relative risk**

Results from the Nurses' Health Study indicate that the magnitude of risk associations with a positive family history is smaller than previously believed, comparable to the CDC data above, except for a relative risk of only 2.3 when both mother and sister (first-degree relatives) had breast cancer.[113] In general, the size of the increased risk with a positive family history is approximately 2 times the normal incidence. In the Nurses' Health Study, there was no interaction between family history and alcohol intake; however, a positive mother or sister history of breast cancer eliminated the protective effects of late menarche, multiple births, and early births.[85]

Using the data from the Cancer and Steroid Hormone Study, the CDC has provided tables which can be used for the purpose of counseling women with a family history of breast cancer.[114] These tables estimate the risks according to the various combinations of affected first- and second-degree relatives and the ages at onset of breast cancer for the affected relatives. The risk is higher with early age of onset and more than one relative with breast cancer. For example, the predicted lifetime risk for a woman with two first-degree relatives (sisters and mother) who developed breast cancer before age 40 is approximately 44%, and with one first-degree relative with breast cancer between ages 30 and 39 years, 17%.

The breast and ovarian cancer gene (*BRCA1*) associated with familial cancer is on the long arm of chromosome 17, localized to 17q12–q21. Although other genetic alterations have been observed in breast tumors, mutations in *BRCA1* are believed to be responsible for approximately 45% of familial breast cancer and 80% of families with both early onset breast and ovarian cancer. Inheritance of this gene can be either maternal or paternal; male carriers are at increased risk for colon and prostate cancers.[115] A second locus, *BRCA2*, on chromosome 13q12–q13, accounts for up to 35% of families with early onset breast cancer (but a lower rate of ovarian cancer), and in males, for prostate cancer, pancreatic cancer, and male breast cancer.[116, 117] Together, *BRCA1* and *BRCA2* account for 80% of families with multiple cases of early-onset breast cancer.[118] About 5–10% of women who develop ovarian cancer have mutations in *BRCA1*.[119, 120]

BRCA1 encodes an 1863 amino acid protein with a zinc finger domain that is probably a tumor suppressor important in DNA transcription. Mutations in many different regions of the *BRCA1* gene cause a loss or reduction in its function.[121, 122] Because not every individual with a mutation in this gene develops cancer, other factors are probably involved, making the accuracy of prediction more difficult and arguing against widespread screening for mutations of this gene. Providing accurate numbers is a difficult task, because breast cancer has a multifactorial etiology with both genetic and environmental factors. The *BRCA1* gene may also play a role in sporadic breast and ovarian cancer, but analysis of tumors has failed to find mutations in sporadic cancers that occur later in life.[123]

High-risk families have a high probability of harboring a mutation in a dominant breast cancer susceptibility gene, transmitted by either parent, and accounting for approximately 5% of breast cancer in the general population. It is estimated that approximately 0.04% to 0.2% of women in the U.S. carry the *BRCA1* susceptibility (and *BRCA2* is less common).[124] Among women of Ashkenazi Jewish descent, the prevalence of *BRCA1* and *BRCA2* mutations is about 2%.[125] The percentage of breast cancer cases in the general population associated with a family history accounts for only a minor part of the overall prevalence. The best estimates initially ranged from 6% to 19% at most.[126] Later more representative studies revealed a lower prevalence, as low as 3% in the general population.[127, 128] In addition, there appears to be great variability in different parts of the world, and the prevalence in minority populations has not been adequately measured.

The presence of ovarian cancer within a family and 3 or more cases of breast cancer within a family are strong predictors of *BRCA1* mutations. Thus, genetic screening should be reserved for patients with high-risk families.

Family History Characteristics Associated With the Presence of *BRCA1*

Early age of onset of breast cancer within a family.
Relatives with ovarian cancer.
3 or more relatives with breast cancer.
Ashkenazi ancestry.

Moderate risk families are characterized by a less striking family history, the absence of ovarian cancer, and an age of onset at the time of diagnosis that is older. High risk families have the presence of multiple cases of breast cancer in close relatives (usually at least 3 cases) that follows an autosomal dominant pattern of inheritance; breast cancer is usually diagnosed before age 45; there may be cases of ovarian cancer in the family as well. Many of the cases, but not all, can be attributed to the susceptibility genes, *BRCA1* and *BRCA2*.

High risk families have the following cumulative breast cancer risk by the age of 80 as determined by the analysis of family histories.[126]

Affected Relative	Age of Affected Relative	Cumulative Breast Cancer Risk by Age 80
One first-degree relative	< 50 years old 50 or more years old	13–21% 9–11%
One second-degree relative	< 50 years old 50 or more years old	10–14% 8–9%
Two first-degree relatives	Both < 50 years old Both 50 years or older	35–48% 11–24%
Two second-degree relatives but both parental or maternal	Both < 50 years old Both 50 years or older	21–26% 9–16%

BRCA1 and *BRCA2* direct DNA screening is now possible. Each child of a carrier has a 50% chance of inheriting the mutation. Although it is recognized that this may be an over estimation, the studies indicate that women who are carrying the *BRCA1* mutation have an 87% cumulative life-time risk of developing breast cancer—about 20% by age 40, 51% by age 50, and 85% by age 70, and a 20–65% risk for ovarian cancer (closer to 20% in more recent studies of less highly selected groups). In addition, the male relatives who are carrying this mutation have approximately a 3-fold increased risk of prostate cancer and 4-fold increased risk of colon cancer. The breast cancer risk is similar for women with *BRCA2* mutations. Breast cancer associated with *BRCA1* mutations is histologically different (more often aneuploid and receptor negative) compared to *BRCA2* mutations and sporadic cancers, and appears to grow faster, but paradoxically, may have a better survival.[129] Outcome results, however, have not been consistent. A well-done Dutch study could not detect a difference in disease-free and overall survival comparing breast cancer cases from families with proven *BRCA1* mutations to patients with sporadic breast cancer.[130]

Because not all families with breast cancer carry mutations of *BRCA1* or *BRCA2*, these families probably have breast cancer susceptibility genes yet to be identified. In addition, the current screening methods do not detect all *BRCA* mutations. ***When 3 or more closely related individuals within a family have been diagnosed with breast cancer, the likelihood that an inherited dominant genetic mutation is present is very high.*** The affected women need not be first-degree relatives, but they must be related either all on the mother's side or the father's side. ***The family presence of just one case of ovarian cancer further increases the likelihood of the BRCA1 mutation.*** Identifying the families that carry the *BRCA2* gene uses the same historical criteria as that for the *BRCA1* gene. In contrast to *BRCA1* families, *BRCA2* families have only a moderately increased incidence of ovarian cancer.

Identification and counseling for families who have the appropriate history but fail to demonstrate BRCA1 or BRCA2 mutations should be exactly the same as when the mutations are found.

Once it has been determined that a family is at high risk for a breast cancer gene mutation, it is recommended that this family be referred to an appropriate laboratory and service that can be identified through the medical genetics department at a regional referral institution. Although blood samples can be mailed by over-night mail, involvement with an appropriate center is highly urged because of the importance of accurate informed consent, counseling, and follow-up care. The way in which information is communicated to patients has a profound impact on decision-making and compliance with surveillance.

A problem exists when it comes to deciding what to do. While we have good data indicating prevalence and risk in these high-risk families, we do not have studies telling us what the risk reduction is from prophylactic surgery, nor do we know the efficacy of increasing surveillance programs for these identified individuals. Because the mutation is present in every cell, and prophylactic mastectomy does not remove all tissue, there is no guarantee that breast cancer will be totally prevented. The same situation applies with prophylactic oophorectomy in that a carcinoma can arise from peritoneal cells. However, prophylactic removal of the bulk of the tissue at risk should be effective.[131] The first follow-up study of high risk women who have undergone prophylactic mastectomy indicated a major reduction in the number of breast cancers in the mastectomy group, although total prevention was not achieved.[132]

Current recommendations from experts in this field are as follows.[126, 133] For an individual identified to be at high risk, clinical breast examination and mammography are recommended every 6–12 months beginning between ages 25 and 35. Evaluation every 6 months is appropriate because the *BRCA1*-related tumors have been demonstrated to be faster growing tumors. Although the evidence for the precise degree of protection offered by prophylactic mastectomy is not available, support should be provided for those women who choose this option. Pelvic examination, serum CA-125 levels, and transvaginal ultrasonography with color Doppler are recommended every 6–12 months for women under age 40. Prophylactic oophorectomy is recommended at the completion of child-bearing, preferably before age 35. It is of benefit to take oral contraceptives to reduce the ovarian cancer risk. A case-control study indicated that the use of oral contraceptives in women with *BRCA1 or BRCA2* mutations was associated with a 50% reduction in the risk of ovarian cancer (increasing with duration of use, from 20% for less than 3 years of use, up to 60% with 6 or more years of use).[134] The magnitude of this protection is identical with that previously observed in the general population. In our view, postmenopausal estrogen therapy is not contraindicated for these women (see Chapter 18).

Dietary Factors

The geographic variation in incidence rates of breast cancer is considerable (the United States has the highest rates and Japan the lowest), and it has been correlated with the amount of animal fat in the diet.[135] Lean women, however, have an increased incidence of breast cancer, although this increase is limited to small, localized, and well-differentiated tumors.[136] Furthermore, studies have failed to find evidence for a positive relationship between breast cancer and dietary total or saturated fat or cholesterol intake.[137–139] On the other hand, there is evidence that dietary fat is a stronger risk factor for postmenopausal breast cancer than for premenopausal breast cancer.[140] Although a cohort study concluded that dietary fat is a determinant of postmenopausal breast cancer, the association did not achieve statistical significance.[141] Thus, the epidemiologic literature provides little support for a major contribution of dietary fat to the risk of breast cancer. Nevertheless, there is a correlation between intra-abdominal fat (android obesity) and the risk of breast cancer, a consequence of excessive caloric consumption, however, not a specific dietary component.[142] Presumably, the connection between android obesity and breast cancer is through the metabolic perturbations associated with excessive body weight.

There is no argument that the incidence of breast cancer is increased in countries associated with affluent, unfavorable diets (high fat content) and a lack of physical exercise. The common denominator may be the peripheral insulin resistance and hyperinsulinemia that become prevalent with aging in affluent, modern societies. This specific metabolic change is becoming a common theme in various clinical conditions, particularly noninsulin-dependent diabetes mellitus, anovulation and polycystic ovaries, hypertension, and dyslipidemia. Hyperinsulinemia is found more often in women with breast cancer.[143] In this subgroup of women, the risk of breast cancer may be unfavorably influenced by hormonal changes (such as a decrease in sex hormone-binding globulin and an increase in unbound, free estradiol). There are, indeed, many reasons to avoid excess body weight. The risk of breast cancer is reduced in women who exercise regularly.[144]

In women, soy consumption produces a reduction in the circulating levels of estradiol.[145] In the parts of the world where soy intake is high, there is a lower incidence of breast, endometrial, and prostate cancers. For example, a case-control study concluded that there was a 54% reduced risk of endometrial cancer, and another case-control study indicated a reduction in the risk of breast cancer, in women with a high consumption of soy and other legumes.[146, 147] It is by no means certain, however, that there is a direct effect of soy intake.[148] Soy intake may be a marker for other factors in lifestyle or diet that are protective.

It is well recognized that the incidence of breast cancer is higher in the U.S. than in China or Japan. It has been further observed that after migration to the U.S., Asian women gradually increase (6-fold) their risk of breast cancer over several generations, eventually reaching the level of white women. Evidence indicates that this reflects a change in diet and lifestyle, with an increase in risk associated with a gain in height and weight.[149, 150] Recent weight gain is especially associated with increased risk. A reduced risk, however, is observed in heavy, younger women.

The effect of body weight on the risk of breast cancer differs in premenopausal and postmenopausal women. In premenopausal women who are overweight, the risk of breast cancer is lower compared with normal weight individuals, and in postmenopausal women, excess weight is associated with either an unchanged or slightly increased risk.[150–152] This is attributed to a more marked increase in total and free estrogen levels in overweight postmenopausal women, in contrast to lower levels with increasing weight in premenopausal women. Postmenopausal obese women have later menopause, higher estrone production rates and free estradiol levels (lower sex hormone-binding globulin), and a slightly greater risk for breast cancer.[153] A large Swedish case-control study suggested that the principal factor is weight gain during adulthood, and that the impact on breast cancer emerges 10 years after menopause.[154] As noted, this weight gain may be the important determinant in the increasing risk experienced by migrants from low-risk parts of the world who move to high-risk areas.

Alcohol in the Diet

There is a modest increase in the risk for breast cancer with the consumption of one or more alcoholic drinks of all forms per day.[155] Almost all of many studies conclude that two drinks daily increase the risk by about 30–40%.[156] It is tempting to speculate that breast cancer and alcohol are linked through estrogen, either a direct or an indirect effect (e.g., on hepatic enzymes) on estrogen metabolism. An effect of alcohol ingestion by premenopausal women was not demonstrated on circulating levels of estrone, estradiol, dehydroepiandrosterone sulfate (DHEAS), or sex hormone-binding globulin in a cross-sectional study that depended upon a questionnaire to assess alcohol intake.[157] However, when alcohol is administered under experimental conditions, circulating estrogen concentrations are raised to high levels.[158, 159] And in a prospective cohort study of premenopausal women in Italy, higher estradiol levels were correlated with an increased alcohol intake over a 1-year period of time.[160]

Specific Endocrine Factors

Adrenal Steroids

Subnormal levels of etiocholanolone (a urinary excretion product of androstenedione) were found from 5 months to 9 years before the diagnosis of breast cancer in women living on the island of Guernsey, off the English coast.[161] A subnormal excretion of this 17-ketosteroid was also found in sisters of patients with breast cancer. A 6-fold increase in the incidence of breast cancer was found between women excreting less than 0.4 mg of etiocholanolone and those excreting over 1 mg/24 hours. Measurement of this 17-ketosteroid might be a useful screening procedure to detect a high-risk group of patients because approximately 25% of the population excretes less than 1 mg/24 hours.

Endogenous Estrogen

Epidemiologic and other information continue to suggest some estrogen-related promoter function. These include the following: 1) the condition is 100 times more common in women than in men; 2) breast cancer invariably occurs after puberty; 3) untreated gonadal dysgenesis and breast cancer are mutually exclusive; 4) a 65% excess rate of breast cancer has been observed among women who have had an endometrial cancer; and 5) breast tumors contain estrogen receptors which are biologically active as indicated by the presence of progesterone receptors in tumor tissue. Taken together, these data suggest an element of estrogen dependence, if not provocation, in many breast cancers.

Estriol generally has failed to produce breast cancer in rodents, and in fact, estriol protects the rat against breast tumors induced by various chemical carcinogens.[162] The hypothesis is that a higher estriol level protects against the more potent effects of estrone and estradiol. This might explain the protective effect of early pregnancies. Women having had an early pregnancy continue to excrete more estriol than nulliparous women. Premenopausal healthy Asiatic women have a lower breast cancer risk than Caucasians and also have a higher rate of urinary estriol excretion.[163] When Asiatic women migrate to the United States, however, the risk of breast cancer increases, and their urinary excretion of estriol decreases, perhaps a consequence of dietary changes as noted above. A major factor in the potency differences among the various estrogens (estradiol, estrone, estriol) is the length of time the estrogen-receptor complex occupies the nucleus. The higher rate of dissociation with the weak estrogen (estriol) can be compensated for by continuous application to allow prolonged nuclear binding and activity. Estriol has only 20–30% affinity for the estrogen receptor compared to estradiol; therefore, it is rapidly cleared from a cell. But if the effective concentration is kept equivalent to that of estradiol, it can produce a similar biologic response.[164] In pregnancy, where the concentration of estriol is very great, it can be an important hormone, not just a metabolite. Thus, higher estriol levels are not necessarily protective. Indeed, antagonism of estradiol occurs only within a vary narrow range of the ratio of estradiol to estriol, a range rarely encountered either physiologically or pharmacologically.[165] Below this range, estradiol is unimpeded, above this range estriol itself exerts estrogenic activity.

Stanley G. Korenman promulgated a most interesting hypothesis concerning the endocrinology of breast cancer.[166, 167] Recognizing that the endocrine changes thought to be related to the promotion or provocation of breast cancer were small, inconsistent, and could hardly account for the differential risk of breast cancer among populations, Korenman concluded that endocrine status is related to breast cancer by influencing the patient's susceptibility to environmental carcinogens. Called the "Open Window Hypothesis," Korenman argued that unopposed estrogen stimulation is the most favorable state for tumor induction (the "open" window). Susceptibility to breast cancer declines with the establishment of normal luteal phase progesterone secretion and becomes very low during pregnancy; the open window is closed.

The two main open window periods are the pubertal years prior to the establishment of regular ovulatory menstrual cycles and the perimenopausal period of waning follicle maturation and ovulation. The prolongation of these open windows by obesity, infertility, delayed pregnancy, earlier menarche, and later menopause would be associated with greater susceptibility. This argument is supported by observational studies indicating that anovulatory and infertile women (exposed to less progesterone) have an increased risk of breast cancer later in life.[168–171] However, the statistical power of these observational studies was limited by small numbers (all fewer than 15 cases).

Although theoretically appealing on the basis of presumed correlation with epidemiologic risks (infertility, late menopause) clinical research has not always confirmed the thesis. Young women at high genetic risk for breast cancer had normal luteal phases, and a group of premenopausal women with breast cancer also had normal luteal phases.[172] Others have failed to find a link between anovulation and the risk of breast cancer.[173–175] Indeed, women with the most irregular menstrual cycles (and thus presumably anovulatory) in the Nurses' Health Study appeared to have a reduced risk of breast cancer.[176]

Studies seeking a correlation between circulating levels of sex hormones and breast cancer have yielded conflicting results. In the Rancho Bernardo cohort, no relationship between estrogen, androgen, and sex hormone-binding globulin levels with the incidence of breast cancer could be demonstrated.[177] Using serum collected earlier in life, no differences in endogenous hormones could be detected in 51 women who subsequently developed breast cancer; including the various estrogens, progesterone, androstenedione, and even sex hormone-binding globulin.[178] On the other hand, in a very large prospective study in Italy, estradiol, testosterone, and sex hormone-binding globulin levels were higher in postmenopausal women who subsequently developed breast cancer.[179] In a British report, women who subsequently developed breast cancer had higher levels of estradiol.[180] Two North American prospective studies also found higher levels of estrogen in women who subsequently developed breast cancer, and most impressively, an increasing risk of breast cancer correlated with increasing levels of free estradiol.[181, 182] In another study, women who developed breast cancer displayed higher levels of non-bound, free estradiol and lower levels of sex hormone-binding globulin (SHBG).[183] In the Nurses' Health Study, an association was reported between an increased risk of breast cancer and higher levels of estradiol, estrone, and dehydroepiandrosterone sulfate; however, no association could be demonstrated with the percent free or bioavailable levels of estradiol, androstenedione, testosterone, or dehydroepiandrosterone.[184]

Bone mass is generally regarded as a marker of estrogen exposure, and women with the highest bone densities have a greater risk of breast cancer compared with women who have low bone densities.[185] Another attempt to link the risk of breast cancer to the endogenous estrogen level focused on prenatal exposure. A reduced risk for breast cancer is observed for women born to mothers with pregnancy-induced hypertension, suggesting that this finding is due to the lower estrogen levels associated with preeclampsia.[186, 187]

The biologic plausibility and epidemiologic support for an estrogen link are impressive arguments. Whether the important factor is the total amount of estrogen, the amount of estrogen unopposed by progesterone, the amount of free (unbound) estradiol, the duration of exposure to estrogen, or some other combination is not known. The discrepancies among the various studies reflect the fact that the differences are very small, and it is a struggle to achieve statistical significance.

Endogenous Progesterone

Because mitotic activity in the breast reaches its peak during the progesterone dominant luteal phase of the menstrual cycle,[188-190] it can be argued that progesterone is the key to influencing the risk of breast cancer. This would be consistent with experimental demonstrations in mice that progesterone is the primary hormonal stimulus for mammary growth and differentiation.[2] However, studies do not support a major role for a progestational influence. Indeed, evidence indicates that with increasing duration of exposure, progesterone can limit breast epithelial growth as it does with endometrial epithelium.[11-13] In vitro studies of normal breast epithelial cells reveal that progestins inhibit proliferation.[191] Human breast tissue specimens removed after the patients were treated with estradiol and progesterone indicate that progesterone inhibits in vivo estradiol-induced proliferation.[13, 192] As noted, women who ultimately develop breast cancer do not have different blood levels of progesterone.[178] In addition, several clinical observations would argue against progesterone as a key factor. Although there is some disagreement, most studies indicate that the high levels of estrogen and progesterone during pregnancy have no adverse impact on the course of breast cancer diagnosed during pregnancy or when pregnancy occurs subsequent to diagnosis and treatment (discussed with references in Chapter 18). Medroxyprogesterone acetate is not associated with an increased risk of breast cancer when used for contraception over long durations (Chapter 23).

Exogenous Estrogen and Progestin

The relationship between the postmenopausal use of exogenous estrogens and the risk of breast cancer has been intensively studied (reviewed with complete references in Chapter 18). At the present time there is no conclusive evidence that estrogen doses known to protect against osteoporosis and cardiovascular disease (0.625 mg conjugated estrogens, 1.0 mg estradiol, or equivalent doses of other products) increase the risk of breast cancer. Some have concluded that a slight increase is noted with long duration of use; however, notable studies have failed to document such an increase. The extensive literature on this subject can be summarized as follows:

> Some epidemiologic case-control and cohort studies conclude that long-term (5 or more years) of current use of postmenopausal hormone therapy is associated with a slight increase in the risk of breast cancer. This conclusion might be due to confounding biases, particularly detection and surveillance bias.

> All epidemiologic studies fail to find an increased risk of breast cancer associated with short-term (less than 5 years) use or past use of postmenopausal hormone therapy.

> The epidemiologic data agree that the addition of a progestin to the treatment regimen neither increases nor decreases the risk observed in individual studies.

> The epidemiologic data indicate that a positive family history of breast cancer should not be a contraindication to the use of postmenopausal hormone therapy.

> Women who develop breast cancer while using postmenopausal hormone therapy have a reduced risk of dying from breast cancer. This is because of two factors: (1). Increased surveillance and early detection; and (2). Acceleration of tumor growth so that tumors appear at a less virulent and aggressive stage.

Thyroid, Prolactin, Various Nonestrogen Drugs

Despite isolated suggestions of increased risk, hypothyroidism, reserpine, and prolactin excess, whether spontaneous or drug-induced, are not related to an enhanced risk of breast cancer.[193, 194]

Oral Contraception and Breast Cancer

The large number of women taking or having taken oral contraceptive steroids, combined with the belief that steroids provoke or promote abnormal breast growth and possibly cancer, has provided a source of major concern for years. The Royal College of General Practitioners, Oxford Family Planning Association, and Walnut Creek studies have indicated no significant differences in breast cancer rates between users and nonusers. However, patients were enrolled in these studies at a time when oral contraceptives were used primarily by married couples spacing out their children. Because this population did not reflect use by younger women for long durations to delay their first pregnancy, case-control studies in the last decade have focused on the contemporary use of oral contraceptives. This subject is reviewed in detail with complete references in Chapter 22.

Long-term use of oral contraception during the reproductive years is not associated with a significant increase in the risk of breast cancer that occurs later in life, after age 45. There is the possibility that a subgroup of young women who use oral contraceptives early and for more than 4 years has a slightly increased risk (a relative risk of less than 1.2) of breast cancer that occurs earlier in life, before age 45.[195] The re-analysis of data from 54 studies indicated that breast cancers that occurred in women who were previous users of oral contraceptives were more localized, with less metastatic disease.[195] Indeed, the risk of metastatic disease in ever users was significantly reduced. Breast cancer before age 45 is relatively rare, and furthermore, the results of these studies may reflect the same problem observed in studies with postmenopausal hormone therapy, detection/surveillance bias. The reduced risk of later metastatic disease and the increased appearance early in life suggest a situation analogous to pregnancy. Thus, breast cells that have already begun malignant transformation may be accelerated in their growth by exposure to oral contraceptives, and appear early in localized form. With the accumulation of greater numbers of older women previously exposed to oral contraceptives, a protective effect may become evident. Overall, the message is reassuring. The statistical effect, if real, is small, and the data are also consistent with explanations other than an etiologic stimulation.

The use of oral contraception does not further increase the risk of breast cancer in women with positive family histories of breast cancer or in women with proven benign breast diseases. There is no evidence that the use of oral contraceptives prior to the diagnosis of breast cancer has an adverse impact on prognosis.[196]

Higher dose oral contraception, used for 2 or more years, protected against benign breast disease, but this protection was limited to current and recent users. It is uncertain whether this same protection is provided by the current low-dose formulations. A French case-control study has indicated a reduction of non-proliferative benign breast disease associated with low-dose oral contraception used before a first full-term pregnancy, but no effect on proliferative disease with use after a pregnancy.[197]

Breast Cancer in Diethylstilbestrol (DES)-Exposed Women

From 1940 to 1970, diethylstilbestrol (DES), a potent synthetic estrogen, was prescribed in high doses for a variety of pregnancy-related complications. Exposure to DES occurred in association with 2 million live births; therefore, the risk for induction of breast cancer during a period of breast differentiation could be significant if DES were a true breast carcinogen. The first study on this subject reported on the follow-up of women who participated in a controlled trial of DES in pregnancy between 1950 and 1952 at the University of Chicago. In this study, an increase in breast cancer risk that did not reach significance was observed with DES exposure.[198] A large collaborative study, involving approximately 6000 women, concluded that there is a small but significant increase in the risk of breast cancer many years later in life in women exposed to DES during pregnancy.[199] A longer follow-up (more than 30 years) of this large cohort of DES-exposed women is now available. Exposure to DES is associated with a significant, but modest (less than two-fold), increase in the risk of breast cancer.[200] Importantly, the relative risk did not increase with duration of follow-up and remained stable over time. This conclusion was confirmed in a prospective study by the American Cancer Society.[201] Certainly it is wise to recommend to DES-exposed women that they adhere religiously to screening for breast cancer, including mammography as discussed below.

Receptors and Clinical Prognosis

There is an excellent correlation between the presence of estrogen receptors and certain clinical characteristics of breast cancer, including response to endocrine therapy.[202] Premenopausal and younger patients are more frequently receptor negative. Patients with receptor positive tumors survive longer and have longer disease-free intervals after mastectomy than those with receptor negative tumors. The presence of estrogen receptors correlates with increased disease-free interval regardless of the presence of positive axillary nodes or the size and location of the tumors. Similarly, patients without axillary lymph node metastases, but with estradiol receptor negative tumors, have the same high rate of recurrence as do patients with axillary lymph node metastases. Patients with tumors that are positive for estrogen receptors are more likely to respond to endocrine treatment.

It appears that patients with estrogen receptors are those with the more slowly growing tumors. Several reports indicate that estrogen receptor status correlates with the degree of differentiation of the primary tumor. A large proportion of highly differentiated Grade I carcinomas are receptor positive, while the reverse is true of Grade III tumors.

Remember that it takes estrogen to make progesterone receptors. Therefore the presence of progesterone receptors proves that the estrogen receptor in the tumor is biologically active. Thus, the presence of progesterone receptors has a correlation with disease-free survival of patients only second to the number of positive nodes.[202] The best prognosis is seen in patients with positive progesterone receptors, even with subsequent disease if the recurrent disease is still progesterone receptor positive. The loss of progesterone receptors is an ominous sign.

Tamoxifen and Breast Cancer

The purpose of adjuvant therapy of breast cancer is to provide treatment in the absence of recognized active disease in order to reduce the risk of future recurrence or to minimize systemic recurrence in the presence of metastatic disease. Tamoxifen is very similar to clomiphene (in structure and actions), both being nonsteroidal compounds structurally related to diethylstilbestrol. Tamoxifen, in binding to the estrogen receptor, competitively inhibits estrogen binding. In vitro, the estrogen binding affinity for its receptor is 100–1000 times greater than that of tamoxifen. Thus, tamoxifen must be present in a concentration 100–1000 times greater than estrogen to maintain inhibition of breast cancer cells. Dose-response studies with tamoxifen have failed to demonstrate an increase in activity with doses larger than the standard, 20 mg daily.[203] In addition, when bound to the estrogen receptor, tamoxifen prevents gene transcription by the TAF-2 pathway. In vitro studies demonstrate that these actions are not cytocidal, but rather cytostatic (and thus tamoxifen use must be long-term). The mechanism of tamoxifen action is discussed in detail in Chapter 2.

We have available a remarkable worldwide overview of 37,000 women involved in tamoxifen randomized trials.[204] Adjuvant treatment with the antiestrogen, tamoxifen, achieves highly significant reductions in recurrence and increases in survival. The beneficial effect of tamoxifen is evident no matter what the age of the patient, in both premenopausal and postmenopausal women, in node positive and node negative disease, and in both estrogen receptor positive and negative tumors (however, the effect of tamoxifen on estrogen receptor negative tumors is small). The impact on recurrence occurs in the first 5 years, but continued impact on survival occurs throughout 10 years. A greater effect is seen with longer treatment (5 years). The 10-year survival difference is even greater than that at 5 years. Adjuvant treatment (which is either tamoxifen, chemotherapy, or ovarian ablation) yields worldwide an extra 100,000 10-year survivors. There is an increased survival at 5 years of approximately 20%, most evident in women over age 50. Response rates in advanced breast cancer are 30–35%, most marked in patients with tumors that are positive for estrogen receptors, reaching 75% in tumors highly positive for estrogen receptors. There is a lower rate (a 47% reduction with 5 years of treatment) of a second primary breast cancer in the contralateral breast in women treated with tamoxifen.

Data from randomized clinical trials document that a treatment duration of 5 years is superior to 2 years.[205] However, the results have indicated that there is little reason to extend tamoxifen treatment of breast cancer patients beyond 5 years.[206, 207] Indeed, the data suggested that survival and recurrence rates worsened with longer therapy, probably due to the emergence of tamoxifen-resistant tumors. There are several possible explanations for resistance, and whichever of these are operative, it is believed that a subpopulation resistant to tamoxifen is present from the beginning, and over time grows to be clinically apparent.[208]

The major disturbing side effect is an increase in hot flushing. In a preliminary report from the prevention trial in England and in the U.S. trial, tamoxifen treatment of postmenopausal women prevented bone loss, but premenopausal women treated with tamoxifen had significant reductions in bone mineral density.[209, 210] Blurred and decreased vision has been reported associated with retinal changes, but it is uncertain whether this is a cause and effect relationship.[211] In a prospective study of 63 patients in Greece, 6.3% developed retinopathy which was reversible except for retinal opacities.[212] In the 2673 patients in the protocols of the Eastern Cooperative Oncology Group, premenopausal women who received tamoxifen and chemotherapy had significantly more venous and arterial thrombosis than those who received chemotherapy without tamoxifen, and in postmenopausal women, tamoxifen alone was associated with more venous thrombi.[213] In summary, the serious side effects of tamoxifen include endometrial cancer (discussed below), venous thrombosis, and cataracts.

Serum protein changes reflect the estrogenic (agonistic) action of tamoxifen. This includes decreases in antithrombin III, cholesterol, and LDL-cholesterol, while HDL-cholesterol and sex hormone-binding globulin (SHBG) levels increase (as do other binding globulins). Because of the significant impact on sex hormone-binding globulin, a marked increase in circulating estrogens has been observed in premenopausal women; however, unbound, free estrogen is actually reduced. For example, in one clinical study of premenopausal women receiving tamoxifen, 20 mg daily, the percent free estradiol *decreased* from 1.72% to 1.47% after 3 months because of the increase in SHBG.[214]

The estrogenic activity of tamoxifen, 20 mg daily, is nearly as potent as 2 mg estradiol in lowering FSH levels in postmenopausal women, 26% vs. 34% with estradiol.[215] The estrogenic actions of tamoxifen include the stimulation of progesterone receptor synthesis, an estrogen-like maintenance of bone and the cardiovascular system, and estrogenic effects on the vaginal mucosa and the endometrium. Indeed, patients with breast cancer who have been treated with tamoxifen have been reported to have less coronary heart disease in some studies, but not all.[204, 210, 216] Tamoxifen increases the frequency of hepatic carcinoma in rats at very large doses. This is consistent with its estrogenic, agonistic action, but this effect is unlikely to be a clinical problem (and it has not been observed) at doses currently used.[204] Tamoxifen causes a decrease in antithrombin III, and there has been a small increase in the incidence of thrombo-embolism observed in tamoxifen-treated patients compared with controls.[206, 213] However, in the world overview of randomized trials, no significant cardiac or vascular increase in mortality was noted in tamoxifen-treated women.[204]

Tamoxifen Breast Cancer Prevention Trials

Women at increased risk for breast cancer participated in a breast cancer prevention trial initiated in the U.S. in 1992. The study compared two groups of women, one treated with placebo and one with 20 mg tamoxifen daily for 5 years. Early in 1998 (after about 4 years of follow-up), the study was unblinded because there were 49% fewer cases of invasive breast cancer and 50% fewer cases of noninvasive breast cancer in the tamoxifen-treated arm of the study.[210] This outcome was not without risk. There was a 2.4-fold increase in postmenopausal endometrial cancer, a 2.8-fold increase in pulmonary embolism, a 1.6-fold increase in venous thrombosis, and a 1.6-fold increase in cataracts. In addition to these side effects, there continues to be concern that, because malignant breast tumors require a relatively long period of time to progress from an abnormal cell to a clinically detectable mass,[217] the impact of tamoxifen may reflect growth deceleration of a pre-existing tumor. A major argument against an effect on pre-existing tumors is the documentation of persistent protection against recurrent disease over 10 years of follow-up in the overview of tamoxifen adjuvant therapy.[204]

Because of the early termination of the American prevention trial, the investigators in tamoxifen prevention trials in Italy and the United Kingdom presented preliminary analyses of their results.[218, 219] Both trials could detect no difference in the frequency of breast cancer between the tamoxifen and placebo arms. A consideration of power calculations indicated that despite the smaller size of these studies it should have been possible to demonstrate an effect comparable to the American trial. A possible explanation is that both the Italian and U.K. trials contained more younger women. This difference could contribute to a lower effect because the impact of tamoxifen in the American trial was confined to estrogen receptor positive cancers in older women. Another possibility, and one that is very worrisome, is that longer durations of treatment as in the European trials could allow the emergence of tamoxifen-resistant, more aggressive tumors (as has been occasionally observed with adjuvant tamoxifen treatment that is longer than 5 years). These European results lend credibility to the argument that estrogen and tamoxifen are exerting promotional (acceleration) and anti-promotional (deceleration) effects on pre-existing tumors, not causing and preventing breast cancer. To answer this, the clinical trials must continue, with long follow-up, especially to document breast cancer mortality in these groups of women. For this reason, the Italian and U.K. investigators both decided to continue their trials. In addition, there is a fourth tamoxifen prevention trial, the International Breast Cancer Intervention Study. In view of the disagreement among the American, Italian, and U.K. trials, the International Study decided to keep their study blinded, and to continue as planned.

These results lead us to recommend tamoxifen prophylaxis (20 mg daily for 5 years) for those women who are diagnosed with ductal carcinoma-in-situ of the breast or who have atypical hyperplasia in a breast biopsy (especially if a positive family history of breast cancer is also present). For others who seek tamoxifen preventive treatment, we advise that the final answers are not in, and that clinical trial results from long-term follow-up will be necessary before fully informed decision making is possible.

Gynecologic Problems With Tamoxifen

Tamoxifen is both an estrogen antagonist and an estrogen agonist. A tissue that is highly sensitive to estrogen, the endometrium, responds to the weak estrogenic action of tamoxifen, which is present in high doses for long durations in women receiving adjuvant treatment for breast cancer. Toremifene has a structure and properties essentially similar to tamoxifen, and we expect the same results, side effects, and problems will be observed when this agent is used in a dose of 60 mg/day to treat breast cancer patients.

The National Surgical Adjuvant Breast and Bowel Project compared the rates of endometrial cancers in tamoxifen and non-tamoxifen treated patients who had breast cancer.[220] The rate of endometrial cancer in the tamoxifen-treated group equaled an increased relative risk of 7.5. Although 88% of the endometrial tumors were stage I, 4 patients died of advanced endometrial cancer. This report from the NSABP finally convinced the breast cancer world that the risk of endometrial cancer is real with tamoxifen treatment. Although the number of deaths from endometrial cancer was small, it was the presence of the 4 deaths that had a major impact. It is worth noting that the incidence of endometrial cancer in the tamoxifen-treated group was estimated to be 6.3 per 1000 patients after 5 years of treatment. This incidence is very similar to what would be expected with unopposed estrogen treatment, a similarity to be expected in that the agonistic estrogenic action of tamoxifen over the long-term should be similar to the relatively low doses of estrogen used for postmenopausal hormone therapy. Similar results have been reported from the Stockholm tamoxifen trial, and an increased rate of postmenopausal endometrial cancer was confirmed in the U.S. Breast Cancer Prevention Trial.[210, 221] In the world overview of randomized trials, the incidence of endometrial cancer quadrupled with 5 years of tamoxifen treatment.[204]

The development of endometrial cancer in women receiving tamoxifen should not be so surprising. We know that duration of exposure to estrogen is more important than the dose of estrogen in influencing progression from proliferative endometrium through hyperplasia to cancer. In addition, women being treated with tamoxifen have been reported to develop atypical hyperplasia of the endometrium, endometrial polyps, ovarian cysts, growth of fibroids, adenomyosis, and rapid exacerbation of endometriosis.[222, 223] In a cohort of postmenopausal women on tamoxifen in the English prevention trial, 16% had atypical hyperplasia of the endometrium at the time of study and 8% had endometrial polyps.[224] In addition, 4 ovarian cysts were detected in the treatment group compared to 2 cysts in the control group. The proper surveillance and management of women being treated with tamoxifen are critical problems.

It is inappropriate to advocate progestational treatment to prevent the endometrial response to tamoxifen. The progestational impact (at the low doses currently used for endometrial protection) on the risk of breast cancer recurrence and the interaction with tamoxifen are not known. Indeed, a relatively high dose of norethindrone (2.5 mg daily for 3 months) was *unable* to exert a protective effect on the endometrium in healthy women participating in the U.K. tamoxifen prevention trial.[225] Periodic endometrial aspiration biopsy, of course, would be sufficient, but this procedure carries with it the potential for a very significant negative effect on patient compliance (with her tamoxifen and with her clinician). It is argued that endometrial assessment should be limited to tamoxifen-treated women who report vaginal bleeding.[226, 227] However, in the U.K. tamoxifen prevention trial, a greater endometrial response to tamoxifen was observed in those women who developed amenorrhea.[228] To be sure, most tamoxifen-treated women who have developed endometrial cancer have been symptomatic with vaginal bleeding, but not all. Furthermore, some of these women have had advanced, invasive disease at the time of presentation. It makes sense to detect abnormal changes as early as possible. The progestin challenge test (discussed in Chapter 18) would be a cost-effective method to detect the presence of stimulated endometrium, and a pilot study has documented its use in tamoxifen-treated women.[229] However, until data are available documenting the reliability of this approach, we favor the use of ultrasonographic measurement of endometrial thickness, with saline instillation when the appearance is not totally benign (also discussed in Chapter 18).[230] Tamoxifen is associated with an ultrasonographic image that is unique, characterized by sonolucent changes that are subendometrial, thus the usefulness of saline instillation.[231]

It is also logical to expect these patients to be at increased risk for the development and progression of endometriosis. There are case reports of women being treated with tamoxifen, 20 mg daily, who required hysterectomy and oophorectomy for severe endometriosis.[232, 233] In our view, an annual pelvic examination is not sufficient; every 6 months is best.

The problem of hot flushing should not be underrated. About 25% of women have vasomotor symptoms on tamoxifen, and those that already had flushing have worse flushing.[234] Alternative treatments are available.

We recommend transdermal clonidine, applied with the 100 mg dose once weekly.[235, 236] Side effects are minimal, and a modest impact can be expected.

Clonidine, bromocriptine, and naloxone given orally are only partially effective for the relief of hot flushes and require high doses with a high rate of side effects. Bellergal (a combination of belladonna alkaloids, ergotamine tartrate, and phenobarbital) treatment is slightly better than a placebo, but it is also a potent sedative.[237] Veralipride, a dopamine antagonist that is active in the hypothalamus, is relatively effective in inhibiting flushing at a dose of 100 mg daily.[238, 239] Mastodynia and galactorrhea are the major side effects, and it should be noted that the effect of increased prolactin secretion on the risk of recurrent breast cancer is unknown. Medroxy-progesterone acetate (10–20 mg daily) and megestrol acetate (20 mg bid) are also effective, but concerns regarding exogenous steroids (especially in patients who have had breast cancer) would apply to progestins as well.[240, 241] Methyldopa, in doses of 500–1000 mg/day, is approximately twice as effective as a placebo, suggesting a role for adrenoreceptors in the hot flush mechanism.[242] Venlafaxine hydrochloride is an antidepressant that inhibits serotonin re-uptake; it effectively reduced hot flush frequency in a dose of 25 mg daily.[243] Vitamin E, 800 IU daily, is only slightly more effective than placebo.[244]

A woman being treated for breast cancer will naturally focus her attention and energy on the cancer itself, especially in the early years of treatment. The same can be said for the specialist who is monitoring the treatment. It falls to the patient's health care manager, her primary clinician, to look at the broader picture. A clinician interacting with patients being treated for breast cancer has an obligation to consider the impact of the patient's treatment on other body systems and functions. Tamoxifen offers the hope of adding many years to a woman's life. Medical intervention by a clinician can help make those years better with good preventive health care.

We recommend the following program for monitoring women during long-term tamoxifen treatment:

All women:	**Careful pelvic examination every 6 months to detect the emergence of endometriosis, ovarian cysts, uterine leiomyomata.**
Postmenopausal women:	**Annual measurement of endometrial thickness by transvaginal ultrasonography. Endometrial biopsy of all women with a two-layer thickness of 5 mm or greater. Saline instillation (sonohysterography) when appearance is not totally benign.**
Premenopausal women:	**Periodic assessment for ovulation; if ovulatory, no further intervention is necessary; however, contraceptive counseling should not be ignored. If anovulatory, an annual endometrial aspiration biopsy; interpretation of endometrial thickness measurements by ultrasonography is uncertain in premenopausal women.**
	Consider the use of the progestin-releasing IUD for both contraception and protection against endometrial change.

An increased risk of endometrial cancer lingers for up to 10 years after discontinuing therapy with estrogen (without the addition of a progestin).[245, 246] It is not known whether a similar persistent increased risk is present in the years after tamoxifen treatment. It would be prudent to investigate any unexpected vaginal bleeding in women who have been previously exposed to tamoxifen.

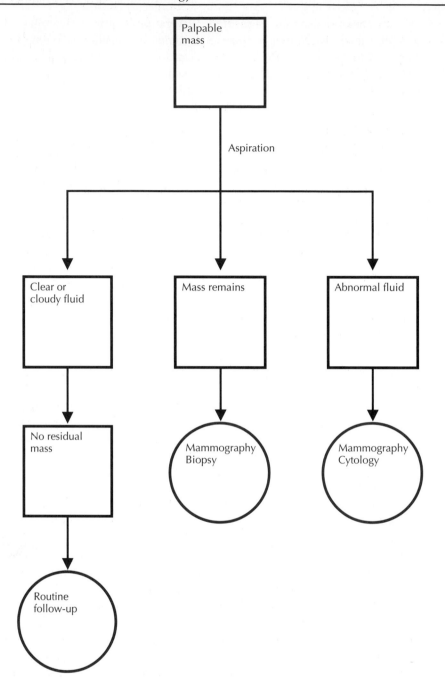

Needle Aspiration

Needle aspiration of breast lumps should be part of the practice of everyone who cares for women.[247] The technique is easy. A small infiltrate of xylocaine is placed in the skin (many clinicians believe that local anesthesia is unnecessary). Holding the lesion between thumb and index fingers with one hand, the other hand passes a 22-gauge needle attached to a 3-finger control syringe into the lesion. Aspiration will reveal the presence of cystic fluid from a cyst. If the mass is solid, the needle should be passed at least 2–4 times (even more if nothing is being obtained) back and forth through the lesion with continuous suction on the syringe. Air is forcibly ejected through the needle on to a cytology slide for smearing and fixing. The usual Pap smear fixative can be used.

The procedure is very cost-effective. When aspiration yields clear or cloudy, green-gray or yellow fluid and the mass disappears, the procedure is both diagnostic and therapeutic. Fluid of any other nature requires cytologic assessment.[248] Failure to obtain material for cytologic evaluation or the persistence of a mass requires biopsy. The mass should not have returned at the follow-up examination 1 month after the aspiration. Locally recurrent cysts should be surgically removed for histologic diagnosis.

Screening Mammography

Mammography is a means of detecting a nonpalpable cancer. Technical advancements have significantly improved the mammographic image and reduced the radiation dose.[249] The doubling time of breast cancer is very variable, but, in general, a tumor doubles in size every 100 days. Thus, it takes a single malignant cell approximately 10 years to grow to a clinically detectable 1 cm mass, but by this time a tumor of 1 cm has already progressed through 30 of the 40 doublings in size which is estimated to be associated with fatal disease.[217] Furthermore, the average size at which a tumor is detected (70–75% of tumors are found by patients themselves) has been (prior to mammography) 2.5 cm, a se which has a 50% incidence of lymph node involvement. To decrease the mortality from breast cancer, we must utilize a technique to find the tumors when they are smaller. Mammography is the answer. Studies of breast self-examination have been disappointing in their failure to demonstrate an impact on breast cancer stage of disease and mortality.[250]

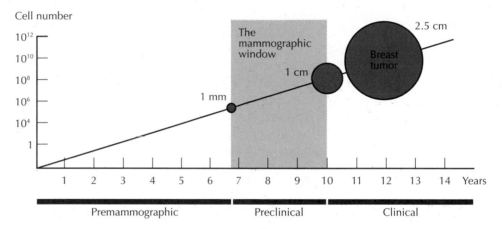

After Wertheimer, et al.[217]

Mammography is the technique of choice. Thermography has a high rate of false positive findings, and, at best, should be considered experimental. Ultrasound can rarely reveal malignant lesions smaller than 1 cm in size. It is useful, however, to guide the aspiration of lesions. CT scanning has 2 serious limitations. The x-ray dose is large, and the slices are too thick to detect early lesions. Finally, magnetic resonance imaging is not practical because of the expense and the long scan times that are necessary.

Mammography is the only method that detecs clustered microcalcifications. These calcifications are less than 1 mm in diameter and are frequently associated with malignant lesions. More than 5 calcifications in a cluster are associated with cancer 25% of the time and require biopsy. Besides microcalcifications, the following mammographic findings usually require surgical evaluation: the appearance of a mass, calcifications associated with a mass, an area of distortion or asymmetrical density, a stellate lesion.

Mammography has a false-negative rate of 5–10%. This means that masses are palpable but not visible. Mammography cannot and should not replace examination by patient and clinician. Cancer commonly presents as a solitary, soli, painless (only 10% of cancers are painful), hard, unilateral, irregular nonmobile mass. A mass requires biopsy regardless of the mammographic picture.

A pattern of dysplasia on the mammogram carries with it an increased risk (2.0–3.5 times normal) of breast cancer. The risk is similar to that seen with the other known risk factors.[251]

The Effectiveness of Mammography

Mammography can reduce breast cancer mortality. In Nijmegan, the breast cancer mortality rate in women 35 and over was redced by 50% by annual mammographic screening.[252] In Utrecht, the relative risk of dying from breast cancer among screened women was reduced by 70%.[253] The first randomized, controlled trials of mammography were begun in Sweden in 1977. Results have demonstrated a 24% reduction in mortality, 29% in women aged 50–69.[254] Most impressively, the results in Sweden were obtained with a screening only every 2–3 years and with only a single mediolateral oblique view. Overall, a 30–40% reduction in mortality can be expected with screening mammography of asymptomatic women over age 50.[255] A greater impact is to be expected with an increased and regular frequency of use combined with state-of-the-art technology.

About 19% more breast cancers occur in women 40–49 than in women aged 50–59, accounting for approximately 20% of all deaths due to breast cancer.[77] But, it has been questioned whether mammography screening is effective for women under 50.[256, 257] The American Breast Cancer Detection Demonstration Project demonstrated that screening was just as effective for women in their 40s as in women over 50.[258] This program that was organized by the American Cancer Society and the National Cancer Institute began operating in 1973 in 28 locations throughout the United States, enrolling more than 280,000 women. Despite the fact that this was not an organized research study with a control group, the massive database permits many valuable conclusions. From 1977 to 1982, similar high survival rates (87%) for women in their 40s compared with women in their 50s verify that screening was just as effective in the younger women. A 5-year survival rate for patients under 50 with breast cancers detected by examination was 77% compared to 95% in those patients with breast cancers detected by mammography.[259] In a randomized trial in Gothenburg, Sweden, women ages 39–49 undergoing mammographic screening every 18 months had a 45% reduction in breast cancer mortality.[260] A meta-analysis of 7 randomized clinical trials concluded that in women aged 40–49 offered mammography screening, there was a 24% reduction in breast cancer mortality.[261]

It takes longer for a significant difference in mortality to appear in 40–49-year-old women compared with women over age 50. There are two explanations. One is that tumors grow faster in younger women, and the other is the greater difficulty in achieving accurate mammography because of the denser, more glandular breasts in younger women compared to the more fatty breasts in older women. Because the breast density changes gradually, rapid tumor growth must be the more critical factor.

Once detected by mammography, the stage of disease and survival expectations are the same comparing women aged 40–49 with women over age 50.[262] However, cancers that are detected between screenings have lower survival rates (at all ages). Therefore another reason that it has been difficult to demonstrate an impact of screening in the age group 40–49 is that because of less than annual screening, more of the cancers are detected late (between screenings). This in turn reflects the faster tumor growth in younger women.[263] Because the randomized clinical trials have screened younger women at 2-year or longer intervals, it is not surprising that screening has been less effective for these faster growing tumors. It is logical that women aged 40–49 should have annual screening mammography.[264, 265]

Younger women without risk factors must understand that approximately 50 out of every 1000 mammograms will require further diagnostic procedures, and the yield will be one invasive cancer and one non-invasive tumor.[266] Although false-positive results are more common among younger women, the difference is not so dramatic that the overall effectiveness of screening is impaired.[264]

There are problems to be anticipated with extensive mammography screening. Small nonpalpable lesions have less than a 5% chance of being malignant, and overall only about 20–30% of biopsy specimens contain carcinoma. That means there will be a large number of biopsies and mammograms performed (including the treatment of clinically irrelevant lesions), which involves costs to the health care system and cost to the individual in terms of stress and anxiety. Nevertheless mammography is the most potent weapon we possess in the battle against breast cancer. Mammography not only lowers mortality, but it also decreases morbidity because less radical surgery is necessary for smaller lesions. Most importantly, the number of unnecessary surgical procedures can be minimized by combining physical examination and mammography with needle aspiration.[267] With the so-called triple approach (examination, mammography or possibly ultrasonography in young women, needle aspiration), the failure to detect a malignancy with at least one of the 3 diagnostic tests is very reliable; open biopsy can be avoided.[268, 269]

It is appropriate to be concerned over the increased cost of annual screening. However, analysis of the increased cost, taking into account the greater efficacy of capturing early tumors comparing annual to biannual screening reveals that the overall benefit is worthwhile, and compares favorably to the cost and benefits of Pap smear screening for cervical cancer.[270, 271]

Postmenopausal women receiving hormone therapy characteristically develop an increase in mammographic density that is often associated with breast tenderness.[272, 273] This increase can be focal, multifocal, or diffuse. The increase in density may be greater with continuous, combined estrogen-progestin regimens.[274] At the present time, these findings have no prognostic or clinical significance other than making it more difficult to interpret mammograms.[275]

There is a special problem with elderly women. Old women are less likely to be screened with mammography, probably due to both patient misconceptions and erroneous physician beliefs. The effectiveness of mammography for women over age 75 has not been established; however, decision analysis of available data predicts a major benefit for elderly women as well.[276] Older women need to be reminded that risk continues to increase with increasing age.

Every woman should be regarded as at risk. Health care professionals who interact with women have the opportunity to initiate an aggressive program of preventive health care. The major deterrent to patient use of mammography is the absence of a strong clinician recommendation. We urge you to follow these guidelines:

Screening for Breast Cancer

All women should be taught self-examination of the breast by age 20. Because of the changes that occur routinely in response to the hormonal sequence of a normal menstrual cycle, breast examination is most effective during the follicular phase of the cycle and should be performed monthly.

All women over the age of 35 should have an annual breast examination.

Women with a first-degree relative with premenopausal breast cancer should begin annual mammography 5 years before the age of the relative when diagnosed.

Annual mammography should be performed in all women over age 39.

References

1. **Enmark E, Pelto-Huikko M, Grandien K, Lagercrantz S, Lagercrantz J, Fried G, Nordenskjöld M, Gustafsson J-Å,** Human estrogen receptor β-gene structure, chromosomal localization, and expression pattern, *J Clin Endocrinol Metab* 82:4258, 1997.

2. **Shyamala G,** Roles of estrogen and progesterone in normal mammary gland development. Insights from progesterone receptor null mutant mice and in situ localization of receptor, *Trends Endocrinol Metab* 8:34, 1997.

3. **Klineberg DL, Niemann W, Flamm E, Cooper P, Babitsky G,** Primate mammary development, *J Clin Invest* 75:1943, 1985.

4. **Christiansen E, Veldhuis JD, Rogol AD, Stumpf P, Evans WS,** Modulating actions of estradiol on gonadotropin-releasing hormone-stimulated prolactin secretion in postmenopausal individuals, *Am J Obstet Gynecol* 157:320, 1987.

5. **Ferguson DP, Anderson TJ,** Morphological evaluation of cell turnover in relation to menstrual cycle in the "resting" human breast, *Br J Cancer* 44:177, 1988.

6. **Longacre TA, Bartow SA,** A correlative morphologic study of human breast and endometrium in the menstrual cycle, *Am J Surg Path* 10:382, 1986.

7. **Going JJ, Anderson TJ, Battersby S, MacIntyre CC,** Proliferative and secretory activity in human breast during natural and artificial menstrual cycles, *Am J Path* 130:193, 1988.

8. **Söderqvist G, Isaksson E, von Schoultz B, Carlström K, Tani E, Skoog L,** Proliferation of breast epithelial cells in healthy women during the menstrual cycle, *Am J Obstet Gynecol* 176:123, 1997.

9. **Potten CS, Watson RJ, Williams GT, Tickle S, Roberts SA, Harris M, Howell A,** The effect of age and menstrual cycle upon proliferative activity of the normal human breast, *Br J Cancer* 58:163, 1988.

10. **Vogel PM, Georgiade NG, Fetter BF, Vogel FS, McCarty KS,** The correlation of histologic changes in the human breast with the menstrual cycle, *Am J Pathol* 104:23, 1981.

11. **Chang K-J, Lee TTY, Linarez-Cruz G, Fournier S, de Ligniéres B,** Influences of percutaneous administration of estradiol and progesterone on human breast epithelial cell cycle in vivo, *Fertil Steril* 63:785, 1995.

12. **Laidlaw IJ, Clarke RB, Howell A, Owen AW, Potten CS, Anderson E,** The proliferation of normal human breast tissue implanted into athymic nude mice is stimulated by estrogen but not progesterone, *Endocrinology* 136:164, 1996.

13. **Foidart J-M, Colin C, Denoo X, Desreux J, Béliard A, Fournier S, de Ligniéres B,** Estradiol and progesterone regulate the proliferation of human breast epithelial cells, *Fertil Steril* 69:963, 1998.

14. **Jernstrom H, Olsson H,** Breast size in relation to endogenous hormone levels, body constitution, and oral contraceptive use in healthy nulligravid women aged 19–25 years, *Am J Epidemiol* 145:571, 1997.

15. **Sinha YN,** Structural variants of prolactin: occurrence and physiological significance, *Endocr Rev* 16:354, 1995.

16. **Ben-Jonathan N, Mershon JL, Allen DL, Steinmetz RW,** Extrapituitary prolactin: distribution, regulation, functions, and clinical aspects, *Endocr Rev* 17:639, 1996.

17. **Brue T, Caruso E, Morange I, Hoffmann T, Evrin M, Gunz G, Benkirane M, Jaquet P,** Immunoradiometric analysis of circulating human glycosylated and nonglycosylated prolactin forms: spontaneous and stimulated secretions, *J Clin Endocrinol Metab* 75:1338, 1992.

18. **Boockfor FR, Hoeffler JP, Frawley LS,** Estradiol induces a shift in cultured cells that release prolactin or growth hormone, *Am J Physiol* 250:E103, 1986.

19. **Maurer RA,** Estradiol regulates the transcription of the prolactin gene, *J Biol Chem* 257:2133, 1982.

20. **Cramer OM, Parker CR, Porter JC,** Estrogen inhibition of dopamine release into hypophyseal portal blood, *Endocrinology* 104:419, 1979.

21. **Snyder JM, Dekowski SA,** The role of prolactin in fetal lung maturation, *Seminars Reprod Endocrinol* 10:287, 1992.

22. **McCoshen JA, Bose R, Embree JE,** Uterine prolactin and labor: modulation by human chorionic gonadotropin affects prostaglandin (PG) E_2 and $PGF_{2\alpha}$ production, *Seminars Reprod Endocrinol* 10:294, 1992.

23. **Ben-Jonathan N,** Dopamine: a prolactin-inhibiting hormone, *Endocr Rev* 6:564, 1985.

24. **de Greef WJ, Voogt JL, Visser TJ, Lamberts SWJ, van der Schoot P,** Control of prolactin release induced by suckling, *Endocrinology* 121:316, 1987.

25. **Bole-Feysot C, Goffin V, Edery M, Binart N, Kelly PA,** Prolactin (PRL) and its receptor: actions, signal transduction pathways and phenotypes observed in PRL receptor knockout mice, *Endocr Rev* 19:225, 1998.

26. **Maaskant RA, Bogic LV, Gilger S, Kelly PA, Bryant-Greenwood GD,** The human prolactin receptor in the fetal membranes, decidua, and placenta, *J Clin Endocrinol Metab* 81:396, 1996.

27. **Kelly PA, Kjiane J, Postel-Vinay M-C, Edery M,** The prolactin/growth hormone receptor family, *Endocr Rev* 12:235, 1991.

28. **Daly DC, Kuslis S, Riddick DH,** Evidence of short-loop inhibition of decidual prolactin synthesis by decidual proteins, Part I, *Am J Obstet Gynecol* 155:358, 1986.

29. **Raabe MA, McCoshen JA,** Epithelial regulation of prolactin effect on amnionic permeability, *Am J Obstet Gynecol* 154:130, 1986.

30. **Tyson JE, Hwang P, Guyda H, Friesen HG,** Studies of prolactin secretion in human pregnancy, *Am J Obstet Gynecol* 113:14, 1972.

31. **Kletzky OA, Marrs RP, Howard WF, McCormick W, Mishell Jr DR,** Prolactin synthesis and release during pregnancy and puerperium, *Am J Obstet Gynecol* 136:545, 1980.

32. **Tyson JE, Friesen HG,** Factors influencing the secretion of human prolactin and growth hormone in menstrual and gestational women, *Am J Obstet Gynecol* 116:377, 1973.

33. **Barberia JM, Abu-Fadil S, Kletzky OA, Nakamura RM, Mishell Jr DR,** Serum prolactin patterns in early human gestation, *Am J Obstet Gynecol* 121:1107, 1975.

34. **Ehara Y, Siler TM, Yen SSC,** Effects of large doses of estrogen on prolactin and growth hormone release, *Am J Obstet Gynecol* 125:455, 1976.

35. **Murphy LJ, Murphy LC, Stead B, Sutherland RL, Lazarus L,** Modulation of lactogenic receptors by progestins in cultured human breast cancer cells, *J Clin Endocrinol Metab* 62:280, 1986.

36. **Simon WE, Pahnke VG, Holzel F,** In vitro modulation of prolactin binding to human mammary carcinoma cells by steroid hormones and prolactin, *J Clin Endocrinol Metab* 60:1243, 1985.

37. **Haslam SZ, Shyamala G,** Progesterone receptors in normal mammary gland: receptor modulations in relation to differentiation, *J Cell Biol* 86:730, 1980.

38. **Lee CS, Oka T,** Progesterone regulation of pregnancy-specific transcription repressor to β-casein gene promoter in mouse mammary gland, *Endocrinology* 131:2257, 1992.

39. **Battin DA, Marrs RP, Fleiss PM, Mishell Jr DR,** Effect of suckling on serum prolactin, luteinizing hormone, follicle-stimulating hormone, and estradiol during prolonged lactation, *Obstet Gynecol* 65:785, 1985.

40. **Stern JM, Konner M, Herman TN, Reichlin S,** Nursing behaviour, prolactin, and postpartum amenorrhoea during prolonged lactation in American and !Kung mothers, *Clin Endocrinol* 25:247, 1986.

41. **Tay CCK, Glasier AF, McNeilly AS,** Twenty-four hour patterns of prolactin secretion during lactation and the relationship to suckling and the resumption of fertility in breast-feeding women, *Hum Reprod* 11:950, 1996.

42. **Dawood MY, Khan-Dawood FS, Wahl RS, Fuchs F,** Oxytocin release and plasma anterior pituitary and gonadal hormones in women during lactation, *J Clin Endocrinol Metab* 52:678, 1981.

43. **McNeilly AS, Robinson KA, Houston MJ, Howe PW,** Release of oxytocin and prolactin in response to suckling, *Br Med J* 286:257, 1983.

44. **Kumar R, Cohen WR, Epstein FH,** Vitamin D and calcium hormones in pregnancy, *New Engl J Med* 302:1143, 1980.

45. **Sowers M, Corton G, Shapiro B, Jannausch ML, Crutchfield M, Smith ML, Randolph JF, Hollis B,** Changes in bone density with lactation, *JAMA* 269:3130, 1993.

46. **Kalkwarf HJ, Specker BL,** Bone mineral loss during lactation and recovery after weaning, *Obstet Gynecol* 86:26, 1995.

47. **Kalkwarf HJ, Specker BL, Bianchi DC, Ranz J, Ho M,** The effect of calcium supplementation on bone density during lactation and after weaning, *New Engl J Med* 337:523, 1997.

48. **Laskey MA, Prentice A, Hanratty LA, Jarjou LM, Dibba B, Beavan SR, Cole TJ,** Bone changes after 3 mo of lactation: influence of calcium intake, breast-milk output, and vitamin D-receptor genotype, *Am J Clin Nutr* 67:685, 1998.

49. **Ritchie LD, Fung EB, Halloran BP, Turnlund JR, Van Loan MD, Cann CE, King JC,** A longitudinal study of calcium homeostasis during human pregnancy and lactation and after resumption of menses, *Am J Clin Nutr* 67:693, 1998.

50. **Pettitt DJ, Forman MR, Hanson RL, Knowler WC, Bennett PH,** Breastfeeding and incidence of non-insulin-dependent diabetes mellitus in Pima Indians, *Lancet* 350:166, 1997.

51. **Dewey KG, Lovelady CA, Nommsen-Rivers LA, McCrory MA, Lönnerdal B,** A randomized study of the effects of aerobic exercise by lactating women on breast-milk volume and composition, *New Engl J Med* 330:449, 1994.

52. **Nishimori K, Young LJ, Guo Q, Wang Z, Insel TR, Matzuk MM,** Oxytocin is required for nursing but is not essential for parturition or reproductive behavior, *Proc Natl Acad Sci USA* 93:11699, 1996.

53. **Auerbach KG, Avery JL,** Induced lactation, *Am J Dis Child* 135:340, 1981.

54. **Campbell OM, Gray RH,** Characteristics and determinants of postpartum ovarian function in women in the United States, *Am J Obstet Gynecol* 169:55, 1993.

55. **Labbok MH, Hight-Laukaran V, Peterson AE, Fletcher V, von Hertzen H, Van Look PFA,** Multicenter study of the lactational amenorrhea method (LAM): I. Efficacy, duration, and implications for clinical application, *Contraception* 55:327, 1997.

56. **Visness CM, Kennedy KI, Gross BA, Parenteau-Carreau S, Flynn AM, Brown JB,** Fertility of fully breast-feeding women in the early postpartum period, *Obstet Gynecol* 89:164, 1997.

57. **Diaz S, Aravena R, Cardenas H, Casado ME, Miranda P, Schiappacasse V, Croxatto HB,** Contraceptive efficacy of lactational amenorrhea in urban Chilean women, *Contraception* 43:335, 1991.

58. **Kremer JAM, Thomas CMG, Rolland R, van der Heijden PF, Thomas CM, Lancranjan I,** Return of gonadotropic function in postpartum women during bromocriptine treatment, *Fertil Steril* 51:622, 1989.

59. **Haartsen JE, Heineman MJ, Elings M, Evers JLH, Lancranjan I,** Resumption of pituitary and ovarian activity postpartum: endocrine and ultrasonic observations in bromocriptine-treated women, *Hum Reprod* 7:746, 1992.

60. **Tyson JE, Carter JN, Andreassen B, Huth J, Smith B,** Nursing mediated prolactin and luteinizing hormone secretion during puerperal lactation, *Fertil Steril* 30:154, 1978.

61. **Sauder SE, Frager M, Case GD, Kelch RP, Marshall JC,** Abnormal patterns of pulsatile luteinizing hormone secretion in women with hyperprolactinemia and amenorrhea: responses to bromocriptine, *J Clin Endocrinol Metab* 59:941, 1984.

62. **Tay CCK, Glasier A, McNeilly AS,** Twenty-four hour secretory profiles of gonadotropins and prolactin in breastfeeding women, *Hum Reprod* 7:951, 1992.

63. **Ishizuka B, Quigley ME, Yen SSC,** Postpartum hypogonadotrophinism: evidence for increased opioid inhibition, *Clin Endocrinol* 20:573, 1984.

64. **Petraglia F, De Leo V, Nappi C, Facchinetti F, Montemagno U, Brambilla F, Genazzani AR,** Differences in the opioid control of luteinizing hormone secretion between pathological and iatrogenic hyperprolactinemic states, *J Clin Endocrinol Metab* 64:508, 1987.

65. **Tay CCK, Glasier AF, McNeilly AS,** Effect of antagonists of dopamine and opiates on the basal and GnRH-induced secretion of luteinizing hormone, follicle stimulating hormone and prolactin during lactational amenorrhea in breastfeeding women, *Hum Reprod* 8:532, 1993.

66. **Zinaman MJ, Cartledge T, Tomai T, Tippett P, Merriam GR,** Pulsatile GnRH stimulates normal cyclic ovarian function in amenorrheic lactating postpartum women, *J Clin Endocrinol Metab* 80:2088, 1995.

67. **Sherman L, Fisher A, Klass E, Markowitz S,** Pharmacologic causes of hyperprolactinemia, *Seminars Reprod Endocrinol* 2:31, 1984.

68. **Davis JRE, Selby C, Jeffcoate C,** Oral contraceptive agents do not affect serum prolactin in normal women, *Clin Endocrinol* 20:427, 1984.

69. **Hwang PLH, Ng CSA, Cheong ST,** Effect of oral contraceptives on serum prolactin: A longitudinal study in 126 normal premenopausal women, *Clin Endocrinol* 24:127, 1986.

70. **Ader DN, Browne MW,** Prevalence and impact of cyclic mastalgia in a United States clinic-based sample, *Am J Obstet Gynecol* 177:126, 1997.

71. **Pye JK, Mansel RE, Hughes LE,** Clinical experience of drug treatments for mastalgia, *Lancet* ii:373, 1985.

72. **Kontostolis E, Stefanidis K, Navrozoglou I, Lolis D,** Comparison of tamoxifen with danazol for treatment of cyclical mastalgia, *Gynecol Endocrinol* 11:393, 1997.

73. **Fentiman IS, Brame K, Caleffi M, Chaudary MA, Hayward JL,** Double-blind controlled trial of tamoxifen therapy for mastalgia, *Lancet* i:287, 1986.

74. **Ernster VL, Mason L, Goodson III WH, Sickles EA, Sacks ST, Selvin S, Dupuy ME, Hawkinson J, Hunt TK,** Effects of caffeine-free diet on benign breast disease: a randomized trial, *Surgery* 91:263, 1982.

75. **Schairer C, Brinton LA, Hoover RN,** Methylxanthines and benign breast disease, *Am J Epidemiol* 124:603, 1986.

76. **Allen S, Froberg D,** The effect of decreased caffeine consumption on benign proliferative breast disease: a randomized trial, *Surgery* 101:720, 1987.

77. **American Cancer Society,** Cancer facts & figures — 1998, *http://www.cancer.org/statistics.html,* 1998.

78. **Feuer EJ, Wun L-M, Boring CC, Flanders WD, Timmel MJ, Tong T,** The lifetime risk of developing breast cancer, *J Natl Cancer Inst* 85:892, 1993.

79. **Harris JR, Lippman ME, Veronesi U, Willett W,** Breast cancer, *New Engl J Med* 327:319, 1992.

80. **Harris JR, Lippman ME, Veronesi U, Willett W,** Breast cancer, *New Engl J Med* 327:390, 1992.

81. **Ewertz M, Duffy SW, Adami H-O, Kvale G, Lund E, Meirk O, Mellemgaard A, Soini I, Tulinius H,** Age at first birth, parity and risk of breast cancer: a meta-analysis of 8 studies from the Nordic countries, *Int J Cancer* 46:597, 1990.

82. **Kalache A, Maguire A, Thompson SG,** Age at last full-term pregnancy and risk of breast cancer, *Lancet* 341:33, 1993.

83. **Pathak DR, Speizer FE, Willett WC, Rosner B, Lipnick RJ,** Parity and breast cancer risk: possible effect on age at diagnosis, *Int J Cancer* 37:21, 1986.

84. **Talamini R, Franceschi S, La Vecchia C, Negri E, Borsa L, Montella M, Falcini F, Conti E, Rossi C,** The role of reproductive and menstrual factors in cancer of the breast before and after menopause, *Eur J Cancer* 32A:303, 1996.

85. **Colditz GA, Rosner BA, Speizer FE, for the Nurses' Health Study Research Group,** Risk factors for breast cancer according to family history of breast cancer, *J Natl Cancer Inst* 88:365, 1996.

86. **Cummings P, Stanford JL, Daling JR, Weiss NS, McKnight B,** Risk of breast cancer in relation to the interval since last full term pregnancy, *Br Med J* 308:1672, 1994.

87. **Lambe M, Hsieh C, Trichopoulos D, Ekbom A, Pavia M, Adami H-O,** Transient increase in the risk of breast cancer after giving birth, *New Engl J Med* 331:5, 1994.

88. **Guinee VF, Olsson H, Moller T, Hess KR, Taylor SH, Fahey T, Gladikov JV, van den Blink JW, Bonichon F, Dische S, et al,** Effect of pregnancy on prognosis for young women with breast cancer, *Lancet* 343:1587, 1994.

89. **Kroman N, Wohlfart J, Andersen KW, Mouriudsen HT, Westergaard U, Melbye M,** Time since childbirth and prognosis in primary breast cancer: population based study, *Br Med J* 315:851, 1997.

90. **Andrieu N, Clavel F, Gairard B, Piana L, Bremond A, Lansac JH, Flamant R, Renaud R,** Familial risk of breast cancer and abortion, *Cancer Detect Prev* 18:51, 1994.

91. **Daling JR, Malone KE, Voigt LF, White E, Weiss NS,** Risk of breast cancer among young women: relationship to induced abortion, *J Natl Cancer Inst* 86:1584, 1994.

92. **Rookus MA, van Leeuwen FE,** Induced abortion and risk for breast cancer: reporting (recall) bias in a Dutch case-control study, *J Natl Cancer Inst* 88:1759, 1996.

93. **Melbye M, Wohlfahrt J, Olsen JH, Frisch M, Westergaard T, Helweg-Larsen K, Andersen PK,** Induced abortion and the risk of breast cancer, *New Engl J Med* 336:81, 1997.

94. **Musey VC, Collins DC, Brogan DR, Santos VR, Musey PI, Martino-Saltzman D, Preedy JRK,** Long term effects of a first pregnancy on the hormonal environment: estrogens and androgens, *J Clin Endocrinol Metab* 64:111, 1987.

95. **Musey VC, Collins DC, Musey PI, Martino-Saltzman D, Preedy JRK,** Long-term effects of a first pregnancy on the secretion of prolactin, *New Engl J Med* 316:229, 1987.

96. **McTiernan A, Thomas DB,** Evidence for a protective effect of lactation on risk of breast cancer in young women: results from a case-control study, *Am J Epidemiol* 124:353, 1986.

97. **Layde PM, Webster LA, Baughman L, Wingo PA, Rubin GL, Ory HW,** The independent associations of parity, age at first full term pregnancy, and duration of breastfeeding with the risk of breast cancer, *J Clin Epidemiol* 42:963, 1989.

98. **United Kingdom National Case-Control Study Group,** Breast feeding and risk of breast cancer in young women, *Br Med J* 307:17, 1993.

99. **Newcomb PA, Storer BE, Longnecker MP, Mittendorf R, Greenberg ER, Clapp RW, Burke KP, Willett WC, MacMahon B,** Lactation and a reduced risk of premenopausal breast cancer, *New Engl J Med* 330:81, 1994.

100. **Ing R, Ho JHC, Petrakis NL,** Unilateral breast-feeding and breast cancer, *Lancet* ii:124, 1977.

101. **Kvåle G, Heuch I,** Lactation and cancer risk: is there a relation specific to breast cancer? *J Epidemiol Comm Health* 2:30, 1987.

102. **London SJ, Colditz GA, Stampfer MJ, Willett WC, Rosner BA, Corsano K, Speizer FE,** Lactation and the risk of breast cancer in a cohort of US women, *Am J Epidemiol* 132:17, 1990.

103. **Berkel H, Birdsell DC, Jenkins H,** Breast augmentation: a risk factor for breast cancer? *New Engl J Med* 326:1649, 1992.

104. **Deapen DM, Brody GS,** Augmentation mammoplasty and breast cancer: a 5-year update of the Los Angeles study, *Plast Reconstr Surg* 89:660, 1992.

105. **Malone KE, Stanford JL, Daling JR, Voigt LF,** Implants and breast cancer, *Lancet* 339:1365, 1992.

106. **Deapen DM, Bernstein L, Brody GS,** Are breast implants anticarcinogenic? A 14-year follow-up of the Los Angeles Study, *Plast Reconstr Surg* 99:1346, 1997.

107. **McLaughlin JK, Nyrén O, Blot WJ, Yin L, Josefsson S, Fraumeni Jr JF, Adami H-O,** Cancer risk among women with cosmetic breast implants: a population-based cohort study in Sweden, *J Natl Cancer Inst* 90:156, 1998.

108. **La Vecchia C, Negri E, Bruzzi P, Dardanoni G, Decarli A, Franceschi S, Palli D, Talamini R,** The role of age at menarche and at menopause on breast cancer risk: combined evidence from four case-control studies, *Ann Oncol* 3:625, 1992.

109. **Dupont WD, Page DL,** Risk factors for breast cancer in women with proliferative breast disease, *New Engl J Med* 312:146, 1985.

110. **London SJ, Connolly JL, Schnitt SG, Colditz GA,** A prospective study of benign breast disease and the risk of breast cancer, *JAMA* 267:941, 1992.

111. **Cancer Committee, College of American Pathologists,** Is 'fibrocystic disease' of the breast precancerous? *Arch Path Lab Med* 110:171, 1986.

112. **Sattin RW, Rubin GL, Webster LA, Huezo CM, Wingo PA, Ory HW, Layde PM,** Family history and the risk of breast cancer, *JAMA* 253:1908, 1985.

113. **Colditz GA, Willett WC, Hunter DJ, Stampfer MJ, Manson JE, Hennekens CH, Rosner BA, Speizer FE,** Family history, age, and risk of breast cancer, *JAMA* 270:338, 1993.

114. **Claus EB, Rich N, Thompson WD,** Autosomal dominant inheritance of early-onset breast cancer: implications for risk prediction, *Cancer* 73:643, 1994.

115. **Ford D, Easton DF, Bishop DT, Naroid SA, Goldgar DE, and the Breast Cancer Linkage Consortium,** Risks of cancer in *BRCA1*-mutation carriers, *Lancet* 343:692, 1994.

116. **Wooster R, Neuhausen SL, Mangion J, Quirk Y, Ford D, Collins N, Nguyen K, Seal S, Tran T, Averill D, et al,** Localization of a breast cancer susceptibility gene, BRCA2, to chromosome 13q12-13, *Science* 265:2088, 1994.

117. **Gayther SA, Mangion J, Russell P, Seal S, Barfoot R, Ponder BA, Stratton MR, Easton D,** Variation of risks of breast and ovarian cancer associated with different germline mutations of the BRCA2 gene, *Nat Genet* 15:103, 1997.

118. **Gayther SA, Ponder BA,** Mutations of the BRCA1 and BRCA2 genes and the possibilities for predictive testing, *Mol Med Today* 3:168, 1997.

119. **Stratton JF, Gayther SA, Russell P, Dearden J, Gore M, Blake P, Easton D, Ponder BA,** Contribution of BRCA1 mutations to ovarian cancer, *New Engl J Med* 336:1125, 1997.

120. **Rubin SG, Blackwood MA, Bandera C, Behbakht K, Benjamin I, Rebbeck TR, Boyd J,** BRCA1, BRCA2, and hereditary nonpolyposis colorectal cancer gene mutations in an unselected ovarian cancer population: relationship to family history and implications for genetic testing, *Am J Obstet Gynecol* 178:670, 1998.

121. **Miki Y, Swensen J, Shattuck-Eidens D, Futreal PA, Harshman K, Tavtigian S, Liu Q, Cochran C, Bennett LM, Ding W, et al,** A strong candidate for the breast and ovarian cancer susceptibility gene *BRCA1*, *Science* 266:66, 1994.

122. **Shattuck-Eidens D, McClure M, Simard J, Labrie F, Narod S, Couch F, Hoskins K, Weber B, Castilla L, Erdos M, et al,** A collaborative survey of 80 mutations in the *BRCA1* breast and ovarian cancer susceptibility gene: implications for presymptomatic testing and screening, *JAMA* 273:535, 1995.

123. **Futreal PA, Liu Q, Shattuck-Eidens D, Cochran C, Harshman K, Tavtigian S, Bennett LM, Haugen-Strano A, Swensen J, Miki Y, et al,** *BRCA1* mutations in primary breast and ovarian carcinomas, *Science* 266:120, 1994.

124. **Krainer M, Silva-Arrieta S, FitzGerald MG, Shaimada A, Ishioka C, Kanamaru R, MacDonald DJ, Unsal H, Finkelstein DM, Bowcock A, Isselbacher KJ, Haber DJ,** Differential contributions of BRCA1 and BRCA2 to early-onset breast cancer, *New Engl J Med* 336:1416, 1997.

125. **Struewing JP, Hartge P, Wacholder S, Baker SM, Berlin M, McAdams M, Timmerman MM, Brody LC, Tucker MA,** The risk of cancer associated with specific mutations of BRCA1 and BRCA2 among Ashkenazi Jews, *New Engl J Med* 336:1401, 1997.

126. **Hoskins KF, Stopfer JE, Calzone KA, Merajver SD, Rebbeck TR, Garber JE, Weber BL,** Assessment and counseling for women with a family history of breast cancer: a guide for clinicians, *JAMA* 273:577, 1995.

127. **Newman B, Mu H, Butler LM, Millikan RC, Moorman PG, King M-C,** Frequency of breast cancer attributable to *BRCA1* in a population-based series of American women, *JAMA* 279:915, 1998.

128. **Malone KE, Daling JR, Thompson JD, O'Brien CA, Francisco LV, Ostrander EA,** *BRCA1* mutations and breast cancer in the general population. Analyses in women before age 35 years and in women before age 45 years with first-degree family history, *JAMA* 279:922, 1998.

129. **Breast Cancer Linkage Consortium,** Pathology of familial breast cancer: differences between breast cancers in carriers of *BRCA1* or *BRCA2* mutations and sporadic cases, *Lancet* 349:1505, 1997.

130. **Verhoog LC, Brekelmans CTM, Seynaeve C, van den Bosch LMC, Dahmen G, van Geel AN, Tilanus-Linthorst MMA, Bartels CCM, Wagner A, van den Ouweland A, Devilee d, Meijers-Heijboer EJ, Klijn JGM,** Survival and tumour characteristics of breast-cancer patients with germline mutations of *BRCA1*, *Lancet* 351:316, 1998.

131. **Schrag D, Kuntz KM, Garber JE, Weeks JC,** Decision analysis — effects of prophylactic mastectomy and oophorectomy on life expectancy among women with *BRCA1* or *BRCA2* mutations, *New Engl J Med* 336:1465, 1997.

132. **Hartmann LC, Schaid DJ, Woods JE, Crotty TP, Myers JL, Arnold PG, Petty PM, Sellers TA, Johnson JL, McDonnell SK, Frost MH, Jenkins RB,** Efficacy of bilateral prophylactic mastectomy in women with a family history of breast cancer, *New Engl J Med* 340:77, 1999.

133. **Burke W, Daly M, Garber J, Botkin J, Kahn MJ, Lynch P, McTiernan A, Offit K, Perlaman J, Petersen G, Thomson E, Varricchio C, for the Cancer Genetics Studies Consortium,** Recommendations for follow-up care of individuals with an inherited predisposition to cancer, *JAMA* 277:997, 1997.

134. **Narod SA, Risch H, Moslehl R, Dørum A, Neuhausen S, Olsson H, Provencher D, Radice P, Evans G, Bishop IS, Brunet J-S, Ponder BAJ, for the Hereditary Ovarian Cancer Clinical Study Group,** Oral contraceptives and the risk of hereditary ovarian cancer, *New Engl J Med* 339:424, 1998.

135. **Carroll KK,** Experimental studies on dietary fat and cancer in relation to epidemiological data, *Prog Clin Biol Res* 222:231, 1986.

136. **Willett WC, Browne ML, Bain C, Lipnick RJ, Stampfer MJ, Rosner B, Colditz GA, Hennekens CH, Speizer FE,** Relative weight and risk of breast cancer among premenopausal women, *Am J Epidemiol* 122:731, 1985.

137. **Jones DY, Schatzkin A, Green SB, Block G, Brinton LA, Ziegler RG, Hoover R, Taylor PR,** Dietary fat and breast cancer in the National Health and Nutrition Examination Survey Epidemiologic Follow-up Study, *J Natl Cancer Inst* 79:465, 1987.

138. **Willett WC, Hunter DJ, Stampfer MJ, Colditz G, Manson JE, Spiegelman D, Rosner B, Hennekens CH, Speizer FE,** Dietary fat and fiber in relation to risk of breast cancer: an 8-year follow-up, *JAMA* 268:2037, 1992.

139. **Hunter DJ, Spiegelman D, Adami H-O, Beeson L, van den Brandt PA, Folsom AR, Fraser GE, Goldbohm A, Graham S, Howe GR, Kushi LH, Marshall JR, McDermott A, Miller AB, Speizer FE, Wolk A, Yaun S-S, Willett W,** Cohort studies of fat intake and the risk of breast cancer — a pooled analysis, *New Engl J Med* 334:356, 1996.

140. **Howe GR, Hirohata R, Hislop TG, Iscovich JM, Yuan JM, Katsouyami K, Lubin F, Marubini E, Modan B, Rohan T, et al,** Dietary factors and risk of breast cancer: Combined analysis of 12 case-control studies, *J Natl Cancer Inst* 82:561, 1990.

141. **Kushi LH, Sellers TA, Potter JD, Nelson CL, Munger RG, Kaye SA, Folsom AR,** Dietary fat and postmenopausal breast cancer, *J Natl Cancer Inst* 84:1092, 1992.

142. **Shapira DV, Clark RA, Wolff PA, Jarrett A, Kumar NB, Aziz NM,** Visceral obesity and breast cancer risk, *Cancer* 74:632, 1994.

143. **Bruning PF, Bonfrèr JMG, van Noord PAH, Hart AAM, De Jong-Bakker M, Nooijen WJ,** Insulin resistance and breast cancer risk, *Int J Cancer* 52:511, 1992.

144. **Thune I, Brenn T, Lund E, Gaard M,** Physical activity and the risk of breast cancer, *New Engl J Med* 336:1269, 1997.

145. **Lu L-JW, Anderson KE, Grady JJ, Nagamani M,** Effects of soya consumption for one month on steroid hormones in premenopausal women: implications for breast cancer risk reduction, *Cancer Epidemiol Biomark Prev* 5:63, 1996.

146. **Goodman MT, Wilkens LR, Hankin JH, Lyu L-C, Wu AH, Kolonel LN,** Association of soy and fiber consumption with the risk of endometrial cancer, *Am J Epidemiol* 146:294, 1997.

147. **Ingram D, Sanders K, Kolybaba M, Lopez D,** Case-control study of phyto-oestrogens and breast cancer, *Lancet* 350:990, 1997.

148. **Messina MJ, Persky V, Setchell KDR, Barnes S,** Soy intake and cancer risk: a review of the *in vitro* and *in vivo* data, *Nutr Cancer* 21:113, 1994.

149. **Wu AH, Ziegler RG, Pike MC, Nomura AMY, West DW, Kolonel LN, Horn-Ross PL, Rosenthal JF, Hoover RN,** Menstrual and reproductive factors and risk of breast cancer in Asian-Americans, *Br J Cancer* 73:680, 1996.

150. **Ziegler RG, Hoover RN, Nomura AM, West DW, Wu AH, Pike MC, Lake AJ, Horn-Ross PL, Kolonel LN, Siiteri PK, Fraumeni Jr JF,** Relative weight, weight change, height, and breast cancer risk in Asian-American women, *J Natl Cancer Inst* 88:650, 1996.

151. **Potischman N, Swanson CA, Siiteri P, Hoover RN,** Reversal of relation between body mass and endogenous estrogen concentrations with menopausal status, *J Natl Cancer Inst* 88:756, 1996.

152. **Yong L-C, Brown CC, Schatzkin A, Schairer C,** Prospective study of relative weight and risk of breast cancer: the breast cancer detection demonstration project follow-up study, 1979 to 1987–1989, *Am J Epidemiol* 43:985, 1996.

153. **Sherman B, Wallace R, Beam J, Schlabaugh L,** Relationship of body weight to menarcheal and menopausal age: implication for breast cancer risk, *J Clin Endocrinol Metab* 52:488, 1981.

154. **Magnusson C, Baron J, Persson I, Wolk A, Bergström R, Trichopoulos D, Adami H-O,** Body size in different periods of life and breast cancer risk in post-menopausal women, *Int J Cancer* 76:29, 1998.

155. **Longnecker MP,** Alcoholic beverage consumption in relation to risk of breast cancer: meta-analysis and review, *Cancer Causes Control* 5:73, 1995.

156. **Smith-Warner SA, Spiegelman D, Yaun S-S, van den Brandt PA, Folsom AR, Goldbohm RA, Graham S, Holmberg L, Howe GR, Marshall JR, Miller AB, Potter JD, Speizer FE, Willett WC, Wolk A, Hunter DJ,** Alcohol and breast cancer in women. A pooled analysis of cohort studies, *JAMA* 279:535, 1998.

157. **Dorgan JF, Reichman ME, Judd JT, Brown C, Longcope C, Schatzkin A, Campbell WS, Franz C, Kahle L, Taylor PR,** The relation of reported alcohol ingestion to plasma levels of estrogens and androgens in premenopausal women, *Cancer Causes Control* 5:53, 1994.

158. **Gavaler JS, Van Thiel DH,** The association between moderate alcoholic beverage consumption and serum estradiol and testosterone levels in normal postmenopausal women: relationship to the literature, *Alcohol Clin Exp Res* 16:87, 1992.

159. **Ginsburg EL, Mello NK, Mendelson JH, Barbieri RL, Teoh SK, Rothman M, Gao X, Sholar JW,** Effects of alcohol ingestion on estrogens in postmenopausal women, *JAMA* 276:1747, 1996.

160. **Muti P, Trevisan M, Micheli A, Krogh V, Bolelli G, Sciajno R, Schünemann HJ, Berrino F,** Alcohol consumption and total estradiol in premenopausal women, *Cancer Epidemiol Biomark Prev* 7:189, 1998.

161. **Bulbrook RD,** Urinary androgen excretion and the etiology of breast cancer, *J Natl Cancer Inst* 48:1039, 1972.

162. **Lemon HM,** Estriol prevention of mammary carcinoma induced by 7,12-dimethylbenz(a)anthracene, *Cancer Res* 35:1341, 1975.

163. **Dickinson LE, MacMahon B, Cole P, Brown JB,** Estrogen profiles of Oriental and Caucasian women in Hawaii, *New Engl J Med* 291:1211, 1974.

164. **Katzenellenbogen BS,** Biology and receptor interactions of estriol and estriol derivatives in vitro and in vivo, *J Steriod Biochem* 20:1033, 1984.

165. **Melamed M, Castraño E, Notides AC, Sasson S,** Molecular and kinetic basis for the mixed agonist/antagonist activity of estriol, *Mol Endocrinol* 11:1868, 1997.

166. **Korenman SG,** Estrogen window hypothesis of the etiology of breast cancer, *Lancet* i:700, 1980.

167. **Korenman SG,** The endocrinology of breast cancer, *Cancer* 46:874, 1980.

168. **Coulam CB, Annegers JF,** Breast cancer and chronic anovulation syndrome, *Surg Forum* 33:474, 1982.

169. **Coulam CB, Annegers JF, Krans JS,** Chronic anovulation syndrome and associated neoplasia, *Obstet Gynecol* 61:403, 1983.

170. **Cowan LD, Gordis L, Tonascia JA, Jones GS,** Breast cancer incidence in women with a history of progesterone deficiency, *Am J Epidemiol* 114:209, 1981.

171. **Ron E, Lunenfeld B, Menczer J, Blumstein T, Katz L, Oelsner G, Serr D,** Cancer incidence in a cohort of infertile women, *Am J Epidemiol* 125:780, 1987.

172. **McFayden IJ, Forrest APM, Prescott RJ, Golder MP, Groom GV, Fahmy DR,** Circulating hormone concentrations in women with breast cancer, *Lancet* i:1000, 1976.

173. **Gammon MD, Thompson WD,** Infertility and breast cancer: a population-based case-control study, *Am J Epidemiol* 132:708, 1990.

174. **Gammon MD, Thompson WD,** Polycystic ovaries and the risk of breast cancer, *Am J Epidemiol* 134:818, 1991.

175. **Anderson KE, Sellers TA, Chen P-L, Rich SS, Hong C-P, Folsom AR,** Association of Stein-Leventhal syndrome with the incidence of postmenopausal breast carcinoma in a large prospective study of women in Iowa, *Cancer* 79:494, 1997.

176. **Garland M, Hunter DJ, Colditz GA, Manson JE, Stampfer MJ, Spiegelman D, Speizer F, Willett WC,** Menstrual cycle characteristics and history of ovulatory infertility in relation to breast cancer risk in a large cohort of US women, *Am J Epidemiol* 147:636, 1998.

177. **Garland CF, Friedlander NJ, Barrett-Connor E, Khaw K-T,** Sex hormones and postmenopausal breast cancer: a prospective study in an adult community, *Am J Epidemiol* 135:1220, 1992.

178. **Helzlsouer KJ, Alberg AJ, Bush TL, Longcope C, Gordon GB, Comstock GW,** A prospective study of endogenous hormones and breast cancer, *Cancer Detect Prev* 18:79, 1994.

179. **Berrino F, Muti P, Micheli A, Bolelli G, Krogh V, Sciajno R, Pisani P, Panico S, Secreto G,** Serum sex hormone levels after menopause and subsequent breast cancer, *J Natl Cancer Inst* 88:291, 1996.

180. **Thomas HV, Key TJ, Allen DS, Moore JW, Dowsett M, Fentiman IS, Wang DY,** A prospective study of endogenous serum hormone concentrations and breast cancer risk in postmenopausal women on the island of Guernsey, *Br J Cancer* 76:401, 1997.

181. **Toniolo PG, Levitz M, Zeleniuch-Jacquotte A, Banerjee S, Koenig KL, Shore RE, Strax P, Pasternack BS,** A prospective study of endogenous estrogens and breast cancer in postmenopausal women, *J Natl Cancer Inst* 87:190, 1995.

182. **Dorgan JF, Longcope C, Stephenson Jr HE, Falk RT, Miller R, Franz C, Kahle L, Campbell WS, Tangrea JA, Schatzkin A,** Relation of prediagnostic serum estrogen and androgen levels to breast cancer risk, *Cancer Epidemiol Biomarkers Prev* 5:533, 1996.

183. **Cuzick J, Wang DY, Bulbrook RD,** The prevention of breast cancer, *Lancet* i:83, 1986.

184. **Hankinson SE, Willett WC, Manson JE, Colditz GA, Hunter DJ, Spiegelman D, Barbieri RL, Speizer FE,** Plasma sex steroid hormone levels and risk of breast cancer in postmenopausal women, *J Natl Cancer Inst* 90:1292, 1998.

185. **Zhang Y, Kel DP, Kreger BE, Cupples LA, Ellison RC, Dorgan JE, Schatzkin A, Levy D, Felson DT,** Bone mass and the risk of breast cancer among postmenopausal women, *New Engl J Med* 336:611, 1997.

186. **Thompson WD, Jacobson HI, Negrini B, Janerich DT,** Hypertension, pregnancy, and risk of breast cancer, *J Natl Cancer Inst* 81:1571, 1989.

187. **Ekbom A, Trichopoulos D, Adami H-O, Hsieh C-C, Lan S-J,** Evidence of prenatal influences on breast cancer risk, *Lancet* 340:1015, 1992.

188. **Key TJA, Pike MC,** The role of oestrogens and progestogens in the epidemiology and prevention of breast cancer, *Eur J Cancer Clin Oncol* 24:29, 1988.

189. **Henderson BE, Ross RK, Judd HL, Krailo MD, Pike MC,** Do regular ovulatory cycles increase breast cancer risk? *Cancer* 56:1206, 1985.

190. **Anderson TJ, Ferguson DJP, Raab GM,** Cell turnover in the "resting" human breast: influence of parity, contraceptive pill, age and laterality, *Br J Cancer* 46:376, 1982.

191. **Gompel A, Malet C, Spritzer P, Lalardrie J-P, Kuttenn F, Mauvais-Jarvis P,** Progestin effect on cell proliferation and 17-hydroxysteroid dehydrogenase activity in normal human breast cells in culture, *J Clin Endocrinol Metab* 63:1174, 1986.

192. **Chang K-J, Lee TTY, Linares-Cruz G, Fournier S, de Ligniéres B,** Influences of percutaneous administration of estradiol and progesterone on human breast epithelial cell cycle in vivo, *Fertil Steril* 63:785, 1995.

193. **Kelsey JH,** A review of the epidemiology of human breast cancer, *Epidemiol Rev* 1:74, 1979.

194. **Kelsey JL, Fischer DB, Holford TR, LiVoisi VA, Mostow ED, Goldenberg IS, White C,** Exogenous estrogens and other factors in the epidemiology of breast cancer, *J Natl Cancer Inst* 67:327, 1981.

195. **Collaborative Group on Hormonal Factors in Breast Cancer,** Breast cancer and hormonal contraceptives: collaborative re-analysis of individual data on 53,297 women with breast cancer and 100,239 women without breast cancer from 54 epidemiological studies, *Lancet* 347:1713, 1996.

196. **Holmberg L, Lund E, Bergstrom R, Adami HO, Merik O,** Oral contraceptives and prognosis in breast cancer: effects of duration, latency, recency, age at first use and relation to parity and body mass index in young women with breast cancer, *Eur J Cancer* 30A:351, 1994.

197. **Charreau I, Plu-Bureau G, Bachelot A, Contesso G, Guinebretiere JM, L''e MG,** Oral contraceptive use and risk of benign breast disease in a French case-control study of young women, *Eur J Cancer Prev* 2:147, 1993.

198. **Bibbo M, Haenszel W, Wied GL, Hubby M, Herbst AL,** A twenty-five year follow-up study of women exposed to DES during pregnancy, *New Engl J Med* 298:763, 1978.

199. **Greenburg ER, Barnes AB, Resseguie L, Barrett JA, Burnside S, Lanza LL, Neff RK, Stevens M, Young RH, Colton T,** Breast cancer in mothers given diethylstilbestrol in pregnancy, *New Engl J Med* 311:1393, 1984.

200. **Colton T, Greenberg ER, Noller K, Resseguie L, Van Bennekom C, Heeren T, Zhang Y,** Breast cancer in mothers prescribed diethylstilbestrol in pregnancy, *JAMA* 269:2096, 1993.

201. **Calle EE, Mervis CA, Thun MJ, Rodriguez C, Wingo PA, Heath Jr CW,** Diethylstilbestrol and risk of fatal breast cancer in a prospective cohort of US women, *Am J Epidemiol* 144:645, 1996.

202. **McGuire WL, Clark GM,** Prognostic factors and treatment decisions in axillary-node-negative breast cancer, *New Engl J Med* 326:1756, 1992.

203. **Tormey DC, Lippmann ME, Edwards BK, Cassidy JG,** Evaluation of tamoxifen doses with and without fluoxymesterone in advanced breast cancer, *Ann Intern Med* 98:139, 1983.

204. **Early Breast Cancer Trialists' Collaborative Group,** Tamoxifen for early breast cancer: an overview of the randomised trials, *Lancet* 351:1451, 1998.

205. **Swedish Breast Cancer Cooperative Group,** Randomized trial of two versus five years of adjuvant tamoxifen for postmenopausal early stage breast cancer, *J Natl Cancer Inst* 88:1543, 1996.

206. **Fisher B, Dignam J, Bryant J, DeCillis A, Wickerham DL, Wolmark N, Costantino J, Redmond C, Fisher ER, Bowman DM, Deschênes L, Dimitrov NV, Margolese RG, Robidoux A, Shibata H, Terz J, Paterson AHG, Feldman MI, Farrar W, Evans J, Lickley HL,** Five versus more than five years of tamoxifen therapy for breast cancer patients with negative lymph nodes and estrogen receptor-positive tumors, *J Natl Cancer Inst* 88:1529, 1996.

207. **Stewart HJ, Forrest AP, Everington D, McDonald CC, Dewar JA, Hawkins RA, Prescott RJ, George WD, on behalf of the Scottish Cancer Trials Breast Group,** Randomized comparison of 5 years of adjuvant tamoxifen with continuous therapy for operable breast cancer, *Br J Cancer* 74:297, 1996.

208. **Horwitz KB,** Hormone-resistant breast cancer or "feeding the hand that bites you," *Prog Clin Biol Res* 387:29, 1994.

209. **Powles TJ, Hickish T, Kanis JA, Tidy A, Ashley S,** Effect of tamoxifen on bone mineral density measured by dual-energy x-ray absorptiometry in healthy premenopausal and postmenopausal women, *J Clin Oncol* 14:78, 1996.

210. **Fisher B, Costantino JP, Wickerham DL, Redmond CK, Kavanah M, Cronin WM, Vogel V, Robidoux A, Dimitrov N, Atkins J, Daly M, Wieand S, Tan-Chiu E, Ford L, Wolmark N, and other National Surgical Adjuvant Breast and Bowel Project Investigators,** Tamoxifen for prevention of breast cancer: report of the National Surgical Adjuvant Breast and Bowel Project P-1 Study, *J Natl Cancer Inst* 90:1371, 1998.

211. **Bentley CR, Davies G, Aclimandos WA,** Tamoxifen retinopathy: a rare but serious complication, *Br Med J* 304:495, 1992.

212. **Pavlidis NA, Petris C, Briassoulis E, Klouvas G, Psilas C, Rempapis J, Petroutsos G,** Clear evidence that long-term low-dose tamoxifen treatment can induce ocular toxicity, *Cancer* 69:2961, 1992.

213. **Saphner T, Tormey DC, Gray R,** Venous and arterial thrombosis in patients who received adjuvant therapy for breast cancer, *J Clin Oncol* 9:286, 1991.

214. **Caleffi M, Fentiman IS, Clark GM, Wang DY, Needham J, Clark K, La Ville A, Lewis B,** Effect of tamoxifen on oestrogen binding, lipid and lipoprotein concentrations and blood clotting parameters in premenopausal women with breast pain, *J Endocrinol* 119:335, 1988.

215. **Helgason S, Wilking N, Carlstrom K, Damber MG, von Schoultz B,** A comparative study of the estrogenic effects of tamoxifen and 17β-estradiol in postmenopausal women, *J Clin Endocrinol Metab* 54:404, 1982.

216. **Costantino JP, Kuller LH, Ives DG, Fisher B, Dignam J,** Coronary heart disease mortality and adjuvant tamoxifen therapy, *J Natl Cancer Inst* 89:776, 1997.

217. **Wertheimer MD, Costanza ME, Dodson TF, D'Orsi C, Pastides H, Zapka JG,** Increasing the effort toward breast cancer detection, *JAMA* 255:1311, 1986.

218. **Veronesi U, Maisonneuve P, Costa A, Sacchini V, Maltoni C, Robertson C, Rotmensz N, Boyle P, on behalf of the Italian Tamoxifen Prevention Study,** Prevention of breast cancer with tamoxifen: preliminary findings from the Italian randomised trial among hysterectomized women, *Lancet* 352:93, 1998.

219. **Powles T, Eeles R, Ashley S, Easton D, Chang J, Dowsett M, Tidy A, Viggers J, Davey J,** Interim analysis of the incidence of breast cancer in the Royal Marsden Hospital tamoxifen randomised chemoprevention trial, *Lancet* 352:98, 1998.

220. **Fisher B, Costantino JP, Redmond CK, Fisher ER, Wickerham DL, Cronin WM, Other NSABP Contributors,** Endometrial cancer in tamoxifen-treated breast cancer patients: findings from the National Surgical Adjuvant Breast and Bowel Project (NSABP) B-14, *J Natl Cancer Inst* 86:527, 1994.

221. **Rutqvist LE, Johansson H, Signomklao T, Johansson U, Fornander T, Wilking N,** Adjuvant tamoxifen therapy for early stage breast cancer and second primary malignancies. Stockholm Breast Cancer Study Group, *J Natl Cancer Inst* 87:645, 1995.

222. **Lahti E, Blanco G, Kauppila A, Apaja-Sarkkinen M, Taskinen PJ, Laatikainen T,** Endometrial changes in postmenopausal breast cancer patients receiving tamoxifen, *Obstet Gynecol* 81:660, 1993.

223. **Cohen I, Rosen DJD, Altaras M, Beyth Y, Shapira J, Yigael D,** Tamoxifen treatment in premenopausal breast cancer patients may be associated with ovarian overstimulation, cystic formations and fibroid overgrowth, *Br J Cancer* 69:620, 1994.

224. **Kedar RP, Bourne TH, Powles TJ, Collins WP, Ashley SE, Cosgrove DO, Campbell S,** Effects of tamoxifen on uterus and ovaries of postmenopausal women in a randomized breast cancer prevention trial, *Lancet* 343:1318, 1994.

225. **Powles TJ, Bourne T, Athanasious S, Chang J, Grubock K, Ashley S, Oakes L, Tidy A, Davey J, Viggers J, Humphries S, Collins W,** The effects of norethisterone on endometrial abnormalities identified by transvaginal ultrasound screening of healthy post-menopausal women on tamoxifen or placebo, *Br J Cancer* 78:272, 1998.

226. **Carlson RW,** Overview from a medical oncologist, *Seminars Oncol* 24(Suppl 1):151, 1997.

227. **Creasman WT,** Endometrial cancer: incidence, prognostic factors, diagnosis, and treatment, *Seminars Oncol* 24(Suppl 1):140, 1997.

228. **Chang J, Powles TJ, Ashley SE, Iveson T, Gregory RK, Dowsett M,** Variation in endometrial thickening in women with amenorrhea on tamoxifen, *Br Cancer Res Treat* 48:81, 1998.

229. **Guerrieri JP, Elkas JC, Nash JD,** Evaluating the endometrium in women on tamoxifen: a pilot study to compare a "gold standard" with an "old standard," *Menopause* 4:6, 1997.

230. **Timmerman D, Deprest J, Bourne T, Van den Berghe I, Collins WP, Vergote I,** A randomized trial on the use of ultrasonography or office hysteroscopy for endometrial assessment in postmenopausal patients with breast cancer who were treated with tamoxifen, *Am J Obstet Gynecol* 179:62, 1998.

231. **Goldstein SR,** Unusual ultrasonographic appearance of the uterus in patients receiving tamoxifen, *Am J Obstet Gynecol* 170:447, 1994.

232. **Ford MRW, Turner MJ, Wood C, Soutter WP,** Endometriosis developing during tamoxifen therapy, *Am J Obstet Gynecol* 158:1119, 1988.

233. **Hajjar LR, Kim W, Nolan GH, Turner S, Raju UR,** Intestinal and pelvic endometriosis presenting as a tumor and associated with tamoxifen therapy: report of a case, *Obstet Gynecol* 82:642, 1993.

234. **Love RR, Cameron L, Connell BL, Leventhal H,** Symptoms associated with tamoxifen treatment in postmenopausal women, *Arch Intern Med* 151:1842, 1991.

235. **Nagamani M, Kelver ME, Smith ER,** Treatment of menopausal hot flushes with transdermal administration of clonidine, *Am J Obstet Gynecol* 156:561, 1987.

236. **Goldberg RM, Loprinzi CL, O'Fallen JR, Veeder MH, Miser AW, Maillard JA, Michalak JC, Dose AM, Rowland Jr KM, Burnham NL,** Transdermal clonidine for ameliorating tamoxifen-induced hot flashes, *J Clin Oncol* 12:155, 1994.

237. **Lebherz TB, French LT,** Nonhormonal treatment of the menopausal syndrome. A double-blind evaluation of an autonomic system stabilizer, *Obstet Gynecol* 33:795, 1969.

238. **David A, Don R, Tajchner G, Weissglas L,** Veralipride: alternative antidopaminergic treatment for menopausal symptoms, *Am J Obstet Gynecol* 158:1107, 1988.

239. **Melis GB, Bambacciani M, Cagnacci A, Paoletti AM, Mais V, Fioretti P,** Effects of the dopamine antagonist veralipride on hot flushes and luteinizing horomone secretion in postmenopausal women, *Obstet Gynecol* 72:688, 1988.

240. **Lobo RA, McCormick W, Singer F, Roy S,** Depomedroxyprogesterone acetate compared with conjugated estrogens for the treatment of postmenopausal women, *Am J Obstet Gynecol* 63:105, 1984.

241. **Loprinzi CL, Michalak JC, Quella SK, O'Fallon JR, Hatfield AK, Nelimark RA, Dose AM, Fischer T, Johnson C, Klatt NE, Bate WW, Rospond RM, Oesterling JE,** Megestrol acetate for the prevention of hot flashes, *New Engl J Med* 331:347, 1994.

242. **Nesheim B-I, Sætre T,** Reduction of menopausal hot flushes by methyldopa: a double blind crossover trial, *Eur J Clin Pharmacol* 20:413, 1981.

243. **Loprinzi CL, Pisansky TM, Fonseca R, Sloan JA, Zahasky KM, Quella SK, Novotny PJ, Rummans TA, Dumesic DA, Perez EA,** Pilot evaluation of venlafaxine hydrochoride for the therapy of hot flashes in cancer survivors, *J Clin Oncol* 16:2377, 1998.

244. **Barton DL, Loprinzi CL, Quella SK, Sloan JA, Veeder MH, Egner JR, Fidler P, Stella PJ, Swan DK, Vaught NL, Novotny P,** Prospective evaluation of vitamin E for hot flashes in breast cancer survivors, *J Clin Oncol* 16:495, 1998.

245. **Shapiro S, Kelly JP, Rosenberg L, Kaufman DW, Helmrich SP, Rosenshein NB, Lewis Jr JL, Knapp RC, Stolley PD, Schottenfeld D,** Risk of localized and widespread endometrial cancer in relation to recent and discontinued use of conjugated estrogens, *New Engl J Med* 313:969, 1985.

246. **Paganini-Hill A, Ross RK, Henderson BE,** Endometrial cancer and patterns of use of oestrogen replacement therapy: a cohort study, *Br J Cancer* 59:445, 1989.

247. **Hindle WH,** Fine needle aspiration, In: Hindle WH, ed. *Breast Disease for Gynecologists,* Appleton & Lange, Norwalk, Connecticut, 1990, p 67.

248. **Donegan WL,** Evaluation of a palpable breast mass, *New Engl J Med* 327:937, 1992.

249. **Kopans LDB, Meyer JE, Sadowsky N,** Breast imaging, *New Engl J Med* 310:960, 1984.

250. **Thomas DB, Gao DL, Self SG, Allison CJ, Tao Y, Mahloch J, Ray R, Qin Q, Presley R, Porter P,** Randomized trial of breast self-examination in Shanghai: methodology and preliminary results, *J Natl Cancer Inst* 89:355, 1997.

251. **Carlile T, Kopecky KJ, Thompson DJ, Whitehead JR, Gilbert Jr FI, Present AJ, Threatt BA, Krook P, Hadaway E,** Breast cancer prediction and the Wolfe classification on mammograms, *JAMA* 254:1050, 1985.

252. **Verbeek ALM, Holland R, Sturmans F, Hendriks JHCL, Miravunac M, Day NE,** Reduction of breast cancer mortality through mass screening with modern mammography, *Lancet* i:1222, 1984.

253. **Collette HJA, Rombach JJ, Day NE, De Waard F,** Evaluation of screening for breast cancer in non-randomized study (the DOM project) by means of a case-control study, *Lancet* i:124, 1984.

254. **Nystrom L, Rutqvist LE, Wall S, Lindgren A, Lindqvist M, Ryden S, Andersson I, Bjurstam N, Fagerberg G, Frisell J, Tabar L, Larsson L-G,** Breast cancer screening with mammography: overview of Swedish randomised trials, *Lancet* 341:973, 1993.

255. **Kerlikowske K, Grady D, Rubin SM, Sandrock C, Ernster VL,** Efficacy of screening mammography: a meta-analysis, *JAMA* 273:149, 1995.

256. **Eddy DM, Hasselblad V, McGivney W, Hendee W,** The value of mammography screening in women under age 50 years, *JAMA* 259:1512, 1988.

257. **Miller AB, Baines CJ, To T, Wall C,** Canadian National Breast Screening Study: 1. Breast cancer detection and death rates among women aged 40 to 49 years, *Can Med Assoc J* 147:1459, 1992.

258. **Seidman H, Gelb SK, Silverberg E, LaVerda N, Lubera JA,** Survival experience in the breast cancer detection demonstration project, *CA* 37:258, 1987.

259. **Stacey-Clear A, McCarthy KA, Hall DA, Pile-Spellman E, White G, Hulka G, Whitman GJ, Mahoney E, Kopans DB,** Breast cancer survival among women under age 50: is mammography detrimental? *Lancet* 340:991, 1992.

260. **Bjurstam N, Björneld L, Duffy SW, Smith TC, Cahlin E, Eriksson O, Hafström L-O, Lingaas H, Mattsson J, Persson S, Rudenstam C-M, Söderbergh JS,** The Gothenburg Breast Screening Trial. First results on mortality, incidence, and mode of detection for women ages 39–49 years at randomization, *Cancer* 80:2091, 1997.

261. **Smart CR, Hendrick RE, Rutledge JH, III, Smith RA,** Benefit of mammography screening in women ages 40-49 years: current evidence from randomized controlled trials, *Cancer* 75:1619, 1995.

262. **Curpen BN, Sickles EA, Sollito RA, Ominsky SH, Galvin HB, Frankel SD,** The comparative value of mammographic screening for women 40-49 years old versus women 50-64 years old, *Am J Roentgenol* 164:1099, 1995.

263. **Kerlikowske K, Grady D, Barclay J, Sickles EA, Ernster V,** Effect of age, breast density, and family history on the sensitivity of first screening mammography, *JAMA* 276:33, 1996.

264. **Kerlikowske K, Grady D, Barclay J, Sickles E, Ernster V,** Likelihood ratios for modern screening mammography: risk of breast cancer based on age and mammographic interpretation, *JAMA* 276:39, 1996.

265. **Report of the Organizing Committee and Collaborators, Falun Meeting,** Breast cancer screening with mammography in women aged 40–49 years, *Int J Cancer* 68:693, 1996.

266. **Kerlikowske K, Grady D, Barclay J, Sickles E, Eaton A, Ernster V,** Positive predictive value of screening mammography by age and family history of breast cancer, *JAMA* 270:2444, 1993.

267. **Hermansen C, Poulsen HS, Jensen J, Langfeldt B, Steenskov V, Frederiksen P, Jensen OM,** Diagnostic reliability of combined physical examination, mammography, and fine-needle puncture ("triple-test") in breast tumors: a prospective study, *Cancer* 60:1866, 1987.

268. **Kaufman Z, Shpitz B, Shapiro M, Roma R, Lew S, Dinbar A,** Triple approach in the diagnosis of dominant breast masses: combined physical examination, mammography, and fine-needle aspiration, *J Surg Oncol* 56:254, 1994.

269. **Vetto J, Pommier R, Schmidt W, Wachtel M, Du Bois P, Jones M, Thurmond A,** Use of the "triple test" for palpable breast lesions yields high diagnostic accuracy and cost savings, *Am J Surg* 169:519, 1995.

270. **Feig SA,** Mammographic screening of women aged 40-49 years: benefit, risk, and cost considerations, *Cancer* 76:2097, 1995.

271. **Lindfors K, Rosenquist C,** The cost-effectiveness of mammographic screening strategies, *JAMA* 274:881, 1995.

272. **Kaufman Z, Garstin WIH, Hayes R, Michell MJ, Baum M,** The mammographic parenchymal patterns of women on hormonal replacement therapy, *Clin Radiol* 43:389, 1991.

273. **McNicholas MMJ, Heneghan JP, Milner MH, Tuinney T, Hourihane JB, MacErlaine DP,** Pain and increased mammographic density in women receiving hormone replacement therapy: a prospective study, *Am J Radiol* 163:311, 1994.

274. **Persson I, Thurfjell E, Holmberg L,** Effect of estrogen and estrogen-progestin replacement regimens on mammographic parenchymal density, *J Clin Oncol* 15:3201, 1997.

275. **Marugg RC, van der Mooren MJ, Hendriks JHCL, Rolland R, Ruijs SHJ,** Mammographic changes in postmenopausal women on hormonal replacement therapy, *Eur Radiol* 7:749, 1997.

276. **Mandelblatt JS, Wheat ME, Monane M, Moshief RD, Hollenberg JP, Tang J,** Breast cancer screening for elderly women with and without comorbid conditions: a decision analysis model, *Ann Intern Med* 116:722, 1992

17 Menopause and the Perimenopausal Transition

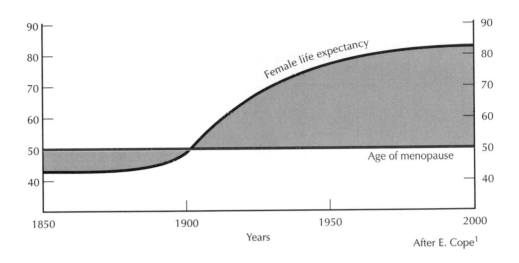

After E. Cope[1]

Throughout recorded history, multiple physical and mental conditions have been attributed to the menopause. Although medical writers often wrote colorfully in the past, unfortunately they were also less than accurate, unencumbered by scientific information and data. A good example of the stereotypical, inaccurate thinking promulgated over the years is the following written in 1887:[2]

> The ovaries, after long years of service, have not the ability of retiring in graceful old age, but become irritated, transmit their irritation to the abdominal ganglia, which in turn transmit the irritation to the brain, producing disturbances in the cerebral tissue exhibiting themselves in extreme nervousness or in an outburst of actual insanity.

The belief that behavioral disturbances are related to manifestations of the female reproductive system is an ancient one that has persisted to contemporary times. This belief regarding the menopause is not totally illogical; there is reason to associate the middle years of life with negative experiences. The events that come to mind are impressive: onset of a major illness or disability (and even death) in a spouse, relative, or friend; retirement from employment; financial insecurity; the need to provide care for very old parents and relatives; and separation from children. And thus, it is not surprising that a middle age event, the menopause, shares in this negative outlook.

The scientific study of all aspects of menstruation has been hampered by the overpowering influence of social and cultural beliefs and traditions. Problems arising from life events have often been erroneously attributed to the menopause. But data (especially more reliable community-based longitudinal data) now establish that the increase in most symptoms and problems in middle-aged women reflects social and personal circumstances, not the endocrine events of the menopause.[3–9] The variability in menopausal reactions makes the cross-sectional study design particularly unsuitable. Longitudinal studies are now documenting what is normal and the variations around normal.

The Massachusetts Women's Health Study, a large and comprehensive prospective, longitudinal study of middle-aged women, provides a powerful argument that the menopause is not and should not be viewed as a negative experience by the vast majority of women.[4, 10] The cessation of menses was perceived by these women (as have the women in other longitudinal studies) as having almost no impact on subsequent physical and mental health. This was reflected by women expressing either positive or neutral feelings about menopause. An exception was the group of women who experienced surgical menopause, but here there is good reason to believe that the reasons for the surgical procedure were more important than the cessation of menses.

Changes in menstrual function are not symbols of some ominous "change." There are good physiologic reasons for changing menstrual function, and understanding the physiology will do much to reinforce a healthy, normal attitude. Attitude and expectations about the menopause are very important. Women who have been frequent users of health services and who expect to have difficulty do experience greater symptoms and higher levels of depression.[5, 9] The symptoms that women report are related to many variables within their lives, and the hormonal change at menopause cannot be held responsible for the common psychosocial and lifestyle problems we all experience. It is time to stress the normalcy of this physiologic event. Menopausal women do not suffer from a disease (specifically a hormone deficiency disease), and postmenopausal hormone therapy should be viewed as specific treatment for symptoms in the short term and preventive pharmacology in the long term.

It can be further argued that physicians have had a biased (negative) point of view, because the majority of women, being healthy and happy, do not seek contact with physicians.[11, 12] It is important, therefore, that clinicians not only are familiar with the facts relative to the menopause but also have an appropriate attitude and philosophy regarding this period of life. Medical intervention at this point of life should be regarded as an opportunity to provide and reinforce a program of preventive health care. The issues of preventive health care for women are familiar ones. They include family planning, cessation of smoking, control of body weight and alcohol consumption, prevention of cardiovascular disease and osteoporosis, maintenance of mental well-being (including sexuality), cancer screening, and treatment of urologic problems.

Growth of the Older Population

We are experiencing a relatively new phenomenon: we can expect to become old. We are on the verge of becoming a rectangular society, one of the greatest achievements of the 20th century. This is a society in which nearly all individuals survive to advanced age and then succumb rather abruptly over a narrow age range centering around the age of 85.

In 1000 BC, life expectancy was only 18 years. By 100 BC, the time of Ceasar, it had reached 25 years. In 1900, in the United States, life expectancy still had reached only 49 years. In 2000, the average life expectancy will be 79.7 years for women and 72.9 for men.[13] Today, once you reach 65, if you are a man you can expect to reach 80.5, if you are a woman, age 84.3. We can anticipate that eventually about two-thirds of the population will survive to 85 or more, and more than 90% will live past age 65—this would be the nearly perfect rectangular society.[14, 15] Currently, Sweden and Switzerland are closest to this demographic composition.

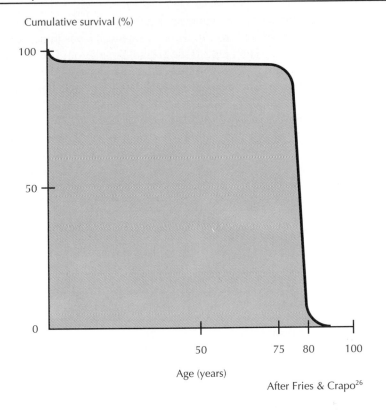

Cumulative survival (%)

Age (years)

After Fries & Crapo[26]

A good general definition of elderly is 65 and older, although it is not until age 75 that a significant proportion of older people show the characteristic decline and problems. Today the elderly population is the largest contributor to illness and human need in the United States.[16] There are more old people (with their greater needs) than ever before.[17] In 1900, there were approximately 3 million Americans 65 and older (about 4% of the total population). By 2030, the elderly population will reach about 57 million (17% of the total population). Soon population aging will replace population growth as the most important social problem.

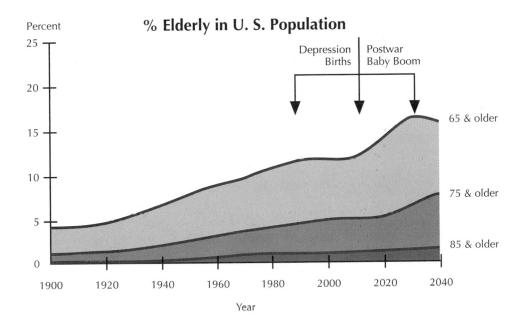

% Elderly in U. S. Population

Percent

Depression Births

Postwar Baby Boom

65 & older

75 & older

85 & older

Year

Two modern phenomena have influenced the rate of change. The first was the post World War II baby boom (1946–1964) that temporarily postponed the aging of the population, but now is causing a faster aging of the general population. The second major influence has been the modern decrease in old age mortality. Our success in postponing death has increased the upper segment of the demographic contour. By 2050, the current developed nations will be rectangular societies. China, by 2050, will contain more people over age 65 (270 million) than the number of people of all ages currently living in the U.S.

Current World Population Changes[18]

	Births	Deaths	Growth
Year	140,773,000	51,315,000	89,458,000
Month	11,731,080	4,276,250	7,454,834
Week	2,707,173	140,589	245,090
Hour	16,070	5,858	10,212
Minute	268	96	170
Second	4.5	1.6	2.8

This is a worldwide development, not limited to affluent societies.[18] The population of the earth will continue to grow until the year 2100 or 2150, when it is expected to stabilize at approximately 11 billion. 95% of this growth will occur in developing countries. The poorest countries today (located in Africa and Asia) will in 2000 account for 87% of the world's population. In most developing countries, the complications associated with pregnancy, abortion, and childbirth are either the first or second most common cause of death, and almost half of all deaths occur in children under age 5. Limiting family size to two children would cut the annual number of maternal deaths by 50% and infant and child mortality also by 50%.[19] Thus, it is appropriate to focus attention on population control; however, even in developing countries this will change. In 1950, only 40% of people 60 and older lived in developing countries. By 2025, more than 70% will live in those countries.

Projected Size of World Population Age 60 and Older[18]

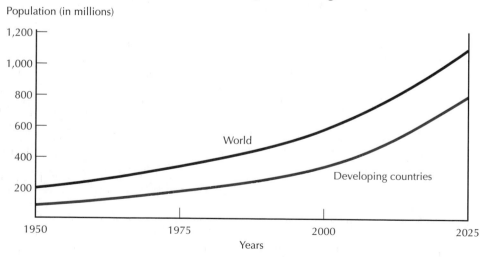

Men per 100 U.S. Women[17]

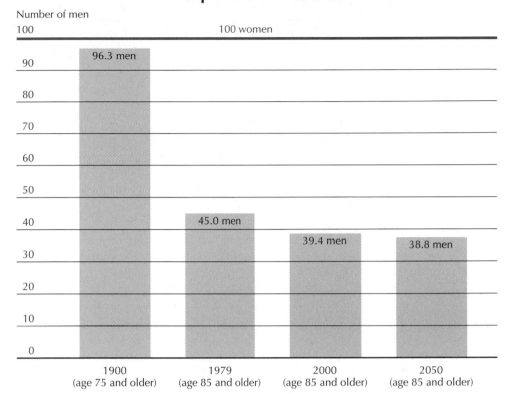

In 1900, older men in the U.S. outnumbered women 102 to 100. In the 1980s, there were only 68 men for every 100 women over the age 65. By age 85, only 40 men are alive for every 100 women. Nearly 90% of white American women can expect to live to age 70. Vital statistics data indicate that this gender difference is similar in both the black and white populations in the U.S.[20] Approximately 55% of girls, but only 35% of boys, live long enough to celebrate their 85th birthday.[21]

Men and women reach old age with different prospects for older age, a sex differential that (it can be argued) is due in significant part to the sex hormone-induced differences in the cholesterol-lipoprotein profile and other cardiovascular factors, and thus the greater incidence of atherosclerosis and earlier death in men.[22] Therefore, the use of postmenopausal estrogen therapy, with its protective effect on atherosclerosis, may, in fact, exaggerate the sex differential in mortality. From a public health point of view, the greatest impact on the sex differential in mortality would be gained by concentrating on lifestyle changes designed to diminish atherosclerosis in men: low cholesterol diet, no smoking, optimal body weight, and active exercise.

The death rate is higher for men at all ages. Coronary heart disease accounts for 40% of the mortality difference between men and women. Another one-third is from lung cancer, emphysema, cirrhosis, accidents, and suicides. It is interesting to note that in our society the mortality difference between men and women is largely a difference in lifestyle. Smoking, drinking, coronary prone behavior, and accidents account for most of the higher male mortality rate over age 65. It has been estimated that perhaps two-thirds of the difference has been due to cigarettes alone. But we should emphasize that this is due to a greater prevalence of smoking in men. Women whose smoking patterns are similar to those of men have a similar increased risk of morbidity and mortality.[23]

The Older U.S. Female Population[17]

Age	1990		2000		2010		2020	
55–64	10.8 mill.	(8.6%)	12.1 mill.	(9.0%)	17.1 mill.	(12.1%)	19.3 mill.	(12.9%)
65–74	10.1	(8.1%)	9.8	(7.3%)	11.0	(7.8%)	15.6	(10.4%)
> 75	7.8	(6.2%)	9.3	(7.0%)	9.8	(6.9%)	11.0	(7.3%)
Total	28.7		31.2		37.9		45.9	

Perhaps because more women are smoking, drinking, and working, the mortality sex difference has begun to lessen. The U.S. Census Bureau projects that the difference in life expectancy between men and women will increase until the year 2050, and then level off.[17] In 2050, life expectancy for women will be 82 years and for men, 76.7 years.[13] There will be 33.4 million women 65 and older, compared with 22.1 million men.

In addition to the growing numbers of elderly people, the older population itself is getting older.[24] For example, in 1984, the 65–74 age group was over 7 times larger than in 1900, but the 75–84 group was 11 times larger and the 85 and older group was 21 times larger. The most rapid increase is expected between 2010 and 2030 when the baby boom generation hits 65. In the next century, the only age groups in the U.S. expected to experience significant growth will be those past age 55. In this elderly age group, women will outnumber men by 2.6 to 1. By the year 2040, there will be 8 million to 13 million people 85 years of age or older; the estimate varies according to pessimistic to optimistic projections regarding disease prevention and treatment.

Unmarried women will be an increasing proportion of the elderly. By 1983, 50% of American women aged 65–74 were unmarried (partly divorced, but largely widowed), and after age 75, 77%![25] Half of men 85 and older live with their wives, but only 10% of elderly women live with their husbands. Because the unmarried tend to be more disadvantaged, there will be a need for more services for this segment of the elderly population. Older unmarried people are more vulnerable, demonstrating higher mortality rates and lower life satisfaction.

The Rectangularization of Life

The lifespan is the biological limit to life, the maximal obtainable age by a member of a species. The general impression is that human lifespan is increasing. Actually lifespan is fixed, and it is a biological constant for each species.[26] In fact, differences in species' lifespans argue in favor of a species-specific genetic basis for longevity. If lifespan were not fixed, it would mean an unlimited increase of our elderly. But a correct analysis of survival reveals that death converges at the same maximal age; what has changed is life expectancy—the number of years of life expected from birth. Life expectancy cannot exceed the lifespan, but it can closely approximate it. Thus the number of old people will eventually hit a fixed limit, but the percentage of a typical life spent in the older years will increase.

Our society has almost eliminated premature death. Diseases of the heart and the circulation, and cancers, are now the leading causes of death. The reason for this is not an increase or an epidemic; it is a result of our success in virtually eliminating infectious diseases. Now the major determinant is chronic disease, affected by genetics, lifestyle, the environment, and aging itself. The major achievement left to be accomplished is in cardiovascular diseases. But even if cancer, diabetes, and all circulatory diseases were totally eliminated, life expectancy would not exceed 90 years.[14]

J. F. Fries describes 3 eras in health and disease.[27] The first era existed until sometime in the early 1900s, and was characterized by acute infectious diseases. The second era, highlighted by cardiovascular diseases and cancer, is now beginning to fade into the third era, marked by problems of frailty (fading eyesight and hearing, impaired memory and cognitive function, decreased strength and reserve). Much of our medical approach is still based on the first era (find the disease and cure it), and now we have conditions that require a combination of medical, psychological, and social approaches. Our focus has been on age-dependent, fatal chronic diseases. The new challenge is with the nonfatal, age-dependent conditions, such as Alzheimer's disease, osteoarthritis, osteoporosis, obesity, and incontinence. It can be argued that health programs in the future should be evaluated by their impact on years free of disability, rather than on mortality.

The Concept of the Compression of Morbidity

Chronic illnesses are incremental in nature. The best health strategy is to change the slope, the rate at which illness develops, thus postponing the clinical illness, and if it is postponed long enough, effectively preventing it. There has been a profound change in public consciousness toward disease. Disease is increasingly seen as something not necessarily best treated by medication or surgery, but by prevention, or more accurately, by postponement.

Postponing illness is expressed by J.F. Fries as the ***compression of morbidity***.[26, 28] We would live relatively healthy lives and compress our illnesses into a short period of time just before death. Is this change really possible? The mean national body weight has decreased by 5 pounds despite a slight increase in the national average height. There has been a decrease in atherosclerosis in the U.S. Reasons include changes in the use of saturated fat, more effective detection and treatment of hypertension, increased exercise, and decreased smoking.

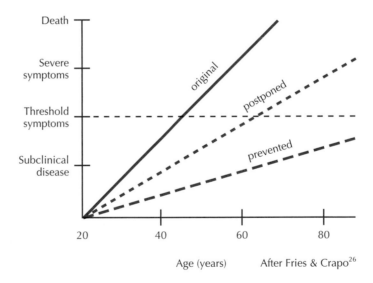

Smoking initiation has decreased markedly in men but, unfortunately, has remained essentially unchanged in women. In addition, female smokers begin smoking at a younger age. More young women (including teenagers) smoke than young men. It is important to note that smoking appears to have a greater adverse effect on women compared with men.[29] Women who smoke only 1 to 4 cigarettes per day have a 2.5-fold increased risk of fatal coronary heart disease.[30]

Physician smokers have declined from a high of 79% to a small minority.[31] It is interesting, and amusing, to note that the greatest decrease has been among pulmonary surgeons, not surprising, while the least decrease has been among proctologists. From the mid 1970s to the early 1990s, smoking among physicians in the U.S. declined from 18.8% to 3.3%. Unfortunately, that still amounted to approximately 18,000 physicians who smoke. The numbers are more discouraging among our professional colleagues. By 1991, (from the 1970s), smoking had declined from

31.7% to 18.3% among registered nurses and from 37.1% to only 27.2% among licensed practical nurses.

In the year 2000, approximately 30% of people in the U.S. who have not obtained a high school diploma will be smokers, but less than 10% of those with higher education will be smoking. Currently, approximately 28% of men and 23% of women are smokers.[32] Cigarette smoking, therefore, continues to be the single most preventable cause of premature death in the U.S. In addition, the use of chewing tobacco, pipe smoking, and cigars contributes significantly to morbidity and mortality.

Physicians and older patients may be skeptical that quitting smoking after decades of smoking could be beneficial. In a longitudinal study of 2674 people, aged 65–74, the mortality rates for exsmokers were no higher than for nonsmokers.[33] The effects are at least partly reversible within one to five years after quitting. Even older patients who already have coronary artery disease have improved survival if they quit smoking.[34] No matter how old you are, if you continue to smoke, you have an increased relative risk of death. But no matter how old you are, if you quit smoking, your risk of death decreases.

Since 1970, the death rate from coronary heart disease has declined approximately 50% in the U.S. Between 1973 and 1987 in the U.S., cardiovascular mortality declined in nearly every age group. In the combined age groups up to 54 years, cardiovascular mortality decreased 42%, and in people 55 to 84 years old, 33%.[29] Despite our progress, we must continue to exert preventive efforts on the risk factors associated with cardiovascular disease, especially obesity, hypertension, and lack of physical activity.

The effort to improve the quality of life has an important value to society; it will decrease the average number of years that people are disabled and a liability. Frailty and disability are now the major health and social problems of society. Most significantly, this is a major financial challenge for health care systems and social programs. With evolution toward a rectangular society, the ratio of beneficiaries to taxpayers grows rapidly, jeopardizing the financial support for health and social programs. Compression of morbidity is at least one attractive solution to this problem.

Menopause as an Opportunity

Clinicians who interact with women at the time of the menopause have a wonderful opportunity and, therefore, a significant obligation. Medical intervention at this point of life offers women years of benefit from preventive health care. This represents an opportunity that should be seized.

It is logical to argue that health programs should be directed to the young. It makes sense to create good lifelong health behavior. While not underrating the importance of good health habits among the young, we would argue that the impact of teaching preventive care is more observable and more tangible at middle age. The prospects of limited mortality and the morbidity of chronic diseases are viewed with belief, understanding, and appreciation during these older years. The chance of illness is higher, but the impact of changes in lifestyle is greater.

The Perimenopausal Transition

Definition of the Perimenopausal Transition

There is only one marker, menstrual irregularity, that is used to define and establish what is called the perimenopausal transition. The ***menopause*** is that point in time when permanent cessation of menstruation occurs following the loss of ovarian activity. Menopause is derived from the Greek words, *men* (month) and *pausis* (cessation). The years prior to menopause that encompass the change from normal ovulatory cycles to cessation of menses are known as the ***perimenopausal transitional*** years, marked by irregularity of menstrual cycles. ***Climacteric*** indicates the period of time when a woman passes from the reproductive stage of life through the perimenopausal transition and the menopause to the postmenopausal years. Climacteric is from the Greek word for ladder.

Menstrual cycle length is determined by the rate and quality of follicular growth and development, and it is normal for the cycle to vary in individual women. Our best information comes from two longitudinal studies (with very similar results): the study of Vollman of more than 30,000 cycles recorded by 650 women and the study of Treloar of more that 25,000 woman-years in a little over 2700 women.[35, 36] The observations of Vollman and Treloar documented a normal evolution in length and variation in menstrual cycles.

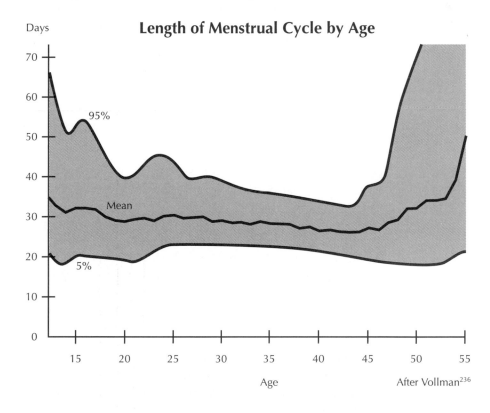

Length of Menstrual Cycle by Age

Days

After Vollman[236]

Age

Menarche is followed by approximately 5–7 years of relatively long cycles at first, and then there is increasing regularity as cycles shorten to reach the usual reproductive age pattern. In the 40s, cycles begin to lengthen again. The highest incidence of anovulatory cycles is under age 20 and over age 40.[37, 38] At age 25, over 40% of cycles are between 25 and 28 days in length; from 25 to 35, over 60% are between 25 and 28 days. The perfect 28-day cycle is indeed the most common mode, but it totaled only 12.4% of Vollman's cycles. Overall, approximately 15% of reproductive age cycles are 28 days in length. Only 0.5% of women experience a cycle less than 21 days long, and only 0.9% a cycle greater than 35 days.[39] Most women have cycles that last from 24 to 35 days, but at least 20% of women experience irregular cycles.[40]

When women are in their 40s, anovulation becomes more prevalent, and prior to anovulation, menstrual cycle length increases, beginning 2 to 8 years before menopause.[36] This period of longer cycles uniformly precedes menopause no matter the age when menses cease, whether menopause is early or late.[41] The duration of the follicular phase is the major determinant of cycle length.[42, 43] This menstrual cycle change prior to menopause is marked by elevated follicle-stimulating hormone (FSH) levels and decreased levels of inhibin, but normal levels of luteinizing hormone (LH) and slightly elevated levels of estradiol.[44–48]

Contrary to older belief (based on the report by Sherman, et al,[42]), *estradiol levels do not gradually wane in the years before the menopause, but remain in the normal range, although slightly elevated, until 6 months to 1 year before follicular growth and development cease.* The Sherman, et al, data were from a small cross-sectional study of one cycle collected from 8 women, age 46–56. More recent longitudinal studies of women as they pass through the perimenopausal transition reveal that estrogen levels do not begin to decline until less than a year before menopause.[48] Indeed, women experiencing the perimenopausal transition actually have higher overall estrogen levels, a response that is logically explained by an increased ovarian follicular response to the increase in FSH secretion during these years.[49]

As noted, most women experience a 2- to 8-year period of time prior to menopause when anovulation becomes prevalent.[36] During this period of time ovarian follicles undergo an accelerated rate of loss until eventually the supply of follicles is finally depleted.[50, 51] In a study of human ovaries, the accelerated loss appeared to begin when the total number of follicles reached approximately 25,000, a number reached in normal women at an age of 37–38.[52] This loss correlates with a subtle but real increase in FSH and decrease in inhibin. The accelerated loss is probably secondary to the increase in FSH stimulation. These changes, including the increase in FSH, reflect the reduced quality and capability of aging follicles, and their reduced secretion of inhibin, the granulosa cell product that exerts an important negative feedback influence over FSH secretion by the pituitary gland. Both inhibin A and inhibin B may be involved. Luteal phase levels of inhibin A and follicular phase levels of inhibin B decrease with aging, and may antedate the rise in FSH.[53, 54, 627]

The inverse and tight relationship between FSH and inhibin indicates that inhibin is a sensitive marker of ovarian follicular competence and, in turn, that FSH measurement is a clinical assessment of inhibin. Thus, the changes in the later reproductive years (the decline in inhibin allowing a rise in FSH) reflect diminishing follicular reactivity and competence as the ovary ages.[45, 46] The decrease in inhibin secretion by the ovarian follicles begins early (around age 35), but accelerates after 40 years of age. This is reflected in the decrease in fecundity that occurs with aging (as discussed in Chapter 26). *Furthermore, the ineffective ability to suppress gonadotropins with postmenopausal hormone therapy is a consequence of the loss of inhibin, and for this reason FSH cannot be used clinically to titer estrogen dosage.*

The perimenopausal years are a time period during which postmenopausal levels of FSH (greater than 20 IU/L) can be seen despite continued menstrual bleeding, while LH levels still remain in the normal range. Occasionally, corpus luteum formation and function occur, and the perimenopausal woman is not safely beyond the risk of an unplanned and unexpected pregnancy until elevated levels of both FSH (>20 IU/L) and LH (>30 IU/L) can be demonstrated.[47] However, even under these circumstances, fluctuations can occur, with a period of ovarian failure followed by resumption of ovarian function.[46] *Because variability is the rule, it would be wise to recommend the use of contraception until the postmenopausal state is definitely established.* According to the *Guinness Book of World Records*, a woman from Portland, Oregon, holds the modern record for the oldest spontaneous pregnancy, conceiving when 57 years and 120 days old.

The Perimenopausal Transition
(mean circulating hormone levels)

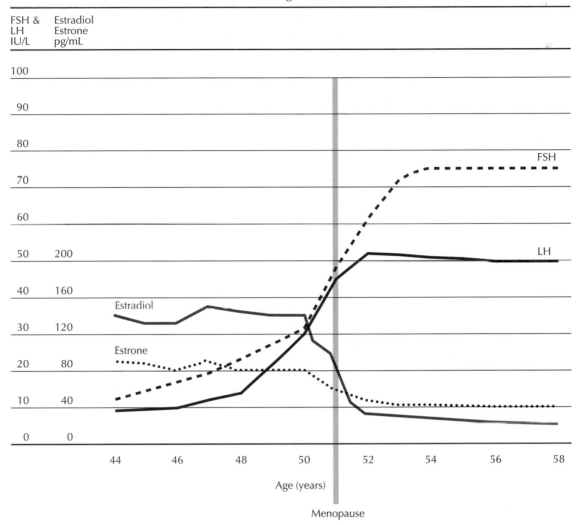

In the longitudinal Massachusetts Women's Health Study, women who reported the onset of menstrual irregularity were considered to be in the perimenopausal period of life.[55] The median age for the onset of this transition was 47.5 years. Only 10% of women ceased menstruating abruptly with no period of prolonged irregularity. The perimenopausal transition from reproductive to postreproductive status was, for most women, approximately 4 years in duration. In the study by Treolar, the average age for entry into the perimenopausal transition was 45.1, and the age range that included 95% of the women was 39–51.[56] The mean duration of the perimenopausal transition was 5.0 years, with a range of 2 to 8 years.

The Perimenopausal Transition[36, 55, 56]

Average age of onset — 46
Age of onset for 95% of women — 39 to 51
Average duration — 5 years
Duration for 95% of women — 2 to 8 years

Preventive Health Screening of Healthy Perimenopausal Women

The most important thing a clinician can offer to the perimenopausal woman is the education she needs and desires to make therapeutic choices. This early educational process will help to build a solid relationship with patients, a relationship they will want to continue as they age.

The following recommendations are derived from our own clinical experience:

- Provide guidance and education to facilitate a patient's decision making.

- Provide time and an appropriate location for sensitive and uninterrupted discussions.

- Use educational materials, especially handouts, but also explain them using your own words.

- Involve family members during counseling and educational visits.

- Be accessible. Consider designating a member of your staff as the menopause resource person. Encourage phone calls.

- Be involved in community and hospital educational programs for the public.

- Use an effective, well-trained counselor for patients who need in-depth help in coping with life's trials and tribulations.

Preventive intervention during the perimenopausal years has three major goals. The overall objective is to prolong the period of maximal physical energy and optimal mental and social activity. A specific goal is to detect as early as possible any of the major chronic diseases, including hypertension, heart disease, diabetes mellitus, and cancer, as well as impairments of vision, hearing, and teeth. Finally, the clinician should help perimenopausal women to smoothly traverse the menopausal period of life. Preventive health care and management of the later reproductive years give clinicians an excellent opportunity to function as a woman's primary care provider.

A complete medical history and physical examination should be performed every 5 years, at about age 40, 45, 50, and 55. Annual visits should include a breast and pelvic examination, Pap test, screening for sexually transmitted diseases when appropriate, a TSH assessment in the 40s and every 2 years beginning at age 60, and hemoccult testing after age 50. Annual screening mammography should begin at age 40 (discussed in Chapter 16). At each visit, appropriate testing is scheduled for specific chronic conditions, indicated immunizations are proved, and counseling covers changing nutritional needs, physical activities, injury prevention, occupational, sexual, marital, and parental problems, urinary function, and use of tobacco, alcohol, and drugs.

The Age of Menopause

Designating the average age of menopause has been somewhat difficult. Based on cross-sectional studies, the median age was estimated to be somewhere between 50 and 52.[57] These studies relied on retrospective memories and the subjective vagaries of the individual being interviewed. Until recently, studies with longitudinal follow-up to observe women and record their experiences as they pass through menopause were hampered by relatively small numbers. The Massachusetts Women's Health Study provides us with data from 2,570 women.[55]

The median age for menopause in the Massachusetts Study was 51.3 years. Only current smoking could be identified as a cause of earlier menopause, a shift of approximately 1.5 years. Those factors that did not affect the age of menopause included the use of oral contraception, socioeconomic status, and marital status. Keep in mind that a median age of menopause means that only half the women have reached menopause at this age. In the classic longitudinal study by Treolar, the ***average*** age of menopause was 50.7, and the range that included 95% of the women was 44 to 56.[58] In a survey in the Netherlands, the average age of menopause was 50.2.[59] About 1% of women will experience menopause before the age of 40.[60]

Clinical impression has suggested that mothers and daughters tend to experience menopause at the same age, and there are two studies indicating that daughters of mothers with an early menopause (before age 46) also have an early menopause.[61–63] There is sufficient evidence to believe that undernourished women and vegetarians experience an earlier menopause.[61, 64] Because of the contribution of body fat to estrogen production, thinner women experience a slightly earlier menopause.[65] Consumption of alcohol is associated with a later menopause.[62] This is consistent with the reports that women who consume alcohol have higher blood and urinary levels of estrogen, and greater bone density.[66–70]

There is no correlation between age of menarche and age of menopause.[58, 59, 61, 71] In most studies, race, parity, and height have no influence on the age of menopause; however, two cross-sectional studies found later menopause to be associated with increasing parity.[55, 59, 61, 65] Two studies have found that irregular menses among women in their early 40s predicts an earlier menopause.[72, 73] A French survey detected no influence of heavy physical work on early menopause (before age 45).[74] An earlier menopause is associated with living at high altitudes,[75] There is reason to believe that premature ovarian failure can occur in women who have previously undergone abdominal hysterectomy or endometrial ablation, presumably because ovarian vascular flow has been compromised.[76, 77] And finally, earlier menopause is associated with growth retardation in late gestation.[78]

Multiple studies have consistently documented that an earlier menopause (an average of 1.5 years earlier) is a consequence of smoking. There is a dose-response relationship with the number of cigarettes smoked and the duration of smoking.[79, 80] Even former smokers show evidence of an impact.

Unlike the decline in age of menarche that occurred with an improvement in health and living conditions, most historical investigation indicates that the age of menopause has changed little since early Greek times.[81, 82] Others (a minority) have disagreed, concluding that the age of menopause did undergo a change, starting with an average age of about 40 years in ancient times.[83] If there has been a change, however, history indicates it has been minimal. Even in ancient writings, an age of 50 is usually cited as the age of menopause.

Sexuality and Menopause

Sexuality is a lifelong behavior with evolving change and development. It begins with birth (maybe before) and ends with death. The notion that it ends with aging is inherently illogical. The need for closeness, caring, and companionship is lifelong. Old people today live longer, are healthier, have more education and leisure time, and have had their consciousness raised in regard to sexuality.

Younger people, especially physicians, underrate the extent of sexual interest in older people. In a random sample of women aged 50 to 82 in Madison, Wisconsin, nearly one-half of the women reported an ongoing sexual relationship.[84] In the Duke longitudinal study on aging, 70% of men in the 67 to 77 age group were sexually active, and 80% reported continuing sexual interest, while 50% of all older women were still interested in sex.[85] In the PEPI trial, 60% of women 55–64 years old were sexually active.[86]

The decline in sexual activity with aging is influenced more by culture and attitudes than by nature and physiology (or hormones). The two most important influences on older sexual interaction are the strength of a relationship and the physical condition of each partner.[86] The single most significant determinant of sexual activity for older women, therefore, is the unavailability of partners due to divorce and the fact that women are outliving men. Given the availability of a partner, the same general high or low rate of sexual activity can be maintained throughout life.[5, 87] Longitudinal studies indicate that the level of sexual activity is more stable over time than previously suggested.[88–90] Individuals who are sexually active earlier in life continue to be sexually active into old age.

There are two main sexual changes in the aging woman. There is a reduction in the rate of production and volume of vaginal lubricating fluid, and there is some loss of vaginal elasticity. The dyspareunia associated with postmenopausal urogenital atrophy includes a feeling of dryness and tightness, vaginal irritation and burning with coitus, and postcoital spotting and soreness. Of course, these changes are effectively prevented by estrogen treatment. Less vaginal atrophy is noted in sexually active women than in inactive women; presumably the activity maintains vaginal vasculature and circulation.

Illness and Sex

It is not uncommon to encounter women who have had surgery that affects sexuality. The list includes vulvectomy, coronary bypass surgery, and surgery of the breast. Sexual problems are not limited, however, to surgical procedures and illnesses of the genitalia. Altered self-image can occur with diseases of any site. However, studies have not found hysterectomy to have a detrimental impact on sexuality.[86, 91]

Sexual counseling, to be effective, must be provided to couples both before and after surgery. It is not unexpected that the surgeon may not be fully capable of providing this counseling. A major contribution from an older woman's primary clinician is to arrange for competent and experienced sexual counseling. Unfortunately, most physicians operate on the principle that if no questions are raised there is no problem. The expert surgeon should be grateful for the help of experts in psychosexual therapy. Seek out the potential for post-treatment sexual morbidity before the treatment. Assess the patient's abilities for coping and her sense of body image. Consider the quality of the patient's relationship, and be sensitive to the absence of a relationship. This entire effort may take some time. The normal state of presurgical anxiety, fear, and denial hampers good communication.

Antihypertensive agents are frequently responsible for male sexual dysfunction, but little information is available regarding female sexual function. However, remember that vaginal lubrication is the female counterpart to the male erection, and, therefore, vaginal dryness is a likely consequence. Adrenergic blocking agents are especially noted to affect libido and potency in men. Similarly, psychotropic drugs of all categories have been associated with inhibition of sexual function. Finally, one should always suspect alcoholism when patients complain of sexual dysfunction.

Hormone Production After Menopause

Shortly after the menopause, one can safely say that there are no remaining ovarian follicles.[92] Eventually there is a 10–20-fold increase in FSH and approximately a 3-fold increase in LH, reaching a maximal level 1–3 years after menopause, after which there is a gradual, but slight, decline in both gonadotropins.[93, 94] Elevated levels of both FSH and LH at this time in life are conclusive evidence of ovarian failure. FSH levels are higher than LH because LH is cleared from the blood so much faster (initial half-lives are about 20 minutes for LH and 3–4 hours for FSH), and perhaps because there is no specific negative feedback peptide for LH like inhibin.

The postmenopausal ovary secretes primarily androstenedione and testosterone. After menopause, the circulating level of androstenedione is about one half that seen prior to menopause.[95] Most of this postmenopausal androstenedione is derived from the adrenal gland, with only a small amount secreted from the ovary, although androstenedione is the principal steroid secreted by the postmenopausal ovary.[96] Dehydroepiandrosterone (DHEA) and its sulfate (DHEAS), originating in the adrenal gland, decline markedly with aging; in the decade after menopause the circulating levels of DHEA are approximately 70% less and levels of DHEAS are about 74% less than the levels in young adult life.[97]

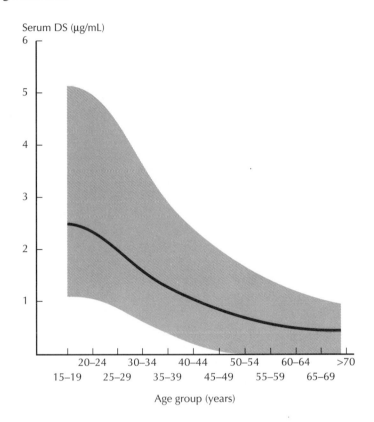

Testosterone production decreases by approximately 25% after menopause, but the postmenopausal ovary in most women, but not all, secretes more testosterone than the premenopausal ovary. With the disappearance of follicles and estrogen, the elevated gonadotropins drive the remaining stromal tissue in the ovary to a level of increased testosterone secretion. Suppression of gonadotropins with gonadotropin-releasing hormone (GnRH) agonist or antagonist treatment of postmenopausal women results in a significant decrease in circulating levels of testosterone, indicating the gonadotropin-dependent postmenopausal ovarian origin.[98–100] The total amount of testosterone produced after menopause, however, is decreased because the amount of the primary source, peripheral conversion of androstenedione, is reduced. The early postmenopausal circulating level of androstenedione decreases approximately 62% from young adult life[97] The menopausal decline in the circulating levels of testosterone is not great, from no change in many women to as much as 15% in others.[48, 94, 97] Nevertheless, compared with young women, the overall androgen exposure of perimenopausal women to androgens is less.[101]

Blood Production Rates of Steroids[102]

	Reproductive age	Postmenopausal	Oophorectomized
Androstenedione	2–3 mg/day	0.5–1.5 mg/day	0.4–1.2 mg/day
Dehydroepiandrosterone	6–8	1.5–4.0	1.5–4.0
Dehydroepiandrosterone sulfate	8–16	4–9	4–9
Testosterone	0.2–0.25	0.05–0.18	0.02–0.12
Estrogen	0.350	0.045	0.045

Changes in Circulating Hormone Levels at Menopause[48, 95, 103]

	Premenopause	Postmenopause
Estradiol	40–400 pg/mL	10–20 pg/mL
Estrone	30–200 pg/mL	30–70 pg/mL
Testosterone	20–80 ng/dL	15–70 ng/dL
Androstenedione	60–300 ng/dL	30–150 ng/dL

The circulating estradiol level after menopause is approximately 10–20 pg/mL, most of which is derived from peripheral conversion of estrone, which in turn is mainly derived from the peripheral conversion of androstenedione.[95, 103, 104] The circulating level of estrone in postmenopausal women is higher than that of estradiol, approximately 30–70 pg/mL. The average postmenopausal production rate of estrogen is approximately 45 µg/24 hours, almost all, if not all, being estrogen derived from the peripheral conversion of androstenedione. The androgen:estrogen ratio changes drastically after menopause because of the more marked decline in estrogen, and an onset of mild hirsutism is common, reflecting this marked shift in the sex hormone ratio. With increasing age, a decrease can be measured in the circulating levels of dehydroepiandrosterone sulfate (DHAS) and dehydroepiandrosterone (DHA), whereas the circulating postmenopausal levels of androstenedione, testosterone, and estrogen remain relatively constant.[94, 95]

Estrogen production by the ovaries does not continue beyond the menopause; however, estrogen levels in postmenopausal women can be significant, principally due to the extraglandular conversion of androstenedione and testosterone to estrogen. The clinical impact of this estrogen will vary from one postmenopausal woman to another, depending on the degree of extraglandular production, modified by a variety of factors.

The percent conversion of androstenedione to estrogen correlates with body weight. Increased production of estrogen from androstenedione with increasing body weight is probably due to the ability of fat to aromatize androgens. This fact and a decrease in the levels of sex hormone-binding globulin (which results in increased free estrogen concentrations) contribute to the well known association between obesity and the development of endometrial cancer. Body weight, therefore, has a positive correlation with the circulating levels of estrone and estradiol.[95] Aromatization of androgens to estrogens is not limited to adipose tissue; however, because almost every tissue tested has this activity.

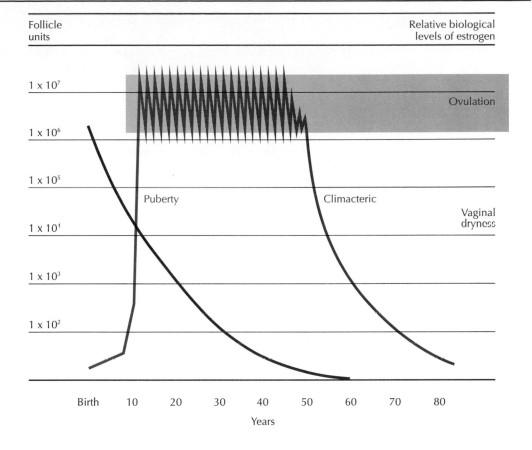

Eventually, the ovarian stroma is exhausted and, despite huge reactive increments in FSH and LH, no further steroidogenesis of importance results from gonadal activity. The postmenopausal ovary weighs less than 10 g, but it can be visualized by ultrasonography.[105]

With increasing age, the adrenal contribution of precursors for estrogen production proves inadequate. In this final stage of estrogen availability, levels are insufficient to sustain secondary sex tissues.

In summary, the symptoms frequently seen and related to decreasing ovarian follicular competence and then estrogen loss in this protracted climacteric are:

1. Disturbances in menstrual pattern, including anovulation and reduced fertility, decreased flow or hypermenorrhea, irregular frequency of menses, and then ultimately, amenorrhea.

2. Vasomotor instability (hot flushes and sweats).

3. Atrophic conditions: atrophy of vaginal epithelium; formation of urethral caruncles; dyspareunia and pruritus due to vulvar, introital, and vaginal atrophy; general skin atrophy; urinary difficulties such as urgency and abacterial urethritis and cystitis.

4. Health problems secondary to long-term deprivation of estrogen: the consequences of osteoporosis and cardiovascular disease.

A precise understanding of the symptom complex the individual patient may display is often difficult to achieve. Some patients will experience severe multiple reactions that may be disabling. Others will show no reactions, or minimal reactions, that go unnoticed until careful medical evaluation.

It is helpful to classify the hormonal problems in 3 categories:

1. Those associated with relative *estrogen excess* such as dysfunctional uterine bleeding, endometrial hyperplasia, and endometrial cancer.

2. Those associated with *estrogen deprivation* such as flushes, atrophic vaginitis, urethritis, and osteoporosis.

3. Those associated with *estrogen-progestin therapy* (Chapter 18).

Problems of Estrogen Excess

Exposure to Unopposed Estrogen

Throughout the perimenopausal period, there is a significant incidence of dysfunctional uterine bleeding. Although the greatest concern provoked by this symptom is endometrial neoplasia, the usual finding is non-neoplastic tissue displaying estrogen effects unopposed by progesterone. This results from anovulation in premenopausal women and from extragonadal endogenous estrogen production or estrogen administration in postmenopausal women.

There are 4 mechanisms that could result in increased endogenous estrogen levels:

1. Increased precursor androgen (functional and nonfunctional endocrine tumors, liver disease, stress).

2. Increased aromatization (obesity, hyperthyroidism, and liver disease).

3. Increased direct secretion of estrogen (ovarian tumors).

4. Decreased levels of SHBG (sex hormone-binding globulin) leading to increased levels of free estrogen.

In all women, whether premenopausal or postmenopausal, whether on or off hormone therapy, specific organic causes (neoplasia, complications of unexpected pregnancy, or bleeding from extrauterine sites) must be ruled out. In addition to careful history and physical examination, dysfunctional uterine bleeding requires evaluation. Transvaginal ultrasonographic measurement of endometrial thickness can be utilized in postmenopausal women to avoid unnecessary biopsies.[106] A total endometrial thickness greater than 4 mm requires biopsy. If the uterus is normal on examination, for reasons of both accuracy and cost-effectiveness, the method of biopsy should be an office aspiration curettage, *NOT* the traditional, more costly and risky, in-hospital dilation and curettage (D and C).

We recommend the use of the plastic endometrial suction device. It is easy to use, requires no cervical dilatation, and is frequently painless. This device is as efficacious as older more painful techniques. Insertion should first be attempted without the use of a tenaculum. In many patients, this is feasible and avoids the sensation of the tenaculum grasping the cervix. Once the suction is applied, the endometrial cavity should be thoroughly curetted in all directions, just as one would with a sharp curette during a D and C. If the cannula fills up with tissue, a second and even a third cannula should be inserted until tissue is no longer obtained. Although most patients report no problems with cramps or pain, the application of suction in some patients stimulates cramping that usually passes within 5–10 minutes. Because cramping occurs in such a small minority of patients, it is not our practice to routinely give an inhibitor of prostaglandin synthesis. For repeat biopsies, in patients known to cramp, it would be helpful to use such an agent at least 20 minutes before the procedure.

Less than 10% of postmenopausal women cannot be adequately evaluated by office biopsy. Most commonly, the reason is the inability to enter the uterine cavity. In such instances, an in-hospital dilatation and curettage (D and C) is in order. ***Furthermore, if the uterus is not normal on pelvic examination, the office endometrial biopsy must yield to an in-hospital D and C with hysteroscopy in order to achieve accuracy of diagnosis.***

If vulva, vagina, and cervix appear normal on inspection, perimenopausal bleeding can be assumed to be intrauterine in origin. Confirmation requires the absence of abnormal cytology on the Pap smear. The principal symptom of endometrial cancer is abnormal vaginal bleeding, but carcinoma will be encountered in patients with bleeding in only about 1–2% of postmenopausal endometrial biopsies.[107, 108] Normal endometrium is found over half the time, polyps in approximately 3%, endometrial hyperplasia about 15% of the time, and atrophic endometrium in the rest of patients with postmenopausal bleeding. Postmenopausal bleeding should always be taken seriously. Approximately 10% of patients who have benign findings at the initial evaluation will subsequently develop significant pathology within 2 years.[108] ***The persistence of abnormal bleeding demands repeated evaluation.***

Additional procedures include the following:

> ***Colposcopy and cervical biopsy*** for abnormal cytology or obvious lesions.

> ***Endocervical assessment by curettage*** for abnormal cytology (the endocervix must always be kept in mind as a source for abnormal cytology).

> ***Hysterogram, hysteroscopy, or ultrasonography with the uterine instillation of saline*** if bleeding persists to determine the presence of endometrial polyps or submucosal fibroids.

Keep in mind that the pathologic reading, "tissue insufficient for diagnosis," when a patient is on estrogen-progestin treatment, often represents atrophic, decidualized endometrium that yields little to the exploring curet. The clinician must be confident in his or her technique, knowing that a full investigation of the intrauterine cavity has been accomplished, then *as long as the patient does not persist in bleeding*, this reading can be interpreted as comforting and benign, the absence of pathology.

In the absence of organic disease, appropriate management of uterine bleeding is dependent on the age of the woman and endometrial tissue findings. In the perimenopausal woman with dysfunctional uterine bleeding associated with proliferative or hyperplastic endometrium (uncomplicated by atypia or dysplastic constituents), periodic oral progestin therapy is mandatory, such as 5–10 mg medroxyprogesterone acetate given daily for at least the first 10 days of each month. If hyperplasia is present, follow-up aspiration curettage after 3–4 months is required, and if progestin is ineffective and histological regression is not observed, formal curettage is an essential preliminary to alternate therapeutic surgical choices. Because hyperplasia with atypia carries with it a risk of cancer (even invasive), hysterectomy is the treatment of choice.

When monthly progestin therapy reverses hyperplastic changes (which it does in 95–98% of cases) and controls irregular bleeding, treatment should be continued until withdrawal bleeding ceases. This is a reliable sign (in effect, a bioassay) indicating the onset of estrogen deprivation and the need for the addition of estrogen. If vasomotor disturbances begin before the cessation of menstrual bleeding, the combined estrogen-progestin program can be initiated as needed to control the flushes.

If contraception is required, the healthy, nonsmoking patient should seriously consider the use of oral contraception. The anovulatory woman cannot be guaranteed that spontaneous ovulation and pregnancy will not occur. The use of a low-dose oral contraceptive will at the same time provide contraception and prophylaxis against irregular, heavy anovulatory bleeding and the risk of endometrial hyperplasia and neoplasia.

Clinicians have been made so wary of providing oral contraceptives to older women that a traditional postmenopausal hormone regimen is often utilized to treat a woman with the kind of irregular cycles usually experienced in the perimenopausal years. This addition of exogenous estrogen without an a contraceptive dose of progestin when a woman is not amenorrheic or experiencing menopausal symptoms is inappropriate and even risky (exposing the endometrium to excessively high levels of estrogen). And most importantly, a postmenopausal hormonal regimen does not inhibit ovulation and provide contraception.[109] The appropriate response is to regulate anovulatory cycles with monthly progestational treatment along with an appropriate contraceptive method or to utilize low-dose oral contraception (see Chapter 15). The oral contraceptive that contains 20 μg estrogen provides effective contraception, improves menstrual cycle regularity, diminishes bleeding, and relieves menopausal symptoms.[110]

A common clinical dilemma is when to change from oral contraception to postmenopausal hormone therapy. It is important to change because even with the lowest estrogen dose oral contraceptive available, the estrogen dose is four-fold greater than the standard postmenopausal dose, and with increasing age, the dose-related risks with estrogen become significant. One approach to establish the onset of the postmenopausal years is to measure the FSH level, beginning at age 50, on an annual basis, being careful to obtain the blood sample on day 6 or 7 of the pill-free week (when steroid levels have declined sufficiently to allow FSH to rise). Friday afternoon works well for patients who start new packages on Sunday. When FSH is greater than 20 IU/L, it is time to change to a postmenopausal hormone program. Because of the variability in FSH levels experienced by women around the menopause, this method is not always accurate.[111] But there is no harm in retesting after another year or two on low-dose oral contraceptives. Some clinicians are comfortable allowing patients to enter their mid-50s on low-dose oral contraception, and then empirically switching to a postmenopausal hormone regimen.

In postmenopausal women, one must view any adnexal mass as cancer until proven otherwise. Surgical intervention is usually necessary, and appropriate consultation must be obtained not only for the surgical procedure but also for suitable preoperative evaluation and preparation. Non-palpable, asymptomatic ovarian cysts are commonly detected by ultrasonography. Cysts that are less than 5 cm in diameter and without septations or solid components have a very low potential for malignant disease and may be managed with serial ultrasound surveillance (at 3 months, 6 months, 12 months and then annually).[112] Surgery is recommended for symptomatic cases, if growth occurs, if internal echoes are obtained, if fluid develops in the pelvis, or if there is a family history of breast or ovarian cancer.

The Impact of Postmenopausal Estrogen Deprivation

The menopause should serve to remind patients and clinicians that this is a time for education. Certainly preventive health care education is important throughout life, but at the time of the menopause, a review of the major health issues can be especially rewarding. Besides the general issues of good health, attention is now being focused (because of their relationship to postmeno-pausal hormone therapy) on cardiovascular disease and osteoporosis.

During the menopausal years, some women will experience severe multiple symptoms, whereas others will show no reactions or minimal reactions that can go unnoticed. The differences in menopausal reactions in symptoms across different cultures is poorly documented, and indeed, it is difficult to do so. Individual reporting is so conditioned by sociocultural factors that it is hard to determine what is due to biological versus cultural variability.[113, 114] For example, there is no word to describe a hot flush in Japanese, Chinese, and Mayan.[115] Nevertheless, there is reason to believe that the nature and prevalence of menopausal symptoms are common to most women, and that variations among cultures and within cultures reflect not physiology, but differences in attitudes, societies, and individual perceptions.[116–119]

Vasomotor Symptoms

The vasomotor flush is viewed as the hallmark of the female climacteric, experienced to some degree by most postmenopausal women. The term "hot flush" is descriptive of a sudden onset of reddening of the skin over the head, neck, and chest, accompanied by a feeling of intense body heat and concluded by sometimes profuse perspiration. The duration varies from a few seconds to several minutes and, rarely, for an hour. The frequency may be rare to recurrent every few minutes. Flushes are more frequent and severe at night (when a woman is often awakened from sleep) or during times of stress. In a cool environment, hot flushes are fewer, less intense, and shorter in duration compared with a warm environment.[120]

In the longitudinal follow-up of a large number of women, fully 10% of the women experienced hot flushes before menopause, while in other studies as many as 15–25% of premenopausal women reported hot flushes.[9, 55, 121, 122] The frequency has been reported to be even higher in premenopausal women diagnosed with premenstrual syndrome.[123] In the Massachusetts Women's Health Study, the incidence of hot flushes increased from 10% during the premenopausal period to about 50% just after cessation of menses.[55] By approximately 4 years after menopause, the rate of hot flushes declined to 20%. In a community-based Australian survey, 6% of premenopausal women, 26% of perimenopausal women, and 59% of postmenopausal women reported hot flushing.[124]

Although the flush can occur in the premenopause, it is a major feature of postmenopause, lasting in most women for 1–2 years but, in some (as many as 25%) for longer than 5 years. In cross-sectional surveys, up to 40% of premenopausal women and 85% of menopausal women report vasomotor complaints.[122] In the U.S., there is no difference in the prevalence of vasomotor complaints in surveys of black and white women.[125, 126] In a massive review of hot flushes, it was concluded that exact estimates on prevalence are hampered by inconsistencies and differences in methodologies, cultures, and definitions.[127]

The physiology of the hot flush is still not understood, but it apparently originates in the hypothalamus and is brought about by a decline in estrogen. However, not all hot flushes are due to estrogen deficiency. Flushes and sweating can be secondary to diseases, including pheochromocytoma, carcinoid, leukemias, pancreatic tumors, and thyroid abnormalities.[128] Unfortunately, the hot flush is a relatively common psychosomatic symptom, and women often are unnecessarily treated with estrogen. ***When the clinical situation is not clear and obvious, estrogen deficiency as the cause of hot flushes should be documented by elevated levels of FSH.***

The Hot Flush

Premenopausal	10–25% of women
Postmenopausal:	
No flushes	15–25%
Daily flushing	15–20%
Duration	1–2 years average 5 plus years: 25%
Other causes:	

    Psychosomatic
    Stress
    Thyroid disease
    Pheochromocytoma
    Carcinoid
    Leukemia
    Cancer

The correlation between the onset of flushes and estrogen reduction is clinically supported by the effectiveness of estrogen therapy and the absence of flushes in hypoestrogen states, such as gonadal dysgenesis. Only after estrogen is administered and withdrawn do hypogonadal women experience the hot flush. Although the clinical impression that premenopausal surgical castrates suffer more severe vasomotor reactions is widely held, this is not borne out in objective study.[129]

Although the hot flush is the most common problem of the postmenopause, it presents no inherent health hazard. The flush is accompanied by a discrete and reliable pattern of physiologic changes.[130] The flush coincides with a surge of LH (not FSH) and is preceded by a subjective prodromal awareness that a flush is beginning. This aura is followed by measurable increased heat over the entire body surface. The body surface experiences an increase in temperature, accompanied by changes in skin conductance, and followed by a fall in core temperature—all of which can be objectively measured. In short, the flush is not a release of accumulated body heat but is a sudden inappropriate excitation of heat release mechanisms. Its relationship to the LH surge and temperature change within the brain is not understood. The observation that flushes occur after hypophysectomy indicates that the mechanism is not dependent on or due directly to LH release. In other words, the same hypothalamic event that causes flushes also stimulates gonadotropin-releasing hormone (GnRH) secretion and elevates LH. This is probably secondary to hypothalamic changes in neurotransmitters that increase neuronal and autonomic activity.[131]

Premenopausal women experiencing hot flushes should be screened for thyroid disease and other illnesses. A comprehensive review of all possible causes is available.[132] Clinicians should be sensitive to the possibility of an underlying emotional problem. Looking beyond the presenting symptoms into the patient's life will be an important service to the patient and her family that eventually will be appreciated. This is far more difficult than simply prescribing estrogen, but confronting problems is the only way of reaching some resolution. Prescribing estrogen inappropriately (in the presence of normal levels of gonadotropins) only temporarily postpones by a placebo response dealing with the underlying issues.

A striking and consistent finding in most studies dealing with menopause and hormonal therapy is a marked placebo response in a variety of symptoms, including flushing. In an English randomized, placebo-controlled study of women being treated with estrogen implants and requesting repeat implants, there was no difference in outcome in terms of psychological and physical symptoms comparing the women who received an active implant to those receiving a placebo.[133]

A significant clinical problem encountered in our referral practice is the following scenario: a woman will occasionally undergo an apparent beneficial response to estrogen, only to have the response wear off in several months. This leads to a sequence of periodic visits to the clinician and ever-increasing doses of estrogen. When a patient reaches a point of requiring large doses of estrogen, a careful inquiry must be undertaken to search for a basic psychoneurotic or psychosocial problem. To help persuade a patient that her symptoms are not due to low levels of estrogen, we find it very helpful and convincing to measure the patient's blood level of estradiol and share the result with her.

Atrophic Changes

With extremely low estrogen production in the late postmenopausal age, or many years after castration, atrophy of vaginal mucosal surfaces takes place, accompanied by vaginitis, pruritus, dyspareunia, and stenosis. Genitourinary atrophy leads to a variety of symptoms that affect the ease and quality of living. Urethritis with dysuria, urgency incontinence, and urinary frequency are further results of mucosal thinning, in this instance, of the urethra and bladder. Recurrent urinary tract infections are effectively prevented by postmenopausal intravaginal estrogen treatment.[134] Vaginal relaxation with cystocele, rectocele, and uterine prolapse, and vulvar dystrophies are not a consequence of estrogen deprivation.

Although it is argued that genuine stress incontinence will not be affected by treatment with estrogen, others contend that estrogen treatment improves or cures stress incontinence in over 50% of patients due to a direct effect on the urethral mucosa.[135, 136] Most cases of urinary incontinence in elderly women are a mixed problem with a significant component of urge incontinence that definitely can be improved by estrogen therapy.

Dysparcunia seldom brings older women to our offices. A basic reluctance to discuss sexual behavior still permeates our society, especially among older patients and physicians. Gentle questioning may lead to estrogen treatment of atrophy and enhancement of sexual enjoyment. Objective measurements have demonstrated that vaginal factors that influence the enjoyment of sexual intercourse can be maintained by appropriate doses of estrogen.[137] Both patient and clinician should be aware that a significant response can be expected by one month, but it takes a long time to fully restore the genitourinary tract (6–12 months), and clinicians and patients should not be discouraged by an apparent lack of immediate response. Furthermore, sexual activity by itself supports the circulatory response of the vaginal tissues and enhances the therapeutic effects of estrogen. Therefore sexually active older women will have less atrophy of the vagina even without estrogen.

A decline in skin collagen content and skin thickness that occurs with aging can be considerably avoided by postmenopausal estrogen therapy.[138–141] The effect of estrogen on collagen is evident in both bone and skin; bone mass and collagen decline in parallel after menopause and estrogen treatment reduces collagen turnover and improves collagen quality.[142, 143] Although it is uncertain whether estrogen treatment can affect physical appearance, at least one study demonstrated not only an increase in facial skin thickness, but an improvement in wrinkles with topical estrogen.[144] More impressively, data from the U.S. First National Health and Nutrition Examination Survey indicated that estrogen use was associated with a lower prevalence of skin wrinkling and dry skin.[145] However, smoking is a major risk factor for facial skin wrinkling, and hormone therapy cannot diminish this impact of smoking.[146]

One of the features of aging in men and women is a steady reduction in muscular strength. Many factors affect this decline, including height, weight, and level of physical activity. However, women currently using estrogen have been reported to demonstrate a lesser decline in muscular strength, although at least one study could detect no impact of estrogen[147–149] This is an important issue because of the potential protective consequences against fractures, as well as a benefit due to the ability to maintain vigorous physical exercise.

Psychophysiologic Effects

The view that menopause has a deleterious effect on mental health is not supported in the psychiatric literature, or in surveys of the general population.[121, 122, 150, 151] The concept of a specific psychiatric disorder (involutional melancholia) has been abandoned. Indeed, depression is less common, not more common, among middle-aged women, and the menopause cannot be linked to psychological distress.[3–9, 152] The longitudinal study of premenopausal women indicates that hysterectomy with or without oophorectomy is not associated with a negative psychological impact among middle-aged women.[153] And longitudinal data from the Massachusetts Women's Health Study document that menopause is not associated with an increased risk of depression.[154] Although women are more likely to experience depression than men, this sex difference begins in early adolescence not at menopause.[155]

The U.S. National Health Examination Follow-up Study includes both longitudinal and cross-sectional assessments of a nationally representative sample of women. This study has found no evidence linking either natural or surgical menopause to psychologic distress.[156] Indeed, the only longitudinal change was a slight decline in the prevalence of depression as women aged through the menopausal transition. Results in this study were the same in estrogen users and non-users.

A negative view of mental health at the time of the menopause is not justified; many of the problems reported at the menopause are due to the vicissitudes of life.[157, 158] Thus, there are problems encountered in the early postmenopause that are seen frequently, but their causal relation with estrogen is unlikely. These problems include fatigue, nervousness, headaches, insomnia, depression, irritability, joint and muscle pain, dizziness, and palpitations. Indeed, men and women at this stage of life both express a multitude of complaints, which do not reveal a gender difference that could be explained by a hormonal cause.[159]

Attempts to study the effects of estrogen on these problems have been hampered by the subjectivity of the complaints (high placebo responses) and the "domino effect" of what reduction of hot flushes does to the frequency of the symptoms. Using a double-blind crossover prospective study format, Campbell and Whitehead concluded many years ago that many symptomatic "improvements" ascribed to estrogen therapy result from relief of hot flushes—a "domino" effect.[160]

A study of 2001 Australian women aged 45–55 focused on the utilization of the health care system by women in the perimenopausal period of life.[11] Users of the health care system in this age group were frequent previous users of health care, less healthy, and had more psychosomatic symptoms and vasomotor reactions. These women were more likely to have had a significant previous adverse health history, including a past history of premenstrual complaints. This study emphasized that perimenopausal women who seek health care help are different from those who do not seek help, and they often embrace hormone therapy in the hope it will solve their problems. Similar findings have been reported in a cohort of British women.[161] It is this population that is seen most often by clinicians, producing biased opinions regarding the menopause among physicians. We must be careful not to generalize to the entire female population the behavior experienced by this relatively small group of women. Most importantly, perimenopausal women who present to clinicians often end up being treated with estrogen inappropriately and unnecessarily. Nevertheless, it is well-established that a woman's quality of life is disrupted by vasomotor symptoms, and estrogen therapy provides impressive improvement.[162, 163] Patients are grateful to be the recipients of this "domino" effect.

Emotional stability during the perimenopausal period can be disrupted by poor sleep patterns. Hot flushing does have an adverse impact on the quality of sleep.[164] Estrogen therapy improves the quality of sleep, decreasing the time to onset of sleep and increasing the rapid eye movement (REM) sleep time.[162, 165, 166] Perhaps flushing may be insufficient to awaken a woman but sufficient to affect the quality of slep, thereby diminishing the ability to handle the next day's problems and stresses. An improvement in insomnia with estrogen treatment can even be documented in postmenopausal women who are reportedly asymptomatic.[166]

Thus, the overall "quality of life" reported by women can be improved by better sleep and alleviation of hot flushing. However, it is still uncertain whether estrogen treatment has an additional direct pharmacologic antidepressant effect or hether the mood response is an indirect benefit of relief from physical symptoms and, consequently, improved sleep. Utilizing various assessment tools for measuring depression, improvements with estrogen treatment have been recorded in oophorectomized women.[167, 168] In the large prospective cohort study of the Rancho Bernardo retirement community, no benefit could be detected in measures of depression in current users of postmenopausal estrogen compared with untreated women.[169] Indeed, treated women had higher depressive symptom scores, presumably reflecting treatment selection bias; symptomatic and depressed women seek hormone therapy. Nevertheless, estrogen therapy is reported to have a more powerful impact on women's well-being beyond the relief of symptoms such as hot flushes.[170] In elderly depressed women, improvements in response to fluoxetine were enhanced by the addition of estrogen therapy.[171]

Cognition and Alzheimer's Disease

Depending on the method of assessment, evidence for beneficial effects of estrogen on cognition can be found in the literature, especially in verbal memory.[172, 173] However, the effects n healthy wome are not impressive, and perhaps of little clinical value. A short-term study failed to document an objective improvement in memory, although a slight improvement in moo was recorded.[174] Another short-term (3 months) randomized, double-blind study could detect no improvement in cognitive performance compared with placebo treatment.[175] On the other hand, estrogen treatment of women immediately after bilateral oophorectomy was associated with improvement in certain, but not all, specific tests of memory, and healthy postmenopausal women taking estrogen scored higher on tests of immediate and delayed recall.[176, 177] In a case-control study of women aged 55–93 years, estrogen users had better recall of proper names, but no improvement in word recall.[178] Women in the Baltimore Longitudinal Study of Aging who were using estrogen performed better in a test of short-term visual memory.[179] In a New York City cohort of women, the use of estrogen was associated with better performance in tests of cognition, and better performance in verbal memory.[180] Perhaps a lack of agreement is due to the variability in test vehicles and the specific aspects of memory function studied. Furthermore, there is impressive individual variability, and when differences have been observed they have not been large, and perhaps of little clinical importance. In addition, any beneficial effects may be attenuated by progestational agents.[173] Fatigue, irritability, headache, and depression are not thought to be estrogen-related phenomena.

Tests of cognitive function in the prospective cohort study of the Rancho Bernardo retirement community failed to support a positive impact of postmenopausal estrogen on mental function in old age.[181] The Rancho Bernardo study has the attribute of being large in size (800 women), which also allowed for testing of duration of use (there was no benefit that resulted from long duration of use). There were too few patients in the Rancho Bernardo cohort with dementia to assess the impact of estrogen on Alzheimer's disease.

Up to 3 times as many women as men develop Alzheimer's disease. Estrogen is capable of protecting central nervous system function by means of multiple mechanisms. For example, estrogen protects against neuronal cytotoxicity induced by oxidation; estrogen reduces the serum concentration of amyloid P component (the glycoprotein found in Alzheimer's neurofibrillary tangles); and estrogen increases synapses and neuronal growth, especially dendritic spine density.[182–184] Progestational agents do not exert similar actions.

Important early findings have indicated that Alzheimer's disease and related dementia occurred less frequently (perhaps as much as 60% less) in estrogen users, and the effect was greater with increasing dose and duration of use.[185, 186] In the Baltimore Longitudinal Study of Aging (a prospective cohort), the risk of Alzheimer's disease was 54% reduced, in a cohort in New York City, the risk was reduced 60%, and in the Italian Longitudinal Study of Aging, the risk was 72% reduced in estrogen users.[187–189] Furthermore, the administration of estrogen to patients with Alzheimer's disease has improved cognitive performance.[190] The presence of estrogen therapy also enhances the beneficial response to tacrine in women with Alzheimer's disease.[191] If this effect of estrogen can be verified in the ongoing clinical trials, the potential impact on this dreadful condition that is more prevalent in women cannot be underrated. This would be another argument in favor of long-term treatment.

Cardiovascular Disease

Diseases of the heart are the leading cause of death for women in the United States, followed by malignant neoplasms, cerebrovascular disease, and motor vehicle accidents. Since 1984, the number of cardiovascular disease deaths for women has exceeded those for men.[32] About 20,000 women under age 65 die of myocardial infarction each year in the U.S. The death rate for coronary heart disease in women is approximately 3 times greater then the rates for breast cancer and lung cancer. Female survivors of a first myocardial infarction face the prospects of a second myocardial infarction in 31%, a stroke in 18%, and sudden death in 6%.

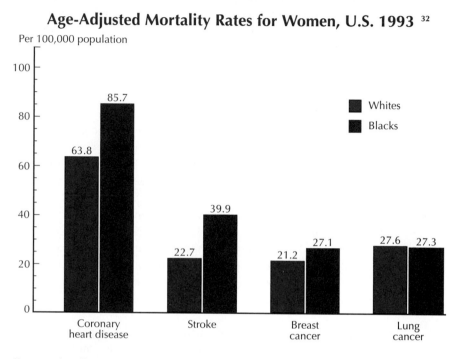

Age-Adjusted Mortality Rates for Women, U.S. 1993 [32]

Most cardiovascular disease results from atherosclerosis in major vessels. The risk factors are the same for men and women: high blood pressure, smoking, diabetes mellitus, and obesity. However, when controlling for these risk factors, men have a risk of developing coronary heart disease over 3.5 times that of women. Even taking into consideration the changing lifestyle of women (e.g., employment outside the home), women still maintain their advantage in terms of risk for coronary heart disease. With increasing age, this advantage is gradually lost, and cardiovascular disease becomes the leading cause of death for both older women and older men.

Cardiovascular disease, especially atherosclerosis, is a consequence of multiple metabolic changes that interact with each other.

1. Adverse changes in the circulating lipid-lipoprotein profile.

2. Oxidation of LDL, producing a modified LDL that is chemotactic for circulating monocytes, that inhibits macrophage motility (thus trapping macrophages in the intima), and that causes cell injury and death in the endothelium.

3. Endothelial injury and dysfunction affecting nitric oxide and prostacyclin production.

4. Macrophage migration and functions, influenced by growth factors and cytokines.

5. Proliferation and migration of smooth muscle cells, also influenced by growth factors and cytokines; these cells become the dominant cell type and the source of the connective tissue matrix in the atherosclerotic lesion, the fibrous plaque.

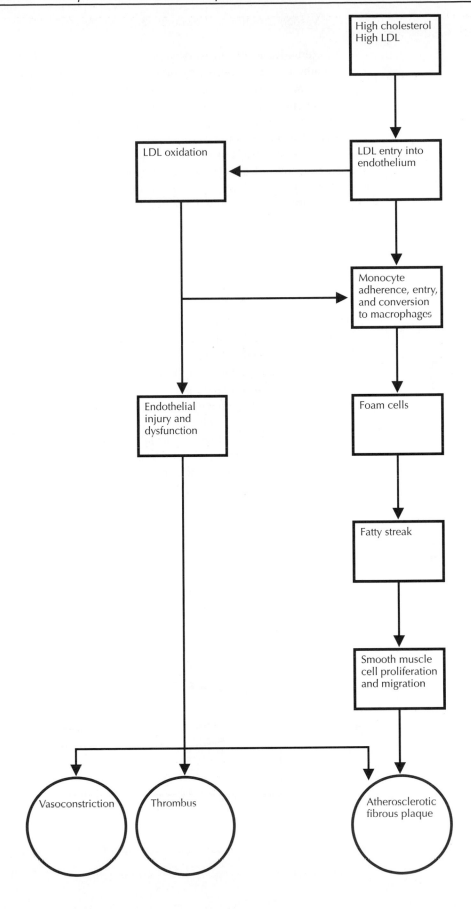

6. Vasoconstriction and thrombogenic events.

7. Remodeling of coronary arteries. An artery is able to respond to a developing atherosclerotic plaque by increasing its overall diameter in an attempt to maintain flow.[192] The mechanism of this adaptive remodeling is not known, but the extent of this process must affect the risk of occlusion and infarction.

The fatty streak in arterial vessels is the precursor to clinically significant lesions. The fatty streak lesion, therefore, antedates the fibrous plaque, developing under the endothelial surface and dominated by fat-laden macrophages (the foam cells). The process is initiated by the aggregation and adherence of circulating monocytes to a site on the arterial endothelium. When the monocytes penetrate through the endothelium and enter the intima, they become loaded with lipids and converted to the foam cells. Modification of LDL, especially oxidation, is crucial in this conversion of monocytes to foam cells. The initial step, adherence of monocytes to endothelium, can be induced by elevated cholesterol and LDL-cholesterol in the circulation.

During the reproductive years, women are "protected" from coronary heart disease. For this reason, women lag behind men in the incidence of coronary heart disease by 10 years, and for myocardial infarction and sudden death, women have had a 20-year advantage. The reasons for this are complex, but a significant contribution to this protection can be assigned to the higher high-density lipoprotein (HDL) levels in younger women, an effect of estrogen. Throughout adulthood, the blood HDL-cholesterol level is about 10 mg/dL higher in women, and this difference continues through the postmenopausal years. Total and low-density (LDL)-cholesterol levels are lower in premenopausal women than in men, although the levels gradually increase with aging and after menopause they rise rapidly.[193–196] After menopause the risk of coronary heart disease doubles for women as the atherogenic lipids about age 60 reach levels greater than those in men. These changes can be favorably reduced by dietary changes.[197, 198] Of course, these lipid changes at menopause (whether natural or surgical) can be reversed with estrogen treatment.[199] At all ages, however, HDL-cholesterol values in women are 10 mg/dL higher than in men.

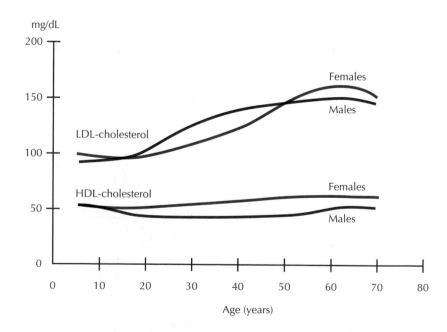

Prospective studies have documented the strong association between total cholesterol and coronary heart disease in women; however, coronary heart disease risk appears at higher total cholesterol levels for women than for men.[200, 201] Women with total cholesterol concentrations greater than 265 mg/dL have rates of coronary heart disease 3 times that of women with low levels. Even in elderly women, a high total cholesterol remains a significant predictor of heart disease; but the strength of the association between the cholesterol level and cardiovascular disease decreases with aging, and by age 80 the cost and benefits may not justify cholesterol intervention.[202] This is the reason for ceasing lipoprotein screening after age 75 in patients with normal lipids. However, this decision should be individualized, taking into account the vigor and health of the patient.

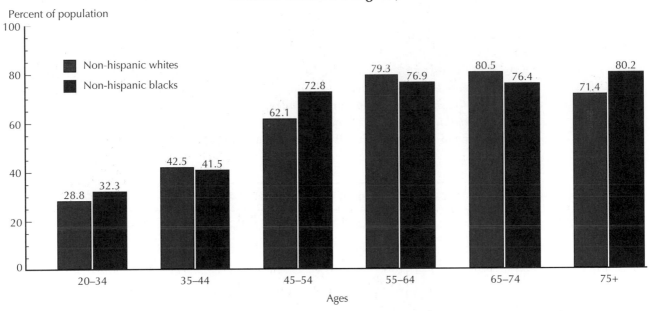

**Percentage of U.S. Women with Blood Cholesterol [32]
Greater than 200 mg/dL, 1991**

The strongest predictor of coronary heart disease in women is a low HDL-cholesterol,[200, 201, 203] The average HDL-cholesterol in women is approximately 55–60 mg/dL. A decrease in HDL-cholesterol of 10 mg/dL increases coronary heart disease risk by 40–50%. In women (and men) who have normal total cholesterol and LDL-cholesterol levels, but low HDL-cholesterol levels, treatment with lovastatin reduced the risk of an acute major coronary event by approximately 37%.[204] Women with very high HDL-cholesterol levels (over 55–60 mg/dL) have virtually no increased risk of heart disease even in the presence of elevated concentrations of total cholesterol. *It is appropriate to be concerned when HDL-cholesterol levels are less than 50 mg/dL.*

The Optimal Cholesterol/Lipoprotein Profile

Total cholesterol	— Less than 200 mg/dL
HDL-cholesterol	— Greater than 50 mg/dL
LDL-cholesterol	— Less than 130 mg/dL
Triglycerides	— Less than 250 mg/dL

In some studies, elevated LDL-cholesterol has been identified as a predictor of coronary heart disease in women, but in others it has not.[205, 206] It should be emphasized that modest elevations in blood pressure markedly increase the risk associated with an elevated LDL-cholesterol or a low HDL-cholesterol.

Triglycerides are also an important risk factor for coronary heart disease in women; however, an increased rate of cardiovascular disease is observed only when increased triglyceride levels are present in association with low HDL-cholesterol levels,[206, 207] If the triglyceride level is greater than 400 mg/dL and the HDL-cholesterol is less than 50 mg/dL, the risk of heart disease is substantially increased. Patients with an elevated triglyceride level and a positive family history for heart disease most likely have an autosomal dominant disorder classified as familial combined hyperlipidemia. This disorder accounts for most myocardial infarctions in women less than 40 years old. Triglyceride levels of 200–400 mg/dL are considered borderline elevated. Triglyceride levels can be elevated because of obesity, smoking, and lack of exercise. Weight loss alone can return elevated triglyceride levels to normal.

The proportion of HDL-cholesterol in the total cholesterol decreases with age in women and results in an age-related increase in the ratio of total cholesterol to HDL-cholesterol, from 3.4 at ages 25–34 years to 4.7 at ages 75–89 years. When the ratio exceeds 7.5, women have the same coronary heart disease risk as men. The optimal ratio is about 3.5, and risk increases significantly above 5.0. *For ease of remembering, consider anything below 4.0 as good and any ratio above 4.0 as unhealthy.* However, attention should not be totally focused on this ratio; the LDL-cholesterol and triglyceride levels cannot be ignored, and the entire lipid profile should be assessed.

Heart Disease Risk Based on Cholesterol/HDL Ratio

Lowest risk	— Less than 2.5
Below average risk	— 2.5–3.7
Average risk	— 3.8–5.6
High risk	— 5.7–8.3
Dangerous	— Greater than 8.3

An important contribution to the gender difference in cardiovascular disease prevalence and age of onset is the favorable effect of estrogen on important endothelial events. Vasodilatory and antithrombotic activities can be attributed to endothelial production of nitric oxide and prostacyclin, a process favorably influenced by estrogen. Hypercholesterolemia adversely affects this important endothelial process, and estrogen protects this important endothelial function in the presence of hypercholesterolemia.[208] Estrogen inhibits the oxidation of LDL, and also protects against the toxic effects of oxidized LDL on the endothelium.

Observational studies and clinical trials indicate that the major determinants of blood lipid levels are the same for both sexes. A diet high in saturated fatty acids and dietary cholesterol unfavorably increases blood lipids. Excess caloric intake and obesity decrease HDL-cholesterol and increase total cholesterol, LDL-cholesterol, and triglycerides. Smoking decreases HDL-cholesterol (and also produces lower estrogen levels and an earlier menopause). Genetic defects of receptor-mediated cholesterol uptake account for only a small percentage of hyperlipidemia in men and women. There is also evidence that men and women who had impaired fetal growth have increased levels of cholesterol and LDL-cholesterol in middle age.[209] The speculation is that impaired liver growth in utero produces a permanent adverse change in cholesterol and lipoprotein metabolism. Reduced fetal growth also leads to insulin resistance and lower HDL-cholesterol levels, most severe in those who become obese.[210]

Another newly appreciated factor is the connection between hormones and fat. Adiposity of the trunk is a risk factor for coronary heart disease in women and is associated with a relatively androgenic hormonal state, hypertension, and disorders of lipid and carbohydrate metabolism.[211] Central fat distribution in women is positively correlated with increases in total cholesterol, triglycerides, and LDL and negatively correlated with HDL.[212] The atherogenic lipid profile associated with abdominal adiposity is at least partly mediated through an interplay with insulin and estrogen.[213] It is worth noting that there is a strong correlation between the magnitude of the worsening in cardiovascular risk factors (lipid and lipoprotein changes, blood pressure, and insulin levels) and the amount of weight gained during the menopausal transition.[214] Attention to weight gain during middle age is one of the most important components of good preventive health care. However, weight gain at menopause is not an effect of hormonal changes, but it reflects diet, exercise, and aging.[214]

In the last 30 years, stroke mortality has declined by 60% and mortality from coronary heart disease by more than 50% in the U.S.[215] Improvements in medical and surgical care can account for some of this decline, but 60–70% of the improvement is due to preventive measures. Excellent data from epidemiologic studies and clinical trials demonstrate a decline in stroke and heart disease morbidity and mortality from smoking cessation, blood pressure reduction, and lowering of cholesterol.[216, 217] It is now recognized that there is a strong and growing scientific basis for preventive medicine and health promotion efforts in clinical practice.

We now have another opportunity. Postmenopausal hormone therapy deserves consideration as a legitimate component of preventive health care for older women. One can argue convincingly that protection against cardiovascular disease is the major benefit of postmenopausal estrogen treatment, and the magnitude of this benefit is considerable. There is a sound rationale for this protection in the link between cardiovascular disease and the sex hormones.

The Evidence for Protection Against Cardiovascular Disease by Estrogen

A review of case-control studies in the literature finds overwhelming support for about a 50% reduced risk of coronary heart disease in estrogen users.[218–231] A population-based case-control study in Rochester, Minnesota, concluded that if all eligible women utilized estrogen, myocardial infarctions could be reduced as much as 45%, an impact comparable with the elimination of smoking or the prevention of hypertension.[231]

One important and large cross-sectional study (1444 cases and 744 controls) compared post-menopausal women undergoing coronary arteriography and therefore utilized an objective end point for coronary disease.[226] The relative risk of coronary disease was decreased 56% in estrogen users after adjustment for age, cigarette smoking, diabetes, cholesterol, and hypertension. Even women over age 70 demonstrated a 44% reduction in risk. In three other studies of women undergoing angiography, a comparison of coronary artery occlusion in users and nonusers of estrogen indicated a significant protective effect of postmenopausal estrogen.[227–229]

In cohort studies, only two produced conflicting data.[232–244] The Walnut Creek Study, one initially with conflicting data, had, in its first report, only 26 women with myocardial infarctions, and only 9 were estrogen users.[235] An update of the Walnut Creek data documented a 50% reduction in death from diseases of the circulatory system when adjusted for all other factors.[245]

The Framingham Heart Study presented data in 1978, and in 1985, which argued that there was a 50% *increased* risk for cardiovascular disease among estrogen users, although there was no difference in fatality rates between users and nonusers.[233, 236] Because of the respect the Framingham Heart Study carries, its impact was significant. Subsequent re-analysis of the Framingham data (eliminating angina as a consideration) by the authors of the study reversed their conclusion.[246] The early reports from the Framingham Heart Study, therefore, stand in lonely opposition to overwhelming evidence that appropriately low doses of estrogen protect postmenopausal women against cardiovascular disease.

In the Nurses' Health Study with 16 years of follow-up, the age-adjusted relative risk of coronary disease in current users of estrogen alone was 40% reduced, and with estrogen and progestin, 61% reduced.[243] No association between use and stroke was observed, but there were relatively few strokes in this cohort. Adjustments for diet, use of vitamins, use of aspirin, and physical activity did not change the conclusions. The beneficial impact was observed to diminish beginning 3 years after discontinuation. It was suggested that higher doses might be harmful because there was an apparent increase in the risk of coronary disease among women taking more than 0.625 mg conjugated estrogens per day. Current postmenopausal hormone users in the Nurses' Health Study have had a 37% reduced risk of mortality, due largely to protection against coronary heart disease, an effect that was still present after adjusting for dietary factors, alcohol intake, vitamin or aspirin use, and exercise.[244]

The Lipid Research Clinics Follow-up Study (a prospective 8.5-year follow-up of 2270 women) demonstrated a 63% reduction in the relative risk of fatal cardiovascular disease in current estrogen users, including a protective effect in current and exsmokers.[237] The National Health and Nutrition Examination Survey Epidemiologic Follow-up Study is a longitudinal study of a cohort derived from the first National Health and Nutrition Examination Survey (NHANES I) conducted from 1971 to 1975.[240] The use of estrogen significantly reduced (40% to 60%) the risk of cardiovascular disease regardless of the age of menopause. Long-term estrogen users (10–25 years) were identified in the Kaiser Permanente Medical Care Program in California and found to have a 46% reduced risk of all-cause mortality, largely due to reductions in cardiovascular disease.[247] Women who used estrogen for more than 15 years had a 30% greater reduction in the risk for mortality than short-term users.

Electron beam tomography (also called ultrafast computed tomography) can assess the presence of coronary artery disease by quantifying the amount of calcium in the coronary arteries, a measure that is known to correlate with the degree of disease and the risk of coronary events. Studies using this technique have demonstrated a lower prevalence of coronary artery calcium in women under age 60, a prevalence comparable to men (of any age) in women older than 60, and less calcium (and therefore less coronary artery disease) in women using postmenopausal hormone therapy compared with nonusers.[248]

An important question has been raised, asking whether estrogen treatment is a marker for variables (such as better diet and better health care) that place postmenopausal estrogen users in a low risk group for cardiovascular disease (the "healthy user" effect). And indeed, women who choose to use hormone therapy have been reported to have a better cardiovascular risk profile than nonusers.[249] This question has been addressed by the Lipid Research Clinics study, the Leisure World Study, and the Nurses' Health Study.[237, 250, 251] These epidemiologists concluded that their evidence strongly indicates that in women receiving estrogen treatment who have the same risk factors for cardiovascular disease as those not receiving treatment the same beneficial effect of estrogen is present. A cohort follow-up study in Southeastern New England documented similar levels of total cholesterol, HDL-cholesterol, body mass index, and blood pressure in estrogen users and non-users, indicating that selection of significantly more healthy women for estrogen use cannot fully explain the beneficial effect of estrogen on the risk of cardiovascular disease.[252] In a comparison of health variables among users and non-users in south Australia, there was no evidence to support the presence of a "healthy user" effect.[253] This issue will not be settled definitively until data are available from the ongoing long-term randomized clinical trials of postmenopausal hormone therapy.

Stroke

The incidence of stroke in women aged 45–64 years (1–2 per 1000 per year) has changed little in the past few decades; however, mortality rates have decreased.[254] In contrast to the uniform results from observational studies of the association between postmenopausal hormone therapy and coronary heart disease, epidemiologic data over the last 20 years regarding estrogen use and stroke have not been consistent. The many studies have indicated either no effect of postmeno-pausal hormone therapy on the risk of stroke or a reduction in risk associated with estrogen or estrogen-progestin use.[234, 235, 237, 243, 255–262]

In a large Danish case-control study, no impact could be detected of either estrogen or combined estrogen and progestin on the risk of non-fatal stroke, both thromboembolic and hemorrhagic.[261] A case-control study from Seattle found about a 50% reduced risk of subarachnoid hemorrhage with the use of postmenopausal hormone therapy, and the effect was even greater among smokers.[260] Positive relationships with duration and recency of use argued in favor of a causal association. In the prospective study of the Leisure World cohort, estrogen therapy was associated with a 46% overall reduction in the risk of death from stroke, with a 79% reduction in recent users.[255] This protection was present in both women with and without hypertension and in both smokers and nonsmokers. This level of protection was similar to that observed in this same Leisure World population for estrogen protection against deaths due to myocardial infarction.[239] The failure to observe protection against stroke in the Nurses' Health Study cohort is in striking contrast to the Leisure World cohort.[243] Indeed, in the Nurses' Health Study cohort, there was a slight increase (not statistically significant) in risk for thromboembolic stroke in current estrogen users. The population-based cohort study in Uppsala, Sweden, documented a 30% reduced incidence of stroke in postmenopausal users of estrogen, and, importantly, women prescribed an estrogen-progestin combination, containing a significant dose of the potent androgenic agent levonorgestrel, also experienced a reduced incidence of stroke.[259] A reduced risk for mortality from stroke in this Swedish study was confined to intracerebral hemorrhage.[263]

Within this confusing mixture of results, there is one consistent observation. The cohort studies (with a sufficient number of cases) that have assessed the impact of hormone use on the risk of death from stroke have all indicated a beneficial impact. For example, the National Health and Nutrition Examination Survey (NHANES) recruited a very large cohort of women in 1971–1975 for epidemiologic analysis. The follow-up longitudinal study of this cohort yielded a U.S. national sample of 1910 white postmenopausal women. Postmenopausal hormone use in this cohort provided a 31% reduction in stroke incidence and a strongly significant 63% reduction in stroke mortality.[258] These relative risks were present even after adjusting for age, hypertension, diabetes, body weight, smoking, socioeconomic status, and previous cardiovascular disease. This study specifically addressed the criticism that one should expect less disease in estrogen users because they are healthier. After adjusting for physical activity as a marker of general health status, the risk estimates remained identical. By virtue of the size of the cohort and the magnitude of the hormone effect, the results of this study provide impressive evidence of the beneficial impact of postmenopausal estrogen on the risk of dying from a stroke.

The epidemiologic evaluation of the association between postmenopausal hormone therapy and stroke is consistent with the possibility that hormone use decreases the severity of strokes, and, thus, reduces the incidence of fatal strokes.

Hypertension

Hypertension is both a risk factor for cardiovascular mortality and a common problem in older people. It is important, therefore, to know that no relationship has been established between hypertension and the doses of estrogen used for postmenopausal therapy. Studies have either shown no effect or a small, but statistically significant, decrease in blood pressure due to estrogen treatment.[264 268] This has been the case in both normotensive and hypertensive women.[269–271] The addition of a progestin does not affect this response.[272, 273] Discontinuing hormone therapy in women with hypertension does not result in a decrease in blood pressure (an expected response if the treatment were raising blood pressure), and in some patients discontinuation is followed by an increase in blood pressure.[274] The acute administration of estrogen to women with hypertension is followed by decreases in blood pressure, pulse rate, and circulating levels of norepinephrine.[275]

The very rare cases of increased blood pressure due to oral estrogen therapy truly represent idiosyncratic reactions. Because of the protective impact of appropriate estrogen treatment on the risk of cardiovascular disease, it can be argued that a woman with controlled hypertension is in need of that specific benefit of estrogen. Indeed, in the Nurses' Health Study, hypertensive women who used postmenopausal hormone therapy did have a reduced risk of coronary heart disease.[243] Blood pressure should be assessed every 6 months in hypertensive women being treated with postmenopausal hormones, and if the blood pressure is labile, every 3 months.

Mechanisms for Estrogen's Protection Against Cardiovascular Disease

A Favorable Impact on Lipids and Lipoproteins

The most important lipid effects of postmenopausal estrogen treatment are the reduction in LDL-cholesterol and the increase in HDL-cholesterol. Although it is now recognized that this is not the sole mechanism for estrogen's beneficial impact on cardiovascular disease, the lipid effects still play a substantial role.[276]

Estrogen increases triglyceride levels and increases LDL catabolism as well as lipoprotein receptor numbers and activity, resulting in decreasing LDL levels.[277–279] The increase in HDL levels, particularly due to the HDL_2 subfraction, is to an important degree the consequence of the inhibition of hepatic lipase activity, which converts HDL_2 to HDL_3. Postmenopausal estrogen therapy with or without added progestin also produces a beneficial reduction in the circulating levels of lipoprotein(a).[280]

LDL particle size gets smaller (potentially a more atherogenic adverse effect) with estrogen treatment, a change that is associated with an increase in the triglyceride content of LDL; however, it is not certain to what degree this change is related to dose nor is the clinical significance understood.[281] The addition of a progestin does not affect this response.[194, 272, 273] Furthermore, although small LDL is more atherogenic because it is more easily oxidized, this change in LDL particle size may be compensated by the antioxidant activity of estrogen, which protects against atherosclerosis by inhibiting lipoprotein oxidation.[282] Indeed, in the monkey, a smaller, more dense LDL is produced in response to estrogen, and this smaller LDL is less atherogenic.[283] In addition, the increase in triglycerides is associated with an increase in a form (buoyant) of very low density lipoprotein (VLDL), a form that is more rapidly transported and thus less likely to be atherogenic.[284] Therefore, estrogen induces a change in LDL toward a smaller more dense particle, but it is in a form with a more rapid turnover in the circulation, allowing less time for oxidation and acquisition of cholesterol.

The changes in circulating apoprotein levels mirror those of the lipoproteins: apolipoprotein B (the principal surface protein of LDL) levels diminish in response to estrogen, and apolipoprotein A-I (the principal apolipoprotein of HDL) increases. The HDL and triglyceride increases induced by estrogen treatment are attenuated if progestins are added in sufficient doses.[272, 285, 286] Both estrogen and exercise favorably affect the lipid and lipoprotein profile; however, in a comparison of exercise and estrogen treatment, combining estrogen and exercise did not produce a synergistic outcome.[287] On the other hand, the concomitant administration of estrogen and an HMG-CoA reductase inhibitor (pravastatin) produced a more favorable change in the lipid profile in hypercholesterolemic women than either treatment alone.[288]

The degree to which estrogen-induced lipid changes contribute to the overall protection against cardiovascular disease exerted by estrogen is uncertain. One analysis suggested that 25% of the estrogen effect could be attributed to lipid changes.[237] Certainly the lipid story is not as important as we once thought it was; nevertheless, it should not be underrated. One study concluded that estrogen-induced lipid changes could reduce the risk of coronary artery disease by about 50% in women who have abnormal lipids.[281]

Direct Antiatherosclerotic Effects

Important studies in monkeys support the protective action of estrogen against atherosclerosis, emphasizing mechanisms independent of the cholesterol-lipoprotein profile. Oral administration of a combination of estrogen and a high dose of progestin to monkeys fed a high-cholesterol diet decreased the extent of coronary atherosclerosis despite a reduction in HDL-cholesterol levels.[289-291] In somewhat similar experiments, estrogen treatment markedly prevented arterial lesion development in rabbits, and this effect was not reduced by adding progestin to the treatment regimen.[292-295] In this same rabbit model, raloxifene also inhibited the development of atherosclerosis, but not as effectively as estrogen.[296] These findings of a direct effect against atherosclerosis suggest that women with already favorable cholesterol profiles would benefit through this additional action. And, in considering the impact of progestational agents, lowering of HDL is not necessarily atherogenic if accompanied by an increased estrogen impact.

The monkey studies have been extended to a postmenopausal model (ovariectomized monkeys). Compared with no hormone treatment, treatment with either estrogen alone or estrogen with progesterone in a sequential manner significantly reduced atherosclerosis, once again independently of the circulating lipid and lipoprotein profile.[297, 298] A direct inhibition of LDL accumulation and an increase in LDL metabolism in arterial vessels could be demonstrated in these monkeys being fed a highly atherogenic diet.[299] However, the daily administration of medroxyprogesterone acetate in this monkey model prevented the beneficial effect of conjugated estrogen on coronary artery atherosclerosis.[300]

In postmenopausal women, the prevalence of atherosclerosis is reduced using either estrogen alone or combined estrogen-progestin therapy as documented in the coronary arteries by CT scanning and in the carotid arteries by ultrasonography.[248, 301, 302]

Thus, estrogen exerts a protective effect directly on the arterial wall independent of its effects on circulating lipoproteins. The presence of sex steroid receptors in arterial endothelium and smooth muscle lends support for the importance of this direct action; however, the mechanisms involved remain unknown.[303] One important mechanism may be coronary artery remodeling. Atherosclerosis is associated with a compensatory change in coronary artery size that increases the magnitude of the lumen (a process called remodeling). It is important to note that the addition of a progestin did not attenuate the beneficial effect of estrogen on coronary remodeling in monkeys.[298] Involvement of estrogen and estrogen receptors is supported by the observation that atherosclerotic coronary arteries in premenopausal women demonstrate diminished expression of estrogen receptors compared with normal premenopausal arteries.[304]

Endothelium-Dependent Vasodilatation and Antiplatelet Aggregation

Endothelium modulates the degree of contraction and function of the surrounding smooth muscle, primarily by the release of endothelium-derived relaxing and contracting factors (EDRFS and EDCFs). In hypertension and other cardiovascular diseases, the release of EDRFs (which is probably one factor, nitric oxide) is blunted, and the release of EDCFs (the most important being endothelin-1) is augmented. The endothelins are a family of peptides that act in a paracrine fashion on smooth muscle cells. Endothelin-1 appears to be exclusively synthesized by endothelial cells. Endothelin-induced vasoconstriction is a consequence of a direct action on vascular smooth muscle cells, an action that is reversed by nitric oxide. Impaired release of nitric oxide, therefore, enhances endothelin action. Hypertension and atherosclerosis are believed to be influenced by the balance among these factors. Women have lower circulating levels of endothelin, and the levels are even lower during pregnancy and decrease in response to oral and transdermal estrogen treatment.[305, 306]

Nitric oxide (and estrogen) also inhibits the adhesion and aggregation of platelets in a synergistic manner with prostacyclin (also a potent vasodilator derived from the endothelium).[307, 308] These

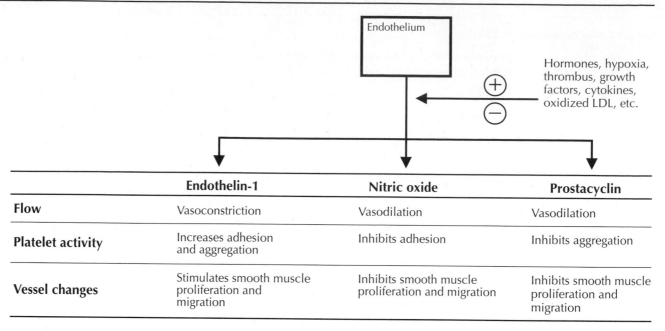

	Endothelin-1	Nitric oxide	Prostacyclin
Flow	Vasoconstriction	Vasodilation	Vasodilation
Platelet activity	Increases adhesion and aggregation	Inhibits adhesion	Inhibits aggregation
Vessel changes	Stimulates smooth muscle proliferation and migration	Inhibits smooth muscle proliferation and migration	Inhibits smooth muscle proliferation and migration

local actions are a likely site for sex steroid involvement; the vasodilating and antiplatelet action of estrogen, especially in the coronary arteries, is a consequence of endothelial responses. In addition, postmenopausal women experience greater stress-induced neuroendocrine and blood pressure responses that are ameliorated by estrogen treatment.[309, 310] However, the addition of medroxyprogesterone acetate (10 mg for 10 days) attenuated the beneficial effects of estrogen on measures of cardiovascular reactivity.[311]

Increased blood flow due to vasodilatation and decreased peripheral resistance can be observed to occur rapidly following the administration of estrogen. This response can be produced by both transdermal and oral administration.[312, 313] The synthesis and secretion of nitric oxide (the potent endothelial vasodilating product) can be directly stimulated by estrogen in in vitro experimental preparations of coronary arteries.[314] In both normal postmenopausal women and women with hypertension, hypercholesterolemia, diabetes mellitus, or coronary artery disease, the intra-arterial infusion of physiologic amounts of estradiol into the forearm potentiates endothelium-dependent vasodilatation, and there is a dose-response effect with enhanced responses limited to the production of high blood levels of estradiol.[315, 316] Nevertheless, comparing brachial artery responses in women who are long-term hormone users (with or without progestin) with non-users, improved endothelium-dependent vasodilatation could be observed with standard doses.[317] In a careful, randomized study, the addition of norethindrone acetate did not reduce the beneficial effect of estrogen on peripheral artery blood flow.[318] However, not all studies agree; a Danish assessment of brachial artery responses demonstrated no difference between postmenopausal women on long-term combined estrogen-progestin therapy compared with postmenopausal women receiving no treatment.[319]

The synthesis of nitric oxide is involved in the regulation of vascular (and gastrointestinal) tone, and in neuronal activity. A family of isozymes (nitric oxide synthases) catalyze the oxidation of l-arginine to nitric oxide and citrulline. The action of nitric oxide synthase in the endothelium is calcium dependent, and its synthesis is mediated specifically by estrogen.[320] In animal experiments, the endothelial basal release of nitric oxide is greater in females, a gender difference that is mediated by estrogen.[314, 321] In women treated with postmenopausal estrogen and either cyproterone acetate or medroxyprogesterone acetate, circulating nitric oxide (as reflected in nitrite-nitrate levels) is increased, a consequence of estrogen-induced nitric oxide production in the endothelium.[322, 323] In contrast, long-term treatment with estradiol and norethindrone acetate was not associated with changes in nitric oxide, endothelin-1, prostacyclin, or thromboxane A_2.[324]

Acetylcholine induces vasoconstriction in coronary arteries; however, the direct administration of estradiol in physiologic doses into the coronary arteries of postmenopausal women with and without coronary heart disease converts acetylcholine-induced vasoconstriction into vasodilatation with increased flow.[325] This favorable vasomotor response to acetylcholine can also be demonstrated in acute experiments with the transdermal administration of estradiol (achieving blood levels of 67–89 pg/mL).[326] This same estrogen-associated response is observed in women with coronary atherosclerosis comparing estrogen users to non-users.[327] This is an endothelium-dependent response, mediated to a significant degree by an increase in nitric oxide.[328] The administration of standard doses of estrogen to women with coronary artery disease reduces the degree of ischemia and delays the onset of signs of myocardial ischemia on electrocardiograms, and increases exercise tolerance.[329–331] In normal women, the standard oral 0.625 mg dose of conjugated estrogens had no effect on hemodynamic responses to treadmill exercise.[332] In the monkey, the vasodilatory response to acetylcholine requires a blood level of estradiol higher than 60 pg/mL.[333]

Endothelium-Independent Vasodilatation

Estrogen causes relaxation in coronary arteries that are denuded of epithelium.[334] This response is not prevented by the presence of inhibitors of nitric oxide synthase or prostaglandin synthase. Thus this vasodilatation is achieved through a mechanism independent of the vascular endothelium, perhaps acting on calcium-mediated events.[335] The vasodilatation produced by sodium nitroprusside is endothelium-independent. In normal postmenopausal women and postmenopausal women with risk factors for atherosclerosis (hypertension, hypercholesterolemia, diabetes mellitus, coronary artery disease), the administration of physiologic levels of estradiol increases forearm vasodilatation induced by sodium nitroprusside.[315]

Inotropic Actions on the Heart and Large Blood Vessels

Estrogen treatment increases left ventricular diastolic filling and stroke volume.[336–338] This effect is probably a direct inotropic action of estrogen that delays the age-related change in compliance that impairs cardiac relaxation.[339] In a 3-month study, medroxyprogesterone acetate (5 mg daily for 10 days each month) did not attenuate the increase in left ventricular output (systolic flow velocity) observed with estrogen treatment.[340] On the other hand, others have detected attenuation of estrogen's beneficial effects on compliance (stiffness) associated with combined estrogen-progestin treatment,[339, 341] And others have not been able to demonstrate an effect of short-term oral estrogen or long-term transdermal estrogen treatment on cardiac structure and function.[342, 343] The reasons for these differences are not apparent.

Improvement of Glucose Metabolism

An age-related decline in the basal metabolic rate begins at menopause, associated with an increase in body fat, especially central (android) body fat.[344, 345] Insulin resistance and circulating insulin levels increase in women after menopause, and impaired glucose tolerance predicts an increased risk of coronary heart disease.[346, 347] Estrogen (with or without progestin) prevents the tendency to increase central body fat with aging.[348–351] This would inhibit the interaction among abdominal adiposity, hormones, insulin resistance, hyperinsulinemia, blood pressure, and an atherogenic lipid profile. Hyperinsulinemia also has a direct atherogenic effect on blood vessels, perhaps secondary to insulin propeptides. In addition to its vasoconstrictive properties, endothelin-1 exerts a mitogenic effect and, therefore, contributes to the atherosclerotic process. Insulin directly stimulates the secretion of endothelin-1 in endothelial cells, and the circulating levels of endothelin-1 are correlated with insulin levels.[352]

Postmenopausal women being treated with oral estrogen have lower fasting insulin levels and a lesser insulin response to glucose, indicating another mechanism for the protection against cardiovascular disease.[353–356] However, not all studies have observed these favorable changes.[357] There is an important dose-response relationship; 0.625 mg conjugated estrogens improved insulin sensitivity, 1.25 mg did not.[358] The addition of a progestational agent can attenuate this beneficial response to oral estrogen, but the clinical impact and variation with dose are unknown.[358, 359] In a 1-year randomized trial comparing unopposed conjugated estrogens to the usual sequential and continuous regimens of conjugated estrogens and medroxyprogesterone acetate, no differences in the treatment groups were observed in the favorable decreases in fasting insulin levels.[355] Nonoral administration of estrogen has little effect on insulin metabolism, unless a dose is administered that is equivalent to 1.25 mg conjugated estrogens.[354, 359] Because a lower oral dose produces a beneficial impact, this suggests that the hepatic first-pass effect is important in this response.

Consistent with this salutary impact of estrogen, the Nurses' Health Study has documented a 20% decreased risk of noninsulin-dependent diabetes mellitus in current users of estrogen.[360] However, in the Rancho Bernardo cohort, no statistically significant difference could be detected comparing hormone users and never users.[361] There was a trend for the lowest incidence of diabetes among those who had received estrogen treatment throughout the period of follow-up, and the highest incidence was among never users, but the investigators believed this reflected the better health status of hormone users. Observational studies examining the incidence of diabetes mellitus are hampered by the biases of "healthy users" and preferential prescribing to women perceived to be at reduced risk of diabetes. Hopefully, the long-term randomized trials will provide reliable information regarding this potential benefit of hormone therapy.

A strong argument can be made that postmenopausal women with diabetes mellitus can benefit from the cardioprotective actions of estrogen. In addition, as noted above, estrogen may improve the metabolic changes associated with diabetes. Indeed, in double-blind, cross-over, placebo-controlled studies of postmenopausal women with noninsulin-dependent diabetes mellitus, estrogen treatment improved all glucose metabolic parameters (including insulin resistance), the lipoprotein profile, and measurements of androgenicity.[362, 363] These changes would reduce the risk of cardiovascular disease; however, long-term studies are yet to be available.

Inhibition of Lipoprotein Oxidation

The oxidation of LDL particles is a step (perhaps the initial step) in the formation of atherosclerosis, and smoking is associated with a high level of lipoprotein oxidation. In animal experiments the administration of large amounts of antioxidants inhibits the formation of atherosclerosis and causes the regression of existing lesions. Vitamin E and beta-carotene (the prohormone of vitamin A) are antioxidants. Studies indicate that the risk of myocardial infarction in smokers is higher in men and women with the lowest carotene levels, and supplementary intake of vitamin E decreases the risk of coronary heart disease.[364–366] The Nurses' Health Study reported a decreased risk of coronary heart disease in women with high carotene levels.[366] Thus, treatment with antioxidants may reduce the risk of cardiovascular disease and the risk of complications in those who already have cardiovascular disease.

Estrogen is an antioxidant. Estradiol directly inhibits LDL oxidation in response to copper, and decreases the overall formation of lipid oxides.[282, 367] Importantly, this antioxidant action of estradiol is associated with physiologic blood levels.[368] In addition, estrogen may regenerate circulating antioxidants (tocopherols and beta-carotene) and preserve these antioxidants within LDL particles. This antioxidant action of estrogen preserves endothelial-dependent vasodilator function by preventing the deleterious effect that oxidized LDL has on endothelial production of vasoactive agents.[369] There is evidence in the monkey in a short-term study that progesterone partially attenuates the inhibition of LDL oxidation by estradiol.[370] However, in an assessment of peroxide formation by platelets, women treated with both estrogen and medroxyprogesterone acetate in a sequential regimen had greater antioxidant activity compared with the days on estrogen alone.[371] And in a 1-year study, the presence of levonorgestrel did not attenuate the antioxidant activity of estradiol.[372]

A Favorable Impact on Fibrinolysis

Menopause is followed by increases in factor VII, fibrinogen, and plasminogen activator inhibitor-1 (PAI-1).[373, 374] These changes produce a relatively hypercoaguable state and are associated with an increased risk of cardiovascular events. Postmenopausal women treated with estrogen have lower fibrinogen and plasminogen levels.

Reduced levels of fibrinogen, factor VII, and plasminogen activator inhibitor-1 (PAI-1) have been observed in premenopausal women compared with postmenopausal women, and oral estrogen alone or combined with a progestin prevents the usual increase in these clotting factors associated with menopause.[357, 375–377] This would be consistent with increased fibrinolytic activity, another possible cardioprotective mechanism probably mediated, at least partially, by nitric oxide and prostacyclin. Platelet aggregation is also reduced by postmenopausal estrogen treatment, and this response is slightly attenuated by medroxyprogesterone acetate.[307] However, in a randomized 1-year trial, the addition of medroxyprogesterone acetate, either sequentially or continuously, produced a more favorable change in coagulation factors compared with unopposed estrogen.[378]

The transdermal and oral routes of administration of estrogen (combined with medroxyprogesterone acetate) have puzzling differences in the reported effects on most hemostatic risk factors, such as factor VII, fibrinogen, PAI-1, and antithrombin III. In at least one study, however, antithrombin III levels were reduced by oral estrogen, but not transdermal administration; however the values remained within the normal range.[379] In regards to PAI-1, studies with transdermal estrogen have provided us with conflicting data; for example, favorable changes in PAI-1 levels as well as no effect.[380, 381] However, in a crossover study designed to compare 100 μg transdermal estradiol with 0.625 mg oral conjugated estrogens (both combined with 2.5 mg medroxyprogesterone acetate daily), only the oral estrogen had a favorable reduction in PAI-1 levels.[381] Appropriate doses of hormone therapy have been reported to not have an adverse impact on clotting factors.[376, 382, 383] However, one study found slightly increased clotting activation with transdermal administration of estradiol, but no change with oral conjugated estrogens.[384] Fibrinopeptide A is an indicator of thrombin generation, and in 3-month studies, no significant alteration was produced by 0.625 mg conjugated estrogens in one and an increase in another.[385, 386] The clotting story is difficult to unravel. Perhaps one contributor to the uncertainty is a possible difference between short-term and long-term effects.[379, 382, 385]

Coagulation and Fibrinolysis Factors

> **Coagulation Factors:**
> > **Factors that favor clotting when increased**
> > > **Fibrinogen**
> > > **Factors VII, VIII, X**
> > **Factors that favor clotting when decreased**
> > > **Antithrombin III**
> > > **Protein C**
> > > **Protein S**
>
> **Fibrinolysis Factors:**
> > **Factors that favor clotting when increased**
> > > **Plasminogen**
> > > **Plasminogen activator inhibitor-1 (PAI-1)**
> > **Factors that favor clotting when decreased**
> > > **Antiplasmin**

Overall, estrogen treatment is associated with favorable changes consistent with an increase in fibrinolysis. The favorable changes in the clotting system may contribute to estrogen's protection of the cardiovascular system by inhibiting arterial thrombosis. How can there be a beneficial effect on arterial thrombosis when there is an increased risk of venous thrombosis (discussed in Chapter 18)? Why is there a difference between venous and arterial clotting? The venous system has low flow with a state of high fibrinogen and low platelets, in contrast to the high-flow state of the arterial system with low fibrinogen and high platelets. Thus, it is understandable why these two different systems can respond in different ways. Decreases in antithrombin III and protein S associated with estrogen treatment, a hypercoagulable change, may have a greater impact on the venous system.[386]

It is important to recognize the importance of the dose-response relationship between estrogen and the risk of arterial thrombosis. We learned from our experience with high-dose oral contraceptives that high doses of estrogen cause arterial thrombosis. Low doses of estrogen may even protect against arterial thrombosis. Thus, we refer to this important dose effect as a ***"narrow therapeutic window."*** (also discussed in Chapter 18) Doses of estrogen greater than those that protect against cardiovascular disease and osteoporosis (equivalent to 0.625 mg conjugated estrogens) should be avoided. At least 3 studies have found that estrogen doses greater than 0.625 mg conjugated estrogens are less beneficial in terms of coronary heart disease and mortality; however, the numbers of patients on the higher doses were relatively small, and these conclusions did not achieve statistical significance.[247, 250, 251]

Inhibition of Vascular Smooth Muscle Growth and Migration — Intimal Thickening

Hypertension and atherosclerosis are associated with increased proliferation of vascular smooth muscle cells. This growth of smooth muscle cells is also characterized by migration into the intima. Arterial intimal thickening is an early indicator of atherosclerosis. The proliferation and migration of human aortic smooth muscle cells in response to growth factors are inhibited by estradiol, and importantly, this inhibition is not prevented by the presence of progestins.[387, 388] Nitric oxide, which is regulated by estrogen, also inhibits smooth muscle proliferation and migration.[389] This smooth muscle response occurs following vascular injury, and this injury-induced reaction is inhibited by estradiol even in a mouse model deficient in the estrogen receptor-alpha, suggesting that the estrogen receptor-beta is an important component of blood vessel cells.[390] Only ER-β, and not ER-α, is expressed in endothelial cells obtained from umbilical veins.[391]

Imaging studies have documented a reduction in intimal thickening in postmenopausal women who are estrogen users compared with nonusers, and this beneficial effect is not compromised by the addition of a progestational agent to the treatment regimen.[341, 392, 393] Thus, postmenopausal hormonal therapy can bring about a reduction in atherosclerosis, and this effect is comparable with that produced by a lipid-lowering drug.[392, 394]

Protection of Endothelial Cells

Endothelial cells can respond to injury by initiating the clotting process or by atherosclerosis. Animals studies indicate that estrogen accelerates healing and recovery of the endothelium in response to injury.[395] This is correlated with inhibition of intimal thickening and recovery of important functions such as nitric oxide production. In vitro studies of human endothelial cells demonstrate that estrogen can inhibit cytokine-induced apoptosis.[396] In the rat, medroxyprogesterone acetate blocked the estrogen-induced healing response after carotid artery injuries.[397]

Inhibition of Macrophage Foam Cell Formation

A feature of atherosclerotic plaque formation is monocytic infiltration into the arterial wall and the formation of macrophage foam cells. In a non-antioxidant activity, estrogen inhibits macrophage foam cell accumulation in atherosclerotic lesions.[398]

Reduction of Angiotensin-Converting Enzyme (ACE) and Renin Levels

Although oral estrogen, but not transdermal estrogen, increases angiotensinogen levels, ACE and renin levels are decreased (with or without progestin) by both routes of administration.[399, 400]

Reduction of P-Selectin Levels

P-selectin is an adhesion glycoprotein that recruits leukocytes to the endothelium and plays a role in attaching platelets to endothelium. It is stored in and mobilized from platelets. Increased P-selectin expression has been demonstrated in atherosclerotic endothelial cells, and premenopausal women have lower circulating levels compared with men. Estrogen treatment lowers circulating levels of P-selectin, a change that should contribute to protection against atherosclerosis.[401]

Reduction of Homocysteine Levels

Increased circulating levels of homocysteine are correlated with increased risks of atherosclerosis and thrombosis. Homocysteine levels increase after menopause, and these levels are significantly lowered by estrogen or estrogen-progestin treatment.[402]

Summary — Estrogen and the Cardiovascular System

The possible beneficial actions of estrogens on cardiovascular disease include all of the following. A study in mice lacking the estrogen receptor-alpha suggests that some (perhaps many or all) of these actions are mediated by the estrogen receptor-beta or by nongenomic actions of estrogen.[390] ER-α and ER-β are both prevalent in coronary and aortic smooth muscle cells from monkeys.[403] Only ER-β is expressed in umbilical vein endothelial cells.[391]

1. **A favorable impact on the circulating lipid and lipoprotein profile, especially a decrease in total cholesterol and LDL-cholesterol and an increase in HDL-cholesterol.**

2. **A direct antiatherosclerotic effect in arteries.**

3. **Augmentation of vasodilating and antiplatelet aggregation factors, specifically nitric oxide and prostacyclin (endothelium-dependent mechanisms).**

4. **Vasodilatation by means of endothelium-independent mechanisms.**

5. **Direct inotropic actions on the heart and large blood vessels.**

6. **Improvement of peripheral glucose metabolism with a subsequent decrease in circulating insulin levels.**

7. **Antioxidant activity.**

8. **Favorable impact on fibrinolysis, at least partially mediated by endothelial nitric oxide and prostacyclin synthesis.**

9. **Inhibition of vascular smooth muscle growth and migration — intimal thickening.**

10. **Protection of endothelial cells from injury.**

11. **Inhibition of macrophage foam cell formation.**

12. **Reduced levels of angiotensin-converting enzyme and renin.**

13. **Reduction of P-selectin levels.**

14. **Reduction of homocysteine levels.**

Cardiovascular Disease and Progestins

Because the public health benefit of estrogen therapy on cardiovascular disease is of such enormous impact, it is vital that we know whether the addition of progestin attenuates estrogen's effects on the cardiovascular system. Conclusions regarding the impact of progestational agents on cardiovascular disease are very much influenced by dose and duration of administration of the progestational agent involved. While short-term studies suggest a negative impact of progestin (i.e., subtracting from the beneficial effect of estrogen), long-term studies indicate that this short-term effect disappears.

In sequential regimens, a review of the literature on this issue suggests a dose-response relationship.[404–412] A decrease in HDL-cholesterol has been noted with 10-day monthly treatment with norethindrone (5 mg), megestrol acetate (5 mg), levonorgestrel (250 µg), and even medroxyprogesterone acetate (10 mg). No significant change was noted with micronized progesterone (200 mg). The lack of an effect noted with micronized progesterone was observed with a dose (200 mg daily) that yields a normal luteal phase blood level of progesterone. A similar "physiologic" dose of synthetic progestins may be free of an adverse impact on HDL-cholesterol. Barrett-Connor and colleagues have been studying the adult residents of Rancho Bernardo, California. The women using both estrogen and progestin demonstrated the same favorable impact on cardiovascular risk factors as estrogen-only users compared with the nonusers.[413] On the other hand, a well-designed study indicated that although the sequential estrogen plus progestin program had a favorable impact on lipids and the lipoprotein profile, the impact (as measured one year later) was less than that achieved by estrogen alone.[414]

Studies with the combination of an estrogen and a low dose of a progestational agent administered continuously (every day without a break) are documenting a favorable impact on total cholesterol and LDL, with attenuation of the estrogen-induced increase in HDL. The various formulations include estradiol and levonorgestrel,[415] estradiol and 1 mg norethindrone acetate,[416] estradiol and dydrogesterone,[417] estradiol valerate and levonorgestrel or cyproterone acetate,[418] ethinyl estradiol and 0.5–1.0 mg norethindrone acetate,[286, 419] and 0.625 conjugated estrogen and 2.5–5.0 mg medroxyprogesterone acetate.[420] Christiansen has documented the maintenance of a favorable lipid profile over a period of 5 years of treatment with continuous, combined estradiol and 1 mg norethindrone acetate.[416]

A large, prospective, 1-year randomized clinical trial compared sequential and combined regimens of conjugated estrogens and medroxyprogesterone acetate with unopposed estrogen.[355] Although the increase in HDL-cholesterol, HDL_2, and apolipoprotein A-I levels was greater with unopposed estrogen, there was still a significant increase with combined estrogen-progestin treatment. Importantly, the decrease in total cholesterol, LDL-cholesterol, apolipoprotein B, and Lp(a) was equivalent, comparing unopposed estrogen with either sequential or daily, combined estrogen-progestin. Fasting glucose and insulin levels were improved in all treatment groups. Similar results have been observed in a 2-year randomized trial with 2 mg estradiol and 1 mg norethindrone acetate.[421] A prospective case-control study indicated that the decrease in Lp(a) achieved by estrogen is attenuated by the addition of a progestin.[422] In a large cross-sectional study of 4958 postmenopausal women, a favorable impact on the lipoprotein profile and fasting insulin levels was observed in users of unopposed estrogen and combined estrogen-progestin compared with nonusers.[285] In Spain, 8 months of uninterrupted treatment with a daily dose of 2.5 mg medroxyprogesterone acetate in a combined estrogen-progestin program produced a favorable effect on the lipoprotein profile not substantially different from that achieved with estrogen alone.[423] Nevertheless, the bulk of evidence indicates that the addition of a progestin attenuates, but does not eliminate, the favorable increase in HDL achieved with estrogen treatment, whereas the beneficial decreases in total cholesterol, LDL, lipoprotein(a), and the apolipoproteins are maintained.[424]

Studies in women of arterial vascular resistance by Doppler ultrasound flow patterns have indicated no detrimental effects of exogenous progesterone or medroxyprogesterone acetate to the beneficial decrease in resistance (and increase in blood flow) produced by estrogen administration.[425, 426]

The Postmenopausal Estrogen/Progestin Interventions (PEPI) Trial

PEPI was a randomized, double-blind, placebo-controlled, 3-year trial of 875 postmenopausal women conducted in 7 clinical centers in the U.S.[272, 427] The participants were randomly assigned to the following treatment groups:

1. Placebo.

2. Estrogen alone, 0.625 mg conjugated estrogens daily.

3. Sequential estrogen and progestin, 0.625 mg conjugated estrogens daily and 10 mg medroxyprogesterone acetate days 1–12.

4. Sequential estrogen and progesterone, 0.625 mg conjugated estrogens daily and 200 mg micronized progesterone days 1–12.

5. Continuous combination estrogen and progestin, 0.625 mg conjugated estrogens and 2.5 mg medroxyprogesterone acetate daily.

The statistical analysis indicated that an increase in HDL-cholesterol levels was greater with unopposed estrogen (mean increase 5.6 mg/dL) and with sequential estrogen and micronized progesterone (mean increase 4.1 mg/dL), than in women receiving estrogen and medroxyprogesterone. However, as in the trials reviewed above,[355, 421] the decrease in LDL-cholesterol was essentially the same in all treatment groups, and significantly improved compared with the placebo group. There were no significant differences in systolic blood pressure, although all groups gradually increased systolic blood pressure with aging. There were no differences in diastolic blood pressure, and no changes with aging. The placebo group demonstrated the well-recognized increase in fibrinogen (a risk factor for cardiovascular disease) that occurs after menopause. All treatments prevented this increase in fibrinogen.

All treatment groups exerted a modestly favorable effect on fasting insulin and glucose levels, and the effect was greater in individuals with elevated fasting insulin concentrations.[428] These changes are consistent with a beneficial impact on insulin resistance, and most notably, the addition of a progestational agent, either medroxyprogesterone acetate or micronized progesterone, did not alter the responses.

The PEPI trial demonstrated a favorable impact on cardiovascular risk factors in women taking estrogen as well as combinations of estrogen and progestins. A major question is whether it is justified to interpret the results as indicating that a combination of estrogen plus micronized progesterone is clinically better because of the HDL-cholesterol responses. Studies have indicated that in women there is a 2–3% decrease in heart disease with a 1 mg increase in HDL-cholesterol. If this is accurate, then potentially the difference between estrogen and micronized progesterone compared with estrogen plus medroxyprogesterone acetate (a 3 mg HDL-cholesterol difference) would amount to a 9% difference in the risk of heart disease. However, the story is not that simple. Many of the beneficial actions of estrogen in terms of cardiovascular disease are dynamic effects on blood flow, atherosclerosis, the clotting system, and insulin levels. Given this complicated and multifactorial impact, the small difference in HDL-cholesterol is reduced in importance. It is worth emphasizing that the PEPI trial revealed the same beneficial effects in all treatment groups on LDL-cholesterol, fibrinogen, insulin levels, and glucose levels. In a Finnish ultrasonographic study, women receiving estradiol valerate and levonorgestrel had as great a reduction in large artery atherosclerotic plaques as those women on unopposed estrogen, despite a similar attenuation in HDL-cholesterol levels as observed in the PEPI trial.[429]

One of the important contributions of PEPI is to provide a good response to the criticism that the reason estrogen users have less cardiovascular disease is because clinicians give estrogen to healthier women. The results of this randomized trial demonstrate that estrogen has a greater impact compared with a placebo group, thus the design compensated for this criticism.

Clinical Events — Epidemiologic Data

The various mechanisms by which estrogen protects the cardiovascular system can be viewed as "surrogate end points," parameters by which the risk of cardiovascular disease can be assessed. A summary of the responses of these surrogate end points to the addition of progestational agents in estrogen regimens indicates a mixed story. This less than clear picture, we would argue, makes it impossible to determine with surrogate end points the overall effect of progestins on actual clinical events; e.g., myocardial infarctions. We must turn to epidemiologic data regarding actual clinical events, and here the data (just now emerging because estrogen and progestin use is relatively recent) are reassuring.

Progestin Effects on Estrogen Actions

ATTENUATION
1. **Increase in HDL and triglyceride levels.**
2. **Measure of acute reactivity; e.g., acute vasodilatation.**
3. **Cardiac inotropic activity; compliance responses.**
4. **Effect of estrogen on coronary atherosclerosis in the monkey.**

NO ATTENUATION
1. **Decrease in cholesterol and LDL.**
2. **Increase in fibrinolysis.**
3. **Inhibition of atherosclerosis (intimal thickening and remodeling).**
4. **Antioxidant activity.**
5. **Reduction in angiotensin converting enzyme (ACE) activity.**

UNCERTAIN
1. **Reduction in hyperinsulinemia.**
2. **Favorable changes in P-seletin.**
3. **Protection of endothelial cells.**
4. **Inhibition of macrophage foam cell formation.**

A report from the ongoing cohort study from Uppsala, Sweden, provided information from the follow-up of approximately 23,000 women who were prescribed hormone therapy.[430] Overall, there was a 30% reduction in myocardial infarction in women prescribed estradiol valerate or conjugated estrogens. What is especially noteworthy was a 50% reduced risk of myocardial infarction in women exposed to a sequential estrogen-progestin regimen consisting of 2 mg estradiol valerate and 10 days each month of levonorgestrel (250 µg). Treatment ith this combined estrogen-progestin product was also associated with a 40% reduced risk of stroke.[259]

In an updated assessment of the Uppsala cohort, reduced mortality rates were documented for ischemic heart disease and intracerebral hemorrhage.[263] Once again, an even greater reduction in the risk of mortality from these conditions was observed in those women taking an estrogen-progestin combination.

In a case-control study from Seattle, unopposed estrogen and sequential estrogen and progestin were associated with a 28% reduction in the risk of myocardial infarction, and the reduction increased with increasing duration of treatment in the current users.[431] There certainly was no evidence of attenuation secondary to the addition of a progestin. A retrospective cohort study by this same Seattle group determined prognosis in women surviving a myocardial infarction and detected a 36% reduced risk of re-infarction in current estrogen users, with a similar result in the one-third of their women on hormone therapy taking both estrogen and a progestin.[432] In a comparison of postmenopausal women in Finland receiving unopposed estrogen or a sequential regimen of estradiol valerate and levonorgestrel (250 µg for 10 days), both treatment groups had an equal reduction in ultrasonographically observed atherosclerotic plaques in the aorta and in the carotid and iliac arteries.[429]

Carotid arterial wall thickening and the prevalence of carotid stenosis can be assessed by ultrasonography. In a study unique because it consisted of women who were 65-years old and older, the same beneficial decreases in carotid atherosclerosis could be documented in users of estrogen alone compared with women who were current users of estrogen and progestin.[302] In this study of elderly long-term users of postmenopausal hormone therapy, the HDL-cholesterol levels were similar in the two groups of women. This raises the possibility that the attenuation of estrogen-induced increases in HDL-cholesterol attributed to progestin treatment may disappear with very long-term use of combined therapy.

As epidemiologic studies gather growing numbers of women on estrogen and progestin, there is consistent reporting of an even greater beneficial impact with combined estrogen and progestin than with estrogen alone. In the Nurses' Health Study report on mortality, the relative risk of death for current users of estrogen-progestin was 54% reduced compared with a 31% reduction with unopposed estrogen.[244] In the 16-year follow-up report of the Nurses' Health Study, the risk of coronary heart disease was reduced 40% in estrogen users and 61% in users of estrogen and progestin.[243] An explanation for this difference is not readily apparent.

The Heart and Estrogen/Progestin Replacement Study (HERS)

The HERS trial was a randomized, double-blind, placebo-controlled clinical trial to determine whether daily treatment with 0.625 mg conjugated estrogens and 2.5 mg medroxyprogesterone acetate would reduce coronary heart disease events in women with pre-existing coronary disease.[433] 2763 women (average age 66.7 years) were enrolled in 20 U.S. clinical centers and randomized to treatment and placebo beginning in February, 1993, and ending in July, 1998. Overall, there were 172 myocardial infarctions and coronary deaths in the hormone group and 176 in the placebo group, obviously no difference. However, over time, differences were recorded:

	Treated	Placebo	Relative Hazard (Risk) & Confidence Interval
Year 1	57 cases	38 cases	1.52 (1.01–2.29)
Year 2	47 cases	48 cases	1.00 (0.67–1.49)
Year 3	35 cases	41 cases	0.87 (0.55–1.37)
Year 4	33 cases	49 cases	0.67 (0.43–1.04)

Thus, there was an increase in events in the first year (mostly in the first 4 months), and after two years of treatment, the appearance of a beneficial impact (although the annual relative risks did not achieve statistical significance, the test for the trend was significant). The authors attribute the increasing beneficial impact noted with increasing duration of treatment to a favorable effect on lipids, a 11% decrease in LDL-cholesterol and an 10% increase in HDL-cholesterol after one year, compared with the levels in the placebo group.

The results of the HERS trial were surprising in view of the overwhelming evidence from observational studies that postmenopausal hormone therapy prevents coronary heart disease. The authors offered two possible explanations for the difference between the HERS trial and previous observational studies. First, they pointed out the common and favorite criticism of the observational studies: selection bias, specifically that healthier women choose to use postmenopausal hormone therapy and therefore develop less coronary heart disease. This issue was addressed earlier in this chapter, noting that several studies have adjusted for this factor and a favorable impact of hormone therapy on coronary heart disease was still present.[237, 250–252]

The authors further emphasized that the HERS trial consisted of older women with significant coronary heart disease, whereas observational studies have focused on primary prevention in younger and healthier women. However, there are observational studies that examined the impact of hormone therapy in women with pre-existing disease, and reported a beneficial effect.[237, 250, 432, 434–436] In the Leisure World study, estrogen users with previous myocardial infarctions, strokes, or hypertension had a 50% reduction in risk for death from a subsequent stroke or myocardial infarction.[250] In the Lipids Research Clinics study, the cardiovascular mortality in women with previous cardiovascular disease was reduced 85%. And most impressively, in women with severe coronary disease (documented by arteriography), estrogen users had a 97% survival rate at 5 years compared with a significantly different 81% rate in nonusers.[434] Estrogen therapy reduces the rate of restenosis in women who have undergone either coronary angioplasty or percutaneous atherectomy.[437] In women who have undergone coronary artery bypass surgery, the 10-year survival rate in estrogen users was 81.4% compared with 65.1% in nonusers.[435] In women who have been treated with estrogen after coronary angioplasty, case-control analysis indicated that the treated women had a better survival rate and experienced fewer subsequent myocardial infarctions.[436]

The HERS trial is also in disagreement with recent reports that estrogen treatment could produce a regression in atherosclerosis. Imaging studies have documented a reduction in intimal thickening in postmenopausal women who are estrogen users compared with nonusers, and this beneficial effect was not compromised by the addition of a progestational agent to the treatment regimen.[341, 392] Thus, postmenopausal hormonal therapy has been reported to bring about a reduction in atherosclerosis, and this effect is comparable to that produced by a lipid-lowering drug.[392, 394]

The size of the HERS trial was determined by power calculations based upon specific assumptions. A comparison of the pre-trial assumptions with the actual outcomes reveals important differences:

	Assumption	Actual
Clinical event rate in the placebo group	5% /year	3.3% /year
Drop-out rate	5% in year 1	18% in year 1
Conversion of placebo to treatment rate	1% /year	1.7% /year
Average follow-up	4.75 years	4.1 years
Recruitment	Paced	Late

These differences between the assumptions and the actual events raise the important question whether the trial achieved sufficient statistical power to provide confident conclusions. The authors indicated that this concern was *"partially"* compensated by an 18% increase in recruitment. But, here too, there was a problem. The reason why the average follow-up was less than expected is that most of the women were enrolled toward the end of the recruitment period. This seriously affected the accuracy of the impact of duration of treatment, an apparent beneficial effect in the HERS trial. Indeed, the late recruitment into HERS would have minimized this effect, and the apparent benefit in years 4 and 5 did not reach statistical significance (although a test for trend was significant). The apparent increasing protection with increasing duration of use is consistent with the preventive effect exerted by hormone therapy in the many observational studies. This is also important information for women who begin hormonal treatment at menopause and are contemplating long-term therapy.

The increase in events recorded in the first year is difficult to understand. The most attractive explanation is to attribute, as the authors did, the increase to prothrombotic effects of estrogen. However, there is a host of evidence that indicates that postmenopausal hormone therapy (with and without progestin) affects clotting factors in a pattern that favors fibrinolysis, an effect that should protect against thrombosis (reviewed earlier in this chapter). It may be that older women with atherosclerosis respond differently than younger, healthier women. In other words, increasing age and disease may change a woman's thrombotic sensitivity to estrogen, perhaps because of the presence of unstable atherosclerotic plaques.

The most disturbing thought about the HERS trial is that the results reflect the impact of the continuous presence of medroxyprogesterone acetate. The clotting factor studies fail to find a detrimental effect of medroxyprogesterone acetate. However, there is reason to believe that the continuous presence of medroxyprogesterone acetate could attenuate and even block the favorable effects of estrogen on atherosclerosis and vasomotor function. There is evidence in the monkey that medroxyprogesterone antagonises the favorable impact of conjugated estrogens on both the process of atherosclerosis and vasodilatation, but progesterone did not interfere with the ability of estrogen to inhibit atherosclerosis.[297, 300, 438, 439] Could attenuation of these estrogen effects make women with coronary heart disease more sensitive to any thrombogenic or ischemic effect of estrogen? In a study of mechanisms involved in the regression of atherosclerosis, conjugated estrogens did exert favorable activity (aortic connective tissue remodeling in response to lipid lowering) in the monkey, but medroxyprogesterone acetate prevented this action.[440]

Do the HERS results indicate a difference between sequential and daily, continuous regimens of estrogen-progestin treatment? The observational data have consistently failed to find any evidence that the addition of a progestational agent to estrogen therapy produced an attenuating impact on protection against clinical coronary events.[243, 244, 263, 430–432] However, this evidence is virtually all derived from experience with sequential regimens because the use of the daily, continuous methods is too recent for epidemiologic study. In our view, the HERS results combined with the experimental data derived from monkeys do raise concern. There are other treatment options, and products with new combinations are around the corner. At this point in time, treatment decisions must be informed clinical judgements, one of the reasons patients turn to their clinicians for assistance, an enduring and rewarding feature of the practice of medicine. All of the available evidence must be included in this decision making, not just the results of the HERS trial, and this evidence must be balanced with individual patient needs.

Protection Against Cardiovascular Disease Is the Major Benefit of Hormone Therapy

The uniformity and consistency of the literature on the effect of postmenopausal hormone therapy on the risk of cardiovascular disease are very impressive. All the population-based case-control studies and (with the re-analysis of the Framingham Heart Study) all of the prospective studies conclude that postmenopausal use of estrogens protects against cardiovascular disease. Sophisticated assessment and analysis (using the methods of information synthesis and meta-analysis) indicate that the effect of estrogen on heart disease is not controversial or ambiguous, but there clearly exists a protective benefit.[441, 442] We have such uniformity and consistency among the epidemiologic studies that the argument is very convincing. There remains, therefore, the important question of the nature and degree of impact due to the addition of progestational agents.

Epidemiologic evidence is accumulating to indicate that a progestational dose that protects the endometrium avoids significant attenuation of estrogen's cardiovascular benefits. These epidemiologic data, however, reflect largely sequential regimens, and soon, we anticipate the appearance of data derived from women using daily, continuous combined methods. Ultimately, the best information will be derived from large, randomized trials, specifically the ongoing Women's Health Initiative in the U.S. (to be completed in 2008) and the WISDOM trial (Women's International Study of Long-Duration Oestrogen use after Menopause) in the U.K. (to be completed in 2011).

In view of the impressive association between estrogen and cardiovascular health in women, it is not illogical to ask whether a little estrogen therapy would be good for men. The normal levels of estrogen in men are important. The experimental suppression of normal physiologic levels of estradiol in young men leads to a significant decrease in apoprotein A-I and HDL-cholesterol, particularly the HDL_2 subfraction.[443] A case report detailed a man with an inability to respond to estrogen because of disruptions in the estrogen receptor gene; this man had osteoporosis, hyperinsulinemia, and low levels of HDL-cholesterol.[444] The long-term administration of estrogen in relatively high doses to male to female transsexuals is associated with improvements in vascular function mediated by many of the mechanisms reviewed in this chapter.[445]

The acute administration of estradiol into the coronary arteries of men, however, did not produce the vasodilatation and increased flow in response to acetylcholine that have been observed in woen studied in a similar fashion.[446] The failure of this acute response y reflect the presence of androgens; e.g., androgen depletion of estrogen receptors. Given the major impact of cardiovascular disease in men, it makes sense that pharmacologic long-term treatment with a small dose of estrogen might have an impressive beneficial impact. Perhaps the administration of phytoestrogens to men will be an acceptable preventive health care approach.

Osteoporosis

Bone is a very active organ. A continuous process, called bone remodeling, involves constant resorption (osteoclastic activity) and bone formation (osteoblastic activity). Both osteoblasts and osteoclasts are derived from bone marrow progenitors, osteoblasts from mesenchymal stem cells and osteoclasts from hematopoietic white cell lineage. Cytokines are involved in this development process, a process regulated by the sex steroids.

The amount of bone at any point of time reflects the balance of the osteoblastic and osteoclastic forces, influenced by a multitude of stimulating and inhibiting agents. Aging and a loss of estrogen both lead to excessive osteoclastic activity. A decrease in calcium intake and/or absorption lowers the serum level of ionized calcium. This stimulates parathyroid hormone (PTH) secretion to mobilize calcium from bone by direct stimulation of osteoclastic activity. Increased PTH also stimulates the production of vitamin D to increase intestinal calcium absorption. Calcium increases and PTH levels return to normal. A deficiency in estrogen is associated with a greater responsiveness of bone to PTH. Thus, for any given level of PTH there is more calcium removed from bone, raising serum calcium which, in turn, lowers PTH and decreases vitamin D and intestinal absorption of calcium.

Osteoporosis, the most prevalent bone problem in the elderly, is decreased bone mass with a normal ratio of mineral to matrix, leading to an increase in fractures. *Osteopenia* is sometimes used to indicate low bone mass, whereas osteoporosis is reserved for low bone mass with fractures. Osteoporosis is a major global public health problem, and it is epidemic in the United States, presently affecting more than 20 million individuals.[447] The increase in osteoporotic fractures in the developed world is partly due to an increase in the elderly population, but not totally. A comparison of bone densities in proximal femur bones in specimens from a period of over 200 years suggested that women lose more bone today, perhaps due to less physical activity and less parity.[448] Other contributing factors include a dietary decrease in calcium and an earlier and greater loss of bone because of the impact of smoking. Our Stone Age predecessors consumed a diet high in calcium, mostly from vegetable sources.[449] However, the impact of the tremendous increase in the elderly population throughout the world cannot be underrated. Because of this demographic change, the number of hip fractures occurring in the world each year will increase approximately 6-fold from 1990 to 2050, and the proportion occurring in Europe and North America will fall from 50% to 25% as the numbers of old people in developing countries increase.[450]

Pathophysiology

Osteoporosis is characterized by microarchitectural deterioration of bone tissue, leading to enhanced bone fragility and a consequent increase in the risk of fractures even with little or no trauma. The skeleton consists of two bone types. Cortical bone (the bone of the peripheral skeleton) is responsible for 80% of total bone, while trabecular bone (the bone of the axial skeleton—the spinal column, the pelvis, and the proximal femur) constitutes a honeycomb structure filled with red marrow and fat, providing greater surface area per unit volume.

The subsequent risk of fracture from osteoporosis will depend on bone mass at the time of menopause and the rate of bone loss following menopause.[451] Although the peak bone mass is influenced by heredity and endocrine factors, it is now recognized that there exists only a relatively narrow window of opportunity for acquiring bone mass. Almost all of the bone mass in the hip and the vertebral bodies will be accumulated in young women by late adolescence (age 18), and the years immediately following menarche (11–14) are especially important.[452, 453] After adolescence, there continues to be only a slight gain in total skeletal mass that ceases around age 30, and in many individuals a decline in bone mass in the hip and spine begins after age 18.[453, 454] After age 30 in most people, there is a slow decline in bone mass density, approximately 0.7% per year. The importance of a normal diet and a normal hormonal environment during adolescence cannot be overrated.

The onset of spinal bone loss begins in the 20s, but the overall change is small until menopause. Bone density in the femur peaks in the mid to late 20s and begins to decrease around age 30. In general, trabecular bone resorption and formation occur four to eight times as fast as cortical bone. Beyond age 30, trabecular resorption begins to exceed formation by about 0.7% per year. This adverse relationship accelerates after menopause and up to 5% of trabecular bone and 1–1.5% of total bone mass loss will occur per year after menopause. This accelerated loss will continue for 10–15 years, after which bone loss is considerably diminished but continues as the aging-related loss. For the first 20 years following cessation of menses, menopause-related bone loss results in a 50% reduction in trabecular bone and a 30% reduction in cortical bone.[455, 456]

When estrogen levels decline, bone remodeling increases. Each remodeling unit is initiated by osteoclast excavation followed by osteoblast refilling. Estrogen exerts a tonic suppression of remodeling and maintains a balance between osteoclastic and osteoblastic activity; in the absence of estrogen, osteoclastic activity predominates, resulting in bone resorption. The precise mechanism of action for sex steroid protection of bones remains unknown; however a growing body of knowledge indicates complex interactions at the molecular level.[457] Increased efficiency of calcium absorption (probably secondary to estrogen-induced enhancement of the availability of vitamin D (1,25-dihydroxycholecalciferol) and a direct role for the estrogen receptors in the osteoblasts are likely important factors. Many estrogen-dependent growth factors and cytokines are involved in bone remodeling.[458] Estrogen modulates the production of bone resorbing cytokines such as interleukin-1 and -6, bone stimulating factors such as insulin-like growth factors I and II, and transforming growth factor-β. Estrogen increases vitamin D receptors in osteoblasts, and this may be a method by which estrogen modulates vitamin D activity in bone.[459] There is little evidence that estrogen affects bone by altering the circulating calcitropic hormones.[460] Thus, the actions of estrogen are primarily direct effects on bone and important effects on vitamin D metabolism, and renal and intestinal handling of calcium.

Estrogen is a critical hormone in both males and females. Males with mutations in the estrogen receptor alpha or who have aromatase deficiencies grow slowly and have markedly reduced bone densities.[444, 461] Analysis of the decline in testosterone and estrogen circulating levels with aging indicates that the amount of bioavailable estrogen circulating in the blood is the most consistent predictor of bone density in men and women.[462] And most impressively, a man with an aromatase deficiency, treated with estrogen, demonstrated that both androgens and estrogens are necessary in order to for males to reach optimal bone mass.[463]

The process is slower in blacks, and bone mass, adjusted for body size, is greater in black women. It is believed that racial differences in bone density are established in childhood and early adolescence.[464, 465] The reasons for this are not entirely clear; it is not simply a difference in estrogen metabolism.[466]

In general, bone mass is increased in black and obese women and decreased in white, Asian, thin, and sedentary women. Despite the greater bone mass (and lower fracture rates) in blacks, the impact of osteoporotic fractures in black women is still considerable. Black women are subject to similar risk factors for osteoporosis (thinness, high alcohol consumption), and, most impor-

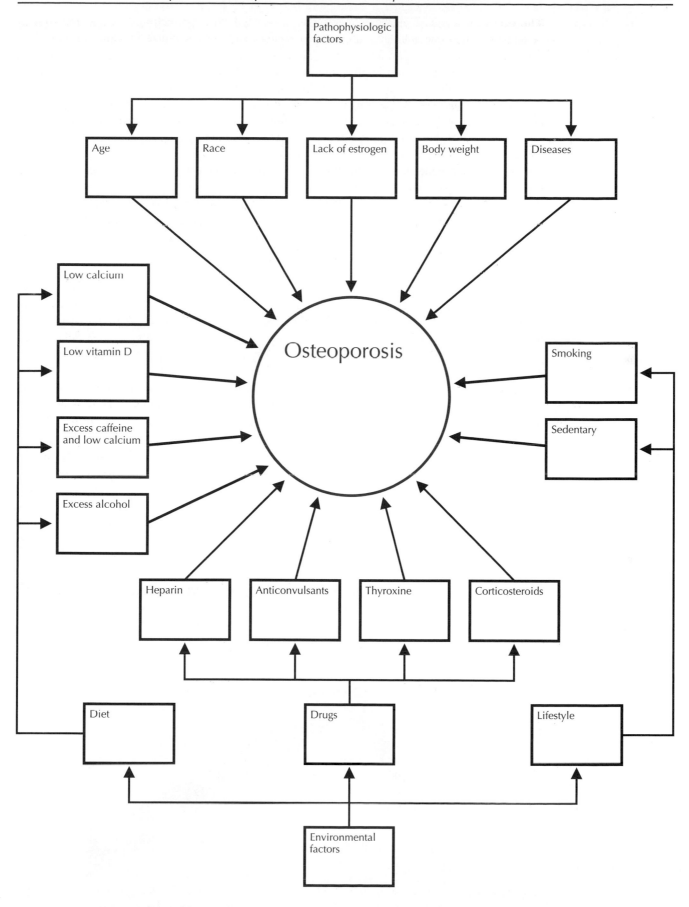

tantly, postmenopausal estrogen therapy is associated with protection.[467] Japanese women demonstrate the same amount and pattern of bone loss after menopause as white women.[468]

Although estrogen plays a principal role in regulating bone density, a genetic susceptibility is important. A study of the premenopausal daughters of women with osteoporosis revealed a reduction in bone mass, suggesting a genetic influence as well as the sharing of a lifestyle that produces a relatively low peak bone mass.[469] Studies of twins and mother-daughter pairs indicate that up to 70% of the variation in bone density is determined by heredity.[470]

Variations in the gene that encodes the vitamin D receptor are prevalent in postmenopausal women with decreased bone densities.[471] The absence of vitamin D receptor gene alleleic polymorphisms has been reported in older women who neither lose significant bone nor respond to calcium supplementation.[472] In addition, low bone density is associated with specific alleles of COLIA1, one of the two genes that encode the two polypeptides of collagen.[473] This opens the way to develop genetic markers to identify individuals at increased risk for osteoporosis, and, ultimately, to develop genetic therapy.

The change in trabecular bone in postmenopausal women is largely attributed to estrogen deficiency; 75% or more of the bone loss that occurs in women during the first 15 years after menopause is attributable to estrogen deficiency rather than to aging itself.[474, 475] Vertebral bone is especially vulnerable, beginning to decline as early as 20 years of age.[476] Vertebral bone mass can be found to be significantly decreased in perimenopausal and early postmenopausal women who have rising FSH and decreasing estrogen levels, while bone loss from the radius is not found until at least a year out from the menopause.[477] This early loss of axial skeleton bone suggests that the hypoestrogenic postmenopausal state is not the only cause of vertebral osteoporosis.[478] One obvious suspect is a decline in dietary intake of calcium in the premenopausal years, nevertheless menopause and the loss of estrogen remain as the major contributors to bone loss. The risk of fracture, therefore, depends upon 2 factors: the bone mass achieved at maturity and the subsequent rate of bone loss. A high rate of bone loss after menopause (the "fast loser") is highly predictive of an increased risk of fracture. The combination of a low bone mass and fast losing is additive, and thus, these individuals are at the highest risk of fracture. Fast losing probably reflects lower endogenous estrogen levels. The bone density, which is the threshold for vertebral fractures, is only slightly below the lower limit of normal for premenopausal women.[479]

Changes in Women's Bone Mass with Age

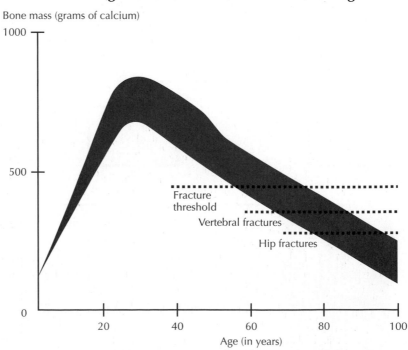

Bone Loss During the Perimenopausal Transition

Should a clinician be concerned about bone loss and consider interventions during the perimenopausal years? Some studies have concluded that calcium supplementation of perimenopausal women retards metacarpal and lumbar bone loss.[480, 481] However, the amount of perimenopausal bone loss is small unless estrogen levels are below normal.[482–484] Healthy women (exercisers and non-exercisers) who are anovulatory or who have inadequate luteal phase function (and thus are exposed to less progesterone) do not have an increase in bone loss.[485, 486] Interventions and treatments to prevent future osteoporosis are not necessary in women who have adequate estrogen levels and who are eating normally.

Signs and Symptoms

The osteoporotic disabilities sustained by the castrate or postmenopausal woman include back pain, decreased height and mobility, and fractures of the vertebral body, humerus, upper femur, distal forearm, and ribs. Back pain is a major clinical symptom of vertebral compression fractures. The pain with a fracture is acute, and then it subsides over 2–3 months, but lingers as chronic low back pain due to increasing lumbar lordosis. The pain will subside within 6 months unless multiple fractures produce a picture of constant pain.

Epidemiologic studies have revealed the following:[487]

1. ***Spinal (vertebral) compression fracture.*** Symptomatic spinal osteoporosis, causing pain, loss of height, postural deformities (the kyphotic Dowager's hump) with consequent pulmonary, gastrointestinal, and bladder dysfunction, is 5 times more common in white women than men. Approximately 50% of women over 65 years of age have spinal compression fractures; about two-thirds are clinically unrecognized. Each complete compression fracture causes the loss of approximately 1 cm in height. The average non-treated postmenopausal white woman can expect to shrink 2.5 inches (6.4 cm). The most common sites for vertebral fractures are the 12th thoracic and the first 3 lumbar vertebrae. These physical changes also have a negative impact on body image and self esteem.

2. ***Colles' fracture.*** There is a 10-fold increase in distal forearm fractures in white women as they progress from age 35 to 60 years. A white woman has approximately a 15% lifetime risk of a forearm fracture. Colles' fractures are the most common fractures among white women until age 75, when hip fractures become more common.

3. ***Head of femur fracture.*** The incidence of hip fractures increases with age in white women, rising from 0.3/1000 to 20/1000 from 45 to 85 years. Eighty percent of all hip fractures are associated with osteoporosis. White women have approximately a 16% lifetime risk of having a hip fracture. This fracture carries an increased risk of morbidity and mortality. Between 15–20% of patients with hip fracture die due to the fracture or its complications (surgical, embolic, cardiopulmonary) within 3 months, and Beals found that only half of hip fracture victims in Portland, Oregon, survived for 1 year.[488] However, most of this increase in mortality is due to underlying conditions and prevention of these fractures would have only a minor impact on longevity.[489] Nevertheless, the survivors are frequently severely disabled and may become permanent invalids. Hip fractures alone occur in more than 300,000 women per year in the U.S. with a mortality of 40,000 annually and an associated cost of billions of dollars.

4. *Tooth Loss.* Oral alveolar bone loss (which can lead to loss of teeth) is strongly correlated with osteoporosis, and the salutary effect of estrogen on skeletal bone mass is also manifested on oral bone.[490] Even in women without osteoporosis, there is a correlation between spinal bone density and number of teeth.[491] Tooth loss is also correlated with the use of cigarettes, a recognized contributor to bone loss.

Diagnostic Tests

Patients with osteoporosis should be screened for other conditions that lead to osteoporosis:

1. Serum parathyroid hormone, calcium, phosphorus, and alkaline phosphatase: for primary hyperparathyroidism.

2. Renal function tests: for secondary hyperparathyroidism with chronic renal failure.

3. Blood count and smear, sedimentation rate, protein electrophoresis: for multiple myeloma, leukemia, or lymphoma.

4. Thyroid function tests: for hyperthyroidism and excessive thyroid hormone treatment.

5. Careful history and, when indicated, appropriate laboratory studies to rule out hypercortisolism, alcohol abuse, and metastatic cancer.

The presence of osteomalacia, to be suspected in all elderly patients with osteoporosis, can be detected by measuring the serum calcium, phosphorous, alkaline phosphatase, and the 1,25-dihydroxyvitamin D levels. These are all normal in patients with osteoporosis.

The effect of excess thyroid hormone on bone is not entirely clear. Although it is recognized that excess thyroxine treatment can cause bone loss, retrospective studies of thyroid function and bone mass have not produced uniform conclusions.[492] In the Study of Osteoporotic Fractures, women with a previous history of hyperthyroidism had an increased risk of subsequent hip fractures, and women taking thyroid hormone also had an increased risk of fracture (which did not reach statistical significance).[493] However, in a prospective assessment of TSH levels in the Study of Osteoporotic Fractures, no association could be detected between low TSH and bone loss.[494] Perhaps abnormal thyroid levels affect bone quality rather than quantity, and until accurate fracture data become available with this issue, it is prudent to maintain TSH levels within the normal range.

Specific Causes of Bone Disease

Drugs	Heparin, anticonvulsants, high intake of alcohol
Chronic disease	Renal and hepatic
Endocrine diseases	Excess glucocorticoids Hyperthyroidism Estrogen deficiency Hyperparathyroidism
Nutritional	Calcium, phosphorous, vitamin D deficiencies

Measuring Bone Density

There is a 50–100% increase in fracture risk for each standard deviation decline in bone mass (approximately 0.1 g/cm bone mass).[495] Measurement of lower bone mass in the hip is even more predictive; a one standard deviation is associated with nearly a 3-fold increase in risk of fracture.[496] Although low bone density reliably predicts the risk of fracture, increases in bone density in response to treatment do not demonstrate a direct correlation with a reduction in fractures. Therefore, a few percentage point differences achieved by various treatments have little clinical meaning.

The impressive correlation between fracture risk and low bone density has raised the question whether it is of value to screen for osteoporosis. Keep in mind that because the rate of bone loss after menopause contributes equally to the risk of fracture as the total bone mass present at the time of the menopause, a normal bone density measurement at the time of menopause does not mean that the patient will not be at risk of fracture later in life. A relatively young woman with a low bone mass could be targeted for appropriate intervention; however, it is not cost-effective to attempt to screen all postmenopausal women with an expensive method, and attention is now returning to the methods of single photon and single-energy x-ray absorptiometry because measurement of bone loss at the heel and radius accurately assess future fracture risk.[497]

Bone density measurements are certainly useful when an individual woman requires the information in order to make an informed decision regarding hormone therapy. Indeed, a decision to use hormone therapy and better maintenance of a hormone program are correlated with patients' knowledge of their bone density measurements.[498, 499] Because smokers have lower estrogen levels on estrogen therapy, it is worthwhile to document the impact of treatment on bone density in order to consider whether dosage is adequate. Patients who have received long-term corticosteroid, thyroxine, anticonvulsant, or heparin treatment deserve bone mass assessment.

There is a percentage of postmenopausal women on hormone therapy (from 5% to 15%, depending upon compliance) who continue to lose bone.[500, 501] Consideration should be given to an occasional measurement of bone density as an effective method of assessment and to motivate compliance.

Summary of Reasons to Measure Bone Mass

1. **To help patients to make decisions regarding hormone therapy.**

2. **To assess response to therapy in selected patients, e.g., smokers, and women with eating disorders.**

3. **To assess bone mass in patients being treated long-term with glucocorticoids, thyroid hormone, anticonvulsants, or heparin.**

4. **To confirm the diagnosis and assess the severity of osteoporosis to aid in treatment decisions, and to monitor efficacy of therapy.**

5. **To assess bone mass in postmenopausal women who present with fractures, who have one or more risk factors for osteoporosis, or who are over age 65.**

Standard x-rays do not provide an early assessment of fracture risk; 30–40% of bone must be lost before radiographic changes become apparent. Photon absorptiometry measures the transmission of photons through bone. Single-photon absorptiometry uses an ^{125}I source of energy or, more recently, miniature x-ray tubes. These methods measure bone density in the radius and the calcaneus and are relatively inexpensive. These measurements correlate with vertebral bone density and predict the risk of future fracture.[497] Dual-energy absorptiometry employs photons from two energy sources. Dual-energy x-ray absorptiometry (DEXA) provides good precision for all sites of osteoporotic fractures, and the radiation dose is much less than for a standard chest x-ray. Whole body scans by DEXA can measure total body calcium, lean body mass, and fat mass. Quantitative computed tomography for bone density measurements can be performed on most commercial computed tomography (CT) systems; however, radiation exposure is higher than with DEXA, and measurements of the femur are not available, although very accurate measurements of the spine are possible.

For high precision, the best information is provided by the DEXA technique (together with sophisticated software to give a precision of 1%), measuring the three sites of greatest interest, the radius, the hip, and the spine.[502] Better accuracy is gained by 3-site assessments because there can be differences among the sites. In other words, a normal value at one site does not preclude a low bone density at another site. Serial measurements are usually at least one year apart. For practical clinical use (and for screening), measurement of the bone density at the radius or calcaneus is sufficient and cost-effective. It is anticipated that ultrasonography will prove to be a low-cost effective method for bone mass assessment.[503] Ultrasonographic measurements of the calcaneus have been reported to be as accurate as femoral neck measurements by DEXA in predicting the risk of hip fractures.[504, 505] Ultrasonometry of the calcaneus can also predict spine and femur fracture risk.

> **T Score — Standard deviations between patient and average peak young adult bone mass. The more negative, the greater the risk of fracture.**
>
> **Z Score — Standard deviations between patient and average bone mass for same age and weight. A Z score lower than –2.0 (2.5% of normal population of same age) requires diagnostic evaluation for causes other than postmenopausal bone loss.**

Definitions Based on Bone Mineral Density

Normal	0 to –1 S.D. from the reference standard (84% of the population)
Osteopenia	–1 to –2.5 S.D.
Osteoporosis	below –2.5 S.D.

Biochemical Markers of Bone Turnover

There are many serum and urinary biochemical markers of bone turnover. Markers of bone formation include serum levels of osteocalcin, total and bone alkaline phosphatase, and procollagen peptide. Bone resorption is indicated by changes in urinary calcium, hydroxyproline, pyridinoline and deoxypyridinoline cross-links of collagen, telopeptides of collagen, and serum cross-linked telopeptides.

The urinary tests use a second morning voided urine specimen, and the immunoassays measure hydroxyproline, pyridinoline, deoxypyridinoline, the collagen cross-linked N-telopeptides, or the collagen cross-linked C-telopeptides.[507] Because of individual variability, marker measurements correlate poorly with bone mineral density; however, changes in these markers quickly indicate responses to estrogen therapy.[508] Therefore, efficacy of therapy (any of the anti-resorptive treatments) can be judged by comparing a baseline value with a single follow-up measurement after 1–3 months of treatment. A lesser decrease in the urinary cross-linked peptides indicates a less than optimal bone response, identifying patients for further evaluation and specific added treatment.[509, 510] How reliable, practical, and cost-effective this approach is for routine clinical use is yet to be determined.

Treatment

Estrogen therapy will stabilize the process of osteoporosis or prevent it from occurring. Besides inhibiting osteoclastic resorption activity, estrogen increases intestinal calcium absorption, increases 1,25-dihydroxyvitamin D (the active form of Vitamin D), increases renal conservation of calcium, and supports the survival of osteoblasts. With estrogen therapy one can expect a 50–60% decrease in fractures of the arm and hip,.[511–514] and when estrogen is supplemented with calcium, an 80% reduction in vertebral compression fractures can be observed.[515] This reduction is seen primarily in patients who have taken estrogen for more than 5 years.[241, 516] ***Protection against fractures wanes with age, and long-term estrogen use is necessary to maximally reduce the risk of fracture after age 75.***

Because most osteoporotic fractures occur late in life, women and clinicians must understand that the short-term use of estrogen immediately after menopause cannot be expected to protect against fractures in the 7th and 8th decades of life. Some long-term protection is achieved with 7–10 years of estrogen therapy after menopause, but the impact is minimal after age 75.[517] In a prospective cohort study of women 65 years of age and older, in the women who had stopped using estrogen, and in those who were over 75 and had stopped using estrogen even if they had used estrogen for more than 10 years, there was no substantial effect on the risk for fractures.[518] The effective impact of estrogen requires initiation within 5 years of menopause and for current use to extend into the elderly years. The protective effect of estrogen rapidly dissipates after treatment is stopped because estrogen withdrawal is followed by rapid bone loss. In the 3- to 5-year period following loss of estrogen, whether after menopause or after cessation of estrogen therapy, there is an accelerated loss of bone.[519–521] In a Swedish case-control study, most of the beneficial effect of hormone therapy was lost 5 years after discontinuing treatment.[514] Maximal protection against osteoporotic fractures, therefore, requires lifelong therapy, and even some long-term protection requires 10 or more years of treatment.[522] Standard doses of estrogen administered transdermally (50 μg) appear to protect against fractures as well as standard oral doses.[514]

For many years, it was believed that estrogen therapy would either prevent or slow bone loss, but not produce a gain in bone density. Modern studies indicate that this is not the case. For example, in the PEPI trial, at the end of 3 years, the women receiving hormone treatment had experienced about a 5% gain in bone mineral density in the spine and 2% in the hip compared with approximately a 2% loss in the placebo group.[501] How long does this gain in bone continue? In a 10-year follow-up study of women receiving estrogen-progestin therapy, the spinal bone density steadily increased, reaching a level 13% over baseline after 10 years of treatment.[523] It is still unknown whether a continuing increase over many years provides additional fracture protection.

The positive impact of hormone therapy on bone has been demonstrated to take place even in women over age 65.[241, 516–518, 524, 525] This is a strong argument in favor of treating very old women who have never been on estrogen. Estrogen use between the ages of 65 and 74 has been documented to protect against fractures.[513]

Studies have demonstrated that a dose of 0.625 mg of conjugated estrogens is necessary to preserve bone density.[526] The conventional wisdom has stated that an estradiol blood level of 40–60 pg/mL is required to protect against bone loss.[527, 528] We now know that any amount of estrogen can have an impact, although it is very likely that some degree of protection is lost when doses are less than the equivalent of 0.625 mg conjugated estrogens.

The rate of bone loss and the incidence of hip and vertebral fracture is inversely related to the circulating estrogen levels in older women.[529, 530] Estradiol levels as low as 10 pg/mL have a beneficial impact on bone density and fracture rates compared with values below 5 pg/mL. ***Thus, any increment in estrogen, even within the usual postmenopausal range, will exert protective effects.*** This explains how a positive effect on bone was observed even with the utilization of the vaginal ring that delivers a very small amount of estradiol with minimal systemic absorption.[531]

A lower dose of 0.3 mg daily of conjugated estrogens or 0.5 mg estradiol prevented loss of vertebral trabecular bone when combined with calcium supplementation (to achieve a total intake of 1500 mg daily).[532–534] In a small study without calcium supplementation, the daily administration of 0.3 mg conjugated estrogens and 2.5 mg medroxyprogesterone acetate produced a slight increase in lumbar bone density with a lesser effect on the hip.[535] A study of women randomized to treatment either with continuous transdermal delivery of estradiol 50 µg daily or oral estrogen demonstrated that both equally prevented postmenopausal bone loss.[536] Major concerns with lower doses include the possibilities that there will be a significant percentage of non-responders and some cardiovascular benefit will be sacrificed. Nevertheless, a lower dose of estrogen may be more acceptable (fewer side effects) in elderly women. Patients electing to be treated with lower doses should have follow-up assessments for response with measurements of either bone density or urinary biochemical markers. After 6 months to one year, we urge patients on lower doses to move up to a standard regimen.

While progestational agents are considered antiestrogenic, they have been reported to act independently, in a manner similar to estrogen, to reduce bone resorption.[537] When added to estrogen, progestins can lead to an apparent synergistic increase in bone formation associated with a positive balance of calcium.[538–541] On the other hand, good studies have failed to find a greater impact on bone, comparing estrogen alone to estrogen plus a progestin.[518] However, the synergistic result of combining estrogen with a progestin is probably determined by the type of progestin, being limited to members of the 19-nortestosterone (norethindrone) family.[286] This could reflect an increase in free estrogen levels because of a reduction in sex hormone-binding globulin. Careful studies indicate that the addition of medroxyprogesterone provides an additional effect on bone only in women with established, significant osteoporosis.[541–543]

In the PEPI trial, at the end of 3 years, there was little difference comparing treatment with estrogen only to the groups receiving combinations of estrogen and medroxyprogesterone acetate or micronized progesterone.[501] Thus, the daily, continuous combination of estrogen-progestin is equally efficacious in maintaining bone density as the standard sequential regimens, although at least one study has indicated a greater response in the lumbar spine with continuous treatment.[544–546]

The addition of testosterone to an estrogen therapy program has been reported to provide no additional beneficial impact on bone or on relief from hot flushes.[547, 548] Others have demonstrated a greater increase in bone density with an estrogen-androgen combination compared with estrogen alone, although the blood estrogen levels achieved were higher than those associated with standard postmenopausal hormone therapy.[549]

Follow-up Assessment of Hormone-Treated Women

Not all women will maintain or gain bone density on postmenopausal hormone therapy; in one study, 12% of treated women lost bone despite apparently good compliance.[500] In the PEPI 3-year clinical trial, where compliance rates were probably maximal, 4% of treated women lost bone in the spine and 6% in the hip.[501]

It is worthwhile to measure the bone density in treated women when they are in their late 60s. The reason why some women fail to respond is unknown. It is further unknown whether these patients will respond to added treatment, such as calcitonin or a bisphosphonate, but it is worth special evaluation, treatment, and surveillance.

Selective Estrogen Agonists/Antagonists (Selective Estrogen Receptor Modulators)

A greater understanding of the estrogen receptor mechanism (Chapter 2) allows us to understand how mixed estrogen agonists-antagonists can have selective actions on specific target tissues. New agents are being developed in an effort to isolate desired actions from unwanted side effects. Raloxifene exerts no proliferative effect on the endometrium but produces favorable responses in bone and lipids.[550, 551] The changes in bone remodeling produced by raloxifene are consistent with an estrogen agonist effect.[552]

Estrogen selective agonists/antagonists (tamoxifen and raloxifene) have been reported to reduce the incidence of breast cancer within 2–3 years of treatment.[553, 554] Short-term clinical trial data indicate that raloxifene has a positive impact on bone density, favorable effects on LDL-cholesterol, fibrinogen, and lipoprotein(a), but no effects on HDL-cholesterol and PAI-1, and raloxifene increases hot flushing.[555, 556] Long-term clinical trial data will be necessary to determine the ultimate impact on clinical events, specifically fractures, coronary heart disease, stress incontinence, and cognition. The MORE study (**M**ultiple **O**utcomes of **R**aloxifene **E**valuation) is a worldwide clinical trial of raloxifene in osteoporotic women. After 2 years, raloxifene treatment was associated with a 44% reduction in vertebral fractures.[557] In a 2-year randomized trial in monkeys, raloxifene exerted no protection against coronary artery atherosclerosis despite changes in circulating lipids similar to those achieved in women.[558] However, a combination of actions (antioxidant activity, some beneficial effects on lipids, a reduction in homocysteine levels) makes it likely there will be some favorable impact on the cardiovascular system.[556, 559, 560] RUTH (**R**aloxifene **U**se for **T**he **H**eart) is both a primary and secondary coronary heart disease prevention trial, started in 1998, that should provide data by 2003. In our view, raloxifene is an option for prevention of osteoporosis, especially for patients reluctant to use hormone therapy, but not a substitute for estrogen.

Calcium Supplementation

There has been considerable confusion over whether calcium supplementation by itself can offer protection against postmenopausal osteoporosis. This is partly due to the fact that calcium studies have been performed in women who were in the very early postmenopausal years, in the midst of the rapid loss of calcium associated with estrogen deficiency, and this estrogen effect overwhelmed any responses to calcium. Studies that involve women beyond this early stage of the postmenopausal period definitely indicate a positive impact of calcium supplementation.[561–563]

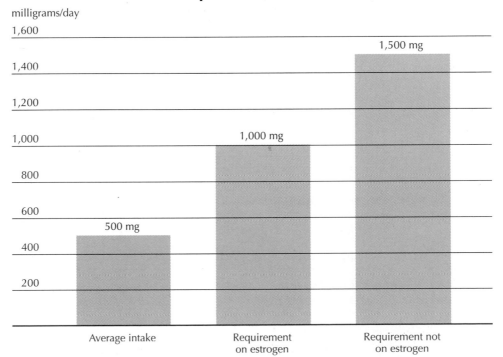

Calcium Requirement for Zero Balance[564]

Calcium absorption decreases with age because of a decrease in biologically active vitamin D and becomes significantly impaired after menopause. A positive calcium balance is mandatory to achieve adequate prevention against osteoporosis. Calcium supplementation (1000 mg per day) reduces bone loss and decreases fractures, especially in individuals with low daily intakes.[564] However, estrogen acts to improve calcium absorption (by increasing the levels of 1,25-dihydroxyvitamin D) and makes it possible to utilize effective supplemental calcium in lower doses. In order to remain in zero calcium balance, women on estrogen therapy require a total of 1000 mg elemental calcium per day.[564–566] Because the average woman receives about 500 mg of calcium in her diet, the minimal daily supplement equals an additional 500 mg. Women not on estrogen require a daily supplement of at least 1000 mg calcium.

Even with the commonly used therapeutic doses of calcium, nearly 40% of postmenopausal women will have inefficient absorption.[567] Estrogen improves calcium absorption and allows the utilization of supplemental calcium in effective doses without the side effects associated with higher doses (constipation and flatulence) that diminish compliance. We must emphasize that although calcium supplementation is important, it cannot provide the same degree of protection against osteoporosis as that achieved by hormonal therapy.[568, 569] Nevertheless, the beneficial impact of estrogen on bone is reduced in the absence of calcium supplementation.[533]

Improved calcium intake in adolescents results in significant increases in bone density and skeletal mass, providing protection against osteoporosis later in life.[570, 571] Calcium supplementation is far more important during adolescence than in the reproductive years when bone formation is minimal. Under age 25, during the years of bone accumulation, the daily calcium intake should be 1500 mg.[564] This amount, 1500 mg/day, is also recommended during pregnancy and lactation. Most calcium comes from dairy products; relying on other foods is not easy because it requires a high intake volume of other foods to provide the same amount of calcium in normal daily servings of dairy products.

Calcium Content of Foods

Yogurt (one cup)	415 mg
Yogurt with fruit (one cup)	345 mg
Juice fortified with calcium (one cup)	300 mg
Milk (one cup)	300 mg plus 100 IU Vitamin D
Ice cream (one cup)	175 mg
Cottage cheese (1 cup)	140 mg
Romano cheese (1 ounce)	300 mg
Parmesan cheese (1 ounce)	335 mg
Cheddar cheese (1 ounce)	205 mg
Swiss cheese (1 ounce)	270 mg
Mozarella cheese (1 ounce)	207 mg
Broccoli, cooked (one cup)	80 mg
Beans, cooked (one cup)	80 mg

There are dozens of calcium supplements on the market, containing calcium carbonate, calcium lactate, calcium phosphate, or calcium gluconate.[572] Calcium carbonate tablets are the cheapest and contain the most elemental calcium (40%). Calcium lactate tablets contain 13% calcium, and calcium gluconate only 9%. The calcium carbonate antacids are excellent, inexpensive sources. One should be aware that aluminum-containing antacids such as Maalox, Mylanta, Gelusil, and Riopan can inhibit gastrointestinal absorption of calcium. Bone meal and dolomite as sources of calcium should be avoided because they can be contaminated with lead. Calcium citrate does not require gastric acid for absorption and is the best choice for older patients with reduced gastric acid production. ***Calcium supplementation is most efficient when single doses do not exceed 500 mg and when taken with a meal.*** Excess calcium supplementation (especially not with meals) is associated with a slight increase in risk for kidney stones.[573]

Vitamin D

Osteoporosis related to aging is due significantly to age-related changes in vitamin D and calcium metabolism. There is an age-related decrease in the ability of the skin and the kidney to synthesize the active form of vitamin D (1,25-dihydroxycholecalcifer, also known as 1,25-dihydroxyvitamin D), and there is a decrease in the ability of the intestine to absorb dietary vitamin D. Exposure of the skin to ultraviolet rays in sunlight stimulates the formation of cholecalciferol (vitamin D_3). Commercial vitamin preparations contain ergocalciferol (vitamin D_2 or calciferol). Vitamin D-fortified milk contains cholecalciferol. Cholecalciferol and ergocalciferol are converted in the liver to calcifediol, which is converted in the kidneys to calcitriol (1,25-dihydroxyvitamin D).

It is now recommended that individuals over age 70 should add 800 units of vitamin D to calcium supplementation. A large randomized trial in Finland documented a reduced rate of fractures in elderly women receiving supplementation of vitamin D_2 (by an annual intramuscular injection), and in France, supplementation of calcium and vitamin D_3 reduced the number of hip fractures by 43%.[568, 574] In postmenopausal women with osteoporosis, treatment with calcitriol (vitamin D) produced a 3-fold reduction in vertebral fractures.[575] And finally, supplementation with 400 IU vitamin D_3 in women age 70 and older restored the markers of vitamin D and calcium metabolism to that observed in young adults, and the bone mineral density at the femoral neck increased.[576]

Because adequate and active vitamin D depends upon cutaneous generation mediated by sun exposure, women who live in cloudy areas during the winter months are relatively vitamin D deficient and lose bone.[577] In far northern and southern areas, the winter sunlight is inadequate to stimulate dermal activation. Vitamin D supplementation is recommended for these women as well but only during the winter and at a lower level, 400 units daily (usually available in over-the-counter multivitamins or in combination with calcium). High doses cause hypercalciuria with a risk of stone formation. If uncertain regarding vitamin D supplementation, the serum level of 1,25-dihydroxyvitamin D can be measured; a level below 15 ng/L is abnormal.[578]

The impact of vitamin D supplementation may be less in younger, early postmenopausal women. In a 2.5-year randomized clinical trial in Finland, supplementation with 300 IU vitamin D_3 did little by itself and added nothing to the beneficial effect of estrogen on bone density.[579] The benefit of vitamin D supplementation is clear in older women, and the lack of side effects with low doses encourages us to recommend vitamin D supplementation as part of the overall program for osteoporosis prevention in younger women.

Bisphosphonates

Bisphosphonates are effective in preventing bone loss by inhibiting bone resorption. The bisphosphonates bind to bone mineral where they remain for many years, making bone less susceptible to osteoclastic action. The most promising of these agents are etidronate, alendronate, clodronate, pamidronate, tiludronate, and risedronate.[580, 581] The first generation of bisphosphonates (etidronate) also inhibited bone mineralization, and therefore intermittent therapy was necessary. The second generation of bisphosphonates allows bone formation to occur while inhibiting bone resorption and makes it possible to use continuous therapy rather than intermittent therapy.

In women with osteoporosis, alendronate (10 mg daily) administration reduced the risk of subsequent non-vertebral fractures by at least 30% (and probably 50%) and vertebral fractures by 90% in the first 3 years of treatment.[582, 583] In normal postmenopausal women, alendronate increased bone density in both the spine and the hip, and the 5 mg dose (the preferred dose for preventive treatment) was more effective than 2.5 mg.[584, 585] The increase in bone density with the 5 mg dose is slightly less than that observed with estrogen-progestin therapy.[584] It is unlikely that a difference of a few percentage points in bone density gain has an impact on the number of fractures ultimately experienced. Alendronate must be taken on an empty stomach with a full glass of water at least 30 minutes before any other food or liquid intake in order to achieve adequate absorption. A failure to remain upright for at least 30 minutes and until after the first food intake of the day after ingesting alendronate can result in esophageal injuries, such as esophagitis, esophageal ulcers, and esophageal erosions with bleeding.[586] Risedronate, 5 mg daily, is as effective as alendronate for the prevention of bone loss and may be better tolerated.[587]

Etidronate given in a cyclic fashion (e.g., 400 mg daily for 2 weeks followed by a 12-week drug-free interval during which calcium supplementation is administered) prevents bone loss and reduces the vertebral fracture rate.[588, 589] In many countries, etidronate is the drug of choice for the treatment of osteoporosis. Although no comparison studies are available, it is probable that the bisphosphonates are comparable in efficacy and safety.

Bisphosphonates are an effective addition to osteoporotic prevention because they are well tolerated if taken correctly. However, unlike estrogens, bisphosphonates are unidimensional, having no effect on cardiovascular disease, hot flushes, or the atrophic changes seen in menopause. A combination of bisphosphonates and estrogen has an additive effect on bone; with alendronate and hormone therapy, there was about a 2% greater gain in bone density in the spine after 2 years of treatment.[590] It is not believed that this addition of several percentage points in bone mineral density will provide a worthwhile gain in fracture protection. Unlike, estrogen, accelerated bone loss does not occur after discontinuation of alendronate therapy.[591] For this reason, long-term treatment may not be necessary.

Calcitonin

Calcitonin regulates plasma calcium by inhibiting bone resorption and can be used in patients for whom hormone therapy is contraindicated. Given by subcutaneous injection in a dose of 100 IU daily to women early after menopause it has the same effectiveness as estrogen in conserving bone density.[592] Studies with intranasal delivery of salmon calcitonin (200 IU dily) indicate it can be similarly effective.[593] Calcitonin treatment should be combined with vitamin D and calcium supplementation. The disadvantages are the high cost and the potential for immunologic reactions to non-human calcitonin. Human calcitonin is available, but recombinant salmon calcitonin is more potent. An oral preparation will soon be available.

Fluoride

The addition of fluoride, a potent stimulator of bone formation, offers significant protection against osteoporosis. The clinical response depends on the formulation and dose. Slow-release sodium fluoride (25 mg bid given 12 of every 14 months) combined with calcium supplementation reduces the vertebral fracture rate with essentially no side effects.[594] Treatments recommended for no longer than 4 years to avoid the toxic accumulation of fluoride in bone.[595] Thus, this treatment is reserved for patients with established postmenopausal osteoporosis.

Tibolone

Tibolone is a steroid, related to the 19-nortestosterone family, that is effective for the treatment of bone and hot flushes in a dose of 2.5 mg per day.[596, 597] A lower dose of 1.25 mg daily also provides bone protection, but it is less effective and there is more vaginal bleeding. Tibolone is metabolized into 3 steroid isomers with varying estrogenic, progestogenic, and adrogenic properties. The metabolites differ in their activities and dominance according to the target tissue. Thus, tibolone provides estrogenic effects on bone and hot flushing, but it induces atrophy of the endometrium.[598] Its beneficial impact on bone (2.5 mg dose) is comparable to standard hormonal therapy.[599] In the endometrium, tibolone is converted locally (by endometrial 3 beta-hydroxysteroid dehydrogenase/isomerase) to its Δ^4 progestational isomer, explaining its nonproliferative effect on the endometrium.[600] Tibolone has an estrogenic effect on the vagina, and women report improvements in the symptoms of vaginal dryness and dyspareunia, and an increase in sexual enjoyment and libido.[601]

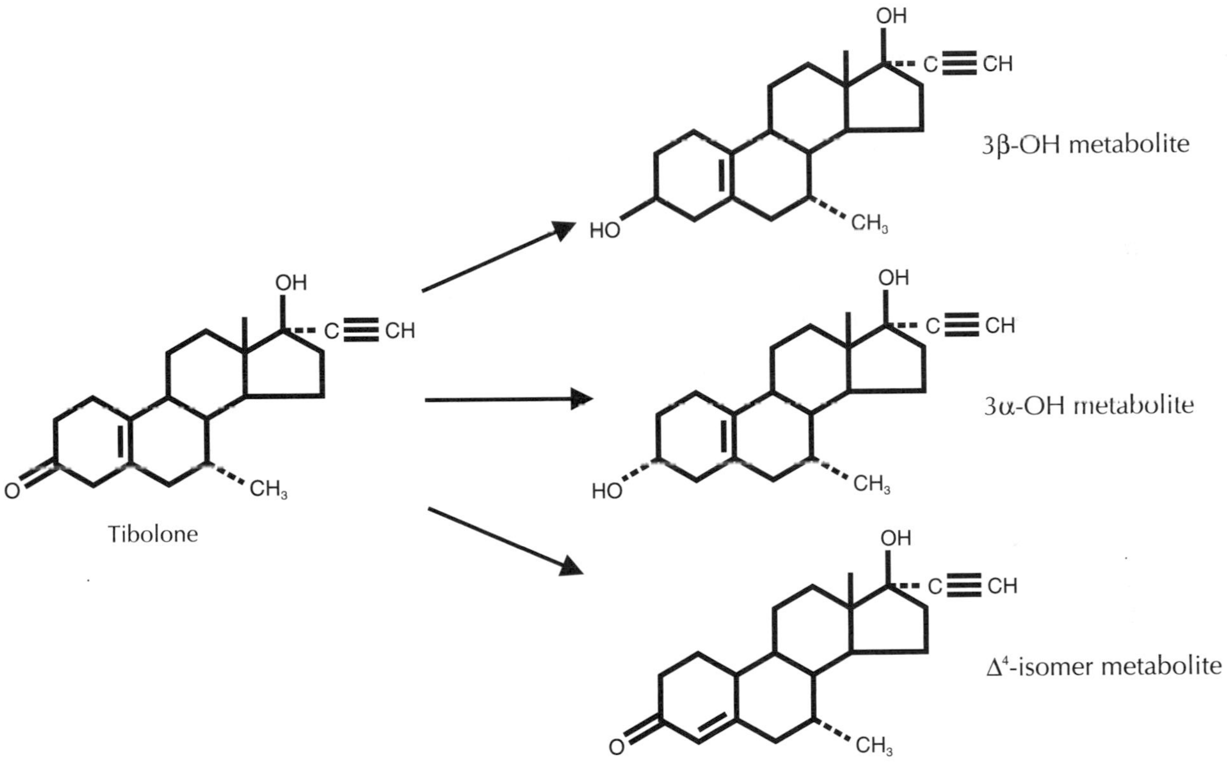

3β-OH metabolite

3α-OH metabolite

Δ^4-isomer metabolite

Tibolone

Although a short-term reduction in HDL-cholesterol is an undesirable consequence; the long-term impact has not been well studied.[602] In a 2-year study, the unfavorable effect on lipoproteins was accompanied by beneficial changes in coagulation factors consistent with enhanced fibrinolysis and unchanged coagulation.[603] Overall, it is possible that some favorable activity on the cardiovascular system is maintained. A major advantage of tibolone (2.5 mg daily) is its low (10–20%) incidence of bleeding. Because tibolone inhibits breast cell proliferation in vitro, it is possible that future studies will indicate that tibolone offers some protection against breast cancer. Tibolone also has a beneficial impact in short-term studies on insulin resistance in normal women and in women with noninsulin-dependent diabetes mellitus.[604, 605]

Thiazides

Older women are often treated with thiazides for hypertension. Thiazides reduce the urinary loss of calcium, induce a positive calcium balance, and treatment is associated with a higher bone density. It is useful to know that estrogen and thiazides are additive; a significantly higher bone density is achieved with combined use.[606]

Growth Hormone

Human growth hormone administration stimulates bone remodeling, but does not produce a significant increase in bone density.[607] The extreme expense and the high incidence of unpleasant side effects further make this option unattractive.

Lifestyle Modifications

Lifestyle can have a beneficial effect on bone density. Physical activity (weight-bearing), as little as 30 minutes a day for 3 days a week, will increase the mineral content of bone in older women.[608] To be effective, exercise must exert a load on bone, especially the spine.[609] Ordinary walking will not suffice.[610] Even brisk walking achieves a significant increase in bone density only in the calcaneus, the site subjected to stress with walking.[611] However, brisk walking may slow the rate of bone loss in the hip.[612] In other words, weight lifting is better for the spine than is ordinary walking, although running probably helps hip bone mass. The activities that are beneficial are running, weight training, aerobics, stair climbing, and sports other than swimming. The effect of weight-bearing exercise on bone density is additive when combined with hormone therapy.[613] Although ordinary walking has little impact on bone density, it is still reasonable to expect walking to have an overall beneficial effect on the risk of fracture. Walking improves the cardiovascular status of patients and reduces body mass. These changes plus the exercise itself will improve balance and decrease the risk of falling. For these reasons, walking, even after adjusting for bone density, is associated with a reduced risk of hip fracture.[493]

The impact of exercise on bone is significantly less than that achieved by hormone therapy.[567] Women require the full combination of pharmacologic therapy, calcium supplementation, and exercise in order to minimize the risk of fractures. For each of these, the beneficial impact lasts only as long as the therapy is continued.

Adverse habits, such as cigarette smoking or excessive alcohol consumption, are associated with an increased risk of osteoporosis. The magnitude of bone loss associated with cigarette smoking is consistent with a 40–45% increase in the risk of hip fracture.[614] Women who smoke also enter menopause earlier, and lose bone at a greater rate in the first years of the postmenopausal period.[615] Studies have indicated that estrogen is associated with lesser protection against fractures in smokers; however, this may be correctable by titering the blood level of estrogen with the dose administered. The lower blood levels of estrogen in smokers have been correlated with an earlier menopause and a reduced bone density, and, therefore, the standard dose of estrogen may not totally counteract the predisposition of smoking toward osteoporosis.[616] The titration of estrogen dosage with circulating blood estradiol levels in smokers makes clinical sense, allowing the use of higher hormonal doses to maintain bone density. Monitoring of bone response with bone density measurements or urinary markers would further aid in achieving maximal effects of therapy.

Clinicians should always remember that exposure to excessive thyroid and glucocorticoid hormones is associated with osteoporosis and an increased rate of fractures. The bone loss associated with glucocorticoid treatment is significantly prevented by estrogen/progestin therapy,[617, 618] and excessive thyroid effects can be avoided by annually monitoring treatment dosage with TSH levels. Specific treatment should also be offered to patients using anticonvulsants.

A high coffee intake has been reported to be associated with an increased risk of osteoporosis.[619] However, this increase in risk is dependent upon dietary calcium intake. In women who drank at least one glass of milk (300 mg calcium) per day throughout most of their lives, increasing caffeinated coffee intake was not associated with a lower bone density.[620] Repeatedly, we see the importance of teaching children and adolescents the merit of an adequate calcium intake; drinking nonfat milk throughout life is good for you. An adequate calcium intake compensates for "calcium robbers," such as caffeine and soft drinks. A British study concluded that an increase of only 300 mL of milk per day in adolescents increases bone density without an increase in weight or body fat.[621]

Remember that not all fractures are solely due to osteoporosis. Drug side effects, impaired vision, neurological dysfunction, and muscular conditions all put patients at risk because more than 90% of fractures occur following a fall.[467] Interventions that reduce the odds of falling and enhance the ability to withstand the impact of a fall are important.[622] This includes patient education regarding hazards in the home, monitoring drug use, adequate nutrition, and a good exercise program. In addition, there is evidence that estrogen with or without added progestin improves muscle strength and balance.[147–149, 623, 624] On the other hand, some studies have not been able to document an increase in muscle strength or improvements in balance.[613, 625] Furthermore, the increase in muscle mass and strength in response to weight-bearing exercise was the same when hormone users were compared with non-users.[626]

Conclusion

The menopause is a physiologic event that brings clinicians and patients together, providing the opportunity to enroll patients in health maintenance. The failure to respond appropriately (by either clinician or patient) easily leads to a loss of the patient from a practice, but equally, if not more, importantly, is the probability that the loss of a patient from a practice means that another woman has lost her involvement in a preventive health care program. Contrary to popular opinion, the menopause is not a signal of impending decline, but, rather, a wonderful phenomenon that can signal the start of something positive, a good health program. Postmenopausal hormone therapy is an option that should be considered by virtually all women as a legitimate part of their preventive health program.

References

1. **Cope E,** Physical changes associated with the post-menopausal years, In: Campbell S, ed. *The Management of the Menopause & Post-Menopausal Years,* University Park Press, Baltimore, 1976, p 33.

2. **Farnham AM,** Uterine disease as a factor in the production of insanity, *Alienst Neurologist* 8:532, 1887.

3. **Hällström T, Samuelsson S,** Mental health in the climacteric. The longitudinal study of women in Gothenburg, *Acta Obstet Gynecol Scand (Suppl)* 130:13, 1985.

4. **McKinlay SM, McKinlay JB,** The impact of menopause and social factors on health, In: Hammond CB, Haseltine FP, Schiff I, eds. *Menopause: Evaluation, Treatment, and Health Concerns,* Alan R. Liss, New York, 1989, p 137.

5. **Matthews KA, Wing RR, Kuller LH, Meilahn EN, Kelsey SF, Costello EJ, Caggiula AW,** Influences of natural menopause on psychological characteristics and symptoms of middle-aged healthy women, *J Consult Clin Psychol* 58:345, 1990.

6. **Koster A,** Change-of-life anticipations, attitudes, and experiences among middle-aged Danish women, *Health Care Women Int* 12:1, 1991.

7. **Holte A,** Influences of natural menopause on health complaints: a prospective study of healthy Norwegian women, *Maturitas* 14:127, 1992.

8. **Kaufert PA, Gilbert P, Tate R,** The Manitoba Project: a re-examination of the link between menopause and depression, *Maturitas* 14:143, 1992.

9. **Dennerstein L, Smith AMA, Morse C, Burger H, Green A, Hopper J, Ryan M,** Menopausal symptoms in Australian women, *Med J Aust* 159:232, 1993.

10. **Avis NE, McKinlay SM,** A longitudinal analysis of women's attitudes toward the menopause: results from the Massachusetts Women's Health Study, *Maturitas* 13:65, 1991.

11. **Morse CA, Smith A, Dennerstein L, Green A, Hopper J, Burger H,** The treatment-seeking woman at menopause, *Maturitas* 18:161, 1994.

12. **Defey D, Storch E, Cardozo S, Diaz O, Fernandez G,** The menopause: women's psychology and health care, *Soc Sci Med* 42:1447, 1996.

13. **Annual Report of the Board of Trustees of the Federal Old-Age and Survivors Insurance and Disability Insurance Trust Funds,** (U.S. Government Printing Office), Report No. Tb1 II.D2, 1995.

14. **Olshansky SJ, Carnes BA, Cassel C,** In search of Methuselah: estimating the upper limits to human longevity, *Science* 250:634, 1990.

15. **Olshansky SJ, Carnes BA, Cassel C,** The aging of the human species, *Scientific American* April:46, 1993.

16. **Rowe JW, Grossman E, Bond E,** Academic geriatrics for the year 2000. An Institute of Medicine report, *New Engl J Med* 316:1425, 1987.

17. **U.S. Bureau of the Census,** (U.S. Government Printing Office), Current Population Reports. Projections of the population of the United States: 1977 to 2050, Report No. Series P25-704, 1993.

18. **Diczfalusy E,** Menopause, developing countries and the 21st century, *Acta Obstet Gynecol Scand* (Suppl)134:45, 1986.

19. **Duke RC, Speidel JJ,** Women's reproductive health: a chronic crisis, *JAMA* 266:1846, 1991.

20. **Miles TP, Bernard MA,** Morbidity, disability, and health status of black American elderly: a new look at the oldest-old, *J Am Geriatr Soc* 40:1047, 1992.

21. **Day JC,** (U.S. Government Printing Office), Bureau of the Census. Current population reports. Population projections of the United States, by age, sex, race, and Hispanic origin: 1993 to 2050, Report No. P25-1104, 1993.

22. **Hazzard WR,** Biological basis of the sex differential in longevity, *J Am Geriatr Soc* 34:455, 1986.

23. **Department of Health and Human Services,** A report of the surgeon general: the health consequences of smoking for women, Rockville, Maryland, 1980.

24. **U.S. Bureau of the Census,** (U.S. Government Printing Office), Current population reports. Special studies. Sixty-five plus in America, Report No. P23-178RV, 1993.

25. **Keith PM,** The social context and resources of the unmarried in old age, *Int J Aging Human Develop* 23:81, 1986.

26. **Fries JF, Crapo LM,** *Vitality and Aging,* W.H. Freeman and Co., San Francisco, 1981.

27. **Fries JF,** The sunny side of aging, *JAMA* 263:2354, 1990.

28. **Fries JF,** Strategies for reduction of morbidity, *Am J Clin Nutr* 55:1257S, 1992.

29. **Davis DL, Dinse GE, Hoel DG,** Decreasing cardiovascular disease and increasing cancer among whites in the United States from 1973 through 1987, *JAMA* 271:431, 1994.

30. **Willett WC, Green A, Stampfer MJ, Speizer FE, Colditz GA, Rosner B, Monson RR, Stason W, Hennekens CH,** Relative and absolute risks of coronary heart disease among women who smoke cigarettes, *New Engl J Med* 317:1303, 1987.

31. **Nelson DE, Giovino GA, Emont SL, Brackbill R, Cameron LL, Peddicord J, Mowery PD,** Trends in cigarette smoking among US physicians and nurses, *JAMA* 271:1273, 1994.

32. **The American Heart Association,** *http://www.amhrt.org* .

33. **Jajich CL, Ostfeld AM, Freeman Jr DH,** Smoking and coronary heart disease mortality in the elderly, *JAMA* 252:2831, 1984.

34. **Hermanson B, Omenn GS, Kronmal RA, Gersh BJ,** Beneficial six-year outcome of smoking cessation in older men and women with coronary artery disease. Results from the CASS registry, *New Engl J Med* 319:1365, 1988.

35. **Vollman RF,** The menstrual cycle, In: Friedman E, ed. *Major Problems in Obstetrics and Gynecology,* W.B. Saunders Co., Philadelphia, 1977.

36. **Treloar AE, Boynton RE, Borghild GB, Brown BW,** Variation of the human menstrual cycle through reproductive life, *Int J Fertil* 12:77, 1967.

37. **Collett ME, Wertenberger GE, Fiske VM,** The effect of age upon the pattern of the menstrual cycle, *Fertil Steril* 5:437, 1954.

38. **Chiazze Jr L, Brayer FT, Macisco Jr JJ, Parker MP, Duffy BJ,** The length and variability of the human menstrual cycle, *JAMA* 203:377, 1968.

39. **Munster K, Schmidt L, Helm P,** Length and variation in the menstrual cycle — a cross-sectional study from a Danish county, *Br J Obstet Gynaecol* 99:422, 1992.

40. **Belsey EM, Pinol APY, and Task Force on Long-Acting Systemic Agents for Fertility Regulation,** Menstrual bleeding patterns in untreated women, *Contraception* 55:57, 1997.

41. **den Tonkelaar I, te Velde ER, Looman CWN,** Menstrual cycle length preceding menopause in relation to age at menopause, *Maturitas* 29:115, 1998.

42. **Sherman BM, West JH, Korenman SG,** The menopausal transition: analysis of LH, FSH, estradiol, and progesterone concentrations during menstrual cycles of older women, *J Clin Endocrinol Metab* 42:629, 1976.

43. **Lenton EA, Landgren B, Sexton L, Harper R,** Normal variation in the length of the follicular phase of the menstrual cycle: effect of chronological age, *Br J Obstet Gynaecol* 91:681, 1984.

44. **Buckler HM, Evans A, Mamlora H, Burger HG, Anderson DC,** Gonadotropin, steroid and inhibin levels in women with incipient ovarian failure during anovulatory and ovulatory 're-bound' cycles, *J Clin Endocrinol Metab* 72:116, 1991.

45. **MacNaughton J, Bangah M, McCloud P, Hee J, Burger HG,** Age-related changes in follicle stimulating hormone, luteinizing hormone, oestradiol and immunoreactive inhibin in women of reproductive age, *Clin Endocrinol* 36:339, 1992.

46. **Hee J, MacNaughton J, Bangah M, Burger HG,** Perimenopausal patterns of gonadotrophins, immunoreactive inhibin, oestradiol and progesterone, *Maturitas* 18:9, 1993.

47. **Metcalf MG, Livesay JH,** Gonadotropin excretion in fertile women: effect of age and the onset of the menopausal transition, *J Endocrinol* 105:357, 1985.

48. **Rannevik G, Jeppsson S, Johnell O, Bjerre B, Yaurell-Borulf Y, Svanberg L,** A longitudinal study of the perimenopausal transition: altered profiles of steroid and pituitary hormones, SHBG and bone mineral density, *Maturitas* 21:103, 1995.

49. **Santoro N, Brown JR, Adel T, Skurnick JH,** Characterization of reproductive hormonal dynamics in the perimenopause, *J Clin Endocrinol Metab* 81:1495, 1996.

50. **Richardson SJ, Senikas V, Nelson JF,** Follicular depletion during the menopausal transition — evidence for accelerated loss and ultimate exhaustion, *J Clin Endocrinol Metab* 65:1231, 1987.

51. **Gougeon A, Echochard R, Thalabard JC,** Age-related changes of the population of human ovarian follicles: increase in the disappearance rate of non-growing and early-growing follicles in aging women, *Biol Reprod* 50:653, 1994.

52. **Faddy MJ, Gosden RG, Gougeon A, Richardson SJ, Nelson JF,** Accelerated disappearance of ovarian follicles in mid-life: implications for forecasting menopause, *Hum Reprod* 7:1342, 1992.

53. **Klein NA, Illingworth PJ, Groome NP, McNeilly AS, Battaglia DE, Soules MR,** Decreased inhibin B secretion is associated with the monotropic FSH rise in older, ovulatory women: a study of serum and follicular fluid leavels of dimeric inhibin A and B in spontaneous menstrual cycles, *J Clin Endocrinol Metab* 81:2742, 1996.

54. **Danforth DR, Arbogast LK, Mroueh J, Kim MH, Kennard EA, Seifer DB, Friedman CI,** Dimeric inhibin: a direct marker of ovarian aging, *Fertil Steril* 70:119, 1998.

55. **McKinlay SM, Brambilla DJ, Posner JG,** The normal menopause transition, *Maturitas* 14:103, 1992.

56. **Treloar AE,** Menstrual cyclicity and the pre-menopause, *Maturitas* 3:249, 1981.

57. **McKinlay SM, Bigano NL, McKinlay JB,** Smoking and age at menopause, *Ann Intern Med* 103:350, 1985.

58. **Treolar AE,** Menarche, menopause and intervening fecundability, *Hum Biol* 46:89, 1974.

59. **van Noord PAH, Dubas JS, Dorland M, Boersma H, te Velde E,** Age at natural menopause in a population-based screening cohort: the role of menarche, fecundity, and lifestyle factors, *Fertil Steril* 68:95, 1997.

60. **Coulam CB, Adamsen SC, Annegers JF,** Incidence of premature ovarian failure, *Obstet Gynecol* 67:604, 1986.

61. **Torgerson DJ, Avenell A, Russell IT, Reid DM,** Factors associated with onset of menopause in women aged 45–49, *Maturitas* 19:83, 1994.

62. **Torgerson DJ, Thomas RE, Campbell MK, Reid DM,** Alcohol consumption and age of maternal menopause are associated with menopause onset, *Maturitas* 26:21, 1997.

63. **Cramer DW, Xu H, Harlow BL,** Family history as a predictor of early menopause, *Fertil Steril* 64:740, 1995.

64. **Baird DD, Tylavsky FA, Anderson JJB,** Do vegetarians have earlier menopause? *Am J Epidemiol* Proceedings of the Society of Epidemiologic Research:907, 1988.

65. **MacMahon B, Worcester J,** Age at menopause U.S. 1960–62, *Vital Health Stat* 19:1, 1966.

66. **Katsouyanni K, Boyle P, Trichopoulos D,** Diet and urine estrogens among postmenopausal women, *Oncology* 48:490, 1991.

67. **Gapstur SM, Potter JD, Sellers TA, Folsom AR,** Increased risk of breast cancer with alcohol consumption in postmenopausal women, *Am J Epidemiol* 136:1221, 1992.

68. **Gavaler JS, Van Thiel DH,** The association between moderate alcoholic beverage consumption and serum estradiol and testosterone levels in normal postmenopausal women: relationship to the literature, *Alcohol Clin Exp Res* 16:87, 1992.

69. **Holbrook TC, Barrett-Connor E,** A prospective study of alcohol consumption and bone mineral density, *Br Med J* 306:1506, 1993.

70. **Ginsburg EL, Mello NK, Mendelson JH, Barbieri RL, Teoh SK, Rothman M, Gao X, Sholar JW,** Effects of alcohol ingestion on estrogens in postmenopausal women, *JAMA* 276:1747, 1996.

71. **Snieder H, MacGregor AJ, Spector TD,** Genes control the cessation of a woman's reproductive life: a twin study of hysterectomy and age at menopause, *J Clin Endocrinol Metab* 83:1875, 1998.

72. **Brambila DJ, McKinlay SM, Johannes CB,** Defining the perimenopause for application in epidemiologic investigations, *Am J Epidemiol* 140:1091, 1994.

73. **Bromberger JT, Matthews KA, Kuller LH, Wing RR, Meilahn EN, Plantinga P,** Prospective study of the determinants of age at menopause, *Am J Epidemiol* 145:124, 1997.

74. **Cassou B, Derriennic F, Monfort C, Dell'Accio P, Touranchet A,** Risk factors of early menopause in two generations of gainfully employed French women, *Maturitas* 26:165, 1997.

75. **Gonzales GF, Villena A,** Age at menopause in Central Andean Peruvian women, *Menopause* 4:32, 1997.

76. **Siddle N, Sarrel P, Whitehead M,** The effect of hysterectomy on the age at ovarian failure: identification of a subgroup of women with premature loss of ovarian function and literature review, *Fertil Steril* 47:94, 1987.

77. **Derksen JGM, Brömann HAM, Wiegerinck MAHM, Vader HL, Heintz APM,** The effect of hysterectomy and endometrial ablation on follicle stimulating hormone (FSH) levels up to 1 year after surgery, *Maturitas* 29:133, 1998.

78. **Cresswell JL, Egger P, Fall CHD, Osmond C, Fraser RB, Barker DJP,** Is the age of menopause determined in-utero? *Early Hum Develop* 49:143, 1997.

79. **Willett W, Stampfer MJ, Bain C, Lipnick R, Speizer FE, Rosner B, Cramer D, Hennekens CH,** Cigarette smoking, relative weight, and menopause, *Am J Epidemiol* 117:651, 1983.

80. **Midgette AS, Baron JA,** Cigarette smoking and the risk of natural menopause, *Epidemiology* 1:474, 1990.

81. **Amundsen DW, Diers CJ,** The age of menopause in classical Greece and Rome, *Hum Biol* 42:79, 1970.

82. **Amundsen DW, Diers CJ,** The age of menopause in medieval Europe, *Hum Biol* 45:605, 1973.

83. **Frommer DJ,** Changing age at menopause, *Br Med J* ii:349, 1964.

84. **Traupman J, Eckels E, Hatfield E,** Intimacy in older women's lives, *Gerontologist* 2:493, 1982.

85. **Pfeiffer E, Verwoerdt A, Davis GC,** Sexual behavior in middle life, *Am J Psychiatr* 128:1262, 1972.

86. **Greendale GA, Hogan P, Shumaker S, for the Postmenopausal Estrogen/Progestin Interventions Trial (PEPI) Investigators,** Sexual functioning in postmenopausal women: the Postmenopausal Estrogen/Progestin Interventions (PEPI) Trial, *J Women's Health* 5:445, 1996.

87. **Martin CE,** Factors affecting sexual functioning in 60–79 year-old married males, *Arch Sex Behav* 10:399, 1981.

88. **George LK, Weiler SJ,** Sexuality in middle and late life, *Arch Gen Psychiatr* 38:919, 1981.

89. **White CB,** Sexual interest, attitudes, knowledge, and sexual history in relation to sexual behavior in the institutionalized aged, *Arch Sex Behav* 11:11, 1982.

90. **Renshaw DC,** Sex, intimacy, and the older woman, *Women Health* 8:43, 1983.

91. **Helström L, Lundberg PO, Sörbom D, Bäckström T,** Sexuality after hysterectomy: a factor analysis of women's sexual lives before and after subtotal hysterectomy, *Obstet Gynecol* 81:357, 1993.

92. **Gosden RG,** Follicular status at menopause, *Hum Reprod* 2:617, 1987.

93. **Chakravarti S, Collins WP, Forecast JD, Newton JR, Oram DH, Studd JWW,** Hormonal profiles after the menopause, *Br Med J* ii:784, 1976.

94. **Jiroutek MR, Chen M-H, Johnston CC, Longcope C,** Changes in reproductive hormones and sex hormone-binding globulin in a group of postmenopausal women measured over 10 years, *Menopause* 5:90, 1998.

95. **Meldrum DR, Davidson BJ, Tataryn IV, Judd HL,** Changes in circulating steroids with aging in postmenopausal women, *Obstet Gynecol* 57:624, 1981.

96. **Grodin JM, Siiteri PK, McDonald PC,** Source of estrogen production in postmenopausal women, *J Clin Endocrinol Metab* 36:207, 1963.

97. **Labrie F, Bélanger A, Cusan L, Gomez J-L, Candas B,** Marked decline in serum concentrations of adrenal C19 sex steroid precursors and conjugated androgen metabolites during aging, *J Clin Endocrinol Metab* 82:2396, 1997.

98. **Dowsett M, Cantwell B, Anshumala L, Jeffcoate SL, Harris SL,** Suppression of postmenopausal ovarian steroidogenesis with the luteinizing hormone-releasing hormone agonist Goserelin, *J Clin Endocrinol Metab* 66:672, 1988.

99. **Andreyko JL, Monroe SE, Marshall LA, Fluker MR, Nerenberg CA, Jaffe RB,** Concordant suppression of serum immunoreactive luteinizing hormone (LH), follicle-stimulating hormone, subunit bioactive LH, and testosterone in postmenopausal women by a potent gonadotropin releasing hormone antagonist (Detirelix), *J Clin Endocrinol Metab* 74:399, 1992.

100. **Sluijmer AV, Heineman MJ, De Jong FH, Evers JL,** Endocrine activity of the postmenopausal ovary: the effects of pituitary down-regulation and oophorectomy, *J Clin Endocrinol Metab* 80:2163, 1995.

101. **Zumoff B, Strain GW, Miller LK, Rosner W,** 24-Hour mean plasma testosterone concentration declines with age in normal premenopausal women, *J Clin Endocrinol Metab* 80:1429, 1995.

102. **Longcope C, Jaffe W, Griffing G,** Production rates of androgens and oestrogens in post-menopausal women, *Maturitas* 3:215, 1981.

103. **Judd HL, Judd GE, Lucas WE, Yen SSC,** Endocrine function of the postmenopausal ovary; concentration of androgens and estrogens in ovarian and peripheral vein blood, *J Clin Endocrinol Metab* 39:1020, 1974.

104. **Judd HL, Shamonki IM, Frumar AM, Lagasse LD,** Origin of serum estradiol in postmenopausal women, *Obstet Gynecol* 59:680, 1982.

105. **Adashi EY,** The climacteric ovary as a functional gonadotropin-driven androgen-producing gland, *Fertil Steril* 62:20, 1994.

106. **Goldstein SR, Zeltser I, Horan CK, Snyder JR, Schwartz LB,** Ultrasonography-based triage for perimenopausal patients with abnormal uterine bleeding, *Am J Obstet Gynecol* 177:102, 1997.

107. **Einerth Y,** Vacuum curettage by the Vabra method. A simple procedure for endometrial diagnosis, *Acta Obstet Gynecol Scand* 61:373, 1982.

108. **Feldman S, Shapter A, Welch WR, Berkowitz RS,** Two-year follow-up of 263 patients with post/perimenopausal vaginal bleeding and negative initial biopsy, *Gynecol Oncol* 55:56, 1994.

109. **Gebbie AE, Glasier A, Sweeting V,** Incidence of ovulation in perimenopausal women before and during hormone replacement therapy, *Contraception* 52:221, 1995.

110. **Casper RF, Dodin S, Reid RL, and Study Investigators,** The effect of 20 µg ethinyl estradiol/1 mg norethindrone acetate (Minnestrin™), a low-dose oral contraceptive, on vaginal bleeding patterns, hot flashes, and quality of life in symptomatic perimenopausal women, *Menopause* 4:139, 1997.

111. **Castracane VD, Gimpel T, Goldzieher JW,** When is it safe to switch from oral contraceptives to hormonal replacement therapy? *Contraception* 52:371, 1995.

112. **Kroon E, Andolf E,** Diagnosis and follow-up of simple ovarian cysts detected by ultrasound in postmenopausal women, *Obset Gynecol* 85:211, 1995.

113. **Beyene Y,** *From Menarche to Menopause: Reproductive Lives of Peasant Women in Two Cultures,* State University of New York Press, Albany, 1989.

114. **Lock M,** *Encounters with Aging: Mythologies of Menopause in Japan and North America,* University of California Press, Berkeley, 1993.

115. **Lock M,** Menopause in cultural context, *Exp Gerontol* 29:307, 1994.

116. **Moore B, Kombe H,** Climacteric symptoms in a Tanzanian community, *Maturitas* 13:229, 1991.

117. **Martin MC, Block JE, Sanchez SD, Arnaud CD, Beyene Y,** Menopause without symptoms: the endocrinology of menopause among rural Mayan Indians, *Am J Obstet Gynecol* 168:1839, 1993.

118. **Robinson G,** Cross-cultural perspectives on menopause, *J Nervous Mental Dis* 184:453, 1996.

119. **Richters JMA,** Menopause in different cultures, *J Psychosom Obstet Gynecol* 18:73, 1997.

120. **Kronnenberg F, Barnard RM,** Modulation of menopausal hot flashes by ambient temerature, *J Therm Biol* 17:43, 1992.

121. **Hunter M,** The South-East England longitudinal study of the climacteric and postmenopause, *Maturitas* 14:17, 1992.

122. **Oldenhave A, Jaszmann LJB, Haspels AA, Everaerd WTAM,** Impact of climacteric on well-being, *Am J Obstet Gynecol* 168:772, 1993.

123. **Hahn PM, Wong J, Reid RL,** Menopausal-like hot flashes reported in women of reproductive age, *Fertil Steril* 70:913, 1998.

124. **Guthrie JR, Dennerstein L, Hopper JL, Burger HG,** Hot flushes, menstrual status, and hormone levels in a population-based sample of midlife women, *Obstet Gynecol* 88:437, 1996.

125. **Schwingl PJ, Hulka BS, Harlow SD,** Risk factors for menopausal hot flashes, *Obstet Gynecol* 84:29, 1994.

126. **Pham KT, Grisso JA, Freeman EW,** Ovarian aging and hormone replacement therapy. Hormonal levels, symptoms, and attitudes of African-American and white women, *J Gen Intern Med* 12:230, 1997.

127. **Kronnenberg F,** Hot flashes: epidemiology and physiology, *Ann NY Acad Sci* 592:52, 1990.

128. **Wilkin JR,** Flushing reactions: consequences and mechanisms, *Ann Intern Med* 95:468, 1981.

129. **Aksel S, Schomberg DW, Tyrey L, Hammond CB,** Vasomotor symptoms, serum estrogens and gonadotropin levels in surgical menopause, *Am J Obstet Gynecol* 126:165, 1976.

130. **Swartzman LC, Edelberg R, Kemmann E,** The menopausal hot flush: symptom reports and concomitant physiological changes, *J Behav Med* 13:15, 1990.

131. **Freedman RR,** Biochemical, metabolic, and vascular mechanisms in menopausal hot flashes, *Fertil Steril* 70:332, 1998.

132. **Mohyi D, Tabassi K, Simon J,** Differential diagnosis of hot flashes, *Maturitas* 27:203, 1997.

133. **Pearce J, Hawton K, Blake F, Barlow D, Rees M, Fagg J, Keenan J,** Psychological effects of continuation versus discontinuation of hormone replacement therapy by estrogen implants: a placebo-controlled study, *J Psychosom Res* 42:177, 1997.

134. **Raz R, Stamm WE,** A controlled trial of intravaginal estriol in postmenopausal women with recurrent urinary tract infection, *New Engl J Med* 329:753, 1993.

135. **Wilson PD, Faragher B, Butler B, Bullock D, Robinson EL, Brown ADG,** Treatment with oral piperazine oestrone sulphate for genuine stress incontinence in postmenopausal women, *Br J Obstet Gynaecol* 94:568, 1987.

136. **Bhatia NN, Bergman A, Karram MM,** Effects of estrogen on urethral function in women with urinary incontinence, *Obstet Gynecol* 160:176, 1989.

137. **Semmens JP, Wagner G,** Effects of estrogen therapy on vaginal physiology during menopause, *Obstet Gynecol* 66:15, 1985.

138. **Castelo-Branco C, Duran M, Gonzalez-Merlo J,** Skin collagen changes related to age and hormone replacement therapy, *Maturitas* 15:113, 1992.

139. **Savvas M, Lausrent GB,** Type III collagen content in the skin of postmenopausal women receiving oestradiol and testosterone implants, *Br J Obstet Gynaecol* 100:154, 1993.

140. **Maheux R, Naud F, Rioux M, Grenier R, Lemay A, Guy J, Langevin M,** A randomized, double-blind, placebo-controlled study on the effect of conjugated estrogens on skin thickness, *Am J Obstet Gynecol* 170:642, 1994.

141. **Callens A, Vaillant L, Lecomte P, Berson M, Gall Y, Lorette G,** Does hormonal skin aging exist? A study of the influence of different hormone therapy regimens on the skin of postmenopausal women using non-invasive measurement techniques, *Dermatol* 193:289, 1996.

142. **Holland EFN, Studd JWW, Mansell JP, Leather AT, Bailey AJ,** Changes in collagen composition and cross-links in bone and skin of osteoporotic postmenopausal women treated with percutaneous estradiol implants, *Obstet Gynecol* 83:180, 1994.

143. **Castelo-Branco C, Pons F, Gratacøs E, Fortuny A, Vanrell JA, Gonzalez-Merlo J,** Relationship between skin collagen and bone changes during aging, *Maturitas* 18:199, 1994.

144. **Creidi P, Faivre B, Agache P, Richard E, Haudiquet V, Sauvanet JP,** Effect of a conjugated oestrogen (Premarin) cream on aging facial skin. A comparative study with a placebo cream, *Maturitas* 19:211, 1994.

145. **Dunn LB, Damesyn M, Moore AA, Reuben DB, Greendale GA,** Does estrogen prevent skin aging? Results from the First National Health and Nutrition Examination Survey (NHANES I), *Arch Dermatol* 133:339, 1997.

146. **Castelo-Branco C, Figueras F, Martínez de Osaba MJ, Vanrell JA,** Facial wrinkling in postmenopausal women. Effects of smoking status and hormone replacement therapy, *Maturitas* 29:75, 1998.

147. **Cauley JA, Petrini AM, LaPorte RE, Sandler RB, Bayles CM, Robertson RJ, Slemenda CW,** The decline of grip strength in the menopause: relationship to physical activity, estrogen use and anthropometric factors, *J Chron Dis* 40:115, 1987.

148. **Phillips SK, Rook KM, Siddle NC, Bruce SA, Woldege RC,** Muscle weakness in women occurs at an earlier age than in men but strength is preserved by hormone replacement therapy, *Clin Sci* 84:95, 1993.

149. **Preisinger E, Alacamlioglu Y, Saradeth T, Resch KL, Holzer G, Metka M,** Forearm bone density and grip strength in women after menopause with and without estrogen replacement therapy, *Maturitas* 21:57, 1995.

150. **Ballinger CB,** Psychiatric aspects of the menopause, *Br J Psychiatr* 156:773, 1990.

151. **Schmidt PJ, Rubinow DR,** Menopause-related affective disorders: a justification for further study, *Am J Psychiatr* 148:844, 1991.

152. **Gath D, Osborn M, Bungay G, Iles S, Day A, Bond A, Passingham C,** Psychiatric disorder and gynaecological symptoms in middle aged women: a community survey, *Br Med J* 294:213, 1987.

153. **Everson SA, Matthews KA, Guzick DS, Meilahn EN, Wing RR, Kuller LH,** Effects of surgical menopause on lipid levels and psychosocial characteristics: the Healthy Women Study, *Health Psychol* 14:435, 1995.

154. **Avis NE, Brambilla D, McKinlay SM, Vass K,** A longitudinal analysis of the association between menopause and depression. Results from the Massachusetts Women's Health Study, *Ann Epidemiol* 4:214, 1994.

155. **Kessler RC, McGonagle KA, Swartz M, Blazer DG, Nelson CB,** Sex and depression in the National Comorbidity Survey I: lifetime prevalence, chronicity and recurrence, *J Affective Disorders* 29:85, 1993.

156. **Busch CM, Zonderman AB, Costa Jr PT,** Menopausal transition and psychological distress in a nationally representative sample: is menopause associated with psychological distress? *J Aging Health* 6:209, 1994.

157. **Dennerstein L, Smith AMA, Morse C,** Psychological well-being, mid-life and the menopause, *Maturitas* 20:1, 1994.

158. **Mitchell ES, Woods NF,** Symptom experiences of midlife women: observations from the Seattle midlife women's health study, *Maturitas* 25:1, 1996.

159. **Van Hall EV, Verdel M, Van Der Velden J,** "Perimenopausal" complaints in women and men: a comparative study, *J Women's Health* 3:45, 1994.

160. **Campbell S, Whitehead M,** Estrogen therapy and the menopausal syndrome, *Clin Obstet Gynecol* 4:31, 1977.

161. **Kuh DL, Wadsorth M, Hardy R,** Women's health in midlife: the influence of the menopause, social factors and health in earlier life, *Br J Obstet Gynaecol* 104:923, 1997.

162. **Wiklund I, Karlberg J, Mattsson L-A,** Quality of life of postmenopausal women on a regimen of transdermal estradiol therapy: a double-blind placebo-controlled study, *Am J Obstet Gynecol* 168:824, 1993.

163. **Daly E, Gray A, Barlow D, McPherson K, Roche M, Vessey M,** Measuring the impact of menopausal symptoms on quality of life, *Br Med J* 307:836, 1993.

164. **Woodward S, Freedman RR,** The thermoregulatory effects of menopausal hot flashes on sleep, *Sleep* 17:497, 1994.

165. **Schiff I, Regestein Q, Tulchinsky D, Ryan KJ,** Effects of estrogens on sleep and psychological state of hypogonadal women, *JAMA* 242:2405, 1979.

166. **Polo-Kantola P, Erkkola R, Helenius H, Irjala K, Polo O,** When does estrogen replacement therapy improve sleep quality? *Am J Obstet Gynecol* 178:1002, 1998.

167. **Dennerstein L, Burrows GD, Hyman GJ, Wood C,** Hormone therapy and affect, *Maturitas* 1:247, 1979.

168. **Sherwin BB,** Affective changes with estrogen and androgen replacement therapy in surgically menopausal women, *J Affective Disorders* 14:177, 1988.

169. **Palinkas LA, Barrett-Connor E,** Estrogen use and depressive symptoms in postmenopausal women, *Obstet Gynecol* 80:30, 1992.

170. **Limouzin-Lamothe M-A, Mairon N, Joyce CRB, Le Gal M,** Quality of life after the menopause: influence of hormonal replacement therapy, *Am J Obstet Gynecol* 170:618, 1994.

171. **Schneider LS, Small GW, Hamilton SH, Bystritsky A, Nemeroff CB, Meyers BS, and the Fluoxetine Collaborative Study Group,** Estrogen replacement and response to fluoxetine in a multicenter geriatric depression trial, *Am J Geriatr Psychiatry* 5:97, 1997.

172. **Sherwin BB,** Estrogen effects on cognition in menopausal women, *Neurol* 48(Suppl 7):S21, 1997.

173. **Rice MM, Graves AB, McCurry SM, Larson EB,** Estrogen replacement therapy and cognitive function in postmenopausal women without dementia, *Am J Med* 103(3A):26S, 1997.

174. **Ditkoff EC, Crary WG, Cristo M, Lobo RA,** Estrogen improves psychological function in asymptomatic postmenopausal women, *Obstet Gynecol* 78:991, 1991.

175. **Polo-Kantola P, Portin R, Polo O, Helenius H, Irjala K, Erkkola R,** The effect of short-term estrogen replacement therapy on cognition: a randomized, double-blind, cross-over trial in postmenopausal women, *Obstet Gynecol* 91:459, 1998.

176. **Phillips SM, Sherwin BB,** Effects of estrogen on memory function in surgically menopausal women, *Psychoneuroendocrinology* 17:485, 1992.

177. **Kampen DL, Sherwin BB,** Estrogen use and verbal memory in healthy postmenopausal women, *Obstet Gynecol* 83:979, 1994.

178. **Robinson D, Friedman L, Marcus R, Tinklenberg J, Yesavage J,** Estrogen replacement therapy and memory in older women, *J Am Geriatr Soc* 42:919, 1994.

179. **Resnick SM, Metter EJ, Zonderman AB,** Estrogen replacement therapy and longitudinal decline in visual memory. A possible protective effect, *Neurology* 49:1491, 1997.

180. **Jacobs DM, Tang MX, Stern Y, Sano M, Marder K, Bell KL, Schofield P, Dooneief G, Gurland B, Mayeux R,** Cognitive function in nondemented older women who took estrogen after menopause, *Neurology* 50:368, 1998.

181. **Barrett-Connor E, Kritz-Silverstein D,** Estrogen replacement therapy and cognitive function in older women, *JAMA* 269:2637, 1993.

182. **Behl C, Skutella T, Lezoualc'h F, Post A, Widmann M, Newton CJ, Holsboer F,** Neuroprotection against oxidative stress by estrogens: structure-activity relationship, *Mol Pharm* 51:535, 1997.

183. **Hashimoto S, Katou M, Dong Y, Murakami K, Terada S, Inoue M,** Effects of hormone replacement therapy on serum amyloid P component in postmenopausal women, *Maturitas* 26:113, 1997.

184. **Wooley CS, Weiland NG, McEwen BS, Schwartzkroin PA,** Estradiol increases the sensitivity of hippocampal CA1 pyramidal cells to NMDA receptor-mediated synaptic input: correlation with dendritic spine density, *J Neurosci* 17:1848, 1997.

185. **Paganini-Hill A, Henderson VW,** Estrogen replacement therapy and risk of Alzheimer disease, *Arch Intern Med* 156:2213, 1996.

186. **Henderson VW,** The epidemiology of estrogen replacement therapy and Alzheimer's disease, *Neurol* 48(Suppl 7):S27, 1997.

187. **Kawas C, Resnick S, Morrison A, Brookmeyer R, Corrada M, Zonderman A, Bacal C, Lingle D, Metter E,** A prospective study of estrogen replacement therapy and the risk of developing Alzheimer's disease: the Baltimore Longitudinal Study of Aging, *Neurol* 48:1517, 1997.

188. **Tang M-X, Jacobs D, Stern Y, Marder K, Schofield P, Gurland B, Andrews H, Mayeux R,** Effect of oestrogen during menopause on risk and age of onset of Alzheimer's disease, *Lancet* 348:429, 1996.

189. **Baldereschi M, Di Carlo A, Lepore V, Bracco L, Maggi S, Grigoletto F, Scarlato G, Amaducci L, for the ILSA Working Group,** Estrogen-replacement therapy and Alzheimer's disease in the Italian Longitudinal Study on Aging, *Neurol* 50:996, 1998.

190. **Henderson V, Paganini-Hill A, Emanuel CK, Dunn ME, Buckwalter G,** Estrogen replacement therapy in older women: comparisons between Alzheimer's disease cases and nondemented control subjects, *Arch Neurol* 51:896, 1994.

191. **Schneider LS, Farlow MR, Henderson VW, Pogoda J,** Effects of estrogen replacement therapy on response to tacrine in patients with Alzheimer's disease, *Neurol* 46:1580, 1996.

192. **Clarkson TB, Prichard RW, Morgan TM, Petrick GS, Klein KP,** Remodeling of coronary arteries in human and nonhuman primates, *JAMA* 271:289, 1994.

193. **Matthews KA, Meilahn E, Kuller LH, Kelsey SF, Caggiula AW, Wing RR,** Menopause and risk factors for coronary heart disease, *New Engl J Med* 321:641, 1989.

194. **Campos H, McNamara JR, Wilson PW, Ordovas JM, Schaefer EJ,** Differences in low density lipoprotein subfractions and apolipoproteins in premenopausal and postmenopausal women, *J Clin Endocrinol Metab* 67:30, 1988.

195. **Jensen J, Nilas L, Christiansen C,** Influence of menopause on serum lipids and lipoproteins, *Maturitas* 12:321, 1990.

196. **Stevenson JC, Crook D, Godsland IF,** Influence of age and menopause on serum lipids and lipoproteins in healthy women, *Atherosclerosis* 98:83, 1993.

197. **van Beresteijn ECH, Korevaar JC, Huijbregts PCW, Schouten EG, Burema J, Kok FJ,** Perimenopausal increase in serum cholesterol: a 10-year longitudinal study, *Am J Epidemiol* 137:383, 1993.

198. **Matthews KA, Wing RR, Kuller LH, Meilahn EN, Plantinga P,** Influence of the perimenopause on cardiovascular risk factors and symptoms of middle-aged healthy women, *Arch Intern Med* 154:2349, 1994.

199. **Bruschi F, Meschia M, Soma M, Perotti D, Paoletti R, Crosignani PG,** Lipoprotein(a) and other lipids after oophorectomy and estrogen replacement therapy, *Obstet Gynecol* 88:950, 1996.

200. **Brunner D, Weisbort J, Meshulam N, Schwartz S, Gross J, Saltz-Rennert H, Altman S, Loebl K,** Relation of serum total cholesterol and high-density lipoprotein cholesterol percentage to the incidence of definite coronary events: twenty-year follow-up of the Donolo-Tel Aviv Prospective Coronary Artery Disease Study, *Am J Cardiol* 59:1271, 1987.

201. **Jacobs Jr DR, Mebane IL, Bangdiwala SI, Criqui MH, Tyroler HA,** High density lipoprotein cholesterol as a predictor of cardiovascular disease mortality in men and women: the follow-up study of the Lipid Research Clinics Prevalence Study, *Am J Epidemiol* 131:32, 1990.

202. **Hulley SB, Newman TB,** Cholesterol in the elderly: is it important? *JAMA* 272:1372, 1994.

203. **Kannel WB,** Metabolic risk factors for coronary heart disease in women: perspective from the Framingham Study, *Am Heart J* 114:413, 1987.

204. **Downs JR, Clearfield M, Weis S, Whitney E, Shapiro DR, Beere PA, Langendorger A, Stein EA, Kruyer W, Gotto Jr AM, for the AFCAPS/TexCAPS Research Group,** Primary prevention of acute coronary events with lovastatin in men and women with average cholesterol levels. Results of AFCAPS/TexCAPS, *JAMA* 279:1615, 1998.

205. **Castelli WP, Garrison RJ, Wilson PWF, Abbott RD, Kalousdian S, Kannel WB,** Incidence of coronary heart disease and lipoprotein cholesterol levels, *JAMA* 256:2835, 1986.

206. **Bass KM, Newschaffer CJ, Klag MJ, Bush TL,** Plasma lipoprotein levels as predictors of cardiovascular deaths in women, *Circulation* 153:2209, 1993.

207. **Castelli WP,** The triglyceride issue: a view from Framingham, *Am Heart J* 112:432, 1986.

208. **Chowienczyk PJ, Watts GF, Cockcroft JR, Brett SE, Ritter JM,** Sex differences in endothelial function in normal and hypercholesterolaemic subjects, *Lancet* 344:305, 1994.

209. **Barker DJP, Martyn CN, Osmond C, Hales CN, Fall CHD,** Growth in utero and serum cholesterol concentrations in adult life, *Br Med J* 307:1524, 1993.

210. **Fall CHD, Osmond C, Barker DJP, Clark PMS, Hales CN, Stirling Y, Meade TW,** Fetal and infant growth and cardiovascular risk factors in women, *Br Med J* 310:428, 1995.

211. **Lapidus L, Bengtsson C, Larsson B, Pennert K, Rybo E, Sjostrom L,** Distribution of adipose tissue and risk of cardiovascular disease and death: a 12 year follow up of participants in the population study of women in Gothenburg, *Br Med J* 289:1257, 1984.

212. **Haarbo J, Hassager C, Riis BJ, Christiansen C,** Relation of body fat distribution to serum lipids and lipoproteins in elderly women, *Atherosclerosis* 80:57, 1989.

213. **Soler JT, Folsom AR, Kaye SA, Prineas RJ,** Associations of abdominal adiposity, fasting insulin, sex hormone binding globulin and estrogen with lipids and lipoproteins in post-menopausal women, *Atherosclerosis* 79:21, 1989.

214. **Wing R, Matthews K, Kuller L, Meilahn EN, Plantinga PL,** Weight gain at the time of menopause, *Arch Intern Med* 151:97, 1990.

215. **National Center for Health Statistics, Division of Vital Statistics,** (National Center for Health Statistics), Public use data tapes for U.S. mortality, 1970 to 1995 and provisional tabulations for 1996, 1997.

216. **Vartiainen E, Puska P, Pekkanen J, Tuomilehto J, Jousilahti P,** Changes in risk factors explain changes in mortality from ischaemic heart disease in Finland, *Br Med J* 309:23, 1994.

217. **Vartiainen E, Sarti C, Tuomilehto J, Kuulasmaa K,** Do changes in cardiovascular risk factors explain changes in mortality from stroke in Finland? *Br Med J* 310:901, 1995.

218. **Rosenberg L, Armstrong B, Jick H,** Myocardial infarction and estrogen therapy in postmenopausal women, *New Engl J Med* 294:1256, 1976.

219. **Pfeffer RI, Whipple GH, Kurosake TT, Chapman JM,** Coronary risk and estrogen use in postmenopausal women, *Am J Epidemiol* 107:479, 1978.

220. **Jick H, Dinan B, Rothman KJ,** Noncontraceptive estrogens and non-fatal myocardial infarction, *JAMA* 239:1407, 1978.

221. **Rosenberg L, Sloane D, Shapiro S, Kaufman D, Stolley PD, Miethinen OS,** Noncontraceptive estrogens and myocardial infarction in young women, *JAMA* 224:339, 1980.

222. **Ross RK, Paganini-Hill A, Mack TM, Arthur M, Henderson BE,** Menopausal oestrogen therapy and protection from death from ischaemic heart disease, *Lancet* i:858, 1981.

223. **Bain C, Willett W, Hennekens CH, Rosner B, Belanger C, Speizer FE,** Use of postmenopausal hormones and risk of myocardial infarction, *Circulation* 64:42, 1981.

224. **Adam S, Williams V, Vessey MP,** Cardiovascular disease and hormone replacement treatment: a pilot case-control study, *Br Med J* 282:1277, 1981.

225. **Szklo M, Tonascia J, Gordis L, Bloom I,** Estrogen use and myocardial infarction risk: a case-control study, *Prev Med* 13:510, 1984.

226. **Sullivan JM, Vander Zwaag R, Lemp GF, Hughes JP, Maddock V, Kroetz FW, Ramanathan KB, Mirvis DM,** Postmenopausal estrogen use and coronary atherosclerosis, *Ann Intern Med* 108:358, 1988.

227. **Gruchow HW, Anderson AJ, Barboriak JJ, Sobocinski KA,** Postmenopausal use of estrogen and occlusion of coronary arteries, *Am Heart J* 115:954, 1988.

228. **McFarland K, Boniface M, Hornung C, Earnhardt W, Humphries J,** Risk factors and noncontraceptive estrogen use in women with and without coronary disease, *Am Heart J* 117:1209, 1989.

229. **Hong MG, Romm PA, Reagan K, Green CE, Rackley CE,** Effects of estrogen replacement therapy on serum lipid values and angiographically defined coronary artery disease in postmenopausal women, *Am J Cardiol* 69:176, 1992.

230. **Psaty BM, Heckbart SR, Atkins D, Lemaitre R, Koepsell TD, Wahl PN, Siscovick DS, Wagner EH,** The risk of myocardial infarction associated with the combined use of estrogens and progestins in postmenopausal women, *Arch Intern Med* 154:1333, 1994.

231. **Beard CM, Kottke TE, Annegers JF, Ballard DJ,** The Rochester Coronary Heart Disease Project: effect of cigarette smoking, hypertension, diabetes, and steroidal estrogen use on coronary heart disease among 40- to 59-year-old women, 1960 through 1982, *Mayo Clin Proc* 64:1471, 1989.

232. **Burch JC, Byrd BF, Vaughn WK,** The effects of long-term estrogen on hysterectomized women, *Am J Obstet Gynecol* 118:778, 1974.

233. **Gordon T, Kannel WB, Hjortland MC, McNamara PM,** Menopause and coronary heart disease: the Framingham Study, *Ann Intern Med* 89:37, 1978.

234. **Hammond CB, Jelovsek FR, Lee KL, Creasman WT, Parker RT,** Effects of long-term estrogen replacement therapy: I. Metabolic effects, *Am J Obstet Gynecol* 133:525, 1979.

235. **Petitti DB, Wingerd J, Pellegrin F, Ramcharan S,** Risk of vascular disease in women: smoking, oral contraceptives, noncontraceptive estrogens, and other factors, *JAMA* 242:1150, 1979.

236. **Wilson PWF, Garrison RJ, Castelli WP,** Postmenopausal estrogen use, cigarette smoking, and cardiovascular morbidity in women over 50, *New Engl J Med* 313:1038, 1985.

237. **Bush TL, Barrett-Connor E, Cowan DK, Criqui MH, Wallace RB, Suchindran CM, Tyroler HA, Rifkind BM,** Cardiovascular mortality and noncontraceptive use of estrogen in women: results from the Lipid Research Clinics Program Follow-up Study, *Circulation* 75:1102, 1987.

238. **Criqui MH, Suarez L, Barrett-Connor E, McPhillips J, Wingard DL, Garland C,** Postmenopausal estrogen use and mortality, *Am J Epidemiol* 128:606, 1988.

239. **Henderson BE, Paganini-Hill A, Ross RK,** Estrogen replacement therapy and protection from acute myocardial infarction, *Am J Obstet Gynecol* 159:312, 1988.

240. **Perlman J, Wolff P, Finucane F, Madans J,** Menopause and the epidemiology of cardiovascular disease in women, *Prog Clin Biol Res* 320:283, 1989.

241. **Lafferty FW, Fiske ME,** Postmenopausal estrogen replacement: a long-term cohort study, *Am J Med* 97:66, 1994.

242. **Folsom AR, Mink PJ, Sellers TA, Hong C-P, Zheng W, Potter JD,** Hormonal replacement therapy and morbidity and mortality in a prospective study of postmenopausal women, *Am J Public Health* 85:1128, 1995.

243. **Grodstein F, Stampfer MJ, Manson JE, Colditz GA, Willett WC, Rosner B, Speizer FE, Hennekens CH,** Postmenopausal estrogen and progestin use and risk of cardiovascular disease, *New Engl J Med* 335:453, 1996.

244. **Grodstein F, Stampfer MJ, Colditz GA, Willett WC, Manson JE, Joffe M, Rosner B, Fuchs C, Hankinson SE, Hunter DJ, Hennekens CH, Speizer FE,** Postmenopausal hormone therapy and mortality, *New Engl J Med* 336:1769, 1997.

245. **Petitti DB, Perlman JA, Sidney S,** Noncontraceptive estrogens and mortality: long-term follow-up of women in the Walnut Creek Study, *Obstet Gynecol* 70:289, 1987.

246. **Eaker ED, Castelli WP,** Coronary heart disease and its risk factors among women in the Framingham Study, In: Eaker E, Packard B, Wenger N, eds. *Coronary Heart Disease in Women,* Haymarket Doyma, New York, 1987, p 122.

247. **Ettinger B, Friedman GD, Bush T, Quesenberry Jr CP,** Reduced mortality associated with long-term postmenopausal estrogen therapy, *Obstet Gynecol* 87:5, 1996.

248. **McLaughlin VV, Hoff JA, Rich S,** Relation between hormone replacement therapy in women and coronary artery disease estimated by electron beam tomography, *Am Heart J* 134:1115, 1997.

249. **Matthews KA, Kuller LH, Wing RR, Meilahn EN, Plantinga P,** Prior to use of estrogen replacement therapy, are users healthier than nonusers? *Am J Epidemiol* 143:971, 1997.

250. **Henderson BE, Paganini-Hill A, Ross RK,** Decreased mortality in users of estrogen replacement therapy, *Arch Intern Med* 151:75, 1991.

251. **Stampfer MJ, Colditz GA, Willett WC, Manson JE, Rosner B, Speizer FE, Hennekens CH,** Postmenopausal estrogen therapy and cardiovascular disease: ten-year follow-up from the Nurses' Health Study, *New Engl J Med* 325:756, 1991.

252. **Derby CA, Hume AL, McPhillips JB, Barbour MM, Carleton RA,** Prior and current health characteristics of postmenopausal estrogen replacement therapy users compared to non-users, *Am J Obstet Gynecol* 173:544, 1995.

253. **MacLennan AH, Wilson DH, Taylor AW,** Hormone replacement therapy: prevalence, compliance and the 'healthy women' notion, *Climacteric* 1:42, 1998.

254. **Falkeborn M, Persson I, Terént A, Bergström R, Lithell H, Naessén T,** Long-term trends in incidence of and mortality from acute myocardial infarction and stroke in women: analyses of total first events and of deaths in the Uppsala health care region, Sweden, *Epidemiology* 7:67, 1996.

255. **Paganini-Hill A, Ross RK, Henderson BE,** Postmenopausal oestrogen treatment and stroke: a prospective study, *Br Med J* 297:519, 1988.

256. **Thompson SG, Meade TW, Greenberg G,** The use of hormonal replacement therapy and the risk of stroke and myocardial infarction in women, *J Epidemiol Comm Health* 43:173, 1989.

257. **Hunt K, Vessey M, McPherson K,** Mortality in a cohort of long-term users of hormone replacement therapy: an updated analysis, *Br J Obstet Gynaecol* 97:1080, 1990.

258. **Finucane FF, Mardans JH, Bush TL, Wolf PH, Kleinman JC,** Decreased risk of stroke among postmenopausal hormone users, *Arch Intern Med* 153:73, 1993.

259. **Falkeborn M, Persson I, Terent A, Adami HO, Lithell H, Bergstrom R,** Hormone replacement therapy and the risk of stroke. Follow-up of a population-based cohort in Sweden, *Arch Intern Med* 153:1201, 1993.

260. **Longstreth Jr WT, Nelson LM, Koepsell TD, van Belle G,** Subarachnoid hemorrhage and hormonal factors in women: a population-based case-control study, *Ann Intern Med* 121:168, 1994.

261. **Pedersen AT, Lidegaard Ø, Kreiner S, Ottesen B,** Hormone replacement therapy and risk of non-fatal stroke, *Lancet* 350:1277, 1997.

262. **Petitti DB, Sidney S, Quesenberry Jr CP, Bernstein A,** Ischemic stroke and use of estrogen and estrogen/progestogen as hormone replacement therapy, *Stroke* 29:23, 1998.

263. **Schairer C, Adami H-O, Hoover R, Persson I,** Cause-specific mortality in women receiving hormone replacement therapy, *Epidemiology* 8:59, 1997.

264. **Lind T, Cameron EC, Hunter WM, Leon C, Moran PF, Oxley A, Gerrard J, Lind UCG,** A prospective, controlled trial of six forms of hormone replacement therapy given to postmenopausal women, *Br J Obstet Gynaecol* 86(Suppl 3):1, 1979.

265. **Pfeffer RI, Kurosaki TT, Charlton SK,** Estrogen use and blood pressure in later life, *Am J Epidemiol* 110:469, 1979.

266. **Lutola H,** Blood pressure and hemodynamics in postmenopausal women during estradiol-17β substitution, *Ann Clin Res* 15(Suppl 38):9, 1983.

267. **Wren BG, Routledge AD,** The effect of type and dose of oestrogen on the blood pressure of postmenopausal women, *Maturitas* 5:135, 1983.

268. **Hassager C, Christiansen C,** Blood pressure during oestrogen/progestogen substitution therapy in healthy post-menopausal women, *Maturitas* 9:315, 1988.

269. **Lip GY, Beevers M, Churchill D, Beevers DG,** Hormone replacement therapy and blood pressure in hypertensive women, *J Hum Hypertens* 8:491, 1994.

270. **Sands RH, Studd JWW, Crook D, Warren JB, Cruickshank J, Coats A,** The effect of estrogen on blood pressure in hypertensive postmenopausal women, *Menopause* 4:115, 1997.

271. **Kornhauser C, Malacara JM, Gray ME, Perez-Luque EL,** The effect of hormone replacement therapy on blood pressure and cardiovascular risk factors in menopausal women with moderate hypertension, *J Hum Hypertens* 11:405, 1997.

272. **The Writing Group for the PEPI Trial,** Effects of estrogen or estrogen/progestin regimens on heart disease risk factors in postmenopausal women: the Postmenopausal Estrogen/Progestin Interventions (PEPI) Trial, *JAMA* 273:199, 1995.

273. **Medical Research Council's General Practice Research Framework,** Randomised comparison of oestrogen versus oestrogen plus progestogen hormone replacement therapy in women with hysterectomy, *Br Med J* 312:473, 1996.

274. **Zarifis J, Lip GYH, Beevers DG,** Effects of discontinuing hormone replacement therapy in patients with uncontrolled hypertension, *Am J Hypertens* 8:1241, 1995.

275. **Mercuro G, Zoncu S, Pilia I, Lao A, Melis GB, Cherchi A,** Effects of acute administration of transdermal estrogen on postmenopausal women with systemic hypertension, *Am J Cardiol* 80:652, 1997.

276. **Manolio T, Furberg C, Shemanski L, Psaty B, O'Leary D, Tracy R, Bush T, for the CHS Collaborative Research Group,** Associations of postmenopausal estrogen use with cardiovascular disease and its risk factors in older women, *Circulation* 88 (Part 1):2163, 1993.

277. **Eriksson M, Berglund L, Rudling M, Henriksson P, Angelin B,** Effects of estrogen on low density lipoprotein metabolism in males. Short-term and long-term studies during hormonal treatment of prostatic cancer, *J Clin Invest* 84:802, 1989.

278. **Walsh BW, Schiff I, Rosner B, Greenberg L, Ravnikar V, Sacks FM,** Effects of postmenopausal estrogen replacement on the concentrations and metabolism of plasma lipoproteins, *New Engl J Med* 325:1196, 1991.

279. **Muesing R, Miller V, LaRosa J, Stoy D, Phillips E,** Effects of unopposed conjugated equine estrogen on lipoprotein composition and apolipoprotein-E distribution, *J Clin Endocrinol Metab* 75:1250, 1992.

280. **Espeland MA, Marcovina SM, Miller V, Wood PD, Wasilauskas C, Sherwin R, Schrott H, Bush TL,** Effect of postmenopausal hormone therapy on lipoprotein(a) concentration, *Circulation* 97:979, 1998.

281. **Granfone A, Campos H, McNamara JR, Schaefer MM, Lemon-Fava S, Ordovas JM, Schaefer EJ,** Effects of estrogen replacement on plasma lipoproteins and apolipoproteins in postmenopausal dyslipidemic women, *Metabolism* 1992:1193, 1992.

282. **Rifici VA, Khachadurian AK,** The inhibition of low-density lipoprotein oxidation by 17-beta estradiol, *Metabolism* 41:1110, 1992.

283. **Manning JM, Edwards IJ, Wagner WD, Wagner JD, Adams MR, Parks JS,** Effects of contraceptive estrogen and progestin on the atherogenic potential of plasma LDLs in Cynomolgus monkeys, *Arterioscler Thromb Vasc Biol* 17:1216, 1997.

284. **Campos H, Walsh BW, Judge H, Sacks FM,** Effect of estrogen on very low density lipoprotein and low density lipoprotein subclass metabolism in postmenopausal women, *J Clin Endocrinol Metab* 82:3955, 1997.

285. **Nabulsi A, Folsom A, White A, Patsch W, Heiss G, Wu K, Szklo M,** Association of hormone-replacement therapy with various cardiovascular risk factors in postmenopausal women, *New Engl J Med* 328:1069, 1993.

286. **Speroff L, Rowan J, Symons J, Genant H, Wilborn W, for the CHART Study Group,** The comparative effect on bone density, endometrium, and lipids of continuous hormones as replacement therapy (CHART Study), *JAMA* 276:1397, 1996.

287. **Lindheim SR, Notelovitz M, Feldman EB, Larsen S, Khan FY, Lobo RA,** The independent effects of exercise and estrogen on lipids and lipoproteins in postmenopausal women, *Obstet Gynecol* 83:167, 1994.

288. **Davidson MH, Testolin LM, Maki KC, von Duvillard S, Drennan KB,** A comparison of estrogen replacement, pravastatin, and combined treatment for the management of hypercholesterolemia in postmenopausal women, *Arch Intern Med* 157:1186, 1997.

289. **Adams MR, Clarkson TB, Koritnik DR, Nash HA,** Contraceptive steroids and coronary artery atherosclerosis in cynomolgus macaques, *Fertil Steril* 47:1010, 1987.

290. **Clarkson TB, Adams MR, Kaplan JR, Shively CA, Koritnik DR,** From menarche to menopause: coronary artery atherosclerosis and protection in cynomolgus monkeys, *Am J Obstet Gynecol* 160:1280, 1989.

291. **Clarkson TB, Shively CA, Morgan TM, Koritnik DR, Adams MR, Kaplan JR,** Oral contraceptives and coronary artery atherosclerosis of cynomolgus monkeys, *Obstet Gynecol* 75:217, 1990.

292. **Kushwaha R, Hazzard W,** Exogenous estrogens attenuate dietary hypercholesterolemia and atherosclerosis in the rabbit, *Metabolism* 30:57, 1981.

293. **Hough JL, Zilversmit DB,** Effect of 17 beta estradiol on aortic cholesterol content and metabolism in cholesterol-fed rabbits, *Arteriosclerosis* 6:57, 1986.

294. **Henriksson P, Stamberger M, Eriksson M, Rudling M, Diczfalusy U, Berglund L, Angelin B,** Oestrogen-induced changes in lipoprotein metabolism: role in prevention of atherosclerosis in the cholesterol-fed rabbit, *Eur J Clin Invest* 19:395, 1989.

295. **Haarbo J, Leth-Espensen P, Stender S, Christiansen C,** Estrogen monotherapy and combined estrogen-progestogen replacement therapy attenuate aortic accumulation of cholesterol in ovariectomized cholesterol-fed rabbits, *J Clin Invest* 87:1274, 1991.

296. **Bjarnason NH, Haarbo J, Byrjalsen I, Kauffman RF, Christiansen C,** Raloxifene inhibits aortic accumulation of cholesterol in ovariectomized, cholesterol-fed rabbits, *Circulation* 96:1964, 1997.

297. **Adams MR, Kaplan JR, Manuck SB, Koritnik DR, Parks JS, Wolfe MS, Clarkson TB,** Inhibition of coronary artery atherosclerosis by 17-beta estradiol in ovariectomized monkeys. Lack of an effect of added progesterone, *Arteriosclerosis* 10:1051, 1990.

298. **Williams JK, Anthony MS, Honoré EK, Herrington DM, Morgan TM, Register TC, Clarkson TB,** Regression of atherosclerosis in female monkeys, *Arterioscler Thromb Vasc Biol* 15:827, 1995.

299. **Wagner JD, St Clair RW, Schwenke DC, Shively CA, Adams MR, Clarkson TB,** Regional differences in arterial low density lipoprotein metabolism in surgically postmenopausal Cynomolgus monkeys: effects of estrogen and progesterone replacement, *Arteriosclerosis Thromb* 12:716, 1992.

300. **Adams MR, Register TC, Golden DL, Wagner JD, Williams JK,** Medroxyprogesterone acetate antagonizes inhibitory effects of conjugated equine estrogens on coronary artery atherosclerosis, *Arterioscler Thromb Vasc Biol* 17:217, 1997.

301. **Shemesh J, Frenkel Y, Leibovitch L, Grossman E, Pines A,** Does hormone replacement therapy inhibit coronary artery calcification? *Obstet Gynecol* 89:989, 1997.

302. **Jonas HA, Kronmal RA, Psaty BM, Manolio TA, Meilahn EN, Tell GS, Tracy RP, Robbins JA, Anton-Culver H, for the CHS Collaborative Research Group,** Current estogen-progestin and estrogen replacement therapy in elderly women: association with carotid atherosclerosis, *Ann Epidemiol* 6:314, 1996.

303. **Ingegno MD, Money SR, Thelmo W, Greene GL, Davidian M, Jaffe BM, Pertschuk L,** Progesterone receptors in the human heart and great vessels, *Lab Invest* 59:353, 1988.

304. **Losordo D, Kearney M, Kim E, Jekanowski J, Isner J,** Variable expression of the estrogen receptor in normal and atherosclerotic coronary arteries of premenopausal women, *Circulation* 89:1501, 1994.

305. **Polderman KH, Stehouwer DC, van Kamp GJ, Dekker GA, Verheugt FW, Gooren LJ,** Influence of sex hormones on plasma endothelin levels, *Ann Intern Med* 118:429, 1993.

306. **Wilcox JG, Hatch IE, Gentzschein E, Stanczyk FZ, Lobo RA,** Endothelin levels decrease after oral and nonoral estrogen in postmenopausal women with increased cardiovascular risk factors, *Fertil Steril* 67:273, 1997.

307. **Bar J, Tepper R, Fuchs J, Pardo Y, Goldberger S, Ovadia J,** The effect of estrogen replacement therapy on platelet aggregation and adenosine triphosphate release in postmenopausal women, *Obstet Gynecol* 81:261, 1993.

308. **Aune B, Øian P, Omsjo P, Østerud B,** Hormone replacement therapy reduces the reactivity of monocytes and platelets in whole blood — a beneficial effect on atherogenesis and thrombus formation? *Am J Obstet Gynecol* 173:1816, 1995.

309. **Saab PG, Matthews KA, Stoney CM, McDonald RH,** Premenopausal and postmenopausal women differ in their cardiovascular and neuroendocrine responses to behavioral stresses, *Psychophysiology* 26:270, 1989.

310. **Lindheim S, Legro R, Bernstein L, Stanczyk F, Vijod M, Presser S, Lobo R,** Behavioral stress responses in premenopausal and postmenopausal women and the effects of estrogen, *Am J Obstet Gynecol* 167:1831, 1992.

311. **Lindheim S, Legro R, Morris R, Wong I, Tran D, Vijod M, Stanczyk F, Lobo R,** The effect of progestins on behavioral stress responses in postmenopausal women, *J Soc Gynecol Invest* 1:79, 1994.

312. **Ganger KF, Vyas S, Whitehead MI, Crook D, Miere H, Campbell S,** Pulsatility index in the internal carotid artery is influenced by transdermal oestradiol and time since menopause, *Lancet* 338:839, 1991.

313. **Hillard TC, Bourne TH, Whitehead MI, Crayford TB, Collins WP, Campbell S,** Differential effects of transdermal estradiol and sequential progestogens on impedance to flow within the uterine arteries of postmenopausal women, *Fertil Steril* 58:959, 1992.

314. **Collins P, Shay J, Jiang C, Moss J,** Nitric oxide accounts for dose-dependent estrogen-mediated coronary relaxation after acute estrogen withdrawal, *Circulation* 90:1964, 1994.

315. **Gilligan DM, Badar DM, Panza JA, Quyyumi AA, Cannon III RO,** Acute vascular effects of estrogen in postmenopausal women, *Circulation* 90:786, 1994.

316. **Gilligan DM, Badar DM, Panza JL, Quyyumi AA, Cannon III RO,** Effects of estrogen replacement therapy on peripheral vasomotor function in postmenopausal women, *Am J Cardiol* 75:264, 1995.

317. **McCrohon JA, Adams MR, McCredie RJ, Robinson J, Pike A, Abbey M, Keech AC, Celermajer DS,** Hormone replacement therapy is associated with improved arterial physiology in healthy post-menopausal women, *Clin Endocrinol* 45:435, 1996.

318. **Lau TK, Wan D, Yim SF, Sanderson JE, Haines CJ,** Prospective, randomized, controlled study of the effect of hormone replacement therapy on peripheral blood flow velocity in postmenopausal women, *Fertil Steril* 70:284, 1998.

319. **Sjorensen KE, Dorup I, Hermann AP, Mosekilde L,** Combined hormone replacement therapy does not protect women against the age-related decline in endothelium-dependent vasomotor function, *Circulation* 97:1234, 1998.

320. **Weiner CP, Lizasoain I, Baylis SA, Knowles RG, Charles IG, Moncada S,** Induction of calcium-dependent nitric oxide synthases by sex hormones, *Proc Natl Acad Sci USA* 91:5212, 1994.

321. **Hayashi T, Fukuto JM, Ignarro L, Chaudhuri G,** Basal release of nitric oxide from aortic rings is greater in female rabbits than in male rabbits: implications for atherosclerosis, *Proc Natl Acad Sci USA* 89:11259, 1992.

322. **Rosselli M, Imthurn B, Keller PJ, Jackson EK, Dubey RK,** Circulating nitric oxide (nitrite/nitrate) levels in postmenopausal women substituted with 17 beta-estradiol and norethisterone acetate. A two-year follow-up study, *Hypertension* 25:848, 1995.

323. **Imthurn B, Rosselli M, Jaeger AW, Keller PJ, Dubey RK,** Differential effects of hormone-replacement therapy on endogenous nitric oxide (nitrite/nitrate) levels in postmenopausal women substituted with 17β-estradiol valerate and cyproterone acetate or medroxyprogesterone acetate, *J Clin Endocrinol Metab* 82:388, 1997.

324. **Ylikorkala O, Cacciatore B, Paakkari I, Tikkanen MJ, Viinikka L, Toivonen J,** The long-term effects of oral and transdermal postmenopausal hormone replacement therapy on nitric oxide, endothelin-1, prostacyclin, and thromboxane, *Fertil Steril* 69:883, 1998.

325. **Gilligan DM, Quyyumi AA, Cannon III RO,** Effects of physiological levels of estrogen on coronary vasomotor function in postmenopausal women, *Circulation* 89:2545, 1994.

326. **Roquél M, Heras M, Roig E, Masotti M, Rigol M, Betriu A, Balasch J, Sanz G,** Short-term effects of transdermal estrogen replacement therapy on coronary vascular reactivity in postmenopausal women with angina pectoris and normal results on coronary angiograms, *J Am Coll Cardiol* 31:139, 1998.

327. **Herrington DM, Braden GA, Williams JK, Morgan TM,** Endothelial-dependent coronary vasomotor responsiveness in postmenopausal women with and without estrogen replacement therapy, *Am J Cardiol* 73:951, 1994.

328. **Guetta V, Quyyumi AA, Prasad A, Panza JA, Waclawiw M, Cannon III RO,** The role of nitric oxide in coronary vascular effects of estrogen in postmenopausal women, *Circulation* 96:2795, 1997.

329. **Rosano GM, Caixeta AM, Chierchia S, Arie S, Lopez-Hidalgo M, Pereira WI, Leonardo F, Webb CM, Pileggi F, Collins P,** Short-term anti-ischemic effect of 17 beta-estradiol in postmenopausal women with coronary artery disease, *Circulation* 96:2837, 1997.

330. **Alpasian M, Shimokawa H, Kuroiwa-Matsumoto M, Harasawa Y, Takeshita A,** Short-term estrogen administration ameliorates dobutamine-induced myocardial ischemia in postmenopausal women with coronary artery disease, *J Am Coll Cardiol* 30:1466, 1997.

331. **Webb CM, Rosano GMC, Collins P,** Oestrogen improves exercise-induced myocardial ischaemia in women, *Lancet* 351:1556, 1998.

332. **Lee M, Giardina E-GV, Homma S, DiTullio MR, Sciacca RR,** Lack of effect of estrogen on rest and treadmill exercise in postmenopausal women without known cardiac disease, *Am J Cardiol* 80:793, 1997.

333. **Williams JK, Shively CA, Clarkson TB,** Determinants of coronary artery reactivity in premenopausal female cynomolgus monkeys with diet-induced atherosclerosis, *Circulation* 90:983, 1994.

334. **Chester AH, Jiang C, Borland JA, Yacoub M, Collins P,** Oestrogen relaxes human epicardial coronary arteries through non-endothelial-dependent mechanisms, *Coron Artery Dis* 6:417, 1995.

335. **Collins P, Rosano GM, Jiang C, Lindsay D, Sarrel PM, Poole-Wilson PA,** Cardiovascular protection by estrogen — a calcium antagonism effect? *Lancet* 341:264, 1993.

336. **Pines A, Fishman EZ, Levo Y, Auerbuch M, Lidor A, Drory Y, Finkelstein A, Hetman-Peri M, Moshkowitz M, Ben-Ari E, Ayalon D,** The effects of hormone replacement therapy in normal postmenopausal women: measurements of Doppler-derived parameters of aortic flow, *Am J Obstet Gynecol* 164:806, 1991.

337. **Pines A, Fishman EZ, Ayalon D, Drory Y, Aveerbuch M, Levo Y,** Long-term effects of hormone replacement therapy on Doppler-derived parameters of aortic flow in postmenopausal women, *Chest* 102:1496, 1992.

338. **Voutilainen S, Hippelainen M, Hulklo S, Karppinen K, Ventila M, Kupri M,** Left ventricular diastolic function by Doppler echocardiography in relation to hormone replacement therapy in healthy postmenopausal women, *Am J Cardiol* 71:614, 1993.

339. **Giraud GD, Morton MJ, Wilson RA, Burry KA, Speroff L,** Effects of estrogen and progestin on aortic size and compliance in postmenopausal women, *Am J Obstet Gynecol* 174:1708, 1996.

340. **Prelevic GM, Beljic T,** The effect of oestrogen and progestogen replacement therapy on systolic flow velocity in healthy postmenopausal women, *Maturitas* 20:37, 1994.

341. **Liang Y-L, Teede H, Shiel L, Thomas A, Craven R, Sachithanandan N, McNeil JJ, Cameron JD, Dart A, McGrath B,** Effects of oestrogen and progesterone on age-related changes in arteries of postmenopausal women, *Clin Exp Pharmacol Physiol* 24:457, 1997.

342. **Pines A, Fisman EZ, Averbuch M, Drory Y, Motro M, Levo Y, et al,** The long-term effects of transdermal estradiol on left ventricular function and dimensions, *Eur J Menopause* 2:22, 1995.

343. **Snabes MC, Payne JP, Kopelen HA, Dunn JK, Young RL, Zoghbi WA,** Physiologic estradiol replacement therapy and cardiac structure and function in normal postmenopausal women: a randomized, double-blind, placebo-controlled, crossover trial, *Obstet Gynecol* 89:332, 1997.

344. **Poehlman ET, Goran MI, Gardner AW, Ades PA, Arciero PJ, Katzman-Rooks SM, Montgovery SM, Toth MJ, Sutherland PT,** Determinants of decline in resting metabolic rate in aging females, *Am J Physiol* 264:E450, 1993.

345. **Trémollieres FA, Pouilles J-M, Ribot CA,** Relative influence of age and menopause on total and regional body composition changes in postmenopausal women, *Am J Obstet Gynecol* 175:1594, 1996.

346. **Walton C, Godsland IF, Proudler A, Wynn V, Stevenson JC,** The effects of the menopause on insulin sensitivity, secretion and elimination in non-obese, healthy women, *Eur J Clin Invest* 23:466, 1993.

347. **Proudler AJ, Godsland IF, Stevenson JC,** Insulin propeptides in conditions associated with insulin resistance in humans and their relevance to insulin measurements, *Metabolism* 43:46, 1994.

348. **Haarbo J, Marslew U, Gotfredsen A, Christiansen C,** Postmenopausal hormone replacement therapy prevents central distribution of body fat after menopause, *Metabolism* 40:1323, 1991.

349. **Ley C, Lees B, Stevenson J,** Sex- and menopause-associated changes in body-fat distribution, *Am J Clin Nutr* 55:950, 1992.

350. **Reubinoff BE, Wurtman J, Rojansky N, Adler D, Stein P, Schenker JG, Brzezinski A,** Effects of hormone replacement therapy on weight, body composition, fat distribution, and food intake in early postmenopausal women: a prospective study, *Fertil Steril* 64:963, 1995.

351. **Gambacciani M, Ciaponi M, Cappagli B, Piaggesi L, De Simone L, Orlandi R, Genazzani AR,** Body weight, body fat distribution, and hormonal replacement therapy in early postmenopausal women, *J Clin Endocrinol Metab* 82:414, 1997.

352. **Ferri C, Pittoni V, Piccoli A, Laurenti O, Cassone MR, Bellini C, Properzi G, Valesini G, De Mattia G, Santucci A,** Insulin stimulates endothelin-1 secretion from human endothelial cells and modulates its circulating levels *in vivo*, *J Clin Endocrinol Metab* 80:829, 1995.

353. **Cagnacci A, Soldani R, Carriero PL, Paoletti AM, Fioretti P, Melis GB,** Effects of low doses of transdermal 17 beta-estradiol on carbohydrate metabolism in postmenopausal women, *J Clin Endocrinol Metab* 74:1396, 1992.

354. **Lindheim S, Duffy D, Kojima T, Vijod M, Stancyzk F, Lobo R,** The route of administration influences the effect of estrogen on insulin sensitivity in postmenopausal women, *Fertil Steril* 62:1176, 1994.

355. **Lobo R, Pickar J, Wild R, Walsh B, Hirvonen E, for The Menopause Study Group,** Metabolic impact of adding medroxyprogesterone acetate to conjugated estrogen therapy in postmenopausal women, *Obstet Gynecol* 84:987, 1994.

356. **Salomaa V, Rasi V, Pekkanen J, Vahtera E, Jauhiainen M, Vartiainen E, Ehnholm C, Tuomilehto J, Myllylä G,** Association of hormone replacement therapy with hemostatic and other cardiovascular risk factors: The FINRISK hemostasis study, *Arterioscler Thromb Vasc Biol* 15:1549, 1995.

357. **Conard J, Gompel A, Pelissier C, Mirabel C, Basdevant A,** Fibrinogen and plasminogen modifications during oral estradiol replacement therapy, *Fertil Steril* 68:449, 1997.

358. **Lindheim S, Presser S, Ditkoff E, Vijod M, Stanczyk F, Lobo R,** A possible bimodal effect of estrogen on insulin sensitivity in postmenopausal women and the attenuating effect of added progestin, *Fertil Steril* 60:664, 1993.

359. **Godsland IF, Ganger K, Walton C, Cust MP, Whitehead MI, Wynn V, Stevenson JC,** Insulin resistance, secretion, and elimination in postmenopausal women receiving oral or transdermal hormone replacement therapy, *Metabolism* 42:846, 1993.

360. **Manson J, Rimm E, Colditz G, Willett W, Nathan D, Arky R, Roxner B, Hennekens C, Speizer F, Stampfer M,** A prospective study of postmenopausal estrogen therapy and subsequent incidence of non-insulin dependent diabetes mellitus, *Ann Epidemiol* 2:665, 1992.

361. **Gabal LL, Goodman-Gruen D, Barrett-Connor E,** The effect of postmenopausal estrogen therapy on the risk of non-insulin-dependent diabetes mellitus, *Am J Public Health* 87:443, 1997.

362. **Andersson B, Mattsson L, Hahn L, Mårin P, Lapidus L, Holm G, Bengtsson B, Björntorp P,** Estrogen replacement therapy decreases hyperandrogenicity and improves glucose homeostasis and plasma lipids in postmenopausal women with noninsulin-dependent diabetes mellitus, *J Clin Endocrinol Metab* 82:638, 1997.

363. **Brussaard HE, Gevers Leuven JA, Frolich M, Kluft C, Krans HMJ,** Short-term oestrogen replacement therapy improves insulin resistance, lipids and fibrinolysis in postmenopausal women with NIDDM, *Diabetologia* 40:843, 1997.

364. **Kardinaal A, Kok F, Ringstad J, Gomez-Aracena J, Mazaev V, Kohlmeier L, Martin B, Aro A, Kark J, Delgado-Rodriquez M, Riemersma R, van't Veer P, Huttunen J, Martin-Moreno J,** Antioxidants in adipose tissue and risk of myocardial infarction: the EURAMIC study, *Lancet* 342:1379, 1993.

365. **Gey KF, Stähelin HB, Eichholzer M,** Poor plasma status of carotene and vitamin C is associated with higher mortality from ischemic heart disease and stroke: Basel Prospective Study, *Clin Invest* 71:3, 1993.

366. **Stampfer MJ, Hennekens CH, Manson JE, Colditz GA, Rosner B, Willett WC,** Vitamin E consumption and the risk of coronary disease in women, *New Engl J Med* 328:1444, 1993.

367. **Knopp R, Zhu X, Bonet B,** Effects of estrogens on lipoprotein metabolism and cardiovascular disease in women, *Atherosclerosis* 110(Suppl 1):S83, 1994.

368. **Sack MN, Rader DJ, Cannon III RO,** Oestrogen and inhibition of oxidation of low-density lipoproteins in postmenopausal women, *Lancet* 343:269, 1994.

369. **Keaney J, Shwaery G, Xu A, Nicholosi R, Loscalzo J, Foxall T, Vita J,** 17β-Estradiol preserves endothelial vasodilator function and limits low-density lipoprotein oxidation in hypercholesterolemic swine, *Circulation* 89:225, 1994.

370. **McKinney KA, Duell PB, Wheaton DL, Hess DL, Patton PE, Spies HG, Burry KA,** Differential effects of subcutaneous estrogen and progesterone on low-density lipoprotein size and susceptibility to oxidation in postmenopausal rhesus monkeys, *Fertil Steril* 68:525, 1997.

371. **Tranquilli AL, Mazzanti L, Cugini AM, Cester N, Garzetti GG, Romanini C,** Transdermal estradiol and medroxyprogesterone acetate in hormone replacement therapy are both antioxidants, *Gynecol Endocrinol* 9:137, 1995.

372. **Samsioe G, Andersson K, Mattsson L-Å,** Relative fatty acid composition of serum lecithin in perimenopausal women using combined hormone replacement therapy, *Menopause* 4:193, 1997.

373. **Meade TW, Dyer S, Howarth DJ, Imeson JD, Stirling Y,** Antithrombin III and procoagulant activity: sex differences and effects of the menopause, *Br J Haematol* 74:77, 1990.

374. **Stefanick ML, Legault C, Tracy RP, Howard G, Kessler CM, Lucas DL, Bush TL,** Distribution and correlates of plasma fibrinogen in middle-aged women. Initial findings of the Postmenopausal Estrogen/Progestin Interventions (PEPI) Study, *Arterioscler Thromb Vasc Biol* 15:2085, 1995.

375. **Meilahn E, Kuller L, Matthews K, Kiss J,** Hemostatic factors according to menopausal status and use of hormone replacement therapy, *Ann Epidemiol* 2:445, 1992.

376. **Scarabin PY, Flu-Bureau G, Bara L, Bonithon-Kopp C, Guize L, Samama M,** Haemostatic variables and menopausal status: influence of hormone replacement therapy, *Thromb Haemost* 70:584, 1994.

377. **Gebara OCE, Mittleman MA, Sutherland P, Lipinska I, Matheney T, Xu P, Welty FK, Wilson PW, Levy D, Muller JE, Tofler GH,** Association between increased estrogen status and increased fibrinolytic potential in the Framingham Offspring Study, *Circulation* 91:1952, 1995.

378. **De Souza MJ, Nulsen JC, Sequenzia LC, Bona RD, Walker FJ, Luciano AA,** The effect of medroxyprogesterone acetate on conjugated equine estrogen-induced changes in coagulation parameters in postmenopausal women, *J Women's Health* 5:121, 1996.

379. **Bonduki CE, Lourenço DM, Baracat E, Haidar M, Noguti MAE, da Motta ELA, Lima GR,** Effect of estrogen-progestin hormonal replacement therapy on plasma antithrombin III of postmenopausal women, *Acta Obstet Gynecol Scand* 77:330, 1998.

380. **Meilahn E, Cauley J, Tracy R, Macy E, Gutai J, Kuller L,** Association of sex hormones and adiposity with plasma levels of fibrinogen and PAI-1 in postmenopausal women, *Am J Epidemiol* 143:159, 1996.

381. **Koh KK, Mincemoyer R, Bui MN, Csako G, Pucino F, Guetto V, Waclawiw M, Cannon III RO,** Effects of hormone-replacement therapy on fibrinolysis in postmenopausal women, *New Engl J Med* 336:683, 1997.

382. **Boschetti C, Corteliaro M, Nencioni T, Bertolli V, Della Volpe A, Zanussi C,** Short- and long-term effects of hormone replacement therapy (transdermal estradiol vs oral conjugated equine estrogens, combined with medroxyprogesterone acetate) on blood coagulation factors in postmenopausal women, *Thromb Res* 62:1, 1991.

383. **Saleh AA, Dorey LG, Dombrowski MP, Ginsburg KA, Hirokawa S, Kowalczyk C, Hirata J, Bottoms S, Cotton DB, Mammen EF,** Thrombosis and hormone replacement therapy in postmenopausal women, *Am J Obstet Gynecol* 169:1554, 1993.

384. **Pinto S, Bruni V, Rosati D, Prisco D, Costanzo M, Giusti B, Abbate R,** Effects of estrogen replacement therapy on thrombin generation, *Thrombosis Res* 85:185, 1997.

385. **Caine YG, Bauer KA, Barzegar S, Ten Cate H, Sacks FM, Walsh BW, Schiff I, Rosenberg RD,** Coagulation activation following estrogen administration to postmenopausal women, *Thromb Haemostas* 68:392, 1992.

386. **Kessler CM, Szymanski LM, Shamsipour Z, Muesing RA, Miller VT, Larosa JC,** Estrogen replacement therapy and coagulation: relationship to lipid and lipoprotein changes, *Obstet Gynecol* 89:325, 1997.

387. **Suzuki A, Mizuno K, Ino Y, Okada M, Kikkawa F, Mizutani S, Tomoda Y,** Effects of 17 beta-estradiol and progesterone on growth-factor-induced proliferation and migration in human female aortic smooth muscle cells in vitro, *Cardiovasc Res* 32:516, 1996.

388. **Okada M, Suzuki A, Mizuno K, Asada Y, Kuwayama T, Tamakoshi K, Mizutani S, Tomoda Y,** Effects of 17 beta-estradiol and progesterone on migration of human monocytic THP-1 cells stimulated by minimally oxidized low-density lipoprotein in vitro, *Cardiovasc Res* 34:529, 1997.

389. **Dubey RK, Jackson EK, Luscher TF,** Nitric oxide inhibits angiotensin II-induced migration of rat aortic smooth muscle cell. Role of cyclic-nucleotides and angiotensin 1 receptors, *J Clin Invest* 96:141, 1995.

390. **Iafrati MD, Karas RH, Aronovitz M, Kim S, Sullivan Jr TR, Lubahn DB, O'Donnell Jr TF, Korach KS, Mendelsohn ME,** Estrogen inhibits the vascular injury response in estrogen receptor alpha-deficient mice, *Nat Med* 3:545, 1997.

391. **Enmark E, Pelto-Huikko M, Grandien K, Lagercrantz S, Lagercrantz J, Fried G, Nordenskjöld M, Gustafsson J-Å,** Human estrogen receptor β-gene structure, chromosomal localization, and expression pattern, *J Clin Endocrinol Metab* 82:4258, 1997.

392. **Espeland MA, Applegate W, Furgerg CD, Lefkowitz D, Rice L, Hunninghake D, the ACAPS Investigators,** Estrogen replacement therapy and progression of intimal-medial thickness in the carotid arteries of postmenopausal women, *Am J Epidemiol* 142:1011, 1995.

393. **Baron YM, Galea MB,** Carotid artery wall thickness in women treated with hormone replacement therapy, *Maturitas* 27:47, 1997.

394. **Akkad A, Hartshorne T, Bell PRF, Al-Azzawi F,** Carotid plaque regression on oestrogen replacement: a pilot study, *Eur J Vasc Endovasc Surg* 11:347, 1996.

395. **Krasinski K, Spyridopoulos I, Asahara T, van der Zee R, Isner JM, Losordo DW,** Estradiol accelerates functional endothelial recovery after arterial injury, *Circulation* 95:1768, 1997.

396. **Spyridopoulos I, Sullivan AB, Kearney M, Isner JM, Losordo DW,** Estrogen-receptor—mediated inhibition of human endothelial cell apoptosis. Estradiol as a survival factor, *Circulation* 95:1505, 1997.

397. **Levine RL, Chen SJ, Durand J, Chen YF, Oparil S,** Medroxyprogesterone attenuates estrogen-mediated inhibition of neointima formation after balloon injury of the rat carotid artery, *Circulation* 94:2221, 1996.

398. **Frazier-Jessen MR, Kovacs EJ,** Estrogen modulcation of JE/monocyte chemoattractant protein-1 mRNA expression in murine macrophages, *J Immunol* 154:1838, 1995.

399. **Proudler AJ, Ahmed AI, Crook D, Fogelman I, Rymer JM, Stevenson JC,** Hormone replacement therapy and serum angiotensin-converting-enzyme activity in postmenopausal women, *Lancet* 346:89, 1995.

400. **Schunkert H, Danser AH, Hense HW, Derkx FH, Kurzinger S, Riegger GA,** Effects of estrogen replacement therapy on the renin-angiotensinogen system in postmenopausal women, *Circulation* 95:39, 1997.

401. **Jilma B, Hildebrandt J, Kapiotis S, Wagner O, Kitzweger E, Müllner C, Monitzer B, Krejcy K, Eichler H-G,** Effects of estradiol on circulating P-selectin, *J Clin Endocrinol Metab* 81:2350, 1996.

402. **Mijatovic V, Kenemans P, Jakobs C, Marchien Van Baal W, Peters-Muller ER, Van Der Mooren MJ,** A randomized controlled study of the effects of 17beta-estradiol-dydrogesterone on plasma homocysteine in postmenopausal women, *Obstet Gynecol* 91:432, 1998.

403. **Register TC, Adams MR,** Coronary artery and cultured aortic smooth muscle cells express mRNA for both the classical estrogen receptor and the newly described estrogen receptor beta, *J Steroid Biochem Mol Biol* 64:187, 1998.

404. **Hirvonen E, Malkonen M, Manninen V,** Effects of different progestogens on lipoproteins during postmenopausal therapy, *New Engl J Med* 304:560, 1981.

405. **Mattsson L, Cullberg L, Samsioe G,** Influence of esterified estrogens and medroxyprogesterone on lipid metabolism and sex steroids, *Horm Metab Res* 14:602, 1982.

406. **Silferstolpe G, Gustafsson A, Samsioe G, Syanborg A,** Lipid metabolic studies in oophorectomized women: effects on serum lipids and lipoproteins of three synthetic progestogens, *Maturitas* 4:103, 1983.

407. **Ylostalo P, Kauppila A, Kivinen S, Tuimala R, Vihkoo R,** Endocrine and metabolic effcts of low-dose estrogen-progestin treatment in climacteric women, *Obstet Gynecol* 62:682, 1983.

408. **Mattsson L, Cullberg G, Samsioe G,** A continuous estrogen-progestogen regimen for climacteric complaints, *Acta Obstet Gynecol Scand* 63:673, 1984.

409. **Ottosson UB, Carlstrom K, Damber JE, von Schoultz B,** Serum levels of progesterone and some of its metabolites including deoxycorticosterone after oral and parenteral administration, *Br J Obstet Gynaecol* 91:1111, 1984.

410. **Wren B, Garrett D,** The effect of low-dose piperazine oestrogen sulphate and low-dose levonorgestrel on blood lipid levels in postmenopausal women, *Maturitas* 7:141, 1985.

411. **Ottosson UB, Johansson BG, von Schoultz B,** Subfractions of high-density lipoprotein cholesterol during estrogen replacement therapy: a comparison between progestogens and natural progesterone, *Am J Obstet Gynecol* 151:746, 1985.

412. **Obel EB, Munk-Jensen N, Svenstrup B, Bennett P, Micic S, Henrik-Nielsen R, Nielsen SP, Gydesen H, Jensen BM,** A two-year double-blind controlled study of the clinical effect of combined and sequential postmenopausal replacement therapy and steroid metabolism during treatment, *Maturitas* 16:13, 1993.

413. **Barrett-Connor E, Wingard DL, Criqui MH,** Postmenopausal estrogen use and heart disease risk factors in the 1980s, *JAMA* 261:2095, 1989.

414. **Sherwin BB, Gelfand MM,** A prospective one-year study of estrogen and progestin in postmenopausal women: effects on clinical symptoms and lipoprotein lipids, *Obstet Gynecol* 73:759, 1989.

415. **Wolfe BM, Huff MW,** Effects of combined estrogen and progestin administration on plasma lipoprotein metabolism in postmenopausal women, *J Clin Invest* 83:40, 1989.

416. **Christiansen C, Riis BJ,** Five years with continuous combined oestrogen/progestogen therapy. Effects on calcium metabolism, lipoproteins, and bleeding pattern, *Br J Obstet Gynaecol* 97:1087, 1990.

417. **Voetberg GA, Netelenbos JC, Kenemans P, Peters-Muller ERA, van de Weijer PHM,** Estrogen replacement therapy continuously combined with four different dosages of dydrogesterone: effect on calcium and lipid metabolism, *J Clin Endocrinol Metab* 79:1465, 1994.

418. **Marslew U, Overgaard K, Riis B, Christiansen C,** Two new combinations of estrogen and progestogen for prevention of postmenopausal bone loss: long-term effects on bone, calcium and lipid metabolism, *Obstet Gynecol* 79:202, 1992.

419. **Williams SR, Frenchek B, Speroff T, Speroff L,** A study of combined continuous ethinyl estradiol and norethindrone acetate for postmenopausal hormone replacement, *Am J Obstet Gynecol* 162:438, 1990.

420. **Weinstein L, Bewtra C, Gallagher JC,** Evaluation of a continuous combined low-dose regimen of estrogen-progestin for treatment of the menopausal patient, *Am J Obstet Gynecol* 162:1534, 1990.

421. **Munk-Jensen N, Ulrich L, Obel E, Nielsen S, Edwards D, Meinertz H,** Continuous combined and sequential estradiol and norethindrone acetate treatment of postmenopausal women: effect on plasma lipoproteins in a two-year placebo-controlled trial, *Am J Obstet Gynecol* 171:132, 1994.

422. **Kim CJ, Min YK, Ryu WS, Kwak JW, Ryoo UH,** Effect of hormone replacement therapy on lipoprotein(a) and lipid levels in postmenopausal women: influence of various progestogens and duration of therapy, *Arch Intern Med* 156:1693, 1996.

423. **Cano A, Fernandes H, Serrano S, Mahiques P,** Effect of continuous oestradiol-medroxyprogesterone administration on plasma lipids and lipoproteins, *Maturitas* 13:35, 1991.

424. **Folsom AR, McGovern PG, Nabulsi AA, Shahar E, Kahn ESB, Winkhart SP, White AD, for the Atherosclerosis Risk in Communities Study Investigators,** Changes in plasma lipids and lipoproteins associated with starting or stopping postmenopausal hormone replacement therapy, *Am Heart J* 132:952, 1996.

425. **de Ziegler D, Bessis R, Frydman R,** Vascular resistance of uterine arteries: physiological effects of estradiol and progesterone, *Fertil Steril* 55:775, 1991.

426. **Penotti M, Nencioni T, Gabrielli L, Farinia M, Castiglioni E, Polvani F,** Blood flow variations in internal carotid and middle cerebral arteries induced by postmenopausal hormone replacement therapy, *Am J Obstet Gynecol* 169:1226, 1993.

427. **Barrett-Connor E, Slone S, Greendale G, Kritz-Silverstein D, Espeland M, Johnson SR, Waclawiw M, Fineberg SE,** The Postmenopausal Estrogen/Progestin Interventions Study: primary outcomes in adherent women, *Maturitas* 27:261, 1997.

428. **Espeland MA, Hogan PE, Fineberg SE, Howard G, Schrott H, Waclawiw MA, Bush TL, for the PEPI investigators,** Effect of postmenopausal hormone therapy on glucose and insulin concentrations, *Diabetes Care* 21:1589, 1998.

429. **Punnonen RH, Jokela HA, Dastidar PS, Nevala M, Laippala PJ,** Combined oestrogen-progestin replacement therapy prevents atherosclerosis in postmenopausal women, *Maturitas* 21:179, 1995.

430. **Falkeborn M, Persson I, Adami HO, Bergstrom R, Eaker E, Lithell H, Mohsen R, Taessen T,** The risk of acute myocardial infarction after oestrogen and oestrogen-progestogen replacement, *Br J Obstet Gynaecol* 99:821, 1992.

431. **Heckbert SR, Weiss NS, Koepsell TD, Lemaitre RN, Smith NL, Siscovick DS, Lin D, Psaty BM,** Duration of estrogen replacement therapy in relation to the risk of incident myocardial infarction in postmenopausal women, *Arch Intern Med* 157:1330, 1997.

432. **Newton KM, LaCroix AZ, McKnight B, Knopp RH, Siscovick DS, Heckbert SR, Weiss NS,** Estrogen replacement therapy and prognosis after first myocardial infarction, *Am J Epidemiol* 145:269, 1997.

433. **Hulley S, Grady D, Bush T, Furberg C, Herrington D, B, Vittinghoff E, for the Heart and Estrogen/progestin Replacement Study (HERS) Research Group,** Randomized trial of estrogen plus progestin for secondary prevention of coronary heart disease in postmenopausal women, *JAMA* 280:605, 1998.

434. **Sullivan JM, Vander Zwaag R, Hughes JP, Maddock V, Kroetz FW, Ramanathan KB, Mirvis DM,** Estrogen replacement and coronary artery disease: effect on survival in postmenopausal women, *Arch Intern Med* 150:2557, 1990.

435. **Sullivan JM, El-Zeky F, Vander Zwaag R, Ramanathan KB,** Effect on survival of estrogen replacement therapy after coronary artery bypass grafting, *Am J Cardiol* 79:847, 1997.

436. **O'Keefe Jr JH, Kim SC, Hall RR, Cochran VC, Lawhorn SL, McCallister BD,** Estrogen replacement therapy after coronary angioplasty in women, *J Am Coll Cardiol* 29:1, 1997.

437. **O'Brien JE, Peterson ED, Keeler GP, Berdan LG, Ohman EM, Faxon DP, Jacobs AK, Topol EJ, Califf RM,** Relation between estrogen replacement therapy and restenosis after percutaneous coronary interventions, *J Am Coll Cardiol* 28:1111, 1996.

438. **Williams JK, Honoré EK, Washburn SA, Clarkson TB,** Effects of hormone replacement therapy on reactivity of atherosclerotic coronary arteries in cynomolgus monkeys, *J Am Coll Cardiol* 24:1757, 1994.

439. **Honoré EK, Williams JK, Anthony MS, Clarkson TB,** Soy isoflavones enhance coronary vascular reactivity in atherosclerotic female macaques, *Fertil Steril* 67:148, 1997.

440. **Register TC, Adams MR, Golden DL, Clarkson TB,** Conjugated equine estrogens alone, but not in combination with medroxyprogesteorne acetate, inhibit aortic connective tissue remodeling after plasma lipid lowering in female monkeys, *Arterioscler Thromb Vasc Biol* 18:1164, 1998.

441. **Speroff T, Dawson N, Speroff L,** Is postmenopausal estrogen use risky? Results from a methodologic review and information synthesis, *Clin Res* 35:362A, 1987.

442. **Grodstein F, Stampfer M,** The epidemiology of coronary heart disease and estrogen replacement in postmenopausal women, *Prog Cardiovasc Dis* 38:199, 1995.

443. **Bagatell CJ, Knopp RH, Rivier JE, Bremner WJ,** Physiological levels of estradiol stimulate plasma high density lipoprotein$_2$ cholesterol levels in normal men, *J Clin Endocrinol Metab* 78:855, 1994.

444. **Smith EP, Boyd J, Frank GR, Takahashi H, Cohen RM, Specker B, Williams TC, Lubahn DB, Korach KS,** Estrogen resistance caused by a mutation in the estrogen-receptor gene in a man, *New Engl J Med* 331:1056, 1994.

445. **New G, Timmins KL, Duffy SJ, Tran BT, O'Brien RC, Harper RW, Meredith IT,** Long-term estrogen therapy improves vascular function in male to female transsexuals, *J Am Coll Cardiol* 29:1437, 1997.

446. **Collins P, Rosano GMC, Sarrel PM, Ulrich L, Adamopoulos S, Beale CM, McNeil J, Poole-Wilson PA,** 17 Beta-estradiol attenuates acetylcholine-induced coronary arterial constriction in women but not in men with coronary heart disease, *Circulation* 92:24, 1995.

447. **Dempster DW, Lindsay R,** Pathogenesis of osteoporosis, *Lancet* 341:797, 1993.

448. **Lees B, Molleson T, Arnett TR, Stevenson JC,** Differences in proximal femur bone density over two centuries, *Lancet* 341:673, 1993.

449. **Eaton SB, Nelson DA,** Calcium in evolutionary perspective, *Am J Clin Nutr* 54:281S, 1991.

450. **Cooper C, Campion G, Melton III LJ,** Hip fractures in the elderly: a world-wide projection, *Osteoporosis Int* 2:285, 1992.

451. **Riis BJ, Hansen MA, Jensen AM, Overgaard K, Christiansen C,** Low bone mass and fast rate of bone loss at menopause: equal risk factors for future fracture: a 15-year follow-up study, *Bone* 19:9, 1996.

452. **Theitz G, Buch B, Rizzoli R, Slosman D, Clavien H, Sizonko PC, Bonjour JPH,** Longitudinal monitoring of bone mass accumulation in healthy adolescents: evidence for a marked reduction after 16 years of age at the levels of lumbar spine and femoral neck in female subjects, *J Clin Endocrinol Metab* 75:1060, 1992.

453. **Matkovic V, Jelic T, Wardlaw GM, Ilich J, Goel PK, Wright JK, Andon MB, Smith KT, Heaney RP,** Timing of peak bone mass in caucasian females and its implication for the prevention of osteoporosis: inference from a cross-sectional model, *J Clin Invest* 93:799, 1994.

454. **Recker RR, Davies KM, Hinders SM, Heaney RP, Stegman MR, Kimmel DB,** Bone gain in young women, *JAMA* 268:2403, 1992.

455. **Ettinger B,** Prevention of osteoporosis: treatment of estradiol deficiency, *Obstet Gynecol* 72:125, 1988.

456. **Lindsay R,** Prevention and treatment of osteoporosis, *Lancet* 341:801, 1993.

457. **Turner RT, Riggs BL, Spelsberg TC,** Skeletal effects of estrogen, *Endocr Rev* 15:275, 1994.

458. **Pacifici R,** Cytokines, estrogen, and postmenopausal osteoporosis — the second decade, *Endocrinology* 130:2659, 1998.

459. **Liel Y, Kraus S, Levy J, Shany S,** Evidence that estrogens modulate activity and increase the number of 1,25-dihydroxyvitamin D receptors in osteoblast-like cells (ROS 17/2.8), *Endocrinology* 130:2597, 1992.

460. **Prince RL,** Counterpoint: estrogen effects on calcitropic hormones and calcium homeostasis, *Endocr Rev* 15:301, 1994.

461. **Carani C, Qin K, Simoni M, Faustini-Fustini M, Serpente S, Boyd J, Korach KS, Simpson ER,** Effect of testosterone and estradiol in a man with aromatase deficiency, *New Engl J Med* 337:91, 1997.

462. **Khosla S, Melton III LJ, Atkinson EJ, O'Fallon WM, Klee GG, Riggs BL,** Relationship of serum sex steroid levels and bone turnover markers with bone mineral density in men and women: a key role for bioavailable estrogen, *J Clin Endocrinol Metab* 83:2266, 1998.

463. **Bilezikian JP, Morishima A, Bell J, Grumbach MM,** Increased bone mass as a result of estrogen therapy in a man with aromatase deficiency, *New Engl J Med* 339:599, 1998.

464. **Ettinger B, Sidney S, Cummings SR, Libanati C, Bikle DD, Tekawa IS, Tolan K, Steiger P,** Racial differences in bone density between young adult black and white subjects persist after adjustment for anthropometric, lifestyle, and biochemical differences, *J Clin Endocrinol Metab* 82:429, 1997.

465. **Nelson DA, Simpson PM, Johnson CC, Barondess DA, Kleerekopper M,** The accumulation of whole body skeletal mass in third- and fourth-grade children: effects of age, ethnicity, and body composition, *Bone* 20:73, 1997.

466. **Kleerekoper M, Nelson DA, Peterson EL, Wilson PS, Jacobsen G, Longcope C,** Body composition and gonadal steroids in older white and black women, *J Clin Endocrinol Metab* 79:775, 1994.

467. **Grisso JA, Kelsey JL, Strom BL, O'Brien LA, Maislin G, LaPann K, Samuelson L, Hoffman S, and the Northeast Hip Fracture Study Group,** Risk factors for hip fracture in black women, *New Engl J Med* 330:1555, 1994.

468. **Iki M, Kajita E, Dohi Y, Nishino H, Kusaka Y, Tsuchida C, Yamamoto K, Ishii Y,** Age, menopause, bone turnover markers and lumbar bone loss in healthy Japanese women, *Maturitas* 25:59, 1996.

469. **Seeman E, Hopper JL, Bach LA, Cooper ME, Parkinson E, McKay J, Jerums G,** Reduced bone mass in daughters of women with osteoporosis, *New Engl J Med* 320:554, 1989.

470. **Slemenda CW, Christian JC, Williams CJ, Norton JA, Johnston Jr CC,** Genetic determinants of bone mass in adult women: a reevaluation of the twin model and the potential importance of gene interaction on heritability estimates, *J Bone Miner Res* 6:561, 1991.

471. **Morrison NA, Qi JC, Tokita A, Kelly PJ, Crofts L, Nguyen TV, Sambrook PN, Eisman JA,** Prediction of bone density from vitamin D receptor alleles, *Nature* 367:284, 1994.

472. **Ferrari S, Rizzoli R, Chevalley T, Slosman D, Eisman JA, Bonjour J-P,** Vitamin-D-receptor-gene polymorphisms and change in lumbar-spine bone mineral density, *Lancet* 345:423, 1995.

473. **Uitterlinden AG, Burger H, Huang Q, Yue F, McGuigan FEA, Grant SFA, Hofman A, van Leeuwen JPTM, Pols HAP, Ralston SH,** Relation of alleles of the collagen type Ia1 gene to bone density and the risk of osteoporotic fractures in postmenopausal women, *New Engl J Med* 338:1016, 1998.

474. **Richelson LS, Wahner HW, Melton III LJ, Riggs BL,** Relative contributions of aging and estrogen deficiency to postmenopausal bone loss, *New Engl J Med* 311:1273, 1984.

475. **Nilas L, Christiansen C,** Bone mass and its relationship to age and the menopause, *J Clin Endocrinol Metab* 65:697, 1987.

476. **Alvioli LV,** Calcium and osteoporosis, *Ann Rev Nutr* 4:471, 1984.

477. **Johnston Jr CC, Hui SL, Witt RM, Appledorn R, Baker RS, Longcope C,** Early menopausal changes in bone mass and sex steroids, *J Clin Endocrinol Metab* 61:905, 1985.

478. **Riggs BL, Wahner HW, Melton III LJ, Richelson LS, Judd HL, Offord KP,** Rates of bone loss in the appendicular and axial skeletons of women, *J Clin Invest* 77:1487, 1986.

479. **Riggs BL, Wahner HW, Dunn WL, Mazess RB, Offord KP, Melton III LJ,** Differential changes in bone mineral density of the appendicular and axial skeleton with aging: relationship to spinal osteoporosis, *J Clin Invest* 67:328, 1981.

480. **Baran D, Sorensen A, Grimes J, Lew R, Karellas A, Johnson B, Roche J,** Dietary modification with dairy products for preventing vertebral bone loss in premenopausal women: a three-year prospective study, *J Clin Endocrinol Metab* 70:264, 1990.

481. **Elders PJM, Lips P, Netelenbos C, Van Ginkel FC, Khoe E, Van Der Vijgh WJF, Van Der Stelt PF,** Long-term effect of calcium supplementation on bone loss in perimenopausal women, *J Bone Miner Res* 9:963, 1994.

482. **Gambacciani M, Spinetti A, Taponeco F, Cappagli B, Maffei S, Manetti P, Piaggesi L, Fioretti P,** Bone loss in perimenopausal women: a longitudinal study, *Maturitas* 18:191, 1994.

483. **Garton M, Martin J, New S, Lee S, Loveridge N, Milne J, Reid D, Reid I, Robins S,** Bone mass and metabolism in women aged 45–55, *Clin Endocrinol* 44:536, 1996.

484. **Guthrie JR, Ebeling PR, Hopper JL, Barrett-Connor E, Dennerstein L, Dudley EC, Burger HG, Wark JD,** A prospective study of bone loss in menopausal Australian-born women, *Osteoporos Int* 8:282, 1998.

485. **Waller K, Reim J, Fenster L, Swan SH, Brumback B, Windham GC, Lasley B, Ettinger B, Marcus R,** Bone mass and subtle abnormalities in ovulatory function in healthy women, *J Clin Endocrinol Metab* 81:663, 1996.

486. **De Souza MJ, Miller BE, Sequenzia LC, Luciano AA, Ulreich S, Stier S, Prestwood K, Lasley BL,** Bone health is not affected by luteal phase abnormalities and decreased ovarian progesterone production in female runners, *J Clin Endocrinol Metab* 82:2867, 1997.

487. **Cummings SR, Kelsey JL, Nevitt MC, O'Dowd KJ,** Epidemiology of osteoporosis and osteoporotic fractures, *Epidemiol Rev* 7:178, 1985.

488. **Beals RK,** Survival following hip fracture: long term follow-up of 607 patients, *J Chronic Dis* 25:235, 1972.

489. **Browner WS, Pressman AR, Nevitt MC, Cummings SR, for the Study of Osteoporotic Fractures Research Group,** Mortality following fractures in older women. The Study of Osteoporotic Fractures, *Arch Intern Med* 156:1521, 1996.

490. **Daniell HW,** Postmenopausal tooth loss: contributions to edentulism by osteoporosis and cigarette smoking, *Arch Intern Med* 143:1678, 1983.

491. **Krall EA, Dawson-Hughes B, Papas A, Garcia RI,** Tooth loss and skeletal bone density in healthy postmenopausal women, *Osteoporosis Int* 4:104, 1994.

492. **Faber J, Gallow AM,** Changes in bone mass during prolonged subclinical hyperthyroidism due to L-thyroxine treatment: a meta-analysis, *Eur J Endocrinol* 130:350, 1994.

493. **Cummings SR, Nevitt MC, Browner WS, Stone K, Fox KM, Ensrud KE, Cauley J, Black D, Voigt TM,** Risk factors for hip fracture in white women. Study of Osteoporotic Fractures Research Group, *New Engl J Med* 332:767, 1995.

494. **Bauer DC, Nevitt MC, Ettinger B, Stone K,** Low thyrotropin levels are not associated with bone loss in older women: a prospective study, *J Clin Endocrinol Metab* 82:2931, 1997.

495. **Johnston Jr CC, Slemenda CW, Melton III LJ,** Clinical use of bone densitometry, *New Engl J Med* 324:1105, 1991.

496. **Cummings SR, Black DM, Nevitt MC, Browner W, Cauley J, Ensrud K, Genant KH, Palermo L, Scott J, Vogt TM,** Bone density at various sites for prediction of hip fractures, *Lancet* 341:72, 1993.

497. **Johnston Jr CC, Slemenda CW,** Identification of patients with low bone mass by single photon absorptiometry and single-energy X-ray absorptiometry, *Am J Med* 98(Suppl 2A):37S, 1995.

498. **Rubin SM, Cummings SR,** Results of bone densitometry affect women's decisions about taking measures to prevent fractures, *Ann Int Med* 116:990, 1992.

499. **Silverman SL, Greenwald M, Klein RA, Drinkwater BL,** Effect of bone density information on decisions about hormone replacement therapy: a randomized trial, *Obstet Gynecol* 89:321, 1997.

500. **Hillard TC, Whicroft SJ, Marsh MS, Ellerington MC, Lees B, Whitehead MI, Stevenson JC,** Long-term effects of transdermal and oral hormone replacement therapy on postmenopausal bone loss, *Osteoporosis Int* 4:341, 1994.

501. **The Writing Group for the PEPI Trial,** Effects of hormone therapy on bone mineral density: results from the Postmenopausal Estrogen/Progestin Interventions (PEPI) Trial, *JAMA* 276:1389, 1996.

502. **Miller PD, Bonnick SL, Rosen CJ,** Consensus of an international panel on the clinical utility of bone mass measurements in the detection of low bone mass in the adult population, *Calcif Tissue Int* 58:207, 1996.

503. **Gregg EW, Kriska AM, Salamone LM, Roberts MM, Anderson SJ, Ferrell RE, Kuller LH, Cauley JA,** The epidemiology of quantitative ultrasound: a review of the relationships with bone mass, osteoporosis and fracture risk, *Osteoporosis Int* 7:89, 1997.

504. **Hans D, Dargent-Molina P, Schott AM, Sebert JL, Cormier C, Kotzkik PO, Delmas PD, Pouilles JM, Breart G, Meunier PJ, for the EPIDOS Prospective Study Group,** Ultrasonographic heel measurements to predict hip fracture in elderly women: the EPIDOS prospective study, *Lancet* 348:511, 1996.

505. **Njeh CF, Boivin CM, Langton CM,** The role of ultrasound in the assessment of osteoporosis: a review, *Osteoporosis Int* 7:7, 1997.

506. **Kanis J, Melton III LJ, Christiansen C, Johnston C, Khaltaev N,** Perspective: the diagnosis of osteoporosis, *J Bone Miner Res* 9:1137, 1994.

507. **Garnero P, Gineyts E, Rious JP, Delmas PD,** Assessment of bone resorption with a new marker of collagen degradation in patients with metabolic bone disease, *J Clin Endocrinol Metab* 79:780, 1994.

508. **Prestwood KM, Pilbeam CC, Burleson JA, Woodiel FN, Delmas PD, Deftos LJ, Raisz LG,** The short term effects of conjugated estrogen on bone turnover in older women, *J Clin Endocrinol Metab* 79:366, 1994.

509. **Chesnut III CH, Bell NH, Clark GS, Drinkwater BL, English SC, Johnston Jr CC, Notelovitz M, Rosen M, Cain DF, Flessland KA, Mallinak NJS,** Hormone replacement therapy in postmenopausal women: urinary N-telopeptide of type I collagen monitors therapeutic effect and predicts response of bone mineral density, *Am J Med* 102:29, 1997.

510. **Rosen CJ, Chesnut III CH, Mallinak NJ,** The predictive value of biochemical markers of bone turnover for bone mineral density in early postmenopausal women treated with hormone replacement or calcium supplementation, *J Clin Endocrinol Metab* 82:1904, 1997.

511. **Weiss NC, Ure CL, Ballard JH, Williams AR, Daling JR,** Decreased risk of fractures of the hip and lower forearm with postmenopausal use of estrogen, *New Engl J Med* 303:1195, 1980.

512. **Ettinger B, Genant HK, Cann CE,** Long-term estrogen replacement therapy prevents bone loss and fractures, *Ann Intern Med* 102:319, 1985.

513. **Kiel DP, Felson DT, Anderson JJ, Wilson PWF, Moskowitz MA,** Hip fracture and the use of estrogen in postmenopausal women: the Framingham Study, *New Engl J Med* 317:1169, 1987.

514. **Michaësson K, Baron JA, Farahmand BY, Johnell O, Magnusson C, Persson P-G, Persson I, Ljunghall S, on behalf of the Swedish Hip Fracture Study Group,** Hormone replacement therapy and risk of hip fracture: population based case-control study, *Br Med J* 316:1858, 1998.

515. **Riggs BL, Seeman E, Hodgson SF, Taves DR, O'Fallon WM,** Effect of the fluoride/calcium regimen on vertebral fracture occurrence in postmenopausal osteoporosis, *New Engl J Med* 306:446, 1982.

516. **Quigley MET, Martin PL, Burnier AM, Brooks P,** Estrogen therapy arrests bone loss in elderly women, *Am J Obstet Gynecol* 156:1516, 1987.

517. **Felson DT, Zhang Y, Hannan MT, Kiel DP, Wilson PWF, Anderson JJ,** The effect of postmenopausal estrogen therapy on bone density in elderly women, *New Engl J Med* 329:1141, 1993.

518. **Cauley JA, Seeley DG, Enbsrud K, Ettinger B, Black D, Cummings SR, for the Study of Osteoporotic Fractures Research Group,** Estrogen replacement therapy and fractures in older women, *Ann Intern Med* 122:9, 1995.

519. **Lindsay R, MacLean A, Kraszewski A, Clark AC, Garwood J,** Bone response to termination of estrogen treatment, *Lancet* i:1325, 1978.

520. **Horsman A, Nordin BEC, Crilly RG,** Effect on bone of withdrawal of estrogen therapy, *Lancet* ii:33, 1979.

521. **Christiansen C, Christiansen MS, Transbol IB,** Bone mass in postmenopausal women after withdrawal of oestrogen/gestagen replacement therapy, *Lancet* i:459, 1981.

522. **Schneider DL, Barrett-Connor EL, Morton DJ,** Timing of postmenopausal estrogen for optimal bone mineral density. The Rancho Bernardo Study, *JAMA* 277:543, 1997.

523. **Eiken P, Kolthoff N, Nielsen SP,** Effect of 10 years' hormone replacement therapy on bone mineral content in postmenopausal women, *Bone* 19:191S, 1996.

524. **Naessén T, Persson I, Thor L, Mallmin H, Ljunghall S, Bergstrom R,** Maintained bone density at advanced ages after long-term treatment with low-dose estradiol implants, *Br J Obstet Gynaecol* 100:454, 1993.

525. **Armamento-Villareal R, Civitelli R,** Estrogen action on the bone mass of postmenopausal women is dependent on body mass and initial bone density, *J Clin Endocrinol Metab* 80:776, 1995.

526. **Lindsay R, Hart DM, Clark DM,** The minimum effective dose of estrogen for postmenopausal bone loss, *Obstet Gynecol* 63:759, 1984.

527. **O'Connell MB,** Pharmacokinetic and pharmacologic variation between different estrogen products, *J Clin Pharmacol* 35(Suppl 9):18S, 1995.

528. **Reginster JY, Sarlet N, Deroisy R, Albert A, Gaspard U, Franchimont P,** Minimal levels of serum estradiol prevent post-menopausal bone loss, *Calcif Tissue Int* 51:340, 1992.

529. **Ettinger B, Pressman A, Sklarin P, Bauer DC, Cauley JA, Cummings SR,** Associations between low levels of serum estradiol, bone density, and fractures among elderly women: The Study of Osteoporotic Fractures, *J Clin Endocrinol Metab* 83:2239, 1998.

530. **Cummings SR, Browner WS, Bauer D, Stone K, Ensrud K, Jamal S, Ettinger B, for the Study of Osteoporotic Fractures Research Group,** Endogenous hormones and the risk of hip and vertebral fractures among older women, *New Engl J Med* 339:733, 1998.

531. **Naessen T, Berglund L, Ulmsten U,** Bone loss in elderly women prevented by ultralow doses of parenteral 17beta-estradiol, *Am J Obstet Gynecol* 177:115, 1997.

532. **Ettinger B, Genant HK, Cann CE,** Postmenopausal bone loss is prevented by treatment with low-dosage estrogen with calcium, *Ann Intern Med* 106:40, 1987.

533. **Ettinger B, Genant HK, Steiger P, Madvig P,** Low-dosage micronized 17β-estradiol prevents bone loss in postmenopausal women, *Am J Obstet Gynecol* 166:479, 1992.

534. **Genant HK, Lucas J, Weiss S, Akin M, Emeky R, McNaney-Flint H, Downs R, Mortola J, Watts N, Yank HM, Banav N, Brennan JJ, Nolan JC, for the Estratab/Osteoporosis Study Group,** Low-dose esterified estrogen therapy: effects on bone, plasma estradiol concentrations, endometrium, and lipid levels, *Arch Intern Med* 157:2609, 1997.

535. **Mizunuma H, Okano H, Soda M, Kagami I, Miyamoto S, Tokizawa T, Honjo S, Ibuki Y,** Prevention of postmenopausal bone loss with minimal uterine bleeding using low dose continuous estrogen/progestin therapy: a 2-year prospective study, *Maturitas* 27:69, 1997.

536. **Stevenson JC, Cust MP, Gangar KF, Hillard TC, Lees B, Whitehead MI,** Effects of transdermal versus oral hormone replacement therapy on bone density in spine and proximal femur in postmenopausal women, *Lancet* 336:1327, 1990.

537. **Prior JC, Vigna YM, Barr SI, Rexworthy C, Lentle BC,** Cyclic medroxyprogesterone treatment increases bone density: a controlled trial in active women with menstrual cycle disturbances, *Am J Med* 96:521, 1994.

538. **Selby PL, Peacock M, Barkworth SA, Brown WB, Taylor GA,** Early effects of ethinyl oestradiol and norethisterone treatment in postmenopausal women on bone resorption and calcium regulating hormones, *Clin Sci* 69:265, 1985.

539. **Christiansen C, Nilas L, Riis BJ, Rodbro P, Deftos L,** Uncoupling of bone formation and resorption by combined oestrogen and progestagen therapy in postmenopausal osteoporosis, *Lancet* ii:800, 1985.

540. **Munk-Jensen N, Nielsen SP, Obel EB, Eriksen PB,** Reversal of postmenopausal vertebral bone loss by oestrogen and progestogen: a double blind placebo controlled study, *Br Med J* 296:1150, 1988.

541. **Gallagher JC, Kable WT, Goldgar D,** Effect of progestin therapy on cortical and trabecular bone: comparison with estrogen, *Am J Med* 90:171, 1991.

542. **Grey A, Cundy T, Evans M, Reid I,** Medroxyprogesterone acetate enhances the spinal bone mineral density response to oestrogen in late post-menopausal women, *Clin Endocrinol* 44:293, 1996.

543. **Adachi JD, Sargeant EJ, Sagle MA, Lamont D, Fawcett PD, Bensen WG, McQueen M, Nazir DJ, Goldsmith CH,** A double-blind randomised controlled trial of the effects of medroxyprogesterone acetate on bone density of women taking oestrogen replacement therapy, *Br J Obstet Gynaecol* 104:64, 1997.

544. **Myers LS, Dixen J, Morrissette D, Carmichael M, Davidson JM,** Effects of estrogen, androgen, and progestin on sexual psychophysiology and behavior in postmenopausal women, *J Clin Endocrinol Metab* 70:1124, 1990.

545. **Fuleihan GE, Brown EM, Curtis K, Berger MJ, Berger BM, Gleason R, LeBoff MS,** Effect of sequential and daily continous hormone replacement therapy on indexes of mineral metabolism, *Arch Intern Med* 152:1904, 1992.

546. **Nielsen SP, Bärenholdt O, Hermansen F, Munkin-Jensen NB,** Magnitude and pattern of skeletal response to long term continuous and cyclic sequential oestrogen/progestin treatment, *Br J Obstet Gynaecol* 101:319, 1994.

547. **Garnett T, Studd J, Watson N, Savvas M, Leather A,** The effects of plasma estradiol levels on increases in vertebral and femoral bone density following therapy with estradiol and estradiol with testosterone implants, *Obstet Gynecol* 79:968, 1992.

548. **Watts NB, Notelovitz M, Timmons MC, Addison WA, Wiita B, Downey LJ,** Comparison of oral estrogens and estrogens plus androgens on bone mineral density, menopausal symptoms, and lipid-lipoprotein profiles in surgical menopause, *Obstet Gynecol* 85:529, 1995.

549. **Davis SR, McCloud P, Strauss BJG, Burger H,** Testosterone enhances estradiol's effects on postmenopausal bone density and sexuality, *Maturitas* 21:227, 1995.

550. **Draper MW, Flowers DE, Huster WJ, Neild JA, Harper KD, Arnaud C,** A controlled trial of raloxifene (LY139481) HCl: impact on bone turnover and serum lipid profile in healthy post-menopausal women, *J Bone Miner Res* 11:835, 1996.

551. **Boss SM, Huster WJ, Neild JA, Glant MD, Eisenhut CC, Draper MW,** Effects of raloxifene hydrochloride on the endometrium of postmenopausal women, *Am J Obstet Gynecol* 177:1458, 1997.

552. **Heaney RP, Draper MW,** Raloxifene and estrogen: comparative bone-remodeling kinetics, *J Clin Endocrinol Metab* 82:3425, 1997.

553. **Fisher B, Costantino JP, Wickerham DL, Redmond CK, Kavanah M, Cronin WM, Vogel V, Robidoux A, Dimitrov N, Atkins J, Daly M, Wieand S, Tan-Chiu E, Ford L, Wolmark N, and other National Surgical Adjuvant Breast and Bowel Project Investigators,** Tamoxifen for prevention of breast cancer: report of the National Surgical Adjuvant Breast and Bowel Project P-1 Study, *J Natl Cancer Inst* 90:1371, 1998.

554. **Cummings SR, Norton L, Eckert S, Grady D, Cauley J, Knickerbocker R, Black DM, Nickelsen T, Glusman J, Krueger K, for the MORE investigators,** Raloxifene reduces the risk of breast cancer and may decrease the risk of endometrial cancer in postmenopausal women. Two-year findings from the Multiple Outcomes of Raloxifene Evaluation (MORE) trial, *http://www.asco.org/*, 1998.

555. **Delmas PD, Bjarnason NH, Mitlak BH, Ravoux A-C, Shah AS, Huster WJ, Draper M, Christiansen C,** Effects of raloxifene on bone mineral density, serum cholesterol concentrations, and uterine endometrium in postmenopausal women, *New Engl J Med* 337:1641, 1997.

556. **Walsh BW, Kuller LH, Wild RA, Paul S, Farmer M, Lawrence JB, Shah AS, Anderson PW,** Effects of raloxifene on serum lipids and coagulation factors in healthy postmenopausal women, *JAMA* 279:1445, 1998.

557. **Ettinger V, Black D, Cummings S, Genant H, Glüer C, Lips P, Knickerbocker R, Eckert S, Nickelsen T, Mitlack B, for the MORE Study Group,** Raloxifene reduces the risk of incident vertebral fractures: 24-month interim analyses, *Osteo Int* 8(Suppl 3):11, 1998.

558. **Clarkson TB, Anthony MS, Jerome CP,** Lack of effect of raloxifene on coronary artery atherosclerosis of postmenopausal monkeys, *J Clin Endocrinol Metab* 83:721, 1998.

559. **Zuckerman SH, Bryan N,** Inhibition of LDL oxidation and myeloperoxidase dependent tyrosyl radical formation by the selective estrogen receptor modulator raloxifene (LY139481 HCL), *Atherosclerosis* 126:65, 1996.

560. **Mijatovic V, Netelenbos C, van der Mooren MJ, de Valk-de Roo GW, Jakobs C, Kenemans P,** Randomized, double-blind, placebo-controlled study of the effects of raloxifene and conjugated equine estrogen on plasma homocysteine levels in healthy postmenopausal women, *Fertil Steril* 70:1085, 1998.

561. **Reid IR, Ames RW, Evans MC, Gamble GD, Sharpe SJ,** Long-term effects of calcium supplementation on bone loss and fractures in postmenopausal women: a randomized controlled trial, *Am J Med* 98:331, 1995.

562. **Recker RR, Hinders S, Davies KM, Heaney RP, Stegman MR, Lappe JM, Kimmel DB,** Correcting calcium nutritional deficiency prevents spine fractures in elderly women, *J Bone Miner Res* 11:1961, 1996.

563. **Dawson-Hughes B, Harris SS, Krall EA, Dallal GE,** Effect of calcium and vitamin D supplementation on bone density in men and women 65 years of age or older, *New Engl J Med* 337:670, 1997.

564. **NIH Consensus Development Panel on Optimal Calcium Intake,** Optimal calcium intake, *JAMA* 272:1942, 1994.

565. **Hasling C, Charles P, Jensen FT, Mosekilde L,** Calcium metabolism in postmenopausal osteoporosis: the influence of dietary calcium and net absorbed calcium, *J Bone Min Res* 5:939, 1990.

566. **Heaney RP, Recker RR,** Distribution of calcium absorption in middle-aged women, *Am J Clin Nutr* 43:299, 1986.

567. **Prince RL, Smith M, Dick IM, Price RI, Webb PG, Henderson NK, Harris MM,** Prevention of postmenopausal osteoporosis: a comparative study of exercise, calcium supplementation, and hormone-replacement therapy, *New Engl J Med* 325:1189, 1991.

568. **Heikinheimo RJ, Inkovaara JA, Harju EJ, Haavisto MV, Kaarela RH, Kataja JM, Kokko AM, Kolho LA, Rajala S,** Annual injection of vitamin D and fractures of aged bones, *Calcif Tissue Int* 51:105, 1992.

569. **Aloia JF, Vaswani A, Yeh JK, Ross PL, Flaster E, Dilmanian FA,** Calcium supplementation with and without hormone replacement therapy to prevent postmenopausal bone loss, *Ann Intern Med* 120:97, 1994.

570. **Lloyd T, Andon MB, Rollings N, Martel JK, Landis JR, Demers LM, Eggli DF, Kiesselhorst K, Kulin HE,** Calcium supplementation and bone mineral density in adolescent girls, *JAMA* 270.841, 1993.

571. **Cadogan J, Eastell R, Jones N, Barker ME,** Milk intake and bone mineral acquisition in adolescent girls: randomised, controlled intervention trial, *Br Med J* 315:1255, 1997.

572. **American Association of Clinical Endocrinologists,** *http://www.aace.com/clin/guides/osteoporosis.html,* 1998.

573. **Curhan GC, Willett WC, Speizer FE, Spiegelman D, Stampfer MJ,** Comparison of dietary calcium with supplemental calcium and other nutrients as factors affecting the risk for kidney stones in women, *Ann Intern Med* 126:497, 1997.

574. **Chapuy MC, Arlot ME, Duboeuf F, Brun J, Crouzet B, Arnaud S, Delmas PD, Meunier PJ,** Vitamin D3 and calcium to prevent hip fractures in elderly women, *New Engl J Med* 327:1637, 1992.

575. **Tilyard MW, Spears GFS, Thomson J, Dovey S,** Treatment of postmenopausal osteoporosis with calcitriol or calcium, *New Engl J Med* 326:357, 1992.

576. **Ooms ME, Roos JC, Bezemer PD, Wim JF, Van Der Vijgh JF, Bouter LM, Lips P,** Prevention of bone loss by vitamin D supplementation in elderly women: a randomized double-blind trial, *J Clin Endocrinol Metab* 80:1052, 1995.

577. **Rosen CJ, Morrison A, Zhou H, Storm D, Hunter SJ, Musgrave K, Chen T, Wen-Wei, Holick MF,** Elderly women in northern New England exhibit seasonal changes in bone mineral density and calciotropic hormones, *Bone Mineral* 25:83, 1994.

578. **Thomas MK, Lloyd-Jones DM, Thadhani RI, Shaw AC, Deraska DJ, Kitch BT, Vamvakas EC, Dick IM, Prince RL, Finkelstein JS,** Hypovitaminosis D in medical inpatients, *New Engl J Med* 338:777, 1998.

579. **Komulainen M, Tuppurainen MT, Kröger H, Heikkinen AM, Puntila E, Alhava E, Honkanen R, Saarikoski S,** Vitamin D and HRT: no benefit additional to HRT alone in prevention of bone loss in early postmenopausal women. A 2.5-year randomized placebo-controlled study, *Osteoprosis Int* 7:126, 1997.

580. **Adami S, Baroni MC, Broggini M, Carratelli L, Caruso I, Gnessi L, Laurenzi M, Lombardi A, Norbiato G, Ortolani S, Ricerca E, Romanini L, Subrizi S, Weinberg J, Yates AJ,** Treatment of postmenopausal osteoporosis with continuous daily oral alendronate in comparison with either placebo or intranasal salmon calcitonin, *Osteoporosis Int* 3(Suppl):S21, 1993.

581. **Watts NB,** Treatment of osteoporosis with bisphosphonates, *Rheum Dis Clin North Am* 20:717, 1994.

582. **Black DM, Cummings SR, Karpf DB, Cauley JA, Thompson DE, Nevitt MC, Bauer DC, Genant HK, Haskell WL, Marcus R, Ott SM, Torner JC, Quandt SA, Reiss TF, Ensrud KE, for the Fracture Intervention Trial Research Group,** Randomised trial of effect of alendronate on risk of fracture in women with existing vertebral fractures, *Lancet* 348:1535, 1996.

583. **Karpf DB, Shapiro DR, Seeman E, Ensrud KE, Johnston Jr CC, Adami S, Harris ST, Santora II AC, Hirsch LJ, Oppenheimer L, Thompson D, for the Alendronate Osteoporosis Treatment Study Groups,** Prevention of nonvertebral fractures by alendronate, *JAMA* 277:1159, 1997.

584. **Hosking D, Chilvers CED, Christiansen C, Ravn P, Wasnich R, Ross P, McClung M, Balske A, Thompson D, Daley M, Yates AJ, for the Early Postmenopausal Intervention Cohort Study Group,** Prevention of bone loss with alendronate in postmenopausal women under 60 years of age, *New Engl J Med* 338:485, 1998.

585. **McClung M, Clemmesen B, Daifotis A, Gilchrist NL, Eisman J, Weinstein RS, Fuleihan GEH, Reda C, Yates AJ, Ravn P, for the Alendronate Osteoporosis Prevention Study Group,** Alendronate prevents postmenopausal bone loss in women without osteoporosis: a double-blind, randomized, controlled trial, *Ann Intern Med* 128:253, 1998.

586. **de Groen PC, Lubbe DF, Hirsch LJ, Daifotis A, Stephenson W, Freedholm D, Pryor-Tillotson S, Seleznick MJ, Pinkas H, Wang KK,** Esophagitis associated with the use of alendronate, *New Engl J Med* 335:1016, 1996.

587. **Mortensen L, Charles P, Bekker PJ, Digennaro J, Johnston Jr CC,** Risedronate increases bone mass in an early postmenopausal population: two years of treatment plus one year of follow-up, *J Clin Endocrinol Metab* 83:396, 1998.

588. **Herd RJ, Balena R, Blake GM, Ryan PJ, Fogelman I,** Prevention of early postmenopausal bone loss by cyclical etidronate: a two-year double-blind placebo-controlled study, *Am J Med* 103:92, 1997.

589. **Meunier PJ, Confavreux E, Tupinon I, Hardouin C, Delmas PD, Balena R,** Prevention of early postmenopausal bone loss with cyclical etidronate therapy (a double-blind, placebo-controlled study and 1-year follow-up), *J Clin Endocrinol Metab* 82:2784, 1997.

590. **American Society for Bone and Mineral Research,** *http://www.asbmr.org/,* 1998.

591. **Stock JL, Bell NH, Chesnut III CH, Ensrud RE, Genant HK, McClung MR, Singes FR, Yood RA, Pryor-Tillotson S, Weil L, Santora 2nd AC,** Increments in bone mineral density of the lumbar spine and hip and suppression of bone turnover are maintained after discontinuation of alendronate in postmenopausal women, *Am J Med* 103:291, 1997.

592. **MacIntyre I, Stevenson JC, Whitehead MI, Wimalawansa SJ, Banks LM, Healy MJ,** Calcitonin for prevention of postmenopausal bone loss, *Lancet* i:900, 1988.

593. **Fioretti P, Gambacciani M, Taponeco F, Melis GB, Capelli N, Spinetti,** Effects of continuous and cyclic nasal calcitonin administration in ovariectomized women, *Maturitas* 15:225, 1992.

594. **Pak CY, Sakhaee K, Adams-Huet B, Piziak V, Peterson RD, Poindexter JR,** Treatment of postmenopausal osteoporosis with slow-release sodium fluoride: final update of a randomized controlled trial, *Ann Intern Med* 123:401, 1995.

595. **Pak CYC, Sakhaee K, Rubin C, Rao S,** Update of fluoride in the treatment of osteoporosis, *Endocrinologist* 8:15, 1998.

596. **Ross LA, Alder EM,** Tibolone and climacteric symptoms, *Maturitas* 21:127, 1995.

597. **Bjarnason NH, Bjarnason K, Haarbo J, Rosenquist C, Christiansen C,** Tibolone: prevention of bone loss in late postmenopausal women, *J Clin Endocrinol Metab* 81:2419, 1996.

598. **Ginsburg J, Prelevic G, Butler D, Okolo S,** Clinical experience with tibolone (Livial) over 8 years, *Maturitas* 21:71, 1995.

599. **Lippuner K, Haenggi W, Birkhaeuser MH, Casez J-P, Jaeger P,** Prevention of postmenopausal bone loss using tibolone or conventional peroral or transdermal hormone replacement therapy with 17β-estradiol and dydrogesterone, *J Bone Miner Res* 12:806, 1997.

600. **Tang B, Markiewicz L, Kloosterboer HJ, Gurpide E,** Human endometrial 3 beta-hydroxysteroid dehydrogenase/isomerase can locally reduce intrinsic estrogenic/progestagenic activity ratios of a steroidal drug (Org OD 14), *J Steroid Biochem Mol Biol* 45:345, 1993.

601. **Rymer J, Chapman MG, Fogelman I, Wilson POG,** A study of the effect of tibolone on the vagina in postmenopausal women, *Maturitas* 18:127, 1994.

602. **Farish E, Barnes JF, Rolton HA, Spowart K, Fletcher CD, Hart DM,** Effects of tibolone on lipoprotein(a) and HDL subfractions, *Maturitas* 20:215, 1994.

603. **Bjarnason NH, Bjarnason K, Haarbo J, Coelingh Bennink HJT, Christiansen C,** Tibolone: influence on markers of cardiovascular disease, *J Clin Endocrinol Metab* 82:1752, 1997.

604. **Cagnacci A, Mallus E, Tuveri F, Cirillo R, Setteneri AM, Melis GB,** Effects of tibolone on glucose and lipid metabolism in postmenopausal women, *J Clin Endocrinol Metab* 82:251, 1997.

605. **Prelevic GM, Beljic T, Balint-Peric L, Ginsburg J,** Metabolic effects of tibolone in postmenopausal women with non-insulin dependent diabetes mellitus, *Maturitas* 28:271, 1998.

606. **Morton DJ, Barrett-Connor EL, Edelstein SL,** Thiazides and bone mineral density in elderly men and women, *Am J Epidemiol* 139:1107, 1994.

607. **Holloway L, Butterfield G, Hintz RL, Gesundheit N, Marcus R,** Effects of recombinant human growth hormone on metabolic indices, body composition, and bone turnover in healthy elderly women, *J Clin Endocrinol Metab* 79:470, 1994.

608. **Chow RK, Harrison JE, Brown CF, Hajek V,** Physical fitness effect on bone mass in postmenopausal women, *Arch Phys Med Rehabil* 67:231, 1986.

609. **Dalsky G, Stocke KS, Ehsani AA, Slatopolsky E, Lee WC, Birjes Jr J,** Weight-bearing exercise training and lumbar bone mineral content in postmenopausal women, *Ann Intern Med* 108:824, 1988.

610. **Cavanagh DJ, Cann CE,** Brisk walking does not stop bone loss in postmenopausal women, *Bone* 9:201, 1988.

611. **Brooke-Wavell K, Jones PRM, Hardman AE,** Brisk walking reduces calcaneal bone loss in post-menopausal women, *Clin Sci* 92:75, 1997.

612. **Ebrahim S, Thompson PW, Baskaran V, Evans K,** Randomized placebo-controlled trial of brisk walking in the prevention of postmenopausal osteoporosis, *Age Ageing* 26:253, 1997.

613. **Kohrt WM, Snead DB, Slatopolsky E, Birge Jr SJ,** Additive effects of weight-bearing exercise and estrogen on bone mineral density in older women, *J Bone Miner Res* 10:1303, 1995.

614. **Hopper JL, Seeman E,** The bone density of female twins discordant for tobacco use, *New Engl J Med* 330:387, 1994.

615. **Krall EA, Dawson-Hughes B,** Smoking and bone loss among postmenopausal women, *J Bone Miner Res* 6:331, 1991.

616. **Jensen J, Christiansen C, Rodbro P,** Cigarette smoking, serum estrogens, and bone loss during hormone replacement therapy early after menopause, *New Engl J Med* 313:973, 1985.

617. **Lukert BP, Johnson BE, Robinson RG,** Estrogen and progesterone replacement therapy reduces glucocorticoid-induced bone loss, *J Bone Miner Res* 7:1063, 1992.

618. **Hall GM, Daniels M, Doyle DV, Spector TD,** Effect of hormone replacement therapy on bone mass in rheumatoid arthritis patients treated with and without steroids, *Arthritis Rheum* 37:1499, 1994.

619. **Kiel DP, Felson DT, Hannan MT, Anderson JJ, Wilson PW,** Caffeine and the risk of hip fracture: the Framingham Study, *Am J Epidemiol* 132:675, 1990.

620. **Barrett-Connor E, Chang JC, Edelstein SL,** Coffee-associated osteoporosis offset by daily milk consumption, *JAMA* 271:280, 1994.

621. **Cadogan J, Eastell R, Jones N, Barker ME,** Milk intake and bone mineral acquisition in adolescent girls: randomised, controlled intervention trial, *Br Med J* 315:1255, 1997.

622. **Greenspan SL, Myers ER, Maitland LA, Resnick NM, Hayes WC,** Fall severity and bone mineral density as risk factors for hip fracture in ambulatory elderly, *JAMA* 271:128, 1994.

623. **Hammar ML, Lindgren R, Berg GE, Möller CG, Niklasson MK,** Effects of hormonal replacement therapy on postural balance among postmenopausal women, *Obstet Gynecol* 88:955, 1996.

624. **Naessen T, Lindmark B, Larsen H-C,** Better postural balance in elderly women receiving estrogens, *Am J Obstet Gynecol* 177:412, 1997.

625. **Armstrong AL, Oborne J, Coupland CAC, MacPherson MB, Bassey EJ, Wallace WA,** Effects of hormone replacement therapy on muscle performance and balance in post-menopausal women, *Clin Sci* 91:685, 1996.

626. **Brown M, Birge SJ, Kohrt WM,** Hormone replacement therapy does not augment gains in muscle strength or fat-free mass in response to weight-bearing exercise, *J Gerontol* 52A:B166, 1997.

627. **Welt CK, McNicholl DJ, Taylor AE, Hall JE,** Female reproductive aging is marked by decreased secretion of dimeric inhibin, *J Clin Endocrinol Metab* 84:105, 1999.

18 Postmenopausal Hormone Therapy

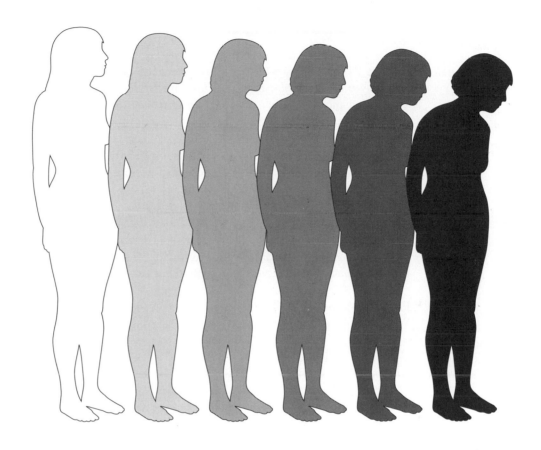

Postmenopausal hormone therapy had its beginning in the effort to alleviate specific symptoms associated with the decline in estrogen production at menopause. There is little question that women who suffer from hot flushes or atrophy of reproductive tract tissues can be relieved of their problems by the use of estrogens. However, in the last decade, the focus of postmenopausal hormone therapy has changed from short-term treatment to the preventive health care benefits associated with long-term treatment. It is almost certain that the long-term disabilities of osteoporosis can be largely prevented by therapy with estrogen and progestin. It is increasingly accepted that appropriate doses of estrogen have a beneficial impact on the risk of cardiovascular disease. The long-term impacts on urinary incontinence and cognition remain to be documented, but there is reason to believe there will be benefits in these areas.

We suggest treatment with estrogen for all women disturbed by the symptoms of hormone deprivation and advocate hormonal prophylaxis against osteoporosis and cardiovascular disease. The decision to use or not to use estrogen belongs to the patient, and it should be based on the information available in this book. The recommendation that hormone therapy be given for the shortest period of time appears to be shortsighted in view of the impressive evidence that sustained therapy has a profound impact on osteoporosis and cardiovascular disease, and that there are more beneficial than potentially harmful effects.

The evidence supporting many of the benefits with postmenopausal hormone therapy is reviewed in the previous chapter (Chapter 17, Menopause and the Perimenopausal Transition) where the effects of hormonal treatment are considered in conjunction with the impact of postmenopausal estrogen deprivation. In this chapter, we will review the clinical aspects of postmenopausal hormone therapy and our methods of patient management.

History[1-3]

Charles Edouard Brown-Sequard, practicing in London, reported in 1889, that he was rejuvenated by the self-administration of testicular extracts, and he suggested that ovarian extracts would have the same effect in women. Efforts to do so around the turn of the century were largely unsuccessful, but in 1897, ovarian extract was reported to be effective for hot flushing.[4] The first American attempt to treat menopausal symptoms is attributed to E.L. Sevringhaus and J. Evans of Madison, Wisconsin, who, in 1929, administered a derivative from the amniotic fluid of cattle.[2, 5] In the 1930s, the ovarian hormones were isolated, and the "estrin" products and the synthetic estrogens, stilbestrol and ethinyl estradiol, were administered to menopausal women.

Allen and Doisy were the first to isolate the estrogenic ovarian hormone. Edgar Allen was born in Colorado, educated at Brown University, and served in France during World War I. In 1933, Allen became the chairman of the Department of Anatomy at Yale University. He died of a heart attack, on patrol off Long Island, for the U.S. Coast Guard, in February 1943.

Edward Doisy was born in Illinois and educated at the University of Illinois and Harvard. During World War I, he was assigned to the Rockefeller Institute in New York City, and then to the Walter Reed Hospital in Washington. Doisy was the first chairman of biochemistry at the St. Louis University School of Medicine. He received the Nobel Prize in Medicine, along with Henrik Dam, in 1943, for his isolation and synthesis of vitamin K. He died in 1986 at the age of 92.

In 1919, Edgar Allen and Edward Doisy, being discharged from the army after World War I, joined the faculty at the Washington University School of Medicine in St. Louis. They became friends playing on a faculty baseball team, and planned their first experiments driving to work together. In 1922, Allen moved to the University of Missouri to be Professor of Anatomy (and Dean in 1930), and Doisy to St. Louis University, but they continued their collaboration. Doisy prepared ovarian extracts and mailed them to Allen for experiments. In 1923 and 1924, Allen and Doisy reported the isolation from pig ovaries and the administration (to animals) of "an ovarian hormone."

In 1926, A.S. Parkes and C.W. Bellerby coined the basic word estrin to designate the hormone (or hormones) that induces estrus in animals. The terminology was extended to include estrone, estradiol, and estriol, although significant amounts of pure estradiol were not isolated until 1936. Doisy and his students (Veler and Thayer) in St. Louis isolated estrone in crystalline form from the urine of pregnant women in 1929. In 1932, at the first meeting of the International Conference on the Standardization of Sex Hormones in London, the pioneering chemists were bemoaning the problem of scarcity, limiting supplies to milligram amounts, when a relatively unknown biochemist, Girard, offered 20 grams of crystalline substance, derived by the use of a new reagent to treat mare's urine.

George W. Corner, at the University of Rochester, invited Willard Myron Allen, an organic chemist but now a medical student at the time in the 1920s, to join him in the study of the corpus luteum. Within 2 years, they had a pure extract, but it was not until 1934 that a crystalline progestin was isolated almost simultaneously in several countries. It took the corpora lutea of 50,000 pigs to yield a few milligrams. At the Second International Conference on Standardization of Sex Hormones in London, Corner and Allen proposed the name progestin. Others proposed luteosterone, and at a cocktail party, the various biochemists agreed to call the chemical progesterone.

Corner was born in Baltimore, graduated from the Johns Hopkins medical school, and completed an internship in gynecology under Howard Kelley. He joined the Department of Anatomy at the University of California, and in 1923 at the age of 34, he became the first professor of anatomy in the new medical school of the University of Rochester. In 1940, Corner became the Director of the Carnegie Laboratory of Embryology in Baltimore. He died in 1981.

Allen was born in Macedon, New York, educated at Hobart College and Brown University, finally receiving his medical degree from the University of Rochester in 1932. He completed a residency in obstetrics and gynecology and served on the faculty in Rochester until he became chairman of obstetrics and gynecology at the Washington University School of Medicine in 1940. He died in 1993.

In the 1930s, the Ayerst Company was extracting estrogens from the urine of pregnant women. Limited by the problems of supply, low activity, plus bad taste and odor, Gordon A. Grant, head of biochemistry for Ayerst, suggested in 1939 that they use urine from horses. The process produced sodium salts from the sulfate esters of the various estrogens, yielding a water-soluble conjugate. Premarin (conjugated estrogens) was ***approved in Canada in 1941 and in the U.S. in 1942*** for the treatment of symptoms associated with menopause.[6] The tablets were and are still designated as variations of 1.25 mg, based on the equivalent amounts of Premarin and estrone (1.25 mg) that could produce the same effect in the Allen–Doisy bioassay (amount required to produce an increase in rat uterine weight). It was not until 1972 that the first quantitative analysis of Premarin was performed, based on gas chromatography.

Composition of Conjugated Estrogens (Premarin)

Sodium estrone sulfate	49.3%
Sodium equilin sulfate	22.4%
Sodium 17α-dihydroequilin sulfate	13.8%
Sodium 17α-estradiol sulfate	4.5%
Sodium Δ8,9-dehydroestrone sulfate	3.5%
Sodium equilenin sulfate	2.2%
Sodium 17β-dihydroequilin sulfate	1.7%
Sodium 17α-dihydroequilenin sulfate	1.2%
Sodium 17β-estradiol sulfate	0.9%
Sodium 17β-dihydroequilenin sulfate	0.5%

Estrogens and progestins used for postmenopausal hormone therapy are among the most commonly prescribed medications in the U.S. Currently, 46% of women who have experienced a natural menopause and 71% of women who have had bilateral oophorectomy report having used postmenopausal hormone therapy.[7] The average duration of use in the U.S. as of 1992 was 6.6 years, but only 20% of users had maintained treatment for at least 5 years.

Selection of Patients for Treatment

Women Under Age 40 (Castrates and Women With Gonadal Dysgenesis)

In these women, the duration of estrogen deprivation is prolonged, and in women after surgical menopause the loss of estrogen is acute. The cyclic use of estrogen is recommended for short-term reduction of vasomotor symptoms and for long-term prophylaxis against cardiovascular disease, osteoporosis, and target organ atrophy. In some young patients, the equivalent of 0.625 mg conjugated estrogens is insufficient to allow menstrual bleeding. Because women of this age ordinarily are exposed to estrogen levels that stimulate endometrial growth and withdrawal bleeding, and for psychological reasons, a higher dose should be considered, if necessary, to maintain withdrawal bleeding until the menopausal time of life. However, in our experience, the doses equivalent to 0.625 mg conjugated estrogens almost always suffice. A standard sequential program is utilized. In those patients castrated because of endometriosis, recurrence of endometriosis has very rarely been a problem with estrogen therapy, but because endometrial cancer has been reported to occur in remaining endometriosis exposed to unopposed estrogen, an estrogen and progestin combination is strongly recommended.

The Perimenopausal Transition Years

After exclusion of other gynecologic causes, dysfunctional uterine bleeding is treated by progestin or oral contraceptive therapy and, if necessary, biopsy surveillance. Vasomotor reactions appearing in women despite the presence of menstrual bleeding should receive careful evaluation. Abnormal thyroid function should be ruled out. If a follicle-stimulating hormone (FSH) level is not greater than 20 IU/L, serious consideration should be directed toward psychosocial reasons for the flushing response.

The risk of fracture from osteoporosis will depend on bone mass at the time of menopause and the rate of bone loss following menopause.[8] Although the peak bone mass is influenced by heredity and endocrine factors, it is now recognized that there exists only a relatively narrow window of opportunity for acquiring bone mass. Almost all of the bone mass in the hip and the vertebral bodies will be accumulated in young women by late adolescence (age 18), and the years immediately following menarche (11–14) are especially important.[9, 10] After adolescence, there continues to be only a slight gain in total skeletal mass that ceases around age 30, and in many individuals a decline in bone mass in the hip and spine begins after age 18.[10, 11] After age 30 in most people, there is a slow decline in bone mass density, about 0.7% per year. The importance of a normal diet and a normal hormonal environment during adolescence cannot be overrated.

Meaningful perimenopausal bone loss that is secondary to a decrease in estrogen is limited to those women with fluctuating hormonal and menstrual function, irregular bursts of follicular function alternating with no ovarian response to gonadotropins, so that these women are exposed to low estrogen over significant periods of time. The bone loss that begins in the 20s is due to a mechanism that is independent of hormones, and longitudinal studies have documented that trivial amounts of bone are lost prior to menopause in women with adequate estrogen levels.

The Early Postmenopause

The long-term postmenopausal use of hormone therapy depends heavily on a woman's own informed assessment, a process that should occur at this point in life. An understanding of hormone therapy is an important component in any preventive health program directed toward the postmenopausal years. As a result of immediate responses in early climacteric symptoms, the patient enters the postmenopausal period of life more confident of herself emotionally, sexually, and physically. In our view, this establishes or cements good patient-clinician interchange and relations. The follow-up of the patient on effective estrogen-progestin therapy is more secure and certain. The practitioner offering estrogen-progestin treatment has a better and more reliable opportunity to act as primary clinician for these aging women. All monitoring of health systems will be improved as a result of this single involvement.

The Late Postmenopause

Atrophic conditions can be effectively treated with local or oral therapy in low maintenance doses. If there is no apparent basis for osteoporosis other than aging and ovarian failure, estrogen-progestin therapy and calcium plus vitamin D supplementation are advisable even for very old women. Further loss of bone can be halted and the risk of fractures reduced. In these older women, an assessment of progress can be obtained by measuring bone density. The impact of initiating hormone therapy in elderly women on the risk of cardiovascular disease has not been ascertained. However, it makes sense that elderly women would benefit from estrogen's dynamic protective mechanisms with an impact on stress incontinence, and probably, on the risk of Alzheimer's disease, as well.

Hormonal Agents and Routes of Administration

The dose of estrogen that is maximally effective in maintaining the axial and peripheral bone mass is equivalent to 0.625 mg conjugated estrogens.[12, 13] The relative potencies of commercially available estrogens become of great importance when prescribing estrogen, and the clinician should be familiar with the potencies in the Table.

Relative Estrogen Potencies[14–18]

Estrogen	FSH levels	Liver proteins	Bone density
Conjugated estrogens	1.0 mg	0.625 mg	0.625 mg
Micronized estradiol	1.0 mg	1.0 mg	1.0 mg
Estropipate (piperazine estrogen sulfate)	1.0 mg	1.25 mg	1.25 mg
Ethinyl estradiol	5.0 µg	2–10 µg	5.0 µg
Estradiol valerate	—	—	1.0 mg
Esterified estrogens	—	—	0.625 mg
Transdermal estradiol	—	—	50 µg

The 17α-ethinyl group of ethinyl estradiol (by resisting metabolism) appears to enhance hepatic effects, for no matter by which route it is administered, liver function is affected.[17] The same is true for conjugated equine estrogens. Contrary to the case with estradiol, the liver appears to preferentially extract ethinyl estradiol and conjugated equine estrogens no matter what the route of administration. Thus, the route of administration appears to influence the metabolic responses only in the case of specific estrogens, most notably estradiol.

At least two studies have been unable to demonstrate prevention of bone loss with the administration of 2 mg estriol daily.[19, 20] A major factor in the potency differences among the various estrogens (estradiol, estrone, estriol) is the length of time the estrogen-receptor complex occupies the nucleus. The higher rate of dissociation with the weak estrogen (estriol) can be compensated for by continuous application to allow prolonged nuclear binding and activity. Estriol has only 20–30% affinity for the estrogen receptor compared to estradiol; therefore, it is rapidly cleared from a cell. But if the effective concentration is kept equivalent to that of estradiol, it can produce a similar biologic response.[21] In pregnancy, where the concentration of estriol is very great, it can be an important hormone, not just a metabolite. Thus, higher estriol levels are not necessarily protective. Because estriol protects the rat against breast tumors induced by various chemical carcinogens,[22] it has been hypothesized that a higher estriol level protects against the more potent effects of estrone and estradiol. Indeed, antagonism of estradiol occurs only within a vary narrow range of the ratio of estradiol to estriol, a range rarely encountered either physiologically or pharmacologically.[23] Below this range, estradiol is unimpeded, above this range estriol itself exerts estrogenic activity.

Esterified estrogens are synthetically prepared from plant precursors and are composed mostly of sodium estrone sulfate with a 6–15% component of sodium equilin sulfate. Estradiol valerate is rapidly hydrolyzed to estradiol, and, therefore, the pharmacology and effects are comparable at similar dosages.[24]

Transdermal Administration

The patches first used for transdermal estrogen administration contained an alcohol reservoir; the estrogen was released through a semipermeable membrane attached to the skin with an adhesive. The current generation of patches has the hormones dissolved and distributed throughout the adhesive matrix. In a study of women who had previously discontinued patches because of skin irritation (contact dermatitis), skin reactions were less common with the newer matrix patches.[25] In addition, the matrix patches are better tolerated in tropical environments.[26] The patches are designated according to the amount of estrogen delivered per day: 50 μg and 100 μg.

The effect of steroids on lipids and lipoproteins is determined by the type of steroid, the dose, and the route of administration. An obstacle to the use of transdermal hormone therapy has been the scarcity of data indicating a beneficial impact on the lipoprotein profile. There has been concern that delivery of estrogen through the skin yields a blood level that might be too low to provide protection against cardiovascular disease, especially because after peak concentrations in the first day after application, there is a progressive decrease that can be relatively rapid. Furthermore, there is marked variation in levels among individuals and within the same individual.

The concentration of estrogen in the portal system after oral administration is 4–5 times higher than that in the periphery.[27] Furthermore, the estradiol:estrone ratio differs in the portal system. Thus, the first-pass effect is either significant for the lipoprotein effects, or it is important only in the short term. For example, short-term studies (6 weeks) could document increased catabolism of LDL and increased production of apoprotein A-I with oral estrogen, but no effect with transdermal estrogen.[28, 29] And a 2-year study in Los Angeles with a transdermal dose (100 μg) detected no significant change in HDL-cholesterol levels.[30] However, English data indicate that the transdermal administration of 50 μg estradiol twice a week is as effective as 0.625 mg oral conjugated estrogens, when combined with a progestin in sequential regimens, on bone density and lipids over a duration of 3 years.[31] Of note, 12% of the women on either the transdermal or oral regimen lost bone from the femoral neck, despite documented adequate compliance. The transdermal administration of 100 μg estradiol combined with a progestin will not only increase bone density, but also reduce the fracture rate in older women who already have significant osteoporosis.[32] However, standard doses of estrogen administered transdermally (50 μg) appear to protect against fractures as well as standard oral doses.[33]

Until data are available documenting the degree of impact of the various routes of administration on actual clinical events (especially cardiovascular disease), the prudent clinical decision is to select the method (an oral program) that has epidemiologic support.

Estradiol Implants

Estradiol pellets are available in doses of 25, 50, and 75 mg for subcutaneous administration twice yearly. The 25 mg pellet provides blood levels in the range of 40–60 pg/mL, levels that are comparable with those obtained with standard oral doses.[34] However, the effect is cumulative, and after several years the blood levels are 2–3 times higher. Significant blood levels of estradiol will persist for up to 2 years after the last insertion. Progestational treatment is necessary, and because of the higher blood levels, a minimal duration of 14 days each month is advised. We believe that the estradiol pellets confer no advantages over the usual treatment regimens. We further recommend that women receiving pellets be monitored with blood estradiol levels, and levels greater than 200 pg/mL (and preferably, 100 pg/mL) should be avoided.

Percutaneous Estrogen

Estradiol delivery can be accomplished by the application of a gel to the skin, usually over the upper arms and shoulders or the abdomen and thighs. The preparation produces blood levels of estradiol of approximately 95–125 pg/mL, levels that are both higher and more variable than the standard oral regimens.[35, 36] As with pellets, we recommend that blood estradiol levels be monitored and maintained at a level below 100–200 pg/mL.

The Narrow Therapeutic Window

There are reasons to believe that the dose of estrogen administered is important in achieving maximal cardiovascular benefits. Hemodynamic responses to estrogen vary according to blood estrogen levels. Relatively normal levels are associated with better left ventricular contraction and performance.[37–39] Very high estradiol levels achieved with large doses of estrogen produce the opposite effects, a decrease in left ventricular size and aortic blood flow.[40] The beneficial effect of postmenopausal estrogen in preventing the hyperinsulinemia associated with aging is present with a dose of 0.625 mg conjugated estrogens, but lost with a dose of 1.25 mg.[41] The effect of estrogen on arterial thrombosis is dose related; we know from our experience with oral contraceptives that high doses of estrogen cause myocardial infarctions and strokes. At least 3 studies have found that estrogen doses greater than 0.625 mg conjugated estrogens are less beneficial in terms of coronary heart disease and mortality; although the numbers of patients on the higher doses were relatively small, and these conclusions did not achieve statistical significance.[42–44] For these reasons, we believe it is important to avoid excessive dosage. We find it helpful to measure the blood level of estradiol in patients who demand ever-increasing doses of estrogen. *Sharing the results of the measurement and the concern regarding high doses helps patients accept the recommendation to keep the blood level of estradiol below 200 pg/mL, and, preferably, below 100 pg/mL.*

Is there a dose of estrogen below which the beneficial effects begin to be lost? This is a difficult question to answer because so few women in epidemiologic studies have taken less than the standard doses. In a 2-year study, the lipid effects associated with 0.3 mg esterified estrogen were not significantly different from the placebo group.[45] In the monkey, the cardiovascular beneficial responses begin to diminish below a circulating blood estradiol level of 60 pg/mL.[46] Therefore, it is likely that some reduction in cardiovascular benefit occurs with less than standard estrogen doses.

Studies have demonstrated that a dose of 0.625 mg of conjugated estrogens is necessary to preserve bone density.[12] The conventional wisdom has stated that an estradiol blood level of 40–60 pg/mL is required to protect against bone loss.[47, 48] We now know that any amount of estrogen can have an impact, although it is very likely that some degree of protection is lost when doses are less than the equivalent of 0.625 mg conjugated estrogens.

The rate of bone loss and the incidence of hip and vertebral fracture is inversely related to the circulating estrogen levels in older women.[49, 50] Estradiol levels as low as 10 pg/mL have a beneficial impact on bone density and fracture rates compared with values below 5 pg/mL. *Thus, any increment in estrogen, even within the usual postmenopausal range, will exert protective effects.* This explains how a positive effect on bone was observed even with the utilization of the vaginal ring that delivers a very small amount of estradiol with minimal systemic absorption.[51]

A lower dose of 0.3 mg daily of conjugated estrogens or 0.5 mg estradiol prevented loss of vertebral trabecular bone when combined with calcium supplementation (to achieve a total intake of 1500 mg daily).[45, 52, 53] In a small study without calcium supplementation, the daily administration of 0.3 mg conjugated estrogens and 2.5 mg medroxyprogesterone acetate produced a slight increase in lumbar bone density with a lesser effect on the hip.[54] A study of women randomized to treatment either with continuous transdermal delivery of estradiol 50 μg daily or oral estrogen demonstrated that both equally prevented postmenopausal bone loss.[55] Major concerns with lower doses include the possibility that there will be a significant percentage of non-responders, and some cardiovascular benefit will be sacrificed. Nevertheless, a lower dose of estrogen may be more acceptable (fewer side effects) in elderly women. Patients electing to be treated with lower doses should have follow-up assessments for bone response with measurements of either bone density or urinary biochemical markers. After 6 months to one year, we urge patients on lower doses to move up to a standard regimen.

Monitoring Estrogen Dosage With Estradiol Blood Levels

Monitoring the estradiol blood level in postmenopausal women receiving hormone therapy is not as straightforward as it would seem. There are two primary difficulties. First, the clinical assays available differ considerably in their technique and quality (laboratory and antibody variations). Second, the various commercial products represent a diverse collection of estrogenic compounds, ranging from estradiol to unique equine estrogens. Although the body interconverts various estrogens into estrone and estradiol, is this process relatively consistent within and between individuals? For example, a highly specific assay for estradiol will detect very low levels of estradiol in women receiving 0.625 mg conjugated equine estrogens; nevertheless, most clinical assays will report a level of 40–100 pg/mL in these women. We find measurement of blood estradiol levels very useful in selected patients, such as the patient who requests ever-increasing doses of estrogen for the treatment of symptoms, which in the presence of very high blood levels of estradiol, can be confidently diagnosed as psychosomatic. What each clinician must do is learn what blood level of estradiol as performed by the local laboratory is associated with the standard doses of hormone therapy (0.625 conjugated estrogens, 1 mg estradiol, 50 μg transdermal estradiol). In our laboratory this range is 40–100 pg/mL estradiol. *Remember that because FSH is regulated by a factor other than estrogen (i.e., inhibin), FSH levels cannot be used to monitor estrogen dosage.* Postmenopausal hormone therapy will produce only a 10–20% decrease in FSH and LH, and there is great individual variability in the responses.[56]

Sequential and Continuous Regimens

The most common sequential method in the U.S. involves oral estrogen administration with 0.625 mg conjugated estrogens or the equivalent doses of a variety of available products. A daily dose of 5 mg medroxyprogesterone acetate (MPA) is added for 14 days of every month. One-year randomized trial data indicate that the 5 mg dose protects the endometrium as well as the 10 mg dose.[57] Unfortunately, progestin withdrawal bleeding occurs in 80–90% of women on a sequential regimen.[58–60] The sequential regimen can also cause adverse symptoms related to the dose of progestin such as breast tenderness, bloating, fluid retention, and depression. Switching from medroxyprogesterone acetate to norethindrone often relieves these complaints.

The Sequential Program for Oral Postmenopausal Hormone Therapy

Daily estrogen: **0.625 mg conjugated estrogens, or**
                     1.25 mg estropipate, or
                     1.0 mg micronized estradiol or
                     equivalent doses of other estrogens.

Monthly progestin: **0.7 mg norethindrone, or**
                     200 mg micronized progesterone, or
                     5 mg medroxyprogesterone acetate, or
                     equivalent doses of other progestins
                     given daily for 2 weeks every month.

Combined with daily calcium supplementation (500 mg with a meal), and vitamin D (400 IU in winter months and 800 IU for women over age 70).

In the sequential regimen, the amount of norethindrone equivalent to 10 mg medroxy-progesterone acetate is 1.0 mg.[61] Norethindrone is available in a dose of 0.35 mg in the progestin-only minipill oral contraceptive. In a 3-year randomized trial, 200 mg micronized progesterone given daily for 12 days each month effectively protected the endometrium against hyperplasia.[60] The lowest effective dose of micronized progesterone and the proper dose for continuous daily administration are not established; however, a short-term (6 months) study indicated 100 mg/day was effective.[62] Micronized progesterone is absorbed irregularly, metabolized rapidly, and peaks in blood levels of progesterone and active metabolites are associated with sedation and other disturbing CNS reactions.

The continuous combined method of treatment evolved to improve patient continuance in the presence of bleeding and other symptoms. The continuous activity of progestin allows the use of lower doses that by virtue of a daily availability inhibit endometrial growth. This approach involves the continuous daily use of the following estrogen-progestin combinations:

The Continuous Combination Program for Oral Postmenopausal Hormone Therapy

Daily estrogen: **0.625 mg conjugated estrogens, or**
                     1.25 mg estropipate, or
                     1.0 mg micronized estradiol, or
                     equivalent doses of other estrogens.

Daily progestin: **0.35 mg norethindrone, or**
                     100 mg micronized progesterone, or
                     2.5 mg medroxyprogesterone acetate, or
                     equivalent doses of other progestins.

Combined with daily calcium supplementation (500 mg with a meal), and vitamin D (400 IU in winter months and 800 IU for women over age 70).

Continuance with hormone therapy programs is notoriously poor.[63, 64] The two most common reasons why women discontinue or do not start hormone treatment are fear of cancer and vaginal bleeding.[65] The current data on breast cancer are reassuring, and the addition of a progestational agent has effectively prevented endometrial cancer. But the persistence of bleeding with the traditional sequential regimen continues to be a barrier to good continuance. To go from 80–90% withdrawal bleeding to 80% no bleeding represents a major accomplishment, and thus, the continuous approach has a significant advantage.

Managing Bleeding During Postmenopausal Hormone Therapy

With sequential therapy, approximately 80–90% of women experience monthly withdrawal bleeding. With continuous, combined estrogen-progestin therapy, one can expect 40–60% of patients to experience breakthrough bleeding during the first 6 months of treatment; however, this percentage decreases to 10–20% after one year.[59, 60, 66] Although this percentage of amenorrhea with continuous, combined therapy is a gratifying accomplishment, the number of women who experience breakthrough bleeding is considerable, and it is a difficult management problem. Indeed, the single most aggravating and worrisome problem with daily, continuous therapy is this breakthrough bleeding.

Why call it breakthrough bleeding? The bleeding experienced by women on continuous, combined therapy is similar to that seen with oral contraceptives: breakthrough bleeding. It originates from an endometrium dominated by progestational influence; hence the endometrium is usually atrophic and yields little, if anything, to the exploring biopsy instrument. Breakthrough bleeding is probably due to a progestational effect on vascular strength and integrity, producing a fragility that is prone to breakdown and bleeding. It is helpful to explain to patients that this bleeding represents tissue breakdown as the endometrium adjusts to its new hormonal stimulation. From our experience with oral contraceptives, we have learned to be comfortable with this type of bleeding. We have learned, that for most patients, the incidence of breakthrough bleeding with oral contraceptives is greatest in the first few months of treatment, and usually disappears in the majority of women. Indeed, this is the same pattern exhibited by postmenopausal women on continuous, combined therapy, and, therefore, the most effective management strategy is patient education and support.

There is no effective method supported by clinical studies, or a large experience, of drug alteration or substitution to manage this breakthrough bleeding. The breakthrough bleeding rate is only slightly better with a higher dose of progestin (5.0 mg medroxyprogesterone acetate) than with the lower dose (2.5 mg).[59, 66] Therefore, there is not a strong reason to use the higher dose, thus minimizing side effects. The best approach is to gain time, because most patients will cease bleeding. This means good educational preparation of the patient beforehand and frequent telephone contact to allay anxiety and encourage persistence.

> **Options for Persistent Bleeding**
> **Sequential therapy**
> **Vaginal hysterectomy**
> **Endometrial ablation**
> **The progestin IUD**

There is a hard core of patients (10–20% at the end of one year) who continue to bleed. The closer a patient is to having been bleeding (either to her premenopausal state or to having been on a sequential method with withdrawal bleeding), the more likely that patient will experience breakthrough bleeding. Some clinicians, therefore, prefer to start patients near the menopause on the sequential method and convert to the continuous method some years later. We prefer to start with the continuous method because those women who achieve amenorrhea are highly appreciative. For the patients who persist in having breakthrough bleeding, it is better to return to the sequential program in order to have expected and orderly withdrawal bleeding instead of the irregularity of breakthrough bleeding.

Some patients may choose to undergo endometrial ablation in order to overcome the problem of breakthrough bleeding. But remember that concern still exists regarding the potential for isolated, residual endometrium to progress to carcinoma without recognition. Another option deserving of consideration is the progestin intrauterine device (IUD). The local release of progestin is effective in suppressing endometrial response and preventing bleeding, but the progesterone-releasing IUD must be replaced every 18 months. The levonorgestrel-releasing IUD can be left in place for

10 years, a decided advantage.[67, 68] Finally, for some patients, vaginal hysterectomy will prove to be an acceptable alternative.

> **Indications for Pretreatment Biopsy**
> **Characteristics associated with a high risk of pathology**
> **Previous unopposed estrogen therapy**
>
> **Indications for Endometrial Biopsy During Treatment**
> **Clinician anxiety**
> **Patient anxiety**
> **Treatment with unopposed estrogen**
> **Endometrial thickness greater than 4 mm**
> **Past history of unopposed estrogen therapy**

It is not essential to routinely perform endometrial biopsies prior to treatment. Endometrial abnormalities in asymptomatic postmenopausal women are very rare.[66, 69, 70] A reasonable economic moderation would be to limit pretreatment biopsies (using the plastic endometrial suction device in the office) to patients at higher risk for endometrial changes: those women with conditions associated with chronic estrogen exposure (obesity, dysfunctional uterine bleeding, anovulation and infertility, hirsutism, high alcohol intake, hepatic disease, metabolic problems such as diabetes mellitus and hypothyroidism) and those women in whom irregular bleeding occurs while on estrogen-progestin therapy. In the absence of abnormal bleeding, a certain amount of trust in the protective effects of the progestin is justified, and routine, periodic biopsies are not necessary. *However, women who elect to be treated with unopposed estrogen require endometrial surveillance at least once a year.*

It is appropriate to perform an endometrial aspiration biopsy when the patient's anxiety over the possibility of pathology requires this response. It is also appropriate to perform a biopsy when the clinician is concerned; with increasing experience with this method, it takes more and more to be concerned. If bleeding persists for 6 months, consider an office hysteroscopy; an impressive number of polyps and intrauterine fibroids will be discovered.

Abnormal endometrium is more frequently encountered in patients on combination estrogen-progestin when the patients have previously been treated for a period of time with unopposed estrogen. Breakthrough bleeding or unscheduled bleeding in these patients requires endometrial surveillance because an increased risk for endometrial cancer persists beyond the period of exposure to unopposed estrogen, and it is unknown how effective the subsequent protective exposure to a progestin will be.[71–73] It is prudent to assess the endometrium in these patients prior to changing from unopposed to combined therapy. Clinicians should maintain a highly anxious state of mind with patients who have been treated previously with unopposed estrogen.

A combined estrogen-progestin program will not totally prevent endometrial cancer.[72] Vigilance on the part of the clinician, however, will detect endometrial cancer at an early stage, a stage that can be treated with excellent results.

It is common for women on a sequential regimen to begin bleeding while in the midst of progestin administration. The timing of withdrawal bleeding in women on a sequential estrogen-progestin program has been suggested as a screening method for biopsy decision making. In women taking a variety of progestins for 12 days each month, bleeding on or before day 10 after the addition of the progestin was associated with proliferative endometrium. Bleeding beginning on day 11 or later was associated with secretory endometrium, presumably indicating less need for biopsy.[74] But does this correlate with the risk of hyperplasia and cancer? According to a study of 413 postmenopausal women, the day of bleeding did *NOT* predict endometrial safety.[75] Late regular withdrawal bleeding on a sequential program does not give 100% assurance that there is no hyperplasia and perhaps endometrial cancer. This uncertainty with the sequential program is another reason to turn to the daily, combined method where irregular bleeding and sonographic measurement of increased endometrial thickness provide us with good indications for endometrial biopsy.

If a patient has recurrent bleeding despite repeated medical therapy, submucous myomas or endometrial polyps must be suspected. Thorough curettage can miss such pathology, and further diagnostic study can be helpful. Either hysterosalpingography with slow instillation of dye and careful fluoroscopic examination or ultrasonography with instillation of saline into the uterine cavity or hysteroscopy may reveal a myoma or polyp. Hysteroscopy can also direct a more accurate biopsy of the endometrium.

Measurement of Endometrial Thickness by Transvaginal Ultrasonography

The thickness of the postmenopausal endometrium as measured by transvaginal ultrasonography in postmenopausal women correlates with the presence or absence of pathology. However, the severity of pathologic change does not correlate with the measured thickness.[76] Endometrial thickness (the two layers of the anterior and posterior walls in the longitudinal axis) under 5 mm is reassuring and allows conservative management.[77, 78] Endometrial thickness greater than 4 mm requires biopsy; it is estimated that 50–75% of bleeding patients on hormone therapy and evaluated by ultrasonography will require biopsy.[76, 79] An endometrial thickness less than 5 mm in women receiving hormone therapy, either a sequential regimen or a daily combination of estrogen-progestin, is reassuring.[78, 80, 81] Because endometrial thickness by ultrasonography in patients on a sequential regimen can be affected by day in the treatment cycle, ultrasonography assessment should be obtained toward the end of the progestin phase or at the beginning of the cycle.[82] When a thick endometrium is associated with atrophic endometrium on biopsy, polyps are often present. Greater accuracy can be gained by the instillation of saline into the uterine cavity during ultrasonography.[83] Doppler velocimetry does not improve the accuracy of discriminating between normal and abnormal endometrium.[84] *A clinician should not be satisfied with "normal" findings on ultrasonography if a patient has persistent bleeding. The pursuit of abnormal bleeding despite "normal" findings should reduce missed cases of pathology to nearly zero.[85] In this circumstance, hysteroscopy is recommended.*

The Progestin Challenge Test

The administration of a progestational agent (e.g., 10 mg medroxyprogesterone acetate for 2 weeks) was developed by R. Don Gambrell Jr. as a means of detecting the presence of estrogen-dependent endometrium in postmenopausal women.[86] A withdrawal bleed would indicate that an endometrial response has occurred to the progestin, a response that requires previous endometrial stimulation by estrogen, and indicates the need for endometrial assessment. In other words, the lack of a withdrawal bleed is reassuring for clinician and patient. Concern with this clinical maneuver has focused on whether there are false-negative and false-positive responses. Several studies are now available that support the efficacy and validity of this method.[87–89] The published data indicate that most, but perhaps not all, women with endometrial proliferation, hyperplasia, and even cancer will respond with a withdrawal bleed after a progestin challenge, and ultrasonography measurement of endometrial thickness will be greater than 4 mm.[90] The problem is that the studies thus far do not consist of very large numbers, and there is a lingering question whether a patient with abnormal endometrium will always bleed in response to progestin treatment and withdrawal.

Progestational Side Effects

Many women do not tolerate treatment with progestational hormones. Typical side effects include breast tenderness, bloating, and depression. These reactions are significant detrimental factors with continuance. However, appropriately designed, placebo-controlled studies fail to document adverse physical or psychological effects with short-term treatment utilizing medroxyprogesterone acetate, except for breast discomfort.[91, 92, 416] This suggests that progestin side effects other than mastalgia are related to duration of treatment or that only studies with large numbers of subjects will detect the small percentage of women who have problems (and both explanations are probably true).

Can the progestational agent be administered less frequently? We are secure in our position, supported by clinical data, that a monthly estrogen-progestin sequential or a daily combination program effectively prevents endometrial hyperplasia. Experience with other regimens is very limited. The administration of medroxyprogesterone acetate every 3 months was associated in one study with longer, heavier menses and unscheduled bleeding, and a 1.5% incidence of hyperplasia at one year, while in another study, overall bleeding was less, but the incidence of hyperplasia was approximately 4%.[93, 94] In yet another study, there was no endometrial hyperplasia encountered by 143 women who completed two years of treatment; however, the progestin administered every 3 months was of high dosage, 20 mg medroxyprogesterone acetate daily for 14 days.[95] Most impressively, the Scandinavian LongCycle Study, a clinical trial scheduled to last 5 years, was canceled after 3 years because of a 12% incidence of endometrial hyperplasia and 4 cases of endometrial cancer.[96] Therefore, if a patient chooses this regimen, more intensive endometrial monitoring is required. In our view, an annual endometrial biopsy is strongly recommended. Indeed, any program that differs from the standard regimen is untested by clinical studies of sufficient length and patient numbers and, therefore, requires periodic surveillance of the endometrium.

Some patients are very sensitive to medroxyprogesterone acetate. In our experience, these patients are often relieved of their symptoms by switching to norethindrone. In a sequential regimen, the dose of norethindrone is 0.7 mg (available in the progestin-only, minipill oral contraceptive; each pill contains 0.35 mg norethindrone). In the continuous, combined regimen, the dose of norethindrone is 0.35 mg daily.

Progesterone can be administered in a vaginal gel that allows the delivery of very low doses that can effectively protect the endometrium with low systemic levels because of a first-pass effect on the uterus.[97] The administration of 90 mg every 2 days produces secretory changes in the endometrium.[98] An application of the 4% commercial preparation twice weekly protects the endometrium and is associated with amenorrhea in most patients. In a sequential regimen, the one applicator of the 4% preparation should be applied daily for at least 10 days each month. No long-term studies are available documenting endometrial safety and metabolic effects.

The only transdermal progestins being used are norethindrone and levonorgestrel.

Progestins Available Worldwide

	Estimated Comparable Doses
21-Carbon derivatives:	
Medroxyprogesterone acetate	5.0 mg
Megestrol acetate	5.0 mg
Cyproterone acetate	1.0 mg
Dydrogesterone	10.0 mg
Chlormadinone acetate	
Medrogestone	
Demegestone	
Promegestone	
Trimegestonel	
Nomegestrol acetate	
19-Nortestosterone Family:	
Norethindrone	0.7 mg
Norethindrone acetate	1.0 mg
Levonorgestrel	0.75 mg
Desogestrel	0.15 mg
Nomegestrol	
Norethynodrel	
Lynestrenol	
Ethnynodiol diacetate	
Gestodene	
Norgestimate	
Dienogest	

The Progestin Intrauterine Device

The contraceptive levonorgestrel-releasing intrauterine device (IUD) has been reconfigured in a smaller model releasing as little as 5 μg of levonorgestrel per 24 hours.[68, 99, 100] The intrauterine presence of the progestin effectively protects the endometrium against hyperplasia and cancer. The local site of action provides endometrial protection and escapes systemic progestin side effects; for example, estrogen's favorable lipid effects are not attenuated.[101] As with the oral continuous, combined regimens, there is irregular breakthrough bleeding in the first 6 months, and after one year, approximately 60–70% of the women are amenorrheic. The levonorgestrel device has the advantage of a 10-year duration of use. The progesterone-releasing device is larger, must be replaced every 18 months, and there have been few studies in postmenopausal women.

Should Progestins Be Administered to Hysterectomized Women?

There are some special conditions that warrant the use of a combined estrogen-progestin regimen in hysterectomized women.

1. *Because adenocarcinoma has been reported in patients with pelvic endometriosis being treated with unopposed estrogen,[102–105] the combined estrogen-progestin program is strongly advised in patients with a past history of endometriosis.* In addition, we have encountered a case of hydronephrosis secondary to ureteral obstruction caused by endometriosis (with atypia) in a woman on unopposed estrogen for years after hysterectomy and bilateral salpingo-oophorectomy for endometriosis.

2. Patients who have had procedures that have the potential to leave residual endometrium (e.g., a supracervical hysterectomy) should be treated with an estrogen-progestin combination. Responsive endometrium may be sequestered in patients who have undergone endometrial ablation,[106, 107] and combined estrogen-progestin treatment is recommended for these women.

3. It has been reported that patients who have had Stage I or Stage II adenocarcinoma of the endometrium can take estrogen without fear of recurrence,[108–111] but the combination of estrogen-progestin is recommended in view of the potential protective action of the progestational agent. Treatment can be initiated immediately postoperatively.

4. The combined estrogen-progestin approach makes sense for patients previously treated for endometrioid tumors of the ovary.[112]

5. There is evidence that the combination of estrogen and progestin has a greater positive impact on bone density than estrogen alone. Thus, in hysterectomized women at high risk for osteoporosis, the combined estrogen-progestin program may offer an important potential advantage. However, this synergistic effect is influenced by the type of progestin, and a greater bone response is probably limited to the 19-nortestosterone (norethindrone) family.[113] Careful studies indicate that the addition of medroxyprogesterone provides an additional effect on bone only in women with established, significant osteoporosis.[114–116]

6. In women with elevated triglyceride levels, the addition of a progestin, especially a 19-nortestosterone progestin, may attenuate a further estrogen-induced increase in triglycerides.

The Addition of Androgens

After menopause, the circulating level of androstenedione is about one half that seen prior to menopause.[117] Most of this postmenopausal androstenedione is derived from the adrenal gland, with only a small amount secreted from the ovary. Testosterone levels do not fall appreciably, and in most women, the postmenopausal ovary, for a few years, actually secretes more testosterone than the premenopausal ovary. The remaining active stromal tissue in the ovary is stimulated by the elevated gonadotropins to this level of increased testosterone secretion. The total amount of testosterone produced, however, is slightly decreased because the primary source, the peripheral conversion of androstenedione, is reduced. Because of this decrease, some argue that androgen treatment is indicated in the postmenopausal period.

The potential benefits of androgen treatment include improvement in psychological well-being and an increase in sexually motivated behavior. These effects, however, have been reported with the administration of relatively large doses of androgen.[118] In a well-designed, placebo-controlled study, lower doses of androgen (but still very pharmacologic—5 mg methyltestosterone) contributed little to actual sexual behavior, although an increase in sexual fantasies and masturbation could be documented.[119]

Any benefit must be balanced by the unwanted effects, in particular, virilization (acne, alopecia, and hirsutism), and a negative impact on the cholesterol-lipoprotein profile. In a short-term study comparing a product with estrogen and a relatively low oral dose of testosterone (1.25 mg methyltestosterone) to estrogen alone, a negative impact on the lipid profile was apparent within 3 months.[120] Over a 2-year period, the administration of estrogen (1.25 mg) combined with 2.5 mg methyltestosterone produced a significant overall adverse impact on the cholesterol-lipoprotein profile.[121] In addition, 30% of the patients experienced acne, and 36% developed facial hirsutism. A lower dose of this combination (0.625 mg esterified estrogens and 1.25 mg methyltestosterone) also significantly lowers HDL-cholesterol.[122] The adverse impact on the lipid profile is less (and may even be avoided) by the parenteral administration of testosterone.[123] Of course, the clinical effects of these metabolic changes are not known.

It should also be remembered that androgens do not protect the endometrium, and the addition of a progestin is still necessary. It is uncertain (and unstudied) how much aromatization of the administered testosterone increases the estrogen impact and whether this might increase the risk of endometrial and/or breast cancer. The addition of androgen does not reduce the amount of breakthrough bleeding women experience with a continuous combination regimen.[124] Adding testosterone to an estrogen therapy program has been reported to provide no additional beneficial impact on bone or on relief from hot flushes.[121, 125] On the other hand, others have demonstrated a greater increase in bone density with an estrogen-androgen combination compared with estrogen alone, although the blood levels achieved were higher than those associated with standard postmenopausal hormone therapy.[123] A greater effect on bone associated with androgen treatment may be indirect, reflecting higher free estrogen levels because of a reduction in sex hormone-binding globulin and/or androgen-induced changes in muscle mass.

There is no doubt that pharmacologic amounts of androgen can increase libido, but these same doses produce unwanted effects.[126] In addition, patients on high doses of androgens often are somewhat addicted to this therapy. Small amounts of androgen supplementation can be provided in situations where the patient and clinician are convinced a depressed libido cannot be explained by psychosocial circumstances. In these cases, the lipid profile should be carefully monitored. Any positive clinical response may well be a placebo effect. After some months or a few years, conversion to a standard program without androgen is recommended.

Selective Estrogen Agonists/Antagonists (Selective Estrogen Receptor Modulators)

A greater understanding of the estrogen receptor mechanism (Chapter 2) allows us to understand how mixed estrogen agonists/antagonists can have selective actions on specific target tissues. New agents are being developed in an effort to isolate desired actions from unwanted side effects. Indeed, in time we can expect to see new agents with progressively better agonist/antagonist profiles, yielding increasingly user friendly drugs.

Raloxifene exerts no proliferative effect on the endometrium but produces favorable responses in bone and lipids.[127, 128] Early results (2–3 years of treatment) indicate that women receiving raloxifene have a reduction in the incidence of estrogen receptor-positive breast cancer.[129] However, because malignant breast tumors require a relatively long period of time to progress from an abnormal cell to a clinically detectable mass,[130] the impact of a specific drug treatment may reflect growth acceleration (as discussed with estrogen therapy) or deceleration of a pre-existing tumor, *not causation or prevention.*

Short-term clinical trial data indicate that raloxifene has a positive impact on bone density, favorable effects on LDL-cholesterol, fibrinogen, and lipoprotein(a), but no effects on HDL-cholesterol and PAI-1, and raloxifene increases hot flushing.[131, 132] Long-term clinical trial data will be necessary to determine the ultimate impact on clinical events, specifically fractures, coronary heart disease, stress incontinence, endometrial cancer, and cognition. The MORE study (**M**ultiple **O**utcomes of **R**aloxifene **E**valuation) is a worldwide clinical trial of raloxifene in osteoporotic women. After 2 years, raloxifene treatment was associated with a 44% reduction in vertebral fractures.[133]

In a 2-year randomized trial in monkeys, raloxifene exerted no protection against coronary artery atherosclerosis despite changes in circulating lipids similar to those achieved in women.[134] In a rabbit model, raloxifene did inhibit aortic atherosclerosis, but not as effectively as estrogen treatment.[135] However, a combination of actions (antioxidant activity, some beneficial effects on lipids, a reduction in homocysteine levels) makes it likely there will be some favorable impact on the cardiovascular system.[132, 136, 137] RUTH (**R**aloxifene **U**se for **T**he **H**eart) is both a primary and secondary coronary heart disease international prevention trial, started in 1998, that should provide data by 2003–05.

At the present time, in our view, raloxifene is an option for prevention of osteoporosis, especially for patients reluctant to use hormone therapy, but not a substitute for estrogen. Remember that women can develop hot flushing on raloxifene, and a 3-fold increase in leg cramping is a problem that is thus far unique for raloxifene.

Does Hormone Therapy Cause Fibroid Tumors to Grow?

Uterine leiomyomas are monoclonal tumors that retain sensitivity to both estrogen and progestin (Chapter 4); and, therefore, it is appropriate to be concerned over whether leiomyomata will grow in response to postmenopausal hormone therapy. As assessed by vaginal ultrasonography, the number and size of uterine leiomyomas increased in women being treated with an intramuscular depot form of estrogen-progestin therapy.[138] However, the hormonal dose in this study was relatively high, certainly higher than standard regimens. At the end of one year, women with small asymptomatic fibroids administered a daily combination of 0.625 mg conjugated estrogens and 2.5 mg medroxyprogesterone acetate had no sonographic evidence of growth in contrast to an increase in size observed with transdermal estradiol (50 μg) and 5 mg medroxyprogesterone acetate daily (a response that may reflect the effect of a higher progestin dose).[139] In follow-up studies with standard doses of estrogen-progestin or tibolone, ultrasonography has detected no changes in uterine or myoma volumes.[140, 141] Clinical experience indicates that fibroid tumors of the uterus almost always are not stimulated to grow by the usual postmenopausal doses of estrogen and progestin. Nevertheless, pelvic examination surveillance is a wise course. For example, a vulvar leiomyoma with growth stimulated by estrogen-progestin treatment has been reported.[142] A case-control study could find no statistically significant increase in the risk of uterine sarcomas associated with estrogen therapy.[143]

Estrogen Therapy and Sleep Apnea

The low prevalence of sleep apnea in premenopausal women and the increased frequency after menopause suggest a hormonal link. In a careful study, however, postmenopausal hormone therapy had no significant effect on sleep disordered breathing in women with more than mild obstructive sleep apnea.[144] The slight rise in basal body temperature induced by a progestational agent may be sufficient to disrupt the quality of sleep in some women, a problem that may be more noticeable with a sequential regimen and with nighttime administration.

Estrogen Therapy and Rheumatic Diseases

No clear conclusion is apparent from the studies of estrogen's effect on rheumatic diseases, especially rheumatoid arthritis. Studies have indicated that exogenous estrogen, either oral contraceptives or postmenopausal therapy, protects against the onset of rheumatoid arthritis, while other studies find no effect.[145–147] These studies have been hampered by small numbers, a problem that will not be overcome unless postmenopausal hormone therapy becomes more widespread. In a randomized, placebo-controlled, clinical trial, maintenance of standard serum estradiol levels was associated with improvements in some measurements of disease activity in patients with rheumatoid arthritis.[148] There has been no evidence that postmenopausal hormone therapy aggravates rheumatoid arthritis or causes a flare in disease activity.

In the Nurses' Health Study, the use of postmenopausal estrogen was associated with approximately a twofold increase in systemic lupus erythematosus, an observation based on 30 cases in past and current users of estrogen.[149] If this epidemiologic association is true, the absolute risk is very small, and, importantly, postmenopausal women with systemic lupus erythematosus may derive substantial benefit from the cardiovascular actions of estrogen. In a follow-up of 60 postmenopausal women with stable systemic lupus erythematosus, no adverse effects of hormone therapy could be detected.[150] Furthermore, patients with systemic lupus erythematosus treated with glucocorticoids are at greater risk for osteoporosis.[151] Nevertheless, there is a concern that exogenous estrogen will increase flares and stimulate thrombosis in patients with systemic lupus erythematosus because of their hypercoaguable state. Postmenopausal hormone therapy can be considered in patients with stable or inactive disease, without renal involvement and high antiphospholipid antibodies. SELENA (Safety of Estrogen in Lupus Erythematosus National Assessment) is an ongoing randomized, controlled, clinical trial of hormone therapy and lupus erythematosus in postmenopausal women, as well as oral contraceptive therapy in premenopausal women.

Bone loss associated with glucocorticoid therapy can be avoided with the usual postmenopausal hormone regimens.[152, 153] These patients are also excellent candidates for bisphosphonate treatment, another effective option that prevents glucocorticoid-induced bone loss.[154, 155] In addition, calcium and vitamin D supplementation has been demonstrated to prevent bone loss associated with low-dose glucocorticoid treatment.[156]

Estrogen Therapy and Osteoarthritis

Osteoarthritis is the most common form of arthritis in older people, and its prevalence increases rapidly in women after menopause. Osteoporosis protects against arthritis,[157] and, therefore, the impact of estrogen therapy on osteoarthritis is a logical concern. Increasing severity of osteoarthritis of the knee has been reported to be associated with increasing bone density and the current use of postmenopausal hormone therapy in middle-aged women.[158] However, a cross-sectional study concluded that current users of estrogen had a reduced prevalence of osteoarthritis of the hip, and there was protection against the severity of osteoarthritis, with a greater effect with longer duration of use.[159] Because there are no known treatments that modify the course of arthritis, this potential benefit of postmenopausal hormone therapy deserves study by a randomized clinical trial.

Estrogen Therapy and Asthma

In some women, changes in asthma activity have been noted to correlate with phases of the menstrual cycle. The impact of postmenopausal hormone therapy on asthma activity has not been well investigated, but there is an indication that estrogen has an adverse effect. A worsening in spirometry assessment could be detected in asthmatics after estrogen therapy; however, the difference was judged to be subclinical, and the patients did not report any changes in their perceptions of symptoms.[160] In a prospective assessment of a cohort of women, the use of postmenopausal hormone therapy (estrogen with or without progestin) was associated with a 50% increase in the risk of developing adult-onset asthma, and the risk was greater with long-term use and with higher doses of estrogen.[161] Because hormonal changes may precipitate asthmatic activity (e.g., catamenial asthma), attention should be directed to the symptomatic pattern and consideration given to the daily, continuous, combined regimen.

Asthma is another condition treated with glucocorticoids and associated with glucocorticoid-induced bone loss.[162] Prevention with hormone therapy or bisphosphonate treatment should be considered.

Estrogen Therapy and the Oral Cavity

Oral complaints are common among postmenopausal women. The administration of estrogen provides significant relief from oral discomfort, burning, bad taste, and dryness.[163] Estrogen therapy is also associated with a reduction in gingival inflammation and bleeding.[164] These changes may reflect epithelial responses to estrogen by the oral mucosa, in a manner similar to that of the vaginal mucosa. Oral alveolar bone loss (which can lead to loss of teeth) is strongly correlated with osteoporosis, and the salutary effect of estrogen on skeletal bone mass should also be manifested on oral bone.[165, 166] In the Leisure World Cohort, tooth loss and edentia were significantly reduced in estrogen users compared with nonusers (with a reduced need for dentures), and this beneficial effect was greater with increasing duration of estrogen use.[167] Approximately a 25% reduced risk of tooth loss in current users of estrogen has been observed in the Nurses' Health Study.[168]

Professional singers have used hormone therapy to prevent what they view as unwanted voice changes associated with menopause.[169] In a 1-year study, objective voice analyses documented a more androgenic change in voice in the early postmenopausal years with a lesser change associated with estrogen treatment, slightly attenuated by the addition of a progestin.[170]

Estrogen Therapy and Vision

There is some evidence that estrogen therapy improves visual acuity (or lessens the decrease occurring during the early postmenopausal years), perhaps due to a beneficial effect on lacrimal fluid.[171] An increased prevalence of keratoconjunctivitis sicca (dry eyes) in menopausal and postmenopausal women is recognized by ophthalmologists, and estrogen therapy offers the potential for symptomatic relief.[172] There is further evidence that postmenopausal estrogen therapy has an effect that protects against lens opacities.[173–175] Estrogen-progestin treatment also lowers intraocular pressure in postmenopausal women with normal eyes or glaucoma.[176, 177]

Estrogen Therapy and Age-Related Hearing Loss

Demineralization of the cochlear capsule occurs with aging and with metabolic bone diseases, such as cochlear otosclerosis. This demineralization is associated with neural hearing loss. Postmenopausal women (age 60–85 years) who have lower than average femoral neck bone mass have an increased risk of having a hearing loss.[178] This association between femoral neck bone mass and age-related hearing loss suggests that prevention of bone loss with estrogen therapy might also prevent to some degree age-related hearing loss. It is possible that this potential action of estrogen could be exerted on the cochlear capsule.

Should Very Old Women Be Started on Hormone Therapy?

The positive impact of hormone therapy on bone has been demonstrated to take place even in women over age 65.[179, 180] This is a strong argument in favor of treating very old women who have never been on estrogen. Estrogen treatment that is not begun until after age 60 can with long-term use achieve bone densities nearly comparable with those in women taking estrogen from menopause, and estrogen use between the ages of 65 and 74 has been documented to protect against hip fractures.[181, 182] Whether estrogen's cardiovascular protection has anything significant to contribute in the elderly has not been addressed. It makes clinical sense, however, that some positive contribution can be expected. Adding a pharmacologic regimen to an old woman's daily life is not a trivial consideration. This judgment requires the conclusion that a relatively youthful and vigorous elderly woman has something to gain from the treatment. Patients with osteoporosis and/or unfavorable lipoprotein profiles would certainly qualify.

If postmenopausal hormone therapy is demonstrated to have a beneficial effect on the risk and severity of Alzheimer's disease, this would become a powerful reason to recommend treatment for very old women.

Older women who have been deficient in estrogen for many years often experience side effects when standard doses of estrogen are initiated. Breast tenderness can be especially disturbing. It is usually better to start older women with lower doses. This can utilize the oral products at half the usual doses (0.3 mg conjugated estrogens or 0.5 mg estradiol) or a transdermal product that delivers relatively low amounts of estrogen. After 6 months, an increase to standard doses is recommended to maximize the bone, cardiovascular, and central nervous system benefits.

How Long Should Postmenopausal Hormone Therapy Be Continued?

The answer to this question is relatively straightforward. A woman should continue her post-menopausal hormone regimen as long as she wants the benefits. Although some estrogen effects will be long-lasting, the full impact is rapidly lost after discontinuation. For example, in the Nurses' Health Study, reduced risk of mortality (largely cardiovascular) was lost by the 5th year after discontinuing treatment.[183]

Can the Diet Produce Variations in Systemic Estrogen Levels?

Oral estrogens have an extensive first-pass metabolism, both in the gastrointestinal tract and the liver. This metabolism consists chiefly of sulfation and hydroxylation. The cytochrome P450 system catalyzes the hydroxylation of estrogen, and antioxidants can inhibit this action. Flavanoids (e.g., naringenin and quercetin) are present in high concentrations in fruits and vegetables, and grapefruit juice inhibits estrogen metabolism, producing an increase in bio-availability that is consistent with an inhibition of hydroxylation.[184, 185] This raises the possibility that dietary interactions with food products could produce a clinical impact. It is well recognized that there is great variability within individuals and between individuals in the pharmacokinetics of exogenously administered estrogen. It is possible that this variability partially reflects the dietary habits of individuals and not intrinsic metabolism. Because of this possibility, it seems prudent to recommend that patients take oral postmenopausal hormone therapy before they go to bed at night. This may minimize any effect of diet on blood levels of steroids.

An effect of alcohol ingestion by premenopausal women was not demonstrated on circulating levels of estrone, estradiol, dehydroepiandrosterone sulfate (DHEAS), or sex hormone-binding globulin in a cross-sectional study that depended on a questionnaire to assess alcohol intake.[186] However, when alcohol is administered under experimental conditions, circulating estrogen concentrations are raised to high levels.[187, 188] And in a prospective cohort study of premenopausal women in Italy, higher estradiol levels were correlated with an increased alcohol intake over a 1-year period of time.[189]

Alternative Treatments for Hot Flushes

When patients with hot flushing cannot take estrogen, we recommend transdermal clonidine, applied with the 100 μg dose once weekly.[190, 191] Side effects are minimal, and a modest impact can be expected.

Clonidine, bromocriptine, and naloxone given orally are only partially effective for the relief of hot flushes and require high doses with a high rate of side effects. Bellergal (a combination of belladonna alkaloids, ergotamine tartrate, and phenobarbital) treatment is slightly better than a placebo, but it is also a potent sedative.[192] Veralipride, a dopamine antagonist that is active in the hypothalamus, is relatively effective in inhibiting flushing at a dose of 100 mg daily.[193, 194] Mastodynia and galactorrhea are the major side effects. Medroxyprogesterone acetate (10–20 mg daily) and megestrol acetate (20 mg bid) are also effective, but concerns regarding exogenous steroids (especially in patients who have had breast cancer) would apply to progestins as well.[195, 196] Methyldopa, in doses of 500–1000 mg/day, is approximately twice as effective as a placebo, suggesting a role for adrenoreceptors in the hot flush mechanism.[197] Venlafaxine hydrochloride is an antidepressant that inhibits serotonin re-uptake; it effectively reduced hot flush frequency in a dose of 25 mg daily.[198] Vitamin E, 800 IU daily, is only slightly more effective than placebo.[199]

Tibolone

Tibolone is a steroid, related to the 19-nortestosterone family, that is effective for the treatment of bone and hot flushes in a dose of 2.5 mg per day.[200, 201] Tibolone is metabolized into 3 steroid isomers with varying estrogenic, progestogenic, and androgenic properties. The metabolites differ in their activities and dominance according to the target tissue. Thus, tibolone provides estrogenic effects on bone and hot flushing, but it induces atrophy of the endometrium.[202] Its beneficial impact on bone (2.5 mg dose) is comparable with standard hormonal therapy.[203] A lower dose of 1.25 mg daily also provides bone protection, but it is less effective and there is more vaginal bleeding. In the endometrium, tibolone is converted locally (by endometrial 3β-hydroxysteroid dehydrogenase/isomerase) to its Δ^4 progestational isomer; hence, tibolone exerts a progestational effect on the endometrium.[204] Tibolone has an estrogenic effect on the vagina, and women report improvements in the symptoms of vaginal dryness and dyspareunia, and an increase in sexual enjoyment and libido.[205]

Although a short-term reduction in HDL-cholesterol is an undesirable consequence with tibolone treatment; the long-term impact on the risk of cardiovascular disease is unknown.[206] In a 2-year study, the unfavorable effect on lipoproteins was accompanied by beneficial changes in coagulation factors consistent with enhanced fibrinolysis and unchanged coagulation.[207] Overall, it is possible that some favorable activity on the cardiovascular system is maintained. A major advantage of tibolone (2.5 mg daily) is its low (10–20%) incidence of bleeding. Because tibolone inhibits breast cell proliferation in vitro, it is possible that future studies will indicate that tibolone offers some protection against breast cancer. Tibolone also has a beneficial impact in short-term studies on insulin resistance in normal women and in women with noninsulin-dependent diabetes mellitus.[208, 209]

"Natural" Therapies

Patients should be questioned regarding the use of "natural" therapies. Some of the herbs that contain estrogen-like compounds include ginseng, agnus castus, red sage, black cohosh, and beth root. The dosage and purity of herbal preparations are unknown, and most importantly, there are no substantial studies documenting either harmful or beneficial effects. [210, 211] Herbs are often contaminated with heavy metals. A rigorous evaluation of one popular herb, dong quai, could detect no effects on vaginal maturation or menopausal symptoms, especially hot flushing.[212] In our view, the use of products without scientific study should be discouraged. We believe it is appropriate to inform a patient that when she uses preparations lacking in data regarding safety and efficacy, she is experimenting with her own body. Of course, every patient has the right to do so, but we have the obligation to provide this admonishment.

Phytoestrogens

Phytoestrogens are classified into 3 groups: isoflavones, coumestans, and lignans.[213, 214] They are present in many plants, especially legumes, and bind to the estrogen receptor. Soybeans, a rich source of phytoestrogens, contain isoflavones, the most common form of phytoestrogens, mainly genistein and daidzein, and a little glycitein. These phytoestrogens are characterized by mixed estrogenic and antiestrogenic actions, depending on the target tissue. Variations in activity may also be due to the fact that the soy phytoestrogens have a greater affinity for the estrogen receptor-beta compared with estrogen receptor-alpha.[215] Estradiol and soy protein produce comparable metabolic changes in the monkey, including favorable lipid changes, improved carbohydrate metabolism, and a decrease in central, android abdominal fat.[216] Human clinical trials have resulted in inconsistent lipid effects.[214] The soybean phytoestrogens do not maintain bone density in the monkey, but do have favorable effects on atherosclerosis and vasomotor responses, although the effect on atherosclerosis is not as robust as that of estrogen.[217–221] Also in the monkey, these phytoestrogens do not stimulate proliferation of breast and endometrial cells.[222]

The daily intake of dietary soy reduces the number of hot flushes in postmenopausal women, although there is significant variability in response, and efficacy appears to be less than that of estrogen.[223] In women, soy consumption produces a reduction in the circulating levels of estradiol, and it is suggested that the replacement of potent estradiol with target specific phytoestrogens may be beneficial.[224] In the parts of the world where soy intake is high, there is a lower incidence of breast, endometrial, and prostate cancers.[225] For example, a case-control study concluded that there was a 54% reduced risk of endometrial cancer, and another case-control study indicated a reduction in the risk of breast cancer, in women with a high consumption of soy and other legumes.[226, 227] It is by no means certain, however, that there is a direct effect of soy intake.[228] Indeed, a study of the impact of administered soy protein on breast secretions in premenopausal and postmenopausal women revealed increased breast secretions with the appearance of hyperplastic epithelial cells.[229] It will require appropriate clinical trials to determine how phytoestrogens compare to estrogens, and the efficacy, safety, and correct dosage (studies thus far recommend a daily intake of 60 g soy protein). In addition, the intake of sufficient soy to produce a clinical response is not easy, handicapped by gastrointestinal symptoms, a major alteration in diet or the use of an unpalatable supplement, and great variability in plant contents and products (due to processing). In addition, individuals demonstrate great variability in absorption and metabolism. A user-friendly preparation needs to be developed that minimizes individual variability in response.

Ipriflavone is a synthetic product with a structure that is very similar to the naturally occurring isoflavones. It prevents postmenopausal bone loss with no major side effect problems.[230, 231] Larger clinical trials are required to determine the variability in response.

Dehydroepiandrosterone (DHEA)

Adrenal androgen production decreases dramatically with aging. The mechanism is not known, but it is not due to the loss of estrogen at menopause, nor can it be reversed with estrogen treatment.[232] The impressive decline (75–85%) in circulating levels of DHEA that occur with aging (greater in men than in women) has stimulated a search for a beneficial impact of DHEA supplementation. Animal studies (in animals that do not even synthesize DHEA) have suggested that DHEA administration enhances the immune system and protects against many conditions associated with aging. Preliminary human studies have indicated significant increases (even at the usual 50 mg/day dose) in testosterone and dihydrotestosterone levels in women (by peripheral conversion in a variety of tissues).[233] Short-term studies of even small doses (25 mg/day) indicate that DHEA administration produces an adverse effect on the lipid profile.[234] What is the impact of a long-term increase in androgens? It is prudent to await the outcome of clinical trials before advocating DHEA supplementation.

Miscellaneous Considerations

A striking and consistent finding in most studies dealing with menopause and hormonal therapy is a marked placebo response in a variety of symptoms, including flushing. A significant clinical problem encountered in our referral practice is the following scenario: a woman will occasionally undergo an apparent beneficial response to estrogen, only to have the response wear off in several months. This leads to a sequence of periodic visits to the clinician and ever-increasing doses of estrogen therapy. When a patient reaches a point of requiring large doses of estrogen, a careful inquiry must be undertaken to search for a basic psychoneurotic or psychosocial problem.

Assessing vaginal cytology is not useful. The vaginal mucosa is too sensitive to estrogen to allow dose-response titering.

High-dose calcium supplementation can unmask asymptomatic hyperparathyroidism. Women receiving calcium supplementation in excess of 500 mg daily should have their blood levels of calcium and phosphorous measured yearly for the first 2 years. If normal, no further surveillance is necessary.

Assessment of the cholesterol-lipoprotein profile should follow the guidelines for general preventive care, with one exception. No further measurements are required in women on postmenopausal hormone therapy, neither before nor during treatment. The one exception is the patient with previous evidence of elevated triglycerides. After 2–4 weeks of hormone treatment, the triglyceride level should be measured to make sure the patient is not the rare individual who responds to estrogen with excessively high triglyceride levels.

The Problems of Estrogen-Progestin Therapy

Metabolic

Patients with high-risk factors need special attention when estrogen therapy is being considered. Metabolic contraindications to estrogen therapy include: chronically impaired liver function, acute vascular thrombosis (with or without emboli), and neurophthalmologic vascular disease. Estrogens may have adverse effects on some patients with seizure disorders, familial hyperlipidemias (very high triglycerides), and migraine headaches.

Pancreatitis and severe hypertriglyceridemia can be precipitated by the administration of oral estrogen to women with elevated triglyceride levels.[235] In women with triglyceride levels between 250 mg/dL and 750 mg/dL, estrogen should be provided with great caution, and a nonoral route of administration is preferred. *The triglyceride response is rapid, and a repeat level should be obtained in 2–4 weeks. If increased, hormone therapy must be discontinued. A level greater than 750 mg/dL represents an absolute contraindication to estrogen treatment.* Although triglyceride levels in the normal range were not affected by progestins in the PEPI trial (see Chapter 17), an exaggerated triglyceride response to estrogen might be attenuated by a progestin, especially a progestin of the 19-nortestosterone family, and, therefore, the daily, combination method of treatment should be considered for women with elevated triglycerides.

Although physiologic and epidemiologic evidence indicates that estrogen use increases the risk of gallbladder disease, the overall impact is not great. The Nurses' Health Study indicated that oral estrogen therapy may carry a 1.5–2.0-fold increased risk of gallbladder disease.[236] The risk of cholecystectomy appeared to increase with dose and duration of use and to persist for 5 or more years after stopping treatment. Others have also reported increased risks of cholecystectomy in past and current users of estrogen.[237, 238] In the HERS clinical trial, the relative risk of gallbladder disease was 1.38; however, this did not achieve statistical significance.[239] At least two case-control studies concluded that estrogen use is not a risk factor for gallstone disease in postmenopausal women, although the statistical power was limited by small numbers.[240, 241] A cross-sectional study of gallstone disease could detect no association with postmenopausal hormone treatment.[242]

The routine, periodic use of blood chemistries is not cost-effective, and careful monitoring for the appearance of the symptoms and signs of biliary tract disease will suffice. It is not certain that this potential problem is limited to oral therapy. Non-oral routes of estrogen administration have been reported to both increase and not increase biliary cholesterol saturation (a lithogenic response).[243, 244]

Weight Gain

The gain in weight that many middle-aged individuals experience is the result of lifestyle, specifically, the balance of dietary intake and exercise. Weight gain in women at menopause is not due to the hormonal changes associated with menopause.[245] Likewise, postmenopausal hormone therapy cannot be blamed for weight gain. The large Rancho Bernardo prospective cohort study and the randomized PEPI clinical trial documented that hormone therapy with or without progestin does not cause an increase in body weight.[246, 247] In fact, in the PEPI trial, the hormone-treated groups actually gained less weight than the placebo group.

Estrogen (with or without progestin) prevents the tendency to increase central body fat with aging.[248–251] This would inhibit the interaction among abdominal adiposity, hormones, insulin resistance, hypcrinsulinemia, blood pressure, and an atherogenic lipid profile.

Venous Thrombosis

It is well recognized that pharmacologic doses of estrogen (oral contraceptives) are associated with an increased risk of venous thrombosis. The impact of the lower doses administered to postmenopausal women has been more difficult to ascertain. Older case-control studies failed to find a link between postmenopausal doses of estrogen and venous thrombosis.[252, 253] However, these studies excluded cases with pre-existing risk factors for thrombosis. A well-designed case-control study of older women unselected for other thrombotic risk factors indicated that postmenopausal doses of estrogen did not increase the risk of venous thrombosis.[254] Others have also failed to find an increase in venous thromboembolism associated with postmenopausal hormone therapy.[255]

The conventional wisdom that the low postmenopausal doses of estrogen do not increase the risk of venous thrombosis was challenged more recently by 4 case-control studies and one cohort study. These studies were larger, but still were limited to 20–40 cases on hormone therapy. In the Nurses' Health Study cohort, the risk of pulmonary embolism was increased 2-fold in the current hormone users.[256] The case-control studies found a 2.1- to 3.6-fold increased risk of deep vein thrombosis in current but not past hormone users.[257–260] The case numbers were too small to enable a reliable analysis of a dose-response effect or the effect of transdermal use. The studies all indicated that the increased risk was confined to early use, and that the risk lowers to a non-significant level after one year. There was no indication that the addition of a progestin changed the risk.

The overall impact of postmenopausal hormone therapy on the clotting cascade is compatible with a favorable effect due to changes consistent with an increase in fibrinolysis.[261–264] However, the favorable impact may be confined to arterial thrombosis. Furthermore, it is always more prudent to make clinical judgments based on epidemiologic event data rather than laboratory tests. However, epidemiologic study of venous thrombosis (deep vein thrombosis and pulmonary embolism) is difficult because of the low incidence of the complication and the problem of diagnostic bias (a clinician is more suspicious of the diagnosis because of the use of estrogen).

The clinching argument on this issue, in our view, is the observation of an increased risk of venous thrombosis in both the HERS secondary prevention study of daily estrogen-progestin therapy for women who already have coronary heart disease and the data obtained with raloxifene.[129, 239] HERS (the Heart and Estrogen-Progestin Replacement Study) recorded a 2.89 relative risk of venous thromboembolism comparable with that reported in the observational studies. The increased risks in these instances were observed in randomized clinical trials, and it is difficult, if not impossible, to not accept these results.

What is the final message for clinicians and patients? First, it should be emphasized that the risk appears to apply only to new starters; women who have been on hormone therapy can be reassured that there is no evidence of an increased risk of venous thrombosis after the initial one year of treatment. The actual risk is very low because of the low frequency of this event. If the relative risk is increased 3-fold, this would increase the incidence of venous thromboembolism by about two cases per 10,000 women per year of hormone use. Furthermore, venous thrombosis carries with it a very low risk of mortality, around 1%, and most of the fatal cases have followed venous thrombosis associated with trauma, surgery, or a major illness.

If a patient has a close family history (parent or sibling) or a previous episode of idiopathic thromboembolism, an evaluation to search for an underlying abnormality in the coagulation system is warranted. The following measurements are recommended, and abnormal results require consultation with a hematologist regarding prognosis and prophylactic treatment. The list of laboratory tests is long, and because this is a dynamic and changing field, the best advice is to consult with a hematologist. When a diagnosis of a congenital condition is made, screening should be offered to other family members.

Hypercoaguable Conditions	Thrombophilia Screening
Antithrombin III deficiency	Antithrombin III
Protein C deficiency	Protein C
Protein S deficiency	Protein S
Factor V Leiden mutation	Activated protein C resistance ratio
Prothrombin gene mutation	Activated partial thromboplastin time
Antiphospholipid syndrome	Hexagonal activated partial thromboplastin time
	Anticardiolipin antibodies
	Lupus anticoagulant
	Fibrinogen
	Prothrombin G mutation (DNA test)
	Thrombin Time
	Homocysteine level
	Complete blood count

A DNA-based test can be used to verify the presence of the factor V Leiden mutation. Other risk factors for thromboembolism that should be considered by clinicians include an acquired predisposition, such as the presence of lupus anticoagulant or malignancy, and immobility or trauma. Varicose veins are not a risk factor unless they are very extensive, and unlike arterial thrombosis, smoking either has no effect or at best is a weak risk factor for venous thromboembolism.

If a patient has a congenital predisposition for venous thrombosis or if she is considered to be at high risk for venous thromboembolism, the clinician and patient can consider the combination of hormone therapy and chronic anticoagulation, in consultation with a hematologist.

There are no studies of venous thromboembolism following surgical procedures in postmenopausal hormone users. *It now seems sensible to recommend appropriate prophylactic anticoagulant treatment in hormone users anticipating immobility with hospitalization, especially if other risk factors are present. Some patients may elect to discontinue hormone treatment 4 weeks prior to major surgery (if extended immobility is to be expected), but this is an empiric, individual decision. Hormone therapy can be resumed when the patient is ambulatory.*

Endometrial Neoplasia

There are two different types of endometrial cancer. The more uncommon form (perhaps 20%) develops rapidly, usually in older women, with a histologic pattern more characteristic of serous carcinomas, in a background of atrophic endometrium. Endometrioid carcinoma develops slowly from a precursor lesion in response to estrogen stimulation. This type is less aggressive, better differentiated, and responds to progestational treatment.

Estrogen normally promotes mitotic growth of the endometrium. Abnormal progression of growth through simple hyperplasia, complex hyperplasia, atypia, and early carcinoma has been associated with unopposed estrogen activity, administered either continuously or in cyclic fashion. Only one year of treatment with unopposed estrogen (0.625 mg conjugated estrogens or the equivalent) will produce a 20% incidence of hyperplasia, largely simple hyperplasia; in the 3-year PEPI trial, 30% of the women on unopposed estrogen developed adenomatous or atypical hyperplasia.[57, 60, 265] Some 10% of women with complex hyperplasia progress to frank cancer, and complex hyperplasia is observed to antedate adenocarcinoma in 25–30% of cases. If atypia is present, 20–25% of cases will progress to carcinoma within a year.[266]

Approximately 40 case-control and cohort studies have estimated that the risk of endometrial cancer in women on estrogen therapy (unopposed by a progestational agent) is increased by a factor of somewhere from 2 to 10 times the normal incidence of 1 per 1000 postmenopausal women per year.[267, 268] The risk increases with the dose of estrogen and with the duration of exposure (reaching a 10-fold increase with 10–15 years of use, and perhaps an incidence of 1 in 10 with very long-term use), lingers for up to 10 years after estrogen is discontinued, and the risk of cancer that has already spread beyond the uterus is increased 3-fold in women who have used estrogen a year or longer.[269, 270] Although most endometrial cancer associated with estrogen use is of low grade and stage, and associated with better survival (probably because of earlier detection), the overall risk of invasive cancer and death is increased. The risk of endometrial hyperplasia and cancer is not reduced by the administration of unopposed estrogen in a cyclic fashion (a period of time each month without treatment).[267, 271]

A short-term study (2 years) has indicated that one-half the usual standard dose of estrogen (in this case, 0.3 mg esterified estrogens) was not associated with an increased incidence of endometrial hyperplasia compared with a placebo group.[272] But we have learned that long-term exposure to low levels of estrogen can induce abnormal endometrial growth, and in our view, lower dose estrogen therapy requires either endometrial assessment annually or the addition of a progestin to the treatment regimen. This is supported by a case-control study from Washington that contained 18 cases and 9 controls who had exclusively used only 0.3 mg/day of unopposed conjugated estrogens.[273] The use of this half-dose estrogen was associated with an overall 5-fold increased risk of endometrial cancer, reaching a relative risk of 9.2 in current users for more than 8 years' duration. Although limited by small numbers, the conclusion is logical and consistent with our understanding of the importance of duration of exposure to any increased level of endometrial estrogen stimulation.

It is now apparent that this risk can be reduced by the addition of a progestational agent to the program.[265] Although estrogen promotes the growth of endometrium, progestins inhibit that growth. This countereffect is accomplished by progestin reduction in cellular receptors for estrogen, and by induction of target cell enzymes that convert estradiol to an excreted metabolite, estrone sulfate. As a result, the number of estrogen receptor complexes that are retained in the endometrial nuclei are decreased in number, as is the overall intracellular availability of the powerful estradiol. In addition, progestational agents suppress estrogen-mediated transcription of oncogenes.

Reports of the clinical impact of adding progestin in sequence with estrogen include both the reversal of hyperplasia and a diminished incidence of endometrial cancer.[274-278] The protective action of progestational agents operates via a mechanism that requires time in order to reach its maximal effect. For that reason, the duration of exposure to the progestin each month is critical. While one standard method incorporated the addition of a progestational agent for the last 10 days of estrogen exposure, most have argued in favor of 12 or 14 days. Studies indicate that the minimal requirement is a monthly exposure of at least 10 days' duration.[71, 279, 280] About 2–3% of women per year develop endometrial hyperplasia when the progestin is administered for less than 10 days monthly.

Important unanswered questions are what will be the actual incidence of endometrial cancer in long-term users of postmenopausal hormone therapy and will there be differences among the various regimens and routes of administration. A case-control study from Seattle reported that the use of combined estrogen-progestin (essentially all sequential and oral) for 5 or more years was associated with an increased relative risk of endometrial cancer, even with 10–21 days of added progestin per month.[73] However, the increased risk was confined to those women who had been previously exposed to unopposed estrogen treatment; remember, after discontinuing unopposed estrogen treatment, the risk of endometrial cancer lingers for up to 10 years, even if a subsequent regimen includes a progestin. In the Swedish prospective cohort in Uppsala, a reduced risk of mortality due to endometrial cancer was observed in women receiving an estrogen-progestin combination; however, there were only 2 deaths, precluding statistical significance.[281] A case-control study from Los Angeles found no increased risk of endometrial cancer with the continuous combined estrogen-progestin regimen or when at least 10 days of progestin were provided in a sequential regimen.[280]

An attractive idea is that protection against endometrial cancer requires shedding of the endometrium. However, we know that at least one-third and up to one-half of the functioning endometrium is not lost during withdrawal bleeding, and it has not been established that endometrial shedding is essential to protect against cancer.[282] It is just as logical to believe that prevention of growth and development of atrophic endometrium are protective. There is good reason to believe that both the sequential regimens (with appropriate dose and duration of progestin administration) and the continuous combined regimens offer protection against endometrial cancer. The degree of protection and comparable performance will ultimately be determined by the long-term randomized clinical trials currently ongoing.

The lowest daily dose of progestin that protects the endometrium has not been established. Currently, the sequential program utilizes 5 or 10 mg medroxyprogesterone acetate and the combined daily method uses 2.5 mg. The dose of norethindrone that is comparable with 2.5 mg medroxyprogesterone acetate is 0.25 mg.[61] Although lower doses of progestational agents are effective in achieving target tissue responses (such as reducing the nuclear concentration of estrogen receptors), the long-term impact on endometrial histology has not yet been firmly established. The question of dose is an issue of major importance, especially in terms of the cardiovascular system and compliance because of progestin-induced side effects.

Although the protective effect of progestin is considerable and predictable, it is unwise to expect all patients on estrogen-progestin therapy to never develop endometrial cancer. Appropriate monitoring of patients cannot be disregarded. Although routine assessments are not cost-effective, interventions directed by clinical responses are prudent and necessary.

Ovarian Cancer

A prospective cohort study concluded that the risk of fatal ovarian cancer is increased with long-term estrogen use.[283] There was no significant increase in the relative risk of fatal ovarian cancer with ever use of postmenopausal estrogen, and the link with long-term use achieved statistical significance only with the 18 cases using estrogen for 11 or more years. By no means is it certain if this association is real. There have been 12 case-control studies of ovarian cancer risk factors, and the pooled analysis of this literature could find no consistent evidence for an association between ovarian cancer and estrogen therapy.[284] A meta-analysis concluded that there is a 14% increased risk of ovarian carcinoma among ever users of hormone therapy, and that there is a 27% increase in risk with more than 10 years of long-term use.[285] We are not impressed by this small increase in a meta-analysis of case-control studies, subject to multiple potential biases. Among the 6 studies included in the analysis of duration of use, only one reported a statistically significant increase in risk with 10 or more years of hormone therapy.

Individual studies have been hampered by relatively small numbers, but the lack of a uniform and consistent association argues against a major impact of postmenopausal estrogen treatment on the risk of ovarian cancer. In a more recent and relatively large case-control study, no indication could be found for an association between postmenopausal hormone therapy and the risk of epithelial ovarian cancer, even with long-term treatment.[286] Another case-control study reported a slightly increased risk, but it was not statistically significant.[287] In a retrospective analysis, no detrimental impact could be detected on prognosis after surgery for ovarian cancer in patients who received postmenopausal hormone therapy after diagnosis.[288]

Cervical Cancer

The association between postmenopausal hormone therapy and cancer of the uterine cervix has not been extensively studied. Evidence from one cohort study and one-case-control study indicates that the postmenopausal use of estrogen does not increase the risk of cervical cancer.[289, 290] Indeed, these studies observed protection against cervical cancer in the estrogen users, but this may reflect detection bias (more examinations and Pap smears in estrogen users). In a follow-up report of 120 women treated for Stage I and II cervical cancer, no adverse effects of hormone therapy on survival or recurrence were observed.[291]

Colorectal Cancer

Most, but not all, cohort and case-control studies have reported a significantly reduced risk of colorectal cancer incidence and mortality in users of postmenopausal estrogen.[292–296] The effect is greatest in current users and most studies have not indicated an increased effect with increasing duration of use; for example, the Nurses' Health Study (which found a 35% reduced risk in current users) could not demonstrate an added benefit with longer duration of current use.[297] A reduction in fatal colon cancer has been documented in current users.[294] There also appears to be a reduced risk of polyps, especially large polyps, among current and recent hormone users.

One can only speculate regarding the mechanism of this benefit. The estrogen-induced change in the bile (a decrease in bile acids with an increase in cholesterol saturation) favors gallstone formation, but may reduce promotion (by bile acids) of colonic cancer. Other possible mechanisms include a direct suppressive effect on mucosal cell growth and an effect on beneficial mucosal secretions. This potential benefit deserves greater attention; colorectal cancer ranks third in women, both in incidence and mortality, more prevalent than cancers of the uterus or ovary.[298]

Malignant Melanoma

The possibility of a relationship between exogenous hormones and cutaneous malignant melanoma has been the subject of many observational studies. Accurate evaluation utilizing the Royal College of General Practitioners and Oxford Family Planning Association prospective cohorts and accounting for exposure to sunlight did not indicate a significant difference in the risk of melanoma comparing users of oral contraceptives to nonusers.[299, 300] Results with the use of postmenopausal estrogen therapy have not indicated a major impact. A slightly increased risk with long-term use of estrogen was noted in one case-control study (a conclusion based on 10–20 cases and not achieving statistical significance), whereas another case-control study could find no association with postmenopausal estrogen treatment.[301, 302] Others have reported slight increases in the risk of malignant melanoma associated with the use of exogenous estrogen, but all failed to reach statistical significance.[289, 303, 304] In an analysis of cancer incidence in a Swedish cohort of women prescribed postmenopausal hormone therapy, no increase in malignant melanoma was observed.[305]

Breast Cancer

The possibility that estrogen use increases the risk of breast cancer must be intensively scrutinized. The American epidemiologic data on the scope of human female breast cancer are astonishing: 1 of every 8 women will develop breast cancer in her lifetime (assuming an 85-year life expectancy). In America, breast cancer is the leading type of cancer in women (29.7%) and now second to lung cancer as the leading cause of cancer death in women (16.1%), about 10 times the number of deaths from endometrial cancer.[298]

Sufficient evidence exists to indicate the possibility of a slightly increased risk of breast cancer associated with long durations (5 or more years) of postmenopausal estrogen use. However, the epidemiologic data on this relationship are by no means consistent and uniform. A review of the epidemiologic studies on postmenopausal hormone therapy and the risk of breast cancer fails to provide definitive evidence regarding this issue. Nevertheless, we believe that patients must consider this possibility in their informed decision making.

Early studies on estrogen use and breast cancer indicated higher risks in special subcategories, such as women with benign breast disease, long duration of use, or natural versus surgical menopause.[306–315] These studies were all limited by a lack of control groups or by relatively small numbers. The CASH (Cancer and Sex Hormone Study of the Centers for Disease Control and Prevention) did not detect an overall increased risk of breast cancer with postmenopausal estrogen use nor a relationship with duration of use up to 20 years or longer,[316] An absence of an effect was evident in all of the following: parity, age at first pregnancy, early or late menopause, menopause by hysterectomy or oophorectomy, family history of breast cancer, presence of benign breast disease, use for many years (20 years or longer), and use of high doses.

A well-publicized study from Uppsala, Sweden, concluded that estrogen use was associated with a slight increase in the risk of breast cancer (relative risk 1.1), and that there was a relationship with duration of use; the relative risk reaching 1.7 after 9 years (although this conclusion did not reach statistical significance).[317, 318] Another conclusion of this study was the indication of increased risk with combined treatment with estrogen-progestin. This conclusion also was not statistically significant, based on only 10 women with breast cancer, and the confidence interval (CI) was impressively wide: 0.9–22.4. In a later report based on an additional 4 years of data, the overall risk of breast cancer associated with the use of the estrogen-progestin sequential product was 0.9 (CI: 0.7–1.1); in those women with 7 to 11 years of follow-up, the relative risk was increased to 1.6 (CI: 1.1–2.1).[319] However, the statistical power of this study continues to be limited, and there is no control group; the relative risk was calculated by using the expected breast cancer incidence in the general population. In a nested case-control study within this Swedish cohort of women, these investigators again reported a moderately increased risk of breast cancer with more than 10 years of postmenopausal hormone therapy.[320]

A Danish case-control study used questionnaires to obtain information on cases and controls and also indicated a slightly increased risk of breast cancer associated with postmenopausal hormone therapy.[321] Interestingly, this report indicated an increased risk only with sequential estrogen and progestin and not with the daily administration of combined estrogen and progestin (however, these conclusions were very limited by the small numbers involved). This study contains statistical problems similar to the Uppsala study (e.g., the relative risk associated with estrogen-progestin use was 1.41, but the confidence interval included 1.0 and was not statistically significant).

The latest reports from the Nurses' Health Study represent 16 years of follow-up (1976–1992).[322, 323] During that period, 1935 cases of breast cancer were identified among more than 69,000 postmenopausal women. The analysis revealed that women who had used estrogen in the past (even for 10 or more years) were not at increased risk of breast cancer. However, the relative risk for current users was 1.46 (CI 1.22–1.74) for 5–9 years of use, and 1.46 (CI 1.20–1.76) for 10 or more years of use.

By virtue of the large numbers in the Nurses' Health Study and the careful analyses by the investigators, reports from this study must be given great credibility. The 16-year follow-up report is disturbing with its finding of an increased risk in current users. Because estrogen users may be examined more frequently, detection bias is a major concern. It is noteworthy that current users had a 14% higher prevalence of mammography compared with never users. Current users were different from never users (history of benign breast disease, birth only once or twice, menarche at age 13 or less, body mass index of 21–23). Another important consideration is the need to adjust for alcohol consumption, an accepted risk factor for breast cancer. In the Iowa

Women's Health Study, an increased risk of breast cancer was observed only in those postmenopausal women who consumed one drink or more of alcohol daily.[324] The concern is that alcohol consumption raises estrogen levels in hormone users to very high concentrations.[187–189] Although each of these factors standing alone would not explain the observed outcome in the Nurses' Health Study, what is the additive effect of all factors? Thus, the finding of an increased relative risk in long-term current users is not definitive and not free of all confounding variables. The size of the statistical risk is not outside the range of influence by biases.

Based on 359 deaths due to breast cancer, the risk of dying of breast cancer in the Nurses' Health Study was 0.80 (CI 0.60–1.07) for past users, 0.99 (CI 0.66–1.48) for current users with less than 5 years of use, and 1.45 (CI 1.01–2.09) with 5 or more years of use. These mortality data raise a question of "prevalence bias," also called by statisticians as interdependence between the probabilities of disease incidence in a population (an issue of competing risks).[325] Is it possible that the protection against cardiovascular disease is so great with long durations of estrogen use that the long-term current users develop a problem that is prevalent with aging, breast cancer. The never users, deprived of the cardiovascular benefit of estrogen, may develop cardiovascular disease before living long enough to experience breast cancer.

A case-control study from Australia, which attempted to control for secular trends in estrogen use, type of menopause, and duration of estrogen use, concluded that there was no evidence for an association between estrogen use and the risk of breast cancer in postmenopausal women.[326]

There is a very helpful study that specifically addressed the relationship between the use of estrogen and benign breast disease.[327] This study is impressive because it is based on 10,366 consecutive breast biopsy specimens with follow-up information on 4227 biopsy specimens in 3303 women (a mean duration of follow-up of 17 years). Analysis indicated that the use of estrogen was associated with a reduced risk of developing breast cancer. Most importantly, in patients with atypical hyperplasia in their biopsies, the use of estrogen did not increase and even lowered the risk of breast cancer. Although the protective effect probably indicates detection/surveillance bias, certainly this is strong evidence that estrogen use does not increase the risk of breast cancer in women with surgically proven benign breast disease, even with atypia.

In a study of 1686 cases and 2077 controls in the eastern U.S., the relative risk for current users was a nonsignificant 1.1 (CI, 0.7–1.6), for a duration of use of 15 or more years, the relative risk was 0.9 (CI, 0.4–1.9).[328] As in the eastern U.S., a study from Toronto found no evidence for an increased risk in either current or recent users or in users for up to 15 years.[329] A case-control study from Washington found no increased risk of breast cancer with past or long-term current use of estrogen alone or with estrogen-progestin.[330] These large case-control studies failed to support the conclusion of the Nurses' Health Study that current users are associated with an increased risk, even with long durations of use. On the other hand, other studies (of smaller size and limited statistical power) have found an increased risk of breast cancer in current users and long-term users.[331, 332] A prospective study from the National Cancer Institute could document only an increase in the risk of *in situ* breast cancer (not invasive disease), possibly reflecting surveillance bias in women taking either estrogen alone or a combination of estrogen and progestin.[333]

The Iowa Women's Health Study, like the Nurses' Health Study, is prospectively following a cohort of women (selected in 1985). After 6 years of follow-up, a statistically significant increase in the risk of breast cancer could not be detected in ever users or current users of hormone therapy.[334] A report through 8 years of follow-up focused on whether postmenopausal hormone therapy increased the risks for breast cancer and mortality in women with a family history of breast cancer.[335] Even in women with a positive family history of breast cancer who were current users of hormone therapy for more than 5 years, there was no significant increase in the rate of breast cancer. A very large case-control study found no increased risk of breast cancer associated with the ever use of estrogen alone or estrogen and progestin combinations, and when long-term use for 15 years or more was examined, again no increase in risk was detected.[336]

Meta-Analyses. Meta-analysis is an increasingly popular statistical method in which many studies are combined and undergo rigorous analysis. The term "meta-analysis" was coined in 1976 to indicate the re-analysis of data to answer new questions.[337] The method was first used in social science, and then in the late 1980s, in medicine. Simply put, the purpose of a meta-analysis is to gain the statistical power that is lacking in individual studies.

An Australian meta-analysis of 23 studies of estrogen use and breast cancer concluded "unequivocally" that estrogen use did not alter the risk of breast cancer.[338] In the meta-analysis by Dupont and Page (Nashville, Tennessee), the authors concluded that "considerable and consistent" evidence exists that a daily dose of 0.625 mg conjugated estrogens taken for several years does not appreciably increase the risk of breast cancer.[339] They found no evidence of an association between the duration of treatment and the risk of breast cancer at this dosage. On the other hand, the data suggested that a daily dose of 1.25 mg conjugated estrogens and higher may increase the risk of breast cancer. This analysis failed to reveal an increased risk in patients with a history of benign breast disease.

A third meta-analysis was from the CDC.[340] This meta-analysis was conducted by using what the authors called a "dose-response curve" for duration of use. The curve for each study analyzed was calculated by plotting breast cancer risk against duration of estrogen use. The combined dose-response slope represented the average change in risk associated with estrogen use over time. The analysis concluded that duration of estrogen use was associated with an increased risk of breast cancer, regardless of whether menopause was natural or surgical. No increase in risk was noted in the first 5 years of use, but after 15 years of use, the risk was increased by 30%. The effect was present irrespective of other risk factors, such as parity or history of benign breast disease. The effect of estrogen therapy on risk of breast cancer was enhanced in women with a positive family history of breast cancer.

A fourth meta-analysis, from Spain, concluded that estrogen is associated with a very small, but statistically significant, increased relative risk of breast cancer and that the increased risk is higher among current users.[341] Confining their analysis to a dose of 0.625 mg conjugated estrogens; however, the Spanish epidemiologists could not detect a statistically significant increased risk. Indeed, this meta-analysis concluded that an estrogen dose of 0.625 mg conjugated estrogens is safe.

A fifth meta-analysis from the epidemiologists associated with the Nurses' Health Study concluded (based on 25 case-control and 6 cohort studies) that there is no increased risk of breast cancer in ever users of estrogen.[342] Current use was associated with an increased risk (which was lost 2 years after using estrogen), and there was a slight increase with more than 10 years of use (but there was no linear trend with increasing duration of use). This observation in long-term users could be influenced by an increased proportion of current users in this group, and the increased risk in current users could be a consequence of detection bias. The statistical power of this meta-analysis was in the ever use category, giving strength to its negative conclusion. This meta-analysis could not detect a link between risk of breast cancer and dosage. Nevertheless, we continue to be concerned with a possible effect of higher doses. The Australia, Nashville, and Spain meta-analyses indicated an increased risk with a daily dose of conjugated estrogens greater than 0.625 mg (or its equivalent).

The Nashville, CDC, and Nurses' Health analyses did not find an enhanced risk in women with a history of benign breast disease. In contrast to the CDC report, the Australia and Nurses' Health analyses found no link between positive family history and estrogen use. The Nashville and Spain investigators did not consider family history.

In a major overview and assessment (yet another meta-analysis) of the world's literature on postmenopausal hormone therapy, commissioned by the American College of Physicians, the authors concluded that long-term use of estrogen was associated with a relative risk of breast cancer of 1.25 (CI, 1.04–1.51).[343] This conclusion, in our view, was not appropriately critical and represents a judgment that extends beyond the statistical power available from the many heterogeneic studies. The heterogeneity of the many studies is an important issue: different drugs, different doses, different methods of diagnosis, different comparison and control groups. The Spanish meta-analysis is the only one to raise the question: perhaps the heterogeneity is too great to allow an accurate meta-analysis of this literature.

A Re-analysis of the World's Literature. A team of epidemiologists invited all investigators who had previously studied the association of postmenopausal hormone use and the risk of breast cancer (51 studies) to submit their original data for a collaborative combined re-analysis, an undertaking more rigorous than a standard meta-analysis. This analysis reached the following conclusions:[344]

- Ever users of postmenopausal hormones had an overall increased relative risk of breast cancer of 1.14

- Current users for 5 or more years had a relative risk of 1.35 (CI = 1.21–1.49), and the risk increased with increasing duration of use.

- Current and recent users had evidence of having only localized disease (no metastatic disease) and ever users had less metastatic disease.

- There was no effect of a family history of breast cancer.

- There was no increase in relative risk in past users.

- The increase in relative risk in current and recent users was greatest in women with lower body weights.

The most compelling reason to believe that long-term use of postmenopausal estrogen increases the risk of breast cancer is the inherent biologic plausibility. Factors known to increase a woman's exposure to estrogen are known to increase the risk of breast cancer; e.g., age of menarche and age of menopause. Indeed, in this report, the authors made a point of demonstrating that the quantitative effect of their conclusion is similar to extending the age of menopause. According to their calculations, current and recent hormone use was associated with a 2.3% increase in breast cancer risk per year and the effect of the age of menopause was equivalent to a 2.8% increase in risk per year of delay. Many clinicians are attracted by the logic in this comparison; however, the steady exposure to postmenopausal estrogen is not exactly the same as extended exposure to cyclic ovarian function.

A strong indication that the conclusion of the re-analysis is subject to bias is the finding that current and recent hormone users had evidence only of localized disease. This is consistent with detection/surveillance bias and hormone acceleration of tumors already present and thus detection at an early, less aggressive stage.

The Influence of Detection/Surveillance Bias and Accelerated Tumor Growth — An Answer to the Paradox of Increased Risk and Decreased Mortality. It is relevant to note that many of the studies that have examined the mortality rates of women who were taking estrogen at the time of breast cancer diagnosis have documented improved survival rates.[305, 345, 346] This undoubtedly reflects earlier diagnosis in users because the greater survival rate in current users is associated with a lower frequency of late-stage disease.[183, 347–349] There is also evidence to suggest that estrogen users develop better differentiated tumors, and that detection/surveillance bias is not the only explanation for better survival.[349, 350] This implies that hormone treatment accelerates the growth of a malignant locus already in place, and it presents clinically at a less virulent and aggressive stage. This conclusion is consistent with the fact that virtually all the studies find that any increase in risk disappears within 5 years of discontinuing hormone therapy.

Increased utilization of mammography by hormone users is a well recognized phenomenon.[351] Indeed, when corrected for use of mammography, an apparent increase in breast cancer in long-term estrogen users in a retrospective cohort study lost its statistical significance.[352] A greater frequency of mammography and breast examinations among hormone users introduces detection/surveillance bias into all observational studies.

If the conclusion of the re-analysis of the world's literature were correct, it would mean that there would be a detectable increase in deaths from breast cancer due to hormone use. However, studies have indicated a *decreased* risk of breast cancer mortality in postmenopausal hormone users. For example, the American Cancer Society 9-year prospective follow-up documented a 16% reduced risk of fatal breast cancer in estrogen users.[346] The mortality data support the contention that accelerated growth of a pre-existing tumor and detection/surveillance bias are influencing the results of observational studies.

Estrogen agonists/antagonists (tamoxifen and raloxifene) have been reported to reduce the incidence of breast cancer within 2–3 years of treatment.[129, 353] Given the length of time it takes for a malignancy to become clinically detectable (approximately 10 years to grow to a 1 cm mass),[130] how is it possible to demonstrate hormonal effects within several years? Do tamoxifen and raloxifene prevent breast cancer and does estrogen increase the risk of breast cancer—or are we only changing the time (age) of diagnosis? Instead of causation/prevention, are we observing acceleration/deceleration of pre-existing tumors?

Causation	**and**	**Prevention**
	OR	
Acceleration	**and**	**Deceleration**
Hormone therapy		Tamoxifen (Chapter 16)
Oral contraceptives (Chapter 22)		Raloxifene
Pregnancy (Chapter 16)		
Return to baseline after therapy		

Why Is There No Definitive Answer Despite Approximately 50 Observational Studies?
Misinterpretation of epidemiologic data should not be attributed to epidemiologic methods, but to their interpreters. When the impact of an association is large, it is relatively easy to demonstrate uniformity and consistency of results with case-control and cohort studies (observational studies). This can be appreciated in the impressive data indicating protection against cardiovascular disease by the use of postmenopausal estrogen. In the case of postmenopausal hormone therapy and the risk of breast cancer, we have neither the comfortable position produced by uniformity and consistency among observational studies nor the results of a randomized clinical trial. The lack of a definitive answer can be attributed to the following:

1. Observational studies lack the ability to overcome recognized and unrecognized biases, unless the studied effect is large. A large effect yields uniformity and consistency of results with case-control and cohort studies (good examples are the benefits of a reduction in the risks of endometrial and ovarian cancer with the use of oral contraception). Therefore, any impact of postmenopausal hormone therapy on the risk of breast cancer is unlikely to be great; otherwise, the observational studies would have achieved uniformity and consistency of results.

2. Most of the available data are derived from a time when hormone dosages and schedules (higher doses and shorter durations) were different compared with current methods—the problem of heterogeneity. In addition to different doses and durations

of exposure, heterogeneity is the result of different study designs, different sources for controls, different geographic locations, different populations, and different drugs.

3.   The method of meta-analysis was developed to combine the results of small, randomized trials.[337] Rapidly (perhaps too rapidly), the method has been extended to observational studies, especially when the results of the individual studies are contradictory. Combining the results of contradictory studies, rather than the results of small (randomized) studies, is precisely when meta-analysis is weakest. Statistical analysis is not an appropriate method to address contradictory results. And even when the technique of meta-analysis is restricted to small randomized trials, because of various subjective and objective problems, the outcomes of subsequent large randomized, controlled trials were not predicted accurately 35% of the time by the previous meta-analyses.[354] The method of meta-analysis is not infallible and does not always yield the truth.

The method of meta-analysis has not overcome the problem of achieving sufficient statistical power. The conclusions of meta-analyses of observational studies are not free of selection bias, detection bias, and the problem of a positive result emerging just by chance when multiple subgroup analyses are performed. Meta-analysis is further limited, not only when the database is subject to biases as is the case with observational studies, but also when there is heterogeneity among the studies (different drugs, doses, durations of exposures, and populations). A meta-analysis can make the problem of bias worse by magnifying the significance level of erroneous results; a meta-analysis does not correct for design flaws in individual studies.

Therefore, our uncertainty will not be resolved by more case-control studies, more cohort studies, or more meta-analyses. Only a properly performed randomized clinical trial will provide us with definitive information.

Where Does That Leave Clinicians and Patients? The lack of agreement, uniformity, and consistency in approximately 50 case-control and cohort studies indicates that the use of postmenopausal hormone therapy cannot be associated with a major impact on the risk of breast cancer, otherwise there would be agreement among the studies. It is helpful to compare this situation with 3 other conditions: the protection against ovarian cancer by oral contraceptives, the protection against coronary heart disease by postmenopausal estrogen use, and the increase in lung cancer due to cigarette smoking. Clinicians believe each of these 3 epidemiologic associations despite the lack of a single randomized clinical trial because all of the studies say the same thing, an impressive agreement and uniformity among observational studies. The results with postmenopausal hormone therapy and the risk of breast cancer indicate either a small impact of estrogen use or the effect of biases that can only be eliminated by large, randomized trials, specifically the ongoing Women's Health Initiative in the U.S. (to be completed in 2008) and the WISDOM trial (Women's International Study of Long-Duration Oestrogen use after Menopause) in the U.K. (to be completed in 2011).

If estrogen use were associated with an increased risk of breast cancer, wouldn't one expect to see an impact on mortality? In the mortality report from the Leisure World follow-up study in California, the risk of breast cancer mortality in hormone users was 19% reduced, and a similar reduction in fatal breast cancer has been documented in the Nurses' Health Study and in the American Cancer Society cohort.[43, 183, 346] This lower relative risk probably is influenced by detection/surveillance bias and by the presence of better differentiated tumors in estrogen users, but certainly there is no evidence that women using estrogen for a long time are dying of breast cancer at a greater rate.

Doses of estrogen known to protect against osteoporosis and cardiovascular disease (0.625 mg conjugated estrogens and 1.0 mg estradiol) are, at the present time, not known to be associated with any clear-cut increased risk of breast cancer. However, because of the concern raised by some studies and reviews that there is a slightly increased risk of breast cancer associated with long-term use of postmenopausal estrogen, this issue requires discussion during the clinician-patient dialogue regarding postmenopausal hormone therapy.

The comfort found in large numbers with epidemiologic research is lost to us when we must make clinical decisions with individual patients. If we wish to minimize the uncertainty from imprecise measurements, we will adopt an appropriate strategy. If we wish to emphasize the possibility or probability of an outcome, we will adopt another. In our view, it is appropriate to emphasize the benefits of postmenopausal hormone therapy, point out the continuing concern regarding the relationship between estrogen use and breast cancer (particularly long-term use), and to ***emphasize the absence of definitive evidence linking such therapy to an increased risk of breast cancer.***

The Risk of Breast Cancer and Estrogen-Progestin Therapy. The addition of a progestational agent to postmenopausal estrogen therapy is now accepted as a standard part of the treatment program. The obvious reason for this combined estrogen-progestin approach is the need to prevent the increased risk of endometrial cancer associated with exposure to unopposed estrogen. Even though this endometrial cancer is not frequently encountered and survival rates are excellent with early disease, the fear of this cancer is a major force in patient continuance, and, therefore, the combined approach is warranted. Clinicians and patients have rapidly turned to the method of a daily combination of estrogen and a progestin, in order to overcome bleeding which is the second major continuance problem.

Only two reports have claimed that the addition of a progestational agent protects against breast cancer.[355, 356] The first was limited by bias in treatment selection (the breast cancer risk factor profiles were not matched in the treated and untreated groups). The second (the Nachtigall study), although it has been the only randomized, placebo-controlled trial, was hampered by small numbers.

At the present time, the available epidemiologic evidence on the impact of combined estrogen-progestin treatment indicates that neither a protective nor a detrimental effect has yet to be convincingly demonstrated; recent studies find that the addition of a progestin does not change the findings with estrogen alone.[323, 330–333] Balancing the information available involving all of the health issues affected by hormone therapy, a combined estrogen-progestin program in appropriate doses continues to offer significant benefits for postmenopausal women. As time goes on, more studies and greater duration of use should provide us with better answers to many of our questions. By virtue of the magnitude of the postmenopausal female population, these questions deserve continuing biologic and epidemiologic research from both the public health and individual points of view.

SUMMARY: Postmenopausal Hormone Therapy and Breast Cancer

- **Some epidemiologic case-control and cohort studies conclude that long-term (5 or more years) of current use of postmenopausal hormone therapy is associated with a slight increase in the risk of breast cancer, a risk that is less than that associated with postmenopausal obesity or daily alcohol consumption. This conclusion might be due to confounding biases, particularly detection/surveillance bias, and accelerated growth of a pre-existing malignancy.**

- **Many observational studies have failed to develop evidence that long-term postmenopausal hormone therapy increases the risk of breast cancer.**

- **All epidemiologic studies fail to find an increased risk of breast cancer associated with short-term (less than 5 years) use or past use of postmenopausal hormone therapy.**

- The epidemiologic data agree that the addition of a progestin to the treatment regimen neither increases nor decreases the risk observed in individual studies.

- The epidemiologic data indicate that a positive family history of breast cancer should not be a contraindication to the use of postmenopausal hormone therapy.

- Women who develop breast cancer while using postmenopausal hormone therapy have a reduced risk of dying from breast cancer. This is because of two factors: (1). Increased surveillance and early detection; and (2). Acceleration of pre-existing tumor growth so that tumors appear at a less virulent and aggressive stage.

Contraindications to Postmenopausal Hormone Therapy

Endometrial Cancer, Endometrioid Tumors, and Endometriosis

Gynecologic oncologists have reported that patients who have had Stage I and Stage II adenocarcinoma of the endometrium can take estrogen without fear of an increased risk of recurrence or a decrease in disease-free interval.[108–111] Nothing is known about the risk in patients with more advanced disease. If a high-risk tumor is estrogen and progesterone receptor negative, it seems reasonable to allow immediate hormone therapy. Because the latent period with endometrial cancer is relatively short, a period of time (5 years) without evidence of recurrence would increase the likelihood of safety on an estrogen program. We recommend that hormone therapy be avoided in patients with high-risk tumors that are receptor-positive until 5 years have elapsed. The combination of estrogen-progestin is recommended in view of the potential protective action of the progestational agent. A similar approach makes sense for patients previously treated for endometrioid tumors of the ovary. In view of the fact that adenocarcinoma has been reported in patients with pelvic endometriosis and on unopposed estrogen, the combined estrogen-progestin program is advised in patients with a past history of endometriosis.[102–104]

Should a Woman Who Has Had Breast Cancer Use Postmenopausal Hormones?

The increasing incidence of breast cancer, together with earlier detection and treatment, is producing a growing pool of patients for whom the question of estrogen treatment is important and at the same time difficult. The problem is easy to articulate: we have no data. There are absolutely no published clinical trials of sufficient size and scope in which the impact of estrogen treatment has been documented when given to women with previously treated breast cancer.

Because there is good reason to believe that breast cancer is hormonally influenced, it is not hard to understand the breast surgeon or medical oncologist who believes that estrogen treatment is foolish and dangerous. Yet, that position is just as unencumbered by data as the position of the clinician who believes that appropriate patients stand to benefit more from estrogen compared with the unknown risk of breast cancer recurrence.

The single most useful prognostic information in women with operable breast cancer has been the histologic status of the axillary lymph nodes. At 10 years, only 25% of patients with positive nodes are free of disease compared with 75% of patients with negative nodes. If more than 3 nodes are involved, the 10-year survival rate drops to 13%. Because of this recognition for the importance of the axillary nodes, the traditional approach to breast cancer (the Halsted surgical approach) was based on the concept that breast cancer is a disease of stepwise progression. There has been an important change in concept. Breast cancer is now viewed as a systemic disease, with spread to local and distant sites at the same time. Breast cancer is best viewed as occultly metastatic (microscopically disseminated) at the time of presentation. Dissemination of tumor cells has occurred by the time of surgery in many patients, and it is concern over the possible response of these cells that fires the debate over this question: should women who have had breast cancer take postmenopausal hormones?

There are two opposing hypotheses that link breast cancer to a hormonal influence: one assigns the critical role to estrogen; the other, to progesterone.

Is Estrogen the Important Influence? When one reviews the various factors associated with breast cancer, many of the factors support a role for increased exposure to estrogen, specifically the importance of age of menarche, age of menopause, obesity, the effect of pregnancy, and added to this list is the therapeutic effect of an antiestrogen, tamoxifen.

Stanley Korenman, therefore, suggested that the endocrine environment does not cause the disease but influences the susceptibility to carcinogens—the so-called estrogen window hypothesis.[357, 358] The two periods of life when the estrogen window is open (this means long periods of unopposed estrogen) are after menarche before ovulation is established and the perimenopausal years. Estrogen shows a significant increase at about Tanner stage 2, ages 8 to 10. Because ovulation occurs on the average 1.5 years after menarche, this window can last 4 to 5 years. It is well recognized that anovulation is common in the perimenopausal years because of the lesser capabilities of the remaining ovarian follicles. Korenman argued that the open window (estrogen exposure) influences the risk of breast cancer and that the window is closed by exposure to progesterone after ovulation and during pregnancy. This argument is supported by observational studies indicating that anovulatory and infertile women (exposed to less progesterone) have an increased risk of breast cancer later in life.[359–361] However, the statistical power of these studies was limited by small numbers (all fewer than 15 cases), and others have failed to find a link between anovulation and the risk of breast cancer.[362–364] In summary, factors that would be associated with an increased risk of breast cancer are those that would prolong the duration of the open window: obesity, infertility due to anovulation, delayed pregnancy, early menarche, late menopause.

Is Progesterone the Important Influence? Some argue that progesterone is the key to influencing the risk of breast cancer because mitotic activity in the breast reaches its peak during the progesterone-dominant luteal phase of the menstrual cycle.[365–367] An earlier age of menarche is sometimes used to buttress the progesterone hypothesis because earlier menarche means an earlier onset of ovulatory cycles. The interaction of estrogen and progesterone on target tissue has been studied mostly in the endometrium, where estrogen clearly stimulates cell growth and progesterone inhibits this estrogen effect. However, there is evidence that progesterone exerts an effect on breast epithelial proliferation similar to its effect on the endometrium.[368–371] With human breast cancer cells, progestins inhibit growth and stimulate differentiation.[372]

Which Hypothesis Is Correct? The hormonal sensitivity of breast cancer appears to be unquestionable, but whether estrogen or progesterone plays a key role is not certain. And perhaps, it is a unique exposure to a combination of factors that is pivotal. Both the estrogen hypothesis and the progesterone hypothesis continue to fuel the debate over these issues. There are specific areas in our clinical experience, however, which are relevant to this consideration.

Pregnancy and Breast Cancer. At one point in time, it was believed that pregnancy (and its impressive levels of estrogens and progesterone) had an adverse impact on the prognosis of breast cancer diagnosed during the pregnancy. It is now believed that there is no difference in survival when pregnant women with breast cancer are matched to nonpregnant women by age and stage of disease, and termination of pregnancy is not associated with improved survival.[373, 374] Pregnant women do have a 2.5-fold higher risk of metastatic disease, but the reason is later diagnosis because the breast changes associated with pregnancy make diagnosis difficult. As with other premenopausal patients, most breast cancers in pregnant women are receptor-negative tumors.[374] Thus, it can be argued that the intense hormonal stimulation of pregnancy (both estrogen and progesterone) has no adverse impact on the course of breast cancer. However, studies do indicate an impact of pregnancy on the risk of subsequent breast cancer. A very large case-control study concluded that pregnancy transiently increases the risk (perhaps for up to 3 years) after a woman's first childbirth, and this is followed by a lifetime reduction in risk.[375] And some have found that a concurrent or recent pregnancy (3–4 years previously) adversely affects survival (even after adjustment for size of tumor and number of nodes).[376] It is argued that breast cells which have already begun malignant transformation are adversely affected (acceleration of growth) by the hormones of pregnancy, whereas normal stem cells become more resistant because of a pregnancy.

Breast Cancer and Subsequent Pregnancy. As with breast cancer diagnosed in already pregnant women, subsequent pregnancy, after diagnosis and treatment, has had no negative impact on prognosis.[377] This, too, would argue against an impact of hormonal stimulation on the risk of recurrent or new disease. But all studies on this subject are retrospective and limited by small numbers. The apparent lack of an adverse impact could be because it is the healthier patients who get pregnant.[378] However, after adjustments for factors that could produce a selection bias, an adverse effect of pregnancy on outcome after breast cancer treatment was still not apparent.[379]

Oral Contraception and the Risk of Breast Cancer. The experience with oral contraceptives over the last 30 years has provided neither definitive evidence that exogenous estrogen and progestin increase the risk of premenopausal breast cancer, nor evidence that exposure to these exogenous hormones offers major protection against breast cancer (Chapter 22). The lack of a major detrimental effect is an effective argument against a major link between breast cancer and exogenous hormone treatment.

Depo-Provera and the Risk of Breast Cancer. Medroxyprogesterone acetate, in large continuous doses, produced breast tumors in beagle dogs. This is an effect unique to the dog (perhaps because in dogs progestins stimulate growth hormone secretion, known to be a mammotrophic agent in dogs) and has not appeared in other animals or in women after years of use. A very large, hospital-based case-control World Health Organization study conducted over 9 years in 3 developing countries has indicated that exposure to Depo-Provera very slightly increased the risk of breast cancer in the first 4 years of use, but there was no evidence for an increase in risk with increased duration of use.[380] The number of cases in the recent use group was not large, and the confidence intervals reflected this. For example, the relative risk for recent users (based on a total of 19 cases) was 1.21, but the confidence interval included 1.0 and, thus, was not statistically significant.

Two earlier population-based case-control studies indicated a possible association between breast cancer and Depo-Provera. One, from Costa Rica, was based on only 19 cases.[381] The other, from New Zealand, did not find an increased relative risk in ever users but did find an indication of increased risk shortly after initiating use in early age (less than age 25).[382] A pooled analysis of the WHO and New Zealand data indicated that the highest risk was in women who had received a single injection.[383]

Certainly the risk, if real, is very slight, and it is equally possible that the suggestions of increased risk have not been free of confounding variables. The results can be interpreted to suggest that the growth of already existing tumors is accelerated. *It is appropriate to emphasize that these studies did not find evidence for an overall increased risk of breast cancer, and the risk did not increase with duration of use.* Thus, experience with exposure to a pure progestational agent does not support the argument that progestational influence will increase the risk of breast cancer; however, this experience reflects the use of very pharmacologic doses of this progestin.

Postmenopausal Hormone Therapy and the Risk of Recurrent Breast Cancer

The argument that postmenopausal hormone therapy should not be given to women who have had breast cancer is a reasonable one. It is based on the recognition of a large body of evidence that indicates that breast cancer is a hormone-responsive tumor. The overriding fear of many clinicians (and patients) is that metastatic cells are present (perhaps being controlled by various host defense factors) that will be susceptible to stimulation by exogenous hormones.[384] However, many women who have had breast cancer are aware of the benefits of postmenopausal hormone treatment (especially protection against cardiovascular disease and osteoporosis) and are asking clinicians to help make this risk-benefit decision. In addition, some women suffer from such severe hot flushing and vaginal dryness that they are willing to consider hormonal treatment. Indeed, estrogen deficiency symptoms are the most common complaints associated with the treatment of breast cancer.[385] Because of the current lack of epidemiologic data, both sides of this debate are strongly influenced by theoretical considerations and clinical experiences, which, unfortunately, often become an obstacle to the patient's own informed choice.

There are reassuring reports that breast cancer survivors using hormone therapy do not experience an obvious increase in recurrent disease. There is a small series in which a combination of 0.625 conjugated estrogens and 0.15 mg norgestrel was given continuously for a short period of time (a maximum of 6 months) to women who had been previously treated for breast cancer.[386] Over the next two years, no patients developed recurrence. Another small series (25 and then 77 women with breast cancer ranging from in situ to stage III disease) received estrogen-progestin therapy for 24 to 82 months; the recurrence rate was not greater than that expected.[387, 388] From this group of patients, 41 breast cancer survivors receiving hormone therapy had the same outcomes when compared with 82 women selected from a cancer registry and not taking hormones.[389] In a report from Australia, 152 women with a history of breast cancer who were given a combination of estrogen and progestin had lower mortality and recurrence rates; however, the dose of progestin was very high (which in itself can be therapeutic) and treatment was not randomized.[390] In a follow-up of 49 women treated with estrogen after treatment for localized breast cancer, only one patient developed recurrent disease.[391] And in another series of 114 women, hormone treatment of disease-free patients was associated with a low rate of recurrence.[392] These patients had both positive and negative nodes and estrogen receptor status. *Although it is reassuring that the results conform to an incidence of recurrent disease no greater than expected, the outcomes may reflect biases in clinician and patient decision making that can only be overcome with a proper long-term, randomized clinical trial.*

A clinical U.S. trial is currently under way, providing estrogen to randomized women who have been treated for stage I or II breast cancer, who have been disease-free for at least 2 years from estrogen receptor negative disease or 10 years if the estrogen receptor status is unknown.[393] Other randomized trials of hormone therapy after breast cancer treatment are underway in Europe; for example, the HABITS study in Sweden.

Because of better treatment and earlier diagnosis, 50–75% of women diagnosed with breast cancer are now cured.[394] Of 100 patients with breast cancer, about 60 will be cured by mastectomy or breast-conserving surgery with radiotherapy and would receive no benefit from adjuvant treatment. Is this group safe for hormone therapy? Of the remaining 40, some will live longer (an average of 2–3 years) because of adjuvant treatment, but only a few. Is the unknown risk with exogenous hormone treatment worth it in this group? Although intuitively it seems that the risk:benefit ratio would be more favorable in the presence of negative nodes, negative receptors, and small tumors, are negative estrogen and progesterone receptor assessments sufficient to conclude that the cancer is not sensitive to hormones? And if the patient is in the high-cure category, does it make any difference what the receptor status is? Receptor status is not absolute; it is always a relative measure. The answers to all of these questions are not known.

Patients and clinicians have to incorporate all of the above considerations into this medical decision. But when all is said and done, patients have to take an unknown risk if they want the benefits of hormone treatment, and clinicians have to take an unknown medical-legal risk. Some patients will choose to take hormones, judging the benefits to be worth the unknown risk. Physicians should support patients in this decision. Other patients will prefer to avoid any unknown risks. These patients, too, deserve support in their decision. Until data are available from appropriate clinical trials, there is no right or wrong decision.

Women With Cardiovascular Disease

Is the woman with a previous history of a cardiovascular event, such as a myocardial infarction or stroke, the very woman who needs the protection of estrogen against cardiovascular disease? There is evidence to support this contention. In the Leisure World study, estrogen users with previous myocardial infarctions, strokes, or hypertension had a 50% reduction in risk for death from a subsequent stroke or myocardial infarction.[43] In the Lipids Research Clinics study, the cardiovascular mortality in women with previous cardiovascular disease was reduced 85%. And most impressively, in women with severe coronary disease (documented by arteriography), estrogen users had a 97% survival rate at 5 years compared with a significantly different 81% rate in nonusers.[395] In women with mild to moderate disease, there was no difference at 5 years, but at 10 years, estrogen users had a 96% survival rate compared with 85% in nonusers.

Estrogen therapy reduces the rate of restenosis in women who have undergone either coronary angioplasty or percutaneous atherectomy.[396] In women who have undergone coronary artery bypass surgery, the 10-year survival rate in estrogen users was 81.4% compared with 65.1% in nonusers.[397] In women who have been treated with estrogen after coronary angioplasty, case-control analysis indicated that the treated women had a better survival rate and experienced fewer subsequent myocardial infarctions.[398] The number of patients on estrogen-progestin was too small in this study for analysis. A retrospective cohort study in Seattle determined prognosis in women surviving a myocardial infarction and detected a 36% reduced risk of re-infarction in current estrogen users, although small numbers prevented the achievement of statistical significance.[399] These studies all indicate reduced risks for adverse clinical events and support the use of postmenopausal hormone therapy in women with coronary heart disease. Furthermore, hormone therapy can improve the state of atherosclerosis; i.e., produce a regression in disease.

Imaging studies have documented a reduction in intimal thickening in postmenopausal women who are estrogen users compared with nonusers, and this beneficial effect is not compromised by the addition of a progestational agent to the treatment regimen.[400, 401] Thus, postmenopausal hormonal therapy can bring about a reduction in atherosclerosis, and this effect is comparable with that produced by a lipid-lowering drug.[400, 402]

The results of the Heart and Estrogen/progestin Replacement Study (HERS), discussed in detail in Chapter 17, are contrary to the many observations reviewed above.[239] However, the inconsistencies with previous biologic studies, concerns regarding the statistical power of HERS, and the disagreement with an impressively large number of observational studies mean that the HERS results are not definitive. Decision making will be easier as the results of more clinical trials become available. Until then, in our opinion, estrogen treatment with the appropriate, standard dose is indicated and safe for patients with cardiovascular disease. We should emphasize, however, that excellent preventive results are obtained with the usual armamentarium of drugs employed by cardiologists for the treatment of coronary heart disease.

In a short-term, randomized, crossover clinical trial, combined conjugated estrogens and medroxyprogesterone acetate raised HDL-cholesterol equally well as simvastatin in women with hypercholesterolemia.[403] Simvastatin achieved a greater reduction in LDL-cholesterol and no effect on lipoprotein(a) and triglyceride levels, while hormone therapy produced a decrease in lipoprotein(a) and an increase in triglycerides. The hormonal effects were even greater in women who had abnormal lipids or atherosclerosis. Thus, both treatments produce beneficial effects, and it is not known whether the differences are clinically important.

The dose of estrogen is very important because it is becoming increasingly apparent that the beneficial cardiovascular effects of estrogen are restricted to a relatively narrow therapeutic window; the benefits may be reduced at doses of estrogen greater than that equivalent to 0.625 mg conjugated estrogens. The HERS results combined with experimental data derived from monkeys (see Chapter 17) make it reasonable to use other progestins than medroxyprogesterone acetate in women with coronary heart disease.

Women With Diabetes Mellitus

A strong argument can be made that postmenopausal women with diabetes mellitus can benefit from the cardioprotective actions of estrogen. In addition, estrogen may improve the metabolic changes associated with diabetes. Indeed, in prospective studies of postmenopausal women with noninsulin-dependent diabetes mellitus, estrogen treatment improved all glucose metabolic parameters, including insulin resistance, the lipoprotein profile, and measurements of androgenicity.[404, 405] These changes should reduce the risk of cardiovascular disease; however, long-term studies are yet to be available. Tibolone also has a beneficial impact in short-term studies on insulin resistance in normal women and in women with noninsulin-dependent diabetes mellitus.[208, 209]

Women With Liver Disease

Osteoporosis is a major consequence of chronic liver disease. Although other bone-preserving agents can be utilized, none provides the multisystem benefits associated with estrogen therapy. In an evaluation of liver chemistries in a group of patients with primary biliary cirrhosis, standard hormone therapy doses produced no adverse changes over a period of one year.[406] We recommend measurement of liver chemistries after one month of treatment, and every 6 months, with continuing hormone therapy in the absence of deterioration.

The Vaginal Administration of Estrogen

Many clinicians believe that estrogen administered intravaginally is not absorbed, and systemic effects can be avoided. However, estrogen is absorbed very readily from a vagina with immature, atrophic mucosa.[407] Indeed the initial absorption is rapid, and relatively high circulating levels of estrogen are easily reached. As the vaginal mucosa cornifies, absorption decreases.[408] This decline takes approximately 3–4 months, after which lesser, but still significant absorption takes place. European studies have demonstrated that vaginal maturation can be achieved with a vaginal ring (which is left in place for 3 months) having incredibly small doses of estrogen, with a low-level of systemic absorption. [409, 410] This is an acceptable method to relieve atrophic vaginal symptoms in women with contraindications to estrogen treatment.

Other Conditions

Close surveillance is indicated for some patients with seizure disorders, familial hyperlipidemias (elevated triglycerides), and migraine headaches. Patients with migraine headaches often improve if a daily, continuous method of treatment is used, eliminating a cyclic change in hormone levels that can serve to trigger headaches.

Conditions that do not represent contraindications include controlled hypertension, diabetes mellitus, smoking, and varicose veins. The belief that estrogen is potentially harmful with each of these clinical situations is derived from old studies of high-dose oral contraceptives. Estrogenn appropriate doses is acceptable in the presence of these conditions.

No other cancers (besides those mentioned above) are known to be adversely affected by hormone therapy. Postmenopausal hormone therapy can be administered to all patients with cervical, ovarian, or vulvar malignancies.

Unusual anecdotal reports include the following:

1. Provocation of chorea by estrogen therapy in a woman with a history of Sydenham's chorea.[411]

2. Exacerbation of pulmonary leiomyomatosis by estrogen therapy.[412]

3. Psychiatric symptoms in response to estrogen in patients with acute intermittent porphyria.[413]

4. Idiosyncratic ocular symptoms associated with estrogen.[414]

5. An infection with *Trichomonas vaginalis* resolved after discontinuation of estrogen-prostin therapy.[415]

Conclusion

We hope we have convinced you that the menopause is a normal life event, not a disease, and that long-term postmenopausal hormone therapy is pharmacologic treatment to obtain preventive health care benefits. We have learned this from the women who revealed what they believe and what they know in the longitudinal studies of the last decade. It only makes sense that trying to convince a woman she has a disease, when she does not believe it, will have a negative impact on the clinician–patient relationship. In addition, w believe our approach yields more willful and stronger decision making that ultimately produces better continuation rates with treatment. Postmenopausal hormone therapy is an option that should be offered to most women as they consider their paths for successful aging, but the attitude and beliefs of the clinician have a major influence on the decisions made by patients. As beneficial as the impact of hormonal therapy may be, we must also emphasize the large improvement in health to be gained by lifestyle changes in smoking cessation, regular exercise, and control of body weight.

References

1. **Medvei VC,** *The History of Clinical Endocrinology,* The Parthenon Publishing Group, New York, 1993.

2. **O'Dowd MJ, Philipp EE,** *The History of Obstetrics and Gynaecology,* The Parthenon Publishing Group, New York, 1994.

3. **Speert H,** *Obstetric & Gynecologic Milestones Illustrated,* The Parthenon Publishing Group, New York, 1996.

4. **Fosbery WHS,** Severe climacteric flushings successfully treated by ovarian extract, *Br Med J* i:1039, 1897.

5. **Servinghaus EL, Evans J,** Clinical observations on the use of an ovarian hormone: amniotin, *Am J Sci* 178:638, 1929.

6. **Harding FE,** The oral treatment of ovarian deficiency with conjugated estrogens — Equine, *West J Surg Obstet Gynecol* 52:31, 1944.

7. **Brett KM, Madans JH,** Use of postmenopausal hormone replacement therapy: estimates from a nationally representative cohort study, *Am J Epidemiol* 145:536, 1997.

8. **Riis BJ, Hansen MA, Jensen AM, Overgaard K, Christiansen C,** Low bone mass and fast rate of bone loss at menopause: equal risk factors for future fracture: a 15-year follow-up study, *Bone* 19:9, 1996.

9. **Theitz G, Buch B, Rizzoli R, Slosman D, Clavien H, Sizonko PC, Bonjour JPH,** Longitudinal monitoring of bone mass accumulation in healthy adolescents: evidence for a marked reduction after 16 years of age at the levels of lumbar spine and femoral neck in female subjects, *J Clin Endocrinol Metab* 75:1060, 1992.

10. **Matkovic V, Jelic T, Wardlaw GM, Ilich J, Goel PK, Wright JK, Andon MB, Smith KT, Heaney RP,** Timing of peak bone mass in caucasian females and its implication for the prevention of osteoporosis: inference from a cross-sectional model, *J Clin Invest* 93:799, 1994.

11. **Recker RR, Davies KM, Hinders SM, Heaney RP, Stegman MR, Kimmel DB,** Bone gain in young women, *JAMA* 268:2403, 1992.

12. **Lindsay R, Hart DM, Clark DM,** The minimum effective dose of estrogen for postmenopausal bone loss, *Obstet Gynecol* 63:759, 1984.

13. **Genant HK, Cann CE, Ettinger B, Gordan GS,** Quantitative computed tomography of vertebral spongiosa: a sensitive method for detecting early bone loss after oophorectomy, *Ann Intern Med* 97:699, 1982.

14. **Mashchak CA, Lobo RA, Dozono-Takano R, Eggena P, Nakamura RM, Brenner PF, Mishell Jr DR,** Comparison of pharmacodynamic properties of various estrogen formulations, *Am J Obstet Gynecol* 144:511, 1982.

15. **Horsman A, Jones M, Francis R, Nordin C,** The effect of estrogen dose on postmenopausal bone loss, *New Engl J Med* 309:1405, 1983.

16. **Field CS, Ory SJ, Wahner HW, Herrmann RR, Judd HL, Riggs BL,** Preventive effects of transdermal 17β-estradiol on osteoporotic changes at surgical menopause: a two-year placebo-controlled trial, *Am J Obstet Gynecol* 168:114, 1993.

17. **Goebelsmann U, Mashchak CA, Mishell Jr DR,** Comparison of hepatic impact of oral and vaginal administration of ethinyl estradiol, *Am J Obstet Gynecol* 151:868, 1985.

18. **Genant HK, Baylink DJ, Gallagher JC, Harris ST, Steiger P, Herber M,** Effect of estrone sulphate on postmenopausal bone loss, *Obstet Gynecol* 76:579, 1990.

19. **Lindsay R, Hart DM, MacLean A, Garwood J, Clarkel AC, Kraszewski A,** Bone loss during oestriol therapy in postmenopausal women, *Maturitas* 1:279, 1979.

20. **Devogelaer JP, Lecart C, Dupret P, De Nayer P, Nagant De Deuxchaisnes C,** Long-term effects of percutaneous estradiol on bone loss and bone metabolism in postmenopausal hysterectomized women, *Maturitas* 28:243, 1998.

21. **Katzenellenbogen BS,** Biology and receptor interactions of estriol and estriol derivatives in vitro and in vivo, *J Steriod Biochem* 20:1033, 1984.

22. **Lemon HM,** Estriol prevention of mammary carcinoma induced by 7,12-dimethylbenz(a)anthracene, *Cancer Res* 35:1341, 1975.

23. **Melamed M, Castraño E, Notides AC, Sasson S,** Molecular and kinetic basis for the mixed agonist/antagonist activity of estriol, *Mol Endocrinol* 11:1868, 1997.

24. **Dusteberg S, Nishino Y,** Pharmacokinetic and pharmacological features of oestradiol valerate, *Maturitas* 4:315, 1982.

25. **Ross D, Rees M, Godfree V, Cooper A, Hart D, Kingsland C, Whitehead M,** Randomised crossover comparison of skin irritation with two transdermal oestradiol patches, *Br Med J* 315:288, 1997.

26. **Bhathena RK, Anklesaria BS, Ganatra AM,** Skin reactions with transdermal estradiol therapy in a tropical environment, *Int J Gynecol Obstet* 60:177, 1998.

27. **Kuhl H,** Pharmacokinetics of oestrogens and progestogens, *Maturitas* 12:171, 1990.

28. **Colvin Jr PL, Auerbach BJ, Koritnik DR, Hazzard WR, Applebaum-Bowden D,** Differential effects of oral estrogen versus 17β-estradiol on lipoproteins in postmenopausal women, *J Clin Endocrinol Metab* 70:1568, 1990.

29. **Walsh BW, Li H, Sacks FM,** Effects of postmenopausal hormone replacement with oral and transdermal estrogen on high density lipoprotein metabolism, *J Lipid Res* 35:2083, 1994.

30. **Pang SC, Greendale GA, Cedars MI, Gambone JC, Lozano K, Eggena P, Judd HL,** Long-term effects of transdermal estradiol with and without medroxyprogesterone acetate, *Fertil Steril* 59:76, 1993.

31. **Hillard TC, Whicroft SJ, Marsh MS, Ellerington MC, Lees B, Whitehead MI, Stevenson JC,** Long-term effects of transdermal and oral hormone replacement therapy on postmenopausal bone loss, *Osteoporosis Int* 4:341, 1994.

32. **Lufkin EG, Wahner HW, O'Fallon WM, Hodgson SF, Kotowicz MA, Lane AW, Judd HL, Caplan RH, Riggs BL,** Treatment of postmenopausal osteoporosis with transdermal estrogen, *Ann Intern Med* 117:1, 1992.

33. **Michaësson K, Baron JA, Farahmand BY, Johnell O, Magnusson C, Persson P-G, Persson I, Ljunghall S, on behalf of the Swedish Hip Fracture Study Group,** Hormone replacement therapy and risk of hip fracture: population based case-control study, *Br Med J* 316:1858, 1998.

34. **Lobo R, March CM, Goebelsmann U, Krauss RM, Mishell Jr DR,** Subdermal estradiol pellets following hysterectomy and oophorectomy, *Am J Obstet Gynecol* 138:714, 1980.

35. **Dupont A, Dupont P, Cusan L, Tremblay M, Rioux J, Cloutier D, Mailloux J, De Lignieres B, Gutkowska J, Boucher H, Belanger A, Moyer DL, Moorjani S, Labrie F,** Comparative endocrinological and clinical effects of percutaneous estadiol and oral conjugated estrogens as replacement therapy in menopausal women, *Maturitas* 13:297, 1991.

36. **Walters KA, Brain KR, Green DM, James VJ, Watkinson AC, Sands RH,** Comparison of the transdermal delivery of estradiol from two gel formulations, *Maturitas* 29:189, 1998.

37. **Pines A, Fishman EZ, Ayalon D, Drory Y, Averbuch M, Levo Y,** Long-term effects of hormone replacement therapy on Doppler-derived parameters of aortic flow in postmenopausal women, *Chest* 102:1496, 1992.

38. **Pines A, Fisman EZ, Averbuch M, Drory Y, Motro M, Levo Y, et al,** The long-term effects of transdermal estradiol on left ventricular function and dimensions, *Eur J Menopause* 2:22, 1995.

39. **Pines A, Fisman EZ, Shapira I, Drory Y, Weiss A, Eckstein N, Levo Y, Averbuch M, Motro M, Rotmensch HH, Ayalon D,** Exercise echocardiography in postmenopausal hormone users with mild hypertension, *Am J Cardiol* 78:1385, 1996.

40. **Pines A, Fisman EZ, Drory Y, Shapira I, Averbuch M, Eckstein N, Motro M, Levo Y, Ayalon D,** The effects of sublingual estradiol on left ventricular action at rest and exercise in postmenopausal women: an echocardiographic assessment, *Menopause* 5:79, 1998.

41. **Lindheim S, Presser S, Ditkoff E, Vijod M, Stanczyk F, Lobo R,** A possible bimodal effect of estrogen on insulin sensitivity in postmenopausal women and the attenuating effect of added progestin, *Fertil Steril* 60:664, 1993.

42. **Stampfer MJ, Colditz GA, Willett WC, Manson JE, Rosner B, Speizer FE, Hennekens CH,** Postmenopausal estrogen therapy and cardiovascular disease: ten-year follow-up from the Nurses' Health Study, *New Engl J Med* 325:756, 1991.

43. **Henderson BE, Paganini-Hill A, Ross RK,** Decreased mortality in users of estrogen replacement therapy, *Arch Intern Med* 151:75, 1991.

44. **Ettinger B, Friedman GD, Bush T, Quesenberry Jr CP,** Reduced mortality associated with long-term postmenopausal estrogen therapy, *Obstet Gynecol* 87:5, 1996.

45. **Genant HK, Lucas J, Weiss S, Akin M, Emeky R, McNaney-Flint H, Downs R, Mortola J, Watts N, Yank HM, Banav N, Brennan JJ, Nolan JC, for the Estratab/Osteoporosis Study Group,** Low-dose esterified estrogen therapy: effects on bone, plasma estradiol concentrations, endometrium, and lipid levels, *Arch Intern Med* 157:2609, 1997.

46. **Williams JK, Honoré EK, Washburn SA, Clarkson TB,** Effects of hormone replacement therapy on reactivity of atherosclerotic coronary arteries in cynomolgus monkeys, *J Am Coll Cardiol* 24:1757, 1994.

47. **O'Connell MB,** Pharmacokinetic and pharmacologic variation between different estrogen products, *J Clin Pharmacol* 35(Suppl 9):18S, 1995.

48. **Reginster JY, Sarlet N, Deroisy R, Albert A, Gaspard U, Franchimont P,** Minimal levels of serum estradiol prevent postmenopausal bone loss, *Calcif Tissue Int* 51:340, 1992.

49. **Cummings SR, Browner WS, Bauer D, Stone K, Ensrud K, Jamal S, Ettinger B, for the Study of Osteoporotic Fractures Research Group,** Endogenous hormones and the risk of hip and vertebral fractures among older women, *New Engl J Med* 339:733, 1998.

50. **Ettinger B, Pressman A, Sklarin P, Bauer DC, Cauley JA, Cummings SR,** Associations between low levels of serum estradiol, bone density, and fractures among elderly women: The Study of Osteoporotic Fractures, *J Clin Endocrinol Metab* 83:2239, 1998.

51. **Naessen T, Berglund L, Ulmsten U,** Bone loss in elderly women prevented by ultralow doses of parenteral 17beta-estradiol, *Am J Obstet Gynecol* 177:115, 1997.

52. **Ettinger B, Genant HK, Cann CE,** Postmenopausal bone loss is prevented by treatment with low-dosage estrogen with calcium, *Ann Intern Med* 106:40, 1987.

53. **Ettinger B, Genant HK, Steiger P, Madvig P,** Low-dosage micronized 17β-estradiol prevents bone loss in postmenopausal women, *Am J Obstet Gynecol* 166:479, 1992.

54. **Mizunuma H, Okano H, Soda M, Kagami I, Miyamoto S, Tokizawa T, Honjo S, Ibuki Y,** Prevention of postmenopausal bone loss with minimal uterine bleeding using low dose continuous estrogen/progestin therapy: a 2-year prospective study, *Maturitas* 27:69, 1997.

55. **Stevenson JC, Cust MP, Gangar KF, Hillard TC, Lees B, Whitehead MI,** Effects of transdermal versus oral hormone replacement therapy on bone density in spine and proximal femur in postmenopausal women, *Lancet* 336:1327, 1990.

56. **Castelo-Blanco C, de Osaba M, Vanrezc JA, Fortuny A, Gonzáez-Merlo J,** Effects of oophorectomy and hormone replacement therapy on pituitary-gonadal function, *Maturitas* 17:101, 1993.

57. **Woodruff JD, Pickar JH, for The Menopause Study Group,** Incidence of endometrial hyperplasia in postmenopausal women taking conjugated estrogens (Premarin) with medroxyprogesterone acetate or conjugated estrogens alone, *Am J Obstet Gynecol* 170:1213, 1994.

58. **Strickland DM, Hammond TL,** Postmenopausal estrogen replacement in a large gynecologic practice, *Am J Gynecol Health* 2:33, 1988.

59. **Archer DF, Pickar JH, Bottiglioni F, for The Menopause Study Group,** Bleeding patterns in postmenopausal women taking continuous combined or sequential regimens of conjugated estrogens with medroxyprogesterone acetate, *Obstset Gynecol* 83:686, 1994.

60. **The Writing Group for the PEPI Trial,** Effects of estrogen or estrogen/progestin regimens on heart disease risk factors in postmenopausal women: the Postmenopausal Estrogen/Progestin Interventions (PEPI) Trial, *JAMA* 273:199, 1995.

61. **King R, Whitehead M,** Assessment of the potency of orally administered progestins in women, *Fertil Steril* 46:1062, 1986.

62. **Gillet JY, Andre G, Faguer B, Ernyl R, Buvat-Herbaut M, Domin MA, Kuhn MJM, Hedon B, Drapier-Faure E, Barrat J, Lopes P, Magnin G, Leng JJ, Bruhat MA, Philippe E,** Induction of amenorrhea during hormone replacement therapy: optimal micronized progesterone dose. A multicenter study, *Maturitas* 19:103, 1994.

63. **Speroff T, Dawson NV, Speroff L, Harber RJ,** A risk-benefit analysis of elective bilateral oophorectomy: effect of changes in compliance with estrogen therapy on outcome, *Am J Obstet Gynecol* 164:165, 1991.

64. **Berman RS, Epstein RS, Lydick EG,** Compliance of women in taking estrogen replacement therapy, *J Women's Health* 5:213, 1996.

65. **Ravnikar VA,** Compliance with hormonal therapy, *Am J Obstet Gynecol* 156:1332, 1987.

66. **Nand S, Webster MA, Baber R, O'Connor V, for the Ogen/Provera Study Group,** Bleeding pattern and endometrial changes during continuous combined hormone replacement therapy, *Obstet Gynecol* 91:678, 1998.

67. **Andersson K, Mattsson L, Rybo G, Stadberg E,** Intrauterine release of levonorgestrel — a new way of adding progestogen in hormone replacement therapy, *Obstet Gynecol* 79:963, 1992.

68. **Raudaskoski TH, Lahti EI, Kauppila AJ, Apaja-Sarkkinen MA, Laatikainen TJ,** Transdermal estrogen with a levonorgestrel-releasing intrauterine device for climacteric complaints: clinical and endometrial responses, *Am J Obstet Gynecol* 172:114, 1995.

69. **Archer DF, McIntyre-Seltman K, Wilborn WH, Dowling EA, Cone F, Creasy GW, Kafrissen ME,** Endometrial morphology in asymptomatic postmenopausal women, *Am J Obstet Gynecol* 165:317, 1991.

70. **Korhonen MO, Symons JP, Hyde BM, Rowan JP, Wilborn WH,** Histologic classification and pathologic findings for endometrial biopsy specimens obtained from 2964 perimenopausal and postmenopausal women undergoing screening for continuous hormones as replacement therapy (CHART 2 Study), *Am J Obstet Gynecol* 176:377, 1997.

71. **Feldman S, Shapter A, Welch WR, Berkowitz RS,** Two-year follow-up of 263 patients with post/perimenopausal vaginal bleeding and negative initial biopsy, *Gynecol Oncol* 55:56, 1994.

72. **McGonigle KF, Karlan BY, Barbuto DA, Leuchter RS, Lagasse LD, Judd HL,** Development of endometrial cancer in women on estrogen and progestin hormone replacement therapy, *Gynecol Oncol* 55:126, 1994.

73. **Beresford SA, Weiss NS, Voigt LF, McKnight B,** Risk of endometrial cancer in relation to use of oestrogen combined with cyclic progestagen therapy in postmenopausal women, *Lancet* 349:458, 1997.

74. **Padwick ML, Psryse-Davies J, Whitehead MI,** A simple method for determining the optimal dosage of progestin in post-menopausal women receiving estrogens, *New Engl J Med* 315:930, 1986.

75. **Sturdee DW, Barlow DH, Ulrich LG, Wells M, Gydesen H, Campbell M, O'Brien K, Vessey M, for the UK Continuous Combined HRT Study Investigators,** Is the timing of with-drawal bleeding a guide to endometrial safety during sequential oestrogen-progestagen replacement therapy? *Lancet* 344:979, 1994.

76. **Langer RD, Pierce JJ, O'Hanlan KA, Johnson SR, Espeland MA, Trabal JF, Barnabei VM, Merino MJ, Scully RE, for the Postmenopausal Estrogen/Progestin Interventions Trial,** Transvaginal ultrasonography compared with endometrial biopsy for the detection of endometrial disease, *New Engl J Med* 337:1792, 1997.

77. **Botsis D, Kassanos D, Pyrgiotis E, Zourlas PA,** Vaginal sonography of the endometrium in postmenopausal women, *Clin Exp Obstet Gynecol* 19:189, 1992.

78. **Karlsson B, Granberg S, Wikland M, Yl"stal P, Torvid K, Marsal K, Valentin L,** Transvaginal ultrasonography of the endometrium in women with postmenopausal bleeding — A Nor-dic multicenter study, *Am J Obstet Gynecol* 172:1488, 1995.

79. **Hänggi W, Bersinger N, Altermatt HJ, Birkhäuser MH,** Com-parison of transvaginal ultrasonography and endometrial biopsy in endometrial surveillance in postmenopausal HRT users, *Maturitas* 27:133, 1997.

80. **Bakos O, Smith P, Heimer G,** Transvaginal ultrasonography for identifying endometrial pathology in postmenopausal women, *Maturitas* 20:181, 1995.

81. **Granberg S, Ylöstalo P, Wikland M, Karlsson B,** Endometrial sonographic and histologic findings in women with and without hormonal replacement therapy suffering from postmenopausal bleeding, *Maturitas* 27:35, 1997.

82. **Levine D, Gosink BB, Johnson LA,** Change in endometrial thickness in postmenopausal women undergoing hormone re-placement therapy, *Radiology* 197:603, 1995.

83. **Goldstein SR, Zeltser I, Horan CK, Snyder JR, Schwartz LB,** Ultrasonography-based triage for perimenopausal patients with abnormal uterine bleeding, *Am J Obstet Gynecol* 177:102, 1997.

84. **Sladkevicius P, Valentin L, Marsal K,** Endometrial thickness and Doppler velocimetry of the uterine arteries as discriminators of endometrial status in women with postmenopausal bleeding: a comparative study, *Am J Obstet Gynecol* 171:722, 1994.

85. **Conoscenti G, Meir YJ, Fischer-Tamaro L, Maieron A, Natale R, D'Ottavio G, Rustico M, Mandruzzato G,** Endometrial as-sessment by transvaginal sonography and histological findings after D & C in women with postmenopausal bleeding, *Ultrasound Obstet Gynecol* 6:108, 1995.

86. **Gambrell Jr RD, Massey FM, Castaneda TA, Ugenas AJ, Ricci A, Wright JM,** Use of the progestogen challenge test to reduce the risk of endometrial cancer, *Obstet Gynecol* 55:732, 1980.

87. **Hanna JH, Brady WK, Hill JM, Phillips Jr GL,** Detection of postmenopausal women at risk for endometrial carcinoma by a progesterone challenge test, *Am J Obstet Gynecol* 147:872, 1983.

88. **Toppozada MK, Ismail AAA, Hamed RSM, Ahmed KS, El-Faras A,** Progesterone challenge test and estrogen assays in menopausal women with endometrial adenomatous hyperplasia, *Int J Gynecol Obstet* 26:115, 1988.

89. **El-Maraghy MA, El-Badawy N, Wafa GA, Bishai N,** Proges-terone challenge test in postmenopausal women at high risk, *Maturitas* 19:53, 1994.

90. **Bortoletto CCR, Baracat EC, Gonçalves WJ, Lima GR, Stávale JN,** Transvaginal ultrasonography and the progestogen challenge test in postmenopausal endometrial evaluation, *Int J Gynecol Obstet* 58:293, 1997.

91. **Kirkham C, Hahn PM, Van Vugtl DA, Carmichael JA, Reid RL,** A randomized, double-blind, placebo-controlled, cross-over trial to assess the side effects of medroxyprogesterone acetate in hormone replacement therapy, *Obstet Gynecol* 78:93, 1991.

92. **Prior JC, Alojado N, McKay DW, Vigna YM,** No adverse effects of medroxyprogesterone treatment without estrogen in postmenopausal women: double-blind, placebo-controlled, cross-over trial, *Obstet Gynecol* 83:24, 1994.

93. **Ettinger B, Selby J, Citron JT, Vangessel A, Ettinger V, Hendrickson MR,** Cyclic hormone replacement therapy using quarterly progestin, *Obstet Gynecol* 83:693, 1994.

94. **Williams DB, Voigt BJ, Fu YS, Schoenfeld MJ, Judd HL,** Assessment of less than monthly progestin therapy in postmeno-pausal women given estrogen replacement, *Obstet Gynecol* 84:787, 1994.

95. **Hirvonen E, Salmi T, Puolakka J, Heikkinen J, Granfors E, Hulkko S, Mäkäräinen L, Nummi S, Pekonen F, Rautio A-M, Sundström H, Telimaa S, Wilen-Rosenqvist G, Virkkunen A, Wahlström T,** Can progestin be limited to every third month only in postmenopausal women taking estrogen? *Maturitas* 21:39, 1995.

96. **Cerin A, Heldaas K, Moeller B,** Adverse endometrial effects of long-cycle estrogen and progestogen replacement therapy. The Scandinavian LongCycle Study Group (Letter), *New Engl J Med* 334:668, 1996.

97. **Miles RA, Press MF, Paulson RJ, Dahmoush L, Lobo RA, Sauer MV,** Pharmacokinetics and endometrial tissue levels of progesterone after administration by intramuscular and vaginal routes: a comparative study, *Fertil Steril* 62:485, 1994.

98. **Ross D, Cooper AJ, Pryse-Davies J, Bergeron C, Collins WP, Whitehead MI,** Randomized, double-blind, dose-ranging study of the endometrial effects of a vaginal progesterone gel in estro-gen-treated postmenopausal women, *Am J Obstet Gynecol* 177:937, 1997.

99. **Andersson J, Rybo G,** Levonorgestrel-releasing intrauterine de-vice in the treatment of menorrhagia, *Br J Obstet Gynaecol* 97:690, 1990.

100. **Wollter-Svensson LO, Stadberg E, Andersson K, Mattsson LA, Odlind V, Persson I,** Intrauterine administration of levonorgestrel 5 and 10 microg/24 hours in perimenopausal hor-mone replacement therapy. A randomized clinical study during one year, *Acta Obstet Gynecol Scand* 76:449, 1997.

101. **Wollter-Svenson L-O, Stadberg E, Andersson K, Mattsson L-Å, Odlind V, Persson I,** Intrauterine administration of levonorgestrel in two low doses in HRT. A randomized clinical trial during one year: effects on lipid and lipoprotein metabolism, *Maturitas* 22:199, 1995.

102. **Heaps JM, Nieberg RK, Berek JS,** Malignant neoplasms arising in endometriosis, *Obstet Gynecol* 75:1023, 1990.

103. **Reimnitz C, Brand E, Nieberg RK, Hacker NF,** Malignancy arising in endometriosis associated with unopposed estrogen re-placement, *Obstet Gynecol* 71:444, 1988.

104. **Gucer F, Pieber D, Arikan MG,** Malignancy arising in extraovarian endometriosis during estrogen stimulation, *Eur J Gynaecol Oncol* 19:39, 1998.

105. **Duun S, Roed-Petersen K, Michelsen JW,** Endometrioid carcinoma arising from endometriosis of the sigmoid colon during estrogenic treatment, *Acta Obstet Gynecol Scand* 72:676, 1993.

106. **Istre O, Holm-Nielsen P, Bourne T, Forman A,** Hormone replacement therapy after transcervical resection of the endometrium, *Obstet Gynecol* 88:767, 1996.

107. **Iqbal PK, Paterson MEL,** Case report: endometrial carcinoma after endometrial resection for menorrhagia, *Br J Obstet Gynaecol* 104:1097, 1997.

108. **Lee RB, Burke TW, Park RC,** Estrogen replacement therapy following treatment for stage 1 endometrial carcinoma, *Gynecol Oncol* 36:189, 1990.

109. **Baker DP,** Estrogen-replacement therapy in patients with previous endometrial carcinoma, *Compr Ther* 16:28, 1990.

110. **Creasman WT,** Estrogen replacement therapy: Is previously treated cancer a contraindication? *Obstet Gynecol* 77:308, 1991.

111. **Chapman JA, DiSaia PJ, Osann K, Roth PD, Gillotte DL, Berman ML,** Estrogen replacement in surgical stage I and II endometrial cancer survivors, *Am J Obstet Gynecol* 175:1195, 1996.

112. **McMeekin DS, Burger RA, Manetta A, DiSaia P, Berman M,** Endometrioid adenocarcinoma of the ovary and its relationship to endometriosis, *Gynecol Oncol* 59:81, 1995.

113. **Speroff L, Rowan J, Symons J, Genant H, Wilborn W, for the CHART Study Group,** The comparative effect on bone density, endometrium, and lipids of continuous hormones as replacement therapy (CHART Study), *JAMA* 276:1397, 1996.

114. **Gallagher JC, Kable WT, Goldgar D,** Effect of progestin therapy on cortical and trabecular bone: comparison with estrogen, *Am J Med* 90:171, 1991.

115. **Grey A, Cundy T, Evans M, Reid I,** Medroxyprogesterone acetate enhances the spinal bone mineral density response to oestrogen in late post-menopausal women, *Clin Endocrinol* 44:293, 1996.

116. **Adachi JD, Sargeant EJ, Sagle MA, Lamont D, Fawcett PD, Bensen WG, McQueen M, Nazir DJ, Goldsmith CH,** A double-blind randomised controlled trial of the effects of medroxyprogesterone acetate on bone density of women taking oestrogen replacement therapy, *Br J Obstet Gynaecol* 104:64, 1997.

117. **Meldrum DR, Davidson BJ, Tataryn IV, Judd HL,** Changes in circulating steroids with aging in postmenopausal women, *Obstet Gynecol* 57:624, 1981.

118. **Sherwin BB, Gelfand MM,** The role of androgen in the maintenance of sexual functioning in oophorectomized women, *Psychosom Med* 49:397, 1987.

119. **Myers LS, Dixen J, Morrissette D, Carmichael M, Davidson JM,** Effects of estrogen, androgen, and progestin on sexual psychophysiology and behavior in postmenopausal women, *J Clin Endocrinol Metab* 70:1124, 1990.

120. **Hickok LR, Toomey C, Speroff L,** A comparison of esterified estrogens with and without methyltestosterone: effects on endometrial histology and serum lipoproteins in postmenopausal women, *Obstet Gynecol* 82:919, 1993.

121. **Watts NB, Notelovitz M, Timmons MC, Addison WA, Wiita B, Downey LJ,** Comparison of oral estrogens and estrogens plus androgens on bone mineral density, menopausal symptoms, and lipid-lipoprotein profiles in surgical menopause, *Obstet Gynecol* 85:529, 1995.

122. **Barrett-Connor E, Timmons C, Young R, Witta B, and the Estratest Working Group,** Interim safety analysis of a two-year study comparing oral estrogen-androgen and conjugated estrogens in surgically menopausal women, *J Women's Health* 5:593, 1996.

123. **Davis SR, McCloud P, Strauss BJG, Burger H,** Testosterone enhances estradiol's effects on postmenopausal bone density and sexuality, *Maturitas* 21:227, 1995.

124. **Bachmann GA, Timmons C, Abernethy WD,** Breakthrough bleeding patterns in two continuous combined estrogen/progestogen hormone replacement therapies, one of which included androgens, *J Women's Health* 5:205, 1996.

125. **Garnett T, Studd J, Watson N, Savvas M, Leather A,** The effects of plasma estradiol levels on increases in vertebral and femoral bone density following therapy with estradiol and estradiol with testosterone implants, *Obstet Gynecol* 79:968, 1992.

126. **Urman B, Pride SM, Ho Yuen B,** Elevated serum testosterone, hirsutism, and virilism associated with combined androgen-estrogen hormone replacement therapy, *Obstet Gynecol* 77:595, 1991.

127. **Draper MW, Flowers DE, Huster WJ, Neild JA, Harper KD, Arnaud C,** A controlled trial of raloxifene (LY139481) HCl: impact on bone turnover and serum lipid profile in healthy postmenopausal women, *J Bone Miner Res* 11:835, 1996.

128. **Boss SM, Huster WJ, Neild JA, Glant MD, Eisenhut CC, Draper MW,** Effects of raloxifene hydrochloride on the endometrium of postmenopausal women, *Am J Obstet Gynecol* 177:1458, 1997.

129. **Cummings SR, Norton L, Eckert S, Grady D, Cauley J, Knickerbocker R, Black DM, Nickelsen T, Glusman J, Krueger K, for the MORE investigators,** Raloxifene reduces the risk of breast cancer and may decrease the risk of endometrial cancer in postmenopausal women. Two-year findings from the Multiple Outcomes of Raloxifene Evaluation (MORE) trial, *http://www.asco.org/,* 1998.

130. **Wertheimer MD, Costanza ME, Dodson TF, D'Orsi C, Pastides H, Zapka JG,** Increasing the effort toward breast cancer detection, *JAMA* 255:1311, 1986.

131. **Delmas PD, Bjarnason NH, Mitlak BH, Ravoux A-C, Shah AS, Huster WJ, Draper M, Christiansen C,** Effects of raloxifene on bone mineral density, serum cholesterol concentrations, and uterine endometrium in postmenopausal women, *New Engl J Med* 337:1641, 1997.

132. **Walsh BW, Kuller LH, Wild RA, Paul S, Farmer M, Lawrence JB, Shah AS, Anderson PW,** Effects of raloxifene on serum lipids and coagulation factors in healthy postmenopausal women, *JAMA* 279:1445, 1998.

133. **Ettinger V, Black D, Cummings S, Genant H, Glüer C, Lips P, Knickerbocker R, Eckert S, Nickelsen T, Mitlack B, for the MORE Study Group,** Raloxifene reduces the risk of incident vertebral fractures: 24-month interim analyses, *Osteoporosis Int* 8(Suppl 3):11, 1998.

134. **Clarkson TB, Anthony MS, Jerome CP,** Lack of effect of raloxifene on coronary artery atherosclerosis of postmenopausal monkeys, *J Clin Endocrinol Metab* 83:721, 1998.

135. **Bjarnason NH, Haarbo J, Byrjalsen I, Kauffman RF, Christiansen C,** Raloxifene inhibits aortic accumulation of cholesterol in ovariectomized, cholesterol-fed rabbits, *Circulation* 96:1964, 1997.

136. **Zuckerman SH, Bryan N,** Inhibition of LDL oxidation and myeloperoxidase dependent tyrosyl radical formation by the selective estrogen receptor modulator raloxifene (LY139481 HCL), *Atherosclerosis* 126:65, 1996.

137. **Mijatovic V, Netelenbos C, van der Mooren MJ, de Valk-de Roo GW, Jakobs C, Kenemans P,** Randomized, double-blind, placebo-controlled study of the effects of raloxifene and conjugated equine estrogen on plasma homocysteine levels in healthy postmenopausal women, *Fertil Steril* 70:1085, 1998.

138. **Frigo P, Eppel W, Asseryanis E, Sator M, Golaszewski T, Gruber D, Lang C, Huber J,** The effects of hormone substitution in depot form on the uterus in a group of 50 perimenopausal women—a vaginosonographic study, *Maturitas* 21:221, 1995.

139. **Sener AB, Seçkin NC, Özmen S, Gökmen O, Dogu N, Ekici E,** The effects of hormone replacement therapy on uterine fibroids in postmenopausal women, *Fertil Steril* 65:354, 1996.

140. **Schwartz LB, Lazer S, Mark M, Nachtigall LE, Horan C, Goldstein SR,** Does the use of postmenopausal hormone replacement therapy influence the size of uterine leiomyomata? A preliminary report, *Menopause* 3:38, 1996.

141. **de Aloysio D, Altieri P, Penacchioni P, Salgarello M, Ventura V,** Bleeding patterns in recent postmenopausal outpatients with uterine myomas: comparison between two regimens of HRT, *Maturitas* 29:261, 1998.

142. **Siegle JC, Cartmell L,** Vulvar leiomyoma associated with estrogen/progestin therapy. A case report, *J Reprod Med* 40:147, 1995.

143. **Schwartz SM, Weiss NS, Daling JR, Gammon MD, Liff JM, Watt J, Lynch CF, Newcomb PA, Armstrong BK, Thoompson WD,** Exogenous sex hormone use correlates of endogenous hormone levels, and the incidence of histologic types of sarcoma of the uterus, *Cancer* 77:717, 1996.

144. **Cistulli PA, Barnes DJ, Grunstein RR, Sullivan CE,** Effect of short term hormone replacement in the treatment of obstructive sleep apnea in postmenopausal women, *Thorax* 46:699, 1994.

145. **Vandenbroucke JP, Witteman JCM, Valkenburg HA, Boersma JW, Cats A, Festen JJM, Hartman AP, Huber-Bruning O, Rasker JJ, Weber J,** Noncontraceptive hormones and rheumatoid arthritis in perimenopausal and postmenopausal women, *JAMA* 255:1299, 1986.

146. **Spector TD, Pregnnan P, Harris P, Studd JWW, Silman AJ,** Does estrogen replacement therapy protect against rheumatoid arthritis? *J Rheumatol* 18:1473, 1991.

147. **Koepsell TD, Dugowson CE, Nelson JL, Voigt LF, Daling JR,** Non-contraceptive hormones and the risk of rheumatoid arthritis in menopausal women, *Int J Epidemiol* 23:1248, 1994.

148. **Hall GM, Daniels M, Huskisson ES, Spector TD,** A randomised controlled trial of the effect of hormone replacement therapy on disease activity in postmenopausal rheumatoid arthritis, *Ann Rheum Dis* 53:112, 1994.

149. **Sanchez-Guerro J, Liang MH, Karlson EW, Hunter DJ, Colditz GA,** Postmenopausal estrogen therapy and the risk for developing systemic lupus erythematosus, *Ann Intern Med* 122:430, 1995.

150. **Arden NK, Lloyd ME, Spector TD, Hughes GRV,** Safety of hormone replacement therapy (HRT) in systemic lupus erythematosus (SLE), *Lupus* 3:11, 1994.

151. **Formiga F, Moga I, Nolla JM, Pac M, Mitjavila F, Roig-Escofet D,** Loss of bone mineral density in premenopausal women with systemic lupus erythematosus, *Ann Rheum Dis* 54:274, 1995.

152. **Hall GM, Daniels M, Doyle DV, Spector TD,** Effect of hormone replacement therapy on bone mass in rheumatoid arthritis patients treated with and without steroids, *Arthritis Rheum* 37:1499, 1994.

153. **Hall GM, Spector TD, Delmas PD,** Markers of bone metabolism in postmenopausal women with rheumatoid arthritis. Effects of corticosteroids and hormone replacement therapy, *Arthritis Rheum* 38:902, 1995.

154. **Diamond T, McGuigan L, Barbagallo S, Bryant C,** Cyclical etidronate plus ergocalciferol prevents glucocorticoid-induced bone loss in postmenopausal women, *Am J Med* 98:459, 1995.

155. **Saag KG, Emkey R, Schnitzer TJ, Brown JP, Hawkins F, Goemaere S, Thamsborg G, Liberman UA, Delmas PD, Malice M-P, Czachur M, Daifotis AG, for the Glucocorticoid-Induced Osteoporosis Intervention Study Group,** Alendronate for the prevention and treatment of glucocorticoid-induced osteoporosis, *New Engl J Med* 339:292, 1998.

156. **Buckley LM, Leib E, Cartularo KS, Vacek PM, Cooper SM,** Calcium and vitamin D_3 supplementation prevents bone loss in the spine secondary to low-dose corticosteroids in patients with rheumatoid arthritis. A randomized, double-blind, placebo-controlled trial, *Ann Intern Med* 125:961, 1996.

157. **Nevitt MC, Lane NE, Scott JC, Hochberg MC, Pressman AR, Genant HK, Cummings SR,** Radiographic osteoarthritis of the hip and bone mineral density, *Arthritis Rheum* 38:907, 1995.

158. **Sowers MF, Hochberg M, Crabbe JP, Muhich A, Crutchfield M, Updike S,** Association of bone mineral density and sex hormone levels with osteoarthritis of the hand and knee in premenopausal women, *Am J Epidemiol* 143:38, 1996.

159. **Nevitt MC, Cummings SR, Lane NE, Hochberg MC, Scott JC, Pressman AR, Genant HK, Cauley JA, for the Study of Osteoporotic Fractures Research Group,** Association of estrogen replacement therapy with the risk of osteoarthritis of the hip in elderly white women, *Arch Intern Med* 156:2073, 1996.

160. **Lieberman D, Kopernik G, Porath A, Lazer S, Heimer D,** Subclinical worsening of bronchial asthma during estrogen replacement therapy in asthmatic post-menopausal women, *Maturitas* 21:153, 1995.

161. **Troisi RJ, Speizer FE, Willett WC, Trichopoulos D, Rosner B,** Menopause, postmenopausal estrogen preparations and the risk of adult-onset asthma, *Am J Respir Crit Care Med* 152:1183, 1995.

162. **Toogood JH, Baskerville JC, Markov AE, Hodsman AB, Fraher LJ, Jennings B, Haddad RG, Drost D,** Bone mineral density and the risk of fracture in patients receiving long-term inhaled steroid therapy for asthma, *J Allergy Clin Immunol* 96:157, 1995.

163. **Volpe A, Lucenti V, Forabosco A, et al,** Oral discomfort and hormone replacement therapy in the post-menopause, *Maturitas* 13:1, 1990.

164. **Norderyd OM, Grossi SG, Machtei EE, Zambon JJ, Hausmann E, Dunford RG, Genco RJ,** Periondontal status of women taking postmenopausal estrogen supplementation, *J Periodontol* 64:957, 1993.

165. **Daniell HW,** Postmenopausal tooth loss: contributions to edentulism by osteoporosis and cigarette smoking, *Arch Intern Med* 143:1678, 1983.

166. **Krall EA, Dawson-Hughes B, Papas A, Garcia RI,** Tooth loss and skeletal bone density in healthy postmenopausal women, *Osteoporosis Int* 4:104, 1994.

167. **Paganini-Hill A,** The benefits of estrogen replacement therapy on oral health. The Leisure World Cohort, *Arch Intern Med* 155:2325, 1995.

168. **Grodstein F, Colditz GA, Stampfer MJ,** Post-menopausal hormone use and tooth loss: a prospective study, *JADA* 127:372, 1996.

169. **Harris TM,** The pharmacological treatment of voice disorders, *Folia Phoniatr* 44:143, 1992.

170. **Lindholm P, Vilkman E, Raudaskoski T, Suvanto-Luukkonen E, Kauppila A,** The effect of postmenopause and postmenopausal HRT on measured voice values and vocal symptoms, *Maturitas* 28:47, 1997.

171. **Metka M, Enzelsberger H, Knogler W, Schurz B, Aichmair H,** Ophthalmic complaints as a climacteric symptom, *Maturitas* 14:3, 1991.

172. **Kramer P, Lubkin V, Potter W, Jacobs M, Labay G, Silverman P,** Cyclic changes in conjunctival smears from menstruating females, *Ophthalmology* 97:303, 1990.

173. **Klein BEK, Klein R, Ritter LL,** Is there evidence of an estrogen effect on age-related lens opacities? *Arch Ophthalmol* 112:85, 1994.

174. **Benitez del Castillo JM, del Rio T, Garcia-Sanchez J,** Effects of estrogen use on lens transmittance in postmenopausal women, *Ophthalmology* 104:970, 1997.

175. **Cumming RG, Mitchell P,** Hormone replacement therapy, reproductive factors, and cataracts. The Blue Mountains Eye Study, *Am J Epidemiol* 145:242, 1997.

176. **Sator MO, Joura EA, Frigo P, Kurz C, Metka M, Hommer A, Huber JC,** Hormone replacement therapy and intraocular pressure, *Maturitas* 28:55, 1997.

177. **Sator MO, Akramian J, Joura EA, Nessmann A, Wedrich A, Gruber D, Metka M, Huber JC,** Reduction of intraocular pressure in a glaucoma patient undergoing hormone replacement therapy, *Maturitas* 29:93, 1998.

178. **Clark K, Sowers MR, Wallace RB, Jannausch ML, Lemke J, Anderson CV,** Age-related hearing loss and bone mass in a population of rural women aged 60 to 85 years, *Ann Epidemiol* 5:8, 1995.

179. **Quigley MET, Martin PL, Burnier AM, Brooks P,** Estrogen therapy arrests bone loss in elderly women, *Am J Obstet Gynecol* 156:1516, 1987.

180. **Cauley JA, Seeley DG, Enbsrud K, Ettinger B, Black D, Cummings SR, for the Study of Osteoporotic Fractures Research Group,** Estrogen replacement therapy and fractures in older women, *Ann Intern Med* 122:9, 1995.

181. **Schneider DL, Barrett-Connor EL, Morton DJ,** Timing of postmenopausal estrogen for optimal bone mineral density. The Rancho Bernardo Study, *JAMA* 277:543, 1997.

182. **Kiel DP, Felson DT, Anderson JJ, Wilson PWF, Moskowitz MA,** Hip fracture and the use of estrogen in postmenopausal women: the Framingham Study, *New Engl J Med* 317:1169, 1987.

183. **Grodstein F, Stampfer MJ, Colditz GA, Willett WC, Manson JE, Joffe M, Rosner B, Fuchs C, Hankinson SE, Hunter DJ, Hennekens CH, Speizer FE,** Postmenopausal hormone therapy and mortality, *New Engl J Med* 336:1769, 1997.

184. **Schubert W, Cullberg G, Edgar B, Hedner T,** Inhibition of 17β-estradiol metabolism by grapefruit juice in ovariectomized women, *Maturitas* 20:155, 1995.

185. **Weber A, Jägger R, Börmer A, Lomger G, Vollanth R, Matthey K, Balogh A,** Can grapefruit juice influence ethinylestradiol bioavailability? *Contraception* 63:41, 1996.

186. **Dorgan JF, Reichman ME, Judd JT, Brown C, Longcope C, Schatzkin A, Campbell WS, Franz C, Kahle L, Taylor PR,** The relation of reported alcohol ingestion to plasma levels of estrogens and androgens in premenopausal women, *Cancer Causes Control* 5:53, 1994.

187. **Gavaler JS, Van Thiel DH,** The association between moderate alcoholic beverage consumption and serum estradiol and testosterone levels in normal postmenopausal women: relationship to the literature, *Alcohol Clin Exp Res* 16:87, 1992.

188. **Ginsburg EL, Mello NK, Mendelson JH, Barbieri RL, Teoh SK, Rothman M, Gao X, Sholar JW,** Effects of alcohol ingestion on estrogens in postmenopausal women, *JAMA* 276:1747, 1996.

189. **Muti P, Trevisan M, Micheli A, Krogh V, Bolelli G, Sciajno R, Schünemann HJ, Berrino F,** Alcohol consumption and total estradiol in premenopausal women, *Cancer Epidemiol Biomark Prev* 7:189, 1998.

190. **Nagamani M, Kelver ME, Smith ER,** Treatment of menopausal hot flushes with transdermal administration of clonidine, *Am J Obstet Gynecol* 156:561, 1987.

191. **Goldberg RM, Loprinzi CL, O'Fallen JR, Veeder MH, Miser AW, Maillard JA, Michalak JC, Dose AM, Rowland Jr KM, Burnham NL,** Transdermal clonidine for ameliorating tamoxifen-induced hot flashes, *J Clin Oncol* 12:155, 1994.

192. **Lebherz TB, French LT,** Nonhormonal treatment of the menopausal syndrome. A double-blind evaluation of an autonomic system stabilizer, *Obstet Gynecol* 33:795, 1969.

193. **David A, Don R, Tajchner G, Weissglas L,** Veralipride: alternative antidopaminergic treatment for menopausal symptoms, *Am J Obstet Gynecol* 158:1107, 1988.

194. **Melis GB, Bambacciani M, Cagnacci A, Paoletti AM, Mais V, Fioretti P,** Effects of the dopamine antagonist veralipride on hot flushes and luteinizing horomone secretion in postmenopausal women, *Obstet Gynecol* 72:688, 1988.

195. **Lobo RA, McCormick W, Singer F, Roy S,** Depo medroxyprogesterone acetate compared with conjugated estrogens for the treatment of postmenopausal women, *Am J Obstet Gynecol* 63:1, 1984.

196. **Loprinzi CL, Michalak JC, Quella SK, O'Fallon JR, Hatfield AK, Nelimark RA, Dose AM, Fischer T, Johnson C, Klatt NE, Bate WW, Rospond RM, Oesterling JE,** Megestrol acetate for the prevention of hot flashes, *New Engl J Med* 331:347, 1994.

197. **Nesheim BI, Sætre T,** Reduction of menopausal hot flushes by methyldopa: a double blind crossover trial, *Eur J Clin Pharmacol* 20:413, 1981.

198. **Loprinzi CL, Pisansky TM, Fonseca R, Sloan JA, Zahasky KM, Quella SK, Novotny PJ, Rummans TA, Dumesic DA, Perez EA,** Pilot evaluation of venlafaxine hydrochoride for the therapy of hot flashes in cancer survivors, *J Clin Oncol* 16:2377, 1998.

199. **Barton DL, Loprinzi CL, Quella SK, Sloan JA, Veeder MH, Egner JR, Fidler P, Stella PJ, Swan DK, Vaught NL, Novotny P,** Prospective evaluation of vitamin E for hot flashes in breast cancer survivors, *J Clin Oncol* 16:495, 1998.

200. **Ross LA, Alder EM,** Tibolone and climacteric symptoms, *Maturitas* 21:127, 1995.

201. **Bjarnason NH, Bjarnason K, Haarbo J, Rosenquist C, Christiansen C,** Tibolone: prevention of bone loss in late postmenopausal women, *J Clin Endocrinol Metab* 81:2419, 1996.

202. **Ginsburg J, Prelevic G, Butler D, Okolo S,** Clinical experience with tibolone (Livial) over 8 years, *Maturitas* 21:71, 1995.

203. **Lippuner K, Haenggi W, Birkhaeuser MH, Casez J-P, Jaeger P,** Prevention of postmenopausal bone loss using tibolone or conventional peroral or transdermal hormone replacement therapy with 17β-estradiol and dydrogesterone, *J Bone Miner Res* 12:806, 1997.

204. **Tang B, Markiewicz L, Kloosterboer HJ, Gurpide E,** Human endometrial 3 beta-hydroxysteroid dehydrogenase/isomerase can locally reduce intrinsic estrogenic/progestagenic activity ratios of a steroidal drug (Org OD 14), *J Steroid Biochem Mol Biol* 45:345, 1993.

205. **Rymer J, Chapman MG, Fogelman I, Wilson POG,** A study of the effect of tibolone on the vagina in postmenopausal women, *Maturitas* 18:127, 1994.

206. **Farish E, Barnes JF, Rolton HA, Spowart K, Fletcher CD, Hart DM,** Effects of tibolone on lipoprotein(a) and HDL subfractions, *Maturitas* 20:215, 1994.

207. **Bjarnason NH, Bjarnason K, Haarbo J, Coelingh Bennink HJT, Christiansen C,** Tibolone: influence on markers of cardiovascular disease, *J Clin Endocrinol Metab* 82:1752, 1997.

208. **Cagnacci A, Mallus E, Tuveri F, Cirillo R, Setteneri AM, Melis GB,** Effects of tibolone on glucose and lipid metabolism in postmenopausal women, *J Clin Endocrinol Metab* 82:251, 1997.

209. **Prelevic GM, Beljic T, Balint-Peric L, Ginsburg J,** Metabolic effects of tibolone in postmenopausal women with non-insulin dependent diabetes mellitus, *Maturitas* 28:271, 1998.

210. **Taylor M,** Alternatives to conventional hormone replacement therapy, *Comp Ther* 23:514, 1997.

211. **Israel D, Youngkin EQ,** Herbal therapies for perimenopausal and menopausal complaints, *Pharmacotherapy* 17:970, 1997.

212. **Hirata JD, Swiersz LM, Zell B, Small R, Ettinger B,** Does dong quae have estrogenic effects in postmenopausal women? A double-blind, placebo-controlled trial, *Fertil Steril* 68:981, 1997.

213. **Murkies AL, Wilcox G, Davis SR,** Phytoestrogens, *J Clin Endocrinol Metab* 83:297, 1998.

214. **Tham DM, Gardner CD, Haskell WL,** Potential health benefits of dietary phytoestrogens: a review of the clinical, epidemiological, and mechanistic evidence, *J Clin Endocrinol Metab* 83:2223, 1998.

215. **Kuiper GGJM, Carlsson B, Grandien K, Enmark E, Häggblad J, Nilsson S, Gustafsson J,** Comparison of the ligand binding specificity and transcript tissue distribution of estrogen receptors α and β, *Endocrinology* 138:863, 1997.

216. **Wagner JD, Cefalu WT, Anthony MS, Litwak KN, Zhang L, Clarkson TB,** Dietary soy protein and estrogen replacement therapy improve cardiovascular risk factors and decrease aortic cholesteryl ester content in ovariectomized Cynomolgus monkeys, *Metabolism* 46:698, 1997.

217. **Jayo MJ, Anthony MS, Register TC, Rankin S, Vest T, Clarkson TB,** Dietary soy isoflavones and bone loss: a study in ovariectomized monkeys (abstract), *J Bone Min Res* 11(Suppl 1):S228, 1996.

218. **Anthony MS, Clarkson TB, Hughes Jr CL, Morgan TM, Burke GL,** Soybean isoflavones improve cardiovascular risk factors without affecting the reproductive system of peripubertal Rhesus monkeys, *J Nutr* 126:43, 1996.

219. **Anthony MS, Clarkson TB, Bullock BC, Wagner JD,** Soy protein versus soy phytoestrogens in the prevention of diet-induced coronary artery atherosclerosis of male cynomolgus monkeys, *Arterioscler Thromb Vasc Biol* 17:2524, 1997.

220. **Honoré EK, Williams JK, Anthony MS, Clarkson TB,** Soy isoflavones enhance coronary vascular reactivity in atherosclerotic female macaques, *Fertil Steril* 67:148, 1997.

221. **Anthony MS, Clarkson TB,** Comparison of soy phytoestrogens and conjugated equine estrogens on atherosclerosis progression in postmenopausal monkeys (abstract), *Circulation* 90:829, 1998.

222. **Clarkson TB, Anthony MS, Williams JK, Honore EK, Cline JM,** The potential of soybean phytoestrogens for postmenopausal hormone replacement therapy, *Proc Soc Exp Biol Med* 217:365, 1998.

223. **Albertazzi P, Pansini F, Bonaccorsi G, Zanotti L, Forini E, Aloysio D,** The effect of dietary soy supplementation on hot flushes, *Obstet Gynecol* 91:6, 1998.

224. **Lu L-JW, Anderson KE, Grady JJ, Nagamani M,** Effects of soya consumption for one month on steroid hormones in premenopausal women: implications for breast cancer risk reduction, *Cancer Epidemiol Biomark Prev* 5:63, 1996.

225. **Adlercreutz H, Mazur W,** Phyto-oestrogens and western diseases, *Ann Med* 29:95, 1997.

226. **Goodman MT, Wilkens LR, Hankin JH, Lyu L-C, Wu AH, Kolonel LN,** Association of soy and fiber consumption with the risk of endometrial cancer, *Am J Epidemiol* 146:294, 1997.

227. **Ingram D, Sanders K, Kolybaba M, Lopez D,** Case-control study of phyto-oestrogens and breast cancer, *Lancet* 350:990, 1997.

228. **Messina MJ, Persky V, Setchell KDR, Barnes S,** Soy intake and cancer risk: a review of the *in vitro* and *in vivo* data, *Nutr Cancer* 21:113, 1994.

229. **Petrakis NL, Barnes S, King EB, Lowenstein J, Wiencke J, Lee MM, Miike R, Kirk M, Coward L,** Stimulatory influence of soy protein isolate on breast secretion in pre- and postmenopausal women, *Cancer Epidemiol Biomark Prev* 5:785, 1996.

230. **Melis GB, Paoletti AM, Cagnacci A,** Ipriflavone prevents bone loss in postmenopausal women, *Menopause* 3:27, 1996.

231. **Gennari C, Agnusdei D, Crepaldi G, Isaia G, Mazzuoli G, Ortolani S, Bufalino L, Passeri M,** Effect of ipriflavone—a synthetic derivative of natural isoflavones—on bone mass loss in the early years after menopause, *Menopause* 5:9, 1998.

232. **Slayden SM, Crabbe L, Bae S, Potter HD, Azziz R, Parker Jr CR,** The effect of 17β-estradiol on adrenocortical sensitivity, responsiveness, and steroidogenesis in postmenopausal women, *J Clin Endocrinol Metab* 83:519, 1998.

233. **Morales A, Nolan J, Nelson J, Yen SSC,** Effects of replacement dose of dehydroepiandrosterone in men and women of advancing age, *J Clin Endocrinol Metab* 78:1360, 1994.

234. **Casson PR, Santoro N, Elkind-Hirsch KE, Carson SA, Hornsby PJ, Abraham G, Buster J,** Postmenopausal dehydroepiandrosterone (DHEA) administration increases insulin-like growth factor-I (IGF-I) and decreases high density lipoprotein (HDL): a six month trial, *Fertil Steril* 70:107, 1998.

235. **Glueck CJ, Lang J, Hamer T, Tracy T,** Severe hypertriglyceridemia and pancreatitis when estrogen replacement therapy is given to hypertriglyceridemic women, *J Lab Clin Med* 123:59, 1994.

236. **Grodstein F, Colditz GA, Stampfer MJ,** Postmenopausal hormone use and cholecystectomy in a large prospective study, *Obstet Gynecol* 83:5, 1994.

237. **Petitti DB, Sidney S, Perlamn JA,** Increased risk of cholecystectomy in users of supplemental estrogen, *Gastroenterolgoy* 94:91, 1988.

238. **La Vecchia C, Negri E, D'Avanzo B, Parazzini F, Genitle A, Franceschi S,** Oral contraceptives and noncontraceptive oestrogens in the risk of gallstone disease requiring surgery, *J Epidemiol Community Health* 46:234, 1992.

239. **Hulley S, Grady D, Bush T, Furberg C, Herrington D, B, Vittinghoff E, for the Heart and Estrogen/progestin Replacement Study (HERS) Research Group,** Randomized trial of estrogen plus progestin for secondary prevention of coronary heart disease in postmenopausal women, *JAMA* 280:605, 1998.

240. **Scragg RK, McMichael AJ, Seamark RF,** Oral contraceptives, pregnancy and endogenous estrogen in gallstone disease — a case-control study, *Br Med J* 288:1795, 1984.

241. **Kakar F, Weiss NS, Strite SA,** Non-contraceptive estrogen use and the risk of gallstone disease in women, *Am J Public Health* 78:564, 1988.

242. **Jorgensen T,** Gallstones in a Danish population: fertility, period, pregnancies, and exogenous female sex hormones, *Gut* 29:433, 1988.

243. **van Erpecum KJ, van Berge Henegouwen GP, Verschoor L, Stoelwinder B, Willekens FLH,** Different hepatobiliary effects of oral and transdermal estradiol in postmenopausal women, *Gasteroenterology* 100:482, 1991.

244. **Uhler ML, Marks JW, Voigt BJ, Judd HL,** Comparison of the impact of transdermal *versus* oral estrogens on biliary markers of gallstone formation in postmenopausal women, *J Clin Endocrinol Metab* 83:410, 1998.

245. **Wing R, Matthews K, Kuller L, Meilahn EN, Plantinga PL,** Weight gain at the time of menopause, *Arch Intern Med* 151:97, 1990.

246. **Kritz-Silverstein D, Barrett-Connor E,** Long-term postmenopausal hormone use, obesity, and fat distribution in older women, *JAMA* 27:46, 1996.

247. **Espeland MA, Stefanick ML, Kritz-Silverstein D, Fineberg SE, Waclawiw MA, James MK, Greendale GA, for the Postmenopausal Estrogen/Progestin Interventions Study Investigators,** Effect of postmenopausal hormone therapy on body weight and waist and hip girths, *J Clin Endocrinol Metab* 82:1549, 1997.

248. **Haarbo J, Marslew U, Gotfredsen A, Christiansen C,** Postmenopausal hormone replacement therapy prevents central distribution of body fat after menopause, *Metabolism* 40:1323, 1991.

249. **Ley C, Lees B, Stevenson J,** Sex- and menopause-associated changes in body-fat distribution, *Am J Clin Nutr* 55:950, 1992.

250. **Reubinoff BE, Wurtman J, Rojansky N, Adler D, Stein P, Schenker JG, Brzezinski A,** Effects of hormone replacement therapy on weight, body composition, fat distribution, and food intake in early postmenopausal women: a prospective study, *Fertil Steril* 64:963, 1995.

251. **Gambacciani M, Ciaponi M, Cappagli B, Piaggesi L, De Simone L, Orlandi R, Genazzani AR,** Body weight, body fat distribution, and hormonal replacement therapy in early postmenopausal women, *J Clin Endocrinol Metab* 82:414, 1997.

252. **Boston Collaborative Drug Surveillance Program,** Surgically confirmed gallbladder disease, venous thromboembolism, and breast tumors in relation to postmenopausal estrogen therapy, *New Engl J Med* 290:15, 1974.

253. **Petitti DB, Wingerd J, Pellegrin F, Ramcharan S,** Risk of vascular disease in women: smoking, oral contraceptives, noncontraceptive estrogens, and other factors, *JAMA* 242:1150, 1979.

254. **Devor M, Barrett-Connor E, Renvall M, Feigal DJ, Ramsdell J,** Estrogen replacement therapy and the risk of venous thrombosis, *Am J Med* 92:275, 1992.

255. **Lowe G, Greer I, Cooke T, and Thromboembolic Risk Factors (THRIFT) Consensus Group,** Risk and prophylaxis for venous thromboembolism in hospital patients, *Br Med J* 305:567, 1992.

256. **Grodstein F, Stampfer MJ, Goldhaber SZ, Manson JE, Colditz GA, Speizer FE, Willett WC, Hennekens CH,** Prospective study of exogenous hormones and risk of pulmonary embolism in women, *Lancet* 348:983, 1996.

257. **Daly E, Vessey MP, Hawkins MM, Carson JL, Gough P, Marsh S,** Risk of venous thromboembolism in users of hormone replacement therapy, *Lancet* 348:977, 1996.

258. **Jick H, Derby L, Myers M, Vasilakis C, Newton K,** Risk of hospital admission for idiopathic venous thromboembolism among users of postmenopausal oestrogens, *Lancet* 348:981, 1996.

259. **Gutthann SP, Rodríguez LAG, Castellsague J, Oliart AD,** Hormone replacement therapy and risk of venous thromboembolism: population based case-control study, *Br Med J* 314:796, 1997.

260. **Varas-Lorenzo C, Garcia-Rodriguez LA, Cattaruzzi C, Troncon MG, Agostinis L, Perez-Gutthann S,** Hormone replacement therapy and the risk of hospitalization for venous thromboembolism: a population-based study in Southern Europe, *Am J Epidemiol* 147:387, 1998.

261. **Meilahn E, Kuller L, Matthews K, Kiss J,** Hemostatic factors according to menopausal status and use of hormone replacement therapy, *Ann Epidemiol* 2:445, 1992.

262. **Scarabin PY, Flu-Bureau G, Bara L, Bonithon-Kopp C, Guize L, Samama M,** Haemostatic variables and menopausal status: influence of hormone replacment therapy, *Thromb Haemost* 70:584, 1994.

263. **Gebara OCE, Mittleman MA, Sutherland P, Lipinska I, Matheney T, Xu P, Welty FK, Wilson PW, Levy D, Muller JE, Tofler GH,** Association between increased estrogen status and increased fibrinolytic potential in the Framingham Offspring Study, *Circulation* 91:1952, 1995.

264. **Conard J, Gompel A, Pelissier C, Mirabel C, Basdevant A,** Fibrinogen and plasminogen modifications during oral estradiol replacement therapy, *Fertil Steril* 68:449, 1997.

265. **The Writing Group for the PEPI Trial,** Effects of hormone replacement therapy on endometrial histology in postmenopausal women: the Postmenopausal Estrogen/Progestin Interventions (PEPI) Trial, *JAMA* 275:370, 1996.

266. **Kurman RJ, Kaminski PT, Norris HJ,** The behavior of endometrial hyperplasia. A long-term study of "untreated" hyperplasia in 170 patients, *Cancer* 56:402, 1985.

267. **Grady D, Gebretsadik T, Kerlikowske K, Ernster V, Petitti D,** Hormone replacement therapy and endometrial cancer risk: a meta-analysis, *Obstet Gynecol* 85:304, 1995.

268. **Weiss NS, Hill DA,** Postmenopausal estrogen and the incidence of gynecologic cancer, *Maturitas* 23:235, 1996.

269. **Shapiro S, Kelly JP, Rosenberg L, Kaufman DW, Helmrich SP, Rosenshein NB, Lewis Jr JL, Knapp RC, Stolley PD, Schottenfeld D,** Risk of localized and widespread endometrial cancer in relation to recent and discontinued use of conjugated estrogens, *New Engl J Med* 313:969, 1985.

270. **Paganini-Hill A, Ross RK, Henderson BE,** Endometrial cancer and patterns of use of oestrogen replacement therapy: a cohort study, *Br J Cancer* 59:445, 1989.

271. **Schiff I, Sela HK, Cramer D, Tulchinsky D, Ryan KJ,** Endometrial hyperplasia in women on cyclic or continuous estrogen regimens, *Fertil Steril* 37:79, 1982.

272. **Notelovitz M, Varner RE, Rebar RW, Fleischmann R, McIlwain HH, Schwartz SL, Sperling M, Wilborn W, Yang H-M, Silfen SL,** Minimal endometrial proliferation over a two-year period in postmenopausal women taking 0.3 mg of unopposed esterified estrogens, *Menopause* 4:80, 1997.

273. **Cushing KL, Weiss NL, Voigt LF, McKnight B, Beresford SAA,** Risk of endometrial cancer in relation to use of low-dose, unopposed estrogens, *Obstet Gynecol* 91:35, 1998.

274. **Thom MH, White PJ, Williams RM, Sturdee PW, Paterson MEL, Wade-Evans T, Studd JWW,** Prevention and treatment of endometrial disease in climacteric women receiving estrogen, *Lancet* ii:455, 1979.

275. **Whitehead MI, Townsend PT, Pryse-Davies J, Ryder TA, King RJB,** Effects of estrogen and progestins on the biochemistry and morphology of the postmenopausal endometrium, *New Engl J Med* 305:1599, 1981.

276. **Gambrell Jr RD, Babgnell CA, Greenblatt RB,** Role of estrogens and progesterone in the etiology and prevention of endometrial cancer: a review, *Am J Obstet Gynecol* 146:696, 1983.

277. **Persson I, Adami H-O, Bergkvist L, Lindgren A, Pettersson, Hoover R, Schairer C,** Risk of endometrial cancer after treatment with oestrogens alone or in conjunction with progestogens: results of a prospective study, *Br Med J* 298:147, 1989.

278. **Voigt LF, Weiss NS, Chu JR, Daling J, McKnight B, van Belle G,** Progestagen supplementation of exogenous oestrogens and risk of endometrial cancer, *Lancet* 338:274, 1991.

279. **Varma TR,** Effect of long-term therapy with estrogen and progesterone on the endometrium of postmenopausal women, *Acta Obstet Gynecol Scand* 64:41, 1985.

280. **Pike MC, Peters RK, Cozen W, Probst-Hensch NM, Felix JC, Wan PC, Mack TM,** Estrogen-progestin replacement therapy and endometrial cancer, *J Natl Cancer Inst* 89:1110, 1997.

281. **Schairer C, Adami H-O, Hoover R, Persson I,** Cause-specific mortality in women receiving hormone replacement therapy, *Epidemiology* 8:59, 1997.

282. **Flowers CE, Wilborn WH, Hyde BM,** Mechanisms of uterine bleeding in postmenopausal patients receiving estrogen alone or with a progestin, *Obstet Gynecol* 61:135, 1983.

283. **Rodriguez C, Calle EE, Coates RJ, Miracle-McMahill HL, Thun MJ, Heath Jr CW,** Estrogen replacement therapy and fatal ovarian cancer, *Am J Epidemiol* 141:828, 1995.

284. **Whittemore AS, Harris R, Itnyre J, and the Collaborative Ovarian Cancer Group,** Characteristics relating to ovarian cancer risk: collaborative analysis of 12 US case-control studies. II: Invasive epithelial ovarian cancers in white women, *Am J Epidemiol* 136:1184, 1992.

285. **Garg PP, Kerlikowske K, Subak L, Grady D,** Hormone replacement therapy and the risk of epithelial ovarian carcinoma: a meta-analysis, *Obstet Gynecol* 92:472, 1998.

286. **Hempling RE, Wong C, Piver MS, Natarajan N, Mettlin CJ,** Hormone replacement therapy as a risk factor for epithelial ovarian cancer: results of a case-control study, *Obstet Gynecol* 89:1012, 1997.

287. **Risch HA,** Estrogen replacement therapy and risk of epithelial ovarian cancer, *Gynecol Oncol* 63:254, 1996.

288. **Eeles RA, Tan S, Whitelaw E, Fryatt I, A'Hern RP, Shepherd JH, Harmer CL, Blake PR, Chilvers CED,** Hormone replacement therapy and survival after surgery for ovarian cancer, *Br Med J* 302:259, 1991.

289. **Adami H-O, Persson I, Hoover R, Schairer C, Bergkvist L,** Risk of cancer in women receiving hormone replacement therapy, *Int J Cancer* 44:833, 1989.

290. **Parazzini F, La Vecchia C, Negri E, Franceschi S, Moroni S, Chatenoud L, Bolis G,** Case-control study of oestrogen replacement therapy and risk of cervical cancer, *Br Med J* 315:85, 1997.

291. **Ploch E,** Hormonal replacement therapy in patients after cervical cancer treatment, *Gynecol Oncol* 26:169, 1987.

292. **Chute CG, Willett WC, Colditz GA, Stampfer MJ, Rosner B, Speizer FE,** A prospective study of reproductive history and exogenous estrogens on the risk of colorectal cancer in women, *Epidemiology* 2:201, 1991.

293. **Jacobs EJ, White E, Weiss NS,** Exogenous hormones, reproductive history, and colon cancer, *Cancer Causes Control* 5:359, 1994.

294. **Calle EE, Miracle-McMahill ML, Thun MJ, Heath Jr CW,** Estrogen replacement therapy and risk of fatal colon cancer in a prospective cohort of postmenopausal women, *J Natl Cancer Inst* 87:517, 1995.

295. **Kampman E, Potter JD, Slattery ML, Caan BJ, Edwards S,** Hormone replacement therapy, reproductive history, and colon cancer: a multicenter, case-control study in the United States, *Cancer Causes Control* 8:146, 1997.

296. **Troisi R, Schairer C, Chow W-H, Schatzkin A, Brinton LA, Fraumeni Jr JF,** A prospective study of menopausal hormones and risk of colorectal cancer (United States), *Cancer Causes Control* 8:130, 1997.

297. **Grodstein F, Martinez E, Platz EA, Giovannucci E, Colditz GA, Kautsky M, Fuchs C, Stampfer MJ,** Postmenopausal hormone use and risk for colorectal cancer and adenoma, *Ann Intern Med* 128:705, 1998.

298. **American Cancer Society,** Cancer facts & figures — 1998, *http://www.cancer.org/statistics.html*, 1998.

299. **Green A,** Oral contraceptives and skin neoplasia, *Contraception* 43:653, 1991.

300. **Hannaford PC, Villard-Mackintosh L, Vessey MP, Kay CR,** Oral contraceptives and malignant melanoma, *Br J Cancer* 63:430, 1991.

301. **Holly EA, Cress RD, Ahn DK,** Cutaneous melanoma in women: ovulatory life, menopause, and use of exogenous hormones, *Cancer Epidemiol Biomark Prev* 3:661, 1994.

302. **White E, Kirkpatrick CS, Lee JAH,** Case-control study of malignant melanoma in Washington State. I. Constitutional factors and sun exposure, *Am J Epidemiol* 139:857, 1994.

303. **Holman CDJ, Armstrong BK, Heenan PJ,** Cutaneous malignant melanoma in women: exogenous sex hormones and reproductive factors, *Br J Cancer* 50:673, 1984.

304. **Osterland A, Tucker MA, Stone BJ, Jensen OM,** The Danish case-control study of cutaneous malignant melanoma. III. Hormonal and reproductive factors in women, *Int J Cancer* 42:821, 1988.

305. **Persson I, Yuen J, Bergkvist L, Schairer C,** Cancer incidence and mortality in women receiving estrogen and estrogen-progestin replacement therapy—long-term follow-up of a Swedish cohort, *Int J Cancer* 67:327, 1996.

306. **Brinton LA, Hoover R, Fraumeni Jr JF,** Menopausal oestrogens and breast cancer risk: an expanded case-control study, *Br J Cancer* 54:825, 1986.

307. **Hiatt RA, Bawol R, Friedman GD, Hoover R,** Exogenous estrogen and breast cancer after bilateral oophorectomy, *Cancer* 54:139, 1984.

308. **Hoover R, Gray Sr LA, Cole P, MacMahon B,** Menopausal estrogens and breast cancer, *New Engl J Med* 295:401, 1976.

309. **Hoover R, Glass A, Finkle WE, Azevedo D, Milne K,** Conjugated estrogens and breast cancer risk in women, *J Natl Cancer Inst* 67:815, 1981.

310. **Hulka BS, Chambless LE, Deubner DC, Wilkinson WE,** Breast cancer and estrogen replacement therapy, *Am J Obstet Gynecol* 143:638, 1982.

311. **Jick H, Walker AM, Watkins RN, D'Ewart DC, Hunter JR, Danford A, Madsen S, Dinan BJ, Rothman KJ,** Replacement estrogens and breast cancer, *Am J Epidemiol* 112:586, 1980.

312. **Kaufman DW, Miller DR, Rosenberg L, Helmrich SP, Stolley P, Schottenfeld D, Shapiro S,** Noncontraceptive estrogen use and the risk of breast cancer, *JAMA* 252:63, 1984.

313. **Kelsey JL, Fischer DB, Holford TR, LiVoisi VA, Mostow ED, Goldenberg IS, White C,** Exogenous estrogens and other factors in the epidemiology of breast cancer, *J Natl Cancer Inst* 67:327, 1981.

314. **Lawson DH, Jick H, Hunter JR, Madsen S,** Exogenous estrogens and breast cancer, *Am J Epidemiol* 114:710, 1981.

315. **Ross RK, Paganini-Hill A, Gerkins VR, Mack TM, Pfeffer R, Arthur M, Henderson BE,** A case-control study of menopausal estrogen therapy and breast cancer, *JAMA* 243:1635, 1980.

316. **Wingo PA, Layde PM, Lee NC, Rubin G, Ory HW,** The risk of breast cancer in postmenopausal women who have used estrogen replacement therapy, *JAMA* 257:209, 1987.

317. **Bergkvist L, Adami H-O, Persson I, Hoover R, Schairer C,** The risk of breast cancer after estrogen and estrogen-replacement, *New Engl J Med* 321:293, 1989.

318. **Bergkvist L, Adami H-O, Persson I, Bergstrom R, Krusemo UB,** Prognosis after breast cancer diagnosis in women exposed to estrogen and estrogen-progestogen replacement therapy, *Am J Epidemiol* 130:221, 1989.

319. **Persson I, Yuen J, Bergkvist L, Adami H-O, Hoover R, Schairer C,** Combined oestrogen-progestogen replacement and breast cancer risk, *Lancet* 340:1044, 1992.

320. **Persson I, Thurfjell E, Bergstrom R, Holmberg L,** Hormone replacement therapy and the risk of breast cancer. Nested case-control study in a cohort of Swedish women attending mammography screening, *Int J Cancer* 72:758, 1997.

321. **Ewertz M,** Influence of non-contraceptive exogenous and endogenous sex hormones on breast cancer risk in Denmark, *Int J Cancer* 42:832, 1988.

322. **Colditz GA, Stampfer MJ, Willett WC, Hunter DJ, Manson JE, Hennekens CH, Rosner BA, Speizer FE,** Type of postmenopausal hormone use and risk of breast cancer: 12-year follow-up from the Nurses' Health Study, *Cancer Causes Control* 3:433, 1992.

323. **Colditz GA, Hankinson SE, Hunter DJ, Willett WC, Manson J, Hennekens C, Rosner B, Speizer FE,** The use of estrogens and progestins and the risk of breast cancer in postmenopausal women, *New Engl J Med* 332:1589, 1995.

324. **Gapstur SM, Potter JD, Sellers TA, Folsom AR,** Increased risk of breast cancer with alcohol consumption in postmenopausal women, *Am J Epidemiol* 136:1221, 1992.

325. **Vrieze OJ, Kuipers J, Boes G,** Scenario analysis in public health and competing risks, *Stat Appl* 1:371, 1990.

326. **Rohan TE, McMichael AJ,** Non-contraceptive exogenous oestrogen therapy and breast cancer, *Med J Aust* 148:217, 1988.

327. **Dupont WD, Page DL, Rogers LW, Parl FF,** Influence of exogenous estrogens, proliferative breast disease, and other variables on breast cancer risk, *Cancer* 63:948, 1989.

328. **Kaufman DW, Palmer JR, De Mouzon J, Rosenberg L, Stolley PD, Warshaver ME, Shapiro S,** Estrogen replacement therapy and the risk of breast cancer: results from the case-control surveillance study, *Am J Epidemiol* 134:1375, 1991.

329. **Palmer JR, Rosenberg L, Clarke EA, Miller DR, Shapiro S,** Breast cancer risk after estrogen replacement therapy: results from the Toronto Breast Cancer Study, *Am J Epidemiol* 134:1386, 1991.

330. **Stanford JL, Weiss NS, Voigt LF, Daling JR, Habel LA, Rossing MA,** Combined estrogen and progestin hormone replacement therapy in relation to risk of breast cancer in middle-aged women, *JAMA* 274:137, 1995.

331. **Yang CP, Daling JR, Band PR, Gallagher RP, White E, Weiss NS,** Noncontraceptive hormone use and risk of breast cancer, *Cancer Causes Control* 3:475, 1992.

332. **Risch HA, Howe GR,** Menopausal hormone usage and breast cancer in Saskatchewan: a record-linkage cohort study, *Am J Epidemiol* 139:670, 1994.

333. **Schairer C, Byrne C, Keyl PM, Brinton LA, Sturgeon SR, Hoover RN,** Menopausal estrogen and estrogen-progestin replacement therapy and risk of breast cancer (United States), *Cancer Causes Control* 5:491, 1994.

334. **Folsom AR, Mink PJ, Sellers TA, Hong C-P, Zheng W, Potter JD,** Hormonal replacement therapy and morbidity and mortality in a prospective study of postmenopausal women, *Am J Public Health* 85:1128, 1995.

335. **Sellers TA, Mink PJ, Cerhan JR, Zheng W, Anderson KE, Kushi LH, Folsom AR,** The role of hormone replacement therapy in the risk for breast cancer and total mortality in women with a family history of breast cancer, *Ann Intern Med* 127:973, 1997.

336. **Newcomb PA, Longnecker MP, Storer BE, Mittendorf R, Baron J, Clapp RW, Bogdan G, Willett WC,** Long-term hormone replacement therapy and risk of breast cancer in postmenopausal women, *Am J Epidemiol* 142:788, 1995.

337. **Petitti DB,** *Meta-Analysis, Decision Analysis, and Cost-Effectiveness Analysis: Methods for Quantitative Synthesis in Medicine,* Oxford University Press, New York, 1994.

338. **Armstrong BK,** Oestrogen therapy after the menopause — boon or bane? *Med J Aust* 148:213, 1988.

339. **Dupont WD, Page DL,** Menopausal estrogen replacement therapy and breast cancer, *Arch Intern Med* 151:67, 1991.

340. **Steinberg KK, Thacker SB, Smith SJ, Stroup DF, Zack MM, Flancers WD, Berkelman RL,** A meta-analysis of the effect of estrogen replacement therapy on the risk of breast cancer, *JAMA* 265:1985, 1991.

341. **Sillero-Arenas M, Delgado-Rodriguez M, Rodigues-Canteras R, Bueno-Cavanillas A, Galvez-Vargas R,** Menopausal hormone replacement therapy and breast cancer: a meta-analysis, *Obstet Gynecol* 79:286, 1992.

342. **Colditz GA, Egan KM, Stampfer MJ,** Hormone replacement therapy and risk of breast cancer: results from epidemiologic studies, *Am J Obstet Gynecol* 168:1473, 1993.

343. **Grady D, Rubin SM, Petitti DB, Fox CS, Black D, Ettinger B, Ernster VL, Cummings SR,** Hormone therapy to prevent disease and prolong life in postmenopausal women, *Ann Intern Med* 117:1016, 1992.

344. **Collaborative Group on Hormonal Factors in Breast Cancer,** Breast cancer and hormone replacement therapy: collaborative reanalysis of data from 51 epidemiological studies of 52,705 women with breast cancer and 108,411 women without breast cancer, *Lancet* 350:1047, 1997.

345. **Hunt K, Vessey M, McPherson K, Coleman M,** Long-term surveillance of mortality and cancer incidence in women receiving hormone replacement therapy, *Br J Obstet Gynaecol* 94:620, 1990.

346. **Willis DB, Calle EE, Miracle-McMahill HL, Heath Jr CW,** Estrogen replacement therapy and risk of fatal breast cancer in a prospective cohort of postmenopausal women in the United States, *Cancer Causes Control* 7:449, 1996.

347. **Hunt K, Vessey M, McPherson K,** Mortality in a cohort of long-term users of hormone replacement therapy: an updated analysis, *Br J Obstet Gynaecol* 97:1080, 1990.

348. **Strickland DM, Gambrell Jr RD, Butzin CA, Strickland K,** The relationship between breast cancer survival and prior postmenopausal estrogen use, *Obstet Gynecol* 80:400, 1992.

349. **Bonnier P, Romain S, Giacalone PL, Laffargue F, Martin PM, Piana L,** Clinical and biologic prognostic factors in breast cancer diagnosed during postmenopausal hormone replacement therapy, *Obstet Gynecol* 85:11, 1995.

350. **Magnusson C, Holmberg L, Norden T, Lindgren A, Persson I,** Prognostic characteristics in breast cancers after hormone replacement therapy, *Breast Cancer Res Treat* 38:325, 1996.

351. **LaCroix AZ, Burke W,** Breast cancer and hormone replacement therapy, *Lancet* 350:1042, 1997.

352. **Ettinger B, Quesenberry C, Schroeder DA, Friedman G,** Long-term postmenopausal estrogen therapy may be associated with increased risk of breast cancer: a cohort study, *Menopause* 4:125, 1997.

353. **Fisher B, Costantino JP, Wickerham DL, Redmond CK, Kavanah M, Cronin WM, Vogel V, Robidoux A, Dimitrov N, Atkins J, Daly M, Wieand S, Tan-Chiu E, Ford L, Wolmark N, and other National Surgical Adjuvant Breast and Bowel Project Investigators,** Tamoxifen for prevention of breast cancer: report of the National Surgical Adjuvant Breast and Bowel Project P-1 Study, *J Natl Cancer Inst* 90:1371, 1998.

354. **LeLorier J, Grégoire G, Benhaddad A, Lapierre J, Derderian F,** Discrepancies between meta-analyses and subsequent large randomized, controlled trials, *New Engl J Med* 337:536, 1997.

355. **Gambrell Jr RD, Maier RC, Sanders BI,** Decreased incidence of breast cancer in postmenopausal estrogen-progestogen users, *Obstet Gynecol* 62:435, 1983.

356. **Nachtigall MJ, Smilen SW, Nachtigall RAD, Nachtigall RH, Nachtigall LI,** Incidence of breast cancer in a 22-year study of women receiving estrogen-progestin replacement therapy, *Obstet Gynecol* 80:827, 1992.

357. **Korenman SG,** Estrogen window hypothesis of the etiology of breast cancer, *Lancet* i:700, 1980.

358. **Korenman SG,** The endocrinology of breast cancer, *Cancer* 46:874, 1980.

359. **Coulam CB, Annegers JF, Krans JS,** Chronic anovulation syndrome and associated neoplasia, *Obstet Gynecol* 61:403, 1983.

360. **Cowan LD, Gordis L, Tonascia JA, Jones GS,** Breast cancer incidence in women with a history of progesterone deficiency, *Am J Epidemiol* 114:209, 1981.

361. **Ron E, Lunenfeld B, Menczer J, Blumstein T, Katz L, Oelsner G, Serr D,** Cancer incidence in a cohort of infertile women, *Am J Epidemiol* 125:780, 1987.

362. **Gammon MD, Thompson WD,** Infertility and breast cancer: a population-based case-control study, *Am J Epidemiol* 132:708, 1990.

363. **Gammon MD, Thompson WD,** Polycystic ovaries and the risk of breast cancer, *Am J Epidemiol* 134:818, 1991.

364. **Anderson KE, Sellers TA, Chen P-L, Rich SS, Hong C-P, Folsom AR,** Association of Stein-Leventhal syndrome with the incidence of postmenopausal breast carcinoma in a large prospective study of women in Iowa, *Cancer* 79:494, 1997.

365. **Key TJA, Pike MC,** The role of oestrogens and progestogens in the epidemiology and prevention of breast cancer, *Eur J Cancer Clin Oncol* 24:29, 1988.

366. **Henderson BE, Ross RK, Judd HL, Krailo MD, Pike MC,** Do regular ovulatory cycles increase breast cancer risk? *Cancer* 56:1206, 1985.

367. **Anderson TJ, Ferguson DJP, Raab GM,** Cell turnover in the "resting" human breast: influence of parity, contraceptive pill, age and laterality, *Br J Cancer* 46:376, 1982.

368. **Gompel A, Malet C, Spritzer P, Lalardrie J-P, Kuttenn F, Mauvais-Jarvis P,** Progestin effect on cell proliferation and 17-hydroxysteroid dehydrogenase activity in normal human breast cells in culture, *J Clin Endocrinol Metab* 63:1174, 1986.

369. **Chang KJ, Lee TT, Linarez-Cruz G, Fournier S, de Ligniéres B,** Influences of percutaneous administration of estradiol and progesterone on human breast epithelial cell cycle in vivo, *Fertil Steril* 63:785, 1995.

370. **Laidlaw IJ, Clarke RB, Howell A, Owen AW, Potten CS, Anderson E,** The proliferation of normal human breast tissue implanted into athymic nude mice is stimulated by estrogen but not progesterone, *Endocrinology* 136:164, 1996.

371. **Foidart J-M, Colin C, Denoo X, Desreux J, Béliard A, Fournier S, de Ligniéres B,** Estradiol and progesterone regulate the proliferation of human breast epithelial cells, *Fertil Steril* 69:963, 1998.

372. **Kester HA, van der Leede BM, van der Saag PT, van der Burg B,** Novel progesterone target genes identified by an improved differential display technique suggest that progestin-induced growth inhibition of breast cancer cells coincides with enhancement of differentiation, *J Biol Chem* 272:16637, 1997.

373. **Zemlickis D, Lishner M, Degendorger P, Panzarella T, Burke B, Sutcliffe SB, Koren G,** Maternal and fetal outcome after breast cancer in pregnancy, *Am J Obstet Gynecol* 166:781, 1992.

374. **Saunders CM, Baum M,** Breast cancer and pregnancy: a review, *J Roy Soc Med* 86:162, 1993.

375. **Lambe M, Hsieh C, Trichopoulos D, Ekbom A, Pavia M, Adami H-O,** Transient increase in the risk of breast cancer after giving birth, *New Engl J Med* 331:5, 1994.

376. **Guinee VF, Olsson H, Moller T, Hess KR, Taylor SH, Fahey T, Gladikov JV, van den Blink JW, Bonichon F, Dische S, et al,** Effect of pregnancy on prognosis for young women with breast cancer, *Lancet* 343:1587, 1994.

377. **Ribeiro G, Jones DA, Jones M,** Carcinoma of the breast associated with pregnancy, *Br J Surg* 73:607, 1986.

378. **Sankila R, Heinavaara S, Hakulinen T,** Survival of breast cancer patients after subsequent term pregnancy: "healthy mother effect," *Am J Obstet Gynecol* 170:818, 1994.

379. **Kroman N, Jensen M-B, Melbye M, Wohlfahrt J, Mouridsen HT,** Should women be advised against pregnancy after breast-cancer treatment? *Lancet* 350:319, 1997.

380. **WHO Collaborative Study of Neoplasia and Steroid Contraceptives,** Breast cancer and depot-medroxyprogesterone acetate: a multinational study, *Lancet* 338:833, 1991.

381. **Lee NC, Rosero-Bixby L, Oberle MW, Grimaldo C, Whatley AS, Rovira EZ,** A case-control study of breast cancer and hormonal contraception in Costa Rica, *J Natl Cancer Inst* 79:1247, 1987.

382. **Paul C, Skegg DCG, Spears GFS,** Depot medroxyprogesterone (Depo-Provera) and risk of breast cancer, *Br Med J* 299:7591, 1989.

383. **Skegg DCG, Noonan EA, Paul C, Spears GFS, Meirik O, Thomas DB,** Depot medroxyprogesterone acetate and breast cancer: a pooled analysis of the World Health Organization and the New Zealand studies, *JAMA* 273:799, 1995.

384. **Spicer D, Pike MC, Henderson BE,** The question of estrogen replacement therapy in patients with a prior diagnosis of breast cancer, *Oncology* 4:49, 1990.

385. **Canney PA, Hatton MQF,** The prevalence of menopausal symptoms in patients treated for breast cancer, *Clin Oncol* 6:297, 1994.

386. **Stoll BA, Parbhoo S,** Treatment of menopausal symptoms in breast cancer patients, *Lancet* i:1278, 1988.

387. **Wile AG, Opfell RW, Margileth DA,** Hormone replacement therapy in previously treated breast cancer patients, *Am J Surg* 165:372, 1993.

388. **DiSaia PJ, Odicino F, Grosen EA, Cowan B, Pecorelli S, Wile AG,** Hormone replacement therapy in breast cancer (letter), *Lancet* 342:1232, 1993.

389. **DiSaia PJ, Grosen EA, Kurosaki T, Gildea M, Cowan B, Anton-Culver H,** Hormone replacement therapy in breast cancer survivors: a cohort study, *Am J Obstet Gynecol* 174:1494, 1996.

390. **Dew J, Eden JA, Beller E, Magarey C, Schwartz P, Crea P, Wren BG,** A cohort study of hormone replacement therapy given to women previously treated for breast cancer, *Climacteric* 1:137, 1998.

391. **Vassilopoulou-Sellin R, Theriault R, Klein MJ,** Estrogen replacement therapy in women with prior diagnosis and treatment for breast cancer, *Gynecol Oncol* 65:89, 1997.

392. **Decker DA, Pettinga JE, Cox TC, Burdakin JH, Jaiyesimi IA, Benitez PR,** Hormone replacement therapy in breast cancer survivors, *Breast J* 3:63, 1997.

393. **Vassilopoulou-Sellin R, Theriault RL,** Randomized prospective trial of estrogen replacement therapy in women with a history of breast cancer, *J Natl Cancer Inst* 16:153, 1994.

394. **Henderson IC,** Breast cancer therapy — The price of success, *New Engl J Med* 326:1774, 1992.

395. **Sullivan JM, Vander Zwaag R, Hughes JP, Maddock V, Kroetz FW, Ramanathan KB, Mirvis DM,** Estrogen replacement and coronary artery disease: effect on survival in postmenopausal women, *Arch Intern Med* 150:2557, 1990.

396. **O'Brien JE, Peterson ED, Keeler GP, Berdan LG, Ohman EM, Faxon DP, Jacobs AK, Topol EJ, Califf RM,** Relation between estrogen replacement therapy and restenosis after percutaneous coronary interventions, *J Am Coll Cardiol* 28:1111, 1996.

397. **Sullivan JM, El-Zeky F, Vander Zwaag R, Ramanathan KB,** Effect on survival of estrogen replacement therapy after coronary artery bypass grafting, *Am J Cardiol* 79:847, 1997.

398. **O'Keefe Jr JH, Kim SC, Hall RR, Cochran VC, Lawhorn SL, McCallister BD,** Estrogen replacement therapy after coronary angioplasty in women, *J Am Coll Cardiol* 29:1, 1997.

399. **Newton KM, LaCroix AZ, McKnight B, Knopp RH, Siscovick DS, Heckbert SR, Weiss NS,** Estrogen replacement therapy and prognosis after first myocardial infarction, *Am J Epidemiol* 145:269, 1997.

400. **Espeland MA, Applegate W, Furgerg CD, Lefkowitz D, Rice L, Hunninghake D, the ACAPS Investigators,** Estrogen replacement therapy and progression of intimal-medial thickness in the carotid arteries of postmenopausal women, *Am J Epidemiol* 142:1011, 1995.

401. **Liang Y-L, Teede H, Shiel L, Thomas A, Craven R, Sachithanandan N, McNeil JJ, Cameron JD, Dart A, McGrath B,** Effects of oestrogen and progesterone on age-related changes in arteries of postmenopausal women, *Clin Exp Pharmacol Physiol* 24:457, 1997.

402. **Akkad A, Hartshorne T, Bell PRF, Al-Azzawi F,** Carotid plaque regression on oestrogen replacement: a pilot study, *Eur J Vasc Endovasc Surg* 11:347, 1996.

403. **Darling GM, Johns JA, McCloud PI, Davis SR,** Estrogen and progestin compared with simvastatin for hypercholesterolemia in postmenopausal women, *New Engl J Med* 337:595, 1997.

404. **Andersson B, Mattsson L, Hahn L, Mårin P, Lapidus L, Holm G, Bengtsson B, Björntorp P,** Estrogen replacement therapy decreases hyperandrogenicity and improves glucose homeostasis and plasma lipids in postmenopausal women with noninsulin-dependent diabetes mellitus, *J Clin Endocrinol Metab* 82:638, 1997.

405. **Brussaard HE, Gevers Leuven JA, Frolich M, Kluft C, Krans HMJ,** Short-term oestrogen replacement therapy improves insulin resistance, lipids and fibrinolysis in postmenopausal women with NIDDM, *Diabetologia* 40:843, 1997.

406. **Crippin JS, Jorgensen RA, Dickson ER, Lindor KD,** Hepatic osteodystrophy in primary biliary cirrhosis: effects of medical treatment, *Am J Gastroenterol* 89:47, 1994.

407. **Rigg LA, Hermann H, Yen SSC,** Absorption of estrogens from vaginal creams, *New Engl J Med* 298:195, 1978.

408. **Pschera H, Hjerpe A, Carlström K,** Influence of the maturity of the vaginal epithelium upon the absorption of vaginally administered estradiol-17β and progesterone in postmenopausal women, *Gynecol Obstet Invest* 27:204, 1989.

409. **Johnston A,** Estrogens — pharmacokinetics and pharmacodynamics with special reference to vaginal administration and the new estradiol formulation — Estring®, *Acta Obstet Gynecol Scand* 75(Suppl 163):16, 1996.

410. **Henriksson L, Stjernquist M, Boquist L, Cedergren I, Selinus I,** A one-year multicenter study of efficacy and safety of a continuous, low-dose, estradiol-releasing vaginal ring (Estring) in postmenopausal women with symptoms and signs of urogenital aging, *Am J Obstet Gynecol* 174:85, 1996.

411. **Steiger MJ, Quinn NP,** Hormone replacement therapy induced chorea, *Br Med J* 302:762, 1991.

412. **Thomas JM,** Hormone-replacement therapy and pulmonary leiomyomatosis (Letter), *New Engl J Med* 327:1956, 1992.

413. **Wetterberg L, Olsson MB, Alm-Agvald I,** Estrogen treatment caused acute attacks of porphyria, *Lakartidningen* 92:2197, 1995.

414. **Gurwood AS, Gurwood I, Gubman DT, Brzezicki LJ,** Idiosyncratic ocular symptoms associated with the estradiol transdermal estrogen replacement patch system, *Optom Vis Sci* 72:29, 1995.

415. **Sharma R, Pickering J, McCormack WM,** *Trichomoniasis* in a postmenopausal women cured after discontinuation of estrogen replacement therapy, *Sex Trans Dis* 2:543, 1997.

416. **Greendale GA, Reboussin BA, Hogan P, Barnabei VM, Shumaker S, Johnson S, Barrett-Connor E,** Symptom relief and side effects of postmenopausal hormones: results from the Postmenopausal Estrogen/Progestin Interventions trial, *Obstet Gynecol* 92:982, 1998.

19   Obesity

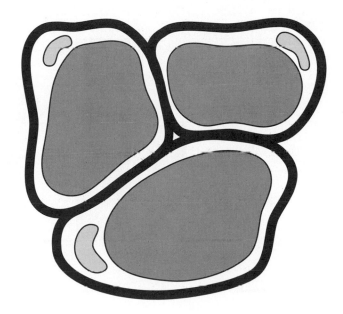

Because approximately one-third of American adults are obese, the unrewarding fight against obesity is all too common, not only with our patients but also with ourselves.[1] About 25% of U.S. women are overweight, and an additional 25% are obese.[2] Unfortunately, for over 100 years the incidence of obesity has been increasing in the United States and Europe, a reflection of an affluent society with an increasingly sedentary life combined with high caloric foods.[1, 3, 4] This change in lifestyle has produced an increasing prevalence of obesity that is similar in adults and children.[5]

The lack of success in treating obesity is not due to an unawareness of the implications of obesity; there is a clear-cut, well recognized relationship between mortality and weight.[6, 7] The death rate from diabetes mellitus, for example, is approximately 4 times higher among obese diabetics than among those who control their weight. The death rate from appendicitis is double, presumably from anesthetic and surgical complications. Even the rate of accidents is higher, perhaps because fat people are awkward or because their view of the ground or floor is obstructed. The Nurses' Health Study estimates that 23% of all deaths in nonsmoking middle-aged women are attributable to being overweight.[7]

The incidence of hypertension, heart disease, noninsulin-dependent diabetes mellitus, gout, gallbladder disease, colorectal cancer, endometrial cancer, postmenopausal breast cancer, and osteoarthritis is elevated in overweight people.[8] Being overweight in adolescence is even a more powerful predictor of cardiovascular adverse health effects than being overweight as an adult.[9]

When the personal and social problems encountered by obese people are also considered, it is no wonder that a clinician without a weight problem cannot comprehend why fat individuals remain overweight. The frequency with which a practitioner encounters the obese patient whose weight does not decrease despite a sworn adherence to a limited-calorie diet makes one question if there is something physiologically different about this patient. Is the problem due to lack of discipline and cheating on a diet, or does it also involve a pathophysiologic factor? Is the physiology of obese people unusual, or are they simply gluttons? *Modern studies of obesity strongly indicate that this is a multifactorial problem, and that lack of willpower and laziness are not the simple answers.*

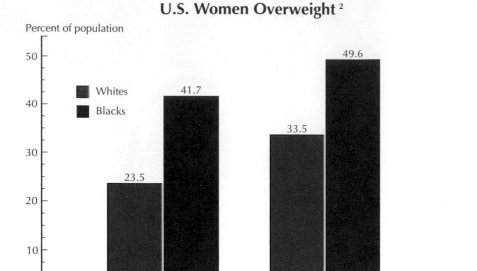

U.S. Women Overweight [2]

Percent of population

Whites
Blacks

23.5 41.7 33.5 49.6

1960–62   1988–91

Definition of Obesity

Obesity is an excess storage of triglycerides in adipose cells. There is a difference between obesity and overweight.[10] Obesity is an excess of body fat. Overweight is a body weight in excess of some standard or ideal weight. The ideal weight for any adult is believed to correspond to his or her ideal weight from age 20 to 30. The following formulas give ideal weight in pounds:

Women: 100 + (4 x (height in inches minus 60))
Men: 120 + (4 x (height in inches minus 60))

At a weight close to ideal weight, individuals may be overweight, but not overfat. This is especially true of individuals engaged in regular exercise. An estimate of body fat, therefore, is more meaningful than a measurement of height and weight.

The most accurate method of determining body fat is to determine the density of the body by underwater measurement (hydrodensitometry). It certainly is not practical to measure density by submerging individuals in water in our offices; therefore, skinfold measurements with calipers have become popular as an index of body fat, or expensive imaging techniques can be utilized. These latter methods are not necessary for clinical practice. It is far simpler to utilize the body mass index nomogram, a method that has been found to correspond closely to densitometry measurements.[11]

The body mass index (the Quetelet index) is the ratio of weight divided by the height squared (in metric units):

BMI = kilograms/meters^2

To use the nomogram for body mass index (BMI), read the central scale by aligning a straightedge between height and body weight. Over the last 30 years, the mean body mass index has increased in the U.S., and now averages 26.3.[1] A body mass index of 27 or more warrants treatment.[12] A body mass index of about 30 is roughly equivalent to 30% excess body weight, the point at which excess mortality begins (approximately 10–12% of people in the U.S. have a body mass index of 30 or greater). Above age 40, the risk from obesity itself is comparable to that associated with major health problems such as hypertension and heavy smoking. A "good" BMI for most people

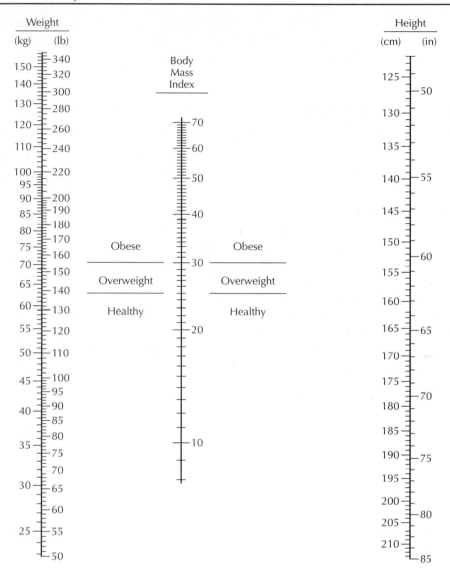

is in the range of 20 to 24. Mortality is minimal although still increased at a body mass index of approximately 22 and lowest in middle-aged women with a body mass index below 19.[7]

Overweight: BMI = 25–29.9
Obesity: BMI = 30 and higher

A person is obese when the amount of adipose tissue is sufficiently high (20% or more over ideal weight) to detrimentally alter biochemical and physiological functions and to shorten life expectancy. Obesity is associated with four major risk factors for atherosclerosis: hypertension, diabetes, hypercholesterolemia, and hypertriglyceridemia. Overweight individuals have a higher prevalence of hypertension at every age, and the risk of developing hypertension is related to the amount of weight gain after age 25.[13] The two in combination (hypertension and obesity) increase the risk of heart disease, cerebrovascular disease, and death. The Nurses' Health Study has documented a continuing correlation between the body mass index and cardiovascular disease, diabetes, and cancer.[7, 14, 15] In other words, even a modest gain in adult weight, even in a range not considered to be overweight, increases the risk of cardiovascular and metabolic diseases. However, at any given BMI level, the presence of an increase in abdominal fat, metabolic risk factors, or a strong family history of diabetes, hypertension, and heart disease increases the risk to good health.

It is well documented that women have a greater prevalence of obesity compared with men. One reason may be the fact that women have a lower metabolic rate than men, even when adjusted for differences in body composition and level of activity.[16] Another reason that more women gain weight with age is the postmenopausal loss of the increase in metabolic rate that is associated with the luteal phase of the menstrual cycle.[17] The difference between men and women is even greater in older age.

Unfortunately, the basal metabolic rate decreases with age.[18, 19] After age 18, the resting metabolic rate declines about 2% per decade. The age-related decline in basal metabolic rate is not observed in women who continue to be involved in a regular endurance exercise program.[20] A 30-year-old individual will inevitably gain weight if there is no change in caloric intake or exercise level over the years. The middle-age spread is both a biologic and a psychosociologic phenomenon. It is, therefore, important for both our patients and ourselves to understand adipose tissue and the problem of obesity.

Physiology of Adipose Tissue

Adipose tissue serves three general functions:

1. Adipose tissue is a storehouse of energy.

2. Fat serves as a cushion from trauma.

3. Adipose tissue plays a role in the regulation of body heat.

Each cell of adipose tissue can be regarded as a package of triglyceride, the most concentrated form of stored energy. There are 8 calories per gram of triglyceride compared to 1 calorie per gram of glycogen. The total store of tissue and fluid carbohydrate in adults (about 300 calories) is inadequate to meet between-meal demands. The storage of energy in fat tissue allows us to do other things besides eating. Our energy balance, therefore, is essentially equivalent to our fat balance. Thus, obesity is a consequence of the fat imbalance inherent in high caloric diets.

The mechanism for mobilizing energy from fat involves various enzymes and neurohormonal agents. Following ingestion of fat and its breakdown by gastric and pancreatic lipases, absorption of long-chain triglycerides and free fatty acids takes place in the small bowel. Chylomicrons (microscopic particles of fat) transferred through lymph channels into the systemic venous circulation are normally removed by hepatic parenchymal cells where a new lipoprotein is released into the circulation. When this lipoprotein is exposed to adipose tissue, lipolysis takes place through the action of lipoprotein lipase, an enzyme derived from the fat cells themselves. The fatty acids that are released then enter the fat cells where they are reesterified with glycerophosphate into triglycerides. Because alcohol diverts fat from oxidation to storage, body weight is directly correlated with the level of alcohol consumption.[21]

Glucose serves three important functions:

1. Glucose supplies carbon atoms in the form of acetyl coenzyme A (acetyl CoA).

2. Glucose provides hydrogen for reductive steps.

3. Glucose is the main source of glycerophosphate.

The production and availability of glycerophosphate (required for reesterification of fatty acids and their storage as triglycerides) are considered rate limiting in lipogenesis, and this process depends on the presence of glucose.

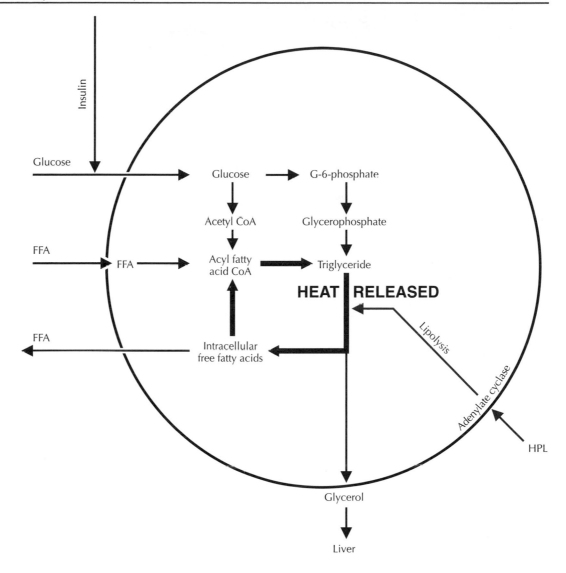

After esterification, subsequent lipolysis results in the release of fatty acids and glycerol. In the cycle of lipolysis and reesterification, energy is freed as heat. A low variable level of lipolysis takes place continuously; its basic function is to provide body heat.

The chief metabolic products produced from fat are the circulating free fatty acids. Their availability is controlled by adipose tissue cells. When carbohydrate is in short supply, a flood of free fatty acids can be released. The free fatty acids in the peripheral circulation are almost wholly derived from endogenous triglycerides that undergo rapid hydrolysis to yield free fatty acid and glycerol. The glycerol is returned to the liver for resynthesis of glycogen.

Free fatty acid release from adipose tissue is stimulated by physical exercise, fasting, exposure to cold, nervous tension, and anxiety. The release of fatty acids by lipolysis varies from one anatomic site to another. Omental, mesenteric, and subcutaneous fat is more labile and easily mobilized than fat from other sources. Areas from which energy is not easily mobilized are retrobulbar and perirenal fat where the tissue serves a structural function. Adipose tissue lipase is sensitive to stimulation by both epinephrine and norepinephrine. Other hormones that activate lipase are ACTH, thyroid-stimulating hormone (TSH), growth hormone, thyroxine (T_4), 3,5,3'-triiodothyronine (T_3), cortisol, glucagon, as well as vasopressin and human placental lactogen (HPL).

Lipase enzyme activity is inhibited by insulin, which appears to be alone as the major physiologic antagonist to the array of stimulating agents. When both glucose and insulin are abundant,

Glucose abundant

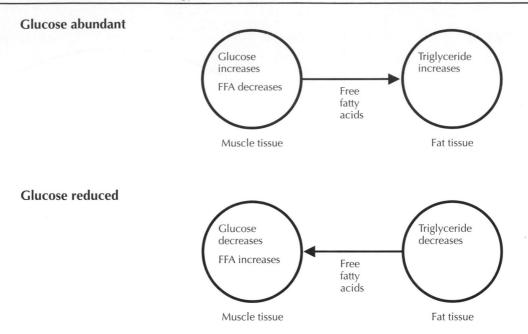

Glucose reduced

transport of glucose into fat cells is high, and glycerophosphate production increases to esterify fatty acids.

The carbohydrate and fat composition of the fuel supply is constantly changing, depending on stresses and demands. Because the central nervous system and some other tissues can utilize only glucose for energy, a homeostatic mechanism for conserving carbohydrate is essential. When glucose is abundant and easily available, it is utilized in adipose tissue for producing glycerophosphate to immobilize fatty acids as triglycerides. The circulating level of free fatty acids in muscle will, therefore, be low, and glucose will be used by all of the tissues.

When carbohydrate is scarce, the amount of glucose reaching the fat cells declines, and glycerophosphate production is reduced. The fat cell releases fatty acids, and their circulating levels rise to a point where glycolysis is inhibited. Thus, carbohydrate is spared in those tissues capable of using lipid substrates. If the rise of fatty acids is great enough, the liver is flooded with acetyl CoA. This is converted into ketone bodies, and clinical ketosis results.

In the simplest terms, when a person eats, glucose is available, insulin is secreted, and fat is stored. In starvation, the glucose level falls, insulin secretion decreases, and fat is mobilized.

If only single large meals are consumed, the body learns to convert carbohydrate to fat very quickly. Epidemiologic studies with schoolchildren demonstrate a positive correlation between fewer meals and a greater tendency toward obesity.[17] The person who does not eat all day and then stocks up at night is perhaps doing the worst possible thing.

Clinical Obesity

Leptin and the Ob Gene (the Lep Gene in Humans)

The hypothalamic location of the appetite center was established in 1940 by the demonstration that bilateral lesions of the ventromedial nucleus produce experimental obesity in rats. Such lesions lead to hyperphagia and decreased physical activity. Interestingly, this pattern is similar to that seen in human beings — the pressure to eat is reinforced by the desire to be physically inactive. The ventromedial nucleus was thought to represent an integrating center for appetite and hunger information. Destruction of the ventromedial nucleus was believed to result in a loss of satiety signals, leading to hyperphagia. Overeating and obesity, however, are not due to ventromedial nucleus damage but rather to destruction of the nearby ventral noradrenergic bundle.[22] Hypothalamic noradrenergic terminals are derived from long fibers ascending from hindbrain cell bodies. Lesions of the ventromedial nucleus produced by radiofrequency current fail to cause obesity. These lesions lead to overeating and obesity only when they extend beyond the ventromedial nucleus. Selective destruction of the ventral noradrenergic bundle results in hyperphagia. A sudden onset of hyperphagia can be due to a hypothalamic lesion. Possible causes include tumors, trauma, inflammatory processes, and aneurysms.

Signals arriving at these CNS centers originate in peripheral tissues. Opiates, substance P, and cholecystokinin play a role in mediating taste, the gatekeeper for feeding, while peptides released from the stomach and intestine act as satiety signals.[23] Neuropeptides that inhibit appetite include corticotropin-releasing hormone (CRH), neurotensin, and cyclo(HisPro), a peptide derived by proteolysis of thyrotropin-releasing hormone.[24] Although recent attention has focused on leptin and the ob gene, keep in mind that the control of food intake and energy expenditure is very complex, and no agent or system functions in isolation.

The word leptin is derived from the Greek word, "leptos," which means thin. ***Leptin is a 167-amino acid peptide secreted in adipose tissue, that circulates in the blood bound to a family of proteins, and acts on the central nervous system neurons that regulate eating behavior and energy balance.*** Rat studies in the 1950s suggested the existence of a hormone in adipose tissue that regulated body weight through an interaction with the hypothalamus.[25, 26] But it was not until 1994 that the ob gene was identified, the gene responsible for obesity in the mouse.[27] In the human, this gene is known as the Lep gene.

There are 4 recessive gene mutations known in mice, and one dominant (Ay/Ay).[28] Fat/fat mice are obese and remain insulin sensitive; the mutation decreases carboxypeptidase E, an enzyme that is involved in the conversion of prohormones to hormones; e.g., proinsulin to insulin. The biology of tub is yet unknown.

Genetic Rodent Models of Obesity

	Single Gene Mutations	Gene Product	Rodent Chromosome	Human Chromosome
Mice:	ob/ob	Leptin	6	7
	db/db	Leptin receptor	4	1
	fat/fat	Carboxypeptidase E	8	11
	tub/tub	Phosphodiesterase	7	4
	Ay/Ay	Agouti protein	2	20
Rats:	fa/fa	Leptin receptor	5	1

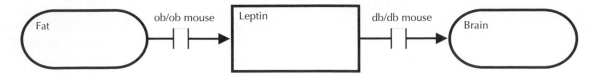

Ob/ob and db/db mice were described over 30 years ago. The ob/ob mutation arose spontaneously in the Jackson Laboratory mouse colony in 1949. The ob/ob mouse is homozygous for a mutation of the ob gene on chromosome 6, and the db/db mouse, discovered in 1966, is homozygous for a mutation of the db gene on chromosome 4.[28, 29] These mice have been the subject of over 1000 publications. The product of the ob gene is leptin, and in the human, the Lep gene is located on chromosome 7q31,3. Db is the *diabetes* gene, and this is the locus of the mouse leptin receptor gene. Thus, the ob/ob mouse is obese because it does not produce leptin, and the db mouse is obese because it cannot respond to leptin; its leptin levels are very high (the mutation alters the leptin receptor).

The Leptin Receptor

The leptin receptor belongs to the cytokine receptor family.[29] There are two major forms, a short form and a long form, OB-R_S and OB-R_L. The extracellular domain is very large with 816 amino acids. The intracellular domain of the short form contains 34 amino acids, and in the long form, about 303 amino acids. The short form has many variations, whereas the long form is the likely signaling receptor. The only place that the long form is expressed in greater amounts than the short forms is in the hypothalamus, in the arcuate, ventromedial, paraventricular, and dorsomedial nuclei.[30, 31]

High levels of the short form leptin receptors in the choroid plexus suggest a transport role for the short form from blood into the cerebrospinal fluid to diffuse into the brain.[32] However, a separate transport mechanism has also been demonstrated for leptin.[33]

The class I cytokine receptor family (to which the long form belongs) acts by proteins that phosphorylate the receptor after binding and STAT proteins that are activated after phosphorylation, and then translocate to the nucleus and stimulate gene transcription. The long-form receptor works through STAT proteins, but gene knockouts specific for STAT proteins are not obese, indicating the presence of other pathways. These signaling mechanisms are the subjects of intense molecular biology studies.

The db gene encodes the leptin receptor. The db mutation converts the long form to the short from. The db/db mouse has a single G for T nucleotide substitution within the C terminal untranslated end of the short intracellular domain of the ob receptor. This results in a new splice site that creates an abnormal exon inserted into the mRNA that encodes the long intracellular domain of the ob receptor. As a result, the long-form mRNA in db/db mice encodes a protein with most of the intracellular domain truncated to be similar to the short form of the ob receptor. The fa/fa mutation is a glutamine for proline substitution in the extracellular domain, and in contrast to the db/db mouse, the fa/fa rat will respond to leptin, but only if it is delivered into the brain.[34]

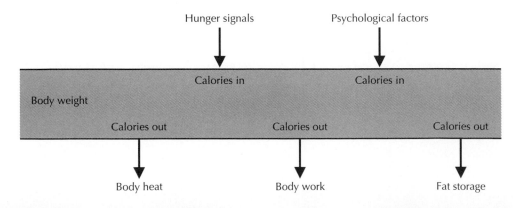

The Physiologic Feedback Loop

Energy expenditure is composed of the basal metabolic rate, diet and temperature-induced heat production, and the energy necessary for physical activity. Leptin induces weight loss in mice due to decreased appetite and food consumption and an increase in heat production and activity.[35] Leptin placed in the lateral ventricle of the rodent brain causes this weight loss, associated with a decrease in the hypothalamic peptide, neuropeptide Y (NPY) expression and secretion. NPY is a 36-amino acid polypeptide that is a potent stimulator of eating when injected directly into the rodent brain.[36] NPY has a tyrosine at both ends, hence the use of Y to stand for tyrosine. NPY stimulates food intake, decreases heat production, and increases insulin and cortisol secretion.

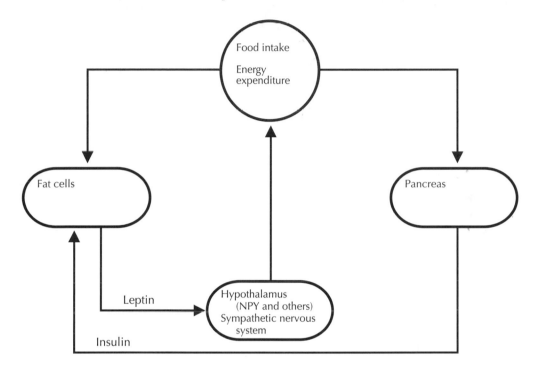

In rodents, insulin increases the expression of the ob gene, but there is controversy in humans.[35] In humans, there is no surge of leptin after meals, and the acute administration of insulin does not stimulate an increase in leptin levels. However, an increase in ob gene expression occurs in humans with chronic insulin stimulation, a situation that would be similar to overeating.[37] In addition, at least one study has found an acute increase in leptin levels following the induction of hyperinsulinemia (but only in women, not in men).[38] It is likely that insulin is at least one regulator of the ob gene and its secretion of leptin. Thus, this is a physiologic feedback loop to maintain weight and energy.

The Ay/Ay rodent becomes fat late in life. The Agouti gene encodes a protein produced by hair follicles. This protein binds to a melanocortin receptor in melanocytes in the skin, thus preventing melanocyte-stimulating hormone action. Agouti rats have high levels of this protein and have yellow instead of black fur. Melanocortins have been demonstrated in the hypothalamus, produced in the arcuate nucleus. Melanocortins binding to the brain receptor influence appetite.[39, 40] Knockout mice for the melanocortin receptor become obese, and these mice have high NPY expression. Ay/Ay rodents make an excess of Agouti protein, blocking melanocortin action. Thus, too little melanocortin could be another pathway for obesity. The importance of this pathway is evident in the report of mutations within the proopiomelanocortin (POMC) gene characterized by deficiencies in both melanocyte-stimulating hormone (MSH) and adrenocorticotrophin (ACTH), yielding individuals with obesity, adrenal insufficiency, and red hair pigmentation.[41]

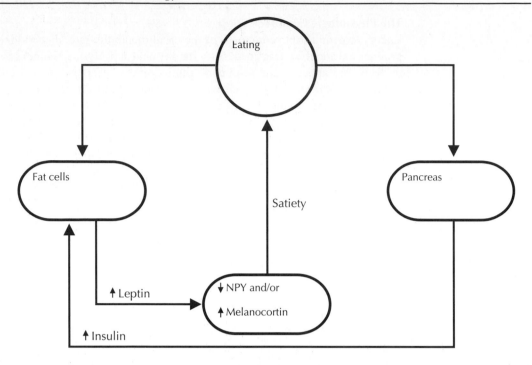

Fasting and exercise decrease leptin secretion and increase NPY gene expression in the arcuate nucleus, followed by release of NPY by neuronal projections into the paraventricular nucleus. The neurons that respond to NPY originate in the arcuate nucleus and project into the paraventricular and dorsomedial nuclei. The arcuate nucleus lies outside the blood-brain barrier (there is no blood-brain barrier in the medial basal hypothalamus) and can be reached by leptin in the circulation. The NPY neurons stimulate feeding and inhibit heat production by inhibiting sympathetic nervous activity. In ob/ob mice with no leptin, NPY levels are high in the hypothalamus, and leptin treatment lowers NPY and restores everything to normal.[30]

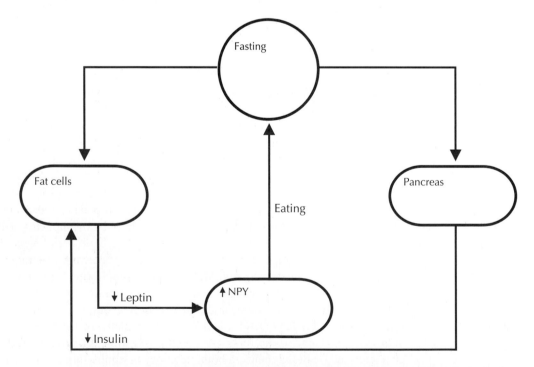

In rodents, caloric restriction increases the expression of NPY in the arcuate nucleus and the release of NPY in the paraventricular nucleus. Leptin and insulin decrease during fasting, allowing an increase in the expression of the NPY gene. Because an increase in metabolism is unwanted during fasting, CRH decreases; however, there is an increase in cortisol that is a consequence of an NPY-induced hypothalamic signal, not yet identified. Fasting decreases leptin more than expected by the decrease in fat content, indicating the presence of other control mechanisms.[42]

In normal mice, leptin decreases NPY.[43] In most animal models, the NPY content in the hypothalamus is high with obesity, and brain infusions of NPY cause obesity and increased ob gene expression.[44] Knockout mice deficient in NPY maintain normal weight and respond to leptin, indicating that NPY is part of a redundant system, not an absolute requirement.[45]

In the human, the ob gene, known as the Lep gene, does not appear to be acutely regulated.[46] Feeding increases leptin levels, but slowly, correlating with insulin levels.[37, 47] Insulin provides negative feedback to the brain in a manner similar to leptin, including an effect on NPY.[36] The hyperphagia of diabetes mellitus reflects a deficiency in this insulin action. In fa/fa rats (obese because of a mutation in the leptin receptor), insulin does not affect neuropeptide Y expression, indicating that the inhibition of NPY exerted by insulin is mediated through the leptin-signaling system.[48]

CRH inhibits food intake and increases energy expenditure; thus, it is expected that weight loss would decrease CRH. In addition, leptin stimulates CRH gene expression, and therefore, lower leptin levels with fasting should lower CRH levels.[48] And indeed, CRH secretion is not increased after acute weight loss; however, it is well recognized that cortisol secretion is increased with stress and exercise. This may be due to a hypothalamic effect of NPY on ACTH secretion by the pituitary.[48] The specific food and energy response associated with CRH may also be mediated by urocortin, a CRH-related peptide.[49] Urocortin is very potent in reducing food intake, perhaps activating the energy system without activating the overall CRH mechanism. These relationships are further confused by evidence that glucocorticoids stimulate leptin synthesis and secretion in humans.[50]

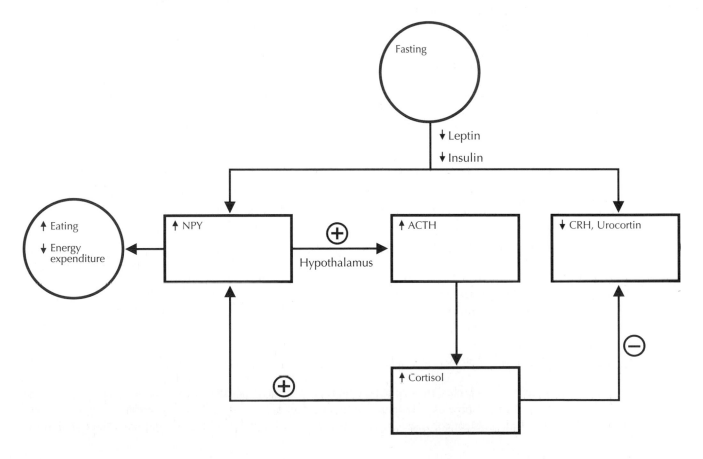

Leptin in Obese People

Most studies have indicated that nearly all obese individuals have elevated leptin levels, probably due to an increase in Lep gene expression and partly due to greater production because of larger fat cells.[51–53] The greater weight of these individuals represents the leptin level at which stability is achieved, when leptin resistance is overcome. In lean individuals, leptin levels are similar in men and women, but in women, as weight increases, leptin increases 3 times more rapidly than in men.[38] Higher levels in women suggest a greater resistance to leptin, correlating with a greater prevalence of obesity in women.[54]

The incidence of obesity in black women is almost twice that of white women.[55] Obese postmenopausal black women have 20% lower leptin levels than white women.[56] These lower leptin levels correlate with a lower resting metabolic rate in the black women. The lower levels may indicate a greater sensitivity to the leptin mechanism in black women.

In obese individuals, fat cells produce leptin normally and a prevalent genetic failure has not been identified. ***Thus it is hypothesized that obesity is due to resistance to leptin.***[57] This may be due to a transport problem of leptin into the brain, as indicated by the finding that leptin level differences between obese and lean individuals are greater in blood than in cerebrospinal fluid.[58, 59] At least in the mouse, this resistance is present only in the periphery in that leptin administered in the brain still works.[60]

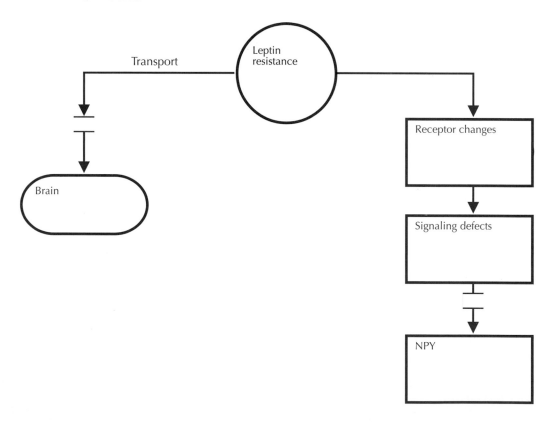

Only a small percentage of humans are expected to have mutations in the leptin receptor and be refractory to leptin agonist treatment.[61] Diet-induced obesity in mice responds to leptin treatment, and it is expected that the majority of overweight humans would also. However, in genetically normal animals, leptin treatment does not always reduce weight by reducing food intake.[62] A crucial question is what happens within physiologic range changes in leptin.

In obese individuals, the majority of leptin is unbound and presumably active, consistent with the resistance hypothesis.[63] In lean individuals, the majority of circulating leptin is bound. Another important subject for research is the regulation of leptin binding to proteins in the circulation.

Why Is Weight Loss So Hard To Maintain?

The average adult eats nearly 1 million calories per year.[28] When life was tougher, leptin served the purpose of meeting the threat of starvation. During periods of food availability, individuals with leptin defects could consume large amounts and store excess fat. Today, with no shortage of food, these individuals who survived during food shortages in the past now become obese, and succumb to the complications of obesity. But the most vexing problem is that 90% to 95% of people who lose weight subsequently regain it.[64]

Weight loss in obese and lean people produces the same response, decreased leptin and insulin. The obese person tends to regain weight because the lower leptin started from a different set point and is now lower than what the body views as required to be stable in terms of the amount of fat. When energy expenditure, food intake, and body weight are in balance, leptin is at a level consistent with a set point determined by this balance. With weight loss and loss of fat, leptin decreases, causing an increase in appetite and a decrease in energy. This is great when you lose weight with an illness, but not good for an overweight person trying to lose weight. Whenever a perturbation occurs, leptin levels change to restore the original status quo, making it difficult for overweight people to maintain weight loss. Thus, there is hope for leptin agonist treatment of these individuals.

Circulating levels of leptin are correlated with the percent body fat.[51] In other words increased body fat increases the expression of the Lep gene in fat cells. The amount of leptin in the circulation, therefore, is a measure of the amount of adipose tissue in the body. For this reason, neither baseline levels nor initial changes in leptin predict whether weight loss can be maintained.[65]

A *reduction* of 10% in body weight is associated with a 53% reduction in serum leptin.[51] This would stimulate an effort to regain the weight. The key question is what happens if an individual can successfully maintain the lower weight. In a longitudinal study of obese people, when weight loss was maintained, leptin levels remained low.[66]

Therefore, whenever a perturbation occurs, leptin levels change to restore the original status quo. Thus, these acute responses work against attempts to lose weight. A change in energy intake causes a change in leptin levels.[48] The body then changes appetite and energy expenditure to conform to the new leptin level. A 10% *increase* in body weight is associated with a 300% increase in serum leptin.[67] The basic purpose is to conserve energy during periods of fasting and to avoid obesity during periods of excess. When caloric intake is reduced, the basal metabolic rate is reduced in a regulatory compensatory adaptation that makes maintenance of weight loss difficult.

Congenital Leptin Deficiency

The Lep gene (ob gene in mice) has been sequenced from hundreds of obese individuals and mutations have been rare, and mutations in the leptin receptor have also not been detected in obese people.[57, 68]

The first definitive demonstration of a congenital leptin deficiency in humans was reported in two severely obese Pakistani children who were cousins. [69] Despite their mass of fat, their serum leptin levels were very low, and the molecular biology study of a fat biopsy revealed a homozygous deletion of a single guanine in the leptin gene. This mutation results in the introduction of 14 aberrant amino acids into the leptin peptide followed by a premature truncation. All four parents were heterozygotes. These children had normal birth weights, but immediately began gaining excessive weight with marked increases in appetites. In contrast to ob/ob mice, they did not have elevated cortisol levels; however they were hyperinsulinemic. Three obese members of a Turkish family have been reported with an amino acid substitution that impairs intracellular transport of leptin.[70] It is noteworthy that these individuals also displayed suppression of gonadal function.

An obese individual has been reported with a mutation in prohormone convertase (an enzyme that participates in the conversion of prohormones into hormones as does the carboxypeptidase E enzyme deficient in the fat/fat mouse).[71] However, a single gene mutation responsible for obesity will probably be discovered only in individuals such as these with extremely severe obesity. Nevertheless, linkages to obesity have been described to regions near the leptin gene or the leptin receptor gene, perhaps indicating differences in regulatory elements of these genes.[72]

It is expected that only a small percentage of obese humans will have mutations in the leptin receptor or the Lep gene.

Leptin and Reproduction

Several observations support a role for leptin in reproductive physiology.

1.   Leptin administration accelerates the onset of puberty in rodents.[73]

2.   Leptin levels increase at puberty in boys.[74]

3.   Low leptin levels are present in athletes and in patients with anorexia and delayed puberty.[75]

4.   The ob/ob mouse undergoes normal sexual development, but remains prepubertal and never ovulates, but fertility is restored with leptin administration.[73]

Leptin levels are greater in females than in males, and in premenopausal women compared with postmenopausal women.[61] In girls, leptin levels are higher and decrease with increasing Tanner stages of puberty.[76] Thus with puberty, there is increasing sensitivity to leptin. Or in another way to look at this relationship, decreasing leptin during puberty may allow greater food intake for growth by lowering the satiety signal.

The effect of leptin on reproduction can be viewed as an additional role in maintaining responses to stress. Weight loss is known to be associated with an increased adrenal response and a decrease in thyroid function; these endocrine changes, along with suppression of the estrous cycle, occur in fasted mice and are reversed by treatment with leptin.[77]

The puzzle is why CRH is elevated in stress amenorrhea (especially that associated with weight loss) in contrast to fasting in normal and obese individuals. One possibility is that the decrease in leptin and increase in NPY associated with stress-related weight loss is the expected response, but it is inadequate to suppress the stress-induced increase in CRH. The blunted patterns in amenorrheic athletes support this. The increase in CRH and resulting hypercortisolism further increase metabolism and weight loss.

Athletes with cyclic menses demonstrate a normal diurnal rhythm in leptin levels. However, amenorrheic athletes do not have a diurnal pattern.[78] Both cycling athletes and amenorrheic athletes have low leptin levels (3-fold reduction) that correlate with reduced body fat, but the levels are further lowered by hypoinsulinemia and hypercortisolemia. In addition, amenorrheic athletes have a blunted leptin response to the increase in insulin following meals.

In postmenopausal women, leptin levels decrease with endurance training, and hormone therapy has no effect.[79] This indicates that the gender difference (higher levels in women) is due to a difference in fat content, not a hormonal difference.

Because of the tight connection between insulin and leptin levels in mice, and the now well recognized prevalence of hyperinsulinemia in women with polycystic ovaries, it makes sense to examine leptin levels in these women.

Although an initial study reported increased leptin levels in women with polycystic ovaries, the study has been criticized for not adjusting for body weight.[80] At least 3 studies, controlling for weight, detected no differences in leptin levels comparing women with and without polycystic ovaries.[81-83] In women with polycystic ovaries, the relationship between leptin and body weight is maintained. Thus, in contrast to the rodent model, hyperinsulinemia and insulin resistance do not affect leptin levels in these women.

However, a role for leptin in the changes associated with polycystic ovaries should not yet be discounted. There may be subtle differences that have biologic consequences. At least one study demonstrated a correlation between leptin levels and 24-hour insulin levels in women with polycystic ovaries.[81] Furthermore, the drug that lowers insulin resistance, troglitazone, inhibits transcription of the Lep gene and may be especially suited for obese women with polycystic ovaries.[84]

Is it possible that leptin has a target tissue role in reproduction? An isoform of leptin has been identified in the ovary, and leptin exerts specific actions on steroidogenesis as studied in vitro.[85, 86] Leptin inhibits the synergistic action of insulin-like growth factor-I (IGF-I) on FSH-stimulated estradiol production (but not progesterone) in rat granulosa cells, and also inhibits FSH stimulation of IGF-I production. In addition, leptin is expressed in human granulosa and cumulus cells, and is present in mature human oocytes and follicular fluid; thus, leptin appears to be secreted by the ovarian follicle.[87] A rise in maternal serum leptin levels after the administration of human chorionic gonadotropin and before ovum retrieval was correlated with a higher pregnancy rate.[87] Leptin, therefore, probably is involved in a multitude of important metabolic and developmental functions.

The leptin story has restored credibility to the critical weight hypothesis originally proposed by Rose Frisch in the 1970s.[88] The critical weight hypothesis states that the onset and regularity of menstrual function necessitate maintaining weight above a critical level, and, therefore, above a critical amount of body fat. It has always been a mystery how total body fat could talk with the brain. A mystery no longer! Fat talks to the brain via leptin, and the leptin system affects reproduction.

There is a difference, however, between ordinary weight loss and stress-induced (e.g., exercise or psychologic problems such as anorexia) weight loss. In ordinary weight loss, corticotropin-releasing hormone (CRH) secretion is reduced, and the hypercortisolism is believed to be mediated through NPY signals in the hypothalamus. In stress-induced weight loss, CRH secretion is increased.

CRH directly inhibits hypothalamic GnRH secretion, probably by augmenting endogenous opioid secretion. Women with hypothalamic amenorrhea (including exercisers and women with eating disorders) demonstrate hypercortisolism (due to increased CRH and ACTH, perhaps augmented by NPY stimulation of ACTH secretion), suggesting that this is the pathway by which stress interrupts reproductive function.[89] In regards to reproduction, the final pathway is suppression of GnRH, a response to multiple inputs indicating the availability of metabolic fuel. The clinical presentation (inadequate luteal phase, anovulation, amenorrhea) will depend on the degree of GnRH suppression.

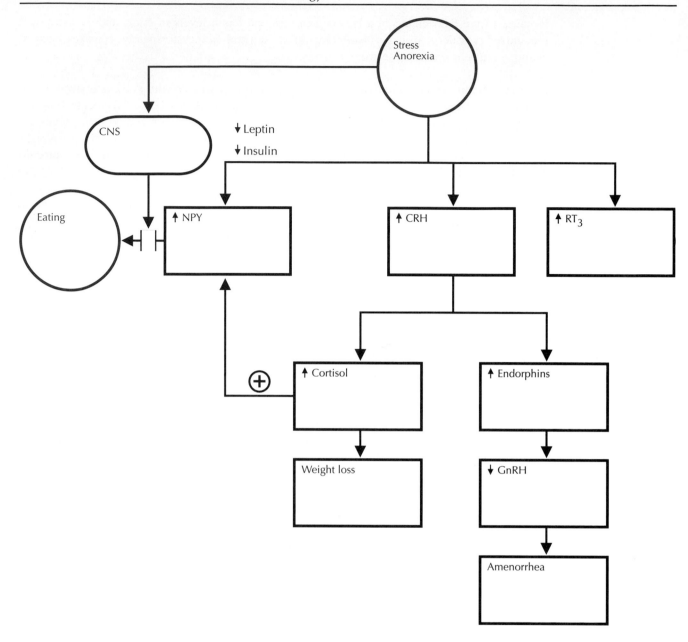

A unifying hypothesis focuses on energy balance.[90] When available energy is excessively diverted, as in exercise, or when insufficient, as with eating disorders, reproduction is suspended in order to support essential metabolism for survival. Thus reproduction may not be directly affected by the level of body fat, rather body fat is a marker of the metabolic energy state, and the extremely low leptin levels in anorexic patients are an appropriate attempt to restore appetite, an attempt that fails to overcome the stress-induced increase in CRH and its consequences. This is consistent with the finding that NPY stimulates GnRH secretion and amplifies gonadotropin response to GnRH in the rodent.[91] From a teleological point of view, there is sense to these relationships; the responses that assist the body to withstand stress also inhibit menstrual function because a stressful period is not the ideal time for reproduction.

Leptin Summary
Because of the high levels of leptin present in overweight people, the purpose of leptin function may be limited to an effect at low levels. A low circulating level of leptin may serve as a signal that fat stores are not sufficient for growth and reproduction. Thus low levels would ordinarily stimulate hyperphagia, reduce energy expenditure, and suppress gonadotropin secretion and reproduction. The high levels of leptin and the apparent resistance to leptin action associated with excess body weight and fat would then reflect not resistance, but a lack of physiologic effect.

Although the leptin mechanism offers the potential for new treatments for obesity, it is not around the corner. Leptin, a polypeptide, cannot be administered orally, and in view of high levels in overweight people, another method must be found to attack the lack of effect or the apparent resistance to leptin. Thus far, it appears that genetic defects in the Lep gene are uncommon; nevertheless, for affected individuals, a leptin agonist may be therapeutic. Even if this complex system yields new treatments, it is unlikely that we will be able to ignore eating appropriately and exercising adequately.

Inherited Aspects of Obesity

Fat cells develop from connective tissue early in fetal life. An important question is whether new fat cells are produced by metaplasia in the adult, or whether an individual achieves a total complement during a certain period of life. In other words, is excess fat stored by increasing the size of the fat cell, or by increasing the number of cells? The possibility arises that there is an inherited increase in the total number of fat cells, which just wait to be packed full of storage fat. Furthermore, the total number of fat cells may depend on an infant's nutritional state during the neonatal period and perhaps in utero as well.

Studies of fat obtained at surgery indicate that the mean fat cell volume is increased 3-fold in obese people, but an increase in the number of fat cells is seen only in the grossly obese. When patients diet, the fat cells decrease in size but not in number. Hypercellular obesity may be a more difficult problem to overcome, because an individual may be saddled with a permanent increase in fat cells.

Some researchers think that, at some period in a person's life, a fixed number of fat cells is obtained. Adolescence, infancy, and intrauterine life seem particularly critical.[92, 93] This premise is not solidly established, because there is no certain way to identify an empty fat cell, and potential fat cells cannot be recognized. Nevertheless, a hyperplastic type of obesity (more fat cells) may be associated with childhood and have a poor prognosis; a hypertrophic type (enlarged fat cells) that is responsive to dieting may occur in adults.

There certainly appears to be a genetic component. The weights of adopted children in Denmark correlated with the body weights of their biologic parents but not with their adoptive parents.[94] This would suggest that the genetic influence is even more important in childhood than environmental factors. Other work suggests that the familial occurrence of obesity can be attributed in part to a genetically related reduced rate of energy expenditure.[95] In studies of identical and fraternal twins reared apart, approximately 70% of the variance in the body mass index could be assigned to genetic influences and the remaining 30% to environmental effects.[96] After the age of 3, obesity in childhood predicts obesity in adulthood, and parental obesity doubles the risk of adult obesity in both obese and nonobese children.[97]

Some argue that each individual has a set point, a level regulated by a signal between the fat cells and the brain (the leptin system). According to this argument, previously obese people who have successfully lost weight have to maintain themselves in a state of starvation (at least as far as their fat cells are concerned).

Genetics and biochemistry are against many obese people. It is best to recognize that an obese individual who has suffered with the problem lifelong does have a disorder, a disorder which is not well understood. However, for each individual, the extent to which the genetic predisposition is expressed depends on environmental influences. The prevalence of obesity is inversely related to the level of physical activity and education and directly related to parity.[98] Thus, socioeconomic and behavioral factors are important determinants of body weight, and surely each individual will reflect varying impacts of genetics and environment.

Endocrine Changes

The most important endocrine change in obesity is elevation of the basal blood insulin level. The circulating insulin level is proportional to the volume of body fat. Increases in body fat change the body's secretion and sensitivity to insulin, appropriately so because insulin acts to reduce food intake by inhibiting the expression of neuropeptide Y as well as affecting other agents that influence appetite.[48] The effect on neuropeptide Y is believed to be mediated via the leptin signaling system.

Overweight individuals are characterized by insulin resistance. The key factors that affect insulin resistance are the amount of fat tissue in the body, the caloric intake per day, the amount of carbohydrates in the diet, and the amount of daily exercise. At least one mechanism for the increased resistance to insulin observed with increasing weight is down-regulation of insulin receptors brought about by the increase in insulin secretion. The increase in insulin resistance affects the metabolism of carbohydrate, fat, and protein. Circulating levels of free fatty acids increase as a result of inadequate insulin suppression of the fat cell. Insulin resistance results in decreased catabolism of triglycerides, yielding a decrease in HDL-cholesterol and an increase in LDL-cholesterol. This, of course, is a major mechanism for the development of atherosclerosis. Hyperinsulinemia is also directly associated with hypertension. The hyperinsulinemia associated with obesity is reversible with weight loss.

The simplest way to assess insulin resistance is to measure the ratio of fasting glucose to fasting insulin. A ratio lower than 4.5 is characteristic of insulin resistance.[99] This method has limitations, the most notable being the variation due to assay precision and pulsatile secretion of insulin. It is more reliable to measure the insulin response to 1 g/kg glucose; the maximal response should not be greater than 150 µU/mL. However, if a patient is obese, one can assume the patient is insulin-resistant.

Genetics plays a greater role in the development of maturity onset diabetes than juvenile onset.[100] It is impossible to predict exactly who eventually will develop diabetes because the tendency is recessive, and it will not develop in every generation in a family. But weight is a good tip-off. As weight increases, the frequency of occurrence of diabetes increases. Both gestational diabetes and insulin-dependent diabetes are more common in overweight pregnant patients.

Contrary to popular misconception, hypothyroidism does not cause obesity. Weight gain due to hypothyroidism is confined to the fluid accumulation of myxedema. There is no place, therefore, for thyroid hormone administration in the treatment of obesity when the patient is euthyroid.

Obese people are relatively unable to excrete both salt and water, especially while dieting. During dieting, this seems to be mediated by increased output of aldosterone and vasopressin. Because water produced from fat outweighs the fat, people on diets often show little initial weight loss. The early use of a diuretic may encourage a patient to persist with dieting.

The basic question is whether metabolic changes observed in obesity represent adaptive responses to a markedly enlarged fat organ or whether they are representative of a metabolic or hormonal defect. The former is true. These changes are secondary responses; they are totally reversible with weight loss. Four-year follow-up in a group of patients who did not regain their weight after dieting revealed persistently normal insulin and glucose responses; patients who regained their weight showed further deterioration in these metabolic factors.[101]

Anatomic Obesity

Gynoid obesity (the pear shape) refers to fat distribution in the lower body (femoral and gluteal regions), whereas android obesity (the apple shape) refers to central body distribution. Gynoid fat is more resistant to catecholamines and more sensitive to insulin than abdominal fat; thus, extraction and storage of fatty acids easily occur, and fat is accumulated more readily in the thighs and buttocks. This fat is associated with minimal fatty acid flux, and, therefore, the negative consequences of fatty acid metabolism are less. Gynoid fat is principally stored fat. The clinical meaning of all this is that women with gynoid obesity are less likely than women with android obesity to develop diabetes mellitus and coronary heart disease.[102]

During pregnancy, lipoprotein lipase activity increases in gynoid fat, further promoting fat storage and explaining the tendency for women to gain thigh and hip weight during pregnancy. Also, because this fat is more resistant to mobilization, it is harder to get rid of. This difficulty is related to the adrenergic receptor concentration in the fat cells, the regulation of which remains a mystery.

Android obesity refers to fat located in the abdominal wall and visceral-mesenteric locations. This fat is more sensitive to catecholamines and less sensitive to insulin and, thus, more active metabolically. It more easily delivers triglyceride to other tissues to meet energy requirements. This fat distribution is associated with hyperinsulinemia, impaired glucose tolerance, diabetes mellitus, an increase in androgen production rates, decreased levels of sex hormone-binding globulin, and increased levels of free testosterone and estradiol.[103, 104] In addition, women with central obesity have decreased cortisol levels, a finding that would be consistent with increased leptin levels.[105, 106] These metabolic changes improve with weight loss.[106]

It is central body obesity that is associated with cardiovascular risk factors, including hypertension and adverse cholesterol-lipoprotein profiles.[107] The waist:hip ratio is a variable strongly and inversely associated with the level of HDL_2, the fraction of HDL-cholesterol most consistently linked with protection from cardiovascular disease.[108] The adverse impact of excess weight in adolescence can be explained by the fact that deposition of fat in adolescence is largely central in location.[9, 109] Weight loss in women with lower body obesity is mainly cosmetic, whereas loss of central body weight is more important for general health in that an improvement in cardiovascular risk is associated with loss of central body fat. At any given level of body mass index (BMI), an increase in central, android fat increases the risk of cardiovascular disease.

It is somewhat surprising that leptin expression and circulating levels are not influenced by android, central obesity.[110, 111] This indicates that leptin is regulated only by subcutaneous fat.

The waist:hip ratio is a means of estimating the degree of upper to lower body obesity; the ratio accurately predicts the amount of intra-abdominal fat (which is greater with android obesity).[112, 113] However, studies have demonstrated that the more easily determined circumference of the waist is a better predictor of central, android abdominal fat.[114, 115] *A waist circumference greater than 100 cm (about 40 inches) in men and 90 cm (about 35 inches) in women is predictive of abnormal endocrinologic and metabolic function and is associated with an increased risk of cardiovascular disease.[114]*

Management of Obesity

In addition to not smoking cigarettes, weight reduction is the most important health measure available for reducing the risk of cardiovascular disease.[116] After adjusting for age and smoking, the Nurses' Health Study documented a 3-fold increase in risk for coronary disease among women with a body mass index of 29 or greater.[117] Even women who are mildly or moderately overweight have a substantial increase in coronary risk. In the Nurses' Health Study, 40% of coronary events could be attributed to excessive body weight, and in the heaviest women, 70%. But most importantly, weight loss is followed by a decrease in mortality from all causes, and, especially, a decrease in cardiovascular and cancer mortality.[118]

For most patients, after a routine evaluation to rule out pathology such as diabetes mellitus, the clinician is left with the frustrating task of prescribing a diet. But it is not enough to just prescribe a diet or prescribe an anorectic drug. An effective weight loss program requires commitment from both patient and clinician.

Clinician and patient should agree on the goal of a diet program. Although the clinician may want the patient to reach ideal weight, the patient may be satisfied with less. Motivation is improved when the goals meet both personal and medical objectives. It is realistic to lose 4–5 pounds in the first month and 20–30 pounds in 4–5 months. To achieve a respectable rate of weight loss, intake must be 500–1000 calories below energy expenditure.[119] But as weight is lost, energy requirements decrease; therefore unless energy intake decreases, the rate of weight loss will slow. Clinicians and patients need to establish reasonable goals, and only modest changes in diet and activity are necessary.

Despite various fads and diet books, the best diet continues to be a limitation of calories to between 900 and 1200 calories per day, the actual amount depending on what the individual patient will accept and pursue. When energy intake is less than this, it is very difficult to obtain the recommended levels of vitamins and minerals. A daily vitamin and mineral supplement should be used with very low calorie diets. There is no evidence supporting the contention that changing the relative proportions of carbohydrates, protein, and fat without reducing overall caloric intake will produce effective weight loss.[120]

> Ideal Diet: Carbohydrates — 50%
> Protein   — 15–20%
> Fat   — <30%

The discouraging aspect is that to lose a pound of fat, the equivalent to a 3500-calorie intake must be expended. Dieting has to be slow and steady to be effective. Successful programs include behavior modification, frequent visits to the clinician, and involvement of family members. Behavior modification starts with daily recording of activity and behavior related to food intake, followed by the elimination of inappropriate cues (other than hunger) that lead to eating.

Careful studies (performed in hospitalized subjects on metabolic wards) have indicated that the carbohydrate and fat composition of the diet has no effect on the rate of weight loss.[121] Restriction of calories remains the important principle, recognizing that reduction in fat intake is the most effective method of weight loss. Substituting one of the liquid formulas for meals has been successful in many individuals. Unbalanced formulations, however, have the same side effects as seen with total starvation (carbohydrate-deprived regimens). Adequate carbohydrate is necessary for utilization of amino acids. In addition, electrolyte problems have been encountered, and there is an initial diuretic phase that can lead to postural hypotension.

The protein-sparing modified fast is a ketogenic regimen providing approximately 800 calories per day. Unsupplemented liquid protein diets have been associated with deaths due to cardiac arrhythmias. The low-calorie diets that use protein and carbohydrate supplemented with minerals and vitamins as the sole source of nutrition are safer but should be used only for severe obesity and under medical supervision.[122] These diets are still potentially dangerous. The other disadvantage to the semistarvation diet is that short-term success does not guarantee long-term weight maintenance. It is reported that at best only one-fourth to one-third of individuals who lose weight by a semistarvation ketogenic regimen plus behavior modification therapy will have significant long-term weight reduction.[123] On the other hand, for that one-fourth to one-third, this represents a major accomplishment and is worth doing. Unfortunately, repeated dieting and recidivism have a negative impact. With each episode, the body learns to become more efficient, so that with each diet, weight comes off more slowly and is regained more rapidly.

It is not unusual to encounter patients who claim to be unable to lose weight despite following a diet with less than 1200 calories per day. In a study of such patients, it was discovered that underreporting of actual food intake and overreporting of physical activity are both common.[124] While it may not be true for all patients, certainly some individuals do eat more than they think and exercise less than they report to their clinicians. This is not a deliberate conscious attempt to deceive the clinician. These patients truly believe their resistance to weight loss is genetic and not due to their own personal behavior. They are astonished and distressed to learn the results of accurate recording of dietary intake and physical exercise. The use of a dietitian to record a typical week's worth of eating and exercise is worthwhile. This kind of knowledge proves to be a powerful lever in providing the motivation to make the changes in lifestyle that can yield loss of weight.

As an index of the general lack of success with diets, a summary of 10 studies (approximately 1200 patients) revealed that only 30% lose 20 pounds or more, and only 4% lose 40 pounds or more.[125] Although most efforts yield short-term success, maintenance of weight loss is uncommon. Commercial organizations are no more successful than physician-directed programs or nonprofit self-help groups.[126, 127] Approximately 90% to 95% of people who lose weight subsequently regain it.[64] Thus, it is obvious why gimmicks abound in this area of patient management. A more reasonable attitude is to emphasize how much can be gained with only a little weight loss. A weight loss of 5–10% of body weight will produce beneficial effects on the risks of cardiovascular disease and diabetes mellitus.[128, 129]

Unfortunately, smoking cessation is associated with an increase in being overweight.[130] And, of course, the link between smoking and weight control is exploited by the tobacco industry in its advertising. This should only increase the importance of our efforts to keep young people from starting smoking and to educate middle-aged people regarding the dangers of smoking.

Anorectics are useful as short-term therapy to control hunger, especially at the beginning of a diet and at a plateau or relapse stage. Compared with amphetamines (which modulate both dopaminergic and noradrenergic neurotransmission), there is far less abuse associated with the catecholamine congeners that affect only noradrenergic neurotransmission. Fenfluramine and dexfenfluramine have no effects on either dopaminergic or noradrenergic neurotransmission, but they increase serotonin release and partially inhibit serotonin reuptake, thus depleting serotonin in the CNS by making it more available for metabolism. However, circulating levels of serotonin become elevated. All of these agents act on the central nervous system to depress appetite.

Because of CNS and cardiovascular side effects (e.g., insomnia, nervousness, euphoria, hypertension, and tachycardia) and the lack of long-term data, the noradrenergic agents should be reserved for short-term use for individuals who wish to lose a small amount of weight. Noradrenergic agents should not be used in individuals with cardiovascular disease. Dexfenfluramine is the d-enantiomer of fenfluramine, the active component of the racemic mixture of d,l-fenfluramine. It was reasoned that lower doses of a noradrenergic agent and a serotonergic agent, when combined, would yield better results, and this proved to be true, but only in a small number of patients.[131] The combination of phentermine and fenfluramine became popular, although weight is promptly regained when treatment is stopped. The popularity of the serotonergic agents received a setback with reports of increased risks due to high circulating levels of serotonin (even with short-term therapy) of the rare but life-threatening conditions, primary pulmonary hyperten-

Weight Loss Drugs

Noradrenergic Agents (affecting the catecholaminergic system):

Diethylpropion	25 mg before meals; 75 mg in morning in slow release form
Phentermine	8 mg before meals; 15 or 37.5 mg in morning
Phendimetrazine	35 mg before meals; 105 mg slow release form daily
Mazindol	1–3 mg 1–3 times daily

Serotonergic Agents:

Fenfluramine	20–40 mg before meals; 60 mg daily in slow release form
Dexfenfluramine	15 mg before meals

Noradrenergic and Serotonergic Agent:

Sibutramine	10–15 mg daily

Lipase Inhibitor:

Orlistat	120 mg tid

sion and cardiac valvular disease, either with the combination or with either agent (including dexfenfluramine) alone, and these products were withdrawn from the U.S. market.[132–134] Symptoms associated with pulmonary hypertension include the onset of dyspnea, changes in exercise tolerance, angina, syncope, and lower extremity edema. Patients who develop valvular disease are usually symptomatic with dyspnea and evidence of congestive heart failure. Minor side effects of serotonergic drugs include diarrhea, polyuria, dry mouth, sleep disturbance, and somnolence. Patients who have used fenfluramine or dexfenfluramine should be examined, and those who have a heart murmur or who used the drugs for long durations or at high doses should be studied with echocardiography.[135]

Sibutramine (10 or 15 mg daily) blocks the neuronal uptake of both norepinephrine and serotonin, and is an effective appetite suppressant with mild side effects (dry mouth, constipation, and insomnia), but it can increase blood pressure.[136] Orlistat (120 mg tid with meals) inhibits pancreatic lipase and increases fecal fat loss.[137, 138] Orlistat is associated with annoying gastrointestinal side effects (increased defecation of oily stools). There is some loss of the fat soluble vitamins, and a vitamin supplement should be taken at bedtime.

Because weight is regained after discontinuing drug treatment, long-term therapy has been championed. However, very little information is available regarding the long-term use of appetite-suppressing drugs. Although the serotonergic agents produce neurotoxicity in animal brains, it is uncertain whether long-term depletion of brain serotonin has adverse neuropsychological effects (e.g., on mood and memory).[139] Short-term studies indicate only a modest efficacy with variable responses.[64] Most of the weight loss occurs in the first 6 months and is limited to 5–10 kg (11–22 lbs). Nevertheless, long-term treatment may enable some individuals to sustain weight loss and to more effectively make beneficial changes in diet and lifestyle. It is recommended that treatment with appetite-suppressing drugs should be limited to individuals who have failed to lose weight with conventional methods and who demonstrate significant comorbidities, such as android obesity, coronary heart disease, insulin resistance, and hypertension.[64] *Attainment of a normal body weight is unlikely with drug treatment; however, a 5% to 10% weight loss will have an important beneficial impact on risk factors for disease.*[64]

Over-the-counter products contain phenylpropanolamine as the active ingredient. This drug is a sympathomimetic derived from ephedrine and can act synergistically with caffeine to produce amphetamine-like reactions. ***It should be noted that phenylpropanolamine taken in combination with a dopamine agonist (e.g. bromocriptine) or a monoamine oxidase inhibitor can precipitate a hypertensive crisis.*** Appetite-suppressing drugs of all kinds are contraindicated in patients taking monoamine oxidase inhibitors and patients with glaucoma.

Surgical treatment and starvation should be reserved for patients who are morbidly obese. Both methods involve many potential problems and require close monitoring.

Controlled studies have not demonstrated the effectiveness of thyroid preparations or human chorionic gonadotropin.[140] Indeed, adding thyroid hormone increases the loss of lean body mass rather than fat tissue. It is clear that adjunctive drug measures are not successful unless the patient is also motivated either to limit caloric intake or to increase the exercise level in what will be a lifelong battle.

A regular pattern of physical exercise reduces the risk of myocardial infarction in all people.[141] Both weight loss and increased physical activity, through an unknown mechanism, lower the level of low density lipoprotein (LDL), and increase the level of high density lipoprotein (HDL).[142] A further benefit of strenuous or prolonged exercise is an inhibition of appetite that lasts many hours and that is associated with an increase in the resting metabolic rate for 2–48 hours. There is one study, however, that indicates a rebound increase in appetite 1–2 days after exercise.[143] The optimal program includes, therefore, a *daily* period of exercise. A combination of diet and exercise is better than either alone, and those who exercise are more successful in maintaining weight loss.[127, 144, 145] The best time for exercise is before meals or about 2 hours after eating. It is probably wise to take a day off at least once a week to give muscles and joints a rest.

Unfortunately one cannot burn up significant calories quickly; it takes 18 minutes of running to compensate for the average hamburger.[146]

Activity	Calories per Hour
Sleeping	90
Office work	240
Walking	240
Golf	300
Housework	300
Bicycling	360
Swimming	360
Tennis	480
Bowling	510
Running slowly	750 (ca. 120/mile)
Cross country skiing	840
Running fast	960 (ca. 160/mile)

Most frustrating is the problem of some patients who limit caloric intake yet do not lose weight. In fact, as the weights of certain patients increase, the number of calories required to remain in equilibrium decreases, due to a combination of reduced activity and a change in metabolism, now known to be appropriate consequences of changes in leptin levels. The Vermont study demonstrated that the normal person with induced obesity requires 2700 calories to remain in equilibrium; spontaneously obese patients require only about 1300 calories.[147] Others argue that virtually everyone can lose weight on a diet of 1000 calories per day in that the maintenance requirement for a sedentary adult is about 1.5 times the resting metabolic rate (about 1000–1500 calories per day).[148] Nevertheless, an individual who has been overweight requires about 15% fewer calories to maintain weight than an individual who has never been obese.[149] The clinician must be careful to avoid a condemning or punitive attitude and understand that it is possible to significantly restrict caloric intake and not lose weight.

Patients appear doomed to frustration and despair unless the clinician can motivate them to increase physical activity. In all individuals, dieting is more effective when combined with physical exercise, but this is especially true in chronically obese patients. In other words, the lifestyle of an obese person must be changed to overcome the desire to be inactive (walk instead of riding). Only by significantly increasing caloric expenditure will the input-output equilibrium be disturbed.

The obese person feels trapped. Obesity leads to characteristic behavioral manifestations, including passive personality, frequent periods of depression, decreased self-respect, and a sense of being hopelessly overwhelmed by problems. But just as the endocrine and metabolic changes are secondary to obesity, many of the psychosocial attributes surrounding obesity are also secondary.[150]

Maintenance of a newly gained lower weight requires constant preventive attention. Motivation to change and emotional support during the change are important. They can be provided by friends, relatives, clinicians, or self-help organizations. If the vicious circle of failed diets, resignation to fate, guilt, and shame can be broken, a more effective, happier person will emerge.

References

1. **Kuczmarski RJ, Flegal KM, Campbell SM, Johnson CL,** Increasing prevalence of overweight among US adults. The National Health and Nutrition Examination Surveys, 1960 to 1991, *JAMA* 272:205, 1994.

2. **Flegal KM, Carroll MD, Kuczmarski RJ, Johnson CL,** Overweight and obesity in the United States: prevalence and trends, 1960–1994, *Int J Obes* 22:39, 1998.

3. **Harlan WR, Landis JR, Flegal KM, Davis CS, Miller ME,** Secular trends in body mass in the United States, 1960–1980, *Am J Epidemiol* 128:1065, 1988.

4. **Prentice AM, Jebb SA,** Obesity in Britain: gluttony or sloth? *Br Med J* 311:437, 1995.

5. **Roiano RP, Flegal KM, Kuczmarski RJ, Campbell SM, Johnson CL,** Overweight prevalence and trends for children and adolescents. The National Health and Nutrition Examination Surveys, 1963 to 1991, *Arch Pediatr Adolesc Med* 149:1085, 1995.

6. **Sjostrom LV,** Mortality of severely obese subjects, *Am J Clin Nutr* 55(Suppl 2):516S, 1992.

7. **Manson JE, Willett WC, Stampfer MJ, Coditz GA, Hunter DJ, Hankinson SE, Hennekens CH, Speizer FE,** Body weight and mortality among women, *New Engl J Med* 333:677, 1995.

8. **Pi-Sunyer FX,** Medical hazards of obesity, *Ann Intern Med* 110:655, 1993.

9. **Must A, Jacques PF, Dallal GE, Bajema CJ, Dietz WH,** Long-term morbidity and mortality of overweight adolescents: a follow-up of the Harvard Growth Study of 1922 to 1935, *New Engl J Med* 327:1350, 1992.

10. **Ravussin E, Swinburn BA,** Pathophysiology of obesity, *Lancet* 340:404, 1992.

11. **Thomas AE, McKay DA, Cutlip MB,** A nomograph method for assessing body weight, *Am J Clin Nutr* 29:302, 1976.

12. **Van Itallie TB,** Health implications of overweight and obesity in the United States, *Ann Intern Med* 103:983, 1985.

13. **Stamler R, Stamler J, Riedlinger WF, Algera G, Roberts RH,** Weight and blood pressure: findings in hypertension screening of 1 million Americans, *JAMA* 240:1607, 1978.

14. **Colditz GA, Willett WC, Rotnitzky A, Manson JE,** Weight gain as a risk factor for clinical diabetes mellitus in women, *Ann Intern Med* 122:481, 1995.

15. **Willett WC, Manson JE, Stampfer MJ, Colditz GA, Rosner B, Speizer FE, Hennekens CH,** Weight change and coronary heart disease in women: risk within the "normal" range, *JAMA* 273:461, 1995.

16. **Ferraro R, Lillioja S, Fontvieille A-M, Rising R, Bogardus C, Ravussin E,** Lower sedentary metabolic rate in women compared with men, *J Clin Invest* 90:780, 1992.

17. **Fabry P, Hejda S, Cerny K,** Effects of meal frequency in school children. Changes in weight-height proportion and skinfold thickness, *Am J Clin Nutr* 18:358, 1966.

18. **Fukagawa NA, Bandini LG, Young JB,** Effect of age on body composition and resting metabolic rate, *Am J Physiol* 259:E233, 1990.

19. **Vaughan L, Zurlo F, Ravussin E,** Aging and energy expenditure, *Am J Clin Nutr* 53:821, 1991.

20. **Van Pelt RE, Jones PP, Davy KP, Desouza CA, Tanaka H, Davy BM, Seals DR,** Regular exercise and the age-related decline in resting metabolic rate in women, *J Clin Endocrinol Metab* 82:3208, 1997.

21. **Suter PM, Schutz Y, Jequier E,** The effect of ethanol on fat storage in healthy subjects, *New Engl J Med* 326:983, 1992.

22. **Gold RM,** Hypothalamic obesity: the myth of the ventromedial nucleus, *Science* 182:488, 1973.

23. **Leibowitz SF,** Brain peptides and obesity: pharmacologic treatment, *Obes Res* 3(Suppl 4):573S, 1995.

24. **Wilber JF,** Neuropeptides, appetite regulation, and human obesity, *JAMA* 266:257, 1991.

25. **Kennedy GC,** The role of depot fat in the hypothalamic control of food intake in the rat, *Proc Roy Soc* 140:578, 1953.

26. **Hervey GR,** The effects of lesions in the hypothalamus in parabiotic rats, *J Physiol* 145:336, 1958.

27. **Zhang Y, Proenca R, Maffei M, Barone M, Leopold L, Friedman J,** Positional cloning of the mouse obese gene and its human homologue, *Nature* 372:425, 1994.

28. **Campfield LA, Smith FJ, Burn P,** The OB protein (leptin) pathway — a link between adipose tissue mass and central neural networks, *Horm Metab Res* 28:619, 1996.

29. **Tartaglia LA,** The leptin receptor, *J Biol Chem* 272:6093, 1997.

30. **Stephens TW, Basinski M, Bristow PK, Bue-Valleskey JM, Burgett SG, Craft L, Hale J, Hoffman J, Hsiung HM, Kriauciunas A, et al,** The role of neuropeptide Y in the antiobesity action of the *obesity* gene product, *Nature* 377:530, 1995.

31. **Mercer JG, Hoggard N, Williams LM, Lawrence CB, Hannah LT, Trayburn P,** Localization of leptin receptor mRNA and the long form splice variant (Ob-Rb) in mouse hypothalamus and adjacent brain regions by in situ hybridization, *FEBS Lett* 387:113, 1996.

32. **Devos R, Richards JG, Campfield LA, Tartaglia LA, Guisez Y, Van der Heyden J, Travernier J, Plaetinck G, Burn P,** OB protein binds specifically to the chorioid plexus of mice and rats, *Proc Natl Acad Sci USA* 93:5668, 1996.

33. **Banks WA, Kastin AJ, Huang W, Jaspan JB, Maness LM,** Leptin enters the brain by a saturable system independent of insulin, *Peptides* 17:305, 1996.

34. **Cusin I, Rohner-Jeanrenaud F, Stricker-Krongrad A, Jeanrenaud B,** The weight-reducing effect of an intracerebroventricular bolus injection of letpin in genetically obese *fa/fa* rats. Reduced sensitivity compared with lean animals, *Diabetes* 45:1446, 1996.

35. **Caro JF, Sinha MK, Kolaczynski JW, Zhang PL, Considine RV,** Leptin: the tale of an obesity gene, *Diabetes* 45:1455, 1996.

36. **Schwartz MW, Seeley RJ,** The new biology of body weight regulation, *J Am Diet Assoc* 97:54, 1997.

37. **Kolaczynski JW, Nyce MR, Considine RV, Boden G, Nolan JJ, Henry R, Mudaliar SR, Olefsky J, Caro JF,** Acute and chronic effect of insulin on leptin production in humans: studies in vivo and in vitro, *Diabetes* 45:699, 1996.

38. **Kennedy A, Gettys TW, Watson P, Wallace P, Ganaway E, Pan Q, Garvey WT,** The metabolic significance of leptin in humans: gender-based differences in relationship to adiposity, insulin sensitivity, and energy expenditure, *J Clin Endocrinol Metab* 82:1293, 1997.

39. **Fan W, Boston BA, Kesterson RA, Hruby VJ, Cone RD,** Role of melanocortinergic neurons in feeding and the agouti obesity syndrome, *Nature* 385:165, 1997.

40. **Huszar D, Lynch CA, Fairchild-Huntress V, Dunmore JH, Fang Q, Berkemeier LR, Gu W, Kesterson RA, Boston BA, Cone RD, Smith FJ, Campfield LA, Burn P, Lee F,** Targeted disruption of the melanocortin-4 receptor results in obesity in mice, *Cell* 88:131, 1997.

41. **Krude H, Biebermann H, Luck W, Horn R, Brabant G, Gruters A,** Severe early-onset obesity, adrenal insufficiency and red hair pigmentation caused by POMC mutations in humans, *Nat Genet* 19:155, 1998.

42. **Wiegle DS, Duell PB, Connor WE, Steiner RA, Soules MR, Kuijper JL,** Effect of fasting, refeeding, and dietary fat restriction on plasma leptin levels, *J Clin Endocrin Metab* 82:561, 1997.

43. **Schwartz MW, Baskin DG, Bukowski TR, Kuijper JL, Foster D, Lasser G, Prunkard DE, Porte D, Woods SC, Seeley RJ, Weigle DS,** Specificity of leptin action on elevated blood glucose levels and hypothalamic neuropeptide Y gene expression in *ob/ob* mice, *Diabetes* 45:531, 1996.

44. **Rohner-Jeanrenaud F,** A neuroendocrine reappraisal of the dual-centre hypothesis: its implications for obesity and insulin resistance, *Int J Obesity* 19:517, 1995.

45. **Erickson JC, Klegg KE, Palmiter PD,** Sensitivity to leptin and susceptibility to seizures of mice lacking neuropeptide Y, *Nature* 381:415, 1996.

46. **Saladin R, Staels B, Auwerx J, Briggs M,** Regulation of *ob* gene expression in rodents and humans, *Horm Metab Res* 28:638, 1996.

47. **Malmstrom R, Taskinen MR, Karonen SL, Ykijarvinen H,** Insulin increases plasma leptin concentrations in normals and patients with NIDDDM, *Diabetologia* 39:993, 1996.

48. **Schwartz MW, Seeley RJ,** Neuroendocrine responses to starvation and weight loss, *New Engl J Med* 336:1802, 1997.

49. **Spina M, Merlo-Pich E, Chan RKW, Basso AM, Rivier J, Vale W, Koob GF,** Appetite-suppressing effects of urocortin, a CRF-related neuropeptide, *Science* 273:1561, 1996.

50. **Masuzaki H, Ogawa Y, Hosoda K, Miyawaki T, Hanaoka I, Hiraoka J, Yasuno A, Nishimura H, Yoshimasa Y, Nishi S, Nakao K,** Glucocorticoid regulation of leptin synthesis and secretion in humans: elevated plasma leptin levels in Cushing's syndrome, *J Clin Endocrinol Metab* 82:2542, 1997.

51. **Considine RV, Sinha MK, Heiman ML, Krauciunas A, Stephens TW, Nyce MR, Ohannesian JP, Marco CC, McKee LJ, Bauer TL, Caro JF,** Serum immunoreactive-leptin concentrations in normal-weight and obese humans, *New Engl J Med* 334:292, 1995.

52. **Lonnqvist F, Arner P, Norfors L, Schalling M,** Overexpression of the obese (ob) gene in adipose tissue of human obese subjects, *Nature Med* 9:950, 1995.

53. **Hamilton B, Paglia D, Kwan A, Deitel M,** Increased obese mRNA expression in omental fat cells from massively obese humans, *Nat Med* 9:953, 1995.

54. **Saad MF, Damani S, Gingerich RL, Riad-Gabriel MG, Khan A, Boyadjian R, Jinagouda SD, El-Tawil K, Rude RK, Kamdar V,** Sexual dimorphism in plasma leptin concentration, *J Clin Endocrinol Metab* 82:579, 1997.

55. **Kumanyika SK,** Obesity in minority populations: an epidemiologic assessment, *Obes Res* 2:166, 1994.

56. **Nicklas BJ, Toth MJ, Goldberg AP, Poehlman ET,** Racial differences in plasma leptin concentrations in obese postmenopausal women, *J Clin Endocrinol Metab* 82:315, 1997.

57. **Considine RV, Considine EL, Williams CJ, Nyce MR, Zhang PL, Opentanova I, Ohannesian JP, Koaczynsi JW, Bauer TL, Moore JH, Caro JF,** Mutation screening and identification of a sequence variation in the human Ob gene coding, *Biochem Biophys Res Commun* 220:735, 1996.

58. **Schwartz MH, Peskind E, Raskind M, Boyko EJ, Porte Jr D,** Cerebrospinal fluid leptin levels: relationship to plasma levels and to adiposity in humans, *Nat Med* 2:589, 1996.

59. **Caro JF, Kolaczynski JW, Nyce MR, Ohannesian JP, Opentanova I, Goldman WH, Lynn RB, Zhang P-L, Sinha MK, Considine RV,** Decreased cerebrospinal-fluid/serum leptin ratio in obesity: a possible mechanism for leptin resistance, *Lancet* 348:159, 1996.

60. **Van Heek M, Compton DS, France CF, Tedesco RP, Fawzi AB, Graziano MP, Sybertz EJ, Strader CD, Davis Jr HR,** Diet-induced obese mice develop peripheral, but not central, resistance to leptin, *J Clin Invest* 99:385, 1997.

61. **Rosenbaum M, Nicolson M, Hirsch J, Heymsfield SB, Gallagher D, Chu F, Leibel R,** Effects of gender, body composition, and menopause on plasma concentrations of leptin, *J Clin Endocrinol Metab* 81:3424, 1996.

62. **Levin N, Nelson C, Gurney A, Vandlen R, de Sauvage F,** Decreased food intake does not completely account for adiposity reduction after ob protein infusion, *Proc Natl Acad Sci USA* 93:1726, 1996.

63. **Sinha MK, Opentanova I, Ohannesian JP, Kolaczynski JW, Heiman ML, Hale J, Becker GW, Bowsher RR, Stephens TW, Caro JF,** Evidence of free and bound leptin in human circulation. Studies in lean and obese subjects and during short-term fasting, *J Clin Invest* 98:1277, 1996.

64. **National Task Force on the Prevention and Treatment of Obesity,** Long-term pharmacotherapy in the management of obesity, *JAMA* 276:1907, 1996.

65. **Wing RR, Sinha MK, Considine RV, Lang W, Caro JF,** Relationship between weight loss maintenance and changes in serum leptin levels, *Horm Metab Res* 28:698, 1996.

66. **Saris WHM, Kempen KR, Campfield LA, Tenenbaum R,** Responses of plasma OB protein concentration to weight cycling in obese women, *Obes Res* 4(Suppl 1):40s, 1996.

67. **Kolaczynski JW, Ohannesian J, Considine RV, Marco CC, Caro JF,** Response of leptin to short term and prolonged overfeeding in humans, *J Clin Endocrinol Metab*, in press.

68. **Considine RV, Considine EL, Williams CJ, Hyde TM, Caro JF,** The hypothalamic leptin receptor in humans: identification of incidental sequence polymorphisms and absence of the ob/ob mouse and fa/fa rat mutations, *Diabetes* 45:992, 1996.

69. **Montague CT, Farooqi IS, Whitehead JP, Soos MA, Rau H, Wareham NJ, Sewter CP, Digby JE, Mohammed SN, Hurst JA, Cheetham CH, Earley AR, Barnett AH, Prins JB, O'Rahilly SO,** Congenital leptin deficiency is associated with severe early-onset obesity in humans, *Nature* 387:903, 1997.

70. **Strobel A, Issad T, Camoin M, Ozata M, Strosberg AD,** A leptin mutation associated with hypogonadism and morbid obesity, *Nat Genet* 18:213, 1998.

71. **Jackson RS, Creemers JWM, Ohagi S, Raffin-Sanson ML, Sanders L, Montague CT, Hutton JC, O'Rahilly S,** Obesity and impaired prohormone processing associated with mutations in the human prohormone convertase 1 gene, *Nat Genet* 16:303, 1997.

72. **Chagnon YC, Perusse L, Lamothe M, Chagnon M, Nadeau A, Dionne FT, Gagnon J, Cheung WK, Leibel RL, Bouchard G,** Suggestive linkages between markers on human 1p32-p22 and body fat and insulin levels in the Quebec Family Study, *Obes Res* 5:115, 1997.

73. **Chehab FF, Mounzih K, Lu R, Lim ME,** Early onset of reproductive function in normal female mice treated with leptin, *Science* 275:88, 1997.

74. **Mantzoros CS, Flier JS, Rogol AD,** A longitudinal assessment of hormonal and physical alterations during normal puberty in boys. V. Rising leptin levels may signal the onset of puberty, *J Clin Endocrinol Metab* 82:1066, 1997.

75. **Hanaoka I, Hosoda K, Ogawa Y, Masuzaki H, Miyawaki T, Natsui K, Hiraoka J, Matsuoka N, Yasuno A, Satoh N, Matsuda J, Shintani M, Azuma Y, Kou T, Nishimura H, Yoshimasa Y, Nishi S, Nakao K,** Decreased plasma leptin levels in anorexia nervosa, P2-539, The Endocrine Society Annual Meeting, 1997.

76. **Hassink SG, Sheslow DV, de Lancey E, Opentanova I, Considine RV, Caro JF,** Serum leptin in children with obesity: relationship to gender and development, *Pediatrics* 98:201, 1996.

77. **Ahima RS, Prabakren D, Mantzoros C, Ou D, Lowell B, Maratzoros-Flier E, Flier J,** Role of leptin in the neuroendocrine response to fasting, *Nature* 382:250, 1996.

78. **Laughlin GA, Yen SSC,** Hypoleptinemia in women athletes: absence of a diurnal rhythm with amenorrhea, *J Clin Endocrinol Metab* 82:318, 1997.

79. **Kohrt WM, Landt M, Birge Jr SJ,** Serum leptin levels are reduced in response to exercise training, but not hormone replacement therapy in older women, *J Clin Endocrinol Metab* 81:3980, 1996.

80. **Brzechffa PR, Jakimiuk J, Agarwal SK, Weitsman SR, Buyalos RP, Magoffin DA,** Serum immunoreactive leptin concentrations in women with polycystic ovary syndrome, *J Clin Endocrinol Metab* 81:4166, 1996.

81. **Laughlin GA, Yen SSC,** Serum leptin levels in women with polycystic ovary syndrome: the role of insulin resistance/hyperinsulinemia, *J Clin Endocrinol Metab* 82:1692, 1997.

82. **Mantzoros CS, Dunaif A, Flier JS,** Leptin concentrations in the polycystic ovary syndrome, *J Clin Endocrinol Metab* 82:1687, 1997.

83. **Rouru J, Anttila L, Koskinen P, Penttilä T-A, Irjala K, Huupponen R, Koulu M,** Serum leptin concentrations in women with polycystic ovary syndrome, *J Clin Endocrinol Metab* 82:1697, 1997.

84. **Nolan JJ, Olefsky JM, Nyce MR, Considine RV, Caro JF,** Effect of troglitazone on leptin production: studies in vitro and in human subjects, *Diabetes* 45:1276, 1996.

85. **Cioffi JA, Shafer AW, Zupancic TJ, Smith-Gbur J, Mikhail A, Platika D, Snodgress HR,** Novel B219/OB receptor isoforms: possible role of leptin in hemapoesis and reproduction, *Nat Med* 2:585, 1996.

86. **Zachow RJ, Magoffin DA,** Direct intraovarian effects of leptin: impairment of the synergistic action of insulin-like growth factor-I on follicle-stimulating hormone-dependent estradiol-17β production by rat ovarian granulosa cells, *Endocrinology* 138:847, 1997.

87. **Cioffi JA, Van Blerkom J, Antczak M, Shafer A, Wittmer S, Snodgrass HR,** The expression of leptin and its receptors in pre-ovulatory human follicles, *Mol Hum Reprod* 3:467, 1997.

88. **Frisch RE,** Body fat, menarche, and reproductive ability, *Seminars Reprod Endocrinol* 3:45, 1985.

89. **Dorn LD, Chrousos GP,** The neurobiology of stress: understanding regulation of affect during female biological transitions, *Seminars Reprod Endocrinol* 15:19, 1997.

90. **Wade GN, Schneider JE, Li H-Y,** Control of fertility by metabolic cues, *Am J Physiol* 270(Endocrinol Metab 33):E1, 1996.

91. **Kalra SP, Allen LG, Sahu A, Kalra PS, Crowley WR,** Gonadal steroids and neuropeptide Y-opioid-LHRH axis: interactions and diversities, *J Steroid Biochem* 30:185, 1988.

92. **Charney E, Goodman HC, McBride M, Lyon B, Pratt R,** Childhood antecedents of adult obesity, *New Engl J Med* 295:6, 1976.

93. **Garn SM, LaVelle M, Rosenberg KR, Hawthorne VM,** Maturational timing as a factor in female fatness and obesity, *Am J Clin Nutr* 43:879, 1986.

94. **Stunkard AJ, Sorensen TIA, Teasdale TW, Chakraborty R, Schull WJ, Schulsinger F,** An adoptive study of human obesity, *New Engl J Med* 314:193, 1986.

95. **Ravussin E, Lillioja S, Knowler WC, Christin L, Freymond D, Abbott WGH, Boyce V, Howard BV, Bogardus C,** Reduced rate of energy expenditure as a risk factor for body-weight gain, *New Engl J Med* 318:467, 1988.

96. **Stunkard AJ, Harris JR, Pederson NL, McClearn GE,** The body-mass index of twins who have been reared apart, *New Engl J Med* 322:1483, 1990.

97. **Whitaker RC, Wright JA, Pepe MS, Seidel KD, Dietz WH,** Predicting obesity in young adulthood from childhood and parental obesity, *New Engl J Med* 337:869, 1997.

98. **Rissanen AM, Heliovaara M, Knekt P, Reunanen A, Aromaa A,** Determinants of weight gain and overweight in adult Finns, *Eur J Clin Nutr* 45:419, 1991.

99. **Legro RS, Finegood D, Dunaif A,** A fasting glucose to insulin ratio is a useful measure of insulin sensitivity in women with polycystic ovary syndrome, *J Clin Endocrinol Metab* 83:2694, 1998.

100. **Fanda OP, Soeldner SS,** Genetic, acquired, and related factors in the etiology of diabetes mellitus, *Arch Intern Med* 137:461, 1977.

101. **Hewing R, Liebermeister H, Daweke H, Gries FA, Gruneklee D,** Weight regain after low calorie diet: long term pattern of blood sugar, serum lipids, ketone bodies, and serum insulin levels, *Diabetologia* 9:197, 1973.

102. **Stern MP, Haffner SM,** Body fat distribution and hyperinsulinemia as risk factors for diabetes and cardiovascular disease, *Arteriosclerosis* 6:123, 1986.

103. **Peiris AN, Sothmann MS, Aiman EJ, Kissebah AH,** The relationship of insulin to sex hormone binding globulin: role of adiposity, *Fertil Steril* 52:69, 1989.

104. **Kirschner MA, Samojlik E, Drejda M, Szmal E, Schneider G, Ertel N,** Androgen-estrogen metabolism in women with upper body versus lower body obesity, *J Clin Endocrinol Metab* 70:473, 1990.

105. **Pasquali R, Cantobelli S, Casimirri F, Capelli M, Bortoluzzi L, Flamia R, Labate AMM, Barbara L,** The hypothalamic-pituitary-adrenal axis in obese women with different patterns of body fat distribution, *J Clin Endocrinol Metab* 77:341, 1993.

106. **Wabitsch M, Hauner H, Heinze E, Bockmann A, Benz R, Mayer H, Teller W,** Body fat distribution and steroid hormone concentrations in obese adolescent girls before and after weight reduction, *J Clin Endocrinol Metab* 80:3469, 1995.

107. **Lapidus L, Bengtsson C, Larsson B, Pennert K, Rybo E, Sjostrom L,** Distribution of adipose tissue and risk of cardiovascular disease and death: a 12 year follow up of participants in the population study of women in Gothenburg, *Br Med J* 289:1257, 1984.

108. **Ostlund Jr RE, Staten M, Kohrt W, Schultz J, Malley M,** The ratio of waist-to-hip circumference, plasma insulin level, and glucose intolerance as independent predictors for the HDL_2 cholesterol level in older adults, *New Engl J Med* 322:229, 1990.

109. **Deutsch MI, Mueller WH, Malina RM,** Androgyny in fat patterning is associated with obesity in adolescents and young adults, *Ann Hum Biol* 12:275, 1985.

110. **Takahashi M, Funahashi T, Shimomura I, Miyaoka K, Matsuzawa Y,** Plasma leptin levels and body fat distribution, *Horm Metab Res* 28:751, 1996.

111. **Montague CT, Prins JB, Sanders L, Digby JE, O'Rahilly S,** Depot- and sex-specific differences in human leptin mRNA expression: implications for the control of regional fat distribution, *Diabetes* 46:342, 1997.

112. **Ashwell M, Chinn S, Stailey S, Garrow JS,** Female fat distribution — a simple classification based on two circumference measurements, *Int J Obesity* 6:143, 1982.

113. **Ashwell M, Cole TJ, Dixon AK,** Obesity: new insight into the anthropometric classification of fat distribution shown by computed tomography, *Br Med J* 290:1692, 1985.

114. **Pouliot MC, Despres JP, Lemieux S, Moorjani S, Bouchard C, Tremblay A, Nadeau A, Lupren PJ,** Waist circumference and abdominal sagittal diameter: best simple anthropometric indexes of abdominal visceral adipose tissue accumulation and related cardiovascular risk in men and women, *Am J Cardiol* 73:460, 1994.

115. **Lean MEJ, Han TS, Durenberg P,** Predicting body composition by densitometry from simple anthropometric measurements, *Am J Clin Nutr* 63:4, 1996.

116. **Gordon T, Kannel WB,** Obesity and cardiovascular disease: the Framingham study, *Clin Endocrinol Metab* 5:367, 1976.

117. **Manson JE, Colditz GA, Stampfer MJ, Willett WC, Rosner B, Monson RR, Speizer FE, Hennekens CH,** A prospective study of obesity and risk of coronary heart disease in women, *New Engl J Med* 322:882, 1990.

118. **Williamson DF, Pamuk E, Thun M, Flanders D, Byers T, Heath C,** Prospective study of intentional weight-loss and mortality in never-smoking overweight US white women aged 40-64, *Am J Epidemiol* 141:1128, 1995.

119. **Garrow JS,** Treatment of obesity, *Lancet* 340:409, 1992.

120. **Leibel RL, Hirsch J, Appel BE, Checani GC,** Energy intake required to maintain body weight is not affected by wide varition in diet composition, *Am J Clin Nutr* 55:350, 1992.

121. **Gordon ES,** Metabolic aspects of obesity, *Adv Metab Disord* 4:229, 1970.

122. **Council on Scientific Affairs, AMA,** Treatment of obesity in adults, *JAMA* 260:2547, 1988.

123. **Wadden TA, Stunkard AJ, Brownell KD,** Very low calorie diets: their efficacy, safety, and future, *Ann Intern Med* 99:675, 1983.

124. **Lichtman SW, Pisarska K, Berman ER, Pestone M, Dowling H, Offenbacher E, Weisel H, Heshka S, Matthews DE, Heymsfield SB,** Discrepancy between self-reported and actual caloric intake and exercise in obese subjects, *New Engl J Med* 327:1893, 1992.

125. **Bray GA, Davidson MB, Drenick EJ,** Obesity: a serious symptom, *Ann Intern Med* 77:787, 1972.

126. **Volkmar FR, Stunkard AJ, Woolston J, Bailey RA,** High attrition rates in commercial weight reduction programs, *Arch Intern Med* 141:426, 1981.

127. **Grodstein F, Levine R, Troy L, Spencer T, Colditz GA, Stampfer MJ,** Three-year follow-up of participants in a commercial weight loss program. Can you keep it off? *Arch Intern Med* 156:1302, 1996.

128. **Williamson DF, Pamuk E, Thun M, Flanders D, Byers T, Heath C,** Prospective study of intentional weight loss and mortality in never-smoking overweight US white women aged 40–64 years, *Am J Epidemiol* 141:1128, 1995.

129. **Sjöström CD, Lissner L, Sjöström L,** Relationships between changes in body composition and changes in cardiovascular risk factors: the SOS Intervention Study, *Obes Res* 5:519, 1997.

130. **Flegal KM, Troiano RP, Pamuk ER, Kuczmarski RJ, Campbell SM,** The influence of smoking cessation on the prevalence of overweight in the United States, *New Engl J Med* 333:1165, 1995.

131. **Weintraub M,** Long-term weight control study: conclusions, *Clin Pharmacol Ther* 51:642, 1992.

132. **Abenhaim L, Moride Y, Brenot F, Rich S, Benichou J, Kurz X, Higenbottom T, Oakley C, Wouters E, Aubier M, Simonneau G, Begaud B,** Appetite-suppressant drugs and the risk of primary pulmonary hypertension, *New Engl J Med* 335:609, 1996.

133. **Connolly HM, Crary JL, McGoon MD, Hensrud DD, Edwards BS, Edwards WD, Schaff HV,** Valvular heart disease associated with fenfluramine-phentermine, *New Engl J Med* 337:581, 1997.

134. **Graham DJ, Green L,** Further cases of valvular heart disease associated with fenfluramine-phentermine, *New Engl J Med* 337:635, 1997.

135. **Devereux RB,** Appetite suppressants and valvular heart disease, *New Engl J Med* 339:765, 1998.

136. **Bray GA, Ryan DH, Gordon D, Heidingsfelder S, Cerise F, Wilson K,** A double-blind randomized placebo-controlled trial of sibutramine, *Obes Res* 4:263, 1996.

137. **Drent ML, van der Veen EA,** First clinical studies with Orlistat: a short review, *Obes Res* 3(Suppl 4):623S, 1995.

138. **Sjöström L, Rissanen A, Andersen T, Boldrin M, Golay A, Koppeschaar HPF, Krempf M, for the European Multicentre Orlistat Study Group,** Randomised placebo-controlled trial of orlistat for weight loss and prevention of weight regain in obese patients, *Lancet* 352:167, 1998.

139. **McCann UD, Seiden LS, Rubin LJ, Ricaurte GA,** Brain serotonin neurotoxicity and primary pulmonary hypertension from fenfluramine and dexfenfluramine: a systematic review of the evidence, *JAMA* 278:666, 1997.

140. **Rivlin RS,** Drug therapy: therapy of obesity with hormones, *New Engl J Med* 292:26, 1975.

141. **Paffenbarger Jr RS, Wing AL, Hyde RT,** Physcial activity as an index of heart attack risk in college alumni, *Am J Epidemiol* 108:161, 1978.

142. **Weisweiler P,** Plasma lipoproteins and lipase and lecithin: cholesterol acyltransferase activities in obese subjects before and after weight reduction, *J Clin Endocrinol Metab* 65:969, 1987.

143. **Edholm OG, Fletcher JG, Widdowson EM, McCance RA,** The energy expenditure and food intake of individual men, *Br J Nutr* 9:286, 1955.

144. **Safer DJ,** Diet, behavior modification, and exercise: a review of obesity treatments from a long-term perspective, *South Med J* 84:1470, 1991.

145. **Skender ML,** Comparison of a 2-year weight loss trends in behavioral treatments of obesity: diet, exercise, and combination internventions, *J Am Diet Assoc* 96:342, 1996.

146. **Konishi F,** Food energy equivalents of various activities, *J Am Diet Assoc* 46:186, 1965.

147. **Sims EAH, Danforth Jr E, Horton ES, Bray GA, Glennon JA, Salans LB,** Endocrine and metabolic effects of experimental obesity in man, *Recent Prog Horm Res* 29:457, 1973.

148. **Welle SL, Amatruda JM, Forbes GB, Lockwood DH,** Resting metabolic rates of obese women after rapid weight loss, *J Clin Endocrinol Metab* 59:41, 1984.

149. **Leibel RL, Rosenbaum M, Hirsch J,** Changes in energy expenditure resulting from altered body weight, *New Engl J Med* 332:621, 1995.

150. **Solow C, Siberfarb PM, Swift K,** Psychosocial effects of intestinal bypass surgery for severe obesity, *New Engl J Med* 290:300, 1974.

20   Reproduction and The Thyroid

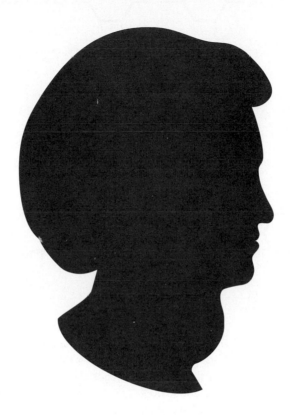

Thomas Wharton, in 1656, gave the thyroid gland its modern name (meaning oblong shield) because he believed the function of the thyroid was to fill vacant spaces and contribute to the shape and beauty of the neck, especially in women.[1] For unknown reasons, thyroid disease is more common in women than in men. Because most thyroid disease is autoimmune in nature, an increased susceptibility to autoimmune diseases, perhaps secondary to the female endocrine environment, is a likely contributing factor.

The clinical objective is to detect and treat thyroid disease before the symptoms and signs are significant and intense. Subtle thyroid disease is easily diagnosed by the sensitive laboratory assessments now available. Therefore, the key to early diagnosis is to maintain a high index of suspicion and to readily screen for the presence of abnormal thyroid function.

Normal Thyroid Physiology

Thyroid hormone synthesis depends in large part on an adequate supply of iodine in the diet. In the small intestine, iodine is absorbed as iodide that is then transported to the thyroid gland. Plasma iodide enters the thyroid under the influence of thyroid-stimulating hormone (TSH), the anterior pituitary thyrotropin hormone. Within the thyroid gland, iodide is oxidized to elemental iodine, which is then bound to tyrosine. Monoiodotyrosine and diiodotyrosine combine to form thyroxine (T_4) and triiodothyronine (T_3). These iodinated compounds are part of the thyroglobulin molecule, the colloid that serves as a storage depot for thyroid hormone. TSH induces a proteolytic process that results in the release of iodothyronines into the bloodstream as thyroid hormone.

Removal of one iodine from the phenolic ring of T_4 yields T_3, while removal of an iodine from the nonphenolic ring yields reverse T_3 (RT_3) which is biologically inactive. In a normal adult, about one third of the T_4 secreted each day is converted in peripheral tissues, largely liver and kidney, to T_3, and about 40% is converted to the inactive, reverse T_3. About 80% of the T_3 generated is derived outside the thyroid gland, chiefly in the liver and kidney. T_3 is 3–5 times more potent than T_4, and virtually all the biologic activity of T_4 can be attributed to the T_3 generated from it. Although T_4 is secreted at 20 times the rate of T_3, it is T_3 that is responsible for most if not all the thyroid action in the body. T_3 is more potent than T_4 because the nuclear thyroid receptor has a ten-fold greater affinity for T_3 than T_4. While T_4 may have some intrinsic activity of its own, it serves mainly as a prohormone of T_3. It is hard to think of a body process or function that doesn't require thyroid hormone for its normal operation, not only metabolism but also development, steroidogenesis, and most specific tissue activities.

Carbohydrate calories appear to be the primary determinant of T_3 levels in adults. A reciprocal relationship exists between T_3 and RT_3. Low T_3 and elevated RT_3 are seen in a variety of illnesses such as febrile diseases, burn injuries, malnutrition, and anorexia nervosa. The metabolic rate is determined to a large degree by the relative production of T_3 and RT_3. During periods of stress, when a decrease in metabolic rate would conserve energy, the body produces more RT_3 and less T_3, and metabolism slows. Upon recovery, this process reverses, and metabolic rate increases.

Circulating thyroid hormones are present in the circulation mainly bound to proteins. Approximately 70% of thyroid hormones are bound to thyroxine-binding globulin (TBG), which, therefore, is the major determining factor in the total thyroid hormone concentration in the circulation. The remaining 30% is bound to thyroxine-binding prealbumin and albumin. The binding proteins have a greater affinity for T_4 and thus allow T_3 to have greater entry into cells. TBG is synthesized in the liver, and this synthesis is increased by estrogens.

The nuclear receptor for thyroid hormone is a member of the super family that includes the steroid hormone receptors (Chapter 2).[2] The thyroid hormone receptor exists in several forms, the products of 2 genes located on different chromosomes. The α receptor is on chromosome 17, and the β receptor is on chromosome 3. The nuclear T_3 receptor is truly ubiquitous, indicating the widespread actions of thyroid hormone throughout the body. Mutations in the gene for the thyroid receptor lead to the synthesis of a receptor that actually antagonizes normal receptors, a syndrome of thyroid resistance characterized by elevated thyroid hormone levels. TSH is elevated as well because of the impairment in thyroid hormone action.

The thyroid axis is stimulated by the hypothalamic factor, thyrotropin-releasing hormone (TRH) and inhibited by somatostatin and dopamine. Thyroid hormones regulate TSH by suppressing TRH secretion, but primarily affecting the pituitary sensitivity to TRH (by reducing the number of TRH receptors). Pituitary secretion of TSH is very sensitive to changes in the circulating levels of thyroid hormone; a slight change in the circulating level of T_4 will produce a many-fold greater response in TSH. TSH-secreting cells are regulated by T_4, but only after the T_4 is converted to T_3 in the pituitary cells. Although modulation of thyroid hormone occurs at the pituitary level, this function is permitted by the hypothalamic releasing hormone, TRH. Although some tissues depend mainly on the blood T_3 for their intracellular T_3, the brain and the pituitary depend on their own intracellular conversion of T_4. The measurement of T_4 and TSH, therefore, provides the most accurate assessment of thyroid function.

The TSH response to TRH is influenced mainly by the thyroid hormone concentration in the circulation; however, lesser effects are associated with dopamine agonists (inhibition), glucocorticoids (inhibition), and dopamine antagonists (stimulation). Estrogen increases the TRH receptor content of the pituitary; hence, the TSH response to TRH is greater in women than in men, and greater in women taking combined oral contraceptives.

TRH also stimulates prolactin secretion by the pituitary. The smallest doses of TRH that are capable of producing an increase in TSH, also increase prolactin levels, indicating a physiologic role for TRH in the control of prolactin secretion. However, except in hypothyroidism, normal physiologic changes as well as abnormal prolactin secretion can be understood in terms of dopaminergic inhibitory control, and TRH need not be considered.

Functional Changes With Aging

Thyroxine metabolism and clearance decrease in older people, and thyroxine secretion decreases in compensation to maintain normal serum thyroxine concentrations.[3] With aging, conversion of T_4 to T_3 decreases, and TSH levels increase. The TSH response to TRH is normal in older women. TBG concentrations decrease slightly in postmenopausal women but not enough to alter measurements in serum.

Thyroid Function Tests

Free Thyroxine (FT$_4$)
Assays that measure free T_4 are usually displacement assays using an antibody to T_4. The result is not affected by changes in TBG and binding. The free T_4 level has a different range of normal values from laboratory to laboratory.

Total Thyroxine (TT$_4$)
The total thyroxine, both the bound portion to TBG and the free unbound portion, is measured by displacement assays, and in the absence of hormone therapy or other illnesses, estimates the thyroxine concentration in the blood. However, the free T_4 is unaffected by factors that influence TBG and is preferred.

Free Thyroxine Index (FTI or T$_7$)
The free thyroxine index is calculated from the TT$_4$ and the T_3 resin uptake measurements. This test too has been replaced by the free T_4 assay.

Total T$_3$ and Reverse T$_3$

Both of these thyronines can be measured by sensitive immunoassays. However, in most clinical circumstances they add little to what is learned by the free T$_4$ and TSH measurements. The clinical situations where measurement will be useful will be discussed under the specific diseases and indicated on the algorithm.

Thyroid-Stimulating Hormone (TSH)

TSH is measured by highly sensitive assays utilizing monoclonal antibodies, usually in a technique that uses two antibodies, one directed at the α-subunit and one directed at the β-subunit of TSH. The normal levels vary from laboratory to laboratory, but the sensitive TSH assay can detect concentrations as low as 0.01 μU/L. TSH is a very sensitive indicator of thyroid hormone action at the tissue level because it is dependent upon the pituitary exposure to T$_4$. In the absence of hypothalamic or pituitary disease, the sensitive TSH assays will provide the best indication of excess or deficient thyroxine; slight changes in T$_4$ are reflected in a many-fold greater response in TSH. Nearly all women with elevated TSH levels have hypothyroidism. Transient changes in TSH can be caused by systemic illnesses, major psychiatric disturbances, and pharmacologic treatment with glucocorticoid agents or dopamine.

Radioactive Iodine Uptake

Because the thyroid gland is the only tissue that utilizes iodine, radioisotopes of iodine can be used as a measure of thyroid gland activity and to localize activity within the gland.

The Laboratory Evaluation. The algorithm represents a cost-effective and accurate clinical strategy.[4] For screening purposes, or when there is a relatively low clinical suspicion of thyroid disease, the initial step is to measure the TSH by a sensitive assay. A normal TSH essentially excludes hypothyroidism or hyperthyroidism. A high TSH requires the measurement of free T$_4$ to confirm the diagnosis of hypothyroidism.

If the initial TSH is low, especially less than 0.08 μU/mL, then measurement of a high T$_4$ will confirm the diagnosis of hyperthyroidism. If the T$_4$ is normal, the T$_3$ level is measured, since some patients with hyperthyroidism will have predominantly T$_3$ toxicosis. If the T$_3$ is normal, it implies that thyroxine secretion is autonomous from TSH, and this is called subclinical hyperthyroidism. Some of these patients will eventually have increased T$_4$ or T$_3$ levels with true hyperthyroidism.

Hypothyroidism

In most cases of hypothyroidism, a specific cause is not apparent. It is believed that the hypothyroidism is usually secondary to an autoimmune reaction, and when goiter formation is present, it is called Hashimoto's thyroiditis.[5] Unless abnormal thyroid function can be documented by specific laboratory assessment, empiric treatment with thyroid hormone is not indicated, and it is especially worth emphasizing that thyroid hormone treatment does not help infertility in euthyroid women. It is uncertain whether hypothyroidism can be a cause of recurrent miscarriages, but an assessment of thyroid function is worthwhile in these patients.

Hypothyroidism increases with aging and is more common in women.[6] Up to 45% of thyroid glands from women over age 60 show evidence of thyroiditis.[7] The incidence of antithyroglobulin antibodies is 7.4% in women over age 75 years, while 16.9% of women age 60 and 17.4% of women over age 75 have elevated TSH levels. In women admitted to geriatric wards, 2–4% have clinically apparent hypothyroidism. ***Therefore, hypothyroidism is frequent enough to warrant consideration in most older women, justifying screening even in asymptomatic older women. We recommend that older women be screened with the highly sensitive TSH assay every 5 years beginning at age 35, then every 2 years beginning at age 60, or with the appearance of any symptoms suggesting hypothyroidism.***[8]

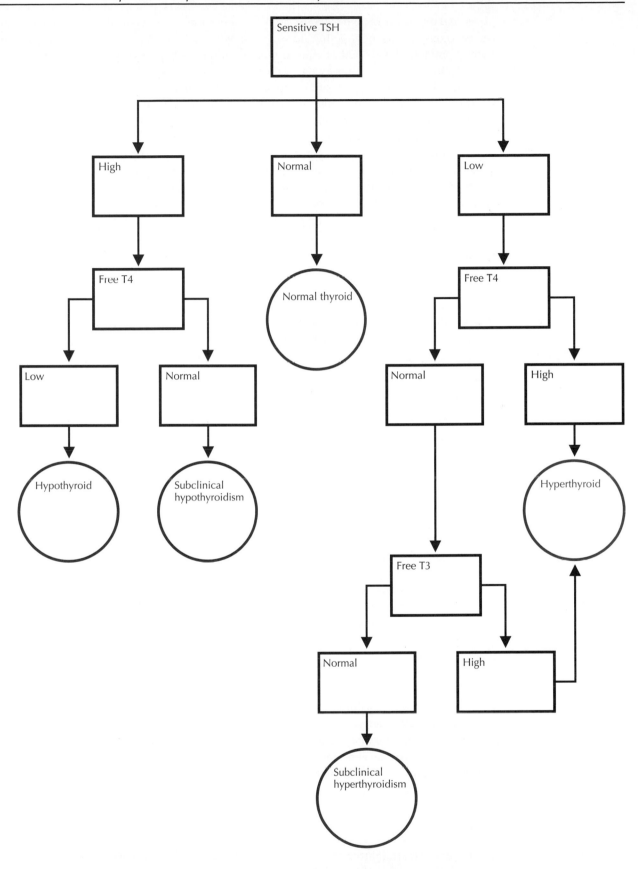

Menstrual irregularities and bleeding problems are common in hypothyroid women. Amenorrhea can be a consequence of hypothyroidism, either with TRH-induced increases in prolactin or with normal prolactin levels. Other clinical manifestations of hypothyroidism include constipation, cold intolerance, psychomotor retardation, carpal tunnel syndrome, and decreased exercise tolerance. However, patients often appear asymptomatic. Close evaluation can reveal mental slowness, decreased energy, fatigue, poor memory, somnolence, slow speech, a low-pitched voice, water retention, periorbital edema, delayed reflexes, or a low body temperature and bradycardia. Hypothyroidism can cause hypertension, cognitive abnormalities, pericardial effusion, asymmetric septal myocardial hypertrophy, myopathy, neuropathy, ataxia, anemia, elevated cholesterol and LDL-cholesterol, or hyponatremia. Myxedematous infiltration can produce enlarged, cystic ovaries.[9] The increase in cholesterol is due to impaired LDL-cholesterol clearance secondary to a decrease in cell membrane LDL receptors. The mechanism for this LDL effect is attributed to a thyroid response element in the LDL receptor gene.[10]

Serum enzymes may be elevated because of decreased clearance, including creatine phosphokinase (CPK), aspartate aminotransferase (AST,SGOT), alanine aminotransferase (ALT, SGPT), lactic dehydrogenase (LDH), and alkaline phosphatase, triggering a fruitless search for other organ disease. It is worth screening for hypothyroidism in any women with abnormal menses or with complaints of fatigue and depression. In addition, patients should be screened who have elevated levels of cholesterol and LDL-cholesterol.

Diagnosis of Hypothyroidism

With primary thyroid failure, the circulating thyroid hormone levels fall, stimulating the pituitary to increase TSH output. Elevated TSH and low T_4 confirm the diagnosis. Hypothyroidism can occur due to pituitary failure in which case the TSH will be inappropriately low for the T_4. The most common cause will be autoimmune thyroid disease (elevated titers of antithyroid antibodies) in areas with normal iodine intake. However, making an etiologic diagnosis in women adds little to the clinical management.

Subclinical Hypothyroidism

In early hypothyroidism, with undetectable symptoms or signs, a compensated state can be detected by an elevated TSH (usually 5–20 µU/L) and normal T_4 (called subclinical hypothyroidism). Many of these patients (but not all) will eventually become clinically hypothyroid with low T_4 concentrations. A good reason to treat subclinical hypothyroidism is to avoid the development of a goiter. Furthermore, some patients in retrospect (after treatment) recognize improved physical and mental well-being. Patients with subclinical hypothyroidism have alterations in energy metabolism in skeletal muscle.[11] An improvement in impaired cognitive function and emotional behavior has been documented with thyroxine treatment of subclinical hypothyroidism.[12] In those patients who are asymptomatic, it is worth measuring antithyroid antibodies. A positive test identifies those who are likely to become clinically hypothyroid, at a rate of approximately 20% per year. With only very slight elevations of TSH (less than 10 µU/L), it is reasonable not to treat and to check thyroid function every 6 months to detect further deterioration. Patients with an abnormal cholesterol-lipoprotein profile can show improvement with thyroxine treatment, usually within one month of therapy.[13]

Treatment of Hypothyroidism

Initial therapy is straightforward with synthetic thyroxine, T_4, given daily. Mixtures of T_4 and T_3, such as desiccated thyroid, provide T_3 in excess of normal thyroid secretion. It is better to provide T_4 and allow the peripheral conversion process to provide the T_3.[14, 15] "Natural" thyroid preparations are not better, and in fact are potentially detrimental. Patients taking biological preparations should be switched to synthetic thyroxine. Because of a risk of coronary heart disease in older women, the initial dose should be 25–50 µg per day for 4 weeks, at which time the dose is increased by 25 µg daily every 4 weeks according to the clinical and biochemical assessment. Usually the dose required will be close to 1.5 µg/lb body weight, but it may be less in very old women.[16] The average final dose required in the elderly is approximately 70% of that in younger patients. ***Patients who have been on thyroid hormone for a long time may have their medication discontinued. Recovery of the hypothalamic-pituitary axis usually requires 6–8 weeks at which time the TSH and free T_4 levels can be measured.***

Evaluation of Therapy

When the patient appears clinically euthyroid, evaluation of TSH levels will provide the most accurate assessment of the adequacy of thyroid hormone replacement. A patient being treated with thyroid hormone should be evaluated once every year with the sensitive TSH assay. Thyroid hormone requirements tend to decrease with age. If the sensitive TSH assay is low, then the free T_4 should be measured to help adjust the thyroxine dose.[17] ***The full response of TSH to changes in T_4 is relatively slow; a minimum of 6–8 weeks is necessary between changes in dosage and assessment of TSH.***

Hyperthyroidism

The two primary causes of hyperthyroidism are Graves' disease (toxic diffuse goiter) and Plummer's disease (toxic nodular goiter).[18] Plummer's disease is usually encountered in postmenopausal women who have had a long history of goiter. Twenty percent of hyperthyroid patients are over 60, and 25% of older women with hyperthyroidism present with an apathetic or atypical syndrome.

Graves' disease is characterized by the triad of hyperthyroidism, exophthalmos, and pretibial myxedema and is believed to be caused by autoantibodies that have TSH properties and, therefore, bind to and activate the TSH receptor. Menstrual changes associated with hyperthyroidism are unpredictable, ranging from amenorrhea to oligomenorrhea to normal cycles (hence, the amenorrhea in a thyrotoxic woman can be due to pregnancy).

The classic symptoms of thyrotoxicosis are nervousness, heat intolerance, weight loss, sweating, palpitations, and diarrhea. These symptoms are associated with typical findings on physical examination: proptosis, lid lag, tachycardia, tremor, warm and moist skin, and goiter. Women in the reproductive years usually present with the classic picture. In postmenopausal women, symptoms are often concentrated in a single organ system, especially the cardiovascular or central nervous system. Goiter is absent in 40%. Sinus tachycardia occurs in less than half, but atrial fibrillation occurs in 40% and is resistant to cardioversion or spontaneous reversion to sinus rhythm. In old women, there is often a coexistent disease, such as an infection or coronary heart disease that dominates the clinical picture.

The triad of weight loss, constipation, and loss of appetite, suggesting gastrointestinal malignancy, occurs in about 15% of older patients with hyperthyroidism. Ophthalmopathy is rare in older patients. Hyperthyroidism in older women is sometimes described as "apathetic hyperthyroidism" because the clinical manifestations are different. The clinician should consider the diagnosis in older patients with "failure to thrive," in patients who are progressively deteriorating for unexplained reasons, and in patients with heart disease, unexplained weight loss, and mental or psychologic changes.

Psychologic changes are not unusual in hyperthyroid women. Women who complain of emotional lability and nervousness should be screened for hyperthyroidism.

Diagnosis of Hyperthyroidism

The diagnosis of hyperthyroidism requires laboratory testing. A suppressed TSH with a high T_4 or a high T_3 confirms the diagnosis. Hyperthyroidism caused by high levels of T_3 is more common in older women. Most patients should have a radioactive iodine thyroid uptake and scan after laboratory confirmation of the diagnosis. If the uptake is suppressed then drug therapy is indicated. The scan will indicate whether the patient has a diffuse toxic goiter, a solitary hot nodule, or a hot nodule in a multinodular gland. Toxic multinodular goiters occur more frequently in the elderly. TSH hypersecretion as a cause of hyperthyroidism is extremely rare; the combination of a normal or elevated TSH and elevated thyroid hormone will be the clue to this possibility.

Subclinical Hyperthyroidism

By definition, patients with subclinical hyperthyroidism have normal T_4 and T_3 levels, but subnormal concentrations of TSH. TSH levels can be suppressed to 0.1–0.5 µU/L by general illnesses and drugs such as glucocorticoids, dopamine, and anticonvulsants; however, this suppression does not extend below 0.1 µU/L. Values below 0.1 µU/L are regarded as nondetectable, and patients with overt hyperthyroidism usually have undetectable TSH. Subclinical hyperthyroidism is half as common in older people as subclinical hypothyroidism (excluding the most common cause, treatment with excessive doses of thyroxine). Keep in mind that the dose of thyroxine required to treat hypothyroidism declines with age (because of the decrease in metabolic clearance with age); all patients being treated with thyroid hormone should have their TSH levels assessed every year. Atrial fibrillation is a common cardiovascular problem associated with subclinical hyperthyroidism.[19] If subclinical hyperthyroidism persists, it should be treated, especially in postmenopausal women, because of the cardiac complications and the loss of bone associated with excess thyroid hormone. TSH levels that are low but not undetectable (0.1–5.0 µU/L) need not be treated, but TSH measurement is warranted every 6 months. Progression to overt hyperthyroidism is uncommon.

Treatment of Hyperthyroidism

There are multiple objectives of therapy: control of thyroid hormone effects on peripheral tissues by pharmacologic blockade of beta-adrenergic receptors, inhibition of thyroid gland secretion and release of thyroid hormone, and specific treatment of nonthyroidal systemic illnesses which can exacerbate hyperthyroidism or be adversely affected by hyperthyroidism.[20] Antithyroid drugs are usually administered first to achieve euthyroidism, then definitive therapy is accomplished by radioactive iodine treatment. Of course, it is important to make sure a woman is not pregnant before treatment with radioactive iodine, and pregnancy should be postponed for several months after treatment. Monitoring treatment response requires a full 8-week interval for stabilization of the hypothalamic-pituitary-thyroid system.

Antithyroid Drugs

The drug of choice in most circumstances will be methimazole because it has fewer adverse effects. The drug inhibits organification of iodide and decreases production of T_4 and T_3. The oral dose is 10–20 mg daily. The onset of effect takes 2–4 weeks. Remember that the half-life of thyroxine is about one week, and the gland usually has large stores of T_4. Maximal effect occurs at 4–8 weeks. The dose can be titrated down once the disease is controlled to a maintenance dose of 5–10 mg daily. The major side effects are rash, gastrointestinal symptoms, and agranulocytosis (an idiosyncratic reaction). Propranolol and other beta-blockers are effective in rapidly controlling the effects of thyroid hormone on peripheral tissues. The dose is usually 20–40 mg, every 12 hours, orally, and the dose is titrated to maintain a heart rate of about 100 beats/minute. The drug may cause bronchospasm, worsening congestive heart failure, fatigue, and depression. Rarely inorganic iodine will be needed to block release of hormone from the gland. Lugol's solution, 2 drops in water daily, is sufficient. The onset of effect is 1–2 days, with maximal effect in 3–7 days. There may be an escape from protection in 2–6 weeks, and the drug can cause rash, fever, and parotitis. Iodine precludes radioiodine administration for several months.

After the symptoms are controlled, and the patient is euthyroid, a dose of radioactive iodine can be selected, the thiouracil withheld temporarily, and definitive therapy accomplished. Patients with solitary nodules will be treated in the same fashion. Some patients with hot nodules in multinodular glands will require surgery because of the size of the gland and because the hyperthyroidism tends to recur in new nodules after the ablation of the original hot nodule. This can result in repetitive treatments with substantial doses of radioactive iodine, and surgery may be preferable. All patients definitively treated for hyperthyroidism must be monitored for the onset of hypothyroidism.

Osteoporosis and Excessive Thyroxine

Because postmenopausal women are at increased risk for osteoporosis, and frequently develop hyperthyroidism or receive levothyroxine treatment for hypothyroidism, the clinician needs to understand how thyroid hormone affects bones.[21] Thyroid hormone excess alters bone integrity via direct effects on bone and gut absorption and indirectly through the effects of vitamin D, calcitonin, and parathyroid hormone.

Thyroid hormone increases bone mineral resorption. In addition, total and ionized calcium increase in hyperthyroid women, leading to increases in serum phosphorous, alkaline phosphatase, and bone Gla protein (osteocalcin), a marker of bone turnover. Parathyroid hormone decreases in response to the increased serum calcium, and this results in decreased hydroxylation of vitamin D. Intestinal calcium and phosphate absorption decrease, while urinary hydroxyproline and calcium excretion increase. The net effect is increased bone resorption and a subsequent decrease in bone density — osteoporosis.[22]

These effects become more clinically important in prolonged exposure to excessive thyroid hormone.[23] Women who have had hyperthyroidism experience postmenopausal fractures earlier than usual.[24]

The major concern is that mild chronic excess thyroid hormone replacement, especially in postmenopausal women, might increase the risk of osteoporosis, and indeed this subsequently was documented.[25] Bone density has been found to be reduced (9%) in premenopausal women receiving enough thyroxine to suppress TSH for 10 years or more.[26] A meta-analysis of the literature on this subject concluded that premenopausal women treated for long durations did not suffer a clinically significant loss of bone (probably because of the protective presence of estrogen); however, postmenopausal women lose an excess of bone if thyroid treatment results in TSH levels below the normal range.[27]

Thus, exposure to excessive thyroxine must be added to the risk factors for osteoporosis. It makes sense to monitor patients (both premenopausal women and especially postmenopausal women) receiving thyroxine with the sensitive TSH assay to ensure that levothyroxine doses are "physiologic." Some patients who require TSH suppressive doses of thyroxine, such as patients with nodules, goiters, and cancer, must be considered at increased risk of osteoporosis. It would be wise to assess bone density in women on long-term thyroid treatment and in women receiving high-dose thyroxine suppression of TSH. The use of hormone therapy, exercise programs, and possibly biphosphate treatment must be seriously considered for these patients. In a cross-sectional study of elderly women, the bone loss associated with long-term thyroid treatment was avoided in those women also taking estrogen.[28]

Thyroid Nodules

The major concern with thyroid nodules is the potential for thyroid cancer.[29] Single nodules are 4 times more common in women, and carcinoma of the thyroid is nearly 3 times more common in women than in men. The incidence rises steadily from the age of 55. Mortality from thyroid cancer occurs predominantly in the middle-aged and the elderly. There are 4 major types of primary thyroid carcinoma: papillary, follicular, anaplastic, and medullary. In solitary nodules that are "cold" (those that do not take up radioactive iodine or pertechnetate on thyroid scan), 12% prove to be malignant. This also means that the majority are benign. Surgical excision of nodules can result in vocal cord paralysis, hypoparathyroidism, and other complications. Therefore, the goal is to select patients for curative surgery who have the greatest likelihood of having cancer in the nodule.

Epidemiologic and Clinical Data

The major risk factors for thyroid cancer are family history of this disease and a history of irradiation to head or neck. In those who have received thyroid irradiation, about one-third will have thyroid abnormalities, and about one-third of those with abnormalities will have thyroid cancer (about 10% overall). The carcinogenic risk has been estimated to be 1% per 100 rads in 20 years. A rapidly growing nodule, a hard nodule, the presence of palpable regional lymph nodes, or vocal cord paralysis greatly increase the probability of thyroid cancer.

Thyroid nodules in multinodular thyroid glands, not previously exposed to thyroid irradiation, have no greater risk of thyroid carcinoma than normal glands. Therefore, predominant thyroid nodules in multinodular glands should be followed and, if a nodule grows, then biopsy or surgery should be considered.

Diagnostic Strategy

In patients with a thyroid nodule, laboratory assessment of thyroid function is essential. When abnormal thyroid function is present, the nodule is almost always benign. Detection of a thyroid nodule is followed by clinical characterization of the nodule, examination of the lymph nodes, and inquiry regarding rapid growth, family history, and history of thyroid irradiation. In the presence of any of these findings, surgery is recommended for excision of the nodule. If none of these is present, proceed directly to fine needle aspiration biopsy or thyroid scan.

If a scan is chosen, hot nodules are evaluated independently. Cold nodules require a surgical diagnosis. If the patient prefers, one can treat with suppressive doses of levothyroxine and evaluate over time. Unfortunately, many of these thyroid nodules do not regress with thyroid treatment, but it is very reassuring if they do. Growth or lack of disappearance with thyroid suppression is an indication for fine needle aspiration biopsy. Thyroid ultrasound can be utilized to more accurately establish size for comparison over time.

Although accounting for only 5% of thyroid cancers, medullary carcinoma is associated with early spread and poor survival rates. Medullary carcinoma of the thyroid is unique in having the serum calcitonin as a very sensitive and specific tumor marker. Measuring the serum calcitonin is recommended for older patients with solitary nodules in order to achieve earlier diagnosis of medullary carcinoma.[30]

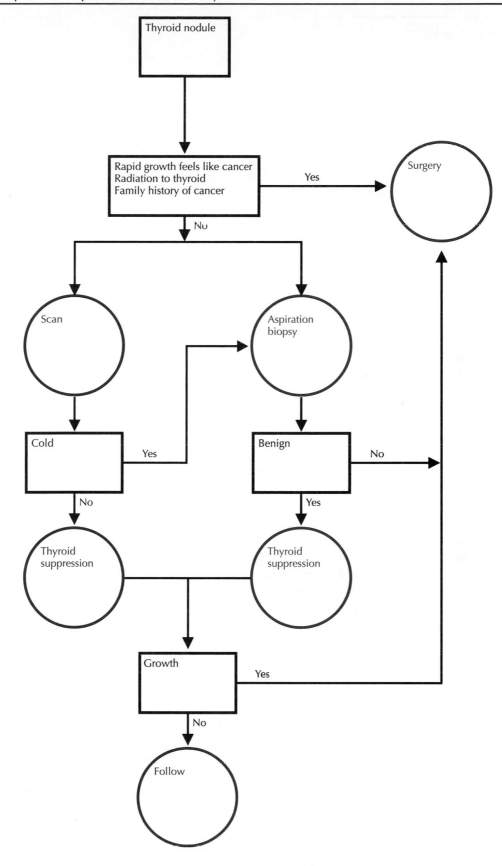

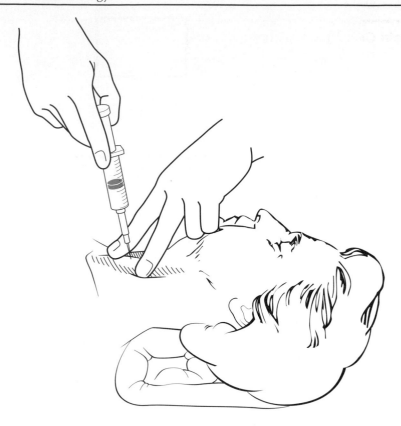

Fine-Needle Aspiration

Fine-needle aspiration biopsy has a 83% sensitivity and 92% specificity in diagnosing thyroid malignancy.[31] When "indeterminate" by biopsy, about one-third prove to be malignant at thyroidectomy. If the fine-needle aspiration biopsy reveals suspicious cells or is indeterminate, a subtotal thyroidectomy should be performed for diagnosis and treatment. If the aspiration biopsy is benign some would repeat the biopsy in one year to avoid false negatives. Most would provide thyroid hormone suppressive therapy (aiming for a TSH level below 0.1 µU/L) for one year with close observation for growth of the nodule.[32] Growth or lack of disappearance indicates the need for biopsy or surgery. If the nodule shrinks during suppression, after one year a choice is made between no treatment or maintenance of the TSH level at the lower end of normal. In some cases, especially in older women, nodules can be followed with no therapy and little risk. If the nodule increases in size, suppressive therapy is recommended. One of the reasons many are treated with levothyroxine is because of the known growth-promoting effects of TSH in carcinoma of the thyroid and the hope that TSH suppression will inhibit the growth of early carcinoma.

The method for fine-needle aspiration biopsy requires no anesthetic. Using sterile technique and a 23-gauge needle on a 10 mL syringe, the nodule is fixed with two fingers of one hand and the nodule entered. Aspiration is performed with the syringe while several passes are made through a vertical distance of about 2 mm in the nodule. Suction is stopped when biopsy material becomes visible in the hub of the needle. The contents of the needle should be expelled onto a slide and fixed for pathology. Gentle pressure is applied over the nodule for 10 minutes. Occasionally, a patient will have some bleeding into the nodule or surrounding tissues, but it is usually self-limiting.

The Thyroid Gland and Pregnancy

In response to the metabolic demands of pregnancy, there is an increase in the basal metabolic rate (which is mainly due to fetal metabolism), iodine uptake, and the size of the thyroid gland caused by hyperplasia and increased vascularity.[33] However, a pregnant woman is euthyroid with normal levels of TSH, free T_4, and free T_3; thyroid nodules and goiter require evaluation. During pregnancy, iodide clearance by the kidney increases. For this reason (plus the iodide losses to the fetus), the prevalence of goiter is increased in areas of iodine deficiency.[34] This is not a problem in the U.S., and any goiter should be regarded as pathologic. In many parts of the world, iodine is not sufficiently available in the environment, and pregnancy increases the risk of iodine deficiency.

The increase in thyroid activity in pregnancy is compensated by an marked increase in the circulating levels of TBG in response to estrogen; therefore, a new equilibrium is reached with an increase in the bound portion of the thyroid hormone. The mechanism for the estrogen effect on TBG is an increase in hepatic synthesis and an increase in glycosylation of the TBG molecule that leads to decreased clearance.

The increase in thyroid activity is attributed to the thyrotropic substances secreted by the placenta: a chorionic thyrotropin and the thyrotropic activity in human chorionic gonadotropin (HCG).[35] It has been calculated that HCG contains approximately 1/4000th of the thyrotropic activity of human TSH. In conditions with very elevated HCG levels, the thyrotropic activity can be sufficient to produce hyperthyroidism, and this can even be encountered in normal pregnancy.[36]

TBG levels reach a peak (twice nonpregnant levels) at about 15 weeks, which is maintained throughout the rest of pregnancy.[37] T_4 undergoes a similar change, but T_3 increases more markedly. Because of the increase in TBG, free T_4 and T_3 levels actually decrease, although they remain within the normal range.[38] There is an inverse relationship between maternal circulation levels of TSH and HCG.[37] TSH reaches a nadir at the same time that HCG reaches a peak at 10 weeks of pregnancy. TSH levels then increase as HCG levels drop to their stable levels throughout the rest of pregnancy. These changes support a role for HCG stimulation of the maternal thyroid gland during early pregnancy.[37, 39, 40] It is well recognized that patients who have conditions associated with very high levels of HCG (trophoblastic disease, HCG-secreting cancers) can

Maternal Thyroid Hormones

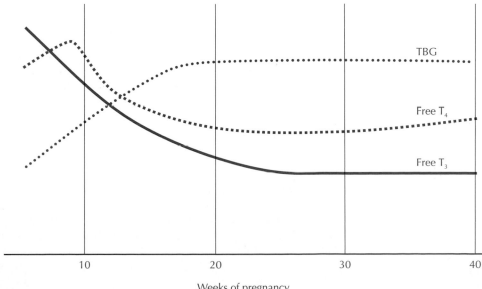

Weeks of pregnancy

Maternal TSH and HCG

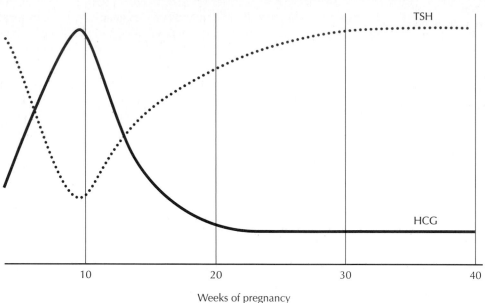

Weeks of pregnancy

develop hyperthyroidism. The thyroid-stimulating activity of HCG is explained by the molecular homology between HCG and TSH, and between their receptors.

In normal pregnancies, placental transfer of TSH, T_4, and T_3 is severely limited in both directions. Indeed, the placenta is essentially impermeable to these substances no matter whether the fetus is euthyroid or hypothyroid. Slight transfer of T_4 and T_3 can occur, however, when maternal levels are very high or when fetal levels are substantially lower than the maternal levels.

The majority of patients with hyperemesis gravidarum have laboratory values consistent with hyperthyroidism, and the severity of the hyperemesis correlates with the degree of hyperthyroidism.[41, 42] These patients have higher levels of HCG, and the transient hyperthyroidism and severity of the hyperemesis may be mediated by the thyrotropic and steroidogenic activity of the HCG. These clinical manifestations in normal pregnancies may be linked to a specific subpopulation of HCG molecules with greater thyrotropic bioactivity (because highly purified, standard HCG has only trivial TSH-like activity).[43] Specifically, HCG with reduced sialic acid content is increased in pregnant patients with hyperemesis and hyperthyroidism.[44]

Thyroid Physiology in the Fetus and the Neonate

The human fetal thyroid gland develops the capacity to concentrate iodine and synthesize hormone between 8 and 10 weeks of gestation, the same time that the pituitary begins to synthesize TSH.[45, 46] Some thyroid development and hormone synthesis are possible in the absence of the pituitary gland, but optimal function requires TSH. By 12–14 weeks, development of the pituitary-thyroid system is complete. Function is minimal, however, until an abrupt increase in fetal TSH occurs at 20 weeks. As with gonadotropin and other pituitary hormone secretion, this thyroid function correlates with the maturation of the hypothalamus and the development of the pituitary portal vascular system, which makes releasing hormone available to the pituitary gland.

Fetal TSH increases and reaches a plateau at 28 weeks and remains at relatively high levels to term. The free T_4 concentration increases progressively. At term, fetal T_4 levels exceed maternal levels. Thus, a state of fetal thyroidal hyperactivity exists near term.

Fetal Thyroid Hormones

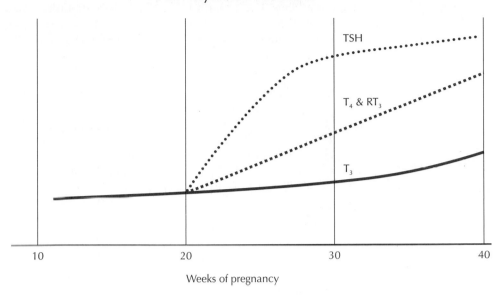

Weeks of pregnancy

The major thyroid hormone secreted by the fetus is T_4. However, total T_3 and free T_3 levels are low throughout gestation, and levels of RT_3 are elevated, paralleling the rise in T_4. Like T_3, this compound is derived predominantly from conversion of T_4 in peripheral tissues. The increased production of T_4 in fetal life is compensated by rapid conversion to the inactive RT_3, allowing the fetus to conserve its fuel resources.

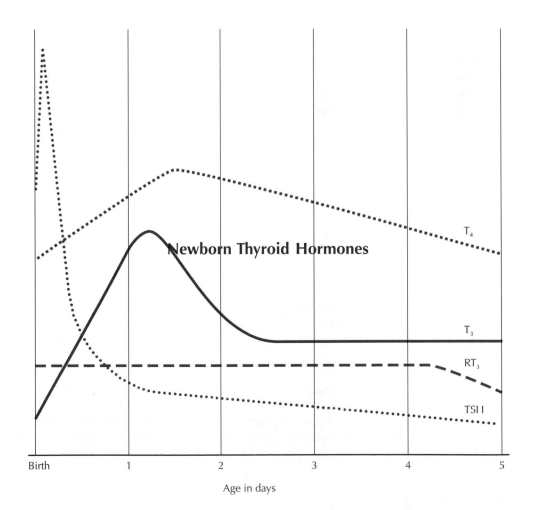

Newborn Thyroid Hormones

Age in days

With delivery, the newborn moves from a state of relative T_3 deficiency to a state of T_3 thyrotoxicosis. Shortly after birth serum TSH concentrations increase rapidly to a peak at 30 minutes of age. They fall to baseline values by 48–72 hours. In response to this increase in TSH, total T_4 and free T_4 increase to peak values by 24–48 hours of age. T_3 levels increase even more, peaking by 24 hours of age. By 3–4 weeks, the thyroidal hyperactivity has disappeared.

The postnatal surge in TSH is accompanied by a prolactin surge, suggesting that both are increased in response to TRH. The TRH surge is thought to be a response to rapid neonatal cooling. A puzzle is the fact that the early increase in T_3 is independent of TSH and is tied in some way to cutting of the umbilical cord. Delaying cord cutting delays the increase in T_3, but TSH levels still reach their peak at 30 minutes. In some way cord cutting augments peripheral (largely liver) conversion of T_4 to T_3. The later increases in T_3 and T_4 (after 2 hours) are due to increased thyroid gland activity. These thyroid changes after birth probably represent defense mechanisms against the sudden entry into the cold world. The high RT_3 levels during pregnancy continue during the first 3–5 days of life, and then fall gradually to normal levels by 2 weeks.

Summary of Fetal and Newborn Thyroid Changes

1. **TSH and T_4 appear in the fetus at 10–13 weeks. Levels are low until an abrupt rise at 20 weeks.**

2. **T_4 rises rapidly and exceeds maternal values at term.**

3. **T_3 levels rise, but concentrations are relatively low, similar to hypothyroid adults.**

4. **RT_3 levels exceed normal adult levels.**

5. **The fetal pattern of low T_3 and high RT_3 is similar to that seen with calorie malnutrition.**

6. **After delivery, TSH peaks at 30 minutes of age, followed by a T_3 peak at 24 hours and a T_4 peak at 24–48 hours. The T_3 increase is independent of the TSH change.**

7. **High RT_3 levels persist for 3–5 days after delivery, then reach normal values by 2 weeks.**

Newborn Screening for Hypothyroidism

The incidence of neonatal hypothyroidism is about one in 4000 live births, and newborn screening programs exist in most of the world. The problem is that congenital hypothyroidism is not clinically apparent at birth. Fortunately, infants with congenital hypothyroidism have low T_4 and high TSH concentrations easily detected in blood, and early treatment before 3 months of age is usually associated with normal mental development.[47] Less than normal development can be a consequence of a delay in treatment or extremely low thyroid hormone production in the fetus.

There is a familial tendency for hypothyroidism, and if the diagnosis is made in the antepartum period, intra-amniotic injections of thyroxine can raise fetal levels of thyroid hormone.[48] Ultrasonographic examination of patients with polyhydramnios should include a search for a fetal goiter. In addition, the fetus should be monitored for goiter formation in women treated with antithyroid drugs for hyperthyroidism during pregnancy. Amniotic fluid iodothyronines and TSH reflect fetal plasma levels, and abnormal values may allow prenatal diagnosis of fetal hypothyroidism by amniocentesis.[48, 49] However, fetal cord blood sampling is advocated for accurate diagnosis.[50] Treatment of fetal hypothyroidism is important because there is a concern that prenatal hypothyroidism can affect some aspects of development; e.g., the full function of physical skills. Although transfer of thyroid hormone from mother to fetus is limited, even a small amount provides protection, especially to the brain, for a fetus with hypothyroidism.

Hyperthyroidism in Pregnancy

Untreated thyrotoxicosis in pregnancy is associated with a higher risk of preeclampsia, heart failure, intrauterine growth retardation, and stillbirth.[51] Heart failure is a consequence of the demands of pregnancy superimposed upon the hyperdynamic cardiovascular state induced by the increased thyroid hormone.[52]

The most common cause of thyrotoxicosis in pregnancy is Graves' disease. However, the clinician should always keep in mind that trophoblastic disease can cause hyperthyroidism due to the TSH property inherent in human chorionic gonadotropin. The maternal changes with pregnancy can make diagnosis difficult. Tachycardia upon awakening from sleep and a failure to gain weight should make a clinician suspicious. Hyperemesis gravidarum is a common presentation of hyperthyroidism in pregnancy. Laboratory assessment is unaffected by pregnancy and should follow our algorithm.

The choice of treatment is between surgery and antithyroid drugs. However prior to surgery, the thyroid gland has to be controlled with medical therapy. Most women can be successfully treated with thioamide drugs.[51] Propylthiouracil and methimazole are equally safe and effective for pregnant women; however, propylthiouracil is preferred in breastfeeding patients because it is less concentrated in breast milk.[53]

The aim of treatment should be to maintain mild hyperthyroidism in the mother to avoid thyroid dysfunction in the fetus. Treatment of maternal hyperthyroidism with propylthiouracil, even with moderate doses of 100–200 mg daily, suppresses T_4 and increases TSH levels in newborns.[54] The infants are clinically euthyroid, however, and their laboratory measurements are normal by the 4th to 5th day of life. In addition, follow-up assessment has indicated unimpaired intellectual development in children whose mothers received propylthiouracil during pregnancy.[55] Nevertheless, pregnant women with thyrotoxicosis should be treated with as low a dose of antithyroid drugs as possible. With proper antithyroid drug treatment, very few, if any, deleterious effects are experienced by mother, fetus, or neonate.[56] Although small amounts of antithyroid drugs are transmitted in breast milk, the amount has no impact on neonatal thyroid function, and breast-feeding should be encouraged. Poor control of maternal hyperthyroidism is associated with increased risks of preeclampsia and low-birth-weight infants.[57]

Maternal TSH-like autoantibodies can cross the placenta and cause fetal thyrotoxicosis and demise. Some have advocated fetal cord blood sampling in women with Graves' disease who are euthyroid but who have positive titers of TSH-like antibodies to assess the fetal thyroid status.[58] The fetus can be treated by treating the mother. Neonates have to be observed closely until antithyroid drugs are cleared (a few days) and the true thyroid state can be assessed.

Thyroid Storm

This life-threatening augmentation of thyrotoxicosis is usually precipitated by stress such as labor, cesarean section, or infection. Stress should be limited as much as possible in patients with uncontrolled thyrotoxicosis.

Hypothyroidism in Pregnancy

Serious hypothyroidism is rarely encountered during pregnancy. Patients with this degree of illness probably do not get pregnant. Patients with mild hypothyroidism probably never have a laboratory assessment for thyroid function during pregnancy and go undetected. Preeclampsia, intrauterine growth retardation, and fetal distress are more frequent in women with significant hypothyroidism.[59–61] There is also reason to believe that patients with hypothyroidism have an increased rate of spontaneous abortion.[62] The mechanism may be impaired ability of important organs such as the endometrium and the corpus luteum. Women being treated for hypothyroidism require an increase (20–50%) in thyroxine during pregnancy.[63, 64] *TSH should be monitored monthly in the first trimester and again in the postpartum period, and dosage should be adjusted to keep the TSH level in the normal range.*

Postpartum Thyroiditis

Autoimmune thyroid disease is suppressed to some degree by the immunologic changes of pregnancy. Thus, there is a relatively high incidence of postpartum thyroiditis (5–10%), usually 3–6 months after delivery, manifested by either hyperthyroidism or hypothyroidism, although commonly transient hyperthyroidism is followed by hypothyroidism.[65] This condition is due to a destructive thyroiditis associated with thyroid microsomal autoantibodies.[66] Women at high risk for postpartum thyroiditis are those with a personal or family history of autoimmune disease, and those with a previous postpartum episode. Women with insulin-requiring diabetes mellitus are at particularly high risk.[67]

Most importantly, the symptoms in these women are often attributed to anxiety or depression, and the obstetrician must have a high index of suspicion for hypothyroidism. The symptoms usually last 1–3 months, and almost all women return to normal thyroid function. Postpartum thyroiditis tends to recur with subsequent pregnancies, and eventually hypothyroidism remains.[68] The symptoms of hyperthyroidism in this condition are not responsive to antithyroid medication, and patients are usually not treated or given beta-adrenergic blocking agents (e.g., propranolol in a dose sufficient to reduce the resting pulse to less than 100 per minute). Because spontaneous remission is common, patients who are treated with hypothyroidism should be reassessed one year after gradual withdrawal of thyroxine. Patients who return to normal should undergo periodic laboratory surveillance of their thyroid status.

References

1. **Medvei VC,** *The History of Clinical Endocrinology,* The Parthenon Publishing Group, New York, 1993.

2. **Brent GA,** The molelcular basis of thyroid hormone action, *New Engl J Med* 331:947, 1994.

3. **Melmed S, Hershman J,** The thyroid and aging, In: Korcnman SG, ed. *Endocrine Aspects of Aging,* Elsevier Science Publishing, New York, 1982, p 33.

4. **Surks MI, Chopra IJ, Mariash CN, Nicoloff JT, Solomon DH,** American Thyroid Association guidelines for use of laboratory tests in thyroid disorders, *JAMA* 263:1529, 1990.

5. **Lindsay RS, Toft AD,** Hypothyroidism, *Lancet* 349:413, 1997.

6. **Robuschi G, Safran M, Braverman LE, Gnudi A, Roti E,** Hypothyroidism in the elderly, *Endocr Rev* 8:142, 1987.

7. **Felicetta JV,** Thyroid changes with aging: significance and management, *Geriatrics* 42:86, 1987.

8. **Danese MD, Powe NR, Sawin CT, Ladenson PW,** Screening for mild thyroid failure at the periodic health examination. A decision and cost-effectiveness analysis, *JAMA* 276:285, 1996.

9. **Hansen KA, Tho SPT, Hanly M, Moretuzzo RW, McDonough PG,** Massive ovarian enlargement in primary hypothyroidism, *Fertil Steril* 67:169, 1997.

10. **Wiseman SA, Powell JT, Humphries SE, Press M,** The magnitude of the hypercholesterolemia of hypothyroidism is associated with variation in the low density lipoprotein receptor gene, *J Clin Endocrinol Metab* 77:108, 1993.

11. **Monzani F, Caraccio N, Siciliano G, Manca L, Murri L, Ferrannini E,** Clinical and biochemical features of muscle dysfunction in subclinical hypothyroidism, *J Clin Endocrinol Metab* 82:3315, 1997.

12. **Monzani F, Del Guerra P, Caraccio N, Pruneti CA, Pucci E, Luisi M, Baschieri L,** Subclinical hypothyroidism: neurobehavioral features and beneficial effect of L-thyroxine treatment, *Clin Investigator* 71:367, 1993.

13. **Kinlaw III WB,** Thyroid disorders and cholesterol: identifying the realm of clinical relevance, *Endocrinologist* 5:147, 1995.

14. **Cooper DS,** Thyroid hormone treatment: new insights into an old therapy, *JAMA* 261:2694, 1989.

15. **Toft AD,** Thyroxine therapy, *New Engl J Med* 331:174, 1994.

16. **Rosenbaum RL, Barzel US,** Levothyroxine replacement dose for primary hypothyroidism decreases with age, *Ann Intern Med* 96:53, 1982.

17. **Watts NB,** Use of a sensitive thyrotropin assay for monitoring treatment with levothyroxine, *Arch Intern Med* 149:309, 1989.

18. **Lazarus JH,** Hyperthyroidism, *Lancet* 349:339, 1997.

19. **Sawin CT, Geller A, Wolf PA, Belanger AJ, Baker E, Bacharach P, Wilson PWF, Benjamin EJ, D'Agostino RB,** Low serum thyrotropin concentrations as a risk factor for atrial fibrillation in older persons, *New Engl J Med* 331:1249, 1994.

20. **Franklyn JA,** The management of hyperthyroidism, *New Engl J Med* 330:1731, 1994.

21. **Cooper DS,** Thyroid hormone and the skeleton, *JAMA* 259:3175, 1988.

22. **Wartofsky L,** Osteoporosis and therapy with thyroid hormone, *Endocrinologist* 1:57, 1991.

23. **Diamond T, Nery L, Hales I,** A therapeutic dilemma: suppressive doses of thyroxine significantly reduce bone mineral measurements in both premenopausal and postmenopausal women with thyroid carcinoma, *J Clin Endocrinol Metab* 72:1184, 1991.

24. **Solomon BL, Wartofsky L, Burman KD,** Prevalence of fractures in postmenopausal women with thyroid disease, *Thyroid* 3:17, 1993.

25. **Barsony J, Lakatos P, Foldes J, Feher T,** Effect of vitamin D_3 loading and thyroid hormone replacement therapy on the decreased serum 25-hydroxyvitamin D level in patients with hypothyroidism, *Acta Endocrinol* 113:329, 1986.

26. **Ross DS, Neer RM, Ridgway EC, Daniels GH,** Subclinical hyperthyroidism and reduced bone density as a possible result of prolonged suppression of the pituitary-thyroid axis with L-thyroxine, *Am J Med* 82:1167, 1987.

27. **Faber J, Gallow AM,** Changes in bone mass during prolonged subclinical hyperthyroidism due to L-thyroxine treatment: a meta-analysis, *Eur J Endocrinol* 130:350, 1994.

28. **Schneider DL, Barrett-Connor EL, Morton DJ,** Thyroid hormone use and bone mineral density in elderly women: effects of estrogen, *JAMA* 271:1245, 1994.

29. **Mazzaferri EL,** Management of a solitary thyroid nodule, *New Engl J Med* 328:553, 1993.

30. **Pacini F, Fontanelli M, Fugazzola L, Elisei R, Romei C, Di Coscio G, Miccoli P, Pinchera A,** Routine measurement of serum calcitonin in nodular thyroid diseases allows the preoperative diagnosis of unsuspected sporadic medullary thyroid carcinoma, *J Clin Endocrinol Metab* 78:826, 1994.

31. **Gharib H, Goellner JR,** Fine-needle aspiration biopsy of the thyroid: an appraisal, *Ann Intern Med* 118:282, 1993.

32. **Cooper DS,** Thyroxine suppression therapy for benign disease, *J Clin Endocrinol Metab* 80:331, 1995.

33. **Glinoer D,** The regulation of thyroid function in pregnancy: pathways of endocrine adaptation from physiology to pathology, *Endocr Rev* 18:404, 1997.

34. **Smyth PPA, Hetherton AMT, Smith DF, Radcliff M, O'Herlihy C,** Maternal iodine status and thyroid volume during pregnancy: correlation with neonatal iodine intake, *J Clin Endocrinol Metab* 82:2840, 1997.

35. **Kennedy RL, Darne J,** The role of hCG in regulation of the thyroid gland in normal and abnormal pregnancy, *Obstet Gynecol* 78:298, 1991.

36. **Kimura M, Amino N, Tamaki H, Ito E, Mitsuda N, Miyai K, Tanizawa O,** Gestational thyrotoxicosis and hyperemesis gravidarum: possible role of hCG with higher stimulating activity, *Clin Endocrinol* 38:345, 1993.

37. **Glinoer D, DeNayer P, Bourdoux P, Lemone M, Robyn C, Van Steirteghem A, Kinthaert J, Lejeune B,** Regulation of maternal thyroid during pregnancy, *J Clin Endocrinol Metab* 71:276, 1990.

38. **Berghout A, Ended E, Ross A, Hogerzeil HV, Smits NJ, Wiersinga WM,** Thyroid function and thyroid size in normal pregnant women living in an iodine replete area, *Clin Endocrinol* 41:375, 1994.

39. **Kimura M, Amino N, Tamaki H, Mitsuda N, Miyai K, Tanizawa O,** Physiologic thyroid activation in normal early pregnancy is induced by circulating hCG, *Obstet Gynecol* 75:775, 1990.

40. **Ballabio M, Poshyachinda M, Ekins RP,** Pregnancy-induced changes in thyroid function: role of human chorionic gonadotropin as putative regulator of maternal thyroid, *J Clin Endocrinol Metab* 73.824, 1991.

41. **Goodwin TM, Montoro M, Mestman JH,** Transient hyperthyroidism and hyperemesis gravidarum: clinical aspects, *Am J Obstet Gynecol* 167:648, 1992.

42. **Goodwin TM, Montoro M, Mestman JH, Pekary AE, Hershman JM,** The role of chorionic gonadotropin in transient hyperthyroidism of hyperemesis gravidarum, *J Clin Endocrinol Metab* 75:1333, 1992.

43. **Yamazaki K, Sato K, Shizume K, Kanaji Y, Ito Y, Obara T, Nakagawa T, Koizumi T, Nishimura R,** Potent thyrotropic activity of human chorionic gonadotropin variants in terms of ^{125}I incorporation and *de novo* synthesized thyroid hormone release in human thyroid follicles, *J Clin Endocrinol Metab* 80:473, 1995.

44. **Tsuruta E, Tada H, Tamaki H, Kashiwai T, Asahio K, Takeoka K, Mitsuda N, Amino N,** Pathogenic role of asialo human chorionic gonadotropin in gestational thyrotoxicosis, *J Clin Endocrinol Metab* 80:350, 1995.

45. **Thorpe-Beeston JG, Nicolaides KH, McGregor AM,** Fetal thyroid function, *Thyroid* 2:207, 1992.

46. **Burrow GN, Fisher DA, Larsen PR,** Maternal and fetal thyroid function, *New Engl J Med* 331:1072, 1994.

47. **Fisher DA,** Clinical review 19: management of congenital hypothyroidism, *J Clin Endocrinol Metab* 72:523, 1991.

48. **Perelman AH, Johnson RL, Clemons RD, Finberg HJ, Clewell WH, Trujillo L,** Intrauterine diagnosis and treatment of fetal goitrous hypothyroidism, *J Clin Endocrinol Metab* 71:618, 1990.

49. **Klein AH, Murphy BEP, Artal R, Oddie TH, Fisher DA,** Amniotic fluid thyroid hormone concentrations during human gestation, *Am J Obstet Gynecol* 136:626, 1980.

50. **Davidson KM, Richards DS, Schatz DA, Fisher DA,** Successful in utero treatment of fetal goiter and hypothyroidism, *New Engl J Med* 324:543, 1991.

51. **Davis LE, Lucas MJ, Hankins GDV, Roark ML, Cunningham FG,** Thyrotoxicosis complicating pregnancy, *Am J Obstet Gynecol* 160:63, 1989.

52. **Easterling TR, Chmucker BC, Carlson KL, Millard SP, Benedetti TJ,** Maternal hemodynamics in pregnancies complicated by hyperthyroidism, *Obstet Gynecol* 78:348, 1991.

53. **Wing DA, Millar LK, Koonings PP, Montoro MN, Mestman JH,** A comparison of propylthiouracil versus methimazole in the treatment of hyperthyroidism in pregnancy, *Am J Obstet Gynecol* 170:90, 1994.

54. **Cheron RG, Kaplan MM, Larsen PR, Selenkow HA, Crigler Jr JF,** Neonatal thyroid function after propylthiouracil therapy for maternal Graves' disease, *New Engl J Med* 304:525, 1981.

55. **Burrow GN, Klatskin EH, Genel M,** Intellectual development in children whose mothers received proplythiouracil during pregnancy, *Yale J Biol Med* 51:151, 1978.

56. **Mitsuda N, Tamaki H, Amino N, Hosono T, Miyaki K, Tanizasa O,** Risk factors for developmental disorders in infants born to women with Graves' disease, *Obstet Gynecol* 80:359, 1992.

57. **Millar LK, Wing DA, Leung AS, Koonings PP, Montoro MN, Mestman JH,** Low birth weight and preeclampsia in pregnancies complicated by hyperthyroidism, *Obstet Gynecol* 84:946, 1994.

58. **Wenstrom KD, Weinger CP, Williamson RA, Grant SS,** Prenatal diagnosis of fetal hyperthyroidism using funipuncture, *Obstet Gynecol* 76:513, 1990.

59. **Davis LE, Leveno KL, Cunningham FG,** Hypothyroidism complicating pregnancy, *Obstet Gynecol* 72:108, 1988.

60. **Leung AS, Millar LK, Koonings PP, Montoro M, Mestman JH,** Perinatal outcome in hypothyroid pregnancies, *Obstet Gynecol* 81:349, 1993.

61. **Wasserstrum N, Anania CA,** Perinatal consequences of maternal hypothyroidism in early pregnancy and inadequate replacement, *Clin Endocrinol* 42:353, 1995.

62. **Maruo T, Katayama K, Matuso H, Anwar M, Mochizuki M,** The role of maternal thyroid hormones in maintaining early pregnancy in threatened abortion, *Acta Endocrinol* 127:118, 1992.

63. **Mandel SJ, Larsen PR, Seely EW, Brent GA,** Increased need for thyroxine during pregnancy in women with primary hypothyroidism, *New Engl J Med* 323:91, 1990.

64. **Kaplan MM,** Monitoring thyroxine treatment during pregnancy, *Thyroid* 2:147, 1992.

65. **Roti E, Emerson CH,** Clinical review 29: postpartum thyroiditis, *J Clin Endocrinol Metab* 74:3, 1992.

66. **Vargas MT, Bariones-Urbina R, Gladman D, Papsin FR, Walfish PG,** Antithyroid microsomal autoantibodies and HLA-DR5 are associated with postpartum thyroid dysfunction: evidence supporting an autoimmune pathogenesis, *J Clin Endocrinol Metab* 67:327, 1988.

67. **Alvarez-Marfany M, Roman SH, Drexler AZ, Robertson C, Stagnaro-Green A,** Long-term prospective study of postpartum thyroid dysfunction in women with insulin dependent diabetes mellitus, *J Clin Endocrinol Metab* 79:10, 1994.

68. **Walfish PG, Chan YYC,** Postpartum hyperthyroidism, *Clin Endocrinol Metab* 14:417, 1985.

Part III

Contraception

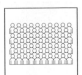

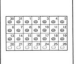

21 Family Planning, Sterilization, and Abortion

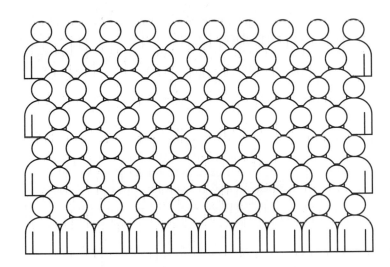

As societies become more affluent, fertility decreases. This decrease is in response to the use of contraception and abortion. During her reproductive lifespan, the average !Kung woman, a member of an African tribe of hunter-gatherers, experienced 15 years of lactational amenorrhea, 4 years of pregnancy, and only 48 menstrual cycles.[1] In contrast, a modern urban woman will experience 420 menstrual cycles. Contemporary women undergo earlier menarche and start having sexual intercourse earlier in their lives than in the past. Even though breastfeeding has increased in recent years, its duration is relatively brief, and its contribution to contraception in the developed world is trivial. Therefore, it is more difficult today to limit the size of a family unless some method of contraception is utilized.

More young women (under age 25) in the United States become pregnant than do their contemporaries in other Western countries.[2, 3] The teenage pregnancy rates in 5 northern European countries and Canada range from 13 to 53% of the U.S. rate. The differences disappear almost completely after age 25. This is largely because American men and women after age 25 utilize surgical sterilization at a great rate.

It is not true that young American women want to have these higher pregnancy rates. About 78% of all pregnancies among American teenagers are unintended.[4] American teenagers abort nearly half of their pregnancies, and this proportion is similar to that seen in other countries.[4] American women age 20–34 have the highest proportion of pregnancies aborted compared with other countries, indicating an unappreciated, but real, problem of unintended pregnancy existing beyond the teenage years. A decrease in unintended pregnancies (about 16%) and the abortion rate in the U.S. in the 1990s is due to better use of contraception; however, the rates are still relatively high. About half of all pregnancies in the U.S. are estimated to be unplanned, and more than half of these are aborted.[4]

Delaying marriage prolongs the period in which women are exposed to the risk of unintended pregnancy. This, however, cannot be documented as a major reason for the large differential between young adults in Europe and the U.S. The available evidence also indicates that a difference in sexual activity is not an important explanation. The major difference between American women and European women is that American women under age 25 are less likely to use any form of contraception.[2] Significantly the use of oral contraceptives (the main choice of younger women) is lower in the U.S. than in other countries.

Why are Americans different? The cultures in areas such as the United Kingdom and the Scandinavian countries are certainly very similar with similar rates of sexual experience. A major difference must be attributed to the availability of contraception. In the rest of the world, contraceptive services can be obtained from more accessible resources and relatively inexpensively. Major problems are the enormous diversity of people and the unequal distribution of income in the U.S. These factors influence the ability of our society to effectively provide education regarding sex and contraception and to effectively make contraception services available.

Contraception is not new, but its widespread development and application are new. The era of modern contraception dates from 1960 when oral contraception was first approved by the U.S. Food and Drug Administration, and intrauterine devices were re-introduced. For the first time, contraception did not have to be a part of the act of coitus. However, national family planning services and research were not funded by the U.S. Congress until 1970, and the last U.S. law prohibiting contraception was not reversed until 1973.

Efficacy of Contraception

A clinician's anecdotal experience with contraceptive methods is truly insufficient to provide the accurate information necessary for patient counseling. The clinician must be aware of the definitions and measurements used in assessing contraceptive efficacy and must draw on the talents of appropriate experts in this area to summarize the accurate and comparative failure rates for the various methods of contraception. The publications by Trussell et al., summarized below, accomplish these purposes and are highly recommended.[5-7]

Definition and Measurement

Contraceptive efficacy is generally assessed by measuring the number of unplanned pregnancies that occur during a specified period of exposure and use of a contraceptive method. The two methods that have been used to measure contraceptive efficacy are the Pearl index and life-table analysis.

The Pearl Index

The Pearl index is defined as the number of failures per 100 woman-years of exposure. The denominator is the total months or cycles of exposure from the onset of a method until completion of the study, an unintended pregnancy, or discontinuation of the method. The quotient is multiplied by 1200 if the denominator consists of months or by 1300 if the denominator consists of cycles.

With most methods of contraception, failure rates decline with duration of use. The Pearl index is usually based on a lengthy exposure (usually one year) and, therefore, fails to accurately compare methods at various durations of exposure. This limitation is overcome by using the method of life-table analysis.

Life-Table Analysis

Life-table analysis calculates a failure rate for each month of use. A cumulative failure rate can then compare methods for any specific length of exposure. Women who leave a study for any reason other than unintended pregnancy are removed from the analysis, contributing their exposure until the time of the exit.

Failure Rates During the First Year of Use, United States[7]

Method	Percent of Women with Pregnancy	
	Lowest Expected	Typical
No method	85.0%	85.0%
Combination Pill	0.1	3.0
Progestin only	0.5	3.0
IUDs		
Progesterone IUD	1.5	2.0
Levonorgestrel IUD	0.6	0.8
Copper T 380A	0.1	0.1
Norplant	0.05	0.05
Female sterilization	0.05	0.05
Male sterilization	0.1	0.15
Depo-Provera	0.3	0.3
Spermicides	6.0	26.0
Periodic abstinence		25.0
Calendar	9.0	
Ovulation method	3.0	
Symptothermal	2.0	
Post–ovulation	1.0	
Withdrawal	4.0	19.0
Cervical cap		
Parous women	26.0	40.0
Nulliparous women	9.0	20.0
Sponge		
Parous women	9.0	28.0
Nulliparous women	6.0	18.0
Diaphragm and spermicides	6.0	20.0
Condom		
Male	3.0	14.0
Female	5.0	21.0

Contraceptive failures do occur and for many reasons. Thus, "method effectiveness" and "use effectiveness" have been used to designate efficacy with correct and incorrect use of a method. It is less confusing to simply compare the very best performance (the lowest expected failure rate) with the usual experience (typical failure rates) as noted in the table of failure rates during the first year of use. The lowest expected failure rates are determined in clinical trials, where the combination of highly motivated subjects and frequent support from the study personnel yields the best results. It should be noted that slightly more than half of the unintended pregnancies in the U.S. are due to contraceptive failures.[4]

Changes in Contraceptive Use by U.S. Women 15–44 [8–11]

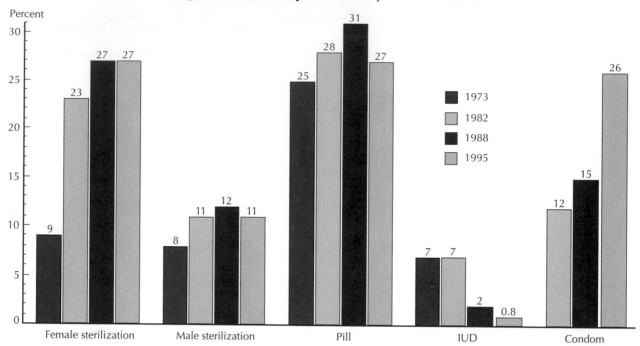

Contraceptive Use in the United States

The National Survey of Family Growth is conducted by the National Center for Health Statistics of the Centers for Disease Control and Prevention. Data are available from 1972, 1976, 1982, 1988 and 1995.[8–11] The samples are very large, and, therefore, the estimates are very accurate.

The percent of married couples using sterilization as a method of contraception more than doubled from 1972 to 1988, and has remained stable since then. The use of oral contraception reached a high in 1992, and then decreased in 1995, especially among Hispanic and black Americans. Approximately 10.7 million American women used oral contraceptives in 1988, and 10.4 million in 1995. Among never married women, oral contraception has been the leading method of birth control, but from 1988 to 1995, oral contraceptive use decreased in women younger than 25 and rose among women aged 30–44. A part of the decrease in oral contraceptive use is due to the new availability and use of implant (about 0.5 million women in 1995) and injectable methods (about 1.0 million women in 1995). However, the greater impact is due to an increase in condom use, especially by never married and formerly married women, women younger than 25, black women, and Hispanic women; indeed, the recent increase in overall contraceptive use is due to the increase in condom use which rose from 5.1 million women aged 15–44 in 1988 (15%) to 7.9 million in 1995 (20%). This increase occurred in all race and ethnic groups. These changes reflect the concern regarding sexually transmitted diseases, including human immunodeficiency (HIV). About one-third of condom users in 1995 were using more than one method, especially younger and never married women!

In 1982, 56% of U.S. women, 15–44 years of age, were using contraception, and this increased in 1995 to 64% (about 39 million women). In 1995, contraceptive sterilization (male and female) was utilized by 38% (15 million) of these women (the next leading method was oral contraception, 27%) The number of reproductive age women using the intrauterine device (IUD) decreased by two-thirds from 1982 to 1988, and further decreased in 1995, from 7.1% to 2% to 0.8%, respectively. IUD use is concentrated in the U.S. in married women over age 35. In 1982 more than 2 million women used the IUD and a similar number used the diaphragm, but in 1995 only 0.3 million women used the IUD and 0.7 million women (1.9%) used the diaphragm. The decrease in IUD use since 1982 has been especially marked in Hispanic and black women.

Contraceptive Methods in Women 15–44 in 1995 [10,11]

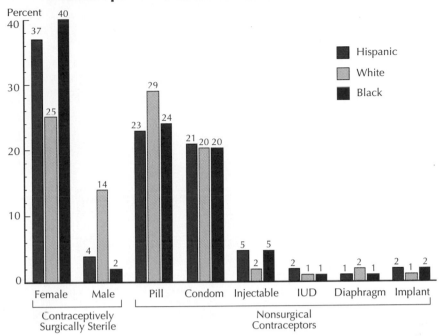

The oral contraceptive is the most popular method among teenagers. However, studies have repeatedly documented that the use of the implant and injectable methods is associated with lower discontinuation rates and a lower rate of repeat pregnancies following delivery.[12, 13] This warrants a renewed effort to extend the use of these methods.

Contraceptive Use by Age in 1995 [10,11]

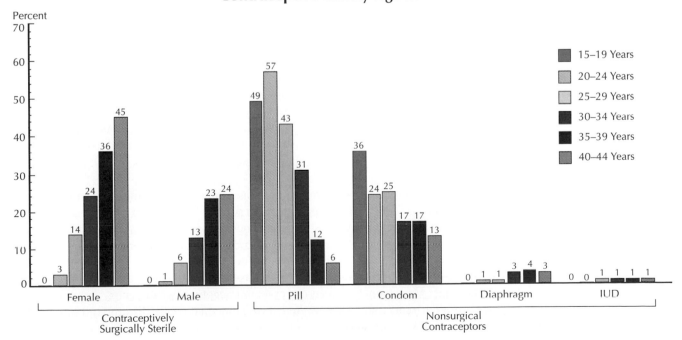

Contraception Relative Five-Year Costs

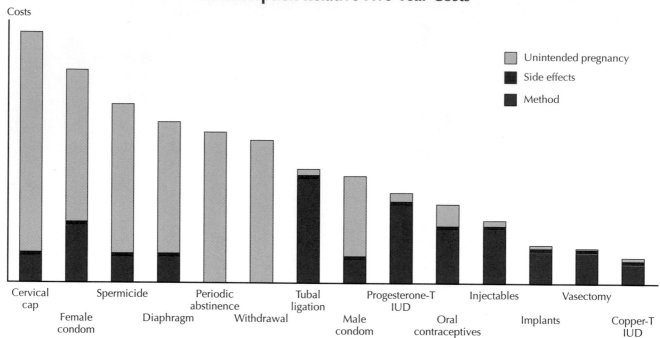

After Trussell, et al [170]

In 1995, 95% of those who were at risk of getting pregnant were using some method of contraception, whereas 36% of women of reproductive age were not using a method of contraception for the following reasons:

- 11% — no sexual experience,
- 9% — pregnant or trying to get pregnant,
- 6% — not sexually active,
- 5% — sterilized for medical reasons,
- 5% — at risk for an unintended pregnancy (this percentage steadily decreased over the last decade).

U.S. couples have made up for the lack of contraceptive choices by greater reliance on voluntary sterilization. Between 1973 and 1982, oral contraception and sterilization changed places as the most popular contraceptive method among women over the age of 30. Approximately one-half of American couples choose sterilization within 15 to 20 years of their last wanted birth. During the years of maximal fertility, oral contraceptives are the most common method peaking at age 20–24. The use of condoms is the second most widely used method of reversible contraception, rising from about 9% in the mid 1980s to approximately 20% of couples in 1995.[11]

The pattern of contraceptive use in Canada in 1995 was similar to that of the U.S., with a slightly higher percentage of oral contraceptive use (38.2% of women 15–44 years of age) and a slightly lower utilization of sterilization (32.5%).[14] Canada, too, has seen an increase in condom use and a decrease in use of the IUD. In France, 36.3% of reproductive aged women used oral contraceptives (in 1994), and although IUD use has slightly decreased (only among younger women), French women use the IUD at a rate that is more than 16-fold greater compared with North American women.[15] Most French women use oral contraceptives when young, and then turn to the IUD in their older years (only 4.1% of French women relied on sterilization in 1994 — male sterilization is virtually nonexistent).

World Population

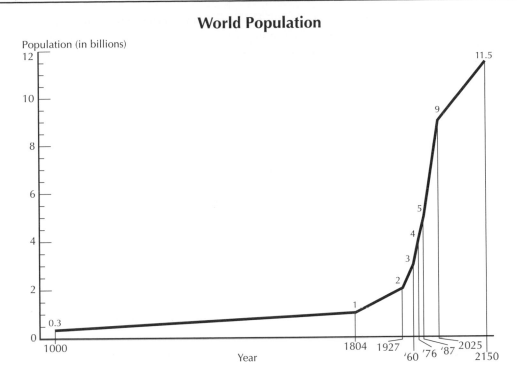

The Impact of the Worldwide Use of Contraception

The world population is expected to stabilize at between 11 and 12 billion around 2150, with a fertility rate of 2.1 children per woman.[16] Approximately 95% of the growth will occur in developing countries, so that by 2100, 13% of the population will live in developed countries, a decrease from the current 25%.[17]

WORLD POPULATION

1 billion	—	**achieved in 1800–1850**
2 billion	—	**achieved in 1930**
3 billion	—	**achieved in 1960**
4 billion	—	**achieved in 1976**
5 billion	—	**achieved in 1987**
9 billion	—	**in 2025**
11.5 billion	—	**in 2150**

Throughout the world, 45% of married women of reproductive age practice contraception. However, there is significant variation from area to area; e.g., 69% in east Asia but only 11% in Africa. Female sterilization and the IUD are most popular in developing countries, whereas oral contraceptives and condoms are most popular in developed countries. Less than 15% of women of reproductive age in the world are using oral contraceptives, and more than half live in the U.S., Brazil, France, and Germany.

The 76% of the world's population living in developing countries account for:

— 85% of all births,
— 95% of all infant and childhood deaths,
— 99% of all maternal deaths.

The problem in the developing world is self-evident. The ability to regulate fertility has a significant impact on infant, child, and maternal mortality and morbidity. A pregnant woman has a 200 times greater chance of dying living in a developing country than in a developed country.[18] The health risks associated with pregnancy and childbirth in the developing world are far greater than risks secondary to the use of modern contraception.[19]

In recent years, there has been an appropriate shift from a narrow focus on contraception to a broader view that encompasses the impact of poverty, emphasizes overall well-being and the rights of individuals, endorses gender equality, and examines the interactions among these issues.[20] It is not enough to simply limit fertility; contraception is only one component of reproductive health.

The Impact of Use and Non-use

Inadequate access to contraception is associated with a high induced abortion rate. Effective contraceptive use largely, although not totally, replaces the resort to abortion.[21] The combination of restrictive abortion laws and the lack of safe abortion services continues to make unsafe abortion a major cause of morbidity and mortality throughout the world. Both safe and unsafe abortions can be minimized by maximizing contraceptive services. However, the need for safe abortion services will persist. Contraceptive failures account for about half of the 1.33 million annual induced abortions in the U.S.

In the U.S. in the late 1980s, $1 spent on public funding for family planning saved an average of $4.40 spent on medical, welfare, and nutritional services.[22] States with higher family planning expenditures have fewer induced abortions, low-birthweight newborns, and premature births.[23] The investment in family planning leads to short-term reductions in expenditures on maternal and child health services and after 5 years, a reduction in costs for education budgets. Cutting back on publicly funded family planning services impacts largely on poor women, increasing the number of unintended births and abortions. In California, in the 1980s, there was an average of $7.70 saved for every $1 spent to provide contraceptive services.[24]

There is a gap between the low levels of unintentional pregnancy that can be achieved and the actual levels being obtained, most of which are in couples using reversible contraception. A major thrust, in addition to providing services, must include education and counseling of couples about effective contraception.

STDs and Contraception

The interaction between clinician and patient for the purpose of contraception provides an opportunity to control sexually transmitted diseases (STDs). The World Health Organization estimates that in the year 2000, over 13 million women will be infected with the human immunodeficiency virus (HIV).[25] The modification of unsafe sexual practices reduces the risk of unplanned pregnancy and the risk of infections of the reproductive tract. A patient visit for contraception is an excellent time for STD screening; if an infection is symptomatic, it should be diagnosed and treated during the same visit in which contraception is requested. A positive history for STDs should trigger both screening for asymptomatic infections and counseling for safer sexual practices. Attention should be given to the contraceptive methods that have the greatest influence on the risk of STDs.

The Future

From 1970 to 1986, the number of births in women over 30 quadrupled; since 1990, the fertility rate among women over 30 has remained relatively stable.[26] As more and more couples defer pregnancy until later in life, the use of sterilization under age 35 will decline, and the need for reversible contraception will increase. Between 1988 and 1995, oral contraceptive use decreased in women younger than 25 and increased in women aged 30–44.[11] These numbers changed because clinicians and patients have come to understand and accept that low-dose oral contraception is safe for healthy, nonsmoking older women.

The need for reversible contraception in women over the age of 30 is growing, not diminishing. The highest number of births in the U.S. occurred between 1947 and 1965 — the post-World War II baby boom (a demographic phenomenon shared by all parts of the developed world). The entire cohort of women born in this period will not reach their 45th birthday until around 2010. For approximately a 20-year period, therefore, there will be an unprecedented number of women in the later childbearing years. The number of women aged 35–49 increased 61% between 1982 and 1995. The proportion of births accounted for by this group of women will increase by about 72%, from 5% in 1982 to 8.6% in 2000.[27] This group of women is not only increasing in number, but it is changing its fertility pattern.

The deferment of marriage is a significant change in our society. In 1960, 28% of women aged 20–24 were single; in 1985, 58.5%. In 1960, 10% of women aged 25–29 were single; in 1985, 26%. But only 16% of the decline in the total fertility rate is accounted for by the increase in the average age at first marriage. Eighty-three percent of the decline in total fertility rate is accounted for by changes in marital fertility rates. In other words postponement of pregnancy in marriage is the more significant change.[28] This combination of increasing numbers, deferment of marriage, and postponement of pregnancy in marriage is responsible for the fact that we will be seeing more and more older women who will need reversible contraception. In short, there will continue to be longer duration of use in younger women and greater use in older women, a pattern that began in 1990.

Change in U.S. Female Demographics 1985–2000 [27]

Age	1985	1990	1995	2000	% Change 1985–2000
15–24	19.5 mill.	17.4 mill.	16.7 mill.	17.7 mill.	-9.2%
25–29	10.9	10.6	9.3	8.6	-21.1
30–34	10.0	11.0	10.8	9.4	-6.0
35–44	16.2	19.1	21.1	21.9	+35.2
Total 15–44	56.6	58.1	57.9	57.6	+1.8

One solution to the problem of a restricted number of contraceptive choices for American women is to develop new methods. There are many obstacles to the development of new methods, including the attitudes of the American public (besides America's traditionally conservative, religion-oriented views toward sex and family, polarization is produced by responses evoked by specific issues such as sterilization and induced abortion), the funding available for research, the time and cost required to meet federal regulations, and the problems of product liability.[29] However, experts in the field remain optimistic, citing the many needs and opportunities for improvements and new developments.[30]

Fortunately, clinicians and patients have recognized that low-dose oral contraception is very safe for healthy, nonsmoking older women. Between 1988 and 1995, the use of oral contraceptives doubled among women aged 35–39, and increased 6-fold in women over age 40.[11] However, as the above statistics indicate, its use is still not sufficient to meet the need. Besides fulfilling a need, this population of women has a series of benefits to be derived from oral contraception that tilt the risk:benefit ratio to the positive side (Chapter 22).

The growing need for reversible contraception would also be served by increased utilization of the IUD. The decline in IUD use in the U.S. is in direct contrast to the experience in the rest of the world, a complicated response to publicity and litigation. An increased risk of pelvic infection with contemporary IUDs in use is limited to the act of insertion and the transportation of pathogens to the upper genital tract. This risk is effectively minimized by careful screening with preinsertion cultures and the use of good technique. A return to IUD use by American couples is both warranted and desirable.

A major problem in the U.S. is the prevalence of misconceptions. More than half of women, even well-educated women, are not accurately aware of the efficacy or the benefits and side effects associated with contraception.[31, 32] Unfortunately, a significant percentage of women still do not know that there are many health benefits with the use of oral contraception. Misconceptions regarding contraception have, in many instances, achieved the stature of myths. Myths are an obstacle to good utilization and can only be dispelled by accurate and effective educational efforts.

Contraceptive advice is a component of good preventive health care. The clinician's approach is a key. This is an era of informed choice by the patient. Patients deserve to know the facts and need help in dealing with the state of the art and the uncertainty. But there is no doubt that patients, especially young patients, are influenced in their choice by their clinicians' advice and attitude. Although the role of a clinician is to provide the education necessary for the patient to make proper choices, one should not lose sight of the powerful influence exerted by the clinician in the choices ultimately made. In the 1970s, we approached the patient with great emphasis on risk. At the turn of the century, the approach should be different, highlighting the benefits and the greater safety of appropriate contraception.

If one attempts to sum the impact of the benefits of contraception on public health, as some have done with models focusing on hospital admissions, there is no doubt that the benefits outweigh the risks. The impact can be measured in terms of both morbidity and mortality. But the impact on public health is of little concern during the clinician–patient interchange in the medical office. Here personal risk is paramount, and compliance with effective contraception requires accurate information presented in a positive, effective fashion.

Sterilization

Contraceptive methods today are very safe and effective, however, we remain decades away from a perfect method of contraception for either women or men. Because reversible contraceptive methods are not perfect, more than a third of American couples use sterilization instead, and sterilization is now the predominant method of contraception in the world.[33]

Over the past 20 years, nearly one million Americans each year have undergone a sterilization operation, and recently, more women than men. By 1995, 38% of reproductive aged women relied on contraceptive sterilization: 27% had tubal occlusion (11 million women), and 11% depended on their partners' vasectomies (4 million men).[11] This same trend has occurred in Great Britain, where by age 40, over 20% of men and women have had a sterilization procedure.[34] In Spain and Italy, sterilization rates are very low, but the use of oral contraceptives and the IUD is very high.[35]

History

James Blundell proposed in 1823, in lectures at Guy's Hospital in London, that tubectomy ought to be performed at cesarean section to avoid the need for repeat sections.[36] He also proposed a technique for sterilization, which he later described so precisely that he must actually have performed the operation, although he never wrote about it. The first report was published in 1881 by Samuel Lungren of Toledo, Ohio, who ligated the tubes at the time of cesarean section, as Blundell had suggested 58 years earlier.[37] The Madlener procedure was devised in Germany in 1910 and reported in 1919. Because of many failures, the Madlener technique was supplanted in the U.S. by the method of Ralph Pomeroy, a prominent physician in Brooklyn, New York. This method, still popular today, was not described to the medical profession by Pomeroy's associates

The Pomeroy

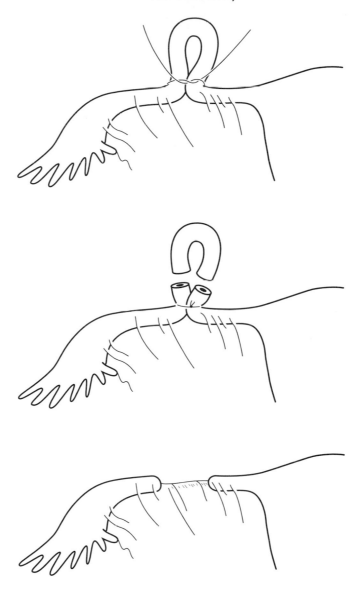

until 1929, 4 years after Pomeroy's death. Frederick Irving of the Harvard Medical School described his technique in 1924, and the Uchida method was not reported until 1946.

Few sterilizations were performed until the 1930s when "family planning" was first suggested as an indication for surgical sterilization by Baird in Aberdeen. He required women to be over 40 and to have had 8 or more children. Mathematical formulas of this kind persisted through the 1960s. In 1965, Sir Dugald Baird delivered a remarkable lecture, entitled "The Fifth Freedom," calling attention to the need to alleviate the fear of unwanted pregnancies, and the important role of sterilization.[38] By the end of the 1960s, sterilization was a popular procedure.

Laparoscopic methods were introduced in the early 1970s. The annual number of vasectomies began to decline, and the number of tubal occlusion operations increased rapidly. By 1973, more sterilization operations were performed for women than for men. This is accurately attributed to dramatic decreases in costs, hospital time, and pain due to the introduction of laparoscopy and minilaparotomy methods. The use of laparoscopy for tubal occlusion increased from only 0.6% of sterilizations in 1970 to more than 35% by 1975.[39] Since 1975, minilaparotomy, a technique popular in the less developed world, has been increasingly performed in the U.S. These methods

The Irving

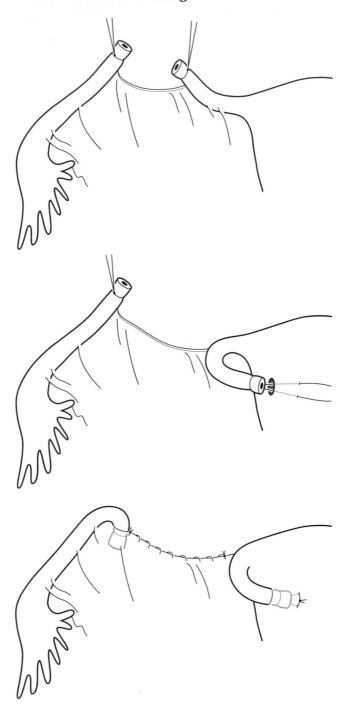

have allowed women to undergo sterilization operations at times other than immediately after childbirth or during major surgery.

Laparoscopy and minilaparotomy have led to a profound change in the convenience and cost of sterilization operations for women. In 1970, the average woman stayed in the hospital 6.5 days for a tubal sterilization. By 1975, this had declined to 3 days, and today, women rarely remain in the hospital overnight. The shorter length of stay achieved from 1970 to 1975 represented a savings of more than $200 million yearly in health care costs and a tremendous increase in convenience for women eager to return to work and their families.[40] Unlike some advances in technology, laparoscopy and minilaparotomy sterilization are technical innovations that have resulted in large savings in medical care costs.

The Uchida

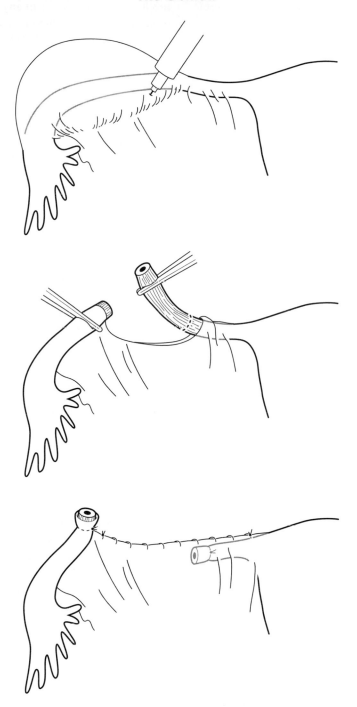

The great majority of sterilization procedures are accomplished in hospitals by physicians in private practice, but a rapidly increasing proportion is performed outside of hospitals in ambulatory surgical settings, including physicians' offices. In either hospital or outpatient settings, female sterilization is a very safe operation. Deaths specifically attributed to sterilization now account for a fatality rate of only 1.5 per 100,000 procedures, a mortality rate that is lower than that for childbearing (about 10 per 100,000 births in the U.S.).[41] When the risk of pregnancy from contraceptive method failure is taken into account, sterilization is the safest of all contraceptive methods.

Vasectomy has long been more popular in the U.S. than anywhere else in the world, but why don't more men use it? One explanation is that women have chosen laparoscopic sterilization in increasing numbers. Another is that men have been frightened by reports, often from animal data, of associations with autoimmune diseases, atherosclerosis, and most recently, prostatic cancer. Large epidemiologic studies have failed to confirm any definite adverse consequences.[42] When patients consider sterilization, we can assure them that vasectomy has not been demonstrated to have any harmful effects on men's health.[43] In addition, vasectomy is less expensive than tubal sterilization, morbidity is less, and mortality is essentially zero.

Efficacy of Sterilization

Laparoscopic and minilaparotomy sterilizations are not only convenient, they are almost as effective at preventing pregnancy as were the older, more complex operations. Vasectomy is also highly effective once the supply of remaining sperm in the vas deferens is exhausted. After 6 weeks or 15 ejaculations, essentially all men are sterile.

Failure Rates During the First Year, United States[6]

Method	Percent of Women with Pregnancy Lowest Expected	Typical
Female sterilization	0.2%	0.4%
Male sterilization	0.1%	0.15%

Besides the specific operation used, the skill of the operator and characteristics of the patient make important contributions to the efficacy of female sterilization. Up to 50% of failures are due to technical errors. The methods using complicated equipment, such as spring-loaded clips and silastic rings, fail for technical reasons more commonly than do simpler procedures such as the Pomeroy tubal ligation.[44] Minilaparotomy failures, therefore, occur much less frequently from technical errors.

It is hardly surprising that more complicated techniques of tubal occlusion have higher technical failure rates. What is surprising is the finding that characteristics of the patient influence the likelihood of failure even when technical problems are controlled for in analytical adjustments. In a careful study of this issue, two patient characteristics, age and lactation, demonstrated a significant impact.[45] Patients younger than 35 years were 1.7 times more likely to become pregnant, and women who were not breastfeeding following sterilization were 5 times more likely to become pregnant. These findings probably reflect the greater fecundity of younger women and the contraceptive contribution of lactation.

Significant numbers of pregnancies after tubal occlusion are present before the procedure. For this reason, some clinicians routinely perform a uterine evacuation or curettage prior to tubal occlusion. It seems more reasonable (and cost-effective) to exclude pregnancy by careful history taking, physical examination, and an appropriate pregnancy test prior to the sterilization procedure.[46]

Because method, operator, and patient characteristics all influence sterilization failures, it is difficult to predict which individual will experience a pregnancy after undergoing a tubal occlusion. Therefore, during the course of counseling, all patients should be made aware of the possibility of failure as well as the intent to cause permanent, irreversible sterility. It is important to avoid giving patients the impression that the tubal occlusion procedure is foolproof or guaranteed. Individual clinicians must be cautious judging their own success in accomplishing sterilization because failure is infrequent and many patients who become pregnant after sterilization never reveal the failure to the original surgeon.

Ectopic pregnancies can occur following tubal occlusion, and the incidence is much higher with some types of tubal occlusion.[47–49] Bipolar tubal coagulation is more likely to result in ectopic pregnancy than is mechanical occlusion.[44, 50] The probable explanation is that microscopic fistulae in the coagulated segment connecting to the peritoneal cavity permit sperm to reach the ovum. Ectopic pregnancies following tubal ligation are more likely to occur 2 or more years after sterilization, rather than immediately after. In the first year after sterilization, about 6% of pregnancies will be ectopic, but the majority of pregnancies that occur 2–3 years after occlusion will be ectopic.[51] Overall, however, the risk of an ectopic pregnancy in sterilized women is lower than if they had not been sterilized. Nevertheless, approximately one-third of the pregnancies that occur after tubal sterilization are ectopic.[52]

Vaginal procedures have higher failure rates than laparoscopy or minilaparotomy, but the principal disadvantage is a higher rate of infection. Intraperitoneal infection is a rare complication of minilaparotomy or laparoscopic techniques, but in vaginal procedures, abscess formation approaches 1%.[53] This risk can be reduced by the use of prophylactic antibiotics administered intraoperatively, but open laparoscopy is usually easier and safer than vaginal sterilization even in obese women.

Sterilization and Ovarian Cancer — A Benefit of Sterilization

Evidence from the Nurses' Health Study indicated that tubal sterilization was associated with a 67% reduced risk of ovarian cancer.[54] In the prospective mortality study, conducted by the American Cancer Society, women who had undergone tubal sterilization experienced about a 30% reduction in the risk of fatal ovarian cancer.[55] In addition, case-control data have consistently supported this finding.[56–58] The mechanism for such an effect is not clear, but this information is worth sharing with patients.

Female Sterilization Techniques

Because laparoscopy permits direct visualization and manipulation of the abdominal and pelvic organs with minimal abdominal disruption, it offers many advantages. Hospitalization is not required; most patients return home within a few hours, and the majority return to full activity within 24 hours. Discomfort is minimal, the incision scars are barely visible, and sexual activity need not be restricted. In addition, the surgeon has an opportunity to inspect the pelvic and abdominal organs for abnormalities. The disadvantages of laparoscopic sterilization include the cost, the expensive, fragile equipment, the special training required, and the risks of inadvertent bowel or vessel injury.

Laparoscopic sterilization can be achieved with any of these methods:

1.   Occlusion and partial resection by unipolar electrosurgery.

2.   Occlusion and transection by unipolar electrosurgery.

3.   Occlusion by bipolar electrocoagulation.

4.   Occlusion by mechanical means (clips or silastic rings).

All of these methods can use an operating laparoscope alone, or the diagnostic laparoscope with operating instruments passed through a second trocar, or both the operating laparoscope and secondary puncture equipment. All can be used with the "open" laparoscopic technique in which the laparoscopic instrument is placed into the abdominal cavity under direct vision to avoid the risk of bowel or blood vessel puncture on blind entry. Patient acceptance and recovery are approximately the same with all methods.

It is now apparent that the long-term failure rates for all methods are higher than previous estimates; overall, 1.85% of sterilized women experience a failure within 10 years.[59] *As much as one-third of these failures are ectopic pregnancies.*[52] The higher failure rates with silastic rings, clips, and bipolar coagulation reflect the greater degree of skill required for these methods. The methods with a greater percentage of failures occurring many years after the procedure are unipolar coagulation, bipolar coagulation, and the silastic ring. Because of the effect of declining fecundity with increasing age, younger sterilized women are more likely to have a failure, including ectopic pregnancy, compared with older women. For these reasons, women seeking sterilization should consider the use of the copper IUD or implants, reversible methods that offer very low failure rates.

Female Tubal Sterilization Methods, 10-Year Cumulative Failure Rates[59]

Unipolar coagulation	0.75%
Postpartum tubal excision	0.75
Silastic (Falope or Yoon) ring	1.77
Interval tubal exclusion	2.01
Bipolar coagulation	2.48
Hulka-Clemens clip	3.65

Tubal Occlusion by Electrosurgical Methods

If electrons from an electrosurgical generator are concentrated in one location, heat within the tissue increases sharply and desiccates the tissue until resistance is so high that no more current can pass. Unipolar methods of sterilization create a dense area of current under the grasping forceps of the unipolar electrode. In order to complete the circuit, however, these electrons must spread through the body and be returned to the generator via a return electrode (the ground plate) that has a broad surface to minimize the density of the current to avoid burns as the electrons leave the body. "Unipolar" refers to the method that requires the patient ground plate.

With the unipolar method, if tissue resistance is high and the electrical pressure (voltage) relatively low, current may cease to flow or may search out alternate pathways with lower resistance. When the voltage is increased, the electrons have more "push" to find another pathway, therefore, the surgeon must use the lowest possible voltage necessary to completely coagulate. The return electrode (the ground plate) must be in good contact with the patient.

Unipolar electrosurgery can create a unique electrical "capacitance" problem when an operating laparoscope is used with unipolar forceps. A capacitor is any device that can hold an electric charge, and can exist wherever an insulated material separates two conductors that have different potentials. This property of capacitance explains some of the inadvertent bowel burns that have occurred with laparoscopic sterilization.[60] The operating laparoscope is a hollow metal tube surrounding an active electrode, the forceps used to grasp and coagulate the tubes. When current passes through the active electrode, the laparoscope itself becomes a capacitor. Up to 70% of the current passed through the active electrode can be induced into the laparoscope. Should bowel or other structures touch a laparoscope, which is insulated from the abdominal incision (for example, by a fiberglass cannula), the stored electrons will be discharged at high density directly into the vital organ. This potential hazard is eliminated by using a metal trocar sleeve rather than a nonconductive sleeve-like fiberglass. Because there is little pressure behind the electrons from a low-voltage generator, not enough heat is generated to burn the skin as the capacitance current leaks out into the patient's body through the sleeve. Even if the active electrode comes in direct contact with the laparoscope, as when a two-incision technique is used, the current will leak harmlessly through the metal trocar sleeve. The risk of inadvertent coagulation of bowel or other organs cannot be completely eliminated because all body surfaces offer a path back to the ground plate.

The unipolar electrosurgical technique is straightforward. The isthmic portion of the fallopian tube is grasped and elevated away from the surrounding structures, and the electrical energy applied until the tissue blanches, swells, and then collapses. The tube is then grasped, moving toward the uterus, recoagulated, and the steps repeated until 2–3 cm of tube have been coagulated. Some surgeons advise against cornual coagulation for fear it may increase the risk of ectopic pregnancy due to fistula formation.

The coagulation and transection technique is performed in a similar fashion with the same instruments. In order to transect the tube, however, an instrument designed to cut tissue must be utilized. The transection of tissue increases the risk of possible bleeding and does not, by itself, reduce the failure rate over coagulation alone. The specimens obtained by this method are usually coagulated beyond microscopic recognition, and therefore will not provide pathological evidence of successful sterilization.

The bipolar method of sterilization eliminates the ground plate required for unipolar electrosurgery and uses a specially designed forceps. One jaw of the forceps is the active electrode, and the other jaw is the ground electrode. Current density is great at the point of forceps contact with tissue, and the use of a low-voltage, high-frequency current prevents the spread of electrons. By eliminating the return electrode, the chance of an aberrant pathway through bowel or other structures is greatly reduced. There is, however, a disadvantage with this technique. Because electron spread is decreased, more applications of the grasping forceps are necessary to coagulate the same length of tube than with unipolar coagulation. As desiccation occurs at the point of high current density, tissue resistance increases, and the coagulated area eventually provides resistance to flow of the low-voltage current. Should the resistance increase beyond the voltage's capability to push electrons through the tissue, incomplete coagulation of the endosalpinx can result.[61] In addition, the desiccated tissue can adhere to the bipolar forceps, making it difficult to remove from the surface of the tube.

The bipolar method can be used with either a single-incision operating laparoscope or with dual incision instruments. The forceps are, however, more delicate than unipolar equipment and must be kept meticulously clean. Damage to the instruments can alter the ability to coagulate, and inadequate or incomplete electrocoagulation is the main cause of failure.

Bipolar cautery is safer than unipolar cautery with regard to burns of abdominal organs, but most studies indicate higher failure rates. Although the bipolar forceps will not burn tissues that are not actually grasped, care must be taken to avoid coagulating structures adherent to the tubes. For example, the ureter can be damaged when the tube is adherent to the pelvic side wall.

Tubal Occlusion With Clips and Rings
Female sterilization by mechanical occlusion eliminates the safety concerns with electrosurgery. However, mechanical devices are subject to flaws in material, defects in manufacturing, and errors in design, all of which can alter efficacy. Three mechanical devices have been widely used and have low failure rates with long-term follow-up: the Hulka-Clemens (spring) clip, the Filshie Clip, and the silastic (Falope or Yoon) ring. Each of the three requires an understanding of its mechanical function, a working knowledge of the intricate applicator necessary to apply the device, meticulous attention to maintenance of the applicators, and skillful tubal placement. These devices are less effective when used immediately postpartum on dilated tubes.

The Hulka-Clemens Spring Clip

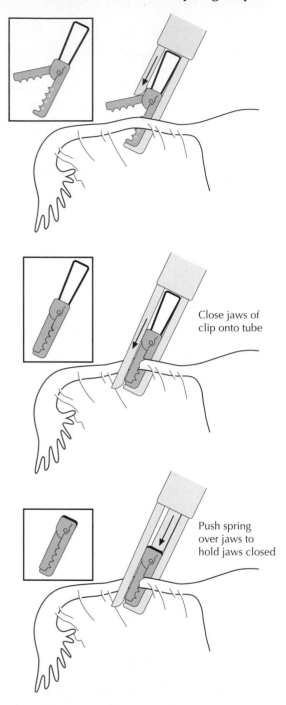

Close jaws of
clip onto tube

Push spring
over jaws to
hold jaws closed

Hulka-Clemens Spring Clip. The spring clip consists of two plastic jaws made of Lexan, hinged by a small metal pin 2 mm from one end. Each jaw has teeth on the opposed surface, and a stainless steel spring is pushed over the jaws to hold them closed over the tube. A special laparoscope for one incision application is most commonly used, although the spring clip can also be used in a two-incision procedure. The spring clip should be applied at a 90 degree angle to include some mesosalpinx at the proximal isthmus of a stretched fallopian tube. The spring clip destroys 3 mm of tube and has one-year pregnancy rates of 2 per 1000 women, but the highest 10-year cumulative failure rate.[44, 59]

The Filshie Clip

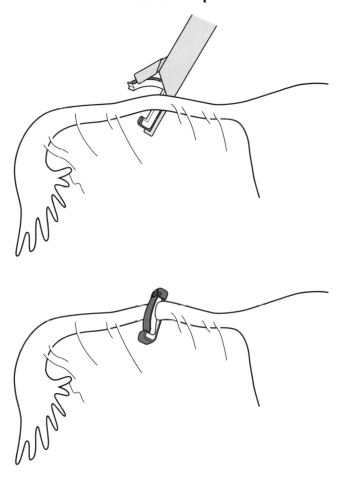

Complications unique to spring clip sterilization result from mechanical difficulties. Should the clip be dislodged or dropped into the abdomen during the procedure, it should be retrieved. Usually, it can be removed laparoscopically, but sometimes laparotomy is necessary. Should incomplete occlusion or incorrect alignment of the clip occur, a second clip can be applied without hazard. This clip offers a good chance for reanastomosis, better than electrosurgical methods that destroy more tube.

Filshie Clip. The Filshie clip is made of titanium lined with silicone rubber. The hinged clip is locked over the tube using a special applicator through a second incision or operating laparoscope. The rubber lining of the clip expands on compression to keep the tube blocked. Only 4 mm of the tube is destroyed. Failure rates one year after the procedure with the newest model approximate 1 per 1000 women.[49] Because the Filshie clip is longer, it is reported to occlude dilated tubes more readily than does the spring clip. Both the spring clip and the Filshie clip provide good chances for tubal reanastomosis.

The Silastic (Falope-Yoon) Ring

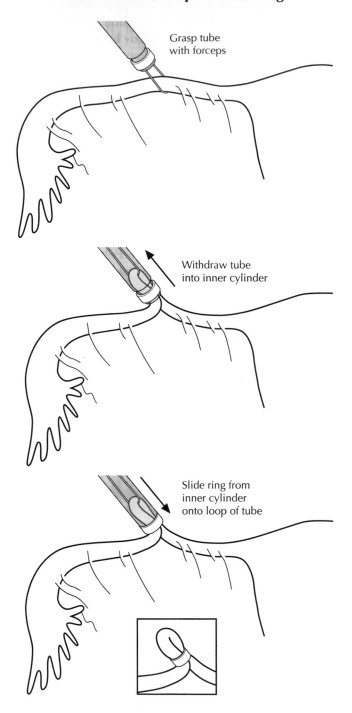

Grasp tube
with forceps

Withdraw tube
into inner cylinder

Slide ring from
inner cylinder
onto loop of tube

Silastic (Falope or Yoon) Ring. This nonreactive silastic rubber band has an elastic memory of 100% if stretched to no more than 6 mm for a brief time (a few minutes at most). A special applicator, 6 mm in diameter, can be placed through a second cannula or through a standard offset operating laparoscope. The applicator is designed to grasp a knuckle of tube and release the silastic band onto a 2.5 cm loop of tube. The avascular loop of tube can be resected with biopsy forceps to provide a pathology specimen, but this is rarely performed (it does not increase efficacy). Ten to 15% of patients experience severe postoperative pelvic cramping from the tight bands (which can be alleviated by the application of a local anesthetic to the tube before or after banding).

The ring applicator consists of two concentric cylinders. Within the inner cylinder is a forceps for grasping, elevating, and retracting a segment of the tube. The silastic ring is stretched around the exposed end of the inner cylinder by means of a special ring loader and ring guide. The outer cylinder moves the ring from the inner cylinder on to the tube, a loop of which is held within the inner cylinder by the forceps.

As with application of clips, the ring should be placed at the junction of the proximal and middle third of each fallopian tube. Once the tube is grasped, it is gently withdrawn into the inner cylinder by slowly squeezing the pistol-like handle of the applicator. A final strong pull is needed to slide the ring from the inner applicator cylinder onto the loop of tube. Necrosis occurs promptly and a 2–3 cm segment of the tube is destroyed. Failure rates are about 1% after two years, and the 10-year cumulative rate is only better with unipolar coagulation and postpartum tubal excision.[59]

Mesosalpingeal bleeding is the most common complication of silastic ring application. It usually occurs when the forceps grabs not only the tube but also a vascular fold of mesosalpinx. The mesosalpinx can also be torn on the edge of the stainless steel cylinder as the tube is drawn into the applicator. If bleeding is noted, application of the silastic band often controls it. If the placement of additional bands or electrocoagulation fails to stop bleeding, laparotomy may be required.

Silastic rings are occasionally placed on structures other than the tube. If this mistake is recognized, the band can usually be removed from the round ligament or mesosalpingeal folds by grasping the band with the tongs of the applicator and applying gradual, increasing traction. If a gentle attempt fails, removal is not necessary. If rings are inadvertently discharged into the peritoneal cavity, they can safely be left behind.

Patients should be prepared for the use of electrosurgical instruments in case bands or clips cannot be applied (because of adhesions or bleeding).

Minilaparotomy

Tubal ligation, accomplished through a small suprapubic incision, "minilaparotomy," is the most frequent method of interval female sterilization around the world. In the U.S. and most of the developed world, laparoscopy is more popular, but minilaparotomy is gaining in favor because of its safety, simplicity, and adaptability to ambulatory surgical settings (particularly when local anesthesia is used).[62, 63]

The fallopian tubes can be occluded through the minilaparotomy incision with bands or clips, but a simple Pomeroy tubal ligation is the method most commonly used. Patient characteristics, such as obesity, previous pelvic infection, or previous surgery, are the principal determinants of complications.[64]

Minilaparotomy is accomplished through an incision that usually measures 3–5 cm in length. Tubal ligation through a suprapubic incision can be accomplished for obese patients, but the incision will necessarily exceed the usual length. Forceful retraction increases the pain associated with the procedure and the time of recovery. For these reasons, we believe that minilaparotomy for ambulatory tubal occlusion should be limited to patients who are not obese (usually less than 150–160 pounds, 70 kg).

Patients who are likely to have adhesions from previous surgery or pelvic infection will probably have a shorter operating and recovery time (and less pain) with open laparoscopic tubal occlusion. In addition, the wide view provided by the laparoscope will make possible a precise description of the pelvic abnormalities that may be useful should the patient develop chronic pelvic pain or recurrent infection.

Tubal occlusion is difficult to accomplish through a minilaparotomy if the uterus is immobile. Laparoscopic tubal occlusion, on the other hand, does not require extreme uterine elevation or rotation and is a better choice for a patient with a uterus fixed in position.

The Vaginal Approach

Although vaginal techniques are still used for tubal sterilization, high rates of infection and occasional pelvic abscesses following these operations have caused most clinicians to abandon them.[53] An apparent advantage in obese patients is sometimes deceptive because omental fat can block access to the fallopian tubes. Open laparoscopy is usually easier and safer in obese women.

Counseling for Sterilization

All patients undergoing a surgical procedure for permanent contraception should be aware of the nature of the operation, its alternatives, efficacy, safety, and complications. The operation can be described using drawings or pelvic models, as well as films, slides, or video tapes. The description of the operation should emphasize its similarities to and differences from laparoscopy and pelvic surgery, especially hysterectomy or ovariectomy which may be confused with simple tubal ligation. Women who undergo tubal sterilization by any method are 4–5-fold more likely to have a hysterectomy; no biologic explanation is apparent, and this may reflect patient attitudes toward surgical procedures.[65] Alternatives, including vasectomy, oral contraception, long-acting hormone methods, barrier methods, and IUDs, should be reviewed. It should be emphasized to the patient that tubal ligation is not intended to be reversible, that it cannot be guaranteed to prevent intrauterine or ectopic pregnancy, and that failures can occur long after the sterilization procedure. Informed consent is best obtained at a time when a patient is not distracted or distraught; e.g., not immediately before or after an induced abortion.

Sexuality

There is no detrimental effect on sexuality specifically due to sterilization procedures.[66] Indeed, sexual life is usually positively affected. Many couples are less inhibited and more spontaneous in lovemaking when they don't have to worry about an unwanted pregnancy.

Menstrual Function

The effects of tubal sterilization on menstrual function are less clear, and, therefore, more difficult to explain. The first well-controlled studies of this issue demonstrated no change in menstrual patterns, volume, or pain.[67, 68] Subsequently these same authors reported an increase in dysmenorrhea and changes in menstrual bleeding.[69, 70] However, these authors failed to agree in their findings (a change found by one group was not confirmed by the other). Adding to the confusion, the incidence of hysterectomy for bleeding disorders in women after tubal sterilization was reported to be increased by some,[71] but not by others.[72] In a large cohort of women in a group health plan, hospitalization for menstrual disorders was significantly increased; however, the authors believed this reflected bias by patient and physician preference for surgical treatment.[73] In the U.S. prospective long-term follow-up study of sterilization, the increased risk of hysterectomy after sterilization was concentrated in women who were treated for gynecologic disorders before tubal sterilization.[65] These discordant reports do not make patient counseling about the long-term effects of tubal sterilization an easy task.

It is possible that extensive electrocoagulation of the fallopian tubes can change ovarian steroid production. Perhaps this is why menstrual changes were detected with longer (4 years) follow-up, while no changes have been noted with the use of rings or clips.[73–75] However, attempts to relate poststerilization menstrual changes with extent of tissue destruction fail to find a correlation, and an increase in hospitalization for menstrual disorders after unipolar cautery cannot be documented.[73, 75] Still another long-term follow-up study (3–4.5 years) failed to document any significant changes in menstrual cycles.[76] This inconsistency can reflect differences in sterilization techniques, as well as the fact that a surgical solution is more likely to be chosen if continuing fertility is no longer an issue.

More studies with careful attention to the type of tubal occlusion procedure will be necessary. The best answer for now is that some women experience menstrual changes, but most do not.

Reversibility

An important objective of counseling is to help couples make the right decision about an irreversible decision to become sterile. The active participation of both partners is a critical factor.[77] Not all couples are pleased following sterilization; in one series, 2% of U.S. women expressed regret one year later and 2.7% after two years.[78] At the two-year mark, the main factors associated with regret were age less than 30 and sterilization at the convenient time of a cesarean section. In Europe where tubal sterilization is less common, the most important risk factor for regret was an unstable marriage.[79] A change in marital status is undoubtedly an important reason for a desire to reverse sterilization.[80]

Young women in unstable relationships need special attention in counseling, and both partners should participate in the counseling. Furthermore, for many couples tubal occlusion at the time of cesarean section or immediately after a difficult labor and delivery is not the best time for the procedure. It is important to know that sterilized women have not been observed to develop psychological problems at a greater than expected rate.[81, 82]

Microsurgery for tubal anastomosis is associated with excellent results if only a small segment of the tube has been damaged. Pregnancy rates correlate with the length of remaining tube, a length of 4 cm or more is optimal. Thus, the pregnancy rates are lowest with electrocoagulation, and reach 70–80% with clips, rings, and surgical methods such as the Pomeroy.[83, 84] About 2 per 1000 sterilized women will eventually undergo tubal anastomosis.[80]

Male Sterilization: Vasectomy

Vasectomy is safer, easier, less expensive, and has a lower failure rate than female sterilization.[85] The operation is almost always performed under local anesthesia, usually by a urologist in a private office.[86] Surgeons who do more than 10 operations yearly have lower complication rates.[87]

Hematomas and infection occur rarely, and are easily treated with heat, scrotal support, and antibiotics. Most men will develop sperm antibodies following vasectomy, but no long-term sequelae have been observed, including no increased risk of cardiovascular disease.[43, 88] Adverse psychological and sexual effects have not been reported. Since the other constituents of semen are made downstream from the testes, men do not notice a decreased volume or velocity of ejaculate.

Prostate cancer is the most frequent cancer among men, with a lifetime risk of 1 in 11 in the United States. An increased risk of prostate cancer after vasectomy has been reported in several cohort and case-control studies.[89–92] However, there is disagreement because other studies could not support an association between prostate or testicular cancer risk and vasectomy.[93–96] In a very large mixed racial/ethnic (black and white; Chinese-Americans and Japanese-Americans) case-control study of prostate cancer, no statistically significant increase in risk could be identified after vasectomy, including no effect of age at vasectomy or years since vasectomy.[97] Reviews of 6 cohort studies and 5 case-control studies concluded that there is no increased risk of cancer of the testis following vasectomy, and consideration of the studies examining the possible association between prostate cancer and vasectomy (6 cohort and 7 case-control studies), found the evidence to be equivocal and weak.[98, 99] A meta-analysis of the literature concluded there is no increased risk of prostate cancer in men who have undergone vasectomy.[100] Observational studies cannot totally avoid potential biases, and the disagreement in regards to prostate cancer is consistent with either no effect or an effect too small to escape confounding biases. It is worth noting that the countries with the highest vasectomy rates (China and India) do not have the highest rates of prostate cancer. Screening for prostate cancer should be no different in men who have had a vasectomy.

Vasectomy reversal is associated with pregnancy rates as high as 70–80%.[101] The prospect for pregnancy diminishes with time elapsed from vasectomy, decreasing significantly to 30% after 10 years; the best results are achieved when reversal is performed within 3 years after vasectomy.[102]

Induced Abortion

Contraception is more effective and convenient than ever, but our modern methods are far from perfect. Even the most conscientious couples can experience contraceptive failure. In the past, failure of contraception meant another, sometimes unwanted, birth or recourse to dangerous, secret abortion. The most ancient medical texts indicate that abortion has been practiced for thousands of years. Induced abortion did not become illegal until the 19th century, as a result of changes in the teachings of the Catholic Church (life begins at fertilization), and in the U.S., the efforts of the American Medical Association to have greater regulation of the practice of medicine.

In the 1950s, vacuum aspiration led to much safer abortion, and beginning in Asia, induced abortion was gradually legalized in the developed countries of the world. This trend reached the U.S. from Western Europe in the late 1960s when California, New York, and other states rewrote their abortion laws. The U.S. Supreme Court followed the lead of these states in 1973 in the "Roe versus Wade" decision that limited the circumstances under which "the right of privacy" could be restricted by local abortion laws. By 1980, legal abortion became the most common surgical procedure performed in the U.S.

The number of abortions performed in the United States has been decreasing since a peak was reached in 1990, totaling 1.33 million in 1993 and 1.21 million in 1995.[103–105] This is partly because the number of pregnancies in the U.S. has been decreasing and the proportion of reproductive age women under age 30 is also decreasing.[106] About one-third of pregnancies not ending in miscarriage or stillbirth are terminated by abortion. The proportion of abortions performed in hospitals has steadily declined, reaching 7% in 1992. The proportion handled by specialized abortion clinics has increased, while the percentage of abortions performed by physicians in their own offices has remained low, about 3–5% of all abortions. More than 50% of abortions are obtained by women younger than 25 (about 20% under the age of 20), with the rate peaking at ages 18–19, and about 80% are unmarried.[103, 105, 107]

A concern in the U.S. is the fact that the decline in the annual number of induced abortions has been greater than the decline in the annual number of births.[105] Possible explanations include a reduction in unintended pregnancies (better contraception) and a greater willingness to experience a pregnancy; however, another possibility is reduced access to abortion services.

American teenagers are especially dependent on abortion compared with their European counterparts who are better educated about sex and use contraception more often and more effectively. In 1993, 20% of women who obtained legal abortions were adolescents.[104] In addition, from ages 20–34, American women have the highest proportion of pregnancies aborted compared with other countries, indicating an unappreciated, but real problem, of unintended pregnancy occurring beyond the teenage years. The lack of perfect contraception and imperfect use of contraception will keep abortion with us.

Public health authorities have demonstrated that the legalization of abortion reduced maternal morbidity and mortality more than any single development since the advent of antibiotics to treat puerperal infections and blood banking to treat hemorrhage. The number of American women reported as dying from abortion declined from nearly 300 deaths in 1961, to only 6 in 1985 and

11 in 1991, or about *0.8 deaths for every 100,000 legal abortions.*[108] For comparison, in 1990, the maternal death rate for childbirth in the U.S. was 10 per 100,000 births, and for ectopic pregnancy, approximately 50 per 100,000 cases.[108–110]

The most important determinants of abortion mortality are duration of gestation and type of anesthesia: later abortions and general anesthesia are more hazardous.[111–113] As with mortality, morbidity rates vary primarily with duration of pregnancy, but other factors are important as well, including type of operation, age of patient, type of anesthesia, operator's skill, and method of cervical dilatation. More experienced surgeons and younger, healthier women are less likely to have complications.

Major and minor complications in a series of 170,000 first-trimester abortion patients were as follows:[114]

Major Complications (Hospitalization Required)

Retained tissue	— 27.7 per 100,000 induced abortions
Sepsis	— 21.2
Uterine perforation	— 9.4
Hemorrhage	— 7.1
Inability to complete	— 3.5
Intrauterine plus tubal pregnancy	— 2.4

Minor Complications (Managed in Clinic or Office)

Mild infection	— 462.0 per 100,000 induced abortions
Reaspiration same day	— 180.8
Reaspiration later	— 167.8
Cervical stenosis	— 16.5
Cervical tear	— 10.6
Underestimated gestation	— 6.5
Convulsive seizure	— 4.0

The possibility that abortion can result in longer-term complications has been examined in over 150 studies.[115] There is no evidence for any adverse consequences of vacuum aspiration abortion for subsequent fertility,[116, 117] pregnancies,[118, 119] or increased risk for ectopic pregnancy.[120, 121] It is not yet clear if second-trimester abortions or several first-trimester abortions can affect the outcome of later pregnancies. However, multiple induced abortions do not increase the risk of a subsequent ectopic pregnancy.[122] The long-term effects of second-trimester abortion may depend on the method used.[123] A French study disagrees with these conclusions, finding a slightly increased risk of ectopic pregnancy in women with a prior induced abortion and no previous ectopic pregnancy.[124]

The psychological sequelae of elective abortion have been studied and debated. The unequivocal evidence indicates that depression is less frequent among women postabortion compared with postpartum, that women denied abortion experience resentment for years, and that the children born after abortion is denied have social, occupational, and interpersonal difficulties lasting into early adulthood.[125]

Conflicting results have been reported in over 20 studies examining the risk of breast cancer associated with the number of abortions (especially induced abortions) experienced by individual patients.[126, 127] Concern for an adverse effect has been based on the theoretical suggestion that a full-term pregnancy protects against breast cancer by invoking complete differentiation of breast cells, but abortion increases the risk by allowing breast cell proliferation in the first-trimester of pregnancy, but not allowing the full differentiation that occurs in later pregnancy. In these studies there has been a major problem of recall bias; women who develop breast cancer are more likely to truthfully reveal their history of induced abortion than healthy women. In studies that avoided recall bias (e.g., by deriving data from national registries instead of personal interviews), the risk of breast cancer was identical in women with and without induced abortions.[128, 129]

Safe abortion is still unavailable to many women in parts of Asia, Africa, and Latin America.[130] Therefore many women resort to clandestine, unsafe abortions, accounting for about 20% of the world's maternal mortality. These deaths are preventable. Family planning services that provide effective contraceptive choices as well as access to safe abortion early in pregnancy are essential in order for societies to achieve desired fertility rates and a healthy female population.

Preoperative Care of Abortion Patients

Approximately 90% of the 1.2 million induced abortions performed in the U.S. yearly are performed during the first-trimester of pregnancy.[103, 131] During the first-trimester, abortion morbidity and mortality rates are less than one tenth those of abortions performed in the later midtrimester.[108] The vast majority of these operations occur in free-standing abortion clinics, although in recent years, physicians have performed larger numbers in their offices where women are less subject to the harassment that has plagued clinics.[103] The safety of outpatient abortion under local anesthesia is well established.

The care of the patient who has decided to terminate a pregnancy begins with the diagnosis of intrauterine pregnancy and an accurate estimate of gestational age. Failure to accomplish this is the most common source of abortion complications and subsequent litigation. Tests for pregnancy, including vaginal ultrasound, should be used when accuracy is difficult.

Nearly all women who want to terminate a pregnancy in the first-trimester are good candidates for an outpatient procedure under local anesthesia. Possible exceptions include patients with severe cardiorespiratory disease, severe anemias or coagulopathies, mental disorders severe enough to preclude cooperation, and excessive concern about operative pain that is not alleviated by reassurance.

Abortions should not be undertaken for women who have known uterine anomalies or leiomyomata or who have previously had difficult first-trimester abortion procedures, unless ultrasonography is immediately available and the surgeon is experienced in its intraoperative use. Previous cesarean section or other pelvic surgery is not a contraindication to outpatient first-trimester abortion.

Counseling Abortion Patients

Counseling has played a critical role in the development of efficient and acceptable abortion services.[132] Whether abortion is accomplished in a clinic, a physician's office, or a surgical center, the functions of a counselor must be fulfilled to ensure quality patient care. These include help with decision making, provision of information about the procedure, obtaining informed consent, provision of emotional support for the patient and her family before, during, and after the operation, and providing information about contraception.[133] Referral opportunities should be provided for prenatal care or adoption for women who choose to carry an unplanned pregnancy to term. These responsibilities can be performed by a physician, nurse, psychologist, social worker, or a trained lay person. An informed consent document should unequivocally state the possibilities of common adverse outcomes, such as incomplete abortion, infection, uterine perforation, the need for laparotomy, ectopic pregnancy, and failed abortion. The counselor should document that all preoperative responsibilities have been discharged.

Methods for First-Trimester Abortions

The most widely used technique for first-trimester abortions is vacuum curettage (99% of legal induced abortions in 1995).[105] The procedure is performed using local anesthesia (a paracervical block). Cervical dilatation is accomplished with tapered Pratt dilators. Some surgeons recommend the preoperative insertion of cervical tents. These are osmotic dilators of dried seaweed or synthetic hydrophilic substances that are left in place from a few hours (synthetic) to overnight (seaweed).[134] Mifepristone (RU486), the progesterone antagonist, produces preoperative cervical dilatation equally effectively, and the ease of its single oral dosage makes it a more attractive choice. After the procedure, the patient is observed for 1–2 hours before returning home.

Aspiration abortion is safe and effective, but it is not available everywhere, and some women find it difficult to undergo a surgical procedure or to go to a clinic where they may be subject to loss of privacy or harassment. Nonsurgical methods might make abortion available to more women and improve the circumstances under which pregnancies are terminated. Two such methods have undergone clinical testing. The progesterone antagonist mifepristone (RU486) and the antimetabolite methotrexate have both been demonstrated to induce abortion early in pregnancy when combined with a prostaglandin.

France and China were the first countries to approve the marketing of the medical abortifacient mifepristone (now available in Great Britain and Sweden as well), a synthetic relative of the progestational agents in oral contraceptives. Mifepristone acts primarily, but not totally, as an antiprogestational agent.

Both progesterone and mifepristone form hormone-responsive element-receptor complexes that are similar, but the mifepristone complex has a slightly different conformational change (in the hormone-binding domain) that prevents full gene activation. The agonistic activity of this progestin antagonist is due to its ability to activate certain, but not all, of the transcription activation functions on the progesterone receptor. The dimethyl (dimethylaminophenyl) side chain at carbon 11 is the principal factor in its antiprogesterone action. There are three major characteristics of its action that are important: a long half-life, high affinity for the progesterone receptor, and active metabolites.

A single 600 mg oral dose of mifepristone is followed a day later by the administration of a prostaglandin analogue. Several analogues have been used, but the most widely available and best tolerated is misoprostol, 800 mg administered vaginally.[135] The combination allows a reduction in dosage of both agents. When administered in the first 8 weeks of pregnancy, this medical termination carries success and complication rates similar to that achieved with vacuum curettage.[136] Misoprostol is a stable, orally active synthetic analogue of prostaglandin E_1, available commercially for the treatment of peptic ulcer. Combined with mifepristone, it provides an effective, simple, inexpensive, completely oral or vaginal method.[137, 138] In the large U.S. trial of 600 mg mifepristone followed by 400 mg misoprostol orally, there was a 1% failure rate under 7 weeks of pregnancy and 9% from 8 weeks to 9 weeks.[139] Based on worldwide experience, the regimen with the least side effects and cost, but equally good efficacy, is a combination of a lower dose of oral mifepristone (200 mg), 36–48 hrs later by the vaginal administration of 800 mg misoprostol.[140]

It is likely that abortion with mifepristone is the result of multiple actions. Although mifepristone does not induce labor, it does open and soften the cervix (this may be an action secondary to endogenous prostaglandins). Its major action is its blockade of progesterone receptors in the endometrium. This leads to a disruption of the embryo and the production of prostaglandins. The disruption of the embryo and perhaps a direct action on the trophoblast lead to a decrease in human chorionic gonadotropin (HCG) and a withdrawal of support from the corpus luteum. The success rate is dependent on the length of pregnancy — the more dependent the pregnancy is on progesterone from the corpus luteum, the more likely the progesterone antagonist, mifepristone, will result in abortion. The combined mifepristone-prostaglandin analogue method is usually restricted to pregnancies that are not beyond 9 weeks gestation. However, a regimen using a higher dose of misoprostol (administered vaginally) achieved a 95% complete abortion rate in women at 9–13 weeks' gestation.[141] Other progesterone antagonists have been developed, but only mifepristone has undergone extensive abortion trials. It seems unlikely that mifepristone could have serious adverse effects, and there have been none reported.

Mifepristone is most noted for its abortifacient activity and the political controversy surrounding it. However, the combination of its agonistic and antagonistic actions can be exploited for many uses, including contraception, therapy of endometriosis, induction of labor, treatment of Cushing's syndrome, and, potentially, treatment of various cancers.

Lack of progesterone antagonists in the U.S. prompted use of methotrexate as an abortifacient in the same dose used to treat ectopic pregnancy, 50 mg intramuscularly per square meter of body surface area.[142] Later, a single 75 mg intramuscular dose was demonstrated to be as effective.[143] Methotrexate has also been administered orally, in does of 25 or 50 mg.[144] As with mifepristone, a prostaglandin is added to promote expulsion of the uterine contents, and again vaginal misoprostol is the most useful analogue. The first trials demonstrated that if the prostaglandin (800 mg misoprostol vaginally) was given a week after the injectin of methotrexate, this method could be almost as effective as mifepristone.[145] Like mifepristone, efficacy diminishes with advancing gestation beyond 7 weeks (since the last menstrual period).[146–148] Because methotrexate takes longer to act than mifepristone, the prostaglandin is used a week after the initial treatment, and is repeated a day later if expulsion has not occurred. Methotrexate is easily available and inexpensive. It has been used in low doses to treat psoriasis and rheumatoid arthritis, as well as ectopic pregnancy, without adverse effects. It is, however, a known teratogen that can be deadly in high doses, and its use as an abortifacient results in prolonged bleeding and a prolonged time to abortion (up to a month in some cases). Mifepristone is preferred by clinicians who have experience with both methods. There are no direct comparison studies of methotrexate and mifepristone.

Another new approach uses the combination of tamoxifen and misoprostol. The administration of tamoxifen (20 mg daily for 4 days) followed by misoprostol (800 mg vaginally, with a second dose if necessary 24 hours later) was associated with a 92% rate of complete abortion in 100 women with pregnancies less than 9 weeks gestational age.[149]

The use of prostaglandin alone has also been pursued.[150] Relatively high success rates have been reported with multiple dosing,[151] but the most effective regimen and the best method of administration remain to be determined. The administration of 800 mg misoprostol daily for 3 days has been reported to be very effective late in the first-trimester (10–12 weeks).[152]

One word of caution regarding misoprostol, the synthetic prostaglandin E_1 analogue; it is now recognized that infants born to pregnant women exposed to misoprostol have an increased risk of abnormal vascular developmet resulting in Möbius's syndrome (congenital facial paralysis with or without limb defects) and defects such as equinovarus and arthogryposis.[153, 154] Although the risk is low, this possibility must be considered in decision making when the various methods for first-trimester abortion are considered.

Careful prospective follow-up assessments can detect no health differences in women who have medical abortions compared with women who have abortions by vacuum aspiration.[155]

Complications of Abortions

Postoperative complications of elective abortions are classified as either immediate or delayd. Uterine perforation and uterine atony are examples of immediate complications. Delayed complications can occur several hours to several weeks after the operation. These usually present according to the major complaint: bleeding, pain, and continuing symptoms of pregnancy.

Bleeding

By far the most common cause of unusually heavy postabortal bleeding is retained products of conception. Rates in large series vary from 0.2 to 0.6%.[114] Patients with retained products of conception occasionally present several weeks after an abortion, but most report excessive bleeding within one week. Severe pain or pelvic tenderness suggests that infection is also present. Treatment is prompt aspiration of the uterus with the largest cannula that will pass the cervix.

Infection

Infection is sometimes marked by uterine bleeding; although without retained products of conception, the volume of blood loss is usually modest. Fever and uterine tenderness are the most common signs of postabortal endometritis, occurring in about 0.5% of cases.[114] Some studies indicate that prophylactic antibiotics reduce the risk of postabortal infection.[156, 158] Most clinicians agree that women at risk of pelvic infection benefit from the use of prophylactic antibiotics prior to induced abortion; others state that women who have not had a previous delivery should receive prophylaxis, while still others believe that all abortion patients would benefit from prophylactic antibiotics.[158, 159] A meta-analysis of antibiotics at the time of induced abortion unequivocally concluded that prophylactic antibiotics should be routinely used without exceptions.[160] Because both gonorrhea and chlamydia, as well as other organisms, can cause postabortion infections, a tetracycline seems the best drug for prophylaxis. Doxycycline, 100 mg an hour before the abortion and 200 mg 30 minutes afterward, is the most convenient and comprehensive regimen.[161] Tetracycline, 500 mg once before and once after the operation, is also acceptable. Metronidazole, 400 mg an hour before and 4–8 hours afterward, has been tested and is effective treatment for patients with bacterial vaginosis detected at the time of abortion.[162, 163]

Patients who present with uterine tenderness, fever, and bleeding require uterine aspiration as well as antibiotic treatment. Patients who have fevers above 38°C (101°F) and signs of peritoneal inflammation, as well as uterine tenderness, require hospitalization and intravenous antibiotics active against anaerobes, gonorrhea, and chlamydia. Outpatient treatment with doxycycline, 100 mg bid for 14 days, should be reserved for patients whose signs and symptoms are confined to the uterus.

Dysfunctional Uterine Bleeding Following Abortion

Women may present with uterine bleeding but without signs or symptoms of retained products of conception or infection. When these two diagnoses have been ruled out by absence of fever, a closed cervix, and a nontender uterus, the bleeding itself can be treated hormonally. Curettage is rarely necessary unless bleeding is excessive.

Ectopic Pregnancy

Failure to diagnose ectopic pregnancy at the time of induced abortion can cause a patient to return with complaints of persistent bleeding with or without pelvic pain. Careful examination of the uterine aspirate for villi at the time of abortion should make a missed ectopic pregnancy an unusual cause of delayed bleeding. If, however, a patient presents with this possibility, quantitative measurement of chorionic gonadotropin and vaginal ultrasonography should be used for accurate diagnosis and management.

Cervical Stenosis

Patients who experience amenorrhea or hypomenorrhea and cyclic uterine pain after first-trimester abortion may have stenosis of the internal os. This condition occurs in about 0.02% of cases and is more common among women whose abortions are performed in the early first-trimester with a minimum of cervical dilatation and a small diameter, flexible plastic cannula. Possibly, the tip of this type of cannula abrades the internal os, and the minimal dilatation allows the abraded areas to heal in contact. The condition is easily treated with cervical dilatation with Pratt dilators under paracervical block.

Other Late Complications

Amenorrhea, usually without pain, can also be caused by Asherman's syndrome, destruction and scarification of the endometrium. This condition is very rare and usually follows endometrial infection. This problem is best diagnosed and treated at hysteroscopy.

Sensitization of Rh-negative women should be prevented. Approximately 4% of these women become sensitized following an induced abortion (the later the abortion the higher the proportion). Subsequent hemolytic disease of the newborn can be prevented by administering 50 mg Rh immunoglobulin to all Rh-negative, Du-negative women undergoing early abortion. The standard dose is administered for second-trimester abortion.

Abortion in the Second-Trimester

Second-trimester abortions can be accomplished surgically or medically. The surgical procedure is termed dilatation and evacuation (D & E). Several approaches have been used for the medical termination of pregnancy. These include the vaginal, intramuscular, or intra-amniotic administration of prostaglandins and the intra-amniotic injection of hypertonic saline or urea. The D & E procedure is safer and less expensive than the medical methods and is better tolerated (and thus preferred) by patients.[164–166]

In 1994, only 4% of induced abortions occurred at 16–20 weeks of gestation and 1% at 21 weeks or later.[131] In 1994, 94% of second-trimester abortions were performed by D & E.

The training, experience, and skills of the surgeon are the primary factors that limit the gestational age at which abortion can be safely performed. Advanced gestational age by itself incurs increased risks for all types of complications. These are multiplied when the duration of pregnancy is discovered, after beginning uterine evacuation, to be beyond the experience and skill of the surgeon or capacity of the equipment. Uterine perforation, infection, bleeding, amniotic fluid embolism, and anesthetic reactions are increased as gestational age increases.[164]

When errors in estimating gestational age require the surgeon to use unfamiliar instruments or techniques that are not frequently practiced, the increased duration of the procedure can cause problems. Efforts to sedate or relieve pain by administering additional drugs increase the risk of toxic reactions or overdosage. If a change from local to general anesthesia is undertaken, the patient is at much greater risk of anesthetic complications. Finally, if complications caused by advanced gestational age necessitate transfer of the patient to physicians who are not familiar with uterine evacuation techniques, the patient may undergo unnecessarily extensive surgery, such as hysterectomy, with all the risks inherent in emergency procedures.

Preoperative cervical dilatation with osmotic dilators makes first-trimester abortion safer and easier and is essential for second-trimester abortion. Local anesthesia instead of general anesthesia also makes abortion safer.[167, 168] Some patients are not good candidates for surgical procedures of any kind under local anesthesia, and others may have special reasons to prefer that an abortion be performed under general anesthesia. Patient requests should be seriously considered, but the clinician also has a responsibility to inform the patient of the risks and benefits of local versus general anesthesia.

In the United Kingdom, prostaglandin analogues are favored for a noninvasive method of second-trimester abortion. A combination of the progesterone antagonist, mifepristone, (a single oral 200 mg dose of mifepristone administered 36 hours before prostaglandin treatment) and an E prostaglandin analogue (misoprostol) administered orally or vaginally is highly effective, and the combination allows a lesser dose of both agents, which results in fewer side effects.[169] In addition, this combination does not require the use of cervical laminaria for dilatation.

References

1. **Djerassi C,** *The Politics of Contraception, Vol. I. The Present,* Stanford Alumni Association, Stanford, California, 1979.

2. **Westoff CF,** Unintended pregnancy in America and abroad, *Fam Plann Perspect* 20:254, 1988.

3. **Spitz AM, Velebil P, Koonin LM, Strauss LT, Goodman KA, Wingo P, Wilson JB, Morris L, Marks JS,** Pregnancy, abortion, and birth rates among US adolescents—1980, 1985, and 1990, *JAMA* 275:989, 1996.

4. **Henshaw SK,** Unintended pregnancy in the United States, *Fam Plann Perspect* 30:24, 1998.

5. **Trussell J, Hatcher RA, Cates Jr W, Stewart FH, Kost K,** A guide to interpreting contraceptive efficacy studies, *Obstet Gynecol* 76:558, 1990.

6. **Trussell J, Hatcher RA, Cates Jr W, Stewart FH, Kost K,** Contraceptive failure in the United States: an update, *Stud Fam Plann* 21:51, 1990.

7. **Trussell J,** Contraceptive efficacy, In: Hatcher RA, Trussell J, Stewart F, et al, eds. *Contraceptive Technology,* 17th ed, Irvington Publishers, New York, NY, 1998.

8. **Mosher WD, Pratt WF,** (National Center for Health Statistics), Contraceptive use in the United States, 1973–88, Advance data from vital and health statistics, Report No. 182, 1990.

9. **Mosher WD,** (National Center for Health Statistics), Use of family planning services in the United States: 1982 and 1988, Advance data from vital and health statistics, Report No. 184, 1990.

10. **Abma JC, Chandra A, Mosher WD, Peterson L, Piccinino L,** (Centers for Disease Control and Prevention, National Center For Heath Statistics), Fertility, family planning, and women's health: new data from the 1995 National Survey of Family Growth, Report No. 19, Series 23, 1997.

11. **Piccinino LJ, Mosher WD,** Trends in contraceptive use in the United States: 1982–1995, *Fam Plann Perspect* 30:4, 1998.

12. **Polaneczky M, Slap G, Forke C, Rappaport A, Sondheimer S,** The use of levonorgestrel implants (Norplant) for contraception in adolescent mothers, *New Engl J Med* 331:1201, 1994.

13. **Polaneczky M, Guarnaccia M, Alon J, Wiley J,** Early experience with the contraceptive use of depo-medroxyprogesterone acetate in an inner-city population, *Fam Plann Perspect* 28:174, 1996.

14. **Boroditsky R, Fisher W, Sand M,** The 1995 Canadian Contraceptive Study, *J Soc Obstet Gynaecol Can* 18:1, 1996.

15. **Toulemon L, Leridon H,** Contraceptives practices and trends in France, *Fam Plann Perspect* 30:114, 1998.

16. **United Nations,** Long-range world population projections: two centuries of population growth, 1950-2150, 1992.

17. **Diczfalusy E,** Menopause, developing countries and the 21st century, *Acta Obstet Gynecol Scand* (Suppl)134:45, 1986.

18. **Diczfalusy E,** The worldwide use of steroidal contraception, *Int J Fertil* 34(Suppl):56, 1989.

19. **DaVanzo J, Parnell AM, Foege WH,** Health consequences of contraceptive use and reproductive patterns: summary of a report from the US National Research Council, *JAMA* 265:2692, 1991.

20. **Garcia-Moreno C, Türmen T,** International perspectives on women's reproductive health, *Science* 269:790, 1995.

21. **Potts M, Rosenfield A,** The fifth freedom revisited: I. Background and existing programs, *Lancet* 336:1227, 1990.

22. **Forrest JD, Singh S,** Public-sector savings resulting from expenditures for contraceptive services, *Fam Plann Perspect* 22:6, 1990.

23. **Meier KJ, McFarlane DR,** State family planning and abortion expenditures: their effect on public health, *Am J Public Health* 84:1468, 1994.

24. **Forrest JD, Singh S,** The impact of public-sector expenditures for contraceptive services in California, *Fam Plann Perspect* 22:161, 1990.

25. **World Health Organization,** *Women's Health,* Geneva, 1994.

26. **Ventura SJ,** (Monthly Vital Statistics Report, Vol. 43), Advance report of final natality statistics, 1992, Report No. 5, Supplement, 1994.

27. **Spencer G,** (Current Population Reports 1989), Projections of the population of the United States by age, sex and race: 1988-2080, Current Population Reports 1989, Report No. 1018, Series P-25, 1989.

28. **Westoff CF,** Fertility in the United States, *Science* 234:554, 1986.

29. **Mastroianni Jr L, Donaldson PJ, Kane TT,** eds, *Developing New Contraceptives: Obstacles and Opportunities,* National Academy Press, Washington, DC, 1990.

30. **Harrison PF, Rosenfield A,** eds, *Contraceptive Research and Development: Looking to the Future,* National Academy Press, Washington, D.C., 1996.

31. **Peipert JF, Gutmann J,** Oral contraceptive risk assessment: a survey of 247 educated women, *Obstet Gynecol* 82:112, 1993.

32. **Murphy P, Kirkman A, Hale RW,** A national survey of women's attitudes toward oral contraception and other forms of birth control, *Women's Health Issues* 5:94, 1995.

33. **Parker-Mauldin W, Segal S,** Prevalence of contraceptive use: trends and issues, *Stud Fam Plann* 6:335, 1988.

34. **Murphy M,** Sterilisation as a method of contraception: recent trends in Great Britain and their implications, *J Biosoc Sci* 27:31, 1995.

35. **Riphagen FE, Fortney JA, Koelb S,** Contraception in women over forty, *J Biosoc Sci* 20:127, 1988.

36. **Speert H,** *Obstetric & Gynecologic Milestones Illustrated,* The Parthenon Publishing Group, New York, 1996.

37. **Lungren SS,** A case of cesarean section twice successfully performed on the same patient, with remarks on the time, indications, and details of the operation, *Am J Obstet* 14:78, 1881.

38. **Baird D,** The Fifth Freedom, *Br Med J* i:234, 1966.

39. **Centers for Disease Control and Prevention,** Surgical sterilization surveillance: tubal sterilization 1976–1978, Report No. 1981.

40. **Layde PM, Ory HW, Peterson HB, Scally MJ, Greenspan JR, Smith JC, Fleming D,** The declining lengths of hospitalization for tubal sterilizations, *JAMA* 245:714, 1981.

41. **Escobedo LG, Peterson HB, Grubb GS, Franks AL,** Case fatality rates for tubal sterilization in U.S. hospitals, *Am J Obstet Gynecol* 160:147, 1989.

42. **Peterson HB, Huber DH, Belker AM,** Vasectomy: an appraisal for the obstetrician-gynecologist, *Obstet Gynecol* 76:568, 1990.

43. **Giovannucci E, Tosteson TD, Speizer FE, Vessey MP, Colditz GA,** A long-term study of mortality in men who have undergone vasectomy, *New Engl J Med* 326:1392, 1992.

44. **Chi I-c, Laufe L, Gardner SD, Tolbert M,** An epidemiologic study of risk factors associated with pregnancy following female sterilizations, *Am J Obstet Gynecol* 136:768, 1980.

45. **Cheng M, Wong YM, Rochat R, Ratnam SS,** Sterilization failures in Singapore: An examination of ligation techniques and failure rates, *Stud Fam Plann* 8:109, 1977.

46. **Lichterg E, Laff S, Friedman E,** Value of routine dilatation and curretage at the time of interval sterilization, *Obstet Gynecol* 67:763, 1986.

47. **WHO Special Programme of Research, Develpment and Research Training in Human Reproduction, Task Force on Intrauterine Devices for Fertility Regulation,** A multinational case-control study of ectopic pregnancy, *Clin Reprod Fertil* 3:131, 1985.

48. **Holt V, Chu J, Daling JR, Stergachis AS, Weiss NS,** Tubal sterilization and subsequent ectopic pregnancy, *JAMA* 266:242, 1991.

49. **Chick PH, Frances M, Paterson PJ,** A comprehensive review of female sterilisation tubal occlusion methods, *Clin Reprod Fertil* 3:81, 1985.

50. **McCausland A,** High rate of ectopic pregnancy following laparoscopic tubal coagulation failure, *Am J Obstet Gynecol* 136:977, 1980.

51. **Chi I-c, Laufe LE, Atwed R,** Ectopic pregnancy following female sterilization procedures, *Adv Plann Parenthood* 16:52, 1981.

52. **Peterson HB, Xia Z, Hughes JM, Wilcox LS, Tylor LR, Trussell J, for the U.S. Collaborative Review of Sterilization Working Group,** The risk of ectopic pregnancy after tubal sterilization, *New Engl J Med* 336:762, 1997.

53. **Miesfeld R, Gaarontans R, Moyers T,** Vaginal tubal sterilization. Is infection a significant risk? *Am J Obstet Gynecol* 137:183, 1980.

54. **Hankinson SE, Hunter DJ, Colditz GA, Willett WC, Stampfer MJ, Rosner B, Hennekens CH, Speizer FE,** Tubal sterilization, hysterectomy, and risk of ovarian cancer. A prospective study, *JAMA* 270:2813, 1993.

55. **Miracle-McMahill HL, Calle EE, Kosinski AS, Rodriguez C, Wingo PA, Thun MJ, Heath Jr CW,** Tubal ligation and fatal ovarian cancer in a large prospective cohort study, *Am J Epidemiol* 145:349, 1997.

56. **Mori M, Harabuchi I, Miyake H, Casagrande JT, Henderson BE, Ross RK,** Reproductive, genetic, and dietary risk factors for ovarian cancer, *Am J Epidemiol* 128:771, 1988.

57. **Irwin KL, Weiss NS, Lee NC, Peterson HB,** Tubal sterilization, hysterectomy, and the subsequent occurrence of epithelial ovarian cancer, *Am J Epidemiol* 134:362, 1991.

58. **Whittemore AS, Harris R, Itnyre J, and the Collaborative Ovarian Cancer Group,** Characteristics relating to ovarian cancer risk: collaborative analysis of 12 US case-control studies. II: Invasive epithelial ovarian cancers in white women, *Am J Epidemiol* 136:1184, 1992.

59. **Peterson HB, Xia Z, Hughes JM, Wilcox LS, Tylor LR, Trussell J, for the U.S. Collaborative Review of Sterilization Working Group,** The risk of pregnancy after tubal sterilization: findings from the U.S. Collaborative Review of Sterilization, *Am J Obstet Gynecol* 174:1161, 1996.

60. **Centers for Disease Control and Prevention,** Deaths following female sterilization with unipolar electrocoagulating devices, *MMWR* 30:150, 1981.

61. **Soderstrom RM, Levy BS, Engel T,** Reducing bipolar sterilization failures, *Obstet Gynecol* 74:60, 1989.

62. **McCann M, Cole L,** Laparoscopy and minilaparotomy: two major advances in female sterilization, *Stud Fam Plann* 11:119, 1980.

63. **Ruminjo JK, Lynam PF,** A fifteen-year review of female sterilization by minilaparotomy under local anesthesia in Kenya, *Contraception* 55:249, 1997.

64. **Layde PM, Peterson HB, Dicker RC, DeStefano F, Ruben GL, Ory HW,** Risk factors for complications of interval tubal sterilization by laparotomy, *Obstet Gynecol* 62:180, 1983.

65. **Hillis SD, Marchbanks PA, Tylor LR, Peterson HB, for the U.S. Collaborative Review of Sterilization Working Group,** Higher hysterectomy risk for sterilized than nonsterilized women: findings from the U.S. Collaborative Review of Sterilization, *Obstet Gynecol* 91:241, 1998.

66. **Kjer J,** Sexual adjustment to tubal sterilization, *Eur J Obstet Gynecol* 35:211, 1990.

67. **Rulin MC, Turner JH, Dunworth R, Thompson D,** Post tubal sterilization syndrome: a misnomer, *Obstet Gynecol* 151:13, 1985.

68. **DeStefano F, Huezo CM, Peterson HB, Rubin GL, Layde PM, Ory HW,** Menstrual changes after tubal sterilization, *Obstet Gynecol* 62:673, 1983.

69. **Rulin MC, Davidson AR, Philliber SG, Graves WL, Cushman LF,** Changes in menstrual symptoms among sterilized and comparison women: a prospective study, *Obstet Gynecol* 79:749, 1989.

70. **DeStefano F, Perlman J, Peterson HB, Diamond E,** Long-term risk of menstrual disturbances after tubal sterilization, *Am J Obstet Gynecol* 152:835, 1985.

71. **Kjer J, Knudsen L,** Hysterectomy subsequent to laparoscopic sterilization, *Eur J Obstet Gynecol* 35:63, 1990.

72. **Stergachis A, Shy KK, Gouthaus LC, Wagner EH, Hecht JA, G A, Normand EH, Raboud J,** Tubal sterilization and the long-term risk of hysterectomy, *JAMA* 264:2893, 1990.

73. **Shy KK, Stergachis A, Grothaus LG, Wagner EH, Hecht J, Anderson G,** Tubal sterilization and risk of subsequent hospital admission for menstrual disorders, *Am J Obstet Gynecol* 166:1698, 1992.

74. **Thranov I, Hertz JB, Kjer JJ, Andresen A, Micic S, Nielsen J, Hancke S,** Hormonal and menstrual changes after laparoscopic sterilization by Falope-rings or Filshie-clips, *Fertil Steril* 57:751, 1992.

75. **Wilcox LS, Martinez-Schnell B, Peterson HB, Ware JH, Hughes JM,** Menstrual function after tubal sterilization, *Am J Epidemiol* 135:1368, 1992.

76. **Rulin MC, Davidson AR, Philliber SG, Graves WL, Cushman LF,** Long-term effect of tubal sterilization on menstrual indices and pelvic pain, *Obstet Gynecol* 82:118, 1993.

77. **Miller WB, Shain RN, Pasta DJ,** Tubal sterilization or vasectomy: how do married couples make the decision? *Fertil Steril* 56:278, 1991.

78. **Grubb G, Refoser H, Layde PM, Rubin GL,** Regret after decision to have a tubal sterilization, *Fertil Steril* 44:248, 1985.

79. **Vemer HM, Colla P, Schoot DC, Willensen WN, Bierkens PB, Rolland R,** Women regretting their sterilization, *Fertil Steril* 46:724, 1986.

80. **Wilcox LS, Chu SY, Peterson HB,** Characteristics of women who considered or obtained tubal reanastomosis: results from a prospective study of tubal sterilization, *Obstet Gynecol* 75:661, 1990.

81. **Vessey M, Huggins G, Lawless M, McPherson K, Yeates D,** Tubal sterilization: findings in a large prospective study, *Br J Obstet Gynaecol* 90:203, 1983.

82. **WHO,** Mental health and female sterilization: report of a WHO collaborative study, *J Biosoc Sci* 16:1, 1984.

83. **Siegler AM, Hulka J, Peretz A,** Reversibility of female sterilization, *Fertil Steril* 43:499, 1985.

84. **Dubuisson JB, Chapron C, Nos Z, Morice P, Aubriot FX, Garnier P,** Sterilisation reversal: fertility results, *Hum Reprod* 10:1145, 1995.

85. **Smith GL, Taylor GP, Smith KF,** Comparative risks and costs of male and female sterilization, *Am J Public Health* 75:370, 1985.

86. **Marquette CM, Koonin LM, Antarsh L, Gargiullo PM, Smith JC,** Vasectomy in the United States, 1991, *Am J Public Health* 85:644, 1995.

87. **Kendrick JS, Gonzales B, Huber DH, Grubb GS, Rubin G,** Complications of vasectomies in the United States, *J Fam Pract* 25:245, 1987.

88. **Schuman LM, Coulson AH, Mandel JS, Massey Jr FJ, O'Fallon WM,** Health status of American men — a study of post-vasectomy sequelae, *J Clin Endocrinol* 46:697, 1993.

89. **Giovanucci E, Ascherio A, Rimm EB, Colditz GA, Stampfer MJ, Willett WC,** A prospective cohort study of vasectomy and prostate cancer in US men, *JAMA* 269:873, 1993.

90. **Giovanucci E, Tosteson TD, Speizer FE, Ascherio A, Vessey MP, Colditz GA,** A retrospective cohort study of vasectomy and prostate cancer in US men, *JAMA* 269:878, 1993.

91. **Hayes RB, Pottern LM, Greenberg R, Schoenberg J, Swanson GM, Liff J, Schwartz AG, Brown LM, Hoover RN,** Vasectomy and prostate cancer in US blacks and whites, *Am J Epidemiol* 137:263, 1993.

92. **Hsing AW, Wang RT, Gu FL, Lee M, Wang T, Leng TJ, Spitz M, Blot WJ,** Vasectomy and prostate cancer risk in China, *Cancer Epidemiol Biomark Prev* 3:285, 1994.

93. **Sidney S, Quesenberry Jr CP, Sadler MC, Guess HA, Lydick EG, Cattolica EV,** Vasectomy and the risk of prostate cancer in a cohort of multiphasic health-checkup examinees: second report, *Cancer Causes Control* 2:113, 1991.

94. **Moller H, Knudsen LB, Lynge E,** Risk of testicular cancer after vasectomy: cohort study of over 73,000 men, *Br Med J* 309:295, 1994.

95. **Rosenberg L, Palmer JR, Zauber AG, Warshauer E, Strom BL, Harlap S, Shapiro S,** The relation of vasectomy to risk of cancer, *Am J Epidemiol* 140:431, 1994.

96. **Zhu K, Stanford JL, Daling JR, McKnight B, Stergachis A, Brawer MK, Weiss NS,** Vasectomy and prostate cancer: a case-control study in a health maintenance organization, *Am J Epidemiol* 144:717, 1996.

97. **John EM, Whittemore AS, Wu AH, Kolonel LN, Hislop TG, Howe GR, West DW, Hankin J, Dreon DM, The C-Z, Burch JD, Paffenbarger Jr RS,** Vasectomy and prostate cancer: results from a multiethnic case-control study, *J Natl Cancer Inst* 87:662, 1995.

98. **Lynge E, Knudsen LB, Müller H,** Vasectomy and testis and prostate cancer, *Fertil Control Rev* 3:8, 1994.

99. **Healey B,** Does vasectomy cause prostate cancer? *JAMA* 269:2620, 1993.

100. **Bernal-Delgado E, Latour-Pérez J, Pradas-Arnal F, Gómez-López LI,** The association between vasectomy and prostate cancer: a systematic review of the literature, *Fertil Steril* 70:191, 1998.

101. **Hendry WF,** Vasectomy and vasectomy reversal, *Br J Urol* 73:337, 1994.

102. **Belker AM, Thomas AJ, Fuchs EF, Konnak JM, Sharlip ID,** Results of 1,469 microsurgical vasectomy reversals by the vasovasostomy group, *J Urol* 145:505, 1991.

103. **Henshaw SK, Van Vort J,** Abortion services in the United States, 1991 and 1992, *Fam Plann Perspect* 26:100, 1994.

104. **Centers for Disease Control,** Abortion surveillance: preliminary data—United States, 1993, *MMWR* 45:235, 1996.

105. **Centers for Disease Control,** Abortion surveillance: preliminary analysis—United States, 1995, *MMWR* 46:1133, 1998.

106. **Deardorff KE, Montgomery P, Hollmann FW,** (U.S. Department of Commerce, Economics and Statistics Administration, Bureau of the Census), U.S. population estimates by age, sex, race, and Hispanic origin: 1990 to 1995, Report No. PPL-41, 1996.

107. **Henshaw SK,** Induced abortions: a world review, 1990, *Fam Plann Perspect* 22:76, 1990.

108. **Lawson H, Frye A, Atrash H, Smith J, Schulman H, Ramick M,** Abortion mortality, United States, 1972 through 1987, *Am J Obstet Gynecol* 171:1365, 1994.

109. **Lawson H, Atrash H, Saftlas A,** Ectopic pregnancy surveillance, United States, 1970-1986, *MMWR* 38:11, 1989.

110. **Berg CJ, Atrash HK, Koonin LM, Tucker M,** Pregnancy-related mortality in the United States, 1987-1990, *Obstet Gynecol* 88:161, 1996.

111. **Grimes DA, Schulz KF, Cates Jr W, Tyler Jr CW,** Local versus general anesthesia: which is safer for performing suction curettage abortions, *Am J Obstet Gynecol* 135:1030, 1979.

112. **Peterson HB, Grimes DA, Cates Jr W, Rubin GL,** Comparative risk of death from induced abortion at 12 weeks' gestation performed with local versus general anesthesia, *Am J Obstet Gynecol* 141:763, 1981.

113. **Buehler J, Schulz K, Grimes D, Mogue C,** The risk of serious complications from induced abortion: do personal characteristics make a difference? *Am J Obstet Gynecol* 153:14, 1985.

114. **Hakim-Elahi E, Tovell H, Burnhill M,** Complications of first trimester abortions: a report of 170,000 cases, *Obstet Gynecol* 76:129, 1990.

115. **Hogue C,** Impact of abortion on subsequent fertility, *Clin Obstet Gynecol* 13:96, 1986.

116. **Stubblefield P, Monson R, Schoenbaum S, Wolfson CE, Cookson DJ, Ryan KJ,** Fertility after induced abortion: a prospective follow-up study, *Obstet Gynecol* 62:186, 1984.

117. **Daling J, Weiss N, Voigt I, Spadoni LR, Soderstrom R, Moore DE, Stadel BV,** Tubal infertility in relation to prior induced abortion, *Fertil Steril* 43:389, 1985.

118. **Schoenbaum S, Monson R, Stubblefield P, Darney PD, Ryan KJ,** Outcome of the delivery following an induced or spontaneous abortion, *Am J Obstet Gynecol* 136:19, 1980.

119. **Frank PI, McNamee R, Hannaford PC, Kay CR, Hirsch S,** The effect of induced abortion on subsequent pregnancy outcome, *Br J Obstet Gynaecol* 98:1015, 1991.

120. **Daling J, Chow W, Weiss N, Metch BT, Soderstrom R,** Ectopic pregnancy in relation to previous induced abortion, *JAMA* 253:1005, 1985.

121. **Atrash HK, Strauss LT, Kendrick JS, Skjeldestad FE, Ahn YW,** The relation between induced abortion and ectopic pregnancy, *Obstet Gynecol* 89:512, 1997.

122. **Skjeldestad FE, Gargiullo PM, Kendrick JS,** Multiple induced abortions as risk factor for ectopic pregnancy. A prospective study, *Acta Obstet Gynecol Scand* 76:691, 1997.

123. **MacKenzie I, Fox A,** A prospective self-controlled study of fertility after second trimester prostaglandin-induced abortion, *Am J Obstet Gynecol* 158:1137, 1988.

124. **Tharaux-Deneux C, Bouyer J, Job-Spira N, Coste J, Spira A,** Risk of ectopic pregnancy and previous induced abortion, *Am J Public Health* 88:401, 1998.

125. **Dagg PKB,** The psychological sequelae of therapeutic abortion — denied and completed, *Am J Psychiatr* 148:578, 1991.

126. **Andrieu N, Clavel F, Gairard B, Piana L, Bremond A, Lansac JH, Flamant R, Renaud R,** Familial risk of breast cancer and abortion, *Cancer Detect Prev* 18:51, 1994.

127. **Daling JR, Malone KE, Voigt LF, White E, Weiss NS,** Risk of breast cancer among young women: relationship to induced abortion, *J Natl Cancer Inst* 86:1584, 1994.

128. **Rookus MA, van Leeuwen FE,** Induced abortion and risk for breast cancer: reporting (recall) bias in a Dutch case-control study, *J Natl Cancer Inst* 88:1759, 1996.

129. **Melbye M, Wohlfahrt J, Olsen JH, Frisch M, Westergaard T, Helweg-Larsen K, Andersen PK,** Induced abortion and the risk of breast cancer, *New Engl J Med* 336:81, 1997.

130. **Kulczycki A, Potts M, Rosenfield A,** Abortion and fertility regulation, *Lancet* 347:1663, 1996.

131. **Koonin L, Smith J, Ramick M,** Abortion surveillance—United States, 1993 and 1994, *MMWR* 46(SS-4):23, 1997.

132. **Landy U, Lewit S,** Administrative, counseling, and medical practices in National Abortion Federation facilities, *Fam Plann Perspect* 14:257, 1982.

133. **Landy U,** Abortion counseling — a new component of medical care, *Clinics Obstet Gynecol* 13:33, 1986.

134. **Darney PD, Atkinson E, Hirabayashi K,** Uterine perforation during second trimester abortion by cervical dilation and instrumental extraction: a review of 15 cases, *Obstet Gynecol* 75:441, 1990.

135. **El-Rafaey HJ, Rajasekar D, Abdalla M, Calder L, Templeton A,** Induction of abortion with mifepristone (RU 486) and oral or vaginal misoprostol, *New Engl J Med* 332:983, 1995.

136. **Silvestre L, Dubois C, Renault M, Rezvani Y, Baulieu EE, Ulmann A,** Voluntary interruption of pregnancy with Mifepristone (RU 486) and a prostaglandin analogue, *New Engl J Med* 322:645, 1990.

137. **Thong KJ, Baird DT,** Induction of abortion with mifepristone and misoprostol in early pregnancy, *Br J Obstet Gynaecol* 99:1004, 1992.

138. **Peyron R, Aubeny E, Targosz V, Silvestre L, Renault M, Elkik F, Leclerc P, Ulmann A, Baulieu EE,** Early termination of pregnancy with mifepristone (RU 486) and the orally active prostaglandin misoprostol, *New Engl J Med* 328:1509, 1993.

139. **Spitz IM, Bardin CW, Benton L, Robbins A,** Early pregnancy termination with mifepristone and misoprostol in the United States, *New Engl J Med* 338:1241, 1998.

140. **Ashok PW, Penney GC, Flett GMM, Templeton A,** An effective regimen for early medical abortion: a report of 2000 consecutive cases, *Hum Reprod* 13:2962, 1998.

141. **Ashok PW, Flett GM, Templeton A,** Termination of pregnancy at 9–13 weeks' amenorrhoea with mifepristone and misoprostol, *Lancet* 352:542, 1998.

142. **Creinin MD, Vittinghoff E, Keder L, Darney PD, Tiller G,** Methotrexate and misoprostol for early abortion: a multicenter trial. I. Safety and efficacy, *Contraception* 53:321, 1996.

143. **Creinin MD,** Medical aboriton with methotrexate 75 mg intramuscularly and vaginal misoprostol, *Contraception* 56:367, 1997.

144. **Creinin MD,** Oral methotrexate and vaginal misoprostol for early abortion, *Contraception* 54:15, 1996.

145. **Creinin M, Darney P,** Methotrexate and misoprostol for early abortion, *Contraception* 48:339, 1993.

146. **Creinin MD, Vittinghoff E,** Methotrexate and misoprostol vs misoprostol alone for early abortion. A randomized controlled trial, *JAMA* 272:1190, 1994.

147. **Creinin MD, Park M,** Acceptablility of medical abortion with methotrexate and misoprostol, *Contraception* 52:41, 1995.

148. **Hauskenecht RU,** Methotrexate and misoprostol to terminate early pregnancy, *New Engl J Med* 333:538, 1995.

149. **Mishell Jr DR, Jain JK, Byrne JD, Lacarra MDC,** A medical method of early pregnancy termination using tamoxifen and misoprostol, *Contraception* 58:1, 1998.

150. **Koopersmith TB, Mishell Jr DR,** The use of misoprostol for termination of early pregnancy, *Contraception* 53:237, 1996.

151. **Carbonell JLL, Varela L, Velazco A, Fernádez C,** The use of misoprostol for termination of early pregnancy, *Contraception* 55:165, 1997.

152. **Carbonell Esteve JL, Varela L, Velazco A, Cabezas E, Tanda R, Sánchez C,** Vaginal misoprostol for late first trimester abortion, *Contraception* 57:329, 1998.

153. **Pastuszak AL, Schüler L, Speck-Martins CE, Coelho K-EFA, Cordello SM, Vargas F, Brunoni D, Schwarz IVD, Larrandaburu M, Safattle H, Meloni VFA, Koren G,** Use of misoprostol during pregnancy and Möbius' syndrome in infants, *New Engl J Med* 338:1881, 1998.

154. **Gonzalez CH, Marques-Dias MJ, Kim CA, Sugayama SMM, Da Paz JA, Huson SM, Holmes LB,** Congenital abnormalities in Brazilian children associated with misoprostol use in first trimester of pregnancy, *Lancet* 351:1624, 1998.

155. **Howie FL, Henshaw RC, Naji SA, Russell IT, Templeton AA,** Medical abortion or vacuum aspiration? Two year follow-up of a patient preference trial, *Br J Obstet Gynaecol* 104:829, 1997.

156. **Brewer C,** Prevention of infection after abortion with a supervised single dose of doxycycline, *Br Med J* 281:780, 1980.

157. **Hodgson JE, Major B, Portmann K, Quattlebaum FW,** Prophylactic use of tetracycline for first trimester abortions, *Obstet Gynecol* 45:574, 1975.

158. **Park T-X, Flock M, Schulz KF, Grimes DA,** Preventing febrile complications of suction curettage abortion, *Am J Obstet Gynecol* 152:252, 1985.

159. **Darj E, Stralin E, Nilsson S,** The prophylactic effect of doxycycline on postoperative infection rate after first trimester abortion, *Obstet Gynecol* 70:755, 1987.

160. **Sawaya GF, Grady D, Kerlikowske K, Grimes DA,** Antibiotics at the time of induced abortion: the case for universal prophylaxis based on a meta-analysis, *Obstet Gynecol* 87:884, 1996.

161. **Levallois P, Rioux J,** Prophylactic antibiotics for suction curettage abortion: results of a clinical controlled trial, *Am J Obstet Gynecol* 158:100, 1988.

162. **Heisterberg L, Petersen K,** Metronidazole prophylaxis in elective first trimester abortion, *Obstet Gynecol* 65:371, 1985.

163. **Larsson PG, Platz-Christensen JJ, Thejls H, Forsum U, Pahlson C,** Incidence of pelvic inflammatory disease after first trimester legal abortion in women with bacterial vaginosis after treatment with metronidazole: a double-blind, randomized study, *Am J Obstet Gynecol* 166:100, 1992.

164. **Peterson WF, Berry FN, Grace MR, Gulbranson CL,** Second trimester abortion by dilatation and evacuation: an analysis of 11,747 cases, *Obstet Gynecol* 62:185, 1983.

165. **Kafrissen M, Schulz K, Grimes D, Cates Jr W,** Midtrimester abortion: intra amniotic instillation of hyperosmolar urea and prostaglandin $F_{2\alpha}$ v dilatation and evacuation, *JAMA* 251:916, 1984.

166. **Ferris LE, McMain-Klein M, Colodny N, Fellows GF, Lamont J,** Factors associated with immediate abortion complications, *Can Med Assoc J* 154:1677, 1996.

167. **Mackay T, Schulz K, Grimes D,** Safety of local versus general anesthesia for second trimester dilatation and evacuation abortion, *Obstet Gynecol* 66:661, 1985.

168. **Atrash H, Chelk T, Hogue C,** Legal abortion and general anesthesia, *Am J Obstet Gynecol* 158:420, 1988.

169. **Webster D, Penney GC, Templeton A,** A comparison of 600 and 200 mg mifepristone prior to second trimester abortion with the prostaglandin misoprostol, *Br J Obstet Gynaecol* 103:706, 1996.

170. **Trussell J, Leveque JA, Koenig JD, London R, Borden S, Henneberry J, LaGuardia KD, Stewart F, Wilson TG, Wysocki S, Strauss M,** The economic value of contraception: a comparison of 15 methods, *Am J Public Health* 85:494, 1995.

Oral Contraception

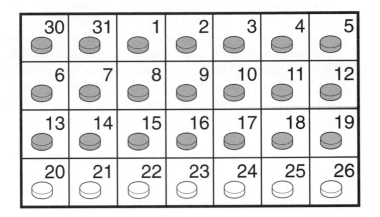

C ontraception is commonly viewed as a modern event, a recent development in human history. On the contrary, efforts to limit reproduction predate our ability to write about it. It is only oral contraception with synthetic sex steroids that is recent.

History[1–3]

It wasn't until the early 1900s, that inhibition of ovulation was observed to be linked to pregnancy and the corpus luteum. Ludwig Haberlandt, professor of physiology at the University of Innsbruck, Austria, was the first to demonstrate that ovarian extracts given orally could prevent fertility (in mice). In the 1920s, Haberlandt and a Viennese gynecologist, Otfried Otto Fellner, were administering steroid extracts to a variety of animals and reporting the inhibition of fertility. By 1931, Haberlandt was proposing the administration of hormones for birth control. An extract was produced, named Infecundin, ready to be used, but Haberlandt's early death in 1932, at age 47, brought an end to this effort. Fellner disappeared after the annexation of Austria to Hitler's Germany.

The concept was annunciated by Haberlandt, but steroid chemistry wasn't ready. The extraction and isolation of a few milligrams of the sex steroids required starting points measured in gallons of urine or thousands of pounds of organs. Edward Doisy processed 80,000 sow ovaries to produce 12 mg of estradiol.

Russell Marker

The supply problem was solved by an eccentric chemist, Russell E. Marker, who completed his thesis, but not his course work, for his Ph.D. Marker, born in 1902 near Hagerstown, Maryland, received his Bachelor's degree in organic chemistry and his Master's degree in colloidal chemistry from the University of Maryland. After leaving the University of Maryland, Marker worked with the Ethyl Gasoline Corporation, and in 1926, developed the process of octane rating, based on the discovery that knocking in gasoline was due to hydrocarbons with an uneven number of carbons.

From 1927 to 1935, Marker worked at the Rockefeller Institute, publishing a total of 32 papers on configuration and optical rotation as a method of identifying compounds. He became interested in solving the problem of producing abundant and cheap amounts of progesterone, but he was told to continue with his work in optical technology. In 1935, he moved to Pennsylvania State University at a reduced salary, but with the freedom to pursue any field of research. At that time, it required the ovaries from 2500 pregnant pigs to produce 1 mg of progesterone. In 1939, Marker devised the method (called the Marker degradation) to convert a sapogenin molecule into a progestin. Marker became convinced that the solution to the problem of obtaining large quantities of steroid hormones was to find plants (in the family that includes the lily, the agave, and the yam) that contained sufficient amounts of diosgenin, a plant steroid (a sapogenin) that could be used as a starting point for steroid hormone production. This conviction was strengthened with his discovery that a species of *Trillium,* known locally as Beth's root, was collected in North Carolina and used in the preparation of Lydia Pinkham's Compound, popular at the time to relieve menstrual troubles. The active ingredient in Beth's root was diosgenin, but the rhizome was too small to provide sufficient amounts for commercial production. Marker's search for an appropriate plant took him to California, Arizona, and Texas.

On a visit to Texas A & M University, Marker found a picture of a large dioscorea (*Dioscorea mexicana)* in a book that he just happened to pick up and browse through while spending the night at the home of a retired botanist. After returning to Pennsylvania, he decided to go to Veracruz, Mexico (it took 3 days by train), to search for this dioscorea. He made several attempts in 1941 and early 1942, but was frustrated first by the lack of a plant-collecting permit from the Mexician government and then by his failure to find the plant. He remembered that the book with the picture reported that this dioscorea was known locally as "cabeza de negro," black tubers that grew near Orizaba and Cordoba. Marker took a bus to Cordoba, and near Orizaba, an Indian who owned a small store brought him two plants. Each tuber was 9–12 inches high and consisted of white material like a turnip, used by local Mexicans as a poison to catch fish.

Marker managed to get one bag of tubers back to Pennsylvania State University and isolated diosgenin. Unable to obtain support from the pharmaceutical industry, Marker used his life savings, and in 1942, he returned to Veracruz, collected the roots of the Mexican yam, and prepared a syrup from the roots. Back in Pennsylvania with his 5-gallon cans of syrup, Marker worked out the degradation of diosgenin to progesterone. One 5-gallon can yielded 3 kg of progesterone. United States pharmaceutical companies still refused to back Marker, and even the University refused, despite Marker's urging, to patent the process.

In 1943, Marker resigned from Pennsylvania State University and went to Mexico where he collected the roots of *Dioscorea mexicana,* 10 tons worth! Looking through the yellow pages in a Mexico City telephone directory, Marker found a company called Laboratorios Hormona, owned by a lawyer, Emeric Somlo, and a physician, Frederick Lehman. Marker arranged a meeting, and the three agreed to form a Mexican company to produce hormones. In an old pottery shed in Mexico City (the laboratories of Laboratorios Hormona), in two months, he prepared several pounds of progesterone (worth $300,000) with the help of four young women who had little education and spoke no English (Marker did not speak Spanish). The two partners and Marker formed a company in 1944 that they called Syntex (from *synthesis* and *Mexico*). In 1944, Marker produced over 30 kg of progesterone. The price of progesterone fell from $200 to $50 a gram.

During this time, Marker received expenses, but he was not given his share of the profits or the 40% share of stock due to him. Failing to reach a settlement, Marker left Syntex after only one year and started a new company in Texcoco, called Botanica-Mex. He changed to *Dioscorea barbasco,* which gave a greater yield of diosgenin, and the price of progesterone dropped to $10 a gram, and later to $5. This company was allegedly harassed (legally and physically) by Syntex, and in 1946, sold, eventually reaching ownership by Organon of Holland, which still uses it.

In 1949, Marker retired to Pennsylvania to devote the rest of his life to making replicas of antique works in silver, a successful business that allowed him, in the 1980s, to endow scientific lectureships at both Pennsylvania State University and the University of Maryland. However, he took his know-how with him. Fortunately for Syntex, he had published a scientific description of his process, and there still was no patent on his discoveries. Syntex recruited George Rosenkranz, a Hungarian immigrant living in Cuba, to reinstitute the commercial manufacture of progesterone (and testosterone) from Mexican yams, a task that took him (with the help of the women left behind by Marker) 2 years.

In 1970, the Mexican government recognized Marker and awarded him the Order of the Aztec Eagle; he declined. In 1984, Pennsylvania State University established the annual Marker Lectures in Science, and in 1987, the Russell and Mildred Marker Professorship of Natural Product Chemistry. In 1987, Marker was granted an honorary Doctorate in Science from the University of Maryland, the degree he failed to receive in 1926. At the age of 92, Russell Earl Marker died in Wernersville, Pennsylvania, in 1995, from complications after a broken hip.

Carl Djerassi[4]

The Djerassi family lived in Bulgaria for hundreds of years after escaping Spain during the Inquisition. Carl Djerassi, the son of a Bulgarian physician, was born in Vienna (as was his physician mother). Djerassi, at the age of 16, and his mother emigrated to the United States in 1939. A Jewish refugee aid organization placed Djerassi with a family in Newark, New Jersey. With a scholarship to Tarkio College in Tarkio, Missouri, he was exposed to middle America, where he earned his way giving talks to church groups about Bulgaria and Europe. His education was further supported by another scholarship from Kenyon College in Ohio, where he pursued chemistry. After a year working for CIBA, Djerassi received his graduate degree from the University of Wisconsin. Returning to CIBA and being somewhat unhappy, he responded to an invitation to visit Syntex. Rosenkranz proposed that Djerassi head a research group to concentrate on the synthesis of cortisone.

In 1949, it was discovered that cortisone relieved arthritis, and the race was on to develop an easy and cheap method to synthesize cortisone. Carl Djerassi, at age 26, joined Syntex to work on this synthesis using the Mexican yam plant steroid diosgenin as the starting point. This was quickly achieved (in 1951), but soon after, an even better method of cortisone production using micro-biologic fermentation was discovered at Upjohn. This latter method used progesterone as the starting point, and, therefore, Syntex found itself as the key supplier to other companies for this important process, at the rate of 10 tons of progesterone per year and a price of 48 cents per gram.

Djerassi and other Syntex chemists then turned their attention to the sex steroids. They discovered that the removal of the 19-carbon from yam-derived progesterone increased the progestational activity of the molecule. Ethisterone had been available for a dozen years, and the Syntex chemists reasoned that removal of the 19-carbon would increase the progestational potency of this orally active compound. In 1951, norethindrone was synthesized; the patent for this drug is the first patent for a drug listed in the National Inventor's Hall of Fame in Akron, Ohio. A closely related compound, norethynodrel, was actually the first orally active progestational agent to receive a patent, assigned to Frank Colton, a chemist at G.D. Searle & Company.

Gregory Pincus

Gregory Goodwin (Goody) Pincus was born in 1903 in New Jersey, the son of Russian Jewish immigrants who lived on a farm colony founded by a German-Jewish philanthropic organization. Pincus was the oldest of 6 children and grew up in a home of intellectual curiosity and energy, but even his family regarded him as a genius.

Pincus graduated from Cornell and went to Harvard to study genetics, joining Hudson Hoagland and B.F. Skinner as graduate students of W.J. Crozier in physiology, receiving degrees in 1927. Crozier's hero was Jacques Loeb who discovered artificial parthenogenesis working with sea urchin eggs. Most importantly, Loeb was a strong believer in applying science to improve human life. Thus, Crozier, influenced by Loeb, taught Pincus, Hoagland, and Skinner (respectively, in reproductive biology, neurophysiology, and psychology) to apply science to human problems. This was to be the cornerstone of Pincus's own philosophy.

Hoagland, after a short stay at Harvard, spent a year in Cambridge, England, and then moved to Clark University in Worcester, Massachusetts, to be the chair of biology at the age of 31. Pincus went to England and Germany, and returned to Harvard as an assistant professor of physiology.

Pincus performed pioneering studies of meiotic maturation in mammalian oocytes, in both rabbit and human oocytes. In 1934, Pincus reported the achievement of in vitro fertilization of rabbit eggs, earning him a headline in the New York Times that alluded to Haldane and Huxley. An article in Colliers depicted him as an evil scientist. By 1936, Harvard had cited Pincus's work as one of the university's outstanding scientific achievements of all time, but Harvard denied him tenure in 1937.

At Clark University, Hudson Hoagland was in constant conflict with the president of the university, Wallace W. Atwood, the senior author of a widely used textbook on geography. In 1931, the Department of Biology consisted of one faculty member and his graduate student, and their chair, Hudson Hoagland. Hoagland, upset and angry over Harvard's refusal to grant tenure to his friend (suspecting that this was because of anti-Semitism), invited Pincus to join him.

Hoagland secured funds for Pincus from philanthropists in New York City, enough for a laboratory and an assistant. This success impressed the two men, especially Hoagland, planting the idea that it would be possible to support research with private money.

Min-Chueh Chang received his Ph.D. degree from Harvard on an infamous day, December 7, 1941, and thus he was forced to remain in this country. He was drawn to Pincus because of Pincus's book, *The Eggs of Mammals,* published in 1936, a book that had a major impact on biologists at that time. The successful recruitment of M-C Chang by Hoagland and Pincus was to pay great dividends.

Soon Hoagland had put together a group of outstanding scientists, but because of his on-going antagonism with President Atwood, the group was denied faculty status. Working in a converted barn, they were totally supported by private funds. By 1943, 12 of Clark's 60 faculty were in the Department of Biology.

Frustrated by the politics of academia, Hoagland and Pincus (who both enjoyed stepping outside of convention) had a vision of a private research center devoted to their philosophy of applied science. Indeed, the establishment of the Worcester Foundation for Experimental Biology, in 1944, can be attributed directly to Hoagland and Pincus, their friendship for each other, their confidence, enthusiasm, ambition, and drive. It was their spirit that turned many members of Worcester society into financial supporters of biologic science. Hoagland and Pincus accomplished what they set out to do. They created and sustained a vibrant, productive scientific institution in which it was a pleasure to work.

Although named the Worcester Foundation for Experimental Biology, the Foundation was located in the summer of 1945 across Lake Quinsigamond in a house on an estate in Shrewsbury. The Board of Trustees was chaired by Harlow Shapley, a distinguished astronomer, vice-chaired by Rabbi Levi Olan, and included 3 Nobel laureates and a group of Worcester businessmen.

From 1945 to the death of Pincus in 1967, the staff grew from 12 to 350 (scientists and support people), 36 of whom were independently funded and 45 were postdoctoral fellows. The annual budget grew from $100,000 to $4.5 million. One hundred acres of adjoining land were acquired, and the campus grew to 11 buildings. In its first 25 years, approximately 3000 scientific papers were published.

But in those early years, Pincus was the animal keeper, Mrs. Hoagland the bookkeeper, M-C Chang was the night watchman, and Hoagland mowed the lawn. During the years of World War II, Pincus and Hoagland combined their interests in hormones and neurophysiology to focus on stress and fatigue in industry and the military.

The initial discoveries that led to an oral contraceptive can be attributed to M-C Chang (also the first to describe the capacitation process of sperm). In 1951, he confirmed the work of Makepeace (in 1937) demonstrating that progesterone could inhibit ovulation in rabbits. When norethindrone and norethynodrel became available, Chang found them to be virtually 100% effective in inhibiting ovulation when administered orally to rabbits.

Katherine Dexter McCormick was a very rich woman; in 1904, she married Stanley McCormick, the son of Cyrus McCormick, the founder of International Harvester. She was also intelligent, the second woman to graduate from the Massachusetts Institute of Technology, socially conscious, and a generous contributor to family planning efforts. McCormick's husband suffered from schizophrenia, and she established the Neuroendocrine Research Foundation at Harvard to study schizophrenia. This brought her together with Hoagland who told her of the work being done by Chang and Pincus.

Pincus attributed his interest in contraception to his growing appreciation for the world's population problem, and to a 1951 visit with Margaret Sanger, at that time president of the Planned Parenthood Federation of America. At that visit, Sanger expressed hope that a method of contraception could be derived from the laboratory work being done by Pincus and Chang.

In 1952, Margaret Sanger brought Pincus and Katherine McCormick together. During this meeting, Pincus formulated his thoughts derived from his mammalian research. He envisioned a progestational agent in pill form as a contraceptive, acting like progesterone in pregnancy. Sanger and McCormick provided a research grant for further animal research. By the time of her death, McCormick had contributed more than $2 million to the Worcester Foundation, and left another $1 million in her will. In his book, *The Control of Fertility*, published in 1965, Pincus wrote: "This book is dedicated to Mrs. Stanley McCormick because of her steadfast faith in scientific inquiry and her unswerving encouragement of human dignity."[5]

It was Pincus who made the decision to involve a physician because he knew human experiments would be necessary. John Rock, chief of gynecology and obstetrics at Harvard, met Pincus at a scientific conference and discovered their mutual interest in reproductive physiology. Rock and his colleagues pursued Pincus's work. Using oocytes from oophorectomies, they reported in vitro fertilization in 1944, probably the first demonstration of fertilization of human oocytes in vitro. Rock was interested in the work with progestational agents, not for contraception however, but because he hoped the female sex steroids could be used to overcome infertility.

Sanger and McCormick needed some convincing that Rock's Catholicism would not be a handicap, but they were eventually won over because of his stature. Rock was a physician who literally transformed his personal values in response to his recognition of the problems secondary to uncontrolled reproduction. With the help of Luigi Mastroianni, the first administration of synthetic progestins to women was to Rock's patients in 1954. Of the first 50 patients to receive 10–40 mg of synthetic progestin (a dose extrapolated from the animal data) for 20 days each month, all failed to ovulate during treatment (causing Pincus to begin referring to the medication as "the pill"), and 7 of the 50 became pregnant after discontinuing the medication (pleasing Rock who all along was motivated to treat infertility).

Pincus and Chang decided to announce their findings at the International Planned Parenthood meeting in Tokyo, in the fall of 1955. Rock refused to join in this effort, believing that Pincus and Chang were moving too fast. Despite this disagreement (which apparently was spirited and strong), it was done, and the Tokyo presentation generated worldwide publicity.

In 1956, with Celso-Ramon Garcia and Edris Rice-Wray, working in Puerto Rico, the first human trial was performed. The initial progestin products were contaminated with about 1% mestranol. In the amounts being used, this added up to 50–500 µg of mestranol, a sufficient amount of estrogen to inhibit ovulation by itself. When efforts to provide a more pure progestin lowered the estrogen content and yielded breakthrough bleeding, it was decided to retain the estrogen for cycle control, thus establishing the principle of the combined estrogen-progestin oral contraceptive. Early clinical trials were conducted by J.W. Goldzieher in San Antonio and E.T. Tyler in Los Angeles.

Pincus, a longtime consultant to Searle, picked the Searle compound for extended use, and with great effort, convinced Searle that the commercial potential of an oral contraceptive warranted the risk of possible negative public reaction. Pincus also convinced Rock, and together they pushed the U.S. Food and Drug Administration for acceptance of oral contraception. In 1957, Enovid was approved for the treatment of miscarriages and menstrual disorders, and in 1960, for contraception. Neither Pincus nor the Worcester Foundation got rich on the pill; alas, there was no royalty agreement.

The Pill did bring Pincus fame and travel. There is no doubt that he was very much aware of the accomplishment and its implications. As he traveled and lectured in 1957, he said: "How a few precious facts obscurely come to in the laboratory may resonate into the lives of men everywhere, bring order to disorder, hope to the hopeless, life to the dying. That this is the magic and mystery of our time is sometimes grasped and often missed, but to expound it is inevitable."[5]

Pincus was the perfect person to bring oral contraception into the public world, at a time when contraception was a private, suppressed subject. Difficult projects require people like Pincus. A scientific entrepreneur, he could plow through distractions. He could be hard and aggressive with his staff. He could remain focused. He hated to lose, even in meaningless games with his children. Yet he combined a gracious, charming manner with his competitive hardness. He was filled with the kind of self-confidence that permits an individual to forge ahead, to translate vision into reality. Pincus died in 1967 (as did Katherine McCormick at the age of 92), of aplastic anemia that some have argued was caused by his long-term exposure to solvents and chemicals. Rock died in 1984, at the age of 94, and Chang, in 1991, was buried at the age of 82, in Shrewsbury, near his laboratory and close to the grave of Pincus.

Pincus wrote his book, *The Control of Fertility*, in 1964–65, only because "a break came in the apparent dam to publication on reproductive physiology and particularly its subdivisions concerned with reproductive behavior, conception, and contraception."[5]

> "We have conferred and lectured in many countries of the world, seen at first hand the research needs and possibilities in almost every European, Asiatic, Central, and South American country. We have faced the hard fact of overpopulation in country after country, learned of the bleak demographic future, assessed the prospects for the practice of efficient fertility control. This has been a saddening and a heartening experience; saddening because of the sight of continuing poverty and misery, heartening because of the dedicated colleagues and workers seeking to overcome the handicap of excess fertility and to promote healthy reproductive function. Among these we have made many friends, found devoted students."[5]

Syntex, a wholesale drug supplier, was without marketing experience or organization. By the time Syntex had secured arrangements with Ortho for a sales outlet, Searle marketed Enovid in 1960 (150 µg mestranol and 9.85 mg norethynodrel). Ortho-Novum, using norethindrone from Syntex, appeared in 1962. Wyeth Laboratories introduced norgestrel in 1968, the same year in which the first reliable prospective studies were initiated. It was not until the late 1970s that a dose-response relationship between problems and the amount of steroids in the pill was appreciated. As a result, health care providers and patients, over the years, have been confronted by a bewildering array of different products and formulations. The solution to this clinical dilemma is relatively straightforward: the theme of this chapter, use the lowest doses that provide effective contraception.

Pharmacology of Steroid Contraception

The Estrogen Component of Combination Oral Contraceptives

Estradiol is the most potent natural estrogen and is the major estrogen secreted by the ovaries. The major obstacle to the use of sex steroids for contraception was inactivity of the compounds when given orally. A major breakthrough occurred in 1938 when it was discovered that the addition of an ethinyl group at the 17 position made estradiol orally active. Ethinyl estradiol is a very potent oral estrogen and is one of the two forms of estrogen in every oral contraceptive. The other estrogen is the 3-methyl ether of ethinyl estradiol, mestranol.

Ethinyl estradiol   Mestranol

Mestranol and ethinyl estradiol are different from natural estradiol and must be regarded as pharmacologic drugs. Animal studies have suggested that mestranol is weaker than ethinyl estradiol, because mestranol must first be converted to ethinyl estradiol in the body. Indeed, mestranol will not bind to the cellular estrogen receptor. Therefore, unconjugated ethinyl estradiol is the active estrogen in the blood for both mestranol and ethinyl estradiol. In the human body, differences in potency between ethinyl estradiol and mestranol do not appear to be significant, certainly not as great as indicated by assays in rodents. This is now a minor point because all of the low-dose oral contraceptives contain ethinyl estradiol.

The metabolism of ethinyl estradiol (particularly as reflected in blood levels) varies significantly from individual to individual, and from one population to another.[6] There is even a range of variability at different sampling times within the same individual. Therefore, it is not surprising that the same dose can cause side effects in one individual and none in another.

The estrogen content (dosage) of the pill is of major clinical importance. Thrombosis is one of the most serious side effects of the pill, playing a key role in the increased risk of death (in the past with high doses) from a variety of circulatory problems. This side effect is related to estrogen, and it is dose related. Therefore, the dose of estrogen is a critical issue in selecting an oral contraceptive.

The Progestin Component of Combination Oral Contraceptives

The discovery of ethinyl substitution and oral potency led (at the end of the 1930s) to the preparation of ethisterone, an orally active derivative of testosterone. In 1951, it was demonstrated that removal of the 19-carbon from ethisterone to form norethindrone did not destroy the oral activity, and most importantly, it changed the major hormonal effect from that of an androgen to that of a progestational agent. Accordingly, the progestational derivatives of testosterone were designated as 19-nortestosterones (denoting the missing 19-carbon). The androgenic properties of these compounds, however, were not totally eliminated, and minimal anabolic and androgenic potential remains within the structure.

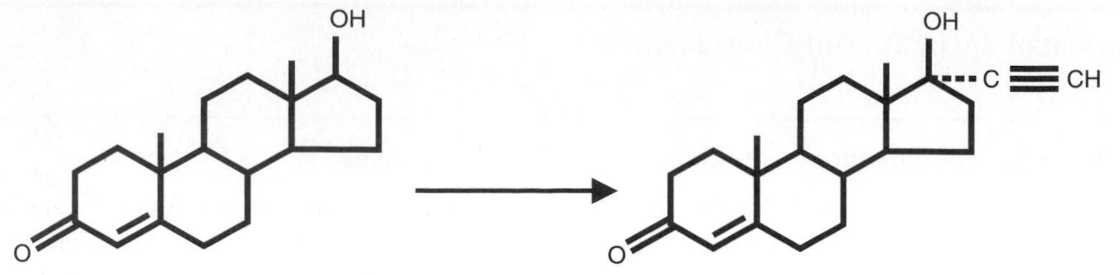

Testosterone → Ethisterone

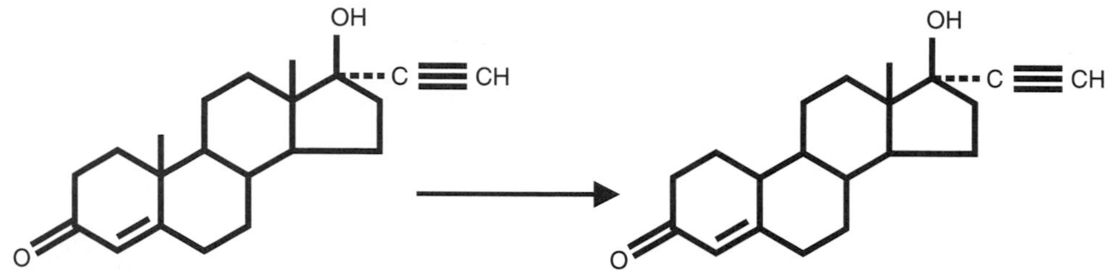

Ethisterone → Norethindrone

The "impurity" of 19-nortestosterone, i.e., androgenic as well as progestational effects, was further complicated in the past by a belief that they were metabolized within the body to estrogenic compounds. This question was restudied, and it was argued that the previous evidence for metabolism to estrogenic compounds was due to an artifact in the laboratory analysis. More recent studies indicate that norethindrone can be converted to ethinyl estradiol; however, the rate of this conversion is so low that insignificant amounts of ethinyl estradiol can be found in the circulation or urine following the administration of the commonly used doses of norethindrone.[7] Any estrogenic activity, therefore, would have to be due to a direct effect. In animal and human studies, however, only norethindrone, norethynodrel, and ethynodiol diacetate have estrogen activity, and it is very slight due to weak binding to the estrogen receptor.[8] Clinically, androgenic and estrogenic activities of the progestin component are, therefore, insignificant due to the low dosage in the current oral contraceptives. As with the estrogen component, serious side effects have been related to the high doses of progestins used in old formulations, not the particular progestin, and routine use of oral contraceptives should now be limited to the low-dose products.

The norethindrone family contains the following 19-nortestosterone progestins: norethindrone, norethynodrel, norethindrone acetate, ethynodiol diacetate, lynestrenol, norgestrel, norgestimate, desogestrel, and gestodene.

Most of the progestins closely related to norethindrone are converted to the parent compound. Thus the activity of norethynodrel, norethindrone acetate, ethynodiol diacetate, and lynestrenol is due to rapid conversion to norethindrone.

Norgestrel is a racemic equal mixture of the dextrorotatory enantiomer and the levorotatory enantiomer. These enantiomers are mirror images of each other and rotate the plane of polarized light in opposite directions. The dextrorotatory form is known as d-norgestrel, and the levorotatory form is l-norgestrel (known as levonorgestrel). Levonorgestrel is the active isomer of norgestrel.

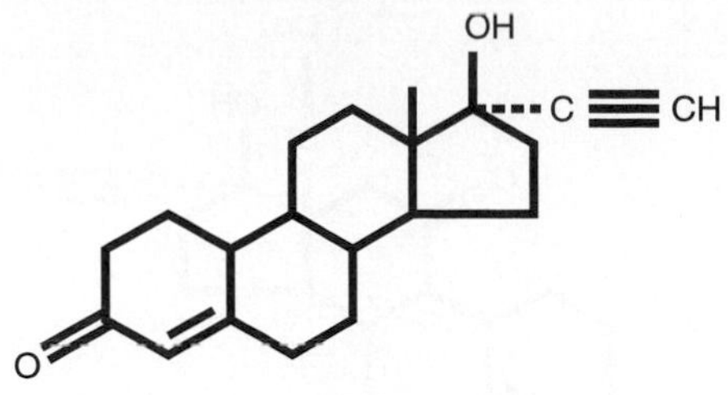

Norethindrone

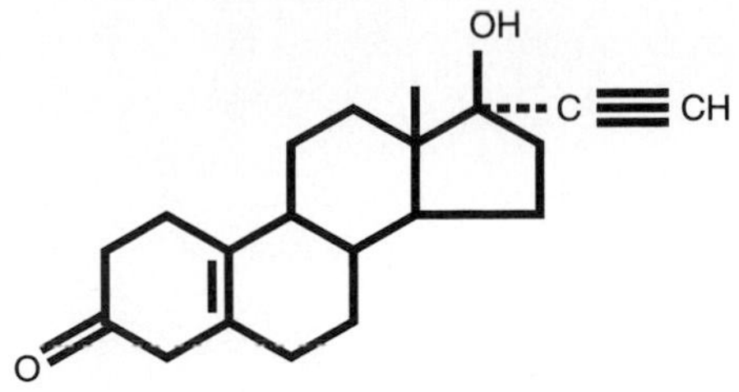

Norethynodrel

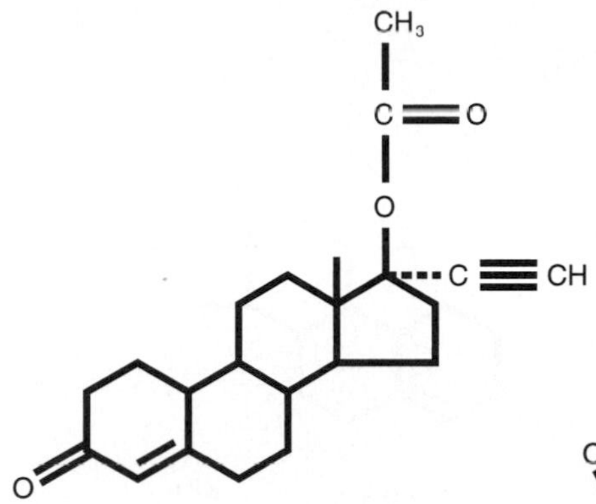

Norethindrone acetate

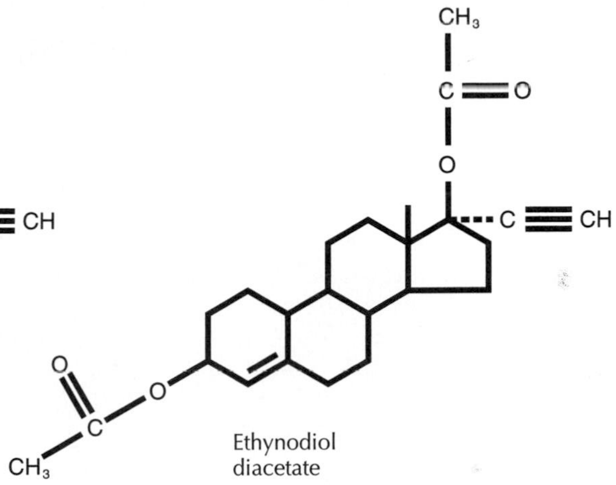

Ethynodiol diacetate

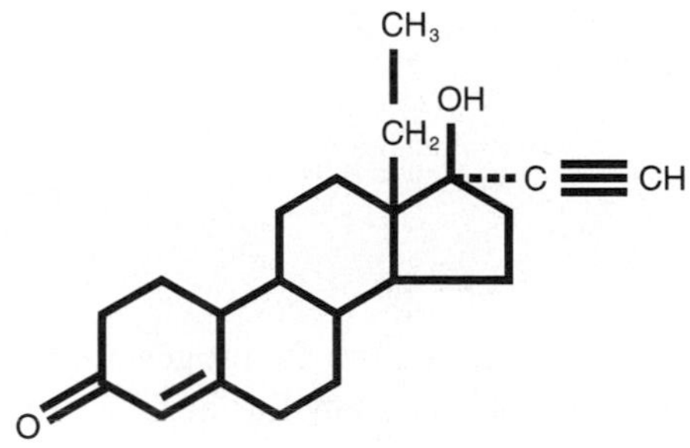

Levonorgestrel

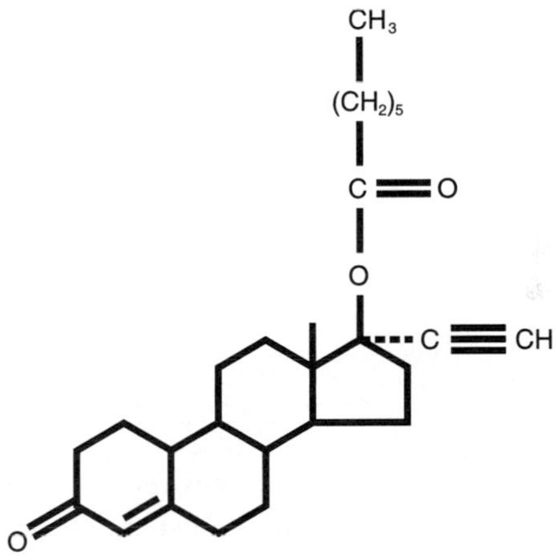

Norethindrone enanthate

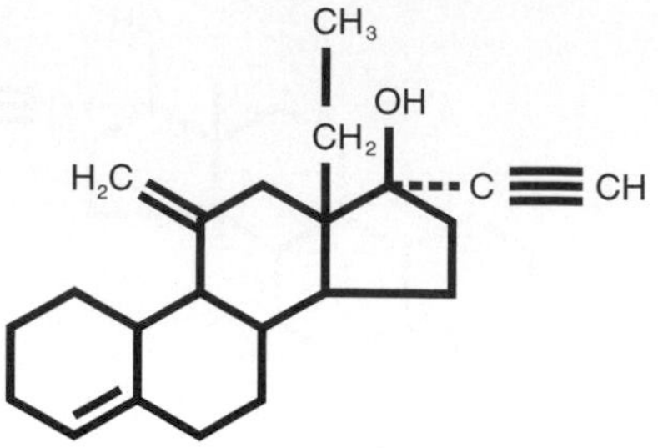

Desogestrel

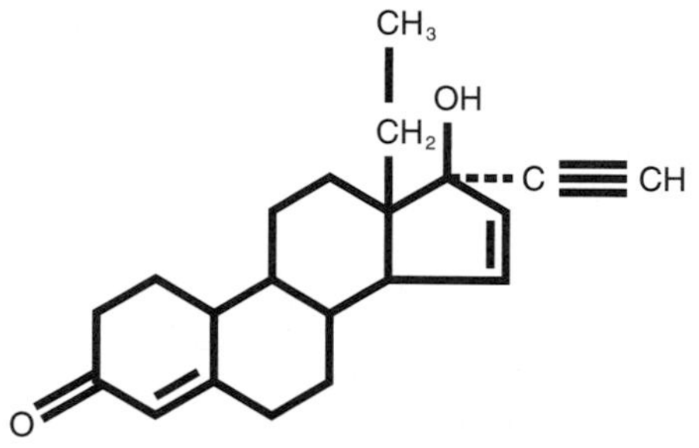

Gestodene

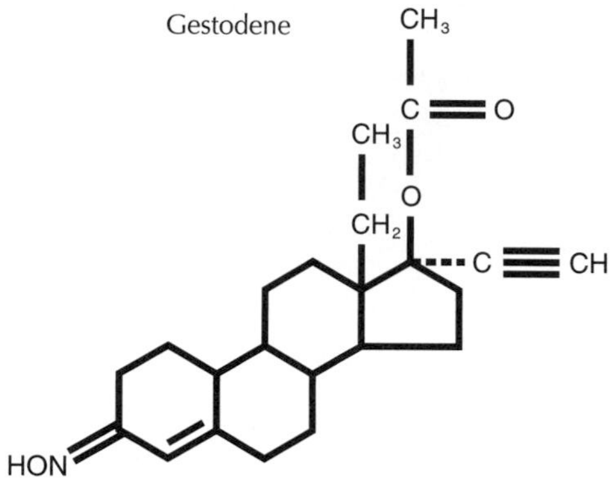

Norgestimate

Desogestrel undergoes two metabolic steps before the progestational activity is expressed in its active metabolite, 3-keto-desogestrel. This metabolite differs from levonorgestrel only by a methylene group in the 11 position. Gestodene differs from levonorgestrel by the presence of a double bond between carbons 15 and 16; thus, it is Δ-15 gestodene. It is metabolized into many derivatives with progestational activity, but not levonorgestrel. Several metabolites contribute to the activity of norgestimate, including 17-deacetylated norgestimate, 3-keto norgestimate, and levonorgestrel. Although norgestimate is a "new" progestin, epidemiologists have included it in the oral contraceptive second generation family because its activity is believed to be largely due to levonorgestrel and levonorgestrel metabolites, although this may not be totally accurate.[9, 10]

Definitions Used in Epidemiologic Studies

Low-Dose Oral Contraceptives — Products containing less than 50 μg ethinyl estradiol

First Generation Oral Contraceptives — Products containing 50 μg or more of ethinyl estradiol

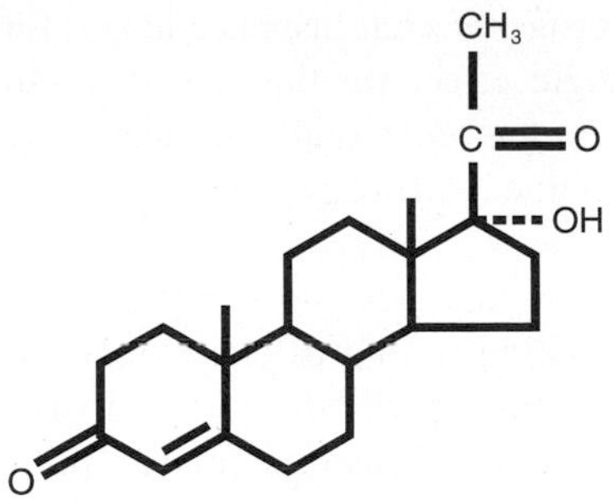

17α-Hydroxyprogesterone

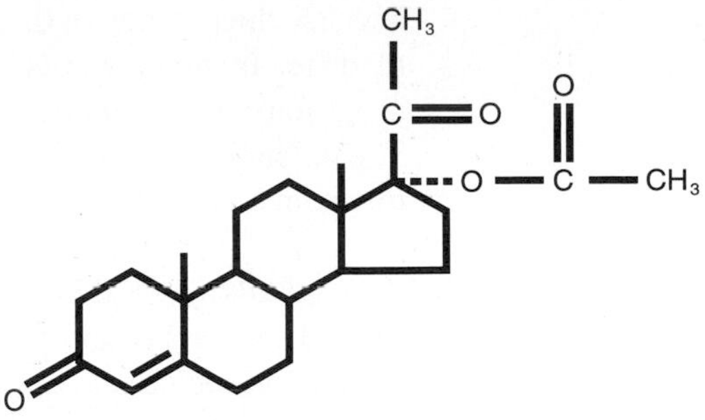

17-Acetoxy progesterone

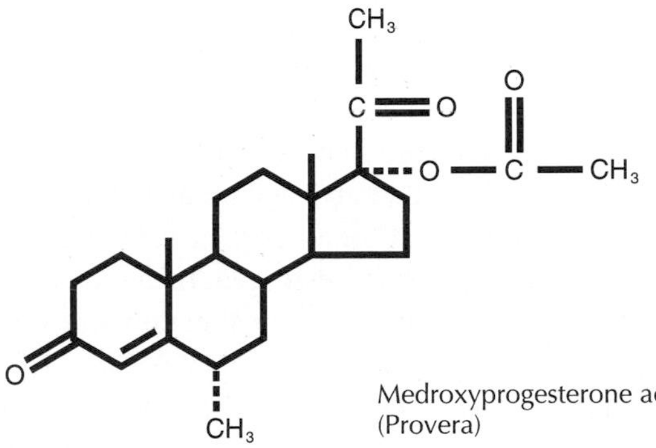

Medroxyprogesterone acetate
(Provera)

Second Generation Oral Contraceptives — Products containing levonorgestrel, norgestimate, and other members of the norethindrone family and 30 or 35 μg ethinyl estradiol

Third Generation Oral Contraceptives — Products containing desogestrel or gestodene with 20 or 30 μg ethinyl estradiol

A second group of progestins became available for use when it was discovered that acetylation of the 17-hydroxy group of 17-hydroxyprogesterone produced an orally active but weak progestin. An addition at the 6 position is necessary to give sufficient progestational strength for human use, probably by inhibiting metabolism. Derivatives of progesterone with substituents at the 17 and 6 positions include the widely used medroxyprogesterone acetate.

Potency

For many years, clinicians, scientists, medical writers, and even the pharmaceutical industry have attempted to assign potency values to the various progestational components of oral contraceptives. An accurate assessment, however, has been difficult to achieve for many reasons. Progestins act on numerous target organs (e.g., the uterus, the mammary glands, and the liver), and potency varies depending upon the target organ and end point being studied. In the past, animal assays, such as the Clauberg test (endometrial change in the rabbit) and the rat ventral prostate assay, were used to determine progestin potency. Although these were considered acceptable methods at the time, a better understanding of steroid hormone action and metabolism, and a recognition that animal and human responses differ, have led to greater reliance on data collected from human studies.

Historically, this has been a confusing issue because publications and experts used potency ranking to provide clinical advice. There is absolutely no need for confusion. Oral contraceptive progestin potency is no longer a consideration when it comes to prescribing oral contraception, because the potency of the various progestins has been accounted for by appropriate adjustments of dose. In other words, the biologic effect (in this case the clinical effect) of the various progestational components in current low-dose oral contraceptives is approximately the same. The potency of a drug does not determine its efficacy or safety, only the amount of a drug required to achieve an effect.

Clinical advice based on potency ranking is an artificial exercise that has not stood the test of time. There is no clinical evidence that a particular progestin is better or worse in terms of particular side effects or clinical responses. Thus oral contraceptives should be judged by their clinical characteristics: efficacy, side effects, risks, and benefits. Our progress in lowering the doses of the steroids contained in oral contraceptives has yielded products with little serious differences. Potency is no longer an important clinical issue.

New Progestins

Probably the greatest influence on the effort that yielded the new progestins was the belief throughout the 1980s that androgenic metabolic effects were important, especially in terms of cardiovascular disease. Cardiovascular side effects are now known to be due to a dose-related stimulation of thrombosis by estrogen. In the search to find compounds that minimize androgenic effects, however, the pharmaceutical companies succeeded.

The new progestins include desogestrel, gestodene, and norgestimate, and even newer progestins are in development.[11] In regard to cycle control (breakthrough bleeding and amenorrhea), the new formulations are comparable with previous low-dose products. All progestins derived from 19-nortestosterone have the potential to decrease glucose tolerance and increase insulin resistance. The impact on carbohydrate metabolism of the previous low-dose formulations was very minimal, and the impact of the new progestins is negligible. Most changes are not statistically significant, and when they are, they are so subtle as to be of no clinical significance. The decreased androgenicity of the progestins in the new products is reflected in increased sex hormone-binding globulin and decreased free testosterone concentrations to a greater degree than the older oral contraceptives. This difference may be of greater clinical value in the treatment of acne and hirsutism, but appropriate comparative clinical studies to document a better response have not been performed.

The new progestins, because of their reduced androgenicity, predictably do not adversely affect the cholesterol-lipoprotein profile. Indeed, the estrogen-progestin balance of combined oral contraceptives containing one of the new progestins may even promote favorable lipid changes. Thus, the new formulations have the potential to offer protection against cardiovascular disease, an important consideration as we enter an era of women using oral contraceptives for longer durations and later in life. But one must be cautious regarding the clinical significance of subtle changes, and it will be difficult to accumulate data with these rare events.

New Formulations

The multiphasic preparation alters the dosage of both the estrogen and progestin components periodically throughout the pill-taking schedule. The aim of these new formulations is to alter steroid levels in an effort to achieve lesser metabolic effects and minimize the occurrence of breakthrough bleeding and amenorrhea, while maintaining efficacy. We are probably at or very near the lowest dose levels that can be achieved without sacrificing efficacy. Metabolic studies with the multiphasic preparations indicate no differences or slight improvements over the metabolic effects of low-dose monophasic products.

Mechanism of Action

The combination pill, consisting of estrogen and progestin components, is given daily for 3 of every 4 weeks. The combination pill prevents ovulation by inhibiting gonadotropin secretion via an effect on both pituitary and hypothalamic centers. The progestational agent in the pill primarily suppresses luteinizing hormone (LH) secretion (and thus prevents ovulation), while the estrogenic agent suppresses follicle-stimulating hormone (FSH) secretion (and thus prevents the selection and emergence of a dominant follicle). Therefore, the estrogenic component significantly contributes to the contraceptive efficacy. However, even if follicular growth and development were not sufficiently inhibited, the progestational component would prevent the surge-like release of LH necessary for ovulation.

The estrogen in the pill serves two other purposes. It provides stability to the endometrium so that irregular shedding and unwanted breakthrough bleeding can be minimized; and the presence of estrogen is required to potentiate the action of the progestational agents. The latter function of estrogen has allowed reduction of the progestational dose in the pill. The mechanism for this action is probably estrogen's effect in increasing the concentration of intracellular progestational receptors. Therefore, a minimal pharmacologic level of estrogen is necessary to maintain the efficacy of the combination pill.

Because the effect of a progestational agent will always take precedence over estrogen (unless the dose of estrogen is increased many, many-fold), the endometrium, cervical mucus, and perhaps tubal function reflect progestational stimulation. The progestin in the combination pill produces an endometrium that is not receptive to ovum implantation, a decidualized bed with exhausted and atrophied glands. The cervical mucus becomes thick and impervious to sperm transport. It is possible that progestational influences on secretion and peristalsis within the fallopian tubes provide additional contraceptive effects. Even if there is some ovarian follicular activity (especially with the lowest dose products), these actions serve to ensure good contraceptive efficacy.[12]

Efficacy

In view of the multiple actions of oral contraceptives, it is hard to understand how the omission of a pill or two can result in a pregnancy. Indeed, careful review of failures suggests that pregnancies usually occur because initiation of the next cycle is delayed allowing escape from ovarian suppression. Strict adherence to 7 pill-free days is critical in order to obtain reliable, effective contraception. For this reason, the 28-day pill package, incorporating 7 pills that do not contain steroids, is a very useful aid to ensure adherence to the necessary schedule. The most prevalent problems that can be identified associated with apparent oral contraceptive failures are vomiting and diarrhea.[13, 14] *Even if no pills have been missed, patients should be instructed to use a backup method for at least 7 days after an episode of gastroenteritis.*

The contraceptive effectiveness of the new progestin oral contraceptives, multiphasic formulations, and lowest estrogen dose products are unequivocally comparable with older low-dose (less than 50 μg estrogen) and higher dose monophasic combination birth control pills.[12] While carefully monitored studies with motivated subjects achieve an annual failure rate of 0.1%, typical usage is associated with a 3.0% failure rate during the first year of use.[15] Efficacy decreases slightly when the estrogen component is removed, and only a small dose of the progestin is administered (the progestin-only minipills).

Failure Rates During the First Year of Use, United States[16]

Method	Percent of Women with Pregnancy	
	Lowest Expected	**Typical**
No method	85.0%	85.0%
Combination Pill	0.1	3.0
Progestin only	0.5	3.0
IUDs		
Progesterone IUD	1.5	2.0
Levonorgestrel IUD	0.6	0.8
Copper T 380A	0.1	0.1
Norplant	0.05	0.05
Female sterilization	0.05	0.05
Male sterilization	0.1	0.15
Depo-Provera	0.3	0.3
Spermicides	6.0	26.0
Periodic abstinence		25.0
Calendar	9.0	
Ovulation method	3.0	
Symptothermal	2.0	
Post–ovulation	1.0	
Withdrawal	4.0	19.0
Cervical cap		
Parous women	26.0	40.0
Nulliparous women	9.0	20.0
Sponge		
Parous women	9.0	28.0
Nulliparous women	6.0	18.0
Diaphragm and spermicides	6.0	20.0
Condom		
Male	3.0	14.0
Female	5.0	21.0

Metabolic Effects of Oral Contraception

Cardiovascular Disease

In October, 1995, the United Kingdom Committee on Safety of Medicines sent a letter to all U.K. physicians and pharmacists stating that women taking oral contraceptives containing desogestrel or gestodene should be urged to complete their current cycle and to continue a formulation with these progestins only if prepared to accept an increased risk of venous thromboembolism. The Committee on Safety of Medicines took this action because of observational studies that indicated a two-fold increase in the risk of venous thromboembolism when desogestrel- and gestodene-containing contraceptives were compared with products with other progestins (mostly levonorgestrel). This action and the studies on which it was based immediately became controversial. The controversy went beyond the validity of the epidemiologic data. The publicity surrounding these events reverberated throughout Europe, leading to an immediate overall decrease in oral contraceptive use, an increase in unwanted pregnancies, and an increase in induced abortions.[17, 18]

The controversy involving new progestin oral contraceptives that began in late 1995, continued through 1996, and began to reach resolution in 1997. The fundamental question is whether oral contraceptives containing desogestrel and gestodene have a different risk of thrombosis compared with oral contraceptives containing older progestins. Thrombosis can be divided into two major categories, venous thromboembolism and arterial thrombosis. Venous thromboembolism includes both deep vein thrombosis and pulmonary embolism. Arterial thrombosis includes acute myocardial infarction and stroke.

The Coagulation System

The goal of the clotting mechanism is to produce thrombin, which converts fibrinogen to a fibrin clot. Thrombin is generated from prothrombin by factor Xa in the presence of factor V, calcium, and phospholipids. The vitamin K-dependent factors include factors VII, IX, and X, as well as prothrombin. Antithrombin III is one of the body's natural anticoagulants, an irreversible inhibitor of thrombin and factors IXa, Xa, and XIa. Protein C and protein S are two other major inhibitors of coagulation and are also vitamin K-dependent. Protein C, and its helper, Protein S, inhibit clotting at the level of factors V and VIII. Tissue plasminogen activator (t-PA) is produced by endothelial cells and released when a clot forms. Both t-PA and plasminogen bind to the fibrin clot. The t-PA converts the plasminogen to plasmin which lyses the clot by degrading the fibrin. Deficiencies of antithrombin III, protein C, and protein S are inherited in an autosomal dominant pattern, accounting for 10–15% of familial thrombosis. A mutation in the prothrombin gene and the factor V Leiden mutation are the most common inherited causes of venous thromboembolism.[19]

An inherited resistance to activated protein C has been identified as the basis for about 50% of cases of familial venous thrombosis, due in almost all cases to a gene alteration recognized as the factor V Leiden mutation.[20, 21] The factor V Leiden mutation is found in approximately 30% of individuals who develop venous thromboembolism.[22] Activated protein C inhibits coagulation by degrading factors V and VIII. One of the 3 cleavages sites in factor V is the precise site of a mutation (known as the factor V Leiden mutation) that substitutes glutamine instead of arginine at this site (adenine for guanine at nucleotide 1691 in the gene).[22] This mutation makes factor V resistant to degradation (and activation in fibrinolysis). The entire clotting cascade is then resistant to the actions of the protein C system.

Coagulation and Fibrinolysis Factors

Coagulation Factors:
    Factors that favor clotting when increased
        Fibrinogen
        Factors VII, VIII, X
    Factors that favor clotting when decreased
        Antithrombin III
        Protein C
        Protein S

Fibrinolysis Factors:
    Factors that favor clotting when increased
        Plasminogen
        Plasminogen activator inhibitor-1 (PAI-1)
    Factors that favor clotting when decreased
        Antiplasmin

Heterozygotes for the factor V Leiden mutation have an 8-fold increased risk of venous thrombosis, and homozygotes, an 80-fold increased risk, and this risk appears to be further enhanced by oral contraceptive use. The highest prevalence (3–4% of the general population) of factor V Leiden is found in Europeans, and its occurrence in populations not of European descent is very rare, perhaps explaining the low frequency of thromboembolic disease in Africa, Asia, and in native Americans.[23] The mutation is believed to have arisen in a single ancestor approximately 21,000 to 34,000 years ago.[24] It has been suggested that this was a useful adaptation in heterozygotes in response to life-threatening bleeding, such as with childbirth.

The next most common inherited disorder (after the factor V Leiden mutation) is a mutation, a guanine to adenine change, in the gene encoding prothrombin.[19, 25] The prevalence of this abnormality in the white population is estimated to range from 0.7% to 4%.[26]

The administration of pharmacologic amounts of estrogen as in high-dose oral contraceptives causes an increase in the production of clotting factors such as factor V, factor VIII, factor X, and fibrinogen.[27] Some studies of the blood coagulation system have concluded that both monophasic and multiphasic low-dose oral contraceptives have no significant clinical impact on the coagulation system. Slight increases in thrombin formation are offset by increased fibrinolytic activity.[28, 29] Other studies of formulations containing 30 and 35 µg of ethinyl estradiol indicate an increase in clotting factors associated with an increase in platelet activity.[30] However, these changes are essentially all within normal ranges and their clinical significance is unknown. Smoking produces a shift to hypercoagulability.[31] A 20 µg estrogen formulation has been reported to have no effect on clotting parameters, even in smokers.[31, 32] One study comparing a 20 µg product with a 30 µg product found similar mild pro-coagulant and fibrinolytic activity, although there was a trend toward increased fibrinolytic activity with the lower dose.[33]

There is no evidence of an increase in risk of cardiovascular disease among past users of oral contraception.[34–36] In the Nurses' Health Study and the Royal College of General Practitioners' Study, long-term past use of oral contraceptives was not associated with an increase in overall mortality.[37, 393] Part of the concern for a possible lingering effect of oral contraceptive use was based on a presumed adverse impact on the atherosclerotic process, which would then be added to the effect of aging and, thus, would be manifested later in life. Instead, the findings have been consistent with the contention that cardiovascular disease due to oral contraception is secondary to acute effects, specifically estrogen-induced thrombosis, a dose-related event.

Venous Thromboembolism — The Conventional Wisdom

Older epidemiologic evaluations of oral contraceptives and vascular disease indicated that venous thrombosis was an effect of estrogen, limited to current users, with a disappearance of the risk by 3 months after discontinuation.[38, 39] Thromboembolic disease was believed to be a consequence of the pharmacologic administration of estrogen, and the level of risk was believed to be related to the estrogen dose.[40–42] Smoking was documented to produce an additive increase in the risk of arterial thrombosis, [43–45] but had no effect on the risk of venous thromboembolism.[46, 47]

Is there still a risk of venous thromboembolism with the current low-dose (less than 50 μg ethinyl estradiol) formulations of oral contraceptives? In the first years of oral contraception, the available products, containing 80 and 100 μg ethinyl estradiol (an extremely high dose), were associated with a 6-fold increased risk of venous thrombosis.[48] Because of the increased risks for venous thrombosis, myocardial infarction, and stroke, lower dose formulations (less than 50 μg estrogen) came to dominate the market, and clinicians became more careful in their screening of patients and prescribing of oral contraception. Two forces, therefore, were at work simultaneously to bring greater safety to women utilizing oral contraception: (1). the use of lower dose formulations, and (2). the avoidance of oral contraception by high-risk patients. Because of these two forces, the Puget Sound study in the United States documented a reduction in venous thrombosis risk to 2-fold.[49] The new studies also reflect the importance of these two forces, but they still indicate an increased risk.

The Hierarchy of Epidemiologic Studies

I. Clinical Reports

A case report: An anecdotal report that serves to bring attention to a possible problem or condition.

A case series: A collection of similar cases that suggests more than a chance or coincidental occurrence.

II. Observational Studies (Non-experimental Studies: Observation Without Intervention)

Cross-sectional studies: A description of a group of individuals at one point in time.

Advantages: A reliable method to estimate prevalence, quick and inexpensive.

Disadvantages: Cannot assess changes over time and very susceptible to sampling error (the group is not representative of the actual population of interest).

Example: The Health and Nutritional Examination Survey

Case-control studies: A retrospective comparison of a group of individuals with a condition or problem compared with a carefully selected control group. Subjects are selected according to specific inclusion and exclusion criteria. The exposure history of those with disease and those with no disease is collected and compared.

Advantages: Relatively quick and inexpensive because of small sample sizes.

Disadvantages: Subject to biases and errors.

Example: WHO Collaborative Study of Cardiovascular Disease and Steroid Hormone Contraception

Cohort studies: A prospective follow-up over a long period of time of a large group of individuals. Also referred to as longitudinal or follow-up studies. Exposure information is collected from all subjects who are disease-free, and subjects are followed over time to determine who develops disease.

Advantages: A relatively accurate estimation because of large numbers, can evaluate changes over time, avoids recall bias.

Disadvantages: Expensive, lengthy in time, and subject to biases (particularly surveillance bias).

Example: The Nurses' Health Study

III. Randomized Controlled Trials

A true clinical experiment in which an intervention is compared with a standard treatment, no treatment, or a placebo, with allocation to treatment by chance. More than one comparison can be made within a study.

Advantages: Provides scientific, epidemiologic proof.

Disadvantages: Very expensive and time-consuming. Only a limited number of hypotheses can be evaluated in any one study.

Example: The Women's Health Initiative

Possible Confounders and Biases of Importance

Confounders: Factors associated with the disease and the exposure, such as age, body weight, smoking, family history, duration of oral contraceptive use, preferential prescribing, healthy user effect.

Biases: Errors due to study design.

Detection or Surveillance Bias: Systematic errors in methods of ascertainment, diagnosis, or verification of cases. Not everyone in the study population has equal access to or utilization of medical interventions and diagnostic tests.

Publication Bias: Negative (null) studies and studies that confirm old results tend not to be published. An important source of bias in meta-analysis.

Reporting or Recall Bias: Inaccurate memory and dishonesty introduce errors.

Selection Bias: Differences in characteristics between those selected for study and those who are not, such as preferential prescribing, family history, preferential referral of patients, healthy user effect. For case-control studies, the source of the controls is important. Hospital-based controls are less likely to be representative of the general population than population-based controls. It is best to choose controls by random selection, but this is not always possible. Selection bias in a cohort study can result in differences between exposed and unexposed groups.

> *Information or observer bias:* A flaw in measuring exposure or outcome that produces different results between comparison groups. Nonresponse or patients lost to follow-up can produce differences in cohort studies.

A Guide to Epidemiologic Terms Commonly Used

Relative Risk:

The ratio of the risk among those exposed to the risk among the unexposed or the ratio of the cumulative incidence rate in the exposed and the unexposed. Also called risk ratio.

Odds Ratio:

The odds ratio is the measure of association calculated in case-control studies when the prevalence of disease events is low; the estimate and interpretation are similar to relative risk.

Confidence Interval (CI):

The range of relative risk that would include 95% of the subjects being studied; the range of relative risks within which the true magnitude of effect lies, given the study data, with a certain degree of assurance. To be statistically significant, a reduced relative risk (a beneficial effect) requires the larger number (the right hand number) to be less than 1.0. An increased relative risk (an adverse effect), to be statistically significant, requires the smaller number (the left hand number) to be greater than 1.0. The tighter (more narrow) the range, the more precise the conclusion. The wider the CI, the more imprecise the conclusion, usually because of small numbers of study subjects.

Attributable risk:

The difference in actual incidence between exposed and unexposed groups, providing a realistic estimate of the change in incidence in a given population. A modest increase in relative risk will produce only a small number of cases when clinical events are rare, such as venous thromboembolism and arterial thrombosis in young women.

Venous Thromboembolism — The Controversial Studies

The World Health Organization (WHO) Collaborative Study of Cardiovascular Disease and Steroid Hormone Contraception was a hospital-based, case-control study with subjects collected from 21 centers in 17 countries in Africa, Asia, Europe, and Latin America.[50] As part of this study, the risk of *idiopathic* venous thromboembolism associated with a formulation containing 30 μg ethinyl estradiol and levonorgestrel (doses ranging from 125 μg to 250 μg) was compared with the risk with preparations containing 20 or 30 μg ethinyl estradiol and either desogestrel or gestodene (data from 10 centers in 9 countries).[51] There were only 9 cases and 3 controls using combined oral contraceptives with other progestins, precluding precise analysis. The users of the levonorgestrel formulation had an increased odds ratio (an estimation of relative risk used in case-control studies) of 3.5 compared with nonusers. Current users of a desogestrel product had an increased risk of 9.1 compared with nonusers, and with gestodene, the odds ratio was also 9.1. Thus, the increased risk for desogestrel and gestodene was 2.6 times that of levonorgestrel, when adjusted for body weight and height. Also of note, the increased risk for the desogestrel formulation containing 20 μg ethinyl estradiol was 38.2, a number that is obviously not reliable because it was based upon only 8 cases and 1 control; the confidence interval (CI) of 4.5–325 reflected this imprecision. Overall, these increased risks were lower than those estimated by earlier case-control studies of higher dose oral contraceptives.

The second case-control study (from an international team of epidemiologists and called *the Transnational Study on Oral Contraceptives and the Health of Young Women*) analyzed 471 cases of deep vein thrombosis and/or venous thromboembolism from the United Kingdom and Germany.[52] Second generation oral contraceptives were defined as products containing 35 µg or less of ethinyl estradiol and a progestin other than desogestrel or gestodene. Comparing users of second generation products to nonusers, the odds ratio was 3.2 (CI = 2.3–4.3). Comparing users of desogestrel and gestodene products to users of second generation oral contraceptives, the risk of venous thromboembolism was 1.5-fold greater.

The third study was from Boston University, but the data were derived from *the General Practice Research Database*, a computerized system involving the general practitioners in the U.K.[53] Using this cohort, the authors calculated the death rate from pulmonary embolism, stroke, and acute myocardial infarction in the users of levonorgestrel, desogestrel, and gestodene low-dose oral contraceptives. Over a 3-year period, they collected a total of 15 unexpected idiopathic cardiovascular deaths in users of these products, a *nonsignificant change*, and no difference in the risk comparing desogestrel and gestodene with levonorgestrel. The risk estimates for venous thromboembolism (adjusted for smoking and body size) were about 2 times greater for desogestrel and for gestodene, compared with levonorgestrel uses. There were only 4 cases and 9 controls using the 20 µg ethinyl estradiol and desogestrel product, and although the risk was similar to that associated with the 30 µg ethinyl estradiol and desogestrel product, this is too small a number for analysis.

Similar results were reported when women with deep vein thrombosis in the *Leiden Thrombophilia Study* in the Netherlands were re-analyzed for their use of oral contraceptives.[54] As expected, the risk of deep vein thrombosis was markedly higher in women who were carriers of the factor V Leiden mutation and in women with a family history of thrombosis.

Smoking, well recognized as a risk factor for arterial thrombosis, did not affect the risk estimates in these studies. This is not a new observation; older studies of venous thromboembolism also failed to identify smoking as a risk factor.[46, 47]

Venous Thromboembolism — Subsequent Studies

The publication of the 4 reports in late 1995 and early 1996 was followed by a flood of letters to editors, as well as reviews and editorials, highlighting confounding and bias problems in these studies.[55–57] Some prominent figures were convinced the reports of increased risks with desogestrel and gestodene were real;[58, 59] others were skeptical, pointing out possible confounding biases. Subsequently, re-analysis and new studies revealed confounders and biases in the initial studies. Thus, a consistent picture gradually emerged with consideration of proper analysis of the generated data, and the adjustment for confounding biases not initially apparent.

In Denmark, Lidegaard and colleagues performed a hospital-based, case-control study of women with confirmed diagnoses of venous thromboembolism in 1994 and 1995 (in Denmark, all women with this diagnosis are hospitalized, and therefore, very few, if any, cases were missed).[60] A 2—fold increased risk of venous thromboembolism was found in current users of oral contraceptives, regardless of estrogen doses ranging from 20 to 50 µg. The increased risk was concentrated in the first year of use. *Because there were more short-term users of the new progestins and more long-term users of the older progestins, adjustment for duration of use resulted in no significant differences between the different types of progestins.* Those factors associated with an increased risk of thromboembolism included coagulation disorders, treated hypertension during pregnancy, family history of venous thromboembolism, and an increasing body mass index. Notably, conditions not associated with an increased risk of venous thromboembolism included smoking, migraine, diabetes, hyperlipidemia, parity, or age at first birth. There was still insufficient strength in this study to establish the absence or presence of a dose-response relationship comparing the 20 µg estrogen dose to higher doses.

A case-control study using 83 cases of venous thromboembolism derived from the computer records of general practices in the U.K. concluded that the increased risk associated with oral contraceptives was the same for all types, and that the pattern of risk with specific oral contraceptives suggested confounding because of "preferential prescribing" (defined below).[61] *In this study, matching cases and controls by exact year of birth eliminated differences between different types of oral contraceptives.* A similar analysis based on 42 cases from a German database again found no difference between new progestin and older progestin oral contraceptives.[62] Thus, in these two studies, more precise adjustments for age eliminated a confounding bias.

A re-analysis of the Transnational Case-Control Study considered the duration and patterns of oral contraceptive use.[63] This re-analysis focused on first-time users of second and third generation oral contraceptives. *Statistical analysis with adjustment for duration of use in 105 cases who were first-time users could find no differences between second and third generation products.*

Evaluation of the Studies

An immediate problem with the initial studies was how to reconcile the results with the conventional wisdom that thrombosis is an estrogen dose-related complication. Furthermore, progestational agents, and desogestrel and gestodene in particular, have no significant impact on clotting parameters.[11] Therefore, there was inherent biologic implausibility surrounding the new studies.

The initial reports resurrected the claim by Kuhl in 1988 and 1989 that gestodene could cause more thrombosis because it affected ethinyl estradiol metabolism, resulting in higher estrogen levels.[64, 65] Other laboratories, however, could not replicate Kuhl's findings.[66, 67]

Former users discontinue oral contraceptives for a variety of reasons, and often are switched to what clinicians perceive to be "safer" products (*"preferential prescribing"*).[68–70] Individuals who do well with a product tend to remain with that product. Thus, at any one point in time, individuals on an older product will be relatively healthy and free of side effects (*"healthy user effect"*). This is also called *attrition of susceptibles* because higher risk individuals with problems are gradually eliminated from the group.[56] *Comparing users of older and newer products, therefore, can involve disparate cohorts of individuals.*

Because desogestrel- and gestodene-containing products were marketed as less androgenic and therefore "better" (a marketing claim not substantiated by epidemiologic studies), clinicians chose to provide these products to higher risk patients and older women.[68, 69] In addition, clinicians switched patients perceived to be at greater risk for thrombosis from older oral contraceptives to the newer formulations with desogestrel and gestodene. Furthermore, these products were prescribed more often to young women who were starting oral contraception for the first time (these young women will not have experienced the test of pregnancy or previous oral contraceptive use to help identify those who have a congenital predisposition to venous thrombosis). These changing practice patterns exert different effects over the lifetime of a product, and analytical adjustments are extremely difficult. The Transnational Group believed it accomplished an appropriate adjustment by focusing on first-time users and duration of use.[63] It is also unlikely that the "healthy user effect" will be dominant in first-time users. And, of course, this analysis found no differences between second and third generation oral contraceptives.

The challenge for a clinician is to make a decision: is an observational study with statistically significant results clinically (biologically) real? This controversy illustrates how difficult this can be. When faced with results from observational studies, clinicians want to see uniformity, consistency, agreement—all arguing in favor of a real clinical effect. Examples are the protective effect of oral contraceptives on the risk of ovarian cancer, and the benefits of postmenopausal estrogen therapy on cardiovascular disease. The initial studies were impressive in their agreement. All indicated increased relative risks associated with desogestrel and gestodene compared with levonorgestrel. Nevertheless, all of the early studies, somewhat similar in design, were influenced by the same unrecognized biases. *Persistent errors will produce consistent conclusions.*

The apparent differences associated with the new progestins, it is now apparent, were due to the marketing and preferential prescribing of new products, which influenced the characteristics of the patients for whom the new products were prescribed. Most impressive and important is the fact that there is no evidence of an increase in mortality due to venous thromboembolism since the introduction of new progestin oral contraceptives.[53, 71]

Venous Thromboembolism and the Factor V Leiden Mutation

The new studies indicate that a risk of idiopathic venous thrombosis persists with low-dose oral contraceptives, at a level of approximately 3–4-fold greater than the normal, general incidence.[51–54, 72] However, an inherited resistance to activated protein C, the factor V Leiden mutation, may account for a significant portion of the patients who experience venous thrombosis while taking oral contraceptives.

Relative Risk and Actual Incidence of Venous Thromboembolism[73,74]

Population	Relative Risk	Incidence per 100,000 per year
Young women — general population	1	4–5
Pregnant women	12	48–60
High-dose oral contraceptives	6–10	24–50
Low-dose oral contraceptives	3–4	12–20
Leiden mutation carrier	6–8	24–40
Leiden carrier and oral contraceptives	30	120–150
Leiden mutation — homozygous	80	320–400

An inherited resistance to activated protein C, the factor V Leiden mutation, is the most common inherited coagulation problem, transmitted in an autosomal dominant fashion.[20, 75] Heterozygotes have a 6- to 8-fold increased risk of venous thromboembolism, and homozygotes an 80-fold increased risk. Oral contraceptive users who have this mutation have been reported to have a 30-fold increased risk of venous thrombosis.[76, 77] There is no known association between the factor V Leiden mutation and arterial thrombosis.[78]

Should screening for the factor V Leiden mutation (or for other inherited clotting disorders) be routine prior to prescribing contraceptives? The carrier frequencies of the Leiden mutation in the American population (the percentages are similar in men and women) are as follows:[74]

Caucasian Americans	5.27%
Hispanic Americans	2.21%
Native Americans	1.25%
Black Americans	1.23%
Asian Americans	0.45%

These estimates are consistent with the European assessments, indicating that this is a trait carried in people of European origin. In the United States, of the approximately 10 million women currently using oral contraceptives, about 450,000 are likely to carry the factor V Leiden mutation. However, because the incidence rate of venous thromboembolism is so low (4–5 per 100,000 young women per year),[73, 74] the number of women required to be screened to prevent one death is prohibitively large. The prevalence of all deficiencies is only about 0.5% in the asymptomatic population, and only one-third of patients at risk are detected by the present tests.[79]

Furthermore, because only a small number of women even with the Leiden mutation (less than 1 in 1000) have a clinical event, the finding of a positive screening test, especially considering the high rate of false positive tests, would be a barrier to the use of oral contraceptives, and a subsequent increase in unwanted pregnancies (which has an even greater risk of venous thromboembolism) would likely follow. *Most experts believe that screening for inherited disorders should be pursued only in women with a previous episode of venous thromboembolism or a close positive family history (parent or sibling) of venous thrombosis.*

This aspect of the oral contraceptive venous thromboembolism controversy received a transfusion of energy with the publication of a report from the Netherlands, utilizing a laboratory test for resistance to activated protein C to compare differences in oral contraceptive non-users, users of second generation oral contraceptives, and users of third generation oral contraceptives.[80] Women who used any oral contraceptive had a decreased sensitivity to activated protein C compared with nonusers, and women who used third generation oral contraceptives were even less sensitive, and less than users of second generation products. This was presented as an explanation for the epidemiologic data indicating greater risks of venous thromboembolism associated with desogestrel and gestodene, and an editorial in the April 19, 1997, issue of Lancet concluded that this report was the "nail in the coffin" confirming the epidemiologic evidence.[59]

Subsequent epidemiologic reports not only removed the nails from the coffin, but returned the coffin to its maker. A closer look at the report from the Netherlands finds considerable overlap in the results among all the groups tested, and many of the oral contraceptive users had results comparable with the nonusers. It is always prudent to avoid making clinically meaningful conclusions from acquired changes in a single laboratory test (especially when the clinical meaning of a laboratory test is uncertain). Furthermore, the results could not be corroborated by another laboratory.[81]

Arterial Thrombosis

Because the incidence of cerebral thrombotic attacks (thrombotic strokes and transient ischemic attacks) among young women is higher than venous thromboembolism and myocardial infarction, and death and disability are more likely, stroke is the most important possible side effect. A very low incidence of stroke in young women carries with it little increase in absolute risk. However, because the incidence of cerebral thrombotic attacks is higher in women over age 40, we should do our best, as the following paragraphs will indicate, to make sure oral contraceptive users over age 40 are in good health and without significant risk factors for cardiovascular disease (especially hypertension, migraine with aura, diabetes mellitus, and smoking).

It has been difficult to establish arterial thrombosis dose-response relationships with estrogen because these events are so rare. Nevertheless, the estrogen dose is important for the risk of myocardial infarction and thrombotic strokes.[82, 83] Thus, a rationale for advocating low-dose estrogen oralontraceptives continues to be valid. It is acknowledged that the apparent higher risk of venous thromboembolism associated with 20 μg products in the WHO and Transnational studies reflects small numbers as well as preferential prescribing and healthy user effects.

Arterial Thrombosis — Myocardial Infarction

A population-based, case-control study analyzed 187 cases of myocardial infarction in users of low-dose oral contraceptives in the Kaiser Permanente Medical Care Program.[84] *There was no statistically significant increase in the odds ratio for myocardial infarction in current oral contraceptive users compared with past or never users.*

In the Transnational case-control study of myocardial infarctions collected from 16 centers in Austria, France, Germany, Switzerland, and the United Kingdom, the results were as follows:[85, 86]

	Cases	Controls	Odds Ratio	Confidence Interval
Any OC use	57	156	2.35	1.42–3.89
50 μg estrogen OCs	14	22	4.32	1.59–11.74
Old progestin OCs	28	71	2.96	1.54–5.66
New progestin OCs	7	49	0.82	0.29–2.31

These data were interpreted as indicating no *increased* risk of myocardial infarction associated with oral contraceptives containing desogestrel or gestodene. However, the *reduced* risk with the new progestin oral contraceptives was also emphasized (the comparison of third generation products to second generation products yielded a reduced risk that was statistically significant), suggesting a possible saving of deaths from myocardial infarction with desogestrel and gestodene. The problem is that the small actual incidence makes it difficult to acquire sufficient numbers. The conclusion was based on only 7 cases and 49 controls using third generation oral contraceptives and 28 cases and 71 controls using second generation products, and, in our view, the power is too limited to make any conclusion regarding the new progestin oral contraceptives. This is a good example of a conclusion that may be statistically significant, but clinically not real.

The Transnational study found that cigarette smoking carried a higher risk for myocardial infarction than oral contraceptives, and *that nonsmoking users of oral contraceptives had no evidence of an increased risk.*[85] In addition, there was an indication that patient screening is important in minimizing the impact of hypertension on the risk of myocardial infarction.

In the WHO multicenter study, there were 368 cases of acute myocardial infarction.[87] Factors associated with an increased risk of myocardial infarction included smoking, a history of hypertension (including hypertension in pregnancy), diabetes, rheumatic heart disease, abnormal blood lipids, and a family history of stroke or myocardial infarction. Duration of use and past use of oral contraceptives did not affect risk. Although there was about a 5-fold overall increased odds ratio of myocardial infarction in current users of oral contraceptives, essentially all cases occurred in women with cardiovascular risk factors. There was no apparent effect of increasing age on risk; however, there were only 12 cases among oral contraceptives users ls than 35 years old. There was no apparent relationship with estrogen dose, and there was no apparent influence of type or dose of progestin. However, the rare occurrence of this condition produced such small numbers that there was insufficient statistical power to accurately assess the effects of progestin type, and estrogen and progestin doses. *The conclusion of this study was that the risk of myocardial infarction in women who use oral contraceptives is increased only in smokers.*

In a Danish case-control study of acute myocardial infarction in young women, a statistically significant increase in risk was noted only in current users of 50 μg ethinyl estradiol.[83] There was a progressive increase in risk with the number of cigarettes smoked, (accounting for 80% of the acute myocardial infarctions in young women), increasing body mass index, treated hypertension, treated hypertension in pregnancy, diabetes mellitus, hyperlipidemia, frequent migraine, and family history of myocardial infarction. However, only family history of myocardial infarction and smoking affected the risk associated with oral contraceptives; no influence on oral contraceptive risk was apparent with diabetes, hypertension, and heart disease. No differences could be demonstrated according to type of progestin.

Incidence of Myocardial Infarction in Reproductive Age Women[87]

Overall incidence[88]	5 per 100,000 per year
Women less than age 35	
Nonsmokers	4 per 100,000 per year
Nonsmokers and OCs	4 per 100,000 per year
Smokers	8 per 100,000 per year
Smokers and OCs	43 per 100,000 per year
Women 35-years-old and older	
Nonsmokers	10 per 100,000 per year
Nonsmokers and OCs	40 per 100,000 per year
Smokers	88 per 100,000 per year
Smokers and OCs	485 per 100,000 per year

Note: The above incidences are estimates based on oral contraceptive use paired with cardiovascular risk factors prevalent in the general population. Effective screening would produce smaller numbers. The increased risks in the smokers and OC groups reflect the impact of undetected cardiovascular risk factors, especially hypertension.

Arterial Thrombosis — Stroke

Older case-control and cohort studies indicated an increased risk of cerebral thrombosis among current users of high-dose oral contraceptives.[89–91] However, thrombotic stroke did not appear to be increased in healthy, nonsmoking women with the use of oral contraceptives containing less than 50 μg ethinyl estradiol.[90, 91] A case-control study of all 794 women in Denmark who suffered a cerebral thromboembolic attack during 1985–1989 concluded that there was an almost two-fold increased relative risk associated with oral contraceptives containing 30–40 μg estrogen, and the risk was significantly influenced by both smoking and the dose of estrogen in additive (not synergistic) fashion.[45] A case-control analysis of data collected by the Royal College of General Practitioners' Oral Contraception Study concluded that current users were at increased risk of stroke (with a persisting effect in former users); however, this outcome was limited mainly to smokers and to formulations with 50 μg or more of estrogen.[91]

A population-based, case-control study of 408 strokes from the California Kaiser Permanente Medical Care Program found no increase in risk for either ischemic stroke or hemorrhagic stroke.[92] The identifiable risk factors for ischemic stroke were smoking, hypertension, diabetes, elevated body weight, and low socioeconomic status. The risk factors for hemorrhagic stroke were the same plus greater body mass and heavy use of alcohol. *Current users of low-dose oral contraceptives did not have an increased risk of ischemic or hemorrhagic stroke compared with former users and with never users.* There was no evidence for an adverse effect of increasing age or for smoking (for hemorrhagic stroke, there was a suggestion of a positive interaction between current oral contraceptive use and smoking, but the numbers were small, and the result was not statistically significant).

The Transnational study also analyzed their data for ischemic stroke in a case-control study of 220 ischemic strokes in the United Kingdom, Germany, France, Switzerland, and Austria.[93] Overall, there was a 3-fold increase in the risk of ischemic stroke associated with the use of oral contraceptives, with higher risks observed in smokers (more than 10 cigarettes per day), in women with hypertension, and in users of higher dose estrogen products. No differences were observed comparing second and third generation progestins. A case-control study from the state of Washington concluded that there is no increased risk of stroke in current users of low-dose oral contraceptives.[94]

The World Health Organization data on stroke come from the same collaborative study that yielded the publications on venous thromboembolism. The results with stroke were published as two separate reports, one on ischemic stroke and the other on hemorrhagic stroke.[95, 96]

This hospital-based, case-control study from 21 centers in 17 countries accumulated 697 cases of ischemic stroke, 141 from Europe and 556 from developing countries.[95] The overall odds ratio for ischemic stroke indicated about a 3-fold increased risk. In Europe, however, the risk was statistically significant only for higher-dose products, and **NOT** statistically significant for products with less than 50 µg ethinyl estradiol. In developing countries, there was no difference in risk with low-dose and higher dose oral contraceptives. This is believed to be due to the strong influence of hypertension. In Europe, it was uncommon for women with a history of hypertension to be using oral contraceptives; however, this was not the case in developing countries. Duration of use and type of progestin had no impact, and past users did not have an increased risk, but smoking 10 or more cigarettes daily exerted a synergistic effect with oral contraceptives, increasing the risk of ischemic stroke, approximating the effect of hypertension and oral contraceptives. The risk was greater in women 35 years and older; however, this, too, was believed to be due to an effect of hypertension. *Thus, the conclusion of this study was that the risk of ischemic stroke is extremely low, concentrated in those who use higher dose products, smoke, or have hypertension.*

In the WHO study on hemorrhagic stroke, there were 1068 cases.[96] Current use of oral contraceptives was associated with a slightly increased risk of hemorrhagic stroke only in developing countries, not in Europe. This again probably reflects the presence of hypertension, because the greatest increased risk (about 10- to 15-fold) was identified in current users of oral contraceptives who had a history of hypertension. Current cigarette smoking also increased the risk in oral contraceptive users, but not as dramatically as hypertension. For hemorrhagic stroke, the dose of estrogen had no effect on risk, and neither did duration of use or type of progestin. *This study concluded that the risk of hemorrhagic stroke due to oral contraceptives is increased only slightly in older women, probably occurring only in women with risk factors such as hypertension.*

A second Danish case-control study included thrombotic strokes and transitory cerebral ischemic attacks analyzed together as cerebral thromboembolic attacks.[82] In this study, the 219 cases during 1994 and 1995 included 146 cases of cerebral infarction and 73 cases of transient ischemic attacks. Only users of 2nd generation oral contraceptives (levonorgestrel, norgestrel, and norgestimate) had a statistically significant increased risk (about 2.5-fold). There was a dose-response relationship with estrogen in the dose ranges of 20, 30–40, and 50 µg ethinyl estradiol, although the number of 20 µg users (5 cases, 22 controls) was not sufficient to establish a lower risk at this lower dose. This analysis claimed a reduced risk associated with desogestrel and gestodene; however, the odds ratio did not achieve statistical significance. Risk was increased with smoking, treated hypertension, diabetes, heart diseases, frequent migraine, a family history of myocardial infarction, but not duration of use, or family history of venous thromboembolism.

Incidence of Stroke in Reproductive Age Women [88, 92, 95, 96]

Incidence of ischemic stroke	5 per 100,000 per year
	1–3 per 100,000 per year in women under age 35
	10 per 100,000 per year in women over age 35
Incidence of hemorrhagic stroke	6 per 100,000 per year
Excess cases per year due to OCs, including smokers and hypertensives	2 per 100,000 per year in low-dose OC users
	1 per 100,000 per year in low-dose OC users under age 35
	8 per 100,000 per year in high-dose OC users

Arterial Thrombosis — Current Assessment

There has been no evidence with respectable statistical power that the new progestins have an appreciable difference in risk for arterial disease, an event that is already *NOT* increased with low-dose older type progestin oral contraceptives. It is possible that as these studies continue and acquire greater statistical power, a difference will emerge, but even if this is the case, the difference will be minor and likely unmeasureable. Conclusions based on a limited number of cases are premature, and a critical attitude toward arterial thrombosis is appropriate just as such an approach finally revealed explanations for the initial findings with venous thrombosis.

Most importantly, the new studies fail to find any substantial risk of ischemic or hemorrhagic stroke with low-dose oral contraceptives in healthy, young women. The WHO study did find evidence for an adverse impact of smoking in women under age 35; the Kaiser study did not. This difference is explained by the confounding effect of hypertension, the major risk factor identified. In the WHO study, a history of hypertension was based on whether a patient reported ever having had high blood pressure (other than in pregnancy) and not validated by medical records. In the Kaiser study, women were classified as having hypertension if they reported using antihypertensive medication (less than 5% of oral contraceptive users had treated hypertension, and there were no users of higher dose products). In the WHO study, the effect of using oral contraceptives in the presence of a high-risk factor is apparent in the different odds ratios when European women who received good screening from clinicians were compared with women in developing countries who received little screening; therefore, more women with cardiovascular risk factors in developing countries were using oral contraceptives.

Over the years, there has been recurring discussion over whether to provide oral contraceptives over the counter on a non-prescription basis. The data in the WHO report make an impressive argument against such a move. The increased risk of myocardial infarction was most evident in developing countries where 70% of the cases received their oral contraceptives from a non-clinical source. Deprived of screening, women with risk factors in developing countries were exposed to greater risk.

Oral contraceptives containing less than 50 μg ethinyl estradiol do not increase the risk of myocardial infarction or stroke in healthy, nonsmoking women, regardless of age. The effect of smoking in women under age 35 is, as we have long recognized, not detectable in the absence of hypertension. After age 35, the subtle presence of hypertension makes analysis difficult, but the Kaiser study indicates that increasing age and smoking by themselves have little impact on the risk of stroke in low-dose oral contraceptive users. The screening of patients in the Kaiser program was excellent, resulting in few women with hypertension using oral contraceptives. *The new studies indicate that hypertension should be a major concern, especially in regards to the risk of stroke.* Certainly, women with uncontrolled hypertension should not use oral contraceptives. Generally, family planning experts have believed that well-treated hypertension should not be a contraindication for oral contraceptive use. The new data do not help us with this problem because it is impossible to accurately categorize hypertensive patients in the studies into groups representing successful and unsuccessful treatment. Nevertheless, the outstanding safety of low estrogen dose oral contraceptives in these studies supports the continued use of low-dose oral contraceptives in treated and well-controlled hypertensive women.

Smoking

Smoking continues to be a difficult problem, not only for patient management, but for analysis of data as well. In large U.S. surveys in 1982 and 1988, the decline in the prevalence of smoking was similar in users and nonusers of oral contraception; however, 24.3% of 35- to 45-year-old women who used oral contraceptives were smokers![97] In this group of smoking, oral contraceptive-using women, 85.3% smoked 15 or more cigarettes per day (heavy smoking). Despite the widespread teaching and publicity that smoking is a contraindication to oral contraceptive use over the age of 35, more older women who use oral contraceptives smoke and smoke heavily, compared with young women. This strongly implies that older smokers are less than honest with clinicians when requesting oral contraception, and this further raises serious concern over how well this confounding variable can be controlled in case-control and cohort studies. *A former smoker must have stopped smoking for at least 12 consecutive months to be regarded as a nonsmoker. Women who have nicotine in their bloodstream obtained from patches or gum should be regarded as smokers.*

Lipoproteins and Oral Contraception

The balance of estrogen and progestin potency in a given oral contraceptive formulation can potentially influence cardiovascular risk by its overall effect on lipoprotein levels. Oral contraceptives with relatively high doses of progestins (doses not used in today's low-dose formulations) do produce unfavorable lipoprotein changes.[98] The levonorgestrel triphasic exerts no significant changes on HDL-cholesterol, LDL-cholesterol, apoprotein B, and no change or an increase in apoprotein A, while the levonorgestrel monophasic combination (with a higher dose of levonorgestrel) has a tendency to increase LDL-cholesterol and apoprotein B, and to decrease HDL-cholesterol and apoprotein A. The monophasic desogestrel and desogestrel pills have a favorable effect on the lipoprotein profile, while the triphasic norgestimate and gestodene pills produce beneficial alterations in the LDL:HDL and apoprotein B:apoprotein A ratios.[99–102] Like the triphasic levonorgestrel pills, norethindrone multiphasic pills have no significant impact on the lipoprotein profile over 6–12 months.[103] *In summary, studies of low-dose formulations indicate that the adverse effects of progestins are limited to the fixed-dose combination with a dose of levonorgestrel that exceeds that in the multiphasic formulation.*

An important study in monkeys indicated a protective action of estrogen against atherosclerosis, but by a mechanism independent of the cholesterol-lipoprotein profile. Oral administration of a combination of estrogen and progestin to monkeys fed a high-cholesterol, atherogenic diet decreased the extent of coronary atherosclerosis despite a reduction in HDL-cholesterol levels.[104–106] In somewhat similar experiments, estrogen treatment markedly prevented arterial lesion development in rabbits.[107–109] In considering the impact of progestational agents, lowering of HDL is not necessarily atherogenic if accompanied by a significant estrogen impact. These animal studies help explain why older, higher dose combinations, which had an adverse impact on the lipoprotein profile did not increase subsequent cardiovascular disease.[34, 37] The estrogen component provided protection through a direct effect on vessel walls, especially favorably influencing vasomotor and platelet factors such as nitric oxide and prostacyclin.

This conclusion is reinforced by angiographic and autopsy studies. Young women with myocardial infarctions who have used oral contraceptives have less diffuse atherosclerosis than nonusers.[110, 111] Indeed, a case-control study indicated that the risk of myocardial infarction in patients taking older, high-dose levonorgestrel-containing formulations is the same as that experienced with pills containing other progestins.[34]

In the past decade, we have been subjected to considerable marketing hype about the importance of the impact of oral contraceptives on the cholesterol-lipoprotein profile. If indeed certain oral contraceptives had a negative impact on the lipoprotein profile, one would expect to find evidence of atherosclerosis as a cause of an increase in subsequent cardiovascular disease. There is no such evidence. Thus, the mechanism of the cardiovascular complications is undoubtedly a short-term acute mechanism—thrombosis (an estrogen-related effect).

Hypertension

Oral contraceptive-induced hypertension was observed in approximately 5% of users of higher dose pills. More recent evidence indicates that small increases in blood pressure can be observed even with 30 mg estrogen, monophasic pills, including those containing the new progestins. However, an increased incidence of clinically significant hypertension has not been reported.[112–115] The lack of clinical hypertension in most studies may be due to the rarity of its occurrence. The Nurses' Health Study observed an increased risk of clinical hypertension in current users of low-dose oral contraceptives, providing an incidence of 41.5 cases per 10,000 women per year.[116] Therefore, an annual assessment of blood pressure is still an important element of clinical surveillance, even when low-dose oral contraceptives are used. Postmenopausal women in the Rancho Bernardo Study who had previously used oral contraceptives (probably high-dose products) had slightly higher (2–4 mm Hg) diastolic blood pressures.[117] Because past users do not demonstrate differences in incidence or risk factors for cardiovascular disease, it is unlikely this blood pressure difference has an important clinical effect.

Variables such as previous toxemia of pregnancy or previous renal disease do not predict whether a woman will develop hypertension on oral contraception.[118] Likewise, women who have developed hypertension on oral contraception are not more predisposed to develop toxemia of pregnancy.

The mechanism for an effect on blood pressure is thought to involve the renin angiotensin system. The most consistent finding is a marked increase in plasma angiotensinogen, the renin substrate, up to 8 times normal values (on higher dose pills). In nearly all women, excessive vasoconstriction is prevented by a compensatory decrease in plasma renin concentration. If hypertension does develop, the renin-angiotensinogen changes take 3–6 months to disappear after stopping combined oral contraception.

One must also consider the effects of oral contraceptives in patients with preexisting hypertension or cardiac disease. In our view, with medical control of the blood pressure and close follow-up (at least every 3 months), the patient and her clinician may choose low-dose oral contraception. Close follow-up is also indicated in women with a history of preexisting renal disease or a strong family history of hypertension or cardiovascular disease. It seems prudent to suggest that patients with marginal cardiac reserve should utilize other means of contraception. Significant increases in cardiac output and plasma volume have been recorded with oral contraceptive use (higher dose pills), probably a result of fluid retention.

Cardiovascular Disease — Summary

The outpouring of epidemiologic data in the last few years allows the construction of a clinical formulation that is evidence-based. The following conclusions are consistent with the recent reports.

SUMMARY: Oral Contraceptives and Thrombosis

- **Pharmacologic estrogen increases the production of clotting factors.**

- **Progestins have no significant impact on clotting factors.**

- **Past users of oral contraceptives do not have an increased incidence of cardiovascular disease.**

- **All low-dose oral contraceptives, regardless of progestin type, have an increased risk of venous thromboembolism. The actual risk of venous thrombosis with low-dose oral contraceptives is lower in the new studies compared with previous reports. Some have argued that this is due to preferential prescribing and the healthy user effect. However, it is also logical that the lower risk reflects better screening of patients and lower estrogen doses.**

- **Smoking has no effect on the risk of venous thrombosis.**

- **Smoking and estrogen have an additive effect on the risk of arterial thrombosis. Why is there a difference between venous and arterial clotting? The venous system has low flow with a state of high fibrinogen and low platelets, in contrast to the high-flow state of the arterial system with low fibrinogen and high platelets. Thus, it is understandable why these two different systems can respond in different ways.**

- **Hypertension is a very important additive risk factor for stroke in oral contraceptive users.**

- **Low-dose oral contraceptives (less than 50 μg ethinyl estradiol) do not increase the risk of myocardial infarction or stroke in healthy, nonsmoking women, regardless of age.**

- **Almost all myocardial infarctions and strokes in oral contraceptive users occur in users of high-dose products, or users with cardiovascular risk factors over the age of 35.**

- **Arterial thrombosis (myocardial infarction and stroke) has a dose-response relationship with the dose of estrogen, but there are insufficient data to determine whether there is a difference in risk with products that contain 20, 30 or 35 μg ethinyl estradiol.**

The recent studies reinforce the belief that the risks of arterial and venous thrombosis are a consequence of the estrogen component of combination oral contraceptives. Current evidence does not support an advantage or disadvantage for any particular formulation, except for the greater safety associated with any product containing less than 50 μg ethinyl estradiol. Although it is logical to expect the greatest safety with the lowest dose of estrogen, the rare occurrence of arterial and venous thrombosis in healthy women makes it unlikely that there will be any measurable differences in the attributable incidence of clinical events with all low-dose products.

The new studies emphasize the importance of good patient screening. The occurrence of arterial thrombosis is essentially limited to older women who smoke or have cardiovascular risk factors, especially hypertension. The impact of good screening is evident in the repeated failure to detect an increase in mortality due to myocardial infarction or stroke in several studies.[53, 88] Although the risk of venous thromboembolism is slightly increased, the actual incidence is still relatively rare, and the mortality rate is about 1% (probably less with oral contraceptives, because most deaths from thrombocmbolism are associated with trauma, surgery, or a major illness). The minimal risk of venous thrombosis associated with oral contraceptive use does not justify the cost of routine screening for coagulation deficiencies. Nevertheless, the importance of this issue is illustrated by the increased risk of a very rare event, cerebral sinus thrombosis, in women who have an inherited predisposition for clotting and use oral contraceptives.[19, 119]

If a patient has a close family history (parent or sibliing) or a previous episode of idiopathic thromboembolism, an evaluation to search for an underlying abnormality in the coagulation system is warranted.[77] The following measurements are recommended, and abnormal results require consultation with a hematologist regarding prognosis and prophylactic treatment. The list of laboratory tests is long, and because this is a dynamic and changing field, the best advice is to consult with a hematologist. If a diagnosis of a congenital deficiency is made, screening should be offered to other family members.

Hypercoaguable Conditions	Thrombophilia Screening
Antithrombin III deficiency	Antithrombin III
Protein C deficiency	Protein C
Protein S deficiency	Protein S
Factor V Leiden mutation	Activated protein C resistance ratio
Prothrombin gene mutation	Activated partial thromboplastin time
Antiphospholipid syndrome	Hexagonal activated partial thromboplastin time
	Anticardiolipin antibodies
	Lupus anticoagulant
	Fibrinogen
	Prothrombin G mutation (DNA test)
	Thrombin Time
	Homocysteine level
	Complete blood count

Combination oral contraception is contraindicated in women who have a history of idiopathic venous thromboembolism, and also in women who have a close family history (parent or sibling) of idiopathic venous thromboembolism. These women will have a higher incidence of congenital deficiencies in important clotting measurements, especially antithrombin III, protein C, protein S, and resistance to activated protein C.[120] Such a patient who screens negatively for an inherited clotting deficiency might still consider the use of oral contraceptives, but this would be a difficult decision with unknown risks for both patient and clinician, and it seems more prudent to consider other contraceptive options. Other risk factors for thromboembolism that should be considered by clinicians include an acquired predisposition such as the presence of lupus anticoagulant or malignancy, and immobility or trauma. Varicose veins are not a risk factor unless they are very extensive.[48]

The conclusion once again is that low-dose oral contraceptives are very safe for healthy, young women. By effectively screening for the presence of smoking and cardiovascular risk factors, especially hypertension, in older women, we can limit, if not eliminate, any increased risk for arterial disease associated with low-dose oral contraceptives. And it is very important to emphasize that there is no increased risk of cardiovascular events associated with duration (long-term) use.

Carbohydrate Metabolism

With the older high-dose oral contraceptives, an impaired glucose tolerance test was present in many women. In these women, plasma levels of insulin as well as the blood sugar were elevated. Generally, the effect of oral contraception is to produce an increase in peripheral resistance to insulin action. Most women can meet this challenge by increasing insulin secretion, and there is no change in the glucose tolerance test, although 1-hour values may be slightly elevated.

Insulin sensitivity is affected mainly by the progestin component of the pill.[121] The derangement of carbohydrate metabolism may also be affected by estrogen influences on lipid metabolism, hepatic enzymes, and elevation of unbound cortisol. The glucose intolerance is dose-related, and once again effects are less with the low-dose formulations. *Insulin and glucose changes with low-dose monophasic and multiphasic oral contraceptives are so minimal, that it is now believed they are of no clinical significance.*[115, 122–124] This includes long-term evaluation with hemoglobin A1c.

The observed changes in studies of oral contraception and carbohydrate metabolism are in the nondiabetic range. In order to measure differences, investigators have resorted to analysis by measuring the area under the curve for glucose and insulin responses during glucose tolerance tests. A highly regarded cross-sectional study utilizing this technique reported that even lower dose formulations have detectable effects on insulin resistance.[121] The reason this is important is that it is now recognized that hyperinsulinemia due to insulin resistance is a contributor to cardiovascular disease. However, there are several critical questions that remain unanswered. Can the results from a cross-sectional study be duplicated in a study of sufficient size with patients serving as their own controls? Is a statistically significant hyperinsulinemia, detected in a study, clinically meaningful?

Because long-term, follow-up studies of large populations have failed to detect any increase in the incidence of diabetes mellitus or impaired glucose tolerance (even in past and current users of high-dose pills),[117, 125, 126] the concern now appropriately focuses on the slight impairment as a potential risk for cardiovascular disease. If slight hyperinsulinemia were meaningful, wouldn't you expect to see evidence of an increase in cardiovascular disease in past users who took oral contraceptives when doses were higher? As we have emphasized before, there is no such evidence. The data strongly indicate that the changes in lipids and carbohydrate metabolism that have been measured are not clinically meaningful.

It can be stated definitively that oral contraceptive use does not produce an increase in diabetes mellitus.[125–128] The hyperglycemia associated with oral contraception is not deleterious and is completely reversible. Even women who have risk factors for diabetes in their history are not affected. In women with recent gestational diabetes, no significant impact on glucose tolerance could be demonstrated over 6–13 months comparing the use of low-dose monophasic and multiphasic oral contraceptives with a control group, and no increase in the risk of overt diabetes mellitus could be detected with long-term follow-up.[129, 130] A high percentage of women with previous gestational diabetes develop overt diabetes and associated vascular complications. Until overt diabetes develops, it is appropriate for these patients to use low-dose oral contraception.

In clinical practice, it may, at times, be necessary to prescribe oral contraception for the overt diabetic. No effect on insulin requirement is expected with low-dose pills.[131] According to the older epidemiologic data, the use of oral contraceptives increases the risk of thrombosis in women with insulin-dependent diabetes mellitus; therefore, women with diabetes have been encouraged to use other forms of contraception. However, this effect in women under age 35 who are otherwise healthy is probably very minimal with low-dose oral contraception, and reliable protection against pregnancy is a benefit for these patients that outweighs the small risk. A case-control study could find no evidence that oral contraceptive use by young women with insulin-dependent diabetes mellitus increased the development of retinopathy or nephropathy.[132] In a 1-year study of women with insulin-dependent diabetes mellitus who were using a low-dose oral contraceptive, no deterioration could be documented in lipoprotein or hemostatic biochemical markers for cardiovascular risk.[133]

The Liver

The liver is affected in more ways and with more regularity and intensity by the sex steroids than any other extragenital organ. Estrogen influences the synthesis of hepatic DNA and RNA, hepatic cell enzymes, serum enzymes formed in the liver, and plasma proteins. Estrogenic hormones also affect hepatic lipid and lipoprotein formation, the intermediary metabolism of carbohydrates, and intracellular enzyme activity. Nevertheless, an extensive analysis of the prospective cohorts of women in the Royal College of General Practitioners' Oral Contraception Study and the Oxford-Family Planning Association Contraceptive Study could detect no evidence of an increased incidence or risk of serious liver disease among oral contraceptive users.[134]

The active transport of biliary components is impaired by estrogens as well as some progestins. The mechanism is unclear, but cholestatic jaundice and pruritus were occasional complications of higher dose oral contraception, and are similar to the recurrent jaundice of pregnancy, i.e., benign and reversible. The incidence with lower dose oral contraception is unknown, but it must be a very rare occurrence.

The only absolute hepatic contraindication to oral contraceptive use is acute or chronic cholestatic liver disease. Cirrhosis and previous hepatitis are not aggravated. Once recovered from the acute phase of liver disease, a woman can use oral contraception.

Data from the Royal College of General Practitioners' prospective study indicated that an increase in the incidence of gallstones occurred in the first years of oral contraceptive use, apparently due to an acceleration of gallbladder disease in women already susceptible.[135] In other words, the overall risk of gallbladder disease was not increased, but in the first years of use, disease was activated or accelerated in women who were vulnerable because of asymptomatic disease or a tendency toward gallbladder disease. The mechanism appears to be induced alterations in the composition of gallbladder bile, specifically a rise in cholesterol saturation that is presumably an estrogen effect.[136] The Nurses' Health Study reported no significant increase in the risk of symptomatic gallstones among ever-users, but slightly elevated risks among current and long-term users.[137] Although oral contraceptive use has been linked to an increased risk of gallbladder disease, the epidemiologic evidence has been inconsistent. Indeed an Italian case-control study and a report from the Oxford Family Planning Association cohort found no increase in the risk of gallbladder disease in association with oral contraceptive use and no interaction with increasing age or body weight.[138, 139] Keep in mind that even though some studies found a statistically significant modest increase in the relative risk of gallbladder disease, even if the effect were real, it is of little clinical importance because the actual incidence of this problem is very low.

Other Metabolic Effects

Nausea, breast discomfort, and weight gain continue to be disturbing effects, but their incidence is significantly less with low-dose oral contraception. Fortunately, these effects are most intense in the first few months of use and, in most cases, gradually disappear. Weight gain usually responds to dietary restriction, but for some patients, the weight gain is an anabolic response to the sex steroids, and discontinuation of oral contraception is the only way that weight loss can be achieved. This must be rare with low-dose oral contraception because data in published studies fail to indicate a difference in body weight between users and nonusers.[140, 141]

There is no association between oral contraception and peptic ulcer disease or inflammatory bowel disease.[142, 143] Oral contraception is not recommended for patients with problems of gastrointestinal malabsorption because of the possibility of contraceptive failure.

Chloasma, a patchy increase in facial pigment, was, at one time, found to occur in approximately 5% of oral contraceptive users. It is now a rare problem due to the decrease in estrogen dose. Unfortunately, once chloasma appears, it fades only gradually following discontinuation of the pill and may never disappear completely. Skin-blanching medications may be useful.

Hematologic effects include an increased sedimentation rate, increased total iron-binding capacity due to the increase in globulins, and a decrease in prothrombin time. The continuous use of oral contraceptives may prevent the appearance of symptoms in porphyria precipitated by menses. Changes in vitamin metabolism have been noted: a small nonharmful increase in vitamin A and decreases in blood levels of pyridoxine (B_6) and the other B vitamins, folic acid, and ascorbic acid. Despite these changes, routine vitamin supplements are not necessary for women eating adequate, normal diets.

Mental depression is very rarely associated with oral contraceptives. In studies with higher dose oral contraceptives, the effect was due to estrogen interference with the synthesis of tryptophan that could be reversed with pyridoxine treatment. It seems wiser, however, to discontinue oral contraception if depression is encountered. Though infrequent, a reduction in libido is occasionally a problem and may be a cause for seeking an alternative method of contraception.

Adverse androgenic voice changes were occasionally encountered with the use of the first very high-dose oral contraceptives. Vocal virilization can be a serious and devastating problem for some women, especially when vocal performance is important. Careful study of women on low-dose oral contraceptives indicates that this is no longer a side effect of concern.[144]

The Risk of Cancer

Endometrial Cancer

The use of oral contraception protects against endometrial cancer. Use for at least 12 months reduces the risk of developing endometrial cancer by **50%**, with the greatest protective effect gained by use for more than 3 years.[145–147] This protection persists for 20 or more years after discontinuation (the actual length of duration of protection is unknown) and is greatest in women at highest risk: nulliparous and low parity women.[148] This protection is equally protective for all 3 major histologic subtypes of endometrial cancer: adenocarcinoma, adenoacanthoma, and adenosquamous cancers. Finally, protection is seen with all monophasic formulations of oral contraceptives, including pills with less than 50 μg estrogen.[145] There are no data as yet with multiphasic preparations or the new progestin formulations, but because these products are still dominated by their progestational component, there is every reason to believe that they will be protective.

Ovarian Cancer

Protection against ovarian cancer, the most lethal of female reproductive tract cancers, is one of the most important benefits of oral contraception. Because this cancer is detected late and prognosis is poor, the impact of this protection is very significant. Indeed, a decline in mortality from ovarian cancer has been observed in several countries since the early 1970s, perhaps an effect of oral contraceptive use.[149] The risk of developing epithelial ovarian cancer of all histologic subtypes in users of oral contraception is reduced by **40%** compared with that of nonusers.[147, 150–152] This protective effect increases with duration of use and continues for at least 10–15 years after stopping the medication. This protection is seen in women who use oral contraception for as little as 3 to 6 months (although at least 3 years of use are required for a notable impact), reaches an 80% reduction in risk with more than 10 years of use, and is a benefit associated with all monophasic formulations, including the low-dose products.[153] The protective effect of oral contraceptives is especially observed in women at high risk of ovarian cancer (nulliparous women and women with a positive family history).[154] Continuous use of oral contraception for 10 years by women with a positive family history for ovarian cancer can reduce the risk of epithelial ovarian cancer to a level equal to or less than that experienced by women with a negative family history.[154] Again, the multiphasic and new progestin products have not been in use long enough to yield any data on this issue, but because ovulation is effectively inhibited by these formulations, protection against ovarian cancer should be exerted. The same magnitude of protection has been observed in a case-control study of women with *BRCA1 or BRCA2* mutations.[155]

Cancer of the Cervix

Studies have indicated that the risk for dysplasia and carcinoma in situ of the uterine cervix increases with the use of oral contraception for more than one year.[156–160] Invasive cervical cancer may be increased after 5 years of use, reaching a two-fold increase after 10 years. It is well recognized, however, that the number of partners a woman has had and age at first coitus are the most important risk factors for cervical neoplasia. Other confounding factors include exposure to human papillomavirus, the use of barrier contraception (protective), and smoking. These are difficult factors to control, and, therefore, the conclusions regarding cervical cancer are not definitive. An excellent study from the Centers for Disease Control and Prevention (CDC) concluded there is no increased risk of invasive cervical cancer in users of oral contraception, and an apparent increased risk of carcinoma in situ is due to enhanced detection of disease (because oral contraceptive users have more frequent Pap smears).[159] In the World Health Organization Study of Neoplasia and Steroid Contraceptives, a Pap smear screening bias was identified, nevertheless the evidence still suggested an increased risk of cervical carcinoma in situ with long-term oral contraceptive use.[160]

A case-control study of patients in Panama, Costa Rica, Colombia, and Mexico concluded that there was a significantly increased risk for invasive adenocarcinoma.[161] Similar results were obtained in a case-control study in Los Angeles and in the World Health Organization Collaborative Study.[162, 163] In Los Angeles, the relative risk of adenocarcinoma of the cervix increased from 2.1 with ever use to 4.4 with 12 or more years of oral contraceptive use.[162] Because the incidence of adenocarcinoma of the cervix (10% of all cervical cancers) has increased in young women over the last 20 years, there is concern that this increase reflects the use of oral contraception.[164] Oral contraceptives increase cervical ectopia, but whether this increases the risk of cervical adenocarcinoma is unclear.

This concern obviously is an important reason for annual Pap smear surveillance. Fortunately, steroid contraception does not mask abnormal cervical changes, and the necessity for prescription renewals offers the opportunity for improved screening for cervical disease. It is reasonable to perform Pap smears every 6 months in women using oral contraception for 5 or more years who are also at higher risk because of their sexual behavior (multiple partners, history of sexually transmitted diseases). Oral contraceptive use is appropriate for women with a history of cervical intraepithelial neoplasia (CIN), including those who have been surgically treated.

Liver Adenomas

Hepatocellular adenomas can be produced by steroids of both the estrogen and androgen families. Actually, there are several different lesions, peliosis, focal nodular hyperplasia, and adenomas. Peliosis is characterized by dilated vascular spaces without endothelial lining, and may occur in the absence of adenomatous changes. The adenomas are not malignant; their significance lies in the potential for hemorrhage. The most common presentation is acute right upper quadrant or epigastric pain. The tumors may be asymptomatic, or they may present suddenly with hemato-peritoneum. There is some evidence that the tumors and focal nodular hyperplasia regress when oral contraception is stopped.[165, 166] Epidemiologic data have not supported the contention that mestranol increased the risk more than ethinyl estradiol.

The risk appears to be related to duration of oral contraceptive use and to the steroid dose in the pills. This is reinforced by the rarity of the condition ever since low-dose oral contraception became available. The ongoing prospective studies have accumulated many woman-years of use and have not identified an increased incidence of such tumors.[134] In our view it is not even worth mentioning during the informed consent (choice) process.

No reliable screening test or procedure is currently available. Routine liver function tests are normal. Computed tomography (CT) scanning or magnetic resonance imaging (MRI) is the best means of diagnosis; angiography and ultrasonography are not reliable. Palpation of the liver should be part of the periodic evaluation in oral contraceptive users. If an enlarged liver is found, oral contraception should be stopped, and regression should be evaluated and followed by imaging.

Liver Cancer

Oral contraception has been linked to the development of hepatocellular carcinoma.[167, 168] However, the very small number of cases, and, thus, the limited statistical power, requires great caution in interpretation. The largest study on this question, the WHO Collaborative Study of Neoplasia and Steroid Contraceptives, found no association between oral contraception and liver cancer.[169] Even case-control analysis of oral contraceptives containing cyproterone acetate (known to be toxic to the liver in high doses) could detect no evidence of an increased risk of liver cancer.[170] In the United States, Japan, Sweden, England, and Wales, the death rates from liver cancer have not changed over the last 3 decades despite introduction and use of oral contraception.[171, 172]

Breast Cancer

Because of its prevalence and its long latent phase, concern over the relationship between oral contraception and breast cancer continues to be an issue in the minds of both patients and clinicians. Unfortunately, the issue is not totally resolved and probably will not be until another decade passes, allowing data to emerge from the modern era of lower dose oral contraception.

Worth emphasizing is the protective effect of higher dose oral contraception on benign breast disease, an effect that became apparent after 2 years of use.[173] After 2 years there was a progressive reduction (about 40%) in the incidence of fibrocystic disease of the breast. Women who used oral contraception were one-fourth as likely to develop benign breast disease as nonusers, but this protection was limited to current and recent users. It is still uncertain whether this same protection is provided by the lower dose products. A French case-control study indicated a reduction of nonproliferative benign breast disease associated with low-dose oral contraceptives used before a first full-term pregnancy, but no effect on proliferative disease or with use after a pregnancy.[174]

The Royal College of General Practitioners,[175] Oxford Family Planning Association,[176, 177] and Walnut Creek[178] cohort studies (and more recently, the Nurses' Health Study)[179] indicated no significant differences in breast cancer rates between users and nonusers. However, patients were enrolled in these studies at a time when oral contraception was used primarily by married couples spacing out their children. Beginning in the 1980s, oral contraception was primarily being used by women early in life, for longer durations, and to delay an initial pregnancy (remember, a full-term pregnancy early in life protects against breast cancer).

Over the last decade, case-control studies have focused on the use of oral contraception early in life, for long duration, and to delay a first, full-term pregnancy. Because the cohort of women who have used oral contraception in this fashion is just now beginning to reach the ages of postmenopausal breast cancer, the studies have had to focus on the risk of breast cancer diagnosed before age 45 (only 13% of all breast cancer). The results of these studies have not been clear-cut. Some studies have indicated an overall increased relative risk of early, premenopausal breast cancer,[180–187] while others indicated no increase in overall risk.[188–190] The most impressive finding indicates a link in most studies,[191–196] but not all,[197–201] of early breast cancer before age 40 with women who used oral contraception for long durations of time.

A collaborative group composed of an enormous number of epidemiologists and cancer investigators from around the world re-analyzed data from 54 studies in 26 countries, a total of 53,297 women with breast cancer and 100,239 without breast cancer, in order to assess the relationship between the risk of breast cancer and the use of oral contraceptives.[202] Oral contraceptives were grouped into 3 categories: low, medium, and high dose (which correlated with <50µg, 50 µg, and >50 µg of estrogen). At the time of diagnosis, 9% of the women with breast cancer were under age 35, 25% were 35–44, 33% were 45–54, and 33% were age 55 and older. A similar percentage of women with breast cancer (41%) and women without breast cancer (40%) had used combined oral contraceptives at some time in their lives. Overall, the relative risk (RR) of breast cancer in ever users of oral contraceptives was very slightly elevated and statistically significant: RR = 1.07; CI = 1.03–1.10.

The relative risk analyzed by duration of use was barely elevated and not statistically significant (even when long-term use, virtually continuous, was analyzed). Women who had begun use as teenagers had about a 20% statistically significant increased relative risk. In other words, recent users who began use before age 20 had a higher relative risk compared with recent users who began at later ages. The evidence was strong for a relationship with time since last use, an elevated risk being significant for current users and in women who had stopped use 1–4 years before (recent use). No influence on this risk was observed with the following: a family history of breast cancer, age of menarche, country of origin, ethnic groups, body weight, alcohol use, years of education, and the design of the study. There was no variation according to specific type of estrogen or progestin in the various products. Importantly, there was no statistically significant effect of low, medium, or high dose preparations. Ten or more years after stopping use, there was no increased risk of breast cancer. Indeed, the risk of metastatic disease compared with localized tumors was reduced: Relative Risk = 0.88; CI = 0.81–0.95.

Oral Contraceptives and the Risk of Breast Cancer
Re-analysis of the World's Data [202]

Current users	RR = 1.24, 95% CI 1.15–1.33
1–4 years after stopping	RR = 1.16, 95% CI 1.08–1.23
5–9 years after stopping	RR = 1.07, 95% CI 1.02–1.13

Data were limited for progestin-only methods. The re-analysis indicated that the results were similar to those with combined oral contraceptives, but a close look at the numbers reveals that not one relative risk reached statistical significance.

Overall, this massive statistical exercise yielded good news. No major adverse impact of oral contraceptives emerged. ***Even though the data indicated that young women who begin use before age 20 have higher relative risks of breast cancer during current use and in the 5 years after stopping, this is a time period when breast cancer is very rare; and, thus, there would be little impact on the actual number of breast cancers.*** The difference between localized disease and metastatic disease was statistically greater and should be observable. Thus many years after stopping oral contraceptive use, the main effect may be protection against metastatic disease. Breast cancer is more common in older years, and 10 or more years after stopping, the risk was not increased.

What other explanation could account for an increased risk associated only with current or recent use, no increase with duration of use, and a return to normal 10 years after exposure? The slightly increased risk could be influenced by detection/surveillance bias (more interaction with the health care system by oral contraceptive users). It is also possible that this situation is analogous to that of pregnancy. Recent studies indicate that pregnancy transiently increases the risk of breast cancer (for a period of several years) after a woman's first childbirth, and this is followed by a lifetime reduction in risk.[203] And some have found that a concurrent or recent pregnancy adversely affects survival.[204, 205] It is argued that breast cells that have already begun malignant transformation are adversely affected by the hormones of pregnancy, while normal stem cells become more resistant because of a pregnancy. It is possible that early and recent use of oral contraceptives also accelerates the growth of a pre-existing malignancy, explaining the limitation of the finding to current and recent use and the increase in localized disease. With the accumulation of greater numbers of older women previously exposed to oral contraceptives, a protective effect may become evident. In a case-control study of women in Toronto, Canada, age 40–69 years, those women who had used oral contraceptives for 5 or more years, 15 or more years previously, had a 50% reduced risk of breast cancer.[206]

Conclusion

Adding up the benefits of oral contraception, the possible slight increase in risk of breast cancer is far outweighed by positive effects on our public health. But the impact on public health is of little concern during the private clinician–patient interchange in the office. Here personal risk receives highest priority; fear of cancer is a motivating force, and compliance with effective contraception requires accurate information. For these reasons, we provide the following summary of our assessment of the impact of oral contraceptives on the risk of breast cancer.

SUMMARY: Oral Contraceptives and the Risk of Breast Cancer

- **Current and recent use of oral contraceptives may be associated with about a 20% increased risk of early premenopausal breast cancer, essentially limited to localized disease and a very small increase in the actual number of cases (so small, there would be no major impact on incidence figures). This finding may be due to detection/surveillance bias and accelerated growth of already present malignancies, a situation similar to the effects of pregnancy and postmenopausal hormone therapy on the risk of breast cancer (as reviewed in Chapter 18). Further comfort can be derived from the fact that the increase in breast cancer in American women was greater in older women from 1973 to 1994, those who did not have the opportunity to use oral contraception.[207] In women under 50 years of age, there was only a slight increase during this same time period.**

- **Previous oral contraceptive use may be associated with a reduced risk of metastatic breast cancer later in life, and possibly with a reduced risk of postmenopausal breast cancer.**

- **Oral contraceptive use does not further increase the risk of breast cancer in women with positive family histories of breast cancer or in women with proven benign breast disease.**

- **The clinician should not fail to take every opportunity to direct attention to all factors that affect breast cancer. Breastfeeding and control of alcohol intake are good examples, and are also components of preventive health care. Especially important is this added motivation to encourage breastfeeding. The protective effect of breastfeeding is exerted (although it is probably a small one; see Chapter 16) on premenopausal breast cancer, the cancer of concern to younger women using oral contraception.**

Other Cancers

The Walnut Creek study suggested that melanoma was linked to oral contraception; however, the major risk factor for melanoma is exposure to sunlight. More recent and accurate evaluation utilizing both the Royal College General Practitioners and Oxford Family Planning Association prospective cohorts and accounting for exposure to sunlight did not indicate a significant difference in the risk of melanoma comparing users to nonusers.[208, 209] There is no evidence linking oral contraceptive use to kidney cancer, gallbladder cancer, or pituitary tumors.[210] Long-term oral contraceptive use may slightly increase the risk of molar pregnancy, but there is no convincing evidence of a cause-and-effect association.[211] Although previous studies have not been in agreement, the Nurses' Health Study reports about a 40% reduced risk of colorectal cancer associated with 8 years of previous use of oral contraceptives (most likely higher dose products).[212]

Endocrine Effects

Adrenal Gland

Estrogen increases the cortisol-binding globulin (CBG). It had been thought that the increase in plasma cortisol while on oral contraception was due to increased binding by this globulin and not an increase in free active cortisol. Now it is apparent that free and active cortisol levels are also elevated. Estrogen decreases the ability of the liver to metabolize cortisol, and in addition, progesterone and related compounds can displace cortisol from transcortin, and thus contribute to the elevation of unbound cortisol. The effects of these elevated levels over prolonged periods of time are unknown, but no obvious impact has become apparent. To put this into perspective, the increase is not as great as that which occurs in pregnancy, and, in fact, it is within the normal range for nonpregnant women.

The adrenal gland responds to adrenocorticotropic hormone (ACTH) normally in women on oral contraceptives; therefore, there is no suppression of the adrenal gland itself. Initial studies indicated that the response to metyrapone (an 11β-hydroxylase blocker) was abnormal, suggesting that the pituitary was suppressed. However, estrogen accelerates the conjugation of metyrapone by the liver; and, therefore, the drug has less effect, thus explaining the subnormal responses initially reported. The pituitary-adrenal reaction to stress is normal in women on oral contraceptive pills.

Thyroid

Estrogen increases the synthesis and circulating levels of thyroxine-binding globulin, Prior to the introduction of new methods for measuring free thyroxine levels, evaluation of thyroid function was a problem. Measurement of TSH (thyroid-stimulating hormone) and the free thyroxine level in a woman on oral contraception provide an accurate assessment of a patient's thyroid state. Oral contraception affects the total thyroxine level in the blood as well as the amount of binding globulin, but the free thyroxine level is unchanged.

Oral Contraception and Reproduction

The impact of oral contraceptives on the reproductive system is less than initially thought. Early studies that indicated adverse effects have not stood the test of time and the scrutiny of multiple, careful studies. There are two major areas that deserve review: (1). Inadvertent use of oral contraceptives during the cycle of conception and during early pregnancy, and (2). Reproduction after discontinuing oral contraception.

Inadvertent Use During the Cycle of Conception and During Early Pregnancy

One of the reasons, if not the major reason, why a lack of withdrawal bleeding while using oral contraceptives is such a problem is the anxiety produced in both patient and clinician. The patient is anxious because of the uncertainty regarding pregnancy, and the clinician is anxious because of the concerns stemming from the retrospective studies that indicated an increased risk of congenital malformations among the offspring of women who were pregnant and using oral contraception.

Organogenesis does not occur in the first 2 embryonic weeks (first 4 weeks since last menstrual period); however, teratogenic effects are possible between the third and eighth embryonic weeks (5 to 10 weeks since LMP).

Initial positive reports linking the use of contraceptive steroids to congenital malformations have not been substantiated. Many suspect a strong component of recall bias in the few positive studies due to a tendency of patients with malformed infants to recall details better than those with normal children. Other confounding problems have included a failure to consider the reasons for the administration of hormones (e.g., bleeding in an already abnormal pregnancy), and a failure to delineate the exact timing of the treatment (e.g., treatment was sometimes confined to a period of time during which the heart could not have been affected).

An association with cardiac anomalies was first claimed in the 1970s.[213, 214] This link received considerable support with a report from the U.S. Collaborative Perinatal Project; however, subsequent analysis of these data uncovered several methodologic shortcomings.[215] Simpson, in a very thorough and critical review in 1990, concluded that there was no reliable evidence implicating sex steroids as cardiac teratogens.[216] In fact, in his review, Simpson found no relationship between oral contraception and the following problems: hypospadias, limb reduction anomalies, neural tube defects, and mutagenic effects which would be responsible for chromosomally abnormal fetuses. Even virilization is not a practical consideration because the doses required (e.g., 20–40 mg norethindrone per day) are in excess of anything currently used. These conclusions reflect use of combined oral contraceptives as well as progestins alone.

In the past there was a concern regarding the VACTERL complex. VACTERL refers to a complex of vertebral, anal, cardiac, tracheoesophageal, renal, and limb anomalies. While case-control studies indicated a relationship with oral contraception, prospective studies have failed to observe any connection between sex steroids and the VACTERL complex.[217] A meta-analysis of 26 prospective studies of the risk of birth defects with oral contraceptive ingestion during pregnancy concluded that there was no increase in risk for major malformations, congenital heart defects, or limb reduction defects.[218]

Women who become pregnant while taking oral contraceptives or women who inadvertently take birth control pills early n pregnancy should be advised that the risk of a significant congenital anomaly is no greater than the general rate of 2–3%. This recommendation can be extended to those pregnant woman who have been exposed to a progestational agent such as medroxyprogesterone acetate or 17-hydroxyprogesterone caproate.[219, 220]

Reproduction After Discontinuing Oral Contraception

Fertility

The early reports from the British prospective studies indicated that former users of oral contraception had a delay in achieving pregnancy. In the Oxford Family Planning Association study, former use had an effect on fertility for up to 42 months in nulligravida women and for up to 30 months in multigravida women.[221] Presumably, the delay is due to lingering suppression of the hypothalamic-pituitary reproductive system.

A later analysis of the Oxford data indicated that the delay was concentrated in women age 30–34 who have never given birth.[222] At 48 months, 82% of these women had given birth compared with 89% of users of other contraceptive methods, not a big difference. No effect was observed in women younger than 30 or in women who had previously given birth. Childless women age 25–29 experienced some delay in return to fertility, but by 48 months, 91% had given birth compared with 92% in users of other methods. It should be noted that after 72 months the proportions of women who remained undelivered were the same in both groups of women.

This delay has been observed in the United States as well. In the Boston area, the interval from cessation of contraception to conception was 13 months or greater for 24.8% of prior oral contraceptive users compared with 10.6% for former users of all other methods (12.4% for intrauterine device {IUD} users, 8.5% for diaphragm uses, and 11.9% for other methods).[223] Oral contraceptive users had a lower monthly percentage of conceptions for the first 3 months, and somewhat lower percentage from 4 to 10 months. It took 24 months for 90% of previous oral contraceptive users to become pregnant, 14 months for IUD users, and 10 months for diaphragm users. Similar findings in Connecticut indicate that this delay lasts at least a year, and the effect is greater with higher dose preparations.[224] Despite this delay, there is no evidence that infertility is increased by the use of oral contraception. In fact, in young women, previous oral contraceptive use is associated with a lower risk of primary infertility.[225]

Spontaneous Miscarriage

There is no increase in the incidence of spontaneous miscarriage in pregnancies after the cessation of oral contraception. Indeed, the rate of spontaneous miscarriages and stillbirths is slightly less in former pill users, about 1% less for spontaneous miscarriages and 0.3% less for stillbirths.[226] A protective effect of previous oral contraceptive use against spontaneous miscarriage has been observed to be more apparent in women who become pregnant after age 30.[227]

Pregnancy Outcome

There is no evidence that oral contraceptives cause changes in individual germ cells that would yield an abnormal child at a later time.[216] There is no increase in the number of abnormal children born to former oral contraceptive users, and there is no change in the sex ratio (a sign of sex-linked recessive mutations).[226, 228] These observations are not altered when analyzed for duration of use. Initial observations that women who had previously used oral contraception had an increase in chromosomally abnormal fetuses have not been confirmed. Furthermore, as noted above, there is no increase in the miscarriage rate after discontinuation, something one would expect if oral contraceptives induce chromosomal abnormalities because these are the principal cause of spontaneous miscarriage.

In a 3-year follow-up of children whose mothers used oral contraceptives prior to conception, no differences could be detected in weight, anemia, intelligence, or development.[229] Former pill users have no increased risks for the following: perinatal morbidity or mortality, prematurity, and low birth weight.[230, 231] Dizygous twinning has been observed to be nearly two-fold (1.6% versus 1.0%) increased in women who conceive soon after cessation of oral contraception.[226] This effect was greater with longer duration of use.

The only reason (and it is a good one) to recommend that women defer attempts to conceive for a month or two after stopping the pill is to improve the accuracy of gestational dating by allowing accurate identification of the last menstrual period.

Breastfeeding

Oral contraception has been demonstrated to diminish the quantity and quality of lactation in postpartum women. Also of concern is the potential hazard of transfer of contraceptive steroids to the infant (a significant amount of the progestational component is transferred into breast milk);[232] however, no adverse effects have thus far been identified. Women who use oral contraception have a lower incidence of breastfeeding after the 6th postpartum month, regardless of whether oral contraception is started at the first, second, or third postpartum month.[233–235]

In adequately nourished breastfeeding women, no impairment of infant growth can be detected; presumably, compensation is achieved either through supplementary feedings or increased suckling.[236] In an 8-year follow-up study of children breastfed by mothers using oral contraceptives, no effect could be detected on diseases, intelligence, or psychological behavior.[237] This study also found that mothers on birth control pills lactated a significantly shorter period of time than controls, a mean of 3.7 months versus 4.6 months in controls.

Because the above considerations indicate that oral contraception shortens the duration of breastfeeding, it is worthwhile to consider the contraceptive effectiveness of lactation. The contraceptive effectiveness of lactation, i.e., the length of the interval between births, depends on the level of nutrition of the mother (if low, the longer the contraceptive interval), the intensity of suckling, and the extent to which supplemental food is added to the infant diet. If suckling intensity and/or frequency is diminished, contraceptive effect is reduced. Only amenorrheic women who exclusively breastfeed (full breastfeeding) at regular intervals, including nighttime, during the first 6 months have the contraceptive protection equivalent to that provided by oral contraception (98% efficacy); with menstruation or after 6 months, the chance of ovulation increases.[238, 239] With full or nearly full breastfeeding, approximately 70% of women remain amenorrheic through 6 months and only 37% through one year; nevertheless with exclusive breastfeeding, the contraceptive efficacy at one year is high, at 92%.[239] Fully breastfeeding women commonly have some vaginal bleeding or spotting in the first 8 postpartum weeks, but this bleeding is not due to ovulation.[240]

Supplemental feeding increases the chance of ovulation (and pregnancy) even in amenorrheic women.[241] Total protection is achieved by the exclusively breastfeeding woman for a duration of only 10 weeks.[240] Half of women studied who are not fully breastfeeding ovulate before the 6th week, the time of the traditional postpartum visit; a visit during the 3rd postpartum week is strongly recommended for contraceptive counseling.

It is apparent that although lactation provides a contraceptive effect, it is variable and not reliable for every woman. Furthermore, because frequent suckling is required to maintain full milk production, women who use oral contraception and also breastfeed less frequently (e.g., because they work outside their home) have two reasons for decreased milk volume. This combination can make it especially difficult to continue nursing.

Initiation of Oral Contraception in the Postpartum Period

The individual woman is in need of contraception early in the postpartum period. In a careful study of 22 postpartum, nonbreastfeeding women, the mean time from delivery to the first menses was 45 ± 10.1 days, and no woman ovulated before 25 days after delivery.[242] A high proportion of the first cycles (81.8%) and the subsequent cycles (37%) were not normal; however, this is certainly not predictable in individual women. Others have documented a mean delay of 7 weeks before resumption of ovulation, but half of the women studied ovulated before the 6th week, the time of the traditional postpartum visit. *The obstetrical tradition of scheduling the postpartum visit at 6 weeks should be changed. A 3-week visit would be more productive in avoiding postpartum surprises.*

The Rule of 3's:

In the presence of FULL breastfeeding, a contraceptive method should be used beginning in the *3rd postpartum month*.

With PARTIAL breastfeeding or NO breastfeeding, a contraceptive method should begin during the *3rd postpartum week*.

After the termination of a pregnancy of less than 12 weeks, oral contraception can be started immediately. After a pregnancy of 12 or more weeks, oral contraception has traditionally been started 2 weeks after delivery to avoid an increased risk of thrombosis during the initial postpartum period. We believe that oral contraception can be started immediately after a second-trimester abortion or premature delivery.

Because of the concerns regarding the impact of oral contraceptives on breastfeeding, a useful alternative is to combine the contraceptive effect of lactation with the progestin-only minipill. This low dose of progestin has no negative impact on breast milk, and some studies document an increase in milk quantity and nutritional quality.[243] Highly effective (near total) protection can be achieved with the combination of lactation and the minipill. Because of the slight positive impact on lactation, the minipill can be started soon after delivery, but at least a 3-day postpartum delay is recommended to allow the decline in pregnancy levels of estrogen and progesterone and the establishment of lactation.[244] In addition, use of the progestin-only minipill has been reported to be associated with a 3-fold increased risk of diabetes mellitus in lactating women with recent gestational diabetes.[130] This special group of women should consider other methods of contraception.

Other Considerations

Prolactin-Secreting Adenomas

Because estrogen is known to stimulate prolactin secretion and to cause hypertrophy of the pituitary lactotrophs, it is appropriate to be concerned over a possible relationship between oral contraception and prolactin-secreting adenomas. Case-control studies have uniformly concluded that no such relationship exists.[245, 246] Data from both the Royal College of General Practitioners and the Oxford Family Planning Association studies indicated no increase in the incidence of pituitary adenomas.[210, 247] Previous use of oral contraceptives is not related to the size of prolactinomas at presentation and diagnosis.[247, 248] Oral contraception can be prescribed to patients with pituitary microadenomas without fear of subsequent tumor growth.[249, 250] *We have routinely prescribed oral contraception to patients with pituitary microadenomas and have never observed evidence of tumor growth.*

Postpill Amenorrhea

The approximate incidence of "postpill amenorrhea" is 0.7–0.8%, which is equal to the incidence of spontaneous secondary amenorrhea,[231, 251, 252] and there is no evidence to support the idea that oral contraception causes secondary amenorrhea. If a cause-and-effect relationship exists between oral contraception and subsequent amenorrhea, one would expect the incidence of infertility to be increased after a given population discontinues use of oral contraception. In those women who discontinue oral contraception in order to get pregnant, 50% conceive by 3 months, and after 2 years, a maximum of 15% of nulliparous women and 7% of parous women fail to conceive.[231] rates comparable with those quoted for the prevalence of spontaneous infertility. Attempts to document a cause-and-effect relationship between oral contraceptive use and secondary amenorrhea have failed.[253] Although patients with this problem come more quickly to our attention because of previous oral contraceptive use and follow-up, there is no cause-and-effect relationship. Women who have not resumed menstrual function within 12 months should be evaluated as any other patient with secondary amenorrhea.

Use During Puberty

Should oral contraception be advised for a young woman with irregular menses and oligo-ovulation or anovulation? The fear of subsequent infertility should not be a deterrent to providing appropriate contraception. Women who have irregular menstrual periods are more likely to develop secondary amenorrhea whether they use oral contraception or not. The possibility of subsequent secondary amenorrhea is less of a risk and a less urgent problem for a young woman than leaving her unprotected. The need for contraception takes precedence

There is no evidence that the use of oral contraceptives in the pubertal, sexually active girl impairs growth and development of the reproductive system.[225] Again, the most important concern is and should be the prevention of an unwanted pregnancy. For most teenagers, oral contraception, dispensed in the 28-day package for better compliance, is the contraceptive method of choice.

Infections and Oral Contraception

Viral STDs

The viral STDs include human immunodeficiency virus (HIV), human papillomavirus (HPV), herpes simplex virus (HSV), and hepatitis B (HBV). At the present time, no known associations exist between oral contraception and the viral STDs. Of course, significant prevention includes barrier methods of contraception. Thus far, most studies have found no association between oral contraceptive use and HIV seropositivity, and some have indicated a protective effect.[254–256] *For women not in a stable, monogamous relationship, a dual approach is recommended, combining the contraceptive efficacy and protection against PID offered by oral contraception with the use of a barrier method (and spermicide) for prevention of viral STDs.*

Bacterial STDs

Sexually transmitted diseases (STDs) are one of the most common public health problems in the United States. It was estimated in 1995, that 7.6% of reproductive age U.S. women reported having been treated for pelvic inflammatory disease (PID).[257] This upper genital tract infection is usually a consequence of STDs. The best estimate of subsequent tubal infertility is derived from an excellent Swedish report; approximately 12% after one episode of PID, 23% after 2 episodes, and 54% after 3 episodes.[258] Because pelvic infection is the single greatest threat to the reproductive future of a young woman, the now recognized protection offered by oral contraception against pelvic inflammatory disease is highly important.[259–261] ***The risk of hospitalization for PID is reduced by approximately 50–60%, but at least 12 months of use are necessary, and the protection is limited to current users.***[259, 262] Furthermore, if a patient does get a pelvic infection, the severity of the salpingitis found at laparoscopy is decreased.[263, 264] The mechanism of this protection remains unknown. Speculation includes thickening of the cervical mucus to prevent movement of pathogens and bacteria-laden sperm into the uterus and tubes, and decreased menstrual bleeding, reducing movement of pathogens into the tubes as well as a reduction in "culture medium."

The argument has been made that this protection is limited to gonococcal disease, and chlamydial infections may even be enhanced. Fifteen of 17 published studies by 1985 reported a positive association of oral contraceptives with lower genital tract chlamydial cervicitis.[265] Because lower genital tract infections caused by chlamydia are on the rise (now the most prevalent bacterial STD in the U.S.) and the rate of hospitalization for PID is also increased, it is worthwhile for both patients and clinicians to be alert for symptoms of cervicitis or salpingitis in women on oral contraception who are at high risk of sexually transmitted disease (multiple sexual partners, a history of STD, or cervical discharge). The mechanism for the association between chlamydial cervicitis and oral contraceptives may be the well recognized extension of the columnar epithelium from the endocervix out over the cervix (ectopia) that occurs with oral contraceptive use.[266]

Despite this potential relationship between oral contraception and chlamydial infections, it should be emphasized that there is no evidence for an impact of oral contraceptives increasing the incidence of tubal infertility.[267] In fact, a case-control study indicated that oral contraceptive users with chlamydia infection are protected against symptomatic PID.[268] A case-control study has suggested that oral contraceptive users are more likely to harbor unrecognized endometritis, and that this would explain the discrepancy between the observed rates between lower and upper tract infection.[269] However, this would not explain the lack of an association between oral contraceptive use and tubal infertility. Thus, the influence of oral contraception on the upper reproductive tract may be different than on the lower tract. These observations on fertility are derived mostly, if not totally, from women using oral contraceptives containing 50 µg of estrogen. The continued progestin dominance of the lower dose formulations, however, should produce the same protective impact, and evidence indicates that this is so.[262]

Other Infections

In the British prospective studies of high-dose oral contraceptives, urinary tract infections were increased in users of oral contraception by 20%, and a correlation was noted with estrogen dose. An increased incidence of cervicitis was also reported, an effect related to the progestin dose. The incidence of cervicitis increased with the length of time the pill was used, from no higher after 6 months to 3 times higher by the 6th year of use. A significant increase in a variety of viral diseases, e.g., chickenpox, was observed, suggesting steroid effects on the immune system. The prevalence of these effects with low-dose oral contraception is unknown.

Oral contraception appears to protect against bacterial vaginosis and infections with *Trichomonas*.[270, 271] Evidence is lacking to convincingly implicate oral contraception with vaginal infections with *Candida* species;[270] however, clinical experience is sometimes impressive when recurrence and cure repeatedly follow use and discontinuation of oral contraception.

Patient Management

Absolute Contraindications to the Use of Oral Contraception

1. Thrombophlebitis, thromboembolic disorders (including a close family history, parent or sibling, suggestive of an inherited susceptibility for venous thrombosis), cerebral vascular disease, coronary occlusion, or a past history of these conditions, or conditions predisposing to these problems.

2. Markedly impaired liver function. Steroid hormones are contraindicated in patients with hepatitis until liver function tests return to normal.

3. Known or suspected breast cancer.

4. Undiagnosed abnormal vaginal bleeding.

5. Known or suspected pregnancy.

6. Smokers over the age of 35.

Relative Contraindications Requiring Clinical Judgment and Informed Consent

1. *Migraine headaches.* In retrospective studies of low-dose pills, it is not clear whether migraine headaches are associated with an increased risk of stroke. Some women report an improvement in their headaches, and in our view, a trial of the lowest dose oral contraceptives is warranted. Oral contraceptives should be avoided in women who have migraine with complex or prolonged aura, or if additional stroke factors are present (older age, smoking, hypertension).[272]

2. *Hypertension.* A woman under 35 who is otherwise healthy and whose blood pressure is well controlled by medication can elect to use oral contraception. We recommend the use of the lowest estrogen dose products.

3. *Uterine leiomyoma.* This is not a contraindication with low-dose oral contraceptives. There is evidence that the risk of leiomyomas was decreased by 31% in women who used higher dose oral contraception for 10 years.[273] However, case-control studies with lower dose oral contraceptives have found neither a decrease nor an increase in risk, although the Nurses' Health Study reported a slightly increased risk when oral contraceptives were first used in early teenage years.[274-276] The administration of low-dose oral contraceptives to women with leiomyomata does not stimulate fibroid growth, and is associated with a reduction in menstrual bleeding.[277]

4. *Gestational diabetes.* Low-dose formulations do not produce a diabetic glucose tolerance response in women with previous gestational diabetes, and there is no evidence that combined oral contraceptives increase the incidence of overt diabetes mellitus.[129, 130] We believe that women with previous gestational diabetes can use oral contraception with annual assessment of the fasting glucose level.

5. *Elective surgery.* The recommendation that oral contraception should be discontinued 4 weeks before elective major surgery to avoid an increased risk of postoperative thrombosis is based on data derived from high-dose pills. If possible, it is safer to follow this recommendation when a period of immobilization is to be expected. It is prudent to maintain contraception right up to the performance of a sterilization procedure, and this short, outpatient operation carries very minimal risk.

6. **Epilepsy.** Oral contraceptives do not exacerbate epilepsy, and in some women, improvement in seizure control has occurred.[278] Antiepileptic drugs, however, may decrease the effectiveness of oral contraception.

7. **Obstructive jaundice in pregnancy.** Not all patients with this history will develop jaundice on oral contraception, especially with the low-dose formulations.

8. **Sickle cell disease or sickle C disease.** Patients with sickle cell trait can use oral contraception. The risk of thrombosis in women with sickle cell disease or sickle C diseases is theoretical (and medicolegal). We believe effective protection against pregnancy in these patients warrants the use of low-dose oral contraception.

9. **Diabetes mellitus.** Effective prevention of pregnancy outweighs the small risk of complicating vascular disease in diabetic women who are under age 35 and otherwise healthy.

10. **Gallbladder disease.** Oral contraceptives do not cause gallstones, but may accelerate the emergence of symptoms when gallstones are already present.

Clinical Decisions

Surveillance

In view of the increased safety of low-dose preparations for healthy young women with no risk factors, such patients need be seen only every 12 months for exclusion of problems by history, measurement of the blood pressure, urinalysis, breast examination, palpation of the liver, and pelvic examination with Pap smear. Women with risk factors should be seen every 6 months by appropriately trained personnel for screening of problems by history and blood pressure measurement. Breast and pelvic examinations are necessary only yearly. It is worth emphasizing that better continuation is achieved by reassessing new users within 1–2 months. It is at this time that subtle fears and unvoiced concerns need to be confronted and resolved.

Oral contraception is safer than most people think it is, and the low-dose preparations are extremely safe. Health care providers should make a significant effort to get this message to our patients (and our colleagues). We must make sure our patients receive adequate counseling, either from ourselves or our professional staff. The major reason why patients discontinue oral contraception is fear of side effects.[279] Let's take time to put the risks into proper perspective, and to emphasize the benefits as well as the risks.

Laboratory surveillance should be used only when indicated. Routine biochemical measurements fail to yield sufficient information to warrant the expense. Assessing the cholesterol-lipoprotein profile and carbohydrate metabolism should follow the same guidelines applied to all patients, users and nonusers of contraception. The following is a useful guide as to who should be monitored with blood screening tests for glucose, lipids, and lipoproteins:

Young women, at least once.
Women 35 years or older.
Women with a strong family history of heart disease, diabetes mellitus, or hypertension.
Women with gestational diabetes melllitus.
Women with xanthomatosis.
Obese women.
Diabetic women.

Choice of Pill

The therapeutic principle remains: utilize the formulations that give effective contraception and the greatest margin of safety. You and your patients are urged to choose a low-dose preparation containing less than 50 µg of estrogen, combined with low doses of new or old progestins. Current data support the view that there is greater safety with preparations containing less than 50 µg of estrogen. The arguments in this chapter indicate that all patients should begin oral contraception with low-dose products, and that patients on higher dose oral contraception should be changed to the low-dose preparations. Stepping down to a lower dose can be accomplished immediately with no adverse reactions such as increased bleeding or failure of contraception.

The multiphasic preparations do have a reduced progestin dosage compared with some of the existing monophasic products; however, based on currently available information there is little difference between the low-dose monophasics and the multiphasics.

The pharmacologic effects in animals of various formulations have been used as a basis for therapeutic recommendations in selecting the optimal oral contraceptive pill. *These recommendations (tailor-making the pill to the patient) have not been supported by appropriately controlled clinical trials. All too often this leads to the prescribing of a pill of excessive dosage with its attendant increased risk of serious side effects.* It is worth repeating our earlier comments on potency. Oral contraceptive potency (specifically progestin potency) is no longer a consideration when it comes to prescribing birth control pills. The potency of the various progestins has been accounted for by appropriate adjustments of dose. Clinical advice based on potency is an artificial exercise that has not stood the test of time. The biologic effect of the various progestational components in current low-dose oral contraceptives is approximately the same. Our progress in lowering the doses of the steroids contained in oral contraceptives has yielded products with little serious differences.

Pill Taking

Effective contraception is present during the first cycle of pill use, provided the pills are started no later than the 5th day of the cycle, and no pills are missed. Thus, starting oral contraception on the first day of menses ensures immediate protection. In the United States, most clinicians and patients prefer the Sunday start packages, beginning on the first Sunday following menstruation. This can be easier to remember, and it usually avoids menstrual bleeding on weekends. It is probable, but not totally certain, that even if a dominant follicle should emerge in occasional patients after a Sunday start, an LH surge and ovulation would still be prevented.[280] Some clinicians prefer to advise patients to use added protection in the first week of use.

Occasionally patients would like to postpone a menstrual period; e.g., for a wedding, holiday, or vacation. This can be easily achieved by omitting the 7-day hormone-free interval. Simply start a new package of pills the next day after finishing the series of 21 pills in the previous package. Remember, when using a 28-pill package, the patient would start a new package after using the 21 *active* pills.

There is no rationale for recommending a pill-free interval "to rest." The serious side effects are not eliminated by pill-free intervals. This practice all too often results in unwanted pregnancies.

How important is it to take the oral contraceptive at the same time every day? Although not well studied, there is reason to believe precise pill taking minimizes breakthrough bleeding. In addition, compliance is improved by a fixed schedule that is habit-forming.

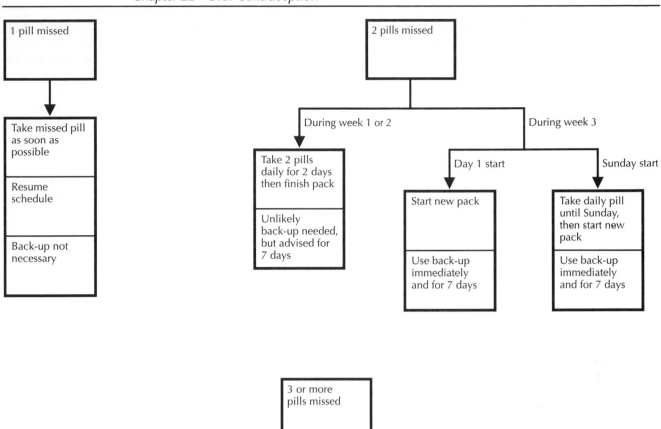

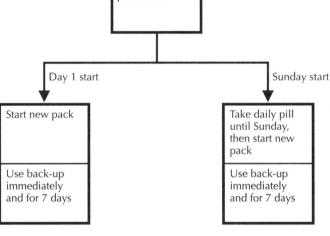

What To Do When Pills Are Missed

Irregular pill taking is a common occurrence. Using an electronic monitoring device to measure compliance, it was apparent that consistency of pill taking is even worse than what patients report; only 33% of women were documented to have missed no pills in cycle 1, and by cycle 3, about one-third of the women missed 3 or more pills with many episodes of consecutive days of missed pills.[281] These data indicate that women become less careful over time, emphasizing the importance of repeatedly reviewing with patients what to do when pills are missed.

If a woman misses 1 pill, she should take that pill as soon as she remembers and take the next pill as usual. No backup is needed.

If she misses 2 pills in the first two weeks, she should take two pills on each of the next two days; it is unlikely that a back-up method is needed, but the official consensus is to recommend backup for the next 7 days.

If 2 pills are missed in the third week, or if more than 2 active pills are missed at any time, another form of contraception should be used as backup immediately and for 7 days; if a Sunday starter, keep taking a pill every day until Sunday, and on Sunday start a new package; if a non-Sunday starter, start a new package the same day.

Studies have questioned whether missing pills has an impact on contraception. One study demonstrated that skipping 4 consecutive pills at varying times in the cycle did not result in ovulation.[280] Studies in which women deliberately lengthen their pill-fee interval up to 11 days have failed to show signs of ovulation.[282, 283] So far there is no evidence that moving to lower doses has had an impact on the margin of error. The studies have involved small numbers of women and given the large individual variation, it still is possible that some women might be at risk with a small increase in the pill-free interval. However, the progestational effects on endometrium and cervical mucus serve to ensure good contraceptive efficacy.[12] We may well prove that current recommendations are too conservative, and that a woman's chance of getting pregnant with missing pills is nearly zero. Nevertheless, this conservative advice is the safest message to convey.

The most prevalent problems that can be identified associated with apparent oral contraceptive failures are vomiting and diarrhea.[13, 14] *Even if no pills have been missed, patients should be instructed to use a backup method for at least 7 days after an episode of gastroenteritis.*

Clinical Problems

Breakthrough Bleeding

A major continuation problem is breakthrough bleeding. Breakthrough bleeding gives rise to fears and concerns; it is aggravating, and even embarrassing. Therefore, on starting oral contraception, patients need to be fully informed about breakthrough bleeding.

There are two characteristic breakthrough bleeding problems: irregular bleeding in the first few months after starting oral contraception, and unexpected bleeding after many months of use. Effort should be made to manage the bleeding problem in a way that allows the patient to remain on low-dose oral contraception. *There is no evidence that the onset of bleeding is associated with decreased efficacy, no matter what oral contraceptive formulation is used, even the lowest dose products.* Indeed, in a careful study, breakthrough bleeding did not correlate with changes in the blood levels of the contraceptive steroids.[284]

The most frequently encountered breakthrough bleeding occurs in the first few months of use. The incidence is greatest in the first 3 months, ranging from 10–30% in the first month to less than 10% in the third. Breakthrough bleeding rates are higher with the lowest dose oral contraceptives, but not dramatically.[285] However, breakthrough bleeding is further increased in women who smoke and use formulations with 20 µg ethinyl estradiol.[286] Breakthrough bleeding is best managed by encouragement and reassurance. This bleeding usually disappears by the third cycle in the majority of women. If necessary, even this early pattern of breakthrough bleeding can be treated as outlined below. It is helpful to explain to the patient that this bleeding represents tissue breakdown as the endometrium adjusts from its usual thick state to the relatively thin state allowed by the hormones in oral contraceptives.

Breakthrough bleeding that occurs after many months of oral contraceptive use is a consequence of the progestin-induced decidualization. This endometrium and blood vessels within the endometrium tend to be fragile and prone to breakdown and asynchronous bleeding.

There are two recognized factors (both preventable) that are associated with a greater incidence of breakthrough bleeding. Consistency of use and smoking increase spotting and bleeding, but inconsistency of pill taking is more important and has a greater effect in later cycles, whereas smoking exerts a general effect from beginning to later cycles.[287] Reinforcement of consistent pill taking can help minimize breakthrough bleeding. Cervical infection can be another cause of breakthrough bleeding; the prevalence of cervical chlamydial infections is higher among oral contraceptive users who report breakthrough bleeding.[288]

If bleeding occurs just before the end of the pill cycle, it can be managed by having the patient stop the pills, wait 7 days and start a new cycle. If breakthrough bleeding is prolonged or if it is aggravating for the patient, regardless of the point in the pill cycle, control of the bleeding can be achieved with a short course of exogenous estrogen. Conjugated estrogen, 1.25 mg, or estradiol, 2 mg, is administered daily for 7 days when the bleeding is present, no matter where the patient is in her pill cycle. The patient continues to adhere to the schedule of pill taking. Usually, one course of estrogen solves the problem, and recurrence of bleeding is unusual (but if it does recur, another 7-day course of estrogen is effective).

Responding to irregular bleeding by having the patient take 2 or 3 pills is not effective. The progestin component of the pill will always dominate; hence, doubling the number of pills will also double the progestational impact and its decidualizing, atrophic effect on the endometrium and its destabilizing effect on endometrial blood vessels. The addition of extra estrogen while keeping the progestin dose unchanged is logical and effective. This allows the patient to remain on the low-dose formulation with its advantage of greater safety. Breakthrough bleeding, in our view, is not sufficient reason to expose patients to the increased risks associated with higher dose oral contraceptives. Any bleeding that is not handled by this routine requires investigation for the presence of pathology.

There is no evidence that any oral contraceptive formulations that are approximately equivalent in estrogen and progestin dosage are significantly different in the rates of breakthrough bleeding. Clinicians often become impressed that switching to another product effectively stops the breakthrough bleeding. It is more likely that the passage of time is the responsible factor, and bleeding would have stopped regardless of switching and regardless of product.

Amenorrhea

With low-dose pills, the estrogen content is not sufficient in some women to stimulate endometrial growth. The progestational effect dominates to such a degree that a shallow atrophic endometrium is produced, lacking sufficient tissue to yield withdrawal bleeding. It should be emphasized that permanent atrophy of the endometrium does not occur, and resumption of normal ovarian function will restore endometrial growth and development. Indeed, there is no harmful, permanent consequence of amenorrhea while on oral contraception.

The major problem with amenorrhea while on oral contraception is the anxiety produced in both patient and clinician because the lack of bleeding may be a sign of pregnancy. The patient is anxious because of the uncertainty regarding pregnancy, and the clinician is anxious because of the medicolegal concerns stemming from the old studies which indicated an increased risk of congenital abnormalities among the offspring of women who inadvertently used oral contraception in early pregnancy. We reviewed this problem earlier, and emphatically stated that there is no association between oral contraception and an increased risk of congenital malformation, and there is no increased risk of having abnormal children.

The incidence of amenorrhea in the first year of use with low-dose oral contraception is less than 2%. This incidence increases with duration, reaching perhaps 5% after several years of use. It is important to alert patients upon starting oral contraception that diminished bleeding and possibly no bleeding may ensue.

Amenorrhea is a difficult management problem. A pregnancy test will allow reliable assessment for the presence of pregnancy even at this early stage. However, routine, repeated use of such testing is expensive and annoying, and may lead to discontinuation of oral contraception. *A simple test for pregnancy is to assess the basal body temperature during the END of the pill-free week; a basal body temperature less than 98 degrees (36.6°C) is not consistent with pregnancy, and oral contraception can be continued.*

Many women are reassured with an understanding of why there is no bleeding and are able to continue on the pill despite the amenorrhea. Some women cannot reconcile themselves to a lack of bleeding, and this is an indication for trying other formulations (a practice unsupported by any clinical trials, and, therefore, the expectations are uncertain). But again, this problem does not warrant exposing patients to the greater risks of major side effects associated with higher dose products.

Some clinicians have observed that the addition of extra estrogen for 1 month (1.25 mg conjugated estrogens or 2 mg estradiol daily throughout the 21 days while taking the oral contraceptive) will rejuvenate the endometrium, and withdrawal bleeding will resume, persisting for many months.

Weight Gain

The complaint of weight gain is frequently cited as a major problem with compliance. Yet, studies of the low-dose preparations fail to demonstrate a significant weight gain with oral contraception, and no major differences among the various products.[140, 141, 289] This is obviously a problem of perception. The clinician has to carefully reinforce the lack of association between low-dose oral contraceptives and weight gain and focus the patient on the real culprit: diet and level of exercise. Most women gain a moderate amount of weight as they age, whether they take oral contraceptives or not.

Acne

Low-dose oral contraceptives improve acne regardless of which product is used.[122, 290–292] The low progestin doses (including levonorgestrel formulations) currently used are insufficient to stimulate an androgenic response.

Ovarian Cysts

Anecdotal reports suggested that functional ovarian cysts are encountered more frequently and suppress less easily with multiphasic formulations. This observation failed to withstand careful scrutiny.[293] Functional ovarian cysts occurred less frequently in women on higher dose oral contraception.[294] This protection is reduced with the current lower dose products to the point where little effect can be measured.[295–298] Thus, the risk of such cysts is not eliminated; and, therefore, clinicians can encounter such cysts in patients taking any of the oral contraceptive formulations.

Drugs That Affect Efficacy

There are many anecdotal reports of patients who conceived on oral contraceptives while taking antibiotics. There is little evidence, however, that antibiotics such as ampicillin, metronidazole, quinolone, and tetracycline, which reduce the bacterial flora of the gastrointestinal tract, affect oral contraceptive efficacy. Studies indicate that while antibiotics can alter the excretion of contraceptive steroids, plasma levels are unchanged, and there is no evidence of ovulation.[299, 300]

A review of a large number of patients derived from dermatology practices failed to find an increased rate of pregnancy in women on oral contraceptives and being treated with antibiotics (tetracyclines, penicillins, cephalosporins).[301]

There is good reason to believe that drugs, which stimulate the liver's metabolic capacity, can affect oral contraceptive efficacy. On the other hand, a search of a large database failed to discover any evidence that lower dose oral contraceptives are more likely to fail or to have more drug interaction problems when other drugs are used.[302]

To be cautious, patients on medications that affect liver metabolism should choose an alternative contraceptive. These drugs are as follows:

> Rifampin
> Phenobarbital
> Phenytoin (Dilantin)
> Primidone (Mysoline)
> Carbamazepine (Tegretol)
> *Possibly* ethosuximide, griseofulvin, and troglitazone.

Other Drug Interactions

Although not extensively documented, there is reason to believe that oral contraceptives potentiate the action of diazepam (Valium), chlordiazepoxide (Librium), tricyclic antidepressants, and theophylline.[303] Thus, lower doses of these agents may be effective in oral contraceptive users. Because of an influence on clearance rates, oral contraceptive users may require larger doses of acetaminophen and aspirin.[304]

Migraine Headaches

True migraine headaches are more common in women, while tension headaches occur equally in men and women. There have been no well done studies to determine the impact of oral contraception on migraine headaches. Patients may report that their headaches are worse or better.

Studies with high-dose pills indicated that migraine headaches were linked to a risk of stroke. More recent studies reflecting the use of low-dose formulations yield mixed results. One failed to find a further increase in stroke in patients with migraine who use oral contraception, another concluded that the use of oral contraception by migraineurs was associated with a 4-fold increase of the already increased risk of ischemic stroke.[305, 306] Because 20–30% of women experience migraine headaches, one would expect the study populations in the most recent studies of thrombosis to have included substantial numbers of migraineurs. An adverse effect of low-dose oral contraceptives on stroke risk in migraineurs should have manifested itself in the data. The lack of an increased risk of stroke in these studies is reassuring.

Because of the seriousness of this potential complication, the onset of visual symptoms or severe headaches requires a response. If the patient is at a higher dose, a move to a low-dose formulation may relieve the headaches. Switching to a different brand is worthwhile, if only to evoke a placebo response. True vascular headaches (classic migraine with aura) are an indication to avoid or discontinue oral contraception. Oral contraceptives should be avoided in women who have migraine with complex or prolonged aura, or if additional stroke factors are present (older age, smoking, hypertension).[272]

Clues To Severe Vascular Headaches:
- Headaches that last a long time.
- Dizziness, nausea, or vomiting with headaches.
- Scotomata or blurred vision.
- Episodes of blindness.
- Unilateral, unremitting headaches.
- Headaches that continue despite medication.

In some women, a relationship exists between their fluctuating hormone levels during a menstrual cycle and migraine headaches, with the onset of headaches characteristically coinciding with menses. We have had personal success (anecdotal to be sure) alleviating headaches by eliminating the menstrual cycle, either with the use of *daily* oral contraceptives or the daily administration of a progestational agent (such as 10 mg medroxyprogesterone acetate) or the use of depot-medroxyprogesterone acetate. Some women with migraine headaches have extremely gratifying responses. Women who experience an exacerbation of their headaches with oral contraception should consider one of the progestin-only methods.

Summary: Oral Contraceptive Use and Medical Problems

Gestational Diabetes. There is no contraindication to combined oral contraceptive use following gestational diabetes.[129, 130] There is a concern with breastfeeding women using the progestin-only minipill (discussed later in this chapter).

Diabetes Mellitus. Oral contraception can be used by diabetic women less than 35 years old who do not smoke and are otherwise healthy (especially an absence of diabetic vascular complications). A case-control study could find no evidence that oral contraceptive use by young women with insulin-dependent diabetes mellitus increased the development of retinopathy or nephropathy.[132] In a one-year study of women with insulin-dependent diabetes mellitus who were using a low-dose oral contraceptive, no deterioration could be documented in lipoprotein or hemostatic biochemical markers for cardiovascular risk.[133]

Hypertension. Low-dose oral contraception can be used in women less than age 35 years old with hypertension well controlled by medication, and who are otherwise healthy and do not smoke. We recommend the lowest estrogen dose formulations.

Pregnancy-Induced Hypertension. Women with pregnancy-induced hypertension can use oral contraception as soon as the blood pressure is normal in the postpartum period.

Hemorrhagic Disorders. Women with hemorrhagic disorders and women taking anticoagulants can use oral contraception. Inhibition of ovulation can avoid the real problem of a hemorrhagic corpus luteum in these patients. A reduction in menstrual blood loss is another benefit of importance.

Gallbladder Disease. Oral contraception use may precipitate a symptomatic attack in women known to have stones or a positive history for gallbladder disease and, therefore, should either be used very cautiously or not at all.

Obesity. An obese woman who is otherwise healthy can use low-dose oral contraception.

Hepatic Disease. Oral contraception can be utilized when liver function tests return to normal. Follow-up liver function tests should be obtained after 2–3 months of use.

Seizure Disorders. There is no impact of oral contraceptives on pattern or frequency of seizures. The concern is that anticonvulsant-induced hepatic enzyme activity can increase the risk of contraceptive failure. Some clinicians advocate the use of higher dose (50 mg estrogen) products;

however, no studies have been performed to demonstrate that this higher dose is necessary.

Mitral Valve Prolapse. Oral contraception use is limited to nonsmoking patients who are asymptomatic (no clinical evidence of regurgitation). There is a small subset of patients with mitral valve prolapse who are at increased risk of thromboembolism. Patients with atrial fibrillation, migraine headaches, or clotting factor abnormalities should consider progestin-only methods or the IUD (prophylactic antibiotics should cover IUD insertion if mitral regurgitation is present).

Systemic Lupus Erythematosus. Oral contraceptive use can exacerbate systemic lupus erythematous, and the vascular disease associated with lupus, when present, represents a contraindication to estrogen-containing oral contraceptives.[307] The progestin-only methods are a good choice. However, in patients with stable or inactive disease, without renal involvement and high antiphospholipid antibodies, low-dose oral contraception can be considered.[308] SELENA (Safety of Estrogen in Lupus Erythematosus National Assessment) is an on-going randomized, controlled clinical trial of oral contraceptive therapy in premenopausal women with systemic lupus erythematosus (as well as postmenopausal hormone therapy).

Migraine Headaches. Low-dose oral contraception (the lowest estrogen dose formulation) can be tried with careful surveillance in women with common migraine headaches. Daily administration can prevent menstrual migraine headaches. Oral contraception is best avoided in women with classic migraine headaches associated with neurologic symptoms.

Sickle Cell Disease. Patients with sickle cell trait can use oral contraception. The risk of thrombosis in women with sickle cell disease or sickle C diseases is theoretical (and medicolegal). We believe effective protection against pregnancy in these patients warrants the use of low-dose oral contraception. In the only long-term (10 years) follow-up report of women with sickle cell disease and using oral contraceptives, no apparent adverse effects were observed (at a time when higher dose products were prevalent).[309] Keep in mind that depot-medroxyprogesterone acetate used for contraception is associated with inhibition of sickling and improvement in anemia in patients with sickle cell disease.[310]

Benign Breast Disease. Benign breast disease is not a contraindication for oral contraception; with 2 years of use, the condition may improve.

Congenital Heart Disease or Valvular Heart Disease. Oral contraception is contraindicated only if there is marginal cardiac reserve or a condition that predisposes to thrombosis.

Hyperlipidemia. Because low-dose oral contraceptives have negligible impact on the lipoprotein profile, hyperlipidemia is not an absolute contraindication, with the exception of very high levels of triglycerides (which can be made worse by estrogen). If vascular disease is already present, oral contraception should be avoided. If other risk factors are present, especially smoking, oral contraception is not recommended. Dyslipidemic patients who begin oral contraception should have their lipoprotein profiles monitored monthly for a few visits to ensure no adverse impact. If the lipid abnormality cannot be held in control, an alternative method of contraception should be used.[311] Oral contraceptives containing desogestrel, noregestimate, or gestodene can increase HDL levels, but it is not known if this change is clinically significant.

Depression. Low-dose oral contraceptives have minimal, if any, impact on mood.

Smoking. Oral contraception is absolutely contraindicated in smokers over the age of 35. In patients 35 years old and younger, heavy smoking (15 or more cigarettes per day) is a relative contraindication. The relative risk of cardiovascular events is increased for women of all ages who smoke and use oral contraceptives; however, because the actual incidence of cardiovascular events is so low at a young age, the real risk is very low for young women, although it increases with age. An ex-smoker (for at least one year) should be regarded as a nonsmoker. Risk is only linked to active smoking. Is there room for judgment? Given the right circumstances, low-dose oral contraceptives might be appropriate for a light smoker or the user of a nicotine patch. A 20 µg estrogen formulation may be a better choice for smoking women, regardless of age (because this dose of estrogen has no impact on clotting factors and platelet activation).[31, 32]

Pituitary Prolactin-Secreting Adenomas. Low-dose oral contraception can be used in the presence of microadenomas.

Infectious Mononucleosis. Oral contraception can be used as long as liver function tests are normal.

Ulcerative Colitis. There is no association between oral contraception and ulcerative colitis. Women with this problem can use oral contraceptives.[143] Oral contraceptives are absorbed mainly in the small bowel.

An Alternative Route of Administration

Occasionally, a situation may be encountered when an alternative to oral administration of contraceptive pills is required. For example, patients receiving chemotherapy can either have significant nausea and vomiting, or mucositis, both of which would prevent oral drug administration. The low-dose oral contraceptives can be administered vaginally. Initially, it was claimed that two pills must be placed high in the vagina daily in order to produce contraceptive steroid blood levels comparable with the oral administration of one pill.[312] However, a large clinical trial has demonstrated typical contraceptive efficacy with one pill administered vaginally per day.[313]

Athletes and Oral Contraception

Because athletes are often amenorrheic and hypoestrogenic, oral contraceptives provide not only confidence against the risk of an unwanted pregnancy, but also estrogen support against bone loss. This is a situation where bone density measurements are worthwhile. A low bone density can help motivate an athlete to take hormone therapy, and a subsequent bone density measurement that reveals a failure of response to estrogen can indicate the presence of a hidden eating disorder.

Competing athletes are often concerned that oral contraceptives could reduce exercise performance. A rationale for the concern can be traced to the physiologic increase in ventilation during pregnancy, mediated by progesterone. Thus, progestin enhancement of ventilatory response could consume energy otherwise available for athletic performance. Indeed, reports have generated conflicting data as measured by laboratory testing. However, experimental studies that simulate athletic events can find no adverse effects on oxygen uptake or respiratory rate.[314] One study documented decreased soreness, both perceived and with palpation, after exercise in women using oral contraceptives.[315] Oral contraceptive use has no effect on prevalence or severity of low back pain, a common problem among female athletes.[316]

Oral contraceptives have a lot to offer with no serious drawbacks for athletes. In athletes who wish to avoid menstrual bleeding, oral contraceptives can be administered on a daily basis, with no breaks, preventing withdrawal bleeding.

The Noncontraceptive Benefits of Oral Contraception

The noncontraceptive benefits of low-dose oral contraception can be grouped into two main categories: benefits that incidentally accrue when oral contraception is specifically utilized for contraceptive purposes and benefits that result from the use of oral contraceptives to treat problems and disorders.

The noncontraceptive incidental benefits can be listed as follows:

Effective Contraception.
   -**less need for induced abortion.**
   -**less need for surgical sterilization.**
Less Endometrial Cancer.
Less Ovarian Cancer.
Fewer Ectopic Pregnancies.
More Regular Menses.
   -**less flow.**
   -**less dysmenorrhea.**
   -**less anemia.**
Less Salpingitis.
Probably Less Endometriosis.
Possibly Less Benign Breast Disease.
Possibly Less Rheumatoid Arthritis.
Possibly Protection against Atherosclerosis.
Possibly Increased Bone Density.
Possibly Fewer Fibroids.
Possibly Fewer Ovarian Cysts.

Many of these benefits have been previously discussed. Protection against pelvic inflammatory disease is especially noteworthy and a major contribution to not only preservation of fertility but to lower health care costs. Also important is the prevention of ectopic pregnancies. Ectopic pregnancies have increased in incidence (partly due to an increase in STDs) and represent a major cost for our society and a threat to both fertility and life for individual patients.

Of course, prevention of benign and malignant neoplasia is an outstanding feature of oral contraception. High-dose oral contraceptive use decreased the incidence of benign breast disease diagnosed clinically as well as fibrocystic disease and fibroadenomas diagnosed by biopsy; hopefully, the same impact will become evident with current lower dose formulations. A 40% reduction in ovarian cancer and a 50% reduction in endometrial cancer represent substantial protection. Studies with higher dose formulations documented in long-term users a 31% reduction in uterine leiomyomata and, in current users, a 78% reduction in corpus luteum cysts and a 49% reduction in functional ovarian cysts.[294] The impact of low-dose preparations on these problems remains to be accurately measured and may be less. Case-control studies with low-dose oral contraceptives have found no impact on the risk of uterine fibroids, neither increased nor decreased.[274, 275] Epidemiologic studies have indicated that a progressive decline in the incidence of ovarian cysts is proportional to the steroid doses in oral contraceptives.[295, 296] Current low-dose monophasic and multiphasic formulations provide no protection against functional ovarian cysts.[295–298] This apparent weaker protection afforded by the current low-dose formulations makes it very likely that clinicians will encounter such cysts in their patients on oral contraceptives.

The low-dose contraceptives are as effective as higher dose preparations in reducing menstrual flow and the prevalence and severity of dysmenorrhea.[317, 318] The use of oral contraception is associated with a lower incidence of endometriosis, although the protective effect is probably limited to current or recent use.[319–321] These benefits involving two common gynecologic problems have an important, positive impact on compliance.

An Austrian study concluded that osteoporosis occurs later and is less frequent in women who have used long-term oral contraception.[322] Cross-sectional studies of postmenopausal women indicate that prior use of oral contraception is associated with higher levels of bone density and that the degree of protection is related to duration of exposure.[323, 324] However, other studies reflecting modern use of low-dose products indicate little impact of oral contraceptive use on bone.[325–327] These measurements of bone density are not as important as the clinical outcome: fractures. The available evidence suggests that any favorable effects on bone density are not clinically important. In the Royal College of General Practitioners Study, the overall risk of fractures in ever users of oral contraceptives was actually slightly increased.[328] Similar results have been observed in the Oxford Family Planning Association Study.[329] It is likely that the increased risk reflects lifestyle effects among oral contraceptive users, but thus far, there is no evidence of a protective effect against fractures. However, previous oral contraceptive users are just now becoming elderly and reaching the age of greatest fracture prevalence. Future studies of postmenopausal women may eventually reveal a beneficial effect on osteoporotic fractures.

The literature on rheumatoid arthritis has been controversial, with studies in Europe finding evidence of protection and studies in North America failing to demonstrate such an effect. An excellent Danish case-control study was designed to answer criticisms of shortcomings in the previous literature.[330] Ever use of oral contraception reduced the relative risk of rheumatoid arthritis by 60%, and the strongest protection was present in women with a positive family history. One meta-analysis concluded that the evidence consistently indicated a protective effect, but that rather than preventing the development of rheumatoid arthritis, oral contraception may modify the course of disease, inhibiting the progression from mild to severe disease; whereas a later meta-analysis concluded there was no evidence of a protective effect.[331, 332]

Oral contraceptives are frequently utilized to manage the following problems and disorders:

> **Definitely Beneficial:**
> -**dysfunctional uterine bleeding.**
> -**dysmenorrhea.**
> -**mittelschmerz.**
> -**endometriosis prophylaxis.**
> -**acne and hirsutism.**
> -**hormone therapy for hypothalamic amenorrhea.**
> -**prevention of menstrual porphyria.**
> -**control of bleeding (dyscrasias, anovulation).**
> **Possibly Beneficial:**
> -**functional ovarian cysts.**
> -**premenstrual syndrome.**

Oral contraceptives have been a cornerstone for the treatment of anovulatory, dysfunctional uterine bleeding. For patients who need effective contraception, oral contraceptives are a good choice to provide hormone therapy for amenorrheic patients, as well as to treat dysmenorrhea. Oral contraceptives are also a good choice to provide prophylaxis against the recurrence of endometriosis in a woman who has already undergone more vigorous treatment with surgery or the GnRH analogues. To protect against endometriosis, oral contraceptives should be taken daily, with no break and no withdrawal bleeding.

The low-dose oral contraceptives are effective in treating acne and hirsutism. Suppression of free testosterone levels is comparable with that achieved with higher dosage.[290, 333] The beneficial clinical effect is the same with low-dose preparations containing levonorgestrel, previously recognized to cause acne at high dosage.[290, 334] Formulations with desogestrel, gestodene, and norgestimate are associated with greater increases in sex hormone-binding globulin and significant decreases in free testosterone levels. Comparison studies with oral contraceptives containing these progestins can detect no differences in effects on various androgen measurements among the various products.[335] Theoretically, these products would be more effective in the treatment of acne and hirsutism; however, this is yet to be documented by clinical studies. It is likely that all low-dose formulations, through the combined effects of an increase in sex hormone-binding globulin and a decrease in testosterone production, produce an overall similar clinical response, especially over time (a year or more).

Oral contraceptives have long been used to speed the resolution of ovarian cysts, but the efficacy of this treatment has not been established. Randomized trials have been performed with women who develop ovarian cysts after induction of ovulation.[336, 337] No advantage for the contraceptive treatment could be demonstrated. The cysts resolved completely and equally fast in both treated and non-treated groups. Of course, these were functional cysts secondary to ovulation induction, and this experience may not apply to spontaneously appearing cysts. Two short-term (5 and 6 weeks) randomized studies could document no greater effect of oral contraceptive treatment on resolution of spontaneous ovarian cysts when compared with expectant management.[338, 339] Clinical experience (untested by studies) leads us to believe that oral contraception does provide protection in women against the recurrent formation of ovarian cysts.

Continuation: Failure or Success?

Despite the fact that oral contraception is highly effective, hundreds of thousands of unintended pregnancies (close to 1 million) occur each year in the United States because of the failure of oral contraception. Worldwide, literally millions of unintended pregnancies result from poor compliance. In general, unmarried, poor, and minority women are more likely to have failures, reaching rates of 10–20%.[340, 341] Overall, the failure rate with actual use ranges from 3 to 6%. This difference between the theoretical efficacy and actual use reflects compliance and noncompliance. Noncompliance includes a wide variety of behavior: failure to fill the initial prescription, failure to continue on the medication, and incorrectly taking oral contraception. Compliance (continuation) is an area in which personal behavior, biology, and pharmacology come together. Oral contraceptive continuation reflects the interaction of these influences. Unfortunately, women who discontinue oral contraception often utilize a less effective method or, worse, fail to substitute another method.

There are 3 major factors that affect continuation:

1. The experience of side effects, such as breakthrough bleeding and amenorrhea, and perceived experience of "minor" problems, such as headaches, nausea, breast tenderness, and weight gain. Multiple side effects dramatically and progressively increase the likelihood of discontinuation.[342, 343] Because these complaints respond well even to placebo treatment,[344] it is reasonable to expect a favorable response to sensitive and attentive counseling.

2. Fears and concerns regarding cancer, cardiovascular disease, and the impact of oral contraception on future fertility.

3. Nonmedical issues, such as inadequate instructions on pill taking, complicated pill packaging, and difficulties arising from the patient package insert.

The information in this chapter is the foundation for good continuation, but the clinician must go beyond the presentation of information and develop an effective means of communicating that information. We recommend the following approach to the clinician–patient encounter as one way to improve continuation with oral contraception.

1. Explain how oral contraception works.

2. Review briefly the risks and benefits of oral contraception, but be careful to put the risks in proper perspective, and to emphasize the safety and noncontraceptive benefits of low-dose oral contraceptives.

3. Show and demonstrate to the patient the package of pills she will use.

4. Explain how to take the pills:
-When to start.
-The importance of developing a daily routine to avoid missing pills.
-What to do if pills are missed (Identify a backup method).

5. Review the side effects that can affect continuation: amenorrhea, breakthrough bleeding, headaches, weight gain, nausea, etc., and what to do if one or more occurs.

6. Explain the warning signs of potential problems: abdominal or chest pain, trouble breathing, severe headaches, visual problems, leg pain or swelling.

7. Ask the patient to be sure to call if another clinician prescribes other medications.

8. Ask the patient to repeat critical information to make sure she understands what has been said. Ask if the patient has any questions.

9. Schedule a return appointment in 1–2 months to review understanding and address fears and concerns; a visit at 3 months is too late because most questions and side effects occur early.[343] Inconsistent use of oral contraceptives is more common in women who are new starters.[341]

10. Make sure a line of communication is open to clinician or office personnel. Ask the patient to call for any problem or concern before she stops taking the oral contraceptives.

The Progestin-Only Minipill

The minipill contains a small dose of a progestational agent and must be taken daily, in a continuous fashion.[345, 346] There is no evidence for any difference in clinical behavior among the available minipill products.

Minipills available worldwide:

1. Micronor, Nor-QD, Noriday, Norod -------- 0.350 mg norethindrone.

2. Microval, Noregeston, Microlut ------------ 0.030 mg norgestrel.

3. Ovrette, Neogest ----------------------------- 0.075 mg levonorgestrel.

4. Exluton -- 0.500 mg lynestrenol.

5. Femulen -- 0.500 mg ethynodial diacetate.

6. CerazetteR --------------------------------------- 0.075 mg desogestrel.

Mechanism of Action

After taking a progestin-only minipill, the small amount of progestin in the circulation (about 25% of that in combined oral contraceptives) will have a significant impact only on those tissues very sensitive to the female sex steroids, estrogen and progesterone. The contraceptive effect is more dependent upon endometrial and cervical mucus effects, because gonadotropins are not consistently suppressed. The endometrium involutes and becomes hostile to implantation, and the cervical mucus becomes thick and impermeable. Approximately 40% of patients will ovulate normally. Tubal physiology may also be affected, but this is speculative.

Because of the low dose, the minipill must be taken every day at the same time of day. The change in the cervical mucus requires 2–4 hours to take effect, and, most importantly, the impermeability diminishes 22 hours after administration, and by 24 hours sperm penetration is essentially unimpaired.

Ectopic pregnancy is not prevented as effectively as intrauterine pregnancy. Although the overall incidence of ectopic pregnancy is not increased (it is still much lower than the incidence in women not using a contraceptive method), when pregnancy occurs, the clinician must suspect that it is more likely to be ectopic. A previous ectopic pregnancy should not be regarded as a contraindication to the minipill.

There are no significant metabolic effects (lipid levels, carbohydrate metabolism, and coagulation factors remain unchanged),[347] and there is an immediate return to fertility on discontinuation (unlike the delay seen with the combination oral contraceptive). Only one disturbing observation has been reported; progestin-only oral contraception was associated with about a 3-fold incrased risk of diabetes mellitus in lactating women with recent gestational diabetes (an observation that is difficult to explain).[130] Because this increased risk is not observed with the use of combined oral contraceptives, it is speculated that the low levels of estrogen associated with breastfeeding allow an unimpeded progestin effect on insulin resistance.

Efficacy

Failure rates have been documented to range from 1.1 to 9.6 per 100 women in the first year of use.[348] The failure rate is higher in younger women (3.1 per 100 woman-years) compared with women over age 40 (0.3 per 100 woman-years).[349] In motivated women, the failure rate is comparable to the rate (less than 1 per 100 woman-years) with combination oral contraception.[350–352]

Pill Taking

The minipill should be started on the first day of menses, and a backup method must be used for the first 7 days because some women (very few) ovulate as early as 7–9 days after the onset of menses. The pill should be keyed to a daily event to ensure regular administration at the same time of the day. If pills are forgotten or gastrointestinal illness impairs absorption, the minipill should be resumed as soon as possible, and a back-up method should be used immediately and until the pills have been resumed for at least 2 days. If 2 or more pills are missed in a row and there is no menstrual bleeding in 4–6 weeks, a pregnancy test should be obtained. ***If more than 3 hours late in taking a pill, a backup method should be used for 48 hours.***

Problems

In view of the unpredictable effect on ovulation, it is not surprising that irregular menstrual bleeding is the major clinical problem. The daily progestational impact on the endometrium also contributes to this problem. Patients can expect to have normal, ovulatory cycles (40%), short, irregular cycles (40%), or a total lack of cycles ranging from irregular bleeding to spotting and amenorrhea (20%). This is the major reason why women discontinue the minipill method of contraception.[352]

Women on progestin-only contraception develop more functional, ovarian follicular cysts.[353] Nearly all, if not all, regress. This is not a clinical problem of any significance. Women who have experienced frequent ovarian cysts would be happier with methods that effectively suppress ovulation (combined oral contraceptives and depot-medroxyprogesterone acetate).

The levonorgestrel minipill may be associated with acne. The mechanism is similar to that seen with Norplant. The androgenic activity of levonorgestrel decreases the circulating levels of sex hormone-binding globulin (SHBG). Therefore free steroid levels (levonorgestrel and testosterone) will be increased despite the low dose. This is in contrast to the action of combined oral contraception where the effect of the progestin is countered by the estrogen-induced increase in SHBG.

The incidence of the other minor side effects is very low, probably at the same rate that would be encountered with a placebo.

Clinical Decisions

There are two situations where excellent efficacy, probably near total effectiveness, is achieved: lactating women and women over age 40. In lactating women, the contribution of the minipill is combined with prolactin-induced suppression of ovulation, adding up to very effective protection.[354] In breastfeeding, overweight, Latina women with prior gestational diabetes, the progestin-only minipill was associated with a 3-fold increased risk of non-insulin dependent diabetes mellitus.[130] It is not known whether this might be a risk in all women who have experienced gestational diabetes; a prudent course would be to advise other methods for this special group of women. In women over age 40, reduced fecundity adds to the minipill's effects.

There is another reason why the minipill is a good choice for the breastfeeding woman. There is no evidence for any adverse effect on breastfeeding as measured by milk volume and infant growth and development.[236, 355, 356] In fact, there is a modest positive impact; women using the minipill breastfeed longer and add supplementary feeding at a later time.[243] Because of the slight positive impact on lactation, the minipill can be started soon after delivery, but at least a 3-day postpartum delay is recommended to allow the decline in pregnancy levels of estrogen and progesterone and the establishment of lactation.[244]

The minipill is a good choice in situations where estrogen is contraindicated, such as patients with serious medical conditions (diabetes with vascular disease, severe systemic lupus erythematosus, cardiovascular disease). It should be noted that the freedom from estrogen effects, although likely, is presumptive. Substantial data, for example on associations with vascular disease, blood pressure, and cancer, are not available because relatively small numbers have chosen to use this method of contraception. On the other hand, it is logical to conclude that any of the progestin effects associated with the combination oral contraceptives can be related to the minipill according to a dose-response curve; all effects should be reduced. The World Health Organization case-control study could find no indication for increased risks of stroke, myocardial infarction, or venous thromboembolism with oral progestin-only contraceptives.[357] No impact can be measured on the coagulation system.[358, 359] The minipill can probably be used in women with previous episodes of thrombosis, and the package insert in the United States has been revised, eliminating vascular disease as a contraindication.

The minipill is a good alternative for the occasional woman who reports diminished libido on combination oral contraceptives, presumably due to decreased androgen levels. The minipill should also be considered for the few patients who report minor side effects (gastrointestinal upset, breast tenderness, headaches) of such a degree that the combination oral contraceptive is not acceptable.

Because of the relatively low doses of progestin administered, patients using medications that increase liver metabolism should avoid this method of contraception. These drugs include the following:

Rifampin.
Phenobarbital.
Phenytoin (Dilantin).
Primidone (Mysoline).
Carbamazepine (Tegretol).
Possibly ethosuximide, griseofulvin, and troglitazone.

Do the noncontraceptive benefits associated with combination oral contraception apply to the minipill? Studies are unable to help us with this issue, again because of the relatively small numbers of users. However, the progestin impact on cervical mucus, endometrium, and ovulation leads one to think the benefits will be present (reduced risks of pelvic infection, endometrial cancer, and ovarian cancer), but probably at reduced levels.

Good efficacy with the minipill requires regularity, taking the pill at the same time each day. There is less room for forgetting, and, therefore, the minipill is probably not a good choice for a disorganized adult or for the average adolescent.

Emergency Postcoital Contraception

The use of large doses of estrogen to prevent implantation was pioneered by Morris and van Wagenen at Yale in the 1960s. The initial work in monkeys led to the use of high doses of diethylstilbestrol (25–50 mg/day) and ethinyl estradiol in women.[360] It was quickly appreciated that these extremely large doses of estrogen were associated with a high rate of gastrointestinal side effects. Yuzpe developed a method utilizing a combination oral contraceptive, resulting in an important reduction in dosage.[361] The following treatment regimens have been documented to be effective:

Ovral: 2 tablets followed by 2 tablets 12 hours later.

Alesse: 5 tablets followed by 5 tablets 12 hours later.

Lo Ovral, Nordette, Levlen, Triphasil, Trilevlen: 4 tablets followed by 4 tablets 12 hours later.

Levonorgestrel in a dose of 0.75 mg given twice, 12 hours apart, is more successful and better tolerated than the combination oral contraceptive method, but this dose is equivalent to 10 pills of the levonorgestrel progestin-only minipill.[362, 363] In some countries, special packages of 0.75 mg levonorgestrel are available for emergency contraception. Greater efficacy and fewer side effects make low-dose levonorgestrel the treatment of choice.

In the United States, a kit is available containing 4 tablets, each containing 50 µg ethinyl estradiol and 0.250 mg levonorgestrel, to be used in the usual fashion, 2 tablets followed by 2 tablets 12 hours later.

This method has been more commonly called postcoital contraception, or the "morning after" treatment. Emergency contraception is a more accurate and appropriate name, indicating the intention to be one-time protection. It is an important option for patients, and should be considered when condoms break, sexual assault occurs, if diaphragms or cervical caps dislodge, or with the lapsed use of any method. In studies at abortion units, 50–60% of the patients would have been suitable for emergency contraception and would have used it if readily available.[364, 365] In the U.S., it is estimated that emergency contraception could annually prevent 1.7 million unintended pregnancies and the number of induced abortions would decrease by about 40% to 800,000 per year.[366]

Many women do not know of this method, and it has been difficult to obtain.[365, 367] In Europe and New Zealand, special packages with printed instructions are marketed specifically for emergency contraception, and this is now available in the U.S. Even if women are aware of this method, accurate and detailed knowledge is lacking.[368] A favorable attitude toward this method requires knowledge and availability. Information can be obtained from the following web site maintained by the Office of Population Research at Princeton University: http://opr.princeton.edu/ec/.

Clinicians should consider providing emergency contraceptive kits to patients (a kit can be a simple envelope containing instructions and the appropriate number of oral contraceptives) to be taken when needed. It would be a major contribution to our efforts to avoid unwanted pregnancies, for all patients without contraindications to oral contraceptives to have emergency contraception available for use when needed. In our view, this would be much more effective in reducing the need for abortion than waiting for patients to call. In a study of such an approach, self-administration by appropriately screened and educated women was found to be effective and free of unwanted effects.[369]

Mechanism and Efficacy

The mechanism of action is not known with certainty, but it is believed with justification that this treatment combines delay of ovulation with a local effect in the endometrium.[370, 371] The efficacy has been confirmed in large clinical trials and summarized in complete reviews of the literature.[372–374] Treatment with high doses of estrogen or with levonorgestrel yields a failure rate of approximately 1%, with the combination oral contraceptive, about 2–3%. The failure rate is lowest with high doses of ethinyl estradiol given within 72 hours (0.1%), but the side effects make the combination oral contraceptive a better choice. In general clinical use, the method can reduce the risk of pregnancy by about 75%; this degree of reduction in probability of conception (given the relatively low chance, about 8%, for pregnancy associated with one act of coitus[375]) yields the 2% failure rate measured in clinical studies (in other words, 98% effective).[376, 377] Results with levonorgestrel will be even better, 99% effective.

Treatment Method

Treatment should be initiated as soon after exposure as possible, and the standard recommendation is that it be no later than 72 hours. Careful assessment of the reported experience with emergency contraception indicated that the method is equally effective when started on the first, second, or third day after intercourse (which would allow user-friendly scheduling), and that efficacy might extend beyond 72 hours.[378] Data from randomized, clinical trials, however, support the importance of timing, finding a reduction in efficacy after 72 hours.[363] Because of possible, but unlikely, harmful effects of these high doses to a fetus, an already existing pregnancy should be ruled out prior to use of postcoital hormones. Furthermore, the patient should be offered induced abortion if the method fails. This patient encounter also provides an important opportunity to screen for STDs.

The combination oral contraceptive method delivers significantly less steroid hormone, and this reduction in the total dose and the number of doses reduces the side effects and limits them to a shorter time period. It is worth adding an antiemetic, oral or suppository, to the treatment; the long-acting nonprescription agent, meclizine, is recommended, to be taken one hour before the emergency contraception treatment. Side effects reflect the high doses used: nausea (50%), vomiting (20%), breast tenderness, headache, and dizziness. If a patient vomits within an hour after taking pills, additional pills must be administered as soon as possible. Although short-term treatment with combined oral contraceptives has been documented to have no effect on clotting factors, the usual contraindications for oral contraception apply to this use.[379] ***In view of the high dose of estrogen, emergency contraception with combined oral contraceptives should not be provided to women with either a personal or close family history (parent or sibling) of***

idiopathic thrombotic disease. For women with a contraindication to exogenous estrogen, the progestin-only minipill can be used for emergency contraception; e.g., administering 10 levonorgestrel tablets (75 µg), for each of the two doses, or in some countries using the special commercial package.

A 3-week follow-up visit should be scheduled to assess the result, and to counsel for routine contraception.

Could other combination oral contraceptive products be used? Because other doses and other formulations have never been tested, the efficacy is unknown. It would not be appropriate to expose patients to an unknown failure rate.

The use of danazol for emergency contraception is not effective.[380] Mifepristone (RU486), the progesterone antagonist, has been without failures and with lower side effects in clinical trials.

The 3 major problems with the available methods of emergency contraception are the high rate of side effects, the need to start treatment within 72 hours after intercourse, and the small, but important, failure rate. Mifepristone in a single oral dose of 600 mg is associated with markedly less nausea and vomiting and an efficacy rate of nearly 100%.[380, 381] Mifepristone is used for emergency contraception in China in a dose as low as 50 mg. Clinical studies have indicated that doses as low as 5 mg or 10 mg daily are effective. Because the next menstrual cycle is delayed after mifepristone, contraception should be initiated immediately after treatment. Ironically, mifepristone, around which swirls the abortion controversy, can make an effective contribution to preventing unwanted pregnancies and induced abortions.

Another method of emergency contraception is the insertion of a copper IUD, up to 5 days after unprotected intercourse. The failure rate (in a small number of studies) is very low, 0.1%.[372, 373] This method definitely prevents implantation, but it is not suitable for women who are not candidates for intrauterine contraception, e.g., multiple sexual partners, rape victim.

Oral Contraception for Older Women

Women of the post-World War II generation have faced a unique evolutionary change. They were the first to be able to exercise control over their fertility, and then as they aged and deferred pregnancy, they had to deal with the problem of unintended infertility. After World War II, the U.S. total fertility rate reached a modern high of 3.8 births per woman. The last women born in this period will not reach their 45th birthday until around 2010. For approximately a 20-year period, therefore, there will be an unprecedented number of women in the later child-bearing years. The aging of the World War II population boom is giving current times a greater number of women who are delaying marriage and childbirth. This demographic change has 3 specific impacts on couples.

1. A need for effective contraception.

2. The problem of achieving pregnancy later in life.

3. The problem of being pregnant later in life.

This combination of increasing numbers, deferment of marriage, and postponement of pregnancy in marriage is responsible for the fact that we will be seeing more and more older women who will need reversible contraception. This is underscored by the fact that from ages 20–44, American women have the highest proportion of pregnancies aborted compared to other countries, indicating an unappreciated, but real, problem of unintended pregnancy existing beyond the teenage years, especially after age 35. More than half of all pregnancies in the U.S. are estimated to be unplanned, and more than half of these are aborted.[382] The best way to minimize the number of induced abortions is effective contraception.

From 1970 to 1986, the number of births in women over 30 quadrupled; however, since 1990, the fertility rate among women over 30 has remained relatively stable.[383] As more and more couples defer pregnancy until later in life, the use of sterilization under age 35 will decline, and the need for reversible contraception will increase. Between 1988 and 1995, oral contraceptive use decreased in women younger than 25 and increased in women aged 30–44.[384] These numbers changed because clinicians and patients have come to understand and accept that low-dose oral contraception is safe for healthy, nonsmoking older women.

Oral Contraception for the Transition Years

The years from age 35 to menopause can be referred to as the transition years. Preventive health care for women is especially important during the transition years. The issues of preventive health care are familiar ones. They include contraception, cessation of smoking, prevention of heart disease and osteoporosis, maintenance of mental well-being (including sexuality), and cancer screening. Management of the transition years should be significantly oriented to preventive health care, and the use of low-dose oral contraception can now legitimately be viewed as a component of preventive health care. A discussion of the noncontraceptive health benefits of low-dose oral contraception is especially important with patients in their transition years. This group of women appreciates and understands decisions made with the risk:benefit ratio in mind.

During this period of time, there are several medical needs that must be addressed: the need for contraception, the management of persistent anovulation, and finally, menopausal and postmenopausal hormone therapy.

At approximately 40 years of age, the frequency of ovulation decreases. This initiates a period of waning ovarian function called the climacteric that will last several years, carrying a woman through decreased fertility and menopause to the postmenopausal years. Prior to menopause, the remaining follicles perform less well. As cycles become irregular, vaginal bleeding occurs at the end of an inadequate luteal phase or after a peak of estradiol without subsequent ovulation and corpus luteum formation. Eventually, many women will live through a period of anovulation. Occasionally, corpus luteum formation and function occur, and therefore the older woman is not totally safe from the threat of an unplanned and unexpected pregnancy.

Fortunately clinicians and patients have recognized that low-dose oral contraception is very safe for healthy, nonsmoking older women. However, their use is still not sufficient to meet the need. Besides fulfilling a need, we would argue that this population of women has a series of benefits to be derived from oral contraception that tilts the risk:benefit ratio to the positive side. The benefits of oral contraceptives reviewed in this chapter are especially pertinent for older women. A case-control study could find no evidence for an increased risk of breast cancer in women who used oral contraceptives *after age 40*.[385]

Despite the widespread teaching and publicity that smoking is a contraindication to oral contraceptive use over the age of 35, more older women who use oral contraceptives smoke and smoke heavily, compared with young women.[97] This strongly implies that older smokers are less than honest with clinicians when requesting oral contraception. *A former smoker must have stopped smoking for at least 12 consecutive months to be regarded as a nonsmoker. Women who have nicotine in their bloodstream obtained from patches or gum should be regarded as smokers.* Smokers over age 35 should continue to be advised that combined oral contraceptives are not a good choice, regardless of the number of cigarettes smoked. In view of the unreported high rate of smoking in older women who use oral contraceptives, clinicians should consider using 20 μg estrogen products for women over age 35.

A product containing 20 μg ethinyl estradiol and 150 μg desogestrel has been demonstrated in multicenter studies of women over age 30 to have the same efficacy and side effects as pills containing 30 and 35 μg of estrogen.[386–388] In a randomized study of women over age 30, this formulation was associated with the virtual elimination of any effects on coagulation factors.[389] Indeed, the 20 μg formulation has no significant impact on the measurements of clotting factors, even in smokers.[31, 32, 389, 390]

Although it is true that the implied safety of the lowest estrogen dose remains to be documented by epidemiologic studies, it seems clinically prudent to maximize the safety margin in this older age group of women. Although there may be some increase in breakthrough bleeding, we believe that older women who understand the increased safety implicit in the lowest estrogen dose are more willing to endure breakthrough bleeding and maintain continuation. With avoidance of risk factors and use of lowest dose pills, health risks are probably negligible for healthy nonsmoking women. For healthy nonsmoking women, no specific laboratory screening is necessary, beyond that which is usually incorporated in a program of preventive health care.

We should also mention the progestin-only minipill. Because of reduced fecundity, the minipill achieves near total efficacy in women over age 40. Therefore, the progestin-only minipill is a good choice for older woman, and especially for those women in whom estrogen is contraindicated. Older women are more accepting of irregular menstrual bleeding when they understand its mechanism, and, thus, are more accepting of the progestin-only minipill.

Anovulation and Bleeding. Throughout the transitional period of life there is a significant incidence of dysfunctional uterine bleeding due to anovulation. While the clinician is usually alerted to this problem because of irregular bleeding, clinician and patient often fail to diagnose anovulation when bleeding is not abnormal in schedule, flow, or duration. As a woman approaches menopause, a more aggressive attempt to document ovulation is warranted. A serum progesterone level measured approximately one week before menses is simple enough to obtain and worth the cost. The prompt diagnosis of anovulation (serum progesterone less than 300 ng/dL) will lead to appropriate therapeutic management that will have a significant impact on the risk of endometrial cancer.

In an anovulatory woman with proliferative or hyperplastic endometrium (unaccompanied by atypia), periodic oral progestin therapy is mandatory, such as 10 mg medroxyprogesterone acetate given daily the first 10 days of each month. If hyperplasia is already present, follow-up aspiration office curettage after 3–4 months is required. If progestin treatment is ineffective and histological regression is not observed, more aggressive treatment is warranted. Monthly progestin treatment should be continued until withdrawal bleeding ceases or menopausal symptoms are experienced. These are reliable signs (in effect, a bioassay) indicating the onset of estrogen deprivation and the need for the addition of estrogen in a postmenopausal hormone program.

If contraception is desired, the clinician and patient should seriously consider the use of oral contraception. The anovulatory woman cannot be guaranteed that spontaneous ovulation and pregnancy will not occur. The use of a low-dose oral contraceptive will at the same time provide contraception and prophylaxis against irregular, heavy anovulatory bleeding and the risk of endometrial hyperplasia and neoplasia. In some patients, oral contraceptive treatment achieves better regulation of menses than monthly progestin administration.

Clinicians have been made so wary of providing oral contraceptives to older women that a traditional postmenopausal hormone regimen is often utilized to treat a woman with the kind of irregular cycles usually experienced in the transitional years. This addition of exogenous estrogen when a woman is not amenorrheic or experiencing menopausal symptoms is inappropriate, and even risky (exposing the endometrium to excessively high levels of estrogen). *And something that is often unappreciated, the standard doses of estrogen and progestin in a postmenopausal regimen will not suppress gonadotropins and prevent ovulation.* [391] The appropriate response is to regulate anovulatory cycles with monthly progestational treatment or to utilize low-dose oral contraception.

When to Change From Oral Contraception to Postmenopausal Hormone Therapy

A common clinical dilemma is when to change from oral contraception to postmenopausal hormone therapy. It is important to change because even with the lowest estrogen dose oral contraceptive available, the estrogen dose is four-fold greater than the standard postmenopausal dose, and with increasing age, the dose-related risks with estrogen become significant. One approach to establish the onset of the postmenopausal years is to measure the FSH level, beginning at age 50, on an annual basis, being careful to obtain the blood sample on day 6 or 7 of the pill-free week (when steroid levels have declined sufficiently to allow FSH to rise). Friday afternoon works well for patients who start new packages on Sunday. When FSH is greater than 20 IU/L, it is time to change to a postmenopausal hormone program. Because of the variability in FSH levels experienced by women around the menopause, this method is not always accurate.[392] But there is no harm in retesting after another year or two on low-dose oral contraceptives. Some clinicians are comfortable allowing patients to enter their midfifties on low-dose oral contraception, and then empirically switching to a postmenopausal hormone regimen.

Concluding Thoughts

In the 1970s, as epidemiologic data first became available, we emphasized in our teaching and in our communication with patients the risks and dangers associated with oral contraceptives. In the 1990s, with better patient screening and epidemiologic data documenting the effects of low-dose products, we appropriately emphasized the benefits and safety of modern oral contraceptives. In the new millennium, we can with confidence promote the idea that the use of oral contraceptives yields an overall improvement in individual health, and from a public health point of view, the collection of effects associated with oral contraceptives leads to a decrease in the cost of health care.

Contraceptive advice is a component of good preventive health care, and the clinician's approach is a key factor. This is an era of informed choice by the patient. Patients deserve to know the facts and need help in dealing with the state of the art and those issues clouded by uncertainty. But there is no doubt that patients are influenced in their choices by their clinician's advice and attitude. Although the role of a clinician is to provide the education necessary for the patient to make proper choices, one should not lose sight of the powerful influence exerted by the clinician in the choices ultimately made. Emphasizing the safety and benefits of oral contraceptives, and the contribution of oral contraceptives to individual and public health, allows a clinician to present oral contraception with a very positive attitude, an approach that makes an important contribution to a patient's ability to make appropriate health choices.

References

1. **Halberstam D,** *The Fifties,* Ballantine Books, New York, 1993.

2. **Perone N,** The progestins, In: Goldzieher JW, ed. *Pharmacology of the Contraceptive Steroids,* Raven Press, Ltd., New York, 1994, p 5.

3. **Asbell B,** *The Pill: A Biography of the Drug that Changed the World,* Random House, New York, 1995.

4. **Djerassi C,** *The Pill, Pygmy Chimps, and Degas' Horse,* Basic Books, 1992.

5. **Pincus G,** *The Control of Fertility,* Academic Press, New York, 1965.

6. **Goldzieher JW,** Selected aspects of the pharmacokinetics and metabolism of ethinyl estrogens and their clinical implications, *Am J Obstet Gynecol* 163:318, 1990.

7. **Stanczyk FZ, Roy S,** Metabolism of levonorgestrel, norethindrone, and structurally related contraceptive steroids, *Contraception* 42:67, 1990.

8. **Edgren RA,** Progestagens, In: Givens J, ed. *Clinical Uses of Steroids,* Yearbook, Chicago, 1980, p 1.

9. **Kuhnz W, Blode H, Maher M,** Systemic availability of levonorgestrel after single oral administration of a noregestimate-containing combination oral contraceptive to 12 young women, *Contraception* 49:255, 1994.

10. **Stanczyk FZ,** Pharmacokinetics of the new progestogens and influence of gestodene and desogestrel on ethinylestradiol metabolism, *Contraception* 55:273, 1997.

11. **Speroff L, DeCherney A,** Evaluation of a new generation of oral contraceptives, *Obstet Gynecol* 81:1034, 1993.

12. **Rossmanith WG, Steffens D, Schramm G,** A comparative randomized trial on the impact of two low-dose oral contraceptives on ovarian activity, cervical permeability, and endometrial receptivity, *Contraception* 56:23, 1997.

13. **Sparrow MJ,** Pill method failures, *N Z Med J* 100:102, 1987.

14. **Hansen TH, Lundvall F,** Factors influencing the reliability of oral contraceptives, *Acta Obstet Gynecol Scand* 76:61, 1997.

15. **Trussell J, Hatcher RA, Cates Jr W, Stewart FH, Kost K,** Contraceptive failure in the United States: an update, *Stud Fam Plann* 21:51, 1990.

16. **Trussell J,** Contraceptive efficacy, In: Hatcher RA, Trussell J, Stewart F, et al, eds. *Contraceptive Technology,* 17th ed, Irvington Publishers, New York, NY, 1998.

17. **Child TJ, Rees M, MacKenzie IZ,** Pregnancy terminations after oral contraception scare, *Lancet* 347:1260, 1996.

18. **Skjeldestad FE,** Increased number of induced abortions in Norway after media coverage of adverse vascular events from the use of third-generation oral contraceptives, *Contraception* 55:11, 1997.

19. **Martinelli I, Sacchi E, Landi G, Taioli E, Duca F, Mannucci PM,** High risk of cerebral-vein thrombosis in carriers of a prothrombin-gene mutation and in users of oral contraceptives, *New Engl J Med* 338:1793, 1998.

20. **HaJJar KA,** Factor V Leiden: an unselfish gene? *New Engl J Med* 331:1585, 1994.

21. **Svensson PJ, Dahlbäck B,** Resistance to activated protein C as a basis for venous thrombosis, *New Engl J Med* 330:517, 1994.

22. **Zöller B, Hillarp A, Berntorp E, Dahlbäck B,** Activated protein C resistance due to a common factor V gene mutation is a major risk factor for venous thrombosis, *Ann Rev Med* 48:45, 1997.

23. **Rees DC, Cox M, Clegg JB,** World distribution of factor V Leiden, *Lancet* 346:1133, 1995.

24. **Zivelin A, Griffin JH, Xu X, Pabinger I, Samama M, Conard J, Brenner B, Eldor A, Seligsohn U,** A single genetic origin for a common Caucasian risk factor for venous thrombosis, *Blood* 89:397, 1997.

25. **Poort SR, Rosendaal FR, Reitsma PH, Bertina RM,** A common genetic variation in the 3'-untranslated region of the prothrombin gene is associated with elevated plasma prothrombin levels and an increase in venous thrombosis, *Blood* 88:3698, 1996.

26. **Rosendaal FR, Doggen CJM, Zivelin A, Arruda VR, Aiach M, Siscovick DS, Hillarp H, Watzke HH, Bernardi F, Cumming AM, Preston FE, Reitsma PH,** Geographic distribution of the 20210 G to A prothrombin variant, *Thromb Haemost* 79:706, 1998.

27. **Meade TW,** Oral contraceptives, clotting factors, and thrombosis, *Am J Obstet Gynecol* 142:758, 1982.

28. **Jespersen J, Petersen KR, Skouby SO,** Effects of newer oral contraceptives on the inhibition of coagulation and fibrinolysis in relation to dosage and type of steroid, *Am J Obstet Gynecol* 163:396, 1990.

29. **Notelovitz M, Kitchens CS, Khan FY,** Changes in coagulation and anticoagulation in women taking low-dose triphasic oral contraceptives: a controlled comparative 12-month clinical trial, *Am J Obstet Gynecol* 167:1255, 1992.

30. **Schlit AF, Grandjean P, Donnez J, Lavenne E,** Large increase in plasmatic 11-dehydro-TXB$_2$ levels due to oral contraceptives, *Contraception* 51:53, 1995.

31. **Fruzzetti F, Ricci C, Fioretti P,** Haemostasis profile in smoking and nonsmoking women taking low-dose oral contraceptives, *Contraception* 49:579, 1994.

32. **Basdevant A, Conard J, Pelissier C, Guyene T-T, Lapousterle C, Mayer M, Guy-Grand B, Degrelle II,** Hemostatic and metabolic effects of lowering the ethinyl-estradiol dose from 30 mcg to 20 mcg in oral contraceptives containing desogestrel, *Contraception* 48:193, 1993.

33. **Winkler UH, Schindler AE, Endrikat J, Düsterberg B,** A comparative study of the effects of the hemostatic system of two monophasic gestodene oral contraceptives containing 20 µg and 30 µg ethinylestradiol, *Contraception* 53:75, 1996.

34. **Croft P, Hannaford PC,** Risk factors for acute myocardial infarction in women: evidence from the Royal College of General Practitioners' oral contraception study, *Br Med J* 298:165, 1989.

35. **Rosenberg L, Palmer JR, Lesko SM, Shapiro S,** Oral contraceptive use and the risk of myocardial infarction, *Am J Epidemiol* 131:1009, 1990.

36. **Stampfer MJ, Willett WC, Colditz GA, Speizer FE, Hennekens CH,** Past use of oral contraceptives and cardiovascular disease: a meta-analysis in the context of the Nurses' Health Study, *Am J Obstet Gynecol* 163:285, 1990.

37. **Colditz GA, and the Nurses' Health Study Research Group,** Oral contraceptive use and mortality during 12 years of follow-up: the Nurses' Health Study, *Ann Intern Med* 120:821, 1994.

38. **Böttiger LE, Boman G, Eklund G, Westerholm B,** Oral contraceptives and thromboembolic disease: effects of lowering oestrogen content, *Lancet* i:1097, 1980.

39. **Gerstman BB, Piper JM, Tomita DK, Ferguson WJ, Stadel BV, Lundin FE,** Oral contraceptive estrogen dose and the risk of deep venous thromboembolic disease, *Am J Epidemiol* 133:32, 1991.

40. **Vessey M, Mant D, Smith A, Yeates D,** Oral contraceptives and venous thromboembolism: findings in a large prospective study, *Br Med J* 292:526, 1986.

41. **Helmrich SP, Rosenberg L, Kaufman DW, Strom B, Shapiro S,** Venous thromboembolism in relation to oral contraceptive use, *Obstet Gynecol* 69:91, 1987.

42. **Thorogood M, Mann J, Murphy M, Vessey M,** Risk factors for fatal venous thromboembolism in young women: a case-control study, *Int J Epidemiol* 21:48, 1992.

43. **Rosenberg L, Hennekens CH, Rosner B, Belanger C, Rothman KH, Speizer FE,** Oral contraceptive use in relation to nonfatal myocardial infarction, *Am J Epidemiol* 11:59, 1980.

44. **Royal College of General Practitioners Oral Contraceptive Study,** Incidence of arterial disease among oral contraceptive users, *J Roy Coll Gen Pract* 33:75, 1983.

45. **Lidegaard Ø,** Oral contraception and risk of a cerebral thromboembolic attack: results of a case-control study, *Br Med J* 306:956, 1993.

46. **Lawson DH, Davidson JF, Jick H,** Oral contraceptive use and venous thromboembolism: absence of an effect of smoking, *Br Med J* ii:729, 1977.

47. **Petitti DB, Wingerd J, Pellegrin F, Ramcharan S,** Oral contraceptives, smoking, and other factors in relation to risk of venous thromboembolic disease, *Am J Epidemiol* 108:480, 1978.

48. **Royal College of General Practitioners,** Oral contraceptive study: oral contraceptives, venous thrombosis, and varicose veins, *J Roy Coll Gen Pract* 28:393, 1978.

49. **Porter JB, Hershel J, Walker AM,** Mortality among oral contraceptive users, *Obstet Gynecol* 70:29, 1987.

50. **WHO Collaborative Study of Cardiovascular Disease and Steroid Hormone Contraception,** Venous thromboembolic disease and combined oral contraceptives: results of international multicentre case-control study, *Lancet* 348:1575, 1995.

51. **WHO Collaborative Study of Cardiovascular Disease and Steroid Hormone Contraception,** Effect of different progestagens in low oestrogen oral contraceptives on venous thromboembolic disease, *Lancet* 348:1582, 1995.

52. **Spitzer WO, Lewis MA, Heinemann LAJ, Thorogood M, MacRae KD, on behalf of the Transnational Research Group on Oral Contraceptives and the Health of Young Women,** Third generation oral contraceptives and risk of venous thromboembolic disorders: an international case-control study, *Br Med J* 312:83, 1996.

53. **Jick H, Jick SS, Gurewich V, Myers MW, Vasilakis C,** Risk of idiopathic cardiovascular death and nonfatal venous thromboembolism in women using oral contraceptives with differing progestagen components, *Lancet* 348:1589, 1995.

54. **Bloemenkammp KWM, Rosendaal FR, Helmerhorst FM, Büller HR, Vandenbroucke JP,** Enhancement by factor V Leiden mutation of risk of deep-vein thrombosis associated with oral contraceptives containing a third-generation progestagen, *Lancet* 348:1593, 1995.

55. **Speroff L,** Oral contraceptives and venous thromboembolism, *Int J Gynecol Obstet* 54:45, 1996.

56. **Lewis MA, Heinemann LAJ, MacRae KD, Bruppacher R, Spitzer WO,** The increased risk of venous thromboembolism and the use of third generation progestagens: role of bias in observational research, *Contraception* 54:5, 1996.

57. **Lidegaard Ø, Milsom I,** Oral contraceptives and thrombotic diseases: impact of new epidemiologic studies, *Contraception* 53:135, 1996.

58. **McPherson K,** Third generation oral contraception and venous thromboembolism. The published evidence confirms the Committee on Safety of Medicine's concerns, *Br Med J* 312:68, 1996.

59. **Vandenbroucke JP, Rosendaal FR,** End of the line for "third-generation-pill" controversy, *Lancet* 349:1113, 1997.

60. **Lidegaard Ø, Edström B, Kreiner S,** Oral contraceptives and venous thromboembolism. A case-control study, *Contraception* 5:291, 1998.

61. **Farmer RDT, Lawrenson RA, Thompson CR, Kennedy JG, Hambleton IR,** Population-based study of risk of venous thromboemboism associated with various oral contraceptives, *Lancet* 349:83, 1997.

62. **Farmer RDT, Todd J-C, Lewis MA, MacRae KD, Williams TJ,** The risks of venous thromboembolic disease among German women using oral contraceptives: a database study, *Contraception* 57:67, 1998.

63. **Suissa S, Blais L, Spitzer WO, Cusson J, Lewis M, Heinemann L,** First-time use of newer oral contraceptives and the risk of venous thromboembolism, *Contraception* 56:141, 1997.

64. **Kuhl H, Jung-Hoffman C, Heidt F,** Alterations in the serum levels of gestodene and SHBG during 12 cycles of treatment with 30 micrograms ethinylestradiol and 75 micrograms gestodene, *Contraception* 38:477, 1988.

65. **Jung-Hoffman C, Kuhl H,** Interaction with the phamacokinetics of ethinylestradiol and progestogens contained in oral contraceptives, *Contraception* 40:299, 1989.

66. **Hümpel M, Täuber U, Kuhnz W, Pfeffer M, Brill K, Heithecker R, Louton T, Steinberg B, Seifert W, Schütt B,** Protein binding of active ingredients and comparison of serum ethinyl estradiol, sex hormone-binding globulin, corticosteroid-binding globulin, and cortisol levels in women using a combination of gestodene/ethinyl estradiol (Femovan) or a combination of desogestrel/ethinyl estradiol (Marvelon) and single dose ethinyl estradiol bioequivalence from both oral contraceptives, *Am J Obstet Gynecol* 163:329, 1990.

67. **Dibbelt L, Knuppen R, Jütting G, Heimann S, Klipping CO, Parikka-Olexik H,** Group comparison of serum ethinyl estradiol, SHBG and CBG levels in 83 women using two low-dose oral contraceptives for three months, *Contraception* 43:1, 1991.

68. **Heinemann LAJ, Lewis MA, Assman A, Gravens L, Guggenmoos-Holzmann I,** Could preferential prescribing and referral behaviour of physicians explain the elevated thrombosis risk found to be associated with third generation oral contraceptives? *Pharmacoepidemiol Drug Saf* 5:285, 1996.

69. **Jamin C, de Mouzon J,** Selective prescribing of third generation oral contraceptives (OCs), *Contraception* 54:55, 1996.

70. **Van Lunsen WH,** Recent oral contraceptive use patterns in four European countries: evidence for selective prescribing of oral contraceptives containing third generation progestogens, *Eur J Contracept Reprod Health* 1:39, 1996.

71. **Farmer R, Lewis M,** Oral contraceptives and mortality from venous thromboembolism, *Lancet* 348:1095, 1996.

72. **Farmer RDT, Preston TD,** The risk of venous thromboembolism associated with low estrogen oral contraceptives, *J Obstet Gynaecol* 15:195, 1995.

73. **Vandenbroucke JP, van der Meer FJM, Helmerhorst FM, Rosendaal FR,** Factor V Leiden, *Br Med J* 313:1127, 1996.

74. **Ridker PM, Miletich JP, Hennekens CH, Buring JE,** Ethnic distribution of factor V Leiden in 4047 men and women: implications for venous thromboembolism screening, *JAMA* 277:1305, 1997.

75. **Vensson PJ, Dahlbäck B,** Resistance to activated protein C as a basis for venous thrombosis, *New Engl J Med* 330:517, 1994.

76. **Hellgren M, Svensson PJ, Dahlbäck B,** Resistance to activated protein C as a basis for venous thromboembolism associated with pregnancy and oral contraceptives, *Am J Obstet Gynecol* 173:210, 1995.

77. **Vandenbroucke JP, Koster T, Briët E, Reitsma PH, Bertina RM, Rosendaal FR,** Increased risk of venous thrombosis in oral-contraceptive users who are carriers of factor V Leiden mutation, *Lancet* 344:1453, 1994.

78. **Ridker PM, Hennekens CH, Lindpaintner K, Stampfer MJ, Eisenberg PR, Miletich JP,** Mutation in the gene coding for coagulation factor V and the risk of myocardial infarction, stroke, and venous thrombosis in apparently healthy men, *New Engl J Med* 332:912, 1995.

79. **Winkler UH,** Blood coagulation and oral contraceptives. A critical review, *Contraception* 57:203, 1998.

80. **Rosing J, Tans G, Nicolaes GAF, Thomassen MCLGD, van Oerle R, van der Ploeg PMEN, Heijnen P, Hamulyak K, Hemker HC,** Oral contraceptives and venous thrombosis: different sensitivities to activated protein C in women using second- and third-generation oral contraceptives, *Br J Haematol* 97:233, 1997.

81. **Schramm W, Heinemann LAJ,** Oral contraceptives and venous thromboembolism: acquired APC resistance? (Letter), *Br J Haematol* 98:491, 1997.

82. **Lidegaard Ø, Kreiner S,** Cerebral thrombosis and oral contraceptives. A case-control study, *Contraception* 57:303, 1998.

83. **Lidegaard Ø, Edström B,** Oral contraceptives and myocardial infarction. A case-control study (abstract), *Eur J Contracept Reprod Health Care* 1(Suppl):72, 1996.

84. **Sidney S, Petitti DB, Quesenberry CP, Klatsky AL, Ziel HK, Wolf S,** Myocardial infarction in users of low-dose oral contraceptives, *Obstet Gynecol* 88:939, 1996.

85. **Lewis MA, Heinemann LAJ, Spitzer WO, MacRae KD, Bruppacher R, for the Transnational Research Group on Oral Contraceptives and the Health of Young Women,** The use of oral contraceptives and the occurrence of acute myocardial infarction in young women. Results from the Transnational Study on Oral Contraceptives and the Health of Young Women, *Contraception* 56:129, 1997.

86. **Lewis MA, Spitzer WO, Heinemann LAJ, MacRae KD, Bruppacher R,** Lowered risk of dying of heart attack with third generation pill may offset risk of dying of thromboembolism, *Br Med J* 315:679, 1997.

87. **WHO Collaborative Study of Cardiovascular Disease and Steroid Hormone Contraception,** Acute myocardial infarction and combined oral contraceptives: results of an international multicentre case-control study, *Lancet* 349:1202, 1997.

88. **Petitti DB, Sidney S, Quesenberry Jr CP, Bernstein A,** Incidence of stroke and myocardial infarction in women of reproductive age, *Stroke* 28:280, 1997.

89. **Jick H, Porter J, Rothman KJ,** Oral contraceptives and nonfatal stroke in healthy young women, *Ann Int Med* 89:58, 1978.

90. **Vessey MP, Lawless M, Yeates D,** Oral contraceptives and stroke: findings in a large prospective study, *Br Med J* 289:530, 1984.

91. **Hannaford PC, Croft PR, Kay CR,** Oral contraception and stroke: evidence from the Royal College of General Practitioners' Oral Contraception Study, *Stroke* 25:935, 1994.

92. **Petitti DB, Sidney S, Bernstein A, Wolf S, Quesenberry C, Ziel HK,** Stroke in users of low-dose oral contraceptives, *New Engl J Med* 335:8, 1996.

93. **Heinemann LAJ, Lewis MA, Spitzer WO, Thorogood M, Guggenmoos-Holzmann I, Bruppacher R, and the Transnational Research Group on Oral Contraceptives and the Health of Young Women,** Thromboembolic stroke in young women. A European case-control study on oral contraceptives, *Contraception* 57:29, 1998.

94. **Schwartz SM, Siscovick DS, Longstreth Jr WT, Psaty BM, Beverly RK, Raghunathan TE, Lin D, Koepsell TD,** Use of low-dose oral contraceptives and stroke in young women, *Ann Intern Med* 127:596, 1997.

95. **WHO Collaborative Study of Cardiovascular Disease and Steroid Hormone Contraception,** Ischaemic stroke and combined oral contraceptives: results of an international, multicentre case-control study, *Lancet* 348:498, 1996.

96. **WHO Collaborative Study of Cardiovascular Disease and Steroid Hormone Contraception,** Haemorrhagic stroke, overall stroke risk, and combined oral contraceptives: results of an international, multicentre, case-control study, *Lancet* 348:505, 1996.

97. **Barrett DH, Anda RF, Escobedo LG, Croft JB, Williamson DF, Marks JS,** Trends in oral contraceptive use and cigarette smoking, *Arch Fam Med* 3:438, 1994.

98. **Wahl P, Walden C, Knopp R, Hoover J, Wallace R, Heiss R, Refkind B,** Effect of estrogen/progestin potency on lipid/lipoprotein cholesterol, *New Engl J Med* 308:862, 1983.

99. **Burkman RT, Robinson JC, Kruszon-Moran D, Kimball AW, Kwiterovich P, Burford RG,** Lipid and lipoprotein changes associated with oral contraceptive use: a randomized clinical trial, *Obstet Gynecol* 71:33, 1988.

100. **Patsch W, Brown SA, Grotto Jr AM, Young RL,** The effect of triphasic oral contraceptives on plasma lipids and lipoproteins, *Am J Obstet Gynecol* 161:1396, 1989.

101. **Gevers Leuven JA, Dersjant-Roorda MC, Helmerhorst FM, de Boer R, Neymeyer-Leloux A, Havekes L,** Estrogenic effect of gestodene-desogestrel-containing oral contraceptives on lipoprotein metabolism, *Am J Obstet Gynecol* 163:358, 1990.

102. **Kloosterboer HJ, Rekers H,** Effects of three combined oral contraceptive preparations containing desogestrel plus ethinyl estradiol on lipid metabolism in comparison with two levonorgestrel preparations, *Am J Obstet Gynecol* 163:370, 1990.

103. **Notelovitz M, Feldmand EB, Gillespy M, Gudat J,** Lipid and lipoprotein changes in women taking low-dose, triphasic oral contraceptives: a controlled, comparative, 12-month clinical trial, *Am J Obstet Gynecol* 160:1269, 1989.

104. **Adams MR, Clarkson TB, Koritnik DR, Nash HA,** Contraceptive steroids and coronary artery atherosclerosis in cynomolgus macaques, *Fertil Steril* 47:1010, 1987.

105. **Clarkson TB, Adams MR, Kaplan JR, Shively CA, Koritnik DR,** From menarche to menopause: coronary artery atherosclerosis and protection in cynomolgus monkeys, *Am J Obstet Gynecol* 160:1280, 1989.

106. **Clarkson TB, Shively CA, Morgan TM, Koritnik DR, Adams MR, Kaplan JR,** Oral contraceptives and coronary artery atherosclerosis of cynomolgus monkeys, *Obstet Gynecol* 75:217, 1990.

107. **Kushwaha R, Hazzard W,** Exogenous estrogens attenuate dietary hypercholesterolemia and atherosclerosis in the rabbit, *Metabolism* 30:57, 1981.

108. **Hough JL, Zilversmit DB,** Effect of 17 beta estradiol on aortic cholesterol content and metabolism in cholesterol-fed rabbits, *Arteriosclerosis* 6:57, 1986.

109. **Henriksson P, Stamberger M, Eriksson M, Rudling M, Diczfalusy U, Berglund L, Angelin B,** Oestrogen-induced changes in lipoprotein metabolism: role in prevention of atherosclerosis in the cholesterol-fed rabbit, *Eur J Clin Invest* 19:395, 1989.

110. **Engel JH, Engel E, Lichtlen PR,** Coronary atherosclerosis and myocardial infarction in young women — role of oral contraceptives, *Eur Heart J* 4:1, 1983.

111. **Jugdutt BI, Stevens GF, Zacks DJ, Lee SJK, Taylor RF,** Myocardial infarction, oral contraception, cigarette smoking, and coronary artery spasm in young women, *Am Heart J* 106:757, 1983.

112. **Kovacs L, Bartfai G, Apro G, Annus J, Bulpitt C, Belsey E, Pinol A,** The effect of the contraceptive pill on blood pressure: a randomized controlled trial of three progestogen-oestrogen combinations in Szeged, Hungary, *Contraception* 33:69, 1986.

113. **Nichols M, Robinson G, Bounds W, Newman B, Guillebaud J,** Effect of four combined oral contraceptives on blood pressure in the pill-free interval, *Contraception* 47:367, 1993.

114. **Qifang S, Deliang L, Ziurong J, Haifang L, Zhongshu Z,** Blood pressure changes and hormonal contraceptives, *Contraception* 50:131, 1994.

115. **Darney P,** Safety and efficacy of a triphasic oral contraceptive containing desogrestrel: results of three multicenter trials, *Contraception* 48:323, 1993.

116. **Chasan-Taber L, Willett WC, Manson JE, Spiegelman D, Hunter DJ, Curhan G, Colditz GA, Stampfer MJ,** Prospective study of oral contraceptives and hypertension among women in the United States, *Circulation* 94:483, 1996.

117. **Brady WA, Kritz-Silverstein D, Barrett-Connor E, Morales AJ,** Prior oral contraceptive use is associated with higher blood pressure in older women, *J Women's Health* 7:221, 1998.

118. **Pritchard JA, Pritchard SA,** Blood pressure response to estrogen-progestin oral contraceptives after pregnancy-induced hypertension, *Am J Obstet Gynecol* 129:733, 1977.

119. **de Bruijn SFTM, Stam J, Koopman MMW, Vandenbroucke JP, for the Cerebral Venous Sinus Thrombosis Study Group,** Case-control study of risk of cerebral sinus thrombosis in oral contraceptive users who are carriers of hereditary prothrombotic conditions, *Br Med J* 316:589, 1998.

120. **Pabinger I, Schneider B, and the GTH Study Group,** Thrombotic risk of women with hereditary antithrombin III, protein C, and protein S deficiency taking oral contraceptive medication, *Thromb Haemost* 5:548, 1994.

121. **Godsland IF, Crook D, Simpson R, Proudler T, Gelton C, Lees B, Anyaoku V, Devenport M, Wynn V,** The effects of different formulations of oral contraceptive agents on lipid and carbohydrate metabolism, *New Engl J Med* 323:1375, 1990.

122. **van der Vange N, Kloosterboer HJ, Haspels AA,** Effect of seven low-dose combined oral contraceptive preparations on carbohydrate metabolism, *Am J Obstet Gynecol* 156:918, 1987.

123. **Bowes WA, Katta LR, Droegemueller W, Braight TG,** Triphasic randomized clinical trial: Comparison of effects on carbohydrate metabolism, *Am J Obstet Gynecol* 161:1402, 1989.

124. **Gaspard UJ, Lefebvre PJ,** Clinical aspects of the relationship between oral contraceptives, abnormalities in carbohydrate metabolism, and the development of cardiovascular disease, *Am J Obstet Gynecol* 163:334, 1990.

125. **Hannaford PC, Kay CR,** Oral contraceptives and diabetes mellitus, *Br Med J* 299:315, 1989.

126. **Rimm EB, Manson JE, Stampfer MJ, Colditz GA, Willett WC, Rosner B, Hennekens CH, Speizer FE,** Oral contraceptive use and the risk of type 2 (non-insulin-dependent) diabetes mellitus in a large prospective study of women, *Diabetologia* 35:967, 1992.

127. **Duffy TJ, Ray R,** Oral contraceptive use: Prospective follow-up of women with suspected glucose intolerance, *Contraception* 30:197, 1984.

128. **Chasan-Taber L, Colditz GA, Willett WC, Stampfer MJ, Hunter BJ, Colditz GA, Spiegelman D, Manson JE,** A prospective study of oral contraceptives and NIDDM among U.S. women, *Diabetes Care* 20:330, 1997.

129. **Kjos SL, Shoupe D, Douyan S, Friedman RL, Bernstein GS, Mestman JH, Mishell Jr DR,** Effect of low-dose oral contraceptives on carbohydrate and lipid metabolism in women with recent gestational diabetes: results of a controlled, randomized, prospective study, *Am J Obstet Gynecol* 163:1822, 1990.

130. **Kjos SL, Peters RK, Xiang A, Thomas D, Schaefer U, Buchanan TA,** Contraception and the risk of type 2 diabetes in Latino women with prior gestational diabetes, *JAMA* 280:533, 1998.

131. **Skouby SO, Malsted-Pedersen L, Kuhl C, Bennet P,** Oral contraceptives in diabetic women: metabolic effects of compounds with different estrogen/progestogen profiles, *Fertil Steril* 46:858, 1986.

132. **Garg SK, Chase HP, Marshall G, Hoops SL, Holmes DL, Jackson WE,** Oral contraceptives and renal and retinal complications in young women with insulin-dependent diabetes mellitus, *JAMA* 271:1099, 1994.

133. **Petersen KR, Skouby SO, Sidelmann J, Mølsted-Petersen L, Jespersen J,** Effects of contraceptive steroids on cardiovascular risk factors in women with insulin-dependent diabetes mellitus, *Am J Obstet Gynecol* 171:400, 1994.

134. **Hannaford PC, Kay CR, Vessey MP, Painter R, Mant J,** Combined oral contraceptives and liver disease, *Contraception* 55:145, 1997.

135. **Royal College of General Practitioners' Oral Contraception Study,** Oral contraceptives and gallbladder disease, *Lancet* ii:957, 1982.

136. **Bennion LJ, Ginsberg RL, Garnick MB, Bennett PH,** Effects of oral contraceptives on the gallbladder bile of normal women, *New Engl J Med* 294:189, 1976.

137. **Grodstein F, Colditz GA, Hunter DJ, Manson JE, Willett WC, Stampfer MJ,** A prospective study of symptomatic gallstones in women: relation with oral contraceptives and other risk factors, *Obstet Gynecol* 84:207, 1994.

138. **La Vecchia C, Negri E, D'Avanzo B, Parazzini F, Genitle A, Franceschi S,** Oral contraceptives and noncontraceptive oestrogens in the risk of gallstone disease requiring surgery, *J Epidemiol Community Health* 46:234, 1992.

139. **Vessey M, Painter R,** Oral contraceptive use and benign gallbladder disease; revisited, *Contraception* 50:167, 1994.

140. **Carpenter S, Neinstein LS,** Weight gain in adolescent and young adult oral contraceptive users, *J Adol Health Care* 7:342, 1986.

141. **Reubinoff BE, Wurtman J, Rojansky N, Adler D, Stein P, Schenker JG, Brzezinski A,** Effects of hormone replacement therapy on weight, body composition, fat distribution, and food intake in early postmenopausal women: a prospective study, *Fertil Steril* 64:963, 1995.

142. **Vessey MP, Villard-Mackintosh L, Painter R,** Oral contraceptives and pregnancy in relation to peptic ulcer, *Contraception* 46:349, 1992.

143. **Lashner BA, Kane SV, Hanauer SB,** Lack of association between oral contraceptive use and ulcerative colitis, *Gastroenterology* 99:1032, 1990.

144. **Wendler J, Siegert C, Schelhorn P, Klinger G, Gurr S, Kaufmann J, Aydinlik S, Braunschweig T,** The influence of Microgynon® and Diane-35®, two sub-fifty ovulation inhibitors, on voice function in women, *Contraception* 52:343, 1995.

145. **The Cancer and Steroid Hormone Study of the CDC and NICHD,** Combination oral contraceptive use and the risk of endometrial cancer, *JAMA* 257:796, 1987.

146. **Schlesselman JJ,** Oral contraceptives and neoplasia of the uterine corpus, *Contraception* 43:557, 1991.

147. **Vessey MP, Painte R,** Endometrial and ovarian cancer and oral contraceptives — findings in a large cohort study, *Br J Cancer* 71:1340, 1995.

148. **Jick SS, Walker AM, Jick H,** Oral contraceptives and endometrial cancer, *Obstet Gynecol* 82:931, 1993.

149. **Mant JWF, Vessey MP,** Ovarian and endometrial cancers, *Cancer Surveys* 19:287, 1994.

150. **The Cancer and Steroid Hormone Study of the CDC and NICHD,** The reduction in risk of ovarian cancer associated with oral-contraceptive use, *New Engl J Med* 316:650, 1987.

151. **Hankinson SE, Colditz GA, Hunter DJ, Spencer TL, Rosner B, Stampfer MJ,** A quantitative assessment of oral contraceptive use and risk of ovarian cancer, *Obstet Gynecol* 80:708, 1992.

152. **Whittemore AS, Harris R, Itnyre J, and the Collaborative Ovarian Cancer Group,** Characteristics relating to ovarian cancer risk: collaborative analysis of 12 US case-control studies. II: Invasive epithelial ovarian cancers in white women, *Am J Epidemiol* 136:1184, 1992.

153. **Rosenberg L, Palmer JR, Zauber AG, Warshauer ME, Lewis Jr JL, Strom BL, Harlap S, Shapiro S,** A case-control study of oral contraceptive use and invasive epithelial ovarian cancer, *Am J Epidemiol* 139:654, 1994.

154. **Gross TP, Schlesselman JJ,** The estimated effect of oral contraceptive use on the cumulative risk of epithelial ovarian cancer, *Obstet Gynecol* 83:419, 1994.

155. **Narod SA, Risch H, Moslehi R, Dørum A, Neuhausen S, Olsson H, Provencher D, Radice P, Evans G, Bishop lS, Brunet J-S, Ponder BAJ, for the Hereditary Ovarian Cancer Clinical Study Group,** Oral contraceptives and the risk of hereditary ovarian cancer, *New Engl J Med* 339:424, 1998.

156. **Brinton LA,** Oral contraceptives and cervical neoplasia, *Contraception* 43:581, 1991.

157. **Delgado-Rodriguez M, Sillero-Arenas M, Martin-Moreno JM, Galvez-Vargas R,** Oral contraceptives and cancer of the cervix uteri. A meta-analysis, *Acta Obstet Gynecol Scand* 71:368, 1992.

158. **Gram IT, Macaluso M, Stalsberg H,** Oral contraceptive use and the incidence of cervical intraepithelial neoplasia, *Am J Obstet Gynecol* 167:40, 1992.

159. **Irwin KL, Rosero-Bixby L, Oberle MW, Lee NC, Whatley AS, Fortney JA, Bonhomme MG,** Oral contraceptives and cervical cancer risk in Costa Rica: detection bias or causal association? *JAMA* 259:59, 1988.

160. **Ye Z, Thomas DB, Ray RM, and the WHO Collaborative Study of Neoplasia and Steroid Contraceptives,** Combined oral contraceptives and risk of cervical carcinoma in situ, *Int J Epidemiol* 24:19, 1995.

161. **Brinton LA, Reeves WC, Brenes MM, Herrero R, de Britton RC, Gaitan E, Tenorio F, Garcia M, Rawls WE,** Oral contraceptive use and risk of invasive cervical cancer, *Int J Epidemiol* 19:4, 1990.

162. **Ursin G, Peters RK, Hendeson BE, d'Ablaing III G, Monroe KR, Pike MC,** Oral contraceptive use and adenocarcinoma of cervix, *Lancet* 344:1390, 1994.

163. **Thomas DB, Ray RM, and the World Health Organization Collaborative Study of Neoplasia and Steroid Contraceptives,** Oral contraceptives and invasive adenocarcinomas and adenosquamous carcinomas of the uterine cervix, *Am J Epidemiol* 144:281, 1996.

164. **Schwartz SM, Weiss NS,** Increased incidence of adenocarcinoma of the cervix in young women in the United States, *Am J Epidemiol* 124:1045, 1986.

165. **Cherqui D, Rahmouni A, Charlotte F, Boulahdour H, Metreau JM, Meignan M, Fagniez PL, Zafrani ES, Mathieu D, Dhumeaux C,** Management of focal nodular hyperplasia and hepatocellular adenoma in young women: a series of 41 patients with clinical radiological and pathological correlations, *Hepatology* 22:1674, 1995.

166. **Côté C,** Regression of focal nodular hyperplasia of the liver after oral contraceptive discontinuation, *Clin Nuc Med* 9:587, 1997.

167. **Neuberger J, Forman D, Doll R, Williams R,** Oral contraceptives and hepatocellular carcinoma, *Br Med J* 292:1355, 1986.

168. **Palmer JR, Rosenberg L, Kaufman DW, Warshauer ME, Stolley P, Shapiro S,** Oral contraceptive use and liver cancer, *Am J Epidemiol* 130:878, 1989.

169. **WHO Collaborative Study of Neoplasia and Steroid Contraceptives,** Combined oral contraceptives and liver cancer, *Int J Cancer* 43:254, 1989.

170. **The Collaborative MILTS Project Team,** Oral contraceptives and liver cancer. Results of the Multicentre International Liver Tumor Study (MILTS), *Contraception* 56:275, 1997.

171. **Mant JWF, Vessey MP,** Trends in mortality from primary liver cancer in England and Wales 1975–92: influence of oral contraceptives, *Br J Cancer* 72:800, 1995.

172. **Waetjen LE, Grimes DA,** Oral contraceptives and primary liver cancer: temporal trends in three countries, *Obstet Gynecol* 88:945, 1996.

173. **Brinton LA, Vessey MP, Flavel R, Yeates D,** Risk factors for benign breast disease, *Am J Epidemiol* 113:203, 1981.

174. **Charreau I, Plu-Bureau G, Bachelot A, Contesso G, Guinebretiere JM, L''e MG,** Oral contraceptive use and risk of benign breast disease in a French case-control study of young women, *Eur J Cancer Prev* 2:147, 1993.

175. **Royal College of General Practitioners Oral Contraceptive Study,** Further analyses of mortality in oral contraceptive users, *Lancet* i:541, 1981.

176. **Vessey M, Baron J, Doll R, McPherson K, Yeates D,** Oral contraceptives and breast cancer: final report of an epidemiological study, *Br J Cancer* 47:455, 1982.

177. **Vessey M, McPherson K, Villard-Mackintosh L, Yeates D,** Oral contraceptives and breast cancer: latest findings in a large cohort study, *Br J Cancer* 59:613, 1989.

178. **Ramcharan S, Pellegrin FA, Ray RM, Hsu J-P,** The Walnut Creek Contraceptive Drug Study. A prospective study of the side effects of oral contraceptives, *J Reprod Med* 25:360, 1980.

179. **Romieu I, Willett WC, Colditz GA, Stampfer MJ, Rosner B, Hennekens CH, Speizer FE,** Prospective study of oral contraceptive use and risk of breast cancer in women, *J Natl Cancer Inst* 81:1313, 1989.

180. **McPherson K, Neil A, Vessey MP,** Oral contraceptives and breast cancer, *Lancet* ii:414, 1983.

181. **La Vecchia C, Decarli A, Fasoli M, Franceschi S, Gentile A, Negri E, Parazzini F, Tognomi G,** Oral contraceptives and cancers of the breast and of the female genital tract. Interim results from a case-control study, *Br J Cancer* 54:311, 1986.

182. **Meirik O, Dami H, Christoffersen T, Lund E, Bergstrom R, Bergsjo P,** Oral contraceptive use and breast cancer in young women, *Lancet* ii:650, 1986.

183. **Kay CR, Hannaford PC,** Breast cancer and the pill — further report from the Royal College of General Practitioners' oral contraceptive study, *Br J Cancer* 58:675, 1988.

184. **Miller DR, Rosenberg L, Kaufman DW, Stolley P, Warshauer ME, Shapiro S,** Breast cancer before age 45 and oral contraceptive use: new findings, *Am J Epidemiol* 129:269, 1989.

185. **UK National Case-Control Study Group,** Oral contraceptive use and breast cancer risk in young women, *Lancet* i:973, 1989.

186. **WHO Collaborative Study of Neoplasia and Steroid Contraceptives,** Breast cancer and combined oral contraceptives: results from a multinational study, *Br J Cancer* 61:110, 1990.

187. **La Vecchia C, Negri E, Franceschi S, Talamini R, Amadori D, Filiberti R, Conti E, Montella M, Veronesi A, Parazzini F, Ferraroni M, Decarli A,** Oral contraceptives and breast cancer: a cooperative Italian study, *Int J Cancer* 60:163, 1995.

188. **Hennekens CH, Speizer FE, Lipnik RJ, Rosner B, Bain C, Belanger C, Stampfer MJ, Willett W, Peto R,** Case-control study of oral contraceptive use and breast cancer, *J Natl Cancer Inst* 72:39, 1984.

189. **Rosenberg L, Miller DR, Kaufman DW, Helmrich SP, Stolley PD, Schoffenfeld D, Shapiro S,** Breast cancer and oral contraceptive use, *Am J Epidemiol* 119:167, 1984.

190. **Stadel BV, Rubin GL, Webster LA, Schlesselmann JJ, Wingo PA,** Oral contraceptives and breast cancer in young women, *Lancet* ii:970, 1985.

191. **Pike MC, Krailo MD, Henderson BE, Duke A, Roy S,** Breast cancer in young women and use of oral contraceptives: possible modifying effect of formulation and age at use, *Lancet* ii:926, 1983.

192. **Wingo PA, Lee NC, Ory HW, Beral V, Peterson HB, Rhodes P,** Age-specific differences in the relationship between oral contraceptive use and breast cancer, *Obstet Gynecol* 78:161, 1991.

193. **Ursin G, Aragaki CC, Paganini-Hill A, Siemiatycki J, Thompson WD, Haile RW,** Oral contraceptives and premenopausal bilateral breast cancer: a case-control study, *Epidemiology* 3:414, 1992.

194. **Rookus MA, Leeuwen FE, for the Netherlands Oral Contraceptives and Breast Cancer Study Group,** Oral contraceptives and risk of breast cancer in women aged 20-54 years, *Lancet* 344:844, 1994.

195. **White E, Malone KE, Weiss NS, Daling JR,** Breast cancer among young U.S. women in relation to oral contraceptive use, *J Natl Cancer Inst* 86:505, 1994.

196. **Brinton LA, Daling JR, Liff JM, Schoenberg JB, Malone KE, Stanford JL, Coates RJ, Gammon MD, Hanson L, Hoover RN,** Oral contraceptives and breast cancer risk among younger women, *J Natl Cancer Inst* 87:827, 1995.

197. **Cancer and Steroid Hormone Study, CDC and NICHD,** Oral contraceptive use and the risk of breast cancer, *New Engl J Med* 315:405, 1986.

198. **Schlesselman JJ, Stadel BV, Murray P, Shenghan L,** Breast cancer risk in relation to type of estrogen contained in oral contraceptives, *Contraception* 36:595, 1987.

199. **Stanford JL, Brinton LA, Hoover RN,** Oral contraceptives and breast cancer: results from an expanded case-control study, *Br J Cancer* 60:375, 1989.

200. **Murray P, Schlesselman JJ, Stadel BV, Shenghan L,** Oral contraceptives and breast cancer risk in women with a family history of breast cancer, *Am J Obstet Gynecol* 73:977, 1989.

201. **Schildkraut JM, Hulka BS, Wilkinson WE,** Oral contraceptives and breast cancer: a case-control study with hospital and community controls, *Obstet Gynecol* 76:395, 1990.

202. **Collaborative Group on Hormonal Factors in Breast Cancer,** Breast cancer and hormonal contraceptives: collaborative reanalysis of individual data on 53,297 women with breast cancer and 100,239 women without breast cancer from 54 epidemiological studies, *Lancet* 347:1713, 1996.

203. **Lambe M, Hsieh C, Trichopoulos D, Ekbom A, Pavia M, Adami H-O,** Transient increase in the risk of breast cancer after giving birth, *New Engl J Med* 331:5, 1994.

204. **Guinee VF, Olsson H, Moller T, Hess KR, Taylor SH, Fahey T, Gladikov JV, van den Blink JW, Bonichon F, Dische S, et al,** Effect of pregnancy on prognosis for young women with breast cancer, *Lancet* 343:1587, 1994.

205. **Kroman N, Wohlfart J, Andersen KW, Mouriudsen HT, Westergaard U, Melbye M,** Time since childbirth and prognosis in primary breast cancer: population based study, *Br Med J* 315:851, 1997.

206. **Rosenberg L, Palmer JR, Clarke EA, Shapiro S,** A case-control study of the risk of breast cancer in relation to oral contraceptive use, *Am J Epidemiol* 136:1437, 1992.

207. **American Cancer Society,** Cancer facts & figures — 1998, *http://www.cancer.org/statistics.html*, 1998.

208. **Green A,** Oral contraceptives and skin neoplasia, *Contraception* 43:653, 1991.

209. **Hannaford PC, Villard-Mackintosh L, Vessey MP, Kay CR,** Oral contraceptives and malignant melanoma, *Br J Cancer* 63:430, 1991.

210. **Milne R, Vessey M,** The association of oral contraception with kidney cancer, colon cancer, gallbladder cancer (including extrahepatic bile duct cancer) and pituitary tumors, *Contraception* 43:667, 1991.

211. **Berkowitz RS, Bernstein MR, Harlow BL, Rice LW, Lage JM, Goldstein DP, Cramer DW,** Case-control study of risk factors for partial molar pregnancy, *Am J Obstet Gynecol* 173:788, 1995.

212. **Martinez ME, Grodstein F, Giovannucci E, Colditz GA, Speizer FE, Hennekens C, Rosner B, Willett WC, Stampfer MJ,** A prospective study of reproductive factors, oral contraceptive use, and risk of colorectal cancer, *Cancer Epidemiol Biomarkers Prev* 6:1, 1997.

213. **Janerich DT, Dugan JM, Standfast SJ, Strite L,** Congenital heart disease and prenatal exposure to exogenous sex hormones, *Br Med J* i:1058, 1977.

214. **Nora JJ, Nora AH, Blu J, Ingram J, Foster D,** Exogenous progestogen and estrogen implicated in birth defects, *JAMA* 240:837, 1978.

215. **Heinonen OP, Slone D, Monson RR, Hook ER, Shapiro S,** Cardiovascular birth defects in antenatal exposure to female sex hormones, *New Engl J Med* 296:67, 1976.

216. **Simpson JL, Phillips OP,** Spermicides, hormonal contraception and congenital malformations, *Adv Contraception* 6:141, 1990.

217. **Michaelis J, Michaelis H, Gluck E, Koller S,** Prospective study of suspected associations between certain drugs administered during early pregnancy and congenital malformations, *Teratology* 27:57, 1983.

218. **Bracken MB,** Oral contraception and congenital malformations in offspring: a review and meta-analysis of the prospective studies, *Obstet Gynecol* 76:552, 1990.

219. **Ressequie LJ, Hick JF, Bruen JA, Noller KL, O'Fallon WM, Kurland LT,** Congenital malformations among offspring exposed in utero to progestins, Olsted County, Minnesota, 1936-1974, *Fertil Steril* 43:514, 1985.

220. **Katz Z, Lancet M, Skornik J, Chemke J, Mogilemer B, Klinberg M,** Teratogenicity of progestogens given during the first trimester of pregnancy, *Obstet Gynecol* 65:775, 1985.

221. **Vessey MP, Wright NH, McPherson K, Wiggins P,** Fertility after stoping different methods of contraception, *Br Med J* i:265, 1978.

222. **Vessey MP, Smith MA, Yates D,** Return of fertility after discontinuation of oral contraceptives: influence of age and parity, *Br J Fam Plann* 11:120, 1986.

223. **Linn S, Schoenbaum SC, Monson RR, Rosner B, Ryan KJ,** Delay in conception for former 'pill' users, *JAMA* 247:629, 1982.

224. **Bracken MB, Hellenbrand KG, Holford TR,** Conception delay after oral contraceptive use: the effect of estrogen dose, *Fertil Steril* 53:21, 1990.

225. **Bagwell MA, Coker AL, Thompson SJ, Baker ER, Addy CL,** Primary infertility and oral contraceptive steroid use, *Fertil Steril* 63:1161, 1995.

226. **Rothman KJ,** Fetal loss, twinning, and birth weight after oral-contraceptive use, *New Engl J Med* 297:468, 1977.

227. **Ford JH, MacCormac L,** Pregnancy and lifestyle study: the long-term use of the contraceptive pill and the risk of age-related miscarriage, *Hum Reprod* 10:1397, 1995.

228. **Rothman KJ, Liess J,** Gender of offspring after oral-contraceptive use, *New Engl J Med* 295:859, 1976.

229. **Magidor S, Poalti H, Harlap S, Baras M,** Long-term follow-up of children whose mothers used oral contraceptives prior to contraception, *Contraception* 29:203, 1984.

230. **Vessey M, Doll R, Peto R, Johnson B, Wiggins P,** A long-term follow-up study of women using different methods of contraception — an interim report, *J Biosoc Sci* 8:373, 1976.

231. **Royal College of General Practitioners,** The outcome of pregnancy in former oral contraceptive users, *Br J Obstet Gynaecol* 83:608, 1976.

232. **Betrabet SS, Shikary ZK, Toddywalla VS, Toddywalla SP, Patel D, Saxena BN,** Transfer of norethisterone (NET) and levonorgestrel (LNG) from a single tablet into the infant's circulation through the mother's milk, *Contraception* 35:517, 1987.

233. **Diaz S, Peralta O, Juez G, Herreros C, Casado ME, Salvatierra AM, Miranda P, Durn E, Croxatto HB,** Fertility regulation in nursing women: III. Short-term influence of a low-dose combined oral contraceptive upon lactation and infant growth, *Contraception* 27:1, 1982.

234. **Croxatto HB, Diaz S, Peralta O, Juez G, Herreros C, Casado ME, Salvatierra AM, Miranda P, Durn E,** Fertility regulation in nursing women: IV. Long-term influence of a low-dose combined oral contraceptive initiated at day 30 postpartum upon lactation and child growth, *Contraception* 27:13, 1983.

235. **Peralta O, Diaz S, Juez G, Herreros C, Casado ME, Salvatierra AM, Miranda P, Durn E, Croxatto HB,** Fertility regulation in nursing women: V. Long-term influence of a low-dose combined oral contraceptive initiated at day 90 postpartum upon lactation and infant growth, *Contraception* 27:27, 1983.

236. **WHO, Special Programme of Research, Development, and Research Training in Human Reproduction, Task Force on Oral Contraceptives,** Effects of hormonal contraceptives on milk volume and infant growth, *Contraception* 30:505, 1984.

237. **Nilsson S, Melbin T, Hofvander Y, Sundelin C, Valentin J, Nygren KG,** Long-term follow-up of children breast-fed by mothers using oral contraceptives, *Contraception* 34:443, 1986.

238. **Campbell OM, Gray RH,** Characteristics and determinants of postpartum ovarian function in women in the United States, *Am J Obstet Gynecol* 169:55, 1993.

239. **Labbok MH, Hight-Laukaran V, Peterson AE, Fletcher V, von Hertzen H, Van Look PFA,** Multicenter study of the lactational amenorrhea method (LAM): I. Efficacy, duration, and implications for clinical application, *Contraception* 55:327, 1997.

240. **Visness CM, Kennedy KI, Gross BA, Parenteau-Carreau S, Flynn AM, Brown JB,** Fertility of fully breast-feeding women in the early postpartum period, *Obstet Gynecol* 89:164, 1997.

241. **Diaz S, Aravena R, Cardenas II, Casado ME, Miranda P, Schiappacasse V, Croxatto HB,** Contraceptive efficacy of lactational amenorrhea in urban Chilean women, *Contraception* 43:335, 1991.

242. **Gray RH, Campbell OM, Zacur HA, Labbok MH, MacRae SL,** Postpartum return of ovarian activity in nonbreastfeeding women monitored by urinary assays, *J Clin Endocrinol Metab* 64:645, 1987.

243. **McCann MF, Moggia AV, Hibbins JE, Potts M, Becker C,** The effects of a progestin-only oral contraceptive (levonorgestrel 0.03 mg) on breast-feeding, *Contraception* 40:635, 1989.

244. **Kennedy KI, Short RV, Tully MR,** Premature introduction of progestin-only contraceptive methods during lactation, *Contraception* 55:347, 1997.

245. **Pituitary Adenoma Study Group,** Pituitary adenomas and oral contraceptives: a multicenter case-control study, *Fertil Steril* 39:753, 1983.

246. **Shy FKK, McTiernan AM, Daling JR, Weiss NS,** Oral contraceptive use and the occurrence of pituitary prolactinomas, *JAMA* 249:2204, 1983.

247. **Wingrave SJ, Kay CR, Vessey MP,** Oral contraceptives and pituitary adenomas, *Br Med J* 280:685, 1980.

248. **Hulting A-L, Werner S, Hagenfeldt K,** Oral contraceptives do not promote the development or growth of prolactinomas, *Contraception* 27:69, 1983.

249. **Corenblum B, Donovan L,** The safety of physiological estrogen plus progestin replacement therapy and oral contraceptive therapy in women with pathological hyperprolactinemia, *Fertil Steril* 59:671, 1993.

250. **Testa G, Vegetti W, Motta T, Alagna F, Bianchedi D, Carlucci C, Bianchi M, Parazzini F, Crosignani PG,** Two-year treatment with oral contraceptives in hyperprolactinemic patients, *Contraception* 58:69, 1998.

251. **Furuhjelm M, Carlstrom K,** Amenorrhea following use of combined oral contraceptives, *Acta Obstet Gynecol Scand* 52:373, 1973.

252. **Shearman RP, Smith ID,** Statistical analysis of relationship between oral contraceptives, secondary amenorrhea and galactorrhea, *J Obstet Gynaecol Br Commonw* 79:654, 1972.

253. **Jacobs HS, Knuth UA, Hull MGR, Franks S,** Post "pill" amenorrhea — cause or coincidence? *Br Med J* ii:940, 1977.

254. **Costello Daly C, Helling-Giese GE, Mati JK, Hunter DJ,** Contraceptive methods and the transmission of HIV: implications for family planning, *Genitourin Med* 70:110, 1994.

255. **Taneepanichskul S, Phuapradit W, Chaturachinda K,** Association of contraceptives and HIV-1 infection in Thai female commercial sex workers, *Aust N Z J Obstet Gynaecol* 37:86, 1997.

256. **Kapiga SH, Lyamuya EF, Lwihula GK, Hunter DJ,** The incidence of HIV infection among women using family planning methods in Dar-es-Salaam, Tanzania, *AIDS* 12:75, 1998.

257. **Abma JC, Chandra A, Mosher WD, Peterson L, Piccinino L,** (Centers for Disease Control and Prevention, National Center For Heath Statistics), Fertility, family planning, and women's health: new data from the 1995 National Survey of Family Growth, Report No. 19; Series 23, 1997.

258. **Westrom I,** Incidence, prevalence, and trends of acute pelvic inflammatory disease and its consequences in industrialized countries, *Am J Obstet Gynecol* 138:880, 1980.

259. **Eschenbach DA, Harnisch JP, Holmes KK,** Pathogenesis of acute pelvic inflammatory disease: role of contraception and other risk factors, *Am J Obstet Gynecol* 128:838, 1977.

260. **Rubin GL, Ory WH, Layde PM,** Oral contraceptives and pelvic inflammatory disease, *Am J Obstet Gynecol* 140:630, 1980.

261. **Senanayake P, Kramer DG,** Contraception and the etiology of pelvic inflammatory diseases: new perspectives, *Am J Obstet Gynecol* 138:852, 1980.

262. **Panser LA, Phipps WR,** Type of oral contraceptive in relation to acute, initial episodes of pelvic inflammatory disease, *Contraception* 43:91, 1991.

263. **Svensson L, Westrom L, Mardh P,** Contraceptives and acute salpingitis, *JAMA* 251:2553, 1984.

264. **Wolner-Hanssen P,** Oral contraceptive use modifies the manifestations of pelvic inflammatory disease, *Br J Obstet Gynaecol* 93:619, 1986.

265. **Cates Jr W, Washington AE, Rubin GL, Peterson HB,** The pill, chlamydia and PID, *Fam Plann Perspect* 17:175, 1985.

266. **Critchlow CW, Wölner-Hanssen P, Eschenbach DA, Kiviat NB, Koutsky LA, Stevens CE, Holmes KK,** Determinants of cervical ectopia and of cervicitis: age, oral contraception, specific cervical infection, smoking, and douching, *Am J Obstet Gynecol* 173:534, 1995.

267. **Cramer DW, Goldman MB, Schiff I, Belisla S, Albrecht B, Stadel B, Gibson M, Wilson E, Stillman R, Thompson I,** The relationship of tubal infertility to barrier method and oral contraceptive use, *JAMA* 257:2446, 1987.

268. **Wolner-Hanssen P, Eschenbach DA, Paavonen J, Kiviat N, Stevens CE, Critchlow C, DeRouen T, Holmes KK,** Decreased risk of symptomatic chlamydial pelvic inflammatory disease associated with oral contraceptive use, *JAMA* 263:54, 1990.

269. **Ness RB, Keder LM, Soper DE, Amortegui AJ, Gluck J, Wiesenfeld H, Sweet RL, Rice PA, Peipert JF, Donegan SP, Kanbour-Shakir A,** Oral contraception and the recognition of endometritis, *Am J Obstet Gynecol* 176:580, 1997.

270. **Barbone F, Austin H, Louv WC, Alexander WJ,** A follow-up study of methods of contraception, sexual activity, and rates of trichomoniasis, candidiasis, and bacterial vaginosis, *Am J Obstet Gynecol* 163:510, 1990.

271. **Shoubnikova M, Hellberg D, Nilsson S, Mårdh P-A,** Contraceptive use in women with bacterial vaginosis, *Contraception* 55:355, 1997.

272. **Becker WJ,** Migraine and oral contraceptives, *Can J Neurol Sci* 24:16, 1997.

273. **Ross RK, Pike MC, Vessey MP, Bull D, Yeates D, Casagrande JT,** Risk factors for uterine fibroids: Reduced risk associated with oral contraceptives, *Br Med J* 293:359, 1986.

274. **Parazzini F, Negri E, La Vecchia C, Fedele L, Rabaiotti M, Luchini L,** Oral contraceptive use and risk of uterine fibroids, *Obstet Gynecol* 79:430, 1992.

275. **Samadi AR, Lee NC, Flanders D, Boring III JR, Parris EB,** Risk factors for self-reported uterine fibroids: a case-control study, *Am J Public Health* 86:858, 1996.

276. **Marshall LM, Spiegelman D, Goldman MB, Manson JE, Colditz GA, Barbieri RL, Stampfer MJ, Hunter DJ,** A prospective study of reproductive factors and oral contraceptive use in relation to the risk of uterine leiomyomata, *Fertil Steril* 70:432, 1998.

277. **Friedman AJ, Thomas PP,** Does low-dose combination oral contraceptive use affect uterine size or menstrual flow in premenopausal women with leiomyomas? *Obstet Gynecol* 85:631, 1995.

278. **Mattson RH, Cramer JA, Darney PD, Naftolin F,** Use of oral contraceptives by women with epilepsy, *JAMA* 256:238, 1986.

279. **Milsom I, Sundell G, Andersch B,** A longitudinal study of contraception and pregnancy outcome in a representative sample of young Swedish women, *Contraception* 43:111, 1991.

280. **Letterie GS, Chow GE,** Effect of "missed" pills on oral contraceptive effectiveness, *Obstet Gynecol* 79:979, 1992.

281. **Potter L, Oakley D, de Leon-Wong E, Cañamar R,** Measuring compliance among oral contraceptive users, *Fam Plann Perspect* 28:154, 1996.

282. **Killick SR, Bancroft K, Oelbaum S, Morris J, Elstein M,** Extending the duration of the pill-free interval during combined oral contraception, *Adv Contracep* 6:33, 1990.

283. **Elomaa K, Rolland R, Brosens I, Moorrees M, Deprest J, Tuominen J, Lähteenmäki P,** Omitting the first oral contraceptive pills of the cycle does not automatically lead to ovulation, *Am J Obstet Gynecol* 179:41, 1998.

284. **Jung-Hoffman C, Kuhl H,** Intra- and interindividual variations in contraceptive steroid levels during 12 treatment cycles: no relation to irregular bleedings, *Contraception* 42:423, 1990.

285. **Endrikat J, Müller U, Düsterberg B,** A twelve-month comparative clinical investigation of two low-dose oral contraceptives containing 20 µg ethinylestradiol/75 µg gestodene and 30 µg ethinylestradiol/75 µg gestodene, with respect to efficacy, cycle control, and tolerance, *Contraception* 55:131, 1997.

286. **Rosenberg MJ, Waugh MS, Stevens CM,** Smoking and cycle control among oral contraceptive users, *Am J Obstet Gynecol* 174:628, 1996.

287. **Rosenberg MJ, Waugh MS, Higgins JE,** The effect of desogestrel, gestodene, and other factors on spotting and bleeding, *Contraception* 53:85, 1996.

288. **Krettek SE, Arkin SI, Chaisilwattana P, Monif GR,** *Chlamydia trachomatis* in patients who used oral contraceptives and had intermenstrual spotting, *Obstet Gynecol* 81:728, 1993.

289. **Moore LL, Valuck R, McDougall C, Fink W,** A comparative study of one-year weight gain among users of medroxyprogesterone acetate, levonorgestrel implants, and oral contraceptives, *Contraception* 52:215, 1995.

290. **Lemay A, Dewailly SD, Grenier R, Huard J,** Attenuation of mild hyperandrogenic activity in postpubertal acne by a triphasic oral contraceptive containing low doses of ethynyl estradiol and d,l-norgestrel, *J Clin Endocrinol Metab* 71:8, 1990.

291. **Mango D, Ricci S, Manna P, Miggiano GAD, Serra GB,** Clinical and hormonal effects of ethinyl estradiol combined with gestodene and desogestrel in young women with acne vulgaris, *Contraception* 53:163, 1996.

292. **Redmond GP, Olson WH, Lippman JS, Kafrissen ME, Jones TM, Jorizzo JL,** Norgestimate and ethinyl estradiol in the treatment of acne vulgaris: a randomized, placebo-controlled trial, *Obstet Gynecol* 89:615, 1997.

293. **Grimes DA, Hughes JM,** Use of multiphasic oral contraceptives and hospitalizations of women with functional ovarian cysts in the United States, *Obstet Gynecol* 73:1037, 1989.

294. **Vessey M, Metcalfe A, Wells C, McPherson K, Westhoff C, Yeates C,** Ovarian neoplasms, functional ovarian cysts, and oral contraceptives, *Br Med J* 294:1518, 1987.

295. **Lanes SF, Birmann B, Walker AM, Singer S,** Oral contraceptive type and functional ovarian cysts, *Am J Obstet Gynecol* 166:956, 1992.

296. **Holt VL, Daling JR, McKnight B, Moore D, Stergachis A, Weiss NS,** Functional ovarian cysts in relation to the use of monophasic and triphasic oral contraceptives, *Obstet Gynecol* 79:529, 1992.

297. **Young RL, Snabes MC, Frank ML, Reilly M,** A randomized, double-blind, placebo-controlled comparison of the impact of low-dose and triphasic oral contaceptives on follicular development, *Am J Obstet Gynecol* 167:678, 1992.

298. **Grimes DA, Godwin AJ, Rubin A, Smith JA, Lacarra M,** Ovulation and follicular development associated with three low-dose oral contraceptives: a randomized controlled trial, *Obstet Gynecol* 83:29, 1994.

299. **Neely JL, Abate M, Swinker M, D'Angio R,** The effect of doxycycline on serum levels of ethinyl estradiol, norethindrone, and endogenous progesterone, *Obstet Gynecol* 77:416, 1991.

300. **Murphy AA, Zacur HA, Charache P, Burkman RT,** The effect of tetracycline on levels of oral contraceptives, *Am J Obstet Gynecol* 164:28, 1991.

301. **Helms SE, Bredle DL, Zajic J, Jarjoura D, Brodell RT, Krishnarao I,** Oral contraceptive failure rates and oral antibiotics, *J Am Acad Dermatol* 36:705, 1997.

302. **Szoka PR, Edgren RA,** Drug interactions with oral contraceptives: compilation and analysis of an adverse experience report database, *Fertil Steril* 49(Suppl):31S, 1988.

303. **Mitchell MC, Hanew T, Meredith CG, Schenker S,** Effects of oral contraceptive steroids on acetaminophen metabolism and elimination, *Clin Pharmacol Ther* 34:48, 1983.

304. **Gupta KC, Joshi JV, Hazari K, Pohujani SM, Satoskjar RS,** Effect of low estrogen combination oral contraceptives on metabolism of aspirin and phenylbutazone, *Int J Clin Pharmacol Ther Toxicol* 20:511, 1982.

305. **Tzourio C, Tehindrazanarierelo A, Iglésias S, Alpérovitch A, Chgedru F, d'Anglejan-Chatillon J, Bousser M-G,** Case-control study of migraine and risk of ischaemic stroke in young women, *Br Med J* 310:830, 1995.

306. **Lidegaard Ø,** Oral contraceptives, pregnancy and the risk of cerebral thromboembolism: the influence of diabetes, hypertension, migraine and previous thrombotic disease, *Br J Obstet Gynaecol* 102:153, 1995.

307. **Jungers P, Dougados M, Pelissier L, Kuttenn F, Tron F, Lesavre P, Bach JF,** Influence of oral contraceptive therapy on the activity of systemic lupus erythematosus, *Arthritis Rheum* 25:618, 1982.

308. **Petri M, Robinson C,** Oral contraceptives and systemic lupus erythematosus, *Arthritis Rheum* 40:797, 1997.

309. **Lutcher CL, Milner PF,** Contraceptive-induced vascular occlusive events in sickle cell disorders — fact or fiction? (abstract), *Clin Res* 34:217A, 1986.

310. **DeCeular K, Gruber C, Hayes R, Serjeant GR,** Medroxyprogesterone acetate and homozygous sickle-cell disease, *Lancet* ii:229, 1982.

311. **Knopp RH, LaRosa JC, Burkman Jr RT,** Contraception and dyslipidemia, *Am J Obstet Gynecol* 168:1994, 1993.

312. **Sullivan-Nelson M, Kuller JA, Zacur HA,** Clinical use of oral contraceptives administered vaginally: a case report, *Fertil Steril* 52:864, 1989.

313. **Coutinho EM, de Souza JC, da Silva AR, de Acosta OM, Flores JG, Gu ZP, Ladipo OA, Adekunle AO, Otolorin EO, Shaaban MM, Abul Oyoom M, et al,** Comparative study on the efficacy and acceptability of two contraceptive pills administered by the vaginal route: an international multicenter clinical trial, *Clin Pharmacol Ther* 53:65, 1993.

314. **Bryner RW, Toffle RC, Ullrich IH, Yeater RA,** Effect of low dose oral contraceptives on exercise performance, *Br J Sports Med* 30:36, 1996.

315. **Thompson HS, Hyatt JP, De Souza MJ, Clarkson PM,** The effects of oral contraceptives on delayed onset muscle soreness following exercise, *Contraception* 56:59, 1997.

316. **Brynhildsen J, Lennartsson H, Klemetz M, Dahlquist P, Hedin B, Hammar M,** Oral contraceptive use among female elite athletes and age-matched controls and its relation to low back pain, *Acta Obstet Gynecol Scand* 76:873, 1997.

317. **Milsom E, Sundell G, Andersch B,** The influence of different combined oral contraceptives on the prevalence and severity of dysmenorrhea, *Contraception* 42:497, 1990.

318. **Larsson G, Milsom I, Lindstedt G, Rybo G,** The influence of a low-dose combined oral contraceptive on menstrual blood loss and iron status, *Contraception* 46:327, 1992.

319. **Vessey MP, Villard-Mackintosh L, Painter R,** Epidemiology of endometriosis in women attending family-planning clinics, *Br Med J* 306:182, 1993.

320. **Parazzini F, Ferraroni M, Bocciolone L, Tozzi L, Rubessa S, La Vecchia C,** Contraceptive methods and risk of pelvic endometriosis, *Contraception* 49:47, 1994.

321. **Sangi-Haghpeykar H, Poindexter III AN,** Epidemiology of endometriosis among parous women, *Obstet Gynecol* 85:983, 1995.

322. **Enzelsberger H, Metka M, Heytmanek G, Schurz B, Kurz C, Kusztrich M,** Influence of oral contraceptive use on bone density in climacteric women, *Maturitas* 9:375, 1988.

323. **Kleerekoper M, Brienza RS, Schultz LR, Johnson CC,** Oral contraceptive use may protect against low bone mass, *Arch Intern Med* 151:1971, 1991.

324. **Kritz-Silverstein D, Barrett-Connor E,** Bone mineral density in postmenopausal women as determined by prior oral contraceptive use, *Am J Public Health* 83:100, 1993.

325. **Mais V, Fruzzetti F, Aiossa S, Paoletti AM, Guerriero S, Melis GB,** Bone metabolism in young women taking a monophasic pill containing 20 μg ethinylestradiol, *Contraception* 48:445, 1993.

326. **Polatti F, Perotti F, Filippa N, Gallina D, Nappi RE,** Bone mass and long-term monophasic oral contraceptive treatment in young women, *Contraception* 51:221, 1995.

327. **Hartard M, Bottermann P, Bartenstein P, Jeschke D, Schwaiger M,** Effects on bone mineral density of low-dosed oral contraceptives compared to and combined with physical activity, *Contraception* 55:87, 1997.

328. **Cooper C, Hannaford P, Croft P, Kay CR,** Oral contraceptive pill use and fractures in women: a prospective study, *Bone* 14:41, 1993.

329. **Vessey M, Mant J, Painter R,** Oral contraception and other factors in relation to hospital referral for fracture. Findings in a large cohort study, *Contraception* 57:231, 1998.

330. **Hazes JMW, Dijkmans BAC, Vandenbroucke JP, De Vries RRP, Cats A,** Reduction of the risk of rheumatoid arthritis among women who take oral contraceptives, *Arthritis Rheum* 33:173, 1990.

331. **Spector TD, Hochberg MC,** The protective effect of the oral contraceptive pill on rheumatoid arthritis: an overview of the analytical epidemiological studies using meta-analysis, *J Clin Epidemiol* 43:1221, 1990.

332. **Pladevall-Vila M, Delclos GL, Varas C, Guyer H, Brugués-Tarradellas J, Anglada-Arisa A,** Controversy of oral contraceptives and risk of rheumatoid arthritis: meta-analysis of conflicting studies and review of conflicting meta-analyses with special emphasis on analysis of heterogeneity, *Am J Epidemiol* 144:1, 1996.

333. **van der Vange N, Blankenstein MA, Kloosterboer HJ, Haspels AA, Thijssen JHH,** Effects of seven low-dose combined oral contraceptives on sex hormone binding globulin, corticosteroid binding globulin, total and free testosterone, *Contraception* 41:345, 1990.

334. **Palatsi R, Hirvensalo E, Liukko P, Malmiharju T, Mattila L, Riihiluoma P, Ylöstalo P,** Serum total and unbound testosterone and sex hormone binding globulin (SHBG) in female acne patients treated with two different oral contraceptives, *Acta Derm Venereol* 64:517, 1984.

335. **Coenen CMH, Thomas CMG, Borm GF, Rolland R,** Changes in androgens during treatment with four low-dose contraceptives, *Contraception* 53:171, 1996.

336. **Steinkampf MP, Hammond KR, Blackwell RE,** Hormonal treatment of functional ovarian cysts: a randomized, prospective study, *Fertil Steril* 54:775, 1990.

337. **Ben-Ami M, Geslevich Y, Battino S, Matilsky M, Shalev E,** Mangement of functional ovarian cysts after induction of ovulation. A randomized prospective study, *Acta Obstet Gynecol Scand* 72:396, 1993.

338. **Turan C, Zorlu CG, Ugur M, Ozcan T, Kaleli B, Gokmen O,** Expectant management of functional ovarian cysts: an alternative to hormonal therapy, *Int J Gynaecol Obstet* 47:257, 1994.

339. **Nezhat CH, Nezhat F, Borhan S, Seidman DS, Nezhat CR,** Is hormonal treatment efficacious in the management of ovarian cysts in women with histories of endometriosis? *Hum Reprod* 11:874, 1996.

340. **Jones EF, Forrest JD,** Contraceptive failure in the United States: revised estimates from the 1982 National Survey of Family Growth, *Fam Plann Perspect* 21:103, 1989.

341. **Peterson LS, Oakley D, Potter LS, Darroch JE,** Women's efforts to prevent pregnancy: consistency of oral contraceptive use, *Fam Plann Perspect* 30:19, 1998.

342. **Rosenberg MJ, Waugh MS, Meehan TE,** Use and misuse of oral contraceptives: risk indicators for poor pill taking and discontinuation, *Contraception* 51:283, 1995.

343. **Rosenberg MJ, Waugh MS,** Oral contraceptive discontinuation: a prospective evaluation of frequency and reasons, *Am J Obstet Gynecol* 179:577, 1998.

344. **Villegas-Salas E, Ponce de León R, Juárez-Perez MA, Grubb GS,** Effect of vitamin B6 on the side effects of a low-dose combined oral contraceptive, *Contraception* 55:245, 1997.

345. **Chi I,** The safety and efficacy issues of progestin-only oral contraceptives — an epidemiologic perspective, *Contraception* 47:1, 1993.

346. **McCann MF, Potter LS,** Progestin-only oral contraception: a comprehensive review, *Contraception* 50(Suppl 1):S9, 1994.

347. **Ball MJ, Gillmer AE,** Progestagen-only oral contraceptives: comparison of the metabolic effects of levonorgestrel and norethisterone, *Contraception* 44:223, 1991.

348. **Trussell J, Kost K,** Contraceptive failure in the United States: a critical review of the literature, *Stud Fam Plann* 18:237, 1987.

349. **Vessey MP, Lawless M, Yeates D, McPherson K,** Progestogen-only contraception: findings in a large prospective study with special reference to effectiveness, *Br J Fam Plann* 10:117, 1985.

350. **Sheth A, Jain U, Sharma S, Adatia A, Patankar S, Andolsek L, Pretnar-Darovec A, Belsey MA, Hall PE, Parker RA, Ayeni S, Pinol A, Li Hoi Foo C,** A randomized, double-blind study of two combined and two progestogen-only oral contraceptives, *Contraception* 25:243, 1982.

351. **Bisset AM, Dingwall-Fordyce I, Hamilton MJK,** The efficacy of the progestogen-only pill as a contraceptive method, *Br J Fam Plann* 16:84, 1990.

352. **Broome M, Fotherby K,** Clinical experience with the progestogen-only pill, *Contraception* 42:489, 1990.

353. **Tayob Y, Adams J, Jacobs HS, Guillebaud J,** Ultrasound demonstration of increased frequency of functional ovarian cysts in women using progestogen-only oral contraception, *Br J Obstet Gynaecol* 92:1003, 1985.

354. **Dunson TR, McLaurin VL, Grubb GS, Rosman AW,** A multicenter clinical trial of a progestin-only oral contraceptive in lactating women, *Contraception* 47:23, 1993.

355. **WHO Task Force for Epidemiological Research on Reproductive Health, Special Programme of Research, Development and Research Training in Human Reproduction,** Progestogen-only contraceptives during lactation. I. Infant growth, *Contraception* 50:35, 1994.

356. **WHO Task Force for Epidemiological Research on Reproductive Health, Special Programme of Research, Development and Research Training in Human Reproduction,** Progestogen-only contraceptives during lactation. II. Infant development, *Contraception* 50:55, 1994.

357. **World Health Organization Collaborative Study of Cardiovascular Disease and Steroid Hormone Contraception,** Cardiovascular disease and use of oral and injectable progestogen-only contraceptives and combined injectable contraceptives. Results of an international, multicenter, case-control study, *Contraception* 57:315, 1998.

358. **Fotherby K,** The progestogen-only pill and thrombosis, *Br J Fam Plann* 15:83, 1989.

359. **Winkler UH, Howie H, Bühler K, Korver T, Geurts TBP, Coelingh Bennink HJT,** A randomized controlled double-blind study of the effects on hemostasis of two progestogen-only pills containing 75 μg desogestrel or 30 μg levonorgestrel, *Contraception* 1998:385, 1998.

360. **Morris JM, van Wagenen G,** Compounds interfering with ovum implantation and development. III. The role of estrogens, *Am J Obstet Gynecol* 96:804, 1966.

361. **Yuzpe AA, Smith RP, Rademaker AW,** A multicenter clinical investigation employing ethinyl estradiol combined with dl-norgestrel as a postcoital contraceptive agent, *Fertil Steril* 37:508, 1982.

362. **Ho PC, Kwan MSW,** A prospective randomized comparison of levonorgestrel with the Yuzpe regimen in post-coital contraception, *Hum Reprod* 8:389, 1993.

363. **Task Force on Postovulatory Methods of Fertility Regulation,** Randomised controlled trial of levonorgestrel versus the Yuzpe regimen of combined oral contraceptives for emergency contraception, *Lancet* 352:428, 1998.

364. **Burton R, Savage W, Reader F,** The "morning after pill." Is this the wrong name for it? *Br J Fam Plann* 15:119, 1990.

365. **Young L, McCowan LM, Roberts HE, Farquhar CM,** Emergency contraception — why women don't use it, *N Z Med J* 108:145, 1995.

366. **Harper CC, Ellerton CE,** The emergency contraceptive pill: a survey of knowledge and attitudes among students at Princeton, *Am J Obstet Gynecol* 173:1438, 1995.

367. **Delbanco SF, Mauldon J, Smith MD,** Little knowledge and limited practice: emergency contraceptive pills, the public, and the obstetrician-gynecologist, *Obstet Gynecol* 89:1006, 1997.

368. **Trussell J, Stewart F, Guest F, Hatcher RA,** Emergency contraceptive pills: a simple proposal to reduce unintended pregnancies, *Fam Plann Perspect* 24:269, 1992.

369. **Glasier A, Baird D,** The effects of self-administering emergency contraception, *New Engl J Med* 339:1, 1998.

370. **Young DC, Wiehle RD, Joshi SG, Poindexter III AN,** Emergency contraception alters progesterone-associated endometrial protein in serum and uterine luminal fluid, *Obstet Gynecol* 84:266, 1994.

371. **Swahn ML, Westlund P, Johannisson E, Bygdeman M,** Effect of postcoital contraceptive methods on the endometrium and the menstrual cycle, *Acta Obstet Gynecol Scand* 75:738, 1996.

372. **Fasoli M, Parazzini F, Cecchetti G, La Vecchia C,** Post-coital contraception: an overview of published studies, *Contraception* 39:459, 1989.

373. **Haspels AA,** Emergency contraception: a review, *Contraception* 50:101, 1994.

374. **Glasier A,** Emergency postcoital contraception, *New Engl J Med* 337:1058, 1997.

375. **Wilcox AJ, Weinberg CR, Baird DD,** Timing of sexual intercourse in relation to ovulation — effects on the probability of conception, survival of the pregnancy, and sex of the baby, *New Engl J Med* 333:1517, 1995.

376. **Trussell J, Ellertson C, Stewart F,** The effectiveness of the Yuzpe regimen of emergency contraception, *Fam Plann Perspect* 28:58, 1996.

377. **Trussell J, Rodríguez G, Ellertson C,** New estimates of the effectiveness of the Yuzpe regimen of emergency contraception, *Contraception* 57:363, 1998.

378. **Trussell J, Ellertson C, Rodriguez G,** The Yuzpe regimen of emergency contraception: how long after the morning after? *Obstet Gynecol* 88:150, 1996.

379. **Webb A, Taberner D,** Clotting factors after emergency contraception, *Adv Contracept* 9:75, 1993.

380. **Webb AMC, Russell J, Elstein M,** Comparison of Yuzpe regimen, danazol, and mifepristone (RU486) in oral postcoital contraception, *Br Med J* 305:927, 1992.

381. **Glasier A, Thong KJ, Dewar M, Mackie M, Baird DT,** Mifepristone (RU 486) compared with high-dose estrogen and progestogen for emergency postcoital contraception, *New Engl J Med* 327:1041, 1992.

382. **Henshaw SK,** Unintended pregnancy in the United States, *Fam Plann Perspect* 30:24, 1998.

383. **Ventura SJ,** (Monthly Vital Statistics Report, Vol. 43), Advance report of final natality statistics, 1992, Report No. 5, Supplement, 1994.

384. **Piccinino LJ, Mosher WD,** Trends in contraceptive use in the United States: 1982–1995, *Fam Plann Perspect* 30:4, 1998.

385. **Paul C, Skegg DC, Spears GF,** Oral contraceptive use and risk of breast cancer in older women, *Cancer Causes Control* 6:485, 1995.

386. **Kirkman RJE, Pedersen JH, Fioretti P, Roberts HE,** Clinical comparison of two low-dose oral contraceptives, Minulet and Mercilon, in women over 30 years of age, *Contraception* 49:33, 1994.

387. **Fioretti P, Fruzzetti F, Navalesi R, Ricci C, Moccoli R, Cerri FM, Orlandi MC, Melis GB,** Clinical and metabolic study of a new pill containing 20 mcg ethinylestradiol plus 0.150 mg desogestrel, *Contraception* 35:229, 1987.

388. **Steffensen K,** Evaluation of an oral contraceptive containing 0.150 mg desogestrel and 0.020 mg ethinylestradiol in women aged 30 years or older, *Acta Obstet Gynecol Scand Suppl* 144:23, 1987.

389. **Melis GB, Fruzzetti F, Nicoletti I, Ricci C, Lammers P, Atsma WJ, Fioretti P,** A comparative study on the effects of a monophasic pill containing desogestrel plus 20 µg ethinylestradiol, a triphasic combination containing levonorgestel and a monophasic combination containing gestodene on coagulatory factors, *Contraception* 43:23, 1991.

390. **Gordon EM, Williams SR, Frenchek B, Mazur CH, Speroff L,** Dose-dependent effects of postmenopausal estrogen/progestin on antithrombin III and factor XII, *J Lab Clin Med* 111:52, 1988.

391. **Gebbie AE, Glasier A, Sweeting V,** Incidence of ovulation in perimenopausal women before and during hormone replacement therapy, *Contraception* 52:221, 1995.

392. **Castracane VD, Gimpel T, Goldzieher JW,** When is it safe to switch from oral contraceptives to hormonal replacement therapy? *Contraception* 52:371, 1995.

393. **Beral V, Hermon C, Kay C, Hannaford P, Darby S, Reeves G,** Mortality associated with oral contraceptive use: 25 year follow up of cohort of 46,000 women from Royal College of General Practitioners' oral contraception study, *Br Med J* 318:96, 1999.

23 Long-Acting Methods of Contraception

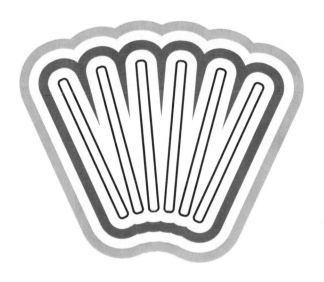

The high rate of unintended pregnancies and the relatively high failure rates with the typical use of reversible methods of contraception are strong indications of a need for long-acting contraceptive methods that simplify compliance. Two effective and popular methods are available, the Norplant system and depot-medroxyprogesterone acetate (Depo-Provera). Once-a-month injectable contraceptives are used in many parts of the world, and are a new option for U.S. women.

Norplant is a "sustained-release" system using Silastic tubing permeable to steroid molecules to provide stable circulating levels of synthetic progestin over years of use. Norplant was first introduced into clinical trials in Chile in 1972. Assessment of this method was completed in more than 45 countries, and in 1990, Norplant was approved for marketing in the U.S., the 20th country of approximately 60 to do so.[1]

The progestin in Norplant, circulating at levels one-fourth to one-tenth of those obtained with combined oral contraceptives, prevents conception by suppressing ovulation and thickening cervical mucus to inhibit sperm penetration so that fertilization rarely occurs.[2] Because serum levels of progestin remain low and because no estrogen is administered, this long-acting contraceptive method does not cause any serious health effects.[1] This method does, however, cause some bothersome side effects attributable to sustained administration of progestin, such as changes in menstrual pattern, weight gain, headache, and effects on mood.

Injectable medroxyprogesterone acetate (Depo-Provera) is a long-acting (3–6 months) agent that has been part of the contraceptive programs of many countries for more than 20 years. This experience has demonstrated it to be safe, effective, and acceptable. It is not a "sustained-release" system, but its action is the same.

The long-acting progestin methods (including Norplant and Depo-Provera) are as effective as sterilization and IUDs, and more effective than oral and barrier contraception.[3] An important reason for this high efficacy in actual use is the nature of the delivery systems themselves which require little effort on the part of the user. Because compliance does not require frequent resupply or instruction in use, as with oral contraception, theoretical (lowest expected) effectiveness is very close to the actual or typical (use) effectiveness.

Sustained-release methods require less of the user, but they demand more of the clinician. Norplant involves minor operative procedures for placement and for discontinuation. Clinicians have a special responsibility to become skillful in the operations required to remove implants and to be available to women when those skills are required to terminate use. Disturbances of menstrual patterns and other side effects prompt many more questions from patients about these methods than about use of the familiar oral, intrauterine, and barrier contraceptives.[4]

The Norplant System

The Norplant subdermal implant system is a long-acting, low-dose, reversible, progestin-only method of contraception for women. It was developed by the Population Council. The implants are manufactured, under license of the Population Council, by Huhtamaki Oy/Leiras Pharmaceuticals in Finland.

The currently available Norplant system consists of 6 capsules, each measuring 34 mm in length with a 2.4 mm outer diameter and containing 36 mg crystalline levonorgestrel. The capsules are made of flexible, medical grade silastic (polydimethylsiloxane and methylvinyl siloxane copolymer) tubing that is sealed shut with silastic medical adhesive (polydimethylsiloxane). The cavity of the capsule has an inner diameter of 1.57 mm, with an inner length of 30 mm. The 6 capsules contain a total of 216 mg levonorgestrel, which is very stable and has remained unchanged in capsules examined after more than 9 years of use.

The implants come packaged in heat-sealed pouches that have a shelf life of 5 years from the date of manufacture and have an additional 5 to 7 years of effective life once inserted. Storage at room temperature with uncontrolled humidity has not altered their composition or lifespan after 4 years, but, optimally, the implants should be stored in a cool, dry area away from direct sunlight. The implants can be ethylene oxide sterilized, but cannot be sterilized by ionizing radiation, dry heat, or autoclaving.

The components of Norplant are not new. The silastic in the tubing has been used in surgical applications such as prosthetic devices, heart valves, and drainage tubes, since the 1950s, and in the most common method of female sterilization (Fallope Rings) since 1970. The progestin, levonorgestrel, has been widely used in oral contraceptives since the 1960s. The toxicology, teratogenicity, and pharmacology of levonorgestrel have been well studied. What is relatively new is the way the system delivers a sustained level of levonorgestrel for a long time — in ongoing trials, up to 7 years, although currently approved for 5 years.

Mechanism of Action

The release rate of the capsule is determined by its total surface area and the thickness of the capsule wall. The levonorgestrel diffuses through the wall of the tubing into the surrounding tissues where it is absorbed by the circulatory system and distributed systemically, avoiding an initial high level in the circulation as with orally or injected steroids. Within 24 hours after insertion, plasma concentrations of levonorgestrel range from 0.4 to 0.5 ng/mL, high enough to prevent conception; however, a study of cervical mucus changes indicates that a backup method should be used for 3 days after insertion.[5, 6]

The capsules release approximately 85 μg of levonorgestrel per 24 hours during the first 6–12 months of use. This rate declines gradually to 50 μg daily by 9 months and 30 μg per day for the

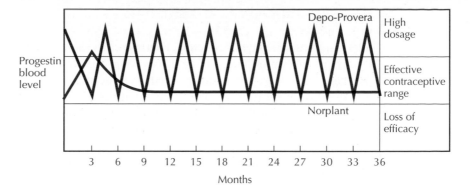

remaining duration of use. The 85 μg of hormone released by the implants during the first few months of use is about equivalent to the daily dose of levonorgestrel delivered by the progestin-only, minipill oral contraceptive, and 25–50% of the dose delivered by low-dose combined oral contraceptives.

Mean plasma concentrations below 0.20 ng/mL are associated with increased pregnancy rates. After 6 months of use, daily levonorgestrel concentrations are about 0.35 ng/mL; at 2.5 years, the levels decrease to 0.25–0.35 ng/mL. Until the 5-year mark, mean levels remain above 0.25 ng/mL.[7]

Body weight affects the circulating levels of levonorgestrel. The greater the weight of the user, the lower the levonorgestrel concentrations at any time during Norplant use. The greatest decrease over time occurs in women weighing more than 70 kg (154 pounds), but even for heavy women, the release rate is high enough to prevent pregnancy at least as reliably as oral contraceptives.

Levonorgestrel levels may also be affected by the levels of sex hormone-binding globulin (SHBG). Levonorgestrel has a high affinity for SHBG. In the week after Norplant insertion, SHBG levels decline rapidly, and then return to approximately half of preinsertion levels by 1-year of use. This effect on SHBG is not uniform and may account for some of the individual variations in plasma levonorgestrel concentrations.[8]

The mechanism by which Norplant prevents conception is only partially explained. There are 3 probable modes of action, which are similar to those attributed to the contraceptive effect of the progestin-only minipills.

1. The levonorgestrel suppresses at both the hypothalamus and the pituitary the luteinizing hormone (LH) surge necessary for ovulation. As determined by progesterone levels in many users over several years, approximately one-third of all cycles are ovulatory.[7, 9] During the first 2 years of use, only about 10% of women are ovulatory, but by 5 years of use, more than 50% are. In those cycles that are ovulatory, there is a high incidence of luteal insufficiency.

2. The constant level of levonorgestrel has a marked effect on the cervical mucus. The mucus thickens and decreases in amount, forming a barrier to sperm penetration.[5,10]

3. The levonorgestrel suppresses the estradiol-induced cyclic maturation of the endometrium, and eventually causes atrophy. These changes could prevent implantation should fertilization occur; however, no evidence of fertilization can be detected in Norplant users.[11]

Specific Advantages

Norplant is a safe, highly effective, continuous method of contraception that requires little user effort or motivation and, unlike long-acting injectable contraception, is rapidly reversible. Because this is a progestin-only method, it can be utilized by women who have contraindications for the use of estrogen-containing oral contraceptives. The sustained release of low doses of progestin avoids the high initial dose delivered by injectables and the daily hormone surge associated with oral contraceptives. Norplant is not a coitus-related contraceptive method. The use effectiveness closely approximates the theoretical effectiveness. Norplant is an excellent choice for a breastfeeding woman (there is no effect on breastfeeding) and can be inserted immediately postpartum, but at least a 3-day postpartum delay is recommended to allow the decline in pregnancy levels of estrogen and progesterone and the establishment of lactation.[12]

General Advantages

One of the major advantages of sustained-release methods is the high degree of efficacy, nearly equivalent to the theoretical effectiveness. In couples for whom elective abortion is unacceptable in the event of an unplanned pregnancy, the high efficacy rate is especially important. There are no forgotten pills, broken condoms, or lost diaphragms. For women who are at high risk of medical complications should they become pregnant, these methods present a significant safety advantage. Users should be reassured that Norplant use has not been associated with changes in carbohydrate or lipid metabolism, coagulation, liver or kidney function, or immunoglobulin levels. Since many women wanting Norplant will have had negative experiences with other contraceptives, it is important that the differences between this method and previous methods be explained.

Norplant is a good method for breastfeeding women. There are no effects on breast milk quality or quantity, and infants grow normally.[13, 14] Another advantage of Norplant is that it allows women to plan their pregnancies precisely; return of fertility after removal is prompt, in contrast to the 18-month delay in ovulation that can follow Depo-Provera injections.[15, 16] In addition, anemia is less likely in Norplant users.[17]

Disadvantages

There are some disadvantages associated with the use of the Norplant system. Norplant causes disruption of bleeding patterns in up to 80% of users, especially during the first year of use, and some women or their partners find these changes unacceptable.[4] Endogenous estrogen is nearly normal, and unlike the combined oral contraceptives, progestin is not regularly withdrawn to allow endometrial sloughing. Consequently, the endometrium sheds at unpredictable intervals.

The implants must be inserted and removed in a surgical procedure performed by trained personnel. Women cannot initiate or discontinue the method without the assistance of a clinician. The incidence of complicated removals is approximately 5%, an incidence that can be best minimized by good training and experience in Norplant insertion.[18] Because the insertion and removal of Norplant require minor surgical procedures, initiation and discontinuation costs will be higher than with oral contraceptives or barrier methods.

The implants can be visible under the skin. This sign of the use of contraception may be unacceptable for some women, and for some partners.[4] Norplant is not known to provide protection against sexually transmitted diseases (STDs) such as herpes, human papillomavirus, HIV, gonorrhea, or chlamydia. Users at risk for STDs must consider adding a barrier method to prevent infection.

The cost of implants plus fees for insertion total an amount that seems high to many patients unless they compare it with the total cost of using other methods for up to 5 years.[19] Nevertheless, short-term use is expensive compared with the relatively low initial costs of other reversible methods, and most women cannot be expected to use long-acting methods for their full duration of action.

Sustained-release, progestin-only methods do not increase the risk of developing STDs, but it is not known whether they provide any protection. Women who have multiple partners, or whose partners do, should use condoms as well. All users must be aware of the possible menstrual changes. It is important to stress that all of the menstrual changes are expected, that they do not cause or represent illness, and that most women revert back to a more normal pattern with increasing duration of use.

Cultural factors can influence the acceptability of menstrual changes. Hispanic users of Norplant, for example, are very accepting of irregular or prolonged bleeding.[4] Some cultures restrict a woman from participating in religious activity, household activities, or sexual intercourse while menstruating.

Insertion and removal of implants will be a new experience for most women. As with any new experience, women will approach it with varying degrees of apprehension and anxiety. In reality, most patients are able to watch in comfort as implants are inserted or removed. Women should be told that the incisions used for the procedures are very small and heal quickly, leaving small scars that are usually difficult to see because of their location and size.

Prospective users should be allowed to see and touch implants. Women should be reassured that the implants will not be damaged or move if the skin above them is accidentally injured. Normal activity cannot damage or displace the implants. Most women become unaware of their presence. A few women report sensing the implants if they have been touched or manipulated for a prolonged period of time, or after vigorous exercise. The implants can be visible in slender women with good muscle tone. Darker-skinned users may notice further darkening of the skin directly over the implants; this resolves after removal.

Indications

The Norplant system is indicated for use by women of reproductive age who are sexually active and desire continuous contraception. Norplant should be considered for women who:

1. Desire spacing of future pregnancies.

2. Desire a highly effective, long-term method of contraception.

3. Experience serious or minor estrogen-related side effects with oral contraception.

4. Have difficulty remembering to take pills every day, have contraindications or difficulty using IUDs, or desire a non-coitus-related method of contraception.

5. Have completed their childbearing but do not desire permanent sterilization.

6. Have a history of anemia with heavy menstrual bleeding.

7. Are considering sterilization, but are not yet ready to undergo surgery.

8. Women with chronic illnesses, whose health will be threatened by pregnancy.

Absolute Contraindications

Norplant use is contraindicated in women who have:

1. *ACTIVE* thrombophlebitis or thromboembolic disease.

2. Undiagnosed genital bleeding.

3. *ACUTE* liver disease.

4. Benign or malignant liver tumors.

5. Known or suspected breast cancer.

Relative Contraindications

Based on clinical judgment and appropriate medical management, Norplant *MAY BE USED* by women with a history of or current diagnosis of the following conditions:

1. Heavy cigarette smoking (15 or more daily) in women older than 35 years.

2. History of ectopic pregnancy.

3. Diabetes mellitus. Because multiple studies have failed to observe a significant impact on carbohydrate metabolism, Norplant, in our view, is particularly well suited for diabetic women.

4. Hypercholesterolemia

5. Hypertension.

6. History of cardiovascular disease, including myocardial infarction, cerebral vascular accident, coronary artery disease, angina, or a previous thromboembolic event. Patients with artificial heart valves.

7. Gallbladder disease

8. Chronic disease, such as immunocompromised patients.

Norplant is not contraindicated in the following situations, but other methods are probably preferable:

1. Severe acne

2. Severe vascular or migraine headaches.

3. Severe depression.

4. Concomitant use of medications that induce microsomal liver enzymes (phenytoin, phenobarbital, carbamazepine, rifampin). In this case, we do not recommend the use of Norplant because of a likely increased risk of pregnancy due to lower blood levels of levonorgestrel.[1, 20]

Efficacy

Norplant is a highly effective method of birth control. In studies conducted in 11 countries, totaling 12,133 woman-years of use, the pregnancy rate was 0.2 pregnancies per 100 woman-years of use.[1, 15] All but one of the pregnancies that occurred during this evaluation were present at the time of implant insertion. If these luteal phase insertions are excluded from analysis, the first-year pregnancy rate was 0.01 per 100 woman-years. In adolescents, Norplant implants provide better protection against unwanted pregnancy, compared with oral contraceptives, and an important factor is the better continuation rate with Norplant.[21]

The overall pregnancy rate after 2 years of use in 9 countries was 0.2 per 100 woman-years of use.[1] The pregnancy rate achieved in the U.S. trials during the second year of use was higher (2.1 per 100 woman-years). Two factors account for this difference. First, users in the U.S. weighed, on the average, more than study participants in other countries. Clinical trials have demonstrated a direct correlation between weight greater than 70 kg (154 pounds) and an increased risk of pregnancy, but even for heavy women, pregnancy rates are lower than with oral contraception. Second, two different types of silastic tubing were used in the manufacture of Norplant capsules.[23] The first type contained a larger proportion of inert filler and was more dense, while the second type contained less filler and was less dense. Higher pregnancy rates have been observed among women using the more dense capsules, and in the U.S. trials, capsules were more often of the more dense variety. The less dense tubing is now the only one used in the manufacture of Norplant and has a 15% higher release rate than denser tubing. The 5-year pregnancy rate with the less dense (soft) tubing is comparable to that of tubal ligation.[24]

Pregnancy Rates According to Years of Use[1, 15]

First Year	Second Year	Third Year	Fourth Year	Fifth Year
0.2%	0.2%	0.9%	0.5%	1.1%

Using the less dense tubing, there now are no weight restrictions for Norplant users, but heavier women (more than 70 kg) may experience slightly higher pregnancy rates in the fourth and fifth years of use compared with lighter women. Even in the later years, however, pregnancy rates for heavier women using Norplant are lower than with oral contraception. The differences in pregnancy rates by weight are probably due to the dilutional effect of larger body size on the low, sustained serum levels of levonorgestrel. Heavier women should not rely on Norplant beyond the 5-year limit. For slender women the duration of Norplant's efficacy may extend well past the fifth year of use. In some extended trials, no pregnancies have occurred into the 7th year.

Failure Rates During the First Year of Use, United States[7]

Method	Percent of Women with Pregnancy	
	Lowest Expected	Typical
No method	85.0%	85.0%
Combination Pill	0.1	3.0
Progestin only	0.5	3.0
IUDs		
Progesterone IUD	1.5	2.0
Levonorgestrel IUD	0.6	0.8
Copper T 380A	0.1	0.1
Norplant	0.05	0.05
Female sterilization	0.05	0.05
Male sterilization	0.1	0.15
Depo-Provera	0.3	0.3
Spermicides	6.0	26.0
Periodic abstinence		25.0
Calendar	9.0	
Ovulation method	3.0	
Symptothermal	2.0	
Post–ovulation	1.0	
Withdrawal	4.0	19.0
Cervical cap		
Parous women	26.0	40.0
Nulliparous women	9.0	20.0
Sponge		
Parous women	9.0	28.0
Nulliparous women	6.0	18.0
Diaphragm and spermicides	6.0	20.0
Condom		
Male	3.0	14.0
Female	5.0	21.0

Ectopic Pregnancy

The ectopic pregnancy rate during Norplant use has been 0.28 per 1000 woman-years.[1] *Although the risk of developing an ectopic pregnancy during use of Norplant is low, when pregnancy does occur, ectopic pregnancy should be suspected. because approximately 30% of Norplant pregnancies are ectopic.*

Ectopic Pregnancy Rates per 1000 Woman-Years [1, 25, 26]

Non-contraceptive users, all ages	3.0–4.5
Copper T-380 IUD	0.20
Norplant	0.28

Menstrual Effects

Menstrual bleeding patterns are highly variable among users of Norplant. Some alteration of menstrual patterns will occur during the first year of use in approximately 80% of users, later decreasing to about 40%, and by the fifth year, to about 33%.[27, 28] The changes include alterations in the interval between bleeding, the duration and volume of menstrual flow, and spotting. Oligomenorrhea and amenorrhea also occur, but are less common, less than 10% after the first year and diminishing thereafter. Irregular and prolonged bleeding usually occurs during the first year. Although bleeding problems occur much less frequently after the second year, they can occur at any time.[28, 29] Studies of the endometrium in Norplant users experiencing abnormal bleeding indicate the presence of enlarged venous sinusoids (fragile vessels) and a reduction in the expression of a protein factor (perivascular stromal cell tissue factor) involved in the initiation of hemostasis.[30]

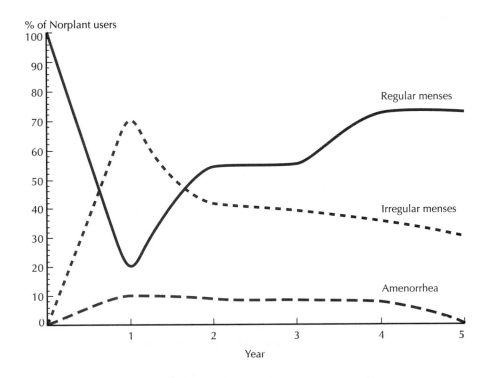

Despite an increase in the number of spotting and bleeding days over preinsertion menstrual patterns, hemoglobin concentrations rise in Norplant users because of a decrease in the average amount of menstrual blood loss.[17, 31]

Patients who can no longer tolerate the presence of prolonged bleeding will benefit from a short course of oral estrogen: conjugated estrogens, 1.25 mg, or estradiol, 2 mg, administered daily for 7 days. A therapeutic dose of one of the prostaglandin inhibitors given during the bleeding will help to diminish flow, but estrogen is the most effective.[32] Another approach is to administer an estrogen-progestin oral contraceptive for 1–3 months.[33]

Although the Norplant system is very effective, pregnancy must be considered in women reporting amenorrhea who had been ovulating previously, as evidenced by regular menses prior to an episode of amenorrhea. A sensitive urine pregnancy test should be obtained. Women who remain amenorrheic throughout their use of Norplant are unlikely to become pregnant.[28] It is important to explain to patients the mechanism of the amenorrhea: the local progestational effect causing decidualization and atrophy.

Metabolic Effects

Exposure to the sustained, low dose of levonorgestrel delivered by the implants is not associated with significant metabolic changes. Studies of carbohydrate metabolism,[34, 35] liver function,[36–38] blood coagulation,[38–41] immunoglobulin levels,[34, 42] serum cortisol levels,[43] and blood chemistries[34, 37] have failed to detect changes outside of normal ranges.

No major impact on the lipoprotein profile can be demonstrated.[2, 36, 44] Minor changes are transient, and with prolonged duration of use, lipoproteins return to preinsertion levels. Long-term exposure to the low dose of levonorgestrel released by Norplant is unlikely to affect users' risk of atherogenesis, just as prolonged exposure to combined oral contraception has not (see Chapter 22). There are no clinically important effects on carbohydrate metabolism.[35, 45] No effect on insulin sensitivity can be detected.[46]

Measurements of bone density in adolescents reveal that Norplant does not affect the teenage gain in bone; similar gains were recorded in Norplant users and control subjects.[47] In older women, an increase in forearm bone density was documented after 6 months of Norplant use.[48]

Effects on Future Fertility

Circulating levels of levonorgestrel become too low to measure within 48 hours after removal of Norplant. Most women resume normal ovulatory cycles during the first month after removal. The pregnancy rates during the first year after removal are comparable with those of women not using contraceptive methods and trying to become pregnant. There are no long-term effects on future fertility, nor are there any effects on sex ratios, rates of ectopic pregnancy, spontaneous miscarriage, stillbirth, or congenital malformations.[1, 15] The return of fertility after Norplant removal is prompt, and pregnancy outcomes are within normal limits. The rate and outcome of subsequent pregnancies are not influenced by duration of use.

For women who are spacing their pregnancies, the difference between Norplant and Depo-Provera in the timing of the return to fertility can be critical. Norplant allows precise timing of pregnancy because the return of ovulation after Norplant removal is so prompt. Depo-Provera, on the other hand, can cause up to 18 months' delay in return to fertility. By that time, 90% of users of either method will have ovulated, but in the first several months, the difference is dramatic. By 3 months after removal, half of Norplant users will have ovulated, but 10 months must elapse before half of Depo-Provera users are ovulatory.

Side Effects

The occurrence of serious side effects is very rare, no different in incidence than that observed in the general population. In addition to the menstrual changes, the following side effects have been reported: headache, acne, weight change, mastalgia, hyperpigmentation over the implants, hirsutism, depression, mood changes, anxiety, nervousness, ovarian cyst formation, and galactorrhea.[1, 15, 27, 29, 49]

It is difficult, of course, to be certain which of these effects were actually caused by the levonorgestrel. For example, careful study fails to reveal a relationship between Norplant use and depressive symptoms.[50] Although most of these side effects are minor in nature, they can cause patients to discontinue the method. Patients often find common side effects tolerable after assurance that they do not represent a health hazard.[4] Many complaints respond to reassurance; others can be treated with simple therapies. The most common side effect experienced by users is headache; approximately 20% of women who discontinue use do so because of headache.[4, 49]

Stroke, thrombotic thrombocytopenic purpura, thrombocytopenia, and pseudotumor cerebri have been reported with Norplant.[51] However, it is by no means established that the incidence of these problems is increased, and there is little reason to suspect a cause-and-effect relationship. In the follow-up study conducted by the World Health Organization in 8 countries, no significant excess of cardiovascular events or malignant disease has been observed.[52]

Weight Change

Women using Norplant more frequently complain of weight gain than of weight loss, but findings are variable. In the Dominican Republic, 75% of those who changed weight lost, while in San Francisco, two-thirds gained. Assessment of weight change in Norplant users is confounded by changes in exercise, diet, and aging. Although an increase in appetite can be attributed to the androgenic activity of levonorgestrel, it is unlikely that the low levels with Norplant have any clinical impact. Counseling for weight changes should include dietary review and focus on dietary changes. Indeed, a 5-year follow-up of 75 women with Norplant implants could document no increase in the body mass index (nor was there a correlation between irregular bleeding and body weight).[53]

Mastalgia

Bilateral mastalgia, often occurring premenstrually, is usually associated with complaints of fluid retention. After pregnancy has been ruled out, reassurance and therapy aimed at symptomatic relief are indicated. This symptom decreases with increasing duration of Norplant use. Most Norplant users respond to treatment and do not elect to remove the implants. Careful assessments of the relationship between methylxanthines and mastalgia have failed to demonstrate a link. The most effective treatments are the following: danazol (200 mg/day), vitamin E (600 units/day), bromocriptine (2.5 mg/day), or tamoxifen (20 mg/day), but there are no studies of these treatments in Norplant users.

Galactorrhea

Galactorrhea is more common among women who have had insertion of the implants on discontinuation of lactation. Pregnancy and other possible causes should be ruled out by performing a pregnancy test and a thorough breast examination. Patients should be reassured that this is a common occurrence among implant and oral contraceptive users. Decreasing the amount of breast and nipple stimulation during sexual relations might alleviate the symptom, but if amenorrhea accompanies persistent galactorrhea, a prolactin level should be obtained.

Acne

Acne, with or without an increase in oil production, is the most common skin complaint among Norplant users. The acne is caused by the androgenic activity of the levonorgestrel that produces a direct impact and also causes a decrease in sex hormone-binding globulin (SHBG) levels leading to an increase in free steroid levels (both levonorgestrel and testosterone). This is in contrast to combined oral contraceptives that contain levonorgestrel, where the estrogen effect on SHBG (an increase) produces a decrease in unbound, free androgens. Common therapies for complaints of acne include dietary change, practice of good skin hygiene with the use of soaps or skin cleansers, and application of topical antibiotics (e.g., 1% clindamycin solution or gel, or topical erythromycin). Use of local antibiotics helps most users to continue Norplant.

Ovarian Cysts

Unlike oral contraception, the low serum progestin levels maintained by Norplant do not suppress follicle-stimulating hormone (FSH), which continues to stimulate ovarian follicle growth in most users. The LH peak during the first two years of use, on the other hand, is usually abolished so that these follicles do not ovulate.[9] However, some continue to grow and cause pain or be palpated at the time of pelvic examination.[54] Adnexal masses are approximately 8 times more frequent in Norplant users compared with normally cycling women. Because these are simple cysts (and most regress spontaneously within one month of detection), they need not be sonographically or laparoscopically evaluated. Further evaluation is indicated if they became large and painful or fail to regress. Regular ovulators are less likely to form cysts so the situation is likely to improve after two years of Norplant use.

Herpes Simplex

Some users have complained of outbreaks of genital herpes simplex lesions occurring more frequently than prior to insertion. Most commonly, the lesions develop during periods of prolonged spotting or bleeding with the wearing of sanitary napkins. Use of vaginal tampons for bleeding and suppression of the virus with oral acyclovir (200 mg tid for up to 6 months) have been sucessful in dealing with this problem.

Cancer

Levonorgestrel and silastic have been thoroughly evaluated in animals and humans for their carcinogenic effects, and none has been found. Epidemiologic evaluation awaits long-term use by large numbers of women. We can speculate on possible effects of Norplant based on our experience with oral contraceptives and Depo-Provera. The risk of endometrial cancer ought to be reduced. A study of the endometrial effects of Norplant failed to find any evidence of hyperplasia, even when levonorgestrel levels were low and endogenous estradiol production was normal.[55] The risk of ovarian cancer is also probably reduced, but not as much as with methods that completely suppress ovulation. Breast and cervical cancer effects will be as difficult to assess because of confounding variables as they are with oral contraception and Depo-Provera. The low dose of Norplant, however, would be unlikely to have effects different from other hormonal contraceptives.

Patient Evaluation

The usual personal and family medical history and physical examination should concentrate on factors that might contraindicate use of the various contraceptive options. If a patient elects to use Norplant, a detailed description of the method, including effectiveness, side effects, risks, benefits, as well as insertion and removal procedures, should be provided. Before insertion, the patient should read and sign a written consent for the surgical placement of Norplant. It should include a review of the potential complications of the procedure which include reaction to the local anesthetic, infection, expulsion of the implants, superficial phlebitis, bruising, and the possibility of a subsequent difficult removal.

Insertion can be performed at any time during the menstrual cycle as long as pregnancy can be ruled out. If the patient's last menstrual period was abnormal, if she has recently had sexual intercourse without contraception, or if there are reasons to suspect pregnancy, a sensitive urine pregnancy test should be performed. Based on cervical mucus changes, a backup method need be used no more than 3 days after insertion.[6] Norplant can be inserted immediately postpartum (after 3 days in breastfeeding women), but certainly should be initiated no later than the third postpartum week in non-breastfeeding women and the 3rd postpartum month in breastfeeding women. Acne and headache are less common in women who receive Norplant immediately postpartum, and there is no difference in post-pregnancy weight loss compared with women who receive it 4–6 weeks later.[56]

Patients should be questioned about allergies to local anesthetics, antiseptic solutions, and tape. A discussion about the technique of insertion and anticipated sensations is an important part of preparing the patient for the experience. All patients approach insertion with some degree of apprehension that can be decreased by detailed explanations and preparation.[23, 57]

Selection of the site for placement of Norplant is based on both functional and aesthetic factors. Various sites (the upper leg, forearm, and upper arm) have been used in clinical trials. The nondominant, upper, inner arm is usually the best site. This area is easily accessible to the clinician with minimal exposure of the patient. It is well protected during most normal activities. It is not highly visible, and immigration of the implants from this site has not been documented. The site of placement does not affect circulating levonorgestrel levels.

Reasons for Termination

Although Norplant is a 5-year method, only approximately 30% of women continue use for that long (although in some cultures 5-year continuation rates reach 65–70%). Discontinuation occurs at a rate of 10–15% yearly, about the same as for intrauterine contraception, but lower than for barrier or oral contraception.[1, 23, 29] Bothersome side effects, such as menstrual changes, headache, or weight change, are the primary reasons for termination of implant use.[4, 49, 58] Users who cannot tolerate these symptoms request removal in the first two years of use while women who want another pregnancy, the most common personal reason for removal, are more likely to terminate use in the third or fourth year.

Menstrual changes are the most common cause for discontinuation of Norplant in the first year of use. An unspoken concern for many patients and their partners is the fact that bleeding irregularity interferes with sexual interactions. The next most common reasons for discontinuing Norplant are headache, weight change, mood change, anxiety or nervousness, depression, ovarian cyst formation, and lower abdominal pain. Presence of ovarian cysts is not usually an indication for removal of Norplant and is almost never a reason for surgery. Most will resolve spontaneously within 4 weeks. Skin conditions, including rashes, dermatitis, and acne, account for about 0.8% of terminations.

User Acceptance of Norplant

Overall, interview surveys throughout the world have indicated that women perceive sustained-release methods, Norplant in particular, as highly acceptable methods of contraception.[57, 59–61] The most popular feature of Norplant is the ease of use. Approximately 20% of U.S. patients report that friends and relatives notice their implants. This may be a greater problem in warmer climates with less encompassing clothing. Only 25% of the women who report that the implants were noticed were bothered by this attention.[4]

In the U.S., the primary motivations for Norplant use have been problems with previous contraceptive methods and ease of Norplant use. Although fear of pain during Norplant insertion is a prominent source of anxiety for many women, the actual pain experienced does not match the expectations. The level of satisfaction has been high in self-motivated and well-informed users.[24] Teenagers provide an example of well-documented success. Their one-year pregnancy rates are much lower, and continuation rates much higher than that with oral contraceptives.[62–65] However, teenage discontinuation of the method due to side effects (especially irregular bleeding and weight gain) is more common with Norplant.[21]

Studies of women's attitudes toward sustained-release contraceptives indicate that the great majority of women find them highly acceptable and perceive them as desirable alternatives to conventional contraceptives, although not everyone finds Norplant preferable.[66, 67] Around the world, women who have used Norplant say they have recommended Norplant to friends and would like to use it again.[4, 15, 49]

Counseling Women

Frank information about negative factors such as irregular bleeding and possible weight changes will avoid surprise and disappointment, and encourage women to continue use long enough to enjoy the positive attributes such as convenience, safety, and efficacy. Open discussion of side effects will lead to public and media awareness of the disadvantages as well as the advantages of these methods. Helping women decide if they are good candidates for use of Norplant, for example, before they invest too much time and money in this long-acting contraceptive, is a very important objective of good counseling.

Common patient questions regarding Norplant are as follows:

— Is it effective?

— How is it inserted and removed; how long do these procedures take; does it hurt; and will it leave scars?

— Will the implants be visible under the skin?

— Will the implants be uncomfortable or restrict movement of the arm?

— Will the implants move in the body?

— Will the implants be damaged if they are touched or bumped?

— Will this contraceptive change sexual drive and enjoyment?

— What are the short- and long-term side effects?

— Are there any effects on future fertility?

— What do the implants look and feel like?

— What happens if pregnancy occurs during use?

— How long will it take for the method to be effective after insertion?

— Can a partner tell if this method is being used?

LNG ROD — The Two Rod System

The two-implant system, "Norplant-2," uses levonorgestrel suspended in a silastic matrix and covered with a silastic membrane. Bleeding, pregnancy, and continuation rates were like those of the 6-capsule system, but insertion and removal were easier.[15] However, the manufacturer of the elastomer used in Norplant-2 ceased production. A new system is composed of 2 levonorgestrel rods, called LNG ROD, encased in silicone rubber tubing, sealed at each end with silastic adhesive.[68] Each rod measures 2.5 mm in diameter and 4.3 cm in length, contains 75 mg levonorgestrel, and releases the drug at the same dose as Norplant.[69] A 3-year clinical trial indicates that the performance and side effects are similar to Norplant, but removal is faster and easier.[68]

New Developments in Implant Contraception

The newer progestins (desogestrel, gestodene, nestorone, nomegestrol, and norgestimate) are less androgenic than levonorgestrel and are useful in contraceptive implants. An example is Implanon, a single implant 4 cm long, that contains 60 mg of 3-keto desogestrel in a core of ethinyl vinyl acetate wrapped with a membrane of the same material. The hormone is released at a rate of about 60 μg per day. Implanon is designed to provide contraception for 2–3 years after which the implant should be removed. Efficacy and side effects are similar to those with Norplant.[38, 70, 71] Another single implant contraceptive is Uniplant, containing 38 mg nomegestrol acetate in a 4 cm silastic tube with a 100 μg per day release rate. It provides contraception for one year.[72–74]

Biodegradable implants deliver sustained levels of progestin for variable periods of time from a vehicle that dissolves in body tissues. The utility of implant contraception would be improved by the elimination of the need for surgical removal. Two types are under evaluation: Capronor and norethindrone pellets.

Capronor is a single capsule, biodegradable, levonorgestrel-releasing subdermal implant composed of the polymer E-caprolactone. Implants measure 0.24 cm in diameter and either 2.5 or 4 cm in length, providing contraception for one year. The shorter capsule contains 16 mg levonorgestrel, and the longer contains 26 mg. Levonorgestrel escapes from caprolactone at a rate 10 times faster than from silastic. The shorter implant maintains circulating levels of levonorgestrel of 0.2–0.3 ng/mL, while the longer implant maintains higher levels equivalent to those found in Norplant users. The longer capsule suppresses ovulation in a higher proportion (about 50%) of cycles than reported with Norplant, but the shorter implant allows ovulation in most users. The higher release rate allows the use of a smaller implant. Experience is still too limited to report pregnancy rates, but the longer implant should provide contraception comparable to Norplant.

When exposed to tissue fluids, E-caprolactone slowly breaks down into E-hydroxycaproic acid, and then finally to carbon dioxide and water. The capsule remains intact during the first 12 months of use, allowing easy removal. After 12 months, the capsule begins to disappear.

Capronor shares the advantages of Norplant with convenience of use and few metabolic effects. There is no adverse impact on the lipoprotein profile. Removal is easier and quicker. The disadvantages are also similar to Norplant: changes in menstrual patterns and the other side effects typical of low-dose, continuous progestin systems. Biodegradable implants could continue to release small, noncontraceptive amounts of hormone after their period of use as a contraceptive has expired. Although it is unlikely that such low serum levels of progestin would be harmful to users or to their pregnancies, this question needs to be resolved. The degrading implants can be removed in the event of pregnancy.[75]

Anuelle is a biodegradable norethindrone pellet that, when injected subdermally, is expected to maintain circulating concentrations of this progestin at contraceptive levels for up to 3 years. The pellets are composed of 10% pure cholesterol and 90% norethindrone, and are about the size of a grain of rice. This method is currently under development to determine the correct size and number of pellets and the cholesterol:hormone ratio necessary to obtain the release rates that provide contraception. Preliminary trials of 2, 3, and 4 pellets have demonstrated that bleeding patterns are disrupted during the first few months of use, then return to normal patterns. Users of 4 and 5 pellets are more likely to be amenorrheic and anovulatory.[76]

Depo-Provera (Depot-Medroxyprogesterone Acetate)

Depo-Provera (depot-medroxyprogesterone acetate) is the most thoroughly studied progestin-only contraceptive. Although its approval for contraception in the U.S. is recent (1992), it has been available in some countries since the mid-1960s. Much of our knowledge of the safety, efficacy, and acceptability of long-acting hormonal contraception comes from Indonesia, Sri Lanka, Thailand, and Mexico where Depo-Provera has been used and studied for decades. The long-delayed approval as a contraceptive in the U.S. was based on political and economic considerations, not scientific ones.[77]

Depo-Provera comes as microcrystals, suspended in an aqueous solution. The correct dose for contraceptive purposes is 150 mg intramuscularly (gluteal or deltoid) every 3 months. A comparative trial established that the 100 mg dose is significantly less effective.[78] The contraceptive level is maintained for at least 14 weeks, providing a safety margin for one of the most effective contraceptives available, about 1 pregnancy per 100 women after 5 years of consistent use.[78, 79]

Depo-Provera is not a "sustained-release" system; it relies on higher peaks of progestin to inhibit ovulation and thicken cervical mucus. The difference between serum levels of progestins in a sustained-release system like Norplant and a depot system like Depo-Provera is illustrated in the diagram.

Mechanism of Action

The mechanism of action of Depo-Provera is different from the other lower dose, progestin-only methods because, in addition to thickening of the cervical mucus and alteration of the endometrium, the circulating level of the progestin is high enough to effectively block the LH surge, and, therefore, ovulation does not occur. Suppression of FSH is not as intense as with the combination oral contraceptive, therefore follicular growth is maintained sufficiently to produce estrogen levels comparable to those in the early follicular phase of a normal menstrual cycle.[80] Symptoms of estrogen deficiency, such as vaginal atrophy or a decrease in breast size, do not occur.

The injection should be given within the first 7 days of the current menstrual cycle, otherwise a back-up method is necessary for 1 week.[81–83] The duration of action can be shortened if attention is not paid to proper administration. The injection must be given deeply in muscle by the Z-track technique and not massaged. It is prudent to avoid locations at risk for massage by daily activities.

Efficacy

The efficacy of this method is equal to that of sterilization. and better than that of all the other temporary methods.[84] Because serum concentrations are relatively high, efficacy is not influenced by weight or by the use of medications that stimulate hepatic enzymes. On the contrary, Depo-Provera is an excellent contraceptive choice for women taking antiepileptic drugs because the high progestin levels raise the seizure threshold.[85]

Indications

1.   At least one year of birth spacing desired.

2.   Highly effective long-acting contraception not linked to coitus.

3.   Estrogen-free contraception needed.

4. Breastfeeding.

5. Sickle cell disease.

6. Seizure disorder.

7. Private, coitally independent method desired.

Absolute Contraindications

1. Pregnancy.

2. Unexplained genital bleeding.

3. Severe coagulation disorders.

4. Previous sex steroid-induced liver adenoma.

Relative Contraindications

1. Liver disease.

2. Severe cardiovascular disease.

3. Rapid return to fertility desired.

4. Difficulty with injections.

5. Severe depression.

Advantages

Like other sustained-release forms of contraception, Depo-Provera is not associated with compliance problems and is not related to the coital event. Continuation rates are better and repeat pregnancy rates are reduced compared with oral contraceptive use in teenagers.[86] Depo-Provera is useful for women whose ability to remember contraceptive requirements is limited. It should be considered for women who lead disorganized lives or who are mentally retarded.

The freedom from the side effects of estrogen allows Depo-Provera to be considered for patients with congenital heart disease, sickle cell anemia, patients with a previous history of thromboembolism, and women over age 30 who smoke or have other risk factors. The absolute safety in regard to thrombosis is mainly theoretical; it has not been proven in a controlled study. However, an increased risk of thrombosis has not been observed in epidemiologic evaluation of Depo-Provera users, and a World Health Organization case-control study could find no evidence for increased risks of stroke, myocardial infarction, or venous thromboembolism.[79, 87]

A further advantage exists for patients with sickle cell disease because evidence indicates an inhibition of in vivo sickling with hematologic improvement during treatment.[88] Both the frequency and the intensity of painful sickle cell crises are reduced.[89]

Another advantage is the finding that Depo-Provera increases the quantity of milk in nursing mothers, a direct contrast to the effect seen with combination oral contraception. The concentration of the drug in the breast milk may be negligible, and no effects of the drug on infant growth and development have been observed,[90–92] In a careful study of male infants being breastfed by women treated with Depo-Provera, no metabolites of depot-medroxyprogesterone acetate could be detected in the infant's urine and no alterations could be observed in the infant levels of FSH, LH, testosterone, and cortisol.[93] Because of the slight positive impact on lactation, Depo-Provera can be administered soon after delivery, but at least a 3-day postpartum delay is recommended to allow the decline in pregnancy levels of estrogen and progesterone and the establishment of lactation.[12]

As noted, Depo-Provera should be considered in patients with seizure disorders; an improvement in seizure control can be achieved probably because of the sedative properties of progestins.[85]

Other benefits associated with Depo-Provera use include a decreased risk of endometrial cancer comparable with that observed with oral contraceptives,[94] and probably the same benefits associated with the progestin impact of oral contraceptives: reduced menstrual flow and anemia, less PID, less endometriosis, fewer uterine fibroids,[95] and fewer ectopic pregnancies. A failure to document a reduced risk of ovarian cancer by the World Health Organization probably reflects the study's low statistical power and the high parity in the Depo-Provera users.[96]

Depo-Provera, like oral contraception, may reduce the risk of pelvic inflammatory disease; however, the only study was hampered by small numbers.[97] Suppression of ovulation means that ectopic pregnancies are abolished and ovarian cysts are rare.

The greater the number of choices women have, the more likely they are to find a contraceptive that works well for them. For some women the primary advantages of Depo-Provera are privacy and ease of use. No one but the user need know about the injection, and the 3-month schedule can be easy to maintain for women who don't mind injections. In some societies, injections are respected as efficacious; in these situations, Depo-Provera is the most popular contraceptive despite bleeding changes and other side effects.

Summary of Advantages

1. Easy to use, no daily or coital action required.

2. Safe, no serious health effects.

3. Very effective, as effective as sterilization and intrauterine and implant contraception.

4. Free from estrogen-related problems.

5. Private, use not detectable.

6. Enhances lactation.

7. Has noncontraceptive benefits.

Problems With Depo-Provera

Major problems with Depo-Provera are irregular menstrual bleeding, breast tenderness, weight gain, and depression.[78, 79] By far, the most common problem is the change in menstrual bleeding. Up to 25% of patients discontinue in the first year because of irregular bleeding.[62] The bleeding is rarely heavy; in fact, hemoglobin values rise in Depo-Provera users. The incidence of irregular bleeding is 70% in the first year, and 10% thereafter. Bleeding and spotting decrease progressively with each re-injection so that after 5 years, 80% of users are amenorrheic (compared with

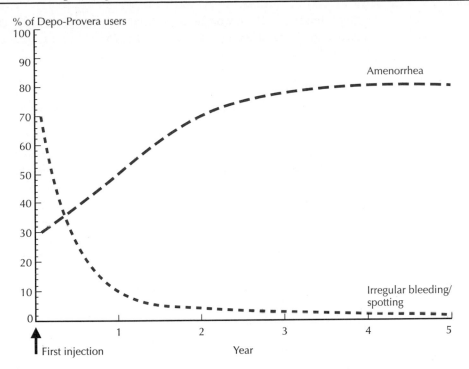

10% of Norplant users).[98] Irregular bleeding can be disturbing and annoying, and for many patients, it inhibits sexuality.

If necessary, the bleeding can be treated with exogenous estrogen, 1.25 mg conjugated estrogens, or 2 mg estradiol, given daily for 7 days. A nonsteroidal anti-inflammatory product given for a week is also effective, and another option is to administer an oral contraceptive for 1–3 months. Giving the Depo-Provera injection earlier (more frequently) does not change the bleeding pattern.[99] Most women can wait for amenorrhea without treatment if they know what to expect with time.

About one-third of patients discontinue Depo-Provera by the end of one year, 50% by the end of two years, and about 80% by the end of three years.[100] In a large international study, the most common medical reasons for discontinuing Depo-Provera during the first two years of use were the following:[79]

1.	Headaches	— 2.3%
2.	Weight gain	— 2.1%
3.	Dizziness	— 1.2%
4.	Abdominal pain	— 1.1%
5.	Anxiety	— 0.7%

In western societies, depression, fatigue, decreased libido, and hypertension are also encountered. Whether medroxyprogesterone acetate causes these side effects is difficult to know since they are very common complaints in nonusers as well.[101] When studied closely, no increase in depressive symptoms can be observed, even in women with significant complaints of depression prior to treatment.[102]

Even attempts to document a greater weight gain specifically associated with Depo-Provera are unable to do so.[103–105] As with oral contraception, the weight gain may not be hormone-induced, but reflect lifestyle and aging. Remember if symptoms are truly due to the progestin, unlike pills and implants, Depo-Provera takes 6–8 months to be gone after the last injection. Clearance is slower in heavier women.

Approximately half of women who discontinue Depo-Provera can expect normal menses to return in 6 months after the last injection, but 25% will wait a year before resumption of a normal pattern.[98]

Breast Cancer

Medroxyprogesterone acetate, in large continuous doses, produced breast tumors in beagle dogs (perhaps because in dogs progestins stimulate growth hormone secretion, known to be a mammotrophic agent in dogs).[106] This is an effect unique with dogs, and has not appeared in women after years of use. A very large, hospital-based case-control WHO study conducted over 9 years in 3 developing countries indicated that exposure to Depo-Provera is associated with a very slightly increased risk in breast cancer in the first 4 years of use, but there was no evidence for an increase in risk with increased duration of use.[107] The results were interpreted to suggest that growth of already existing tumors is enhanced. The number of cases with recent use was not large, and the confidence intervals reflected this. Another possible explanation for this finding is the combination of detection/surveillance bias and accelerated growth of an already present tumor, a situation similar to those described with oral contraceptives (Chapter 22) and postmenopausal hormone therapy (Chapter 18).

Two earlier population-based case-control studies indicated a possible association between breast cancer and Depo-Provera. One, from Costa Rica, was based on only 19 cases.[108] The other, from New Zealand, did not find an increased relative risk in ever users but did find an indication of increased risk shortly after initiating use at an early age, less than age 25.[109] A pooled analysis of the WHO and New Zealand data indicated that the highest risk was in women who had received a single injection.[110] The risk, if real, is very slight, and it is equally possible that the suggestions of increased risk based on a small number of cases have not been free of confounding variables. Because recent use appears to be the key factor, it is appropriate to emphasize that these studies did not find evidence for an overall increased risk of breast cancer, and the risk did not increase with duration of use. However, clinicians should consider informing patients that Depo-Provera might accelerate the growth of an already present occult cancer. We would expect such tumors to be detected at an earlier stage and grade of disease and be associated with a better outcome.

Other Cancers

An increased risk of cervical dysplasia cannot be documented even with long-term use (4 or more years).[111] No increase in adenocarcinoma or adenosquamous carcinoma could be detected in the WHO study.[112] The WHO study has not detected an increased risk of invasive squamous cell cancer of the cervix in Depo-Provera users; however, the risk of cervical carcinoma *in situ* was slightly elevated in the WHO case-control study, and it is not certain whether this is a real finding or a consequence of unrecognized biases.[113, 114] In New Zealand, a modest increase in the risk of cervical dysplasia among users of Depo-Provera could be attributed to an increased prevalence of known risk factors for dysplasia among women who choose this method of contraception.[111] Nevertheless, it is prudent to insist on annual Pap smear surveillance in all users of contraception, no matter what method. Women at higher risk because of their sexual behavior (multiple partners, history of STDs) should have Pap smears every 6 months.

As noted, Depo-Provera is associated with a reduction in the risk of endometrial cancer, and there is probably a modest reduction in the risk of ovarian cancer. There is no evidence that liver cancer risk is changed by the use of Depo-Provera.[115]

Metabolic Effects

The impact of Depo-Provera on the lipoprotein profile is uncertain. While some fail to detect an adverse impact, and claim that this is due to the avoidance of a first-pass through effect in the liver,[116] others have demonstrated a decrease in HDL-cholesterol and increases in total cholesterol and LDL-cholesterol.[116, 117] In a multicenter clinical trial by the World Health Organization, a transient adverse impact was present only in the few weeks after injection when blood levels were high.[118] The clinical impact of these changes, if any, have yet to be reported. It seems prudent to monitor the lipid profile annually in women using Depo-Provera for long durations. The emergence of significant adverse changes in LDL-cholesterol and HDL-cholesterol warrant reconsideration of contraceptive choice.

There are no clinically significant changes in carbohydrate metabolism or in coagulation factors.[119, 120]

Concern has been raised because the blood levels of estrogen with this method of contraception are relatively lower over a period of time compared with a normal menstrual cycle, and, therefore, patients might lose bone to some degree, and, indeed, bone loss has been documented in cross-sectional studies.[47, 121, 122] This bone loss has also been observed in women receiving a high oral dose of medroxyprogesterone acetate, 50 mg daily.[123] However, bone density measurements in women who stopped using Depo-Provera indicated that the loss was regained even after long-term use. [124] Furthermore, a cross-sectional study in Thailand found no bone loss in long-term (greater than 3 years) users of Depo-Provera.[125] And most importantly, longitudinal, prospective studies of bone fail to document bone loss in users of Depo-Provera. Loss of forearm bone density could not be detected despite 3 years of Depo-Provera use, suggesting that previous adverse findings could be explained by inadequate control of factors that affect bone, such as smoking and alcohol intake.[126] A small prospective study documented stable forearm bone density over a 6-month period of time.[48] This concern will require ongoing surveillance of past users, but at the present time, this should not be a reason to avoid this method of contraception. *It is unlikely that bone loss occurs sufficiently to raise the risk of osteoporosis later in life.*

Effect on Future Fertility

The delay in becoming pregnant after ceasing use of Depo-Provera is a problem unique to injectable contraception; all the other temporary methods allow a more prompt return to fertility.[127] However, medroxyprogesterone acetate does not permanently suppress ovarian function, and the concern that infertility with suppressed menstrual function may be caused by Depo-Provera has not been supported by epidemiologic data. The pregnancy rate in women discontinuing the injections because of a desire to become pregnant is normal.[128] By 18 months after the last injection, 90% of Depo-Provera users have become pregnant, the same proportion as for other methods.[129] The delay to conception is about 9 months after the last injection, and the delay does not increase with increasing duration of use. Because of this delay, women who want to conceive promptly after discontinuing their contraceptive should not use Depo-Provera. Suppressed menstrual function persisting beyond 12 months after the last injection is not due to the drug and deserves evaluation.

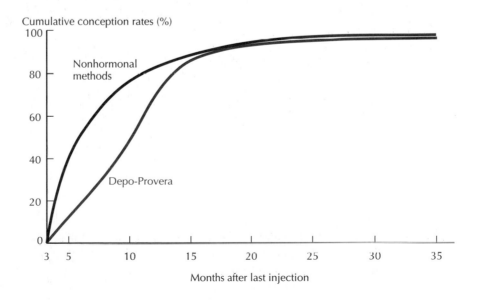

Accidental pregnancies occurring at the time of the initial injection of Depo-Provera have been reported to be associated with higher neonatal and infant mortality rates, probably due to an increased risk of intrauterine growth retardation.[130, 131] The timing of the first injection is, therefore, very important. To ensure effective contraception, the first injection should be administered within the first 5 days of the menstrual cycle (before a dominant follicle emerges), or a back-up method is necessary for 2 weeks.

Short-Term Injectable Contraceptives

Monthly or every other month injectable combinations of estrogen and progestin are not new, having been developed over several decades.[132] This method of contraception is popular in China, Latin America, and Eastern Asia. A preparation widely used in China consists of 250 mg 17α-hydroxyprogesterone caproate and 5 mg estradiol valerate, known as Chinese Injectable No.1.

Cyclo-Provera (or Cyclofem)

Cyclo-Provera consists of 25 mg depot-medroxyprogesterone acetate and 5 mg estradiol cypionate and is administered monthly as a deep intramuscular injection. This method is as effective as Depo-Provera, but avoids the problems of menstrual irregularity and heavy bleeding, as well as amenorrhea.[133–136] In addition, the method is rapidly reversible. Besides the need for a monthly injection, another disadvantage is the likelihood that the combination of estrogen and progestin will inhibit lactation. The requirement for a monthly injection can be made more convenient by the utilization of an automatic device for self-administration.[137] Approximately 80% of women who are amenorrheic on Depo-Provera will develop vaginal bleeding if switched to Cyclo-Provera.[138]

Norethindrone Enanthate

Norethindrone enanthate is given in a dose of 200 mg intramuscularly every 2 months. This progestin acts in the same way as Depo-Provera, and has the same problems.[79] A combination (Mesigyna) of norethindrone enanthate (50 mg) with estradiol valerate (5 mg) given monthly provides effective contraception with good cycle control.[139] Compared with Cyclofem (25 mg medroxyprogesterone acetate and 5 mg estradiol cypionate), Mesigyna has less bleeding problems.[140] Fertility returns rapidly (by one month) after discontinuation with once-a-month methods.[141]

Dihydroxyprogesterone Acetophenide and Estradiol Enanthate

The combination of 150 mg dihydroxyprogeserone acetophenide with 10 mg estradiol enanthate (various brand names) is the most widely used injectable contraceptive in Latin America. As with Mesigyna and Cyclofem, the monthly regimen allows regular, and even reduced, cyclic bleeding.[142] A lower dose (90 mg dihydroxyprogesterone acetophenide and 6 mg estradiol enanthate) provides the same effective contraception as the higher dose with similar bleeding patterns.[143]

New Developments in Injectable Contraception

Microspheres or microcapsules have been studied for several years.[144, 145] They consist of a biodegradable copolymer and one or more hormones. Like other injectable contraceptives, they are easy to administer and are highly effective. Unlike implants, injectables do not require surgical skills of the clinician and can be discontinued by the patient simply by declining to have another injection. Unlike implants, the microspheres cannot be removed once they are injected.

If a woman experiences side effects or becomes pregnant, the hormone will remain in her body until completely metabolized. For this reason, the duration of action of the norethindrone capsules has been limited to a few months.

The carrier of the microsphere is composed of a polymer commonly used in biodegradable suture, poly-dl-lactide-co-glycolide. The size of the microspheres varies from 0.06 to 0.1 mm in diameter, and each is composed of about 50% norethindrone dispersed within the polymer. The release of norethindrone occurs initially by diffusion and later by degradation of the carrier. The size of the microspheres, the amount of hormone contained within the carrier, and the quantity of microspheres delivered by injection determine the daily dose of norethindrone delivered. Injections currently under evaluation contain a total dose of either 65 mg or 100 mg norethindrone, and the amount released daily is approximately the same as that delivered by low-dose oral contraception, but circulating levels are more stable.

The microspheres come preloaded in a syringe and are put into suspension with the addition of 2.5 mL of dextran diluent and vigorously agitated. The mixture must be shaken until all of the microspheres are in suspension, and again immediately prior to injection. The microspheres are deposited in the gluteal muscle using a 21-gauge needle and Z-track intramuscular injection technique.

As with other progestin-only methods of contraception, menstrual changes occur and are the most common cause of discontinuation during the first year of use. Users may experience amenorrhea or persistent or irregular spotting or bleeding. In contrast to Depo-Provera, hormone levels decline rapidly after the microspheres have degraded, so that contraceptive effectiveness ends promptly at the predicted time. Most users will resume ovulatory cycles within 2–3 months after the predicted duration of the injection. If pregnancy occurs shortly after expiration of the norethindrone microspheres, the fetus will not be exposed to significant levels of norethindrone.

Microsphere preparations containing norethindrone combined with ethinyl estradiol are also under development. It is hoped that the addition of estrogen at a low dose will lead to fewer menstrual irregularities.

Long-Acting Methods for Older Women

The long-acting methods of hormonal contraception deserve consideration in those situations where combination estrogen-progestin is unacceptable because of health problems (where estrogen is contraindicated), or where oral contraception has already proved to be unsuccessful. These methods are especially advantageous for smokers and for women with a history of thromboembolic disease. Progestin-only contraception is a good choice for women with hypertriglyceridemia, for diabetic women (even if they are older and smoke), and for women with severe migraine headaches or hypertension.

Older women, as they approach the menopause, may be more comfortable with the irregular bleeding or amenorrhea associated with these methods. However, the irregular bleeding patterns can cause more concern in some women regarding possible pathology. Postmenopausal hormone treatment can be initiated if menopausal symptoms develop or when annual measurement of the FSH level, beginning at age 50, indicates a rise above 20 IU/L (progestins do not suppress FSH secretion, and, therefore, this measurement can be obtained even while the patient has therapeutic circulating levels of progestin).

References

1. **Sivin I,** International experience with Norplant and Norplant-2 contraceptives, *Stud Fam Plann* 19:81, 1988.

2. **Roy S, Mishell Jr DR, Robertson D, Krauss RM, Lacarra M, Duda MJ,** Long-term reversible contraception with levonorgestrel-releasing Silastic rods, *Am J Obstet Gynecol* 148:1006, 1984.

3. **Trussell J, Hatcher RA, Cates Jr W, Stewart FH, Kost K,** Contraceptive failure in the United States: an update, *Stud Fam Plann* 21:51, 1990.

4. **Darney PD, Elizabeth A, Tanner S, MacPherson S, Hellerstein S, Alvardo A,** Acceptance and perceptions of Norplant among users in San Francisco, USA, *Stud Fam Plann* 21:152, 1990.

5. **Brache V, Faundes A, Johansson E, Alvarez F,** Anovulation, inadequate luteal phase, and poor sperm penetration in cervical mucus during prolonged use of Norplant implants, *Contraception* 31:261, 1985.

6. **Dunson TR, Blumenthal PD, Alvarez F, Brache V, Cochon L, Dalberth B, Glover L, Remsburg R, Vu K, Katz D,** Timing of onset of contraceptive effectiveness in Norplant implant users. Part I. Changes in cervical mucus, *Fertil Steril* 69:258, 1998.

7. **Brache V, Alvarez-Sanchez F, Faundes A, Tejada AS, Cochon L,** Ovarian endocrine function through five years of continuous treatment with Norplant subdermal contraceptive implants, *Contraception* 41:169, 1990.

8. **Affandi B, Cekan S, Boonkasemanti R, Samil RS, Diczfalusy E,** The interaction between sex hormone binding globulin and levonorgestrel released from Norplant, an implantable contraceptive, *Contraception* 35:135, 1987.

9. **Alvarez F, Brache V, Tejada AS, Faundes A,** Abnormal endocrine profile among women with confirmed or presumed ovulation during long-term Norplant use, *Contraception* 33:111, 1986.

10. **Croxatto HB, Diaz S, Salvatierra AM, Morales P, Ebensperger C, Brandeis A,** Treatment with Norplant subdermal implants inhibits sperm penetration through cervical mucus in vitro, *Contraception* 36:193, 1987.

11. **Segal SJ, Alvarez-Sanchez F, Brache V, Faundes A, Vilja P, Tuohimaa P,** Norplant implants: the mechanism of contraceptive action, *Fertil Steril* 56:273, 1991.

12. **Kennedy KI, Short RV, Tully MR,** Premature introduction of progestin-only contraceptive methods during lactation, *Contraception* 55:347, 1997.

13. **Shaaban MM, Salem HT, Abdullah KA,** Influence of levonorgestrel contraceptive implants, Norplant, initiated early postpartum, upon lactation and infant growth, *Contraception* 32:623, 1985.

14. **Diaz S, Herreros C, Juez G, Casado ME, Salvatierra AM, Miranda P, Peralta O, Croxatto HB,** Fertility regulation in nursing women: influence of Norplant levonorgestrel implants upon lactation and infant growth, *Contraception* 32:53, 1985.

15. **Sivin I, Stern J, Diaz S, Pavez M, Alvarez F, Brache V, Mishell Jr DR, Lacarra M, McCarthy T, Holma P, Darney P, Klaisle C, Olsson S-E, Odlind V,** Rates and outcomes of planned pregnancy after use of Norplant capsules, Norplant II rods, or levonorgestrel-releasing or copper TCu 380Ag intrauterine contraceptive devices, *Am J Obstet Gynecol* 166:1208, 1992.

16. **Diaz S, Pavez M, Cardenas H, Croxatto HB,** Recovery of fertility and outcome of planned pregnancies after the removal of Norplant subdermal implants or copper-T IUDs, *Contraception* 35:569, 1987.

17. **Fakeye O, Balogh S,** Effect of Norplant contraceptive use on hemoglobin, packed cell volume, and menstrual bleeding patterns, *Contraception* 39:265, 1989.

18. **Dunson TR, Amatya RN, Krueger SL,** Complications and risk factors associated with the removal of Norplant implants, *Obstet Gynecol* 85:543, 1995.

19. **Trussell J, Leveque JA, Koenig JD, London R, Borden S, Henneberry J, LaGuardia KD, Stewart F, Wilson TG, Wysocki S, Strauss M,** The economic value of contraception: a comparison of 15 methods, *Am J Public Health* 85:494, 1995.

20. **Haukkamaa M,** Contraception by Norplant subdermal capsules is not reliable in epileptic patients on anticonvulsant treatment, *Contraception* 33:559, 1986.

21. **Berenson AB, Wiemann CM, Rickerr VI, McCombs SL,** Contraceptive outcomes among adolescents prescribed Norplant implants versus oral contraceptives after one year of use, *Am J Obstet Gynecol* 176:586, 1997.

22. **Trussell J,** Contraceptive efficacy, In: Hatcher RA, Trussell J, Stewart F, et al, eds. *Contraceptive Technology,* 17th ed, Irvington Publishers, New York, NY, 1998.

23. **Darney PD, Klaisle CM, Tanner S, Alvarado AM,** Sustained-release contraceptives, *Curr Prob Obstet Gynecol Fertil* 13:95, 1990.

24. **Sivin I, Mishell Jr DR, Darney P, Wan L, Christ M,** Levonorgestrel capsule implants in the United States: a 5-year study, *Obstet Gynecol* 92:337, 1998.

25. **Centers for Disease Control and Prevention,** Ectopic pregnancy — United States, 1988-1989, *MMWR* 41:591, 1992.

26. **Franks AL, Beral V, Cates Jr W, Hogue CJ,** Contraception and ectopic pregnancy risk, *Am J Obstet Gynecol* 163:1120, 1990.

27. **Sivin I, Alvarez-Sanchez F, Diaz S, Holma P, Coutinho E, McDonald O, Robertson DN, Stern J,** Three-year experience with Norplant subdermal contraception, *Fertil Steril* 39:799, 1983.

28. **Shoupe D, Mishell Jr DR, Bopp B, Fiedling M,** The significance of bleeding patterns in Norplant implant users, *Obstet Gynecol* 77:256, 1991.

29. **Sivin I, Diaz S, Holma P, Alvarez-Sanchez F, Robertson DN,** A four-year clinical study of Norplant implants, *Stud Fam Plann* 14:184, 1983.

30. **Runic R, Schatz F, Krey L, Demopoulos R, Thung S, Wan L, Lockwood CJ,** Alterations in endometrial stromal cell tissue factor protein and messenger ribonucleic acid expression in patients experiencing abnormal uterine bleeding while using Norplant-2 contraception, *J Clin Endocrinol Metab* 82:1983, 1997.

31. **Nilsson C, Holma P,** Menstrual blood loss with contraceptive subdermal levonorgestrel implants, *Fertil Steril* 35:304, 1981.

32. **Diaz S, Croxatto HB, Pavez M, Belhadj H, Stern J, Sivin I,** Clinical assessment of treatments for prolonged bleeding in users of Norplant implants, *Contraception* 42:97, 1990.

33. **Alvarez-Sanchez F, Brache V, Thevenin F, Cochon L, Faundes A,** Hormonal treatment for bleeding irregularities in Norplant implant users, *Am J Obstet Gynecol* 174:919, 1996.

34. **Croxatto HB, Diaz S, Robertson D, Pavez M,** Clinical chemistries in women treated with levonorgestrel implant (Norplant) or a TCu 200 IUD, *Contraception* 27:281, 1983.

35. **Konje JC, Otolorin EO, Ladipo OA,** Changes in carbohydrate metabolism during 30 months on Norplant, *Contraception* 44:163, 1991.

36. **Shaaban MM, Elwan SI, El-Sharkawy MM, Farghaly AS,** Effect of subdermal levononorgestrel contraceptive implants, Norplant, on liver functions, *Contraception* 30:407, 1984.

37. **Singh K, Viegas OAC, Liew D, Singh P, Ratnam SS,** Two-year follow-up of changes in clinical chemistry in Singaporean Norplant acceptors: metabolic changes, *Contraception* 39:129, 1989.

38. **Egberg N, van Beek A, Gunnervik C, Hulkko S, Hirvonen E, Larsson-Cohn U, Bennink HC,** Effects on the hemostatic system and liver function in relation to Implanon® and Norplant®, *Contraception* 58:93, 1998.

39. **Shaaban MM, Elwan SI, El-Kabsh MY, Farghaly SA, Thabet N,** Effect of levonorgestrel contraceptive implants, Norplant, on bleeding and coagulation, *Contraception* 30:421, 1984.

40. **Singh K, Viegas OAC, Koh SCL, Ratnam SS,** Effect of long-term use of Norplant implants on haemostatic function, *Contraception* 45:203, 1992.

41. **Viegas OAC, Koh SLC, Ratnam SS,** The effects of reformulated 2-rod Norplant implant on haemostasis after three years, *Contraception* 54:219, 1996.

42. **Abdulla K, Elwan SI, Salem HS, Shaaban MM,** Effect of early postpartum use of the contraceptive impants, Norplant, on the serum levels of immunoglobulin of the mothers and their breastfed infants, *Contraception* 32:261, 1985.

43. **Bayad M, Ibrahim I, Fayad M, et al,** Serum cortisol in women users of subdermal levonorgestrel implants, *Contracept Delivery Syst* 4:133, 1983.

44. **Otubu JAM, Towobola OA, Aisien AO, Ogunkeye OO,** Effects of Norplant contraceptive subdermal implants on serum lipids and lipoproteins, *Contraception* 47:149, 1993.

45. **Koopersmith TB, Lobo RA,** Insulin sensitivity is unaltered by the use of the Norplant subdermal implant contraceptive, *Contraception* 51:197, 1995.

46. **Harper MA, Meis PJ, Steele L,** A prospective study of insulin sensitivity and glucose metabolism in women using a continuous subdermal levonorgestrel implant system, *J Soc Gynecol Invest* 4:86, 1997.

47. **Cromer BA, Blair JM, Mahan JD, Zibners L, Naumovski Z,** A prospective comparison of bone density in adolescent girls receiving depot medroxyprogesterone acetate (Depo-Provera), levonorgestrel (Norplant), or oral contraceptives, *J Pediatr* 129:671, 1996.

48. **Naessen T, Olsson SE, Gudmundson J,** Differential effects on bone density of progestogen-only methods for contraception in premenopausal women, *Contraception* 52:35, 1995.

49. **Gu S, Du M, Zhang L, Liu YL, Wang SH, Sivin I,** A 5-year evaluation of Norplant contraceptive implants in China, *Obstet Gynecol* 83:673, 1994.

50. **Westhoff C, Truman C, Kalmuss D, Cushman L, Rulin M, Heartwell S, Davidson A,** Depressive symptoms and Norplant® contraceptive implants, *Contraception* 57:241, 1998.

51. **Wysowski DK, Green L,** Serious adverse events in Norplant users reported to the Food and Drug Administration's MedWatch Spontaneous Reporting System, *Obstet Gynecol* 85:538, 1995.

52. **Fraser IS, Tiitinen A, Affandi B, Brache V, Croxatto HB, Diaz S, Ginsburg J, Gu S, Holma P, Johansson E, Meirik O, Mishell Jr DR, Nash HA, von Schoultz B, Sivin I,** Norplant® consensus statement and background review, *Contraception* 57:1, 1998.

53. **Pasquale SA, Knuppel RA, Owens AG, Bachmann GA,** Irregular bleeding, body mass index and coital frequency in Norplant contraceptive users, *Contraception* 50:109, 1994.

54. **Faundes A, Brache V, Tejada AS, Cochon L, Alvarez-Sanchez F,** Ovulatory dysfunction during continuous administration of low-dose levonorgestrel by subdermal implants, *Fertil Steril* 56:27, 1991.

55. **Darney PD, Taylor RN, Klaisle C, Bottles K, Zaloudek C,** Serum concentrations of estradiol, progesterone, and levonorgestrel are not determinants of endometrial histology or abnormal bleeding in long-term Norplant implant users, *Contraception*, in press.

56. **Phemister DA, Lauarent S, Harrison Jr FNH,** Use of Norplant contraceptive implants in the immediate postpartum period: safety and tolerance, *Am J Obstet Gynecol* 172:175, 1995.

57. **Zimmerman M, Haffey J, Crane E, Szumowski D, Alvarez F, Bhiromrut P, Brache V, Lubis F, Salah M, Shaaban MM, Shawly B, Sidiip S,** Assessing the acceptability of Norplant implants in four countries: findings from focus group research, *Stud Fam Plann* 21:92, 1990.

58. **Gu S, Sivin I, Du M, Zhang L, Ying-Lin L, Meng F, Wu S, Wang P, Gao Y, He X, Qi L, Chen C, Liu Y, Wang D,** Effectiveness of Norplant implants through seven years: a large-scale study in China, *Contraception* 52:99, 1995.

59. **Salah M, Ahmed A, Abo-Eloyoun M, Shaaban MM,** Five-year experience with Norplant implants in Assiut, Egypt, *Contraception* 35:543, 1987.

60. **Bashayake S, Thapa S, Balogh A,** Evaluation of safety, efficacy, and acceptability of Norplant implants in Sri Lanka, *Stud Fam Plann* 19:39, 1988.

61. **Dugoff L, Jones III OW, Allen-Davis J, Hurst BS, Schlaff WD,** Assessing the acceptability of Norplant contraceptive in four patient populations, *Contraception* 52:45, 1995.

62. **Cromer BA, Smith RD, Blair JM, Dwyer J, Brown RT,** A prospective study of adolescents who choose among levonorgestrel implant (Norplant), medroxyprogesterone acetate (Depo-Provera), or the combined oral contraceptive pill as contraception, *Pediatrics* 94:687, 1994.

63. **Cullins VE, Remsburg RE, Blumenthal PD, Huggins GR,** Comparison of adolescent and adult experience with Norplant levonorgestrel contraceptive implants, *Obstet Gynecol* 83:1026, 1994.

64. **Polaneczky M, Slap G, Forke C, Rappaport A, Sondheimer S,** The use of levonorgestrel implants (Norplant) for contraception in adolescent mothers, *New Engl J Med* 331:1201, 1994.

65. **Berenson AB, Wiemann CM,** Use of levonorgestrel implants versus oral contraceptives in adolescence: a case-control study, *Am J Obstet Gynecol* 172:1128, 1995.

66. **Gao J, Wang SL, Wu SC, Sun BL, Allonen H, Luukkainen T,** Comparison of the clinical performance, contraceptive efficacy and acceptability of levonorgestrel-releasing IUD and Norplant implants in China, *Contraception* 41:485, 1990.

67. **Ollila E, Sihvo S, Merilainen J, Hemminki E,** Experience of Finnish women with Norplant insertions and removals, *Br J Obstet Gynaecol* 104:488, 1997.

68. **Sivin I, Viegas O, Campodonico I, Diaz S, Pavez M, Wan L, Koetsawang S, Kiriwat O, Anant MP, Holma P, el din Abdalla K, Stern J,** Clinical performance of a new two-rod levonorgestrel contraceptive implant: a three-year randomized study with Norplant® implants as controls, *Contraception* 55:73, 1997.

69. **Sivin I, Lähteenmäki P, Ranta S, Darney P, Klaisle C, Wan L, Mishell Jr DR, Lacarra M, Viegas OAC, Bilhareus P, Koetsawang S, Piya-Anant M, Diaz S, Pavez M, Alvarez F, Brache V, LaGuardia K, Nash H, Stern J,** Levonorgestrel concentrations during use of levonorgestrel rod (LNG ROD) implants, *Contraception* 55:81, 1997.

70. **Olsson S-E, Odlind V, Johansson E,** Clinical results with subcutaneous implants containing 3-keto desogestrel, *Contraception* 42:1, 1990.

71. **Diaz S, Pavez M, Moo-Young AJ, Bardin CW, Croxatto HB,** Clinical trial with 3-keto-desogestrel subdermal implants, *Contraception* 44:393, 1991.

72. **Coutinho EM,** One year contraception with a single subdermal implant containing nomegestrel acetate (Uniplant), *Contraception* 47:94, 1993.

73. **Haukkamaa M, Laurikka-Routti M, Heikinheimo O, Moo-Young A,** Contraception with subdermal implants releasing the progestin ST-1435: a dose-finding study, *Contraception* 45:49, 1992.

74. **Diaz S, Schiappacasse V, Pavez M, Zepeda A, Moo-Young AJ, Brandeis A, Lahteenmaki P, Croxatto HB,** Clinical trial with Nestorone subdermal contraceptive implants, *Contraception* 51:33, 1995.

75. **Darney PD, Klaisle CM, Monroe SE, Cook CE, Phillips N, Schindler A,** Evaluation of a 1-year levonorgestrel-releasing contraceptive implant: side effects, release rates, and biodegradability, *Fertil Steril* 58:137, 1992.

76. **Singh M, Saxena BB, Raghubanshi RS, Ledger WJ, Harman SM, Leonard RJ,** Biodegradable norethindrone (NET:cholesterol) contraceptive implants: phase II-A: a clinical study in women, *Contraception* 55:23, 1997.

77. **Rosenfield A, Maine D, Rochat R, Shelton J, Hatcher R,** The Food and Drug Administration and medroxyprogesterone acetate: what are the issues? *JAMA* 249:2922, 1983.

78. **WHO,** A multicentered phase III comparative clinical trial of depot-medroxyprogesterone acetate given three-monthly at doses of 100 mg or 150 mg: I. Contraceptive efficacy and side effects, *Contraception* 34:223, 1986.

79. **WHO,** Multinational comparative clinical evaluation of two long-acting injectable contraceptive steroids: norethisterone enanthate and medroxyprogesterone acetate. Final report, *Contraception* 28:1, 1983.

80. **Fraser IS, Weisberg EA,** A comprehensive review of injectable contaception with special emphasis on depot medroxyprogesterone acetate, *Med J Aust* 1(Suppl):3, 1981.

81. **Siriwongse T, Snidvonga W, Tantayaporn P, Leepipalboon S,** Effect of depot-medroxyprogesterone acetate on serum progesterone levels, when administered on various cycle days, *Contraception* 26:487, 1982.

82. **Petta C, Faúndes A, Dunson TR, Ramos M, DeLucio M, Faúndes D, Bahamondes L,** Timing of onset of contraceptive effectiveness in Depo-Provera users. I. Changes in cervical mucus, *Fertil Steril* 69:252, 1998.

83. **Petta CA, Faúndes A, Dunson TR, Ramos M, DeLucio M, Faúndes D, Bahamondes L,** Timing of onset of contraceptive effectiveness in Depo-Provera users. II. Effects on ovarian function, *Fertil Steril* 70:817, 1998.

84. **Harlap S, Kost K, Forrest JD,** *Preventing Pregnancy, Protecting Health: A New Look at Birth Control Choices in the United States,* The Alan Guttmacher Institute, New York, 1991.

85. **Mattson RH, Cramer JA, Caldwell BV, Siconolfi BC,** Treatment of seizures with medroxyprogesterone acetate: preliminary report, *Neurol* 34:1255, 1984.

86. **Polaneczky M, Guarnaccia M, Alon J, Wiley J,** Early experience with the contraceptive use of depo-medroxyprogesterone acetate in an inner-city population, *Fam Plann Perspect* 28:174, 1996.

87. **World Health Organization Collaborative Study of Cardiovascular Disease and Steroid Hormone Contraception,** Cardiovascular disease and use of oral and injectable progestogen-only contraceptives and combined injectable contraceptives. Results of an international, multicenter, case-control study, *Contraception* 57:315, 1998.

88. **DeCeular K, Gruber C, Hayes R, Serjeant GR,** Medroxyprogesterone acetate and homozygous sickle-cell disease, *Lancet* ii:229, 1982.

89. **de Abood M, de Castillo Z, Guerrero F, Espino M, Austin KL,** Effect of Depo-Provera® or Microgynon® on the painful crises of sickle-cell anemia patients, *Contraception* 56:313, 1997.

90. **Jimenez J, Ochoa M, Soler MP, Portales P,** Long-term follow-up of children breast-fed by mothers receiving depot-medroxyprogesterone acetate, *Contraception* 30:523, 1984.

91. **Zacharias S, Aguilena J, Assanzo JR, Zanatu J,** Effects of hormonal and non-hormonal contracepters on lactation and incidence of pregnancy, *Contraception* 33:203, 1986.

92. **Pardthaisong T, Yenchit C, Gray R,** The long-term growth and development of children exposed to Depo-Provera during pregnancy or lactation, *Contraception* 45:313, 1992.

93. **Virutamasen P, Leepipatpaiboon S, Kriengsinyot R, Vichaidith P, Muia PN, Sekadde-Kigondu CB, Mati JKG, Forest MG, Dikkeschei LD, Wolthers BG, d'Arcangues C,** Pharmacodynamic effects of depot-medroxyprogesterone acetate (DMPA) administered to lactating women on their male infants, *Contraception* 54:153, 1996.

94. **WHO Collaborative Study of Neoplasia and Steroid Contraceptives,** Depot-medroxyprogesterone acetate (DMPA) and risk of endometrial cancer, *Int J Cancer* 49:186, 1991.

95. **Lumbiganon P, Rugpao S, Phandhu-fung S, Laopaiboon M, Vudhikamraksa N, Werawatkul Y,** Protective effect of depot-medroxyprogesterone acetate on surgically treated uterine leiomyomas: a multicentre case-control study, *Br J Obstet Gynaecol* 103:909, 1996.

96. **WHO Collaborative Study of Neoplasia and Steroid Contraceptives,** Depot-medroxyprogesterone acetate (DMPA) and risk of epithelial ovarian cancer, *Int J Cancer* 49:191, 1991.

97. **Gray RH,** Reduced risk of pelvic inflammatory disease with injectable contraceptives, *Lancet* i:1046, 1985.

98. **Gardner JM, Mishell Jr DR,** Analysis of bleeding patterns and resumption of fertility following discontinuation of a long-acting injectable contraceptive, *Fertil Steril* 21:286, 1970.

99. **Harel Z, Biro FM, Kollar LM,** Depo-Provera in adolescents: effects of early second injection or prior oral contraception, *J Adolesc Health* 16:379, 1995.

100. **Smith RD, Cromer BA, Hayes JR, et al,** Medroxyprogesterone acetate (Depo-Provera) use in adolescents: uterine bleeding and blood pressure patterns, patient satisfaction, and continuation rates, *Adolesc Pediatr Gynecol* 8:24, 1995.

101. **Westhoff C, Wieland D, Tiezzi L,** Depression in users of depo-medroxyprogesterone acetate, *Contraception* 51:351, 1995.

102. **Westhoff C, Truman C, Kalmuss D, Cushman L, Davidson A, Rulin M, Heartwell S,** Depressive symptoms and Depo-Provera, *Contraception* 57:237, 1998.

103. **Moore LL, Valuck R, McDougall C, Fink W,** A comparative study of one-year weight gain among users of medroxyprogesterone acetate, levonorgestrel implants, and oral contraceptives, *Contraception* 52:215, 1995.

104. **Mainwaring R, Hales HA, Stevenson K, Hatasaka HH, Poulson AM, Jones KP, Peterson CM,** Metabolic parameters, bleeding, and weight changes in U.S. women using progestin only contraceptives, *Contraception* 51:149, 1995.

105. **Taneepanichskul S, Reinprayoon D, Khaosaad P,** Comparative study of weight change between long-term DMPA and IUD acceptors, *Contraception* 58:149, 1998.

106. **Jordan A,** Toxicology of depot medroxyprogesterone acetate, *Contraception* 49:18901, 1994.

107. **WHO Collaborative Study of Neoplasia and Steroid Contraceptives,** Breast cancer and depot-medroxyprogesterone acetate: a multinational study, *Lancet* 338:833, 1991.

108. **Lee NC, Rosero-Bixby L, Oberle MW, Grimaldo C, Whatley AS, Rovira EZ,** A case-control study of breast cancer and hormonal contraception in Costa Rica, *J Natl Cancer Inst* 79:1247, 1987.

109. **Paul C, Skegg DCG, Spears GFS,** Depot medroxyprogesterone (Depo-Provera) and risk of breast cancer, *Br Med J* 299:7591, 1989.

110. **Skegg DCG, Noonan EA, Paul C, Spears GFS, Meirik O, Thomas DB,** Depot medroxyprogesterone acetate and breast cancer: a pooled analysis of the World Health Organization and the New Zealand studies, *JAMA* 273:799, 1995.

111. **The New Zealand Contraception and Health Study Group,** History of long-term use of depot-medroxyprogesterone acetate in patients with cervical dysplasia; case-control analysis nested in a cohort study, *Contraception* 50:443, 1994.

112. **Thomas DB, Ray RM, Contraceptives and the WHO Collaborative Study of Neoplasia and Steroid Contraception,** Depot-medroxyprogesterone acetate (DMPA) and risk of invasive adenocarcinomas and adenosquamous carcinomas of the uterine cervix, *Contraception* 52:307, 1995.

113. **WHO Collaborative Study of Neoplasia and Steroid Contraception,** Depot-medroxyprogesterone acetate (DMPA) and risk of invasive squamous cell cervical cancer, *Contraception* 45:299, 1992.

114. **Thomas DB, Ye Z, Ray RM, and the WHO Collaborative Study of Neoplasia and Steroid Contraception,** Cervical carcinoma *in situ* and use of depot-medroxyprogesterone acetate (DMPA), *Contraception* 51:25, 1995.

115. **WHO,** Depo-medroxyprogesterone acetate (DMPA) and cancer; memorandum from a WHO meeting, *Bull World Health Organization* 64:375, 1986.

116. **Garza-Fores J, De la Cruz DL, Valles de Bourges V, Sanchez-Nuncio R, Martinez M, Fuziwara JL, Perez-Palacios G,** Long-term effects of depot-medroxyprogesterone acetate on lipoprotein metabolism, *Contraception* 44:61, 1991.

117. **Enk L, Landgren BM, Lindberg U-B, Silverstolpe G, Crona N,** A prospective, one-year study on the effects of two long acting injectable contraceptives (depot-medroxyprogesterone acetate and norethisterone enanthate) on serum and lipoprotein lipids, *Horm Metab Res* 24:85, 1992.

118. **WHO,** A multicentre comparative study of serum lipids and apolipoproteins in long-term users of DMPA and a control group of IUD users, *Contraception* 47:177, 1993.

119. **Fahmy K, Khairy M, Allam G, Gobran F, Allush M,** Effect of depo-medroxyprogesterone acetate on coagulation factors and serum lipids in Egyptian women, *Contraception* 44:431, 1991.

120. **Fahmy K, Abdel-Razik M, Shaaraway M, Al-Kholy G, Saad S, Wagdi A, Al-Azzony M,** Effect of long-acting progestagen-only injectable contraceptives on carbohydrate metabolism and its hormonal profile, *Contraception* 44:419, 1991.

121. **Cundy T, Evans M, Roberts H, Wattie D, Ames R, Reid IR,** Bone density in women receiving depot medroxyprogesterone acetate for contraception, *Br Med J* 303:13, 1991.

122. **Cundy T, Cornish J, Roberts H, Elder H, Reid IR,** Spinal bone density in women using depot medroxyprogesterone contraception, *Obstet Gynecol* 92:569, 1998.

123. **Cundy T, Farquhar CM, Cornish J, Reid IR,** Short-term effects of high dose oral medroxyprogesterone acetate on bone density in premenopausal women, *J Clin Endocrinol Metab* 81:1014, 1996.

124. **Cundy T, Cornish J, Evans MC, Roberts H, Reid IR,** Recovery of bone density in women who stop using medroxyprogesterone acetate, *Br Med J* 308:247, 1994.

125. **Virutamasen P, Wangsuphachart S, Reinprayoon D, Kriengsinyot R, Leepipatpaiboon S, Gua C,** Trabecular bone in long-term depot-medroxyprogesterone acetate users, *Asia Oceania J Obstet Gynaecol* 20:269, 1994.

126. **Taneepanichskul S, Intaraprasert S, Theppisai U, Chaturachinda K,** Bone mineral density in long-term depot medroxyprogesterone acetate acceptors, *Contraception* 56:1, 1997.

127. **Garza-Flores J, Cardenas S, Rodriguez V, Cravioto MC, Diaz-Sanchez V, Perez-Palacios G,** Return to ovulation following the use of long-acting injectable contraceptives: a comparative study, *Contraception* 31:361, 1985.

128. **Pardthaisong T,** Return of fertility after use of the injectable contraceptive Depo Provera: up-dated analysis, *J Biosoc Sci* 16:23, 1984.

129. **Schwallie P, Assenze J,** The effect of depo medroxyprogesterone acetate on pituitary and ovarian function, and the return of fertility following its discontinuation. A review, *Contraception* 10:181, 1974.

130. **Pardthaisong T, Gray RH,** In utero exposure to steroid contraceptives and outcome of pregnancy, *Am J Epidemiol* 134:795, 1991.

131. **Gray RH, Pardthaisong T,** In utero exposure to steroid contraceptives and survival during infancy, *Am J Epidemiol* 134:804, 1991.

132. **Newton JR, d'Arcangues C, Hall PE,** A review of 'once-a-month' combined injectable contraceptives, *J Obstet Gynaecol* 14(Suppl 1):S1, 1994.

133. **WHO Special Programme of Research Development and Research Training in Human Reproduction, Task Force on Long-Acting Systemic Agents for Fertility Regulation,** A multicentered phase III comparative study of two hormonal contraceptive preparations given once-a-month by intramuscular injection, *Contraception* 40:531, 1989.

134. **Cuong DT, Huong M,** Comparative phase III clinical trial of two injectable contraceptive preparations, depot-medroxyprogesterone acetate and Cyclofem in Vietnamese women, *Contraception* 54:169, 1996.

135. **Hall P, Bahamondes L, Diaz J, Petta C,** Introductory study of the once-a-month, injectable contraceptive Cyclofem® in Brazil, Chile, Columbia, and Peru, *Contraception* 56:353, 1997.

136. **Garza-Flores J, Morales del Olmo A, Fuziwara JL, Figueroa JG, Alonso A, Monroy J, Perez M, Urbina-Fuentes M, Guevara SJ, Cedeno E, Barrios R, Ferman JJ, Medina LM, Velezquez E, Perez-Palacios G,** Introduction of Cyclofem® once-a-month injectable contraceptive in Mexico, *Contraception* 58:7, 1998.

137. **Bahamondes L, Marchi NM, Nakagava HM, de Melo MLR, de Lourdes Cristofoletti M, Pellini E, Scozzafave RH, Petta C,** Self-administration with UniJect® of the once-a-month injectable contraceptive Cyclofem®, *Contraception* 56:301, 1997.

138. **Piya-Anant M, Koetsawang S, Patrasupapong N, Dinchuen P, d'Arcangues C, Piaggio G, Pinol A,** Effectiveness of Cyclofem® in the treatment of depot medroxyprogesterone acetate induced amenorrhea, *Contraception* 57:23, 1998.

139. **Kesseru EV, Aydinlik S, Etcheparreborda JJ,** Multicentered, phase III clinical trial of norethisterone enanthate 50 mg plus estradiol valerate 5 mg as a monthly injectable contraceptive; final three-year report, *Contraception* 50:329, 1994.

140. **Sang GW, Shao QX, Ge RS, Chen JK, Song S, Fang KJ, He ML, Luo SY, Chen SF, Chen XB, Li MX, Wu SC, Sun GL, Zhou HE, Zhang SF, Zhu LL, Ye BL, Zhang JH, Ma FL, Jiang BY, Zhou ZQ, Dong QH, Shenm HC, Liu YX, Shao JY, Wang SX, Ming HD, Zhu ZR, Cheng HZ, Chen SH, Yu HY, Zhang ZY, Qing YN, Wang XY, Hall PE, d'Arcangues C, Snow RC,** A multicentred phase III comparative clinical trial of Mesigyna, Cyclofem, and injectable no. 1 given monthly by intramuscular injection to Chinese women. I. Contraceptive efficacy and side effects, *Contraception* 51:167, 1995.

141. **Bahamondes L, Lavín P, Ojeda G, Petta C, Diaz J, Maradiegue E, Monteiro I,** Return of fertility after discontinuation of the once-a-month injectable contraceptive Cyclofem®, *Contraception* 55:307, 1997.

142. **Martínez GH, Castañeda A, Correa JE,** Vaginal bleeding patterns in users of Perlutal®, a once-a-month injectable contraceptive consisting of 10 mg estradiol enanthate combined with 150 mg dihydroxyprogesterone acetophenide. A trial of 5462 woman-months, *Contraception* 58:21, 1998.

143. **Coutinho EM, Spinola P, Barbosa I, Gatto M, Tomaz G, Morais K, Yazlle ME, de Souza RN, Neto JSP, de Barros Leal W, Leal C, Hippolito SB, Abranches AD,** Multicenter, double-blind, comparative clinical study on the efficacy and acceptability of a monthly injectable contraceptive combination of 150 mg dihydroxyprogesterone acetophenide and 10 mg estradiol enanthate compared to a monthly injectable contraceptive combination of 90 mg dihydroxyprogesterone acetophenide and 6 mg estradiol enanthate, *Contraception* 55:175, 1997.

144. **Beck L, Pope V,** Long-acting injectable norethindrone contraceptive system: review of clinical studies, *Res Front Fertil Reg* 3:1, 1984.

145. **Grubb GS, Welch JD, Cole L, Goldsmith A, Rivera R,** A comparative evaluation of the safety and contraceptive effectiveness of 65 mg and 100 mg of 90-day norethindrone (NET) injectable microspheres: a multicenter study, *Fertil Steril* 51:803, 1989.

24 The Intrauterine Device (IUD)

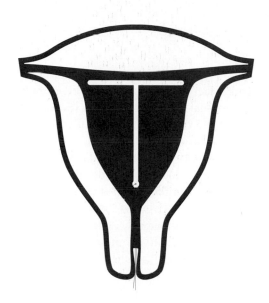

A frequently told, but not well-documented story, assigns the first use of IUDs to caravan drivers who allegedly used intrauterine stones to prevent pregnancies in their camels during long journeys.

The forerunners of the modern IUD were small stem pessaries used in the 1800s, small button-like structures that covered the opening of the cervix and which were attached to stems extending into the cervical canal.[1] It is not certain whether these pessaries were used for contraception, but this seems to have been intended. In 1902, a pessary that extended into the uterus was developed by Hollweg in Germany and used for contraception. This pessary was sold for self-insertion, but the hazard of infection was great, earning the condemnation of the medical community.

In 1909, Richter in Germany, reported success with a silkworm catgut ring having a nickel and bronze wire protruding through the cervix.[2] Shortly after, Pust combined Richter's ring with the old button-type pessary, and replaced the wire with a catgut thread.[3] This IUD was used during World War I in Germany, although the German literature was quick to report infections with its insertion and use. In the 1920s, Gräfenberg removed the tail and pessary because he believed this was the cause of infection. He reported his experience in 1930, using rings made of coiled silver and gold, and then steel.[4]

The Gräfenberg ring was short-lived, falling victim to Nazi political philosophy that was bitterly opposed to contraception. The non-Aryan Gräfenberg was finally sent to jail, but he managed to flee Germany, dying in New York City in 1955. He never received the recognition that was his just due.

The Gräfenberg ring was associated with a high rate of expulsion. This was solved by Ota in Japan who added a supportive structure to the center of his gold or silver plated ring in 1934.[5] Ota also fell victim to World War II politics, being sent into exile, but his ring continued to be used.

The Gräfenberg and Ota rings were essentially forgotten by the rest of the world throughout the World War II period. An awareness of the explosion in population and its impact began to grow in the first two decades after World War II. In 1959, reports from Japan and Israel by Ishihama

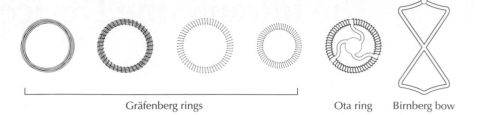

Gräfenberg rings   Ota ring   Birnberg bow

and Oppenheimer once again stirred interest in the rings.[6, 7] The Oppenheimer report was in the American Journal of Obstetrics and Gynecology, and several American gynecologists were stimulated to use rings of silver or silk, and others to develop their own devices.

In the 1960s and 1970s, the IUD thrived. Techniques were modified and a plethora of types introduced. The various devices developed in the 1960s were made of plastic (polyethylene) impregnated with barium sulfate so that they would be visible on an x-ray. The Margulies Coil, developed by Lazer Margulies, in 1960, at Mt. Sinai Hospital in New York City, was the first plastic device with a memory, allowing the use of an inserter and reconfiguration of the shape when it was expelled into the uterus. The Coil was a large device (sure to cause cramping and bleeding), and its hard plastic tail proved risky for the male partner.

In 1962, the Population Council, at the suggestion of Alan Guttmacher, who that year became president of the Planned Parenthood Federation of America, organized the first international conference on IUDs in New York City. It was at this conference that Jack Lippes of Buffalo presented experience with his device, which fortunately as we will see, had a single filament thread as a tail. The Margulies Coil was rapidly replaced by the Lippes Loop, which quickly became the most widely prescribed IUD in the United States in the 1970s.

The 1962 conference also led to the organization of a program established by the Population Council, under the direction of Christopher Tietze, to evaluate IUDs, the Cooperative Statistical Program. The Ninth Progress Report in 1970 was a landmark comparison of efficacy and problems with the various IUDs being used.[8]

Many other devices came along, but, with the exception of the four sizes of Lippes Loops and the two Saf-T-Coils, they had limited use. Stainless steel devices incorporating springs were designed to compress for easy insertion, but the movement of these devices allowed them to embed in the uterus, making them too difficult to remove. The Majzlin Spring is a memorable example.

The Dalkon Shield was introduced in 1970. Within 3 years, a high incidence of pelvic infection was recognized. There is no doubt that the problems with the Dalkon Shield were due to defective construction, pointed out as early as 1975 by Tatum.[9] The multifilamented tail (hundreds of fibers enclosed in a plastic sheath) of the Dalkon Shield provided a pathway for bacteria to ascend protected from the barrier of cervical mucus.

Although sales were discontinued in 1975, a call for removal of all Dalkon Shields was not issued until the early 1980s. The large number of women with pelvic infections led to many lawsuits against the pharmaceutical company, ultimately causing its bankruptcy. Unfortunately, the Dalkon Shield problem tainted all IUDs, and ever since, media and the public in the U.S. have inappropriately regarded all IUDs in a single, generic fashion.

About the time of the introduction of the Dalkon Shield, the U.S. Senate conducted hearings on the safety of oral contraception. Young women who were discouraged from using oral contraceptives following these hearings turned to IUDs, principally the Dalkon Shield, which was promoted as suitable for nulliparous women. Changes in sexual behavior in the 1960s and 1970s, and failure to use protective contraception (condoms and oral contraceptives), led to an epidemic

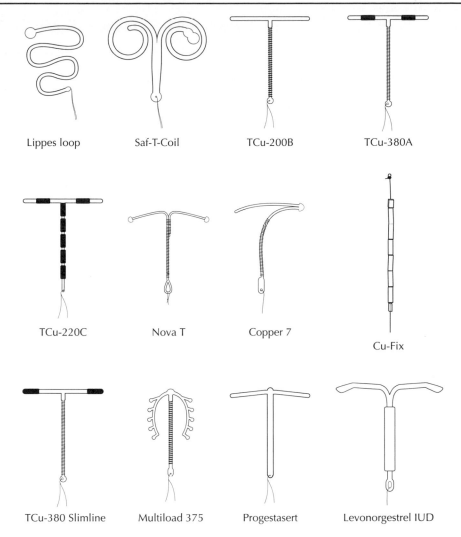

Lippes loop   Saf-T-Coil   TCu-200B   TCu-380A

TCu-220C   Nova T   Copper 7   Cu-Fix

TCu-380 Slimline   Multiload 375   Progestasert   Levonorgestrel IUD

of sexually transmitted diseases (STDs) and pelvic inflammatory disease (PID) for which IUDs were held partially responsible.[10]

The first epidemiologic studies of the relationship between IUDs and PID used as controls women who depended on oral contraception or barrier methods, and who were, therefore, at reduced risk of PID compared with non-contraceptors and IUD users.[11, 12] In addition, these first studies failed to control for the characteristics of sexual behavior that are now accepted as risk factors for PID (multiple partners, early age at first intercourse, and increased frequency of intercourse).[13] The Dalkon Shield magnified the risk attributed to IUDs because its high failure rate in young women who were already at risk of STDs led to septic spontaneous abortions and, in some cases, death.[14] Reports of these events led the American public to regard all IUDs as dangerous, including those that, unlike the Dalkon Shield, had undergone extensive clinical trials and post-marketing surveillance.

The 1980s saw the decline of IUD use in the United States as manufacturers discontinued marketing in response to the burden of litigation. Despite the fact that most of the lawsuits against the copper devices were won by the manufacturer, the cost of the defense combined with declining use affected the financial return. It should be emphasized that this action was the result of corporate business decisions related to concerns for profit and liability, not for medical or scientific reasons. It was not until 1988 that the IUD was returned to the U.S. market. The number of reproductive age women using the intrauterine device decreased by two-thirds from 1982 to 1988, and further decreased in 1995, from 7.1% to 2% to 0.8%, respectively.[15] Nevertheless, in the rest of the world, the IUD is the most widely used method of reversible contraception; currently, over 100 million women use the IUD.

Use of the IUD in the U.S. and the World[15, 16]

	U.S.A.	China	Total World
1981	2.2 million women	42 million	60 million
1988	0.7 million women	59 million	83 million
1995	0.3 million women	75 million	106 million

The reason for the decline in the U.S. was the consumer fear of IUD-related pelvic infection. The final blow to the IUD in the U.S. came in 1985 with the publication of two reports indicating that the use of IUDs was associated with tubal infertility.[17, 18] Later, better controlled studies identified the Dalkon Shield as a high-risk device, and failed to demonstrate an association between PID and other IUDs, except during the period shortly after insertion. Efforts to point out that the situation was different for the copper IUDs, and that, in fact, pelvic inflammatory disease was not increased in women with a single sexual partner,[19] failed to prevent the withdrawal of IUDs from the American market and the negative reaction to IUDs by the American public.

Ironically, the IUD declined in the country that developed the modern IUD. It is time for a revival!

The Modern IUD

The addition of copper to the IUD was suggested by Jaime Zipper of Chile, whose experiments with metals indicated that copper acted locally on the endometrium.[20] Howard Tatum combined Zipper's suggestion with the development of the T-shape to diminish the uterine reaction to the structural frame, and produced the copper-T. The first copper IUD had copper wire wound around the straight shaft of the T, the TCu-200 (200 mm^2 of exposed copper wire), also known as the Tatum-T.[21] Tatum's reasoning was that the T-shape would conform to the shape of the uterus in contrast to the other IUDs that required the uterus to conform to their shape. Furthermore, the copper IUDs could be much smaller than those of simple, inert plastic devices and still provide effective contraception. Studies indicate that copper exerts its effect before implantation of a fertilized ovum; it may be spermicidal, or it may diminish sperm motility or fertilizing capacity. The addition of copper to the IUD and reduction in the size and structure of the frame improved tolerance, resulting in fewer removals for pain and bleeding.

The Cu-7 with a copper wound stem was developed in 1971 and quickly became the most popular device in the U.S. Both the Cu-7 and the Tatum-T were withdrawn from the U.S. market in 1986 by G. D. Searle and Company.

IUD development continued, however. More copper was added by Population Council investigators, leading to the TCu-380A (380 mm^2 of exposed copper surface area) with copper wound around the stem plus a copper sleeve on each horizontal arm).[22] The "A" in TCu-380A is for arms, indicating the importance of the copper sleeves. Making the copper solid and tubular increased effectiveness and the lifespan of the IUD. The TCu-380A has been in use in more than 30 countries since 1982, and in 1988, it was marketed in the U.S. as the "ParaGard."

The "Progestasert" was developed by the Alza Corporation at the same time that the copper IUDs were developed. This T-shaped device releases 65 µg of progesterone per day for at least one year. The progesterone diminishes the amount of cramping and the amount of blood loss; thus, it is especially useful for women who have heavy periods and cramping. The short lifespan can be and has been solved by using a more potent progestin, such as levonorgestrel.

Efforts continue to develop IUDs that address the main problems of bleeding and cramping. The IUDs of the future will possibly be medicated and frameless.

Types of IUDs

Unmedicated IUDs

The Lippes Loop, made of plastic (polyethylene) impregnated with barium sulfate, is still used throughout the world (except in the U.S.). Flexible stainless steel rings are widely used in China, but not elsewhere.[23]

Copper IUDs

The first copper IUDs were wound with 200 to 250 mm^2 of wire, and two of these are still available (except in the U.S.), the TCu-200 and the Multiload-250. The more modern copper IUDs contain more copper, and part of the copper is in the form of solid tubular sleeves, rather than wire, increasing efficacy and extending lifespan. This group of IUDs is represented in the U.S. by the TCu-380A (the ParaGard), and in the rest of the world, by the TCu-220C, the Nova T, and the Multiload-375. The modern generation of IUDs in China includes a stainless steel ring with copper wire that also releases indomethacin (very effective with a low expulsion rate and less blood loss), a V-shaped copper IUD, and a copper IUD shaped like the uterine cavity.[23] The Sof-T is a copper IUD used only in Switzerland.

The TCu-380A is a T-shaped device with a polyethylene frame holding 380 mm^2 of exposed surface area of copper. The pure electrolytic copper wire wound around the 36 mm stem weighs 176 mg, and copper sleeves on the horizontal arms weigh 66.5 mg. A polyethylene monofilament is tied through the 3 mm ball on the stem, providing two white threads for detection and removal. The ball at the bottom of the stem helps reduce the risk of cervical perforation. The IUD frame contains barium sulfate, making it radiopaque. The TCu-380Ag is identical to the TCu-380A, but the copper wire on the stem has a silver core to prevent fragmentation and extend the lifespan of the copper. The TCu-380 Slimline has the copper sleeves flush at the ends of the horizontal arms to facilitate easier loading and insertion. The performance of the TCu-380Ag and the TCu-380 Slimline is equal to that of the TCu-380A.[24, 25]

The Multiload-375 has 375 mm^2 of copper wire wound around its stem. The flexible arms were designed to minimize expulsions. This is a popular device in many parts of the world. The Multiload-375 and the TCu-380A are similar in their efficacy and performance.[26]

The Nova T is similar to the TCu-200, containing 200 mm^2 of copper; however, the Nova T has a silver core to the copper wire, flexible arms, and a large, flexible loop at the bottom to avoid injury to cervical tissue. There was some concern that the efficacy of the Nova T decreased after 3 years in WHO data; however, results from Finland and Scandinavia indicate low and stable pregnancy rates over 5 years of use.[26]

Hormone-Releasing IUDs

The Progestasert is a T-shaped IUD made of ethylene/vinyl acetate copolymer containing titanium dioxide. The vertical stem contains a reservoir of 38 mg progesterone together with barium sulfate dispersed in silicone fluid. The horizontal arms are solid and made of the same copolymer. Two blue-black, monofiliment strings are attached at a hole in the base of the stem. Progesterone is released at a rate of 65 µg per day.

The LNG-20, manufactured by Leiras in Finland, releases *in vitro* 20 µg of levonorgestrel per day.[27] This T-shaped device has a collar attached to the vertical arm, which contains 52 mg levonorgestrel dispersed in polydimethylsiloxane and released at a rate of 15 µg per day *in vivo*.

The levonorgestrel IUD lasts up to 10 years and reduces menstrual blood loss and pelvic infection rates.[28–30]

Future IUDs

Modifications of the copper IUD are being studied throughout the world. The Ombrelle-250 and Ombrelle-380, designed to be more flexible in order to reduce expulsion and side effects, have been marketed in France. A frameless IUD, the FlexiGard (also known as the Cu-Fix or the GyneFix), consists of 6 copper sleeves (330 mm^2 of copper) strung on a surgical nylon (polypropylene) thread that is knotted at one end. The knot is pushed into the myometrium during insertion with a notched needle that works like a miniature harpoon. Because it is frameless, it has a low rate of removal for bleeding or pain, but a more difficult insertion may yield a higher expulsion rate.[31, 32] However, when inserted by experienced clinicians, the expulsion rate is very low, and the device is especially suited for nulligravid and nulliparous women.[33]

Mechanism of Action

The contraceptive action of all IUDs is mainly in the uterine cavity. Ovulation is not affected, nor is the IUD an abortifacient.[34, 35] It is currently believed that the mechanism of action for IUDs is the production of an intrauterine environment that is spermicidal.

Nonmedicated IUDs depend for contraception on the general reaction of the uterus to a foreign body. It is believed that this reaction, a sterile inflammatory response, produces tissue injury of a minor degree, but sufficient enough to be spermicidal. Very few, if any, sperm reach the ovum in the fallopian tube. Normally cleaving, fertilized ova cannot be obtained by tubal flushing in women with IUDs in contrast to noncontraceptors, indicating the failure of sperm to reach the ovum, and thus fertilization does not occur.[36] If this action should fail, the inflammatory response would also prevent implantation. In women using copper IUDs, sensitive assays for human chorionic gonadotropin (HCG) do not find evidence of fertilization.[37, 38] This is consistent with the fact that the copper IUD protects against both intrauterine and ectopic pregnancies (see below).

The copper IUD releases free copper and copper salts that have both a biochemical and morphological impact on the endometrium, and also produce alterations in cervical mucus and endometrial secretions. There is no measurable increase in the serum copper level. Copper has many specific actions, including the enhancement of prostaglandin production and the inhibition of various endometrial enzymes. The copper IUD is associated with an enhanced inflammatory response, marked by production in the endometrium of cytokine peptides known to be cytotoxic.[39] An additional spermicidal effect probably takes place in the cervical mucus.

The progestin-releasing IUDs add the endometrial action of the progestin to the foreign body reaction. The endometrium becomes decidualized with atrophy of the glands. The progesterone IUD (serum progesterone levels are not increased) probably has two mechanisms of action: inhibition of implantation and inhibition of sperm capacitation and survival. The levonorgestrel IUD produces serum concentrations of the progestin about half those of Norplant so that ovarian follicular development and ovulation are also partially inhibited; after the first year, cycles are ovulatory in 85% of women, regardless of their bleeding patterns.[40] Finally, the progestin IUDs thicken the cervical mucus, creating a barrier to sperm penetration. The progestin IUDs decrease menstrual blood loss (about 40–50%) and dysmenorrhea; with the levonorgestrel IUD, bleeding can be reduced by 90% one year after insertion.[41] Average hemoglobin and iron levels increase over time compared with preinsertion values.

Following removal of IUDs, the normal intrauterine environment is rapidly restored. *In large studies, there is no delay, regardless of duration of use, in achieving pregnancy at normal rates, which belies the assertion that IUD use is associated with infection leading to infertility.*[42–45] There has been no significant difference in cumulative pregnancy rates between parous and nulliparous or nulligravid women.[44, 45]

Efficacy of IUDs

Intrauterine Pregnancy

The TCu-380A is approved for use in the United States for 10 years. However, the TCu 380A has been demonstrated to maintain its efficacy over at least 12 years of use.[46] The TCu-200 is approved for 4 years and the Nova T for 5 years. The progesterone-releasing IUD must be replaced every year because the reservoir of progesterone is depleted in 12–18 months. The levonorgestrel IUD can be used for at least 7 years, and probably 10.[26] The progesterone IUD has a slightly higher failure rate, but the levonorgestrel device that releases 15–20 mg levonorgestrel per day is as effective as the new copper IUDs.[25, 28, 47, 48]

The nonmedicated IUDs never have to be replaced. The deposition of calcium salts on the IUD can produce a structure that is irritating to the endometrium. If bleeding increases after a nonmedicated IUD has been in place for some time, it is worth replacing it. Some clinicians (as do we) recommend replacing all older IUDs with the new, more effective copper IUDs.

First Year Clinical Trial Experience in Parous Women[49]

Device	Pregnancy Rate	Expulsion Rate	Removal Rate
Lippes Loop	3%	12–20%	12–15%
Cu–7	2–3	6	11
TCu–200	3	8	11
TCu–380A	0.5–0.8	5	14
Progesterone IUD	1.3–1.6	2.7	9.3
Levonorgestrel IUD	0.2	6	17

Considering all IUDS together, the actual use failure rate in the first year is approximately 3%, with a 10% expulsion rate, and a 15% rate of removal, mainly for bleeding and pain. With increasing duration of use and increasing age, the failure rate decreases, as do removals for pain and bleeding. The performance of the TCu-380A in recent years, however, has proved to be superior.

Ten-Year Experience with Paragard, TCu-380A
Rate per 100 users per year

| | Year | | | | | | | | | |
	1	2	3	4	5	6	7	8	9	10
Pregnancy	0.7	0.3	0.6	0.2	0.3	0.2	0.0	0.4	0.0	0.0
Expulsion	5.7	2.5	1.6	1.2	0.3	0.0	0.6	1.7	0.2	0.4
Bleeding/pain removal	11.9	9.8	7.0	3.5	3.7	2.7	3.0	2.5	2.2	3.7
Medical removals	2.5	2.1	1.6	1.7	0.1	0.3	1.0	0.4	0.7	0.3
Continuation	76.8	78.3	81.2	86.2	89.0	91.9	87.9	88.1	92.0	91.8
Number starting each year	4,932	3,149	2,018	1,121	872	621	563	483	423	325

Data from Population Council (n = 3,536) and WHO (n = 1,396) trials.

In careful studies, with attention to technique and participation by motivated patients, the failure rate with the TCu-380A and the other newer copper IUDs is less than one per 100 women per year.[26, 49, 50] The cumulative net pregnancy rate after 7 years of use is 1.5 per 100 woman-years, and after 12 years, only 1.9 per 100 women (not a single pregnancy was reported after 8 years of use).[46, 51] In developing countries, the failure rate with IUDs is less than that with oral contraception.[52] Failure rates are slightly higher in younger (less than age 25), more fertile women.

Women use IUDs longer than other reversible methods of contraception. The IUD continuation rate is higher than that with oral contraception, condoms, or diaphragms. This may reflect the circumstances surrounding the choice of an IUD (older, parous women).

Expulsion

Approximately 5% of patients spontaneously expel the TCu-380A within the first year. This event can be associated with cramping, vaginal discharge, or uterine bleeding. However, in some cases, the only observable change is lengthening or absence of the IUD strings. Patients should be cautioned to request immediate attention if expulsion is suspected. A partially expelled IUD should be removed. If pregnancy or infection is not present, a new IUD can be inserted immediately (in this instance, antibiotic prophylaxis is recommended).

Ectopic Pregnancy

The previous use of an IUD does not increase the risk of a subsequent ectopic pregnancy.[45, 53, 54] The current use of an IUD, other than the progesterone-releasing device, offers some protection against ectopic pregnancy.[53-58] The largest study, a WHO multicenter study, concluded that IUD users were 50% less likely to have an ectopic pregnancy when compared with women using no contraception.[53] This protection is not as great as that achieved by inhibition of ovulation with oral contraception. Therefore, when an IUD user becomes pregnant, the pregnancy is more likely to be ectopic. However, the actual occurrence of an ectopic pregnancy in an IUD user is a rare event.

The lowest ectopic pregnancy rates are seen with the most effective IUDs, like the TCu-380A (90% less likely compared with noncontraceptors).[59] The rate is about one-tenth the ectopic pregnancy rate associated with the Lippes Loop or with devices with less copper such as the TCu-200.[59] The progesterone-releasing IUD has a higher rate, probably because its action is limited to a local effect on the endometrium,[56] while very few ectopic pregnancies have been reported with the levonorgestrel IUD, presumably because it is associated with a partial suppression of gonadotropins with subsequent disruption of normal follicular growth and development, and, in a significant number of cycles, inhibition of ovulation.[25, 30, 48, 59, 60]

The risk of ectopic pregnancy does not increase with increasing duration of use with the TCu-380A or the levonorgestrel IUD.[25, 51] In a 7-year prospective study, not a single ectopic pregnancy was encountered with the levonorgestrel IUD.[25] In 8000 woman-years of experience in randomized multicenter trials, there has been only a single ectopic pregnancy reported with the TCu-380A (which is one-tenth the rate with the Lippes Loop or TCu-200).[25]

The protection against ectopic pregnancy provided by the TCu-380A and the levonorgestrel IUD makes these IUDs acceptable choices for contraception in women with previous ectopic pregnancies.

Ectopic Pregnancy Rates per 1000 Woman-Years [59, 61]

Non-contraceptive users, all ages	3.00–4.50
Progesterone IUD (based on small numbers, thus probably the same as non-contraceptive users)	6.80
Levonorgestrel IUD	0.20
TCu-380A IUD	0.20

Side Effects

With effective patient screening and good insertion technique, the copper and medicated IUDs are not associated with an increased risk of infertility after their removal. Even if IUDs are removed for problems, subsequent fertility rates are normal.[44, 45, 48]

The symptoms most often responsible for IUD discontinuation are increased uterine bleeding and increased menstrual pain. Within one year, 5–15% of women discontinue IUD use because of these problems. Smaller copper and progestin IUDs have reduced the incidence of pain and bleeding considerably, but a careful menstrual history is still important in helping a woman consider an IUD. Women with prolonged, heavy menstrual bleeding or significant dysmenorrhea may not be able to tolerate copper IUDs but may benefit from a progestin IUD.[41] Because bleeding and cramping are most severe in the first few months after IUD insertion, treatment with a nonsteroidal anti-inflammatory (NSAID) agent (an inhibitor of prostaglandin synthesis) during the first several menstrual periods can reduce bleeding and cramping and help a patient through this difficult time. Even persistent heavy menses can be effectively treated with NSAIDs.[62] NSAID treatment should begin at the onset of menses and be maintained for 3 days. A copper IUD is available in China that also releases a small amount of indomethacin; this device is associated with markedly less bleeding.[63]

It is not unusual to have a few days of intermenstrual spotting or light bleeding. Although aggravating, this does not cause significant blood loss. Such bleeding deserves the usual evaluation for cervical or endometrial pathology. These changes can be objectionable for women who are prevented from having intercourse while bleeding.

Following insertion of a modern copper IUD, menstrual blood loss increases by about 55%, and this level of bleeding continues for the duration of IUD use.[64] This is associated with a slight (1–2 day) prolongation of menstruation. Over a year's time, this amount of blood loss does not result in changes (e.g., serum ferritin) indicative of iron deficiency. Assessment for iron depletion and anemia should be considered, however, in long-term users and in women susceptible to iron deficiency anemia.

Because of a decidualizing, atrophic impact on the endometrium, amenorrhea can develop over time with the progestin-containing IUDs. With the levonorgestrel IUD, 70% of patients are oligomenorrheic and 30% amenorrheic within 2 years. For some women, the lack of periods is so disconcerting that they request removal. On the other hand, this effect on menstruation is manifested by an increase in blood hemoglobin levels.[25, 49] Sufficient progestin reaches the systemic circulation from the levonorgestrel-containing IUD so that androgenic side effects, such as acne and hirsutism, can occur. More extensive clinical studies are needed to assess the impact of this IUD on the lipoprotein profile; however, it is unlikely that the low dose of levonorgestrel has an important effect on cardiovascular risk.

Some women report an increased vaginal discharge while wearing an IUD. This complaint deserves examination for the presence of vaginal or cervical infection. Treatment can be provided with the IUD remaining in place.

Long-term use of the IUD is associated with impressive safety and lack of side effects. In a 7-year prospective study, the use of either the copper IUD or the levonorgestrel IUD beyond 5 years led to no increase in pelvic infection, no increase in ectopic pregnancy rates, no increase in anemia, and no increase in abnormal Pap smears.[25] Duration of use does not affect pregnancy rates or outcome.

The presence of copper may yield some benefits. There are epidemiologic data indicating that both the copper IUD and the inert IUD reduce the risks of endometrial cancer and invasive cervical cancer.[65–69] Presumably, this protective effect is due to induced biochemical alterations that affect cellular responses.

The copper IUD is not affected by magnetic resonance imaging, and therefore, the copper IUD need not be removed prior to MRI, and neither patients nor workers need be excluded from MRIs or the MRI environment.[70, 71]

Infections

IUD-related bacterial infection is now believed to be due to contamination of the endometrial cavity at the time of insertion. Mishell's classic study indicated that the uterus is routinely contaminated by bacteria at insertion.[72] Infections that occur 3–4 months after insertion are believed to be due to acquired STDs, not the direct result of the IUD. The early, insertion-related infections, therefore, are polymicrobial, derived from the endogenous cervicovaginal flora, with a predominance of anaerobes.

A review of the World Health Organization data base derived from all of the WHO IUD clinical trials concluded that the risk of pelvic inflammatory disease was 6 times higher during the 20 days after the insertion compared with later times during follow-up, but, most importantly, PID was extremely rare beyond the first 20 days after insertion.[73] In nearly 23,000 insertions, however, only 81 cases of PID were diagnosed, and a scarcity of PID was observed in those situations where STDs are rare. There was no statistically significant difference comparing the copper IUD to the inert Lippes Loop or progestin-containing IUDs. These data confirm earlier studies that the risk of infection is highest immediately after insertion and that PID risk does not increase with long-term use.[14, 19] The problem of infection can be minimized with careful screening and the use of aseptic technique. Even women with insulin-dependent diabetes mellitus do not have an increased risk for infection.[74, 75]

Doxycycline (200 mg) or azithromycin (500 mg) administered orally one hour prior to insertion can provide protection against insertion-associated pelvic infection, but prophylactic antibiotics are probably of little benefit for women at low risk for STDs.

Compared with oral contraception, barrier methods, and hormonal IUDs, there is no reason to think that nonmedicated or copper IUDs can confer protection against STDs.[76] However, the levonorgestrel-releasing IUD has been reported to be associated with a protective effect against pelvic infection, and the copper IUD is associated with lower titers of anti-chlamydial antibody.[29, 77] In vitro, copper inhibits chlamydial growth in endometrial cells.[78] Thus, the association between IUD use and pelvic infection (and infertility) is now seriously questioned.[79] Women who use IUDs must be counseled to use condoms along with the IUD whenever they have intercourse with a partner who could be an STD carrier. Because sexual behavior is the most important modifier of the risk of infection, clinicians should ask prospective IUD users about numbers of partners, their partner's sexual practices, the frequency and age of onset of intercourse, and history of STDs.[80] Women at low risk are unlikely to have pelvic infections while using IUDs.[19]

It is not certain that the IUD is inappropriate for women who are at increased risk of bacterial endocarditis (previous endocarditis, rheumatic heart disease, or the presence of prosthetic heart valves). The bacteriologic contamination of the uterine cavity at insertion is short-lived.[72] Three studies have attempted to document bacteremia during IUD insertion or removal.[81–83] Only one of the three could find blood culture evidence of bacteremia, and it was present transiently in only a few patients.[83] In our view, the IUD is acceptable for patients at risk of bacterial endocarditis, *but antibiotic prophylaxis (amoxicillin 2 g) should be provided one hour before insertion or removal.*

Asymptomatic IUD users whose cervical cultures show gonorrheal or chlamydia infection should be treated with the recommended drugs without removal of the IUD. If, however, there is evidence that an infection has ascended to the endometrium or fallopian tubes, treatment must be instituted and the IUD removed promptly. Vaginal bacteriosis should be treated (metronidazole, 500 mg bid for 7 days), but the IUD need not be removed unless pelvic inflammation is present. There is no evidence that the prevalence of bacterial vaginosis is influenced by IUD use.[84]

For simple endometritis, in which uterine tenderness is the only physical finding, doxycycline (100 mg bid for 14 days) is adequate. If tubal infection is present, as evidenced by cervical motion tenderness, abdominal rebound tenderness, adnexal tenderness or masses, or elevated white blood count and sedimentation rate, parenteral treatment is indicated with removal of the IUD as soon as antibiotic serum levels are adequate. The previous presence of an IUD does not alter the treatment of PID. IUD-associated pelvic infection is more likely to be caused by non-STD organisms.[85]

Appropriate outpatient management of less severe infections:
Cefoxitin (2 g IM) plus probenecid (1 g orally), or
Ceftriaxone (250 mg IM) plus doxycycline (100 mg bid orally), for 14 days.

Severe infections require hospitalization and treatment with:
Cefoxitin (2 g IV q 6 h), or
Cefotetan (2 g IV q 12 h)
Plus doxycycline (100 mg bid orally or IV)
Followed by 14 days of an oral regimen of antibiotics.

The following is an alternative regimen:
Clindamycin (900 mg IV q 8 h), plus
Gentamicin (2 mg/kg IV or IM followed by 1.5 mg/kg q 8 h).

There is a suggestion (in cross-sectional studies) that IUD use increases the risk of HIV transmission from man to woman, especially when the IUD is inserted or removed during exposure to the infected man.[86, 87] However, this is not a strong suggestion, because the risk with IUD use was ascertained compared with other contraceptive methods (which can protect against transmission), and the many and various influencing factors are difficult to adjust and control. In the only longitudinal study, no association was observed between IUD use and HIV acquisition by women.[88] In the only study reported, no evidence for female-to-male HIV transmission with IUD use was detected.[89] HIV-infected women who utilize IUDs for contraception *do not* have a greater incidence of complications (including pelvic inflammatory disease).[90]

Actinomyces

The significance of actinomycosis infection in IUD users is unclear. There are several reports of IUD users with unilateral pelvic abscesses containing *Actinomyces*.[91, 92] However, *Actinomyces* are found in Pap smears of up to 30% of plastic IUD wearers when cytologists take special care to look for the organisms. The rate is much lower (less than 1%) with copper devices and varies with duration of use.[91–94] Furthermore, *actinomyces* are commonly present in the normal vagina.[95] The clinician must decide whether to remove the IUD and treat the patient, treat with the IUD in place, or simply remove the IUD. These patients are almost always asymptomatic and without clinical signs of infection. If uterine tenderness or a pelvic mass is present, the IUD should always be removed after the initiation of treatment with oral penicillin G, 500 mg qid that should continue for a month. If *Actinomyces* are present on the Pap smear of an asymptomatic well woman, in our view, it is not necessary to administer antibiotic treatment or to remove the IUD. Although it has been recommended that the IUD should be removed in this instance and replaced when a repeat Pap smear is negative, there is no evidence to support this recommendation. Another anarobic, gram-positive rod, *Eubacterium nodatum*, resembles *Actinomyces* and has also been reported to be associated with colonization of an IUD.[96] *E. nodatum* can be mistaken for *Actinomyces* on Pap smears. Our recommendations can be applied to both *E. nodatum* and *Actinomyces*.

Pregnancy With an IUD In Situ

Spontaneous Miscarriage

Spontaneous miscarriage occurs more frequently among women who become pregnant with IUDs in place, a rate of approximately 40–50%. Because of this high rate of spontaneous miscarriage, IUDs should always be removed if pregnancy is diagnosed and the string is visible. Use of instruments inside the uterus should be avoided if the pregnancy is desired, unless sonographic guidance can help avoid rupture of the membranes.[97] After removal of an IUD with visible strings, the spontaneous miscarriage rate is approximately 30%.[98, 99] Combining ultrasonography guidance with carbon dioxide hysteroscopy, an IUD with a missing tail can be identified and removed during early pregnancy.[100] *If the IUD is easily removed without trauma or expelled during the first trimester, the risk of spontaneous miscarriage is not increased.*[101, 102]

Septic Abortion

In the past, if the IUD could not be easily removed from a pregnant uterus, the patient was offered induced abortion because it was believed that the risk of life-threatening septic, spontaneous miscarriage in the second trimester was increased 20-fold if the pregnancy continued with the IUD in utero. However, this belief was derived from experiences with the Dalkon Shield. There is no evidence that there is an increased risk of septic abortion if pregnancy occurs with an IUD in place other than the Shield.[102, 103] There have been no deaths in the United States since 1977 among women pregnant with an IUD.[104]

If a patient plans to terminate a pregnancy that has occurred with an IUD in place, the IUD should be removed immediately. If there is no evidence of infection, the IUD can safely be removed in a clinic or office.

If an IUD is in an infected, pregnant uterus, removal of the device should be undertaken only after antibiotic therapy has been initiated, and equipment for cardiovascular support and resuscitation is immediately available. These precautions are necessary because removal of an IUD from an infected, pregnant uterus can lead to septic shock.

Congenital Anomalies

There is no evidence that exposure of a fetus to medicated IUDs is harmful. The risk of congenital anomalies is not increased among infants born to women who become pregnant with an IUD in place.[102, 105] A case-control study did not find an increased incidence of IUD use in pregnancies resulting in limb reduction deformities.[106]

Preterm Labor and Birth

The incidence of preterm labor and delivery is increased approximately 4-fold when an IUD is left in place during pregnancy.[102, 107–109]

Other Complications

Obstetrical complications at delivery (such as hemorrhage, stillbirth, and difficulties wth placenta removal) have been reported only with the Dalkon Shield in situ.

IUD Insertion

Patient Selection

Patient selection for successful IUD use requires attention to menstrual history and the risk for STDs. Age and parity are not the critical factors in selection; the risk factors for STDs are the most important consideration. Women who have multiple sexual partners, whose partners have multiple partners, who are drug or alcohol dependent, and who are not in a stable sexual relationship are at greater risk of pelvic infection at the time of IUD insertion and at greater risk of acquiring a sexually transmitted disease after IUD insertion.[17–19] It would be appropriate for these women to use condoms for STD protection and an IUD for effective contraception. Current, recent, or recurrent PID is a contraindication for IUD use. Hormonal and barrier methods are better choices for these women. Nulliparous and nulligravid women can safely use the IUD if both sexual partners are monogamous. In a national U.S. survey, only 13% of adults had more than one sexual partner in the previous year.[110] Most women are good candidates for the IUD.

Patients with heavy menstrual periods should be cautioned regarding the increase in menstrual bleeding associated with the copper IUD. Women who are anticoagulated or have a bleeding disorder are obviously not good candidates for the copper IUD, but might benefit from a progestin IUD.

There are other conditions that can compromise success. Women who have abnormalities of uterine anatomy (bicornuate uterus, submucous myoma, cervical stenosis) may not accommodate an IUD. The IUD is not a good choice when the uterine cavity is distorted by leiomyomata. According to conventional wisdom, the few individuals who have allergies to copper or have Wilson's disease (a prevalence of about 1 in 200,000) should not use copper IUDs; however, no cases of difficulty have ever been recorded and it is doubtful, considering the low exposure to copper, that there would be a problem. The amount of copper released into the circulation per day is less than that consumed in a normal diet.[111]

Immunosuppressed patients should not use IUDs. Patients at risk for endocarditis should be treated with prophylactic antibiotics at insertion and removal. In our view, cervical dysplasia does not preclude IUD insertion or continued use.

Because many older women have diabetes mellitus, it is worth emphasizing that no increase in adverse events has been observed with copper IUD use in women with either insulin-dependent or noninsulin-dependent diabetes.[74, 75, 112] Indeed, the IUD can be an ideal choice for a woman with diabetes, especially if vascular disease is present.

The IUD should not be dismissed just because the patient is an adolescent. Although the clinical performance of the IUD in a study of parous adolescents was not as good as in older women, it was still similar or slightly better than other reversible methods used by adolescents.[113] Given appropriate screening, counseling, and care, the IUD can provide long-term effective contraception for adolescents.

A careful speculum and bimanual examination is essential prior to IUD insertion. It is important to know the position of the uterus; undetected extreme posterior uterine position is the most common reason for perforation at the time of IUD insertion. However, perforation is rare; the incidence is estimated to be less than 1 per 3000 insertions.[114] A very small or large uterus, determined by examination and sounding, can preclude insertion. For successful IUD use, the uterus should preferably not sound less than 6 cm or more than 9 cm.

Preferably, the absence of cervical or vaginal infection should be established before insertion. If this is not feasible, insertion should definitely be delayed if a mucopurulent discharge of the cervix or a significant vaginitis (including vaginal bacteriosis) is present.

Key Points in Patient Counseling

Prospective IUD users should be aware of the following important possibilities:

1. Protection against unwanted pregnancy begins immediately after insertion.

2. Menses can be longer and heavier (except with hormonal IUDs); tampons can be used.

3. There is a slightly increased risk of pelvic infection in the first few months after insertion.

4. Protection against infections transmitted through the vaginal mucosa requires the use of condoms.

5. Ectopic pregnancies can still occur.

6. The IUD can be spontaneously expelled; monthly palpation of the IUD strings is important to avoid unwanted pregnancies. If the strings are not felt or something hard is palpable (suggestive of the IUD frame), a clinician should be notified as soon as possible. Backup contraception should be provided until the patient can be examined.

Timing

An IUD can be safely inserted at any time after delivery, spontaneous miscarriage or induced abortion, or during the menstrual cycle. Expulsion rates were higher when the older, large plastic IUDs were inserted sooner than 8 weeks postpartum, however studies indicate that the copper IUDs can be inserted between 4 and 8 weeks postpartum without an increase in pregnancy rates, expulsion, uterine perforation, or removals for bleeding and/or pain.[115, 116] Insertion can even occur immediately after a vaginal delivery; it is not associated with an increased risk of infection, uterine perforation, postpartum bleeding, or uterine subinvolution.[117] Postvaginal delivery insertion is not recommended if intrauterine infection is present, and a slightly higher expulsion rate is to be expected compared with insertion 4–8 weeks postpartum. The IUD can also be inserted at cesarean section; the expulsion rate is slightly lower than that with insertion immediately after vaginal delivery.[118]

Insertion of an IUD in breastfeeding women is relatively easier, and is associated with a lower removal rate for bleeding or pain.[117] Reports disagree whether perforation is more common in lactating women.[117, 119, 120]

An IUD can be inserted immediately after a first-trimester abortion, but after a second-trimester abortion, it is recommended to wait until uterine involution occurs.[121, 122]

Insertions can be more difficult if the cervix is closed between menses. The advantages of insertion during or shortly after a menstrual period include a more open cervical canal, the masking of insertion-related bleeding, and the knowledge that the patient is not pregnant. These relative advantages may be outweighed by the risk of unintended pregnancy if insertion is delayed to await menstrual bleeding. In addition, there is evidence that the expulsion rate and termination rates for pain, bleeding, and pregnancy are lower if insertions are performed after day 11 of the menstrual cycle, and the infection rate may be lower with insertions after the 17th cycle day.[123]

Technique for the TCu-380A and the Progestasert

Inserting an IUD requires only a few minutes, has few complications, and is rarely painful, but preoperative examination, medication, and the right equipment will ensure a good experience for your patient. After introducing a vaginal spectrum, the cervix is cleaned with chlorhexadine or povidone-iodine. Leave the antiseptic-soaked cotton-tipped applicator in the cervical canal during the procedures prior to insertion of the IUD. Place a paracervical block by injecting one mL of local anesthetic (1% chloroprocaine) into the cervical lip (anterior if the uterus is anterior in the pelvis and posterior if it lies posteriorly). Inclusion of atropine, 0.4 mg, in the anesthetic will reduce the incidence of vasovagal reactions. After one minute, grasp the cervical lip with the tenaculum ratcheting it only to the first position in a slow, deliberate fashion. Use the tenaculum to move the cervix to the patient's right, revealing the left lateral vaginal fornix. Place the needle tip in the cervical mucosa at 3 o'clock, 1–2 cm lateral to the cervical os, advance it about 1.5 inches (4 cm) under the mucosa and inject about 4 mL of anesthetic, leaving an additional 1 mL behind under the mucosa as the needle is withdrawn. Now deflect the cervix to the patient's left and inject local anesthetic at 9 o'clock in similar fashion. *Wait 2–3 minutes before proceeding.* A very common mistake is to not allow sufficient time for anesthetic action.

Many women can tolerate IUD insertion, especially at the time of menses, without a paracervical block. For some women, however, insertion is less painful with local anesthetic and with administration of a nonsteroidal anti-inflammatory agent 30 minutes to one hour prior to the procedure. If a paracervical block is not used, having the patient cough just as the tenaculum is applied reduces pain and the chance of a vasovagal reaction.

Sound and measure the depth of the uterus (the insertion tube can be used for this purpose). The IUD is loaded into its insertion tube immediately prior to insertion. The arms of the TCu 380A must be folded manually, either with sterile gloves or through the sterile wrapper, and maneuvered into the end of the insertion tube, just enough to hold them in place during insertion. The insertion tube is advanced into the uterus to the correct depth as marked on the tube either by a sliding plastic flange (TCu-380A) or printed gradations (Progestasert). The flange should be twisted to be in the same plane as the horizontal arms. When the insertion tube and IUD reach the fundus, withdraw a few mm. Check to make sure that the transverse arm of the IUD is in the horizontal plane so that the tips of the T will rest in the cornual regions of the endometrial cavity. Placement in the vertical plane increases the risk of expulsion and pregnancy.[124] To release the Progestasert, remove the thread-retaining plug, and withdraw the insertor tube. To release the TCu-380A, advance the solid rod until the resistance of the IUD is felt, fix the rod against the tenaculum which is held in traction, and withdraw the insertion tube while the solid insertion rod is held against the stem of the T, releasing the transverse arms into high fundal position. Remove the solid rod and finally the inserter tube taking care not to pull on the strings. You can ensure that the TCu-380A is in a high fundal position if, after removing the solid rod, you push the insertor tube up against the cross arm of the T prior to withdrawing it completely from the cavity. Trim the strings to about 4 cm from the external os, and record their length in the chart. Shorter strings can cause unpleasant bristle-like sensations. With the Progestasert, the shorter string verifies correct placement; the longer thread should be trimmed.

Patients with newly inserted IUDs should attempt to feel the strings before they leave the examining room. Giving them the cut ends of the strings as a sample of what to feel is helpful. Palpation should be performed monthly by the patient to verify continuing presence of the IUD after each menstrual flow. Patients should return within 3 months, preferably after the first menses, to confirm the presence of the IUD and to provide support, because bleeding changes and expulsion are most likely to occur during this time. Caution the patient that the first 2 menses are typically heavier. As with all office procedures, patients should be provided a 24-hour phone number for urgent questions or concerns, and especially to report unusual pain, bleeding, or vaginal discharge.

Prophylactic Antibiotics

Doxycycline (200 mg) administered orally one hour prior to insertion can provide protection against insertion-associated pelvic infection, but three double-blind randomized studies, two conducted in Africa and one in Turkey, found no significant advantage in the treated groups.[125–127] Azithromycin in a dose of 500 mg has also been used prophylactically, presumably offering more protection because of a longer half-life.[128] However, a randomized trial in low-risk women could find no effect on the subsequent rate of IUD removal or morbidity when 500 mg azithromycin was administered 1 hour before IUD insertion.[129] In women at low risk for STDs, the incidence of infection is so low that there is little benefit to be expected with prophylactic antibiotics.

Summary: IUD Use and Medical Conditions

1. A woman with a previous ectopic pregnancy can use a copper IUD or the levonorgestrel IUD.

2. Women with heavy menses and dysmenorrhea, including women who have a bleeding disorder or are anticoagulated, should consider a progestin-releasing IUD.

3. Women at risk for bacterial endocarditis should receive prophylactic antibiotics at insertion and removal.

4. Current, recent, or recurrent PID is a contraindication for IUD use.

5. Women with diabetes mellitus, either insulin-dependent or noninsulin-dependent, can use IUDs.

6. IUD insertion is relatively easier in breastfeeding women, and the rates of expulsion and uterine perforation are not increased.

IUD Removal

Removal of an IUD can usually be accomplished by grasping the string with a ring forcep or uterine dressing forcep and exerting firm traction. If strings cannot be seen, they can often be extracted from the cervical canal by rotating two cotton-tipped applicators or a Pap smear cytobrush in the endocervical canal. If further maneuvers are required, a paracervical block should be administered. Oral administration of a nonsteroidal anti-inflammatory drug beforehand will reduce uterine cramping.

If IUD strings cannot be identified or extracted from the endocervical canal, a light plastic uterine sound should be passed into the endometrial cavity after administration of a paracervical block. A standard metal sound is too heavy and insensitive for this purpose. The IUD can frequently be felt with the sound and localized against the anterior or posterior wall of the uterus. The device can then be removed using a Facit polyp or alligator-type forcep directed to where the device was felt, taking care to open the forcep widely immediately on passing it through the internal cervical os so that the IUD can be caught between the jaws. If removal is not easily accomplished using this forcep, direct visualization of the IUD with sonography or hysteroscopy can facilitate removal. Sonography is less painful and more convenient, and should be tried first.

Fertility returns promptly and pregnancies after removal of an IUD occur at a normal rate, sooner than after oral contraception.[42–45, 47, 48] Pregnancy outcome after IUD removal is assocated with a normal incidence of spontaneous miscarriage and ectopic pregnancy.[48]

If a patient wishes to continue use of an IUD, a new device can be placed immediately after removal of the old one. In this case, antibiotic prophylaxis is advised.

Embedded IUDs

If removal is not easily accomplished, direct visualization of the IUD with sonography or hysteroscopy can be helpful. Sonography is safer and less expensive.[97, 130] Transvaginal ultrasonography provides the best image to confirm the location of the IUD, but there is little room for the removal procedure. A better approach is to fill the bladder and use an abdominal sector transducer to image the uterine cavity as the forceps are introduced. Open the forceps widely and see if the IUD moves when the forceps close on it. If it moves, close the forceps tightly and extract the IUD. If unsuccessful, re-introduce the forceps in a different plane, keeping one jaw of the open forceps firmly against first the anterior and then the posterior uterine wall. If this approach is not successful, hysteroscopy is indicated.

Finding a Displaced IUD

When an IUD cannot be found, besides expulsion, one has to consider perforation of the uterus into the abdominal cavity (a very rare event) or embedment into the myometrium. All IUDs are radiopaque, but localizing them radiographically requires 2–3 views, is time-consuming and expensive, and does not allow intrauterine direction of instruments. A quick, real-time sonographic scan in the office is the best method to locate a lost IUD, whether or not removal is desired. If the IUD cannot be visualized with ultrasonography, abdominal x-rays are necessary because the IUD can be high and hidden.

If the IUD is identified perforating the myometrium or in the abdominal cavity, it should be removed using operative laparoscopy, usually under general anesthesia. If the IUD is in the uterine cavity, but cannot be grasped with a forcep under sonographic guidance, hysteroscopy is the best approach. Both routes may be helpful if an IUD is partially perforated.

Copper in the abdominal cavity can lead to adhesion formation, making laparoscopic removal difficult.[131] Although inert perforated devices without closed loops were previously allowed to remain in the abdominal cavity, current practice is to remove any perforated IUD. Because IUD perforations usually occur at the time of insertion, it is important to check for correct position by identifying the string within a few weeks after insertion. Uterine perforation itself is unlikely to cause more than transient pain and bleeding, and can go undetected at the time of IUD insertion. If you believe perforation has occurred, prompt sonography is indicated so that the device can be removed before adhesion formation can occur.

This problem should be put into perspective. With the new generation of IUDs (copper and medicated), adhesion formation appears to be an immediate reaction which does not progress, and rarely leads to serious complications.[132] In appropriate situations (where the risk of surgery is considerable), clinician and patient may elect not to remove the translocated IUD. However, a case has been reported of sigmoid perforation occurring 5 years after insertion, and the general consensus continues to favor removal of a perforated IUD immediately upon diagnosis.[133]

IUD Myths

We hope the information in this chapter will lay to rest 4 specific myths associated with IUDs. For emphasis, the following sentences provide the correct responses to what we believe are common misconceptions among clinicians:

1. **IUDs are *NOT* abortifacients.**

2. **An increased risk of infection with the modern IUD is related *ONLY* to the insertion.**

3. **The modern IUD *HAS NOT* exposed clinicians to litigation.**

4. **IUDs *DO NOT* increase the risk of ectopic pregnancy.**

The IUD for Older Women

The IUD is a good reversible contraceptive choice for older women. An older woman is more likely to be mutually monogamous and less likely to develop PID, and for those women who have already had their children, concern with fertility and problems with cramping and bleeding are both lesser issues. If protection from STDs is not a concern, insertion of a copper IUD can provide very effective contraception until the menopause without the need to do anything other than check the string occasionally. On the other hand, because alterations of bleeding patterns become more common in this age group, it may be necessary to remove an IUD.

References

1. **Huber SC, Piotrow PT, Orlans B, Dommer G,** Intrauterine devices, *Pop Reports, Series B* No. 2, 1975.

2. **Richter R,** Ein mittel zur verhutung der konzeption, *Deutsche Med Wochenschrift* 35:1525, 1909.

3. **Pust K,** Ein brauchbarer frauenschutz, *Deutsche Med Wochenschrift* 49:952, 1923.

4. **Gräfenberg E,** An intrauterine contraceptive method, In: Sanger M, Stone HM, eds. *The Practice of Contraception: Proceedings of the 7th International Birth Control Conference, Zurich, Switzerland,* Williams & Wilkins, Baltimore, 1930, p 33.

5. **Ota T,** A study on birth control with an intra-uterine instrument, *Jap J Obstet Gynecol* 17:210, 1934.

6. **Ishihama A,** Clinical studies on intrauterine rings, especially the present state of contraception in Japan and the experiences in the use of intra-uterine rings, *Yokohama Med Bull* 10:89, 1959.

7. **Oppenheimer W,** Prevention of pregnancy by the Graefenberg ring method: A re-evaluation after 28 years' experience, *Am J Obstet Gynecol* 78:446, 1959.

8. **Tietze C,** Evaluation of intrauterine devices. Ninth progress report of the cooperative statistical program, *Stud Fam Plann* 1:1, 1970.

9. **Tatum HJ, Schmidt FH, Phillips DM, McCarty M, O'Leary WM,** The Dalkon shield controversy, structural and bacteriologic studies of IUD tails, *JAMA* 231:711, 1975.

10. **Kessel E,** Pelvic inflammatory disease with intrauterine device use: A reassessment, *Fertil Steril* 51:1, 1989.

11. **Eschenbach DA, Harnisch JP, Holmes KK,** Pathogenesis of acute pelvic inflammatory disease: role of contraception and other risk factors, *Am J Obstet Gynecol* 128:838, 1977.

12. **Kaufman DW, Shapiro S, Rosenberg L, Monson RR, Miettinen OS, Stolley PD, Slone D,** Intrauterine contraceptive device use and pelvic inflammatory disease, *Am J Obstet Gynecol* 136:159, 1980.

13. **Kaufman DW, Watson J, Rosenberg L, Helmrich SP, Miettinen OS, Stolley PD, Shapiro S,** The effect of different types of intrauterine devices on the risk of pelvic inflammatory disease, *JAMA* 250:759, 1983.

14. **Lee NC, Rubin GL, Ory HW, Burkman RT,** Type of intrauterine device and the risk of pelvic inflammatory disease, *Obstet Gynecol* 62:1, 1983.

15. **Piccinino LJ, Mosher WD,** Trends in contraceptive use in the United States: 1982–1995, *Fam Plann Perspect* 30:4, 1998.

16. **Population Crisis Committee,** Access to birth control: A world assessment, Population Briefing Paper, Report No. 19, 1986.

17. **Daling JR, Weiss NS, Metch BJ, Chow WH, Soderstrom RM, Moore DE, Spadoni LR, Stadel BV,** Primary tubal infertility in relation to the use of an intrauterine device, *New Engl J Med* 312:937, 1985.

18. **Cramer DW, Schiff I, Schoenbaum SC, Gibson M, Belisle S, Albrecht B, Stillman RJ, Berger MJ, Wilson E, Stadel BV, Seible M,** Tubal infertility and the intrauterine device, *New Engl J Med* 312:941, 1985.

19. **Lee NC, Rubin GL, Borucki R,** The intrauterine device and pelvic inflammatory disease revisited: new results from the Women's Health Study, *Obstet Gynecol* 72:1, 1988.

20. **Zipper JA, Medel M, Prage R,** Suppression of fertility by intrauterine copper and zinc in rabbits: A new approach to intrauterine contraception, *Am J Obstet Gynecol* 105:529, 1969.

21. **Tatum HJ,** Milestones in intrauterine device development, *Fertil Steril* 39:141, 1983.

22. **Sivin I, Tatum HJ,** Four years of experience with the TCu 380A intrauterine contraceptive device, *Fertil Steril* 36:159, 1981.

23. **Sujuan G, Liuqu Z, Yuhao W, Feng L,** Chinese IUDs, In: Bardin CW, Mishell Jr DR, eds. *Proceedings from the Fourth International Conference on IUDs,* Butterworth-Heinemann, Boston, 1994, p 308.

24. **Sivin I, Diaz S, Pavéz M, Alvarez F, Brache V, Diaz J, Odlind V, Olsson S-E, Stern J,** Two-year comparative trial of the gyne T 380 slimline and gyne T 380 intrauterine copper devices, *Contraception* 44:481, 1991.

25. **Sivin I, Stern J, International Committee for Contraception Research,** Health during prolonged use of levonorgestrel 20 µg/d and the copper TCu 380 Ag intrauterine contraceptive devices: a multicenter study, *Fertil Steril* 61:70, 1994.

26. **Chi I-c,** The TCu-380A (AG), MLCu375, and Nova-T IUDs and the IUD daily releasing 20 µg levonorgestrel — four pillars of IUD contraception for the nineties and beyond? *Contraception* 47:325, 1993.

27. **Luukkainen T, Allonen H, Haukkamaa M, Lahteenmake P, Nilsson CG, Toivonen J,** Five years' experience with levonorgestrel-releasing IUDs, *Contraception* 33:139, 1986.

28. **Sivin I, Stern J, Coutinho E, Mattos CER, El Mahgoub S, Diaz S, Pavéz M, Alvarez F, Brache V, Thevinin F, Diaz J, Faundes A, Diaz MM, McCarthy T, Mishell Jr DR, Shoupe D,** Prolonged intrauterine contraception: a seven-year randomized study of the levonorgestrel 20 mcg/day (LNg 20) and the copper T380 Ag IUDs, *Contraception* 44:473, 1991.

29. **Toivonen J, Luukkainen T, Alloven H,** Protective effect of intrauterine release of levonorgestrel on pelvic infection: three years' comparative experience of levonorgestrel and copper-releasing intrauterine devices, *Obstet Gynecol* 77:261, 1991.

30. **Bilian X, Liying Z, Xuling Z, Mengchun J, Luukkainen T, Allonen H,** Pharmacokinetic and pharmacodynamic studies of levonorgestrel-releasing intrauterine device, *Contraception* 41:353, 1990.

31. **UNDP, UNFPA, and WHO Special Programme of Research, Development and Research Training in Human Reproduction,, World Bank: IUD Research Group,** The TCu 380A IUD and the frameless IUD "the Flexigard:" interim three-year data from an International Multicenter Trial, *Contraception* 52:77, 1995.

32. **Rosenberg MJ, Foldesy R, Mishell Jr DR, Speroff L, Waugh MS, Burkman R,** Performance of the TCu380A and Cu-Fix IUDs in an international randomized trial, *Contraception* 53:197, 1996.

33. **Van Kets H, Van der Pas H, Thiery M, Wildemeersch D, Vrijens M, Van Trappen Y, Temmerman M, DePypere H, Delbarge W, Dhont M, Defoort P, Schacht EH, Bátárl I, Barri P, Martinez F, Iglesias Cortit LH, Creatsas G, Shangchun W, Xiaoming C, Zuan-chong F, Yu-ming W, Andrade A, Reinprayoon D, Pizarro E,** The GyneFix® implant system for interval, postabortal and postpartum contraception: a significant advance in long-term reversible contraception, *Eur J Contraception Reprod Health Care* 2:1, 1997.

34. **Sivin I,** IUDs are contraceptives, not abortifacients: a comment on research and belief, *Stud Fam Plann* 20:355, 1989.

35. **Ortiz ME, Croxatto HB,** The mode of action of IUDs, *Contraception* 36:37, 1987.

36. **Alvarez F, Gulloff E, Brache V, Hess R, Fernandez E, Salvatierra AM, Guerrero B, Zacharias S,** New insights on the mode of action of intrauterine contraceptive devices in women, *Fertil Steril* 49:768, 1988.

37. **Segal SJ, Alvarez-Sanchez F, Adejuwon CA, Brache De Mejla V, Leon P, Faundes A,** Absence of chorionic gonadotropin in sera of women who use intrauterine devices, *Fertil Steril* 44:214, 1985.

38. **Wilcox AJ, Weinberg CR, Armstrong EG, Canfield RE,** Urinary human chorionic gonadotropin among intrauterine device users: Detection with a highly specific and sensitive assay, *Fertil Steril* 47:265, 1987.

39. **Ämmälä M, Nyman T, Strengell L, Rutanen E-M,** Effect of intrauterine contraceptive devices on cytokine messenger ribonucleic acid expression in the human endometrium, *Fertil Steril* 63:773, 1995.

40. **Nilsson CG, Lahteenmaki P, Luukkainen T,** Ovarian function in amenorrheic and menstruating users of a levonorgestrel-releasing intrauterine device, *Fertil Steril* 41:52, 1984.

41. **Andersson J, Rybo G,** Levonorgestrel-releasing intrauterine device in the treatment of menorrhagia, *Br J Obstet Gynaecol* 97:690, 1990.

42. **Vessey MP, Lawless M, McPherson K, Yeates D,** Fertility after stopping use of intrauterine contraceptive device, *Br Med J* 283:106, 1983.

43. **Belhadj H, Sivin I, Diaz S, Pavéz M, Tejada A-S, Brache V, Alvarez F, Shoupe D, Breaux H, Mishell Jr DR, McCarthy T, Yo V,** Recovery of fertility after use of the levonorgestrel 20 mcg/day or copper T 380Ag intrauterine device, *Contraception* 34:261, 1986.

44. **Skjeldestadt FE, Bratt H,** Fertility after complicated and non-complicated use of IUDs. A controlled prospective study, *Adv Contracept* 4:179, 1988.

45. **Wilson JC,** A prospective New Zealand study of fertility after removal of copper intrauterine devices for conception and because of complications: a four-year study, *Am J Obstet Gynecol* 160:391, 1989.

46. **United Nations Development Programme/United Nations Population Fund/World Health Organization/World Bank, Special Programme of Research, Development and Research Training in Human Reproduction,** Long-term reversible contraception. Twelve years of experience with the TCu380A and TCu220C, *Contraception* 56:341, 1997.

47. **Sivin I, Stern J, Diaz J, Diaz MM, Faundes A, Mahgoub SE, Diaz S, Pavéz M, Coutinho E, Mattos CER, McCarthy T, Mishell Jr DR, Shoupe D, Alvarez F, Brache V, Jimenez E,** Two years of intrauterine contraception with levonorgestrel and with copper: a randomized comparison of the TCu 380Ag and levonorgestrel 20 mcg/day devices, *Contraception* 35:245, 1987.

48. **Sivin I, Stern J, Diaz S, Pavez M, Alvarez F, Brache V, Mishell Jr DR, Lacarra M, McCarthy T, Holma P, Darney P, Klaisle C, Olsson S-E, Odlind V,** Rates and outcomes of planned pregnancy after use of Norplant capsules, Norplant II rods, or levonorgestrel-releasing or copper TCu 380Ag intrauterine contraceptive devices, *Am J Obstet Gynecol* 166:1208, 1992.

49. **Sivin I, Schmidt F,** Effectiveness of IUDs: a review, *Contraception* 36:55, 1987.

50. **Petta CA, Amatya R, Farr G,** Clinical evaluation of the TCu 380A IUD at six Latin American centers, *Contraception* 50:17, 1994.

51. **WHO Special Programme of Research, Development and Research Training in Human Reproduction, Task Force on the Safety and Efficacy of Fertility Regulating Methods,** The TCu 380A, TCu 220C, Multiload 250, and Nova T IUDs at 3, 5, and 7 years of use, *Contraception* 42:141, 1990.

52. **Farr G, Amatya R,** Contraceptive efficacy of the copper T 380A and copper T 200 intrauterine devices: results from a comparative clinical trial in six developing countries, *Contraception* 49:231, 1994.

53. **WHO Special Programme of Research, Development and Research Training in Human Reproduction, Task Force on Intrauterine Devices for Fertility Regulation,** A multinational case-control study of ectopic pregnancy, *Clin Reprod Fertil* 3:131, 1985.

54. **Marchbanks PA, Annegers JE, Coulam CB, Strathy JH, Kurland LT,** Risk factors for ectopic pregnancy. A population based study, *JAMA* 259:1823, 1988.

55. **Ory HW,** Ectopic pregnancy and intrauterine contraceptive devices: new perspectives, *Obstet Gynecol* 57:2, 1981.

56. **Edelman DA, Porter CW,** The intrauterine device and ectopic pregnancy, *Contraception* 36:85, 1987.

57. **Makinen JL, Erkkola RU, Laippala PJ,** Causes of the increase in incidence of ectopic pregnancy — a study on 1017 patients from 1966 to 1985 in Turku, Finland, *Am J Obstet Gynecol* 160:642, 1989.

58. **Skjeldestad FE,** How effectively do copper intrauterine devices prevent ectopic pregnancy? *Acta Obstet Gynecol Scand* 76:684, 1997.

59. **Sivin I,** Dose- and age-dependent ectopic pregnancy risks with intrauterine contraception, *Obstet Gynecol* 78:291, 1991.

60. **Barbosa I, Bakos O, Olsson S-E, Odlind V, Johansson EDB,** Ovarian function during use of a levonorgestrel-releasing IUD, *Contraception* 42:51, 1990.

61. **Franks AL, Beral V, Cates Jr W, Hogue CJ,** Contraception and ectopic pregnancy risk, *Am J Obstet Gynecol* 163:1120, 1990.

62. **Cameron IT, Haining R, Lumsden M-A, Thomas VR, Smith SK,** The effects of mefenamic acid and norethisterone on measured menstrual blood loss, *Obstet Gynecol* 76:85, 1990.

63. **Zhao G, Minshi L, Pengdi Z, Ruhua X, Jiedong W, Renqing X,** A preliminary morphometric study on the endometrium from patients treated with indomethacin-releasing copper intrauterine device, *Hum Reprod* 12:1563, 1997.

64. **Milsom I, Andersson K, Jonasson K, Lindstedt G, Rybo G,** The influence of the Gyne-T 380S IUD on menstrual blood loss and iron status, *Contraception* 52:175, 1995.

65. **Castellsague X, Thompson WD, Dubrow R,** Intra-uterine contraception and the risk of endometrial cancer, *Int J Cancer* 54:911, 1993.

66. **Lassise DL, Savitz DA, Hamman RF, Baron AE, Brinton LA, Levines RS,** Invasive cervical cancer and intrauterine device use, *Int J Epidemiol* 20:865, 1991.

67. **Parazzini F, La Vecchia C, Negri E,** Use of intrauterine device and risk of invasive cervical cancer, *Int J Epidemiol* 21:1030, 1992.

68. **Hill DA, Weiss NS, Voigt LF, Beresford SAA,** Endometrial cancer in relation to intra-uterine device use, *Int J Cancer* 70:278, 1997.

69. **Sturgeon SR, Brinton LA, Berman ML, Mortel R, Twiggs LB, Barrett RJ, Wilbanks GD, Lurain JR,** Intrauterine device use and endometrial cancer risk, *Int J Epidemiol* 26:496, 1997.

70. **Mark AS, Hricak H,** Intrauterine contraceptive devices: MR imaging, *Radiology* 162:311, 1987.

71. **Pasquale SA, Russer TJ, Foldesy R, Mezrich RS,** Lack of interaction between magnetic resonance imaging and the copper-T380A IUD, *Contraception* 55:169, 1997.

72. **Mishell Jr DR, Bell JH, Good RG, Moyer DL,** The intrauterine device: a bacteriologic study of the endometrial cavity, *Am J Obstet Gynecol* 96:119, 1966.

73. **Farley MM, Rosenberg MJ, Rowe PJ, Chen J-H, Meirik O,** Intrauterine devices and pelvic inflammatory disease: an international perspective, *Lancet* 339:785, 1992.

74. **Skouby SO, Molsted-Pedersen L, Kosonen A,** Consequences of intrauterine contraception in diabetic women, *Fertil Steril* 42:568, 1984.

75. **Kimmerle R, Weiss R, Bergert M, Kurz K,** Effectiveness, safety, and acceptability of a copper intrauterine deivce (Cu Safe 300) in type I diabetic women, *Diabetes Care* 16:1227, 1993.

76. **Buchan H, Villard-Mackintosh L, Vessey M, Yeates D, McPherson K,** Epidemiology of pelvic inflammatory disease in parous women with special reference to intrauterine device use, *Br J Obstet Gynaecol* 97:780, 1990.

77. **Mehanna MTR, Rizk MA, Ramadan M, Schachter J,** Chlamydial serologic characteristics among intrauterine contraceptive device users: does copper inhibit chlamydial infection in the female genital tract? *Am J Obstet Gynecol* 171:691, 1994.

78. **Kleinman D, Insler V, Sarov I,** Inhibition of Chlamydia trachomatis growth in endometrial cells by copper: possible relevance for the use of copper IUDs, *Contraception* 39:665, 1989.

79. **Kronmal RA, Whitney CW, Mumford SD,** The intrauterine device and pelvic inflammatory disease: the Women's Health Study reanalyzed, *J Clin Epidemiol* 44:109, 1991.

80. **Lee NC, Rubin GL, Grimes DA,** Measures of sexual behavior and the risk of pelvic inflammatory disease, *Obstet Gynecol* 77:425, 1991.

81. **Everett ED, Reller LB, Droegemueller W, Greer BE,** Absence of bacteremia after insertion or removal of intrauterine device, *Obstet Gynecol* 47:207, 1976.

82. **Hall SM, Jamieson JR, Witcomb MA,** Bacteraemia after insertion of intrauterine devices, *S Afr Med J* 50:12321, 1976.

83. **Murray S, Hickey JB, Houang E,** Significant bacteremia associated with replacement of intrauterine contraceptive device, *Am J Obstet Gynecol* 156:698, 1987.

84. **Shoubnikova M, Hellberg D, Nilsson S, Mårdh P-A,** Contraceptive use in women with bacterial vaginosis, *Contraception* 55:355, 1997.

85. **Jossens MOR, Schachter J, Sweet RL,** Risk factors associated with pelvic inflammatory disease of differing microbial etiologies, *Obstet Gynecol* 83:989, 1994.

86. **European Study Group,** Risk factors for male to female transmission of HIV, *Br Med J* 298:411, 1989.

87. **Musicco M, Nicolosi A, Saracco A, Lazzarin A,** IUD use and man to woman sexual transmission of HIV-1, In: Bardin CW, Mishell Jr DR, eds. *Proceedings from the Fourth International Conference on IUDs,* Butterworth-Heinemann, Boston, 1994, p 179.

88. **Kapiga SH, Lyamuya EF, Lwihula GK, Hunter DJ,** The incidence of HIV infection among women using family planning methods in Dar-es-Salaam, Tanzania, *AIDS* 12:75, 1998.

89. **European Study Group on Heterosexual Transmission of HIV,** Comparison of female to male and male to female transmission of HIV in 563 stable couples, *Br Med J* 304:809, 1992.

90. **Sinei SK, Morrison CS, Sekadde-Kigondu C, Allen M, Kokonya D,** Complications of use of intrauterine devices among HIV-1-infected women, *Lancet* 351:1238, 1998.

91. **Chapin DS, Sullinger JC,** A 43-year old woman with left buttock pain and a presacral mass, *New Engl J Med* 323:183, 1990.

92. **Keebler C, Chatwani A, Schwartz R,** Actinomycosis infection associated with intrauterine contraceptive devices, *Am J Obstet Gynecol* 145:596, 1983.

93. **Duguid HLD,** Actinomycosis and IUDs, *Int Plann Parenthood Fed Med Bull* 17:3, 1983.

94. **Petitti DB, Yamamoto D, Morgenstern N,** Factors associated with actinomyces-like organisms on Papanicolaou smear in users of IUDs, *Am J Obstet Gynecol* 145:338, 1983.

95. **Persson E, Holmberg K, Dahlgren S, Nielsson L,** Actinomyces Israelii in genital tract of women with and without intrauterine contraception devices, *Acta Obstet Gynecol Scand* 62:563, 1983.

96. **Hill GB,** *Eubacterium nodatum* mimics Actinomyces in intrauterine device-associated infections and other settings within the female genital tract, *Obstet Gynecol* 79:534, 1992.

97. **Stubblefield P, Fuller A, Foster S,** Ultrasound-guided intrauterine removal of intrauterine contraceptive devices in pregnancy, *Obstet Gynecol* 72:961, 1988.

98. **Lewit S,** Outcome of pregnancy with intrauterine device, *Contraception* 2:47, 1970.

99. **Alvior Jr GT,** Pregnancy outcome with removal of intrauterine device, *Obstet Gynecol* 41:894, 1973.

100. **Assaf A, Gohar M, Saad S, El-Nashar A, Abdel Aziz A,** Removal of intrauterine devices with missing tails during early pregnancy, *Contraception* 45:541, 1992.

101. **Foreman H, Stadel BV, Schlesselman S,** Intrauterine device usage and fetal loss, *Obstet Gynecol* 58:669, 1981.

102. **United Kingdom Family Planning Research Network,** Pregnancy outcome associated with the use of IUDs, *Br J Fam Plann* 15:7, 1989.

103. **Williams P, Johnson B, Vessey M,** Septic abortion in women using intrauterine devices, *Br Med J* iv:263, 1975.

104. **Atrash HK, Frye A, Hogue CJR,** Incidence of morbidity and mortality with IUD in situ in the 1980s and 1990s, In: Bardin CW, Mishell Jr DR, eds. *Proceedings from the Fourth International Conference on IUDs,* Butterworth-Heinemann, Boston, 1994, p 76.

105. **Guillebaud J,** IUD and congenital malformation, *Br Med J* i:1016, 1975.

106. **Layde PM, Goldberg MF, Safra MJM, Oakley GP,** Failed intrauterine device contraception and limb reduction deformities: a case-control study, *Fertil Steril* 31:18, 1979.

107. **Tatum HJ, Schmidt FH, Jain AK,** Management and outcome of pregnancies associated with the copper-T intrauterine contraceptive device, *Am J Obstet Gynecol* 127:869, 1976.

108. **Vessey M, Doll R, Peto R, Johnson B, Wiggins P,** A long-term follow-up study of women using different methods of contraception — an interim report, *J Biosoc Sci* 8:373, 1976.

109. **Chaim W, Mazor M,** Pregnancy with an intrauterine device in situ and preterm delivery, *Arch Gynecol Obstet* 252:21, 1992.

110. **Leigh BC, Temple MT, Trocki KF,** The sexual behavior of US adults: results from a national survey, *Am J Pub Health* 83:1400, 1993.

111. **Newton J, Tacchi D,** Long-term use of copper intrauterine devices, *Br J Fam Plann* 16:116, 1990.

112. **Kjos SL, Ballagh SA, La Cour M, Xiang A, Mishell Jr DR,** The copper T380A intrauterine device in women with Type II diabetes mellitus, *Obstet Gynecol* 84:1006, 1994.

113. **Diaz J, Pinto-Neto AM, Bahamondes L, Diaz M, Arce XE, Castro S,** Performance of the copper T 200 in parous adolescents: are copper IUDs suitable for these women? *Contraception* 48:23, 1993.

114. **Edelman D, Van Os W,** Safety of intrauterine contraception, *Adv Contracept* 6:207, 1990.

115. **Mishell Jr DR, Roy S,** Copper intrauterine contraceptive device event rates following insertion 4 to 8 weeks post partum, *Am J Obstet Gynecol* 143:29, 1982.

116. **Zhuang L, Wang H, Yang P,** Observations of the clinical efficacies and side effects of six different timings of IUD insertions, *Clin J Obstet Gynecol* 22:350, 1987.

117. **Chi I-c, Farr G,** Postpartum IUD contraception—A review of an international experience, *Adv Contracept* 5:127, 1989.

118. **Zhou S, Chi I-c,** Immediate postpartum IUD insertions in a Chinese hospital — A two-year follow-up, *Int J Gynaecol Obstet* 35:157, 1991.

119. **Chi I-c, Potts M, Wilkens L, Champion C,** Performance of the TCu-380A device in breastfeeding and non-breastfeeding women, *Contraception* 39:603, 1989.

120. **Andersson K, Ryde-Blomqvist E, Lindell K, Odlind V, Milsom I,** Perforations with intrauterine devices. Report from a Swedish survey, *Contraception* 57:251, 1998.

121. **Nielsen NC, Nygren K-G, Allonen H,** Three years of experience after post-abortal insertion of Nova-T and Copper-T-200, *Acta Obstet Gynecol Scand* 63:261, 1984.

122. **Querido L, Ketting E, Haspels AA,** IUD insertion following induced abortion, *Contraception* 31:603, 1985.

123. **White MK, Ory HW, Rooks JB, Rochat RW,** Intrauterine device termination rates and the menstrual cycle day of insertion, *Obstet Gynecol* 55:220, 1980.

124. **Anteby E, Revel A, Ben-Chetrit A, Rosen B, Tadmor O, Yagel S,** Intrauterine device failure: relation to its location within the uterine cavity, *Obstet Gynecol* 81:112, 1993.

125. **Sinei SKA, Schulz KF, Laptey PR, Grimes D, Arnsi J, Rosenthal S, Rosenberg M, Rivon G, Njage P, Bhullar V, Ogendo H,** Preventing IUCD-related pelvic infection: The efficacy of prophylactic doxycycline at insertion, *Br J Obstet Gynaecol* 97:412, 1990.

126. **Lapido OA, Farr G, Otolorin E, Konje JC, Sturgen K, Cox P, Champion CB,** Prevention of IUD-related pelvic infection: the efficacy of prophylactic doxycycline at IUD insertion, *Adv Contracept* 7:43, 1991.

127. **Zorlu CG, Aral K, Cobanoglu O, Gurler S, Gokmen O,** Pelvic inflammatory disease and intrauterine devices: prophylactic antibiotics to reduce febrile complications, *Adv Contracept* 9:299, 1993.

128. **Walsh TL, Bernstein GS, Grimes DA, Frezieres R, Bernstein L, Coulson AH, IUD Study Group,** Effect of prophylactic antibiotics on morbidity associated with IUD insertion: results of a pilot randomized controlled trial, *Contraception* 50:319, 1994.

129. **Walsh T, Grimes D, Frezieres R, Nelson A, Bernstein L, Coulson A, Bernstein G, for the IUD Study Group,** Randomised controlled trial of prophylactic antibiotics before insertion of intrauterine devices, *Lancet* 351:1005, 1998.

130. **Sachs BP, Gregory K, McArdle C, Pinshaw A,** Removal of retained intrauterine contraceptive devices in pregnancy, *Am J Perinatol* 9:139, 1992.

131. **Gorsline J, Osborne N,** Management of the missing intrauterine contraceptive device: Report of a case, *Am J Obstet Gynecol* 153:228, 1985.

132. **Adoni A, Chetrit AB,** The management of intrauterine devices following uterine perforation, *Contraception* 43:77, 1991.

133. **Gronlund B, Blaabjerg J,** Serious intestinal complication five years after insertion of a Nova-T, *Contraception* 44:517, 1991.

25 Barrier Methods of Contraception

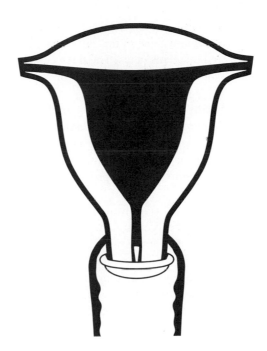

The use of vaginal contraceptives is probably as ancient as homo sapiens. References to sponges and plugs appear in the earliest of writings. Substances with either barrier or spermicidal properties (or both) have included honey, alum, spices, oils, tannic acids, lemon juice, and even crocodile dung. However, the diaphragm and the cervical cap were not invented until the late 1800s, the same time period that saw the beginning of investigations with spermicidal agents.

Intravaginal contraception was widespread in isolated cultures throughout the world. The Japanese used balls of bamboo paper; Islamic women used willow leaves; and the women in the Pacific Islands used seaweed. References can be found throughout ancient writings to sticky plugs, made of gumlike substances, to be placed in the vagina prior to intercourse. In preliterate societies, an effective method had to have been the result of trial and error, with some good luck thrown in.

How was contraceptive knowledge spread? Certainly, until modern times, individuals did not consult physicians for contraception. Contraceptive knowledge was folklore, undoubtedly perpetuated by the oral tradition. The social and technical circumstances of ancient times conspired to make communication of information very difficult. But even when knowledge was lacking, the desire to prevent conception was not. Hence, the widespread use of potions, body movements, and amulets; all of which can be best described as magic.

Egyptian papyri dating from 1850 BC refer to plugs of honey, gum, acacia, and crocodile dung. The descriptions of contraceptive techniques by Soranus are viewed as the best in history until modern times.[1] Soranus of Ephesus lived from 98 to 138, and has often been referred to as the greatest gynecologist of antiquity. He studied in Alexandria, and practiced in Rome. His great text was lost for centuries, and was not published until 1838.

Soranus gave explicit directions how to make concoctions that probably combined a barrier with spermicidal action. He favored making pulps from nuts and fruits (probably very acidic and spermicidal) and advocated the use of soft wool placed at the cervical os. He described up to 40 different combinations.

The earliest penis protectors were just that, intended to provide prophylaxis against infection. Gabriello Fallopius, one of the early authorities on syphilis, described, in 1564, a linen condom that covered the glans penis. The linen condom of Fallopius was followed by full covering with animal skins and intestines, but use for contraception cannot be dated to earlier than the 1700s.

There are many versions accounting for the origin of the word, "condom." Most attribute the word to a Dr. Condom, a physician in England in the 1600s. The most famous story declares that Dr. Condom invented the sheath in response to the annoyance displayed by Charles II at the number of his illegitimate children. All attempts to trace this physician have failed. This origin of the word can neither be proved nor disproved.

By 1800, condoms were available at brothels throughout Europe, but nobody wanted to claim responsibility. The French called the condom the English cape; the English called condoms French letters.

Vulcanization of rubber dates to 1844, and by 1850, rubber condoms were available in the U.S. The vulcanization of rubber revolutionized transportation and contraception. The introduction of liquid latex and automatic machinery ultimately made reliable condoms both plentiful and affordable.

Diaphragms first appeared in publication in Germany in the 1880s. A practicing German gynecologist, C. Haase, wrote extensively about his diaphragm, using a pseudonym of Wilhelm P.J. Mensinga. The Mensinga diaphragm retained its original design with little change until modern times.

The cervical cap was available for use before the diaphragm. A New York gynecologist, E.B. Foote, wrote a pamphlet describing its use around 1860. By the 1930s, the cervical cap was the most widely prescribed method of contraception in Europe. Why was the cervical cap not accepted in the U.S.? The answer is not clear. Some blame the more prudish attitude towards sexuality as an explanation for why American women had difficulty learning self-insertion techniques.

Scientific experimentation with chemical inhibitors of sperm began in the 1800s. By the 1950s, more than 90 different spermicidal products were being marketed, and some of them were used in the first efforts to control fertility in India.[2] With the availability of the intrauterine device and the development of oral contraception, interest in spermicidal agents waned, and the number of products declined.

In the last decades of the 1800s, condoms, diaphragms, pessaries, and douching syringes were widely advertised; however, they were not widely utilized. It is only since 1900 that the knowledge and application of contraception have been democratized, encouraged, and promoted. And it is only since 1960, that contraception teaching and practice became part of the program in academic medicine, but not without difficulty.

In the 1960s, Duncan Reid, chair of obstetrics at Harvard Medical School, organized and cared for women in a clandestine clinic for contraception. Called "Dr. Reid's Clinic," women of Boston were able to receive contraceptives not available elsewhere in the city.

In 1961, C. Lee Buxton, chair of obstetrics and gynecology at Yale Medical School, and Estelle Griswold, the 61-year-old executive director of Connecticut Planned Parenthood, opened four Planned Parenthood clinics in New Haven, in a defiant move against the current Connecticut law. In an obvious test of the Connecticut law, Buxton and Griswold were arrested at the Orange Street clinic, in a pre-arranged scenario scripted by Buxton and Griswold at the invitation of the district attorney. Found guilty, and fined $100, imprisonment was deferred because the obvious goal was a decision by the United States Supreme Court. Buxton was forever rankled by the trivial amount of the fine. On June 7, 1965, the Supreme Court voted 7–2 to overturn the Connecticut law on the basis of a constitutional right of privacy. It was not until 1972 and 1973 that the last state laws prohibiting the distribution of contraceptives were overthrown.

Failure Rates During the First Year of Use, United States[7]

Method	Percent of Women with Pregnancy Lowest Expected	Typical
No method	85.0%	85.0%
Combination Pill	0.1	3.0
Progestin only	0.5	3.0
IUDs		
Progesterone IUD	1.5	2.0
Levonorgestrel IUD	0.6	0.8
Copper T 380A	0.1	0.1
Norplant	0.05	0.05
Female sterilization	0.05	0.05
Male sterilization	0.1	0.15
Depo-Provera	0.3	0.3
Spermicides	6.0	26.0
Periodic abstinence		25.0
Calendar	9.0	
Ovulation method	3.0	
Symptothermal	2.0	
Post–ovulation	1.0	
Withdrawal	4.0	19.0
Cervical cap		
Parous women	26.0	40.0
Nulliparous women	9.0	20.0
Sponge		
Parous women	9.0	28.0
Nulliparous women	6.0	18.0
Diaphragm and spermicides	6.0	20.0
Condom		
Male	3.0	14.0
Female	5.0	21.0

Risks and Benefits Common to all Barrier Methods

Barrier (condoms and diaphragms) and spermicide methods provide protection (about a 50% reduction) against sexually transmitted diseases (STDs) and pelvic inflammatory disease (PID).[4–8] This includes infections with chlamydia, gonorrhea, herpes simplex, cytomegalovirus, human papillomavirus, and human immunodeficiency virus (HIV); however, only the condom has been proven to prevent HIV infection. STD protection has a beneficial impact on the risk of tubal infertility and ectopic pregnancy.[6,9] There have been no significant clinical studies on STDs and cervical caps or the female condom, but these methods should be effective. Women who have never used barrier methods of contraception are almost twice as likely to develop cancer of the cervix.[9,10] The risk of toxic shock syndrome is increased with female barrier methods, but the actual incidence is so rare that this is not a significant clinical consideration.[11] Women who have had toxic shock syndrome, however, should be advised to avoid barrier methods.

Barrier Methods and Preeclampsia. An initial case-control study indicated that methods of contraception that prevented exposure to sperm were associated with an increased risk of preeclampsia.[12] This was not confirmed in a careful analysis of two large prospective pregnancy studies.[13] This latter conclusion was more compelling in that it was derived from a large prospective cohort data base.

The Diaphragm

The first effective contraceptive method under a woman's control was the vaginal diaphragm. Distribution of diaphragms led to Margaret Sanger's arrest in New York City in 1918. This was still a contentious issue in 1965 when the Supreme Court's decision in Griswold v. Connecticut ended the ban on contraception in that state. By 1940, one-third of contracepting American couples were using the diaphragm. This decreased to 10% by 1965 after the introduction of oral contraceptives and intrauterine devices, and fell to about 1.9% in 1995. (Chapter 21).

Efficacy

Failure rates for diaphragm users vary from as low as 2% per year of use to a high of 23%. The typical use failure rate after one year of use is 18–20%.[3, 14] Older, married women with longer use achieve the highest efficacy, but young women can use diaphragms very successfully if they are properly encouraged and counseled. There have been no adequate studies to determine whether efficacy is different with and without spermicides.[15]

Side Effects

The diaphragm is a safe method of contraception that rarely causes even minor side effects. Occasionally, women report vaginal irritation due to the latex rubber or the spermicidal jelly or cream used with the diaphragm. Less than 1% discontinue diaphragm use for these reasons. Urinary tract infections are 2–3-fold more common among diaphragm users than among women using oral contraception.[16, 17] Possibly, the rim of the diaphragm presses against the urethra and causes irritation which is perceived as infectious in origin, or true infection may result from touching the perineal area or incomplete emptying of the bladder. It is more probable that spermicides used with the diaphragm can increase the risk of bacteriuria with *E coli*, perhaps due to an alteration in the normal vaginal flora.[18] Clinical experience suggests that voiding after sexual intercourse is helpful, and if necessary, a single postcoital dose of a prophylactic antibiotic can be recommended. Postcoital prophylaxis is effective, using trimethoprim-sulfamethoxazole (1 tablet postcoitus), nitrofurantoin (50 or 100 mg postcoitus), or cephalexin (250 mg postcoitus).

Improper fitting or prolonged retention (beyond 24 hours) can cause vaginal abrasion or mucosal irritation. There is no link between the normal use of diaphragms and the toxic shock syndrome.[19] It makes sense, however, to minimize the risk of toxic shock by removing the diaphragm after 24 hours and during menses.

Benefits

Diaphragm use reduces the incidence of cervical gonorrhea,[20] pelvic inflammatory disease,[21] and tubal infertility.[4, 9] This protection may be due in part to the simultaneous use of a spermicide. There are no data, as of yet, regarding the effect of diaphragm use on the transmission of the AIDS virus (HIV). An important advantage of the diaphragm is low cost. Diaphragms are durable, and with proper care, can last for several years.

Choice and Use of the Diaphragm

There are three types of diaphragms, and most manufacturers produce them in sizes ranging from 50 to 105 mm diameter, in increments of 2.5 to 5 mm. Most women use sizes between 65 and 80 mm.

The diaphragm made with a *flat metal spring* or a *coil spring* remains in a straight line when pinched at the edges. This type is suitable for women with good vaginal muscle tone and an adequate recess behind the pubic arch. However, many women find it difficult to place the posterior edge of these flat diaphragms into the posterior cul-de-sac, and over the cervix.

Arcing diaphragms are easier to use for most women. They come in two types. The All-Flex type bends into an arc no matter where around the rim the edges are pinched together. The hinged type must be pinched between the hinges in order to form a symmetrical arc. The hinged type forms a narrower shape when pinched together, and, thus, may be easier for some women to insert. The arcing diaphragms allow the posterior edge of the diaphragm to slip more easily past the cervix and into the posterior cul-de-sac. Women with poor vaginal muscle tone, cystocele, rectocele, a long cervix, or an anterior cervix of a retroverted uterus use arcing diaphragms more successfully.

Fitting

Successful use of a diaphragm depends on proper fitting. The clinician must have available aseptic fitting rings or diaphragms themselves in all diameters. These devices should be scrupulously disinfected by soaking in a bleach solution. At the time of the pelvic examination, the middle finger is placed against the vaginal wall and the posterior cul-de-sac, while the hand is lifted anteriorly until the pubic symphysis abuts the index finger. This point is marked with the examiner's thumb to approximate the diameter of the diaphragm. The corresponding fitting ring or diaphragm is inserted, the fit to be assessed by both clinician and patient.

If the diaphragm is too tightly pressed against the pubic symphysis, a smaller size is selected. If the diaphragm is too loose (comes out with a cough or bearing down), the next larger size is selected. After a good fit is obtained, the diaphragm is removed by hooking the index finger under the rim behind the symphysis and pulling. It is important to instruct the patient in these procedures during and after the fitting. The patient should then insert the diaphragm, practice checking for proper placement, and attempt removal.

Timing

Diaphragm users need additional instruction about the timing of diaphragm use in relation to sexual intercourse and the use of spermicide. None of this advice has been rigorously assessed in clinical studies; therefore, these recommendations represent the consensus of clinical experience.

The diaphragm should be inserted no longer than 6 hours prior to sexual intercourse. About a tablespoonful of spermicidal cream or jelly should be placed in the dome of the diaphragm prior to insertion, and some of the spermicide should be spread around the rim with a finger. The diaphragm should be left in place for approximately 6 hours (but no more than 24 hours) after coitus. Additional spermicide should be placed in the vagina before each additional episode of sexual intercourse while the diaphragm is in place.

Reassessment

Weight loss, weight gain, vaginal delivery, and even sexual intercourse can change vaginal caliber. The fit of a diaphragm should be assessed every year at the time of the regular examination.

Care of the Diaphragm

After removal, the diaphragm should be washed with soap and water, rinsed, and dried. Powders of any sort need not and should not be applied to the diaphragm. It is wise to use water to periodically check for leaks. Diaphragms should be stored in a cool and dark location.

The Cervical Cap

The cervical cap was popular in Europe long before its re-introduction into the United States. There are several types of cervical caps, but only the cavity rim (Prentif) cap is approved in the U.S. U.S. trials have demonstrated the cervical cap to be about as effective as the diaphragm, but somewhat harder to fit (it comes in only four sizes) and more difficult to insert (it must be placed precisely over the cervix).[22, 23] Efficacy is significantly reduced in parous women.

The cervical cap has several advantages over the diaphragm. It can be left in place for a longer time (up to 48 hours), and it need not be used with a spermicide. However, a tablespoonful of spermicide placed in the cap before application is reported to increase efficacy (to a 6% failure rate in the first year) and to prolong wearing time by decreasing the incidence of foul-smelling discharge (a common complaint after 24 hours).[23]

The size of the cervix varies considerably from woman to woman, and the cervix changes in individual women in response to pregnancy or surgery. Proper fitting can be accomplished in about 80% of women. Women with a cervix that is too long or too short, or with a cervix that is far forward in the vagina, may not be suited for cap use. However, women with vaginal wall or pelvic relaxation, who cannot retain a diaphragm, may be able to use the cap.

Those women who can be fitted with one of the 4 sizes must first learn how to identify the cervix, and then how to slide the cap into the vagina, up the posterior vaginal wall and onto the cervix. After insertion, and after each act of sexual intercourse, the cervix should be checked to make sure it is covered.

To remove the cap (at least 8 hours after coitus), pressure must be exerted with a finger tip to break the seal. The finger is hooked over the cap rim to pull it out of the vagina. Bearing down or squatting or both can help to bring the cervix within reach of the finger.

The cervical cap can be left in place for 2 days, but some women experience a foul-smelling discharge by 2 days. Like the diaphragm, it must be left in place for at least 8 hours after sexual intercourse in order to ensure that no motile sperm are left in the vagina.

The most common cause of failure is dislodgment of the cap from the cervix during sexual intercourse. There is no evidence that cervical caps cause toxic shock syndrome or dysplastic changes in the cervical mucosa.[24] It seems likely (although not yet documented) that cervical caps would provide the same protection from sexually transmitted diseases as the diaphragm.

The Fem Cap, made of nonallergic silicone rubber, is shaped like a sailor's hat, a design that allows a better fit over the cervix and in the vaginal fornices.[25] This cap may be easier to fit and use, and provides better efficacy. There are two sizes, one for nulliparous women and a larger size for women who have had a vaginal delivery.

The Contraceptive Sponge

The vaginal contraceptive sponge is a sustained-release system for a spermicide. The sponge also absorbs semen and blocks the entrance to the cervical canal. The "Today" sponge is a dimpled polyurethaned disc impregnated with one gram of nonoxynol-9. Approximately 20% of the nonoxynol-9 is released over the 24 hours the sponge is left in the vagina. Production of the "Today" sponge in the U.S. ceased in 1995, and availability awaits a new manufacturer. "Protectaid" is a polyurethane sponge available in Canada and Hong Kong that contains 3 spermicides and a dispersing gel.[26] The spermicidal agents are sodium cholate, nonoxynol-9, and benzalkonium chloride. This combination exerts antiviral actions in vitro.[27] The dispersing agent, polydimethysiloxane, forms a protective coating over the entire vagina, providing sustained protection.

To insert, the Today sponge is moistened with water (squeezing out the excess) and placed firmly against the cervix. There should always be a lapse of at least 6 hours after sexual intercourse before removal, even if the sponge has been in place for 24 hours before intercourse (maximal wear time, therefore, is 30 hours). It can be inserted immediately before sexual intercourse or up to 24 hours beforehand. It is removed by hooking a finger through the ribbon attached to the back of the sponge. The Protectaid sponge can be inserted up to 12 hours before intercourse, and it is easier to remove than the Today sponge. Obviously, the sponge is not a good choice for women with anatomical changes that make proper insertion and placement difficult.

In most studies, the effectiveness of the sponge exceeds that of foam, jellies, and tablets, but it is lower than that associated with diaphragm or condom use.[14, 28] Some studies indicated higher failure rates (twice as high) in parous women, suggesting that one size may not fit all users.[29]

Discontinuation rates are generally higher among sponge users, compared to diaphragm and spermicide use. For some women, however, the sponge is preferred because it provides continuous protection for 24 hours regardless of the frequency of coitus. In addition, it is easier to use and less messy.

Side effects associated with the sponge include allergic reactions in about 4% of users. Another 8% complain of vaginal dryness, soreness, or itching. Some women find removal difficult. There is no risk of toxic shock syndrome, and in fact, the nonoxynol-9 retards staphylococcal replication and toxin production. There has been some concern that the sponge may damage the vaginal mucosa and enhance HIV transmission.[30]

Spermicides

Jellies, creams, foams, melting suppositories, foaming tablets, foaming suppositories, and soluble films are used as vehicles for chemical agents that inactivate sperm in the vagina before they can move into the upper genital tract. Some are used together with diaphragms, caps, and condoms, but even used alone, they can provide protection against pregnancy.

Various chemicals and a wide array of vehicles have been used vaginally as contraceptives for centuries. The first commercially available spermicidal pessaries were made in England in 1885 of cocoa butter and quinine sulfite. These or similar materials were used until the 1920s when effervescent tablets that released carbon dioxide and phenyl mercuric acetate were marketed. Modern spermicides, introduced in the 1950s, contain surface active agents that damage the sperm cell membranes (this same action occurs with bacteria and viruses, explaining the protection against STDs). The agents currently used are nonoxynol-9, octoxynol-9, benzalkonium chloride, and menfegol. Most preparations contain 60–100 mg of these agents in each vaginal application, with concentrations ranging from 2–12.5%.

Representative Products:

Vaginal Contraceptive Film – VCF (70 mg nonoxynol-9)

Foams —	**Delfen (nonoxynol-9, 12.5%)**
	Emko (nonoxynol-9, 8%)
	Koromex (nonoxynol-9, 12.5%)
Jellies and Creams —	**Conceptrol (nonoxynol-9, 4%)**
	Delfen (nonoxynol-9, 12.5%)
	Ortho Gynol (nonoxynol-9, 3%)
	Ramses (nonoxynol-9, 5%)
	Koromex Jellly (nonoxynol-9, 3%)

Suppositories —   **Encare (nonoxynol-9, 2.27%)**
Koromex Inserts (nonoxynol-9, 125 mg)
Semicid (nonoxynol-9, 100 mg)

"Advantage 24" is a contraceptive gel that adheres to the vaginal mucosa and provides longer availability of nonoxynol-9; it is intended to be effective for 24 hours. Although available without prescription, adequate clinical trial data are not available. Allendale-N9 is a new vaginal contraceptive film that contains more nonoxynol-9 than VCF.[31] An Allendale film has also been developed that contains benzalkonium chloride instead of nonoxynol-9.[32] In addition to spermicidal activity, benzalkonium chloride is microbicidal and demonstrates activity against HIV.[33] Benzalkonium chloride is available for contraceptive use in the form of a suppository, in a sponge, or as a cream in several countries.

Efficacy

Only periodic abstinence demonstrates as wide a range of efficacy in different studies as do the studies of spermicides. Efficacy seems to depend more on the population studied than the agent used. Efficacy ranges from less than 1% failure to nearly one-third in the first year of use. Failure rates of approximately 20–25% during a year's use are most typical.[3, 14] There are no comparative studies to indicate which preparations, if any, are better or worse.

Spermicides require application 10–30 minutes prior to sexual intercourse. Jellies, creams, and foams remain effective for as long as 8 hours, but tablets and suppositories are good for less than one hour. If ejaculation does not occur within the period of effectiveness, the spermicide should be reapplied. Reapplication should definitely take place for each coital episode.

Vaginal douches are ineffective contraceptives even if they contain spermicidal agents. Postcoital douching is too late to prevent the rapid ascent of sperm (within seconds) to the fallopian tubes.

Advantages

Spermicides are relatively inexpensive and widely available in many retail outlets without prescription. This makes spermicides popular among adolescents and others who have infrequent or unpredictable sexual intercourse. In addition, spermicides are simple to use.

Spermicides provide protection against sexually transmitted diseases. In vitro studies have demonstrated that contraceptive spermicides kill or inactivate most STD pathogens, including HIV. Spermicides have been reported to prevent HIV seroconversion as well as to have no effect.[34—37] Clinical studies indicate reductions in the risk of gonorrhea,[38—40] pelvic infections,[21] and chlamydial infection.[38, 40] There is little difference in the incidence of trichomoniasis, candidiasis, or bacterial vaginosis among spermicide users.[41] ***It is probably that spermicides do not provide additional protection against STDs over that associated with condoms, and, therefore, spermicides should not be used without condoms if a primary objective is to prevent infection with HIV, gonorrhea, or chlamydia.***[42]

Side Effects

No serious side effects or safety problems have arisen in all the years that spermicides have been used. The only serious question raised was that of a possible association between spermicide use and congenital abnormalities or spontaneous miscarriages. Epidemiologic analysis, including a meta-analysis, concluded that there is insufficient evidence to support these associations.[43—45] Spermicides are not absorbed through the vaginal mucosa in concentrations high enough to have systemic effects.[46] Vaginal and cervical mucosal damage (de-epithelialization without inflammation) has been observed with nonoxynol-9, and the overall impact on HIV transmission, although unknown, is of concern.[47, 48]

The principal minor problem is allergy that occurs in 1–5% of users, related to either the vehicle or the spermicidal agent. Using a different product often solves the problem. Spermicide users also have an altered vaginal floral promoting the colonization of *E. coli*, leading to a greater susceptibility to urinary tract infections as noted with diaphragm/spermicide users.[17, 49]

The Search for Contraceptives to Prevent STDs

Research is underway to develop microbicides and contraceptives to prevent STDs. The ideal agent would be a topical microbicide that would prevent infection and be spermicidal. The road is long, extending from in vitro work to clinical application. An acceptable agent must avoid damage to vaginal epithelial cells and disruption of vaginal flora, and the delivery system must be user-friendly. However, it is unlikely that any new agent can match the latex condom, which is nearly 100% effective in blocking bacteria and viruses.

Condoms

Although awareness of condoms as an effective contraceptive method as well as protectors against STDs has increased tremendously in recent years, a great deal remains to be accomplished in order to reach the appropriate level of condom use. Contraceptive efficacy and STD prevention must be linked together and publicly promoted. The male condom is the only contraceptive proven to prevent HIV infection.

There are three specific goals: correct use, consistent use, and affordable, easy availability. If these goals are met, the early 2000s will see the annual manufacture of 20 billion condoms per year.

Various types of condoms are available. Most are made of latex; polyurethane and silicone rubber condoms are also now manufactured. "Natural skin" (lamb's intestine) condoms are still obtainable (about 1% of sales). Latex condoms are 0.3–0.8 mm thick. Sperm that are 0.003 mm in diameter cannot penetrate condoms. The organisms which cause STDs and AIDS also do not penetrate latex condoms, but they can penetrate condoms made from intestine.[50, 51] Condom use (latex) also probably prevents transmission of human papillomavirus (HPV), the cause of condylomata acuminata. Because spermicides provide significant protection against STDs, condoms and spermicides used together offer more protection than either method used alone. The use of spermicides or spermicide-coated condoms, however, increases the incidence of *E. coli* bacteriuria and urinary tract infections in women because of the spermicide-induced alteration in vaginal flora.[18, 52] Consistent use of condoms when one partner is HIV seropositive is highly effective in preventing HIV transmission (there was no seroconversion in 124 couples who used condoms consistently compared to 12.7% conversion after 24 months in couples with inconsistent use.[53] Women who are partners of condom users are less likely to be HIV-positive.[54]

Polyurethane condoms are expected to protect against STDs and HIV, based upon in vitro efficacy as a barrier to bacteria and viruses. They are odorless, may have greater sensitivity, and are resistant to deterioration from storage and lubricants. Those individuals who have the infrequent problem of latex allergy can use polyurethane condoms. Breakage and slippage have been reported to be comparable with latex condoms.[55] However, in a randomized, well-designed study, the polyurethane condom had a 6-fold higher breakage rate.[56]

Condoms can be straight or tapered, smooth or ribbed, colored or clear, lubricated or nonlubricated. These are all marketing ventures aimed at attracting individual notions of pleasure and enjoyment.[57] Condoms that incorporate a spermicidal agent coating the inner and outer surfaces logically promise greater efficacy, but this remains to be determined. Some women are allergic to the spermicide, and it is a concern (not documented) that mucosal lesions can promote HIV transmission should a condom break.

An often repeated concern is the alleged reduction in penile glans sensitivity that accompanies condom use.[57] This has never been objectively studied, and it is likely that this complaint is perception (or excuse) not based on reality. A clinician can overcome this obstruction by advocating the use of thinner (and more esoteric) condoms, knowing that any difference is also more of perception than reality.

As is true for most contraceptive methods, older, married couples experienced in using condoms and strongly motivated to avoid another pregnancy are much more effective users than young, unmarried couples with little contraceptive experience. This does not mean that condoms are not useful contraceptives for adolescents, who are likely to have sex unexpectedly or infrequently. The recent decline in the teen pregnancy rate partly reflects wider use of condoms by teens concerned about avoiding HIV infection.

Prospective users need instructions if they are to avoid pregnancy and STDs. A condom must be placed on the penis before it touches a partner. Uncircumcised men must pull the foreskin back. Prior to unrolling the condom to the base of the penis, air should be squeezed out of the reservoir tip with a thumb and forefinger. The tip of the condom should extend beyond the end of the penis to provide a reservoir to collect the ejaculate (a half-inch of pinched tip). If lubricants are used, they must be water based. Oil-based lubricants (such as Vaseline) will weaken the latex. Couples should be concerned that any vaginal medication can compromise condom integrity. After intercourse, the condom should be held at the base as the still erect penis is withdrawn. Semen must not be allowed to spill or leak. The condom should be handled gently because fingernails and rings can penetrate the latex and cause leakage. If there is evidence of spill or leakage, a spermicidal agent should be quickly inserted into the vagina.

Summary — Key Steps for Maximal Condom Efficacy

1. **Use condoms for every act of coitus.**

2. **Place the condom before vaginal contact.**

3. **Withdraw while the penis is still erect.**

4. **Hold the base of the condom during withdrawal.**

5. **Use a spermicide or a condom lubricated with a spermicide.**

These instructions should be provided to new users of condoms who are likely to be reluctant to ask questions. Most condoms are acquired without medical supervision, and therefore, clinicians should use every opportunity to inform patients about their proper use.

Inconsistent use explains most condom failures. Incorrect use accounts for additional failures, and also, condoms sometimes break. Breakage rates range from 1–8 per 100 episodes of vaginal intercourse (and somewhat higher for anal intercourse), and slippage rates range from 1% to 5%.[58, 59] With experienced couples, condom failure due to breakage and slippage (sufficient to increase the risk of pregnancy or STDs) occurs at a rate of about 1%.[60] In a U.S. survey, one pregnancy resulted for every 3 condom breakages.[61] Concomitant use of spermicides lowers failure rates in case of breakage.

Breakage is a greater problem for couples at risk for STDs. An infected man transmits gonorrhea to a susceptible woman approximately two-thirds of the time.[62] If the woman is infected, transmission to the man occurs one-third of the time.[63] The chances of HIV infection after a single sexual exposure ranges from one in 1000 to one in 10.[64, 65]

Condom breakage rates depend on sexual behavior and practices, experience with condom use, the condition of the condoms, and manufacturing quality. Condoms remain in good condition for up to 5 years unless exposed to ultraviolet light, excessive heat or humidity, ozone, or oils. Condom manufacturers regularly check samples of their products to make sure they meet national standards. These procedures limit the proportion of defects to less than 0.1% of all condoms distributed. Contraceptive failure is more likely to be due to nonuse or incorrect use.

When a condom breaks, or if there is reason to believe spillage or leakage occurred, a woman should contact a clinician within 72 hours. Emergency contraception, as discussed in Chapter 22, should be provided. Couples who rely on condoms for contraception should be educated regarding emergency contraception, and an appropriate supply of oral contraceptives should be kept available for self-medication (see Chapter 22).

For the immediate future, prevention of STDs and control of the AIDS epidemic will require a great increase in the use of condoms. We must all be involved in the effort to promote condom use. Condom use must be portrayed in the positive light of STD prevention. The main motivation for condom use among women continues to be prevention of pregnancy, not prevention of STDs.[54, 66] An important area of concentration is the teaching of the social skills required to ensure use by a reluctant partner. We believe that bans on condom advertising should be eliminated. Using scare tactics about STDs in order to encourage condom use is not sufficient. A more positive approach can yield better compliance. It is useful to emphasize that prevention of STDs will preserve future fertility.

We suggest that clinicians consider making free condoms available in their office. Manufacturers will sell condoms at a bulk rate, from $50–$100 per 1000, depending on style and lubrication.

> **U.S. CONDOM MANUFACTURERS:**
> **Ansell Health Care (telephone: 800–327–8659)**
> **Carter Products (telephone: 609–655–6000)**
> **Meyer Laboratories (telephone: 800–426–6366)**
> **Okamoto USA (telephone: 800–283–7546)**
> **Schmid Laboratories (telephone: 800–829–0987)**

The Female Condom

The female condom is a pouch made of polyurethane, which lines the vagina.[67] An internal ring in the closed end of the pouch covers the cervix and an external ring remains outside the vagina, partially covering the perineum. The female condom is prelubricated with silicone, and a spermicide need not be used. The female condom should be an effective barrier to STD infection;[68] however, high cost and acceptability are major problems. The devices are more cumbersome than condoms, and studies have indicated relatively high rates of problems such as slippage.[69] Women who have successfully used barrier methods and who are strongly motivated to avoid STDs are more likely to choose the female condom. With careful use, the efficacy rate should be similar to that of the diaphragm and the cervical cap.[70–72]

	Diaphragm	Cap	Sponge	Female Condom
Insertion before coitus, no longer than:	6 hrs.	6 hrs.	24 hrs.	8 hrs.
After coitus, should be left in place for:	6 hrs.	8 hrs.	6 hrs.	6 hrs.
Maximal wear time:	24 hrs.	48 hrs.	30 hrs.	8 hrs.

Future Developments

New barrier devices are being pursued, such as sponges incorporating several spermicides and cervical caps made of different materials. Chemical agents are being investigated that can combine spermicidal and antimicrobial actions, and vaginal spermicidal films of different materials and containing other spermicidal agents are being tested. Disposable diaphragms that release spermicide are in development.

Lea's Shield is a vaginal barrier contraceptive composed of silicone.[73, 74] This soft, pliable device comes in one size and fits over the cervix, held in place by the pressure of the vaginal wall around it. There is a collapsible valve that communicates with a 9 mm opening in the bowl that fits over the cervix. This valve allows equalization of air pressure during insertion and drainage of cervical secretions and discharge, permitting a snug fit over the cervix. A thick U-shaped loop attached to the anterior side of the bowl is used to stabilize the device during insertion and for removal. The thicker part of the device is shaped to fill the posterior fornix, thus contributing to its placement and stability over the cervix. The addition of a spermicide, placed in the bowl, is recommended to enhance STD protection. Lea's Shield is designed to remain in place for 48 hours after intercourse. Pregnancy rates are similar to other barrier methods, and no serious adverse effects have been reported.[75]

References

1. **Himes NE,** *Medical History of Contraception,* Williams & Wilkins, Baltimore, 1936.

2. **Gamble CJ,** Spermicidal times as aids to the clinician's choice of contraceptive materials, *Fertil Steril* 8:174, 1957.

3. **Trussell J,** Contraceptive efficacy, In: Hatcher RA, Trussell J, Stewart F, et al, eds. *Contraceptive Technology,* 17th ed, Irvington Publishers, New York, NY, 1998.

4. **Grimes DA, Cates Jr W,** Family planning and sexually transmitted diseases, In: Holmes KK, Mardh P-A, Sparling PF, eds. *Sexually Transmitted Diseases,* 2nd ed, McGraw-Hill, New York, 1990, p 1087.

5. **Cramer DW, Goldman MB, Schiff I, Belisla S, Albrecht B, Stadel B, Gibson M, Wilson E, Stillman R, Thompson I,** The relationship of tubal infertility to barrier method and oral contraceptive use, *JAMA* 257:2446, 1987.

6. **Rosenberg MJ, Davidson AJ, Chen J-H, Judson FN, Douglas JM,** Barrier contraceptives and sexually transmitted diseases in women: a comparison of female-dependent methods and condoms, *Am J Pub Health* 82:669, 1992.

7. **Cates Jr W, Stone K,** Family planning, sexually transmitted diseases and contraceptive choice: a literature update: part I, *Fam Plann Perspect* 24:75, 1992.

8. **Rowe PJ,** You win some and you lose some — contraception and infections, *Aust N Z Obstet Gynaecol* 34:299, 1994.

9. **Kost K, Forrest JD, Harlap S,** Comparing the health risks and benefits of contraceptive choices, *Fam Plann Perspect* 23:54, 1991.

10. **Coker AL, Hulka BS, McCann MF, Walton LA,** Barrier methods of contraception and cervical intraepithelial neoplasia, *Contraception* 45:1, 1992.

11. **Schwartz B, Gaventa S, Broome CV, Reingold AL, Hightower AW, Perlman JA, Wolf PH,** Nonmenstrual toxic shock syndrome associated with barrier contraceptives: report of a case-control study, *Rev Infect Dis* 11(Suppl):S43, 1989.

12. **Klonoff-Cohen HS, Savitz DA, Cefalo RC, McCann MF,** An epidemiologic study of contraception and preeclampsia, *JAMA* 262:3143, 1989.

13. **Mills JL, Klebanoff MA, Graubard BI, Carey JC, Berendes HW,** Barrier contraceptive methods and preeclampsia, *JAMA* 265:70, 1991.

14. **Trussell J, Hatcher RA, Cates Jr W, Stewart FH, Kost K,** Contraceptive failure in the United States: an update, *Stud Fam Plann* 21:51, 1990.

15. **Craig S, Hepburn S,** The effectiveness of barrier methods of contraception with and without spermicide, *Contraception* 26:347, 1982.

16. **Fihn SD, Latham RH, Roberts P, Running K, Stamm WE,** Association between diaphragm use and urinary tract infection, *JAMA* 254:240, 1985.

17. **Hooton TM, Scholes D, Hughes JP, Winter C, Roberts PL, Stapleton AE, Stergachis A, Stamm WE,** A prospective study of risk factors for symptomatic urinary tract infection in young women, *New Engl J Med* 335:468, 1996.

18. **Hooton TM, Hillier S, Johnson C, Roberts P, Stamm WE,** Escherichia coli bacteriuria and contraceptive method, *JAMA* 265:64, 1991.

19. **Centers for Disease Control,** Toxic shock syndrome, United States, 1970–1982, *MMWR* 31:201, 1982.

20. **Keith L, Berger G, Moss W,** Prevalence of gonorrhea among women using various methods of contraception, *Br J Venereal Dis* 51:307, 1975.

21. **Kelaghan J, Rubin GL, Ory HW, Layde PM,** Barrier method contraceptives and pelvic inflammatory disease, *JAMA* 248:184, 1982.

22. **Bernstein G, Kilzer LH, Coulson AH, Nakamara RM, Smith GC, Bernstein R, Frezieres R, Clark VA, Coan C,** Studies of cervical caps, *Contraception* 26:443, 1982.

23. **Richwald GA, Greenland S, Gerber MM, Potik R, Kersey L, Comas MA,** Effectiveness of the cavity-rim cervical cap: results of a large clinical study, *Obstet Gynecol* 74:143, 1989.

24. **Gollub EL, Sivin I,** The Prentif cervical cap and pap smear results: a critical appraisal, *Contraception* 40:343, 1989.

25. **Shihata AA, Trussell J,** New female intravaginal barrier contraceptive device, *Contraception* 44:11, 1991.

26. **Courtot AM, Nikas G, Gravanis A, Psychoyos H,** Effects of cholic acid and "Protectaid" formulations on human sperm motility and ultrastructure, *Hum Reprod* 9:1999, 1994.

27. **Psychoyos A, Creatsas G, Hassan E,** Spermicidal and antiviral properties of cholic acid: contraceptive efficacy of a new vaginal sponge (Protectaid®) containing sodium cholate, *Hum Reprod* 8:866, 1993.

28. **Edelman DA, McIntyre SL, Harper J,** A comparative trial of the Today contraceptive sponge and diaphragm: a preliminary report, *Am J Obstet Gynecol* 150:869, 1984.

29. **McIntyre SL, Higgins JE,** Parity and use-effectiveness with the contraceptive sponge, *Am J Obstet Gynecol* 155:796, 1986.

30. **Costello Daly C, Helling-Giese GE, Mati JK, Hunter DJ,** Contraceptive methods and the transmission of HIV: implications for family planning, *Genitourin Med* 70:110, 1994.

31. **Mauck CK, Baker JM, Barr SP, Johanson WM, Archer DF,** A phase I comparative study of three contraceptive films containing nonoxynol-9. Postcoital testing and coloposcopy, *Contraception* 56:97, 1997.

32. **Mauck CK, Baker JM, Barr SP, Abercrombie TJ, Archer DF,** A phase I comparative study of contraceptive films containing benzalkonium chloride and nonoxynol-9. Postcoital testing and coloposcopy, *Contraception* 56:89, 1997.

33. **Mendez F, Castro A,** Prevention of sexual transmission of AIDS/STD by a spermicide containing benzalkonium chloride, *Arch AIDS Res* 4:115, 1990.

34. **Hicks DR, Martin LS, Getchell JP, Health JL, Francis DP, McDougal JS, Curran JW, Voeller B,** Inactivation of HTLV-III/LAV-infected cultures of normal human lymphocytes by nonoxynol-9 in vitro, *Lancet* ii:1422, 1985.

35. **Kreiss J, Ngugi E, Holmes K, Ndinya-Achola J, Waiyaki P, Roberts PL, Ruminjo I, Sajabi R, Kimata J, Fleming TR, Anzala A, Holton D, Plummer F,** Efficacy of nonoxynol-9 contraceptive sponge use in preventing heterosexual acquisition of HIV in Nairobi prostitutes, *JAMA* 268:477, 1992.

36. **Zekeng L, Feldblum PJ, Oliver RM, Kaptue L,** Barrier contraceptive use and HIV infection among high risk women in Cameroon, *AIDS* 7:725, 1993.

37. **Wittkowski KM, Susser E, Kietz K,** The protective effect of condoms and nonoxynol-9 against HIV infection, *Am J Public Health* 88:590, 1998.

38. **Louv WC, Austin H, Alexander WJ, Stagno S, Cheeks J,** A clinical trial of nonoxynol-9 as a prophylaxis for cervical Neisseria gonorrhoeae and Chlamydia trachomatis infections, *J Infect Dis* 158:518, 1988.

39. **Austin H, Louv WC, Alexander WJ,** A case-control study of spermicides and gonorrhea, *JAMA* 251:2822, 1984.

40. **Niruthisard S, Roddy RE, Chutivongse S,** Use of nonoxynol-9 and reduction in rate of gonococcal and chlamydial cervical infections, *Lancet* 339:1371, 1992.

41. **Barbone F, Austin H, Louv WC, Alexander WJ,** A follow-up study of methods of contraception, sexual activity, and rates of trichomoniasis, candidiasis, and bacterial vaginosis, *Am J Obstet Gynecol* 163:510, 1990.

42. **Roddy RE, Zekeng L, Ryan KA, Tamoufém U, Weir SS, Wong EL,** A controlled trial of nonoxynol 9 film to reduce male-to-female transmission of sexually transmitted diseases, *New Engl J Med* 339:504, 1998.

43. **Louik C, Mitchell AA, Werler MM, Hanson JW, Shapiro S,** Maternal exposure to spermicides in relation to certain birth defects, *New Engl J Med* 317:474, 1987.

44. **Bracken MB, Vita K,** Frequency of non-hormonal contraception around conception and association with congenital malformations in offspring, *Am J Epidemiol* 117:281, 1983.

45. **Einarson TR, Koren G, Mattice D, Schechter-Tsafiri O,** Maternal spermicide use and adverse reproductive outcome: a meta-analysis, *Am J Obstet Gynecol* 162:655, 1990.

46. **Malyk B,** Preliminary results: serum chemistry values before and after the intravaginal administration of 5% nonoxynol-9 cream, *Fertil Steril* 35:647, 1981.

47. **Niruthisard S, Roddy RE, Chutivonge S,** The effects of frequent nonoxynol-9 use on vaginal and cervical mucosa, *Sex Transm Dis* 268:521, 1991.

48. **Roddy RE, Cordero M, Cordero C, Fortney JA,** A dosing study of nonoxynol-9 and genital irritation, *AIDS* 4:165, 1993.

49. **Hooton TM, Fennell CL, Clark AM, Stamm WE,** Nonoxynol-9: differential antibacterial activity and enhancement of bacterial adherence to vaginal epithelial cells, *J Infect Dis* 164:1216, 1991.

50. **Stone KM, Grimes DA, Magder LS,** Primary prevention of sexually transmitted diseases. A primer for clinicians, *JAMA* 255:1763, 1986.

51. **Van de Perre P, Jacobs D, Sprecher-Goldberger S,** The latex condom, an efficient barrier against sexual transmission of AIDS-related viruses, *AIDS* 1:49, 1987.

52. **Fihn SD, Boyko EJ, Normand EH, Chen C-L, Grafton JR, Hunt M, Yarbro P, Scholes D, Stergachis A,** Association between use of spermicide-coated condoms and *Escherichia coli* urinary tract infection in young women, *Am J Epidemiol* 144:512, 1996.

53. **DeVincenzi I, for the European Study Group on Heterosexual Transmission of HIV,** A longitudinal study of human immunodeficiency virus transmission by heterosexual partners, *New Engl J Med* 331:341, 1994.

54. **Diaz T, Schable B, Chu SY, and the Supplement to HIV and AIDS Surveillance Project Group,** Relationship between use of condoms and other forms of contraception among human immunodeficiency virus-infected women, *Obstet Gynecol* 86:277, 1995.

55. **Rosenberg MJ, Waugh MS, Solomon HM, Lyszkowski ADL,** The male polyurethane condom: a review of current knowledge, *Contraception* 53:141, 1996.

56. **Frezieres RG, Walsh TL, Nelson AL, Clark VA, Coulson AH,** Breakage and acceptability of a polyurethane condom: a randomized, controlled study, *Fam Plann Perspect* 30:73, 1998.

57. **Grady WR, Klepinger DH, Billy JOG, Tanfer K,** Condom characteristics: the perceptions and preferences of men in the United States, *Fam Plann Perspect* 25:67, 1993.

58. **Trussell J, Warner DL, Hatcher RA,** Condom slippage and breakage rates, *Fam Plann Perspect* 24:20, 1992.

59. **Sparrow MJ, Lavill K,** Breakage and slippage of condoms in family planning clients, *Contraception* 50:117, 1994.

60. **Rosenberg MJ, Waugh MS,** Latex condom breakage and slippage in a controlled clinical trial, *Contraception* 56:17, 1997.

61. **Population Information Program,** (The Johns Hopkins University), Population Reports, Condoms, now more than ever, Report No. H-81, 1990.

62. **Platt R, Rice PA, McCormack WM,** Risk of acquiring gonorrhea and prevalence of abnormal adnexal findings among women recently exposed to gonorrhea, *JAMA* 250:3205, 1983.

63. **Hooper RR, Reynolds GM, Jones OG, Zaidi A, Wiesner RJ, Latimer KP, Lester A, Campbell AF, Harrison WO, Karney WW, Holmes KK,** Cohort study of venereal disease. I. The risk of gonorrhea transmission from infected women to men, *Am J Epidemiol* 108:136, 1978.

64. **Anderson RM, Medley GF,** Epidemiology of HIV infection and AIDS: incubation and infectious periods, survival and vertical transmissions, *AIDS* 2(Suppl 1):557, 1988.

65. **Cameron DW, Simonsen JN, D'Costa LJ, Ronald AR, Maitha GM, Gakinya MN, Cheang M, et al,** Female to male transmission of human immunodeficiency virus type 1: risk factors for seroconverison in men, *Lancet* ii:403, 1989.

66. **Fleisher JM, Senie RT, Minkoff H, Jaccard J,** Condom use relative to knowledge of sexually transmitted disease prevention, method of birth control, and past or present infection, *J Community Health* 19:395, 1994.

67. **Soper DE, Brockwell NJ, Dalton JP,** Evaluation of the effects of a female condom on the female lower genital tract, *Contraception* 44:21, 1991.

68. **Drew WL, Blair M, Miner RC, Conant M,** Evaluation of the virus permeability of a new condom for women, *Sex Transm Dis* 17:110, 1990.

69. **Bounds W, Guillebaud J, Newman GB,** Female condom (Femidom). A clinical study of its use-effectiveness and patient acceptability, *Br J Fam Plann* 18:36, 1992.

70. **Trussell J, Sturgen K, Strickler J, Dominik R,** Comparative contraceptive efficacy of the female condom and other barrier methods, *Fam Plann Perspect* 26:66, 1994.

71. **Farr G, Gabelnick H, Sturgen K, Dorflinger L,** Contraceptive efficacy and acceptability of the female condom, *Am J Public Health* 84:1960, 1994.

72. **Trussell J,** Contraceptive efficacy of the Reality® female condom, *Contraception* 58:147, 1998.

73. **Hunt WL, Gabbay L, Potts M,** Lea's Shield®, a new barrier contraceptive; preliminary clinical evaluations, three-day tolerance study, *Contraception* 50:551, 1994.

74. **Archer DF, Mauck CK, Viniegra-Sibal A, Anderson FD,** Lea's Shield®: a phase I postcoital study of a new contraceptive barrier device, *Contraception* 52:167, 1995.

75. **Mauck C, Glover LH, Miller E, Allen S, Archer DF, Blumenthal P, Rosenzweig BA, Dominik R, Sturgen K, Cooper J, Fingerhut F, Peacock L, Gabelnick HL,** Lea's Shield®: a study of the safety and efficacy of a new vaginal barrier contraceptive used with and without spermicide, *Contraception* 53:329, 1996.

Part IV

Infertility

26   Female Infertility

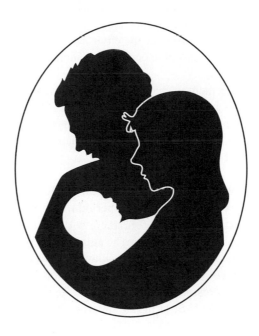

Infertility is defined as one year of unprotected coitus without conception. It affects approximately 10–15% of couples in the reproductive age group, which makes it an important component of the practices of many physicians.[1] *Fecundability* is the probability of *achieving a pregnancy* within one menstrual cycle (about 25% in normal couples); *fecundity* is the ability to *achieve a live birth* within one menstrual cycle.

There have been 3 striking changes in infertility practice during the past 2 decades. First was the introduction of in vitro fertilization and other assisted reproductive technologies (ART) that have enlarged the possibilities for successful treatment and provided an opportunity to study basic reproductive processes. ART refers to all techniques involving direct retrieval of oocytes from the ovary (Chapter 31). Second, and partially because of the media attention focused on ART, the public has become more aware of potential treatments, and this has generated a marked increase in patient visits for infertility. The third change is the increase in the proportion of women over 35 seeking medical attention for infertility. One of every five women in the United States is having a first child after 35, a marked increase over earlier figures. This reflects both a later age for marriage and postponement of pregnancy in marriage as women, by choice or by circumstances, commit to the work place. There also has been a slight increase in the proportion of couples considered infertile. More importantly, there is an increasing number of infertile couples due to the aging of the large post World War II population boom generation.

The Epidemiology of Infertility in the U.S.

The first United States census was in 1790. At that time, the birth rate was 55 per 1000 population; 200 years later, it is 15.5 per 1000 population, a decrease from 8 births per woman to 1.2.[2] There are some obvious and some speculative explanations for the decline in U.S. fertility.

Popular Explanations for the Decline in U.S. Fertility
- Changing roles and aspirations for women.
- Postponement of marriage.
- Delayed age of childbearing.
- Increasing use of contraception.
- Liberalized abortion.
- Concern over the environment.
- Unfavorable economic conditions.

The deferment of marriage and postponement of pregnancy in marriage are the most significant changes in modern society. Only 16% of the decline in the total fertility rate in the U.S. is accounted for by the increase in the average age at first marriage; 83% of the decline in the total fertility rate is accounted for by a change in marital fertility rates (avoiding pregnancy in the first years of marriage).[1, 3]

After World War II, the U.S. total fertility rate reached a modern high of 3.8 births per woman. The last women born in this period won't be reaching their 45th birthdays until around 2010. For the next decade, therefore, there will continue to be an unprecedented number of women in the later child-bearing years. The aging of the World War II population boom is giving current times a greater number of women who are delaying marriage and childbirth. The proportion of births accounted for by this older group of women increased by about 72% from 1982 to 2000.[4] These couples, pressed for time, have a desire to get pregnancies accomplished in a shorter time period. In 1996, the U.S. birth rate for women aged 30–34 was the highest since 1966, for women aged 35–39, the highest since 1968, and for women aged 40–44, the highest since 1971.[5]

Concern With Infertility

In 1995, approximately one in 6 women of reproductive age reported that they had sought professional help during their lifetimes because of infertility.[2] A sharp escalation of demand for infertility services began in 1981. From approximately 600,000 visits in 1968, the total increased to nearly 1 million in the early 1970s, then in the early 1980s, the total went over 2 million visits. In 1995, 15% of reproductive age women (9.3 million) reported some use of an infertility service, compared with 12% (6.8 million women) in 1988.[2] Approximately 1% of 60.2 million women of reproductive age used one of the methods of assisted reproductive technology, and 3% used ovulation drugs.

There was no significant change in the proportion of U.S. infertile couples in the 1980s.[6] However, the overall percentage of infertile women increased from 8.4% in 1982 and 1988 to 10.2% (6.2 million) in 1995.[2, 7] Although this increase is significantly due to the increase in older women who were born in the years after World War II, there is also an increase across all age groups, partly reflecting the effect of sexually transmitted diseases and partly an increasing concern for infertility.

Why then is there this increasing concern for infertility? First, there is an increasing number of infertile couples. As noted, the aging of the post World War II generation is yielding a greater number of women who are delaying marriage and childbirth. From 1982 to 1995, the number of childless women aged 35–44 years increased by about 1 million, from 1.9 million in 1982 to 2.8 million in 1995.[2] In addition, there is a greater awareness of modern treatments and a greater ability to afford health care. The impact of widespread publicity is significant. There is an increased availability of services, and there is a greater knowledge of the diagnosis and management of infertility among clinicians. Finally, infertility is now more socially acceptable as a problem.

The post World War II generation has faced a unique evolutionary change. They were the first to be able to exercise control over their fertility, and then as they aged and deferred pregnancy, they had to deal with the problem of unintended infertility. Because many couples defer pregnancy and then desire their families within a condensed interval of time, there is a sudden urgency regarding fertility. These factors have combined to substantially increase the number of couples seeking and using infertility services. Nevertheless, in the 1995 U.S. National Survey of Family Growth, the majority of women (56%) with impaired fecundity had not obtained any professional services.[2]

Aging and Fertility

Age alone impacts on fertility; aging of the reproductive system plays a role and spontaneous abortion provides another factor. The majority of early spontaneous abortions after age 35 are due to autosomal trisomies, the incidence of which increases with maternal age. The risk of clinically recognized spontaneous abortion increases from about 10% under age 30, to 18% in the late 30s, and 34% in the early 40s.[8] Indeed, once pregnancy is achieved by an older woman, the greatest obstacle to successful delivery is the risk of spontaneous loss. The frequency of both euploid (normal) and aneuploid (abnormal) abortuses increases with maternal age. The overall abortion risk (recognized and unrecognized) in women over age 40 is approximately 75%! [9, 10] Studies of oocytes from older women have suggested that older oocytes have impaired meiotic spindle formation or function that could cause the failure of proper chromosome migration.[11]

In addition, as women enter their 30s, there is a greater likelihood of being affected by a number of diseases, for example endometriosis, that can interfere with fertility. Cumulative exposures to occupational or environmental hazards also could lessen fertility as a woman ages. Another factor that has contributed to infertility at all ages is the spread of sexually transmitted diseases with their damaging effect on the fallopian tubes.

What is the exact impact of age on fertility? The classic study is that of the Hutterites who live in the Dakotas, Montana, and the adjacent parts of Canada. The sect originated in Switzerland in the 1500s, and practically all of the living Hutterites came to South Dakota in the 1870s. Four colonies of 443 Hutterites grew, by 1950, to 93 colonies containing 8,542 Hutterites. Contraception is condemned, and because of the communal arrangement of their society, there is no incentive to limit the size of families. All families are provided for equally.

In the 1950s, Christopher Tietze analyzed the fertility rates of the Hutterites.[12] Only 5 of 209 women had no children for an infertility rate of 2.4%. The average age of the women at the last pregnancy was 40.9 years, and there was a definite decrease in fertility with age. Eleven percent of the women bore no children after age 34; 33% of the women were infertile by age 40, and 87% were infertile at age 45.

The fertility of the Hutterites has become legendary. Their fertility rate is an example of how high fertility can be when a population is healthy, stable, and not using contraception. Based on the Hutterite data, it can be concluded that a population that marries around age 22, has some lactational amenorrhea, and some age-related and parity-related decline in coital frequency, can produce 11 live births per married woman. Hypothetically, if marriage were earlier, there were no lactational amenorrhea, and no sterilization or decline in coitus, the total fertility rate would be about 15 live births per woman.[13]

The French studied the pregnancy rate in a donor insemination program, including only women with azoospermic husbands.[14] These women were less likely to have infertility factors than those women married to oligospermic males. Below the age of 31 the pregnancy rate over one year was 74%. This decreased to 62% at ages 31 to 35 and to 54% when the women were older than 35. Because donor insemination was used, the effect of reduced coital frequency in older couples did not influence the results. An American study with donor insemination has demonstrated a similar relationship with age.[15] Of note was the requirement for more treatment cycles to achieve pregnancy in older women, 9–10 cycles rather than the usual 6. In a donor insemination program in the Netherlands, the probability of having a healthy baby decreased 3.5% per year after age

30.[16] A woman age 35 had 50% the chance of having a healthy baby compared to a woman age 25. In a study of almost 3000 donor insemination cycles in one center, the cumulative conception rates after 3, 6, and 12 cycles were 21%, 40%, and 62% for patients less than 30 years old, compared with 17%, 26%, and 44% for women 30 years and older.[17]

The decline of fertility among married couples with advancing age has been repeatedly documented.[18] It is safe to say that about one-third of women who defer pregnancy until the mid to late 30s will have an infertility problem, as will at least half of women over age 40. In programs of assisted reproductive technologies, delivery rates in women over age 40 are one-third to one-half of those in younger women, and many programs have only rare successful pregnancies in women over age 40.[19-21]

The oldest spontaneous pregnancy in modern times (according to The Guiness Book of World Records) occurred in a woman from Portland, Oregon, who delivered when she was 57 years and 120 days old. In older times, a Scottish woman was reputed to have delivered 6 children after the age of 47, the last at age 62![22]

There are changes in the male reproductive system with aging.[23] A decline in testosterone and an increase in gonadotropins are associated with a decrease in sperm production and the number of normal sperm. There are reasons to believe that the quality of sperm decreases. A paternal age greater than 40 is associated with a 20% greater chance of birth defects in the offspring.[24] These changes in the male with aging are modest, but significant, although the capacity to fertilize is maintained.[25] A short report in 1935 told of a North Carolina farmer born in 1840.[26] Over a period of 30 years, his first wife had 16 children. At age 93, he remarried to a 27-year-old widow; one year later, a child was born. Reading the detailed physical examination provided in this report, it is obvious that this 94-year-old man was very unattractive, with leathery, wrinkled skin and no teeth. It is by no means certain that he was the father of the child.

Endocrine Changes With Aging

The early fetal mitotic multiplication of germ cells produces a total of 6–7 million oogonia by 16–20 weeks of pregnancy. From this point in time, the germ cell content will irretrievably decrease. At the onset of puberty, the germ cell mass has already been reduced to approximately 300,000 units. Over the next 35–40 years of reproductive life, during which time only 400–500 oocytes will ovulate, these units will be depleted by atresia to a point at menopause when only a few hundred remain.

In the last 10–15 years before menopause, there is an acceleration of follicular loss.[27] This accelerated loss begins when the total number of follicles reaches approximately 25,000, a number reached in normal women at age 37–38.[28] This loss correlates with a subtle but real increase in follicle-stimulating hormone (FSH) and decrease in inhibin. These changes reflect the reduced quality and capability of aging follicles. These subtle changes (which influence fertility) are not associated with any noteworthy and observable changes, other than an alteration in menstrual cycle characteristics.

Prior to the menopause, there is a period with shorter follicular phases, with increased FSH levels, but normal luteinizing hormone (LH) levels and luteal phases.[29, 30] The menstrual periods for 10–15 years before the menopause are regular, but there is a steady decrease in cycle length due to the shortened follicular phase. Cycle lengths are the shortest (with the least variability) in the late 30s, a time when subtle but real increases in FSH and decreases in inhibin are occurring.[31-34] For a period of several years (as much as 10 years in some women) prior to menopause, the cycles lengthen again.

Women who present with "incipient" ovarian failure have elevated FSH levels and decreased levels of inhibin, but normal levels of estradiol.[35, 36] The rise in FSH during the later years is in response to declining inhibin production.[37–40] Inhibin levels are lower in the follicular phase in women 45–49 years old compared to younger women. The specific inhibin involved in this feedback effect on FSH during the follicular phase is inhibin B.[41, 42] In addition, a decline in luteal phase inhibin A can contribute to a greater rise in FSH during the luteal-follicular transition.[43, 179] This decline in inhibin begins early, but accelerates after 40 years of age. The rise in FSH is very apparent after age 40, but there is no change in LH levels until menopause. The changes in the later reproductive years reflect either lesser follicular competence as the better primordial follicles respond early in life, leaving the lesser follicles for later, or the fact that the total follicular pool is reduced in number (or both factors). Arguing in favor of a role for a reduced follicular pool is the observation that follicular fluid obtained from preovulatory follicles of older women contains amounts of inhibin A and B that are similar to that measured in follicular fluid from young women.[44]

These endocrine changes and the decline in ovarian follicles are correlated with a decrease in ovarian volume.[45] A measurement of volume by ultrasonography that is equal to or less than 3 cm^3 predicts a poor response to ovulation induction.[46]

Testing the Ovarian Reserve

The measurement of baseline hormonal levels provides important and helpful prognostic information. Because FSH levels increase with age, elevated FSH levels on cycle day 3 (greater than 12 IU/L, but especially greater than 20 IU/L) are associated with poor performance with in vitro fertilization.[47] A cycle day 3 FSH level that is 25 IU/L or more, or an age of 44 years or more, are both independently associated with a chance of pregnancy close to zero during ovulation induction or with assisted reproductive technologies.[48] *Values can vary between laboratories, significantly due to differences in antibodies and standards used to measure gonadotropin levels.[49] With the most recent assays, day 3 values above 10 IU/L are abnormal and are comparable with values greater than 20 IU/L with older assays.*

Women with one ovary have higher day 3 FSH levels that correlate with reduced outcomes in in vitro fertilization.[50] It is not certain whether this reflects the loss of the other ovary or the factors that were responsible for the unilateral oophorectomy.

Keep in mind that there is no abrupt change at 40, and therefore, these changes can apply to younger women. The age of change is determined by the rate of oocyte loss, a rate that is genetically programed in most women. An elevated FSH at any age is correlated with fewer available oocytes, and advancing age adds the factor of lesser oocyte quality. An elevated estradiol level on day 3 (greater than 80 pg/mL) is also predictive of difficulty in achieving pregnancy;[51, 52] premature estradiol elevations are associated with a hurried recruitment of follicles in response to increased FSH secretion, changes characteristic of the years preceding menopause. When both FSH and estradiol are elevated on day 3, ovarian response to stimulation is very poor.

The Clomiphene Challenge Test.

Navot and colleagues developed the clomiphene challenge test as a bioassay of FSH response (which in turn reflects ovarian follicular inhibin capability).[53] Clomiphene is administered in a dose of 100 mg/day on days 5–9. The level of FSH on day 10 is compared with the baseline level on day 3. An exaggerated FSH response of 26 IU/L or more was two standard deviations above the control values in this study, and this increase in FSH was associated with a significant prospect for failure to achieve pregnancy. *Remember that there is a wide variety of FSH assays (the newer assays provide numbers that are approximately 70% of the older results), and clinicians must become familiar with the values provided by their own laboratories.* There is a high incidence of abnormal responses in women over age 35, and 85% of women with increased FSH levels respond poorly to ovarian stimulation.[54] In a general infertility population, about 10% of women have an abnormal response to the clomiphene challenge test. As expected, the percentage increased with increasing age (from 3% under age 30 to 26% over age 39), and women with unexplained infertility had a 38% incidence of abnormal tests.[55] This test of ovarian reserve is more sensitive than just measuring basal FSH levels in predicting the potential for pregnancy in both assisted and natural reproduction. An abnormal response to the clomiphene challenge test indicates a poor prognosis no matter the woman's age.[49] However, because age alone is an important factor (presumably due to other age-related oocyte conditions of quality), older women with normal hormone levels and normal responses to clomiphene still have diminished chances of pregnancy.

We believe it is worthwhile to screen all infertile women beginning at age 30, women of any age with unexplained infertility, and women who respond poorly to ovulation induction with the clomiphene challenge test and a day 3 estradiol level. For practical purposes, equivalent results can be expected on days 2, 3, and 4 of the cycle. Far less certain is the need for these tests in the woman over 40, because even normal tests do not provide reassurance of adequate ovarian reserve. An abnormal test in a woman over 40, however, can be used to bolster advice to consider ovum donation. Although an abnormal test at any age indicates a very poor prognosis, it does not indicate an absolute inability to achieve pregnancy. Testing the ovarian reserve is just another part of the decision making process for patients and clinicians.

Assisted Reproduction in Older Couples

Experience has repeatedly demonstrated a reduction in IVF pregnancy rates when the oocytes are of advanced age. When embryos from the same cohort of young donated oocytes were simultaneously transferred to young and older recipients, however, the pregnancy rates were similar.[56] The high rate of implantation and pregnancy in older women receiving donated younger oocytes argues that uterine factors are not involved with the decline in fecundity with aging. Uterine factors that could suffer with age include responses of the endometrium to implantation, capillary permeability and hyperemia, and decidual differentiation.

The reproductive endocrine group at the University of Southern California has concluded that the problems of decreased fecundability and increased pregnancy wastage can be attributed to the effect of aging on oocytes. In 100 consecutive patients in an oocyte donor program, there was no decline in success over the age range from 40 to 50.[57] Furthermore, excellent outcomes have been achieved in women aged 50–62.[58, 59] There are two important observations regarding these older women. First, the older recipients of young oocytes received extensive medical screening, infectious disease screening, reproductive function assessment, and psychological assessment. The good obstetrical outcomes in these patients must reflect, to an important degree, the youthful good health of this older group of patients. Second, the stimulation protocol utilized a 100 mg dose of progesterone.

Meldrum reported a lesser percentage of delivered pregnancies in women over 40 compared with women under 40 going through an identical donor oocyte-IVF program.[19] However, he then achieved pregnancy rates in women over 40 similar to those in women under 40 by increasing the progesterone dose in the stimulation protocol from 50 mg to 100 mg per day. Meldrum argued that this age-related decline in endometrial receptivity for progesterone might be due to an age-related decline in estrogen receptors as demonstrated in animal studies. Others have also concluded that hormone treatment produces a better endometrium and corrects any uterine factor,[60] On the other hand, the uterine factor must not be a major obstacle in older women because in a carefully designed study, good quality ova derived from the same cohort yielded similar pregnancy rates in younger and older recipient women (even though the progesterone dose was 50 mg per day).[56] A pregnancy rate in older women of approximately 40–50% per cycle can be achieved in a donor oocyte program. A cumulative birth rate per patient can reach 90% with 4 or more cycles.[57–61]

The experience with donor oocyte programs argues strongly that the age-related decline in fecundity is primarily due to aging oocytes. These results further point out that the increased risks of spontaneous abortion and chromosomal anomalies associated with older age are also due primarily to aging oocytes. In a large series, the rate of spontaneous abortion in recipients correlated with the age of the donors. The abortion rate increased from 14% in recipients who received oocytes from donors aged 20–24 years to 44.5% when the recipient received oocytes from donors older than age 35.[60] Pregnancy wastage directly correlates with the age of the woman who produces the oocytes.

We know that we can establish pregnancy in women over age 50, now we have to consider whether this feat is a wise accomplishment. We have little control over natural events, but moral and social questions do arise when we have the opportunity to assist a woman to achieve a pregnancy. There can be no objection to the use of these procedures to achieve pregnancies in women who undergo ovarian failure at an early age. But when are couples too old to have a child? It can be argued that the risk involved in the pregnancy (a relatively high incidence of hypertension and gestational diabetes),[59] and the risks involved in raising a teenager when you are yourself a senior citizen are issues that patients and clinicians must resolve. On the other hand, couples over 40 may be ideal parents: high degree of motivation, increased maturity and wisdom, better financial circumstances. They are more able and willing to devote attention to their children. Certainly it is a wise precaution to discourage the use of these techniques by women who are not biologically young and healthy no matter what their age. Besides the health and medical circumstances of the individuals involved, it seems appropriate to also consider the provisions for child rearing. In our view, Paulson and Sauer put it well when they stated that "It seems unlikely that these children will be so disturbed that they would prefer not to have been born than to have suffered this indignity."[62]

Clinicians can appropriately advise older women that there is no time to waste, and serious consideration should be given to an early resort to hormonal stimulation for both oocyte response and support of the endometrium. Older couples should be provided the option of oocyte donation from young donors instead of standard assisted reproductive technologies.

The Role of the Physician

When is a medical success really a success? Approximately one-half of couples presenting after one year of infertility can be expected to become pregnant spontaneously in the following year. In an English study, only 20% of women who had failed to have a birth within the first two years of marriage never had a child.[18] In a life-table analysis of 58 untreated apparently normal infertile couples, 74% were pregnant by two years; however, normal couples achieve this rate in 9 months.[63] Overall, approximately 40% of couples become pregnant after discontinuation of treatment, and 35% of couples never treated can expect to become pregnant.[64] Therefore, achieving pregnancy is not the only measure of success. One of the important missions for the infertility physician is to speed up the period of time required to achieve pregnancy. For couples in their 30's, the recommendation to seek help promptly is valid — the sooner a problem is detected, the better. Because the incidence of spontaneous pregnancy is significant until 3 years have passed, it is appropriate to require 3 years of infertility in women less than 30 years old before making a diagnosis of infertility Because age is an important determinant, evaluation and therapy should not be deferred in older women.

In response to the needs of infertile individuals, physicians should have four goals in mind:

1. The first goal is to seek out and to correct the causes of infertility. With proper evaluation and therapy, the majority of women will become pregnant.

2. The second goal is to provide accurate information and to dispel the misinformation commonly gained from friends and mass media.

3. The third goal is to provide emotional support for the couple during a trying period. The inability to conceive generates a feeling in many couples that they have lost control over a very significant segment of their lives. The burden is aggravated by

the manipulations that couples have to undergo during the infertility investigation, including the need to have intercourse on schedule. Couples need to have an opportunity to ventilate their concerns and dispel some of their fears. A valuable adjunct to the efforts of the physician are support groups for infertile couples such as those organized by RESOLVE. Meetings in groups allows individuals to realize that their problems are not unique, and it enables them to obtain information on how others cope with infertility. It must be emphasized that, while severe anxieties can interfere with ovulation and frequency of intercourse, there is no substantial evidence that infertility is caused by the usual anxieties besetting a couple trying to conceive.

4. An often neglected goal is that of counseling a couple concerning the proper time to discontinue investigation and treatment, to consider adoption, and/or to move on to the assisted reproductive technologies. This is especially important in the 10–15% of couples with no known cause for their infertility.

Counseling also should be an ongoing process during the infertility investigation and treatment. At least every 3 months the physician and couple should review the status of their care and outline the anticipated management; thereby, changes in plans due to medical, emotional, or financial reasons can be instituted in a timely fashion.

The Female Infertility Investigation

Infertility problems, once thought to be refractory to treatment, have progressively responded to newer therapies. Occlusive tubal disease now is bypassed by in vitro fertilization. Even the most unpromising cases of male infertility can be overcome by the intracytoplasmic injection of sperm. The deleterious effects of aging on female reproduction can be neutralized by the use of ovum donation from younger women.

There are, however, many cases of infertility that yield to less intrusive and less expensive therapy. Even this area has undergone major changes, with a decreased emphasis on diagnosis, and rapid movement toward empiric therapy with superovulation and intrauterine insemination (IUI).

We find it very helpful to mail a detailed questionnaire to our patients prior to their initial visit. The questionnaire is very complete, providing information that ranges from previous medical events and sexuality to recreational, social, and vocational activities. Patients often write comments regarding their past history and their feelings that are difficult to express during an office interview.

There are advantages to having the male present during the initial interview. He may contribute valuable historical and attitudinal information. It also gives the physician the opportunity to emphasize that both partners are involved in the infertility investigation. A male who has been acquainted at its inception with the clinician's treatment of the infertility problem will be less reluctant, as time progresses, to ask for clarification of any aspect of the testing and treatment. This can prevent misunderstandings engendered when the male partner's only source of information is the woman. Early in the clinician-couple interaction, frequency of coitus, and possible sexual problems should be ascertained.

Failure to ovulate is the major problem in approximately 40% of female infertility; another 40% is due to tubal pathology and pelvic pathology, and less than 10% is due to problems such as anatomic abnormalities or thyroid disease. It should be noted that induced abortions do not influence subsequent pregnancy rates.[65] Fetal wastage is definitely higher in diethylstilbestrol-exposed women, and while there is still some uncertainty, evidence suggests that primary infertility is also more common.[66] Besides the well-known impact of smoking on pregnancy, there

Causes of Infertility

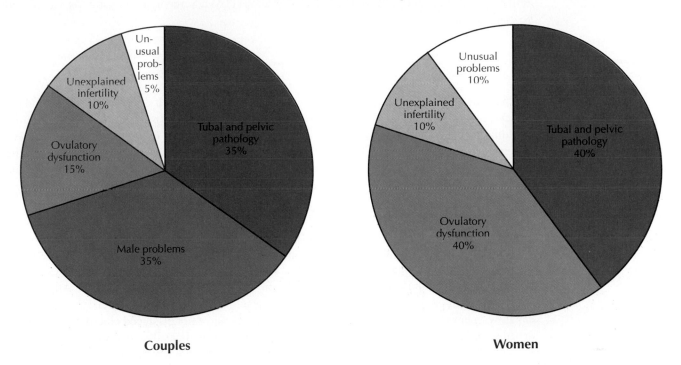

Couples   **Women**

is good evidence that fecundity is reduced in men and women who smoke, and the risk is greater with smoking at an early age.[67–69] There is a dose-response relationship between the number of cigarettes smoked and how long it takes to achieve pregnancy.[70] Marijuana inhibits the secretion of GnRH and can suppress reproductive function in both men and women, and cocaine use is known to reduce spermatogenesis.[71, 72] Studies have failed to confirm an adverse impact of caffeine on fertility, although high levels of intake may be associated with a delay in conception.[69, 73, 74]

Couples need to be aware that there is a normal time requirement to achieve pregnancy. In each ovulatory cycle, normal couples have only about a 30% chance of becoming pregnant. Guttmacher's classic table has been a standard since 1956.

Time Required for Conception in Couples Who Will Attain Pregnancy [75]

Time of Exposure	% Pregnant
3 months	57%
6 months	72%
1 year	85%
2 years	93%

Because the male factor accounts for approximately 35% of infertility, examination of the semen should be an early diagnostic step in the investigation. If abnormal, further diagnostic procedures in the woman should be deferred until decisions are reached regarding the man (see Chapter 29). If the semen is normal, attention is directed to the woman.

Laboratory testing should be directed by clinical judgment. However, there are a few specific recommendations. Women with a negative rubella titer should be immunized and attempts for pregnancy delayed for 3 months. When personnel are exposed to sperm and/or oocytes, many states now mandate tests for syphilis, antihepatitis B core, hepatitis B surface antigen, antihepatitis C, and antibody to HIV 1/2 (AIDS) and HTLV-I. Screening for cystic fibrosis should be considered.

The Postcoital Test

The postcoital test provides information regarding both the receptivity of cervical mucus and the ability of sperm to reach and survive in the mucus. Estrogen levels peak just prior to ovulation, and this provides maximal stimulation of the cervical glands. An outpouring of clear, watery mucus is fostered, which may be of sufficient quantity to be noted by the woman. Earlier in the cycle, when estrogen output is lower, and starting 2 to 3 days after ovulation when progesterone levels increase and counteract the estrogen, the mucus is thick, viscid, and opaque.

The postcoital test is performed around the time of the expected luteinizing hormone (LH) surge as determined by a previous basal body temperature chart or by the length of prior cycles. Timing also can be obtained with ultrasonography and LH monitoring, but this usually is not necessary. Between 2 and 8 hours after coitus, cervical mucus is removed with a nasal polyp forceps or tuberculin syringe and examined for macroscopic and microscopic characteristics. Attempts to refine the postcoital test by studying individual fractions from different levels in the cervical canal, with emphasis on the sample from the internal os, have not produced convincing evidence of value. Sperm distribution is uniform throughout the cervical canal, and selective sampling at the level of the internal os is not necessary.[76] A less than 2-hour interval between coitus and examination has been recommended as giving maximal information, but this early evaluation may be deceptive because complement dependent reactions in mucus, which can immobilize sperm may not be apparent for a few hours. Others have suggested that a 16- to 24-hour interval provides a better assessment of sperm longevity, and a study has indicated that there is no drop in the number of sperm at any time during the first 24 hours.[77] There are other indications, however, that the number of sperm does decrease after 8 hours, and this is more in keeping with our experience. Therefore, we suggest that the couple have coitus in the morning or late at night, and that the test be performed 2 to 8 hours later. It is also suggested that the couple abstain from intercourse for 48 hours prior to the postcoital test.

The need for scheduling the postcoital test at precise times in the cycle may produce problems for the couple who cannot have sex on demand. This may further burden a couple already troubled by the need to cope with their infertility and the loss of control involved in the infertility investigation. A physician must be sympathetic to this problem, and on occasion, precise timing must be sacrificed and the woman told to come to the office following unscheduled intercourse.

The stretchability (*spinnbarkeit*) of the mucus at midcycle should be 8–10 cm or more. This characteristic can be assessed as the mucus is pulled from the cervix, or alternatively, by placing the mucus on a slide, covering it with a coverslip and then lifting the coverslip. At midcycle the mucus contains 95–98% water and should be watery, thin, clear, acellular, and abundant. When dried on a slide, it should form a distinct fern pattern.

If the mucus is thick rather than thin, opaque instead of clear, the proximity of the test to ovulation should be determined by the onset of the next period (or by the temperature chart if one is being taken during that cycle). The best time for the postcoital test is the day prior to the first temperature elevation. If poor mucus quality is related to inaccurate timing, the test should be repeated in a subsequent cycle with scheduling based on urinary LH testing. Poor mucus at midcycle can be a physical barrier that decreases sperm penetration. In one study 54% of women with good mucus became pregnant, compared to 37% with poor mucus, a statistically significant difference.[78] In all likelihood some of these poor tests were reflections of inaccurate timing, and pregnancies do occur even with poor mucus at ovulation time.[79] It remains our impression, however, that poor mucus is associated with a decreased chance for fertility.

Fern Pattern

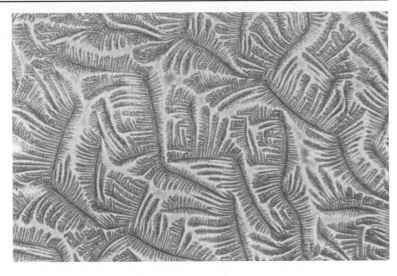

Lack of Fern

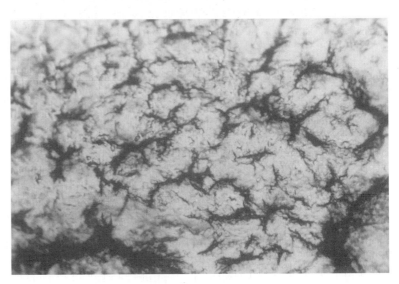

Treatment of poor mucus has been attempted by giving 0.625 mg of conjugated estrogens daily for the 8 or 9 days preceding the expected time of ovulation. In a 28-day cycle that would be between days 5 and 13. There is no advantage to continuing the hormone treatment through the luteal phase of the cycle. If the initial treatment with estrogen fails to produce a change in the mucus, the dose is increased to 1.25 mg/day. In refractory cases, 5 mg of conjugated estrogens can be given starting a few days prior to expected ovulation. However, evidence for the value of estrogen therapy is lacking, and it has no demonstrable benefit for the poor mucus which is, on occasion, associated with the use of clomiphene citrate.[80] If there is evidence of chronic cervicitis with thick yellowish mucus, culture for chlamydia is important, and, where appropriate, systemic antibiotics should be used. On rare occasions, the cervix is treated with electrocautery or cryosurgery.

The most logical approach to overcome the barrier of thick cervical mucus is the method we prefer, the use of intrauterine insemination (IUI) of washed sperm (discussed below and in Chapter 29). If poor mucus is the sole problem, IUI for 3–4 cycles is associated with a cumulative pregnancy rate of 40–50%.[81]

In addition to providing an evaluation of mucus, the postcoital test also gives information concerning the male. Absence of sperm requires a review of the couple's coital technique. Repeated cancellations of appointments for the postcoital test may be a clue that there are sexual problems that have not been uncovered by the interview. However, most often the stress of performance for the scheduled postcoital test is responsible for the failure to achieve coitus. Most importantly, absence of sperm necessitates a detailed review of the semen specimen.

One of the most difficult problems in infertility is the postcoital test that repeatedly shows no sperm or only dead sperm despite good mucus. The patient should be cautioned that lubricants, such as K-Y Jelly and Surgilube, have a spermicidal effect in vitro and should not be used by infertile couples. If lubrication is necessary, vegetable oil can be used without interfering with sperm movement. As noted earlier, re-examination of the semen to check sperm count and motility is a necessity if the postcoital test is poor.

If the semen is normal, the pH of the cervical mucus at midcycle should be determined. Good results have been reported using a precoital douche of 1 tablespoon of sodium bicarbonate in 1 quart of water when a poor postcoital test was associated with a pH below 7.[82] Cervical cultures should be obtained for chlamydia if the mucus is yellowish, and sperm antibody testing should be performed in cases where there are no sperm or mostly nonmotile sperm. In addition, sperm antibody testing (Chapter 29) is mandatory when, in a postcoital test with good mucus, the sperm are found shaking in place but not moving progressively. This shaking movement is a common finding in immunologic infertility.

In vitro cross testing, utilizing donor or bovine mucus and donor sperm, can help to determine whether the poor postcoital test is due to factors in the mucus or to defects in the sperm. However, in clinical practice this type of testing has little value because the next step is treatment with IUI regardless of results with cross testing.

A postcoital test cannot be considered a substitute for a semen analysis. While 21 or more sperm/ high power field (HPF) is almost always associated with a sperm count above 20 million/mL, the postcoital test gives little information concerning the morphology of sperm in the ejaculate. There are considerably fewer abnormal forms in the cervical mucus compared to the ejaculate. This may represent a filtering effect of the cervical mucus or may indicate that abnormal forms do not have the motility to penetrate the cervical mucus.

The postcoital test has had a role in the infertility investigation for over 100 years.[83] The postcoital examination first received prominence in the late 1800s in the writings of J. Marion Sims who was primarily interested in how long sperm survived in the mucus. Sims' son, Harry, reported to the American Gynecological Society in 1888 the details and purpose of the postcoital test, essentially as still performed today. The major impetus to general clinical use can be attributed to a book published in 1913 by Max Hühner, entitled *Sterility in the Male and Female*. Hühner, born in Berlin and a graduate of the College of Physicians and Surgeons of Columbia University, was a urologist in New York City. His second book, *A Practical Treatise on Disorders of the Sexual Function in the Male and Female*, was published in 1916 and went through 3 editions and a Spanish translation; this was followed by a third book in 1937. Thus, the postcoital test is also known as the Sims-Hühner test.

The postcoital test has always had its detractors because of limited correlations with fertility, the inability to establish universally agreed upon normal values, and controversies concerning the proper treatment of a poor postcoital test. One study could find no difference in the subsequent pregnancy rates among groups having no sperm, no motile sperm, 1–5 motile sperm, 6–10 motile sperm, and 11 or more motile sperm.[79] Another study indicated that there was a statistically significant increase in the percentage of pregnancies only when there were more than 20 sperm/ HPF.[78] Moreover, in a study of postcoital tests in *fertile* couples, 20% had either no sperm or less than one sperm/HPF.[84] A newer argument raised against use of the postcoital test is that widespread use of intrauterine inseminations (IUI) combined with superovulation has made the assessment of sperm-cervical mucus interactions merely an academic exercise. In this view, whether the postcoital test is normal or abnormal, the treatment is the same.

Given the array of negative assessments of the postcoital test, what can be said in its defense beyond that it provides an opportunity to observe interactions of sperm and a product of the female reproductive tract. If the mucus is clear and abundant with good spinnbarkeit, the patient has a better chance for pregnancy than if it is thick and sparse. If sperm are found in the mucus, it is reasonable assurance that coital technique is adequate. Additional reassurance is provided by the finding of motile sperm in the postcoital test. If live sperm are found in the cervical mucus, the pH is not hostile and the pregnancy rate is higher than if the sperm are all immotile. If there are more than 20 sperm/HPF, the male, in all likelihood, has a sperm count above 20 million/mL, and the couple has a significantly better chance for pregnancy than if the postcoital test contains fewer than 20 sperm/HPF. A poor result in the postcoital test can raise a suspicion of an immunologic problem. A poor result also can suggest the need for intrauterine inseminations. Individuals with progressively motile sperm in the postcoital test have significantly higher pregnancy rates.[85] In addition, sperm numbers in the postcoital test correlate with the length of time it takes to become pregnant. We believe there is still a limited usefulness for the postcoital test. When postcoital tests repeatedly reveal no sperm, only sperm shaking in place, only immotile sperm, or only a few motile sperm, despite good mucus, and when the mucus is repeatedly poor, timed IUI, without the risks and expense of superovulation, is appropriate therapy for 3–4 cycles.

What constitutes a poor postcoital test in terms of sperm numbers is controversial. Intrauterine insemination has been reported to enhance the chances for pregnancy when there were 3 or fewer sperm/HPF in the postcoital test but not when there were 5 or more sperm/HPF.[86] We continue to support a minimum level of one motile progressive sperm/HPF as compatible with normality. The finding of no sperm, all dead sperm or a large proportion of shaking sperm suggests a possible immunologic factor. These findings, specifically immotile or absent sperm, also should prompt inquiry concerning use of vaginal lubricants. If there are no motile sperm in the postcoital test, the pH of the mucus should be determined.

Hysterosalpingography

A history of pelvic inflammatory disease, septic abortion, ruptured appendix, tubal surgery, or ectopic pregnancy alerts the physician to the possibility of tubal damage. Pelvic inflammatory disease is unquestionably the major contributor to tubal infertility and ectopic pregnancies. Westrom's classic studies with laparoscopically confirmed pelvic inflammatory disease indicated that the incidence of subsequent tubal infertility is approximately 12% after one episode of pelvic infection, 23% after two episodes, and 54% after three episodes.[87] The risk of ectopic pregnancy is increased 6–7-fold after pelvic infection. Almost one-half of patients who are eventually found to have tubal damage and/or pelvic adhesions, however, have no history of antecedent disease. Many of these women will have elevated anti-Chlamydia antibodies, suggestive of prior infection. There have been a few reports of damaged tubes showing histologic evidence of viral infection which could explain the absence of traditional causes of tubal damage.

Tubal disease is diagnosed by the hysterosalpingogram (HSG) and by laparoscopy. The HSG is performed 2 to 5 days after cessation of a menstrual flow. If there is a history suggestive of pelvic inflammatory disease, a sedimentation rate is obtained prior to the HSG and, if elevated, antibiotic therapy is given. The procedure is than postponed for a month when a repeat sedimentation rate is obtained. Only if this is normal is the HSG scheduled. If masses or tenderness are revealed by the pelvic examination at any time, the HSG should be bypassed and the pelvis evaluated by laparoscopy. If there is a documented history of pelvic inflammatory disease, the risk of a serious reinfection following HSG is too high, and it should be replaced by laparoscopy. If an HSG is performed in a patient who is at questionable risk for infection, a water-soluble rather than an oil dye should be used because of the faster absorption. The overall risk of infection with HSG is probably less than 1%, although in a high-risk population serious infection can occur in approximately 3% of cases.[88] Clinically apparent infections were not present in 398 women who had nondilated tubes on HSG; however, 11% of those with dilated tubes developed pelvic inflammatory disease following an HSG.[89] Doxycycline, 200 mg after the procedure, can be administered if the tubes are dilated, followed by 100 mg bid for 5 days. Many clinicians routinely administer prophylactic antibiotics (doxycycline, 100 mg bid for 5 days, beginning 2 days before the procedure).

HSG should be performed under image intensification fluoroscopy, and a minimal number of films taken. Too often, multiple oblique views are taken to delineate small filling defects in the uterus that are of no clinical significance. In our experience, the oblique films are of little help even in diagnosing tubal patency. Only 3 films are usually required — a preliminary before dye is injected, a film showing spill of dye from one or both tubes, and a delayed film to show spread of dye through the peritoneal cavity. The dye can be injected either using a classic Jarcho cannula with a single-tooth tenaculum, or its more modern variants through a cannula contained within a suction apparatus that attaches to the cervix, or by using a pediatric Foley catheter threaded through the cervix into the uterus. Use of a prostaglandin synthesis inhibitor 30 minutes prior to the procedure can decrease the pain many women experience with HSG.

The dye should be injected slowly so that abnormalities of the uterine cavity are not missed. This is of special importance in diethylstilbestrol-exposed women, many of whom have abnormalities of uterine contour. Usually no more than 3 to 6 mL of dye are required to fill the uterus and tubes. If the patient complains of cramping, the injection of dye should be stopped for a few minutes and fluoroscopy temporarily discontinued. Spasm is rare with Ethiodol, an oil dye that is our preferred medium; if it does occur, slow injection with pauses is helpful. If the tubes fill but dye droplets do not spill from the ends of the tubes, the uterus should be pushed up in the abdomen by means of the tenaculum or suction cup. This puts the tubes on stretch and may help to release dye from the fimbriated ends. The droplets seen coming from the tube are the result of mixing of the oil dye and peritoneal fluid. On occasion, injection of dye into a hydrosalpinx will produce a similar pattern, and a delayed film to show loculation of dye is crucial in differentiating this condition from normal spill where the dye is distributed throughout the pelvis.

If dye goes through one tube rapidly and fails to enter the other tube, it usually means that the dye-containing tube presents the path of least resistance. In this situation, the nonfilling tube is usually normal. In our own series, when both tubes were patent on x-ray, the pregnancy rate was only slightly higher (58%) than when there was unilateral patency and nonfilling of the other tube (50%).[90] This finding has been confirmed in a more recent study.[91]

Evidence of distal tubal disease on HSG is usually confirmed when laparoscopy is performed. However, a normal study does not rule out pelvic pathology, especially adhesions or endometriosis. While the diagnostic usefulness of the HSG is established, its value as a therapeutic procedure in infertility is a subject of some controversy. Does an HSG enhance fertility, and, if so, is the effect seen with both oil and water-soluble dyes? A conception rate of 41.3% within 1 year of an HSG with oil media has been reported, whereas the rate was only 27.3% when water-soluble agents were employed.[92] This is in accord with other reports where the great majority of pregnancies that followed HSG occurred within 7 months of the procedure. A review of the question of oil versus aqueous dye noted that in every retrospective study in which increased pregnancy rates were noted after HSG, an oil dye was used.[93]

In a randomized, prospective study of close to 400 women, the pregnancy and live birth rates were increased in women who had their HSG performed with oil dye.[94] Within 9 ovulation cycles following an HSG, the pregnancy rate was 33% in the oil dye group and 17% in the water dye group. However, another prospective, randomized study indicated no difference in subsequent pregnancy rates following HSG with oil or water dye.[95] Nevertheless, most of the evidence indicates that HSG with Ethiodol is a very useful therapeutic as well as diagnostic tool in women with infertility.[96]

The effect of the oil dye on fertility could involve any of a number of mechanisms:

1. It may produce a mechanical lavage of the tubes, dislodging mucus plugs.

2. It may straighten the tubes and thus break down peritoneal adhesions.

3. It may provide a stimulatory effect for the cilia of the tube.

4. It may improve the cervical mucus.

5. The iodine may exert a bacteriostatic effect on the mucous membranes.

6. Ethiodol decreases in vitro phagocytosis by peritoneal macrophages. If the same effect occurs in vivo it could decrease macrophage activity and thus aid fertility by inhibiting the release of cytokines and decreasing phagocytosis of sperm.[97, 98]

The use of an oil medium has been criticized on grounds that it is only slowly absorbed and may cause granuloma formation. Granulomas are found very infrequently, and they also can follow the use of water dyes. An additional fear with oil dye is embolization. However, only 13 cases of dye intravasation were encountered in 533 HSGs performed with Ethiodol.[99] Six of these women had embolization of the dye, but there were no symptoms, and no morbidity was noted. When fluoroscopy is used, venous or lymphatic intravasation can be detected immediately, and injection of dye halted. A common approach is to demonstrate tubal patency with a water soluble dye, then follow with Ethiodol for its fertility-enhancing effects.

HSG is less sensitive than sonohysterography in the identification of uterine polyps or myomas. Sonohysterography involves the injection of saline into the uterine cavity by means of a #8 pediatric Foley catheter with the balloon inflated in the cervix, followed by ultrasonography of the uterus. Similarly, saline or albumin-based fluids can be tracked by ultrasound as they course through the tubes into the peritoneal cavity, providing evidence of tubal patency without the use of x-ray.[100] Sonohysterography with a contrast solution of galactose microbubbles in galactose (Echovist) is being utilized in Europe to provide an overall evaluation of the pelvis, the uterus, and the fallopian tubes.[101, 102]

Hysteroscopy

Hysteroscopy is a technique that complements hysterosalpingography. Direct visualization of the uterine cavity with a hysteroscope is good for differentiating between endometrial polyps and submucous leiomyomas, establishing the definitive diagnosis and treatment of intrauterine adhesions, and for the diagnosis and treatment of intrauterine congenital anomalies. One can argue from a cost-effective point of view that hysterosalpingography and sonohysterography are more useful screening procedures. The hysteroscope should be reserved to pursue abnormalities identified by other techniques, especially when operative intervention is planned.

Falloposcopy

Because of its narrow and tortuous character, it has been difficult to pass probes via the uterine cavity into the fallopian tube. This problem was overcome by the development of self-seeking guidewires and the adaptation of techniques used for coronary angioplasty. Hysteroscopic directed falloposcopy can be utilized to transvaginally examine the entire length of the tubal lumen.[103] This technique requires considerable expertise, but it has verified that the tubal ostium can undergo spasm, and intraluminal debris is present that can be a cause of tubal obstruction. The latter can be cleared by cannulation or balloon tuboplasty, or even be by hysterosalpingography. Visualization of the inner aspect of the tube can also be accomplished from the distal end of the tube at the time of laparoscopy. Falloposcopy, originating at either end of the tube, can provide a good assessment of the tubal lining, indicating the prospect of success with tubal surgery.

Outpatient Canalization of the Tube

Proximal tubal obstruction can be treated by outpatient tubal cannulation or balloon tuboplasty. Transcervical tuboplasty can be performed by either a fluoroscopic or hysteroscopic approach, although most of the experience thus far is with the fluoroscopic technique.[104–106] Discomfort can be minimized with intravenous sedation and a paracervical block. Cannulation and balloon tuboplasty success is achieved in at least one tube in 80–90% of attempts. Approximately 30% of patients will become pregnant in the 3–6 months following the procedure. The advantage of these accomplishments is the avoidance of expensive surgery or assisted reproductive technology.

Disorders of Ovulation

Disorders of ovulation account for approximately 20% of all infertility problems in couples. These can be anovulation or severe oligoovulation. In the latter cases, even though ovulation does occur, its relative infrequency decreases the woman's chances for pregnancy. If periods occur only every 3 or 4 months, for practical purposes it matters little whether these are ovulatory or anovulatory. Anovulatory or oligoovulatory women should be promptly treated with clomiphene citrate to increase the frequency of, or to initiate, ovulation (see Chapter 30), and the drug can be started immediately, even before other areas have been investigated. If anovulation is the only infertility factor, most couples will become pregnant within 3 months of ovulation induction. Women with amenorrhea or hyperandrogenic anovulation should be evaluated and managed according to the clinical approaches detailed in Chapters 11, 12, and 13.

Basal Body Temperature

Women who have menstrual periods at monthly intervals marked by premenstrual symptoms and dysmenorrhea are almost always ovulatory, but not always; 5% are anovulatory. Indirect confirmatory evidence of ovulation can be obtained by use of basal body temperature (BBT) charts. The temperature can be taken orally with a regular thermometer or with special instruments (unnecessarily expensive however) that show a range of only a few degrees and thus are easier to read. The temperature is best taken immediately upon awakening and before any activity. The woman may be surprised to find that the basal temperatures are substantially lower than the usual 98.6° F (37° C). Days when intercourse takes place should be noted on the chart, and this may give the physician an indication that coital frequency is a problem.

Use of the BBT chart has been criticized because a small percentage of women who ovulate have monophasic graphs, and there is often disagreement concerning interpretation of individual charts. Moreover, the time of ovulation predicted by the BBT does not always correlate well with measurements of the LH surge or with perceptions of maximal cervical mucus production. There is a relationship between a nadir in the BBT and the LH surge, but the BBT is reliable in predicting the day of the LH surge only within 2–3 days.[107] Although the nadir is believed to represent the beginning of the LH surge, the occurrence of a nadir is variable and often is not detected. To be used prospectively to predict ovulation, nearly absolute cycle regularity is required, and this occurs infrequently.

Nevertheless, we still find the BBT helpful as a preliminary indicator of ovulation and as a tool for advising patients about the timing of intercourse. Patients should not become fixated on taking their temperatures, and usually several months of charts are sufficient.

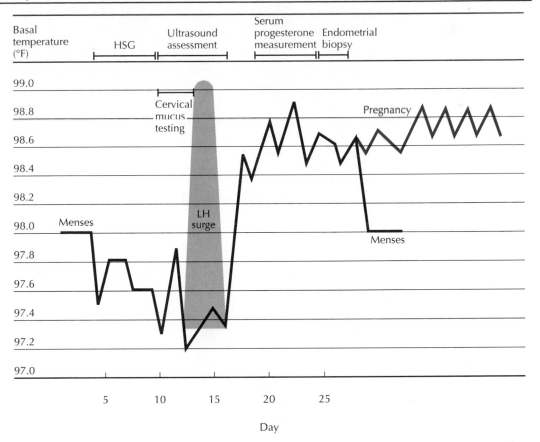

A significant increase in temperature is not noted until 2 days after the LH peak, coinciding with a rise in peripheral levels of progesterone to greater than 4 ng/mL.[108] Physical release of the ovum probably occurs on the day prior to the first temperature elevation. The temperature elevation should be sustained for 11 to 16 days, falling at the time of the subsequent menstrual period.

If an approximate time of ovulation can be determined by temperature charts, a sensible schedule for coitus is every 36 to 48 hours in a period encompassed by 3 to 4 days prior to and 2 days after expected ovulation. It is unwise, however, to demand rigid adherence to a schedule. This may produce psychologic stress sufficient to inhibit sexual relations.

In discussing coital timing, the patients frequently want to know the fertilizable life of the sperm and the egg. The fertilizable life of the human oocyte is unknown, but most estimates range between 12 and 24 hours. However, immature human eggs recovered for in vitro fertilization can be fertilized even after 36 hours of incubation. Equally uncertain is knowledge of the fertilizable lifespan of human sperm. The most common estimate is 48–72 hours, although motility can be maintained after the sperm have lost the ability to fertilize. The extreme intervals that have achieved pregnancy documented after a single act of coitus are 6 days prior to and 3 days after ovulation.[109] The great majority of pregnancies occur when coitus takes place within the 3-day interval just prior to ovulation.[110]

Home urinary LH testing is commonly used to assist diagnostic and therapeutic timing. The postcoital test should be performed within 12 hours of a positive urinary LH test.[111] However, appropriate use of the basal body temperature chart yields results equivalent to those obtained with the more expensive methods of urinary LH assays, and also directs the patients regarding "timing" of further urinary LH testing..[112]

Endometrial Biopsy

A reliable assessment of ovulation can be obtained by endometrial biopsy. Endometrial biopsy is performed 2 to 3 days prior to the expected period, although a biopsy performed in the midluteal phase is superior for diagnosing luteal phase defects.[113] The histology is read by the criteria outlined by Noyes, Hertig, and Rock,[114] Although premenstrual biopsy could interrupt a pregnancy if performed in a conception cycle, the danger is not great.[115] We recommend the use of the plastic endometrial suction curette. It is easy to use, requires cervical dilation only occasionally, and is usually painless.

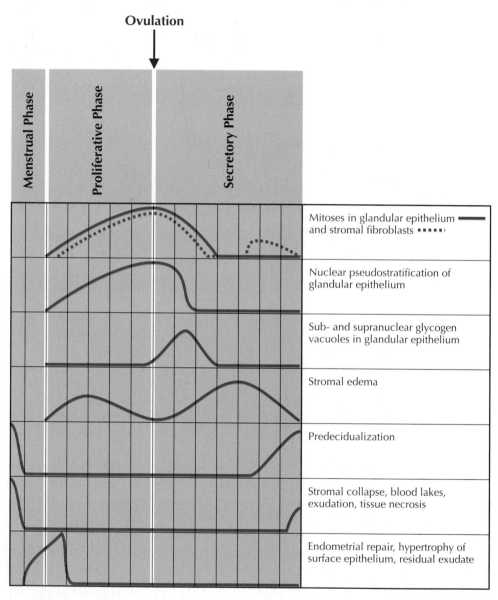

After Noyes, et al [9]

Progesterone Measurements

A serum progesterone level of less than 3 ng/mL is consistent with follicular phase levels.[116] To confirm ovulation, values at the midluteal phase, just at the midpoint between ovulation and the onset of the subsequent menstrual period, should be at least 6.5 ng/mL and preferably 10 ng/mL or more. The consensus of opinion is that a single midluteal phase progesterone level is *insufficient* evidence upon which to judge the adequacy of the luteal phase.[117–122] The progesterone level is subject to the variation associated with pulsatile secretion, but more importantly, there is often poor correlation with the histologic state of the endometrium.

Luteal Phase Defect (Inadequate Luteal Phase)

A luteal phase defect, historically defined as a lag of more than two days in histologic development of the endometrium compared to day of the cycle (presumably due to inadequate progesterone secretion or action), can be found in up to 30% of isolated cycles of normal women, and only if the defect is found repeatedly is it thought to be a possible factor in infertility. Approximately 3 to 4% of infertile women will be diagnosed as having luteal phase defect, and the incidence may be higher (approximately 5%) in women with a history of recurrent abortions.[123]

Although luteal phase defect is often a direct result of decreased hormone production by the corpus luteum, the underlying causes of this dysfunction can be multiple. Decreased levels of FSH in the follicular phase of the cycle, abnormal patterns of LH secretion, decreased levels of LH and FSH at the time of the ovulatory surge, or decreased response of the endometrium to progesterone have been implicated.[121] Elevated prolactin levels and hypothyroidism can be associated with luteal phase defect, emphasizing the importance of assessing prolactin and TSH levels in infertile women with less than normal ovulatory cycles.

The diagnosis should be considered in women with normal cycles and unexplained infertility, women with short luteal phases demonstrated by basal body temperature charts, and women with a history of recurrent spontaneous abortions.

Controversies surrounding the concept of luteal phase defect have revolved around issues of diagnosis, endometrial biopsy versus progesterone levels, and treatment, progesterone versus clomiphene citrate. However, a more fundamental question must be addressed. Is there really such an entity as luteal phase defect, and even if there is, does it play any role in infertility?

As noted above, although measuring progesterone levels has been advocated as a means of diagnosing luteal phase defect, the majority of clinical studies on this subject have used endometrial biopsy as the standard. The endometrium must lag behind the day of the cycle by greater than two days, and the lag must occur in more than one cycle. Whereas it is common to date the cycle day from the onset of the subsequent menstrual period, there is evidence that better dating can be achieved by counting forward from the LH surge.[124, 125]

An important issue is how well can the physician, usually a pathologist, date the endometrium. When the same observer viewed 63 endometrial biopsies on two separate occasions, there was exact agreement in only 15 (24%).[126] Disagreement of more than two days in the dating of the endometrium occurred in six instances (10%). A further problem in establishing luteal phase defect as a clinical entity is the finding in most studies of an out-of-phase biopsy in approximately 20% to 30% of normal cycles and repetitive lags in more than one normal cycle of approximately 5%.[125, 127] These figures suggest that luteal phase defect occurs by chance alone.

The frequency of luteal phase defect in women with infertility, when strictly defined, is no greater than that found by chance in normal cycles.[127] In a series of 1492 biopsies in 1055 women reported by Balasch, there were 26 biopsies in conception cycles.[128] With an in-phase biopsy, 15 of 20 pregnancies went to term but 4 out of 6 pregnancies with out-of-phase biopsies also went to term. Similarly, the term pregnancy rates were almost identical in women treated and untreated for luteal phase defect. There is a window of endometrial hormonally-induced development during which successful embryo transfer with in vitro fertilization can occur.[129] The window extends over a 6-day period, and this indicates that precise synchronization of the endometrium and the embryo may not be needed for successful implantation.

Given the uncertainties surrounding the diagnosis of luteal phase defect, it becomes difficult to justify putting women through the expense and possible pain of endometrial biopsy.

In common practice, again because of the discomfort, the difficulties of precise dating, and the expense associated with endometrial biopsy, attention has turned to measurements of serum progesterone levels as a means of diagnosing, if not luteal phase defect, then at least a "hormone deficiency." Whereas exact normal values for progesterone are in some dispute, many physicians believe that a level of less than 10 ng/mL one week prior to the onset of menstruation or 5–7 days after the LH surge is a good indication of a luteal phase defect. Frequently a diagnosis of "hormone deficiency" is made based on an isolated and not always well timed progesterone level of less than 10 ng/mL. It is also common practice to utilize such a finding as a rationale for treating as if a luteal phase defect were present. Daily progesterone measurements taken throughout the luteal phase could provide strong evidence for a luteal phase defect if the values are low, but such frequent sampling is impractical. An assessment of various approaches for progesterone measurements concluded that the best correlation with endometrial histology is achieved with 3 progesterone levels obtained randomly during days 5–9 after ovulation (normal equal to or greater than a sum of 30 ng/mL or a pooled concentration, a less expensive alternative, greater than 9 ng/mL).[130] Most important, however, is the impressive evidence documenting poor correlation between progesterone measurements and endometrial histology. [117–122]

Other methods of diagnosis include the basal body temperature chart, ultrasonography of follicular size, and salivary progesterone measurements. All have been studied, and all demonstrate poor correlations with multiple progesterone levels and endometrial histology.[130, 131]

Treatment of Luteal Phase Defect

Based on findings that low FSH values prior to ovulation can be associated with luteal phase defect, it would seem reasonable, in selected cases, to use human gonadotropins or clomiphene citrate. Gonadotropin treatment is expensive, has the potential for causing hyperstimulation of the ovaries, and is associated with an increased incidence of multiple births. Because of these effects, gonadotropin treatment is seldom, if ever, used for this indication. Clomiphene citrate is the first choice of many clinicians for the treatment of luteal phase defect. The only significant risk is a 5% (twice normal) chance of multiple births, essentially all twins. The initial dose is 50 mg a day for 5 days starting on day 3, 4, or 5 of the cycle (Chapter 30).

Because there is a suspected deficiency of progesterone in luteal phase defect, exogenous progesterone has been utilized. A vaginal suppository compounded by a pharmacist and containing 25 mg of progesteroe is inserted bid starting approximately 2–3 days after ovulation. Treatment is maintained until menstruation occurs or through the 10th week of a pregnancy. Once pregnancy is diagnosed, a switch can be made to weekly injections of 17-hydroxyprogesterone caproate (250 mg) through the 10th week of pregnancy. Oral micronized progesterone can be utilized in a dose of 100 mg tid; however, the oral administration of progesterone leads to metabolic products that cause somnolence and other CNside effects. Progesterone in a gel that adheres to the vaginal mucosa (Crinone) is available in a prefilled vaginal applicator, applied with one 8% (90 mg progesterone) application daily. Vaginal administration accomplishes targeted delivery to the uterus without producing high circulating levels. Using progesterone therapy, success rates of approximately 50% have been acheved, but good controlled studies are lacking.

There is no difference in pregnancy rates in studies comparing clomiphene and progesterone treatment.[132–134] In our view, this is an argument in favor of clomiphene because of a significant disadvantage associated with progesterone therapy. Progesterone supplementation prolongs the luteal phase and can delay the onset of menses. This is not a problem for the clinician, but for the couple the disappointment at the time of delayed menses or a negative pregnancy test is profound.

Dopamine agonist treatment has been reported to correct luteal phase defect associated with hyperprolactinemia, but its value in women with normal prolactin levels has not been demonstrated. In a subgroup of patients with unexplained infertility, high normal prolactin levels, and expressible galactorrhea, treatment with bromocriptine enhanced fertility compared to similar women treated with pyridoxine.[135] If galactorrhea is present, even if the prolactin is normal, ovulatory dysfunction responds well to dopamine agonist therapy.[136] In the absence of galactorrhea, a prolactin elevation may be subtle (such as an increase in nocturnal peaks), and this could explain occasional good responses to dopamine agonist treatment. In evaluating any therapy it is important to keep in mind that pregnancies can occur without treatment in women who are diagnosed as having luteal phase defect.

Many physicians dispense with the diagnostic evaluation of hormone adequacy and proceed to treatmentith clomiphene citrate. It is a reasonable argument that there may be subtle hormonal abnormalities that cannot be diagnosed with current technology but that can be successfully treated by stimulating the ovaries. Moreover, there is a theoretical advantage in having more than one oocyte in the fallopian tube at the time of fertilization. Randomized placebo-controlled studies support the efficacy of this approach (reviewed with references in Chapter 30). By contrast, some have not found a benefit for the use of clomiphene citrate in unexplained infertility.[137]

We do not object to the empirical use of clomiphene, provided there is a clear understanding of the potential side effects and the uncertain efficacy of the medication.

Luteinized Unruptured Follicle

On occasion, a corpus luteum will form despite the failure of release of the oocyte. Initially it was thought that this problem could be identified at laparoscopy by visualizing an absence of the ovulatory stigma, but now it is apparent that the stigma can be epithelialized rapidly and thus obscured from view.[138] Currently, clinical diagnosis of a luteinized unruptured follicle (LUF) is made on the basis of ultrasound monitoring. The preovulatory growth of the follicle usually is normal but the follicle does not collapse following the LH surge, and there may be increased growth in the luteal phase. The interior of the follicle lacks the echoes often seen in corpora lutea. Whereas these criteria seem straightforward, establishing the diagnosis of LUF is often difficult. Even if ultrasonography is performed daiy, the collapse of the follicle can be missed, and a corpus luteum refilled with blood can be mistaken for a persistent follicle. Therefore, serial ultrasound screening of women with unexplained infertility is of questionable value, not only for the diagnosis of LUF, but also for determining the size of the follicle just prior to rupture. Whereas ovulation usually occurs in the normal cycle when the follicle is 17–23 mm in diameter, some fertile women ovulate from a smaller follicle. In the evaluation of unexplained infertility, a single ultrasound examination in the late follicular phase is of value to detect endometrial polyps and myomas.

It is doubtful that LUF is a significant cause of infertility, and furthermore, the suggested treatments are superovulation, either alone or in conjunction with one of the assisted reproductive technologies, treatment choices that will be empirically offered even without a diagnosis of LUF. Because inhibition of prostaglandin synthesis can cause a luteinized unruptured follicle, patients should be cautioned to avoid the use of nonsteroidal antiinflammatory agents.[139–141]

Mycoplasma

Mycoplasma, a pleuropneumonia-like organism, has been implicated as a possible cause of recurrent abortion and salpingitis. A markedly higher prevalence of T mycoplasma (*ureaplasma urealyticum*) was detected in the cervical mucus and semen of infertile couples compared with a group of fertile couples.[142] Treatment with doxycycline decreased the number of couples with mycoplasma and also was associated with pregnancy in 15 of 52 couples (29%), all of whom had had primary infertility of at least 5 years duration. However, a series of reports from England agreed with these findings in only one respect.[143, 144] They confirmed that treatment with doxycycline could eliminate mycoplasma from the genital tract of the majority of individuals. There was no difference, however, in the frequency of either T strain or *Mycoplasma hominis* between infertile and fertile couples. In a double-blind study, treatment with doxycycline for 28 days had no effect on the rate of conception, and e English group suggested that culturing for mycoplasma in the routine investigation of infertility was unrewarding.[144]

Since those early publications, a number of studies have estaished the widespread distribution of *ureaplasma urealyticum* in both fertile and infertile populations. Some have found higher colonization in infertile couples, whereas others have found no relationship between the organisms and infertility. In a study that received a great deal of media attention, it was reported that 60% of males who were culture positive for *ureaplasma urealyticum* and were cleared of infection by antibiotic treatment achieved a pregnancy.[145] Failure to clear the infection resulted in a 5% pregnant rate. This study suffered from lack of clarity on the criteria for entry into treatment and from any mention of individuals lost to follow-up. The incidence of ureaplasma infection is only significantly higher in those women whose male partners have semen abnormalities.[146]

Ureaplasma urealyticum is widespread, but there is no compelling evidence that it causes infertility. Empiric treatment with antibiotics is not warranted.

Endoscopy

Traditionally, laparoscopy has been the final diagnostic procedure of any infertility investigation. As the success rates with in vitro fertilization improve (Chapter 31), patients and clinicians increasingly believe that turning to the assisted reproductive technologies is appropriate, even without laparoscopy. In most hands, in vitro fertilization will be more successful than treating significant tubal disease through the laparoscope. Mild, asymptomatic endometriosis of prolonged duration may also require in vitro fertilization if superovulation, combined with intrauterine inseminations, does not achieve pregnancy. Considerations of cost and healthcare coverage often influence the types of treatment selected by couples.

If laparoscopy is contemplated after a normal HSG, the endoscopic procedure is usually performed after an interval of 6 months from the x-ray. This allows time for the fertility enhancing effect of the x-ray procedure. An exception can be made for t woman who is at high risk for pelvic infection or the older woman who has no time to wait. The findings at laparoscopy agree with those of HSG in approximately two-thirds of the cases. The major area of disagreement is the failure of the HSG to detect pelvic adhesions or endometriosis. Approximately 50% of apparently normal infertile patients undergoing laparoscopy will have pelvic pathology, usually pelvic adhesions or endometriosis (but ordinarily a degree of endometriosis not requiring treatment).[147] With due care in selection of cases these abnormalities can be treated through the laparoscope either by lysis of adhesions, salpingostomy, or fulguration or vaporization of implants of endometriosis. Patients with significant tubal disease are best advised to proceed to in vitro fertilization.

Laparoscopic Treatment of Distal Tubal Pathology[148]

Lysis of adhesions	50% pregnancy rate
Distal tubal obstruction:	
Mild disease	80% pregnancy rate
Moderate disease	30% pregnancy rate
Severe disease	15% pregnancy rate

Unexplained Infertility

An infertile couple has what is called unexplained infertility when all standard clinical investigations (semen analysis, the postcoital test, assessment of ovulation, demonstration of tubal patency) yield normal results. It is estimated that from 10% to 15% of infertile couples will ultimately reach this clinical diagnosis, and, using normal findings on laparoscopy as a criterion, the prevalence may be less than 10%.[149] Important variables are age of the woman and duration of the infertility.[64]

The average monthly fecundity in normal couples is 30%; the monthly pregnancy rate in couples with unexplained infertility is 1.5–3%. After 3 years of infertility, the prospect of pregnancy decreases by 24% each year.[149] Approximately 60% of couples with unexplained infertility of less than 3 years duration will become pregnant with 3 years of *expectant* management.[150, 151] Because the incidence of spontaneous pregnancy is significant until 3 years have passed, tis appropriate to require 3 years of infertility in women less than 30 years old before making this diagnosis. Because age is an important determinant, further evaluation and therapy should not be deferred in older women.

A meticulous review of available results is essential to avoid overlooking a treatable factor. The use of sperm function tests may be helpful. There is some correlation between absent sperm penetration of hamster eggs and subsequent outcome (see Chapter 29). If these tests are not available, keep in mind that a definite diagnosis of unexplained infertility requires successful fertilization in vitro. Thus, a human egg test (in vitro fertilization) is the ultimate test of sperm fertility, and it is more time and cost efficient to move promptly to asissted reproduction, rather than testing sperm function.

Superovulation and Intrauterine Insemintion

Empiric treatment for suspected endometriosis or with dopamine agonists has no impact on unexplained infertility. However, the methods of assisted reproductive technology and superovulation with intrauterine insemination do increase the prospect of pregnancy. The results with superovulation alone are inferior to those achieved with one of the assisted reproductive techniques, but the overall cost is also less.[152] Studies indicate that subtle hormonal abnormalities do exist in women with unexplained infertility.[153, 154] These changes (elevated gonadotropins and estradiol in the follicular phase and decreased luteal phase progesterone) have been attributed to a reduction in ovarian reserve as usually seen in older women.[154] Thus, there is a rational basis to provide ovarian stimulation.

A cumulative pregnancy rate of 40% can be achieved in couples with unexplained infertility after 6 cycles of superovulation or 3 cycles of in vitro rtilization.[155] In andomized, controlled clinical trials, the monthly pregnancy rates in couples with unexplained infertility is increased 2–3-fold (a monthly fecundity rate of 9%) with clomiphene treatment, and with human gonadotropins, the monthly fecundity rate is approximately 10–15%.[156–158] *Although some studies have failed to yield increased pregnancy rates with the empiric use of clomiphene,[137, 159] we believe couples with unexplained infertility should be offered superovulation or one of the assisted reproductive technologies. However, superovulation should be limited to 3 or 4 cycles.*

The addition of intrauterine insemination of washed sperm (IUI) to clomiphene treatment increased fecundity in couples with unexplained infertility or surgically treated endometriosis, compared with intercourse without hormonal stimulation).[157] As with almost all infertility, success is age-related, with pregnancy rates 3–4-fold greater in women under age 20.[160] Although the combination of IUI with clomiphene may enhance the pregnancy rate in couples with unexplained infertility, *IUI by itself does not.*[161–163]

The combination of IUI with gonadotropin stimulation provides even better results than clomiphene and IUI. In two studies, the pregnancy rate per cycle with gonadotropins and IUI was 19% and 14.3% compared to 4% and 7.7% with clomiphene and IUI respectively.[158, 164] In a meta-analysis of randomized trials comparing gonadotropin stimulation with IUI or with timed intercourse, IUI was associated with approximately a 2-fold greater pregnancy rate.[165] In a randomized trial, superovulation and IUI resulted in a 3-fold greater pregnancy rate compared with intracervical insemination and 2-fold greater compared with either IUI alone or a combination of superovulation and intracervical insemination.[180]

The effectiveness of gonadotropin treatment combined with IUI has been repeatedly demonstrated for a variety of infertility disorders, including endometriosis, cervical factor, and unexplained infertility.[166–168] As with clomiphene, few pregnancies occur after 4 cycles of treatment.

Thus, there exist a number of options for the empiric treatment of unexplained infertility before considering the more complex and costly assisted reproductive technologies (Chapter 31). These options and the timing of their use should always be considered in the context of the known spontaneous cure rate for unexplained infertility. Approximately 60% of couples with unexplained infertility of less than 3 years duration will become pregnant within 3 years of expectant management. However, as time progresses, the monthly fecundity rate decreases, and this can be improved by active management with superovulation and IUI. For older women, decreasing the time to achieve a pregnancy is an important objective.

In a meta-analysis of methods used to treat unexplained infertility, pregnancy rates were estimated to be as follows:

Pregnancy Rate per Cycle [169]

No treatment	1.3–4.1%
IUI	3.8%
Clomiphene	5.6%
Clomiphene & IUI	8.3%
Gonadotropins	7.7%
Gonadotropins & IUI	17.1%
IVF	20.7%

Because it is relatively inexpensive, easy to administer, and not usually burdened with major side effects (except for a 2-fold increase in twinning), clomiphene is usually the first treatment choice. Patient demand for this treatment is substantial, and it is not unreasonable to respond to that demand with 3–4 clomiphene cycles. The uncertainty regarding the efficacy of adding IUI to clomiphene influences us to proceed from clomiphene treatment to the combination of gonadotropins and IUI, with an expectation of achieving a pregnancy rate of 15% per cycle. The combination of clomiphene and IUI is still appropriate in circumstances where cost, time, and avoidance of complications are paramount. The use of IUI alone or gonadotropins without IUI is not recommended for the treatment of unexplained infertility.[162, 170]

The success of treatment is influenced by the number of sperm inseminated. Pregnancies are rare if less than 1–3 million sperm are inseminated.[163, 171] Once this baseline is surpassed, increasing the number of sperm inseminated does not increase the pregnancy rate; although one study achieved higher pregnancy rates with inseminations of greater than 10 million motile sperm.[172, 173] Morphology plays only a minor role. Once the percentage of normal forms exceeds 5–10%, there is no influence on success.[174, 175]

The effects of age remain critical whatever the method of ovarian stimulation. In one series of 136 treatment cycles, no pregnancies were achieved in women who were 43 or older.[176] Despite rare successes in older women, it borders on the exploitive to treat women over age 40 with superovulation and IUI. Indeed, pregnancy rates begin to decline with this treatment around age 35.[160]

Adoption

With proper assessment and therapy, the majority of couples evaluated for infertility will become pregnant. For those who are refractory to the usual treatments, consideration of assisted reproductive technologies or adoption is appropriate. Couples thinking about adoption have a range of choices including social agency adoptions, private adoptions, and international adoptions. In some states, private adoption is not legal; however, where it is legal, it can provide an effective, more rapid alternative to adoption through a social agency. In most cases the biologic mother has the opportunity to know the adopting parents, and this lack of anonymity may direct some individuals away from private adoption. In addition, there is a short time period during which the biologic mother can reclaim the baby. In our experience, this devastating event occurs in approximately 5% of private adoptions.

To facilitate private adoption, patients should be encouraged to "spread the word" that they are interested in adoption. In addition, letters can be directed to obstetricians throughout the country describing the couple and their desire for adoption. Both lawyers and non-lawyers have practices devoted to counseling couples (and individuals) on approaches to private adoption and regarding the adoption laws in individual states.

Myths and Appropriate Goals

It is important for physicians and other health care professionals to dispel the myths that are associated with infertility. Women should not be told that they are infertile because they are too nervous. Unless anxiety interferes with ovulation or coital frequency, there is no present evidence that infertility is caused by the usual anxieties besetting a couple attempting to conceive. Despite many anecdotes to the contrary, adoption does not increase a couple's fertility.[177] The treatment of euthyroid infertile women with thyroid has been shown repeatedly to be worthless. A dilation and curettage (D and C) is not a legitimate part of a routine infertility investigation. It provides minimal information beyond that obtained by endometrial biopsy and is both expensive and potentially hazardous because it subjects the woman to the risk of general anesthesia. There is also no evidence to support the old belief that a woman becomes more fertile following D and C. Quite the contrary, one study indicates a decreased fertility potential for those women undergoing D and C.[178] A retroverted uterus is not a cause for infertility, although it can be found in association with pelvic adhesions or endometriosis that does influence infertility.

The routine ordering of laboratory tests, such as imaging and hormone determinations not indicated by clinical judgment, is ill advised. These may be of value in selected cases but certainly not in every case.

Remember that a substantial number of pregnancies occur in infertile couples without treatment, irrespective of the diagnoses.[64] Thus, the physician should not feel obligated to render a treatment just to do something. The goals of the practitioner should be to accomplish a thorough investigation, to treat any abnormalities that are uncovered or to provide empiric therapy based upon the evidence reviewed in this text, to educate the couple in the workings of the reproductive system, to give the couple some estimate of their fertility potential, to counsel for adoption where appropriate, and to provide emotional support either directly or through staff members or groups like RESOLVE. If these goals are achieved by a sympathetic, understanding clinician, they will satisfy most couples who suffer from infertility.

References

1. **Mosher WD, Pratt WF,** Fecundity and infertility in the United States: incidence and trends, *Fertil Steril* 56:192, 1991.

2. **Abma JC, Chandra A, Mosher WD, Peterson L, Piccinino L,** (Centers for Disease Control and Prevention, National Center For Heath Statistics), Fertility, family planning, and women's health: new data from the 1995 National Survey of Family Growth, Report No. 19; Series 23, 1997.

3. **Westoff CF,** Fertility in the United States, *Science* 234:554, 1986.

4. **Spencer G,** (US Department of Commerce), Projections of the population of the United States, by age, sex, and race: 1983–2080. Current Population Reports — Population Estimates and Projections, Report No. 952, Series P-25, 1984.

5. **Ventura S, Peters KD, Martin JD, Maurer JD,** Births and deaths: United States, 1996, *Monthly Vital Statistics Report* 46, No.1:Suppl.2, 1997.

6. **Mosher WD, Pratt WF,** The demography of infertility in the United States, In: Asch RH, Studd JW, eds. *Annual Progress in Reproductive Medicine,* Parthenon Publishing Group, Pearl River, New York, 1993, p 37.

7. **Stephen EH, Chandra A,** Updated projections of infertility in the United States: 1995–2025, *Fertil Steril* 70:30, 1998.

8. **Warburton D, Kline J, Stein Z, Strobino B,** Cytogenetic abnormalities in spontaneous abortions of recognized conceptions, In: Porter IH, ed. *Perinatal Genetics: Diagnosis and Treatment,* Academic Press, New York, 1986, p 133.

9. **Warburton D,** Reproductive loss: how much is preventable? *New Engl J Med* 316:158, 1987.

10. **Wilcox AJ, Weiberg CR, O'Connor JF, Baird DD, Schlatterer JP, Canfield RE, Armstrong EG, Nisula BC,** Incidence of early loss of pregnancy, *New Engl J Med* 319:189, 1988.

11. **Battaglia DE, Goodwin P, Klein NA, Soules MR,** Influence of maternal age on meiotic spindle assembly in oocytes from naturally cycling women, *Hum Reprod* 11:2217, 1996.

12. **Tietze C,** Reproductive span and rate of reproduction among Hutterite women, *Fertil Steril* 8:89, 1957.

13. **Robinson WC,** Another look at the Hutterites and natural fertility, *Soc Biol* 33:65, 1986.

14. **Federation CECOS, Schwartz D, Mayaux JM,** Female fecundity as a function of age: results of artificial insemination in 2193 nulliparous women with azoospermic husbands, *New Engl J Med* 306:404, 1982.

15. **Virro MS, Shewchuk AB,** Pregnancy outcome in 242 conceptions after artificial insemination with donor sperm and effects of maternal age on the prognosis for successful pregnancy, *Am J Obstet Gynecol* 148:518, 1984.

16. **van Noord-Zaadstra BM, Looman CW, Alsbach H, Habbena JDF, te Velde ER, Karbaat J,** Delaying child-bearing: effect of age on fecundity and outcome of pregnancy, *Br Med J* 302:1361, 1991.

17. **Shenfield F, Doyle P, Valentine A, Steele SJ, Tan S-L,** Effects of age, gravidity and male infertility status on cumulative conception rates following artificial insemination with cryopreserved donor semen: analysis of 2998 cycles of treatment in one centre over 10 years, *Hum Reprod* 8:60, 1993.

18. **Menken J, Trussell J, Larsen U,** Age and infertility, *Science* 233:1389, 1986.

19. **Meldrum DR,** Female reproductive aging — ovarian and uterine factors, *Fertil Steril* 59:1, 1993.

20. **Wood C, Calderon I, Crombie A,** Age and fertility: results of assisted reproductive technology in women over 40 years, *J Assist Reprod Genetics* 9:482, 1992.

21. **Tan SL, Royston P, Campbell S, Jacobs HS, Betts J, Mason B, Edwards RG,** Cumulative conception and livebirth rates after in-vitro fertilisation, *Lancet* 339:1390, 1992.

22. **Kennedy WJ,** *Edinburgh Med J* 27:1086, 1882.

23. **Meacham RB, Murray MJ,** Reproductive function in the aging male, *Urol Cl No Am* 21:549, 1994.

24. **Lian Z, Zack MM, Erickson JD,** Paternal age and the occurrence of birth defects, *Am J Hum Genet* 39:648, 1986.

25. **Gallardo E, Simón C, Levy M, Guanes PP, Remohí J, Pellicer A,** Effect of age on sperm fertility potential: oocyte donation as a model, *Fertil Steril* 66:260, 1996.

26. **Seymour FI, Duffy C, Koerner A,** A case of authenticated fertility in a man of 94, *JAMA* 105:423, 1935.

27. **Gougeon A, Echochard R, Thalabard JC,** Age-related changes of the population of human ovarian follicles: increase in the disappearance rate of non-growing and early-growing follicles in aging women, *Biol Reprod* 50:653, 1994.

28. **Faddy MJ, Gosden RG, Gougeon A, Richardson SJ, Nelson JF,** Accelerated disappearance of ovarian follicles in mid-life: implications for forecasting menopause, *Hum Reprod* 7:1342, 1992.

29. **Metcalf MG, Livesay JH,** Gonadotropin excretion in fertile women: effect of age and the onset of the menopausal transition, *J Endocrinol* 105:357, 1985.

30. **Klein NA, Battaglia DE, Fujimoto VY, Davis GS, Bremmer WJ, Soules MR,** Reproductive aging: accelerated ovarian follicular devlopment associated with a monotropic follicle-stimulating hormone rise in normal older women, *J Clin Endocrinol Metab* 81:1038, 1996.

31. **Lenton EA, Landgren B, Sexton L, Harper R,** Normal variation in the length of the follicular phase of the menstrual cycle: effect of chronological age, *Br J Obstet Gynaecol* 91:681, 1984.

32. **Lee SJ, Lenton EA, Sexton L, Cooke ID,** The effect of age on the cyclical patterns of plasma LH, FSH, oestradiol and progesterone in women with regular menstrual cycles, *Hum Reprod* 3:851, 1988.

33. **Musey VC, Collins DC, Musey PI, Saltzman-Martino D, Preedy JRK,** Age-related changes in the female hormonal environment during reproductive life, *Am J Obstet Gynecol* 157:312, 1987.

34. **Hughes EG, Robertson DM, Handelsman DJ, Hayward S, Healy DL, de Kretser DM,** Inhibin and estradiol responses to ovarian hyperstimulation: effects of age and predictive value for in vitro fertilization outcome, *J Clin Encrinol Metab* 70:358, 1990.

35. **Cameron IT, O'Shea FC, Rolland JM, Hughes EG, de Kretser DM, Healy DL,** Occult ovarian failure: a syndrome of infertility, regular menses, and elevated follicle-stimulating hormone concentrations, *J Clin Endocrinol Metab* 67:1190, 1986.

36. **Buckler HM, Evans A, Mamlora H, Burger HG, Anderson DC,** Gonadotropin, steroid and inhibin levels in women with incipient ovarian failure during anovulatory and ovulatory 'rebound' cycles, *J Clin Endocrinol Metab* 72:116, 1991.

37. **Lenton EA, de Kretser DM, Woodward AJ, Robertson DM,** Inhibin concentrations throughout the menstrual cycles of normal, infertile, and older women compared with those during spontaneous conception cycles, *J Clin Endocrinol Metab* 73:1180, 1991.

38. **McNaughton J, Banah M, McCloud P, Hee J, Burger H,** Age related changes in follicle stimulating hormone, luteinizing hormone, oestradiol and immunoreactive inhibin in women of reproductive age, *Clin Endocrinol* 36:339, 1992.

39. **Pellicer A, Marí M, de los Santos MJ, Simón C, Remohí J, Tarín JJ,** Effects of aging on the human ovary: the secretion of immunoreactive α-inhibin and progesterone, *Fertil Steril* 61:663, 1994.

40. **Burger HG, Cahir N, Robertson DM, Groome NP, Dudley E, Green A, Dennerstein L,** Serum inhibins A and B fall differentially as FSH rises in perimenopausal women, *Clin Endocrinol* 48:809, 1998.

41. **Klein NA, Illingworth PJ, Groome NP, McNeilly AS, Battaglia DE, Soules MR,** Decreased inhibin B secretion is associated with the monotropic FSH rise in older, ovulatory women: a study of serum and follicular fluid levels of dimeric inhibin A and B in spontaneous menstrual cycles, *J Clin Endocrinol Metab* 81:2742, 1996.

42. **Hofmann GE, Danforth DR, Seifer DB,** Inhibin-B: the physiologic basis of the clomiphene citrate challenge test for ovarian reserve screening, *Fertil Steril* 69:474, 1998.

43. **Danforth DR, Arbogast LK, Mroueh J, Kim MH, Kennard EA, Seifer DB, Friedman CI,** Dimeric inhibin: a direct marker of ovarian aging, *Fertil Steril* 70:119, 1998.

44. **Klein NA, Battaglia DE, Miller PB, Branigan EF, Giudice LC, Soules MR,** Ovarian follicular development and the follicular fluid hormones and growth factors in normal women of advanced reproductive age, *J Clin Endocrinol Metab* 81:1946, 1996.

45. **Lass A, Silye R, Abrams D-C, Krausz T, Hovatta O, Margara R, Winston RML,** Follicular density in ovarian biopsy of infertile women: a novel method to assess ovarian reserve, *Hum Reprod* 12:1028, 1997.

46. **Lass A, Skull J, McVeigh E, Margara R, Winston RM,** Measurement of ovarian volume by transvaginal sonography before human menopausal gonadotrophin superovulation for in-vitro fertilization can predict poor response, *Hum Reprod* 12:294, 1997.

47. **Toner JP, Philput CB, Jones GS, Muasher SJ,** Basal follicle-stimulating hormone level is a better predictor of in vitro fertilization performance than age, *Fertil Steril* 55:784, 1991.

48. **Pearlstone AC, Fournet N, Gambone JC, Pang SC, Buyalos RP,** Ovulation induction in women age 40 and older: the importance of basal follicle-stimulating hormone level and chronological age, *Fertil Steril* 58:674, 1992.

49. **Scott Jr RT, Hofmann GE,** Prognostic assessment of ovarian reserve, *Fertil Steril* 63:1, 1995.

50. **Khalifa E, Toner JP, Muasher SJ, Acosta AA,** Significance of basal follicle-stimulating hormone levels in women with one ovary in a program of in vitro fertilization, *Fertil Steril* 57:835, 1992.

51. **Smotrich DB, Widra EA, Gindoff PR, Levy MJ, Hall JL, Stillman RJ,** Prognostic value of day 3 estradiol on in vitro fertilization outcome, *Fertil Steril* 64:1136, 1995.

52. **Buyalos RP, Daneshmand S, Brzechffa PR,** Basal estradiol and follicle-stimulating hormone predict fecundity in women of advanced reproductive age undergoing ovulation induction therapy, *Fertil Steril* 68:272, 1997.

53. **Navot D, Rosenwaks Z, Margalioth EJ,** Prognostic assessment of female fecundity, *Lancet* ii:645, 1987.

54. **Tanbo T, Dale PO, Lunde O, Norman N, Abyholm T,** Prediction of response to controlled ovarian hyperstimulation: a comparison of basal and clomiphene citrate-stimulated follicle-stimulating hormone levels, *Fertil Steril* 57:819, 1992.

55. **Scott Jr RT, Leonardi MR, Hofmann GE, Illions EH, Neal GS, Navot D,** A prospective evaluation of clomiphene citrate challenge test screening of the general infertility population, *Obstet Gynecol* 82:539, 1993.

56. **Navot D, Drews MR, Bergh PA, Guzman I, Karstaedt A, Scott Jr RT, Garrisi GJ, Hofmann GE,** Age-related decline in female fertility is not due to diminished capacity of the uterus to sustain embryo implantation, *Fertil Steril* 61:97, 1994.

57. **Sauer MV, Paulson RJ, Lobo RA,** Reversing the natural decline in human fertility: an extended clinical trial of ooctye donation to women of advanced reproductive age, *JAMA* 268:1275, 1992.

58. **Sauer MV, Paulson RJ, Lobo RA,** Pregnancy after age 50: application of oocyte donation to women after natural menopause, *Lancet* 341:321, 1993.

59. **Borini A, Bafaro G, Violini F, Bianchi L, Casadio V, Flamini C,** Pregnancies in postmenopausal women over 50 years old in an oocyte donation program, *Fertil Steril* 63:258, 1995.

60. **Abdalla HI, Burton G, Kirkland A, Johnson MR, Leonard T, Brooks AA, Studd JW,** Age, pregnancy and miscarriage: uterine versus ovarian factors, *Hum Reprod* 8:1512, 1993.

61. **Legro RS, Wong IL, Paulson RJ, Lobo RA, Sauer MV,** Recipient's age does not adversely affect pregnancy outcome after oocyte donation, *Am J Obstet Gynecol* 172:96, 1995.

62. **Paulson RJ, Sauer MV,** Pregnancies in post-menopausal women: oocyte donation to women of advanced reproductive age: 'How old is too old?' *Hum Reprod* 9:571, 1994.

63. **Barnea ER, Holford TR, McInnes DRA,** Long-term prognosis of infertile couples with normal basic investigations: a life-table analysis, *Obstet Gynecol* 66:24, 1985.

64. **Collins JA, Wrixon W, Janes LB, Wilson EH,** Treatment-independent pregnancy among infertile couples, *New Engl J Med* 309:1201, 1983.

65. **Stubblefield P, Monson R, Schoenbaum S, Wolfson CE, Cookson DJ, Ryan KJ,** Fertility after induced abortion: a prospective follow-up study, *Obstet Gynecol* 62:186, 1984.

66. **Senekjian EK, Potkul RK, Frey K, Herbst A,** Infertility among daughters either exposed or not exposed to diethylstilbestrol, *Am J Obstet Gynecol* 184:493, 1988.

67. **Stillman RJ, Rosenberg MJ, Sachs BP,** Smoking and reproduction, *Fertil Steril* 46:545, 1986.

68. **Laurent SL, Thompson SJ, Addy C, Garrison CZ, Moore EE,** An epidemiologic study of smoking and primary infertility in women, *Fertil Steril* 57:565, 1992.

69. **Hakim RB, Gray RH, Zacur H,** Alcohol and caffeine consumption and decreased fertility, *Fertil Steril* 70:632, 1998.

70. **Bolumar F, Olsen J, Boldsen J,** Smoking reduces fecundity: a European Multicenter Study on Infertility and Subfecundity, *Am J Epidemiol* 143:578, 1996.

71. **Smith CG, Asch RH,** Drug abuse and reproduction, *Fertil Steril* 48:355, 1987.

72. **Bracken MB, Eskenazi B, Sachse K, McSharry J-E, Hellenbrand K, Leon-Summers L,** Association of cocaine use with sperm concentration, motility, and morphology, *Fertil Steril* 53:315, 1990.

73. **Bolumar F, Olsen J, Rebagliato M, Bisanti L,** Caffeine intake and delayed conception: a European multicenter study on infertility and subfecundity. European Study Group on Infertility and Subfecundity, *Am J Epidemiol* 145:324, 1997.

74. **Caan B, Quesenberry Jr CP, Coates AO,** Differences in fertility associated with caffeinated beverage consumption, *Am J Public Health* 88:270, 1998.

75. **Guttmacher AF,** Factors affecting normal expectancy of conception, *JAMA* 161:855, 1956.

76. **Drake TS, Tredway DR, Buchanan GC,** A reassessment of the fractional postcoital test, *Am J Obstet Gynecol* 133:382, 1979.

77. **Gibor Y, Garcia CJ, Cohen MR, Scommegna A,** The cyclical changes in the physical properties of the cervical mucus and the results of the postcoital test, *Fertil Steril* 21:20, 1970.

78. **Jette NT, Glass RH,** Prognostic value of the postcoital test, *Fertil Steril* 23:29, 1972.

79. **Collins JA, So Y, Wilson EH, Wrixon W, Casper RF,** The postcoital test as a predictor of pregnancy among 355 infertile couples, *Fertil Steril* 41:703, 1984.

80. **Bateman BG, Nunley Jr WC, Kolp LA,** Exogenous estrogen therapy for the treatment of clomiphene citrate-induced cervical mucus abnormalities: Is it effective? *Fertil Steril* 54:577, 1990.

81. **Davajan V, Vargyas JM, Kletzky OA, et al,** Intrauterine insemination with washed sperm to treat infertility, *Fertil Steril* 40:419, 1983.

82. **Ansari AH, Gould KG, Ansari VM,** Sodium bicarbonate douching for improvement of the postcoital test, *Fertil Steril* 33:608, 1980.

83. **Speert H,** *Obstetric & Gynecologic Milestones Illustrated,* The Parthenon Publishing Group, New York, 1996.

84. **Kovacs GT, Newman GB, Henson GL,** The postcoital test: What is normal? *Br Med J* i:818, 1978.

85. **Hull MGR, Savage PE, Bromham DR,** Prognostic value of the postcoital test: prospective study based on time-specific conception rates, *Br J Obstet Gynaecol* 89:299, 1982.

86. **Quagliarello J, Arny M,** Intracervical versus intrauterine insemination: correlation of outcome with antecedent postcoital testing, *Fertil Steril* 46:870, 1986.

87. **Westrom I,** Incidence, prevalence, and trends of acute pelvic inflammatory disease and its consequences in industrialized countries, *Am J Obstet Gynecol* 138:880, 1980.

88. **Stumpf PG, March CM,** Febrile morbidity following hysterosalpingography: identification of risk factors and recommendations for prophylaxis, *Fertil Steril* 33:487, 1980.

89. **Pittaway DE, Winfield AC, Maxson W, Daniell J, Herbert C, Wentz AC,** Prevention of acute pelvic inflammatory disease after hysterosalpingography: efficacy of doxycycline prophylaxis, *Am J Obstet Gynecol* 147:623, 1983.

90. **Mackey RA, Glass RH, Olson LE, Vaidya RA,** Pregnancy following hysterosalpingography with oil and water soluble dye, *Fertil Steril* 22:504, 1971.

91. **Mol BWJ, Swart P, Bossuyt PMN, van der Veen F,** Is hysterosalpingography an important tool in predicting fertility outcome? *Fertil Steril* 67:663, 1997.

92. **Gillespie HW,** The therapeutic aspect of hysterosalpingography, *Br J Radiol* 38:301, 1965.

93. **Soules MR, Spadoni LR,** Oil versus aqueous media for hysterosalpingography: a continuing debate based on many opinions and few facts, *Fertil Steril* 38:1, 1982.

94. **Rasmussen F, Lindequist S, Larsen C, Justesen P,** Therapeutic effect of hysterosalpingography: oil versus water soluble contrast media — a randomized prospective study, *Radiology* 179:75, 1991.

95. **Spring D, Barkan M, Pruyn S,** The potential therapeutic effects of contrast media in hysterosalpingography: a randomized, prospective clinical trial, Annual Meeting, Society of Uroradiology, Sante Fe, New Mexico,1997.

96. **Watson A, Vandekerckhove P, Liford R, Vail A, Brosen I, Hughes E,** A meta-analysis of the therapeutic role of oil soluble contrast media at hysterosalpingography: a surprising result? *Fertil Steril* 61:470, 1994.

97. **Boyer P, Territo MC, de Ziegler D, Meldrum DR,** Ethiodol inhibits phagocytosis by pelvic peritoneal macrophages, *Fertil Steril* 46:715, 1986.

98. **Johnson JV, Montoya IA, Olive DL,** Ethiodol oil contrast medium inhibits macrophage phagocytosis and adherence by altering membrane electronegativity and microviscosity, *Fertil Steril* 58:511, 1992.

99. **Bateman BG, Nunley Jr WC, Kitchin JD,** Intravasation during hysterosalpingography using oil-base contrast media, *Fertil Steril* 34:439, 1980.

100. **Chenia F, Hofmeyr GJ, Moolla S, Oratis P,** Sonographic hydrotubation using agitated saline: a new technique for improving fallopian tube visualization, *Br J Radiol* 70:833, 1997.

101. **Dietrich M, Surren A, Hinney B, Osmers R, Kuhn W,** Evaluation of tubal patency by hysterocontrast sonography (HyCoSy, Echovist) and its correlation with laparoscopic findings, *J Clin Ultrasound* 24:523, 1996.

102. **Hamilton JA, Larson AJ, Lower AM, Hasnain S, Grudzinskas JG,** Evaluation of the performance of hysterosalpingo contrast sonography in 500 consecutive, unselected infertile women, *Hum Reprod* 13:1519, 1998.

103. **Kerin JF, Williams DB, San Roman GA, Pearlstone AC, Grundfest WS, Surrey ES,** Falloposcopic classification and treatment of fallopian tube lumen disease, *Fertil Steril* 57:731, 1992.

104. **Novy MJ, Thurmond AS, Patton P, Uchida BT, Rosch J,** Diagnosis of cornual obstruction by transcervical fallopian tube cannulation, *Fertil Steril* 50:434, 1988.

105. **Thurmond AS, Rosch J,** Nonsurgical fallopian tube recanalization for treatment of infertility, *Radiology* 174:371, 1990.

106. **Confino E, Tur-Kaspa I, DeCherney AH, Corfman R, Coulam C, Robinson E, Haas G, Katz E, Vermesh M, Gleicher N,** Transcervical balloon tuboplasty: a multicenter trial, *JAMA* 264:2079, 1990.

107. **Quagliarello J, Arny M,** Inaccuracy of basal body temperature charts in predicting urinary luteinizing hormone surges, *Fertil Steril* 45:334, 1986.

108. **Luciano AA, Peluso J, Koch E, Maier D, Kuslis S, Davison E,** Temporal relationship and reliability of the clinical, hormonal, and ultrasonographic indices of ovulation in infertile women, *Obstet Gynecol* 75:412, 1990.

109. **France JT, Graham FM, Gosling L, Hair P, Knox BS,** Characteristics of natural conception cycles occurring in a prospective study of sex preselection: fertility awareness symptoms, hormone levels, sperm survival, and pregnancy outcome, *Int J Fertil* 37:244, 1992.

110. **Wilcox AJ, Weinberg CR, Baird DD,** Timing of sexual intercourse in relation to ovulation — effects on the probability of conception, survival of the pregnancy, and sex of the baby, *New Engl J Med* 333:1517, 1995.

111. **Nulsen J, Wheeler C, Ausmanas M, Blasco L,** Cervical mucus changes in relationship to urinary luteinizing hormone, *Fertil Steril* 48:783, 1987.

112. **Corsan GH, Blotner MB, Bohrer MK, Sheldon R, Kemmann E,** The utility of a home urinary LH immunoassay in timing the postcoital test, *Obstet Gynecol* 81:736, 1993.

113. **Castelbaum AJ, Wheeler J, Coutifaris CB, Mastrioianni Jr L, Lessey BA,** Timing of the endometrial biopsy may be critical for the accurate diagnosis of luteal phase deficiency, *Fertil Steril* 61:443, 1994.

114. **Noyes RW, Hertig AW, Rock J,** Dating the endometrial biopsy, *Fertil Steril* 1:3, 1950.

115. **Wentz AC, Herbert III CM, Maxon WS, Hill GA, Pittaway DE,** Cycle of conception endometrial biopsy, *Fertil Steril* 46:196, 1986.

116. **Wathen NC, Perry L, Lilford RJ, Chard T,** Interpretation of single progesterone measurement in diagnosis of anovulation and defective luteal phase: observations on analysis of the normal range, *Br Med J* 288:7, 1984.

117. **Cooke ID, Morgan CA, Parry TE,** Correlation of endometrial biopsy and plasma progesterone levels in infertile women, *J Obstet Gynaecol Br Comm* 79:647, 1972.

118. **Shepard MK, Senturia YD,** Comparison of serum progesterone and endometrial biopsy for confirmation of ovulation and evaluation of luteal function, *Fertil Steril* 28:541, 1977.

119. **Rosenfeld DL, Chudow S, Bronson RA,** Diagnosis of luteal phase inadequacy, *Obstet Gynecol* 56:193, 1980.

120. **Cumming DC, Honore LH, Scott JZ, Williams KP,** The late luteal phase in infertile women: comparison of simultaneous endometrial biopsy and progesterone levels, *Fertil Steril* 43:715, 1985.

121. **Soules MR, McLachlan RI, Ek M, Dahl KD, Cohen NL, Bremmer WJ,** Luteal phase deficiency: characterization of reproductive hormones over the menstrual cycle, *J Clin Endocrinol Metab* 69:804, 1989.

122. **Li T-C, Lenton EA, Dockery P, Rogers AW, Cooke ID,** The relation between daily salivary progesterone profile and endometrial development in the luteal phase of fertile and infertile women, *Br J Obstet Gynaecol* 96:445, 1989.

123. **Peters AJ, Lloyd RP, Coulam CP,** Prevalence of out-of-phase endometrial biopsy specimens, *Am J Obstet Gynecol* 166:1738, 1992.

124. **Shoupe D, Mishell Jr DR, Lacarra M, Lobo R, Horenstein J, d'Ablaing G, Moyer D,** Correlation of endometrial maturation with four methods of estimating day of ovulation, *Obstet Gynecol* 73:88, 1989.

125. **Batista MC, Cartledge TP, Merino MJ, Axiotis C, Platia MP, Merriam GR, Loriaux DL, Nieman LK,** Midluteal phase endometrial biopsy does not accurately predict luteal function, *Fertil Steril* 59:294, 1993.

126. **Li T-C, Dockery P, Rogers AW, Cooke ID,** How precise is histologic dating of endometrium using the standard dating criteria? *Fertil Steril* 51:759, 1989.

127. **Wentz AC, Kossoy L, Parker RA,** The impact of luteal phase inadequacy in an infertile population, *Am J Obstet Gynecol* 162:937, 1990.

128. **Balasch J, Fabreques F, Creus M, Vanrell JA,** The usefulness of endometrial biopsy for luteal phase evaluation in infertility, *Hum Reprod* 7:973, 1992.

129. **Navot D, Bergh PA, Williams M, Garrisi GJ, Guzman I, Sandler B, Fox J, Schreiner-Engle P, Hofmann GE, Grunfeld L,** An insight into early reproductive processes through the in vivo model of ovum donation, *J Clin Endocrinol Metab* 72:408, 1991.

130. **Jordan J, Craig K, Clifton DK, Soules MJ,** Luteal phase defect: the sensitivity and specificity of diagnostic methods in common use, *Fertil Steril* 62:54, 1994.

131. **Nakajima ST, Miller PB, Clifton DK, et al,** Luteal phase assessment by serum progesterone, urinary pregnanediol-3-glucuronide, and salivary progesterone levels, *Fertil Steril*, in press.

132. **Balasch J, Vanrell JA, Marquez M, Burzaco I, Gonzalez-Merlo J,** Dehydrogesterone versus vaginal progesterone in the treatment of the endometrial luteal phase deficiency, *Fertil Steril* 37:751, 1982.

133. **Huang K-E,** The primary treatment of luteal phase inadequacy: progesterone versus clomiphene citrate, *Am J Obstet Gynecol* 155:824, 1986.

134. **Murray DL, Reich L, Adashi EY,** Oral clomiphene citrate and vaginal progesterone suppositories in the treatment of luteal phase dysfunction: a comparative study, *Fertil Steril* 51:35, 1989.

135. **DeVane GW, Guzick DS,** Bromocriptine therapy in normoprolactinemic women with unexplained infertility and galactorrhea, *Fertil Steril* 46:1026, 1986.

136. **Padilla SL, Person GK, McDonough PG, Reindollar RH,** The efficacy of bromocriptine in patients with ovulatory dysfunction and normoprolactinemic galactorrhea, *Fertil Steril* 44:695, 1985.

137. **Martinez AR, Bernardos RE, Voorhorst FJ, Vermeiden JPW, Schoemaker J,** Intrauterine insemination does and clomiphene citrate does not improve fecundity in couples with infertility due to male or idiopathic factors: a prospective, randomized, controlled study, *Fertil Steril* 53:847, 1990.

138. **Dhont M, Serreyn R, Duvivier P, Vanluchene E, DeBoever J, Vandekerckhove D,** Ovulation stigma and concentration of progesterone and estradiol in peritoneal fluid: relation with fertility and endometriosis, *Fertil Steril* 41:872, 1984.

139. **O'Grady JP, Caldwell BV, Auletta FJ, Speroff L,** The effects of an inhibitor of prostaglandin synthesis (indomethacin) on ovulation, pregnancy, and pseudopregnancy in the rabbit, *Prostaglandins* 1:97, 1972.

140. **Priddy AR, Killick SR, Elstein M, Morris J, Sullivan M, Patel L, Elder M,** The effect of prostaglandin synthetase inhibitors on human preovulatory follicular fluid prostaglandin, thromboxane, and leukotriene concentrations, *J Clin Endocrinol Metab* 71:235, 1990.

141. **Smith G, Roberts R, Hall C, Nuki G,** Reversible ovulatory failure associated with the development of luteinized unruptured follicles in women with inflammatory arthritis, *Br J Rheumatol* 35:458, 1996.

142. **Gnarpe H, Friberg J,** T-mycoplasmas as a possible cause for reproductive failure, *Nature* 242:120, 1973.

143. **de Louvois J, Blades M, Harrison RF, Hurley R, Stanley VC,** Frequency of mycoplasma in fertile and infertile couples, *Lancet* i:1073, 1974.

144. **Harrison RF, de Louvois J, Blades M, Hurley R,** Doxycycline treatment and human infertility, *Lancet* i:605, 1975.

145. **Toth A, Lesser ML, Brooks C, Labriola D,** Subsequent pregnancies among 161 couples treated for T-mycoplasma genital tract infection, *New Engl J Med* 308:505, 1983.

146. **Cassell GH, Younger JB, Brown MB, Blackwell RE, Davis JK, Marriott P, Stagno S,** Microbiologic study of infertile women at the time of diagnostic laparoscopy, *New Engl J Med* 308:502, 1983.

147. **El-Yahia AW,** Laparoscopic evaluation of apparently normal infertile women, *Aust N Z J Obstet Gynaecol* 34:440, 1994.

148. **Schlaff WD, Hassiakos DK, Damewood MD, Rock JA,** Neosalpingostomy for distal tubal obstruction: prognostic factors and impact of surgical technique, *Fertil Steril* 54:984, 1990.

149. **Crosignani PG, Collins J, Cooke ID, Diczfaluzy E, Rubin B,** Unexplained infertility, *Hum Reprod* 8:977, 1993.

150. **Verkauf BS,** The incidence and outcome of single-factor, multifactorial and unexplained infertility, *Am J Obstet Gynecol* 147:175, 1983.

151. **Collins J, Rowe T,** Age of the female partner is a prognostic factor in prolonged unexplained infertility: a multicenter study, *Fertil Steril* 52:15, 1989.

152. **Crosignani PG, Walters DS, Soliani A,** Addendum to the ESHRE multicentre trial: a summary of the abortion and birth statistics, *Hum Reprod* 7:286, 1992.

153. **Tummon IS, Macklin VM, Radwanska E, Binor Z, Dimowski WP,** Occult ovulatory dysfunction in women with minimal endometriosis or unexplained infertility, *Fertil Steril* 50:716, 1988.

154. **Leach RE, Moghissi KS, Randolph JF, Reame NE, Blacker CM, Ginsburg KA, Diamond MP,** Intensive hormone monitoring in women with unexplained infertility: evidence for subtle abnormalities suggestive of diminished ovarian reserve, *Fertil Steril* 68:413, 1997.

155. **Simon A, Laufer N,** Unexplained infertility: a reappraisal, *Assist Reprod Rev* 3:26, 1993.

156. **Glazener CMA, Coulson C, Lambert PA, Watt EM, Hinton RA, Kelly NG, Hull MGR,** Clomiphene treatment for women with unexplained infertility: placebo-controlled study of hormonal responses and conception rates, *Gynecol Endocrinol* 4:75, 1990.

157. **Deaton JL, Gibson N, Blackmer KM, Nakajima ST, Badger GJ, Brumsted JR,** A randomized, controlled trial of clomiphene citrate and intrauterine insemination in couples with unexplained infertility, *Fertil Steril* 54:1083, 1990.

158. **Karlstrom P-O, Bergh T, Lundkvist O,** A prospective randomized trial of artificial insemination versus intercourse in cycles stimulated with human menopausal gonadotropin or clomiphene citrate, *Fertil Steril* 59:554, 1993.

159. **Fujii S, Fukui A, Fukushi Y, Kagiya A, Sato S, Saito Y,** The effects of clomiphene citrate on normal ovulatory women, *Fertil Steril* 68:997, 1997.

160. **Agarwal SK, Buyalos RP,** Clomiphene citrate with intrauterine insemination: is it effective therapy in women above the age of 35 years? *Fertil Steril* 65:759, 1996.

161. **Serhal PF, Katz M, Little V, Woronowski H,** Unexplained infertility — the value of pergonal superovulation combined with intrauterine insemination, *Fertil Steril* 49:602, 1988.

162. **Chaffkin LM, Nulsen JC, Luciano AA, Metzger DA,** A comparative analysis of the cycle fecundity rates associated with combined human menopausal gonadotropin (hMG) and intrauterine insemination (IUI) versus either hMG or IUI alone, *Fertil Steril* 55:252, 1991.

163. **Nulsen JC, Walsh S, Dumez S, Metzger DA,** A randomized and longitudinal study of human menopausal gonadotropin with intrauterine insemination in the treatment of infertility, *Obstet Gynecol* 82:780, 1993.

164. **Kemmann E, Bohrer M, Shelden R, Fiasconaro G, Beardsley L,** Active ovulation management increases the monthly probability of pregnancy occurrence in ovulatory women who receive intrauterine insemination, *Fertil Steril* 48:916, 1987.

165. **Zeyneloglu HB, Arici A, Olive DL, Duleba AJ,** Comparison of intrauterine insemination with timed intercourse in superovulated cycles with gonadotropins: a meta-analysis, *Fertil Steril* 69:486, 1998.

166. **Dodson WC, Whitesides DB, Hughes Jr CL, Easley III HA, Haney AF,** Superovulation with intrauterine insemination in the treatment of infertility: a possible alternative to gamete intrafallopian transfer and in vitro fertilization, *Fertil Steril* 48:441, 1987.

167. **Dodson WL, Haney AF,** Controlled ovarian hyperstimulation and intrauterine insemination for treatment of infertility, *Fertil Steril* 55:457, 1991.

168. **DiMarzo SJ, Kennedy JF, Young PE, Hebert SA, Rosenberg DC, Villanueva B,** Effects of controlled ovarian hyperstimulation on pregnancy rates after intrauterine insemination, *Am J Obstet Gynecol* 166:1607, 1992.

169. **Guzick DS, Sullivan MW, Adamson GD, Cedars MI, Falk RJ, Peterson EP, Steinkampf MP,** Efficacy of treatment of unexplained infertility, *Fertil Steril* 70:207, 1998.

170. **Hughes EG,** The effectiveness of ovulation induction and intrauterine insemination in the treatment of persistent infertility: a meta-analysis, *Hum Reprod* 12:1865, 1997.

171. **Brasch JG, Rawlins R, Tarchala S, Radwanska E,** The relationship between total motile sperm count and the success of intrauterine insemination, *Fertil Steril* 62:150, 1994.

172. **Berg U, Brucker C, Berg FD,** Effect of motile sperm count after swim-up on outcome of intrauterine insemination, *Fertil Steril* 67:747, 1997.

173. **Van Voorhis BJ, Sparks AET, Allen BD, Stovall DW, Syrop CH, Chapler FK,** Cost-effectiveness of infertility treatments: a cohort study, *Fertil Steril* 67:830, 1997.

174. **Burr RW, Siegberg R, Flaherty SP, Wang X-J, Matthews CJ,** The influence of sperm morphology and the numnbers of motile sperm inseminated on the outcome of intrauterine insemination combined with mild ovarian hyperstimulation, *Fertil Steril* 65:127, 1996.

175. **Karabinus DS, Gelety TJ,** The impact of sperm morphology evaluated by strict criteria on intrauterine insemination success, *Fertil Steril* 67:536, 1997.

176. **Corsan G, Trias A, Trout S, Kemmann E,** Ovulation induction combined with intrauterine insemination in women 40 years of age and older: is it worthwhile? *Hum Reprod* 11:1109, 1996.

177. **Lamb EJ, Leurgans S,** Does adoption affect subsequent fertility? *Am J Obstet Gynecol* 134:138, 1979.

178. **Taylor PJ, Graham G,** Is diagnostic curettage harmful in women with unexplained infertility? *Br J Obstet Gynaecol* 89:296, 1982.

179. **Welt CK, McNicholl DJ, Taylor AE, Hall JE,** Female reproductive aging is marked by decreased secretion of dimeric inhibin, *J Clin Endocrinol Metab* 84:105, 1999.

180. **Guzick DS, Carson SA, Coutifaris C, Overstreet JW, Factor-Litvak P, Staimkampf MP, Hill JA, Mastroianni Jr L, Buster JE, Nakajima ST, Vogel DL, Canfield RE, for the National Cooperative Reproductive Medicine Network,** Efficacy of superovulation and intrauterine insemination in the treatment of infertility, *New Engl J Med* 340:177, 1999.

27 Recurrent Early Pregnancy Losses

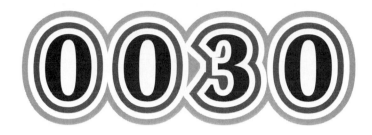

Early pregnancy loss (abortion or miscarriage) is defined as the termination of pregnancy before 20 weeks of gestation (dated from the last menstrual period) or below a fetal weight of 500 g. Approximately 15% of all pregnancies between 4–20 weeks of gestation will undergo clinically recognized spontaneous miscarriages. The true early pregnancy loss rate is closer to 50% because of the high rate of unrecognized miscarriages in the 2–4 weeks immediately following conception. The majority of these very early cases are caused by chromosomal abnormalities in the sperm or the egg.

"Habitual" abortion was classically defined as 3 or more consecutive spontaneous miscarriages. In 1938, Malpas, using theoretical calculations, stated that a woman with a history of 3 consecutive spontaneous miscarriages had a 73% chance of aborting in the next pregnancy.[1] In 1946, Eastman presented statistical calculations indicating that after 3 miscarriages the risk was 83.6%.[2] These early conclusions, based primarily upon intuition rather than clinical studies, established the notion that the chance for a subsequent miscarriage increases dramatically with each successive miscarriage; and that after 3 miscarriages the chances for a successful pregnancy are very low. Studies on the efficacy of many types of treatments used these pessimistic figures for comparison rather than containing their own controls. If treatment increased the salvage rate to 70% it was considered curative. However, clinical studies have indicated that the risk of pregnancy loss after 3 successive spontaneous miscarriages is in fact 30–45%.[3–5] The chance of a successful live birth after 3 consecutive miscarriages without a live birth is 55–60%; with at least one previous normal pregnancy (live birth) in addition to the repetitive miscarriages, the chance is approximately 70%.[4, 5] However, keep in mind that these numbers are derived from younger women, and older women have a risk of pregnancy loss that is twice that of younger women.

The Risk of Recurrent Early Pregnancy Loss in Young Women [4-6]

	Number of Prior Miscarriages	% Risk of Miscarriage in Next Pregnancy
Women who have had at least one liveborn infant:	0	12%
	1	24%
	2	26%
	3	32%
	4	26%
	6	53%
Women who have not had at least one liveborn infant:	2 or more	40–45%

The projections by Malpas and Eastman were theoretical exercises that were not confirmed when appropriate data were collected. Thus, it is not surprising that treatment with a wide range of approaches, including vitamins and psychotherapy, produced successful pregnancies in a reasonable percentage of women with recurrent miscarriages. These cures were not due to the therapy; the claims for success were based on a comparison with the discredited statistics of Malpas and Eastman.

The diagnostic and therapeutic response to a couple with pregnancy loss is not dictated by the number of miscarriages. The response is significantly influenced by the woman's age, the couple's level of anxiety, and factors readily identified in the family and medical history. The degree of response will range from an educational discussion to a full diagnostic evaluation with appropriate treatment. It is helpful to consider recurrent pregnancy losses according to the following categories:

1. Normal statistics,
2. Genetic factors,
3. Environmental factors,
4. Endocrine factors,
5. Anatomic causes,
6. Infectious causes,
7. Thrombophilia,
8. Immunologic problems.

Normal Statistics

The reproductive loss between conception and clinically recognizable pregnancy is significant; about 50% of fertilized ova do not progress to a viable pregnancy.[7, 8] The use of sensitive assays for human chorionic gonadotropin (HCG) suggests that up to 30% of pregnancies are lost between implantation and the 6th week.[9] It is important for physicians and their patients to be aware of the high degree of reproductive loss, especially in older women due in part to the increasing frequency of trisomies with advancing age. However, the frequency of both euploid (normal) and aneuploid (abnormal) abortuses increases with maternal age.

Approximately 80% of spontaneous miscarriages occur in the first 12 weeks of pregnancy, and nearly 70% of these miscarriages in early pregnancy are due to chromosomal anomalies.[10] Clinically recognized miscarriage occurs in only 12% of women younger than age 20, but the incidence increases to 26% in women older than age 40. The overall rate of loss (recognized and unrecognized) in women over age 40 is approximately 75%! An appreciation for these statistics contributes significantly to a couple's ability to cope with an early pregnancy loss.

Once a live embryo is detected by ultrasonography in normal young women or in young women with infertility, the rate of fetal loss is 3–5%. However, in women with recurrent pregnancy loss, the rate of loss after detection of fetal cardiac activity is 4–5 times higher.[11] The rate of spontaneous miscarriage in women with two or more recurrent losses was 22.7% after ultrasound documentation of fetal cardiac activity.[12] Keep in mind that the risk of spontaneous miscarriage is higher in older woman; spontaneous miscarriage occurred in 29% of women 40 or more years old, undergoing in vitro fertilization, after the demonstration of fetal heart motion by ultrasonography.[13]

Genetic Factors

Despite the knowledge that the spontaneous success rate is 55–70%, it is still worth trying to uncover causes for repetitive first-trimester miscarriages. A recognized cause of the problem is a genetic abnormality, and karyotyping of couples will reveal that 3–8% have some abnormality, most frequently a balanced chromosomal rearrangement, a translocation.[14–19] Other abnormalities usually encountered include sex chromosome mosaicism, chromosome inversions, and ring chromosomes. Besides spontaneous miscarriages, these abnormalities are associated with a high risk of malformations and mental retardation. Karyotyping is especially vital if the couple has had a malformed infant or fetus in addition to miscarriages. It is important to emphasize that karyotyping uncovers only a percentage of those pregnancies lost due to genetic abnormalities. There may be single gene defects that are not manifested by chromosomal abnormalities, and it is very likely that a percentage of those patients now considered to have unexplained repetitive pregnancy loss have this type of genetic defect. In addition, karyotyping of blood cells misses abnormalities of meiosis, which can be found in sperm cell lines.

If the karyotype is abnormal, nothing can be done to lessen the chances for another miscarriage, however with many abnormalities there is a 50% chance the next pregnancy will be normal. Amniocentesis or chorionic villus biopsy should be encouraged in any pregnancy in couples with an abnormal karyotype because of the risk of an abnormal child. Today, couples with serious high risk abnormalities may elect to pursue a pregnancy by means of donor sperm or in vitro fertilization with donor oocytes (or both).

As noted, approximately 70% of early spontaneous miscarriages are associated with fetal chromosomal abnormalities.[20, 21] In addition, 30% of second-trimester miscarriages and 3% of stillbirths have abnormal chromosomes. In most cases, the couple is chromosomally normal and the fetal chromosomal abnormality is a random event. The abnormalities include maternal and paternal accidents in gametogenesis, as well as miscues after fertilization. The fetal chromosomal abnormalities in single spontaneous miscarriages are different than those in recurrent miscarriages. Autosomal trisomy is the most frequent anomaly (about 50% of early pregnancy miscarriages), due to nondisjunction or translocation.[22] Trisomies of chromosomes 13, 16, 18, 21, and 22 are the most common. The next most common anomaly (about 25%) is 45,X which is responsible for Turner syndrome when the fetus survives. Of the remaining anomalies, most are polyploidies.

Fetuses that abort later in gestation usually have normal chromosomes. Perhaps in this situation, the responsible factors are external to the fetus. Subtle chromosomal defects, however, may be revealed as our analytic techniques improve.

According to McDonough, treatment of endocrine factors yields a 90% normal child rate; correction of anatomic factors yields a 60–70% rate, but known genetic factors are associated with only a 32% expectation for a normal child.[23]

It is helpful to have a karyotype on a previous miscarriage to determine aneuploidy or euploidy. Once determined, there is an increased likelihood that subsequent miscarriages will be the same, although there is still a chance for women with recurrent pregnancy loss to have a normal pregnancy. If aneuploidy is documented, accurately timed inseminations could be considered based on animal studies relating aneuploidy to aging of ovum and sperm; otherwise the choice is between hoping for the best or donor insemination. Once pregnant, chorionic villus sampling should be considered. If euploidy has been documented, anatomic and endocrine factors should be corrected.

Karyotyping is expensive. A factor that can help in decision making is a positive family history for recurrent miscarriages.[24] Translocations within families are usually associated with a mixed history: some normal pregnancies intermixed with recurrent miscarriages. Karyotyping is indicated when family members can be identified with multiple spontaneous miscarriages or the family has a malformed or mentally retarded child or a child with a known chromosomal abnormality. In any event, we recommend a karyotype when there is a history of 3 consecutive spontaneous early pregnancy losses and no previous normal liveborn.

Environmental Factors

Smoking, alcohol, and heavy coffee consumption have been reported to be associated with an increased risk of recurrent pregnancy losses.[10, 25, 26] The increase in risk is proportional to the number of cigarettes smoked. In these cases, the fetal chromosomes are normal. More recently, the link with caffeine intake could not be supported.[27] Anesthetic gases and tetrachloroethylene (used in dry cleaning) have been implicated as causative agents of miscarriage, but exposure to video terminals is not a factor.[28] Exercise programs do not increase the risk of spontaneous miscarriage, and bed rest will not influence the risk of recurrent miscarriage. Isotretinoin (Accutane) is definitely associated with an increased incidence of spontaneous miscarriage.[29] An increased risk of spontaneous miscarriage has not been documented among laboratory workers or women in the pharmaceutical industry.[30, 31] The use of electric blankets and heated water beds is also not associated with an increased risk of spontaneous miscarriage.[32]

Endocrine Factors

Mild or subclinical endocrine diseases are not causes of recurrent miscarriages. Patients who have significant thyroid disease or uncontrolled diabetes mellitus may suffer spontaneous miscarriages, but it is unlikely that laboratory assessments of thyroid function and carbohydrate metabolism are worthwhile in relatively healthy women.[33–35] Nevertheless, the high frequency of hypothyroidism warrants screening with a measurement of thyrotropin-stimulating hormone (TSH).[18] No convincing evidence exists linking endometriosis with an increased risk of spontaneous miscarriage.[36]

Elevated luteinizing hormone (LH) levels have been associated with an increased risk of miscarriage in women with polycystic ovaries who become pregnant.[37, 38] There is no reason to believe that this is a factor in ovulatory women with recurrent miscarriages. Even in women with polycystic ovaries and a history of 3 or more consecutive early pregnancy losses, suppression of LH secretion with a GnRH agonist prior to ovulation induction yielded no difference in outcome.[39]

An endocrine abnormality that may cause recurrent miscarriages is the inadequate luteal phase. Studies of the role of hormone deficiency as a cause of recurrent miscarriage have largely focused on deficiencies of progesterone or its metabolites. Attempts to implicate low progesterone or pregnanediol levels in early pregnancy as a cause for miscarriage, and, as a corollary, to treat with exogenous progesterone or progestins have been fruitless.[40, 41]

Another approach has been to diagnose an inadequate luteal phase during the nonpregnant state and to initiate treatment with progesterone a few days after ovulation. Jones and Delfs[42] claimed that 30% of women with pregnancy wastage had an inadequate luteal phase, whereas more recent studies have found that 20–25% of women with recurrent miscarriages have an inadequate luteal phase.[14–19] Yet it is by no means certain that progestational treatment makes a difference. Indeed, a meta-analysis of randomized trials of pregnancies treated with progestational agents failed to find any evidence for a positive effect on the maintenance of pregnancy.[41] Nevertheless, clinicians continue to report, as we have noted, a significant incidence of luteal phase inadequacy in their series of patients with recurrent miscarriages.[18, 43, 44]

The uncertainty that plagues physicians in dealing with the inadequate luteal phase in infertility, therefore, is also apparent when considering recurrent miscarriages. If repetitive endometrial biopsies indicate a lag in histologic development of more than 2 days or if the basal body temperature chart shows a luteal phase of less than 11 days, it is reasonable to treat with clomiphene or progesterone (Chapter 26) and with a dopamine agonist if galactorrhea or an elevated prolactin is present. In the absence of galactorrhea or hyperprolactinemia, we prefer clomiphene because this avoids the situation of a prolonged luteal phase due to progesterone treatment, a false expectation of pregnancy, and a more difficult time for the couple in coping with the results of a negative pregnancy test.

Should clomiphene be offered empirically (for 6 cycles) when no other cause for recurrent miscarriages can be identified? Placebo treatment may be useful in maintaining a clinician-patient relationship in which the patient derives needed psychologic sustenance. Furthermore, there is no evidence of any major harmful consequences with clomiphene treatment (see Chapter 30). In view of the difficulty in establishing the diagnosis of an inadequate luteal phase and the uncertainties that surround this diagnosis, we believe there is a place for empirical treatment. It must be remembered, however, that there is a reasonable cure rate in unexplained recurrent miscarriage, even without treatment.

Anatomical Causes

Uterine abnormalities can result in impaired vascularization of a pregnancy and limited space for a fetus due to distortion of the uterine cavity. Approximately 12–15% of women with recurrent miscarriages have a uterine malformation, and this can be best diagnosed by vaginal ultrasonography (especially with saline instillation), and confirmed by magnetic resonance imaging. Hysterosalpingography is relatively inaccurate and decisions should not be based upon hysterosalpingography alone.[45] The various uterine anomalies, including leiomyomata and diethylstilbestrol (DES) exposure, are discussed in detail in Chapter 4. Surgical repair of these defects, often by hysteroscopy, is rewarded with delivery rates in the 70–80% range; however, this high rate of success must be tempered by the realization that it is not derived from randomized clinical trials. The septate uterus is the most frequent anatomic abnormality associated with recurrent early spontaneous miscarriages, and the results with hysteroscopic repair have been impressive.[46] Repeat procedures are occasionally necessary; the surgical result should be evaluated several weeks postoperatively by hysterosalpingography (which is sufficiently accurate for this purpose) or office hysteroscopy. Surgery is unlikely to make a difference in a patient who has successfully delivered a live born term infant. The prophylactic use of cervical cerclage has not been supported by results from randomized trials.[47] However, when there is nothing else to offer, cervical cerclage is worthwhile; e.g., in patients with late losses and müllerian anomalies such as a bicornuate or unicornuate uterus and in DES-exposed women with a hypoplastic cervix.

In addition to müllerian anomalies, another anatomic cause, although uncommon, of recurrent miscarriages is intrauterine synechiae (Asherman's syndrome). If an appropriate predisposing factor, such as uterine curettage or a severe uterine infection, can be identified, diagnostic hysterosalpingography or hysteroscopy should be performed.

Infectious Causes

Despite periodic reports that have implicated specific infectious agents as etiologic factors in recurrent miscarriages, there currently is no hard evidence that bacterial or viral infections cause recurrent pregnancy losses. An impressive incidence of antichlamydial antibody has been reported in women with 3 or more spontaneous miscarriages, but it is not certain whether this an association with *Chlamydia trachomatis* or whether this is a marker of a different immune response in women with recurrent miscarriages.[48] In a prospective study, no association could be detected between antichlamydia antibodies and spontaneous miscarriage.[49]

Claims of effective antibiotic treatment have been derived without benefit of randomized studies. Perhaps an exception is infection with *Ureaplasma urealyticum*.[50] Other organisms that have been implicated, but not substantiated, include *Toxoplasma gondii, Listeria monocytogenes, Mycoplasma hominis,* herpes virus, and cytomegalovirus. It is more cost-effective and time efficient to prescribe both partners a course of doxycycline (100 mg bid for 14 days) or erythromycin (250 mg qid for 14 days) than to pursue multiple and repeated cultures.

Thrombophilia

The major cause of thrombosis in pregnancy is an inherited predisposition for clotting, especially the factor V Leiden mutation. Deficiencies of antithrombin III, protein C, and protein S are inherited in an autosomal dominant pattern, accounting for 10–15% of familial thrombosis. Mutations in the prothrombin gene and the factor V Leiden mutation are the most common inherited causes of venous thromboembolism.[51] An inherited resistance to activated protein C has been identified as the basis for about 50% of cases of familial venous thrombosis, due in almost all cases to a gene alteration recognized as the factor V Leiden mutation.[52, 53] The factor V Leiden mutation is found in approximately 30% of individuals who develop venous thromboembolism.[54] Activated protein C inhibits coagulation by degrading factors V and VIII. One of the 3 cleavages sites in factor V is the precise site of a mutation (known as the factor V Leiden mutation) that substitutes glutamine instead of arginine at this site (adenine for guanine at nucleotide 1691 in the gene).[54] This mutation makes factor V resistant to degradation (and activation in fibrinolysis). The entire clotting cascade is then resistant to the actions of the protein C system.

Heterozygotes for the factor V Leiden mutation have an 8-fold increased risk of venous thrombosis, and homozygotes, an 80-fold increased risk, and this risk appears to be further enhanced by oral contraceptive use. The highest prevalence (3–4% of the general population) of factor V Leiden is found in Europeans, and its occurrence in populations not of European descent is very rare, perhaps explaining the low frequency of thromboembolic disease in Africa, Asia, and in native Americans.[55] The mutation is believed to have arisen in a single ancestor approximately 21,000 to 34,000 years ago.[56] It has been suggested that this was a useful adaptation in heterozygotes in response to life-threatening bleeding, such as with childbirth. The next most common inherited disorder (after the factor V Leiden mutation) is a mutation a guanine to adenine change in the gene encoding prothrombin.[51, 57] The prevalence of this abnormality in the white population is estimated to range from 0.7% to 4%.[58]

In a group of 39 women with recurrent miscarriages, the factor V Leiden mutation was identified in nearly half, and 5 women treated with anticoagulation had normal term deliveries.[59] Others have found an increased incidence of the factor V Leiden mutation in women with second-trimester losses, but either not at all or only a slight increase in women with first-trimester losses.[60–63] In a survey of 500 consecutive women with unexplained recurrent pregnancy losses, von Willebrand's disease, fibrinogen deficiency, deficiencies in antithrombin, protein C, and proteins S, and resistance to activated protein C were not more frequent.[64] In a prospective cohort study, inherited deficiencies were associated with increased risks of late loss, but not for early miscarriage.[65] Elevated homocysteine levels are a risk factor for venous thrombosis, and this condition has also been suggested to be a factor in recurrent early pregnant losses.[66] Overall, these results are less than clear-cut.

In view of the new recognition for the clinical importance of inherited disorders that predispose to venous thrombosis, we believe that women with recurrent miscarriages who have no obvious identified cause should consider hematologic screening. This is definitely necessary in women with a previous episode or a close family history (parent or sibling) of thromboembolism. The list of laboratory tests is long, and because this is a dynamic and changing field, the best advice is to consult with a hematologist. A positive result warrants treatment with low molecular weight heparin after pregnancy is diagnosed.

Hypercoaguable Conditions	**Thrombophilia Screening**
Antithrombin III deficiency	Antithrombin III
Protein C deficiency	Protein C
Protein S deficiency	Protein S
Factor V Leiden mutation	Activated protein C resistance ratio
Prothrombin gene mutation	Activated partial thromboplastin time
Antiphospholipid syndrome	Hexagonal activated partial thromboplastin time
	Anticardiolipin antibodies
	Lupus anticoagulant
	Fibrinogen
	Prothrombin G mutation (DNA test)
	Thrombin Time
	Homocysteine level
	Complete blood count

Immunologic Problems

Autoimmunity (Self Antigens)

In autoimmunity, a humoral or cellular response is directed against a specific component of the host. The lupus anticoagulant and anticardiolipin antibodies are antiphospholipid antibodies, which arise as the result of an autoimmune disease. The lupus anticoagulant is present in a variety of clinical conditions, not just with lupus erythematosus. The antiphospholipid antibodies are directed against platelets and the vascular endothelium and cause thrombosis, spontaneous miscarriage, and fetal wastage. These antibodies block prostacyclin formation, which results in unbalanced thromboxane activity, leading to vasoconstriction and thrombosis.[67] In several series, 10–16% of women with recurrent miscarriages have had antiphospholipid antibodies.[68] These antibodies are also associated with fetal growth retardation and fetal death in addition to recurrent miscarriages, and when present, there is a high rate of second-trimester fetal deaths. The mechanism of pregnancy loss is probably decidual and placental insufficiency due to the thrombotic tendency. Annexin-V is a phospholipid-binding protein that inhibits coagulation; the levels of annexin-V on trophoblasts and endothelial cells are reduced in the presence of antiphospholipid antibodies.[69]

Despite activating thrombosis, the antiphospholipid antibodies prolong the prothrombin time and the partial thromboplastin time. The activated partial thromboplastin time is a relatively sensitive screening test, but we also obtain a kaolin clotting time. The anticardiolipin antibody and lupus anticoagulant can be identified and titered by specific immunoassays; other individual antiphospholipid antibodies have not been associated with recurrent miscarriages.[70] The antiphospholipid antibodies all produce the same clinical impact and have identical effects on clotting tests. Although the prevalence is uncertain, patients with recurrent miscarriages should be screened with the activated partial thromboplastin time, a kaolin clotting time, lupus anticoagulant, and the anticardiolipin antibody.[71–75] It is not clinically helpful to measure antinuclear antibodies, IGA antibodies, or leukocyte antibodies.

Our preferred treatment for significant titers of antiphospholipid antibodies consists of the combination of low-dose aspirin (80 mg daily) and low-dose heparin as soon as pregnancy is diagnosed.[76, 77] Treatment is not always successful.[78] Studies of low-dose aspirin alone do not demonstrate a favorable effect on pregnancy outcome in either women with unexplained recurrent losses or in women with detectable anticardiolipin antibodies.[79, 80] Others advocate the addition of a glucocorticoid in a dose sufficient to restore the clotting studies to normal.[81] However, the addition of glucocorticoids is not very effective in eliminating the anticardiolipin antibody, and in a randomized trial, a combination of prednisone and aspirin (100 mg daily) was no better than placebo treatment.[82] Many of these patients develop preeclampsia, often very severe, but approximately 75% of patients with antiphospholipid antibodies will deliver a viable infant in a treated pregnancy. Because of the risks associated with anticoagulation, aspirin and heparin treatment should be confined to women with recurrent pregnancy losses who have antiphospholipid antibodies. Indeed, it can be argued that treatment should be offered only to women with antiphospholipid antibodies who have experienced both first-trimester and second-trimester losses.[83]

Alloimmunity (Foreign Antigens)

Alloimmunity refers to all causes of pregnancy losses related to an abnormal maternal immune response to antigens on placental or fetal tissues.[68] Normally, maintenance of pregnancy may require the formation of blocking factors (probably complexes of antibody and antigen) that prevent maternal rejection of fetal antigens. It has been argued that couples with repetitive miscarriages have an increased sharing of human leukocyte antigens (HLA), a condition that would not allow the mother to make blocking antibodies.

Immunotherapy to stimulate antibody formation has been offered to produce a favorable maternal immune response in order to protect the developing embryo. Women with recurrent miscarriages have been treated with infusions of their partner's lymphocytes. In one study, 77% of women receiving their husband's cells gave birth compared to 37% receiving their own cells.[84] Critics of this study have contended that success in the control group raises the question of the adequacy of matching in the selection of control patients. Others have claimed good results with transfusion of leukocyte-rich, erythrocyte-rich donor blood (3 transfusions every 4–8 weeks) or with intravenous immunoglobulin or seminal plasma vaginal suppositories.[85–87]

Women have been selected for immunotherapy by HLA typing, but its use is no longer supported. Many investigators have failed to confirm that sharing of HLA antigens is found to a greater degree in couples with recurrent miscarriages.[88–90] This agrees with experiments in animals where sharing of HLA antigens has not been found to affect reproduction. The sharing of genetic loci may be a broader problem that includes genetic loci critical for embryonic development, and the antigens available for measurement serve only as markers for a more fundamental genetic immunologic failure in pregnancy. There is also concern that immunization of mothers may affect placenta and fetus. ***There is no specific immunologic test or clinical method which will predict the need for treatment.***[91]

Immunotherapy remains experimental with potential risks of adverse consequences on the immune systems of mother and child. At least 5 randomized placebo-controlled studies have failed to demonstrate a beneficial effect of immunotherapy.[92–96] In a study of women with 5 or more early miscarriages, paternal leukocyte immunization appeared to have a beneficial effect; suggesting that 25% of multiple aborters (without a live birth) would benefit.[97] In a re-analysis of the world-wide raw data, the difference in birth rate between treatment and control groups amounted to 10%, a difference so small that it may not be clinically significant.[98] Our recommendation is that women with an extreme number of recurrent early pregnancy losses should be referred to a center operating an immunotherapy protocol.[99]

Summary of Immunologic Causes

Women whose recurrent miscarriages are more likely to have an immunologic cause have the following characteristics:[91]

1. Many previous spontaneous miscarriages.
2. No recent full term pregnancies.
3. Less than 35 years old.
4. Aborted conceptus with a normal karyotype.
5. Usually at least one loss after the first-trimester.

Summary of Laboratory Evaluation and Management for Repeated Early Pregnancy Losses

Category	Evaluation	Treatment
Normal Statistics	Numbers review, No lab tests	Education and support
Genetic Factors	Karyotypes of both parents	Counseling Donor gametes where appropriate
Environmental Factors	No lab tests	Counseling
Endocrine Factors	TSH, prolactin, luteal phase assessment	Empiric clomiphene
Anatomic Causes	Vaginal ultrasound with saline instillation, confirmed by MRI	Surgery
Infectious Causes	Cultures if clinically indicated	Empiric doxycycline or erythromycin
Thrombophilia	Screen for inherited predisposition for thrombosis	Low molecular weight heparin anticoagulation
Immunologic	Activated partial thromboplastin time, kaolin clotting time, anticardiolipin antibody, lupus anticoagulant	Low-dose aspirin and heparin

Conclusion

The patient with early miscarriages usually presents as an anxious, frustrated individual on the verge of despair. Evaluation should be spaced over several visits, allowing the clinician to establish communication and rapport with the patient. Frequent communication between the clinician and the patient during the first-trimester of the next pregnancy is essential. The emotional support that the clinician can bring to this interaction will be most useful and in some cases may be therapeutic.[16] It should be emphasized that continued attempts at conception are rewarded with success in the majority of women (70–75%) labeled as recurrent aborters and who have no identifiable cause.[6] Except in the case of a second-trimester loss which is associated with a poor prognosis in the subsequent pregnancy with increased risks for preterm delivery, stillbirth, and neonatal death, approximately 50% of women with histories of recurrent pregnancy losses have no identifiable abnormalities and do well in their next pregnancies.[16–19, 96, 100] All subsequent pregnancies should be closely monitored because there is a higher rate of ectopic pregnancies in women with recurrent miscarriages.[101]

The expectant management of spontaneous early miscarriages is now known to provide an outcome (both medical and psychologic morbidity) equivalent to surgical evacuation of the uterus, with no adverse effect on future fertility.[102–104] For appropriate patients, this approach with effective support can be easier and less distressing.

Finally, the outcome of the assisted reproductive technologies is not certain in women with a large number of recurrent miscarriages. In one series of 12 women, 8 women delivered at term after in vitro fertilization.[105] In addition, in vitro fertilization outcome is not reduced in women with positive antiphospholipid antibodies.[106] However, in another in vitro fertilization experience, although pregnancy rates were good, a high rate of spontaneous miscarriage (50%) occurred in women with 3 or more consecutive losses.[107] Good results have been reported with oocyte donation in women with recurrent losses.[108] These are individual decisions, heavily influenced by psychologic and financial resources.

References

1. **Malpas P,** A study of abortion sequence, *J Obstet Gynaecol Br Emp* 45:932, 1938.

2. **Eastman NJ,** Habitual abortion, In: Meigs JV, Sturgis S, eds. *Progress in Gynecology,* Vol. 1, Grune & Stratton, New York, 1946.

3. **Warburton D, Fraser FS,** Spontaneous abortion risks in man: data from reproductive histories collected in a medical genetics unit, *Am J Hum Genet* 16:1, 1964.

4. **Poland BJ, Miller JR, Jones DC, Trimble BK,** Reproductive counseling in patients who have had a spontaneous abortion, *Am J Obstet Gynecol* 127:685, 1977.

5. **Roman E,** Fetal loss rates and their relation to pregnancy order, *J Epidemiol Community Health* 38:29, 1984.

6. **Clifford K, Rai R, Regan L,** Future pregnancy outcome in unexplained recurrent first trimester miscarriage, *Hum Reprod* 12:387, 1997.

7. **Wramsby H, Fredga F, Liedholm P,** Chromosome analysis of human oocytes recovered from preovulatory follicles in stimulated cycles, *New Engl J Med* 316:121, 1987.

8. **Warburton D,** Reproductive loss: how much is preventable? *New Engl J Med* 316:158, 1987.

9. **Wilcox AJ, Weiberg CR, O'Connor JF, Baird DD, Schlatterer JP, Canfield RE, Armstrong EG, Nisula BC,** Incidence of early loss of pregnancy, *New Engl J Med* 319:189, 1988.

10. **Harlap S, Shiono PH,** Alcohol, smoking, and incidence of spontaneous abortions in the first and second trimester, *Lancet* ii:173, 1980.

11. **van Leeuwen I, Branch DW, Scott JR,** First trimester ultrasonography findings in women with a history of recurrent pregnancy loss, *Am J Obstet Gynecol* 168:111, 1993.

12. **Laufer MR, Ecker JL, Hill JA,** Pregnancy outcome following ultrasound-detected fetal cardiac activity in women with a history of multiple spontaneous abortions, *J Soc Gynecol Invest* 1:138, 1994.

13. **Deaton JL, Honoré GM, Huffman CS, Bauguess P,** Early transvaginal ultrasound following an accurately dated pregnancy: the importance of finding a yolk sac or fetal heart motion, *Hum Reprod* 12:2820, 1997.

14. **Tho PT, Byrd JR, McDonough PG,** Etiologies and subsequent reproductive performance of 100 couples with recurrent abortion, *Fertil Steril* 32:389, 1979.

15. **Harger JH, Archer DF, Marchese SG, Muracca-Clemens M, Garver KL,** Etiology of recurrent pregnancy losses and outcome of subsequent pregnancies, *Obstet Gynecol* 62:574, 1983.

16. **Stray-Pedersen B, Stray-Pedersen S,** Etiologic factors and subsequent reproductive performance in 195 couples with a prior history of habitual abortion, *Am J Obstet Gynecol* 148:140, 1984.

17. **Portnoi M-F, Joye N, van den Akker J, Morlier G, Taillemite JL,** Karyotypes of 1142 couples with recurrent abortion, *Obstet Gynecol* 72:310, 1988.

18. **Plouffe Jr L, White EW, Tho ST, Sweet CS, Layman LC, Whitman GF, McDonough PG,** Etiologic factors of recurrent abortion and subsequent reproductive performance of couples: have we made any progress in the past 10 years? *Am J Obstet Gynecol* 167:313, 1992.

19. **Tulppala M, Palosuo T, Ramsay T, Miettinen A, Salonen R, Ylikorkala O,** A prospective study of 63 couples with a history of recurrent spontaneous abortions: contributing factors and outcome of subsequent pregnancies, *Hum Reprod* 8:7640, 1993.

20. **Boue J, Boue A, Lazar P,** Retrospective and prospective epidemiological studies of 1500 karyotyped spontaneous human abortions, *Teratology* 12:11, 1975.

21. **Guerneri S, Bettio D, Simoni G, Brambat B, Lanzani A, Fraccaro M,** Prevalence and distribution of chromosome abnormalities in a sample of first-trimester internal abortions, *Hum Reprod* 2:735, 1987.

22. **Carr DH,** Chromosome studies in selected spontaneous abortions and early pregnancy loss, *Obstet Gynecol* 37:570, 1971.

23. **McDonough PG,** Repeated first-trimester loss: evaluation and management, *Am J Obstet Gynecol* 153:1, 1985.

24. **Mowbray JF, Underwood J, Gill III TJ,** Familial recurrent spontaneous abortions, *Am J Reprod Immunol* 26:17, 1991.

25. **Armstrong BG, McDonald AD, Sloan M,** Cigarette, alcohol, and coffee consumption and spontaneous abortion, *Am J Public Health* 82:85, 1992.

26. **Windham GC, Voin Behren J, Fenster L, Schaefer C, Swan SH,** Moderate maternal alcohol consumption and risk of spontaneous abortion, *Epidemiology* 8:509, 1997.

27. **Fenster L, Hubbard AE, Swan SH, Windham GC, Waller K, Hiatt RA, Benowitz N,** Caffeinated beverages, decaffeinated coffee, and spontaneous abortion, *Epidemiology* 8:515, 1997.

28. **Schnorr TM, Grajewski BA, Hornung RW, Thun MJ, Egeland GM, Murray WE, Conover DL, Halperin WE,** Video display terminals and the risk of sponaneous abortion, *New Engl J Med* 324:727, 1991.

29. **Lammer EJ, Chen DT, Hoar RM, Agnish ND, Benke PJ, Braun JT, Curry CJ, Fernhoff PM, Grix Jr AW, et al,** Retinoic acid embryopathy, *New Engl J Med* 313:837, 1985.

30. **Heidam LZ,** Spontaneous abortions among laboratory workers, *J Epidemiol Community Health* 38:36, 1984.

31. **Taskinen H, Lindbohm ML, Hemminki K,** Spontaneous abortions among women working in the pharmaceutical industry, *Br J Indust Med* 43:199, 1984.

32. **Belanger K, Leaderer B, Hellenbrand K, Holford TR, McSharry J, Power M-E, Bracken MB,** Spontaneous abortion and exposure to electric blankets and heated water beds, *Epidemiology* 9:36, 1998.

33. **Montoro M, Collea JV, Frasier D, Mestman J,** Successful outcome of pregnancy in women with hypothyroidism, *Ann Intern Med* 94:31, 1981.

34. **Sutherland HW, Pritchard CW,** Increased incidence of spontaneous abortion in pregnancies complicated by maternal diabetes mellitus, *Am J Obstet Gynecol* 155:135, 1986.

35. **Mills JE, Simpson JL, Driscoll SG,** Incidence of spontaneous abortion among normal women and insulin-dependent diabetic women whose pregnancies were identified within 21 days of conception, *New Engl J Med* 319:1617, 1988.

36. **Damewood MD,** The association of endometriosis and repetitive (early) spontaneous abortions, *Seminars Reprod Endocrinol* 7:155, 1989.

37. **Regan L, Owen EJ, Jacobs HS,** Hypersecretion of luteinising hormone, infertility, and miscarriage, *Lancet* 336:1141, 1990.

38. **Tulppala M, Stenman U-H, Cacciatore B, Ylikorkala O,** Polycystic ovaries and levels of gonadotrophins and androgens in recurrent miscarriage: prospective study in 50 women, *Br J Obstet Gynaecol* 100:348, 1993.

39. **Clifford K, Rai R, Watson H, Franks S, Regan L,** Does suppressing luteinising hormone secretion reduce the miscarriage rate? Results of a randomised controlled trial, *Br Med J* 312:1508, 1996.

40. **Sherman RP, Garrett WJ,** Double blind study of effect of 17-hydroxyprogesterone caproate on abortion rate, *Br Med J* i:292, 1963.

41. **Goldstein P, Berrier J, Rosen S, Sacks HS, Chalmers TC,** A meta-analysis of randomized control trials of progestational agents in pregnancy, *Br J Obstet Gynaecol* 96:265, 1989.

42. **Jones GES, Delfs E,** Endocrine patterns in term pregnancies following abortion, *JAMA* 146:1212, 1951.

43. **Stephenson MD,** Frequency of factors associated with habitual abortion in 197 couples, *Fertil Steril* 66:27, 1996.

44. **Li TC,** Recurrent miscarriages: principles of management, *Hum Reprod* 13:478, 1998.

45. **Pellerito JS, McCarthy SM, Doyle MB, Glickman MG, DeCherney AH,** Diagnosis of uterine anomalies: relative accuracy of MR imaging, endovaginal sonography, and hysterosalpingography, *Genitourin Radiol* 183:795, 1992.

46. **Daly DC, Maier D, Soto-Albors C,** Hysteroscopic metroplasty: six years experience, *Obstet Gynecol* 73:201, 1989.

47. **Lazar P, Gueguen S, Dreyfus J, Renaud R, Pontonnier G, Papiernik E,** Multicentered controlled trial of cervical cerclage in women at moderate risk of preterm delivery, *Br J Obstet Gynaecol* 91:731, 1984.

48. **Witkin SS, Ledger WJ,** Antibodies to Chlamydia trachomatis in sera of women with recurrent spontaneous abortions, *Am J Obstet Gynecol* 167:135, 1992.

49. **Osser S, Persson K,** Chlamydial antibodies in women who suffer miscarriage, *Br J Obstet Gynaecol* 103:137, 1996.

50. **Quinn PA, Shewchuk AB, Shuber J, Lie KI, Ryan E, Chipman ML, Nocilla DM,** Efficacy of antibiotic therapy in preventing spontaneous pregnancy loss among couples colonized with genital mycoplasmas, *Am J Obstet Gynecol* 145:239, 1983.

51. **Martinelli I, Sacchi E, Landi G, Taioli E, Duca F, Mannucci PM,** High risk of cerebral-vein thrombosis in carriers of a prothrombin-gene mutation and in users of oral contraceptives, *New Engl J Med* 338:1793, 1998.

52. **Hajjar KA,** Factor V Leiden: an unselfish gene? *New Engl J Med* 331:1585, 1994.

53. **Svensson PJ, Dahlbäck B,** Resistance to activated protein C as a basis for venous thrombosis, *New Engl J Med* 330:517, 1994.

54. **Zöller B, Hillarp A, Berntorp E, Dahlbäck B,** Activated protein C resistance due to a common factor V gene mutation is a major risk factor for venous thrombosis, *Ann Rev Med* 48:45, 1997.

55. **Rees DC, Cox M, Clegg JB,** World distribution of factor V Leiden, *Lancet* 346:1133, 1995.

56. **Zivelin A, Griffin JH, Xu X, Pabinger I, Samama M, Conard J, Brenner B, Eldor A, Seligsohn U,** A single genetic origin for a common Caucasian risk factor for venous thrombosis, *Blood* 89:397, 1997.

57. **Poort SR, Rosendaal FR, Reitsma PH, Bertina RM,** A common genetic variation in the 3'-untranslated region of the prothrombin gene is associated with elevated plasma prothrombin levels and an increase in venous thrombosis, *Blood* 88:3698, 1996.

58. **Rosendaal FR, Doggen CJM, Zivelin A, Arruda VR, Aiach M, Siscovick DS, Hillarp H, Watzke HH, Bernardi F, Cumming AM, Preston FE, Reitsma PH,** Geographic distribution of the 20210 G to A prothrombin variant, *Thromb Haemost* 79:706, 1998.

59. **Brenner B, Mandel H, Lanir N, Younis J, Rothbart H, Ohel G, Blumenfeld Z,** Activated protein C resistance can be associated with recurrent fetal loss, *Br J Haematol* 97:551, 1997.

60. **Rai R, Regan L, Hadley E, Dave M, Cohen H,** Second-trimester pregnancy loss is associated with activated protein C reistance, *Br J Haematol* 92:489, 1996.

61. **Grandone E, Margaglione M, Colaizzo M, d'Addedda M, Cappucci G, Vecchione G, Scianname N, Pavone G, Di Minno G,** Factor V Leiden is associated with repeated and recurrent unexplained fetal losses, *Thromb Haemost* 5:822, 1997.

62. **Balasch J, Reverter JC, Fábregues F, Tàssies D, Rafel M, Creus M, Vanrell JA,** First-trimester abortion is not associated with activated protein C resistance, *Hum Reprod* 12:1094, 1997.

63. **Dizon-Townson D, Kinney S, Branch DW, Ward K,** The factor V Leiden mutation is not a common cause of recurrent miscarriage, *J Reprod Immunol* 34:217, 1997.

64. **Gris JC, Ripart-Neveu S, Maugard C, Tailland ML, Brun S, Courtieu C, Biron C, Hoffet M, Hedon B, Mares P,** Retrospective evaluation of the prevalence of haemostasis abnormalities in unexplained primary early recurrent miscarriages. The Nimes Obstetricians and Haematologists (NOHA) Study, *Thromb Haemost* 77:1096, 1997.

65. **Preston FE, Rosendaal FR, Walker ID, Briet E, Berntorp E, Conard J, Fontcuberta J, Makris M, Mariani G, Noteboom W, Pabinger I, Legnani C, Scharrer I, Schulman S, van der Meer FJ,** Increased fetal loss in women with heritable thrombophilia, *Lancet* 348:913, 1996.

66. **Quere I, Bellet H, Hoffet M, Janbon C, Mares P, Gris J-C,** A woman with five consecutive fetal deaths: case report and retrospective analysis of hyperhomocysteinemia prevalence in 100 consecutive women with recurrent miscarriages, *Fertil Steril* 69:152, 1998.

67. **Tulppala M, Viinikka L, Ylikorkala O,** Thromboxane dominence and prostacyclin deficiency in habitual abortion, *Lancet* 337:879, 1991.

68. **Scott JR, Rote NS, Branch DW,** Immunologic aspects of recurrent abortion and fetal death, *Obstet Gynecol* 70:645, 1987.

69. **Rand JH, Wu XX, Andree HA, Lockwood CJ, Guller S, Scher J, Harpel PC,** Pregnancy loss in the antiphospholipid-antibody syndrome — a possible thrombogenic mechanism, *New Engl J Med* 337:154, 1997.

70. **Branch DW, Silver R, Pierangeli S, van Leeuwen I, Harris EN,** Antiphospholipid antibodies other than lupus anticoagulant and anticardiolipin antibodies in women with recurrent pregnancy loss, fertile controls, and antiphospholipid syndrome, *Obstet Gynecol* 89:549, 1997.

71. **Cowchock S, Smith JB, Gocial B,** Antibodies to phospholipids and nuclear antigens in patients with repeated abortions, *Am J Obstet Gynecol* 155:1002, 1986.

72. **Lockwood CJ, Romero R, Feinberg RF, Clyne LP, Coster B, Hobbins JC,** The prevalence and biologic significance of lupus anticoagulant and anticardiolipin antibodies in a general obstetric population, *Am J Obstet Gynecol* 161:369, 1989.

73. **Balasch J, Lopez-Soto A, Cervera R, Jove I, Casals FJ, Vanrell JA,** Antiphospholipid antibodies in unselected patients with repeated abortion, *Hum Reprod* 5:43, 1990.

74. **Parazzini F, Acaia B, Faden D, Lovotti M, Marelli G, Cortelozzo S,** Antiphospholipid antibodies in recurrent abortion, *Obstet Gynecol* 77:854, 1991.

75. **Infante-Rivard C, David M, Gauthier R, Rivard G-E,** Lupus anticoagulants, anticardiolipin antibodies, and fetal loss, *New Engl J Med* 325:1063, 1991.

76. **Cowchock FS, Reece EA, Balaban D, Branch DW, Plouffe L,** Repeated fetal losses associated with antiphospholipid antibodies: a collaborative randomized trial comparing prednisone with low-dose heparin treatment, *Am J Obstet Gynecol* 166:1318, 1992.

77. **Rai R, Cohen H, Dave M, Regan L,** Randomised controlled trial of aspirin and aspirin plus heparin in pregnant women with recurrent miscarriage associated with phospholipid antibodies (or antiphospholipid antibodies), *Br Med J* 314:253, 1997.

78. **Branch DW, Silver RM, Blackwell JL, Reading JC, Scott JR,** Outcome of treated pregnancies in women with antiphospholipid syndrome: an update of the Utah experience, *Obstet Gynecol* 80:614, 1992.

79. **Kutteh WH,** Antiphospholipid antibody-associated recurrent pregnant loss: treatment with heparin and low-dose aspirin is superior to low-dose aspirin alone, *Am J Obstet Gynecol* 174:1584, 1996.

80. **Tulppala M, Marttunen M, Söderström-Anttila V, Foudila T, Ailus K, Palosuo T, Ylikorkala O,** Low-dose aspirin in prevention of miscarriage in women with unexplained or autoimmune related recurrent miscarriage: effect on prostacyclin and thromboxane A2 production, *Hum Reprod* 12:1567, 1997.

81. **Branch DW, Scott JR, Kochenour NK, Hershgold E,** Obstetric complications associated with the lupus anticoagulant, *New Engl J Med* 313:1322, 1985.

82. **Laskin CA, Bombardier C, Hannah ME, Mandel FP, Ritchie JW, Farewell V, Farine D, Spitzer K, Fielding L, Soloninka CA, Yeung M,** Prednisone and aspirin in women with autoantibodies and unexplained recurrent fetal loss, *New Engl J Med* 337:148, 1997.

83. **Simpson JL, Carson SA, Chesney C, Conley MR, Metzger B, Aarons J, Holmes LB, Jovanovic-Peterson L, Knopp R, Mills JL,** Lack of association between antiphospholipid antibodies and first-trimester spontaneous abortion: prospective study of pregnancies detected within 21 days of conception, *Fertil Steril* 69:814, 1998.

84. **Mowbray JF, Gibbings C, Liddell H, Reginald PW, Underwood JL, Beard RW,** Controlled trial of treatment of recurrent spontaneous abortion by immunization with paternal cells, *Lancet* i:941, 1985.

85. **Unander AM, Lindholm A,** Transfusions of leukocyte-rich erythrocyte concentrates: a successful treatment in selected cases of habitual abortion, *Am J Obstet Gynecol* 154:516, 1986.

86. **Christiansen OB, Mathiesen O, Lauritsen JG, Grunnet N,** Intravenous immnunoglobulin treatment of women with multiple miscarriages, *Hum Reprod* 7:718, 1992.

87. **Stern JJ, Coulam CB, Wagenknecht DR, Peters AJ, Faulk WP, McIntyre JA,** Seminal plasma treatment of recurrent spontaneous abortions, *Am J Reprod Immunol* 27:50, 1992.

88. **Adinolfi M,** Recurrent habitual abortion, HLA sharing and deliberate immunization with partner's cells: a controversial topic, *Hum Reprod* 1:45, 1986.

89. **Eroglu G, Betz G, Torregano C,** Impact of histocompatibility antigens on pregnancy outcome, *Am J Obstet Gynecol* 166:1364, 1992.

90. **Karhukorpi J, Laitinen T, Tiilikainen AS,** HLA-G polymorphism in Finnish couples with recurrent spontaneous miscarriages, *Br J Obstet Gynaecol* 104:1212, 1997.

91. **Cowchuck S,** What's a mother to do? Analysis of trials evaluating new treatments for unexplained recurrent miscarriages and other complaints, *Am J Reprod Immunol* 26:156, 1991.

92. **Ho H-N, Gill III TJ, Hsieh H-J, Hian J-J, Hsieh C-Y,** Immunotherapy for recurrent spontaneous abortions in a Chinese population, *Am J Reprod Immunol* 25:10, 1991.

93. **Cauchi MN, D L, Young DE, Kloss M, Pepperell RJ,** Treatment of recurrent aborters by immunization with paternal cells: controlled trial, *Am J Reprod Immunol* 25:16, 1991.

94. **Christiansen OB, Christiansen BS, Husth M, Mathiesen O, Lauritsen JG, Grunnet N,** Prospective study of anticardiolipin antibodies in immunized and untreated women with recurrent spontaneous abortions, *Fertil Steril* 58:328, 1992.

95. **Illeni MT, Marelli G, Parazzini F, Acaia B, Bocciolone L, Bontempelli M, Faden D, Fedele L, Maffeis A, Radici E,** Immunotherapy and recurrent abortions: a randomized clinical trial, *Hum Reprod* 9:1247, 1994.

96. **Perino A, Vassiliadis A, Vucetich A, Colacurci N, Menato G, Cignitti M, Semprini AE,** Short-term therapy for recurrent abortion using intravenous immunoglobulins: results of a double-blind placebo-controlled Italian study, *Hum Reprod* 12:2388, 1997.

97. **Carp HJA, Toder V, Torchinsky A, Portuguese S, Lipitz S, Gazit E, Mashiach S, and the Recurrent Miscarriage Immunotherapy Trialists Group,** Allogenic leukocyte immunization after five or more miscarriages, *Hum Reprod* 12:250, 1997.

98. **Recurrent Miscarriage Immunotherapy Trialists Group,** Worldwide collaborative observational study and meta-analysis on allogenic leukocyte immunotherapy for recurrent spontaneous abortion, *Am J Reprod Immunol* 32:55, 1994.

99. **Hill JA,** Immunotherapy for recurrent pregnancy loss: "standard of care or buyer beware," *J Soc Gynecol Invest* 4:267, 1997.

100. **Goldenberg RL, Mayberry SK, Copper RL, Dubard MB, Hauth JC,** Pregnancy outcome following a second-trimester loss, *Obstet Gynecol* 81:444, 1993.

101. **Fedele L, Acala B, Parazzini F, Ricciardiello, Cantiani GB,** Ectopic pregnancy and recurrent spontaneous abortion: two associated reproductive failures, *Obstet Gynecol* 73:206, 1989.

102. **Nielsen S, Hahlin M,** Expectant management of first-trimester spontaneous abortion, *Lancet* 345:84, 1995.

103. **Nielsen S, Hahlin M, Möller A, Granberg S,** Bereavement, grieving and psychological morbidity after first trimester spontaneous abortion: comparing expectant management with surgical evacuation, *Hum Reprod* 11:1767, 1996.

104. **Blohm F, Hahlin M, Nielsen S, Milsom I,** Fertility after a randomised trial of spontaneous abortion manged by surgical evacuation or expectant management, *Lancet* 349:995, 1997.

105. **Balasch J, Creus M, Fabregues F, Civico S, Carmona F, Martorell J, Vanrell JA,** In-vitro fertilization treatment for unexplained recurrent abortion: a pilot study, *Hum Reprod* 11:1579, 1996.

106. **Denis AL, Guido M, Adler RD, Bergh PA, Brenner C, Scott Jr RT,** Antiphospholipid antibodies and pregnancy rates and outcome in in vitro patients, *Fertil Steril* 67:1084, 1997.

107. **Raziel A, Herman A, Strassburger D, Soffer Y, Bukovsky I, Ron-El R,** The outcome of in vitro fertilization in unexplained habitual aborters concurrent with secondary infertility, *Fertil Steril* 67:88, 1997.

108. **Remohí J, Gallardo E, Levy M, Valbuena D, de los Santos MJ, Simón C, Pellicer A,** Oocyte donation in women with recurrent pregnancy loss, *Hum Reprod* 11:2048, 1996.

28 Endometriosis

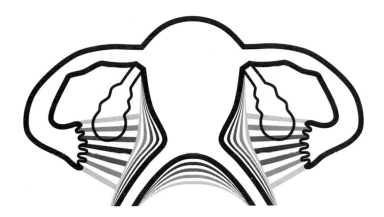

Endometriosis is a disease involving ectopic (outside the uterus) endometrial glands and stroma. In its clinical manifestations, it is a progressive disease that is a vexing problem for both patient and clinician. However, clinical studies over the past 2 decades have provided information for a better understanding of the disease and better decision-making regarding management options. This chapter will review the more recent information regarding treatment as well as what is known concerning the etiology and pathogenesis of endometriosis.

Etiology of Endometriosis

Endometriosis was described in the medical literature in the 1800s, but it was not until the 20th century that its common occurrence was appreciated. Based on clinical observation and examination of histopathologic specimens, John Sampson of Albany, New York, in 1921, suggested that peritoneal endometriosis in the pelvis arose from seedings from ovarian endometriosis. Subsequently, in 1927, he published his classic paper, "Peritoneal Endometriosis Due to Menstrual Dissemination of Endometrial Tissue Into the Peritoneal Cavity," which introduced the term "endometriosis" and established retrograde flow of endometrial tissue through the fallopian tubes and into the abdominal cavity as the probable cause of the disease.[1] The conclusions of Sampson have been validated by the following observations:

1. During laparoscopy, flow of blood from the fimbriated end of the tube has been observed in virtually all menstruating women.[2]

2. Endometriosis is most commonly found in dependent portions of the pelvis, most frequently on the ovaries, the anterior and posterior cul-de-sac, and the uterosacral ligaments, followed by the posterior uterus and posterior broad ligaments.[3–5]

3. Endometrial fragments from the menstrual flow can grow both in tissue culture and following injection beneath the abdominal skin, and can be retrieved from the peritoneal fluid of most menstruating women.[6]

4. Endometriosis developed when the cervices of monkeys were transposed so that menstruation occurred into the peritoneal cavity.[7] The retroperitoneal injection of menstrual endometrium caused peritoneal endometriosis in baboons.[8]

5. A higher incidence of endometriosis is observed in women who have obstructions to the outward flow of the menstrual effluvium.[9]

6. The risk of endometriosis is increased in women with shorter menstrual cycles and longer flows, characteristics that give greater opportunity for ectopic endometrial implantation.[10, 11]

7. Retrograde menstruation has been observed to occur more frequently in baboons with spontaneous endometriosis.[12]

However, there may be other pathways for the development of endometriosis. Endometriosis at sites distant from the pelvis may be due to vascular or lymphatic transport of endometrial fragments.[13] Even the common occurrence of endometriosis on the ovaries can be explained by lymphatic flow from the uterus to the ovary.[14]

Endometriosis can occur in almost every organ of the body.[15] For example, pulmonary endometriosis occurs and can be manifested by asymptomatic nodules or as pneumothorax, hemothorax, or hemoptysis during menses.[16] Urologic endometriosis is of importance because of the possibility for ureteral obstruction.

Extrapelvic endometriosis is occasionally encountered years after surgical removal of the uterus and the ovaries.[17] This endometriosis can be hormone-resistant, and we can only speculate as to why it grows. One possibility is transplantation of endometrial implants during the original surgery, or activation of residual disease. Another possibility is transformation by metaplasia of other tissue or activation of embryonic rest tissue. When the endometriosis is hormone-sensitive, a good possibility is that an ovarian remnant was left behind during the complicated surgery, and this allows continuing hormonal stimulation of residual endometriosis.

There are case reports of endometriosis in men who received treatment with estrogen, and therefore, another possible cause of endometriosis is the transformation of coelomic epithelium into endometrial-type glands as a result of unspecified stimuli. The following arguments can be used to support the coelomic metaplasia theory:[18]

1. Endometriosis occurs in adolescent girls in the absence of müllerian anomalies, and it can be discovered a few years after menarche before many menstrual cycles have been experienced.[19]

2. Endometriosis has been reported in a prepubertal girl.[20]

3. Endometriosis has been encountered in women who never menstruated.[21]

4. Endometriosis in unusual sites, such as thumb, thigh, or knee, can be explained by the fact that mesenchymal limb buds develop adjacent to coelomic epithelium during early embryogenesis.

5. Endometriosis does occur in men, usually associated with high-dose estrogen treatment.[22, 23]

Because many women have reflux seeding of menstrual debris into the peritoneal cavity, and not all develop endometriosis, there may be genetic or immunologic factors that influence the susceptibility of a woman to the disease. Simpson and coworkers reported 6.9% of first-degree relatives of patients with endometriosis had the disease, compared with 1.0% in a control group.[24]

Monozygotic twins are markedly concordant for endometriosis.[25] A worldwide collaborative project (The Oxford Endometriosis Gene Study) has been organized to identify a genetic basis for endometriosis.[26] A web site is available and can be used to provide access to the study for affected families: http://www.medicine.ox.ac.uk/ndog/oxegene/oxegene.htm.

Dmowski and coworkers demonstrated that monkeys with endometriosis had decreased cellular immunity to endometrial tissue, suggesting that specific immunologic defects can render some individuals susceptible to endometriosis.[27] Others have found an increased prevalence of humoral antibodies directed against endometrial and ovarian tissue in the sera of women with endometriosis.[28] In addition, women with endometriosis demonstrate a decrease in various measurements of immune response.[29, 30]

A consideration of the etiologic theories regarding endometriosis leads to the conclusion that all of these mechanisms can contribute to the clinical problem in an individual patient, and the degree of contribution for each probably varies from patient to patient. Endometrial cells can be spread by mechanical means, or perhaps can arise by metaplasia, and progression of the disease is influenced by the individual's immune mechanisms, especially leukocyte and cytokine responses.

Prevalence of Endometriosis

Widely varying figures for the prevalence of endometriosis have been published, and a rough estimate is that 3–10% of women in the reproductive age group and 25–35% of infertile women have endometriosis.[5, 31, 32] About 4 per 1000 women age 15–64 are hospitalized with endometriosis each year, slightly more than those admitted with breast cancer. The common perceptions that endometriosis only occurs in goal-oriented women over the age of 30 and is not found often in black women have now been discredited. Whereas endometriosis essentially does not occur before menarche, there are increasing reports of its occurrence in the teenage years.[33] A number of these cases involve anatomic abnormalities that obstruct the outflow tract.[34] Endometriosis is not confined to nulliparous women, and physicians should be alert to the presence of endometriosis in cases of secondary infertility.

Diagnosis of Endometriosis

Endometriosis should be suspected in any woman complaining of infertility. Suspicion is heightened when there are also complaints of dysmenorrhea and dyspareunia.

Symptoms and Signs

Dysmenorrhea and deep dyspareunia are even more suggestive of endometriosis if the symptoms begin after years of relatively pain-free menses and coitus.[35] It should be recognized, however, that many women who have endometriosis are asymptomatic. A common observation is that some women with extensive endometriosis have little or no pain, whereas others with only minimal endometriosis complain of severe pain. Very severe pain, however, is associated with deeply infiltrating endometriosis.[36–38] Thus, the lack of correlation between pain and visible endometriosis is because the degree of pain is determined by the depth of infiltration. In addition, it has been our observation that midline disease is usually more symptomatic than lesions that are laterally placed.

Pain can be diffuse in the pelvis or it can be more localized, often in the area of the rectum. Symptoms also can arise from rectal, ureteral, or bladder involvement with endometriosis, and can be present throughout the month. Blockage of the ureter can occur, and urinary tract symptoms should be investigated with urologic and radiologic techniques. Low back pain, too, may be due to endometriosis. An association of endometriosis and premenstrual spotting has been suggested, but in most cases menstrual dysfunction is not increased with endometriosis. An association between galactorrhea and endometriosis has been claimed, but baseline elevations of prolactin are not higher in patients with endometriosis than in normal women.[39, 40]

The CA-125 Assay

CA-125 is a cell surface antigen found on derivatives of the coelomic epithelium (which includes endometrium), and it is a useful marker in the monitoring of women with epithelial ovarian carcinoma. In addition, serum CA-125 levels are often elevated in patients with endometriosis and correlate with both the degree of disease and the response to treatment.[41, 42] The sensitivity of this assay is too low to use it as a screening test, but it can be a marker of response to treatment and for recurrence; however, elevated levels which suppress during medical treatment often promptly return to pretreatment concentrations immediately after cessation of therapy, limiting its clinical usefulness.[43] Serum CA-125 determinations may be able to differentiate endometriotic from nonendometriotic benign adnexal cysts, especially when combined with transvaginal ultrasonography.[44, 45] Note that CA-125 levels can be elevated by early pregnancy, acute pelvic inflammatory disease, leiomyomata, and menstruation.

Examination

We recommend that pelvic examination be performed at the time of menses when tenderness is easier to detect. The uterus is often in fixed retroversion and the ovaries may be enlarged. However, retroversion of the uterus is not an etiologic factor, and prophylactic uterine suspension is no longer recommended. Nodularity (which is usually tender) of the uterosacral ligaments and cul-de-sac can be found in one-third of patients with endometriosis. The diagnosis almost always should be confirmed by laparoscopy before treatment is initiated. Minimal findings, such as slight beading and tenderness of the uterosacral ligaments in the young, asymptomatic patient, can be treated initially, however, with combined, low dose oral contraceptives.

The classic chocolate cyst of the ovary is the result of a blood-filled cavity within an endometrioma. Ultrasonography and magnetic resonance imaging can be helpful in diagnosing endometriomas.[46–48] However, neither can diagnose small peritoneal implants or adhesions. Although transvaginal ultrasonography is highly accurate in diagnosing ovarian endometriomas, hemorrhagic cysts account for a significant false positive rate.[45]

The appearance of endometriosis is quite varied. All too often the clinician fails to observe endometrial lesions because of a preconceived expectation limited to the classic blue or black powder burn appearance. Lesions can be red, black, blue, or white and nonpigmented.[49] Biopsies from visibly normal peritoneum can contain endometriosis in 6–13% of infertile women; however, the clinical significence of this presence is uncertain (and, in our view, unlikely to be important).[50] Adhesions, peritoneal defects, and tan, creamy, fresh-appearing endometrium also can be observed. The dark pigmented lesions are later consequences of tissue bleeding responses to cyclic hormones. The ovary is the most common site for both implants and adhesions, followed by widespread distribution, anteriorly and posteriorly, over the broad ligament and cul-de-sac.[3–5]

A Classification System

Because both treatment and prognosis are determined to some extent by the severity of the disease, it is desirable to have a uniform system of classification that takes into account both the extent and severity of the disease. A uniform classification is also crucial for comparing the results of different treatments. The American Society for Reproductive Medicine developed a classification system based on findings at laparoscopy or laparotomy.[51] However, there were weaknesses in the classification system, especially the fact that it was based upon the arbitrary impressions of the clinician. A revised classification system was produced to standardize the documentation of findings in patients who have pelvic pain and endometriosis, and forms are available from the Society.[52] There can be a high intraobserver and interobserver variability in the evaluation of endometriosis using any classification system.[53, 54] Therefore, efforts must continue to provide an accurate method for staging.

Endometriosis and Infertility

When endometriosis involves the ovaries and causes adhesions that block tubal motility and pickup of the egg, there is no question of its role in causing mechanical interference with fertility. Less secure is the information on the role of peritoneal endometriosis on fertility. Many physicians believe that even minimal endometriosis can cause infertility, impairing tubal function or gamete quality. This argument has been weakened by a failure to find benefit from medical treatment of infertility associated with minimal to mild endometriosis.[55–58]

The absence of benefit from therapy, however, could represent a problem with the treatment rather than a lack of association between infertility and endometriosis.[59] Endometriosis diagnosed by laparoscopy is reported in a higher proportion of infertile women (38.5%) compared with fertile women (5.2%).[60] Moreover, fecundity rates in women with endometriosis tend to be lower than the normal fecundity rate.[32, 61, 62] However, the long-term cumulative pregnancy rates are very high in women who have minimal to mild endometriosis and are not treated.[63]

If minimal or mild endometriosis does affect fertility, what are the mechanisms? Certainly, dyspareunia secondary to endometriosis could play a role.

Another mediator could be prostaglandins produced by the implants, which could, in turn, affect tubal motility, or folliculogenesis and corpus luteum function. Patients with endometriosis have been reported to have an increase in both the volume of peritoneal fluid and the concentration of thromboxane B_2 and 6-keto-prostaglandin $F_{1\alpha}$ in the fluid.[64, 65] Others, however, found neither an increase in peritoneal fluid nor an increase in concentration of peritoneal fluid prostaglandin E_2, prostaglandin $F_{2\alpha}$, 15-keto-13,14-dihydroprostaglandin $F_{2\alpha}$, and thromboxane B_2.[66, 67]

Subsequent studies also have provided contradictory information. No elevation in peritoneal fluid prostanoid levels during the proliferative phase in women with endometriosis has been reported, and similarly no peritoneal fluid elevation in 6-keto prostaglandin $F_{1\alpha}$ levels has been observed in the luteal phase.[68, 69] However, others have reported elevated concentrations of prostanoids in the peritoneal fluid of women with endometriosis.[70] These differences could be accounted for by differing levels of prostaglandin synthesis according to different morphologic characteristics of the lesions.[71] In summary, it has not been established that women with endometriosis have higher levels of prostanoids in peritoneal fluid compared to other infertile women. Even if higher levels were found consistently, their role in infertility still would be speculative. Nevertheless, interest in prostaglandins continues. A correlation can be demonstrated between the degree of dysmenorrhea experienced by women with endometriosis and the amount of prostaglandins produced by the endometriosis tissue.[72]

Peritoneal macrophages have been suggested as possible mediators of infertility, and increased activation of macrophages has been found in association with endometriosis.[73, 74] Phagocytosis of sperm by macrophages could be one mechanism of action.[75] However, patients with and without endometriosis have the same number of motile sperm recoverable from the peritoneal cavity. Peritoneal macrophages from women with endometriosis secrete interleukin-1 which is toxic to mouse embryos.[76] In addition, cytokines are elevated in the peritoneal fluid, which could recruit macrophages and lymphocytes and perpetuate the inflammatory reaction.[77] Macrophages and endometrial cells also produce vascular endothelial growth factor (VEGF), an important angiogenic factor involved in endometrial proliferation.[78]

Endometriosis has been implicated as a factor in disordered follicle growth, ovulatory dysfunction, and failure of embryo development. Ultrasonography studies suggest that there is some retardation in growth of follicles in women with endometriosis. Luteinized unruptured follicle syndrome (LUF) in which the oocyte is not released at the time of follicle rupture (or there is a failure of the follicle to rupture) has been suggested as a cause of both unexplained infertility and infertility secondary to endometriosis. Although an unruptured follicle can occur in women, there currently is no impressive evidence that this syndrome is secondary to endometriosis or is even a cause of infertility.[79]

The question of how minimal or mild endometriosis can affect fertility now has been superseded by the question of whether there is *any* effect of mild endometriosis on fertility. More importantly, should endometriosis be treated if the complaint is infertility and not pain? Many articles purporting to show that therapy overcomes endometriosis-associated infertility are flawed by lack of control groups and the failure to use life-table analyses.[66] Moreover, expectant management of mild endometriosis is rewarded with reasonable pregnancy rates that are comparable to those obtained with treatment.[55–58, 80–83] A cumulative pregnancy rate after 5 years of 90% has been reported in women not treated for minimal or mild endometriosis.[63]

Whereas the studies cited above strongly suggest that medical or surgical treatment of mild endometriosis may not be worthwhile, there are those who champion fulguration treatment under laparoscopic visualization.[84] In a randomized trial involving 341 infertile women with minimal or mild endometriosis, comparing diagnostic laparoscopy with laparoscopic resection or ablation of visible endometriosis, the surgically-treated group experienced a 48% pregnancy rate (over 9 months) compared with 35% in the non-treated group.[85] Of note was the observation that this improvement only occurred in women with blue or black lesions, not with red lesions. Furthermore, an argument can be made that active treatment of even mild endometriosis is warranted because endometriosis is often a progressive disease.

The increase (only a modest one) in the pregnancy rate associated with laparoscopic treatment is consistent with the good pregnancy rates associated with expectant management of mild endometriosis. Nevertheless, it is currently recommended that resection or ablation should be immediately performed when minimal or mild endometriosis is diagnosed during laparoscopy for infertility. Moderate and severe endometriosis should be treated surgically at the time of diagnosis. If pregnancy is not achieved after surgery, infertility should be treated first with superovulation and IUI, and then with IVF.[86]

Surgical Treatment of Endometriosis

In contrast to the dispute over the proper treatment of mild endometriosis, there is little doubt that adhesive disease associated with endometriosis, or large (>2 cm) endometriomas, is best treated by surgery. The object of surgery should be to restore normal anatomical relationships and to excise or fulgurate as much of the endometriosis as possible. Removal of severely diseased adnexa when the other side is more normal produces better results than attempts to do major repairs. Presacral neurectomy does not enhance fertility, although many surgeons advocate it to alleviate dysmenorrhea. This may be less compelling now that prostaglandin inhibitors are available to accomplish the same purpose. A careful study of presacral neurectomy concluded that this procedure is only indicated in patients with pain limited to the midline area.[87]

The success of surgery in relieving infertility is directly related to the severity of endometriosis. Patients with moderate disease can expect a pregnancy success of approximately 60%, whereas the comparable figure is 35% in those with severe disease.[88] As noted above, surgical treatment of blue or black lesions yielded a slightly higher (13%) pregnancy rate compared to expectant management in a randomized trial.[85] Of note was the observation that this improvement only occurred in women with blue or black lesions, not with red lesions. There is support for selective use of medical treatment for 2–3 months following laparoscopy and prior to conservative surgery, especially in patients with pain due to major disease.[89] Preoperative treatment aids surgery by softening endometrial implants.

Postoperative use of hormones has been the subject of greater controversy. The highest pregnancy rates following conservative surgery occur in the first year after surgery, and most physicians have been reluctant to use hormones that prevent pregnancy even for a few months. If pregnancy does not occur within 2 years of surgery for endometriosis, the chances are poor that pregnancy will occur. The recurrence rate reported for endometriosis after surgery is 20% within 5 years,[90, 91] and when it does recur, second surgeries to aid fertility have only a limited chance for success. When the objective of laparoscopic surgery is symptomatic relief and not pregnancy, a return of symptoms is delayed with as little as 6 months of postoperative medical treatment.[92]

The type of surgery that we have been discussing is labeled "conservative" to indicate that reproductive function is maintained. When endometriomas are removed a vigorous attempt should be made to leave behind any normal ovarian tissue. Even one-tenth of an ovary can be enough to preserve function and fertility. Conservative surgery can be accomplished by laparoscopy which decreases costs and morbidity, yet provides results that are as efficacious in all stages of disease as laparotomy.[93]

"Conservative" surgery is in contradistinction to "radical" surgery, which includes hysterectomy and usually bilateral salpingo-oophorectomy. When radical surgery is performed, an uninvolved ovary can be preserved in some cases if all of the nonovarian endometriosis is removed by fulguration or excision. However, this does provide a risk for recurrent disease. Patients who undergo hysterectomy with ovarian conservation have a 6-fold increased risk of developing recurrent symptoms compared with women who have oophorectomy.[94]

Medical Treatment of Endometriosis

Although hormonal therapy of infertility associated with endometriosis is not of proven value,[95] medical therapy for dysmenorrhea, dyspareunia, and pelvic pain associated with endometriosis is very successful (although relief may be short-term). ***The various agents used are comparable in terms of efficacy, and choice of treatment is determined by cost and side effects.*** Implants of endometriosis react to steroid hormones in a manner somewhat, but not exactly, similar to normally stimulated endometrium. However, endometriotic tissue displays histologic differences and biochemical differences, including enzyme activity and receptor levels that differ in concentration and response compared to normal endometrium. Nevertheless, estrogen stimulates growth of the implants. For this reason, endometriosis usually regresses following menopause and is usually not found prior to menarche unless there is a blockage of the outflow tract.

Hormonal therapy is designed to interrupt the cycle of stimulation and bleeding. An early approach was the use of massive doses of diethylstilbestrol (DES), which, because of variable success, the risk of affecting the fetus, and side effects of severe bleeding and nausea, is now of only historical interest. Treatment with androgens (methyltestosterone linguets 5–10 mg/day) can provide only transient relief of the pain of endometriosis, and its effect on infertility appears to be negligible. In addition, ovulation can occur while on treatment, and there is a risk of exposure of the fetus to the androgen.

Until the late 1970s the most important alternative to conservative surgery was the use of combination oral contraceptives taken in a continuous fashion.[96] It seems to matter little which low dose monophasic product is used to accomplish the conversion of endometrial implants into decidualized cells associated with a few inactive endometrial glands.[97] At this time the efficacy of the multiphasic formulations is unknown. The usual dose of the combined oral contraceptive is one pill per day continuously for 6–12 months. Estrogen (conjugated estrogens 1.25 mg or estradiol 2.0 mg daily for 1 week) is added if breakthrough bleeding occurs. The treatment with oral contraceptives was called pseudopregnancy because of the amenorrhea and the decidualization of the endometrial tissue induced by the estrogen-progestin combination. It also reflected the commonly held belief that pregnancy can improve endometriosis, a belief that has been disputed. The side effects of treatment are those associated with oral contraceptives (Chapter 22). Pregnancy rates after stopping medication are reported to be in the 40–50% range. Whereas published recurrence rates are not excessive, this therapy, as with all medical treatment for endometriosis, must be viewed as suppressive rather than curative.

Treatment With Danazol

The golden age for danazol has passed. Although its expense and side effects seemed a reasonable tradeoff for an effective treatment, it is now apparent that danazol is no more effective than the other medications used to treat endometriosis. In distinction to the pseudopregnancy induced by oral contraceptives, danazol produces what has been incorrectly termed as pseudomenopause. Danazol is an isoxazole derivative of the synthetic steroid 17α-ethinyltestosterone. It originally was thought to exert its effect solely by inhibition of pituitary gonadotropins. Although danazol can decrease follicle-stimulating hormone (FSH) and luteinizing hormone (LH) in castrated individuals, it does not alter basal gonadotropin concentrations in premenopausal women. It does, however, eliminate the midcycle surge of FSH and LH. Danazol inhibits steroidogenesis in the human corpus luteum.[98] Danazol is metabolized to at least 60 different products, some of which may contribute to its many effects. The multiple effects of danazol produce a high-androgen, low-estrogen environment that does not support the growth of endometriosis, and the amenorrhea that is produced prevents new seeding from the uterus into the peritoneal cavity.[99]

Danazol

The side effects of danazol are related both to the hypoestrogenic environment it creates and to its androgenic properties. The most common side effects are weight gain, fluid retention, fatigue, decreased breast size, acne, oily skin, growth of facial hair, atrophic vaginitis, hot flushes, muscle cramps, and emotional lability. Some of these side effects occur in approximately 80% of women who are taking danazol, but less than 10% find the side effects sufficiently troublesome to warrant discontinuation of the drug. Because danazol has been associated with the development *in utero* of female pseudohermaphroditism, it should not be given if there is the possibility of pregnancy.[100] The androgenic action of danazol can irreversibly deepen the voice.[101, 102] It is worth inquiring whether singing is an important part of your patient's life before prescribing this drug.

Danazol is metabolized largely in the liver, and in some patients it causes hepatocellular damage. Its use, therefore, is contraindicated in women with liver disease. Furthermore, liver enzymes should be monitored during treatment with danazol. The fluid retention that is often associated with danazol makes it dangerous to use when there is severe hypertension, congestive heart failure, or impaired renal function. It can produce increased cholesterol and low-density lipoprotein levels and decreased levels of high-density lipoprotein. It is unlikely that these short-term effects on lipids and lipoproteins are clinically important. The drug has been used to treat autoimmune disease, but it is not known if this action plays a role in its effects on endometriosis.

It should be noted again that medical treatment of mild endometriosis associated with infertility has been called into question because women with untreated mild endometriosis have pregnancy rates equal to women who have received medical treatment for the endometriosis. Thus, danazol treatment of infertility associated with mild endometriosis has no scientific support.

On the other hand, danazol is useful to relieve the pain of endometriosis and to prevent progression of the disease. Pain relief is obtained in 90% of patients. The usual dose is two 200 mg tablets twice a day (although some claim that spacing the drug at 6-hour intervals may be more effective) for 6 months. Dmowski and Cohen reviewed 99 women who completed danazol treatment for a period of 3–18 months (average 6 months) and who were reevaluated an average of 37 months later.[103] During the course of treatment all the patients had symptomatic improvement, and the majority (85%) were clinically improved. At the time of the reevaluation, however, approximately one-third were symptomatic and had clinical findings suggestive of recurrent endometriosis. In the majority of these patients, the symptoms recurred within the first year after discontinuation of the drug.

The success of danazol treatment is greatest in cases of peritoneal endometriosis or those with small lesions of the ovary. Endometriomas larger than 1.0 cm are less likely to respond to danazol, although quite surprising regression of endometriomas larger than 1.0 cm is sometimes seen.

Because of the significant side effects encountered with danazol, and its cost, there has been a trend toward the use of lower doses than the usual 800 mg daily. However, doses below 800 mg may be less effective.[104] The occurrence of amenorrhea appears to be correlated with improved outcome, and this is more consistently obtained at the 800 mg level. Others, however, do not believe that amenorrhea is an important consideration because many of the patients will bleed from an atrophic endometrium.

There is a general perception, but only limited experimental evidence, that danazol is more effective than oral contraceptives for the treatment of endometriosis.[105] Noble and Letchworth compared danazol with a high dose estrogen-progestin combination (Enovid).[106] The dose of both danazol and the oral contraceptive was increased until the patients became amenorrheic. One of 25 patients taking danazol could not complete 5 months of treatment, whereas 7 of 17 (41%) of the group taking oral contraceptives dropped out because of side effects. Danazol was more effective than estrogen-progestin in relieving symptoms, and laparoscopic assessment showed much better results with danazol. Seven of 12 danazol-treated patients became pregnant compared with 4 of the 10 women who had taken oral contraceptives. Unfortunately, the study size was too small to allow statistical analysis.

Treatment With a Progestational Agent

Both oral and injectable medroxyprogesterone acetate have been effective in treating endometriosis by causing decidualization and subsequent atrophy of endometrial tissue.[107] Medroxyprogesterone acetate in an oral dose of 30 mg daily has been demonstrated to be as effective as danazol in treating endometriosis.[82] Similar results have been obtained with higher doses.[108] Although not studied, it is likely that lower doses (10–20 mg daily) would be effective. For this reason and because it is more cost-effective and there are fewer side effects, medroxyprogesterone acetate is often the first choice for medical treatment of endometriosis. High doses of medroxyprogesterone can adversely affect the lipoprotein profile; there is no reason to use a dose greater than 30 mg/day. Megestrol acetate has been administered in a dose of 40 mg daily with good results.[109] These progestin doses suppress luteinizing hormone (LH) secretion, and, therefore, patients can be relatively hypoestrogenic. As a result, some loss in spinal bone can occur, but recovery follows discontinuation of treatment, and there should be no effect on fracture risk.[110]

Side effects include weight gain, fluid retention, and breakthrough bleeding. Breakthrough bleeding is a common occurrence although it is usually cleared by short-term (7 days) administration of estrogen. Depression is a significant problem, and both patient and physician should be alert for its development. The usefulness of depo-medroxyprogesterone acetate (150 mg im every 3 months) in infertile patients is limited by the varying length of time it takes for ovulation to resume after discontinuation of therapy. This is not a problem with oral administration.

Medroxyprogesterone acetate, like danazol, can relieve the symptoms of endometriosis, but it is not effective in treating infertility. In a prospective, randomized clinical trial, there was no difference in pregnancy rates following treatment with medroxyprogesterone acetate (100 mg/day) or placebo.[111]

Treatment With GnRH Agonists

Gonadotropin-releasing hormone (GnRH) has a short half-life because it is rapidly cleaved between amino acids 5–6, 6–7, and 9–10. Analogues of GnRH have been produced by altering the amino acids at these positions. Substitutions of amino acids at the 6 position and/or replacement of the C-terminal glycine-amide (inhibiting degradation) produce agonists. The GnRH agonists are administered intramuscularly, subcutaneously, or by intranasal absorption. After an initial agonistic action (the so-called flare response), down-regulation and desensitization of the pituitary produce a hypogonadotropic, hypogonad state. The depot formulation of leuprolide is administered intramuscularly and monthly. Goserelin comes in a small biodegradable cylinder that is inserted subcutaneously and monthly using a prepackaged syringe.

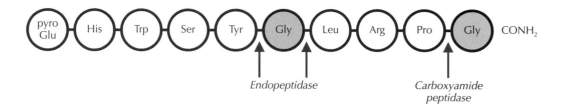

Gonadotropin releasing hormone

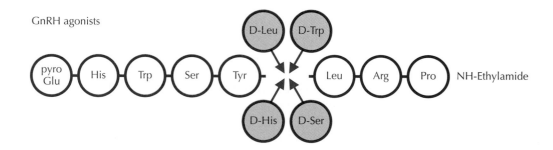

GnRH agonists

A long-acting GnRH agonist can create a pseudomenopause for the treatment of endometriosis.[112, 113] At the end of 2–4 weeks of daily administration of the agonist, estrogen levels will decrease to those found in oophorectomized women. Dosage can be adjusted by monitoring serum estradiol levels; the best therapeutic effect is associated with a range of 20–40 pg/mL. Thus, the "medical oophorectomy" caused by the continuous use of a GnRH agonist has provided a new approach to the treatment of endometriosis. Excellent, large, well-designed studies (with advanced disease in nearly 50% of the patients) have compared GnRH agonist therapy (with various agents) with danazol.[114–118] The results in terms of reduction of disease (as demonstrated by post-treatment laparoscopies) and pregnancy rates have been the same with either treatment. However, GnRH agonist treatment does not have an adverse impact on serum lipids and lipoproteins compared to that observed with danazol.[119] An experimental comparison of agonist and progestin treatment in monkeys concluded that the progestin was just as effective as the agonist.[120]

GnRH Agonists in Clinical Use

Position	1	2	3	4	5	6	7	8	9	10
Native GnRH	pGlu	His	Trp	Ser	Tyr	Gly	Leu	Arg	Pro	Gly-NH$_2$
Leuprolide						D-Leu				NH-Ethylamide
Buserelin						D-Ser (tertiary butanol)				NH-Ethylamide
Nafarelin						D-Naphthylalanine (2)				
Histrelin						D-His (tertiary benzyl)				NH-Ethylamide
Goserelin						D-Ser (tertiary butanol)				Aza-Gly
Deslorelin						D-Trp				NH-Ethylamide
Tryptorelin						D-Trp				

An uneventful pregnancy with delivery of a normal infant has been reported despite GnRH agonist treatment (monthly treatment with a long-acting agonist was continued through the first two months of pregnancy).[121]

As with all other drug therapies of endometriosis, the GnRH agonist provides suppression rather than cure of the disease. The long-term consequences of the hypoestrogenic state on calcium metabolism and bone are of concern. Therefore, treatment is usually limited to 6 months to avoid bone loss, although even during this time period there can be a 6–8% decrease in trabecular bone density. This short-term bone loss is reversed after cessation of therapy, but many patients have not regained the bone that was lost, as much as one year later.[122–124] A study with longer follow-up indicated that bone density was restored by 2 years after 6 months of GnRH agonist treatment.[125] Because long-term therapy carries with it the concern over a lasting impact on the risk of osteoporosis, consideration should be given to add-back therapy. The addition of a 19-nortestosterone progestin as add-back treatment is effective in decreasing bone loss.[126–128] A postmenopausal estrogen-progestin program can be utilized (conjugated estrogens 0.625 mg daily and medroxyprogesterone acetate 2.5 mg daily or any of the other estrogen-progestin combinations available). This combined add-back treatment is effective for endometriosis and prevents the hypoestrogenic symptoms (especially hot flushes and vaginal dryness) associated with GnRH agonist therapy, including loss of bone.[129] Other effective options for add-back therapy to prevent bone loss are tibolone (2.5 mg daily) and bisphosphonate treatment.[130, 131] Endometriosis by itself is not a cause of accelerated bone loss.[132–134]

In well-designed trials, treatment with GnRH agonists has not increased pregnancy rates in women with infertility associated with minimal or mild endometriosis.[95]

Treatment With Gestrinone

Gestrinone, a 19-nortestosterone derivative, decreases the secretion of FSH and LH and has the advantage of requiring only twice a week administration. Used in Europe, it has been as effective as danazol in treating endometriosis.[135] The clinical side effects are also similar to those seen with danazol. As with other hormonal treatments, gestrinone has been ineffective for the infertility associated with endometriosis.[95]

Recurrence of Endometriosis

Endometriosis tends to recur unless definitive surgery (total hysterectomy and bilateral oophorectomy) is performed. The recurrence rate with medical treatment is approximately 5–20% per year (reaching an overall cumulative rate at 5 years as much as 40%). The recurrence rates 5 years after women were treated with various GnRH agonists were 37% for minimal disease and 74% for severe disease.[136] After 7 years, 56% of all treated women had a recurrence. In women treated for pelvic pain, the symptoms usually return rather quickly after cessation of medical therapy.[97, 107] For a period of time after medical treatment, however, the intensity of symptoms is less severe.[115, 137] *It should be emphasized that pain relief, pregnancy rates, and recurrence rates are similar with all methods of medical treatment.* A randomized clinical trial comparing a low-dose oral contraceptive with a GnRH agonist measured no difference in the recurrence of pain.[97] The recurrence rates after treatment with GnRH agonists are similar to those after danazol, and both are greater than that obtained with surgical excision. After conservative laparoscopy, approximately 10% of patients experience a recurrence within 1 year, and 20% within 5 years.[90, 91]

Speculation regarding the reason for recurrence focuses on endometriosis (perhaps microscopic) which escaped detection, incomplete treatment, or reestablishment of primary disease by whatever mechanism is responsible. *The treatment choices and results are no different than when originally confronted.* Successful treatment with total pelvic irradiation has been reported in rare patients who have repeatedly failed standard therapy.[138]

Hormone Treatment After Surgery

Definitive surgery for severe endometriosis, which includes abdominal hysterectomy and bilateral salpingo-oophorectomy as well as resection of all endometriosis, is the only cure for the disease. If oophorectomy is performed, estrogen-progestin therapy at usual doses can be started immediately postoperatively with an essentially negligible risk of inciting growth of residual endometriosis or a return of pain.[139] *The addition of a progestational agent is strongly recommended because of reported cases of adenocarcinoma in endometriosis tissue in women treated with unopposed estrogen, as well as exacerbation of residual disease.*[94, 140–143]

Long-Term Medical Therapy

Long-term medical therapy without surgery is useful in patients with severe symptoms but with little in the way of palpable findings. Before undertaking prolonged therapy, diagnosis should be established by laparoscopy. Prolonged medical therapy also is indicated if symptoms recur after conservative surgery.

Prevention of Infertility

A common clinical problem is the incidental finding at surgery of mild endometriosis in a young woman who has no immediate interest in pregnancy. As previously stated, we favor immediate surgical treatment of visible endometriosis when the opportunity presents itself. Consideration should be given, however, to prophylactic therapy. Combination oral contraceptives to decrease the risk of further seeding are appropriate for treatment of very mild disease, for example a few implants in the cul-de-sac. More advanced disease should be treated with 6 months of medroxyprogesterone acetate, a GnRH agonist, or danazol, followed by oral contraceptives to decrease the risks of progression of the disease. Although not well documented, clinical experience has suggested that continuous oral contraceptives are more effective as prophylaxis than the usual cyclic regimen. Indeed, we favor the continuous regimen without a break for this purpose.

As with all medical treatments, as time passes after treatment, endometriosis emerges. Although spontaneous regression occurs, endometriosis is usually progressive. The risk of endometriosis is reduced in women currently using oral contraceptives; however, effective prophylaxis requires long-term treatment.[144] Nevertheless, treatment of endometriosis does have a beneficial impact on the natural history of the disease. Consideration should be given to the prophylactic use of oral contraceptives in women with impressive family histories of endometriosis.

Endometriosis and Spontaneous Miscarriage

Endometriosis has been purported to be associated with an increased risk of spontaneous miscarriage, a risk that is said to be substantially lessened by either medical or surgical treatment.[145] In appropriately controlled studies, however, the miscarriage rate was in the normal range in women with endometriosis who were not treated, and it is likely that previous studies were flawed by their choice of control miscarriage rates.[85, 146, 147]

Endometriosis and Ovulation

The frequency of anovulation and luteal phase defects is similar in women with and without endometriosis.[148, 149] Thus, a woman need not be ovulating in order to have endometriosis. One report has suggested, however, that the success of ovulation induction in women with endometriosis is enhanced by prior treatment with danazol.[150]

Endometriosis and Assisted Reproduction

The use of superovulation with intrauterine insemination (Chapters 30 and 31) has been reported to increase fecundity rates (as high as 5- or 6-fold) in women with infertility associated with endometriosis.[151–153] However, although superovulation raised fecundity rates, it did not raise cumulative pregnancy rates.[154] This treatment may accelerate the occurrence of pregnancy without changing overall fertility.

Individuals with mild to moderate endometriosis do as well in in vitro fertilization programs as those with tubal disease.[155, 156] Although results with severe endometriosis have been poor in the past, more recent experience (perhaps reflecting improved technique and technology) has yielded good pregnancy rates (Chapter 31).[157, 158]

A Patient Support Organization

The Endometriosis Association is an international organization that provides education and support for women with endometriosis. Their information prepared for teenagers is especially helpful.

Endometriosis Association International Headquarters
8585 N. 76th Place
Milwaukee, WI 53223

http://www.EndometriosisAssn.org

References

1. **Sampson JA,** Peritoneal endometriosis due to the menstrual dissemination of endometrial tissue into the peritoneal cavity, *Am J Obstet Gynecol* 14:422, 1927.

2. **Liu DTY, Hitchchock A,** Endometriosis: its association with retrograde menstruation, dysmenorrhea, and tubal pathology, *Br J Obstet Gynaecol* 93:859, 1986.

3. **Ishimaru T, Masuzaki H,** Peritoneal endometriosis: endometrial tissue implantation as its primary etiologic mechanism, *Am J Obstet Gynecol* 165:210, 1991.

4. **Jenkins S, Olive DL, Haney AF,** Endometriosis: pathogenetic implications of the anatomic distribution, *Obstet Gynecol* 67:335, 1986.

5. **Gruppos Italiano per lo Studio Dell'Endometriosi,** Prevalence and anatomical distribution of endometriosis in women with selected gynaecological conditions: results from a multicentric Italian study, *Hum Reprod* 9:1158, 1994.

6. **Kruitwagen RFPM, Poels LG, Willemsen WNP, Jap PHK, Thomas CMG, Rolland R,** Endometrial epithelial cells in peritoneal fluid during the ealy follicular phase, *Fertil Steril* 55:297, 1991.

7. **Scott RB, TeLinde RW, Wharton Jr LR,** Further studies on experimental endometriosis, *Am J Obstet Gynecol* 66:1082, 1953.

8. **D'Hooghe TM, Bambra CS, Raeymaekers BM, De Jonge I, Lauweryns JM, Koninckx PR,** Intrapelvic injection of menstrual endometrium causes endometriosis in baboons (*Papio cynocephalus* and *Papio anubis*), *Am J Obstet Gynecol* 173:125, 1995.

9. **Olive DL, Henderson DY,** Endometriosis and müllerian anomalies, *Obstet Gynecol* 69:412, 1987.

10. **Cramer DW, Wilson E, Stillman RJ, Berger MJ, Belisle S, Schiff I, Albrecht B, Gibson M, Stadel BV, Schoenbaum SC,** The relation of endometriosis to menstrual characteristics, smoking and exercise, *JAMA* 355:1904, 1986.

11. **Darrow SL, Vena JE, Batt RE, Zielezny MA, Michalek AM, Selman S,** Menstrual cycle characteristics and the risk of endometriosis, *Epidemiology* 4:135, 1993.

12. **Hooghe TMD, Bambra CS, Raeymaekers BM, Koninckx PR,** Increased prevalence and recurrence of retrograde menstruation in baboons with spontaneous endometriosis, *Hum Reprod* 11:2022, 1996.

13. **Javert CT,** Pathogenesis of endometriosis based on endometrial homeoplasia, direct extension, exfoliation and implantation, lymphatic and hematogenous metastasis. Including five case reports of endometrial tissue in pelvic lymph nodes, *Cancer* 2:399, 1949.

14. **Ueki M,** Histologic study of endometriosis and examination of lymphatic drainage in and from the uterus, *Am J Obstet Gynecol* 165:201, 1991.

15. **Rock JA, Markham SM,** Extra pelvic endometriosis, In: Wilson EA, ed. *Endometriosis,* Alan R. Liss, Inc., New York, 1987, p 185.

16. **Foster DC, Stern JL, Buscema J, Rock JA, Woodruff JD,** Pleural and parenchymal pulmonary endometriosis, *Obstet Gynecol* 58:552, 1981.

17. **Metzger DA, Lessey BA, Soper JT, McCarty Jr KS, Haney AF,** Hormone-resistant endometriosis following total abdominal hysterectomy and bilateral salpingo-oophorectomy: correlation with histology and steroid receptor content, *Obstet Gynecol* 78:946, 1991.

18. **Suginami H,** A reappraisal of the coelomic metaplasia theory by reviewing endometriosis occurring in unusual sites and instances, *Am J Obstet Gynecol* 165:214, 1991.

19. **Schifrin BS, Erez S, Moore JG,** Teen-age endometriosis, *Am J Obstet Gynecol* 116:973, 1973.

20. **Clark AH,** Endometriosis in a young girl, *JAMA* 136:690, 1948.

21. **El-Mahgoub S, Yaseen S,** A positive proof for the theory of coelomic metaplasia, *Am J Obstet Gynecol* 137:137, 1980.

22. **Oliker AJ, Harris AE,** Endometriosis of the bladder in a male patient, *J Urol* 106:858, 1971.

23. **Schrodt GR, O AM, Ibanez J,** Endometriosis of the male urinary system: a case report, *J Urol* 124:722, 1980.

24. **Simpson JL, Elias J, Malinak LR, Buttram VC,** Heritable aspects of endometriosis. I. Genetic studies, *Am J Obstet Gynecol* 137:327, 1980.

25. **Hadfield RM, Mardon JH, Barlow DH, Kennedy SH,** Endometriosis in monozygotic twins, *Fertil Steril* 68:941, 1997.

26. **Kennedy S,** Is there a genetic basis to endometriosis? *Seminars Reprod Endocrinol* 15:309, 1997.

27. **Dmowski WP, Steele RW, Baker GF,** Deficient cellular immunity in endometriosis, *Am J Obstet Gynecol* 141:377, 1981.

28. **Mathur S, Peress MR, Williamson HO, Youmans CD, Maney SA, Garvin AJ, Rust PF, Fudenberg HH,** Autoimmunity to endometrium and ovary in endometriosis, *Clin Exp Immunol* 50:259, 1982.

29. **Vigano P, Vercellini P, Di Blasio AM, Colombo A, Candiani GB, Vignali M,** Deficient antiendometrium lymphocyte-mediated cytotoxicity in patients with endometriosis, *Fertil Steril* 56:894, 1991.

30. **Oosterlynck DJ, Meuleman C, Waer M, Vandeputte M, Koninckx PR,** The natural killer activity of peritoneal fluid lymphocytes is decreased in women with endometriosis, *Fertil Steril* 58:292, 1992.

31. **Cramer DW,** Epidemiology of endometriosis, In: Wilson EA, ed. *Endometriosis,* Alan R. Liss, Inc., New York, 1987, p 5.

32. **Olive DL, Schwartz LB,** Endometriosis, *New Engl J Med* 328:1759, 1993.

33. **Sanfillippo JS,** Endometriosis in adolescents, In: Wilson EA, ed. *Endometriosis,* Alan R. Liss, Inc., New York, 1987, p 161.

34. **Huffman JW,** Endometriosis in young teen-age girls, *Pediatr Ann* 10:501, 1981.

35. **Fedele L, Bianchi S, Bocciolone L, Di Nola G, Parazzini F,** Pain symptoms associated with endometriosis, *Obstet Gynecol* 79:767, 1992.

36. **Cornillie FJ, Oosterlynck D, Lauweryns JM, Konickx PR,** Deeply infiltrating pelvic endometriosis: histology and clinical significance, *Fertil Steril* 53:978, 1990.

37. **Koninckx PR, Meuleman C, Demeyere S, Lesaffre E, Cornillie FJ,** Suggestive evidence that pelvic endometriosis is a progressive disease, whereas deeply infiltrating endometriosis is associated with pelvic pain, *Fertil Steril* 55:759, 1991.

38. **Vercellini P, Trespidi L, De Giorgi O, Cortesi I, Parazzini F, Crosignani PG,** Endometriosis and pelvic pain: relation to disease stage and localization, *Fertil Steril* 65:299, 1996.

39. **Arumugam K,** Serum prolactin levels in infertile patients with endometriosis, *Malays J Pathol* 13:43, 1991.

40. **Machida T, Taga M, Minaguchi H,** Prolactin secretion in endometriotic patients, *Eur J Obstet Gynecol Reprod Biol* 72:89, 1997.

41. **Barbieri RL, Niloff JM, Bast Jr RC, Schaetzl E, Kistner RW, Knapp RC,** Elevated serum concentrations of CA-125 in patients with advanced endometriosis, *Fertil Steril* 45:630, 1986.

42. **Pittaway DE,** The use of serial CA-125 concentrations to monitor endometriosis in infertile women, *Am J Obstet Gynecol* 163:1032, 1990.

43. **Franssen AMHW, van der Heijden PFM, Thomas CMG, Doesburg WH, Willemsen WNP, Rolland R,** On the origin and significance of serum CA-125 concentrations in 97 patients with endometriosis before, during, and after buserelin acetate, nafarelin, or danazol, *Fertil Steril* 57:974, 1992.

44. **Pittaway DE, Fayez JA, Douglas JW,** Serum CA-125 in the evaluation of benign adnexal cysts, *Am J Obstet Gynecol* 157:1426, 1987.

45. **Alcázar JL, Laparte C, Jurado M, López-Garcia G,** The role of transvaginal ultrasonography combined with color velocity imaging and pulsed Doppler in the diagnosis of endometrioma, *Fertil Steril* 67:487, 1997.

46. **Friedman H, Vogelzang RL, Mendelson EB, Neiman HL, Cohen M,** Endometriosis detection by US with laparoscopic correlation, *Radiology* 157:217, 1985.

47. **Arrivé L, Hricak H, Martin MC,** Pelvic endometriosis: MR imaging, *Radiology* 171:687, 1989.

48. **Togashi K, Nishimura K, Kimura I, Tsuda Y, Yamashita K, Shibata T, Nakano Y, Konishi J, Konishi I, Mori T,** Endometrial cysts: diagnosis with MR imaging, *Radiology* 180:73, 1991.

49. **Jansen RPS, Russell P,** Nonpigmented endometriosis: clinical, laparoscopic and pathologic definition, *Am J Obstet Gynecol* 155:1154, 1986.

50. **Nisolle M, Paindaveine B, Bourdon A, Berliére M, Casanas-Roux F, Donnez J,** Histologic study of peritoneal endometriosis in infertile women, *Fertil Steril* 53:984, 1990.

51. **The American Fertility Society,** Revised American Fertility Society classification of endometriosis, *Fertil Steril* 43:351, 1985.

52. **The American Society for Reproductive Medicine,** Revised American Society for Reproductive Medicine classification of endometriosis, *Fertil Steril* 67:819, 1997.

53. **Hornstein MD, Gleason RE, Orav J, Haas ST, Friedman AJ, Rein MS, Hill JA, Barbieri RL,** The reproducibility of the revised American Fertility Society classification of endometriosis, *Fertil Steril* 59:1015, 1993.

54. **Damario MA, Rock JA,** Classification of endometriosis, *Seminars Reprod Endocrinol* 15:235, 1997.

55. **Garcia CF, Davis SS,** Pelvic endometriosis: infertility and pelvic pain, *Am J Obstet Gynecol* 129:740, 1977.

56. **Schenken RS, Malinak LR,** Conservative surgery versus expectant management for the infertile patient with mild endometriosis, *Fertil Steril* 37:183, 1982.

57. **Seibel M, Berger MJ, Weinstein FG, Taymor ML,** The effectiveness of danazol on subsequent fertility in minimal endometriosis, *Fertil Steril* 38:534, 1982.

58. **Fedele L, Parazzini F, Radici E, Bocciolone L, Bianchi S, Bianchi C, Candiani GB,** Buserelin acetate versus expectant management in the treatment of infertilty associated with minimal or mild endometriosis: a randomized clinical trial, *Am J Obstet Gynecol* 166:1345, 1992.

59. **Guzick DS,** Clinical epidemiology of endometriosis and infertility, *Obstet Gynecol Clin North Am* 16:43, 1989.

60. **Verkauf BS,** The incidence, symptoms and signs of endometriosis in fertile and infertile women, *J Fla Med Assoc* 74:671, 1987.

61. **Candiani GB, Vercellini P, Fedele L, Colombo A, Candiani M,** Mild endometriosis and infertility: a critical review of epidemiologic data, diagnostic pitfalls, and classification limits, *Obstet Gynecol Survey* 46:374, 1991.

62. **Toma SK, Stovall DW, Hammond MG,** The effect of laparoscopic ablation or Danocrine on pregnancy rates in patients with stage I or II endometriosis undergoing donor insemination, *Obstet Gynecol* 80:253, 1992.

63. **Badawy SZA, Elbakry MM, Samuel F, Dizer M,** Cumulative pregnancy rates in infertile women with endometriosis, *J Reprod Med* 33:757, 1988.

64. **Drake TS, Metz SA, Grunert GM, O'Brien WF,** Peritoneal fluid volume in endometriosis, *Fertil Steril* 34:280, 1980.

65. **Drake TS, O'Brien WF, Ramwell PW, Metz SA,** Peritoneal fluid thromboxane B2 and 6-keto-prostaglandin $F_{1\alpha}$ in endometriosis, *Am J Obstet Gynecol* 140:401, 1981.

66. **Rock JA, Dubin NH, Ghodgaonkar RB, Berquist CA, Erozan YS, Kimball Jr AW,** Cul-de-sac fluid in women with endometriosis: Fluid volume and prostanoid concentration during the proliferative phase of the cycle — days 8 to 12, *Fertil Steril* 37:747, 1982.

67. **Rezai N, Ghodgaonkar RB, Zacur HA, Rock JA, Dubin NH,** Cul-de-sac fluid in women with endometriosis: fluid volume, protein and prostanoid concentration during the periovulatory period — days 13 to 18, *Fertil Steril* 48:29, 1987.

68. **Sgarlatta CS, Hertelendy F, Mikhail G,** The prostanoid content in peritoneal fluid and plasma of women with endometriosis, *Am J Obstet Gynecol* 147:563, 1983.

69. **Mudge TJ, James MJ, Jones WR, Walsh JA,** Peritoneal fluid 6-keto-prostaglandin $F_{1\alpha}$ levels in women with endometriosis, *Am J Obstet Gynecol* 152:901, 1985.

70. **DeLeon FD, Vijayakumar R, Brown M, Rao CV, Yussman MA, Schultz G,** Peritoneal fluid volume, estrogen, progesterone, prostaglandin, and epidermal growth factor concentrations in patients with and without endometriosis, *Obstet Gynecol* 68:189, 1986.

71. **Vernon MW, Beard JS, Graves K, Wilson EA,** Classification of endometriotic implants by morphologic appearance and capacity to synthesize prostaglandin F, *Fertil Steril* 46:801, 1986.

72. **Koike H, Egawa H, Ohtsuka T, Yamaguchi M, Ikenoue T, Mori N,** Correlation between dysmenorrheic severity and prostaglandin production in women with endometriosis, *Prostaglandins Leuk Essential Fatty Acids* 46:133, 1992.

73. **Halme J, Becker W, Wing R,** Accentuated cyclic activation of peritoneal macrophages in patients with endometriosis, *Am J Obstet Gynecol* 148:85, 1984.

74. **Chacho KJ, Chacho MS, Andresen PJ, Scommegna A,** Peritoneal fluid in patients with and without endometriosis: prostanoids and macrophages and their effect on the spermatozoa penetration assay, *Am J Obstet Gynecol* 154:1290, 1986.

75. **Muscato JJ, Haney AF, Weinberg JB,** Sperm phagocytosis by human peritoneal macrophages: a possible cause of infertility and endometriosis, *Am J Obstet Gynecol* 144:503, 1982.

76. **Mori H, Sawairi M, Nakagawa M, Itoh N, Wada K, Tamaya T,** Expression of interleukin-1 IIL-1) beta messenger ribonucleic acid (mRNA) and IL-1 receptor antagonist mRNA in peritoneal macrophages from patients with endometriosis, *Fertil Steril* 57:535, 1992.

77. **Harada T, Yoshioka H, Yoshida S, Iwabe T, Onohara Y, Tanikawa M, Terakawa N,** Increased interleukin-6 levels in peritoneal fluid of infertile patients with active endometriosis, *Am J Obstet Gynecol* 176:593, 1997.

78. **McLaren J, Prentice A, Charnock-Jones DS, Milican SA, Muller KH, Sharkey AM, Smith SK,** Vascular endothelial growth factor is produced by peritoneal fluid macrophages in endometriosis and is regulated by ovarian steroids, *J Clin Invest* 98:482, 1996.

79. **Mahmood TA, Templeton A,** Folliculogenesis and ovulation in infertile women with mild endometriosis, *Hum Reprod* 6:227, 1991.

80. **Portuondo JA, Echanojauregui AD, Herran C, Alijarte I,** Early conception in patients with untreated mild endometriosis, *Fertil Steril* 39:22, 1983.

81. **Olive DL, Stohs GF, Metzger DA, Franklin RR,** Expectant management and hydrotubations in the treatment of endometriosis-associated infertility, *Fertil Steril* 44:35, 1985.

82. **Hull ME, Moghissi KS, Magyar DF, Haves MF,** Comparison of different treatment modalities of endometriosis in infertile women, *Fertil Steril* 47:40, 1987.

83. **Bérubé S, Marcoux S, Langevin M, Maheux R, and The Canadian Collaborative Group on Endometriosis,** Fecundity of infertile women with minimal or mild endometriosis and women with unexplained infertility, *Fertil Steril* 69:1034, 1998.

84. **Tulandi T, Mouchawar M,** Treatment-dependent and treatment-independent pregnancy in women with minimal and mild endometriosis, *Fertil Steril* 56:790, 1991.

85. **Marcoux S, Maheux R, Bérubé S, and the Canadian Collaborative Group on Endometriosis,** Laparoscopic surgery in infertile women with minimal or mild endometriosis, *New Engl J Med* 337:217, 1997.

86. **Adamson GD,** Treatment of endometriosis-associated infertility, *Seminars Reprod Endocrinol* 15:263, 1997.

87. **Candiani GB, Fedele L, Vercellini P, Bianchi S, Di Nola G,** Presacral neurectomy for the treatment of pelvic pain associated with endometriosis: a controlled study, *Am J Obstet Gynecol* 167:100, 1992.

88. **Olive DL, Lee KL,** Analysis of sequential treatment protocols for endometriosis-associated infertility, *Am J Obstet Gynecol* 154:613, 1986.

89. **Donnez J, Lemaire-Rubbers M, Karaman Y, Nisolle-Pochet M, Casanas-Roux F,** Combined (hormonal and microsurgical) therapy in infertile women with endometriosis, *Fertil Steril* 48:239, 1987.

90. **Wheeler JM, Malinak LR,** Recurrent endometriosis: incidence, management, and prognosis, *Am J Obstet Gynecol* 146:247, 1983.

91. **Sutton CJG, Pooley AS, Ewen SP, Haines P,** Follow-up report on a randomized controlled trial of laser laparoscopy in the treatment of pelvic pain associated with minimal to moderate endometriosis, *Fertil Steril* 68:1070, 1997.

92. **Hornstein MD, Hemmings R, Yuzpe AA, Heinrichs WL,** Use of nafarelin versus placebo after reductive laparoscopic surgery for endometriosis, *Fertil Steril* 68:860, 1997.

93. **Adamson GD, Pasta DJ,** Surgical treatment of endometriosis-associated infertility: meta-analysis compared with survival analysis, *Am J Obstet Gynecol* 171:1488, 1994.

94. **Namnoum AB, Hickman TN, Goodman SB, Gehlbach DL, Rock JA,** Incidence of symptom recurrence after hysterectomy for endometriosis, *Fertil Steril* 64:898, 1995.

95. **Hughes EG, Fedorkow DM, Collins JA,** A quantitative overview of controlled trials in endometriosis-associated infertility, *Fertil Steril* 59:963, 1993.

96. **Kistner RW,** Management of endometriosis in the infertile patient, *Fertil Steril* 26:1151, 1975.

97. **Vercellini P, Trespidi L, Colombo A, Vendola N, Marchini M, Crosignani PG,** A gonadotropin-releasing hormone agonist versus a low-dose oral contraceptive for pelvic pain associated with endometriosis, *Fertil Steril* 60:75, 1993.

98. **Barbieri RL, Osathanondh R, Ryan KJ,** Danazol inhibition of steroidogenesis in the human corpus luteum, *Obstet Gynecol* 57:722, 1981.

99. **Barbieri RL, Hornstein MD,** Medical therapy for endometriosis, In: Wilson EA, ed. *Endometriosis,* Alan R. Liss, Inc., New York, 1987, p 111.

100. **Quagliarello J, Alba Greco M,** Danazol and urogenital sinus formation in pregnancy, *Fertil Steril* 43:939, 1985.

101. **Wardle PG, Whitehead MI, Mills RP,** Nonreversible and wide ranging vocal changes after treatment with danazol, *Br Med J* 287:946, 1983.

102. **Mercaitis PA, Peaper RE, Schwartz PA,** Effect of danazol on vocal pitch: a case study, *Obstet Gynecol* 65:131, 1985.

103. **Dmowski WP, Cohen MR,** Antigonadotropin (danazol) in the treatment of endometriosis: evaluation of post-treatment fertility and three-year follow-up data, *Am J Obstet Gynecol* 130:41, 1978.

104. **Dmowski WP, Kapetanakis E, Scommegna A,** Variable effects of danazol on endometriosis at 4 low-dose levels, *Obstet Gynecol* 59:408, 1982.

105. **Barbieri RL, Evans S, Kistner RW,** Danazol in the treatment of endometriosis: analysis of 100 cases with a 4-year follow-up, *Fertil Steril* 37:737, 1982.

106. **Noble AD, Letchworth AT,** Medical treatment of endometriosis: a comparative trial, *Postgrad Med J* 55(Suppl 5):37, 1979.

107. **Vercellini P, Cortesi I, Crosignani PG,** Progestins for synthetic endometriosis: a critical analysis of the evidence, *Fertil Steril* 68:393, 1997.

108. **Kauppila A,** Changing concepts of medical treatment of endometriosis, *Acta Obstet Gynecol Scand* 72:324, 1993.

109. **Schlaff WD, Dugoff L, Damewood MD, Rock JA,** Megestrol acetate for treatment of endometriosis, *Obstet Gynecol* 75:646, 1990.

110. **Cundy T, Farquhar CM, Cornish J, Reid IR,** Short-term effects of high dose oral medroxyprogesterone acetate on bone density in premenopausal women, *J Clin Endocrinol Metab* 81:1014, 1996.

111. **Tellima S,** Danazol and medroxyprogesterone acetate inefficacious in the treatment of infertility in endometriosis, *Fertil Steril* 50:872, 1988.

112. **Meldrum DR,** Clinical management of endometriosis with luteinizing hormone-releasing hormone analogues, *Seminars Reprod Endocrinol* 3:371, 1985.

113. **Lemay A, Sandow J, Bureau M, Maneux R, Fontaine J-Y, Merat P,** Prevention of follicular maturation in endometriosis by subcutaneous infusion of luteinizing hormone-releasing hormone agonist started in the luteal phase, *Fertil Steril* 49:410, 1988.

114. **Henzl MR, Corson SL, Moghissi K, Buttram Jr VC, Berqvist C, Jacobson J,** Administration of nasal nafarelin as compared with oral danazol for endometriosis, *New Engl J Med* 318:485, 1988.

115. **The Nafarelin European Endometriosis Trial Group,** Nafarelin for endometriosis: a large-scale, danazol-controlled trial of efficacy and safety, with 1-year follow-up, *Fertil Steril* 57:514, 1992.

116. **Wheeler JM, Knittle JD, Miller JD,** Depot leuprolide versus danazol in treatment of women with symptomatic endometriosis, *Am J Obstet Gynecol* 167:1367, 1992.

117. **Wheeler JM, Knittle JD, Miller JD, for the Lupron Endometriosis Study Group,** Depot leuprolide acetate versus danazol in the treatment of women with symptomatic endometriosis: a multicenter, double-blind randomized clinical trial. II. Assessment of safety, *Am J Obstet Gynecol* 169:26, 1993.

118. **Rock JA, Truglia JA, Caplan RJ, and the Zoladex Endometriosis Study Group,** Zoladex (goserelin acetate implant) in the treatment of endometriosis: a randomized comparison with danazol, *Obstet Gynecol* 82:198, 1993.

119. **Välimäki M, Nilsson G, Roine R, Ylikorkala O,** Comparison between the effects of nafarelin and danazol on serum lipids and lipoproteins in patients with endometriosis, *J Clin Endocrinol Metab* 69:1097, 1989.

120. **Mann DR, Collins DC, Smith MM, Kessler MJ, Gould KG,** Treatment of endometriosis in monkeys: effectiveness of continuous infusion of a gonadotropin-releasing hormone agonist compared to treatment with a progestational steroid, *J Clin Endocrinol Metab* 63:1277, 1986.

121. **Har-Toov J, Brenner SH, Jaffa A, Yavetz H, Peyser MR, Lessing JB,** Pregnancy during long-term gonadotropin-releasing hormone agonist therapy associated with clinical pseudomenopause, *Fertil Steril* 59:446, 1993.

122. **Henzl MR,** Gonadotropin-releasing analogs: update on new findings, *Am J Obstet Gynecol* 166:757, 1992.

123. **Dawood MY, Ramos J, Khan-Dawood FS,** Depot leuprolide acetate versus danazol for treatment of pelvic endometriosis: changes in vertebral bone mass and serum estradiol and calcitonin, *Fertil Steril* 63:1177, 1995.

124. **Revilla R, Revilla M, Hernández ER, Villa LF, Varela L, Rico H,** Evidence that the loss of bone mass induced by GnRH agonists is not totally recovered, *Mauritas* 22:145, 1995.

125. **Paoletti AM, Serra GG, Cagnacci A, Vacca AM, Guerriero S, Solla E, Melis GB,** Spontaneous reversibility of bone loss induced by gonadotropin-releasing hormone analog treatment, *Fertil Steril* 65:707, 1996.

126. **Cedars M, Lu JKH, Meldrum DR, Judd HL,** Treatment of endometriosis with a long acting gonadotropin-releasing hormone agonist plus medroxyprogesterone acetate, *Obstet Gynecol* 75:641, 1990.

127. **Surrey ES,** Steroidal and nonsteroidal "add-back" therapy: extending safety and efficacy of gonadotropin-releasing hormone agonists in the gynecologic patient, *Fertil Steril* 64:673, 1995.

128. **Gargiulo AR, Hornstein MD,** The role of GnRH agonists plus add-back therapy in the treatment of endometriosis, *Seminars Reprod Endocrinol* 15:273, 1997.

129. **Friedman AJ, Hornstein MD,** Gonadotropin-releasing hormone agonist plus estrogen-progestin "add-back" therapy for endometriosis-related pelvic pain, *Fertil Steril* 60:236, 1993.

130. **Taskin O, Yalcinoglu AI, Kucuk S, Uryan I, Buhur A, Burak F,** Effectiveness of tibolone on hypoestrogenic symptoms induced by goserelin treatment in patients with endometriosis, *Fertil Steril* 67:40, 1997.

131. **Surrey ES, Voigt B, Fournet N, Judd HL,** Prolonged gonadotropin-releasing hormone agonist treatment of symptomatic endometriosis: the role of cyclic sodium ethidronate and low-dose norethindrone "add-back" therapy, *Fertil Steril* 63:747, 1995.

132. **Lane N, Baptista J, Snow-Harter C,** Bone mineral density of the lumbar spine in endometriosis subjects compared to an age-similar control population, *J Clin Endocrinol Metab* 72:510, 1991.

133. **Rico H, Revilla M, Arnanz F, Villa LF, Perera S, Arribas I,** Total and regional bone mass values and biochemical markers of bone remodeling in endometriosis, *Obstet Gynecol* 81:272, 1993.

134. **Ulrich U, Murano R, Skinner MA, Yin H, Chesnut III CH,** Women of reproductive age with endometriosis are not osteopenic, *Fertil Steril* 69:821, 1998.

135. **Fedele L, Bianchi S, Viezzoli T, Arcaini L, Candiani GB,** Gestrinone versus danazol in the treatment of endometriosis, *Fertil Steril* 51:781, 1989.

136. **Waller KG, Shaw RW,** Gonadotropin-releasing hormone analogues for the treatment of endometriosis: long-term follow-up, *Fertil Steril* 59:511, 1993.

137. **Fedele L, Bianchi S, Bocciolone L, Di Nola G, Franchi D,** Buserelin acetate in the treatment of pelvic pain associated with minimal and mild endometriosis: a controlled study, *Fertil Steril* 59:516, 1993.

138. **Thoms Jr WW, Hughes LL, Rock J,** Palliation of recurrent endometriosis with radiotherapeutic ablation of ovarian remnants, *Fertil Steril* 68:938, 1997.

139. **Hickman TN, Namnoum AB, Hinton EL, Zacur HA, Rock JA,** Timing of estrogen replacement therapy following hysterectomy with oophorectomy for endometriosis, *Obstet Gynecol* 91:673, 1998.

140. **Reimnitz C, Brand E, Nieberg RK, Hacker NF,** Malignancy arising in endometriosis associated with unopposed estrogen replacement, *Obstet Gynecol* 71:444, 1988.

141. **Heaps JM, Nieberg RK, Berek JS,** Malignant neoplasms arising in endometriosis, *Obstet Gynecol* 75:1023, 1990.

142. **Duun S, Roed-Petersen K, Michelsen JW,** Endometrioid carcinoma arising from endometriosis of the sigmoid colon during estrogenic treatment, *Acta Obstet Gynecol Scand* 72:676, 1993.

143. **Gucer F, Pieber D, Arikan MG,** Malignancy arising in extraovarian endometriosis during estrogen stimulation, *Eur J Gynaecol Oncol* 19:39, 1998.

144. **Vessey MP, Villard-Mackintosh L, Painter R,** Epidemiology of endometriosis in women attending family-planning clinics, *Br Med J* 306:182, 1993.

145. **Groll M,** Endometriosis and spontaneous abortion, *Fertil Steril* 41:933, 1984.

146. **Metzger DA, Olive DL, Stohs GF, Franklin RR,** Association of endometriosis and spontaneous abortion: effect of control group selection, *Fertil Steril* 45:18, 1986.

147. **FitzSimmons J, Stahl R, Gocial B, Shapiro SS,** Spontaneous abortion and endometriosis, *Fertil Steril* 47:696, 1987.

148. **Pittaway DE, Maxson W, Daniell J, Herbert C, Wentz AC,** Luteal phase defects in infertility patients with endometriosis, *Fertil Steril* 39:712, 1983.

149. **Kusuhara K,** Luteal function in infertile patients with endometriosis, *Am J Obstet Gynecol* 167:274, 1992.

150. **Dmowski WP, Radwanska E, Binor Z, Rana N,** Mild endometriosis and ovulatory dysfunction: effect of danazol treatment on success of ovulation induction, *Fertil Steril* 46:784, 1986.

151. **Dodson WC, Whitesides DB, Hughes Jr CL, Easley III HA, Haney AF,** Superovulation with intrauterine insemination in the treatment of infertility: a possible alternative to gamete intrafallopian transfer and in vitro fertilization, *Fertil Steril* 48:441, 1987.

152. **Chaffkin LM, Nulsen JC, Luciano AA, Metzger DA,** A comparative analysis of the cycle fecundity rates associated with combined human menopausal gonadotropin (hMG) and intrauterine insemination (IUI) versus either hMG or IUI alone, *Fertil Steril* 55:252, 1991.

153. **Tummon IS, Asher LJ, Martin JSB, Tulandi T,** Randomized controlled trial of superovulation and insemination for infertility associated with minimal or mild endometriosis, *Fertil Steril* 68:8, 1997.

154. **Fedele L, Bianchi S, Marchini M, Villa L, Brioschi D, Parazzini F,** Superovulation with human menopausal gonadotropins in the treatment of infertility associated with minimal or mild endometriosis: a controlled randomized study, *Fertil Steril* 58:28, 1992.

155. **Simón C, Gutiérrez A, Vidal A, de los Santos MJ, Tarín JJ, Remohí J, Pellicer A,** Outcome of patients with endometriosis in assisted reproduction: results from in-vitro fertilization and oocyte donation, *Hum Reprod* 9:725, 1994.

156. **Nasseri A, Copperman AB,** Endometriosis and its effects on assisted reproduction technologies: a review, *Assist Repro Rev* 7:71, 1997.

157. **Dmowski WP, Rana N, Michalowska F, J, Papierniak C, El-Roeiy A,** The effect of endometriosis, its stage and activity, and of autoantibodies on in vitro fertilization and embryo transfer success rates, *Fertil Steril* 63:555, 1995.

158. **Olivennes F, feldberg D, Liu H-C, Cohen J, Moy F, Rosenwaks Z,** Endometriosis: a stage-by-stage analysis—the role of in vitro fertilization, *Fertil Steril* 64:392, 1995.

29 Male Infertility

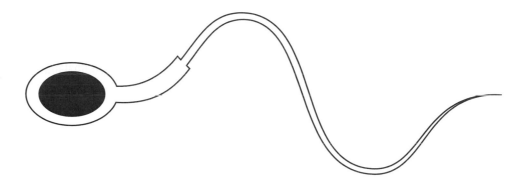

The perception of the degree of male involvement in infertility has undergone a number of revisions during the past 50 years. Initially, infertility was considered primarily a female problem. This notion gave way to the realization that 40–50% of infertility is wholly or in part due to a male factor. More recently, there has been a trend to redefine, in a downward direction, the lower limit of "normal" for a sperm count. Thus, some men who in the past would have been categorized as subfertile now are considered normal.

Despite these changes, there is no doubt that a substantial percentage of infertility is due to deficiencies in the semen. For this reason it is important to be knowledgeable concerning male infertility. It usually depends on the woman's clinician to order and review the results of the initial semen analysis, and to determine the need for urologic consultation. This chapter will consider the analysis of semen and other tests of sperm function, indicate factors responsible for abnormalities of the semen, and consider available treatments for problems of male infertility, including artificial insemination. Influencing the entire field of male infertility is the striking success achieved with intracytoplasmic sperm injection (ICSI), the direct injection of a single spermatozoon or spermatid into the cytoplasm of an oocyte. Men who in the past have been considered hopelessly infertile now have reasonable chances for fertility with the use of ICSI.

Regulation of the Testes

The testes have 2 distinct components, the seminiferous tubules (site of spermatogenesis) and the Leydig cells (source of testosterone). The function of these 2 components requires both pituitary gonadotropins, follicle-stimulating hormone (FSH) and luteinizing hormone (LH). The primary effect of LH is to stimulate the synthesis and secretion of testosterone by Leydig cells (about 5–10 mg per day), an effect that is enhanced by FSH, which also binds to Leydig cells and increases the number of LH receptors on the cells. Increasing levels of testosterone, in turn, inhibit LH secretion, acutely through the hypothalamus and chronically at the pituitary level. This negative feedback action does not require aromatization to estrogen. In men virtually all the estrone and estradiol present is derived from androstenedione and testosterone; there is essentially no direct secretion of estrogen.

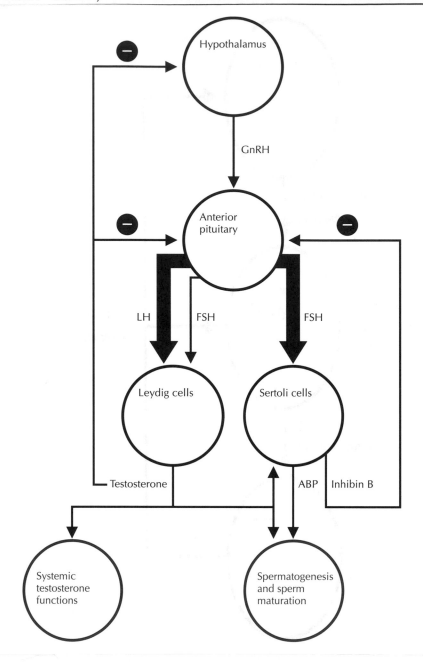

FSH, in conjunction with testosterone, acts on the seminiferous tubules to stimulate spermatogenesis. This effect may be mediated by activation of Sertoli cell function, which is controlled by both FSH and testosterone. FSH binds to Sertoli cells and stimulates the production of several proteins, chief of which is ABP, the androgen-binding protein. Spermatogenesis requires a very high local concentration of testosterone and dihydrotestosterone, 50 times higher than that present in the circulation and greater than can be administered exogenously. The ABP is secreted into the tubule lumen and binds testosterone and dihydrotestosterone as they diffuse into the lumen, concentrating the androgens in the seminiferous epithelium for spermatogenesis and in the epididymis for sperm maturation. Spermatogenesis and fertility can occur in men who have an inactivating mutation in the FSH receptor gene, indicating that testosterone can compensate for a deficiency in FSH.[1]

In contrast to the effects of testosterone on LH, steroid hormones at physiologic levels do not suppress FSH secretion. Orchiectomy is followed, however, by a rise in FSH levels. This phenomenon led to the discovery of inhibin. Inhibin B is synthesized in the Sertoli cells in response to FSH, secreted into the circulation, and specifically inhibits FSH secretion in the pituitary.[2–4] Inhibin has been found in seminal fluid, spermatozoa, Sertoli cells, and Leydig cells.

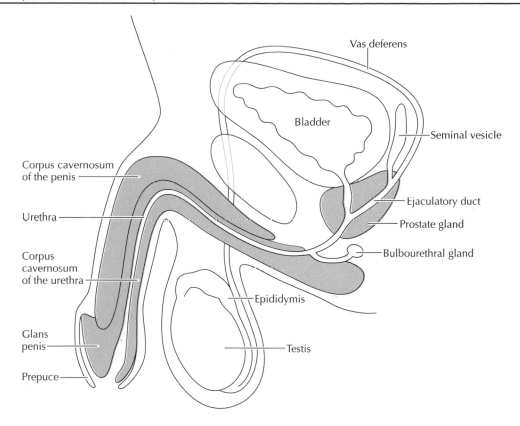

Inhibin A is absent in the circulation of males. The secretion of inhibin B is further modulated by LH, human chorionic gonadotropin (HCG), and testosterone. Undoubtedly, autocrine/paracrine regulation by growth factors and local peptides is involved in a system similar to the complex interaction in the ovarian follicle.[5] The Sertoli cells of the testis are analogous to the granulosa cells of the ovary, and the Leydig cells are comparable to the theca cells.

Leydig cells contain receptors for prolactin. Prolactin at normal levels stimulates testosterone secretion, whereas hypersecretion of prolactin leads to reduced testosterone secretion. Although studies suggest that prolactin synergizes with LH and testosterone in the testes, a role for prolactin has not been established for normal testicular function.

The seminiferous tubules and the intraluminal environment are controlled by the Sertoli cells. Tight junctions between the Sertoli cells effectively seal off the tubules, creating the blood-testis barrier. The seminiferous tubules, therefore, are essentially avascular, and regulatory substances must enter by diffusion. The blood-testis barrier protects the germ cells from antigens, antibodies, and environmental toxins. The Leydig cells are in the connective tissue between the seminiferous tubules.

Developing sperm are enveloped by Sertoli cells that influence the sequential process of spermatogenesis. Spermatogonia undergo mitotic division to form the primary spermatocytes, which, in turn, form the haploid (23 chromosomes) secondary spermatocytes by meiotic division. The secondary spermatocytes proceed through a maturation process to the spermatid stage, ultimately becoming the spermatozoa. One X chromosome is inactivated in female somatic cells; however, in the oocyte both X chromosomes are genetically active. The opposite situation prevails in the male where the single X chromosome is genetically active in somatic cells but inactive in spermatogenesis. Normal spermatogenesis is directed by the genes on the Y chromosome, although many required regulating proteins are derived from autosomal chromosomes.[6]

Most of the testis is composed of the tightly coiled seminiferous tubule, which, if uncoiled, would reach a length of 70 cm. Approximately 74 days are required to produce spermatozoa, about 50 days of which are spent in the tubule. After leaving the testes, sperm take 12–21 days to travel

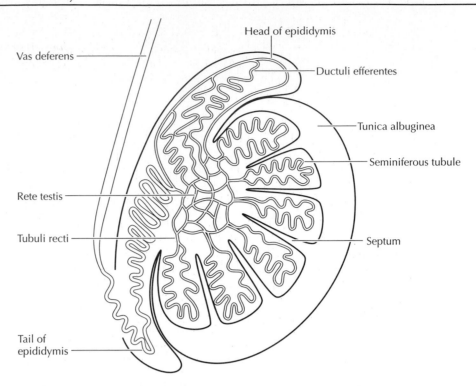

the epididymis (which is 5–6 meters long) and appear in the ejaculate. The vas deferens is 30–35 cm in length, begins at the cauda epididymis and terminates in the ejaculatory duct near the prostate. Because of the long development and transit times the semen analysis can reflect events that occurred weeks earlier. The semen is composed of secretions contributed in a sequential fashion, first the prostatic fluid and contents of the distal vas deferens, followed by seminal vesicle secretions.

Semen Analysis

An abstinence period of 2–3 days prior to semen collection is adequate, although some urologists favor 5 days. Increasing the ejaculatory frequency reduces the volume and count but has no significant impact on quality (morphology and motility). The specimen should be collected directly into a clean container and not into a condom because the latter contains spermicidal agents. Sheathes are available that do not contain a spermicidal agent, and they can be used during intercourse if the man cannot, or will not, obtain a specimen by masturbation. Collection of a specimen by withdrawal runs the risk of losing the first part of the specimen that contains the highest concentration of sperm. Ideally, the specimen should be collected in a private room near the laboratory. If collected at home, the specimen should be protected from the cold and delivered to the laboratory within 1 hour of collection.

Semen liquefaction, which occurs 20–30 minutes after ejaculation, is a necessary prerequisite for doing an accurate analysis. On occasion, a specimen does not undergo normal liquefaction or is abnormally viscid, and, if this is associated with a poor postcoital test, it may be a factor in infertility. Techniques used to break up a viscid specimen in preparation for doing a sperm count or for artificial insemination include mechanically dispersing the gel by running the semen repeatedly through a number 19 needle, collecting the semen as a split ejaculate because the first part may be less gelatinous, or, rarely, treating the semen with a proteolytic enzyme. If the postcoital test is normal, however, poor liquefaction and high viscosity are probably not infertility factors.

It has been suggested that the average sperm count has been decreasing over the past 50 years.[7, 8] Environmental toxins, and specifically chemicals with estrogen-like activity (xenoestrogens), have been blamed for this change. However, many studies have failed to document a decline.[9-12] Most importantly, infertility has not increased significantly during the periods studied, and this argues that even if a decrease in sperm count has occurred, it is not clinically meaningful.

The World Health Organization (WHO) suggests the following for normal values, but these should be viewed as rough guidelines only.[13]

Volume	**2.0 mL or more**
Sperm concentration	**20 million/mL or more**
Motility	**50% or more with forward progression, or 25% or more with rapid progression within 60 minutes of ejaculation**
Morphology	**30% or more normal forms**
White blood cells	**fewer than 1 million/mL**
Immunobead test	**fewer than 20% spermatozoa with adherent particles**
SpermMar test	**fewer than 10% spermatozoa with adherent particles**

Defining male infertility on the basis of sperm count or motility is more complicated than suggested by the above criteria. Whereas it is still true that very poor sperm counts (less than 5 million/mL) and very low motilities (less than 20%) indicate compromised fertility, even these low values or lower can, on occasion, be associated with a pregnancy. Adding to the difficulties of diagnosing male infertility is the variability in count and motility that can be seen in successive semen specimens from the same individual.[14] This is the basis of a fundamental recommendation: at least two, and preferably three, samples should be screened before an individual can be categorized as potentially fertile, subfertile, or infertile (azoospermia). Because it can take 2.5 months for the testes to recover from an insult, it is reasonable to space the specimens over a longer period of time.

There have been conflicting statements in textbooks and articles pertaining to the lower limit of normal for the sperm count. The most commonly cited figures are 60 million/mL, 40 million/mL, 20 million/mL, and 10 million/mL, with the 20 million/mL figure being the generally accepted standard.[15, 16] Confidence in any figure is limited by the inaccuracies inherent in the methods used for counting sperm. When a group of technicians and pathologists used a counting chamber to do a semen analysis on the same pooled specimen, the mean sperm count was 46.7 million/mL with a range of values lying between 10 and 98 million/mL, giving a coefficient of variation of 37.8%.[17] These inconsistent results are not necessarily remedied with computer-assisted semen analysis (CASA). Significant errors can still occur with CASA, especially with specimens containing low numbers where other cells can be miscounted as sperm.[18]

In an attempt to increase the prognostic value of the routine semen analysis, the results of the sperm count and the percentage of motility have been combined to give total motile sperm count (total sperm in the ejaculate x percent motility) or motile sperm per milliliter (sperm per mL x percent motility). The combining of count and motility allows determination of the number or concentration of active sperm and may provide a more informative way to present the data. Males with less than 24 months of infertility and a motile sperm count of greater than 10 million/mL have a higher pregnancy rate than those with 2–10 million/mL motile sperm.[19] Even with motile sperm counts less than 5.1 million/mL, the pregnancy rate was 37.5%.[20] However, with counts between 60.1 and 100 million motile sperm/mL, the pregnancy rate rose to 78.6%. Whereas trends are evident, the overlapping results limit the prognostic power of combining sperm count and sperm motility.

Sperm Morphology

Until recently, the evaluation of sperm morphology was beset with the same variations that plague sperm counts. Katz and Overstreet introduced an overlay to use with video microscopy, which allowed a more standardized assessment of morphology.[21] With this method the coefficient of variation between observers was markedly reduced; 50% of sperm should have normal morphology when assessed with this technique.

Kruger and coworkers championed morphology as the best prognostic indicator for subsequent successful fertilization with in vitro fertilization.[22] They utilized "strict criteria" that shift many sperm out of the normal category, by including as abnormal, sperm with even minor abnormalities as well as those with abnormalities of the acrosome. Using these strict criteria, males with greater than 14% normal forms had normal rates of fertilization with in vitro fertilization, whereas those with less than 4% normal forms had fertilization rates of only 7–8%.[22] Values between 4% and 14% normal forms were associated with intermediate rates of fertilization. Many andrology laboratories have adopted "strict criteria" for the assessment of sperm morphology. In a dissenting study, the usual criteria for assessment of sperm morphology provided better prognostic information than did assessment by strict criteria.[23] Technicians well trained in using strict criteria can provide highly reproducible results, but the standardization may not be possible on a more widespread scale. Interobserver differences in assessing sperm morphology could be decreased with the utilization of computer-assisted morphometric evaluations.[24]

Other Parameters

Whereas the count, motility, and morphology of the specimen constitute the major parameters on which the male's fertility is categorized, there are other characteristics of the semen that may impact on fertility potential. A volume of less than 1 mL may be too small to make contact with the cervix, and a volume greater than 7 mL may dilute the sperm concentration so that insufficient numbers are in close proximity to the cervix.

Round cells in the specimen can be either white cells or immature cells, and these look similar in wet preparations. The WHO standards manual states that a normal ejaculate should not contain more than 5 million round cells per mL (5 per high power field) while the number of leukocytes should not exceed 1 million per mL.[13] There are staining methods, biochemical tests, and immunologic techniques to differentiate immature cells from white cells.[25] In laboratories where these tests are not performed, all round cells are lumped together and reported as white blood cells. It is reasonable to obtain a culture, perhaps by prostatic massage, when the report states that there are 5 or more white cells per high power field, even though some of these may be immature cells, and the presence of white cells does not always correlate with infection.

Repetitive agglutination of sperm (except when it is on pieces of debris) is suggestive of an immunologic effect or an infection. It can, however, be nonspecific and of no significance. Although it is common practice to evaluate the pH of semen because abnormalities may provide a clue to disorders of the accessory glands, in practice this measurement is of little value.

Tests of Sperm Function

Although all of the major elements of the semen analysis (numbers, motility, and morphology) have some bearing on fertility, especially when markedly deficient, the lack of precise correlations has led to a search for tests of the functional capacity of sperm. Despite enthusiasms generated by a variety of assays over the past 4 decades, no test has emerged as a reliable standard for the fertilizing ability of sperm. One problem is that the functional tests individually measure only one aspect of the many functions performed by sperm, whether it is attachment to the zona, penetration of the egg membrane, or the release of enzymes. Recently, there has been a trend in centers of assisted reproductive technologies to dispense with functional tests because the ultimate end point of fertilization of the human egg can now be tested by ICSI. If the functional tests were better prognosticators and less cumbersome to perform, they still could play a role in clinical practice. For example, a couple with unexplained infertility and an abnormal result might consider donor insemination as a therapeutic option.

Sperm Penetration Assay (SPA)

The zona pellucida of most mammalian species presents not only a block to polyspermia but also a barrier to fertilization of an egg by sperm of a different species. However, foreign sperm can fuse with and penetrate an egg if the zona is removed by gentle enzyme digestion. In the sperm penetration assay, eggs are collected from superovulated golden hamsters, the zonae are removed by enzyme digestion, and the denuded eggs are cultured for 2–3 hours with human sperm that have been washed and incubated overnight in culture media.[26] Presence of a swollen sperm head in the egg cytoplasm is evidence of successful penetration. Most laboratories report the percentage of eggs penetrated and compare this figure to the percent penetrated by a known fertile sperm specimen (some laboratories use the criterion of number of sperm penetrations per egg with 2 or more considered normal).

Whereas the concept of the SPA as a measure of sperm fertilizing ability is an attractive one, the practical aspects of the test have hindered its standardization. For example, the source of the albumin used as the protein supplement in the media can influence the result as can use of resuspended compared to swim-up sperm. Moreover, an individual's results in the SPA can vary over time. In addition, different laboratories utilize different cutoff points for the lower limit of normal penetration with the most common points being 0, 10, 14, and 20%.

Equally important has been a continuing controversy over the prognostic value of the test. A meta-analysis concluded that the test was not of value.[27] Other authors, however, have found correlations with eventual fertility. An SPA result of greater than 19% was associated with a pregnancy rate of 48%, whereas below 20% eggs penetrated was associated with a pregnancy rate of 20%.[28] However, even with an SPA of 0%, the pregnancy rate in this series was 16%. Thus, failure of the sperm to penetrate the hamster egg is not an absolute indication that the sperm cannot penetrate the human egg. Because of this limitation of the SPA, attempts have been made to optimize the test with a goal of eliminating these false-negative results. Strategies to eliminate or to lower the number of false-negative tests include treatment of sperm with follicular fluid, test yolk buffer, calcium ionophore, miniaturizing the test, and adjusting the concentration of albumin or the ions in the culture media.[29, 30] With any of these maneuvers an SPA showing no or low penetration is a more accurate (although not 100%) indicator of poor sperm fertilizing ability. If an optimized SPA has zero penetration, the couple should be given the option of considering use of donor sperm or ICSI. In contrast to the problems with low SPAs, normal levels of sperm penetration correlate quite well, although not absolutely, with human fertilization in vivo and in vitro.

If there is a place in clinical practice for the SPA, it is to identify abnormalities of sperm not evident by studies of count, motility, or morphology. In cases of unexplained infertility, this could shorten the time period before pursuing either donor insemination or ICSI.

Human Zona Binding Assay

Whereas the SPA tests the ability of sperm to penetrate or to be engulfed by the egg, it does not test the critical ability to pass through the zona pellucida. The zona is, of course, removed in preparation for the SPA because it is, with rare exceptions, impervious to foreign sperm. Thus, to test zona penetrating or zona binding ability of human sperm requires the use of human zonae. One approach is to use zonae obtained from surgically removed ovarian tissue and slit them in half so that both patient sperm and donor sperm can be tested in parallel on different portions of the same zona.[31] The ratio of the number of sperm bound for the test subject to the number of sperm bound for fertile control sperm has been labeled the hemizona assay index (HZI). A breakpoint at an HZI value of 36 has provided a good correlation with results in human IVF.[32] The limited availability of zonae and the technical requirements of the assay will always restrict its application to a small number of committed laboratories. In the future, the development of materials that mimic the properties of the zona could lead to simpler tests. However, the widespread use of ICSI, which bypasses the zona, renders such tests superfluous, unless they can determine with certainty which couples require ICSI.

In Vitro Tests of Sperm Penetration into Mucus

Some of the vagaries of the postcoital test can be eliminated by use of in vitro testing with bovine cervical mucus or an artificial mucus. A drop of sperm is placed next to mucus on a slide and progression of sperm into the mucus monitored through a microscope. To better standardize the test, tubes filled with bovine cervical mucus, available commercially, can be utilized and the length of mucus traversed by the sperm measured. One problem is that antibody-affected sperm are not handicapped in moving through bovine mucus, whereas they usually move poorly in human cervical mucus. Because couples with poor postcoital tests and those with unexplained infertility will almost always be treated with intrauterine inseminations of washed sperm (IUI), with or without gonadotropins, there is little practical value for the in vitro sperm mucus tests in current practice.

Assessments of Sperm Motility

A sperm quality analyzer uses an electro-optical method to provide an assessment of the number of motile sperm in a specimen and, to some extent, the quality of the motility.[33] This test provides some indication of the functional capacity of the sperm, but it has not gained widespread use.

Measurement of Sperm Velocity

The CASA systems are best at supplying information on sperm velocity and specific movements, such as lateral head displacement. However, it is unlikely that these measurements provide information that cannot be obtained with less expensive methods. The computer printouts of multiple measurements by CASA instruments provide a wealth of information, but little that is of current value for the clinician.

Hypo-osmotic Swelling Test

When sperm are placed in a hypo-osmotic solution of sodium citrate and fructose, a sperm tail with normal membrane function will swell and coil as fluid is transported across the membrane.[34] Conversely, if there is a functional disturbance of the tail membrane, the tail will appear unaffected. This test has been scrutinized by a number of investigators with no clear-cut decision regarding its clinical usefulness. A specific niche has been suggested for the test. Non-motile sperm, but positive with the hypo-osmotic test, may provide better results with ICSI than those obtained with non-motile and hypo-osmotic negative sperm.[35]

Measurement of Adenosine Triphosphate (ATP)

ATP is an important component of sperm metabolism related to tail movement. In one report, levels of ATP in semen were a strong discriminator between populations of fertile and infertile males.[36] A multicenter study sponsored by the World Health Organization concluded, however, that levels of semen ATP could not predict the occurrence of pregnancy when the female was normal and the male partner had a sperm concentration greater than 20 million/mL.[37]

Measurement of the Acrosome Reaction

The acrosome reaction that allows the release of enzymes from the acrosome (see Chapter 7) occurs on or near the zona pellucida. However, a low percentage of sperm will also become reactive while in media or following treatment with a calcium ionophore that induces capacitation. Although the artificial initiation of the acrosome reaction has been correlated with IVF results, the relatively small difference in acrosome-reactive sperm in the different groups indicates that this approach is not clinically important.[38]

Measurement of Acrosin

Acrosin is a proteolytic enzyme associated with the acrosome that may be important for aiding sperm to traverse the zona.[39] Low acrosin concentrations could be associated with infertility. Although theoretically appealing, the test has little application in clinical practice.

Sperm Antibodies

Whereas the previous assays measure sperm function or sperm numbers, sperm antibody tests determine reactions to sperm. It has been known for more than 100 years that animals, both male and female, can be rendered infertile by immunization with sperm.[40] Semen is very antigenic and, fortunately, is normally isolated from the immune system by the blood-testis barrier. Disruption of this anatomic and functional barrier in the seminiferous tubules can lead to antibody formation; hence antibody production in the male can follow vasectomy, testicular torsion, infections, or trauma. In addition, there are women who have allergic reactions to semen manifested by reactions as diverse as irritation of the vagina and cardiovascular collapse following intercourse. The basic question is whether more subtle immunologic reactions can occur that interfere with fertility.

Initial efforts to detect sperm antibodies involved incubating sperm in the sera of both males and females with agglutination being the endpoint. Despite the fact that substantial agglutination of sperm in semen on a repetitive basis is an indication of the presence of antibodies, agglutination in serum often is nonspecific. Thus, testing with serum alone has been abandoned.[41] It is now recognized that sperm antibodies in the circulation of men or women have no influence on fertility.[42, 43]

The two most widely used tests for sperm antibodies use immunologically mediated attachment of particles or beads to sperm that are assessed with a microscope.[44] The immunobead test uses beads labeled with anti-IgG, anti-IgA, or anti-IgM, and, thus, it provides identification of the class of antibodies on the sperm. The site on the sperm where the beads are adherent also can be noted. Anti-IgA usually localizes to the tail and anti-IgG to the head of the sperm. Antibody localized only to the tip of the tail usually is not significant, whereas antibody on the rest of the tail may interfere with sperm motility. Antibodies on the head of the sperm can cause failure of fusion with the egg. A second test, the mixed agglutination test (SpermMar), uses antibody to IgG to bridge antibody-coated sperm and latex particles that have been conjugated with human IgG. The endpoint in this test is clumping, and the reactions against individual segments of the sperm cannot be identified. The SpermMar test can be used on unprepared semen, as opposed to the immunobead test where sperm washing is required.

With the SpermMar test, the diagnosis of immunologic infertility is suggested when 10–39% of motile sperm are attached to the particles, whereas immunologic infertility is very probable when 40% or more of the motile sperm are covered with beads. Using the immunobead test, when over 50% of sperm were antibody-bound, the subsequent pregnancy rate was 15.3%, whereas when the percentage of sperm positive for antibody was less than 50%, the pregnancy rate was 66.7%.[45] Others have used a cut off of 20%, and it is not clear at this time which is the more valid number.[13]

An additional difficulty in diagnosing immunologic infertility is the fluctuations in antibody levels even without therapy. In males receiving a placebo, 58% had a decrease in sperm-bound immunoglobulins.[46]

A high percentage of positive sperm antibody tests is associated with poor postcoital tests, and it would seem cost-effective to initially screen for antibodies only in individuals whose postcoital tests show no sperm, all dead sperm, a high percentage of shaking sperm, or less than 3 motile sperm per high power field. This latter number is somewhat arbitrary, and some may choose to use less than 5 or even less than 1 as the cut off value.

Because both unexplained infertility and immunologic infertility are treated with intrauterine inseminations, the usefulness of sperm antibody testing is limited.

Treatment of Sperm Antibodies

Use of condoms to avoid contact between sperm and the female with antibodies has been abandoned because of lack of efficacy. The current office treatments for sperm antibodies in the male are the use of steroids or, preferably, intrauterine inseminations with prepared specimens.[47, 48] In an alternative, but experimental, treatment, the sperm are separated on Percoll gradients, and then incubated with antibody beads.[49] A population of sperm without antibody can be separated from the mix and utilized for insemination.

Moderate to high doses of corticosteroids have been used to treat sperm antibodies in the male. Reports of efficacy in reducing antibody levels and marginal increases in pregnancy rate have been balanced by sporadic reports of serious side effects such as aseptic necrosis of the femoral head and less severe side effects such as irritability.[50]

A more popular therapeutic approach is the intrauterine insemination of washed spermatozoa in conjunction with gonadotropin treatment (superovulation) of the female.[47, 48, 51] Determination of the efficacy of this treatment has been hindered by difficulties in deciding what constitutes a positive sperm antibody test in the female and reports that lumped together patients who were antibody positive with others who may not have been afflicted with antibodies but who had poor postcoital tests. Nevertheless, the reported pregnancy rates warrant several cycles of IUI-superovulation before considering the more expensive methods of assisted reproduction.

Use of in vitro fertilization is a reasonable final approach to the treatment of sperm antibodies. Success with in vitro fertilization is reduced in couples with sperm antibodies, but once fertilization occurs, the probability of pregnancy is not affected.[52] The results with ICSI are very good, even in the presence of high levels of antisperm antibodies.[53]

Donor insemination should be considered as an alternative to the more expensive methods of assisted reproduction.

Investigation and Treatment of Male Infertility

If the semen analysis is abnormal, inquiry should be made concerning the presence of the following factors, any of which can produce abnormal sperm quality and quantity.

1.   History of testicular injury, surgery, or mumps.

2.   Exposure to excessive heat. A small rise in scrotal temperature can adversely affect spermatogenesis, and a febrile illness can produce striking changes in sperm count and motility. The effect of the illness can be seen in the sperm count and motility even 2–3 months later. This reflects the 74 days required for a spermatozoon to be generated from a primary germ cell. Environmental sources of heat, such as the use of jockey shorts instead of boxer shorts, excessively hot baths, hot tubs, or occupations that require long hours of sitting; e.g., long distance truck driving, may all decrease fertility potential; however, none of these factors has ever been substantiated by clinical study.[54]

3.   Severe allergic reactions.

4.   Exposure to radiation or to industrial or environmental toxins Those who believe there is a downward trend in sperm counts commonly place blame on environmental pollutants or chemicals, including chemicals that mimic the effects of estrogen. A study from Scandinavia did show lower sperm counts in males from an urban area compared to males in rural areas, suggesting an effect of urban pollutants.[55] More direct evidence of a deleterious effect of environmental hazards is difficult to obtain because there is a reluctance of workers to produce the serial semen specimens that would be required for a thorough industrial study. In any case, the clinician should determine if a male with an abnormal semen specimen has had exposure to industrial or environmental toxins.

5.   Heavy marijuana and alcohol use can depress sperm counts and testosterone levels. Marijuana inhibits the secretion of GnRH and can suppress reproductive function in both men and women, and cocaine use is known to reduce spermatogenesis.[56, 57] There is no evidence to indicate that moderate alcohol intake affects fertility.[58] There is good evidence that fecundity is reduced in women who smoke, and this is probably true for men as well, although not all studies agree.[59–61] Studies have failed to confirm an adverse impact of caffeine on fertility, although high levels of intake may be associated with a delay in conception.[62, 63]

   Certain drugs, including cimetidine, spironolactone, nitrofurans, sulfasalazine, erythromycin, tetracyclines, anabolic steroids, and chemotherapeutic agents, can depress sperm quantity and quality. Cephalosporins, penicillins, quinolones, and the combination of sulfamethoxazole and trimethoprim are relatively safe to use when there is concern about effects on sperm.[64] Neurologic ejaculatory dysfunction can be caused by α-blockers, phentolamine, methyldopa, guanethidine, and reserpine. Resumption of spermatogenesis has been reported to occur within 2 years following discontinuation of anabolic steroids; however, it is not known whether all individuals will return to normal function.[65]

6.   Coital frequency. Counts at the lower levels of the normal range may be depressed to below normal levels by ejaculations occurring daily or more frequently. Conversely, abstinence for 10–14 days or more to save up sperm may be counterproductive because the gain in numbers can be offset by the lower motility produced by the increased proportion of older sperm. For most couples, coitus every 36 hours around the time of ovulation will give the optimal chance for pregnancy. However, studies in men with oligospermia fail to detect a decline in sperm numbers with

sequential ejaculations, suggesting that limitations on coital frequency are not necessary.[66, 67]

7. Exposure to diethylstilbestrol in utero has been suggested, but not proven, as a cause of male infertility.[68] Indeed, in the largest follow-up of men born to the women treated with diethylstilbestrol, no impairment of fertility or sexual function was detected.[69]

Urologic Evaluation

In the presence of semen abnormalities, referral is made to an urologist in order to look for an anatomic abnormality, an infection, an endocrine or genetic disorder, or a varicocele. Evaluation by an urologist detects serious medical pathology (such as a tumor) in approximately 1 of every 100 patients.[70]

Anatomic Abnormalities

Examination may reveal a physical impairment such as a marked hypospadias, which can cause sperm to be deposited outside the vagina. In rare cases of diabetes, with some neurologic diseases, or occasionally following prostatectomy or pelvic lymphadenectomy, there can be retrograde ejaculation into the bladder. Pregnancies have been reported after insemination of sperm obtained from alkalinized urine or following treatment with a variety of drugs.[71] Retrograde ejaculation may be only partial, and some men with this condition have small amounts of visible ejaculate.

Obstruction or absence of the vas deferens is a relatively uncommon cause of male infertility. If the ducts are congenitally absent, fructose which is produced in the seminal vesicles will be absent from the semen. Testicular biopsy can differentiate between a block in the outflow tract or primary damage to the testes. Testicular damage or maldevelopment can be found following mumps orchitis, cryptorchidism, or in association with Klinefelter's syndrome. Males with the latter genetic abnormality (XXY) usually have small testes and azoospermia. With blockage of the vas, sperm can be aspirated from the epididymis and vasa efferentia. Successful fertilization in vitro can result in pregnancy.[72]

It is important that any infection in the genitourinary tract, including those caused by mycoplasma and chlamydia, be treated even though the specific effect on male fertility is not established.

Genetic Causes of Male Infertility

There is a high prevalence of Y chromosome submicroscopic deletions in men with oligospermia. A cluster of genes that are deleted in men with azoospermia or oligospermia has been referred to as DAZ ("deleted in azoospermia").[73, 74] Subsequently, at least 3 specific regions on Yq were identified and labeled as "azoospermia factors," AZFa, AZFb, and AZFc (the same region as DAZ).[75] From 7% to 10% of men with severe oligospermia have been reported to have deletions in the AZFb and AZFc regions on the long arm of the Y chromosome.[76, 77] These microdeletions correlate poorly with the numbers of sperm present in the semen analysis. These could be normal genetic variants and not the cause of the infertility; however, these deletions can now be transmitted with the use of ICSI, and it is now appropriate to consider Y chromosome deletion analysis prior to treatment with assisted reproduction. On the other hand, Y chromosome deletions are rare in men participating in an ICSI program. Indeed, the prevalence of overall chromosomal abnormalities is greater in men with abnormal semen than the prevalence of Y chromosome microdeletions.[78, 79] Although these genetic abnormalities are relatively infrequent, and there is uncertainty regarding the role of Y chromosome microdeletions, because of the consequences, there is strong support for genetic screening of all men considering ICSI.[80] Indeed, 90% of couples receiving genetic counseling elect to undergo genetic screening.[81]

Approximately 1–2% of infertile males have the congenital bilateral absence of the vas deferens.[82] Most males with bilateral congenital absence of the vas deferens have at least two mutations in the cystic fibrosis transmembrane conductance regulator gene.[83] Screening for cystic fibrosis mutations should be considered in males with bilateral absent vas deferens who are considering ICSI. A reasonable approach involves screening the female partner; the absence of cystic fibrosis mutations in the female reduces the risk of having a child with cystic fibrosis to a very low level.

Primary ciliary dyskinesia refers to a group of disorders with autosomal inheritance and caused by abnormal or absent motility in ciliary structures. Kartagener syndrome includes sperm immotility, bronchiectasis, sinusitis, and situs inversus.

The presence of azoospermia or severe oligospermia with an intact vas warrants karyotyping. The most frequent diagnosis is Klinefelter syndrome, which occurs in approximately 1 in every 500 males. Among other genetic abnormalities, azoospermia and hypogonadism can result because of a mutation that causes an abnormality in the beta-subunit of LH.[84] An inactivating mutation in the gene for the FSH receptor is associated with varying degrees of suppression of spermatogenesis, indicating that FSH is not absolutely essential for sperm production[1].

Endocrine Disorders

Although endocrine disorders are an uncommon cause for infertility, testing for thyroid, gonadotropins, prolactin, and testosterone may occasionally uncover unsuspected abnormalities. FSH levels are elevated with germ cell aplasia, and testosterone levels are decreased in men who are hypogonadotropic. Hyperprolactinemia is commonly associated with impotence, and in the absence of impotence, measuring a prolactin level is unlikely to aid in the diagnosis.

Infusion of gonadotropin-releasing hormone (GnRH) can stimulate secretion of gonadotropins, and there have been occasional reports of the usefulness of this treatment as well as the administration of gonadotropins in males who have an isolated gonadotropin deficiency. Although nonspecific therapy with thyroid, clomiphene citrate, and human chorionic gonadotropin has been used extensively, there is no compelling evidence that it is beneficial. Clomiphene citrate can elevate the sperm count, but an associated increase in fertility does not occur.[85]

A fundamental problem in most studies of the efficacy of drug therapy in male fertility is the lack of a control group for comparison. Investigators make the erroneous assumption that the spontaneous cure rate of male infertility is zero and that any pregnancy that occurs during or following treatment is due solely to that treatment. A number of studies, however, have attested to the spontaneous cure rate of male infertility. In one study approximately one-third of males, with counts below 10 million/mL and who were not treated, successfully impregnated their partners.[16] In summary, hormone treatment of infertile males who do not have an endocrine disorder is almost always unrewarding, and it does not improve fertility beyond what occurs by chance.

Varicocele

A varicocele is an abnormal tortuosity and dilatation of the veins of the pampiniform plexus within the spermatic cord. Approximately 20% to 40% of infertile males, depending on the zeal of the search, have a varicocele, usually on the left side because of the direct insertion of the spermatic vein into the renal vein. Varicoceles, in all likelihood, exert their effects by raising testicular temperature, an effect mediated by increased arterial blood flow.[86]

Approximately 10–15% of males in a general population have a varicocele on physical examination, but there is no evidence that males with normal semen characteristics need treatment even if a varicocele is present. They should be checked periodically, however, to be sure that there is no deterioration in their semen characteristics.

It has been difficult to perform randomized studies of varicocele repair. A trial in Melbourne, Australia, failed because of poor compliance.[87] Because the authors told their patients that varicocele repair might not make a difference, only 283 of 651 men chose to have it done. In those who had the repair, the only impact on the semen analysis was an improvement in motility from 33.5% to 39.3%, the classically reported finding. The same change, however, was noted in the nonoperated group, and the pregnancy rates in both the operated and nonoperated groups were the same! A small randomized trial in Germany observed a significant increase in sperm concentration in the treated group, but the pregnancy rates were the same in both treated and non-treated groups.[88] However, varicocele is more commonly found in men with abnormal semen, and there is evidence that a varicocele may exert an increasingly deleterious effect over time.[89]

Ligation of varicoceles results in a 30–35% pregnancy rate. Although the beneficial effects of treatment of varicocele have been disputed by some investigators who found equal results without treatment, current clinical practice supports the utilization of varicocele ligation in those males who have infertility and an impaired semen specimen.[86]

Larger varicoceles exert a greater effect than small ones. Very small varicoceles, diagnosed only by ultrasound, are not worth treating. Decreased size of the left testicle together with a varicocele is associated with a worse prognosis with treatment compared with cases in which the testicles are of normal size. Although surgical interruption of the internal spermatic vein is the usual treatment for clinically apparent varicoceles, there is also a nonsurgical approach that utilizes embolization to occlude the vein.[86]

Reactive Oxygen Species

Increased levels of reactive oxygen species can cause damage to the sperm membrane.[90] Substances such as peroxidase and hydrogen peroxide can be released by abnormal sperm and by white blood cells, and when elevated levels of leukocytes are present in the semen (with a negative culture), treatment with vitamin E and glutathione is advocated.[91, 92]

Intrauterine Insemination of Washed Sperm (IUI)

Inseminations of whole semen have a limited role in infertility. They are useful when, either because of physical or psychologic factors, it is not possible to deposit sperm in the vagina by intercourse. In addition they are obviously useful in donor insemination. In the past small amounts of untreated semen were used for intrauterine insemination, but the potential for reactions to the proteins, prostaglandins, and bacteria in semen have made this approach a historical relic. In its place has emerged the use of washed sperm for intrauterine insemination (IUI).

The initial indications for IUI were failure of sperm to penetrate cervical mucus and male infertility. During the past decade the indications for IUI have been liberalized and now it is frequently employed, often in conjunction with the woman's use of clomiphene citrate or gonadotropins. Current controversies revolve around issues of techniques and those of efficacy.

There are a variety of methods that allow the separation of a more promising population of sperm. Most commonly used are washing and swim-up or resuspension of sperm or separation of sperm on density gradients. Other methods include allowing the sperm to swim into hyaluronic acid or filtering the sperm on glass wool. All isolate a population of sperm with a higher percentage of motile forms and with a more uniform morphology than those found in untreated ejaculates. In the swim-up techniques, the semen is washed once or twice with one to three volumes of culture medium. A variety of media is available from commercial suppliers. After washing and centrifugation the supernatant is decanted and the pellet overlaid with 0.5 mL media. At this point the pellet is agitated to resuspend the sperm and the preparation is inseminated into the uterus. Because of the resuspension, the live sperm in the inseminate are accompanied by dead sperm and miscellaneous cellular elements. In the alternative swim-up technique, the unagitated pellet and overlying medium are placed in an incubator at 37° for 30–60 minutes. This provides lower numbers of sperm in the medium portion compared to the resuspension technique, but it achieves a cleaner specimen and for this reason it is the method we prefer. However, with severely oligospermic specimens it may be necessary to use resuspension to obtain sufficient sperm for insemination.

Whereas all sperm separation methods produce specimens with better motility and more uniform morphology, this improvement may not necessarily translate into increased pregnancy rates. When equal numbers of motile sperm separated from good and from poor specimens were used in the sperm penetration assay, sperm separated from the good specimens were superior in achieving penetration.[93] Thus, there may be intrinsic defects in sperm from poor specimens that may affect even the best sperm from that cohort.

At least 1 million motile sperm should be inseminated because lower numbers are seldom associated with success.[94] When more than 15 million motile sperm were inseminated, there was no increase in the pregnancy rate; however, there was an increase in multiple births when the inseminate exceeded 20 million motile sperm.[95] In another study, pregnancy rates were substantially higher when more than 10 million motile sperm were inseminated compared with inseminations of less than 10 million.[96] Others have also reported increased pregnancy rates when higher numbers of donor sperm were inseminated.[97] Important factors in determining the final motile sperm count are the initial sperm count and sperm motility. Combining two ejaculates obtained 4 hours apart can increase the numbers of sperm available from oligospermic specimens.[98]

Empiric therapy, consisting of clomiphene alone, gonadotropin alone, IUI, or IUI combined with clomiphene or gonadotropin, in the female increasingly has been used for treatment of infertility of any origin. The greatest enthusiasm supports IUI combined with gonadotropin, which offers a number of possible advantages. It increases the number of oocytes that have the potential for fertilization and increases the number of sperm reaching the uterine cavity. It raises the woman's hormone levels and eliminates seminal plasma, that may contain factors inimical to sperm. The enthusiasm was fueled not only by these postulated advantages of gonadotropin-IUI but by a series of positive reports that appeared in the literature in the late 1980s and early 1990s. In a population selected for male factor infertility or poor postcoital tests, superovulation combined with IUI increased the monthly probability of pregnancy approximately four times compared to that following IUI timed by the LH surge.[99] The most striking advantage was seen in the subgroup of women who were treated with gonadotropin and HCG rather than clomiphene alone or clomiphene-gonadotropin/HCG combinations. Another study in couples with unexplained infertility demonstrated a pregnancy rate per cycle of 2.7% with IUI alone, 6.1% with gonadotropin alone, but 26.4% when gonadotropin/IUI was used.[100] Very similar experiences have been reported by others (see Chapter 30).[101] Dodson and Haney surveyed the literature and found that gonadotropin and IUI fecundity was 8.7% for male factor and 17% for unexplained infertility.[102] Their own experience, which was included in the survey, was 15% for each category.

Our current formulation concludes that IUI without associated superovulation has little value in the treatment of male infertility. Gonadotropin-IUI marginally increases the pregnancy rate to approximately 7–8% per cycle (from a baseline of 2–3% per cycle) when an abnormality is present in the semen. Several treatment cycles are warranted, except in the presence of severely compromised semen specimens, where an early resort to ICSI is indicated.

The timing of inseminations and the number of inseminations per cycle may influence the ultimate pregnancy rates. Most commonly IUI is timed for the day following the LH surge measured in the urine or at approximately 36 hours after an injection of human chorionic gonadotropin (HCG). Variations on these schedules can still be associated with reasonable pregnancy rates. Increased pregnancy rates have been obtained by doing two IUI's in a cycle, the day of and the day after the LH surge or the ovulatory injection of HCG.[103, 104] Others have reported no difference in results with one or two IUIs.[105] Because of the lesser expense and the greater convenience, we perform one insemination for several cycles before considering multiple inseminations.

Prior down-regulation with GnRH agonist treatment does not enhance results with gonadotropin/IUI.[106] Similarly, intraperitoneal or intratubal inseminations of sperm, although conceptually attractive, have no proven advantage over intrauterine insemination.[107] Moreover, intratubal transfer could increase the risk of infection. Infection with IUI is rare, probably in the range of 1 in 500 inseminations. Multiple pregnancies occur in approximately 20% of cases of gonadotropin/IUI, and the pregnancy loss rate is approximately 20%. Hyperstimulation of the ovaries can be minimized, but not eliminated, by monitoring of ovarian follicle numbers and growth by ultrasound (reviewed in Chapter 30). The cycle should be canceled by withholding HCG if more than 3–4 follicles with diameters of 14 mm or greater are present when the lead follicle size (18 mm or larger) indicates the time for HCG injection. Estrogen monitoring is not usually required, as opposed to IVF cycles where stimulation is more aggressive.

Estrogen monitoring can be helpful if a lead follicle displays an abnormal rate of growth, either too fast or too slow. A value of less than 200 pg/mL per mature follicle raises the suspicion that a follicle does not contain a normal oocyte. If there are excessive numbers of small follicles (10–13 mm) associated with 3 or 4 leading follicles, a high estrogen level (over 2000 pg/mL) indicates an increased risk of hyperstimulation, and HCG administration should not occur.

Treatment of sperm with methylxanthines such as caffeine and pentoxifylline seem to enhance motility. The compounds inhibit cyclic AMP phosphodiesterase which results in an increase in cyclic AMP. Despite some earlier enthusiasm, pentoxiphylline offered no advantage in an IVF program, and a cautionary note was raised because the safety of the compound in early pregnancy has not been established.[108]

Therapeutic Donor Insemination

The combined problems of male infertility and decreased availability of adoptable babies have increased the interest in, and the demand for, therapeutic donor inseminations (TDI). The procedure raises emotional, ethical, and legal questions that must be considered and discussed. The clinician must never do inseminations without the consent of both partners. Increasingly, single women are seeking TDI. McGuire and Alexander[109] reported that children in single head of household families are as psychologically adjusted as those from two-parent households and that TDI should not be denied to single women solely on the basis of their lack of a male partner.

Three points are worth emphasizing.

1. Donor inseminations do not guarantee pregnancy. In the past, the success rate with fresh semen was about 70% over 5–6 cycles. The current use of frozen semen lowers the success rate.[110, 111] The fecundability (chance of getting pregnant per cycle) has been reported to be 18.9% with fresh semen and only 5.0% with frozen semen.[110] However, with exceptionally good frozen specimens, success can approach that achieved with fresh specimens. Over 80% of pregnancies that will occur do so within 6 months with fresh semen and within 12 months with frozen semen. In a summary of nearly 3000 treatment cycles with frozen sperm, the cumulative pregnancy rates were 21% at 3 months, 40% at 6 months, and 62% at 12 months for

women less than 30 years old.[112] For women over the age of 30, the pregnancy rates were 17%, 26%, and 44%, respectively. Because of the risk of acquired immunodeficiency syndrome (AIDS), use of frozen sperm that has been quarantined for 6 months is now accepted clinical practice. The donor is tested for HIV at the time of collection and again at 6 months. In highly selected cases, washed, swim-up sperm for intrauterine insemination from an HIV-infected man has been used to achieve a healthy pregnancy in his partner.[113] Despite an absence of seroconversion of the female partner, the full safety of this approach has not been established. Of course, sperm prepared in this manner should not be used in a donor program.

2.   The couple needs to give some thought to their feelings should the child be born with a congenital anomaly. This will occur in 4–5% of all pregnancies, irrespective of whether they follow intercourse or therapeutic donor insemination.[114]

3.   Both the woman and her partner, or the woman alone if there is no partner, should sign a consent form, The procedure is covered by law in many, but not all, states. It is worthwhile for the clinician to know the legal status of TDI in his or her state so that correct information can be conveyed to patients.

As a rule the donor should be unknown to the couple. However, there has been discussion of sealing personal information on the donor with the understanding that, if he gives permission, the information can be conveyed to children conceived with his sperm, when those children reach adulthood.

The health and fertility of the donor must be unimpeachable, and there should be no family history of genetic diseases. Screening for thalassemia in Mediterranean races, Tay-Sachs heterozygosity in Jews, and sickle cell disease in blacks is a wise precaution. Donors can also be tested for cystic fibrosis. Potential donors who are at high risk for AIDS (homosexuals, bisexuals, intravenous drug users) should be excluded as should individuals who have multiple sexual partners. Similar exclusions include those individuals with histories of herpes, chronic hepatitis, and venereal warts. In addition, testing is recommended for human immunodeficiency virus (HIV), syphilis, hepatitis B antigen, antibody to hepatitis B, hepatitis C, gonorrhea, chlamydia, and cytomegalovirus. As noted above, an initial screening test for HIV, if negative, should be repeated after 6 months. If both results are negative, the semen, which should be cryopreserved and quarantined for the 6 months, can be used. The donor will not be a mirror image of the male partner, but an attempt should be made to match physical characteristics.

Most individuals undergoing TDI consider it a private matter and not subject to discussion with family and friends. If successful in achieving pregnancy, some individuals discuss the origins of the conception with their children, but most people prefer to leave it unsaid.

Use of friends or relatives as donors raises the potential for emotional problems in the future, although we have used a relative when it was requested by a stable, intelligent couple who understood the long-term implications. The related donor must be subjected to the same laboratory screening as all other donors. Requests to mix the partner's sperm with the donor's signifies that the couple may not have made the emotional adjustment to the thought of donor insemination. A partner's semen also may impair the donor's sperm, although this is in dispute.

Donor inseminations are useful in azoospermia, severe oligospermia, or asthenospermia refractory to treatment. They also are useful for the rare woman who has a history of fetal loss due to Rh sensitization. In that case an Rh-negative donor would be used. Genetic diseases may, on occasion, be an indication for donor insemination.

The basal body temperature (BBT) change, the woman's perception of vaginal wetness, and ovulatory pain, if present, are useful guides for timing of inseminations. More precise timing can be accomplished by monitoring of the day of the LH surge with measurements of LH in urine with any of a number of commercially available kits. In our experience approximately 75% of women can successfully use the kits at home to identify their LH surge. Insemination is performed the day after the LH surge is identified. In more difficult cases, monitoring and treatment approaches utilize ultrasound to monitor preovulatory follicle growth and an injection of 5000 or 10,000 IU human chorionic gonadotropin when the dominant follicle reaches 18 mm or greater in diameter.

If the BBT alone is used, an attempt is made to inseminate on the date just before or two days before the temperature rise with the timing based on reviewing 2 months of charts and/or the day of maximal vaginal wetness.

IUI with donor inseminations produces higher pregnancy rates compared with intracervical insemination.[115, 116] However, the multiple pregnancy rate may be slightly higher.[117] One IUI per cycle should be performed for two cycles, and then, if no success, increase to two inseminations per cycle. Double inseminations in a donor program increase the pregnancy rate and shorten the time required to achieve pregnancy.[103, 118] IUI should be performed the day after a positive test with the urinary LH kit, or approximately 36 hours after HCG administration. When two IUIs are performed, they should be timed the day of and the day after the LH kit tests positive, or approximately 18 and 42 hours after HCG administration. A minimum of 6 months of donor inseminations, with or without superovulation, should be completed prior to moving on to in vitro fertilization. In a healthy woman, 3–4 cycles can be concluded prior to hysterosalpingography.

The children born after donor insemination have outcomes comparable to the general population.[114] Interestingly, approximately half of couples do and half do not tell their children of their origins. The divorce rate in families with children conceived with donor insemination is lower than the general rate.[114]

Intracytoplasmic Sperm Injection (ICSI)

ICSI, the direct injection of a single spermatozoon or spermatid into the cytoplasm of an oocyte (described in Chapter 31), was first described in 1992.[119] The results have been nothing short of amazing, with pregnancy rates equal to or slightly surpassing the normal fecundity rate.[120, 121] Pregnancy rates are independent of any semen analysis parameter (number, motility, morphology). All that is required is the DNA material, and this can be derived from a barely moving spermatozoon or in men with no spermatozoa or spermatids in the semen analysis from a spermatid (or spermatocyte) obtained by epididymal aspiration or from a biopsy of the seminiferous tubules.[122–124]

Although ICSI avoids the natural process of sperm selection, the chromosomal abnormality rates in the offspring have been equal to the rate in the general population, with the exception of a slight increase in minor sex chromosome abnormalities (that could pass the male infertility problem to children), and, thus far, growth and development of the children have been normal.

Conclusion

For many years, the outlook for male infertility (with the exception of donor insemination) was very pessimistic. Today, in vitro fertilization with ICSI can overcome even the most grievous cases. The availability and expense of this technology, however, often are out of the reach of many couples. Therefore, less rigorous treatment continues to be an important part of the treatment of male infertility. It is important to identify a urologist in the local community who has both an interest and expertise in male infertility. Even without that resource, the clinician has the ability to offer IUI and superovulation.

References

1. **Tapanainen JS, Aittomäki K, Min J, Vaskivuo T, Huhtaniemi I,** Men homozygous for an inactivating mutation of the follicle-stimulating hormone (FSH) receptor gene present variable suppression of spermatogenesis and fertility, *Nature Genet* 15:205, 1997.

2. **Plymate SR, Paulsen CA, McLachlan RI,** Relationship of serum inhibin levels to serum follicle stimulating hormone and sperm production in normal men and men with varicoceles, *J Clin Endocrinol Metab* 74:859, 1992.

3. **Illingworth PJ, Groome NP, Byrd W, Rainey WE, McNeilly AS, Mather JP, Bremmer WJ,** Inhibin-B: a likely candidate for the physiologically important form of inhibin in men, *J Clin Endocrinol Metab* 81:1321, 1996.

4. **Anderson RA, Wallace EM, Groome NP, Bellis AJ, Wu FCW,** Physiological relationships between inhibin B, follicle stimulating hormone secretion and spermatogenesis in normal men and response to gonadotrophin suppression by exogenous testosterone, *Hum Reprod* 12:746, 1997.

5. **Gnessi L, fabbri A, Spera G,** Gonadal peptides as mediators of development and functional control of the testis: an integrated system with hormones and local environment, *Endocr Rev* 18:541, 1997.

6. **Burgoyne PS,** The role of the mammalian Y chromosome in spermatogenesis, *Development* 101(Suppl):133, 1987.

7. **Carlsen E, Giwercman A, Keidin N, Skakkebaek NE,** Evidence for decreasing quality of semen during past 50 years, *Br Med J* 305:609, 1992.

8. **Auger J, Kunstmann JM, Czyglik F, Jouannet P,** Decline in semen quality among fertile men in Paris during the last 20 years, *New Engl J Med* 332:281, 1995.

9. **Sherins RJ,** Are semen quality and male infertility changing? *New Engl J Med* 332:327, 1995.

10. **Fisch H, Goluboff ET, Olson JH, Feldshuh J, Broder SH, Barad DH,** Semen analysis in 1283 men from the United States over a 25-year period: no decline in quality, *Fertil Steril* 65:1009, 1996.

11. **Paulsen CA, Berman NG, Wang C,** Data from men in greater Seattle area reveals no downward trend in semen quality: further evidence that deterioration of semen quality is not geographically uniform, *Fertil Steril* 65:1015, 1996.

12. **Rasmussen PE, Erb K, Westergaard LG, Laursen ST,** No evidence for decreasing semen quality in four birth cohorts of 1,055 Danish men born between 1950 and 1970, *Fertil Steril* 68:1059, 1997.

13. **World Health Organization,** *Laboratory Manual for the Examination of Human Semen and Sperm — Cervical Mucus Interaction,* Cambridge University Press, Cambridge, 1992.

14. **Sherins RJ, Brightwell D, Sternthal PM,** Longitudinal analysis of semen of fertile and infertile men, In: Troen P, Nankin R, eds. *The Testis in Normal and Infertile Men,* Raven Press, New York, 1977, p 473.

15. **MacLeod J, Gold RA,** The male factor in fertility and infertility. II. Spermatozoan counts in 1000 cases of known fertility and 1000 cases of infertile marriage, *J Urol* 66:436, 1951.

16. **Smith KD, Rodriguez-Rigau LJ, Steinberger E,** Relationship between indices of semen analysis and pregnancy rate in infertile couples, *Fertil Steril* 28:1314, 1977.

17. **Jequier AM, Ukome EB,** Errors inherent in the performance of a routine semen analysis, *Br J Urol* 55:434, 1983.

18. **Neuwinger J, Behre HM, Nieschlag E,** External quality control in the andrology laboratory: an experimental multicenter trial, *Fertil Steril* 54:38, 1990.

19. **Hargreave TB, Elton RA,** Fecundability rates from an infertile population, *Br J Urol* 58:194, 1986.

20. **Steinberger E, Rodriguez-Rigau LJ, Smith KD,** The interaction between the fertility potentials of the two members of an infertile couple, In: Frajese G, Hafez ESE, Conti C, Fabbrini A, eds. *Oligospermia: Recent Progress in Andrology,* Raven Press, New York, 1981, p 9.

21. **Katz DF, Diel L, Overstreet JW,** Differences in the movement of morphologically normal and abnormal human seminal spermatozoa, *Biol Reprod* 26:66, 1982.

22. **Kruger TF, Acosta AA, Simmons KF, Swanson RJ, Matta JF, Oehninger S,** Predictive value of abnormal sperm morphology in in vitro fertilization, *Fertil Steril* 49:112, 1988.

23. **Morgenthaler A, Fung MY, Harris DH, Powers RD, Alper MM,** Sperm morphology and in vitro fertilization outcome: a direct comparison of World Health Organization and strict criteria methodologies, *Fertil Steril* 64:1177, 1995.

24. **Kruger TF, Dutoit TC, Franken DR, Acosta AA, Oehninger SC, Menkveld R, Lombard CJ,** A new computerized method of reading sperm morphology (strict criteria) is as efficient as technician reading, *Fertil Steril* 59:202, 1993.

25. **Eggert-Krause W, Bellmann A, Rohr G, Tilgen W, Runnenbaum B,** Differentiation of round cells in semen by means of monoclonal antibodies and relationship with male fertility, *Fertil Steril* 58:1046, 1992.

26. **Yanagimachi R,** Zona-free hamster eggs: their use in assessing fertilizing capacity and examining chromosomes of human spermatozoa, *Gamete Res* 10:187, 1984.

27. **Mao C, Grimes DA,** The sperm penetration assay: can it discriminate between fertile and infertile men? *Am J Obstet Gynecol* 159:279, 1988.

28. **Margalioth EJ, Feinmesser M, Navot D, Mordel N, Bronson RA,** The long-term predictive value of the zona-free hamster ova sperm penetration assay, *Fertil Steril* 52:490, 1989.

29. **McClure DR, Tom RA, Dandekar PV,** Optimizing the sperm penetration assay with human follicular fluid, *Fertil Steril* 53:546, 1990.

30. **Falk RM, Silverberg KM, Fetterolf PM, Kirschner FK, Rogers BJ,** Establishment of test-yolk buffer enhanced sperm penetration assay limits for fertile males, *Fertil Steril* 54:121, 1990.

31. **Burkman LJ, Coddington CC, Franken DR, Kruger TF, Rosenwaks Z, Hodgen GD,** The hemizona assay (IIZA): development of a diagnostic test for the binding of human spermatozoa to the human hemizona pellucida to predict fertilization potential, *Fertil Steril* 49:688, 1988.

32. **Coddington III CC,** The hemizona assay (HZA) and considerations for its use in assisted reproductive technology, *Seminars Reprod Endocrinol* 10:1, 1992.

33. **Bartoov B, Ben-Barak J, Mayevsky A, Sneider M, Yogev L, Lightman A,** Sperm motility index: a new parameter for human sperm evaluation, *Fertil Steril* 56:108, 1991.

34. **Jeyendran RS, Van der Ven HH, Perez-Peleaz M, Crabo BG, Zaneveld LJD,** Development of an assay to assess the functional integrity of the human sperm membrane and its relationship to other semen characteristics, *J Reprod Fertil* 79:219, 1984.

35. **Casper RF, Meriano JS, Jarvi KA, Cowen L, Lucato ML,** The hypo-osmotic swelling test for selection of viable sperm for intracytoplasmic sperm injection in men with complete asthenozoospermia, *Fertil Steril* 65:972, 1996.

36. **Comhaire FH, Vermeulen L, Schoonjans F,** Reassessment of the accuracy of traditional sperm characteristics and adenosine triphosphate (ATP) in estimating the fertilizing potential of human semen in vivo, *Int J Androl* 10:654, 1987.

37. **WHO Task Force on the Prevention and Management of Infertility,** Adenosine triphosphate in semen and other sperm characteristics: their relevance for fertility prediction in men with normal sperm concentration, *Fertil Steril* 57:877, 1992.

38. **Takahashi K, Wetzels AMM, Goverde HJM, Bastiaans BA, Janssen HJG, Rolland R,** The kinetics of the acrosome reaction of human spermatozoa and its correlation with in vitro fertilization, *Fertil Steril* 57:889, 1992.

39. **Liu DY, Baker HWG,** Inhibition of acrosin activity with a trypsin inhibitor blocks human sperm penetration of the zona pellucida, *Biol Reprod* 48:340, 1993.

40. **Adeghe J-H,** Male subfertility due to sperm antibodies: a clinical overview, *Obstet Gynecol Survey* 48:1, 1992.

41. **Critser JR, Villines PM, Coulam CB, Crister ES,** Evaluation of circulating antisperm antibodies in fertile and patient populations, *Am J Reprod Immunol* 21:137, 1989.

42. **Eggert-Kruse W, Christmann M, Gerhard I, Pohl S, Klinga K, Runnebaum B,** Circulating antisperm antibodies and fertility prognosis: a prospective study, *Hum Reprod* 4:513, 1989.

43. **Collins JA, Burrows EA, Yeo J, Younglai EV,** Frequency and predictive value of antisperm antibodies among infertile couples, *Hum Reprod* 8:592, 1993.

44. **Rajah SV, Parslow JM, Howell RJR, Hendry WF,** Comparison of mixed antiglobulin reaction and direct immunobead test for detection of sperm-bound antibodies in subfertile males, *Fertil Steril* 57:1300, 1992.

45. **Ayvaliotis B, Bronson R, Rosenfeld D, Cooper G,** Conception rates in couples where autoimmunity to sperm is detected, *Fertil Steril* 44:739, 1986.

46. **Haas Jr GG, Manganiello P,** A double-blind placebo-controlled study of the use of methylprednisolone in infertile men with sperm-associated immunoglobins, *Fertil Steril* 47:295, 1987.

47. **Margalioth EJ, Sauter E, Bronson RA, Rosenfeld DL, Schou GM, Cooper GW,** Intrauterine insemination as treatment for antisperm antibodies in the female, *Fertil Steril* 50:441, 1988.

48. **Agarwal A,** Treatment of immunological infertility by sperm washing and intrauterine insemination, *Arch Androl* 29:207, 1992.

49. **Grundy CE, Robinson J, Gordon AG, Hay DM,** Selection of an antibody-free population of spermatozoa from semen samples of men suffering from immunological infertility, *Hum Reprod* 6:593, 1991.

50. **Hendry WF, Hughes L, Scammell G, Pryor JP, Hargreave TB,** Comparison of prednisolone and placebo in subfertile men with antibodies to spermatozoa, *Lancet* 335:85, 1990.

51. **Ombelet W, Vandeput H, Janssen M, Cox A, Vossen C, Pollet H, Steeno O, Bosmans E,** Treatment of male infertility due to sperm surface antibodies: IUI or IVF? *Hum Reprod* 12:1165, 1997.

52. **Rajah SV, Parslow JM, Howell RJ, Hendry WF,** The effects on in-vitro fertilization of autoantibodies to spermatozoa in subfertile men, *Hum Reprod* 8:1079, 1993.

53. **Nagy ZP, Verheyen G, Liu J, Joris H, Janssenswillen C, Wisanto A, Devroey P, Van Steirteghem AC,** Results of 55 intracytoplasmic sperm injection cycles in the treatment of male-immunological infertility, *Hum Reprod* 10:1775, 1995.

54. **Wang C, McDonald V, Leung A, Superlano L, Berman N, Hull L, Swerdloff RS,** Effect of increased scrotal temperature on sperm production in normal men, *Fertil Steril* 68:334, 1997.

55. **Ledholm OP, Ranstam J,** Depressed semen quality: a study over two decades, *Arch Androl* 12:113, 1984.

56. **Smith CG, Asch RH,** Drug abuse and reproduction, *Fertil Steril* 48:355, 1987.

57. **Bracken MB, Eskenazi B, Sachse K, McSharry J-E, Hellenbrand K, Leon-Summers L,** Association of cocaine use with sperm concentration, motility, and morphology, *Fertil Steril* 53:315, 1990.

58. **Olsen J, Bolumar F, Boldsen J, Bisanti L,** Does moderate alcohol intake reduce fecundability? A European multicenter study on infertility and subfecundity, *Alcohol Clin Exp Res* 21:206, 1997.

59. **Stillman RJ, Rosenberg MJ, Sachs BP,** Smoking and reproduction, *Fertil Steril* 46:545, 1986.

60. **Laurent SL, Thompson SJ, Addy C, Garrison CZ, Moore EE,** An epidemiologic study of smoking and primary infertility in women, *Fertil Steril* 57:565, 1992.

61. **Hughes EG, Brennan BG,** Does cigarette smoking impair natural or assisted fecundity, *Fertil Steril* 66:679, 1996.

62. **Bolumar F, Olsen J, Rebagliato M, Bisanti L,** Caffeine intake and delayed conception: a European multicenter study on infertility and subfecundity. European Study Group on Infertility and Subfecundity, *Am J Epidemiol* 145:324, 1997.

63. **Caan B, Quesenberry Jr CP, Coates AO,** Differences in fertility associated with caffeinated beverage consumption, *Am J Public Health* 88:270, 1998.

64. **Schlegel PN, Chang TSK, Marshall FF,** Antibiotics: potential hazard to male fertility, *Fertil Steril* 55:235, 1991.

65. **Gazvani MR, Buckett W, Luckas MJM, Aird IA, Hipkin LJ, Lewis-Jones DI,** Conservative management of azoospermia following steroid abuse, *Hum Reprod* 12:1706, 1997.

66. **Cooper TG, Keck C, Oberdieck U, Nieschlag E,** Effects of multiple ejaculations after extended periods of sexual abstinence on total, motile and normal sperm numbers, as well as accessory gland secretions, from healthy normal and oligozoospermic men, *Hum Reprod* 8:1251, 1993.

67. **Tur-Kaspa I, Maor Y, Levran D, Yonish M, Mashiach S, Dor J,** How often should infertile men have intercourse to achieve conception? *Fertil Steril* 62:370, 1994.

68. **Stillman RJ,** In utero exposure to diethylstilbestrol: adverse effects on the reproductive tract and reproductive performance in male and female offspring, *Am J Obstet Gynecol* 142:905, 1982.

69. **Wilcox AJ, Baird DD, Weinberg CR, Hornsby PP, Herbst AL,** Fertility in men exposed prenatally to diethylstilbestrol, *New Engl J Med* 332:1411, 1995.

70. **Honig SC, Lipshultz LI, Jarow J,** Significant medical pathology uncovered by a comprehensive male infertility evaluation, *Fertil Steril* 62:1028, 1994.

71. **Hershlag A, Schiff SF, DeCherney AH,** Retrograde ejaculation, *Hum Reprod* 6:255, 1991.

72. **Silber SJ, Ord T, Balmaceda J, Patrizio P, Asch RH,** Congenital absence of the vas deferens. The fertilizing capacity of human epididymal sperm, *New Engl J Med* 323:1788, 1990.

73. **Reijo R, Lee T-Y, Salo P, Alagappan R, Brown LG, Rosenberg M, Rozen S, Jaffe T, Straus D, Hovatta O, et al,** Diverse spermatogenic defects in humans caused by Y chromosome deletions encompassing a novel RNA-binding gene, *Nature Genet* 10:383, 1995.

74. **Reijo R, Alagappan RK, Patrizio P, Page DC,** Severe oligozoospermia resulting from deletions of azoospermia factor gene on Y chromosome, *Lancet* 347:1290, 1996.

75. **Vogt PH, Edelmann A, Kirsch S, Henegrin O, Hirschmann P, Kiesewetter F, Kohn FM, Schill WB, Farah S, Ramos C, Hartmann M, Hartschuh W, Meschede D, Behre HM, Castel A, Nieshlag E, Weidner W, Grone HJ, Jung A, Engel W, Haidl G,** Human Y chromosome azoospermia factors (AZF) mapped to different subregions in Yq11, *Hum Mol Genet* 5:933, 1996.

76. **Girardi SK, Mielnik A, Schlegel PN,** Submicroscopic deletions in the Y chromosome of infertile men, *Hum Reprod* 12:1635, 1997.

77. **Pryor JL, Kent-First M, Muallem A, Van Bergen AH, Nolten WE, Meisner L, Roberts KP,** Microdeletions in the Y chromosome of infertile men, *New Engl J Med* 336:534, 1997.

78. **Pandiyan N, Jequier AM,** Mitotic chromosomal anomalies among 1210 infertile men, *Hum Reprod* 11:2604, 1996.

79. **van der Ven K, Montag M, Peschka B, Leygraaf J, Schwanitz G, Haidl G, Krebs D, van der Ven H,** Combined cytogenetic and Y chromosome microdeletion screening in males undergoing intracytoplasmic sperm injection, *Mol Hum Reprod* 3:699, 1997.

80. **Johnson MD,** Genetic risks of intracytoplasmic sperm injection in the treatment of male infertility: recommendations for genetic counseling and screening, *Fertil Steril* 70:397, 1998.

81. **Pauer HU, Hinney B, Michelmann HW, Krasemann EW, Zoll B, Engel W,** Relevance of genetic counselling in couples prior to intracytoplasmic sperm injection, *Hum Reprod* 12:1909, 1997.

82. **Jequier AM, Ansell ID, Bullimore NJ,** Congenital absence of the vasa deferentia presenting with infertility, *J Androl* 6:15, 1985.

83. **De Braekeleer M, Férec C,** Mutations in the cystic fibrosis gene in men with congenital bilateral absence of the vas deferens, *Hum Mol Reprod* 2:669, 1996.

84. **Weiss J, Axelrod L, Whitcomb RW, Harris PE, Crowley WF, Jameson JL,** Hypogonadism caused by a single amino acid substitution in the β-subunit of luteinizing hormone, *New Engl J Med* 326:179, 1992.

85. **WHO,** A double-blind trial of clomiphene citrate for the treatment of idiopathic male infertility, *Int J Androl* 15:299, 1992.

86. **Howards SS,** Varicocele, *Infertil Reprod Med Clin North Am* 3:429, 1992.

87. **Baker HWG, Burger HG, de Kretser DM, Hudson B, Rennie GC, Straffon WGE,** Testicular vein ligation and fertility in men with varicoceles, *Br Med J* 291:1678, 1985.

88. **Nieschlag E, Hertle L, Fischedick A, Abshagen K, Behre HM,** Treatment of varicocele: counselling as effective as occlusion of the vena spermatica, *Hum Reprod* 13:2147, 1998.

89. **Gorelick JI, Goldstein M,** Loss of fertility in men with varicocele, *Fertil Steril* 59:613, 1993.

90. **Aitken RJ,** The role of free oxygen radicals and sperm function, *Int J Androl* 12:95, 1989.

91. **Kessopoulou E, Powers HJ, Sharma KK, Pearson MJ, Russell JM, Cooke ID, Barratt CL,** A double-blind randomized placebo cross-over controlled trial using the antioxidant vitamin E to treat reactive oxygen species associated male infertility, *Fertil Steril* 64:825, 1995.

92. **Lenzi A, Culasso F, Gandini L, Lombardo F, Dondero F,** Placebo-controlled, double-blind, cross-over trial of glutathione therapy in male infertility, *Hum Reprod* 8:1657, 1993.

93. **Syms AJ, Johnson A, Lipshultz LI, Smith RG,** Reduced ability of motile human spermatozoa obtained from oligospermic males to penetrate zona-free hamster eggs, *Fertil Steril* 41:1055, 1984.

94. **Nulsen JC, Walsh S, Dumez S, Metzger DA,** A randomized and longitudinal study of human menopausal gonadotropin with intrauterine insemination in the treatment of infertility, *Obstet Gynecol* 82:780, 1993.

95. **Kerin J, Byrd W,** Supracervical placement of spermatozoa, In: Soules MR, ed. *Controversies in Reproductive Endocrinology and Infertility,* Elsevier, Amsterdam, 1989.

96. **Van Voorhis BJ, Sparks AET, Allen BD, Stovall DW, Syrop CH, Chapler FK,** Cost-effectiveness of infertility treatments: a cohort study, *Fertil Steril* 67:830, 1997.

97. **Shapiro SS,** Strategies to improve efficiency of threapeutic donor insemination, *Infertil Reprod Med Clin North Am* 3:469, 1992.

98. **Tur-Kaspa I, Dudkiewicz A, Confino E, Gleicher N,** Pooled sequential ejaculates: a way to increase the total number of motile sperm from oligospermic men, *Fertil Steril* 54:906, 1990.

99. **Kemmann E, Bohrer M, Shelden R, Fiasconaro G, Beardsley L,** Active ovulation management increases the monthly probability of pregnancy occurrence in ovulatory women who receive intrauterine insemination, *Fertil Steril* 48:916, 1987.

100. **Serhal PF, Katz M, Little V, Woronowski H,** Unexplained infertility — the value of pergonal superovulation combined with intrauterine insemination, *Fertil Steril* 49:602, 1988.

101. **Chaffkin LM, Nulsen JC, Luciano AA, Metzger DA,** A comparative analysis of the cycle fecundity rates associated with combined human menopausal gonadotropin (hMG) and intrauterine insemination (IUI) versus either hMG or IUI alone, *Fertil Steril* 55:252, 1991.

102. **Dodson WL, Haney AF,** Controlled ovarian hyperstimulation and intrauterine insemination for treatment of infertility, *Fertil Steril* 55:457, 1991.

103. **Centola GM, Mattox JH, Raubertas RF,** Pregnancy rates after double versus single insemination with frozen donor semen, *Fertil Steril* 54:1089, 1990.

104. **Silverberg KM, Johnson JV, Olive DL, Burns WN, Schenken RS,** A prospective, randomized trial comparing two different intrauterine insemination regimens in controlled ovarian hyperstimulation cycles, *Fertil Steril* 57:357, 1992.

105. **Ransom MX, Blotner MB, Bohrer M, Corsan G, Kemmann E,** Does increasing frequency of intrauterine insemination improve pregnancy rates significantly during ovulation induction cycles? *Fertil Steril* 61:303, 1994.

106. **Dodson WL, Walmer DK, Hughles Jr CL, Yancy SE, Haney AF,** Adjunctive leuprolide therapy does not improve cycle fecundity in controlled ovarian hyperstimulation and intrauterine insemination of subfertile women, *Obstet Gynecol* 78:187, 1991.

107. **Oei ML, Surrey ES, McCaleb B, Kerin JF,** A prospective, randomized study of pregnancy rates after transuterotubal and intrauterine insemination, *Fertil Steril* 58:167, 1992.

108. **Tournays H, Janssens R, Camus M, Staessen C, Devroey P, Van Steirteghem A,** Pentoxifylline is not useful in enhancing sperm function in cases with previous in vitro fertilization failure, *Fertil Steril* 59:210, 1993.

109. **McGuire M, Alexander NJ,** Artificial insemination of single women, *Fertil Steril* 43:182, 1985.

110. **Richter MA, Haning Jr RV, Shapiro SS,** Artificial donor insemination: fresh versus frozen semen: the patient as her own control, *Fertil Steril* 41:277, 1984.

111. **Subak LL, Adamson GD, Boltz NL,** Therapeutic donor insemination: a prospective randomized trial of fresh versus frozen sperm, *Am J Obstet Gynecol* 166:1597, 1992.

112. **Shenfield F, Doyle P, Valentine A, Steele SJ, Tan S-L,** Effects of age, gravidity and male infertility status on cumulative conception rates following artificial insemination with cryopreserved donor semen: analysis of 2998 cycles of treatment in one centre over 10 years, *Hum Reprod* 8:60, 1993.

113. **Semprini AE, Levi-Setti P, Bozzo M, Ravizza M, Tagliorettie A, Sulpizio P, Albani E, Oneta M, Pardi G,** Insemination of HIV-negative women with processed semen of HIV-positive partners, *Lancet* 340:1317, 1992.

114. **Amuzu B, Laxova R, Shapiro SS,** Pregnancy outcome, health of children, and family adjustment after donor insemination, *Obstet Gynecol* 75:899, 1990.

115. **Byrd W, Edman C, Bradshaw K, Odom J, Carr B, Ackerman G,** A prospective randomized study of pregnancy rates following intrauterine and intracervical insemination using frozen donor sperm, *Fertil Steril* 53:521, 1990.

116. **Hurd WW, Menge AC, Randolph Jr JF, Ohl DA, Ansbacher R, Brown AN,** Comparison of intracervical, intrauterine, and intratubal techniques for donor insemination, *Fertil Steril* 59:339, 1993.

117. **Tur R, Buxaderas C, Martinez F, Busquets A, Coroleu B, Barri PN,** Comparison of the role of cervical and intrauterine insemination techniques on the incidence of multiple pregnancy after artifical insemination with donor sperm, *J Assist Reprod Genet* 14:250, 1997.

118. **Deary AJ, Seaton JEV, Prentice A, Morton NC, Booth AK, Smith SK,** Single versus double insemination: a retrospective audit of pregnancy rates with two treatment protocols in donor insemination, *Hum Reprod* 12:1494, 1997.

119. **Palermo G, Joris H, Devroey P, Van Steirteghem AC,** Pregnancies after intracytoplasmic injection of a single spermatozoon into an oocyte, *Lancet* 340:17, 1992.

120. **Van Steirteghem AC, Nagy Z, Joris H, Liu J, Staessen C, Smitz J, Wisanto A, Devroey P,** High fertilization and implantation rates after intracytoplasmic sperm injection, *Hum Reprod* 8:1061, 1993.

121. **Nagy ZP, Liu J, Joris H, Verheyen G, Tournage H, Camus M, Derde MC, Devroey P, Van Steirteghem AC,** The result of intracytoplasmic sperm injection is not related to any of the three basic sperm parameters, *Hum Reprod* 10:1123, 1995.

122. **Hauser R, Temple-Smith PD, Southwick G, de Kretser DM,** Fertility in cases of hypergonadotrophic azoospermia, *Fertil Steril* 63:631, 1995.

123. **Antinori S, Versaci C, Dani G, Antinori M, Pozza D, Selman HA,** Fertilization with human testicular spermatids: four sucessful pregnancies, *Hum Reprod* 12:286, 1997.

124. **Watkins W, Nieto F, Bourne H, Wutthiphan B, Speirs A, Gordon Baker HW,** Testicular and epididymal sperm in a microinjection program: methods of retrieval and results, *Fertil Steril* 67:527, 1997.

30 Induction of Ovulation

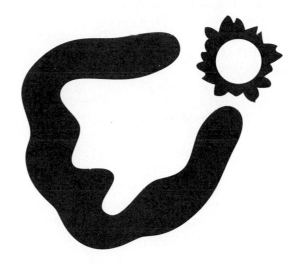

In previous editions of this book, we began this chapter with a statement in celebration of one of the greatest achievements of reproductive endocrinology, the ability to induce ovulation and attain pregnancy in women who in the past had little basis or hope for reversal of their ovulatory dysfunction. As we approach a half century of ovulation induction for infertility, this elation remains justified. A variety of logical strategies, often empirically defined, designed to respond to specific indications do yield excellent results. In many clinical circumstances accurate data confirm the theoretical expectation that treatment can result in pregnancy rates equivalent to those in the normal population.

As the field has matured, however, the initial exuberance has been tempered by the realities of objective review. Results of treatment, despite restriction to a single indication, are not uniform. Complications occur, and escalation to more costly and hazardous treatments is a common occurrence. Perhaps most concerning is the vexingly persistent disparity between rates of successful ovulation (high) and pregnancy (relatively low). This paradox presents two challenges.

1. The informed consent dialogue with the infertile couple does not conclude with the initial outline of strategic options. Helping the couple deal with the frustration of repeated partial success but persistent ultimate failure requires special time, sensitivity, and compassion.

2. The disparity between ovulation and pregnancy rates is an emphatic reminder for the clinician of the imprecision of the diagnosis, "ovulatory dysfunction and/or failure," the inadequacy of the available tests to determine if induction of ovulation has actually occurred, and the existence of more basic inherent defects in the reproductive process not disclosed by our current thorough work up or simply not discovered.

These considerations are all the more reason for the clinician to understand thoroughly the various indications and the many options available for induction of ovulation. This chapter will review the principles which guide the use of clomiphene, human menopausal gonadotropins, purified follicle-stimulating hormone (FSH), recombinant FSH, bromocriptine, and gonadotropin-releasing hormone (GnRH), and consider the results and complications of the medical induction of ovulation. In addition, laparoscopic ovarian surgical procedures (modified wedge resection) and the impact of GnRH agonist therapy will be reviewed.

Despite the specificity of the therapy and the promise of successful results, it is incumbent upon the practitioner to perform the appropriate medical evaluation to ensure that a contraindication to therapy is not overlooked. The reader is referred to Chapter 12 and Chapter 13 for a consideration of anovulation and hirsutism, and Chapter 11 for the evaluation of amenorrhea and galactorrhea.

For reference purposes, we provide the following definitions of ovulatory deficiencies according to the World Health Organization.

Group I: Hypothalamic-Pituitary Failure

This classfication includes patients diagnosed as hypothalamic amenorrhea, and includes stress-related amenorrhea, anorexia nervosa and its variants, Kallmann's syndrome, and isolated gonadotropin deficiency. These patients display hypogonadotropic hypogonadism with low gonadotropin and estrogen levels, normal prolactin concentrations, and a failure to bleed after the administration of a progestational agent (the progestational challenge).

Group II: Hypothalamic-Pituitary Dysfunction

This classification includes normogonadotropic, normoestrogenic, anovulatory, oligoamenorrheic women. The classic anovulatory polycystic ovary syndrome is in this category.

Group III: Ovarian Failure

Patients in this classification are hypergonadotropic hypogonadal individuals with low estrogen levels. All variants of ovarian failure and ovarian resistance are in this category.

For the purposes of this chapter, as well as the expression of our clinical philosophy, hyper-prolactinemic ovulatory dysfunction is treated as a specific treatment entity.

Induction of Ovulation With Clomiphene Citrate

Clomiphene citrate was first synthesized in 1956, introduced for clinical trials in 1960, and approved for clinical use in the United States in 1967.[1, 2] Clomiphene citrate is an orally active nonsteroidal agent distantly related to diethylstilbestrol. Clomiphene is a racemic mixture of its 2 stereochemical isomers, originally described as the cis and trans isomers. This designation is now recognized to have been inaccurate, and the isomers have been relabeled as zuclomiphene and enclomiphene citrate.[3] Clomiphene is available in 50 mg tablets, which contain 38% of the more active zuclomiphene form.

The similarity of clomiphene's structure to an estrogenic substance is the clue to its mechanism of action. Clomiphene exerts only a very weak biologic estrogenic effect. The structural similarity to estrogen is sufficient to achieve uptake and binding by estrogen receptors; however, there are several important different characteristics.[4, 5] Perhaps most importantly, clomiphene occupies the nuclear receptor for long periods of time, for weeks rather than hours. Clomiphene modifies hypothalamic activity by affecting the concentration of the intracellular estrogen receptors. Specifically, the concentration of estrogen receptors is reduced by inhibition of the process of receptor replenishment.

When exposed to clomiphene, the hypothalamic-pituitary axis is blind to the endogenous estrogen level in the circulation. Because receptor capacity is reduced and the true estrogen signal falsely lowered, negative feedback is diminished and the neuroendocrine mechanism for GnRH secretion is activated. When clomiphene is administered to normally cycling women, FSH and luteinizing hormone (LH) pulse frequency (but not amplitude) is increased, suggesting an

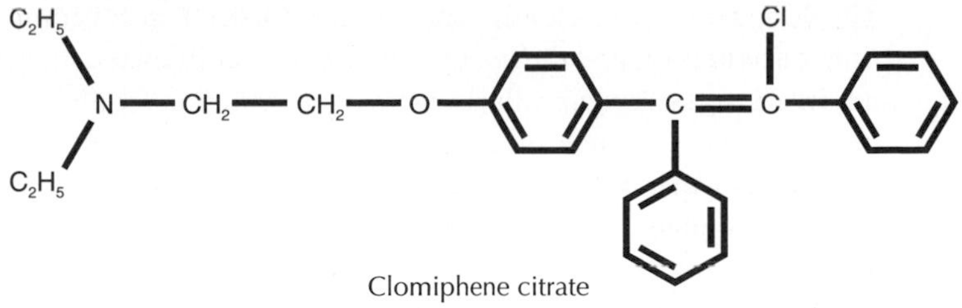

Clomiphene citrate

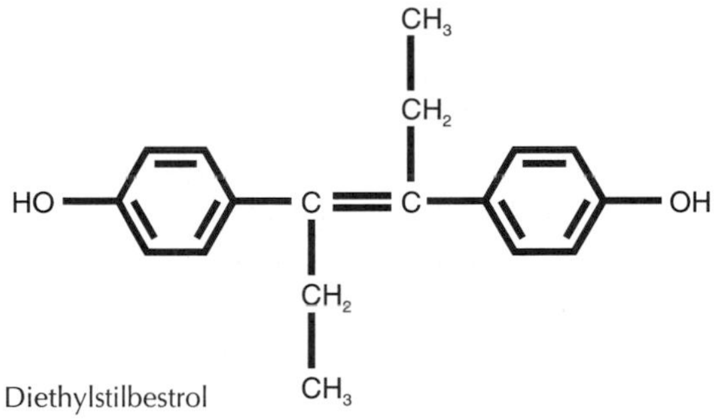

Diethylstilbestrol

increase in GnRH pulse frequency.[6] Anovulatory women, however, respond in a different fashion. Clomiphene stimulates an increase in gonadotropin pulse amplitude, presumably because GnRH pulses are already operating at maximal frequency in anovulatory women with polycystic ovaries.[7] Nevertheless, the experimental data indicate that the primary site of action is the hypothalamus.

During clomiphene administration, circulating levels of FSH and LH rise. The subsequent ovulation that occurs after clomiphene therapy is a manifestation of the hormone and morphologic changes produced by the growing follicles. Clomiphene therapy does not directly stimulate ovulation, but it retrieves and magnifies the sequence of events that are the physiologic features of a normal cycle. The effectiveness of the drug, however, may not be restricted to its ability to cause an appropriate GnRH discharge.

In animal models, clomiphene exerts an estrogenic effect on the pituitary and directly stimulates gonadotropin release, independent of its action on GnRH.[5] In the presence of estrogen, clomiphene influences pituitary response to GnRH in women, preferentially promoting FSH secretion.[8] In addition, clomiphene exerts a direct ovarian effect. In the absence of estrogen, clomiphene is an estrogen agonist, directly enhancing FSH stimulation of LH receptors in granulosa cells.[9] In an important contrast, in the uterus, cervix, and vagina, clomiphene acts primarily as an antiestrogen. Thus vaginal cornification is attenuated, and the effect of estrogen on cervical mucus and endometrium is antagonized, potentially important actions affecting implantation, sperm transport, and early embryonic development.[10] However, no significant effects on luteal phase endometrial morphology could be detected when clomiphene was administered to normal women.[11] Nor could a detrimental impact on cervical mucus be documented in either anovulatory or normal women.[12] In addition, the administration of clomiphene failed to affect endometrial concentrations of estrogen and progesterone receptors in normal ovulatory women.[13] These latter observations indicate that the potential antiestrogenic, adverse effects of clomiphene do not appear when clomiphene is used clinically.

Clomiphene has no progestational, corticotropic, androgenic, or antiandrogenic effects. Clomiphene does not interfere with adrenal or thyroid function. Although the pharmacologic effect of the drug is brief, only 51% of the oral dose is excreted after 5 days, and radioactivity from labeled clomiphene appears in the feces up to 6 weeks after administration. Significant plasma concentrations of the active zu isomer can be detected up to 1 month after treatment with a single dose of 50 mg.[14]

This long half-life of clomiphene presents theoretical concern. The presence of clomiphene at the time of ovulation and during the luteal phase could have unwanted effects. In vitro, clomiphene inhibits progesterone production by luteal granulosa cells in a fashion that suggests that clomiphene in the presence of estrogen, by virtue of its antiestrogenic action, interferes with the induction of LH receptors.[15] Because this inhibition is reversed by human chorionic gonadotropin (HCG), pregnancy and the appearance of HCG may prevent this unwelcome effect.

In rats and rabbits, a dose-dependent increase in the incidence of fetal malformations is seen when clomiphene is given during the period of organogenesis. Clomiphene has been found to cause disruptions of the organization of the uterine mesenchyme and tubal epithelium in human fetal reproductive tissue transplanted to athymic nude mice.[16] Extremely high doses inhibit fetal development. In these experiments, exposure took place at later periods of gestation than those associated with clomiphene exposure when the drug is taken for the induction of ovulation. Although clomiphene therapy should be withheld if there is any possibility of pregnancy, there is no good evidence that clomiphene is teratogenic in humans.[17–19] Furthermore, infant survival and performance after delivery are normal.

Selection of Patients for Clomiphene Treatment

Absent or infrequent ovulation is the chief indication for clomiphene therapy. It is the clinician's responsibility to rule out disorders of pituitary, adrenal, and thyroid origin requiring specific treatment before initiating clomiphene therapy. A complete history and physical examination are mandatory, but only a minimum of laboratory procedures is necessary. Liver function evaluation should precede clomiphene therapy if history and physical examination findings suggest liver disease. The vast majority of patients are healthy women suffering only from infertility secondary to oligoovulation or anovulation.

If periods are infrequent, it is not absolutely necessary to document infrequent or absent ovulation by basal body temperature records or endometrial biopsy. An endometrial biopsy is a wise precaution in a patient who has been anovulatory for a long period of time because of the tendency for these patients to develop hyperplasia and even carcinoma of the endometrium. It is also wise to precede therapy with an evaluation of the semen, to avoid an unnecessary waste of time and effort in the presence of azoospermia. A dedicated effort must be made to detect galactorrhea, and the prolactin level must be measured. Galactorrhea or hyperprolactinemia dictate a different therapeutic approach: dopamine agonist treatment. The remainder of the infertility workup in a patient with no previous medical or surgical problems is deferred until after a trial of clomiphene therapy. Because approximately 75% of pregnancies occur during the first 3 treatment cycles, the infertility workup is pursued only after the patient has responded with 3 months of ovulatory cycles and has not become pregnant.[20] This is appropriate because clomiphene is simple, safe, and cost-effective.

Cases of ovarian failure are unresponsive to any form of ovulation induction. Therefore, the presence of ovarian tissue capable of responding to gonadotropins must be documented. This is only a problem in the patient with amenorrhea, since the presence of menstrual bleeding confirms the function (although perhaps limited) of the hypothalamic-pituitary-ovarian axis. The patient with amenorrhea who fails to produce a withdrawal bleed after a course of a progestational agent (medroxyprogesterone acetate, 10 mg daily for 5 days) must be further evaluated (Chapter 11). A case has been made by others for the usefulness of an ovarian biopsy, perhaps via the laparoscope, to establish the presence of competent ovarian tissue. It is our practice, however, to rely on the immunoassay of gonadotropin levels and the response to a progestin, thus avoiding unnecessary surgical and anesthetic risks, to accurately rule out hypergonadotropic hypogonadism (ovarian failure). Attempts at medical induction of ovulation in these patients would be a waste of time and money.

The patients most likely to respond to clomiphene display some evidence of pituitary-ovarian activity as expressed in the biologic presence of estrogen (spontaneous or withdrawal menstrual bleeding). These are anovulatory women who have gonadotropin and estrogen production, but do not cycle, or women with inadequate luteal phases.

If the mechanism of an inadequate corpus luteum is inadequate FSH stimulation during the follicular phase, it makes sense to treat this condition with clomiphene, and a good response has been observed by ourselves and others.[21] Two randomized trials comparing clomiphene to progesterone treatment for inadequate luteal phases demonstrated equal pregnancy rates with each treatment.[22, 23] Clomiphene does not prolong the luteal phase (as progesterone supplementation does). This is an important advantage, avoiding the anxiety and heightened monthly emotional response of infertile couples.

The patient who is deficient in gonadotropin secretion and, as a result, is hypoestrogenic, cannot be expected to respond to further lowering of the estrogen signal and thus should not respond to clomiphene. However, this principle is not completely applicable to clinical practice. An occasional patient who is, by all criteria, hypoestrogenic will respond. Therefore, any otherwise medically uncomplicated patient with infertility secondary to lack of ovulation is a candidate for clomiphene therapy unless galactorrhea or hyperprolactinemia is present. Hypoestrogenic women respond so rarely, however, that it is appropriate to omit treatment with clomiphene and move to other more productive options.

In addition to anovulation, treatment with clomiphene is indicated to improve the timing and frequency of ovulation and to enhance the possibilities of conception in the patient who ovulates only occasionally. Clomiphene can also be used to regulate the timing of ovulation in women undergoing insemination.

There is one special group in whom clomiphene is indicated in women who ovulate regularly and spontaneously. Certain religious requirements, such as those in Orthodox Judaism, interfere with the normal reproductive process. In the devout Orthodox Jewish couple, intercourse is prohibited in the presence of menstrual flow and for 7 days following its conclusion. In some women menstrual flow is prolonged or the follicular phase is shortened, so that coitus cannot take place until after ovulation. In the usual mode of treatment, medication is begun on day 5 of the cycle. Ovulation can be delayed to a more appropriate time by starting clomiphene later, usually on day 7 or 8 of the cycle. Ovulation can be expected in the interval 5–10 days after the last day of medication. This manipulation has its limitations. Administration too late in the cycle, beyond day 9, may have no effect.

The question is often asked whether the indications for clomiphene therapy should be extended to include the initiation of cyclicity in the oligoamenorrheic patient who does not seek fertility. In our opinion, this is an inappropriate use of clomiphene for several reasons: 1) the effectiveness of clomiphene is restricted to the cycle in which it is used and it should not be expected to induce cyclicity following the conclusion of treatment, 2) the use of clomiphene may aggravate the clinical problems of acne and hirsutism during the treatment cycle by increasing LH stimulation of ovarian steroid production, and 3) the inability to induce cyclicity can be so discouraging to the patient that her acceptance of the drug will be impaired at some future date when it is legitimately offered as a fertility agent for the induction of ovulation.

Clomiphene and Unexplained Infertility

Clomiphene is used for the treatment of unexplained infertility; i.e., women who have prolonged (more than 3 years) infertility but who ovulate spontaneously and repeatedly by all available measures and do not have other abnormalities. While the spontaneous pregnancy rate is high in these patients (cumulative rates approach 50%), patient pressure and physician enthusiasm have led to superovulation induction in these couples. The rationale is appealingly clear. With more than one ovulation, surely there is an increased probability of successful fertilization, and such therapy would reverse (if present) episodic, unpredictable, recurrent, occult ovulatory dysfunction. Despite the high spontaneous pregnancy rate, clomiphene does have value in the empiric treatment of unexplained infertility, particularly prior to undertaking the more expensive and more complicated assisted reproductive technologies. In some studies, but not all, treatment with clomiphene has been associated with higher pregnancy rates. Superovulation for unexplained infertility is discussed in greater detail at the end of this chapter.

How to Use Clomiphene

A program of clomiphene therapy is begun on the 5th day of a cycle following either spontaneous or induced bleeding. It has not been established that a progestin withdrawal bleed is necessary before starting clomiphene treatment; we often omit this step if we are certain that the patient is not pregnant. The initial dose is 50 mg daily for 5 days. There is no advantage to beginning with a higher dose for the following two reasons: 1) in a random distribution of our patients begun with initial doses of either 50 mg or 100 mg daily, the pregnancy rate was identical; and 2) the highest incidence of side effects in our experience occurs at the 50 mg dose, and beginning with 100 mg, patients may develop more serious reactions. About 50% of patients conceive at the 50 mg dose, and another 20% at 100 mg.[20, 24] An occasional patient will be exceptionally sensitive to clomiphene and can achieve pregnancy at the reduced dose of 25 mg.

Beginning clomiphene on the 5th day is a method arrived at empirically; however, we can now offer a rational explanation based on ovarian physiology. The clomiphene-induced increase in gonadotropins during days 5–9 occurs at a time when the dominant follicle is being selected. Beginning clomiphene earlier can be expected to stimulate multiple follicular maturation resulting in a greater incidence of multiple gestation. Indeed, clomiphene is administered earlier in in vitro fertilization programs in order to obtain more than one oocyte. However, in standard ovulation induction protocols, no differences have been observed in the rates of ovulation, pregnancy, or spontaneous miscarriage whether clomiphene was started on day 2, 3, 4, or 5.[25]

If ovulation is not achieved in the very first cycle of treatment, dosage is increased to 100 mg. Thereafter, if ovulation and a normal luteal phase are not achieved in any cycle, dosage is increased in a staircase fashion by 50 mg increments to a maximum of 200–250 mg daily for 5 days. The highest dose is pursued for 3–4 months before considering the patient to be a clomiphene failure. The quantity of drug and the number of cycles go beyond those recommended by manufacturers. However, in our experience those recommendations are inappropriately limiting. We have achieved a 15% pregnancy rate at the 150 mg and 200 mg dose levels.[20]

There is a significant correlation between body weight and the dose of clomiphene required for ovulation.[26–28] One must adhere to the usual regimen, however, because the weight cannot be used to predict prospectively the correct ovulatory dose. In other words, some obese women ovulate at the same low dose that achieves ovulation in thin women. Clomiphene is not stored in adipose tissue, and the increased dose often necessary in obese women is more likely due to a more intense anovulatory state with higher androgen levels producing a more resistant hypothalamic-pituitary-ovarian axis. Increasing the dose of clomiphene will eventually achieve the same level of success in overweight women as can be attained in lean women.[29, 30]

At the present time there is no clinical or laboratory parameter that can predict the dose of clomiphene necessary to achieve ovulation. Androgen and estrogen levels do not show any correlation with the dose of clomiphene that proves successful.[31]

Following the 5-day course of clomiphene, the ovulatory surge of gonadotropins can occur anywhere from 5 to 12 days after the last day of clomiphene administration, but most commonly on cycle day 16 or 17 when clomiphene is administered on days 5–9.[32] Once ovulation is established, the subsequent treatment cycles are uniformly consistent. The patient is advised to

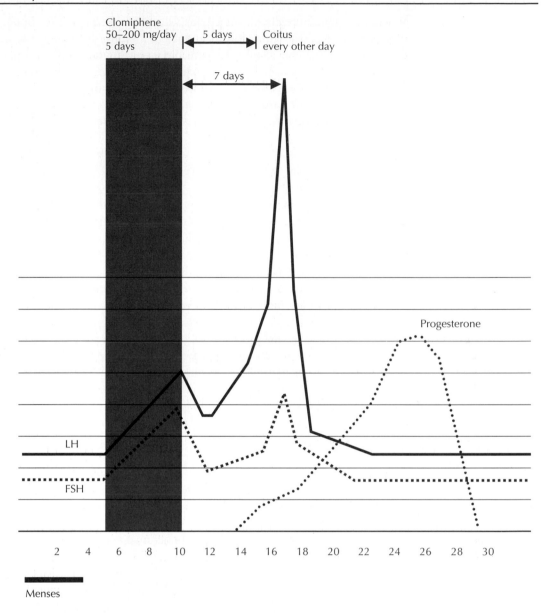

Clomiphene
50–200 mg/day
5 days

5 days

Coitus
every other day

7 days

Progesterone

LH

FSH

2   4   6   8   10   12   14   16   18   20   22   24   26   28   30

Menses

have intercourse every other day for 1 week beginning 5 days after the last day of medication. In view of the role prostaglandins play in the physical expulsion of an oocyte, it is prudent to advise patients involved in programs of ovulation induction to avoid the use of agents that inhibit prostaglandin synthesis.

After the first treatment cycle the patient is evaluated for side effects, residual ovarian enlargement, and basal body temperature changes. We have found it unnecessary to perform a pelvic examination every month because significant ovarian enlargement is encountered infrequently, and it is usually symptomatic. It is more economical, for both patient and clinician, to mail the temperature chart to the office and several days later plan by telephone for the following month. Cysts within a reasonable size range (3–5 cm) do not require a rest from treatment; they do not respond to further stimulation, and they do not impact upon subsequent response.

We recommend basal body temperature charting to follow the response. If an inadequate luteal phase is evident, (temperature elevation less than 11 days duration) the amount of clomiphene is increased to the next dose level. If the patient is already at the maximal level, consider the available options for dealing with clomiphene failure (detailed below). Biphasic changes are taken as an indication of ovulation and success. Maintenance of the temperature elevation beyond the expected time of menses is the earliest practical indication of pregnancy.

When the temperature chart is inconclusive or when the patient is not pregnant despite a period of apparently normal ovulations, an endometrial biopsy is indicated to document the adequacy of the luteal phase. One should also consider ultrasonographic monitoring for treatment failures, looking for follicles which do not reach mature size or the luteinized unruptured follicle syndrome (although it is by no means certain that luteinized unruptured follicles are a factor in infertility). ***For most patients, adding ultrasonography and urinary LH testing to basal body temperature charting does not improve pregnancy rates.***[33]

The additional use of HCG is limited to those cases in which there is a failure to ovulate at the maximal dose level or, when at that level, a short luteal phase is demonstrated. The rationale is to improve on the midcycle LH surge; therefore, 10,000 IU of HCG can be given as a single intramuscular dose on the 7th day after clomiphene when follicular maturation is at its peak. Because premature HCG administration may interfere with normal ovulation by down-regulating LH receptors, more accurate timing of HCG administration may be desirable. This requires either measurement of the blood estradiol level or estimation of follicular size (18–20 mm diameter) by sonography. When HCG is administered, intercourse is advised for that night and for the next 2 days. ***In our experience as well as in others reported in the literature, the addition of HCG has not had a significant impact on the pregnancy rate.***[34]

Care should be taken to review with the patient the pathophysiology of her condition, the principles of treatment, the prolonged course of therapy that may be necessary, and possible complications. Repeated failures accumulate frustration and despair in the couple, making each successive cycle of treatment more difficult. The anxiety and stress may hinder coital performance, and it is not uncommon for a couple to have difficulty performing scheduled intercourse.

Results With Clomiphene

In properly selected patients, 80% can be expected to ovulate, and approximately 40% become pregnant.[20, 24] The percent of pregnancies per induced ovulatory cycle is about 20–25%. The multiple pregnancy rate is approximately 10%, almost entirely twins.[35] There have been rare cases of quintuplet and sextuplet births. In our own experience, with standardization of therapy, the incidence of twins has decreased.

The miscarriage rate is not increased.[19, 36] Most importantly, the incidence of congenital malformations is not increased, and infant survival and performance after delivery are no different from normal.[18, 19, 37]

The discrepancy between ovulation rates and pregnancy rates is mainly due to 2 factors, the presence of other causes of infertility and a lack of persistence. ***In those patients with no other cause of infertility, the cumulative 6-month conception rate approaches a normal rate of 60–75%.***[24, 31, 35] The pregnancy rate per ovulatory cycle equals the normal rate. The pregnancy rate in 70 of our patients who received therapy sufficient to ovulate in at least 3 cycles was 55.7%, the same pregnancy rate after 3 months of exposure in the general population.[20] With additional treatment cycles, the pregnancy rate decreases, although the ovulatory rate remains high. Approximately 15% of patients treated with the higher doses of 150–250 mg will become pregnant.[20] Therefore there may be no need to attribute negative effects of clomiphene on oocyte, endometrium, the corpus luteum, and an early embryo.

If all factors are corrected, and conception has not occurred in 6 months, prognosis is poor. In one large series, only 7.8% of those who had one or more infertility factors in addition to anovulation became pregnant.[24]

Complications With Clomiphene

Side effects do not appear to be dose related, occurring more frequently at the 50 mg dose. Patients requiring the high doses are probably less sensitive to the drug. The most common problems are vasomotor flushes (10%), abdominal distension, bloating, pain, or soreness (5.5%), breast discomfort (2%), nausea and vomiting (2.2%), visual symptoms (1.5%), headache (1.3%), and dryness or loss of hair (0.3%). Patients who are extremely sensitive to the side effects of clomiphene can be successfully treated with half a tablet (25 mg) daily for 5 days, and even with half a tablet daily for 3 days.

A common antiestrogenic effect is an increase in the basal body temperature during the 5-day period of clomiphene administration. This is sometimes incorrectly interpreted as evidence of an early ovulation.

Visual symptoms include blurring vision, scotoma (visual spots or flashes), or abnormal perception. The cause of these symptoms is unknown, but in almost all cases, the visual symptoms have disappeared upon discontinuation of the medication. Usually these symptoms disappear within a few days but may take 1 or 2 weeks. There is one report of 3 women who had a persistence of visual side effects (shimmering, afterimages, and photophobia) after discontinuing treatment.[38] It is likely that this problem is increased with increasing dosage and duration of exposure. Persistence of treatment in the presence of this reaction is not recommended.

Significant ovarian enlargement is associated with longer periods of treatment and is infrequent (5%) with the usual 5-day course. Maximal enlargement of the ovary usually occurs several days after discontinuing the clomiphene (in response to the increase in gonadotropins). If the patient is symptomatic, pelvic examination, intercourse, and undue physical exercise should be avoided because the enlarged ovaries are very fragile. Ovarian enlargement dissipates rapidly and only rarely is a subsequent treatment cycle delayed.

Because of multiple ovulations in some patients, it is possible that the risk of ectopic pregnancy is increased. However, evidence in the literature indicates that this increase at most is only slight.[2, 19]

What to Do With Clomiphene Failures

Patients most likely to not respond to clomiphene are those who are most hyperandrogenic and overweight (and probably insulin resistant).[39] There are several options available for the 10–20% of women who fail to become pregnant with clomiphene up to the highest dose. Knowledge gained from experience with in vitro fertilization provides us with several explanations for failure to respond to clomiphene.[31] These include the effects of excessive LH in the follicular phase, the dysfunctional effects of an untimely LH surge, excess local concentrations of androgens, and hyperinsulinemia. These mechanisms may yield impaired folliculogenesis, increased atresia, poor oocyte quality, precocious or impaired oocyte maturation, low fertilization rates, variable implantation rates, and deficient corpus luteum function. Strategies have developed to mitigate or avoid many of these detrimental effects: the treatment of hyperinsulinemia, the supplemental use of dexamethasone (to reduce androgen burden), GnRH agonists (to eliminate endogenous LH intrusion), pulsatile GnRH therapy (to preserve physiologic interactive feedback mechanisms), and, finally, the use of human gonadotropins. We are also seeing the return of modified ovarian wedge resection by laparoscopic multiple ovarian tissue destruction with cautery or laser techniques.

First, make sure galactorrhea has not been overlooked and a prolactin level has been obtained. The good results with dopamine agonist treatment make it essential that this cause of anovulation be detected. It is worth performing a postcoital test to assess the quality of the cervical mucus. Despite the antiestrogen action of clomiphene the incidence of poor cervical mucus on the postcoital test is only 15%.[24] In the past, estrogen (0.625 to 2.5 mg conjugated estrogens daily) was administered from day 10 to day 16 (for 1 week starting the day after the last day of clomiphene administration) in an effort to improve mucus production. Although high doses of estrogen do not interfere with the gonadotropin response, ovulation, or the pregnancy rate, there is reason to believe that estrogen treatment is ineffective.[40, 41] Another alternative, the one we prefer, is to proceed with intrauterine inseminations of prepared sperm, bypassing the cervix.

After 6 months of clomiphene therapy, and in the absence of any other infertility factors, we proceed to one of the available options.

Treatment of Hyperinsulinemia

Anovulatory women with polycystic ovaries and hyperinsulinemia are more resistant to clomiphene treatment. The best therapy for these women who are obese is weight loss. Both the hyperinsulinemia and the hyperandrogenism can be reduced with weight loss, which is at least more than 5% of the initial weight.[42–47] These metabolic improvements are associated with an impressive rate of resumption of ovulation and pregnancy.[48, 49] In one study, 60 of 67 anovulatory women, who lost from 4 to 15 kg, resumed ovulation.[50] A goal for weight loss that correlates with a good chance of achieving pregnancy, a reduction in insulin levels, and a decrease in free testosterone levels is a body mass index of less than 27 (see the nomogram for calculating body mass index in Chapter 19). It should be emphasized, that only a relatively small percentage of weight (5–10%) need be lost to have a beneficial impact upon insulin resistance and cardiovascular hemodynamic function.[51]

It is reasonable to assume that all overweight, anovulatory women with polycystic ovaries are hyperinsulinemic. Nevertheless we recommend the measurement of the ratio of fasting glucose to fasting insulin in order to provide evidence that lends credence and importance to counseling efforts. *A ratio of less than 4.5 is consistent with insulin resistance.*[52]

All anovulatory women who are hyperandrogenic should be assessed for insulin resistance and glucose tolerance with measurements of:

1.   **The fasting glucose:insulin ratio, followed by**

2.   **The 2-hour glucose level after a 75 g glucose load:**
normal	— **less than 140 mg/dL**
impaired	— **140–199 mg/dL**
noninsulin-dependent diabetes mellitus	— **200 mg/dL and higher**

The best application of drugs, such as metformin and troglitazone, remains to be determined by data from appropriate clinical trials. Metformin improves insulin sensitivity, but the primary effect is a significant reduction in gluconeogenesis, thus decreasing hepatic glucose production. Metformin treatment (500 mg tid) reduces hyperinsulinemia, basal and stimulated LH levels, and free testosterone concentrations in overweight women with polycystic ovaries.[53–55] A significant number of these anovulatory women treated with metformin ovulate and achieve pregnancy.[56, 57] In a group of obese women with polycystic ovaries, 90% of the women treated with metformin and 50 mg clomiphene ovulated compared with 8% in the group treated with placebo and clomiphene.[58] However, there has been controversy, suggesting that the improvement was the result of the weight loss that often accompanies the use of metformin.[59] In a study designed to control the effect of body weight, the administration of metformin was without effect on insulin resistance in extremely overweight women with polycystic ovaries.[60] In another well-designed study, metformin again had no effect on insulin resistance when body weights remained unchanged, and in this study baseline weights and hyperinsulinemia were only modestly increased.[61] In lean, anovulatory women with hyperinsulinemia, metformin treatment reduced hyperandrogenemia although there was no change in body weight; however, a decrease in the waist to hip ratio accompanied a reduction in the hyperinsulinemia.[62] This study indicates that both obese and nonobese patients with hyperinsulinemia respond to metformin treatment. The reasons for the differences among the studies is not apparent. Perhaps only certain patients will respond to metformin, and, thus, patient selection could influence the reported results. Lactic acidosis is a rare complication in patients treated with metformin; however, virtually all cases have occurred in patients with complicated medical problems, such as sepsis, renal insufficiency, and congestive heart failure. Patients who become ill should discontinue metformin treatment, and metformin should not be administered to women who have abnormal renal chemistries.

The thiazolidinediones markedly improve insulin sensitivity and insulin secretion (improved peripheral glucose utilization and β-cell function) without weight changes. Troglitazone (400 mg daily) decreases hyperinsulinemia, and improvements in metabolic abnormalities (decreased androgens, increased SHBG, decreased PAI 1 consistent with improved fibrinolytic capacity, and decreased LH), and a return to ovulation in very obese women have been reported with this agent.[63, 64] Although changes are uncommon, liver function must be monitored during troglitazone treatment. The pharmaceutical company's package information should be consulted for the currently recommended monitoring regimen of serum alanine aminotransferase levels.

There is little doubt that these drugs can produce significant and beneficial improvements in this condition, although metformin may be effective only when weight loss occurs. However, is short-term use better than our standard methods of the induction of ovulation, and are these drugs safe during pregnancy and lactation? How effective are these agents in women who are of normal or only slightly elevated body weight? Appropriate clinical trials are required to answer these questions. In the meantime, clinicians have offered treatment with these agents to patients who have failed to respond to clomiphene. If an ovulatory response does not occur within 3 months, clomiphene treatment, beginning again at the lowest dose, is resumed in addition to the drug therapy for hyperinsulinemia.

The Addition of Dexamethasone to Clomiphene

Patients with hirsutism and high circulating androgen concentrations are more resistant to clomiphene.[65–67] Dexamethasone, 0.5 mg at bedtime to blunt the nighttime peak of ACTH, is added to decrease the adrenal contribution to circulating androgens and, thus, diminish the androgen level in the microenvironment of the ovarian follicles. Higher ovulation and conception rates are achieved with this treatment when the circulating level of dehydroepiandrosterone sulfate (DHAS) is greater than the upper limit of normal. The dexamethasone is maintained daily until pregnancy is apparent. The dose of clomiphene is returned to the starting point of 50 mg and increased in incremental fashion as needed. One report indicated that even non-responders to clomiphene with normal DHAS levels achieved ovulation and pregnancy with the addition of a 10-day course of dexamethasone begun concurrently with clomiphene.[68]

Extended Clomiphene Treatment

Several approaches have been reported for extending clomiphene treatment. We have very little experience with extended clomiphene treatment. In one approach, 250 mg of clomiphene was given for 8 days, followed by 10,000 IU HCG 6 days later. Three pregnancies were achieved out of 25 treatment cycles.[69] In another series, the clomiphene dose was increased every 5 days, with some patients receiving up to 25 days of consecutive treatment, the last 5 days at 250 mg daily.[70] Eight of 21 patients conceived and, in those patients who responded, measurement of gonadotropin revealed sustained elevations in FSH. This latter approach requires estrogen monitoring with discontinuation of the clomiphene when an increase in estrogen is detected. No patient ovulated after more than 21 days of treatment. Extending a dose of 100 mg clomiphene to 10 days has been reported to achieve pregnancies in women previously resistant to a 5-day regimen.[71] A simple approach is to extend the duration of clomiphene treatment until a follicle of 18 mm diameter (on ultrasound) is obtained, then administer HCG.

Pretreatment Suppression

The anovulatory state is a dysfunctional condition. It is reasonable to expect suppression of the contributing factors to be followed by a reassertion of the harmony operating in a normal menstrual cycle, at least for a short time. Clinicians have long advocated (without benefit of careful study) a period of suppression (at least 6 months) with an oral contraceptive, followed immediately by resumption of clomiphene administration. The same principle applies to the use of a GnRH agonist. Spontaneous resumption of ovulation has been reported to follow suppression for 6 months with a combination of a GnRH agonist and an oral contraceptive.[72] Pretreatment suppression has an added attraction. There is reason to believe that women with elevated LH and testosterone levels not only have more difficulty achieving pregnancy, but also experience a higher spontaneous miscarriage rate.[73–75] However, an excellent, randomized trial, testing pituitary suppression in women with polycystic ovaries, elevated LH levels, and recurrent miscarriages, obtained equal and good live birth rates with gonadotropin treatment in both the GnRH agonist-suppressed group and the non-suppressed group.[76]

The Addition of Bromocriptine to Clomiphene

Although the use of bromocriptine to induce ovulation is indicated in the presence of galactorrhea or hyperprolactinemia, its use in the clomiphene failure patient with a normal prolactin and no galactorrhea is controversial. Anovulatory patients with normal levels of prolactin do respond to bromocriptine, but the effectiveness of this treatment has not been established by controlled studies. Nevertheless, the clinical response is occasionally impressive.

Bromocriptine. Elevated prolactin levels interfere with the normal function of the menstrual cycle by suppressing the pulsatile secretion of GnRH. This is manifested clinically by a spectrum, ranging from a subtle inadequate luteal phase to total suppression and hypoestrogenic amenorrhea. Regardless of the prolactin level, we interpret the presence of galactorrhea to indicate excessive prolactin stimulation. We screen all patients with galactorrhea or any ovulatory disorder with an assessment of the prolactin level. After a consideration of the problems of amenorrhea, galactorrhea, and the pituitary adenoma (as discussed in Chapter 11), bromocriptine emerges as the drug of choice for the induction of ovulation in these patients.

Ovulatory dysfunction in the presence of galactorrhea responds well to bromocriptine, even if the prolactin level is normal.[77] Either biologic activity is not being detected by the immunoassay or a random blood sample fails to reveal subtle elevations in prolactin.

Bromocriptine is examined in detail in Chapter 11, but it would be helpful to review pertinent details here. Bromocriptine is a dopamine agonist that directly inhibits pituitary secretion of prolactin. Suppression of prolactin levels restores CNS-pituitary gonadotropin function and also appears to increase ovarian responsiveness. The increase in ovarian responsiveness is seen in patients with normal prolactin levels and no galactorrhea. This is the apparent mechanism for an increase in sensitivity to clomiphene when bromocriptine is added to the therapeutic regimen. In women with persistent anovulation and polycystic ovaries, LH secretion is decreased by bromocriptine treatment, thus providing a rationale for why it might enhance the ovulatory response in these patients.[78]

The gastrointestinal and cardiovascular systems react to the dopaminergic action of bromocriptine, and, therefore, the side effects are mainly nausea, diarrhea, dizziness, headache, and fatigue. Side effects can be minimized by slowly building tolerance toward the usual dose, 2.5 mg bid. We start treatment with an initial dose of 2.5 mg at bedtime. If intolerance occurs, the tablet can be cut in half, and a slower program, developed by the patient, can be followed to work up to the standard dose. Usually, the second dose is added after 1 week, at breakfast or at lunch. In some patients, elevated prolactin levels can be reduced to normal levels with very small doses of bromocriptine, as little as 0.625 or 1.25 mg.[79] Patients extremely sensitive to the side effects of bromocriptine can be treated by administering the drug intravaginally. Usually one 2.5 mg tablet daily will be effective; if the prolactin level is elevated, the dose can be titrated to bring the prolactin level into the normal range.

The usual regimen is to administer bromocriptine daily until it is apparent the patient is pregnant, as usually determined by the basal body temperature chart. Although there has been no evidence of any harmful effects on the fetus, some patients and clinicians prefer to avoid bromocriptine in the luteal phase and, therefore, during early pregnancy. The drug is stopped when a temperature rise occurs and resumed when menses begin.

Ovulatory menses and pregnancy are achieved in 80% of patients with galactorrhea and hyperprolactinemia. Response is rapid, and, therefore, if there is no indication of ovulation (a rise in the basal body temperature) within 2 months, clomiphene is added to the regimen. The starting dose of clomiphene is 50 mg daily for 5 days, given and increased in the usual fashion.

Cabergoline is also an ergot-derived dopamine agonist.[80] Patients resistant to both bromocriptine and quinagolide have been reported to respond to cabergoline.[81] Cabergoline can be administered orally at doses of 0.5 to 3.0 mg only once weekly, although it can be given twice weekly if necessary, with minimal dopamine agonist side effects (headache being the most common complaint).[82–85] *The low rate of side effects and the once weekly dosage make cabergoline an attractive choice for initial treatment, replacing bromocriptine.* The only reservation (a small one) is a more limited experience documenting fetal safety for patients being treated for infertility.[86] Cabergoline can also be administered vaginally for the rare patient who cannot tolerate it orally.[87]

Bromocriptine for Euprolactinemic Women. Clinical experience suggests that successful induction of ovulation and achievement of pregnancy with bromocriptine can occur in the absence of galactorrhea and with a normal prolactin level in women who have failed to respond to clomiphene.[88] Some anovulatory women with normal prolactin levels who ovulated in response to bromocriptine have been found to have elevated nocturnal peaks of prolactin.[89] The mechanism of action may be an increase in follicular responsiveness either due to suppression of prolactin or suppression of LH (a known action of dopamine). A decrease in LH may alter local follicular steroidogenesis in such a way to create a more favorable microenvironment. The method of administration is the same as above. If, after 2 months of treatment, there is no response, clomiphene is reinitiated, working up again from the starting dose of 50 mg daily. A carefully designed study has demonstrated that bromocriptine has nothing to offer for ovulatory women with unexplained infertility.[90] On the other hand, bromocriptine or bromocriptine plus clomiphene treatment of ovulatory women with galactorrhea (and normal prolactin levels) yielded higher pregnancy rates when compared to a control group.[91] Once again the importance of detecting galactorrhea is emphasized.

Ovarian Surgical Procedures

The clomiphene-resistant patient can be treated by an ovarian surgical procedure. This subject is discussed near the end of this chapter.

Induction of Ovulation With Human Gonadotropins

For over 30 years, the only preparation used for gonadotropin treatment consisted of human menopausal gonadotropins, a preparation of gonadotropins extracted from the urine of postmenopausal women. The commercial preparation is still available, with either 75 units of FSH and 75 units of LH per ampule, or in an ampule with twice the amount, 150 units of each gonadotropin. Gonadotropins are inactive orally and, therefore, must be given parenterally; the heavy protein content of the urinary preparation requires intramuscular injections.

A more purified urinary preparation of FSH became available by removing most of the LH in the urinary product. This product still requires intramuscular injection. A more highly purified form is available that can be administered subcutaneously.

Recombinant FSH is now produced in Chinese hamster ovary cells transfected with the human FSH subunit genes.[92] Recombinant FSH is homogeneous and free of contamination by proteins (characteristic of menopausal gonadotropins from urinary extracts); this allows simpler subcutaneous administration.

Because of its structural and biologic similarity to LH, HCG, readily available from human pregnancy urine and placental tissue, is used to simulate the midcycle LH ovulatory surge.

Recombinant HCG and recombinant LH are now available. These preparations will allow patient self-administration by subcutaneous injections. It is unlikely that the results will be different; however, it is possible that the risk of ovarian hyperstimulation will be reduced.

PREPARATION	TRADE NAMES
Human menopausal gonadotropins	Pergonal, Humegon, Menogon, Repronex
Purified urinary FSH	Metrodin, Normegon, Orgafol
Highly purified urinary FSH	Fertinex or Metrodin HP
Recombinant FSH	Puregon, Gonal-F, Follistim
Human chorionic gonadotropin	Pregnyl, Profasi, A.P.L.
Recombinant HCG	Ovidrel
Recombinant LH	LHadi

Selection of Patients for Gonadotropin Treatment

Not only because of its expense but because of its greater complication rate, patients should not receive gonadotropin therapy without a very careful evaluation. An absolute requirement is the demonstration of ovarian competence. Abnormally high serum gonadotropins with a failure to demonstrate withdrawal bleeding indicate ovarian failure and preclude induction of ovulation except in those special cases of ovarian failure discussed in Chapter 11. Successful induction of ovulation and pregnancy has been reported in women with apparent ovarian failure, treated with a combination of estrogen (to suppress FSH to normal levels) and gonadotropins. Our own experience with this approach has been disappointing, and the chance of achieving pregnancy must be very low.

A thorough infertility investigation must be performed. In addition to the demonstration of ovarian competence, tubal and uterine pathology should be ruled out, anovulation documented, and semen analysis obtained. Nongynecologic endocrine problems must be treated. Hypo-gonadotropic function (low serum gonadotropins), including galactorrhea syndromes, requires evaluation for an intracranial lesion, with appropriate imaging and measurement of prolactin levels. It is imperative to take all steps necessary to exclude treatable pathology to which anovulation is secondary.

In our practice we sometimes, but not often, offer a course of clomiphene, not only because of the cost and complications associated with gonadotropin therapy, but also because some apparently hypogonadotropic patients will unpredictably respond to clomiphene. Because some patients cannot tolerate dopamine agonist treatment, it is important to know that hyperprolactinemia has no adverse effect on response to gonadotropins.[93]

How to Use Gonadotropin Therapy

Instruction and counseling of the couple are essential. A thorough understanding of the need for daily treatment and frequent observation is necessary prior to initiating therapy. As part of this instruction, the partner can be taught to administer injections. Daily recording of the basal body temperature and body weight is important for proper management. The couple should be told about the need for scheduled intercourse, the possibility that more than one course of treatment may be necessary, and the expense of the treatment. Above all, the patient must be prepared for the anguish that accompanies failure. Because this is a pressure-packed situation, unexpected impotence is occasionally encountered on the days of scheduled intercourse.

Although there is evidence indicating that recombinant FSH yields better results with in vitro fertilization, there is no clear-cut indication that better results are obtained with any of the gonadotropin preparations when used for ovulation induction.[94] Optimal results are dependent on the experience and judgement of the clinician, not on the preparation used. There is no doubt that some LH is necessary for normal ovarian steroidogenesis (see Chapter 6), and very low day 3 LH levels (less than 3 IU/L) have been reported to predict poor response to gonadotropin stimulation.[95] In this circumstance, perhaps a preparation containing some LH would be a better choice; for example, in patients with amenorrhea due to weight loss and anorexia.

A variable dosage method is used to achieve follicular growth and maturation. Follicle stimulation is achieved by 7–14 days of continuous gonadotropin, beginning with one ampule daily. Response is judged by the degree of estrogen produced by the growing follicles. The patient is monitored periodically with the measurement of the circulating estradiol level and vaginal ultrasound assessment of the number and size of follicles. The patient is seen on the 7th day of treatment, and a decision is made to continue or increase the dose (step up method). After the 7th day, the patient is seen anywhere from daily to every one or two days. Another approach, the step down method, starts with a higher dose (2–3 ampules) and reduces the dose to one ampule after the initial response, theoretically approximating the changes in FSH in a normal ovulatory cycle.

Patients with polycystic ovaries are handled more gingerly because they are more sensitive to gonadotropin stimulation, and, therefore, at greater risk for multiple pregnancy and the ovarian hyperstimulation syndrome. The increased sensitivity to FSH is apparently due to the availability of a larger cohort of small follicles ready to respond to FSH (recruitable follicles).[96] In these patients, monitoring begins on the 4th or 5th day of treatment. Excessive stimulation can be avoided in women with polycystic ovaries by using lower doses of gonadotropin extended over a longer duration of treatment.[97, 98] In addition, good results are inversely correlated with the degree of insulin resistance,[99] and consideration should be given to treatment that improves insulin sensitivity (see elsewhere in this chapter and Chapter 12).

It cannot be emphasized too strongly that dosage administration and the judicious use of estrogen measurements depend upon the experience of the clinician administering gonadotropin therapy. When estradiol and ultrasound monitoring indicate that the patient is ready to receive the ovulatory stimulus, 10,000 units of HCG are given as a single dose intramuscularly. Neither manipulation of HCG dosage nor time of administration has been successful in changing the rates of multiple gestation and hyperstimulation. The patient is advised to have intercourse the day of the HCG injection and for the next 2 days. In view of the fragility of hyperstimulated ovaries, further intercourse as well as strenuous physical exercise should be avoided.

Pregnancy is usually achieved with the administration of gonadotropins for 7–12 days. The best results are obtained when the treatment period covers 10–15 days; when less than 10 days, the spontaneous miscarriage rate is increased.[100] In general there is a direct relationship between dose and body weight; however, the same empiric approach is needed even in obese patients.[101] In some individuals, presumably with extremely hyposensitive ovaries, adequate follicular stimulation requires doses up to 4, 6, and more ampules/day. In this group of amenorrheic women massive doses of gonadotropins are necessary, and with proper monitoring, pregnancy can be achieved safely.

The range between the dose that does not induce ovulation and the dose that results in hyperstimulation is narrow. The situation is made even more difficult because the ovaries may react differently to essentially similar doses from month to month. Close supervision and experience in the use of gonadotropin therapy are necessary to avoid difficulties. There is no reason to avoid consecutive cycles of ovarian stimulation; indeed, an increased cycle fecundity has been observed in consecutive treatment cycles when compared to alternating stimulation and nontreatment.[102, 103]

Estrogen Monitoring

The use of estrogen measurements is necessary to choose the correct moment for administering the ovulatory dose of HCG in order to prevent hyperstimulation. On day 7 of the therapeutic cycle, blood is assayed for estradiol. Depending on the findings, the dosage of gonadotropin is individualized for the duration of the cycle. With experience, the clinician can avoid daily estrogen measurements, although sometimes this is necessary.

What should the blood estradiol level be? Because the blood estradiol is determined on a single sample of blood, the timing of the sampling with relationship to the previous injection of gonadotropin becomes a significant variable. When gonadotropin injections are given between 5 and 8 PM and blood samples are obtained first thing in the morning, an estradiol window of 1000–1500 pg/mL is optimal.[104] The risk of hyperstimulation is significant from 1500 to 2000 pg/mL and, as a general rule, over 2000 pg/mL, HCG should not be given, and the ovarian follicles should be allowed to regress. Careful correlation of estrogen levels with the ultrasonographic picture allows a more aggressive approach. Haning has calculated that an upper limit for estradiol of 3800 pg/mL for anovulatory women (with polycystic ovaries) and 2400 for women with hypothalamic amenorrhea gives a risk of severe hyperstimulation of 5% in pregnant cycles and 1% in nonconception cycles.[105]

Attempting to reproduce the normal midcycle levels of estradiol does not achieve a maximal pregnancy rate, and higher levels are required. The relative safety of this approach was seen in our series, where only 2 of 24 patients with estradiol levels over 1000 pg/mL developed hyperstimulation and it was moderate in both cases.[104] When a patient nears ovulation, timing of the HCG administration can be predicted fairly accurately by plotting the estradiol values on semilogarithmic paper. The rate of increase in estradiol is the same in spontaneous and induced cycles, and does not differ in cycles that result in multiple gestation.[106] The level which is reached at the time of HCG administration is more critical than the slope of increase. Once a linear rise of estradiol is established, there is no need to increase the dose.

Ultrasound Monitoring

Ultrasound assessment of the growth and development of the ovarian follicle indicates the degree of follicular maturity and capability.[107] During normal cycles, the growing cohort of follicles can be first identified by ultrasonography on days 5 to 7 as small sonolucent cysts. The dominant follicle will become apparent by days 8–10. The maximal mean diameter, indicating ovum maturity, of the preovulatory dominant follicle varies from 20 to 24 mm (range 14–28 mm) in normal, spontaneous cycles. Individual women tend to produce the same maximal diameter on repeated cycles. Pregnancies have not been observed with follicles less than 17 mm diameter in normal cycles.[107] Subordinate follicles rarely exceed 14 mm in diameter. In 5–11% of cycles, two dominant follicles develop.

During the 5 days preceding ovum expulsion, the dominant follicle exhibits a linear growth pattern of approximately 2 to 3 mm per day, followed by rapid exponential growth during the last 24 hours prior to ovulation. *Ultrasonographic surveillance of ovaries reveals that mittelschmerz is associated not with follicular rupture but with the rapid expansion of the dominant follicle, thus the pain precedes follicular rupture.*

Ovulation is associated with complete emptying of the follicular contents in 1 to 45 minutes. Fluid can be detected frequently, but not always, in the cul-de-sac. The follicle either disappears or more commonly appears as a smaller, irregular cyst which diminishes in size over the next 4–5 days.

In response to clomiphene treatment, follicles pursue a linear but generally accelerated rate of growth compared to spontaneous cycles.[108] The maximal diameter of clomiphene-induced preovulatory follicles is similar to that seen with spontaneous cycles, 20–24 mm, but ovulation can be successfully induced with HCG administration when the diameter reaches 18–20 mm (by the time of ovulation, the follicle will have grown another 2–3 mm). With gonadotropin therapy, the maximal follicular diameter (15–18 mm) is smaller than that seen during spontaneous and clomiphene-induced cycles. When follicles reach this size, ovulation will occur approximately 36 hours after HCG is administered.

Ultrasound monitoring does not eliminate the risks of multiple gestation and hyperstimulation. It is claimed that a higher pregnancy rate can be achieved when ultrasound is combined with estrogen monitoring.[109] The guiding principle has been to administer HCG when mature follicles correlate with an estrogen level of 200–400 pg per mature follicle (greater than 13 mm diameter). This principle only applies when there are several leading follicles, not when many intermediate (9–16 mm) and small (<9 mm) follicles are present. As a general rule, hyperstimulation is associated with the presence of more follicles. We believe that HCG should not be administered if there are more than 3–5 follicles 13 mm or greater in diameter (offering some protection against multiple gestation and hyperstimulation). Mild hyperstimulation has been associated with an increased number of intermediate size follicles, and severe hyperstimulation with an increase in small follicles.[110, 111] A large number (11 or more) of smaller follicles also should preclude HCG administration.

Measurement of Endometrial Thickness. Ultrasonographic studies in cycles of in vitro fertilization have revealed that successful implantation is correlated with endometrial thickness on the day of HCG administration.[112] This same correlation has been observed in patients in non-IVF patients receiving gonadotropins for ovulation induction.[113] Consistent with the antiestrogenic action of clomiphene, endometrial thickness is reduced in women treated with clomiphene (and reversed with estrogen). In a program utilizing clomiphene and timed administration of HCG for the purposes of intrauterine inseminations, no pregnancies occurred when the endometrial thickness measured less than 6 mm.[114] The chance of pregnancy is greatest, no matter what program of ovarian stimulation is being used, if endometrial thickness is 9–10 mm or more.[115, 116]

The Effect of Persistent Ovarian Cysts. In contrast to results with IVF or GIFT, the presence of a baseline ovarian cyst greater than 10 mm in diameter is associated with decreased fecundity in ovulation induction with gonadotropins.[117] With large cysts, treatment should be either delayed, or cyst suppression with a GnRH agonist or oral contraceptives should be considered, although it has never been proven that such treatment is effective. With this exception, there is no advantage in avoiding multiple successive treatment cycles (such as alternating treatment and nontreatment cycles).[102, 103]

Clomiphene-Gonadotropin Combination

The combination of clomiphene and gonadotropin was explored in order to minimize the amount and the cost of gonadotropin alone. As long as treatment is monitored with estrogen levels, the side effects and complications should not be dissimilar to those with gonadotropin alone. It has not been demonstrated that patients unresponsive to gonadotropin alone would respond to the sequence method, and there is no logical reason to assume that this would be true.

The usual method of treatment is to administer clomiphene 100 mg for 5–7 days, then to immediately proceed with gonadotropin beginning with 2 ampules per day. Estrogen levels are monitored as usual. This method may decrease the amount of gonadotropin required by approximately 50%; however, the same risks of multiple pregnancy and hyperstimulation can be expected. This reduced requirement for gonadotropin is found only in those patients who demonstrate a positive withdrawal bleeding following progestin medication or who have spontaneous menses.[118]

Pulsatile Administration of Gonadotropin

Gonadotropin can be administered in pulsatile fashion, either subcutaneously or intravenously, using an appropriate pump system.[119, 120] The aim is to reproduce the pulsatile pattern of gonadotropin secretion during the normal menstrual cycle. The dose administered intravenously is 6–9 units per pulse every 90 minutes, with adjustments upward according to response. The usual monitoring with estradiol levels and ultrasonography is necessary. It is not certain whether this complicated method is better beyond a decrease in dose and possibly a response in patients unresponsive to the traditional intramuscular regimen.

Results With Gonadotropin Treatment

The most significant aspect of this method of treatment is that it does achieve pregnancy in otherwise untreatable situations. A cumulative conception rate of 90% after 6 treatment cycles can be achieved in women with hypothalamic amenorrhea (this rate exceeds that observed in spontaneously ovulating women), with a 23% rate of spontaneous miscarriage.[121, 122] Women with normogonadotropic anovulation achieve only a slightly lower cumulative conception rate with relatively, but slightly, higher rates of miscarriage; however, with appropriate and careful gonadotropin treatment, these rates equal those in the normal population[123]. A slightly higher rate of spontaneous miscarriage reflects the combination of better detection of early pregnancy loss, advanced maternal age, and the increased incidence of multiple pregnancies. As with clomiphene, there is a normal incidence of congenital malformations, and the children have a normal postnatal development.[18] ***The risk of ectopic pregnancy is increased with ovulation induction, a consequence of multiple oocytes and high hormone levels.[124]*** These patients should be closely monitored in the early weeks of their pregnancies.

Women with polycystic ovaries and moderate obesity require larger doses of gonadotropin and ovulate at a lesser rate compared to leaner women with polycystic ovaries.[125] A comparable pregnancy rate (40%) is achieved. However, spontaneous miscarriage is more frequent, which is consistent with the observation that spontaneous miscarriage is more frequent in obese women.

HCG disappears from the blood with an initial component having a half-life of about 6 hours and a second, slower, component with a half-life of about 24 hours. It is this relatively slow half-life that enables a single injection of 10,000 IU to maintain the corpus luteum until pregnancy takes over. The HCG concentration after the ovulation injection should be less than 50–100 IU/L by day 14 after the injection. A β-subunit assay of HCG at this time or one of the urine assays performed 2–4 weeks after the HCG injection are reliable tests for pregnancy. Additional HCG (during the luteal phase) does not improve pregnancy rates.[126] Luteal supplementation is required only with concurrent treatment with a GnRH agonist.

The rate of serious hyperstimulation is 1–2%. Prior to the present era of more careful monitoring, the multiple pregnancy rate was reported as approximately 30% (triplets or more, 5%). Currently, the multiple pregnancy rate can be as low as 10% with careful monitoring and good medical judgment; however, rates as high as 40% are reported.[109] A striking increase in multiple births in many countries, especially triplets and quadruplets, can be directly attributed to ovulation stimulation for the treatment of infertility.[127–129]

The multiple pregnancies are secondary to multiple ovulations, and, therefore, the siblings are not identical. The rate of spontaneous occurrence of twins is only about 1% and that of triplets 0.010–0.017% of the pregnant population. Dizygotic twinning varies among different populations and is inherited through the mother. The monozygotic twinning rate is about 0.3–0.4%, fairly constant, and uninfluenced by heredity. Surprisingly, induction of ovulation increases the frequency of monozygotic twinning 3-fold.[130] It is not known whether the multiple pregnancy rate with gonadotropin is significantly affected by a maternal history of twinning.

Maternal complications and fetal loss caused by prematurity in the multiple pregnancies have been serious problems. In addition, the miscarriage rate with gonadotropin is somewhat higher (25%) than normal, probably a combination of the effect of age, multiple pregnancies, and recognition of early miscarriages.[131]

After at least one gonadotropin-induced pregnancy, the subsequent spontaneous pregnancy rate reaches 30% after 5 years.[132] Most of the pregnancies occur within 3 years of the gonadotropin-induced pregnancy, and the more endogenous hypothalamic-pituitary-ovarian function a patient has, the more likely a spontaneous pregnancy will occur.[133] This is consistent with a return to normal function in some women after suppression of a dysfunctional state. With time, it is logical to expect the original dysfunctional state to reestablish itself.

Multifetal Pregnancy Reduction. Induced abortion in the case of triplets or more is an option, but it would be surprising if patient and clinician would choose this solution. On the other hand, selective reduction of embryos in multiple pregnancy can be accomplished.[134] Under ultrasound guidance, a gestational sac can be aspirated or a cardiotoxic drug (potassium chloride) can be injected into, or adjacent to, the fetal heart. The transvaginal procedure is best performed between the 8th and 9th weeks of gestation and the transabdominal procedure between the 11th and 12th weeks. A later procedure is worthwhile because the spontaneous disappearance of one or more gestational sacs in multiple gestations can occur, an incidence of approximately 5% after fetal heartbeats have been identified.[135] Selection of which gestational sac to terminate is based solely on technical considerations, such as accessibility. The subsequent risk of losing one or more of the remaining fetuses is 4–9%, and of losing the pregnancy, 10% by experienced clinicians and higher with less experience. Reduction of a monochorionic pregnancy is not advisable because of shared vasculature and the high risk of losing all fetuses. The moral and ethical aspects of fetal reduction are significant, but in view of the potential problems associated with a multiple birth, it is a reasonable alternative for some.

The Hyperstimulation Syndrome

Ovarian hyperstimulation can be life-threatening. In mild cases the syndrome includes ovarian enlargement, abdominal distension, and weight gain. In severe cases, a critical condition develops with ascites, pleural effusion, electrolyte imbalance, and hypovolemia with hypotension and oliguria.[136–138] The ovaries are tremendously enlarged with multiple follicular cysts, stromal edema, and many corpora lutea. Because of this enlargement, torsion of the adnexa is a relatively common complication of this syndrome.[139]

The incidence of clinically important hyperstimulation is striking. Although it might be expected that the mild type would be relatively common, the moderate to severe form appears at an impressive rate (1–2%). Two-thirds of cases occur early in a conception cycle, the remainder in nonconception cycles. For purposes of one of the methods of assisted reproduction, the ovaries are stimulated at an even greater rate than for conventional ovulation induction; however, the incidence of hyperstimulation is no greater, or even lower.[140, 141] For this reason, it has been suggested that follicular aspiration offers partial protection against the hyperstimulation syndrome. Some reports have indicated a higher incidence of hyperstimulation in in vitro fertilization protocols using the combination of gonadotropin and a GnRH agonist.[140] Because support during the luteal phase is required when GnRH agonist treatment is used, the additional HCG administered is responsible for greater stimulation. The use of progesterone for luteal support is probably safer, and therefore, when estradiol levels are high (greater than 2500 pg/mL) and when the follicle number is greater than 15, progesterone supplementation is recommended instead of HCG.

Anovulatory women with polycystic ovaries are at greatest risk for the hyperstimulation syndrome. The use of a GnRH agonist in combined therapy does not eliminate this risk. These patients should be treated slowly with careful titration of dose as described earlier.

The basic disturbance in hyperstimulation is a shift of fluid from the intravascular space into the abdominal cavity, creating a massive third space. The resulting hypovolemia leads to circulatory and excretory problems. The genesis of the ascites is unclear. The very high level of estrogen secretion by the ovaries may be the primary factor, inducing increased local capillary permeability and leakage of fluid from the peritoneal capillaries as well as the ovaries. The leakage of fluid is also critically related to the mass, volume, and surface area of the ovaries. Therefore, the larger the ovaries and the greater the steroid production, the more severe the condition. Or the syndrome may result from overproduction of autocrine/paracrine factors that affect vascular permeability.

A growing body of evidence implicates vascular endothelial growth factor (VEGF) in the pathophysiology of the hyperstimulation syndrome. The origin of VEGF is presumed to be the ovarian follicle, and increased capillary permeability and the severity of the syndrome are correlated with circulating levels of VEGF.[142–144] Other cytokines, especially the interleukin family, are also believed to be involved in the permeability changes, and it is hypothesized that these agents affect the nitric oxide system.[145, 146] Large amounts of angiotensin II are present in the ascites produced by ovarian hyperstimulation, presumably originating from HCG stimulation of the ovarian renin-angiotensin system.[147]

The loss of fluid and protein into the abdominal cavity accounts for the hypovolemia and hemoconcentration. This in turn results in low blood pressure and decreased central venous pressure. The major clinical complications are increased coagulability and decreased renal perfusion. Blood loss as the cause of the clinical picture can be easily ruled out since a hematocrit will reveal hemoconcentration. The decreased renal perfusion leads to increased salt and water reabsorption in the proximal tubule, producing oliguria and low urinary sodium excretion. With less sodium being presented to the distal tubule, there is a decrease in the exchange of hydrogen and potassium for sodium, resulting in hyperkalemic acidosis. A rise in the blood urea nitrogen (BUN) is due to decreased perfusion and increased urea reabsorption. Because it is only filtered, creatinine does not increase as much as the BUN. Thus, the patient is hypovolemic, azotemic, and hyperkalemic. In response to these changes, aldosterone, plasma renin activity, and antidiuretic hormone levels are all elevated.[148]

Treatment is conservative and empiric. When a patient displays excessive weight gain (usually 10 or more pounds), excessive pain, hemoconcentration (hematocrit over 50%, white blood count over 25,000), oliguria, dyspnea, or postural hypotension, she should be hospitalized. Pelvic and abdominal examinations are contraindicated in view of the extreme fragility of the enlarged ovaries. Ovarian rupture and hemorrhage are easily precipitated.

Upon admission, the patient is put on bed rest, with daily body weights, strict monitoring of intake and output, and frequent vital signs. Serial studies of the following are obtained: hematocrit, BUN, creatinine, electrolytes, total proteins with albumin:globulin ratio, coagulation studies, and urinary sodium and potassium. The electrocardiogram is utilized to follow and evaluate hyperkalemia. Fluid and salt restriction is controversial. It is argued that correction of the decreased circulating volume is not necessary as long as the BUN remains stable (an abnormally low urine output can be tolerated).[148] Others believe that plasma expanding agents and electrolyte supplements should be administered.[149] Human albumin (safe from viral contamination) is the volume expander of choice. Potassium exchange resins may be necessary. Diuretics are without effect and, indeed, may be disadvantageous. The fluid in the abdominal cavity is not responsive to diuretic treatment, and diuresis may further contract the intravascular volume and produce hypovolemic shock or thrombosis. Arterial and venous thromboses have been reported in both the upper and lower portions of the body, and anticoagulant therapy should be considered in severely hemoconcentrated patients.[150–152] Although both antihistamines and indomethacin have been demonstrated to ameliorate the hyperstimulation in animal studies, their efficacy and safety in early human pregnancy are unknown. Inhibition of prostaglandin synthesis can worsen renal perfusion.

In severe cases, life-threatening adult respiratory distress syndrome can occur.[153] These patients require intensive care monitoring, including central venous and pulmonary wedge pressures. Adult respiratory distress syndrome is associated with a 50% mortality rate. Chlorpheniramine maleate, an H-1 receptor blocker, appears to maintain membrane stability, allowing the use of fluids and mannitol to retain intravascular volume.[154] With ultrasound guidance to avoid the enlarged ovaries, abdominal paracentesis can relieve severe pulmonary compromise. Aspiration of ascites can also be accomplished (and probably more easily) transvaginally (with ultrasound guidance).[155, 156] With repeated aspirations, it is very important to replace the lost plasma proteins (autotransfusion of the ascitic fluid has been used in a small number of cases). On the average, repeat aspirations are necessary in 3 to 5 days.

In severe cases, transvaginal aspiration of follicular structures should be considered to interfere with the intraovarian mechanism responsible for the clinical picture; progesterone supplementation will be necessary to maintain an on-going pregnancy.[157]

The possibility of ovarian rupture should always be considered, and serial hematocrits may be the only clue to intraperitoneal hemorrhage. Of course, a falling hematocrit accompanied by diuresis is an indication of resolution, not hemorrhage. Laparotomy should be avoided in these precarious patients. If surgery is necessary, only hemostatic measures should be undertaken and the ovaries should be conserved if possible, since a return to normal size is inevitable. If torsion of the adnexa is encountered, unwinding the adnexa (and preserving the ovary in an infertile patient) is possible even when the adnexa are already ischemic.

The key point is that the hyperstimulation syndrome will undergo gradual resolution with time. In a patient who is not pregnant, the syndrome will cover a period of approximately 7 days. In a patient who is pregnant and in whom the ovaries are restimulated by the emerging endogenous HCG production, the syndrome will last 10–20 days.

The syndrome will not develop unless the ovulatory dose of HCG is given. Thus, the major emphasis in recent years has been to utilize monitoring to avoid hyperstimulation. The relationship between estrogen levels and hyperstimulation is not a perfect one. Hyperstimulation has been found with relatively low estrogen levels, and high estrogen is not necessarily followed by hyperstimulation. As a general rule, the more follicles present (on ultrasound examination) the greater the risk for hyperstimulation. But this too is not a perfect correlation. Nevertheless, monitoring is the major available deterrent to a potentially life-threatening situation.

What to Do With Gonadotropin Failures?

At one time, management of the couple who had failed ovulation induction with gonadotropin treatment was difficult, but straightforward. Short of another costly round if funds and emotional reserves were sufficient, nothing was left to offer except adoption. Today, a major option is now available in the assisted reproductive technologies (Chapter 31). Although even more costly and emotionally charged, these methods do offer significant additional opportunities for unsuccessful patients. Nevertheless, guidance to adoption services and emotional support continue to be part of the physician's obligation.

A very important question for patients is: when to stop? All clinicians have been confronted by the dismal and frustrating prospects of a woman who has squandered years in vain repetitive attempts at ovulation induction, only to arrive at age 40 for intervention with one of the methods of assisted reproductive technology. If a properly managed set of 6 gonadotropin cycles is unsuccessful, the prudent counsel is to recommend a turn toward the methods of assisted reproductive technology.

Can Failure to Respond Be Predicted?

Women who present with "incipient" ovarian failure have elevated FSH levels and decreased levels of inhibin, but normal levels of estradiol.[158, 159] The rise in FSH during the later years is in response to declining inhibin production.[160–163] Inhibin levels are lower in the follicular phase in women 45–49 years old compared with younger women. The specific inhibin involved in this feedback effect on FSH during the follicular phase is inhibin B.[164, 165] In addition, a decline in luteal phase inhibin A can contribute to a greater rise in FSH during the luteal-follicular transition.[166] This decline in inhibin begins early, but accelerates after 40 years of age. The rise in FSH is very apparent after age 40, but there is no change in LH levels until menopause. The changes in the later reproductive years reflect either lesser follicular competence, as the better primordial follicles respond early in life, leaving the lesser follicles for later, or the fact that the total follicular pool is reduced in number (or both factors). Arguing in favor of a role for a reduced follicular pool is the observation that follicular fluid obtained from preovulatory follicles of older women contains amounts of inhibin A and B that are similar to that measured in follicular fluid from young women.[167]

These endocrine changes and the decline in ovarian follicles are correlated with a decrease in ovarian volume.[168] A measurement of volume by ultrasonography that is equal to or less than 3 cm^3 predicts a poor response to ovulation induction.[169]

Testing the Ovarian Reserve

The measurement of baseline hormonal levels provides important and helpful prognostic information. Because FSH levels increase with age, elevated FSH levels on cycle day 3 (greater than 12 IU/L, but especially greater than 20 IU/L) are associated with poor performance with in vitro fertilization.[170] A cycle day 3 FSH level that is 25 IU/L or more, or an age of 44 years or more, are both independently associated with a chance of pregnancy close to zero during ovulation induction or with assisted reproductive technologies.[171] *Values can vary between laboratories, significantly due to differences in antibodies and standards used to measure gonadotropin levels.[172] With the most recent assays, day 3 values above 10 IU/L are abnormal and are comparable with values greater than 20 IU/L with older assays.*

Keep in mind that there is no abrupt change at 40, and, therefore, these changes can apply to younger women. The age of change is determined by the rate of oocyte loss, a rate that is genetically programmed in most women. An elevated FSH at any age is correlated with fewer available oocytes, and advancing age adds the factor of lesser oocyte quality. An elevated estradiol level on day 3 (greater than 80 pg/mL) is also predictive of difficulty in achieving pregnancy;[173, 174] premature estradiol elevations are associated with a hurried recruitment of follicles in response to increased FSH secretion, changes characteristic of the years preceding menopause. When both FSH and estradiol are elevated on day 3, ovarian response to stimulation is very poor.

The Clomiphene Challenge Test. Navot and colleagues developed the clomiphene challenge test as a bioassay of FSH response (which in turn reflects ovarian follicular inhibin capability).[175] Clomiphene is administered in a dose of 100 mg/day on days 5–9. The level of FSH on day 10 is compared with the baseline level on day 3. An exaggerated FSH response of 26 IU/L or more was two standard deviations above the control values in this study, and this increase in FSH was associated with a significant prospect for failure to achieve pregnancy. *Remember that there is a wide variety of FSH assays (the newer assays provide numbers that are approximately 70% of the older results), and clinicians must become familiar with the values provided by their own laboratories.* There is a high incidence of abnormal responses in women over age 35, and 85% of women with increased FSH levels respond poorly to ovarian stimulation.[176] In a general infertility population, about 10% of women have an abnormal response to the clomiphene challenge test. As expected, the percentage increased with increasing age (from 3% under age 30 to 26% over age 39), and women with unexplained infertility had a 38% incidence of abnormal tests.[177] This test of ovarian reserve is more sensitive than just measuring basal FSH levels in predicting the potential for pregnancy in both assisted and natural reproduction. An abnormal response to the clomiphene challenge test indicates a poor prognosis no matter the woman's age.[178] However, because age alone is an important factor (presumably due to other age-related oocyte conditions of quality), older women with normal hormone levels and normal responses to clomiphene still have diminished chances of pregnancy.

We believe it is worthwhile to screen all infertile women beginning at age 30, women of any age with unexplained infertility, and women who respond poorly to ovulation induction with the clomiphene challenge test and a day 3 estradiol level. For practical purposes, equivalent results can be expected on days 2, 3, and 4 of the cycle. Far less certain is the need for these tests in the woman over 40, because even normal tests do not provide reassurance of adequate ovarian reserve. An abnormal test in a woman over 40, however, can be used to bolster advice to consider ovum donation. Although an abnormal test at any age indicates a very poor prognosis, it does not indicate an absolute inability to achieve pregnancy.

Regardless of age, women with elevated day 3 FSH levels and/or abnormal responses to the clomiphene challenge test should consider in vitro fertilization with young, donated oocytes. Patients should also be informed that a failure to respond to gonadotropin treatment despite normal screening hormonal levels places them at risk for progressing to ovarian failure in a relatively short time.[179]

GnRH Agonist and Gonadotropin Combined Treatment

Recognizing that women with significant estrogen, androgen, and gonadotropin levels do not respond well to induction of ovulation, attention was turned to a method that could turn off a woman's endogenous reproductive hormone production. The availability of GnRH agonists provided such a method. The thesis underlying the use of a GnRH agonist as an adjunctive therapy in ovulation induction is straightforward: convert normogonadotropic anovulators to a hypogonadotropic hypogonad state by the process of pituitary GnRH receptor desensitization and down-regulation.[180, 181] Premature LH effects on the follicle and the burden of excess local androgen can be diminished and an improved therapeutic response achieved. There is reason to believe that women with anovulatory polycystic ovaries have a higher incidence of spontaneous miscarriage following induction of ovulation with gonadotropin;[73–75] combining the GnRH agonist with gonadotropin not only yields a greater pregnancy rate, but also reduces the miscarriage rate.[182] Furthermore, premature LH release is believed to contribute to the risk of ovarian hyperstimulation in women with polycystic ovaries.[183] Combining a GnRH agonist with gonadotropin treatment could reduce (although not eliminate) the risk of this serious complication.

Leuprolide acetate (Lupron) is administered twice daily (0.5 mg subcutaneously) for 2 weeks.[181] Suppression of gonadotropin secretion is confirmed by measurement of the estradiol level; a concentration less than 25 pg/mL should be achieved before treatment is initiated with gonadotropins. Lupron treatment is maintained throughout the gonadotropin regimen until HCG is administered. It is not unusual to require higher doses of gonadotropin. With this combination, no difference has been observed in the number of follicles recruited, the rate of rise and final estradiol level achieved, or the number of cycles canceled compared with gonadotropin alone. Hyperstimulation is not avoided, but per cycle fecundity appears to be modestly increased. Any of the available GnRH agonists can be used for this purpose. Pituitary suppression can be combined with highly purified or recombinant FSH; it appears that very little LH is necessary for normal responses.[184]

The administration of a GnRH agonist to a woman who has menstrual function will initially produce a stimulatory response, known as the "flare." The magnitude of the flare response depends upon when in the cycle the agonist is administered. During the follicular phase or in anovulatory women, the flare is greater, and enlarged follicular cysts can occur. This response can be minimized by beginning therapy during the midluteal phase or by administering a progestational agent (e.g., 10 mg medroxyprogesterone acetate daily for 10 days) and beginning GnRH agonist treatment after 3 days of progestin.

During the hypoestrogenic period of time, menopausal-like symptoms are common, especially hot flushes. Forewarning and reassurance are usually sufficient to help patients tolerate these short-lived reactions.

Utilization of a GnRH agonist suppresses endogenous LH levels to such a low level that, after ovulation, the corpus luteum requires additional exogenous support. One can administer HCG (2000 IU) twice, 3 days, and 6 days after ovulation, or progesterone supplementation beginning 3 days after ovulation (4 days after the LH surge): intravaginal progesterone suppositories, 25 mg twice per day, intramuscular progesterone, 50 mg per day, or oral micronized progesterone, 300 mg per day. The dose of micronized progesterone is relatively high and should be administered at bedtime to avoid side effects. Progesterone in a gel that adheres to the vaginal mucosa (Crinone) is available in a prefilled vaginal applicator, applied with one 8% (90 mg progesterone) application daily. Vaginal administration accomplishes targeted delivery to the uterus without producing high circulating levels. The pregnancy rates with either HCG or progesterone treatment are the same, but the use of HCG adds to the risk of hyperstimulation.[185, 186]

GnRH Antagonists

More extensive alterations in the GnRH structure yield compounds that bind to the GnRH receptor and totally block any stimulation of the pituitary gonadotropin-secreting cells. GnRH antagonists can be used concomitantly with gonadotropin induction of ovulation to prevent premature LH surges.[187] Because GnRH antagonists are competitive inhibitors, a GnRH agonist could be used for the ovulatory signal, possible avoiding the use of HCG and reducing the risk of ovarian hyperstimulation. The optimal use of GnRH antagonists is currently being explored.

Adding Growth Hormone

As discussed in Chapter 6, the primate ovarian follicular cycle is very dependent upon autocrine/paracrine factors. In view of the critical role played by insulin-like growth factor-I, it was quickly recognized that the addition of growth hormone (which stimulates insulin-like growth factor-I production), usually in a dose of 24 IU given intramuscularly every other day, might facilitate ovulation induction by gonadotropins, and especially, might convert poor responders to good responders. Initial results in poor responders were favorable, although this may be limited to patients with polycystic ovaries.[188, 189] In women with normal responses, however, the addition of growth hormone did not improve results or reduce the total dose of gonadotropin.[190] Thus, in normally responding women, the growth hormone and IGF-I system may be operating at maximal levels. In poorly responding women, concomitant treatment with growth hormone can reduce the amount of gonadotropin necessary, shorten the duration of treatment, and increase the chance of pregnancy. However, not all poorly responding women respond favorably to growth hormone treatment.[191] The effective selection of patients, dosage, and treatment regimens remains to be standardized, and the extreme cost of growth hormone is a significant disadvantage. Another approach is to administer growth hormone-releasing hormone. In a small randomized trial (13 women), the addition of growth hormone-releasing hormone to gonadotropin treatment was associated with a higher pregnancy rate.[192] However, others have administered 500 µg of growth hormone releasing hormone twice daily to poor responders with little effect, although the dosage of gonadotropin may be reduced.[193, 194]

Induction of Ovulation With Gonadotropin-Releasing Hormone (GnRH)

Numerous advantages can be cited in favor of pulsatile GnRH therapy for ovulation induction. GnRH methodology, once established, is simple to use, requires no extensive (or expensive) follicular monitoring, and, relative to its counterparts, is quite safe. Ovarian hyperstimulation and multiple gestations are rare because only "physiologic" levels of FSH should be generated. Because GnRH serves largely a permissive role, the internal feedback mechanisms between the ovary and pituitary should be operative, yielding follicular growth and development similar to a normal menstrual cycle in response to the "turning on" of the system by GnRH.

GnRH is administered constantly in a pulsatile fashion by a programmable portable minipump. Induction of ovulation with the GnRH pump is most effective in women with hypothalamic amenorrhea (absence of menstrual bleeding following a progestin challenge) where endogenous GnRH is dysfunctional or absent. Unfortunately, although it has been successful in some anovulatory women with polycystic ovaries, this success is far less than anticipated, and these patients are at greater risk for hyperstimulation and multiple pregnancy, therefore requiring a lower dose (2.5 µg per bolus).[195, 196] Nevertheless, the GnRH pump is a safer, less expensive alternative for these patients than gonadotropin therapy. The GnRH pump is also effective in women with hyperprolactinemia, providing a good alternative if dopamine agonist treatment cannot be tolerated.

GnRH is available in crystalline form that when reconstituted in the aqueous diluent is stable for at least 3 weeks at room temperature. The pump must be worn constantly around the clock, requiring some ingenuity for bathing and sleeping. GnRH can be administered by either the intravenous or subcutaneous routes. The subcutaneous route requires a higher dose. Failure with subcutaneous administration is associated with a polycystic ovary-like picture, with high LH levels, anovulation, and even symptoms of androgen excess. This is not surprising because subcutaneous administration results in an absorption curve with a broad base without a definite peak. For intravenous administration, heparin is added to the GnRH solution in a concentration of 1000 U/mL. We favor starting with the intravenous route. The needle is left in place until there are signs of local reaction and then changed. Women at risk for bacterial endocarditis should be restricted to the subcutaneous route of administration.

Although some argue in favor of near physiologic duplication of the pulse frequency, similar results can be obtained with empiric 90-minute cycles throughout treatment. The dose for subcutaneous administration is 20 µg per bolus, for intravenous administration, 5 µg per bolus. If the patient fails to respond (assessed by weekly measurement of estradiol), the dose should be increased by 5 µg increments.

After ovulation, the luteal phase is maintained by either continuing the pump or administering HCG (2000 IU intramuscularly at the time of the temperature rise and then every 3 days for 3 doses). In our experience, most patients would rather discontinue the pump.

One of the reasons that the GnRH pump is less expensive is that it reproduces physiologic hormonal events, and intensive monitoring is not necessary. The main problem is knowing with some accuracy when to have intercourse. Usually ovulation occurs by 14 days of treatment, but the range extends from 10 days to 22 days. Intercourse every other day during this period of time can be a formidable challenge. Ultrasonic monitoring of follicular development may be required, or more conveniently, the couple can use one of the urinary LH test kits to detect the LH surge and have intercourse for 2–3 days beginning the day of the color change.

Side effects with the GnRH pump are minimal, principally related to pump functioning and local reactions to the needle placement. The patient must be educated to pay close attention to proper function of the pump and maintenance of the GnRH reservoir. Hyperstimulation and multiple births have been encountered, but this is rare and associated with higher than recommended doses. The risk of dangerous hyperstimulation is essentially zero. Several cases of allergic response with the development of circulating antibodies have been reported.

The pregnancy rate in anovulatory women is 20–30% per treatment cycle, which approximates the pregnancy rate of normal couples.[197, 198] Persistence with repeated cycles is rewarded with high cumulative pregnancy rates, approximately 80% after 6 cycles and 93% after 12 cycles.[199] The miscarriage rate of 20% is typical of all methodologies. The incidence of multiple pregnancy is low (4–5%). The cumulative pregnancy rate in women with polycystic ovaries is approximately 30–40%. If this method is to be used for women with polycystic ovaries, it is recommended that desensitization and down-regulation of the pituitary with a GnRH agonist precede treatment (and retreatment will be necessary with each cycle). This approach can yield a cumulative pregnancy rate of 60%.[200] Even then, obese patients are less likely to respond, and they have higher rates of spontaneous miscarriage.

The safety and simplicity of GnRH administration are powerful attractions. Despite the clear advantages, the GnRH pump has not received wide acceptance by patients. Many are irrationally fearful of the risk of needle displacement or equipment problems associated with the technology. Because of this low acceptance, appropriate pumps for the administration of GnRH are no longer available in many countries.

Ovarian Surgical Procedures

Irving Stein and Michael Leventhal, in 1935, at the Michael Reese Hospital in Chicago, described 7 cases of the syndrome that bears their names.[201] They developed wedge resection of the ovaries when they observed that several of their amenorrheic (anovulatory) patients with polycystic ovaries menstruated after ovarian biopsies. In their original procedure, they removed 50 to 75% of each ovary. They concluded that the thickened surface of the ovary prevented follicles from reaching the surface. For years, the wedge resection was the only method available to induce ovulation in these patients, and it wasn't until 30–40 years later that an accurate understanding of the mechanism was achieved.

The purpose of wedge resection of the ovaries is to remove a significant amount of hormone-producing tissue. Documentation of hormone changes following wedge resection indicates that an important change is a sustained reduction in testosterone levels.[202, 203] This suggests that the barrier to ovulation is the intraovarian, atresia-promoting effects of the high testosterone production. Removal of androgen-producing tissue effectively lowers this barrier, and ovulatory cycles can ensue. The success of wedge resection is directly proportional to the volume of androgen-producing tissue removed. Tissue removal and destruction are the key factors, not the shape and procedure of the "wedge." Indeed, even a unilateral oophorectomy is followed by resumption of ovulation in anovulatory women with polycystic ovaries.[204]

Another contributing factor is a reduction in circulating levels of inhibin, which follows the loss of ovarian tissue.[205] A rise in FSH occurs in the days after wedge resection; successful ovulation reflects the combined effects of increased FSH and the removal of the local androgen obstruction to the emergence of a dominant follicle.

The response to ovarian wedge resection is variable. Some patients resume ovulation permanently. However, most patients return to their anovulatory state. Some patients fail to respond at all. Furthermore, the surgical procedure carries with it the potential problem of postoperative adhesion formation.

The operative risk, the variable response, and the possibility of postoperative adhesion formation are the liabilities of wedge resection. These must be weighed against the excellent results obtained with medical induction of ovulation (approximating the normal conception rate when anovulation is the only fertility problem present). It should truly be a rare patient in whom wedge resection of the ovaries is necessary.

Today, a new type of "wedge resection" is available. Using either cautery, diathermy, or laser vaporization by means of the laparoscope, destruction of ovarian tissue at multiple sites (15–20 per ovary) can achieve spontaneous ovulations or an increased sensitivity to clomiphene, ultimately achieving pregnancy rates equivalent to those with gonadotropin treatment (but without the risks of hyperstimulation and multiple pregnancies).[206–210] These procedures are associated with the same decrease in androgens and inhibin as observed with wedge resection. When clomiphene is reinstituted, 70–80% of patients will ovulate, and approximately 60% will achieve pregnancy. Adhesion formation remains a problem, but perhaps it is less profound than in the traditional surgery.[210, 211] Second look laparoscopy with lysis of adhesions is indicated if pregnancy does not follow successful ovulations. This therapy can be performed at the time of a planned diagnostic laparoscopy in a patient with known anovulation and polycystic ovaries. These procedures are worth considering by patients who are reluctant to pursue the more expensive and difficult methods of the assisted reproductive technologies. These methods are the modern equivalent of the original ovarian wedge resection pioneered by Stein and Leventhal.

Superovulation and IUI for Unexplained Infertility

The methods of assisted reproductive technology and superovulation with intrauterine insemination (IUI) increase the prospect of pregnancy in couples with unexplained infertility. The results with superovulation alone are inferior to those achieved with one of the assisted reproductive techniques, but the overall cost is also less.[212] Studies indicate that subtle hormonal abnormalities do exist in women with unexplained infertility.[213, 214] These changes (elevated gonadotropins and estradiol in the follicular phase and decreased luteal phase progesterone) have been attributed to a reduction in ovarian reserve as usually seen in older women.[214] Thus, there is a rational basis to provide ovarian stimulation.

A cumulative pregnancy rate of 40% can be achieved in couples with unexplained infertility after 6 cycles of superovulation or 3 cycles of in vitro fertilization.[215] In randomized, controlled clinical trials, the monthly pregnancy rates in couples with unexplained infertility is increased 2–3-fold (a monthly fecundity rate of 9%) with clomiphene treatment, and with human gonadotropins, the monthly fecundity rate is approximately 10–15%.[216–218] *Although some studies have failed to yield increased pregnancy rates with the empiric use of clomiphene,[219, 220] we believe couples with unexplained infertility should be offered superovulation or one of the assisted reproductive technologies. However, superovulation should be limited to 3 or 4 cycles.*

The addition of intrauterine insemination of washed sperm (IUI) to clomiphene treatment increased fecundity in couples with unexplained infertility or surgically treated endometriosis, compared with intercourse without hormonal stimulation).[217] As with almost all infertility, success is age-related, with pregnancy rates 3–4-fold greater in women under age 20.[221] Although the combination of IUI with clomiphene may enhance the pregnancy rate in couples with unexplained infertility, ***IUI by itself does not.***[222–224]

The combination of IUI with gonadotropin stimulation provides even better results than clomiphene and IUI. In two studies, the pregnancy rate per cycle with gonadotropins and IUI was 19% and 14.3% compared to 4% and 7.7% with clomiphene and IUI respectively.[218, 225] In a meta-analysis of randomized trials comparing gonadotropin stimulation with IUI or with timed intercourse, IUI was associated with approximately a 2-fold greater pregnancy rate.[226] In a randomized trial, superovulation and IUI resulted in a 3-fold greater pregnancy rate compared with intracervical insemination and 2-fold greater compared with either IUI alone or a combination of superovulation and intracervical insemination.[241]

The effectiveness of gonadotropin treatment combined with IUI has been repeatedly demonstrated for a variety of infertility disorders, including endometriosis, cervical factor, and unexplained infertility.[227–229] As with clomiphene, few pregnancies occur after 4 cycles of treatment.

In summary, a meta-analysis of methods used to treat unexplained infertility, pregnancy rates were estimated to be as follows:

Pregnancy Rate per Cycle [169]

No treatment	1.3–4.1%
IUI	3.8%
Clomiphene	5.6%
Clomiphene & IUI	8.3%
Gonadotropins	7.7%
Gonadotropins & IUI	17.1%
IVF	20.7%

Because it is relatively inexpensive, easy to administer, and not usually burdened with major side effects (except for a 2-fold increase in twinning), clomiphene is usually the first treatment choice. Patient demand for this treatment is substantial, and it is not unreasonable to respond to that demand with 3–4 clomiphene cycles. The uncertainty regarding the efficacy of adding IUI to clomiphene influences us to proceed from clomiphene treatment to the combination of gonadotropins and IUI, with an expectation of achieving a pregnancy rate of 15% per cycle. The combination of clomiphene and IUI is still appropriate in circumstances where cost, time, and avoidance of complications are paramount. The use of IUI alone or gonadotropins without IUI is not recommended for the treatment of unexplained infertility.[223, 231]

The effects of age remain critical whatever the method of ovarian stimulation. In one series of 136 treatment cycles, no pregnancies were achieved in women who were 43 or older.[232] Despite rare successes in older women, it borders on the exploitive to treat women over age 40 with superovulation and IUI. Indeed, pregnancy rates begin to decline with this treatment around age 35.[221]

The incidence of multiple births and ovarian hyperstimulation is higher with this empiric treatment. Patients and clinicians undertaking empiric superovulation should have ready recourse to in vitro fertilization. ***If gonadotropin stimulation is excessive, several choices are available: avoiding HCG administration and cancelling the cycle, aspirating most of the ovarian follicles with ultrasound guidance and proceeding with in vitro fertilization.***

Fertility Drugs and the Risk of Ovarian Cancer

An analysis of 3 case-control studies of ovarian cancer conducted in the U.S. from 1987–1989 concluded that the risk was increased among women who had used fertility drugs and among women who had been exposed to long periods of sexual activity without contraception.[233] However, this conclusion was limited by the small number of cases, and the exact drugs and dosage used by these cases were unknown. Concern over this issue was further fueled by a report that prolonged use of clomiphene (12 or more cycles) was associated with an increased risk of borderline or invasive ovarian tumors.[234] The conclusion in this comparison of a cohort of women with the rate of ovarian tumors in the general population was based on only 5 cases of borderline tumors and 4 cases of invasive tumors. Nevertheless, the idea that superovulation can increase the risk of ovarian cancer is biologically plausible because there is a decreasing risk for invasive epithelial ovarian cancer associated with those conditions marked by a decrease in the number of ovulations: multiparity, increasing duration of breastfeeding, and the use of oral contraception.

It is worth noting that a long-term follow-up of 2632 women in Israel who had received drugs for induction of ovulation did not record an increased incidence of ovarian cancer in the subsequent years.[235] More recently, stimulated by the above reports, several epidemiologic studies appeared with the strength of larger case numbers. A study from Israel indicated an increased risk, but the relative risk was not statistically significant.[236] Two case-control studies from Italy and a Danish case-control study (the largest in size) failed to find a relationship between fertility drugs and the risk of epithelial ovarian cancer.[237–239]

The best evidence does not indicate an increased risk of ovarian cancer with less than 12 months of clomiphene treatment (there is no reason to pursue clomiphene treatment for more than 12 months), or with gonadotropin treatment. Nulliparity and infertility in nulliparous women are associated with a slight increase in the risk of ovarian cancer, but ovarian stimulation with fertility drugs does not change this baseline risk.[240]

References

1. **Greenblatt RB, Barfield WE, Jugck EC, Ray AW,** Induction of ovulation with MRL/41, preliminary report, *JAMA* 178:255, 1961.

2. **Dickey RP, Holtkamp DE,** Development, pharmacology and clinical experience with clomiphene citrate, *Hum Reprod Update* 2:483, 1996.

3. **Ernst S, Hite G, Cantrell JS, Richardson Jr A, Benson HD,** Stereochemistry of geometric isomers of clomiphene: a correction of the literature and a reexamination of structure-activity relationships, *J Pharm Sci* 65:148, 1976.

4. **Clark JH, Markaverich BM,** The agonistic-antagonistic properties of clomiphene: a review, *Pharmacol Ther* 15:467, 1982.

5. **Adashi EY,** Clomiphene citrate-initiated ovulation: a clinical update, *Seminars Reprod Endocrinol* 4:255, 1986.

6. **Kerin JF, Liu JH, Phillipou G, Yen SSC,** Evidence for a hypothalamic site of action of clomiphene citrate in women, *J Clin Endocrinol Metab* 61:265, 1985.

7. **Kettel LM, Roseff SJ, Berga SL, Mortola JF, Yen SSC,** Hypothalmic-pituitary-ovarian response to clomiphene citrate in women with polycystic ovarian syndrome, *Fertil Steril* 59:532, 1993.

8. **de Moura MD, Ferriani RA, de Sa MFS,** Effects of clomiphene citrate on pituitary luteinizing hormone and follicle-stimulating hormone release in women before and after treatment with ethinyl estradiol, *Fertil Steril* 58:504, 1992.

9. **Kessel B, Hsueh AJW,** Clomiphene citrate augments follicle-stimulating hormone-induced luteinizing hormone receptor content in cultured rat granulosa cells, *Fertil Steril* 46:334, 1987.

10. **Birkenfeld A, Beier HM, Schenker JG,** The effect of clomiphene citrate on early embryonic development, endometrium and implantation, *Hum Reprod* 1:387, 1986.

11. **Li T, Warren MA, Murphy C, Sargeant S, Cooke ID,** A prospective, randomised, cross-over study comparing the effects of clomiphene citrate and cyclofenil on endometrial morphology in the luteal phase of normal, fertile women, *Br J Obstet Gynaecol* 99:1008, 1992.

12. **Thompson LA, Barratt CLR, Thornton SJ, Bolton AE, Cooke ID,** The effects of clomiphene citrate and cyclofenil on cervical mucus volume and receptivity over the periovulatory period, *Fertil Steril* 59:125, 1993.

13. **Fritz MA, Holmes RT, Keenan EJ,** Effect of clomiphene citrate treatment on endometrial estrogen and progesterone receptor induction in women, *Am J Obstet Gynecol* 165:177, 1991.

14. **Mikkelson TJ, Kroboth PD, Cameron WJ, Dittert LW, Chungi V, Manberg PJ,** Single-dose pharmacokinetics of clomiphene citrate in normal volunteers, *Fertil Steril* 46:392, 1986.

15. **Lavy G, Diamond MP, Polan ML,** Reversal by human chorionic gonadotropin of the inhibitory effect of clomiphene on progesterone production by granulosa-luteal cells in culture, *Int J Fertil* 34:359, 1989.

16. **Cunha GR, Taguchi O, Namikawa R, Nishizuka Y, Robboy SJ,** Teratogenic effects of clomiphene, tamoxifen, and diethylstilbestrol on the developing human female genital tract, *Hum Pathol* 18:1132, 1987.

17. **Mills JL, Simpson JL, Rhoads GG, Graubard BI, Hoffman H, Conley MR, Lassman M, Cunningham G,** Risk of neural tube defects in relation to maternal fertility and fertility drug use, *Lancet* 336:103, 1990.

18. **Shoham Z, Zosmer A, Insler V,** Early miscarriage and fetal malformations after induction of ovulation (by clomiphene citrate and/or human menotropins), in vitro fertilization, and gamete intrafallopian transfer, *Fertil Steril* 55:1, 1991.

19. **Venn A, Lumley J,** Clomiphene citrate and pregnancy outcome, *Aust N Z J Obstet Gynaecol* 34:56, 1994.

20. **Gorlitsky GA, Kase NG, Speroff L,** Ovulation and pregnancy rates with clomiphene citrate, *Obstet Gynecol* 51:265, 1978.

21. **Downs KA, Gibson M,** Clomiphene citrate therapy for luteal phase defect, *Fertil Steril* 39:34, 1983.

22. **Huang K-E,** The primary treatment of luteal phase inadequacy: progesterone versus clomiphene citrate, *Am J Obstet Gynecol* 155:824, 1986.

23. **Murray DL, Reich L, Adashi EY,** Oral clomiphene citrate and vaginal progesterone suppositories in the treatment of luteal phase dysfunction; a comparative study, *Fertil Steril* 51:35, 1989.

24. **Gysler M, March CM, Mishell Jr DR, Bailey EJ,** A decade's experience with an individualized clomiphene treatment regimen including its effect on the postcoital test, *Fertil Steril* 37:161, 1982.

25. **Wu CH, Winkel CA,** The effect of therapy initiation day on clomiphene citrate therapy, *Fertil Steril* 52:564, 1989.

26. **Shepard MK, Balmaceda JP, Leija CG,** Relationship of weight to successful induction of ovulation with clomiphene citrate, *Fertil Steril* 32:641, 1979.

27. **Lobo RA, Gysler M, March CM, Goebelsmann U, Mishell Jr DR,** Clinical and laboratory predictors of clomiphene response, *Fertil Steril* 37:168, 1982.

28. **Dickey RP, Taylor SN, Curole DN, Rye PH, Lu PY, Pyrzak R,** Relationship of clomiphene dose and patient weight to successful treatment, *Hum Reprod* 12:449, 1997.

29. **Hammond MG, Halme JK, Talbert LM,** Factors affecting the pregnancy rate in clomiphene citrate induction of ovulation, *Obstet Gynecol* 62:196, 1983.

30. **Tiitinen AE, Laatikainen TJ, Seppala MT,** Serum levels of insulin-like growth factor binding protein-1 and ovulatory responses to clomiphene citrate in women with polycystic ovarian disease, *Fertil Steril* 60:58, 1993.

31. **Lunenfeld B, Pariente C, Dor J, Menashe Y, Seppala M, Mortman H, Insler V,** Modern aspects of ovulation induction, *Ann N Y Acad Sci* 626:207, 1991.

32. **Opsahl MS, Robins ED, O'Connor DM, Scott RT, Fritz MA,** Characteristics of gonadotropin response, follicular development, and endometrial growth and maturation across consecutive cycles of clomiphene citrate treatment, *Fertil Steril* 66:533, 1996.

33. **Smith YR, Randolph Jr JF, Christman GM, Ansbacher R, Howe DM, Hurd WW,** Comparison of low-technology and high-technology monitoring of clomiphene citrate ovulation induction, *Fertil Steril* 70:165, 1998.

34. **Agarwal SK, Buyalos RP,** Corpus luteum function and pregnancy rates with clomiphene citrate therapy: comparison of human chorionic gonadotrophin-induced versus spontaneous ovulation, *Hum Reprod* 10:328, 1995.

35. **Kousta E, White DM, Franks S,** Modern use of clomiphene citrate in induction of ovulation, *Hum Reprod Update* 3:359, 1997.

36. **Dickey RP, Taylor SN, Curole DN, Rye PH, Pyrzak R,** Incidence of spontaneous abortion in clomiphene pregnancies, *Hum Reprod* 11:2623, 1996.

37. **Greenland S, Ackerman DL,** Clomiphene citrate and neural tube defects: a pooled analysis of controlled epidemiologic studies and recommendations for future studies, *Fertil Steril* 64:936, 1995.

38. **Purvin VA,** Visual disturbance secondary to clomiphene citrate, *Arch Ophthalmol* 113:482, 1995.

39. **Imani B, Eijkemans MJC, te Velde ER, Habbema JDF, Fauser BCJM,** Predictors of patients remaining anovulatory during clomiphene citrate induction of ovulation in normogonadotropic oligoamenorrheic infertility, *J Clin Endocrinol Metab* 83:2361, 1998.

40. **Taubert H-D, Dericks-Tan JE,** High doses of estrogens do not interfere with the ovulation-inducing effect of clomiphene citrate, *Fertil Steril* 27:375, 1976.

41. **Bateman BG, Nunley Jr WC, Kolp LA,** Exogenous estrogen therapy for the treatment of clomiphene citrate-induced cervical mucus abnormalities: Is it effective? *Fertil Steril* 54:577, 1990.

42. **Pasquali R, Antenucci D, Casimirri F, Venturoli S, Paradisi R, Fabbri R, Balestra V, Melchiondra N, Barbara L,** Clinical and hormonal characteristics of obese amenorrheic hyperandrogenic women before and after weight loss, *J Clin Endocrinol Metab* 68:173, 1989.

43. **Kiddy DS, Hamilton-Fairley D, Seppälä M, Koistinen R, James VHT, Reed MJ, Franks S,** Diet-induced changes in sex hormone binding globulin and free testosterone in women with normal or polycystic ovaries: correlation with serum insulin and insulin-like growth factor-I, *Clin Endocrinol* 31:757, 1989.

44. **Kiddy DS, Hamilton-Fairley D, Bush A, Short F, Anyaoku V, Reed MJ, Franks S,** Improvement in endocrine and ovarian function during dietary treatment of obese women with polycystic ovary syndrome, *Clin Endocrinol* 36:105, 1992.

45. **Guzick DS, Wing R, Smith D, Berga S, Winters SJ,** Endocrine consequences of weight loss in obese, hyperandrogenic anovulatory women, *Fertil Steril* 61:598, 1994.

46. **Andersen P, Selifeflot I, Abdelnoor M, Arnese H, Dale PO, Lovik A, Birkeland K,** Increased insulin sensitivity and fibrinolytic capacity after dietary intervention in obese women with polycystic ovary syndrome, *Metabolism* 44:611, 1995.

47. **Jakubowicz DJ, Nestler JE,** 17α-Hydroxyprogesterone responses to leuprolide and serum androgens in obese women with and without polycystic ovary syndrome after dietary weight loss, *J Clin Endocrinol Metab* 82:556, 1997.

48. **Clark AM, Ledger W, Galletly C, Tomlinson L, Blaney F, Wang X, Norman RJ,** Weight loss results in significant improvement in pregnancy and ovulation rates in anovulatory obese women, *Hum Reprod* 10:2705, 1995.

49. **Hollmann M, Runnebaum B, Gerhard I,** Effects of weight loss on the hormonal profile in obese, infertile women, *Hum Reprod* 11:1884, 1996.

50. **Clark AM, Thornley B, Tomlinson L, Galletley C, Norman RJ,** Weight loss in obese infertile women results in improvement in reproductive outcome for all forms of fertility treatment, *Hum Reprod* 13:1502, 1998.

51. **Muscelli E, Camastra S, Catalano C, Galvan AQ, Ciociaro D, Baldi S, Ferrannini E,** Metabolic and cardiovascular assessment in moderate obesity: effect of weight loss, *J Clin Endocrinol Metab* 82:2937, 1997.

52. **Legro RS, Finegood D, Dunaif A,** A fasting glucose to insulin ratio is a useful measure of insulin sensitivity in women with polycystic ovary syndrome, *J Clin Endocrinol Metab* 83:2694, 1998.

53. **Velázquez EM, Mendoza S, Hamer T, Sosa F, Glueck CJ,** Metformin therapy in polycystic ovary syndrome reduces hyperinsulinemia, insulin resistance, hyperandrogenemia, and systolic blood pressure, while facilitating normal menses and pregnancy, *Metabolism* 43:647, 1994.

54. **Nestler JE, Jakubowicz DJ,** Decreases in ovarian cytochrome P450c17 alpha activity and serum free testosterone after reduction of insulin secretion in polycystic ovary syndrome, *New Engl J Med* 335:617, 1996.

55. **Velázquez EM, Mendoza SG, Wang P, Glueck CG,** Metformin therapy is associated with a decrease in plasma plasminogen activator inhibitor-1, lipoprotein (a), and immunoreactive insulin levels in patients with the polycystic ovary syndrome, *Metabolism* 46:454, 1997.

56. **Veláquez E, Acosta A, Mendoza SG,** Menstrual cyclicity after metformin therapy in polycystic ovary syndrome, *Obstet Gynecol* 90:392, 1997.

57. **Diamanti-Kandarakis E, Kouli C, Tsianateli T, Bergiele A,** Therapeutic effects of metformin on insulin resistance and hyperandrogenism in polycystic ovary syndrome, *Eur J Endocrinol* 138:269, 1998.

58. **Nestler JE, Jakubowicz DJ, Evans WS, Pasquali R,** Effects of metformin on spontaneous and clomiphene-induced ovulation in the polycystic ovary syndrome, *New Engl J Med* 338:1876, 1998.

59. **Crave J-C, Fimbel S, Lejeune H, Cugnardey N, Dechaud H, Pugeat M,** Effects of diet and metformin administration on sex hormone-binding globulin, androgens, and insulin in hirsute and obese women, *J Clin Endocrinol Metab* 80:2057, 1995.

60. **Ehrmann DA, Cavaghan MK, Imperial J, Sturis J, Rosenfield RL, Polonsky KS,** Effects of metformin on insulin secretion, insulin action, and ovarian steroidogenesis in women with polycystic ovary syndrome, *J Clin Endocrinol Metab* 82:524, 1997.

61. **Açbay O, Gündogdu S,** Can metformin reduce insulin resistance in polycystic ovary syndrome? *Fertil Steril* 65:946, 1996.

62. **Nestler JE, Jakubowicz DJ,** Lean women with polycystic ovary syndrome respond to insulin reduction with decreases in ovarian P450c17α activity and serum androgens, *J Clin Endocrinol Metab* 82:4075, 1997.

63. **Dunaif A, Scott D, Finegood D, Quintana B, Whitcomb R,** The insulin-sensitizing agent troglitazone improves metabolic and reproductive abnormalities in the polycystic ovary syndrome, *J Clin Endocrinol Metab* 81:3299, 1996.

64. **Ehrmann DA, Schneider DJ, Sobel BE, Cavaghan MK, Imperial J, Rosenfield RL, Polonsky KS,** Troglitazone improves defects in insulin action, insulin secretion, ovarian steroidogenesis, and fibrinolysis in women with polycystic ovary syndrome, *J Clin Endocrinol Metab* 82:2108, 1997.

65. **Lobo RA, Paul W, March CM, Granger L, Kletzky OA,** Clomiphene and dexamethasone in women unresponsive to clomiphene alone, *Obstet Gynecol* 60:497, 1982.

66. **Daly DC, Walters CA, Soto-Albers CE, Tohan N, Riddick DH,** A randomized study of dexamethasone in ovulation induction with clomiphene citrate, *Fertil Steril* 41:844, 1984.

67. **Hoffman D, Lobo RA,** Serum dehydroepiandrosterone sulfate and the use of clomiphene citrate in anovulatory women, *Fertil Steril* 43:196, 1985.

68. **Trott EA, Plouffe Jr L, Hansen K, Hines R, Brann DW, Mahesh VB,** Ovulation induction in clomiphene-resistant anovulatory women with normal dehydroepiandrosterone sulfate levels: beneficial effects of the addition of dexamethasone during the follicular phase, *Fertil Steril* 66:484, 1996.

69. **Lobo RA, Granger LR, Davajan V, Mishell Jr DR,** An extended regimen of clomiphene citrate in women unresponsive to standard therapy, *Fertil Steril* 37:762, 1982.

70. **O'Herlihy C, Pepperell RJ, Brown JB, Smith MA, Sandri L, McBain JC,** Incremental clomiphene therapy: a new method for treating persistent anovulation, *Obstet Gynecol* 58:535, 1981.

71. **Fluker MR, Wang IY, Rowe TC,** An extended 10-day course of clomiphene citrate (CC) in women with CC-resistant ovulatory disorders, *Fertil Steril* 66:761, 1996.

72. **Genazzani AD, Petraglia F, Battaglia C, Gamba O, Volpe A, Genazzani AR,** A long-term treatment with gonadotropin-releasing hormone agonist plus a low-dose oral contraceptive improves the recovery of the ovulatory function in patients with polycystic ovary syndrome, *Fertil Steril* 67:463, 1997.

73. **Homburg R, Armar NA, Eshel A, Adams J, Jacobs HS,** Influence of serum luteinising hormone concentrations on ovulation, conception, and early pregnancy loss in polycystic ovary syndrome, *Br Med J* 297:1024, 1988.

74. **Regan L, Owen EJ, Jacobs HS,** Hypersecretion of luteinising hormone, infertility, and miscarriage, *Lancet* 336:1141, 1990.

75. **Watson H, Kiddy DS, Hamilton-Fairley D, Scanlon MJ, Barnard C, Collins WP, Bonney RC, Franks S,** Hypersecretion of luteinizing hormone and ovarian steroids in women with recurrent early miscarriage, *Hum Reprod* 8:829, 1993.

76. **Clifford K, Rai R, Watson H, Franks S, Regan L,** Does suppressing luteinising hormone secretion reduce the miscarriage rate? *Br Med J* 312:1508, 1996.

77. **Padilla SL, Person GK, McDonough PG, Reindollar RH,** The efficacy of bromocriptine in patients with ovulatory dysfunction and normoprolactinemic galactorrhea, *Fertil Steril* 44:695, 1985.

78. **Falaschi P, Rocco A, del Pozo E,** Inhibitory effect of bromocriptine treatment on luteinizing hormone secretion in polycystic ovary syndrome, *J Clin Endocrinol Metab* 62:348, 1986.

79. **Soto-Albers CE, Daly DC, Walters CA, Ying YK, Riddick DH,** Titrating the dose of bromocriptine when treating hyperprolactinemic women, *Fertil Steril* 43:485, 1985.

80. **Rains CP, Bryson HM, Fitton A,** Cabergoline. A review of its pharmacological properties and therapeutic potential in the treatment of hyperprolactinemia and inhibition of lactation, *Drugs* 49:255, 1995.

81. **Colao A, Di Sarno A, Sarnacchiaro F, Ferone D, Di Renzo G, Merola B, Annunziato L, Lombardi G,** Prolactinomas resistant to standard dopamine agonists respond to chronic cabergoline treatment, *J Clin Endocrinol Metab* 82:876, 1997.

82. **Ciccarelli E, Giusti M, Miola C, Potenzoni F, Sghedoni D, Camanni F, Giordano G,** Effectiveness and tolerability of long term treatment with cabergoline, a new long-lasting ergoline derivative, in hyperprolactinemic patients, *J Clin Endocrinol Metab* 69:725, 1989.

83. **Webster J, Piscitelli G, Polli A, Ferrari CI, Ismail I, Scanlon MF, for the Cabergoline Comparative Study Group,** A comparison of cabergoline and bromocriptine in the treatment of hyperprolactinemic amenorrhea, *New Engl J Med* 331:904, 1994.

84. **Biller BMK, Molitch ME, Vance ML, Cannistraro KB, Davis KR, Simons JA, Schoenfelder JR, Klibanski A,** Treatment of prolactin-secreting macroadenomas with the once-weekly dopamine agonist cabergoline, *J Clin Endocrinol Metab* 81:2338, 1996.

85. **Colao A, Di Sarno A, Landi ML, Cirillo S, Sarnacchiaro F, Gacciolli G, Pivonello R, Cataldi M, Merola B, Annuziato L, Lombardi G,** Long-term and low-dose treatment with cabergoline induces macroprolactinoma shrinkage, *J Clin Endocrinol Metab* 82:3574, 1997.

86. **Robert E, Musatti L, Piscitelli G, Ferrari CI,** Pregnancy outcome after treatment with the ergot drivative, cabergoline, *Reprod Toxicol* 10:333, 1996.

87. **Motta T, deVincentiis S, Marchinin M, Colombo N, D'Alberton A,** Vaginal cabergoline in the treatment of hyperprolactinemic patients intolerant to oral dopaminergics, *Fertil Steril* 65:440, 1996.

88. **Porcile A, Gallardo E, Venegas E,** Normoprolactinemic anovulation nonresponsive to clomiphene citrate: ovulation induction with bromocriptine, *Fertil Steril* 53:50, 1990.

89. **Suginami H, Hamada K, Yano K, Kuroda G, Matsuura S,** Ovulation induction with bromocriptine in normoprolactinemic anovulatory women, *J Clin Endocrinol Metab* 62:899, 1986.

90. **Weight CS, Steele SJ, Jacobs HS,** Value of bromocriptine in unexplained primary infertility: a double-blind controlled trial, *Br Med J* i:1037, 1979.

91. **DeVane GW, Guzick DS,** Bromocriptine therapy in normoprolactinemic women with unexplained infertility and galactorrhea, *Fertil Steril* 46:1026, 1986.

92. **Germond M, Dessole S, Senn A, Loumaye E, Howles C, Beltrami V,** Successful in-vitro fertilisation and embryo transfer after treatment with recombinant FSH, *Lancet* 339:1170, 1992.

93. **Farine D, Dor J, Lupovici N, Lunenfeld B, Mashiach S,** Conception rate after gonadotropin therapy in hyperprolactinemia and normoprolactinemia, *Obstet Gynecol* 65:658, 1985.

94. **Out HJ, Driessen SGAJ, Mannaerts BMJL, Coelingh Bennink HJT,** Recombinant follicle-stimulating hormone (follitropin beta, Puregon®) yields higher pregnancy rates in in vitro fertilization than urinary gonadotropins, *Fertil Steril* 68:138, 1997.

95. **Noci I, Biagiotti R, Maggi M, Ricci F, Cinotti A, Scarselli G,** Low day 3 luteinizing hormone values are predictive of reduced response to ovarian stimulation, *Hum Reprod* 13:531, 1998.

96. **van der Meer M, Hompes PGA, de Boer JAM, Schats R, Schoemaker J,** Cohort size rather than follicle-stimulating hormone threshold level determines ovarian sensitivity in polycystic ovary syndrome, *J Clin Endocrinol Metab* 83:423, 1998.

97. **Homburg R, Levy T, Ben-Rafael Z,** A comparative prospective study of conventional regimen with chronic low-dose administration of follicle-stimulating hormone for anovulation associated with polycystic ovary syndrome, *Fertil Steril* 63:729, 1995.

98. **White DM, Polson DW, Kiddy D, Sagle P, Watson H, Gilling-Smith C, Hamilton-Fairley D, Franks S,** Induction of ovulation with low-dose gonadotropins in polycystic ovary syndrome: an analysis of 109 pregnancies in 225 women, *J Clin Endocrinol Metab* 81:3821, 1996.

99. **Dale PO, Tanbo T, Haug E, Åbyholm T,** The impact of insulin resistance on the outcome of ovulation induction with low-dose follicle stimulating hormone in women with polycystic ovary syndrome, *Hum Reprod* 13:567, 1998.

100. **Gindoff PR, Jewelewicz R,** Use of gonadotropins in ovulation induction, *N Y State J Med* 85:580, 1985.

101. **Chong AP, Rafael RW, Forte CC,** Influence of weight in the induction of ovulation with human menopausal gonadotropin and human chorionic gonadotropin, *Fertil Steril* 46:599, 1986.

102. **Diamond MP, DeCherney AH, Baretto P, Lunenfeld B,** Multiple consecutive cycles of ovulation inductions with human menopausal gonadotropins, *Gynecol Endocrinol* 3:237, 1989.

103. **Silverberg KM, Klein NA, Burns WN, Schenken RS, Olive DL,** Consecutive versus alternating cycles of ovarian stimulation using human menopausal gonadotrophins, *Hum Reprod* 7:940, 1992.

104. **Haning Jr RV, Levin RM, Behrman HR, Kase NG, Speroff L,** Plasma estradiol window and urinary estriol glucuronide determination for monitoring menotropin induction of ovulation, *Obstet Gynecol* 54:442, 1979.

105. **Haning Jr RV, Boehnlein LM, Carlson IH, Kuzma DL, Zweibel WJ,** Diagnosis-specific serum 17β-estradiol (E2) upper limits for treatment with menotropins using a ^{125}I direct E2 assay, *Fertil Steril* 42:882, 1984.

106. **Wilson EA, Jawad MJ, Hayden TL,** Rates of exponential increase of serum estradiol concentrations in normal and human menopausal gonadotropin-induced cycles, *Fertil Steril* 37:46, 1982.

107. **Ritchie WGM,** Ultrasound in the evaluation of normal and induced ovulation, *Fertil Steril* 43:167, 1985.

108. **Leerentueld R, Van Gent I, Der Stoep M, Wladimiroff J,** Ultrasonographic assessment of Graffian follicle growth under monofollicular and multifollicular conditions in clomiphene citrate stimulated cycles, *Fertil Steril* 43:565, 1985.

109. **March CM,** Improved pregnancy rate with monitoring of gonadotropin therapy by three modalities, *Am J Obstet Gynecol* 156:1473, 1987.

110. **Tal J, Paz B, Samberg I, Lazarov N, Sharf M,** Ultrasonographic and clinical correlates of menotropin versus sequential clomiphene citrate: menotropin therapy for induction of ovulation, *Fertil Steril* 44:342, 1985.

111. **Blankstein J, Shalev J, Sasdon T, Kukia EE, Rabinovici J, Pariente C, Lunenfeld B, Serr DM, Mashiach S,** Ovarian hyperstimulation syndrome: prediction by number and size of preovulatory follicles, *Fertil Steril* 47:597, 1987.

112. **Ueno J, Oehninger S, Brzyski RG, Acosta AA, Philput B, Muasher SJ,** Ultrasonographic appearance of the endometrium in natural and stimulated in-vitro fertilization cycles and its correlation with outcome, *Hum Reprod* 6:901, 1991.

113. **Shoham Z, Di Carlo C, Patel A, Conway GS, Jacobs HS,** Is it possible to run a successful ovulation induction program based solely on ultrasound monitoring? The importance of endometrial measurements, *Fertil Steril* 56:836, 1991.

114. **Dickey RP, Olar TT, Taylor SN, Curole DN, Matulich EM,** Relationship of endometrial thickness and pattern to fecundity in ovulation induction cycles: effect of clomiphene citrate alone and with human menopausal gonadotropin, *Fertil Steril* 59:756, 1993.

115. **Shapiro H, Cowell C, Casper RF,** The use of vaginal ultrasound for monitoring endometrial preparation in a donor oocyte program, *Fertil Steril* 59:1055, 1993.

116. **Isaacs Jr JD, Wells CS, Williams DB, Odem RR, Gast MJ, Strickler RC,** Endometrial thickness is a valid monitoring parameter in cycles of ovulation induction with menotropins alone, *Fertil Steril* 65:262, 1996.

117. **Akin JW, Shepard MK,** The effects of baseline ovarian cysts on cycle fecundity in controlled ovarian hyperstimulation, *Fertil Steril* 59:453, 1993.

118. **March CM, Tredway DR, Mishell Jr DR,** Effect of clomiphene citrate upon amount and duration of human menopausal gonadotropin therapy, *Am J Obstet Gynecol* 125:699, 1976.

119. **Ho Yuen B, Pride SM, Burch-Callegari P, Leroux AM, Moon YS,** Clinical and endocrine response to pulsatile intravenous gonadotropins in refractory anovulation, *Obstet Gynecol* 74:763, 1989.

120. **Nakamura Y, Yoshimura Y, Yamada H, Ubukata Y, Yoshida K, Tamaoka Y, Suzuki M,** Clinical experience in the induction of ovulation and pregnancy with pulsatile subcutaneous administration of human menopausal gonadotropin: a low incidence of multiple pregnancy, *Fertil Steril* 51:423, 1989.

121. **Ho Yuen B, Pride S,** Induction of ovulation with exogenous gonadotropins in anovulatory infertile women, *Seminars Reprod Endocrinol* 8:1861, 1990.

122. **Fluker MR, Urman B, MacKinnon M, Barrow SR, Pride SM, Ho Yuen B,** Exogenous gonadotropin therapy in World Health Organization Groups I and II ovulatory disorders, *Obstet Gynecol* 83:189, 1994.

123. **Balen AH, Braat DDM, West C, Patel A, Jacobs HS,** Cumulative conception and live birth rates after the treatment of anovulatory infertility: safety and efficacy of ovulation induction in 200 patients, *Hum Reprod* 9:1563, 1994.

124. **Fernandez H, Coste J, Job-Spira N,** Controlled ovarian hyperstimulation as a risk factor for ectopic pregnancy, *Obstet Gynecol* 78:656, 1991.

125. **Hamilton-Fairley D, Kiddy D, Watson H, Paterson C, Franks S,** Association of moderate obesity with a poor pregnancy outcome in women with polycystic ovary syndrome treated with low dose gonadotropin, *Br J Obstet Gynaecol* 99:128, 1992.

126. **Keenan JA, Moghissi KS,** Luteal phase support with hCG does not improve fecundity rate in human menopausal gonadotropin-stimulated cycles, *Obstet Gynecol* 79:983, 1992.

127. **Kurinczuk JJ, Pemberton RJ, Binns SC, Parsons DE, Stanley FJ,** Singleton and twin confinements associated with infertility treatments, *Aust N Z J Obstet Gynaecol* 35:27, 1995.

128. **Ho ML, Chen JY, Ling UP, Chen JH, Huang CM, Chang CC, Su PH,** Changing epidemiology of triplet pregnancy: etiology and outcome over twelve years, *Am J Perinatol* 13:269, 1996.

129. **Corchia C, Mastroiacovo P, Lanni R, Mannazzu R, Curro V, Fabris C,** What proportion of multiple births are due to ovulation induction? A register-based study in Italy, *Am J Public Health* 86:851, 1996.

130. **Derom C, Derom R, Vlietink R, Van Den Berghe H, Thiery M,** Increased monozygotic twinning rate after ovulation induction, *Lancet* i:1236, 1987.

131. **Bohrer M, Kemmann E,** Risk factors for spontaneous abortion in menotropin-treated women, *Fertil Steril* 48:571, 1987.

132. **Ben-Rafael Z, Mashiach S, Oelsner G, Farine D, Lunenfeld B, Serr DM,** Spontaneous pregnancy and its outcome after human menopausal gonadotropin/human chorionic gonadotropin-induced pregnancy, *Fertil Steril* 36:560, 1981.

133. **Aboulghar MA, Mansour RT, Serour GI, Rizk P, Riad R,** Improvement of spontaneous pregnancy rate after stopping gonadotropin therapy for anovulatory infertility, *Fertil Steril* 55:722, 1991.

134. **Evans MI, Dommergues M, Timor-Tritsch I, Zador IE, Wapner RJ, Lynch L, Dumez Y, Goldberg JD, Nicolaides KH, Johnson MP, Golbus MS, Boulot P, Aknin AJ, Monteagudo A, Berkowitz RL,** Transabdominal versus transcervical and transvaginal multifetal pregnancy reduction: international collaborative experience of more than one thousand cases, *Am J Obstet Gynecol* 170:902, 1994.

135. **Kol S, Levron J, Lewit N, Drugan A, Itskovitz-Eldor J,** The natural history of multiple pregnancies after assisted reproduction: is spontaneous fetal demise a clinically significant phenomenon? *Fertil Steril* 60:127, 1993.

136. **Engel T, Jewelewicz R, Dyrenfurth I, Speroff L, Vande Wiele RL,** Ovarian hyperstimulation syndrome: report of a case with notes on pathogenesis and treatment, *Am J Obstet Gynecol* 112:1052, 1972.

137. **Navot D, Bergh PA, Laufer N,** Ovarian hyperstimulation syndrome in novel reproductive technologies: prevention and treatment, *Fertil Steril* 58:249, 1992.

138. **Schenker JG,** Prevention and treatment of ovarian hyperstimulation, *Hum Reprod* 8:653, 1993.

139. **Mashiach S, Bider D, Moran O, Goldenberg M, Ben-Rafael Z,** Adnexal torsion of hyperstimulated ovaries in pregnancies after gonadotropin therapy, *Fertil Steril* 53:76, 1990.

140. **Rizk B, Smitz J,** Ovarian hyperstimulation syndrome after superovulation using GnRH agonists for IVF and related procedures, *Hum Reprod* 7:320, 1992.

141. **Morris RS, Paulson RJ, Sauer MV, Lobo RA,** Predictive value of serum oestradiol concentrations and oocyte number in severe ovarian hyperstimulation syndrome, *Hum Reprod* 10:811, 1995.

142. **Neulen J, Yan Z, Raczek S, Weindel K, Keck C, Weich Ha, Marme D, Breckwoldt M,** Human chorionic gonadotropin-dependent expression of vascular endothelial growth factor/vascular permeability factor in human granulosa cells: importance in ovarian hyperstimulation syndrome, *J Clin Endocrinol Metab* 80:1967, 1995.

143. **Abramov Y, Barak V, Nisman B, Schenker JG,** Vascular endothelial growth factor plasma levels correlate to the clinical picture in severe ovarian hyperstimulation syndrome, *Fertil Steril* 67:261, 1997.

144. **Lee A, Christenson LK, Stouffer RL, Burry KA, Patton PE,** Vascular endothelial growth factor levels in serum and follicular fluid of patients undergoing in vitro fertilization, *Fertil Steril* 68:305, 1997.

145. **Revel A, Barak V, Lavy Y, Anteby E, Abramov Y, Schenker JJ, Amit A, Finci-Yeheskel Z, Mayer M, Simon A, Laufer N, Hurwitz A,** Characterization of intraperitoneal cytokines and nitrites in women with severe ovarian hyperstimulation syndrome, *Fertil Steril* 66:66, 1996.

146. **Abramov Y, Schenker JG, Lewin A, Friedler S, Nisman B, Barak V,** Plasma inflammatory cytokines correlate to the ovarian hyperstimulation syndrome, *Hum Reprod* 11:1381, 1996.

147. **Delbaere A, Bergmann PJM, Gervy-Decoster C, Deschodt-Lanckman M, de Maertelaer V, Staroukine M, Camus M, Englert Y,** Increased angiotensin II in ascites during severe ovarian hyperstimulation syndrome: role of early pregnancy and ovarian gonadotropin stimulation, *Fertil Steril* 67:1038, 1997.

148. **Haning Jr RV, Strawn EY, Nolten WE,** Pathophysiology of the ovarian hyperstimulation syndrome, *Obstet Gynecol* 66:220, 1985.

149. **Rizk B, Aboulghar M,** Modern management of ovarian hyperstimulation syndrome, *Hum Reprod* 6:1082, 1991.

150. **Rizk B, Meagher S, Fisher AM,** Severe ovarian hyperstimulation syndrome and cerebrovascular accidents, *Hum Reprod* 5:697, 1990.

151. **Fournet N, Surrey E, Kerin J,** Internal jugular vein thrombosis after ovulation induction with gonadotropins, *Fertil Steril* 56:354, 1991.

152. **Stewart JA, Hamilton PJ, Murdoch AP,** Thromboembolic disease associated with ovarian stimulation and assisted conception techniques, *Hum Reprod* 12:2167, 1997.

153. **Zosmer A, Katz Z, Lancet M, Konichezky S, Schwartz-Shoham Z,** Adult respiratory distress syndrome complicating ovarian hyperstimulation syndrome, *Fertil Steril* 47:524, 1987.

154. **Kirshon B, Doody MC, Cotton DB, Gibbons W,** Management of ovarian hyperstimulation syndrome with chlorpheniramine maleate, mannitol, and invasive hemodynamic monitoring, *Obstet Gynecol* 71:485, 1988.

155. **Padilla SA, Zamaria S, Baramki TA, Garcia JE,** Abdominal paracentesis for the ovarian hyperstimulation syndrome with severe pulmonary compromise, *Fertil Steril* 53:365, 1990.

156. **Aboulghar MA, Mansour RT, Serour GI, Sattar MA, Amin YM, Elattar I,** Management of severe ovarian hyperstimulation syndrome by ascitic fluid aspiration and intensive intravenous fluid therapy, *Obstet Gynecol* 81:108, 1993.

157. **Fakih H, Bello S,** Ovarian cyst aspiration: a therapeutic approach to ovarian hyperstimulation syndrome, *Fertil Steril* 58:829, 1992.

158. **Cameron IT, O'Shea FC, Rolland JM, Hughes EG, de Kretser DM, Healy DL,** Occult ovarian failure: a syndrome of infertility, regular menses, and elevated follicle-stimulating hormone concentrations, *J Clin Endocrinol Metab* 67:1190, 1986.

159. **Buckler HM, Evans A, Mamlora H, Burger HG, Anderson DC,** Gonadotropin, steroid and inhibin levels in women with incipient ovarian failure during anovulatory and ovulatory 're-bound' cycles, *J Clin Endocrinol Metab* 72:116, 1991.

160. **Lenton EA, de Kretser DM, Woodward AJ, Robertson DM,** Inhibin concentrations throughout the menstrual cycles of normal, infertile, and older women compared with those during spontaneous conception cycles, *J Clin Endocrinol Metab* 73:1180, 1991.

161. **McNaughton J, Banah M, McCloud P, Hee J, Burger H,** Age related changes in follicle stimulating hormone, luteinizing hormone, oestradiol and immunoreactive inhibin in women of reproductive age, *Clin Endocrinol* 36:339, 1992.

162. **Pellicer A, Marí M, de los Santos MJ, Simón C, Remohí J, Tarín JJ,** Effects of aging on the human ovary: the secretion of immunoreactive α-inhibin and progesterone, *Fertil Steril* 61:663, 1994.

163. **Burger HG, Cahir N, Robertson DM, Groome NP, Dudley E, Green A, Dennerstein L,** Serum inhibins A and B fall differentially as FSH rises in perimenopausal women, *Clin Endocrinol* 48:809, 1998.

164. **Klein NA, Illingworth PJ, Groome NP, McNeilly AS, Battaglia DE, Soules MR,** Decreased inhibin B secretion is associated with the monotropic FSH rise in older, ovulatory women: a study of serum and follicular fluid leavels of dimeric inhibin A and B in spontaneous menstrual cycles, *J Clin Endocrinol Metab* 81:2742, 1996.

165. **Hofmann GE, Danforth DR, Seifer DB,** Inhibin-B: the physiologic basis of the clomiphene citrate challenge test for ovarian reserve screening, *Fertil Steril* 69:474, 1998.

166. **Danforth DR, Arbogast LK, Mroueh J, Kim MH, Kennard EA, seifer DB, Friedman CI,** Dimeric inhibin: a direct marker of ovarian aging, *Fertil Steril* 70:119, 1998.

167. **Klein NA, Battaglia DE, Miller PB, Branigan EF, Giudice LC, Soules MR,** Ovarian follicular development and the follicular fluid hormones and growth factors in normal women of advanced reproductive age, *J Clin Endocrinol Metab* 81:1946, 1996.

168. **Lass A, Silye R, Abrams D-C, Krausz T, Hovatta O, Margara R, Winston RML,** Follicular density in ovarian biopsy of infertile women: a novel method to assess ovarian reserve, *Hum Reprod* 12:1028, 1997.

169. **Lass A, Skull J, McVeigh E, Margara R, Winston RM,** Measurement of ovarian volume by transvaginal sonography before human menopausal gonadotrophin superovulation for in-vitro fertlization can predict poor response, *Hum Reprod* 12:294, 1997.

170. **Toner JP, Philput CB, Jones GS, Muasher SJ,** Basal follicle-stimulating hormone level is a better predictor of in vitro fertilization performance than age, *Fertil Steril* 55:784, 1991.

171. **Pearlstone AC, Fournet N, Gambone JC, Pang SC, Buyalos RP,** Ovulation induction in women age 40 and older: the importance of basal follicle-stimulating hormone level and chronological age, *Fertil Steril* 58:674, 1992.

172. **Scott Jr RT, Hofmann GE,** Prognostic assessment of ovarian reserve, *Fertil Steril* 63:1, 1995.

173. **Smotrich DB, Widra EA, Gindoff PR, Levy MJ, Hall JL, Stillman RJ,** Prognostic value of day 3 estradiol on in vitro fertilization outcome, *Fertil Steril* 64:1136, 1995.

174. **Buyalos RP, Daneshmand S, Brzechffa PR,** Basal estradiol and follicle-stimulating hormone predict fecundity in women of advanced reproductive age undergoing ovulation induction therapy, *Fertil Steril* 68:272, 1997.

175. **Navot D, Rosenwaks Z, Margalioth EJ,** Prognostic assessment of female fecundity, *Lancet* ii:645, 1987.

176. **Tanbo T, Dale PO, Lunde O, Norman N, Abyholm T,** Prediction of response to controlled ovarian hyperstimulation: a comparison of basal and clomiphene citrate-stimulated follicle-stimulating hormone levels, *Fertil Steril* 57:819, 1992.

177. **Scott Jr RT, Leonardi MR, Hofmann GE, Illions EH, Neal GS, Navot D,** A prospective evaluation of clomiphene citrate challenge test screening of the general infertility population, *Obstet Gynecol* 82:539, 1993.

178. **Scott Jr RT, Opsahl MS, Leonardi MR, Neal GS, Illions EH, Navot D,** Life table analysis of pregnancy rates in a general infertility population relative to ovarian reserve and patient age, *Hum Reprod* 10:1706, 1995.

179. **Farhi J, Homburg R, Ferber A, Orvieto R, Ben Rafael Z,** Non-response to ovarian stimulation in normogonadotrophic, normogonadal women: a clinical sign of impending onset of ovarian failure pre-empting the rise in basal follicle stimulating hormone levels, *Hum Reprod* 12:241, 1997.

180. **Dodson WC,** Gonadotropin releasing analogues as adjunctive therapy in ovulation induction, *Seminars Reprod Endocrinol* 8:198, 1990.

181. **Dodson WC, Hughes CL, Whitesides DB, Haney AF,** The effect of leuprolide acetate on ovulation induction with human menopausal gonadotropins in polycystic ovary syndrome, *J Clin Endocrinol Metab* 65:95, 1987.

182. **Homburg R, Levy T, Berkovitz D, Farchi J, Feldberg D, Ashkenazi J, Ben-Rafael Z,** Gonadotropin-releasing hormone agonist reduces the miscarriage rate for pregnancies achieved in women with polycystic ovarian syndrome, *Fertil Steril* 59:527, 1993.

183. **Mizunuma H, Andoh K, Yamada K, Takagi T, Kamijo T, Ibuki Y,** Prediction and prevention of ovarian hyperstimulation by monitoring endogenous luteinizing hormone release during purified follicle-stimulating hormone therapy, *Fertil Steril* 58:46, 1992.

184. **Devroey P, Mannaerts B, Smitz J, Coelingh Bennink H, Van Steirteghem A,** Clinical outcome of a pilot efficacy study on recombinant human follicle-stimulating hormone (Org 32489) combined with various gonadotrophin-releasing hormone agonist regimens, *Hum Reprod* 9:1064, 1994.

185. **Smitz J, Devroey P, Camus M, Deschacht J, Khan I, Staessen C, Van Waesberghe L, Wisanto A, Van Steirteghem AC,** The luteal phase and early pregnancy after combined GnRH-agonist/hMG treatment for superovulation in IVF and GIFT, *Hum Reprod* 3:585, 1988.

186. **McClure N, Leya J, Radwanska E, Rawlins R, Haning Jr RV,** Luteal phase support and severe ovarian hyperstimulation syndrome, *Hum Reprod* 7:758, 1992.

187. **Albano C, J, Camus M, Riethmüller-Winzen H, Siebert-Weigel M, Diedrich K, Van Steirteghem AC, Devroey P,** Comparison of different doses of gonadotropin-releasing hormone antagonist Cetrorelix during controlled ovarian hyperstimulation, *Fertil Steril* 67:917, 1997.

188. **Ibrahim ZHZ, Lieberman BA, Matson PL, Buck P,** The use of biosynthetic growth hormone to augment ovulation induction with buserelin acetate/human menopausal gonadotrophin in women with a poor ovarian response, *Fertil Steril* 55:202, 1991.

189. **Owen EJ, Shoham Z, Mason BA, Ostergaard H, Jacobs HS,** Cotreatment with growth hormone, after pituitary suppression, for ovarian stimulation in in vitro fertilization: a randomized, double-blind, placebo-control trial, *Fertil Steril* 56:1104, 1991.

190. **Hughes SM, Huang ZH, Matson PL, Buck P, Lieberman BA, Morris ID,** Clinical and endocrinological changes in women following ovulation induction using buserelin acetate/human menopausal gonadotrophin augmented with biosynthetic human growth hormone, *Hum Reprod* 7:770, 1992.

191. **Levy T, Limor R, Villa Y, Eshel A, Eckstein N, Vagman I, Lidor A, Ayalon D,** Another look at co-treatment with growth hormone and human menopausal gonadotrophins in poor ovarian responders, *Hum Reprod* 8:834, 1993.

192. **Tulandi T, Galcone T, Guyda H, Hemmings R, Billiar R, Morris D,** Effects of synthetic growth hormone-releasing factor in women treated with gonadotrophin, *Hum Reprod* 8:525, 1993.

193. **Hugues JN, Torresani T, Herve F, Martin-Point B, Tamboise A, Sanarelli J,** Interest of growth hormone-releasing hormone administration for improvement of ovarian repsonsiveness to gonadotropins in poor responder women, *Fertil Steril* 55:945, 1991.

194. **Volve A, Coukos G, Barreca A, Giordano G, Artini PG, Genazzani AR,** Clinical use of growth hormone-releasing factor for induction of superovulation, *Hum Reprod* 6:1228, 1991.

195. **Bunger CW, Korsen TJM, Hompes PGA, Vankessel H, Schoemaker J,** Ovulation induction with pulsatile LHRH in women with clomiphene resistant polycystic ovary-like disease: clinical results, *Fertil Steril* 46:1045, 1986.

196. **Filicori M, Flamigni C, Meriggiola MC, Ferrari P, Michelacci L, Campaniello E, Valdiserri A, Cognigni G,** Endocrine response determines the clinical outcome of pulsatile gonadotropin-releasing hormone ovulation induction in different ovulatory disorders, *J Clin Endocrinol Metab* 72:965, 1991.

197. **Carr JS, Reid RL,** Ovulation induction with gonadotropin-releasing hormone (GnRH), *Seminars Reprod Endocrinol* 8:174, 1990.

198. **Filicori M, Flamigni C, Dellai P, Cognigni G, Michelacci L, Arnone R, Sambataro M, Falbo A,** Treatment of anovulation with pulsatile gonadotropin-releasing hormone: prognostic factors and clinical results in 600 cycles, *J Clin Endocrinol Metab* 79:1215, 1994.

199. **Braat DD, Schoemaker R, Schoemaker J,** Life table analysis of fecundity of intravenously gonadotropin-releasing hormone-treated patients with normogonadotropic and hypogonadotropic amenorrhea, *Fertil Steril* 55:266, 1991.

200. **Filicori M, Flamigni C, Campaniello E, Meriggiola MC, Michelacci L, Valdiserri A, Ferrari P,** Polycystic ovary syndrome: abnormalities and management with pulsatile gonadotropin-releasing hormone and gonadotropin-releasing hormone analogs, *Am J Obstet Gynecol* 163:1737, 1990.

201. **Stein IF, Leventhal ML,** Amenorrhea associated with bilateral polycystic ovaries, *Am J Obstet Gynecol* 29:181, 1935.

202. **Judd HL, Rigg LA, Anderson DC, Yen SSC,** The effect of ovarian wedge resection on circulating gonadotropin and ovarian steroid levels in patients with polycystic ovary syndrome, *J Clin Endocrinol Metab* 43:347, 1976.

203. **Katz M, Carr PJ, Cohen BM, Milhin RP,** Hormonal effects of wedge resection of polycystic ovaries, *Obstet Gynecol* 51:437, 1978.

204. **Kaaijk EM, Beek JF, Hamerlynck JVTH, van der Veen F,** Unilateral oophorectomy in polycystic ovary syndrome: a treatment option in highly selected cases? *Hum Reprod* 12:2370, 1997.

205. **Kovacs G, Buckler H, Gangah M, Burger H, Healy D, Baker G, Phillips S,** Treatment of anovulation due to polycystic ovarian syndrome by laparoscopic ovarian electrocautery, *Br J Obstet Gynaecol* 98:30, 1991.

206. **Daniell JF, Miller W,** Polycystic ovaries treated by laparoscopic laser vaporization, *Fertil Steril* 51:232, 1989.

207. **Gadir A, Mowafi RS, Alnaser HMI, Alrashid AH, Alonezi OM, Shaw RW,** Ovarian electrocautery versus human menopausal gonadotrophins and pure follicle stimulating hormone therapy in the treatment of patients with polycystic ovarian disease, *Clin Endocrinol* 33:585, 1990.

208. **Naether OGJ, Fischer R, Weise HC, Geiger-Kotzler L, Delfs T, Rudolf K,** Laparoscopic electrocoagulation of the ovarian surface in infertile patients and polycystic ovarian disease, *Fertil Steril* 60:88, 1993.

209. **Armar NA, Lachelin GCL,** Laparoscopic ovarian diathermy: an effective treatment for anti-oestrogen resistant anovulatory infertility in women with polycystic ovarian syndrome, *Br J Obstet Gynaecol* 100:161, 1993.

210. **Campo S,** Ovulatory cycles, pregnancy outcome and complications after surgical treatment of polycystic ovary syndrome, *Obstet Gynecol Survey* 53:297, 1998.

211. **Naether OGJ, Fischer R,** Adhesion formation after laparoscopic electrocoagulation of the ovarian surface in polycystic ovary patients, *Fertil Steril* 60:95, 1993.

212. **Crosignani PG, Walters DS, Soliani A,** Addendum to the ESHRE multicentre trial: a summary of the abortion and birth statistics, *Hum Reprod* 7:286, 1992.

213. **Tummon IS, Macklin VM, Radwanska E, Binor Z, Dimowski WP,** Occult ovulatory dysfunction in women with minimal endometriosis or unexplained infertility, *Fertil Steril* 50:716, 1988.

214. **Leach RE, Moghissi KS, Randolph JF, Reame NE, Blacker CM, Ginsburg KA, Diamond MP,** Intensive hormone monitoring in women with unexplained infertility: evidence for subtle abnormalities suggestive of diminished ovarian reserve, *Fertil Steril* 68:413, 1997.

215. **Simon A, Laufer N,** Unexplained infertility: a reappraisal, *Assist Reprod Rev* 3:26, 1993.

216. **Glazener CMA, Coulson C, Lambert PA, Watt EM, Hinton RA, Kelly NG, Hull MGR,** Clomiphene treatment for women with unexplained infertility: placebo-controlled study of hormonal responses and conception rates, *Gynecol Endocrinol* 4:75, 1990.

217. **Deaton JL, Gibson N, Blackmer KM, Nakajima ST, Badger GJ, Brumsted JR,** A randomized, controlled trial of clomiphene citrate and intrauterine insemination in couples with unexplained infertility, *Fertil Steril* 54:1083, 1990.

218. **Karlstrom P-O, Bergh T, Lundkvist O,** A prospective randomized trial of artificial insemination versus intercourse in cycles stimulated with human menopausal gonadotropin or clomiphene citrate, *Fertil Steril* 59:554, 1993.

219. **Martinez AR, Bernardos RE, Voorhorst FJ, Vermeiden JPW, Schoemaker J,** Intrauterine insemination does and clomiphene citrate does not improve fecundity in couples with infertility due to male or idiopathic factors: a prospective, randomized, controlled study, *Fertil Steril* 53:847, 1990.

220. **Fujii S, Fukui A, Fukushi Y, Kagiya A, Sato S, Saito Y,** The effects of clomiphene citrate on normal ovulatory women, *Fertil Steril* 68:997, 1997.

221. **Agarwal SK, Buyalos RP,** Clomiphene citrate with intrauterine insemination: is it effective therapy in women above the age of 35 years? *Fertil Steril* 65:759, 1996.

222. **Serhal PF, Katz M, Little V, Woronowski H,** Unexplained infertility — the value of pergonal superovulation combined with intrauterine insemination, *Fertil Steril* 49:602, 1988.

223. **Chaffkin LM, Nulsen JC, Luciano AA, Metzger DA,** A comparative analysis of the cycle fecundity rates associated with combined human menopausal gonadotropin (hMG) and intrauterine insemination (IUI) versus either hMG or IUI alone, *Fertil Steril* 55:252, 1991.

224. **Nulsen JC, Walsh S, Dumez S, Metzger DA,** A randomized and longitudinal study of human menopausal gonadotropin with intrauterine insemination in the treatment of infertility, *Obstet Gynecol* 82:780, 1993.

225. **Kemmann E, Bohrer M, Shelden R, Fiasconaro G, Beardsley L,** Active ovulation management increases the monthly probability of pregnancy occurrence in ovulatory women who receive intrauterine insemination, *Fertil Steril* 48:916, 1987.

226. **Zeyneloglu HB, Arici A, Olive DL, Duleba AJ,** Comparison of intrauterine insemination with timed intercourse in superovulated cycles with gonadotropins: a meta-analysis, *Fertil Steril* 69:486, 1998.

227. **Dodson WC, Whitesides DB, Hughes Jr CL, Easley III HA, Haney AF,** Superovulation with intrauterine insemination in the treatment of infertility: a possible alternative to gamete intrafallopian transfer and in vitro fertilization, *Fertil Steril* 48:441, 1987.

228. **Dodson WL, Haney AF,** Controlled ovarian hyperstimulation and intrauterine insemination for treatment of infertility, *Fertil Steril* 55:457, 1991.

229. **DiMarzo SJ, Kennedy JF, Young PE, Hebert SA, Rosenberg DC, Villanueva B,** Effects of controlled ovarian hyperstimulation on pregnancy rates after intrauterine insemination, *Am J Obstet Gynecol* 166:1607, 1992.

230. **Guzick DS, Sullivan MW, Adamson GD, Cedars MI, Falk RJ, Peterson EP, Steinkampf MP,** Efficacy of treatment of unexplained infertility, *Fertil Steril* 70:207, 1998.

231. **Hughes EG,** The effectiveness of ovulation induction and intrauterine insemination in the treatment of persistent infertility: a meta-analysis, *Hum Reprod* 12:1865, 1997.

232. **Corsan G, Trias A, Trout S, Kemmann E,** Ovulation induction combined with intrauterine insemination in women 40 years of age and older: is it worthwhile? *Hum Reprod* 11:1109, 1996.

233. **Whittemore AS, Harris R, Itnyre J, and the Collaborative Ovarian Cancer Group,** Characteristics relating to ovarian cancer risk: collaborative analysis of 12 US case-control studies. II: Invasive epithelial ovarian cancers in white women, *Am J Epidemiol* 136:1184, 1992.

234. **Rossing MA, Daling JR, Weiss NS, Moore DE, Self SG,** Ovarian tumors in a cohort of infertile women, *New Engl J Med* 331:771, 1994.

235. **Ron E, Lunenfeld B, Menczer J, Blumstein T, Katz L, Oelsner G, Serr D,** Cancer incidence in a cohort of infertile women, *Am J Epidemiol* 125:780, 1987.

236. **Shushan A, Paltiel O, Iscovich J, Elchalal U, Peretz T, Schenker JG,** Human menopausal gonadotropin and the risk of epithelial ovarian cancer, *Fertil Steril* 65:13, 1996.

237. **Franceschi S, La Vecchia C, Negri E, Guarneri S, Montella M, Conti E, Parazzini F,** Fertility drugs and risk of epithelial ovarian cancer in Italy, *Hum Reprod* 9:1673, 1994.

238. **Parazzini F, Negri E, La Vecchia C, Moroni S, Franceschi S, Crosignani PG,** Treatment for infertility and risk of invasive epithelial ovarian cancer, *Hum Reprod* 12:2159, 1997.

239. **Mosgaard BJ, Lidegaard Ø, Kjaer SK, Schou G, Andersen AN,** Infertility, fertility drugs, and invasive ovarian cancer: a case-control study, *Fertil Steril* 67:1005, 1997.

240. **Mosgaard BJ, Lidegaard Ø, Andersen AN,** The impact of parity, infertility and treatment with fertility drugs on the risk of ovarian cancer, *Acta Obstet Gynecol Scand* 76:89, 1997.

241. **Guzick DS, Carson SA, Coutifaris C, Overstreet JW, Factor-Litvak P, Staimkampf MP, Hill JA, Mastroianni Jr L, Buster JE, Nakajima ST, Vogel DL, Canfield RE, for the National Cooperative Reproductive Medicine Network,** Efficacy of superovulation and intrauterine insemination in the treatment of infertility, *New Engl J Med* 340:177, 1999.

31   Assisted Reproduction

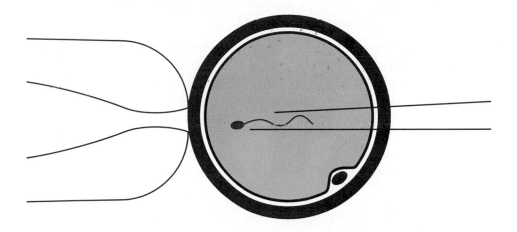

Assisted reproductive technology (ART) refers to all techniques involving direct retrieval of oocytes from the ovary. The first and still most common procedure is in vitro fertilization, but there is an ever increasing list of technologies.

IVF — In Vitro Fertilization: extraction of oocytes, fertilization in the laboratory, transcervical transfer of embryos into the uterus.

GIFT — Gamete Intrafallopian Transfer: the placement of oocytes and sperm into the fallopian tube.

ZIFT — Zygote Intrafallopian Transfer: the placement of fertilized oocytes into the fallopian tube.

TET — Tubal Embryo Transfer: the placement of cleaving embryos into the fallopian tube.

POST — Peritoneal Oocyte and Sperm Transfer: the placement of oocytes and sperm into the pelvic cavity.

In addition, techniques of sperm retrieval and sperm injection are now part of the assisted reproductive technology armamentarium:

ICSI — Intracytoplasmic Sperm Injection (of a single spermatozoon).

TESE — Testicular Sperm Extraction.

MESA — Microsurgical Epididymal Sperm Aspiration.

It has been over two decades since the birth of the first child conceived by in vitro fertilization (IVF). During the intervening years, the number of IVF programs has increased to over 250 in the United States alone, technology has evolved, the success rate has improved dramatically, and indications for IVF have enlarged. In addition, procedures that utilize some, but not all, of the methodology of IVF have become a part of clinical practice.

Numerous volumes have been published which extensively cover all aspects of ART, and we will not duplicate that effort. Rather, this chapter will focus on the evolving techniques with an emphasis on ICSI, and will review briefly the place of ART in the treatment of nontubal disease.

Patient Selection for IVF

The initial experience with in vitro fertilization involved women with tubal disease, but early in the 1980s, the treatment was extended to individuals with male factor infertility, unexplained infertility, endometriosis, and immunologic causes for infertility. In addition, a high degree of success has been obtained using donor oocytes for women with premature ovarian failure or decreased ovarian function.[1] Although it is reasonable to recommend tubal surgery in young women with mild distal tubal disease, IVF is the treatment of choice for patients with more severe distal disease, proximal obstruction (especially after 6 months have elapsed following cannulation or balloon tuboplasty), and for patients who have failed to achieve pregnancy within 2 years after tubal surgery or when tubal obstruction persists after surgery. Large hydrosalpinges can reduce the success rate with IVF, and removal is recommended prior to treatment.[2]

Couples undergoing IVF should be screened for antibodies to HIV-1/2 and HTLV-1, hepatitis B antigen, and antibodies to hepatitis B and C. Testing for chlamydia, syphilis, gonorrhea, and cytomegalovirus should also be considered. Smoking, as always, should be discouraged; smokers require twice as many IVF cycles to achieve pregnancy.[3]

Whereas IVF can overcome a number of the barriers to fertility, it suffers the same limitation as does in vivo fertilization when it comes to age (discussed in Chapter 26). In successful IVF programs, where the delivery rate per oocyte retrieval can be over 30% in women age 35 or younger, the figure is 10% or less in women age 40 and over. Beyond the simple effect of age on oocyte quality, there also is a negative influence on IVF success from decreased ovarian responsiveness. This can be manifested by poor response to exogenous gonadotropin stimulation with abnormal hormone profiles and the retrieval of small numbers of oocytes.

There is no exact definition of a poor responder, but it encompasses those who respond to stimulation with the development of 4 or fewer follicles or with depressed estrogen levels. Pretreatment diagnosis of these individuals can be achieved by measuring basal FSH and estradiol levels, and by using the clomiphene challenge test (see Chapter 26).

Three distinct populations have been identified on the basis of the cycle day three FSH.[4] With FSH values less than 15 IU/L, the pregnancy rate with IVF was 24%, whereas when the FSH values were 15 to 24.9 IU/L, the pregnancy rate was 13.6%. When the FSH was 25 IU/L or higher, the initial pregnancy rate was 10.7%, and the ongoing pregnancy rate was only 3.6%. Remember in all discussions pertaining to specific hormone levels that these may differ between laboratories, depending on which assay system is used. Assays using new standards have an upper limit of normal of 10–12 IU/L compared with the 25 IU/L cited in the above study.

Older women (certainly 40 and older, but perhaps even women in their late 30s) with infertility and younger women with abnormal basal FSH and estradiol values and an abnormal response to a clomiphene challenge should seriously consider an early resort to hormonal stimulation for both multiple oocyte response and better support of the endometrium. Older couples should be provided the option of oocyte donation from young donors instead of standard assisted reproductive technologies.

Stimulation Protocol

The momentous work of Edwards and Steptoe that produced the first birth from IVF was developed over more than 10 years. Success was finally achieved by utilizing a nonstimulated cycle with timing of oocyte retrieval based on measurements of luteinizing hormone (LH) at 3-hour intervals. Nonstimulated cycles are still used as a means of decreasing expenses, but the delivery rate per retrieval is only approximately 6%.[5] The very low success rate associated with nonstimulated cycles led to the use of clomiphene citrate and human menopausal gonadotropins to stimulate the development of multiple ovarian follicles. Injections of human chorionic gonadotropin (HCG), whose biologic activity mimics that of LH, were utilized to allow more certain timing of oocyte retrieval.

In the late 1980's, gonadotropin-releasing hormone agonists (GnRH agonists) were introduced as a means of down-regulating the pituitary to prevent premature ovulation, which in the past had necessitated canceling approximately 15% of IVF cycles prior to egg retrieval. The down-regulating effects of GnRH agonists, as opposed to the stimulatory effects of GnRH, are related to the frequency of administration and the prolonged occupation of GnRH receptors by the agonists. Since their introduction, pregnancy rates have increased because of the opportunity to retrieve cycles that would have been lost to early ovulation and because of the increase in the number of oocytes obtained in GnRH agonist cycles.[6] However, use of an agonist increases the amount of gonadotropins needed to stimulate follicular growth, and, thus, it also increases the expense. Despite this negative aspect, the combination of GnRH agonist and gonadotropin controlled hyperstimulation of the ovary, and substitution of exogenous HCG for the endogenous LH surge, is now utilized by most IVF programs. This approach has another beneficial attribute. Because the fear of premature ovulation is virtually eliminated, there is more flexibility in scheduling the necessary interventions.

Protocols starting standard doses of GnRH agonists in the follicular phase of the cycle preceding the one in which gonadotropin is started have the drawback, because of an initial stimulatory effect, the flare, of the GnRH agonist, of causing a larger number of ovarian cysts and higher androgen levels than cycles in which the agonist is started in the midluteal phase of the cycle.[7] In a further variation, GnRH agonist is started on the second or third day of menses, and gonadotropin is started 2 days later. This "flare" protocol tries to capture the initial stimulatory effect of the GnRH agonist and build on it with gonadotropin before the inhibitory effect of the agonist is established. This flare approach is particularly useful for poor responder patients. To aid timing, a common pretreatment for women with irregular menses uses oral contraceptives for one or two cycles.

Most commonly, the GnRH agonist is started in the midluteal phase, and gonadotropin treatment is started following menses. Ultrasonography is used prior to initiation of gonadotropin treatment to rule out the presence of an ovarian cyst larger than 15 mm. Ovarian cysts form in approximately 10% of women when the GnRH agonist is started in the midluteal phase, but these cysts almost always regress spontaneously in 1–3 weeks. Gonadotropin treatment is postponed until the cysts disappear or decrease to less than 15 mm in size.

GnRH agonist administration is continued for the duration of gonadotropin treatment. Whereas leuprolide (Lupron) injected subcutaneously is the most commonly used GnRH agonist in the United States, equally good results, if not better, have been achieved with the use of nafarelin (Synarel), which is administered as a nasal spray, one inhalation bid.[8] The initial dose of gonadotropin is usually 225–300 IU/daily, except in young women or those with polycystic ovarian disease where a lower dose (75–150 IU/daily) is appropriate. The dose can be adjusted as cycle monitoring proceeds with ultrasonography and estradiol measurements.

Intramuscular injections of urinary menopausal gonadotropins containing both FSH and LH were the mainstays of treatment until the development of a urinary gonadotropin that contained primarily FSH (see Chapter 30). One of the goals in limiting or eliminating LH is to decrease stimulation of the androgenic component of the ovarian response because excessive androgens block ovarian follicular growth and development. However, in clinical practice, there was no clear-cut advantage for the predominately FSH product. Still newer, highly purified urinary FSH products introduced the advantage of being effective with subcutaneous administration. Recombinant FSH also allows subcutaneous administration. Differences comparing recombinant FSH with the urinary hormones include enhanced purity, the need for less medication, the achievement of slightly lower estradiol levels, and a modest increase in the pregnancy rate.[9]

Whichever product or protocol is used, there is a 10–15% cancellation rate because of inadequate follicular response. Measurements of basal FSH and estradiol and the clomiphene challenge test can provide information for discussing with patients the expectations for success. Ideally, a stimulation protocol can be tailored to boost the chances for an adequate response. However, it is evident that most poor responders are resistant to conversion to good responders. The 5 most common changes in protocol designed to accomplish that elusive goal are:

1. Increase the gonadotropin dose or change the mix of FSH-LH and FSH. This is usually not successful. No improvement was noted when the gonadotropin dose was increased from 300 to 450 IU beginning on day 1 or 2 of the cycle.[10]

2. Use of the flare protocol, including the use of a microdose flare (20 μg leuprolide bid), approximately 1/50 the usual dose.[11]

3. Lower the dose of the GnRH agonist to allow some pituitary action, but starting as usual in the midluteal phase.

4. Omit the GnRH agonist and use gonadotropin alone or a combination of clomiphene and gonadotropin. To prevent premature ovulation in the absence of down-regulation by the GnRH agonist, a single dose of a GnRH antagonist can be given at midcycle to prevent the LH surge.

5. A less common approach, limited by expense and availability of drug, is the use of growth hormone in conjunction with gonadotropin. Moreover, results with this combination have been mixed; a double-blind study found no benefit associated with the addition of growth hormone.[12]

Monitoring Ovarian Response

Measurements of serum estradiol and ultrasound imaging of ovarian follicles are used to monitor the ovarian response to stimulation. The minimum goal of stimulation is to achieve the growth of a lead follicle to at least 18 mm diameter, and to have at least 3 or 4 other follicles with diameters of 14 mm or greater, combined with estradiol levels of approximately 200 pg/mL per large (14 mm or greater) follicle. Once this level of stimulation is achieved, a single injection of 5000 or 10,000 IU of HCG is given to induce final follicular maturation. The time interval between HCG injection and retrieval is critical. Whereas 34–36 hours is standard and believed to allow good oocyte maturation, intervals up to 39 hours may allow for better maturation of the oocytes while only marginally increasing the risk for ovulation.[13] The values given for follicle size and estradiol levels on the day of decision for HCG injection are only rough guidelines because ultrasound measurements can differ among observers and machines. In addition, each program must establish, based on its own experience, its criteria for determining the adequacy of follicle size. Moreover, estradiol assays will differ from one laboratory to another, and comparisons, therefore, are difficult. Estradiol levels per follicle can vary widely and still be compatible with successful IVF. Concern has been expressed that elevated levels of progesterone, signifying premature luteinization, just prior to HCG injection can disrupt the cycle. The weight of evidence indicates that the frequently seen modest rise in progesterone does not interfere with pregnancy rates.[14]

To avoid the significant medical risks of hyperstimulation, cancellation of the cycle and avoidance of HCG injection should be strongly considered if the ovaries are markedly hyperstimulated (more than 25 follicles or a total estradiol greater than 4000 pg/mL). (Hyperstimulation is discussed in Chapter 30.) Again, the specific values may not be valid with other assays, and each program must establish which estradiol level is its warning sign. Alternatives to cancellation include proceeding with the regular IVF cycle in the face of markedly elevated estradiol levels, but cryopreserving all the embryos for transfer in subsequent cycles to avoid further HCG stimulation accompanying a pregnancy, or discontinuing the daily gonadotropin injections (coasting) and delaying retrieval until the estradiol level (measured daily) drops to 2500–3000 pg/mL or lower, at which point HCG is administered.[15] However, cycles in which coasting produces very precipitous drops in estradiol to below 1000 pg/mL warrant cancellation. The pregnancy rates with coasting are lower than those obtained with the usual methods.

The risk of hyperstimulation can be decreased by lowering the dose of gonadotropin used to initiate the cycle. The use of FSH as opposed to mixtures of FSH and LH in women with polycystic ovaries is not protective; with all stimulation protocols, the key is careful use of appropriate doses. An important protection against hyperstimulation is the use progesterone after retrieval, rather than HCG injections, to support the luteal phase. Retrieval itself, with aspiration of follicular fluid and granulosa cells, is somewhat, but not absolutely, protective against hyperstimulation.[16]

When follicles are fully developed, the endometrium viewed by ultrasonography should be at least 8 mm wide. If the width is 6 mm or less, there is a reduced chance for pregnancy.[17–19] Although there is some dispute over the significance of the endometrial pattern, most reports indicate a superior pregnancy rate if there is a trilaminar appearance on the day of HCG administration compared to a homogenous whiteout pattern.

Oocyte Retrieval

Ultrasonically guided vaginal oocyte retrieval is performed approximately 34–35 hours after the HCG injection, but as late as 39 hours with the combined use of a GnRH agonist and gonadotropin.[20] The HCG injection allows for confidence in this precise timing. Intravenous analgesia and/or light anesthesia provide an acceptable level of comfort. In all cases, monitoring by a pulse oximeter is mandatory, as is immediate access to emergency resuscitation equipment. A number 16 or 17 long needle is placed down a sterile needle guide that is attached to the upper side of the vaginal ultrasound transducer. A line on the monitor screen indicates the path the needle will traverse once it enters the peritoneal cavity and the ovary. The ultrasound transducer is manipulated to position a follicle along this pathway. Usually only one puncture of each ovary is needed to allow sequential aspiration of the follicles. Accessibility of the ovaries is rarely a problem. Rare complications of the procedure are intra-abdominal bleeding or introduction of infection into the ovary and pelvis.

Oocyte Culture

Oocytes, surrounded by their cumulus masses, are identified under either a dissecting or an invert microscope. Exposure to ambient temperature and room air is minimized. One of the major breakthroughs in IVF was the discovery that sperm need not be added to the eggs immediately after retrieval; oocytes have a higher chance for fertilization if insemination follows retrieval by 4 to 6 hours.[21]

Sperm are prepared by washing, centrifugation, discarding the supernatant, and overlaying the sperm pellet with fresh media. Sperm that swim up into the media are used for insemination, with approximately 50,000 sperm (100,000 or more if the sperm specimen is poor) placed in each petri dish containing an oocyte. Isolation of the most motile sperm can also be accomplished by separating the sperm on columns of liquid albumin, hyaluronate, glass wool, or gradients of silica particles.

A variety of media has been used for embryo culture. Most media for IVF contain a protein source, such as maternal serum, fetal cord serum, albumin and/or serum globulin. All protein components require screening for HIV and hepatitis. Because proteins, on occasion, may be deleterious to embryos, protein free media have been successfully used in limited studies.[22]

Culture of oocytes and embryos on cell monolayers from a variety of sources has been advocated as a means of enhancing development.[23] Pregnancy rates were increased and blastomere fragmentation reduced when human embryos were cultured on outgrowths of bovine tissue.[24] The explanation for the beneficial effect could be the secretion of an "embryotrophic" factor by the somatic cells or their removal of detrimental components from the media. Bavister suggested that greater attention to culture media quality can yield the same gains as those seen with co-culture, and this has been confirmed by recent experience.[25, 26] In addition, co-culture with granulosa cells has not helped couples with previous fertilization failures.[27]

Fertilization

The day after insemination, cumulus cells that remain attached to the zona pellucida are removed, and the egg is examined for evidence of fertilization (the presence of 2 pronuclei). 65–80% of mature oocytes will fertilize. Approximately 6% of oocytes contain 3 or more pronuclei, indicating penetration by more than one sperm. It is important to identify and discard these abnormal embryos at this early stage because they have the potential to cleave and appear normal at later preimplantation stages. If the diagnosis is missed at the pronuclear stage, the embryos will be transferred and the result will be a failure to implant or a spontaneous miscarriage.

A failure to fertilize is sometimes viewed by clinicians as a "human egg test" for that specific couple. However, fertilization failure in one cycle, despite normal sperm and eggs, is not an absolute indication of an insurmountable problem. Indeed, a high rate of fertilization has been reported in subsequent cycles after an initial fertilization failure, although the eventual pregnancy rate is a little lower than the usual rate in IVF programs.[28, 29] To demonstrate a complete failure of fertilization, at least 3 IVF cycles are necessary. Surprisingly the use of ICSI in a cycle following one with unexplained fertilization failure does not always overcome the failure to fertilize.

Extra embryos can be cryopreserved at the pronuclear stage. There is no known limit on duration of cryopreserved embryo storage. About two-thirds of embryos survive the freezing and the subsequent thawing process. The transfer of cryopreserved embryos adds significantly (15% delivery per transfer) to the success rate with a single retrieval and lowers the cost. Older age of the woman is associated with a decrease in pregnancy rates, not only because of a decrease in the number of oocytes and a reduction in oocyte and embryo quality, but also because fewer embryos are available for cryopreservation.[30]

Embryo Transfer

Embryos have been transferred successfully at any stage from the pronuclear to the blastocyst, although most commonly, they are transferred when development is between the 8- and 10-cell stage, approximately 72–80 hours after retrieval. Transfer of more than one embryo increases the chances for pregnancy, but the multiple pregnancy rate with IVF is approximately 35%.

High order multiples can create unfortunate outcomes for the pregnancy, the children, and for subsequent family life. It is not unusual for patients to welcome the prospects for a multiple birth, and they must be informed of the associated risks. To decrease the incidence of multiple birth, programs in the U.K. transfer a maximum of 2 embryos. The guidelines of the American Society for Reproductive Medicine are more liberal, and they are influenced by the age of the woman. The recommendation is for no more than 3 embryos to be transferred in women younger than age 35, no more than 4 at age 35–40, and no more than 5 in women older than age 40. Our preference is to transfer 2 good quality 8–10 cell embryos in women under the age of 35, whereas women between age 35–39 may have 2–3 good quality embryos transferred. It may be reasonable to place higher numbers in women age 40 and older, but this is influenced by the experience of the individual program. At least one study did not experience a decrease in multiple birth risk in older women.[31] While we cite "good quality" of the embryos as a qualification, it must be recognized that this assessment is highly subjective. On occasion, transfer of "poor" quality embryos results in pregnancy. The ability to use fetal reduction to limit the number of continuing fetuses lessens somewhat the concerns over the major hazards of multiple pregnancies. In experienced hands, the risk of losing the entire pregnancy from selective fetal reduction is less than 10%.[32] However, moral concerns and the psychological impact of fetal reduction are important considerations.

Success with culture to the blastocyst stage has raised the hope that high pregnancy rates can be achieved with the transfer of only one blastocyst (reaching this stage in culture is predictive of excellent potential).[26]

Ancillary medications given around the time of transfer, such as prostaglandin inhibitors, tranquilizers, or antibiotics are of no proven value. It is common practice to supplement the luteal phase with progesterone. Several options are available, including progesterone vaginal suppositories, 50–100 mg daily, progesterone in oil, 50–100 mg im daily, one application of vaginal progesterone daily, or oral micronized progesterone, 200 mg tid. An alternative therapy is the use of HCG, 1500 IU every 3 days for 4 doses; however, HCG supplementation increases the risk of ovarian hyperstimulation. The value of luteal phase supplementation can be questioned, but there is no doubt that it provides some psychologic benefit for both patient and physician. An initial quantitative HCG measurement can be obtained 12 days after transfer. If the test is positive, a follow-up test is obtained 3 days later. This will establish the trend of the HCG and provide prognostic information.

A rise in the HCG level indicates pregnancy, whereas a drop indicates a failed cycle. If weekly determinations demonstrate appropriate elevations, ultrasonography 5 weeks after the transfer should reveal a fetal heart beat. If not, repeat ultrasonography can be performed in one week. The presence of a rapid heartbeat is an excellent prognostic sign, and if the woman is under age 30, the chance for a spontaneous miscarriage is near zero; between age 31–35, the risk of spontaneous miscarriage is 4%.[33] If the woman is over age 40, the prognosis is less sanguine, with spontaneous miscarriage rates close to 20%. If the woman has a history of recurrent early pregnancy losses, a positive heartbeat still leaves the chance of a spontaneous miscarriage in the 20–25% range.

Assisted hatching consists of making an opening in the zona pellucida just prior to transfer to help the embryo emerge. This can be accomplished by slitting open the zona with a microneedle, by treating a localized area of the zona with an acid Tyrode's solution, or by using a laser to breech the zona. Assisted hatching has been reported to increase the implantation rate in poor prognosis patients, especially in older women.[34–36] However, two studies, one in women older than age 36, and the other in women older than age 38, could find no benefit with assisted hatching.[37, 38]

IVF Results

Some skepticism has been expressed concerning the pregnancy rates reported by IVF programs.[39] Competition for patients is a motivation for some of the exaggerations and half-truths contained in advertisements and public statements. An associated confusion is generated by the differing criteria that can be used to determine what constitutes a success. A slight unsustained rise in the HCG is properly termed a "chemical pregnancy," and it should not be counted as a success. The most important indicators of success are the delivery rate per retrieval and the delivery rate per cycle initiated. Even these figures cannot be properly evaluated without knowledge of the specific age mix of the treated women. Obviously, a program with a higher percentage of older women should not be expected to do as well as one with mostly younger women. In addition, clinics that transfer large numbers of embryos to each woman can marginally inflate their pregnancy numbers but at a significant price of multiple pregnancies.

Uniform reporting by clinics, monitored by the Society for Assisted Reproductive Technology, has produced yearly statistics available to the public.[40] Results from the U.S. and Canada are published nearly 3 years later, reflecting a significant lag because of the need to await deliveries resulting from cycles initiated and the difficulties in obtaining timely submission of data from 281 programs.

In 1995, the deliveries per retrieval were 22.3% for standard IVF, 27.0% with GIFT, and 27.9% with ZIFT.[40] Women under age 35 had a 27.2% delivery rate per retrieval with IVF compared with 10.5% in women older than age 39. With transfers of donor embryos, the delivery rate was 36.0%, whereas with the transfer of cryopreserved embryos, the delivery rate was 15.2%. These figures for 1995, reported in 1998, are probably already outmoded. Many clinics are achieving delivery rates in the 35% range, especially in women under age 35. The advantages noted for GIFT and ZIFT disappear when comparisons are made within the same program.[41]

Surprisingly, 3% of pregnancies achieved through IVF are ectopic, emphasizing the need for close ultrasonographic and HCG titer surveillance (see Chapter 32). Pregnancies occurring simultaneously in different body sites (heterotropic pregnancies) are a rare condition, occurring in 1 of 30,000 spontaneous pregnancies. The incidence of combined pregnancy among patients who have undergone one of the assisted reproduction procedures is much higher, closer to 1 in 100 pregnancies.[42-44] A case-control study has concluded that the risk of ectopic pregnancy with assisted reproduction is due to the multiple ovulations and high hormone levels secondary to the stimulation protocols.[45]

Twenty percent of clinical pregnancies result in spontaneous miscarriages, which is close to the rate in infertility populations; there is no increase in the rate of congenital malformations.[46] The children experience normal growth and development.[47]

The multiple pregnancy rate is approximately 35% (30% twins, 5% triplets, and about 0.6% higher multiples). This leads to an increase in cesarean sections, prematurity, and perinatal mortality. As noted previously, selective reduction can be offered as an option with multiples greater than two.[32] This can be a difficult decision for some couples, but in view of the potential problems associated with a multiple pregnancy, it is an option deserving consideration.

A major factor influencing IVF results is the gross inefficiency of human reproduction in vivo. A number of studies have attested to the low fecundability of humans. Only 30% of normal women who attempt pregnancy in a given cycle are successful.[48] There is a large loss of embryos prior to or around the time of implantation in vivo, and thus, many women have pregnancy losses without realizing that they have been pregnant because the menstrual period comes at the expected time. It can be concluded that many sperm and many oocytes, even from individuals who are fertile, do not have the ability to contribute to a normal pregnancy. This affects the success of both in vivo and in vitro fertilization.

The chance for success in successive IVF cycles decreases after 3 cycles.[49] However, approximately 50% of women under age 35 have a live birth within 6 cycles of treatment.[50, 51] Most individuals find the emotional, physical, and financial consequences of going beyond 3 to 6 cycles too difficult, and adoption or donor embryos should be considered. Patients should also be aware that occasional spontaneous pregnancies occur even after failure of IVF.

Male Infertility and IVF

The limited effectiveness of treatments for male infertility has provided a sizable number of individuals who desire IVF to overcome problems with sperm. Early experience with male factor infertility in IVF indicated that even placing sperm in the dish with the oocyte still left many sperm specimens with a handicap. Fertilization rates tended to be approximately one-half those achieved with normal sperm, and the pregnancy rates were correspondingly lower. On occasion, however, fertilization occurred with surprisingly few sperm available.

IVF provides the ability to visualize the results of sperm and egg interaction and thus to quickly determine if specific manipulations of the sperm can affect fertilization. A variety of sperm treatments have been attempted. One approach is to increase the number of sperm in the dish with the hope that even with abnormal specimens there will be a few normal sperm that can achieve fertilization. By increasing the numbers in each dish there will be more normal sperm per egg. A second approach is to isolate the best sperm from the specimen, not by the standard swim-up technique, but by using a variety of gradients. In some hands this has provided increased fertilization rates, but others have not found it to be a significant advantage. Similar contradictory results have been reported with drug treatment of the semen; the most popular such treatment has utilized pentoxifylline, which acts by increasing cyclic AMP in cells.[52] The drug must be washed out from the sperm specimen before incubation with the egg because it may have adverse effects. Another treatment that has been used to enhance sperm is incubation in follicular fluid.[53] In men with sperm autoantibodies, in vitro fertilization is correlated with the extent the sperm are covered with antibodies.

Micromanipulation

The early techniques of making a hole in the zona to facilitate sperm entry and the injection of sperm through the zona into the perivitelline space have been superseded by the intracytoplasmic injection of single sperm (ICSI). The pioneering success of Van Steirteghem and his coworkers in Belgium[54] has now been duplicated in many laboratories. The results have surpassed all expectations, with pregnancy rates equal to or slightly surpassing the normal fecundity rate.[55] Pregnancy rates are independent of any semen analysis parameter (number, motility, and morphology).[56]

Sperm for injection have been obtained not only from the ejaculate, but in azoospermia by microsurgery from the epididymis (MESA) or from the testis (TESE).[57] Both percutaneous aspirations and open biopsies have been used. Fine-needle biopsy on occasion will locate small pockets of sperm or spermatids in otherwise hopeless appearing cases, such as the Sertoli cell only syndrome. Even the use of the sperm precursors in ICSI has produced successful pregnancies.[57, 58] The success with spermatids and with immotile sperm, however, is substantially lower than with motile sperm.[59] It is worthwhile, therefore, to vigorously search poor quality ejaculates for motile sperm.

ICSI is the treatment of choice for azoospermia and severe oligospermia (including the absence of sperm because of blockage in the ejaculatory ducts), and it is also indicated when antisperm antibodies are present, for cases of poor fertilization despite normal semen, and as a last resort for refractory unexplained infertility. In the collected 1995 U.S. and Canadian results, the delivery rate per retrieval after ICSI was 23.5%, marginally higher than the 22.3% without ICSI.[40] In women younger than age 34, the pregnancy rate per transfer after ICSI has been reported to be as high as 49%.[60] A pregnancy rate of 14.8% per cycle has even been achieved with ICSI one day after oocytes had failed conventional fertilization.[61] As with regular IVF, ICSI pregnancies, including singletons, have higher than normal rates of preterm delivery, low birth weight, and perinatal mortality.[62]

Concern arose that the gains achieved with ICSI, by bypassing the selection process exerted by the zona pellucida, might exact a price. The zona is a barrier to fertilization by morphologically abnormal sperm that have a higher rate of genetic abnormalities compared with normal shaped sperm. However, even sperm that are normally shaped can harbor genetic aberrations, and there is continuing concern regarding the transmission of genetic abnormalities with ICSI.

Chromosomal analyses of testicular biopsies indicate chromosomal abnormalities iin approximately 5–7% of infertile males.[63] There is a high prevalence of Y chromosome submicroscopic deletions in men with oligospermia. A cluster of genes that are deleted in men with azoospermia or oligospermia has been referred to as DAZ ("deleted in azoospermia").[64, 65] Subsequently, at least 3 specific regions on Yq were identified and labeled as "azoospermia factors," AZFa, AZFb, and AZFc (the same region as DAZ).[66] From 7% to 10% of men with severe oligospermia have been reported to have deletions in the AZFb and AZFc regions on the long arm of the Y chromosome.[67, 68] These microdeletions correlate poorly with the numbers of sperm present in the semen analysis. These could be normal genetic variants and not the cause of the infertility; however, these deletions can now be transmitted with the use of ICSI, and it is now appropriate to consider Y chromosome deletion analysis prior to treatment with assisted reproduction. On the other hand, Y chromosome deletions are rare in men participating in an ICSI program. Indeed, the prevalence of overall chromosomal abnormalities is greater in men with abnormal semen than the prevalence of Y chromosome microdeletions.[69, 70]

Approximately 10% of sperm from fertile males carry an extra chromosome, but the rate of newborns with chromosomal abnormalities is under 1%.[63] Prenatal selection is protective against the majority of abnormalities. Prenatal testing of ICSI pregnancies revealed an incidence of 0.83% of sex chromosome abnormalities and a similarly low figure for autosomal abnormalities.[71] These figures, however, are higher than those reported for spontaneous pregnancies.

Although these genetic abnormalities are relatively infrequent, and there is uncertainty regarding the role of Y chromosome microdeletions, because of the consequences, there is strong support for genetic screening of all men considering ICSI.[72] Indeed, 90% of couples receiving genetic counseling elect to undergo genetic screening.[73] Nevertheless, because of the relative infrequency of the various abnormalities, most IVF programs do not routinely karyotype prospective ICSI patients. However, males with azoospermia and severe oligospermia should have genetic screening because their risk of genetic abnormalities is higher than men with mild sperm impairment. The most frequent diagnosis is Klinefelter syndrome, which occurs in approximately 1 in every 500 males. Among other genetic abnormalities, azoospermia and hypogonadism can result because of a mutation that causes an abnormality in the beta-subunit of LH.[74] An inactivating mutation in the gene for the FSH receptor is associated with varying degrees of suppression of spermatogenesis, indicating that FSH is not absolutely essential for sperm production[75].

Approximately 1–2% of infertile males have congenital bilateral absence of the vas deferens.[76] Most males with bilateral congenital absence of the vas deferens have at least two mutations in the cystic fibrosis transmembrane conductance regulator gene.[77] Screening for cystic fibrosis mutations should be considered in males with bilateral absent vas deferens who are considering ICSI. A reasonable approach involves screening the female partner; the absence of cystic fibrosis mutations in the female reduces the risk of having a child with cystic fibrosis to a very low level.

Delayed mental development at one year of age has been reported in children born as the result of ICSI.[78] 17% of ICSI children had mild or significantly delayed development (memory, problem solving, language skills) compared with 2% of IVF children and 1% of natural conception children. More reassuring are the reports of low rates of neurologic or developmental problems at 2 months of age, and normal mental development at age 2.[79, 80] With the large numbers of ICSI pregnancies, the long-term outcome of ICSI children will soon be apparent.

IVF for Endometriosis

Early experience with IVF in cases of endometriosis suggested that more severe disease exerted an adverse effect on oocyte recruitment, embryo development, and pregnancy rates. With greater experience, however, pregnancy rates (uninfluenced by the severity of the disease) have been achieved that are comparable to those with tubal disease.[81, 82]

IVF for Autoimmunity

ICSI is recommended for cases of sperm autoimmunity, and results are comparable to those obtained with other diagnoses.[83, 84] ICSI bypasses the zona, which is a major barrier to antibody-laden sperm.

Other Techniques

In addition to IVF, individuals with unexplained infertility have been offered a number of tactics to overcome hypothesized problems with gamete transport. For gamete intrafallopian transfer (GIFT), minilaparotomy or laparoscopy is used to aspirate oocytes following hyperstimulation of the ovary. Alternatively, aspiration can be performed more easily through the vagina, and laparoscopy is then used only for oocyte and sperm transfer (transfer via the uterus produces poorer results). After the oocytes are identified in the laboratory, they are taken up into a transfer catheter that contains 100,000 sperm isolated by the swim-up technique. The transfer catheter is guided into the distal 4 cm of a fallopian tube and the contents gently discharged. Two oocytes can be placed in each tube although placement in one tube is more common and equally successful. Extra eggs obtained at retrieval can be fertilized and cryopreserved for future use. Success with GIFT in the collected statistics from the United States and Canada (1995) was 27.0% deliveries per retrieval.[40] In the same year the success with IVF was 22.5% deliveries per retrieval. This difference is believed to be due largely to differences in patient selection. Ectopic pregnancy occurs in approximately 4.2% of GIFT pregnancies, somewhat higher than the 2.6% reported with IVF. The multiple pregnancy rate with GIFT is similar to that of IVF, approximately 35%.

In a variation of GIFT, called ZIFT, oocytes are obtained by vaginal aspiration, fertilized in vitro, and then 1 day later at the pronuclear stage placed in the fallopian tubes by the GIFT technique. The 1995 figures for ZIFT were 27.9% deliveries per retrieval.[40] Whereas these figures continue to reflect an early impression that ZIFT was decidedly superior to IVF, this is not the case in current statistics. Indeed, prospective comparisons within the same clinics demonstrate similar results with uterine (IVF) versus tubal transfers (GIFT or ZIFT).[41, 85]

The choice of method, IVF, GIFT, or ZIFT, can be made on the basis of infertility factors, cost, and risk. If there is tubal damage, GIFT or ZIFT is not a good choice. In rare instances, where there is severe scarring of the cervix, one of the intratubal techniques is preferable. The comfort level of the program with each of the techniques and the program's experience in terms of pregnancy results are important considerations. Use of GIFT or ZIFT can incur greater costs, depending on the setting for the surgery and the anesthesia used.

Other attempts to overcome problems of gamete transport include injections of washed sperm and oocytes into the peritoneal cavity (POST) and cannulation of the fallopian tube via the cervix, as a conduit for injecting sperm directly into the tube.[86] These methods have not gained wide usage. In a technique of limited applicability, because it risks pregnancy in a donor, a fertilized human ovum at the blastocyst stage can be removed by uterine lavage from a donor and placed transcervically in the uterus of an infertile recipient.[87]

Ovum Donation

A technique of proven value is ovum donation for older women, those with premature ovarian failure or women who are unresponsive to gonadotropin stimulation. The donor, who ideally should be under the age of 33 and has been both physically and psychologically screened, is down-regulated with a GnRH agonist, and then stimulated with gonadotropins as in IVF.[88] Following retrieval, the donor's oocytes are fertilized with sperm from the recipient's partner. If the recipient is having periods, indicative of endogenous hormone production, she is down-regulated with a GnRH agonist before starting on at least 10 days of estrogen (a common dose is estradiol, 4–8 mg per day). When ultrasonography indicates adequate endometrial development, progesterone is added to synchronize the endometrium with the egg retrieval. If pregnancy occurs, the hormone supplementation continues for at least 10 weeks, until placental steroidogenesis is firmly established. Success rates are lower in older recipients unless high doses of progesterone are provided for uterine support.[89] A delivery rate in older women of approximately 40–50% per cycle can be achieved in a donor oocyte program. A cumulative birth rate can reach 90% with 4 or more cycles.[90, 91]

Experimental Methods

Oocytes can be matured in vitro and then cryopreserved. This technique would allow young women who require chemotherapy or pelvic irradiation to preserve a possibility for fertility in the future. However, fertilization rates and survival of cryopreservation is low for oocytes compared with the excellent survival obtained with cryopreserved embryos.

Preimplantation Genetic Diagnosis

Diagnosing genetic disorders before implantation provides couples with the option of foregoing the attempt to establish a pregnancy. This avoids the difficult decision whether or not to continue an affected pregnancy when the diagnosis is made at amniocentesis or by chorionic villus biopsy. There are 3 possible approaches for preimplantation diagnosis.[92, 93] The first is the removal of a polar body, but greater accuracy is obtained by studying both polar bodies. The polar body contains only one copy of the gene, but if the copy is found to be normal, it can be presumed that the oocyte contains a normal copy. However, this method is technically very difficult and subject to error if crossing-over occurs and both copies are present in the polar body. A second method is to biopsy cells that are destined to become the placenta. This requires culturing the embryo to the blastocyst stage, and then opening the zona pellucida in the 5–6 day embryo. The disadvantage is the lower pregnancy rate when the embryo is transferred at this later stage. The third method is the removal of a single cell from the 6–8 cell embryo (blastomere biopsy) for DNA amplification by polymerase chain reaction and analysis with fluorescent probes specific for chromosomes 13, 18, 21, and the X and Y chromosomes.[94] The biopsy procedure does not affect development and implantation, and the diagnostic testing is rapid; the biopsy and DNA analysis are accomplished within 8 hours.

Preimplantation genetic diagnosis has successfully detected single gene defects in disorders such as cystic fibrosis, Duchene's muscular dystrophy, sickle cell disease, hemophilia, Tay-Sachs disease, Lesch-Nyhan syndrome, and at least 11 other diseases. These methods can also be used to determine the sex of the embryo for couples who are at risk for transmitting X-linked disorders.

The utilization of molecular biology techniques for preimplantation genetic diagnosis is associated with some significant risks. Polymerase chain reaction amplification does not always succeed. An erroneous diagnosis can occur because of contamination by DNA from surrounding cells or from sperm that are attached to the zona pellucida. This type of genetic diagnosis is only available in a limited number of centers.

Concluding Thoughts

The new reproductive techniques and the technology associated with in vitro fertilization have been presented in a somewhat mechanistic way in this chapter. This should not obscure the fact that, despite the excellent success rates, this is an emotionally trying experience for almost everyone undertaking therapy. Psychological stresses can be acute, and anxiety is accentuated with each step of the process. Failures at every stage are exceptionally difficult for both patients and clinicians. Psychologic counseling services associated with IVF programs, and support groups, such as those organized by RESOLVE, are helpful for almost every couple going through an ART program.

References

1. **Sauer MV, Paulson RJ, Lobo RA,** Pregnancy in women 50 or more years of age: outcomes of 22 consecutively established pregnancies from oocyte donation, *Fertil Steril* 64:11, 1995.

2. **Strandell A, Waldenstrom U, Nilsson L, Hamberger L,** Hydrosalpinx reduces in-vitro-fertilization/embryo transfer pregnancy rates, *Hum Reprod* 9:861, 1994.

3. **Feichtinger W, Papalambrou K, Poehl M, Krischker U, Neumann K,** Smoking and in vitro fertilization: a meta-analysis, *J Assist Reprod Genet* 14:596, 1997.

4. **Scott RT, Toner JP, Muasher SJ, Oehninger S, Robinson S, Rosenwaks Z,** Follicle-stimulating homone levels on cycle day 3 are predictive of in vitro fertilization outcome, *Fertil Steril* 51:651, 1989.

5. **Claman P, Domingo M, Garner P, Leader A, Spence JEH,** Natural cycle in vitro fertilization-embryo transfer at the University of Ottawa: an inefficient therapy for tubal infertility, *Fertil Steril* 60:298, 1993.

6. **Hughes EG, Fedorkow DM, Daya S, Sagle MA, Van de Koppel P, Collins JA,** The routine use of gonadotropin-releasing hormone agonists prior to in vitro fertilization and gamete intrafallopian transfer: a meta-analysis of randomized controlled trials, *Fertil Steril* 58:888, 1992.

7. **Gelety TJ, Pearlstone AC, Surrey ES,** Short-term endocrine response to gonadotropin-releasing hormone agonist initiated in the early follicular, midluteal, or late luteal phase in normally cycling women, *Fertil Steril* 64:1074, 1995.

8. **Martin M, Givens CR, Schriock ED, Glass RH, Dandekar PV,** The choice of GnRH analog influences outcome in in vitro fertilization treatment, *Am J Obstet Gynecol* 170:1629, 1994.

9. **Out HJ, Driessen SGAJ, Mannaerts BMJL, Coelingh Bennink HJT,** Recombinant follicle-stimulating hormone (follitropin beta, Puregon®) yields higher pregnancy rates in in vitro fertilization than urinary gonadotropins, *Fertil Steril* 68:138, 1997.

10. **Karande VC, Jones GS, Veeck LL, Muasher SJ,** High-dose follicle-stimulating hormone stimulation at the onset of the menstrual cycle does not improve the in vitro fertilization outcome in low-responder patients, *Fertil Steril* 53:486, 1990.

11. **Scott RT, Navot D,** Enhancement of ovarian responsiveness with microdoses of gonadotropin-releasing hormone agonist during ovulation induction of in vitro fertilization, *Fertil Steril* 61:880, 1994.

12. **Suikkara A-M, MacLachlan V, Koistinen R, Seppala M, Healy DL,** Double-blind placebo controlled study: human biosynthetic growth hormone for assisted reproductive technology, *Fertil Steril* 65:800, 1996.

13. **Jamieson ME, Fleming R, Kader S, Ross KS, Yates RWS, Coutts JRT,** In vivo and in vitro maturation of human oocytes: effects on embryo development and polyspermic fertilization, *Fertil Steril* 56:93, 1991.

14. **Givens CR, Schriock ED, Dandekar PV, Martin MC,** Elevated serum progesterone levels on the day of human chorionic gonadotropin administration do not predict outcome in assisted reproductive cycles, *Fertil Steril* 62:1011, 1994.

15. **Urman B, Pride SM, Yuen BH,** Management of overstimulated gonadotropin cycles with a controlled drift period, *Hum Reprod* 7:213, 1992.

16. **Aboulghar MA, Mansour RT, Serour GI, Elattar I, Amin Y,** Follicular aspiration does not protect against the development of ovarian hyperstimulation syndrome, *J Assist Reprod Genetics* 9:238, 1992.

17. **Gonen Y, Casper RF,** Prediction of implantation by the sonographic appearance of the endometrium during controlled ovarian stimulation for in vitro fertilization (IVF), *J In Vitro Fertil Embryo Transfer* 7:146, 1990.

18. **Sher G, Herbert C, Maassarani G, Jacob MH,** Assessment of the late proliferative phase endometrium by ultrasonography in patients undergoing in vitro fertilization and embryo transfer (IVF/ET), *Hum Reprod* 6:232, 1991.

19. **Bohrer M, Hock DL, Rhodes GG, Kemmann E,** Sonographic assessment of endometrial pattern and thickness in patients treated with human menopausal gonadotropins, *Fertil Steril* 66:244, 1996.

20. **Tarlatzis BC,** Oocyte collection and quality, *Assist Reprod Rev* 2:16, 1992.

21. **Trounson AO, Mohr LR, Wood C, Leeton JF,** Effect of delayed insemination on in vitro fertilization, culture and transfer of human embryos, *J Reprod Fertil* 64:285, 1982.

22. **Caro CM, Trounson A,** Successful fertilization, embryo development, and pregnancy in human in vitro fertilization (IVF) using a chemically defined culture medium containing no protein, *J In Vitro Fertil Embryo Transfer* 3:215, 1986.

23. **Bongso A, Ng S-C, Sathanathan H, Ng PL, Rauff M, Ratnam S,** Improved quality of human embryos when co-cultured with human ampullary cells, *Hum Reprod* 4:706, 1989.

24. **Weimer KE, Hoffman DI, Maxson WS, Eager S, Muhlberger B, Fiore I, Cuervo M,** Embryonic morphology and rate of implantation of human embryos following co-culture on bovine oviductal epithelial cells, *Hum Reprod* 8:97, 1993.

25. **Bavister BD,** Co-culture for embryo development: Is it really necessary? *Hum Reprod* 7:1339, 1992.

26. **Gardner DK, Vella P, Lane M, Wagley L, Schlenker T, Schoolcraft WB,** Culture and transfer of human blastocysts increases implantation rates and reduces the need for multiple embyo transfers, *Fertil Steril* 69:84, 1998.

27. **Plachot M, Mendelbaum J, Junca AM, Anatoine JM, Salat-Baroux J, Cohen J,** Co-culture with granulosa cells does not increase the fertilization rate in couples with previous fertilization failures, *Hum Reprod* 8:1455, 1993.

28. **Molloy D, Harrison K, Breen T, Hennessey J,** The predictive value of idiopathic failure to fertilize on the first in vitro fertilization attempt, *Fertil Steril* 56:285, 1991.

29. **Lipitz S, Rabinovici J, Ben-Shlomo I, Bider D, Ben-Rafael Z, Mashiach S, Dor J,** Complete failure of fertilization in couples with unexplained infertility: implications for subsequent in vitro fertilization cycles, *Fertil Steril* 59:348, 1993.

30. **Toner JP, Veeck LL, Muasher SJ,** Basal follicle-stimulating hormone level and age affect the chance for and outcome of pre-embryo cryopreservation, *Fertil Steril* 59:664, 1993.

31. **Senöz S, Ben-Chetrit A, Casper RF,** An IVF fallacy: multiple pregnancy rate is lower for older women, *J Assist Reprod Genet* 14:192, 1997.

32. **Evans MI, Dommergues M, Timor-Tritsch I, Zador IE, Wapner RJ, Lynch L, Dumez Y, Goldberg JD, Nicolaides KH, Johnson MP, Golbus MS, Boulot P, Aknin AJ, Monteagudo A, Berkowitz RL,** Transabdominal versus transcervical and transvaginal multifetal pregnancy reduction: international collaborative experience of more than one thousand cases, *Am J Obstet Gynecol* 170:902, 1994.

33. **Smith KE, Buyalos RP,** The profound impact of patient age on pregnancy outcome after early detection of fetal cardiac activity, *Fertil Steril* 65:35, 1996.

34. **Cohen J, Elsner C, Kort H, Malter H, Massey J, Mayer MP, Wiemer K,** Impairment of the hatching process following IVF in the human and improvement of implantation by assisting hatching using micromanipulation, *Hum Reprod* 5:7, 1990.

35. **Stein A, Rufas O, Amit S, Avrech O, Pinkas H, Ovaida J, Fisch B,** Assisted hatching by partial zona dissection of human pre-embryos in patients with recurrent implantation failure after in vitro fertilization, *Fertil Steril* 63:838, 1995.

36. **Hellebaut S, DeSutter P, Dozortzev D, Onghena A, Qian C, Dhont M,** Does assisted hatching improve implantation rates after in vitro fertilization or intracytoplasmic sperm injection in all patients? A prospective randomized study, *J Assist Reprod Genet* 13:19, 1996.

37. **Bider D, Liushits A, Yonish M, Yemini Z, Mashiach S, Dor J,** Assisted hatching by zona drilling of human embryos in women of advanced age, *Hum Reprod* 12:317, 1997.

38. **Lanzendorf SE, Nehchiri F, Mayer JF, Oehninger S, Muasher SJ,** A prospective, randomized, double-blind study for the evaluation of assisted hatching in patients with advanced maternal age, *Hum Reprod* 13:409, 1998.

39. **Soules MR,** The in vitro fertilization pregnancy rate: Let's be honest with one another, *Fertil Steril* 43:511, 1985.

40. **Society for Assisted Reproductive Technology, The American Society for Reproductive Medicine,** Assisted Reproductive Technology in the United States and Canada: 1995 results generated from the American Society for Reproductive Medicine/Society for Assisted Reproductive Technology, *Fertil Steril* 69:389, 1998.

41. **Tanbo T, Dale PO, Aabyholm T,** Assisted fertilization in infertile women with patent fallopian tubes. A comparison of in vitro fertilization, gamete intrafallopian transfer and tubal embryo stage transfer, *Hum Reprod* 5:266, 1990.

42. **Molloy D, Deambrosis W, Keeping D, Hynes J, Harrison K, Hennessey J,** Multiple-sited (heterotropoic) pregnancy after in vitro fertilization and gamete intrafallopian transfer, *Fertil Steril* 53:1068, 1990.

43. **Dor J, Seidman DS, Levran D, Ben-Rafael Z, Ben-Shlomo I, Mashiach S,** The incidence of combined intrauterine and extrauterine pregnancy after in vitro fertilization and embryo transfer, *Fertil Steril* 55:833, 1991.

44. **Savare J, Norup P, Thomsen SG, Hornes P, Maigaard S, Helm P, Petersen K, Andersen AN,** Heterotropic pregnancies after in-vitro fertilization and embryo transfer — a Danish survey, *Hum Reprod* 8:116, 1993.

45. **Fernandez H, Coste J, Job-Spira N,** Controlled ovarian hyperstimulation as a risk factor for ectopic pregnancy, *Obstet Gynecol* 78:656, 1991.

46. **Shoham Z, Zosmer A, Insler V,** Early miscarriage and fetal malformations after induction of ovulation (by clomiphene citrate and/or human menotropins), in vitro fertilization, and gamete intrafallopian transfer, *Fertil Steril* 55:1, 1991.

47. **Olivennes F, Kerbrat V, Rufat P, Blanchat V, Franchin R, Frydman R,** Followup of a cohort of 422 children aged 5 to 13 years conceived by in vitro fertilization, *Fertil Steril* 67:284, 1997.

48. **Zinaman MJ, Clegg ED, Brown CC, O'Connor J, Selevan SG,** Estimates of human fertility and pregnancy loss, *Fertil Steril* 65:503, 1996.

49. **Meldrum DR, Silverberg KM, Bustillo M, Stokes L,** Success rate with repeated cycles of in vitro fertilization-embryo transfer, *Fertil Steril* 69:1005, 1998.

50. **Guzick DS, Wilkes C, Jones Jr HW,** Cumulative pregnancy rates for in vitro fertilization, *Fertil Steril* 46:663, 1986.

51. **Tan SL, Royston P, Campbell S, Jacobs HS, Betts J, Mason B, Edwards RG,** Cumulative conception and livebirth rates after in-vitro fertilisation, *Lancet* 339:1390, 1992.

52. **Yovich JL,** Pentoxifylline: actions and applications in assisted reproduction, *Hum Reprod* 8:1786, 1993.

53. **McClure DR, Tom RA, Dandekar PV,** Optimizing the sperm penetration assay with human follicular fluid, *Fertil Steril* 53:546, 1990.

54. **Palermo G, Joris H, Devroey P, Van Steirteghem AC,** Pregnancies after intracytoplasmic injection of a single spermatozoon into an oocyte, *Lancet* 340:17, 1992.

55. **Van Steirteghem AC, Nagy Z, Joris H, Liu J, Staessen C, Smitz J, Wisanto A, Devroey P,** High fertilization and implantation rates after intracytoplasmic sperm injection, *Hum Reprod* 8:1061, 1993.

56. **Nagy ZP, Liu J, Joris H, Verheyen G, Tournaye H, Camus M, Derde MP, Devroey P, Van Steirteghem AC,** The result of intracytoplasmic sperm injection is not related to any of the three basic sperm parameters, *Hum Reprod* 10:1123, 1995.

57. **Silber SJ, Nagy Z, Liu J, Tournaye H, Lissens W, Ferec C, Liebaers I, Devroey P, Van Steirteghem AC,** The use of epididymal and testicular spermatozoa for intracytoplasmic sperm injection: the genetic implications for male infertility, *Hum Reprod* 10:2031, 1995.

58. **Tesarik J, Mendoza C, Testart J,** Viable embryos from injection of round spermatids into oocytes, *New Engl J Med* 333:525, 1995.

59. **Vandervorst M, Tournaye H, Camus M, Nagy ZP, Van Steirteghem A, Devroey P,** Patients with absolutely immotile spermatozoa and intracytoplasmic sperm injection, *Hum Reprod* 12:2429, 1997.

60. **Oehninger S, Veeck L, Lanzendorf S, Maloney M, Toner J, Muasher S,** Intracytoplasmic sperm injection: achievement of high pregnancy rates in couples with severe male factor infertility is dependent upon female and not male factors, *Fertil Steril* 64:977, 1995.

61. **Morton PC, Yoder CS, Tucker MJ, Wright G, Brockman WDW, Kort HI,** Reinsemination by intracytoplasmic sperm injection of 1-day old oocytes after complete conventional fertilization failure, *Fertil Steril* 68:488, 1997.

62. **Aytoz A, Camus M, Tournaye H, Bonduelle M, Van Steirteghem A, Devroey P,** Outcome of pregnancies after intracytoplasmic sperm injection and the effect of sperm origin and quality on this outcome, *Fertil Steril* 70:500, 1998.

63. **Engel W, Murphy D, Schmid M,** Are there genetic risks associated with microassisted reproduction? *Hum Reprod* 11:2359, 1996.

64. **Reijo R, Lee T-Y, Salo P, Alagappan R, Brown LG, Rosenberg M, Rozen S, Jaffe T, Straus D, Hovatta O, et al,** Diverse spermatogenic defects in humans caused by Y chromosome deletions encompassing a novel RNA-binding gene, *Nature Genet* 10:383, 1995.

65. **Reijo R, Alagappan RK, Patrizio P, Page DC,** Severe oligozoospermia resulting from deletions of azoospermia factor gene on Y chromosome, *Lancet* 347:1290, 1996.

66. **Vogt PH, Edelmann A, Kirsch S, Henegrin O, Hirschmann P, Kiesewetter F, Kohn FM, Schill WB, Farah S, Ramos C, Hartmann M, Hartschuh W, Meschede D, Behre HM, Castel A, Nieshlag E, Weidner W, Grone HJ, Jung A, Engel W, Haidl G,** Human Y chromosome azoospermia factors (AZF) mapped to different subregions in Yq11, *Hum Mol Genet* 5:933, 1996.

67. **Girardi SK, Mielnik A, Schlegel PN,** Submicroscopic deletions in the Y chromosome of infertile men, *Hum Reprod* 12:1635, 1997.

68. **Pryor JL, Kent-First M, Muallem A, Van Bergen AH, Nolten WE, Meisner L, Roberts KP,** Microdeletions in the Y chromosome of infertile men, *New Engl J Med* 336:534, 1997.

69. **Pandiyan N, Jequier AM,** Mitotic chromosomal anomalies among 1210 infertile men, *Hum Reprod* 11:2604, 1996.

70. **van der Ven K, Montag M, Peschka B, Leygraaf J, Schwanitz G, Haidl G, Krebs D, van der Ven H,** Combined cytogenetic and Y chromosome microdeletion screening in males undergoing intracytoplasmic sperm injection, *Mol Hum Reprod* 3:699, 1997.

71. **Bonduelle M, Aytoz A, Van Assche E, Devroey P, Liebaers I, Van Steirteghem A,** Incidence of chromosomal aberrations in children born after assisted reproduction through intracytoplasmic sperm injection, *Hum Reprod* 13:781, 1998.

72. **Johnson MD,** Genetic risks of intracytoplasmic sperm injection in the treatment of male infertility: recommendations for genetic counseling and screening, *Fertil Steril* 70:397, 1998.

73. **Pauer HU, Hinney B, Michelmann HW, Krasemann EW, Zoll B, Engel W,** Relevance of genetic counseling in couples prior to intracytoplasmic sperm injection, *Hum Reprod* 12:1909, 1997.

74. **Weiss J, Axelrod L, Whitcomb RW, Harris PE, Crowley WF, Jameson JL,** Hypogonadism caused by a single amino acid substitution in the β-subunit of luteinizing hormone, *New Engl J Med* 326:179, 1992.

75. **Tapanainen JS, Aittomäki K, Min J, Vaskivuo T, Huhtaniemi I,** Men homozygous for an inactivating mutation of the follicle-stimulating hormone (FSH) receptor gene present variable suppression of spermatogenesis and fertility, *Nat Genet* 15:205, 1997.

76. **Jequier AM, Ansell ID, Bullimore NJ,** Congenital absence of the vasa deferentia presenting with infertility, *J Androl* 6:15, 1985.

77. **De Braekeleer M, Férec C,** Mutations in the cystic fibrosis gene in men with congenital bilateral absence of the vas deferens, *Hum Mol Reprod* 2:669, 1996.

78. **Bowen JR, Gibson FL, Leslie GI,** Medical and developmental outcome at 1 year for children conceived by intracytoplasmic sperm injection, *Lancet* 351:1529, 1998.

79. **Bonduelle M, Legein J, Buysse A, Van Assche E, Wisanto A, Devroey P, Van Steirteghem A, Liebaers I,** Prospective followup study of 423 children born after intracytoplasmic sperm injection, *Hum Reprod* 11:1558, 1996.

80. **Bonduelle M, Joris H, Hofmans K, Liebaers I, Van Steirteghem A,** Mental development of 201 ICSI children at 2 years of age, *Lancet* 351:1553, 1998.

81. **Geber S, Paraschos T, Atkinson G, Margara R, Winston RML,** Results of IVF in patients with endometriosis: the severity of the disease does not affect outcome, or the incidence of miscarriage, *Hum Reprod* 10:1507, 1995.

82. **Olivennes F, Feldberg D, Liu H-C, Cohen J, Moy F, Rosenwaks Z,** Endometriosis: a stage-by-stage analysis—the role of in vitro fertilization, *Fertil Steril* 64:392, 1995.

83. **Nagy ZP, Verheyen G, Liu J, Joris H, Janssenswillen C, Wisanto A, Devroey P, Van Steirteghem AC,** Results of 55 intracytoplasmic sperm injection cycles in the treatment of male-immunological infertility, *Hum Reprod* 10:1775, 1995.

84. **Clarke GN, Bourne H, Baker HWG,** Intracytoplasmic sperm injection for treating infertility associated with sperm autoimmunity, *Fertil Steril* 68:112, 1997.

85. **Balmaceda JP, Alam V, Roszjtein D, Ord T, Snell K, Asch R,** Embryo implantation rates in oocyte donation: a prospective comparison of tubal versus uterine transfers, *Fertil Steril* 57:362, 1992.

86. **Craft I, Djahanbakhch O, McLeod F, Bernard A, Green S, Twigg H, Smith W, Lindsay K, Edmonds K,** Human pregnancy following oocyte and sperm transfer to the uterus, *Lancet* i:1031, 1982.

87. **Sauer MV, Bustillo M, Gorrill MJ, Louw JA, Marshall JR, Buster JE,** An instrument for the recovery of preimplantation uterine ova, *Obstet Gynecol* 71:804, 1988.

88. **Faber BM, Mercan R, Hamacher P, Muasher SJ, Toner JP,** The impact of an egg donor's age and her prior fertility on recipient pregnancy outcome, *Fertil Steril* 68:370, 1997.

89. **Meldrum DR,** Female reproductive aging — ovarian and uterine factors, *Fertil Steril* 59:1, 1993.

90. **Legro RS, Wong IL, Paulson RJ, Lobo RA, Sauer MV,** Recipient's age does not adversely affect pregnancy outcome after oocyte donation, *Am J Obstet Gynecol* 172:96, 1995.

91. **Remohí J, Gartner B, Gallardo E, Yalil S, Simón C, Pellicer A,** Pregnancy and birth rates after oocyte donation, *Fertil Steril* 67:717, 1997.

92. **Dubey AK, Layman LC,** Preimplantation genetic diagnosis, *Assist Reprod Rev* 3:224, 1993.

93. **Handyside AH, Lesko JG, Tarin JJ, Winston RML, Hughes MR,** Birth of a normal girl after in vitro fertilization and preimplantation diagnostic testing for cystic fibrosis, *New Engl J Med* 327:905, 1992.

94. **Verlinsky Y, Munne S, Simpson JL, Kullen A, Ao A, Ray P, Sermon K, Martin R, Strom C, Van Steirteghem A, Veiga A, Drury K, Williams S, Ginsberg N, Wilton L,** Current status of preimplantation diagnosis, *J Assist Reprod Genet* 14:72, 1997.

32 Ectopic Pregnancy

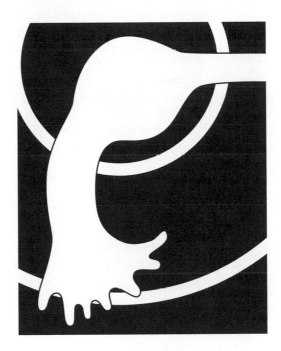

The modern management of ectopic pregnancy is one of medicine's greatest success stories. Ectopic pregnancy has been recognized for a very long time (it was first described in the 11th century), and for a long time, only as a universally fatal event. In medieval times, the ectopic pregnancy was believed to be located outside the uterus because of a violent emotion, usually fright or surprise, experienced by the woman during the coitus of conception.[1] Treatment was so unavailable that the only recourse was speculation.

The first documentation of an unruptured ectopic pregnancy was recorded in 1693 in the results of an autopsy performed on a woman prisoner condemned to death and executed. Previous infertility was linked to ectopic pregnancy in 1752 with the report of an extrauterine pregnancy in a prostitute with 20 years of sterility. In the mid 19th century, pathology reports began to stress pelvic inflammation as a cause of ectopic pregnancy. This knowledge was derived from women who died because of tubal rupture and hemorrhage. Although data were gradually accumulated from autopsies and the pathology was described, treatment remained unavailable.

Because the ectopic fetus was obviously responsible for the death of the mother, physicians recommended measures to kill the fetus. These measures included starvation, purging, bleeding, and even large doses of strychnine. Early attempts to surgically puncture ectopic sacs or to introduce electric current into the fetus were followed by sepsis and maternal death.

Around 1600, there were several isolated reports of abdominal surgical procedures in women with repeat ectopic pregnancies. Then for more than 100 years there was no mention of a surgical operation for this purpose. The first case in the 18th century was reported in France in 1714. The first American surgeon to operate abdominally and successfully (for the removal of a macerated fetus) was John Bard of New York City in 1759. The second successful American operation was performed in 1791 by William Baynham, a country physician in Virginia. In 30 abdominal operations in the first 80 years of the 1800s, only 5 women survived.[1] The survival rate in those not treated (one out of three) was better!

W.W. Harbert of Louisville was the first, in 1849, to suggest surgery early enough to stop fatal bleeding.[2] But the problem was that diagnosis was only certain when it was too late. In 1876, John S. Parry (of the Philadelphia Hospital) wrote:[3]

> ...when one is called to a case of this kind, it is his duty to look upon his unhappy patient as inevitably doomed to die, unless he can by some active measure wrest her from the grave already yawning before her.

Robert Lawson Tait in London, after experiencing the death of several women and at autopsy recognizing that appropriate dissection and ligation of bleeding vessels would be effective, for the first time in 1883, deliberately and successfully performed a laparotomy to ligate the broad ligament and a ruptured tube.[4] By 1885, Tait had accumulated a relatively large number of successful cases.

Asepsis, anesthesia, and antibiotics (and blood transfusions) combined to save the lives of many women. But diagnosis was still difficult, and surgical intervention was relatively late. Even in the first half of the 20th century, the maternal mortality rate in the United States ranged from 200 to 400 per 10,000 cases of ectopic pregnancies. As dramatic as the contribution of immediate salpingectomy coupled with simultaneous blood transfusion was, progress in the last 20 years has been even more impressive. Treatment has shifted from the saving of lives to the preservation of fertility.

The Centers for Disease Control first began to report the incidence of ectopic pregnancies in the U.S. in 1970. In 1970, there were 17,800 ectopic pregnancies, and by 1992, the number had increased to 108,800, a rate increase of 4.5 to 19.7 ectopic pregnancies per 1000 pregnancies.[5] *However, at the same time, the fatality rate decreased from 35.5 to 3.4 per 10,000 ectopic pregnancies, a decrease of 90%.*

The increase in ectopic pregnancies has not been paralleled by a similar increase in sexually transmitted diseases (STDs), and, therefore, the increased incidence of ectopic pregnancies is not due to STDs alone.[6] Ectopic pregnancies do occur in totally normal tubes, suggesting that abnormalities of the conceptus or maternal hormonal changes can function as etiologic factors. The other important contributing factors are reconstructive tubal surgery, assisted reproductive technologies, and, most importantly, earlier and more accurate diagnosis.

Today, management intervention occurs prior to tubal rupture in more than 80% of cases.[7] This can be attributed directly to three diagnostic advances: a highly specific and sensitive immunoassay for human chorionic gonadotropin (HCG), ultrasonography, and the use of laparoscopy.

Etiology and Clinical Presentation

Even though the risk of death from ectopic pregnancy has declined dramatically, ectopic pregnancy is the second leading cause of overall maternal mortality in the United States and the leading cause of pregnancy-related deaths during the first trimester.[8] This represents a combination of a lack of access to appropriate services and misdiagnosis.

Ectopic pregnancy is the great masquerader. The clinical presentation can vary from vaginal spotting to vasomotor shock with hematoperitoneum. The classic triad of delayed menses, irregular vaginal bleeding, and abdominal pain is most commonly *not* encountered. The exact frequency of clinical symptoms and signs is hard to assess. Standard descriptions in texts are based upon older reports and, thus, older methods of diagnosis. Suspicion of the diagnosis and rapid recourse to the methods of early diagnosis represent the best and most rewarding approach. Patients who present because of acute symptoms (frequently in emergency rooms) are usually at a more advanced gestational age compared to asymptomatic infertility patients being followed closely because of their increased risk for ectopic pregnancy.

Differential Diagnosis

- Normal intrauterine pregnancy.
- Ruptured ovarian cyst.
- Bleeding corpus luteum.
- Spontaneous miscarriage.
- Salpingitis.
- Appendicitis.
- Adnexal torsion.
- Endometriosis.
- Diverticulitis.

Relevant factors in a patient's medical history include prior tubal surgery, the use of assisted reproductive technology, exposure to diethylstilbestrol (DES), previous pelvic inflammatory disease, vaginal douching,[9] and the method of contraception. In addition, cigarette smoking is associated with a 2-fold increased risk for ectopic pregnancy.[10] However, most patients presenting with an ectopic pregnancy do not have a recognized risk factor, suggesting dysfunctional problems in tubal transport or impaired implantation due to some abnormality in the conceptus. Nevertheless, pregnancies following tubal surgery or treatment with one of the methods of assisted reproduction should, ideally, be diagnosed immediately and followed closely with HCG titers and ultrasonography.

Previous Pelvic Inflammatory Disease

In Westrom's classic report, women with a history of salpingitis (verified by laparoscopy) had a four-fold increased risk of ectopic pregnancy.[11] Salpingitis damages the endosalpinx, resulting in agglutination of the mucosal folds and adhesion formation. The risk of an ectopic pregnancy increases with each inflammatory episode. Evidence of chlamydial infection (circulating antibodies) is associated with a greater than two-fold increased risk of ectopic pregnancy.[12] A similar increased risk is associated with douching, but the presence of infection may be the reason for the douching.

Prior Tubal Surgery

Women who have had tubal surgery have an increased risk of ectopic pregnancy. High-risk surgery includes any infertility surgery on the tube, but not abdominal or pelvic surgery that avoids the tubes.[13] Women with an ectopic pregnancy treated by conservative surgery have a tenfold increased risk of a subsequent ectopic. Ectopic pregnancies occur after tubal occlusion procedures for sterilization that are not performed immediately postpartum (interval sterilization); the risk with postpartum sterilization is very low, comparable to that observed in oral contraceptive users.[14–16] With interval sterilization, bipolar tubal coagulation is more likely to result in ectopic pregnancy than is mechanical occlusion.[16–18] This is attributed to fistula formation that allows sperm passage, and this may explain the difference in ectopic pregnancy rates between interval and postpartum sterilization because postpartum procedures are mostly by the Pomeroy method. Ectopic pregnancies following tubal ligation usually occur two or more years after the sterilization, rather than immediately after. In the first year after sterilization, about 6% of sterilization failures will be ectopic pregnancies, but the majority of pregnancies that occur 2–3 years after occlusion will be ectopic.[17] Overall, the ectopic risk in women with interval sterilizations is 80% less than that in nonsterilized women; however, the relative risk is 3.7 times that of women using oral contraception and 2.8 times that with barrier methods of contraception.[15] About one-third of pregnancies that occur after tubal sterilization are ectopic.[16]

Estimated Relative Risk of Ectopic Pregnancy [10, 19–21]

Risk Factor	Relative Risk
Tubal surgery	20.0
Previous ectopic	10.0
Previous salpingitis	4.0
Assisted reproduction	4.0
Age <25	3.0
Previous pelvic infection	3.0
Infertility	2.5
Cigarette smoking	2.5
Vaginal douching	2.5

The Use of Assisted Reproductive Technology

Pregnancies occurring *simultaneously* in different body sites *(heterotopic pregnancies)* are a rare condition, occurring in 1 of 30,000 spontaneous pregnancies. The incidence of combined pregnancy among patients who have undergone one of the assisted reproduction procedures (in vitro fertilization, gamete intrafallopian transfer, and even superovulation) is much higher, closer to 1 in 100 pregnancies.[22–24] Close monitoring of pregnancies in these programs is important to prevent a deleterious delay in the treatment of an ectopic pregnancy.

Is the increased risk with these treatment methods due to ovulation induction (with superovulation and elevated levels of hormone influence on the tubes) or due to previous tubal disease? A case-control study has concluded that the risk of ectopic pregnancy was increased four-fold with ovulation induction, but not further increased when ovulation induction was used for in vitro fertilization.[25] This would indicate that the multiple eggs and high hormone levels are the important factors. Retrograde embryo migration is believed to be a major mechanism.

Method of Contraception

The risk of ectopic pregnancy is reduced with all methods of contraception except the progesterone-containing intrauterine device.[14, 26, 27]

The IUD has been traditionally listed as a risk factor for ectopic pregnancy. The previous use of an IUD does not increase the risk of a subsequent ectopic pregnancy.[28] And it should be emphasized that the current use of modern copper-bearing IUDs does *NOT* increase the risk of ectopic pregnancy and, in fact, offers considerable protection.[14, 29–32] The largest study, a World

Ectopic Pregnancy Rates per 1000 Woman-Years [5, 14, 26, 27]

All U.S. women	1.50
Noncontraceptive users	3.00
Copper T-380 IUD	0.20
Progesterone IUD	6.80
Levonorgestrel IUD	0.20
Norplant	0.28

Health Organization multicenter study, concluded that IUD users were 50% less likely to have an ectopic pregnancy when compared to women using no contraception.[14] However, if an IUD user becomes pregnant, the pregnancy is more likely to be ectopic. About 3–4% of IUD pregnancies have been ectopic, making the actual occurrence a rare event.

The lowest ectopic pregnancy rates are seen with the most effective IUDs, like the TCu-380A (90% less likely compared to noncontraceptors).[27] The rate is about one-tenth the ectopic pregnancy rate associated with the Lippes Loop or with devices with less copper such as the TCu-200.[27] The progesterone-releasing IUD has a higher rate, probably because its action is limited to a local effect on the endometrium,[31] while very few ectopic pregnancies have been reported with the levonorgestrel IUD, presumably because it is associated with a partial suppression of gonadotropins with subsequent disruption of normal follicular growth and development, and in a significant number of cycles, inhibition of ovulation.[27, 33–36]

The risk of ectopic pregnancy does not increase with increasing duration of use with the TCu-380A or the levonorgestrel IUD.[33, 37] In a 7-year prospective study, not a single ectopic pregnancy was encountered with the levonorgestrel IUD.[33] In 8000 woman-years of experience in randomized multicenter trials, there has been only a single ectopic pregnancy reported with the TCu-380A (which is one-tenth the rate with the Lippes Loop or TCu-200).[33]

The protection against ectopic pregnancy provided by the TCu-380A and the levonorgestrel IUD makes these IUDs acceptable choices for contraception in women with previous ectopic pregnancies.

The risk of an ectopic pregnancy during use of Norplant is lower than the general rate. However, because of the impressive contraceptive efficacy of Norplant, when pregnancy does occur, ectopic pregnancy should be suspected. With the progestin-only minipill, ectopic pregnancy is not prevented as effectively as intrauterine pregnancy. Although the overall incidence is not increased, the situation is similar to that with Norplant. When pregnancy occurs, an ectopic gestation must be suspected.

Ectopic Sites

Almost all ectopic pregnancies are located in the tube. Although relatively uncommon, ectopic pregnancies in nontubal sites are very susceptible to complications, especially hemorrhage. For example, abdominal pregnancies are often misdiagnosed, and the mortality rate is 17 times greater compared to the overall ectopic rate.[38] Contrary to the experience with tubal pregnancy, recurrence in nontubal sites is rare.

Sites of Ectopic Implantation[39]

Fallopian tube:	
Ampullary segment	80 %
Isthmic segment	12 %
Fimbrial end	5 %
Cornual and interstitial	2 %
Abdominal	1.4%
Ovarian	0.2%
Cervical	0.2%

The Methods of Early Diagnosis

Patients with normal intrauterine pregnancies can present with the same symptoms encountered in patients with unruptured ectopic pregnancies. The best way to diagnose ectopic pregnancy is to be highly suspicious and sensitive to its possibility, and to utilize the new tools of diagnosis: the quantitative measurement of β-HCG and ultrasonography. Laparoscopy is necessary only when the diagnosis is in doubt, or when laparoscopy is the technique selected for surgical treatment.

The Quantitative Measurement of HCG

HCG is secreted by the syncytiotrophoblast and reaches a maximal level of 50,000–100,000 IU/L at 8–10 weeks of gestation. The maternal circulating HCG concentration is approximately 100 IU/L at the time of the expected but missed menses. Virtually 100% (but not absolutely all) of patients suspected of an ectopic pregnancy, but not pregnant, will have a negative blood assay for β-HCG.[40] Contrast this present day sensitivity of the HCG assay with the urinary tests of the past. In the 1960s and early 1970s, the urinary pregnancy tests were positive in only 50% of patients with ectopic pregnancies.

The modern assay for HCG measures the serum level of the HCG beta subunit. β-HCG is the largest gonadotropin β-subunit, containing a larger carbohydrate moiety and 145 amino acid residues, including a unique carboxyl terminal tail piece of 24 amino acid groups. It is this unique part of the HCG structure which allows the production of highly specific antibodies and the utilization of highly specific immunologic assays. In some laboratories, the lower limit of the assay is 4–6 IU/L, but even that level is almost never associated with a false negative. With a detection limit of less than 5 IU/L for the serum β-HCG assay, there should be no false-negative results; however, this situation (very rarely) can be encountered.[41] When the clinical picture is confusing, a definitive diagnosis by laparoscopy is warranted.

A landmark observation was reported from Yale in 1981, documenting that HCG levels approximately double every 2 days in early, normal intrauterine pregnancies, and that a lesser increase is associated with ectopic pregnancies and spontaneous miscarriages.[42] In the first 6 weeks of normal pregnancy, the concentration of HCG in the maternal blood follows a well-recognized pattern.[43] The rate of increase is nonlinear, changing with advancing gestational age and increasing HCG concentrations.[44] However, during the time period when the diagnosis of ectopic pregnancy is most important, from 2 to 4 weeks after ovulation, the relationship between HCG titers and gestational age is linear, approximately doubling every 2 days until the titer is greater than 10,000.[45] Use of the HCG titer requires medical judgment. Some ectopic pregnancies will display a normal rise in titer (at least for awhile), and some normal pregnancies (about 10%) will have an abnormal doubling time.

The Clinical Usefulness of the Quantitative Measurement of β-HCG

1. **Assessment of pregnancy viability.**

   Most of the time, but not always, a normal rate of rise indicates a normal pregnancy. Clinical decisions require serial measurements of HCG.

2. **Correlation with ultrasonography.**

   When the titer exceeds 1000–1500 IU/L, vaginal ultrasonography should identify the presence of an intrauterine gestation. With multiple gestation, a gestational sac will not be apparent until the titer is a little higher.[46] In an asymptomatic patient, repeat ultrasonography 2–3 days later is warranted.

3. **Assessment of treatment results.**

   Declining levels are consistent with effective medical or surgical treatment. Persistent or rising levels indicate the presence of viable trophoblastic tissue.

Vaginal Ultrasonography

The difficulty in diagnosis is establishing the cause of abnormal HCG levels: is it an ectopic pregnancy or a spontaneous miscarriage? The addition of ultrasonography has made an important contribution to this differential diagnosis. A "gestational sac" is an ultrasonographic landmark, located beneath the endometrial surface, and visualized by transvaginal ultrasonography beginning 30–35 days after the last menstrual period.[47, 48] It is a sonolucent center surrounded by a thick echogenic rim, formed by a decidual reaction round the chorionic sac. The yoke sac is the first structure visualized within the gestational sac, at 5 weeks after the last menstrual period. Cardiac motion is first observed at 5.5–6 weeks gestation.

The discriminatory zone is that HCG titer above which a gestational sac can be identified with ultrasonography. Previously, with abdominal ultrasonography, this level was approximately 6000 IU/L. Transvaginal ultrasonography has now established the discriminatory zone at a level that varies from 1000 to 1500 IU/L. This level is achieved approximately one week after the time of expected menses. Institutions must establish their own exact discriminatory zone based on the sensitivity of their immunoassay and their equipment and the ability of their ultrasonographers. Keep in mind that in a multiple pregnancy, the discriminatory zone will be a little higher, requiring an extra 2–3 days for a gestational sac to become visible. Thus, an accurate gestational age is very helpful; failure to demonstrate the presence of a gestational sac 24 or more days after conception (38 or more gestational days) usually indicates an ectopic pregnancy.[49]

Demonstration of a viable intrauterine pregnancy does not absolutely exclude the possibility of an ectopic pregnancy. Along with the increase in incidence of ectopic pregnancy associated with superovulation, dizygotic twinning is more common, and thus a combined intrauterine pregnancy and extrauterine pregnancy (heterotopic pregnancy) is more frequent. ***Heterotopic pregnancy should especially be considered when the pregnancy is the result of one of the methods of assisted reproductive technology.***

Color and pulsed Doppler increases the sensitivity of vaginal ultrasonography. This method adds physiologic information to the anatomic picture of regular ultrasonography. A small intrauterine gestational sac, without the double sac sign (decidua and membranes) or the presence of a yolk sac is hard to distinguish from the pseudosac of an ectopic pregnancy. A pseudogestational sac due to endometrial bleeding occurs in about 10% of ectopic pregnancies.[50] Local vascular changes associated with a true gestational sac differentiate an intrauterine pregnancy from the pseudosac of ectopic pregnancy. Vascular pulses increase with pregnancy and produce a "warm" appearance with color Doppler ultrasonography. In addition, high-velocity arterial flow is detected even with very early pregnancies.

A failed intrauterine pregnancy can be associated with either elevated flow velocity around the trophoblast or very low velocities. Thus, a characteristic peritrophoblastic arterial flow correlates with gestational sac size and HCG levels.[51] Ectopic masses can also be distinguished by the surrounding abnormal color mapping. Doppler ultrasound, therefore, has greater sensitivity and is technically less challenging (and quicker). Although traditional ultrasonography can reveal an adnexal mass, Doppler flow imaging can indicate that the mass is an ectopic pregnancy by documenting abnormal vascular activity of the mass combined with the relatively cool uterine vasculature. This difference between Doppler and standard ultrasonography is greatest in early pregnancy, and thus this greater accuracy can allow earlier initiation of medical treatment.

Important Observations With Vaginal Ultrasonography

1. **Documentation of an intrauterine sac.**
    An experienced ultrasonographer should be able to identify a viable intrauterine pregnancy if the HCG titer is 1000–1500 IU/L or greater. An HCG titer of greater than 1000–1500 IU/L with no intrauterine sac is consistent with an ectopic pregnancy.

2. **Adnexal masses.**
    An ectopic equal to or greater than 2 cm in diameter should be identified by ultrasonography. Vaginal ultrasonography should also establish large ectopics that require different consideration. Currently an ectopic pregnancy with a diameter of 4 cm or more is a relative contraindication to medical treatment.

3. **Adnexal cardiac activity.**
    The presence of cardiac activity in an ectopic pregnancy, detectable when the HCG titer is approximately 15,000–20,000 IU/L, is a relative contraindication to medical treatment.

The Progesterone Level

Single serum progesterone levels have a wide spectrum with considerable overlap between normal and ectopic pregnancies. This measurement must be viewed as an adjunct to HCG levels and ultrasonography. The concentration of the serum progesterone is usually lower in ectopic pregnancies. A value of 25 ng/mL or more is 98% of the time associated with a normal intrauterine pregnancy, while a value of less than 5 ng/mL identifies a nonviable pregnancy, regardless of location.[52] The value of the serum progesterone is to help make a decision regarding the viability of a possible intrauterine pregnancy prior to curettage. In most cases, however, this is a decision

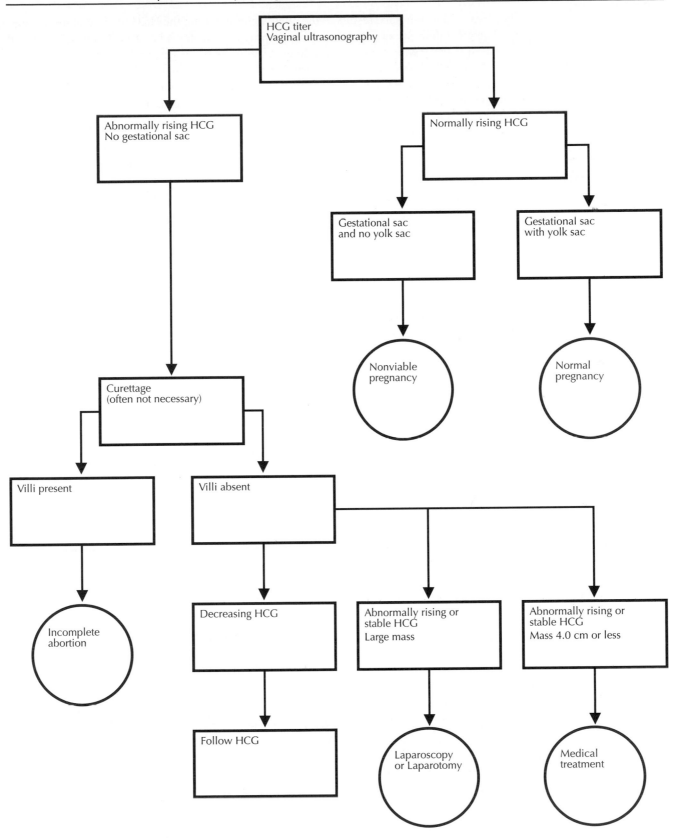

easily made by the combined results of the clinical presentation, the HCG titers, and ultrasonography. The great majority of patients will have a progesterone level between 10 and 20 ng/mL at presentation, significantly limiting the clinical usefulness of progesterone measurement.[53] The value of 25 ng/mL as an indicator of a normal intrauterine pregnancy was established in women with spontaneous ovulations and pregnancies. The appropriate number for women receiving medication for the induction of ovulation is probably higher, and in these cases, the use of the progesterone level is even more limited.

Uterine Curettage

The purpose of uterine curettage is to determine the presence or absence of villi to rule out a nonviable intrauterine pregnancy. In most cases, curettage is helpful when a serum progesterone is less than 5 ng/mL and a non-rising HCG titer is below 1000 IU/L. Curettage with examination of the curettings can be used to prevent unnecessary laparoscopies in patients undergoing spontaneous miscarriages. Floating the curettings in saline will usually identify villi if present, but not always. The saline flotation of curettings has been reported to be incorrect in 6.6% of patients with ectopic pregnancies and incorrect in 11.3% of patients with intrauterine pregnancies.[52] Because of this inaccuracy, permanent sections and follow-up HCG titers are necessary for confirmation.

Culdocentesis

Culdocentesis to seek the presence of unclotted blood was for a period of time a valuable technique to aid in the diagnosis of an ectopic pregnancy. We have progressed to the point where the relative accuracy of culdocentesis is no longer sufficient. Furthermore, the presence of blood in the cul-de-sac does not mean that an ectopic pregnancy has ruptured. Therefore, a positive culdocentesis is of no help in deciding whether to treat medically or surgically. Culdocentesis no longer has a place in the differential diagnosis of ectopic pregnancy.

The Treatment of Ectopic Pregnancy

Expectant Management

Part of the increased incidence of ectopic pregnancy is due to earlier diagnosis detecting ectopic pregnancies, which previously resolved and remained clinically undiagnosed. Not all tubal pregnancies progress to clinical manifestations, and, therefore, expectant management of ectopic pregnancies diagnosed very early is an appropriate choice.[54] Expectant management includes the monitoring of clinical symptoms, HCG titers, and ultrasonography findings. Approximately one-fourth of women presenting with ectopic pregnancy can be managed expectantly, and 70% of this select group of patients will avoid surgery and experience successful outcomes.[55] Success with expectant management decreases with increasing HCG levels; best results are achieved when the initial HCG level is less than 2000 IU/L.[56, 57] The long-term outcome (subsequent intrauterine and ectopic pregnancies) is similar to that with active treatment interventions.[58] The following criteria are reasonable requirements for expectant management:

Criteria for Expectant Management

1. Falling HCG titer.

2. Ectopic pregnancy definitely in the tube.

3. No significant bleeding.

4. No evidence of rupture.

5. Ectopic mass not larger than 4 cm in greatest diameter.

Medical Treatment

Medical treatment of unruptured ectopic pregnancies is appealing for several reasons: less tubal damage, less cost, and, hopefully, enhanced potential for future fertility. Methotrexate, a folic acid antagonist that interferes with DNA synthesis, has a long history of effectiveness against trophoblastic tissue, derived from experience in the treatment of hydatiform moles and choriocarcinoma. Methotrexate was used in the 1960s to treat the difficult problem of trophoblastic tissue left in situ after removal of an abdominal pregnancy. Methotrexate was first used to treat an ectopic pregnancy in Japan in 1982.[59] The first U. S. experience was reported by Ory in 1986.[60] The guidelines for the safe and effective use of methotrexate were established by Stovall and his colleagues.[61, 62]

Criteria for Patient Selection

1. The patient is healthy, hemodynamically stable, reliable, and compliant.

2. Ultrasonography should fail to find an intrauterine pregnancy, and uterine curettage should fail to obtain villi.

3. The ectopic pregnancy measures 4 cm or less in its greatest diameter.

4. There is no evidence of rupture of the ectopic pregnancy.

5. HCG titers greater than 10,000 IU/L and fetal cardiac activity are relative contraindications. However, even patients with fetal cardiac activity have been successfully treated.

Prior to Methotrexate Treatment

1. Administer Rhogam if patient is Rh-negative and greater than 8 weeks gestation.

2. Obtain baseline liver and renal function tests, complete blood and platelet counts.

3. Consider uterine curettage.

Patient Instructions

The following are avoided until HCG titers are negative: alcohol use, sexual intercourse, and the use of folic acid-containing vitamins.

The Multiple Dose Method. The initial protocols for treatment utilized multiple doses of methotrexate together with citrovorum factor (folinic acid) to minimize side effects. Treatment with this method has been reported to be 70–94% successful. Failures have been more common with HCG levels greater than 5000 IU/mL, and thus the presence of fetal cardiac activity is generally a contraindication. Side effects (in 3–4% of patients) include mild stomatitis, gastritis, diarrhea, and transient elevations in liver enzymes. Significant reactions (bone marrow suppression, dermatitis, pneumonitis) have been very rare.[63, 64] The incidence of nonresponders and/or tubal rupture is 3–4%.

In our own experience, the onset of abdominal cramping occurring 3–4 days after the initiation of methotrexate treatment (in approximately 60% of patients) produces some anxious moments. The concern, of course, is that the ectopic pregnancy is rupturing. Although this is always a possibility, the cramping is usually a side effect of the methotrexate and resolves in a day or two. Occasionally, hospitalization is necessary until hemodynamic stability is verified.

Multiple Dose Methotrexate Protocol

Treatment is discontinued when a decline is observed in two consecutive daily HCG titers, or after 4 doses of methotrexate.

Day 1:	Baseline studies.	
	Methotrexate	1.0 mg/kg im.
Day 2:	Citrovorum factor	0.1 mg/kg im.
Day 3:	Methotrexate	1.0 mg/kg im.
Day 4:	Citrovorum factor	0.1 mg/kg im.
	HCG titer.	
Day 5:	Methotrexate	1.0 mg/kg im.
	HCG titer.	
Day 6:	Citrovorum factor	0.1 mg/kg im.
	HCG titer.	
Day 7:	Methotrexate	1.0 mg/kg im.
	HCG titer.	
Day 8:	Citrovorum factor	0.1 mg/kg im.
	HCG titer.	
	Complete blood and platelet counts.	
	Renal and liver function tests.	
Weekly:	HCG titer until negative.	

Approximately 20% of patients will require only one dose of methotrexate, and 20% will require 4 doses.[62, 65, 66] The side effects are encountered in those patients who require multiple doses. Changes in blood counts and liver enzymes are so infrequent and so mild, that daily monitoring is unnecessary.

In terms of subsequent fertility, methotrexate compares favorably with conservative laparoscopic surgery, and the rate of subsequent ectopic pregnancy is lower.[21, 67] In a randomized trial comparing multiple dose methotrexate with laparoscopy, the results were as follows:[68]

	Multiple Dose Methotrexate	Laparoscopy
No further treatment	82%	72%
Treatment for persistent trophoblast	4%	20%

The ultrasonographic picture of a mass persists after HCG titers become negative.[69] The time for resolution of the mass is variable, and often it takes several months. Thus, the persistence of a mass should not be interpreted as a treatment failure.

The Single Dose Method. Experience with the multiple dose method indicated that a significant number of patients responded promptly and did not require several doses. With lesser dosing, fewer side effects could be anticipated, and the use of citrovorum factor could be abandoned. The results with a single dose are very good (80–90%), even with very high HCG titers and the presence of fetal cardiac activity.[65, 70, 71] The HCG titers usually keep rising for 3 days after treatment but by day 7 are declining. Full resolution requires 3 to as much as 6 weeks. Serious side effects are virtually absent. If there is less than a 15% decline on day 7 (the usual assay variation), the treatment protocol is repeated (necessary in approximately 8% of patients).[21]

Single Dose Methotrexate Protocol

Day 1:	Baseline studies.	
	Methotrexate	50 mg/M^2 im.
Day 4:	HCG titer.	
Day 7:	HCG titer	
	Complete blood and platelet count.	
	Liver and renal function tests.	
Weekly:	HCG titer until negative.	

Oral Methotrexate. Experience with the oral method of treatment is not encouraging. One comparison with placebo in the expectant management of ectopic pregnancy found no indication of any effect.[72]

Important Cautions. The medical treatment of ectopic pregnancy requires compulsive compliance. An ectopic pregnancy can exist in the absence of detectable HCG.[73] Although in this instance, the extrauterine pregnancy is usually degenerating and associated with an indolent clinical course, rupture can still occur. Clinicians should always be alert for the possibility of rupture (3–4% of medically treated cases). A satisfying decline in HCG titers does not guarantee against rupture.[74] The average time for HCG to return to nondetectable levels is about 4 weeks.

The risk of tubal rupture is about 10% when the HCG titer is less than 1000 IU/L, and if the ectopic is isthmic, a risk of rupture is still present with a titer of 100 or less. Remember that a negative HCG assay means that HCG is not present in levels greater than the sensitivity of the assay; therefore, trophoblastic tissue can still be present, secreting minimal amounts of HCG (below the limits of the assay). Ectopic pregnancies will continue to adhere to their historical record; always expect behavior that is an exception to the general rule.

Although experience is limited with the medical treatment of relatively large masses (with a fetus present and high levels of HCG), case reports indicate a greater risk of bleeding and problems. Carefully selected cases with HCG titers greater than 10,000 IU/L might warrant medical treatment, but as a general rule these cases deserve surgical treatment.

Special Indications for Methotrexate. Treatment with methotrexate is especially useful when the pregnancy is located in a site (cervix, ovary, or cornua) where surgical treatment carries significant risk.[75–77] Methotrexate treatment is an attractive option when an ectopic pregnancy is in the interstitial portion of the tube or growing in the wall of the uterus (diagnosed by ultrasonography).[78]

Salpingocentesis

Salpingocentesis is the injection of a substance directly into the gestational sac within the tube, either at laparoscopy or under ultrasound guidance. Various substances have been used, including methotrexate, potassium chloride, prostaglandins, and hyperosmotic glucose. The efficacy, safety, and the long-term impact on fertility have not been established. Thus far local injections have been associated with inconsistent results; at least one clinical trial was discontinued because of poor results with tubal injection of methotrexate while another claimed excellent results, especially when the HCG level was under 5000 IU/L.[79–81] Circulating levels of methotrexate are similar when gestational sac injection is compared to intramuscular injection.[82] Thus, local treatment with methotrexate offers no obvious advantage over systemic treatment. Hyperosmotic glucose (a 50% solution) appears to be safe and effective when the HCG titers are less than 2500 IU/L.[83]

Surgical Treatment

With earlier diagnosis, conservative surgery to preserve fertility has replaced the life-saving procedure of salpingectomy. Linear salpingostomy along the antimesenteric border to remove the products of conception is the procedure of choice for ectopic pregnancies in the ampullary portion of the tube. Ectopic pregnancies in the ampulla are usually located between the lumen and the serosa, and thus these are ideal candidates for linear salpingostomy. Segmental excision with either simultaneous or delayed microsurgical anastomosis is the preferred procedure for isthmic pregnancies. Although linear salpingostomy is possible for a small and unruptured gestation, isthmic pregnancies reflect a damaged endosalpinx, and these patients do poorly with linear salpingostomy (with a high rate of recurrent ectopic pregnancy).

Occasionally, an ampullary pregnancy can be expressed through the fimbrial end of the tube (milking the tube), but this procedure is associated with a higher incidence of persistent and recurrent ectopic pregnancy, undoubtedly due to invasion of the tube by the trophoblastic tissue. However, fimbrial expression of an ectopic pregnancy that is easily dislodged is acceptable. Interstitial pregnancy at the utero-tubal junction usually requires surgical excision, and even hysterectomy if bleeding cannot be controlled. The first unruptured ectopic pregnancy treated with methotrexate was an interstitial pregnancy, and this is now the treatment of choice if diagnosis is achieved early enough.

Patients with compromised fertility do better when the tube that contains the ectopic pregnancy is conserved (even when the opposite tube appears to be normal). However, in patients with a history positive for previous tubal disease, the risk of a recurrent ectopic pregnancy in the same tube is very much higher, and in this case, some argue in favor of salpingectomy. When performing a salpingectomy, a cornual wedge excision as prophylaxis against recannulation and a subsequent ectopic pregnancy is no longer considered to be necessary. An effort should be made to retain both ovaries when appropriate as a resource for the future use of in vitro fertilization.

> **Indications for Salpingectomy**
> **Childbearing completed.**
> **Second ectopic pregnancy in the same tube.**
> **Uncontrolled bleeding.**
> **Severely damaged tube.**

These procedures can be accomplished either by laparotomy or laparoscopy. The choice of surgical method and specific procedure is determined by the patient's condition, desire for future fertility, the location, size, and state of the ectopic pregnancy, and the experience of the surgeon. The relative contraindications to laparoscopy include extensive pelvic adhesions, hemato-peritoneum, and an ectopic pregnancy greater than 4 cm diameter. Hemodynamic instability is an absolute contraindication.

Linear salpingostomy through the laparoscope achieves results comparable with those obtained at laparotomy.[84, 85] Hemostasis is the key and several methods are used, including the use of vasopressin, microcautery, and laser. The gains are notable: outpatient versus inpatient cost and a more rapid recovery. Almost all patients can now be successfully treated with conservative surgery. Comparisons of the different types of surgery (laparoscopic salpingostomy, laparotomy salpingostomy, and laparotomy salpingectomy) indicate that the surgical technique chosen is less important in determining future fertility than the causes of the ectopic pregnancy.[86, 87]

Results with Laparoscopic Surgery

Subsequent intrauterine pregnancy	70%
Subsequent tubal patency	84%
Subsequent ectopic pregnancy	12%
Persistent trophoblast	15%

Treatment of an Ectopic Pregnancy After Tubal Ligation

An ectopic pregnancy after a previous tubal ligation is usually located in the segment of tube containing the fimbria. The pregnancy occurs because of small channel recannulation through the ligation site, allowing sperm to migrate toward the oocyte. A prophylactic procedure should be highly considered. Removing both fimbrial segments and fulgurating the proximal segments (either by laparoscopy or laparotomy) will prevent the recurrence of another ectopic pregnancy.

Treatment of Persistent Trophoblastic Tissue

The risk of a persistent ectopic pregnancy with conservative surgery by laparotomy is 5%.[88] Laparoscopic salpingostomy is associated with a higher rate of persistent trophoblastic tissue; approximately 15% of patients will require further treatment.[89] Persistence of ectopic trophoblastic tissue can be associated with hemorrhage and tubal rupture (usually within 2 weeks); however, regression without clinical sequelae is the general rule. For this reason, *weekly HCG measurements are necessary following conservative surgery.* The incidence of persistent trophoblastic tissue is greater (not surprising) with higher HCG titers, and relatively rare with a titer less than 3000 IU/L.[90] The risk of persistent trophoblastic tissue is very significant with a hematosalpinx greater than 6 cm in diameter, an HCG titer greater than 20,000 IU/L, and a hematoperitoneum greater than 2000 mL.[91] Rupture is unlikely for an ampullary pregnancy with an HCG level of 100 or less, but not so for an isthmic pregnancy.

The average time for HCG levels to become undetectable is 4 weeks, but it can take 6 weeks. The need for treatment of persistent trophoblastic tissue can emerge in a few days or not until 1 month later. Although reoperation is always a treatment option, the use of methotrexate is preferable. Prophylactic treatment can be administered with a single dose of methotrexate (1mg/kg), or a single dose of methotrexate (15 mg/m^2) can be administered after diagnosis.[92, 93]

Low and declining HCG levels warrant only close surveillance; only persistent or rising titers require treatment (a small minority of patients). Symptomatic patients, of course, usually demand surgical therapy.

The problem of persistent trophoblastic tissue after surgery makes earlier diagnosis of an ectopic pregnancy even more important. With sufficiently early diagnosis, medical treatment becomes the method of choice.

Rh Sensitization

Despite underutilization of Rhogam in Rh-negative women, no apparent increase in sensitization has been observed.[94, 95] This indicates that ectopic pregnancies do not contain sufficiently large quantities of fetal red blood cells. The use of Rhogam should be considered only for ectopic pregnancies that are older than 8 weeks gestation.

Fertility After Ectopic Pregnancy

Having had one ectopic pregnancy, a woman is at increased risk for another, especially if infectious pathology is present.[21] Nevertheless, after one ectopic pregnancy, the chance of having a live-born infant is 85% with the next pregnancy. After 2 ectopic pregnancies, the risk of ectopic pregnancy is increased nearly 10-fold, and consideration should be given to in vitro fertilization.

References

1. **Graham H,** *Eternal Eve, The History of Gynaecology & Obstetrics,* Doubleday & Company, Inc., Garden City, NY, 1951.

2. **Harbert WW,** A case of extra-uterine pregnancy, *West J Med Surg* 3:110, 1849.

3. **Parry JS,** *Extra-uterine Pregnancy: Its Causes, Species, Pathological Anatomy, Clinical History, Diagnosis, Prognosis, and Treatment,* H. C. Lea, Philadelphia, 1876.

4. **Tait RL,** Five cases of extra-uterine pregnancy operated upon at the time of rupture, *Br Med J* i:1250, 1884.

5. **Centers for Disease Control,** *http://www.cdc.gov* .

6. **Nederlof KP, Lawson HW, Saftlas AF, Atrash HK, Finch EL,** Ectopic pregnancy surveillance, United States, 1970-1987, *MMWR* 39:9, 1990.

7. **Pansky M, Golan A, Bukovsky I, Caspi E,** Nonsurgical management of tubal pregnancy: necessity in view of the changing clincal appearance, *Am J Obstet Gynecol* 164:888, 1991.

8. **Centers for Disease Control,** Abortion surveillance: preliminary analysis—United States, 1995, *MMWR* 46:1133, 1998.

9. **Zhang J, Thomas AG, Leybovich E,** Vaginal douching and adverse health effects: a meta-analysis, *Am J Public Health* 87:1207, 1997.

10. **Saraiya M, Berg CJ, Kendrick JS, Strauss LT, Atrash HK, Ahn YW,** Cigarette smoking as a risk factor for ectopic pregnancy, *Am J Obstet Gynecol* 178:493, 1998.

11. **Westrom L, Joesoef R, Reynolds G, Hagdu A, Thompson SE,** Pelvic inflammatory disease and fertility, *Sex Trans Dis* 19:185, 1992.

12. **Chow JM, Yonekura L, Richwald GA, Greenland S, Sweet RL, Schachter J,** The association between Chlamydia trachomatis and ectopic pregnancy: a matched-pair, case-control study, *JAMA* 263:3164, 1990.

13. **Ni H, Daling J, Chu J, Stergachis A, Voigt L, Weiss N,** Previous abdominal surgery and tubal pregnancy, *Obstet Gynecol* 75:919, 1990.

14. **WHO Special Programme of Research, Development and Research Training in Human Reproduction, Task Force on Intrauterine Devices for Fertility Regulation,** A multinational case-control study of ectopic pregnancy, *Clin Reprod Fertil* 3:131, 1985.

15. **Holt V, Chu J, Daling JR, Stergachis AS, Weiss NS,** Tubal sterilization and subsequent ectopic pregnancy, *JAMA* 266:242, 1991.

16. **Peterson HB, Xia Z, Hughes JM, Wilcox LS, Tylor LR, Trussell J, for the U.S. Collaborative Review of Sterilization Working Group,** The risk of ectopic pregnancy after tubal sterilization, *New Engl J Med* 336:762, 1997.

17. **Chi I-c, Laufe LE, Atwed R,** Ectopic pregnancy following female sterilization procedures, *Adv Plann Parenthood* 16:52, 1981.

18. **McCausland A,** High rate of ectopic pregnancy following laparoscopic tubal coagulation failure, *Am J Obstet Gynecol* 136:977, 1980.

19. **Ankum WM, Mol BWJ, Van der Veen F, Bossuyt PMM,** Risk factors for ectopic pregnancy: a meta-analysis, *Fertil Steril* 65:1093, 1996.

20. **Pisarska MD, Carson SA, Buster JE,** Ectopic pregnancy, *Lancet* 351:1115, 1998.

21. **Skjeldestad FE, Hadgu A, Eriksson N,** Epidemiology of repeat ectopic pregnancy: a population-based prospective cohort study, *Obstet Gynecol* 91:129, 1998.

22. **Molloy D, Deambrosis W, Keeping D, Hynes J, Harrison K, hennessey J,** Multiple-sited (heterotropoic) pregnancy after in vitro fertilization and gamete intrafallopian transfer, *Fertil Steril* 53:1068, 1990.

23. **Dor J, Seidman DS, Levran D, Ben-Rafael Z, Ben-Shlomo I, Mashiach S,** The incidence of combined intrauterine and extrauterine pregnancy after in vitro fertilization and embryo transfer, *Fertil Steril* 55:833, 1991.

24. **Savare J, Norup P, Thomsen SG, Hornes P, Maigaard S, Helm P, Petersen K, Andersen AN,** Heterotropic pregnancies after in-vitro fertilization and embryo transfer — a Danish survey, *Hum Reprod* 8:116, 1993.

25. **Fernandez H, Coste J, Job-Spira N,** Controlled ovarian hyperstimulation as a risk factor for ectopic pregnancy, *Obstet Gynecol* 78:656, 1991.

26. **Franks AL, Beral V, Cates Jr W, Hogue CJ,** Contraception and ectopic pregnancy risk, *Am J Obstet Gynecol* 163:1120, 1990.

27. **Sivin I,** Dose- and age-dependent ectopic pregnancy risks with intrauterine contraception, *Obstet Gynecol* 78:291, 1991.

28. **Wilson JC,** A prospective New Zealand study of fertility after removal of copper intrauterine devices for conception and because of complications: a four-year study, *Am J Obstet Gynecol* 160:391, 1989.

29. **Ory HW,** Ectopic pregnancy and intrauterine contraceptive devices: new perspectives, *Obstet Gynecol* 57:2, 1981.

30. **Marchbanks PA, Annegers JE, Coulam CB, Strathy JH, Kurland LT,** Risk factors for ectopic pregnancy. A population based study, *JAMA* 259:1823, 1988.

31. **Edelman DA, Porter CW,** The intrauterine device and ectopic pregnancy, *Contraception* 36:85, 1987.

32. **Skjeldestad FE,** How effectively do copper intrauterine devices prevent ectopic pregnancy? *Acta Obstet Gynecol Scand* 76:684, 1997.

33. **Sivin I, Stern J, International Committee for Contraception Research,** Health during prolonged use of levonorgestrel 20 μg/d and the copper TCu 380 Ag intrauterine contraceptive devices: a multicenter study, *Fertil Steril* 61:70, 1994.

34. **Sivin I, Stern J, Diaz S, Pavez M, Alvarez F, Brache V, Mishell Jr DR, Lacarra M, McCarthy T, Holma P, Darney P, Klaisle C, Olsson S-E, Odlind V,** Rates and outcomes of planned pregnancy after use of Norplant capsules, Norplant II rods, or levonorgestrel-releasing or copper TCu 380Ag intrauterine contraceptive devices, *Am J Obstet Gynecol* 166:1208, 1992.

35. **Barbosa I, Bakos O, Olsson S-E, Odlind V, Johansson EDB,** Ovarian function during use of a levonorgestrel-releasing IUD, *Contraception* 42:51, 1990.

36. **Bilian X, Liying Z, Xuling Z, Mengchun J, Luukkainen T, Allonen H,** Pharmacokinetic and pharmacodynamic studies of levonorgestrel-releasing intrauterine device, *Contraception* 41:353, 1990.

37. **WHO Special Programme of Research, Development and Research Training in Human Reproduction, Task Force on the Safety and Efficacy of Fertility Regulating Methods,** The TCu 380A, TCu 220C, Multiload 250, and Nova T IUDs at 3, 5, and 7 years of use, *Contraception* 42:141, 1990.

38. **Atrash HK, Friede A, Hogue CJ,** Abdominal pregnancy in the United States: frequency and maternal mortality, *Obstet Gynecol* 69:333, 1987.

39. **Breen JL,** A 21 year survey of 654 ectopic pregnancies, *Am J Obstet Gynecol* 106:1004, 1970.

40. **Schwartz RO, DiPietro DL,** β-HCG as a diagnostic aid for suspected ectopic pregnancy, *Obstet Gynecol* 56:197, 1980.

41. **Maccato ML, Estrada R, Faro S,** Ectopic pregnancy with undetectable serum and urine β-hCG levels and detection of β-hCG in the ectopic trophoblast by immunocytochemical evaluation, *Obstet Gynecol* 81:878, 1993.

42. **Kadar N, Caldwell BV, Romero R,** A method of screening for ectopic pregnancy and its indications, *Obstet Gynecol* 58:162, 1981.

43. **Kadar N, Romero R,** Observations on the long human chorionic gonadotropin-time relationship in early pregnancy and its practical implications, *Am J Obstet Gynecol* 157:73, 1987.

44. **Fritz MA, Guo S,** Doubling time of human chorionic gonadotropin (hCG) in early normal pregnancy: relationship to hCG concentration and gestational age, *Fertil Steril* 47:584, 1987.

45. **Kadar N, Freedman M, Zacher M,** Further observations on the doubling time of human chorionic gonadotropin in early asymptomatic pregnancies, *Fertil Steril* 54:783, 1990.

46. **Keith SC, London SN, Weitzman GA, O'Brien TJ, Miller MJ,** Serial transvaginal ultrasound scans and β-human chorionic gonadotropin levels in early singleton and multiple pregnancies, *Fertil Steril* 59:1007, 1993.

47. **Goldstein SR, Snyder JR, Watson C, Danon M,** Very early pregnancy detection with endovaginal ultrasound, *Obstet Gynecol* 72:200, 1988.

48. **Timor-Tritsch IE, Farine D, Rosen MG,** A close look at early embryonic development with the high-frequency transvaginal transducer, *Am J Obstet Gynecol* 159:676, 1988.

49. **Kadar N, Bohrer M, Kemmann E, Shelden R,** The discriminatory human chorionic gonadotropin zone for endovaginal sonography: a prospective, randomized study, *Fertil Steril* 61:1016, 1994.

50. **Chambers S, Muir B, Haddad N,** Ultrasound evaluation of ectopic pregnancy including correlation with human chorionic gonadotropin levels, *Br J Radiol* 63:246, 1990.

51. **Emerson DS, Cartier MS, Altier LA, Felker RE, Smith WC, Stovall TG, Gray LA,** Diagnostic efficacy of endovaginal color Doppler flow imaging in an ectopic pregnancy screening program, *Radiology* 183:413, 1992.

52. **Stovall TG, Ling FW, Carson SA, Buster JE,** Serum progesterone and uterine curettage in differential diagnosis of ectopic pregnancy, *Fertil Steril* 57:456, 1992.

53. **Gelder MS, Boots LR, Younger JB,** Use of a single random serum progesterone value as a diagnostic aid for ectopic pregnancy, *Fertil Steril* 55:497, 1991.

54. **Garcia AJ, Aubert JM, Sama J, Josimovich JB,** Expectant management of presumed ectopic pregnancies, *Fertil Steril* 48:395, 1987.

55. **Ylostalo P, Cacciatore B, Sjoberg J, Kaariainen M, Tenhunen A, Stenman U-H,** Expectant management of ectopic pregnancy, *Obstet Gynecol* 80:345, 1992.

56. **Trio D, Strobelt N, Picciolo C, Lapinski R, Ghidioni A,** Prognostic factors for successful expectant management of ectopic pregnancy, *Fertil Steril* 63:469, 1995.

57. **Shalev E, Peleg D, Tsabari A, Romano S, Bustan M,** Spontaneous resolution of ectopic tubal pregnancy: natural history, *Fertil Steril* 63:15, 1995.

58. **Rantala M, Mäkinen J,** Tubal patency and fertility outcome after expectant management of ectopic pregnancy, *Fertil Steril* 68:1043, 1997.

59. **Tanaka T, Hayashi H, Kutsuzawa T, Ichinoe K,** Treatment of interstitial ectopic pregnancy with methotrexate: report of a successful case, *Fertil Steril* 37:851, 1982.

60. **Ory SJ, Villanueva AL, Sand PK, Tamura RK,** Conservative treatment of ectopic pregnancy with methotrexate, *Am J Obstet Gynecol* 154:1299, 1986.

61. **Stovall TG, Ling FW, Buster JE,** Outpatient chemotherapy of unruptured ectopic pregnancy, *Fertil Steril* 51:435, 1989.

62. **Stovall TG, Ling FW, Gray LA, Carson SA, Buster JE,** Methotrexate treatment of unruptured ectopic pregnancy: a report of 100 cases, *Obstet Gynecol* 77:749, 1991.

63. **Isaacs JD, McGehee RP, Cowan BD,** Life-threatening neutropenia following methotrexate treatment of ectopic pregnancy: a report of two cases, *Obstet Gynecol* 88:694, 1996.

64. **Horrigan TJ, Fanning J, Marcotte MP,** Methotrexate pneumonitis after systemic treatment for ectopic pregnancy, *Am J Obstet Gynecol* 176:714, 1997.

65. **Stovall TG, Ling FW, Gray LA,** Single-dose methotrexate for treatment of ectopic pregnancy, *Obstet Gynecol* 77:754, 1991.

66. **Stovall TG,** Medical management should be routinely used as primary therapy for ectopic pregnancy, *Clin Obstet Gynecol* 38:346, 1995.

67. **Stovall TG, Ling FW, Buster JE,** Reproductive performance after methotrexate treatment of ectopic pregnancy, *Am J Obstet Gynecol* 162:1620, 1990.

68. **Hajenius PJ, Engelsbel S, Mol BWJ, Van der Veen F, Ankum WB, Bossuyt PM, Hemrika DJ, Lammes FB,** Randomised trial of systemic methotrexate versus laparoscopic salpingostomy in tubal pregnancy, *Lancet* 350:774, 1997.

69. **Brown DL, Felker RE, Stovall TG, Emerson DS, Ling FW,** Serial endovaginal sonography of ectopic pregnancies treated with methotrexate, *Obstet Gynecol* 77:406, 1991.

70. **Sitka CS, Anderson L, Frederiksen C,** Single-dose methotrexate for the treatment of ectopic pregnancy: Northwestern Memoral Hospital three-year experience, *Am J Obstet Gynecol* 174:1840, 1996.

71. **Lipscomb GH, Bran D, McCord ML, Portera JC, Ling FW,** Analysis of three hundred fifteen ectopic pregnancies treated with single-dose methotrexate, *Am J Obstet Gynecol* 178:1354, 1998.

72. **Korhonen J, Stenman UH, Ylostalo P,** Low-dose oral methotrexate with expectant management of ectopic pregnancy, *Obstet Gynecol* 88:775, 1996.

73. **Hochner-Celnikier D, Ron M, Goshen R, Azcut D, Amir G, Yagel S,** Rupture of ectopic pregnancy following disappearance of serum beta subunit of HCG, *Obstet Gynecol* 79:826, 1992.

74. **Tulandi T, Hemmings R, Khalifa R,** Rupture of ectopic pregnancy in women with low and declining serum β-chorionic gonadotropin concentration, *Fertil Steril* 56:786, 1991.

75. **Yankowitz J, Leake J, Huggins G, Gazaway P, Gates E,** Cervical ectopic pregnancy: review of the literature and report of a case treated by single-dose methotrexate therapy, *Obstet Gynecol Survey* 45:405, 1990.

76. **Timor-Tritsch IE, Monteagudo A, Matera C, Veit CR,** Sonographic evolution of cornual pregnancies treated without surgery, *Obstet Gynecol* 79:1044, 1992.

77. **Kung F-T, Chang S-Y, Tsai Y-C, Hwang F-R, Hsu T-Y, Soong Y-K,** Subsequent reproduction and obstetric outcome after methotrexate treatment of cervical pregnancy: a review of original literature and international collaborative follow-up, *Hum Reprod* 12:591, 1997.

78. **Karsdorp VHM, Van der Veen F, Schats R, Boer-Meisel ME, Kenemans P,** Successful treatment with methotrexate of five vital interstitial pregnancies, *Hum Reprod* 7:1164, 1992.

79. **Menard A, Crequat J, Mandelbrot L, Hauuy JP, Madelenat P,** Treatment of unruptured tubal pregnancy by local injection of methotrexate under transvaginal sonographic control, *Fertil Steril* 54:47, 1990.

80. **Mottla GL, Rulin MC, Guzick DS,** Lack of resolution of ectopic pregnancy by intratubal injection of methotrexate, *Fertil Steril* 57:685, 1992.

81. **Fernandez H, Benifla J-L, Lelaidier C, Baton C, Frydman R,** Methotrexate treatment of ectopic pregnancy: 100 cases treated by primary transvaginal injection under sonographic control, *Fertil Steril* 59:773, 1993.

82. **Schiff E, Shalev E, Bustan M, Tsafari A, Mashiach S, Winer E,** Pharmacokinetics of methotrexate after local tubal injection for conservative treatment of ectopic pregnancy, *Fertil Steril* 57:688, 1992.

83. **Lang PF, Tamussino K, Honigl W, Ralph G,** Treatment of unruptured tubal pregnancy by laparoscopic instillation of hyperosmolar glucose solution, *Am J Obstet Gynecol* 166:1378, 1992.

84. **Vermesh M, Presser SC,** Reproductive outcome after linear salpingostomy for ectopic gestation: a prospective 3-year follow-up, *Fertil Steril* 57:682, 1992.

85. **Lundorff P, Thorburn J, Lindblom B,** Fertility outcome after conservative surgical treatment of ectopic pregnancy evaluated in a randomized trial, *Fertil Steril* 57:998, 1992.

86. **Sultana CJ, Easley K, Collins RL,** Outcome of laparoscopic versus traditional surgery for ectopic pregnancies, *Fertil Steril* 57:285, 1992.

87. **dela Cruz A, Cumming DC,** Factors determining fertility after conservative or radical surgical treatment for ectopic pregnancy, *Fertil Steril* 68:871, 1997.

88. **DiMarchi JM, Kosasa TS, Kobara TY, Hale RW,** Persistent ectopic pregnancy, *Obstet Gynecol* 70:555, 1987.

89. **Seifer DB, Gutman JN, Grant WD, Kamps CA, DeCherney AH,** Comparison of persistent ectopic pregnancy after laparoscopic salpingostomy versus salpingostomy at laparotomy for ectopic pregnancy, *Obstet Gynecol* 81:378, 1993.

90. **Lundorff P, Hahlin M, Sjoblom P, Lindblom B,** Persistent trophoblast after conservative treatment of tubal pregnancy: prediction and detection, *Obstet Gynecol* 77:129, 1991.

91. **Pouly JL, Chapron C, Mage G, Manhes H, Wattiez A, Canis M, Gaillard G, Bruhat MA,** The drop in the levels of hCG after conservative laparoscopic treatment of ectopic pregnancy, *J Gynecol Surg* 4:211, 1991.

92. **Hoppe DE, Bekkar BE, Nager CW,** Single-dose systemic methotrexate for the treatment of persistent ectopic pregnancy after conservative surgery, *Obstet Gynecol* 83:51, 1994.

93. **Graczykowski JW, Mishell Jr DR,** Methotrexate prophylaxis for persistent ectopic pregnancy after conservative treatment by salpingostomy, *Obstet Gynecol* 89:118, 1997.

94. **Grimes D, Ross W, Hutchen R,** Rh immunoglobulin utilization after spontaneous and induced abortion, *Obstet Gynecol* 57:261, 1977.

95. **Grant J, Hyslop M,** Underutilization of Rh prophylaxis in the emergency department: A retrospective survey, *Ann Emer Med* 21:181, 1992.

Appendix

Laboratory Values for Selected Measurements in Urine

Substance	Conventional Units	Conversion Factor	SI Units
Cortisol, free	10–90 µg/24 hr	2.759	28–250 nmol/24 hr
Estrogens, total	5–25 µg/24 hr	3.67	18–92 nmol/24 hr
17-Hydroxycorticosteroids	2–6 mg/24 hr	2.759	5.5–15.5 µmol/24 hr
17-Ketosteroids	6.0–15 mEq/24 hr	3.467	21–52.5 µmol/24 hr

SI Prefixes and Their Symbols

10^{9}	giga	G
10^{6}	mega	M
10^{3}	kilo	k
10^{2}	hecto	h
10^{1}	deka	da
10^{-1}	deci	d
10^{-2}	centi	c
10^{-3}	milli	m
10^{-6}	micro	µ
10^{-9}	nano	n
10^{-12}	pico	p
10^{-15}	femto	f
10^{-18}	alto	a

Laboratory Values for Selected Measurements in Blood, Plasma, and Serum

Substance	Conventional Units	Conversion Factor	SI Units
ACTH, adrenocorticotropin hormone 6:00 AM 6:00 PM	10–80 pg/mL <50 pg/mL	0.2202 0.2202	2.2–17.6 pmol/L <11 pmol/L
Androstenedione	60–300 ng/dL	0.0349	2.1–10.5 nmol/L
Calcium, total	8.5–10.5 mg/dL	0.25	2.1–2.6 mmol/L
Cholesterol LDL-cholesterol HDL-cholesterol	<200 mg/dL 60–130 mg/dL 30–70 mg/dL	0.0259 0.0259 0.0259	<5.2 mmol/L 1.6–3.4 mmol/L 0.8–1.8 mmol/L
Cortisol 8:00 AM 4:00 PM 10:00 PM	5–25 µg/dL 3–12 µg/dL <50% of AM value	27.6 27.6 27.6	140–690 nmol/L 80–330 nmol/L <50% of AM value
DHAS, Dehydroepiandrosterone sulfate	80–350 µg/dL	0.0027	2.2–9.5 µmol/L
11-Deoxycortisol	0.05–0.25 µg/dL	28.86	1.5–7.3 nmol/L
11-Deoxycorticosterone	2–10 ng/dL	30.3	60–300 pmol/L
Estradiol	20–400 pg/mL	3.67	70–1500 pmol/L
Estrone	30–200 pg/mL	3.7	110–740 pmol/L
FSH, reproductive years	5–20 mIU/mL	1.0	5–20 IU/L
Glucose, fasting	70–110 mg/dL	0.0556	4.0–6.0 mmol/L
Growth hormone	<10 ng/mL	1.0	<10 µg/L
17-Hydroxyprogesterone	100–300 ng/dL	0.03	3–9 nmol/L
Insulin, fasting	5–20 µU/mL	7.175	35–145 pmol/L
Insulin-like growth factor-I	0.3–2.2 U/mL	1000	300–2200 U/L
LH, reproductive years	5–20 mIU/mL	1.0	5–20 IU/L
Progesterone Follicular phase Secretory phase	<3 ng/mL 5–30 ng/mL	3.18 3.18	<9.5 nmol/L 16–95 nmol/L
Prolactin	1–20 ng/mL	44.4	44.4–888 pmol/L
Testosterone, total	20–80 ng/dL	0.0347	0.7–2.8 nmol/L
Testosterone, free	100–200 pg/dL	0.0347	35–700 pmol/L
TSH, thyroid stimulating hormone	0.35–5.0 µU/mL	1.0	0.35–5.0 mU/L
Thyroxine, free T_4	0.8–2.3 ng/dL	1.29	10–30 nmol/L
Triglycerides	40–250 mg/dL	0.0113	0.5–2.8 mmol/L
Triidothyronine, T_3, total	80–220 ng/dL	0.0154	1.2–3.4 nmol/L
Triidothyronine, T_3, free	0.13–0.55 ng/dL	15.4	2.0–8.5 pmol/L
Triidothyronine, reverse	8–35 ng/dL	15.4	120–540 pmol/L

Index

Page numbers in **bold** denote figures or tables.